Data for reference values in these tables was compiled from multiple sources. These values will vary slightly among laboratories. Laboratories should derive reference ranges for their population and geographic location.

★ TABLE A

Hematology Reference Values in Adults and Children (shown in conventional units; SI units in parentheses)

Age	Hb g/dL (g/L)	Hct % (L/L)	RBC × 10⁶/µL (×10¹²/L)	MCV (fL)	MCH (pg)	MCHC (g/dL)	Reticulocytes % (×10⁹/L)
Adult							
Male	14–17.4 (140–174)	42–52 (0.42–0.52)	4.5–5.5 (4.5–5.5)	80–100	28–34	32–36	0.5–2.5; (18–158)
Female	12.0–16.0 (120–160)	36–46 (0.36–0.46)	4.0–5.0 (4.0–5.0)	80–100	28–34	32–36	0.5–2.5; (18–158)
Critical low limit	**6.6 g/dL, 1.7 SD**	**18%, 5 SD**					
Critical high limit	**19.9 g/dL, 2.7 SD**	**61%, 6 SD**					
Birth	135–200	0.42–0.60	3.9–5.9	98–123	31–37	30–36	1.8–8.0; (220–420)
2 weeks	130–200	0.39–0.65	3.6–5.9	88–123	30–37	28–35	1.0–3.0; (45–135)
							(same up to 1 year)
1 month	110–170	0.33–0.55	3.3–5.3	91–112	29–36	28–36	
2 months	90–130	0.28–0.42	3.1–4.3	84–106	27–34	28–35	
4 months	100–130	0.32–0.44	3.5–5.1	76–97	25–32	29–37	
6 months	110–140	0.31–0.41	3.9–5.5	68–85	24–30	33–37	
9 months	110–140	0.32–0.40	4.0–5.3	70–85	25–30	32–37	
1 year	130–140	0.33–0.41	4.1–5.3	71–84	24–30	32–37	
2–6 years	115–135	0.34–0.41	3.9–5.3	75–87	24–30	31–37	
6–12 years	115–155	0.35–0.45	4.0–5.2	77–95	25–33	31–37	

Reference ranges derived from combined data. Critical limits are the low and high boundaries of life-threatening values. Results that fall below the low critical limit and above the high critical limit are "panic values" or critical results that require emergency notification of physicians. These limits were derived by Dr. George Kost from a national survey of 92 institutions. Kost GJ: Critical limits for urgent clinician notification at US Medical Centers. JAMA. 1990; 263:704.

✪ TABLE B

Age and Race-Specific Reference Ranges for Leukocyte Count and Differential (Compiled from multiple sources. Values may vary among sources and laboratories.)

	Birth	6 Months	4 Years	Adult	Adult of African Descent
Total leukocyte count ($\times 10^9$/L)	9.0–30.0	6.0–18.0	4.5–13.5	4.5–11.0	3.0–9.0
Segmented neutrophil: percent (%)	50–60	25–35	35–45	40–80	45–55
Absolute ($\times 10^9$/L)	4.5–18.0	1.5–6.3	1.5–8.5	1.8-7.0	1.5–5.0
Band neutrophil percent (%)	5–14	0–5	0–5	0–5	0–5
Absolute ($\times 10^9$/L)	0.5–4.2	0–1.0	0–0.7	0–0.7	0–0.7
Lymphocyte percent (%)	25–35	55–65	50–65	25–35	35–45
Absolute ($\times 10^9$/L)	2.0–11.0	4.0–13.5	2.0–8.8	1.0–4.8	1.0–4.8
Monocyte percent (%)	2–10	2–10	2–10	2–10	2–10
Absolute ($\times 10^9$/L)	0.2–3.0	0.1–2.0	0.1–1.4	0.1–0.8	0.1–0.8
Eosinophil percent (%)	0–5	0–5	0–5	0–5	0–5
Absolute ($\times 10^9$/L)	0–1.5	0–0.9	0–0.7	0–0.4	0–0.4
Basophil percent (%)	0–1	0–1	0–1	0–1	0–1
Absolute ($\times 10^9$/L)	0–0.6	0–0.4	0–0.3	0–0.2	0–0.2

✪ TABLE C

Other Hematology Reference Values

Analyte	Reference Value
Immature reticulocyte fraction (IRF)	0.09–0.31
RDW	12–14.6
Platelet count	150–450 $\times 10^9$/L
MPV	6.8–10.2 fL
Sedimentation rate	
Male <50 years	0–15 mm/hr
>50 years	0–20 mm/hr
Female <50 years	0–20 mm/hr
>50 years	0–30 mm/hr
Zeta sedimentation rate	
Male	40–52
Female	40–52
Cerebrospinal fluid	
Erythrocytes	0
Leukocytes	<5/µL

CLINICAL LABORATORY HEMATOLOGY

Second Edition

Shirlyn B. McKenzie, PhD, CLS(NCA), MT(ASCP)SH

Department of Clinical Laboratory Sciences
University of Texas Health Science Center at San Antonio

J. Lynne Williams, PhD, CLS(NCA), MT(ASCP)

Medical Laboratory Sciences Program
Oakland University

Pearson

Boston Columbus Indianapolis New York San Francisco Upper Saddle River
Amsterdam Cape Town Dubai London Madrid Milan Munich Paris Montreal Toronto
Delhi Mexico City Sao Paulo Sydney Hong Kong Seoul Singapore Taipei Tokyo

Library of Congress Cataloging-in-Publication Data

McKenzie, Shirlyn B.

   Clinical laboratory hematology / Shirlyn B. McKenzie,
J. Lynne Williams.—2nd ed.

      p. ; cm.

   Includes bibliographical references and index.

   ISBN-13: 978-0-13-513732-1

   ISBN-10: 0-13-513732-2

  1. Blood—Examination.   2. Hematology.   3. Blood—
Diseases—Diagnosis.   I. Williams, J. Lynne.   II. Title.

   [DNLM: 1. Clinical Laboratory Techniques.   2. Hematology—methods.   3. Hematologic Diseases—diagnosis.
4. Hematopoietic System—physiology.   WH 25 M478c 2010]

   RB45.M385 2010

   616.1'50076—dc22

                                     2009009577

Notice: The authors and the publisher of this volume have taken care that the information and technical recommendations contained herein are based on research and expert consultation, and are accurate and compatible with the standards generally accepted at the time of publication. Nevertheless, as new information becomes available, changes in clinical and technical practices become necessary. The reader is advised to carefully consult manufacturers' instructions and information material for all supplies and equipment before use, and to consult with a healthcare professional as necessary. This advice is especially important when using new supplies or equipment for clinical purposes. The authors and publisher disclaim all responsibility for any liability, loss, injury, or damage incurred as a consequence, directly or indirectly, of the use and application of any of the contents of this volume.

Publisher: Julie Levin Alexander

Publisher's Assistant: Regina Bruno

Editor-in-Chief: Mark Cohen

Development Editor: Melissa Kerian

Assistant Editor: Nicole Ragonese

Director of Marketing: Karen Allman

Executive Marketing Manager: Katrin Beacom

Marketing Specialist: Michael Sirinides

Marketing Assistant: Judy Noh

Managing Production Editor: Patrick Walsh

Production Liaison: Christina Zingone

Production Editor: Jessica Balch, Laserwords Maine

Senior Media Editor: Amy Peltier

Media Project Manager: Lorena Cerisano

Manufacturing Manager: Ilene Sanford

Manufacturing Buyer: Pat Brown

Art Director: Christopher Weigand

Cover Designer: Kevin Kall

Manager, Visual Rights and Permissions: Zina Arabia

Manager, Visual Research: Beth Brenzel

Manager, Cover Visual Research and Permissions:
  Karen Sanatar

Composition: Laserwords Maine

Printing and Binding: Courier/Kendallville

Cover Printer: Lehigh Phoenix

10 9 8 7 6 5 4 3 2 1

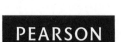

www.pearsonhighered.com

ISBN-13: 978-0-13-513732-1

ISBN-10: 0-13-513732-2

DEDICATION

Dedicated to my family, Gary, Scott, Shawn, Belynda, and Dora; my precious grandchildren, Lauren, Kristen, Weston, Waylon, and Wyatt, and to the memory of my parents, George and Helen Olson.

Shirlyn B. McKenzie

For my parents, David and Mary Williams, who gave their children roots as well as wings; for Lee, Laurie, Roger, and Richard, who sustain my roots; and for Dulaney, Corie, Chris and Ava, whom I love as my own.

J. Lynne Williams

CONTENTS

▶ **Eight HEMATOLOGY PROCEDURES**

▶ **Nine HEMATOLOGY PROCEDURES AND QUALITY ASSESSMENT**

FOREWORD

Clinical Laboratory Hematology is part of Pearson's Clinical Laboratory Science series of textbooks, which is designed to balance theory and practical applications in a way that is engaging and useful to students. The authors of and contributors to *Clinical Laboratory Hematology* present highly detailed technical information and real-life case studies that will help learners envision themselves as members of the health care team, providing the laboratory services specific to hematology that assist in patient care. The mixture of theoretical and practical information relating to hematology provided in this text allows learners to analyze and synthesize this information and, ultimately, to answer questions and solve problems and cases. Additional applications and instructional resources are available at www.pearsonhighered.com/mckenzie.

We hope that this book, as well as the entire series, proves to be a valuable educational resource.

Elizabeth A. Zeibig, PhD, MT(ASCP), CLS(NCA)
Clinical Laboratory Science Series Editor
Pearson Health Science

Vice Chair & Associate Professor
Department of Clinical Laboratory Science
Doisy College of Health Sciences
Saint Louis University

PREFACE

The second edition of *Clinical Laboratory Hematology* continues as a comprehensive, yet easy-to-read text of hematology and hemostasis written for students at all levels in clinical laboratory science programs, including clinical laboratory technicians (CLT)/medical laboratory technicians (MLT), clinical laboratory scientists (CLS)/medical technologists (MT). Other health professional students and practitioners may also benefit from this book, including pathology residents, medical students, physician assistants, and nurse practitioners. The team of authoritative contributing authors updated chapters with cutting edge advancements. The chapters have a striking design that will appeal to today's visually oriented student. To help readers grasp the content more easily, an exciting set of learning features is included in a repetitive format for each chapter. The book-specific online study guide is available at www.pearsonhighered.com/mckenzie with additional learning material and self-assessment items.

ORGANIZATION OF THE BOOK

Understanding hematologic/hemostatic diseases is dependent on a thorough knowledge and understanding of normal processes. Thus, the book begins with a section on normal hematopoiesis and progresses through anemias, nonmalignant and malignant leukocyte disorders. Hemostasis adheres to a similar format with normal hemostasis function discussed first, followed by abnormalities in hemostasis. Hematology and hemostasis laboratory procedures comprise the last section of the book.

Each hematology instructor has his or her idea of the ideal content sequence in which to teach hematology/hemostasis. This edition has a different organization than the first, based on user feedback. The text is divided into sections and may be studied by section or chapter sequence. If the instructor decides to use a different sequence than is used in the book, the background basics that are included in each chapter may help to determine if students have the appropriate background to progress. This gives each instructor flexibility to fit the book to his or her specific course design.

Section One covers an introduction to hematology and hematopoiesis, including a discussion of cell morphology, cell cycle, and its regulation. The cellular processes involved in hematopoiesis and tissue homeostasis have been expanded from one chapter (Chapter 2) in the first edition, to two chapters (Chapters 2 and 3) in this edition. Included in these chapters are discussions of regulation of these processes at the molecular level. Not all educational programs will elect to include Chapter 2, Cellular Homeostasis; alternatively, some may teach it but exclude processes at the molecular level.

Section Two includes chapters on normal hematopoiesis, including a discussion of hematopoietic tissues and organs as well as leukopoiesis, erythropoiesis, and hemoglobin structure and function.

Sections Three through Five cover hematologic disorders. Section Three covers the anemias and begins with an introduction to anemia. Section Four covers nonmalignant disorders of the leukocytes. Section Five is a study of the hematopoietic neoplasms. It begins with an introductory chapter that will help the student understand the classification, terminology, and pathophysiology of these disorders and the laboratory's role in diagnosis and treatment. Some instructors may want to cover the study of bone marrow (Chapter 35), flow cytometry (Chapter 37), cytogenetics (Chapter 38), and molecular genetics (Chapter 39) prior to teaching Section Five, or integrate this material with Section Five.

Section Six is a study of body fluids. Body fluid analysis is often a function of the hematology laboratory, since analysis includes cell counts and review of cell morphology. As much of the analysis includes identification of cells and differentiation of malignant cells from reactive or normal cells, this section has many excellent microphotographs.

Section Seven is a study of hemostasis. It begins with a study of normal hemostasis processes and proceeds to abnormalities associated with bleeding and thrombosis. Due to the high frequency of thrombotic disorders and the rapid discovery of mechanisms responsible for thrombosis, the laboratory's role in diagnosis of thrombotic disorders is expanding. Thus, an entire chapter is devoted to hypercoagulability (thrombophilia). Laboratory testing procedures for evaluation of hemostasis are included in Chapter 40, a chapter that has been expanded significantly from the first edition and written by a CLS coagulation laboratory specialist. Extensive additional material is included on the web page for this chapter, including links to educational videos and detailed laboratory procedures for download.

Section Eight covers hematology and hemostasis procedures. Section Nine is a thorough discussion of quality assessment in the hematology laboratory. Included in this chapter are common abnormal results and alert flags and corrective actions to take. Automation in hematology and hemostasis is supplemented on the Website with extensive use of graphics to illustrate abnormal results using various analyzers and to teach evaluation and interpretation of data.

The text incorporates ethical issues and management issues of test utilization and value, as well as critical testing pathways. This is the soft side of science, but addressing these topics alerts students to issues they will be facing in their work and communities. In many cases the laboratorian is the one who has the breadth of information needed to help make critical decisions involving the laboratory and its effective, efficient, ethical use.

SUITABLE FOR ALL LEVELS OF LEARNING

This book has been designed for both CLT/MLT and CLS/MT students. Using only one textbook is beneficial and economical in laboratory science programs offering both levels of instruction. Use of the book is also helpful to programs that design articulated curricula. The CLS/MT program can be confident of the CLT's/MLT's knowledge level in hematology without doing an extensive CLT/MLT course analysis.

Objectives are divided into two levels: Level I (basic) and Level II (advanced). CLT/MLT instructors reviewed the Level I objectives and generally agreed that most are appropriate for the CLT/MLT body of knowledge. These instructors also indicated that some Level II objectives were approproiate for CLT/MLT students. CLS/MT students should be able to meet both Level I and Level II objectives in most cases, but of course there may be differences among programs. Therefore, both CLT and CLS instructors are encouraged to review both levels of objectives to ensure their appropriateness for the course they teach. Although all chapters are appropriate for the CLS/MT student, if the program has two levels of hematology courses, Level I and Level II, instructors may choose to use the book as for a CLT/MLT program in the first course and the remainder of the book in the second course.

All instructors, regardless of discipline or level, will need to communicate to their students what is expected of them. They may want their students to find the information in the text that allows them to satisfy selected objectives, or they may assign particular sections to read. If not assigned specific sections to read, the CLT/MLT student may read more than expected, which is certainly not a bad thing! The two levels of questions at the end of each chapter are matched to the two levels of objectives.

The case study questions and checkpoints are not delineated by level. All students should try to answer as many of these as possible to assess their understanding of the previous material discussed.

Instructors should select appropriate chapters for their students based on the course goals. Some chapters, such as molecular techniques, cytogenetics, flow cytometry and body fluids may not be included in some hematology courses. Each program will need to assess what fits its particular curriculum.

In all cases the instructor should begin the course with Sections One and Two. The remaining sections can be rearranged and used as the instructor desires. The "Background Basics" feature will help the instructor determine which concepts the student should have mastered before beginning a unit of study. This concept should help instructors customize their courses.

UNIQUE PEDAGOGICAL FEATURES

This text has a number of unique pedagogical features that will help the student assimilate, organize, and understand the information. Each chapter begins with a group of components intended to set the stage for the content to follow.

- **Background Basics** alert students to material that should be learned or reviewed before starting the chapter. In most cases it refers readers to previous chapters to help them find the material if they want to review it.
- **Objectives** are comprised of two levels: Level I for basic or essential information and Level II for more advanced information. These objectives were reviewed by clinical (medical) laboratory technician (CLT/MLT) educators who made recommendations that aimed the Level I objectives to their students. Clinical laboratory science/medical technologist (CLS/MT) educators may expect their students to meet both Level I and Level II objective requirements.
- **Overview** gives the reader an idea of the chapter content and organization.
- **Key terms** alert the student to important terms used in the chapter and found in the glossary.

Each chapter offers students a variety of opportunities to assess their knowledge and ability to apply it.

- **Case Study** is a running case feature that first appears at the beginning of each chapter and focuses the student's attention on the subject matter that the chapter will cover. Throughout the chapter at appropriate places, additional information on the case may be given such as laboratory test results, and then questions are asked. The questions relate to the material presented in preceding sections. Appendix A provides the answers to the Case Study questions.
- **Checkpoints** are integrated throughout the chapter. These questions require the student to pause along the way to recall or apply information covered in preceding sections. The answers are provided in Appendix B.
- A **Summary** concludes the text portion of each chapter in order to help the student bring all the material together.
- **Review Questions** appear at the end of each chapter. The two sets of questions are referenced and organized to correspond to the Level I and Level II objectives. Answers are provided in Appendix C.

The page design features a number of enhancements intended to aid the learning process.

- **Colorful symbols** ✪ ■ are used within the chapter text to help the student quickly cross-reference from the tables and figures to the text.
- A ∞ **symbol** is also used when referring the student to another chapter.
- **Figures and tables** are used liberally to help the student organize and conceptualize information. This is especially important to visual learners.

- Algorithms (critical pathways, reflex testing pathways) are used when appropriate to help illustrate effective, cost-efficient use of laboratory tests in diagnosis.
- The microphotographs displayed in the book are typical of those found in a particular disease or disorder. Students should be aware that cell variations occur and that blood and bone marrow findings will not always mimic those found in textbooks.

A COMPLETE TEACHING AND LEARNING PACKAGE

The book is complemented by a variety of ancillary materials designed to help instructors be more effective and students more successful.

Instructor's Resource Manual—designed to equip faculty with necessary teaching resources, regardless of the level of instruction. Features include suggested learning activities for each chapter, test item writing guide, introduction to Bloom's taxonomy, crossword puzzles, word finds, sample syllabi, and a transition grid to assist instructors in correlating the content of other hematology texts to this text.

Instructor's Resource DVD-ROM (0-13-513737-3)—available upon adoption of the text and gives the instructor access to a number of powerful tools in an electronic format. The following materials are included on the DVD-ROM:

- Test Bank includes questions to allow instructors to design customized quizzes and exams using our award-winning TestGen 7.0 test building engine. The TestGen wizard guides you through the steps to create a simple test with drag-and-drop or point-and-click transfer. You can select test questions either manually or randomly and use online spellchecking and other tools to quickly polish your test content and presentation. You can save your test in a variety of formats both locally and on a network, print up to 25 variations of a single test, and publish your tests in an online course.
- PowerPoint Lectures contain key discussion points and color images for each chapter. This feature provides dynamic, fully designed, integrated lectures that are ready to use, allowing instructors to customize the materials to meet their specific course needs. These ready-made lectures will save you time and ease the transition into use of *Clinical Laboratory Hematology*.
- Image Library contains all of the images from the text. You have permission to copy and paste these images into PowerPoint lectures, printed documents, or website, as long as you are using *Clinical Laboratory Hematology* as your course textbook.
- Electronic version of the Instructor's Resource Manual in PDF and Word formats can be accessed.
- Bonus image library contains microphotographs of normal and abnormal blood cells filed by chapter. These can be downloaded into your digital presentations or used on password protected course Websites.

Companion Website (www.pearsonhighered.com/mckenzie)—This online study guide is completely unique to the market. In addition to providing an array of assessment quizzes, critical thinking questions, and case studies corresponding to each chapter of the book, the website presents additional figures, tables, and information. The quizzes and critical thinking questions have been developed within an automatic grading system that provides users with instant scoring once users submit their answers. Each student's quiz results can be emailed directly to the educator if desired. For procedure chapters, the website also includes detailed laboratory procedures that can be printed for use in the laboratory.

ACKNOWLEDGMENTS

I am grateful to the many contributors who gave their expertise to make this book a comprehensive source of current knowledge in hematology and hemostasis for clinical laboratory science. I am honored to work with so many hematology and hemostasis experts. Thank you for sharing your expertise and for your patience.

We had a great panel of clinical laboratory educators review every chapter for appropriate content. Their reviews were invaluable in helping assure that this book met the needs of both clinical laboratory technicians (medical laboratory technicians) and clinical laboratory scientists (medical technologists) and that it reflects current laboratory practice.

Those who assisted in other tasks are invaluable members of the book's team.

Thank you, Linda Comeaux for updating the accompanying instructor's manual to this book. Thank you to Lynne Williams and Barbara Russell for providing many Power-Points; to Venus Ward and Karen Brown for reviewing and revising questions, case studies and critical thinking questions on the Website; to Demetra Castillo, Victoria Norbury, and John Landis for writing the questions for the test bank. Thank you to my dear friend, Keila Paulsen, for reviewing chapters, providing excellent cell images for the book and Instructor's Resource DVD-ROM, and for offering many helpful suggestions to improve the book. A project of this size benefits greatly from the many contributions of these experts.

A very special thanks is due to my co-editor, Lynne Williams, for her assistance with this edition. She not only edited many chapters but extensively revised chapters she authored. Her knowledge of hematologic disease at the molecular level was invaluable in assuring this new edition is at the cutting edge of hematology.

I am fortunate to have family members who directly or indirectly support all that I take on. A special thanks to my devoted husband who made many sacrifices while providing enormous support during the years it took me to complete this project. He put up with my nights and weekends in isolation to finish this project. Thank you also to the rest of my family who help me appreciate what is really important in life: my sons, Scott and Shawn; their wives, Belynda and Dora; my precious grandchildren who make everything worthwhile, Lauren, Kristen, Weston, Waylon, and Wyatt. I owe a great deal of my success to my parents, George and Helen Olson, who gave me the confidence to do anything I put my mind to. During my writing of this edition, they entered their heavenly home.

Thank you also to Mark Cohen, Melissa Kerian, Nicole Ragonese, and Christina Zingone for their assistance in putting this book together. They provided many of the new ideas on the book's design as well as encouragement along the way that it could be done. Melissa and Nicole provided the gentle prodding and follow through to get the job done. Thank you to Linda Duarte and Jessica Balch for their editorial assistance. You are a great team. And finally, a special thanks to Pearson Health Science for publishing this creation.

SBM

I would like to extend a special "thank-you" to my colleagues in the Medical Laboratory Sciences Program at Oakland University, Wanda Reygaert and Sumit Dinda, who kept the MLS program moving forward and allowed me to focus on the writing and editing of this new edition. Also to the MLS students of the past two years, who tolerated a distracted and often absent-minded professor—you've been my inspiration to try to create a meaningful and useful book to support your educational endeavors.

JWL

REVIEWERS

Linda J. McCown, MS, MT(ASCP), CLS(NCA)
Chair/Associate Professor, Clinical Laboratory Science
University of Illinois at Springfield
Springfield, Illinois

D. Gayle Melberg, MS, MT(ASCP)
Adjunct Faculty, Medical Laboratory Technology
J. Sargeant Reynolds Community College
Richmond, Virginia

Richard Miller, PhD, MBA, MT(ASCP), CLS(NCA)
Program Director/Instructor, Clinical Laboratory Technology
Southwest Georgia Technical College
Thomasville, Georgia

Adriana B. Nunemaker, MLT(ASCP), MAA
Instructor, Medical Laboratory Technology
Laredo Community College
Laredo, Texas

Anna Oller, PhD, MT (ASCP)
Associate Professor, Biology
Central Missouri State University
Warrensburg, Missouri

Evelyn Paxton, MS, MT(ASCP)
Program Director, Clinical Laboratory Technology
Rose State College
Midwest City, Oklahoma

Amira Rodriguez, BS, MT(ASCP)
Instructor, Medical Laboratory Technology
Laredo Community College
Laredo, Texas

Brooke Solberg, MS, MT(ASCP)
Instructor, Clinical Laboratory Science
University of North Dakota
Grand Forks, North Dakota

Deborah Stai, PhD, MT(ASCP), CLS(NCA)
Coordinator, Clinical Laboratory Science
Lake Superior State University
Sault Sainte Marie, Michigan

Stacy E. Walz, BS, MT(ASCP)
Associate Lecturer, Clinical Laboratory Science
University of Wisconsin–Madison
Madison, Wisconsin

Venus J. Ward, PhD, MT(ASCP), CLS(NCA)
Chair/Program Director, Clinical Laboratory Sciences
University of Kansas Medical Center
Kansas City, Kansas

Whitney Williams, PhD, MT(ASCP)
Chair, Clinical Laboratory Science
Arkansas State University
State University, Arkansas

First Edition

Larry Birnbaum, PhD, CLS(NCA), MT(ASCP)
Department Chair, Clinical Laboratory Sciences
The College of St. Scholastica
Duluth, Minnesota

Cynthia C. Cowall, MEd, MT(ASCP)
Assistant Professor, Medical Technology
Salisbury State University
Salisbury, Maryland

Dorothy J. Fike, MS, MT(ASCP)
Associate Professor, Clinical Laboratory Sciences
Marshall University
Huntington, West Virginia

Rena E. Goode, MT(ASCP)
Associate Professor, Medical Laboratory Technician
Ivy Tech State College
Terre Haute, Indiana

Nancy L. McQueen, PhD
Professor, Biology and Microbiology
California State University, Los Angeles
Los Angeles, California

Yasmen Simonian, PhD, CLS(NCA), MT(ASCP)
Chair and Professor, Clinical Laboratory Science
Weber State University
Ogden, Utah

Peggy Simpson, MS, MT(ASCP)
Director, Medical Laboratory Technician
Alamance Community College
Graham, North Carolina

Larry J. Smith, PhD, SH(ASCP)
Director, Coagulation Lab
Memorial Sloan-Kettering Cancer Center
New York, New York

Dan Southern, MS, CLS(NCA), MT(ASCP)
Program Director, Clinical Laboratory Sciences
Western Carolina University
Cullowhee, North Carolina

CONTENT LEVEL REVIEW PANEL

Linda L. Breiwick, BS, CLS(NCA), MT(ASCP)
Program Director, Medical Laboratory Technology
Shoreline Community College
Seattle, Washington

Linda Comeaux, BS, CLS(NCA)
Program Director, Medical Laboratory Technology
Arapahoe Community College
Littleton, Colorado

Mona Gleysteen, MS, CLS(NCA)
Program Director, Clinical Laboratory Technology
Lake Area Technical Institute
Watertown, South Dakota

CONTRIBUTORS

Sue S. Beglinger, MS, CLS(NCA), MT(ASCP)
Program Director, Clinical Laboratory Technology
School of Health Sciences
Madison Area Technical College
Madison, Wisconsin
Chapters 20, 22

Cheryl Burns, MS, CLS(NCA)
Associate Professor, Department of Clinical Laboratory Sciences
University of Texas Health Science Center at San Antonio
San Antonio, Texas
Chapters 34, 36, 41

Shannon Carpenter, MD, MSCI
Pediatric Hematology/Oncology
Children's Mercy Hospital
Kansas City, MO
Chapter 32

Nanette Clare, MD
Senior Associate Dean
Associate Dean for Academic Affairs
School of Medicine
Professor, Pathology
University of Texas Health Science Center at San Antonio
San Antonio, Texas
Chapter 28

Diana L. Cochran-Black, DrPH, MT(ASCP)SH
Assistant Professor, Medical Technology
College of Health Professions
Wichita State University
Wichita, Kansas
Chapter 15

Fiona E. Craig, MD
Associate Professor, Hematopathology
Department of Pathology
University of Pittsburgh School of Medicine
Pittsburgh, Pennsylvania
Chapters 26, 37

Aamir Ehsan, MD
Chief, Pathology and Laboratory Medicine
South Texas Veterans Health Care System
Associate Professor, Pathology
University of Texas Health Science Center at San Antonio
San Antonio, Texas
Chapters 27, 35

Margaret L. Gulley, MD
Professor and Director, Molecular Pathology
Department of Pathology and Laboratory Medicine
University of North Carolina at Chapel Hill
Chapel Hill, North Carolina
Chapter 39

Carol R. Hillman-Wiseman, MS, MT(ASCP)
Administrative Research Coordinator, Special Coagulation
Division of Hematology/Oncology
Children's Hospital of Michigan
Detroit, Michigan
Chapter 40

Joel D. Hubbard, PhD, MT(ASCP)
Associate Professor, Laboratory Sciences and Primary Care
Texas Tech University Health Science Center
Lubbock, Texas
Chapters 5, 12

Beverly Kirby, EdD, CLS(NCA), MT(ASCP)
Associate Professor, Medical Technology
West Virginia University
Morgantown, West Virginia
Chapter 32

Martha Lake, EdD, CLS(NCA), MT(ASCP)
Professor, School of Medicine
Assistant Chair, Professional Programs
Program Director, Medical Technology
West Virginia University
Morgantown, West Virginia
Chapter 16

Rebecca J. Laudicina, PhD, CLS(NCA)
Professor, Allied Health Sciences
Division of Clinical Laboratory Science
University of North Carolina at Chapel Hill
Chapel Hill, North Carolina
Chapters 7, 10, 13

Louann Lawrence, DrPH, CLS(NCA)
Professor and Department Head, Clinical Laboratory
  Sciences
Louisiana State University Health Sciences Center
New Orleans, Louisiana
Chapter 23

Susan Leclair, PhD, CLS(NCA)
Chancellor Professor, Medical Laboratory Science
University of Massachusetts Dartmouth
Dartmouth, Massachusetts
Chapters 24, 25

Shirlyn B. McKenzie, PhD, CLS(NCA), MT(ASCP)SH
Distinguished Teaching Professor Emeritus and Chair Emeritus,
    Department of Clinical Laboratory Sciences
University of Texas Health Science Center at San Antonio
San Antonio, Texas
Chapters 1, 6, 8, 9, 14, 21, 22

Lucia E. More, Lt. Col. USAF, Biomedical Sciences Corps,
    MS, MT(ASCP)
Laboratory Flight Commander
Elmendorf AFB, Alaska
Chapter 41

Barbara O'Malley, MD, FASCP, MT(ASCP)
Associate Director, Transfusion Medicine
Detroit Medical Center
Assistant Clinical Professor, Wayne State University School
    of Medicine
Detroit, MI
Chapters 29, 31

Tim R. Randolph, PhD, CLS(NCA), MT(ASCP)
Associate Professor, Clinical Laboratory Science
Saint Louis University
St. Louis, Missouri
Chapter 11

Wanda C. Reygaert, PhD, MT(ASCP)
Assistant Professor, Medical Laboratory Sciences Program
Oakland University
Rochester, Michigan
Chapter 19

Annette Schlueter, MD, PhD
Associate Professor, Pathology
University of Iowa
Iowa City, Iowa
Chapter 4

Yasmen Simonian, PhD, CLS(NCA), MT(ASCP)
Dean and Presidential Distinguished Professor
Dr. Ezekiel R. Dunke College of Health Professions
Weber State University
Ogden, Utah
Chapter 7

Linda Smith, PhD, CLS(NCA)
Professor and Chair, Department of Clinical Laboratory
    Sciences
University of Texas Health Science Center at San Antonio
San Antonio, Texas
Chapters 17, 18

J. Lynne Williams, PhD, CLS(NCA)
Professor and Director, Medical Laboratory Sciences
Oakland University
Rochester, Michigan
Chapters 2, 3, 24, 25, 30, 33

Kathleen Wilson, MD, FCAP, FACMG
Chief, Division of Genetic Diagnostics
Director, Comparative Genomic Hybridization Laboratory
Associate Professor, McDermott Center for Growth
    and Development
University of Texas Southwestern Medical Center
Dallas, Texas
Chapter 38

ABBREVIATIONS

ADCC – Antibody dependent cell-mediated cytotoxicity
AHG – Antihuman globulin
AIDS – Acquired immune deficiency syndrome
AIHA – Autoimmune hemolytic anemia
AL – Acute leukemia
ALL – Acute lymphoblastic leukemia
AML – Acute myeloid leukemia
ANLL – Acute nonlymphocytic leukemia
APTT – Activated partial thromboplastin time
ARC – AIDS related complex
Band – Nonsegmented neutrophil
BT – Bleeding time
CBC – Complete blood count
CD – Cluster of differentiation
cDNA – Complementary DNA
CFU – Colony forming unit
CGL– Chronic granulocytic leukemia
CLL – Chronic lymphocytic leukemia
CML – Chronic myeloid leukemia
CMML – Chronic myelomonocytic leukemia
CMV – Cytomegalovirus
DAF – Decay accelerating factor
DAT – Direct antiglobulin test
DIC – Disseminated intravascular coagulation
dL – Deciliter
DNA – Deoxyribonucleic acid
DVT – Deep vein thrombosis
EBV – Epstein-Barr virus
EPO – Erythropoietin
ER – Endoplasmic reticulum
FA – Fanconi's anemia
FAB – French-American-British
FFP – Fresh frozen plasma
G6PD – Glucose-6-phosphate dehydrogenase
Hb or Hgb – Hemoglobin
Hct – Hematocrit
HDN – Hemolytic disease of the newborn
HPFH – Hereditary persistance of fetal hemoglobin
HUS – Hemolytic uremic syndrome
IAT – Indirect antiglobulin test
Ig – Immunoglobulin
INR – International normalized ratio
IRF – Immature reticulocyte fraction
ISC – Irreversibly sickled cells
ISI – International sensitivity index
ITP – Immune (formerly idiopathic) thrombocytopenic purpura

L – Liter
LAP – Leukocyte alkaline phosphatase
LCAT – Lecithin:cholesterol acyl transferase
LD – Lactic dehydrogenase
Lymph – Lymphocyte
MAHA – Microangiopathic hemolytic anemia
MCH – Mean corpuscular hemoglobin
MCHC – Mean corpuscular hemoglobin concentration
MCV – Mean corpuscular volume
MDS – Myelodysplastic syndrome
MHC – Major histocompatibility complex
mL – Milliliter
Mono – Monocyte
MPD – Myeloproliferative disorders
MW – Molecular weight
NRBC – Nucleated red blood cell
PAS – Periodic-acid-Schiff
PCH – Paroxysmal cold hemoglobinuria
PCR – Polymerase chain reaction
PDW – Platelet distribution width
PIVKA – Protein-induced by vitamin-K absence (or antagonist)
PK – Pyruvate kinase
PMN – Polymorphonuclear neutrophil
PNH – Paroxsymal nocturnal hemoglobinuria
PT – Prothrombin time
RA – Refractory anemia
RAEB – Refractory anemia with excess blasts
RARS – Refractory anemia with ringed sideroblasts
RBC – Red blood cell
RDW – Red cell distribution width
RER – Rough endoplasmic reticulum
RNA – Ribonucleic acid
RPI – Reticulocyte production index
SCIDS – Severe combined immunodeficiency syndrome
Seg – Segmented neutrophil
SER – Smooth endoplasmic reticulum
SLL – Small lymphocytic lymphoma
TCR – T cell receptor
TIBC – Total iron binding capacity
TRAP – Tartrate resistant acid phosphatase
TTP – Thrombotic thrombocytopenic purpura
VWF – von Willebrand factor
WBC – White blood cell
WHO – World Health Organization

SECTION ONE
INTRODUCTION TO HEMATOLOGY

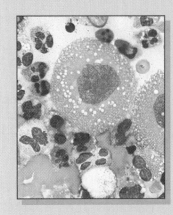

1

Introduction

Shirlyn B. McKenzie, Ph.D.

■ OBJECTIVES—LEVELS I AND II

At the end of this unit of study, the student should be able to:

1. Compare the reference intervals for hemoglobin, hematocrit, erythrocytes, and leukocytes in infants, children, and adults.
2. Identify the function of erythrocytes, leukocytes, and platelets.
3. Describe the composition of blood.
4. Explain the causes of change in the steady state of blood components.
5. Describe clinical pathway, critical pathway, reflex testing, and disease management and identify the laboratory's role in developing these models.
6. Compare capitated payment, prospective payment, and fee-for-service and describe the impact of capitation on the laboratory.

CHAPTER OUTLINE

KEY TERMS

Activated partial thromboplastin time (APTT)
Capitated payment
Complete blood count (CBC)
Diapedese
Erythrocytes
Fee-for-service
Hematocrit
Hematology
Hemoglobin
Hemostasis
Leukocytes
Platelets
Prothrombin time (PT)
RBC indices
Reflex testing
Thrombocytes

BACKGROUND BASICS

Students should complete courses in biology and physiology before beginning this study of hematology.

CASE STUDY

We will address this case study throughout the chapter.
Aaron, a two-year-old male, was seen by his pediatrician because he had a fever of 102 to 104°F over the past 24 hours. Aaron was lethargic. Prior to this, he had been in good health except for two episodes of otitis. Consider why the pediatrician may order laboratory tests and how this child's condition might affect the composition of his blood.

▶ OVERVIEW

The hematology laboratory is one of the busiest areas of the clinical laboratory. Even small, limited-service laboratories usually offer hematology tests. This chapter is an introduction to the composition of blood and the testing performed to identify the presence of disease. It also includes a discussion on the laboratory's role in ensuring cost-effective and diagnostically efficient testing.

▶ INTRODUCTION

Blood has been considered the essence of life for centuries. One of the Hippocratic writings from about 400 B.C. describes the body as being a composite of four humors: black bile, blood, phlegm, and yellow bile. Fahraeus, a twentieth-century Swedish physician, suggested that the theory of the four humors came from the observation of four distinct layers in clotted blood. In the process of clotting, blood separates into a dark-red, almost black, jellylike clot (black bile); a thin layer of oxygenated red cells (blood); a layer of white cells and platelets (phlegm); and a layer of yellowish serum (yellow bile).[1] Health and disease were thought to occur as a result of an upset in the equilibrium of these humors. This may help explain why bloodletting to purge the body of its contaminated fluids was practiced from the time of Hippocrates until the nineteenth century.

The cellular composition of blood was not recognized until the invention of the microscope. With the help of a crude magnifying device that consisted of a biconvex lens, Leeuwenhoek (1632–1723) accurately described and measured the red cells (erythrocytes). The discovery of white blood cells (leukocytes) and platelets (thrombocytes) followed after microscope lenses were improved.

As a supplement to these categorical observations of blood cells, Karl Vierordt in 1852 published the first quantitative results of blood cell analysis.[2] His procedures for quantification were tedious and time consuming. After several years, attempts were made to correlate blood cell counts with various disease states.

Improved methods of blood examination in the 1920s and the increased knowledge of blood physiology and blood-forming organs in the 1930s allowed the study of anemias and other blood disorders to be studied on a rational basis. In some cases, the pathophysiology of hematopoietic disorders was realized only after the patient responded to experimental therapy.

Contrary to early hematologists, modern hematologists recognize that alterations in the components of blood are the *result* of disease, not a *primary* cause of it. Under normal conditions, the production of blood cells in the bone marrow, their release to the peripheral blood, and their survival are highly regulated to maintain a steady state of morphologically normal cells. Quantitative and qualitative hematologic abnormalities may result when an imbalance occurs in this steady state.

▶ COMPOSITION OF BLOOD

Blood is composed of a liquid called *plasma* and of cellular elements, including **leukocytes, platelets,** and **erythrocytes.** The normal adult has about 6 liters of this vital fluid, which composes from 7% to 8% of the total body weight. Plasma makes up about 55% of the blood volume, whereas about 45% of the volume is composed of erythrocytes and 1% of the volume is composed of leukocytes and platelets (**thrombocytes**). Variations in the quantity of these blood elements are often the first sign of disease occurring in body tissue. Changes in diseased tissue often can be detected by laboratory tests that measure deviations from normal in blood constituents. **Hematology** is primarily the study of the formed cellular blood elements.

The principal component of plasma is water, which contains dissolved ions, proteins, carbohydrates, fats, hormones, vitamins, and enzymes. The principal ions necessary for normal cell function include calcium, sodium, potassium, chloride, magnesium, and hydrogen. The main protein constituent of plasma is albumin, which is the most important component in maintaining osmotic pressure. Albumin also acts as a carrier molecule, transporting compounds such as bilirubin and heme. Other blood proteins carry vitamins, minerals, and lipids. Immunoglobulins and complement are specialized blood proteins involved in immune defense. The coagulation proteins responsible for **hemostasis** (arrest of bleeding) circulate in the blood as inactive enzymes until they are needed for the coagulation process. An upset in the balance of these dissolved plasma constituents may indicate a disease in other body tissues.

Blood plasma also acts as a transport medium for cell nutrients and metabolites; for example, hormones manufactured in one tissue are transported by the blood to target tissue in other parts of the body. Bilirubin, the main catabolic residue of hemoglobin, is transported by albumin from the spleen to the liver for excretion. Blood urea nitrogen, a nitrogenous waste product, is carried to the kidneys for filtration and excretion. Increased concentration of these normal catabolites may indicate either increased cellular metabolism or a defect in the organ responsible for their excretion. For example, in liver disease, the bilirubin level in blood increases, indicating the end organ disease. In hemolytic anemia, however, the bilirubin concentration may rise not because of liver disease but because of the increased metabolism of hemoglobin.

When body cells die, they release their cellular constituents into surrounding tissue. Eventually, some of these constituents reach the blood. Many constituents of body cells are specific for the cell's particular function; thus, increased concentration of these constituents in the blood, especially enzymes, may indicate abnormal cell destruction in a specific organ.

Each of the three cellular constituents of blood has specific functions. Erythrocytes contain the vital protein **hemoglobin,** which is responsible for transport of oxygen and carbon dioxide between the lungs and body tissues. There are five major types of leukocytes: neutrophils, eosinophils, basophils, lymphocytes, and monocytes. They are responsible for defending the body against foreign antigens such as bacteria and viruses. Platelets are necessary for maintaining hemostasis. Blood cells circulate through blood vessels, which are distributed throughout every body tissue. Erythrocytes and platelets carry out their functions without leaving the vessels, but leukocytes **diapedese** (pass through vessel walls) to tissues where they defend against invading foreign antigens.

 CASE STUDY *(continued from page 2)*

1. If Aaron was diagnosed with otitis media, what cellular component(s) in his blood would be playing a central role in fighting this infection?

► REFERENCE INTERVALS FOR BLOOD CELL CONCENTRATION

Physiologic differences in the concentration of cellular elements may occur according to race, age, sex, and geographic location; pathologic changes in specific blood cell concentrations may occur as the result of disease or injury. Whites have slightly higher cell counts than blacks: Their leukocyte counts are higher by 0.5×10^9/L, hemoglobin levels by 0.7 g/dL, **hematocrit** by 0.17 L/L, and erythrocyte counts by 0.05×10^{12}/L.[3]

The greatest differences in reference intervals occur between newborns and adults. Generally, newborns have a higher erythrocyte concentration than any other age group. The erythrocytes are also larger than those of adults. For six months after birth, erythrocytes decrease and then slowly increase. Hemoglobin and erythrocyte counts increase in children between the ages of 5 and 17.[3] The leukocyte concentration is also increased at birth but decreases after the first year of life. A common finding in young children is an absolute and relative lymphocytosis. After 12 years of age, males have higher hemoglobin, hematocrit, and erythrocyte levels than females. Tables A through K on the inside covers of this text give hematologic reference intervals for various age groups.

Each individual laboratory must determine reference intervals of hematologic values to account for the physiologic differences of a population in a specific geographical area. Reference values are determined by calculating the mean for a group of healthy individuals and reporting the reference interval as the mean ±2 standard deviations. This interval represents the reference interval for 95% of normal individuals. A value just below or just above this interval is not necessarily abnormal; normal and abnormal overlap. Statistical probability indicates that about 5% of normal individuals will fall outside the ±2 standard deviation range. The farther a value falls from the reference interval, however, the more likely the value is to be abnormal.

 CASE STUDY *(continued)*

2. Aaron's physician ordered a complete blood count (CBC). The results are Hb 115 g/L; Hct 0.34 L/L; RBC 4.0×10^{12}/L; WBC 18×10^9/L. What parameters, if any, are outside the reference intervals? Why do you have to take Aaron's age into account when evaluating these results?

► HEMOSTASIS

Hemostasis is the process of forming a barrier (blood clot) to blood loss when the vessel is traumatized and limiting the barrier to the site of injury. Hemostasis occurs in stages called primary and secondary hemostasis and fibrinolysis. These stages are the result of interaction of platelets, blood vessels, and proteins circulating in the blood. An upset in any of the stages can result in bleeding or abnormal blood clotting (thrombosis). Laboratory testing for abnormalities in hemostasis is usually performed in the hematology section of the laboratory. Alternatively, hemostasis testing may be performed in a separate section of the laboratory.

✓ Checkpoint! 1

What cellular component of blood may be involved in disorders of hemostasis?

► BLOOD COMPONENT THERAPY

Blood components may be used in therapy for various hematologic and nonhematologic disorders. Whole blood collected from donors can be separated into various cellular and fluid components. Only the specific blood component (i.e., platelets for thrombocytopenia or erythrocytes for anemia) needed by the patient will be administered. In addition, the components can be specially prepared for the patient's specific needs (i.e., washed erythrocytes for patients with IgA deficiency to reduce the risk of anaphylactic reactions). Table 1-1 ✪ lists the various components that can be prepared for specific uses. The reader may want to refer back to this table when reading about therapies that use these components in subsequent chapters.

 TABLE 1-1

Blood Components and Their Uses

Component Name	Composition	Primary Use
Whole blood	Red blood cells and plasma	Not used routinely. May be used in selected trauma, autologous transfusions, and neonatal situations; increases oxygen-carrying capacity and volume
Packed red blood cells (PRBC)	PRBC	Symptomatic anemia to increase oxygen-carrying capability
PRBC, washed	PRBC; plasma and most leukocytes and platelets removed	For individuals with repeated allergic reactions to components containing plasma; for IgA-deficient individuals with anaphylatic reactions to products containing plasma
PRBC, leukoreduced	PRBC; WBC removed	Decrease the risk of febrile nonhemolytic transfusion reaction, HLA sensitization, and cytomegalovirus (CMV) transmission
PRBC, frozen, deglycerolized	PRBC frozen in cryoprotective agent, thawed, washed	For individuals with rare blood groups (autologous donation)
PRBC, irradiated	PRBC with lymphocytes inactivated	Reduce risk of graft-vs-host disease
Platelets, pooled*	4–6 units of random donor platelets	Increase platelet count and decrease bleeding when there is a deficiency or abnormal function of platelets
Platelets, single* donor (pheresis)	Equivalent of 4–6 donor platelets collected from single donor	Patients refractory to random platelet transfusion or to increase platelet count due to a deficiency or abnormal function of platelets
Fresh frozen plasma (FFP)	Plasma with all stable and labile coagulation factors; frozen within 8 hours of collection of unit of blood	Patients with multiple coagulation factor deficiencies; DIC; used with packed RBC in multiple transfusions
Cryoprecipitated AHF**	Concentrated F-VIII, fibrinogen, F-XIII, VWF***	Hypofibrinogenemia, hemophilia A, von Willebrand's disease, F-XIII deficiency
Plasma, cryo-poor	Plasma remaining after cryo removed	Thrombotic thrombocytopenic purpura (TTP)
Liquid plasma	Plasma not frozen within 8 hours of collection	Stable coagulation factor deficiency; volume replacement
Granulocytes	Granulocytes	Neutropenic patient who is septic and unresponsive to antimicrobials and who has chance of marrow recovery

*Platelets may also be leukoreduced or irradiated. See PRBC for reasons.
**Cryoprecipitated antihemophilic factor, or cryo.
***von Willebrand factor.
Courtesy of Linda Smith, Ph.D., CLS (NCA); Adapted from the *Circular of information for the use of human blood and blood components.* Prepared jointly by the American Association of Blood Banks, America's Blood Centers, and the American Red Cross (2002).

► THE LABORATORY'S ROLE IN DISEASE MANAGEMENT

In the United States, personal health care spending accounts for about 14% of the gross domestic product (GDP).[4] Yet only 3.5% of the amount spent on personal health care is for laboratory tests. In 2005, 16.6% of hospital outpatient charges under Medicare were for laboratory services.[4]

The rising cost of health care associated with diagnosis and treatment of disease has caused increased scrutiny of the health care system. In an attempt to gain an understanding of these costs and to identify whether medical resources are used inappropriately, researchers studied medical practice patterns. Results revealed overutilization of services and significant variations in diagnosis and treatment of common disorders.[5,6,7] Study of Medicare records reveals variations in the quality of health care across geographical regions as well as disparities in types of procedures performed.[8] Concerns over these rising costs and variations in practice resulted in the implementation of cost-containment strategies by insurers and health care organizations. Many insurers went from a fee-for-service reimbursement to a capitated payment system. **Fee-for-service** plans allow consumers to choose their own health care providers who determine the fees. Under **capitated payment** plans, the insurer contracts with certain health care providers who agree to provide services for a defined population on a per-member fee schedule. The insurer determines who the providers will be.

Under Medicare (the federal health care program for older Americans), payment for inpatient services is based on the prospective payment system (PPS). This payment system reimburses the hospital a fixed amount for services provided to a patient based on medical diagnosis (cost per case). In the capitated payment plan and the PPS plan, every test or service performed is a cost to the provider who will be reimbursed only a fixed amount regardless of the amount of service provided. Laboratory testing on outpatients is based on a fee schedule (Section 1833(h) of the Social Security Act). Payment is the lesser of the amount billed, the fee for a given geographical area, or the national limit. The laboratory uses laboratory test codes—current procedural terminology (CPT)—when billing Medicare.

These managed cost plans are an attempt by third-party payers (insurers) to ensure that services provided are necessary and reasonably priced. The new reimbursement systems place the provider at risk to provide necessary services while controlling overall costs. Thus, laboratory services must be considered a resource to be managed rather than a source of revenue.

The health care system is now interested in managing not only costs but also care. The goal of managed care is to provide quality care while maximizing efficiency and effectiveness. The use of disease management (DM) models is an attempt to meet this goal. Under these models, a protocol is designed to identify patients with a specific disease, and a therapy is developed to maximize clinical outcomes at an acceptable cost. The DM model for a particular disease is based on evidence in the literature and other sources.[9] Thus, DM is a population-level approach to improving health status rather than a patient-focused approach as has dominated the U.S. health care system. DM is designed to improve the value of health care delivery from the perspectives of providers, patients, and insurers. This value concept is broad based and includes the maximization of clinical, economic, quality-of-life, and satisfaction outcomes for the lowest expenditure of time and resources.[10]

Many organizations are creating and adopting new strategies to provide cost-effective and diagnostically efficient health care. These strategies include clinical pathways, also known as *practice guidelines*, and critical pathways (care plans). Sometimes clinical pathways and critical pathways are considered the same and the terms are used interchangeably. Here *clinical pathways* refer to plans and procedures developed by physicians using a foundation of scientific outcomes for diagnosing and treating a particular disease.[7,10] The guidelines indicate tests, procedures, and treatments. *Critical pathways* refer to the care and services provided by an interdisciplinary health care team after treatment decisions have been made. Teams of practitioners who have the knowledge and perspectives to view the total care process develop these pathways.[11] Clinical and critical pathways are usually designed for common and/or high-cost diagnoses. They are not appropriate in complicated cases.

These evolving health care practices require a partnership among physicians, nurses, allied health practitioners, patients, and health care administrators. As the complexity of laboratory testing increases, communication between the physician and clinical laboratory provider must increase. The laboratory provider must be able to correlate laboratory test results with clinical disease states, pathophysiology, and treatment; effectively communicate these results to the physician; and suggest cost-effective follow-up testing when appropriate.[12] The focus should be on changing structure and processes to improve patient outcomes. The goal is optimal utilization of laboratory testing, not necessarily less testing. The laboratory can take proactive approaches to control test utilization. These include:

* Assisting in the development of critical pathways
* Managing the test ordering system
* Instituting sequential testing protocols
* Eliminating incorrect use of tests
* Designing wellness panels

As more outcome studies are performed to determine which processes and treatments are most effective and as information on the value of laboratory testing is documented, the role of laboratory tests in clinical and critical pathways will become more important. Physicians will want to order the appropriate tests under the guidelines.

► LABORATORY TESTING IN THE INVESTIGATION OF A HEMATOLOGIC PROBLEM

A physician's investigation of a hematologic problem includes taking a medical history and performing a physical examination. Clues provided by this preliminary investigation will help guide the physician's choice of laboratory tests to help confirm the diagnosis. The challenge is to select appropriate tests that contribute to a cost-efficient and effective diagnosis. Laboratory testing usually begins with screening tests; based on results of these tests, more specific tests, are ordered. Repeat tests may be ordered to track disease progression, evaluate treatment, identify side effects and complications, or assist in prognosis.

Hematology screening tests include the **complete blood count (CBC),** which quantifies the white blood cells (WBC), red blood cells (RBC), hemoglobin, hematocrit, and platelets and calculates the **RBC indices.** The indices are calculated from the results of the hemoglobin, RBC count, and hematocrit to define the size and hemoglobin content of RBCs. The indices are important parameters in differentiating causes of anemia and help direct further testing. The CBC may also include a WBC differential. This procedure enumerates the five types of WBCs and reports each as a percentage of the total WBC count. A differential is especially helpful if the WBC count is abnormal. When it is, the differential identifies which cell type is abnormally increased or decreased and determines whether immature and/or abnormal forms are present, thus, providing a clue to diagnosis. The morphology of RBCs and platelets is also studied as a routine part of the differential. If a hemostasis problem is suspected, the screening tests include the platelet count, **prothrombin time (PT),** and **activated partial thromboplastin time (APTT).** These tests provide clues that guide the choice of follow-up tests to help identify the problem. Follow-up tests may include not only hematologic tests but also chemical, immunologic, and/or molecular analysis.

Follow-up testing that is done based on results of screening tests is referred to as **reflex testing.** As scientists learn more about the pathophysiology and treatment of hematopoietic disease, the number of tests designed to assist in diagnosis expands. To help physicians select the most cost-effective testing strategies, the laboratory must collaborate with physicians to design reflex testing protocols for common diseases.[13] These protocols are sometimes referred to as *algorithms.*

Throughout this text, readers are urged to use the reflex testing concept in their thought processes when studying the laboratory investigation of a disease. Each hematopoietic disorder is discussed in the following order: pathophysiology, clinical findings, laboratory findings, and treatment. The reader should consider which laboratory tests provide the information necessary to identify the cause of the disorder based on the suspected disorder's pathophysiology. Although it is unusual for the physician to provide a patient history or diagnosis to the laboratory when ordering tests, this information is often crucial to direct investigation and assist in interpretation of the test results. Perhaps with the medical necessity guidelines enforced by Medicare, the laboratory will be provided this information in the future. *Medical necessity* refers to the need for a test to be done given the patient's diagnosis. Medicare carriers determine medical necessity and require that the diagnostic related group (DRG) code accompany the request for reimbursement of tests the laboratory performs. In any case, if laboratory professionals need more patient information in order to perform testing appropriately, they should obtain the patient's chart or call the physician.

✓ Checkpoint! 2

A 13-year-old female was seen by her physician for complaints of a sore throat, lethargy, and swollen lymph nodes. A CBC was performed with the following results: Hb 90 g/L; Hct 0.30 L/L; RBC 3.8×10^{12}/L; WBC 15×10^9/L. Is reflex testing suggested by these results?

SUMMARY

Hematology is the study of the cellular components of blood: erythrocytes, leukocytes, and platelets. Changes in the concentrations of these cells occur from infancy until adulthood. Diseases can upset the steady state concentration of these parameters. A CBC is usually performed as a screening test to determine whether there are quantitative abnormalities in blood cells. The physician may order reflex tests if one or more of the CBC parameters are outside the reference interval.

Changes in the health care system focus on containing costs while maintaining quality of care. The laboratory's role in this system is to work with physicians to optimize utilization of laboratory testing.

REVIEW QUESTIONS

LEVELS I AND II

1. In which group of individuals would you expect to find the highest reference intervals for hemoglobin, hematocrit, and erythrocyte count? (Objective 1)
   a. newborns
   b. males older than 12 years of age
   c. females older than 17 years of age
   d. children between 1 and 5 years of age

2. Which cells are important in transporting oxygen and carbon dioxide between the lungs and body tissues? (Objective 2)
   a. platelets
   b. leukocytes
   c. thrombocytes
   d. erythrocytes

3. Forty-five percent of the volume of blood is composed of: (Objective 3)
   a. erythrocytes
   b. leukocytes
   c. platelets
   d. plasma

4. Alterations in the concentration of blood cells generally are the result of: (Objective 4)
   a. laboratory error
   b. amount of exercise before blood draw
   c. a disease process
   d. variations in analytical equipment

5. Leukocytes are necessary for: (Objective 2)
   a. hemostasis
   b. defense against foreign antigens
   c. oxygen transport
   d. excretions of cellular metabolites

6. Laboratories can use which type of testing to help direct the physician's selection of appropriate testing after screening tests are performed? (Objective 5)
   a. reflexive based on results of screening tests
   b. manual repeat of abnormal results
   c. second test by a different instrument
   d. standing orders for all inpatients

7. Managed care plans use which type of payment system to help contain costs of medical care? (Objective 6)
   a. fee-for-service
   b. cost-per-case
   c. capitation
   d. disease containment

8. A model used to help diagnose and manage the care of the diabetic patient in a cost-effective and diagnostically efficient manner while providing quality care is an example of: (Objective 5)
   a. reflex testing
   b. disease management
   c. capitated payment
   d. critical pathway

9. The payment system that Medicare uses to contain costs is: (Objective 6)
   a. capitated payment
   b. disease management
   c. fee-for-service
   d. PPS

10. Under the capitation payment system, the laboratory is viewed as a: (Objective 6)
    a. revenue center
    b. profit center
    c. loss center
    d. cost center

www.pearsonhighered.com/mckenzie
Use this address to access the interactive Companion Website created for this textbook. Find additional information, tables and figures. Evaluate your command of the chapter information using case studies and critical thinking and multiple choice questions.

REFERENCES

1. Wintrobe MM. *Blood. Pure and Eloquent.* New York: McGraw-Hill; 1980.

2. Vierordt K. Zahlungen der Blutkorperchen des Menschen. *Arch Physiol Heilk,* 1852;11:327.

3. Bao W, Dalferes ER, Srinivasan BR, Webber LS, and Berenson GS. Normative distribution of complete blood count from early childhood through adolescence: The Bogulusa Heart Study. *Prev Med.* 1993;22:825–37.

4. U.S. Dept of Health & Human Services. Medicare and Medicaid Statistical Supplement. Health Care Financing Review. 2007.

5. Wennberg JE. Variations in medical practice and hospital costs. *Conn Med.* 1985;49:444–53.

6. Wennberg JE, Gittelsohn A. Variations in medical care among small areas. *Sci Am.* 1982;246:120–34.

7. Wennberg JE, Gittelsohn A. Small area variations in health care delivery. *Science.* 1973;12:1102–8.

8. Baicker K, Chandra A, Skinner JS, Wennberg JE. Who you are and where you live: How race and geography affect the treatment of Medicare beneficiaries. *Health Affairs.* 2004;var.33–44.

9. Couch JB. Disease management: An overview. In: Couch JB, ed. *The physician's guide to disease management.* Gaithersburg, MD: Aspen Publishers; 1997:1–27.

10. Weingarten S, Graber G. Outcome-validated clinical practice guidelines: A scientific foundation for disease management. In: Couch JB, ed. *The physician's guide to disease management.* Gaithersburg, MD: Aspen Publishers; 1997:57–82.

11. Keiser JF, Howard BJ. Critical pathways: Design, implementation, and evaluation. *Clin Lab Manage Rev.* 1998;12:317–32.

12. Fritsma GA, Ens GE. Reflexive protocols and laboratory-clinician communication. *Clin Hem Rev.* April 1997:2–3.

13. Hernandez JS. Cost-effectiveness of laboratory testing. *Arch Pathol Lab Med.* 2003;127:440–445.

2

Cellular Homeostasis

J. Lynne Williams, Ph.D.

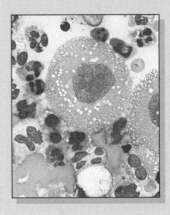

■ OBJECTIVES—LEVEL I

At the end of this unit of study, the student should be able to:

1. Describe the location, morphology, and function of subcellular organelles of a cell.
2. Describe the lipid asymmetry found in the plasma membrane of most hematopoietic cells.
3. Differentiate the parts of the mammalian cell cycle.
4. Define R (restriction point) and its role in cell cycle regulation.
5. Define *apoptosis* and explain its role in normal human physiology.
6. Classify and give examples of the major categories of initiators and inhibitors of apoptosis.
7. List the major events regulated by apoptosis in hematopoiesis.

■ OBJECTIVES—LEVEL II

At the end of this unit of study, the student should be able to:

1. Explain the significance of SNPs, introns, exons, UTRs, post-translational protein modifications.
2. List the components and explain the function of the Ubiquitin-Proteosome system.
3. Define *cyclins* and *Cdks* and their role in cell cycle regulation; describe the associated Cdk partners and function of cyclins D, E, A, and B.
4. Define *CAK* (Cdk-activating kinase) and the two major classes of CKIs (cyclin-dependent kinase inhibitors) and describe their function.
5. Compare the function of cell-cycle checkpoints in cell-cycle regulation.
6. Describe/illustrate the roles of p53 and pRb in cell-cycle regulation.
7. Propose how abnormalities of cell-cycle regulatory mechanisms can lead to malignancy.
8. Define *caspases* and explain their role in apoptosis.
9. Differentiate the extrinsic and intrinsic pathways of cellular apoptosis.
10. Define and contrast the roles of proapoptotic and antiapoptotic members of the Bcl-2 family of proteins.
11. Describe apoptotic regulatory mechanisms.
12. Give examples of diseases associated with increased apoptosis and inhibited (decreased) apoptosis.
13. Define, and give examples of, epigenetics, oncogenes and tumor suppressor genes and their roles in cell biology.
14. Differentiate using morphologic observations, the processes of necrotic cell death and apoptotic cell death.

KEY TERMS

Anti-oncogene/tumor suppressor gene
Apoptosis
Caspase
Cell cycle
Cell-cycle checkpoints
Cyclins/Cdks
Epigenetics
Exon
Genome/genomics
Intron
Mutation
Necrosis
Oncogene
Polymorphism
Post-translational modification
Proteomics
Proteosome
Proto-oncogene
Quiescence (G_0)
Restriction point (R)
Single nucleotide polymorphism (SNP)
Tissue homeostasis
Transcription factors (TFs)
Ubiquitin
Untranslated regions (UTRs)

BACKGROUND BASICS

Level I and Level II
Students should have a solid foundation in basic cell biology principles, including the component parts of a cell and the structure and function of cytoplasmic organelles. They should have an understanding of the segments composing a cell cycle (interphase and mitosis) and the processes that take place during each stage.

▶ OVERVIEW

Not all hematology courses include the material in this chapter. However, it is a review of basic principles of cellular metabolism and homeostasis, which provide the foundation for understanding many of the pathologic abnormalities underlying the hematologic disorders in subsequent chapters. The chapter begins with a review of the basic components and cellular processes of a normal cell and presents the concept of tissue homeostasis. Cellular processes that maintain tissue homeostasis—cell proliferation and cell death—are discussed at the functional and molecular level. The chapter concludes with a discussion of what happens when genes controlling cell proliferation, differentiation, and/or cell death mutate.

▶ INTRODUCTION

The maintenance of an adequate number of cells to carry out the functions of the organism is referred to as **tissue homeostasis.** Tissue homeostasis depends on the careful regulation of several cellular processes, including cellular proliferation, cellular differentiation, and cell death (apoptosis). A thorough understanding of cell structural components as well as the processes of cell division and cell death allows us to understand not only the normal (physiologic) regulation of the cells of the blood but also disease processes in which these events become dysregulated (e.g., cancer).

▶ CELL MORPHOLOGY REVIEW

A basic understanding of cell morphology is essential to the study of hematology because many hematologic disorders are accompanied by abnormalities or changes in morphology of cellular or subcellular components and by changes in cell concentrations.

A cell is an intricate, complex structure consisting of a membrane-bound aqueous solution of proteins, carbohydrates, fats, inorganic materials, and nucleic acids. The nucleus, bound by a double layer of membrane, controls and directs the development, function, and division of the cell. The cytoplasm, where most of the cell's metabolic reactions take place, surrounds the nucleus and is bound by the cell membrane. The cytoplasm contains highly ordered organelles, which are membrane-bound components with specific cellular functions (Figure 2-1a ■). The different kinds of organelles and the quantity of each depend on the function of the cell and the state of maturation.

CELL MEMBRANE

The outer boundary of the cell, the plasma (cell) membrane, is often considered a barrier between the cell and its environment. In fact, it functions to allow the regulated passage of ions, nutrients, and information between the cytoplasm and its extracellular milieu and thus determines the interrelationships of the cell with its surroundings.

The plasma membrane consists of a complex, ordered array of lipids and proteins that serves as the interface between the cell and its environment (Figure 2-1b ■). The plasma membrane is in the form of a phospholipid bilayer punctuated by proteins. The lipids have their polar (hydrophilic) head groups directed toward the outside and inside of the cell and their long-chain (hydrophobic) hydrocarbon tails directed inward. While the plasma membrane has traditionally been described as a "fluid mosaic" structure,[1] it is in fact highly ordered with asymmetric distribution of both membrane lipids and proteins. The lipid and protein compositions of the outside and inside of the membrane differ from

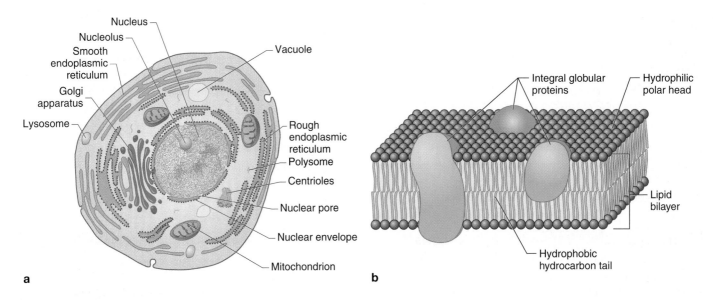

■ FIGURE 2-1   a. Drawing of a cell depicting the various organelles. **b.** The fluid mosaic membrane model proposed by Singer and Nicholson.

one another in ways that reflect the different functions performed at the two surfaces of the membrane.

Four major phospholipids are found in the plasma membrane: phosphatidylethanolamine (PE), phosphatidylserine (PS), phosphatidylcholine (PC), and sphingomyelin (SM) (Web Figure 2-1 ■). Most blood cells have an asymmetric distribution of these phospholipids with PE and PS occurring in the inner layer of the lipid bilayer and PC and SM occurring predominantly in the outer layer. The membrane lipids can freely diffuse laterally throughout their own half of the bilayer, or they may flip-flop from one side of the bilayer to the other in response to certain stimuli as occurs in platelets when activated; ∞ Chapter 29. Membrane lipids including phospholipids, cholesterol, lipoproteins, and lipopolysaccharides contribute to the basic framework of cell membranes and account for the cell's high permeability to lipid-soluble substances. Different mixtures of lipids are found in the membranes of different types of cells.

Although lipids are responsible for the basic structure of the plasma membrane, most of the specific functions of the membrane are carried out by proteins. The proteins of the membrane provide selective permeability and transport of specific substances, structural stability, enzymatic catalysis, and cell-to-cell recognition functions. The membrane proteins are divided into two general groups: integral (transmembrane) proteins and peripheral proteins. The peripheral proteins are located on either the cytoplasmic or on the extracellular half of the lipid bilayer. Some of the integral proteins span the entire lipid bilayer while other integral proteins only partially penetrate the membrane. Some membrane-spanning proteins traverse the membrane once (e.g., erythrocyte glycophorin A) while others criss-cross the membrane multiple times (e.g. erythrocyte Band 3, the cation transporter) (∞ Chapter 5). In

some cells, such as erythrocytes (∞ Chapter 5), peripheral proteins on the cytoplasmic side of the membrane form a lattice network that functions as a cellular cytoskeleton, imparting order on the membrane.

Carbohydrates linked to membrane lipids (glycolipids) or proteins (glycoproteins) may extend from the outer surface of the membrane. Functions of the carbohydrate moieties include specific binding, cell-to-cell recognition, and cell adhesion. The sugar groups are added to the lipid or protein molecules in the lumen of the Golgi apparatus after synthesis by the endoplasmic reticulum. Many of the glycoprotein transmembrane proteins serve as receptors for extracellular molecules such as growth factors. Binding of the specific ligand to a receptor may result in transduction of a signal to the cell's interior without passage of the extracellular molecule through the membrane.

CYTOPLASM

The cytoplasm, or cytosol, is where the metabolic activities of the cell including protein synthesis, growth, motility, and phagocytosis take place. The structural components, called *organelles,* include the mitochondria, lysosomes, endoplasmic reticulum (ER), Golgi apparatus, ribosomes, granules, microtubules, and microfilaments (Table 2-1 ✪). Organelles and other cellular inclusions lie within the cytoplasmic matrix. The composition of the cytoplasm depends on cell lineage and degree of cell maturity. The appearance of cytoplasm in fixed, stained blood cells is important in evaluating the morphology, classifying the cell, and determining the stage of differentiation. Immature or synthetically active blood cells stained with Romanowsky stains (∞ Chapter 34) have very basophilic (blue) cytoplasm due to the large quantity of ribonucleic acid (RNA) they contain.

❂ TABLE 2-1

Cellular Organelles

Structure	Composition	Function
Ribosomes	RNA + proteins	Assemble amino acids into protein
"Free"	Scattered in the cytoplasm	Synthesis of protein destined to remain in cytosol
	Linked by mRNA-forming polyribosomes	
"Fixed"	Ribosomes bound to outer surface of RER	Synthesis of protein destined for export from the cell
Endoplasmic reticulum (ER)	Interconnecting membrane-bound tubules and vesicles	Synthesis and transport of lipid and protein
Rough ER (RER)	Studded on outer surface with ribosomes	Abundant in cells synthesizing secretory protein; protein transported to Golgi
Smooth ER (SER)	Lacks attached ribosomes	Lipid synthesis, detoxification, synthesis of steroid hormones
Golgi apparatus	Stacks of flattened membranes located in juxtanuclear region	Protein from RER is sorted, modified (e.g., glycosylated), and packaged; forms lysosomes
Lysosomes	Membrane-bound sacs containing hydrolytic enzymes	Destruction of carbohydrates, lipids, and proteins (phagocytosed material or metabolites)
Mitochondria	Double-membrane organelle; inner folds (cristae) house enzymes of aerobic metabolism	Oxidative phosphorylation (ATP production) abundant in metabolically active cells
Cytoskeleton	Microfilaments, intermediate filaments, and microtubules	Gives the cell shape, provides strength, and enables movement of cellular structures
Microfilaments	Fine filaments (5–9 nm); polymers of actin	Control shape and surface movement of most cells
Intermediate filaments	Ropelike fibers (~10 nm); composed of number of fibrous proteins	Provide cells with mechanical strength
Microtubules	Hollow cylinders (~25 nm); composed of protein tubulin	Important in maintaining cell shape and organization of organelles; form spindle apparatus during mitosis
Centrosome	"Cell center"; includes centrioles	Microtubule-organizing center; forms poles of mitotic spindle during anaphase
Centrioles	Two cylindrical structures arranged at right angles to each other; consist of nine groups of three microtubules	Enable movement of chromosomes during cell division; self-replicate prior to cell division

 Checkpoint! 1

What is meant by the phrase "lipid asymmetry" when describing cell membranes?

NUCLEUS

The nucleus contains the genetic material, deoxyribonucleic acid (DNA), responsible for the regulation of all cellular functions. The nuclear material, chromatin, consists of DNA and associated structural proteins (histones) packaged into chromosomes. The total genetic information stored in the chromosomes of an organism constitutes its **genome.** The fundamental subunit of chromatin is the nucleosome, a beadlike segment of chromosome composed of about 180 base pairs of DNA wrapped around a histone protein. The linear array of successive nucleosomes gives chromatin a "beads-on-a-string" appearance in electron micrographs. The appearance of chromatin varies, presumably depending on activity. It is generally considered that the dispersed, lightly stained portions of chromatin (euchromatin) represent unwound or loosely twisted regions of chromatin that are transcriptionally active. The condensed, more deeply staining chromatin (heterochromatin) is believed to represent tightly twisted or folded regions of chromatin strands that are transcriptionally inactive. In addition to being less tightly associated with the histones, active chromatin characteristically has "unmethylated" promoter regions and highly acetylated histones (see the later section on "Epigenetics"). The ratio of euchromatin to heterochromatin depends on the cell activity with the younger or more active cells having more euchromatin and a finer chromatin structure. The nuclei of most active cells contain from one to four pale staining nucleoli. The nucleolus (singular) consists of RNA and proteins and is believed to be important in RNA synthesis. The nucleolus of very young blood cells is easily seen with brightfield microscopy on stained smears.

The nuclear contents are surrounded by a double membrane, the nuclear envelope. The outer membrane (cytoplasmic side) is continuous with the ER and has a polypeptide composition distinct from that of the inner membrane. The gap between the two membranes (~50 nm) is called the *perinuclear space*. The nuclear envelope is interrupted at irregular intervals by openings consisting of nuclear pore complexes (NPCs), which provide a means of communication between nucleus and cytoplasm. They constitute envelope-piercing channels that function as selective gates allowing bidirectional movement of molecules. The nucleus exports newly assembled ribosomal subunits while importing proteins such as transcription factors and DNA repair enzymes.

 Checkpoint! 2

Explain the difference between densely staining chromatin and lighter staining chromatin when viewing blood cells under a microscope.

► CELLULAR METABOLISM: DNA DUPLICATION, TRANSCRIPTION, TRANSLATION

Genomics is the study of the entire genome of an organism. *Functional genomics* is the study of the actual gene expression "profile" of a particular cell at a particular stage of differentiation or functional activity (i.e., which genes are actively producing mRNA). Microarray or expression array technology can be used to determine the mRNA profile being produced by a cell or tissue of interest, which would reflect which genes are actively being transcribed. The field of **proteomics** is the study of the composition, structure, function, and interaction of the proteins being produced by a cell. [Genetic nomenclature has specific rules for gene and protein font styles. To differentiate between the gene and its protein, genes are written as italicized capital letters (i.e., *RB*) while the gene's protein product is written with only the first letter capitalized and it is not italicized. This style is used in this text.]

Genes, which contain the genetic information of an individual, constitute regions (loci) of the chromosome on which they are located. Most genes are not composed of continuous stretches of nucleotides. Rather, they are organized into segments called **exons,** which are separated by intervening sequences called **introns.** The nucleotide base pairs of the introns do not code for protein. When a gene is transcribed into RNA, the entire sequence of exons and introns is copied as *pre-messenger RNA* (sometimes called *heteronuclear RNA/ hnRNA*). Subsequently, the nucleotides corresponding to the intron sequences are spliced out, resulting in the shorter, mature mRNA. However, not all of the mature mRNA will be translated into protein. Both the 5′ and the 3′ ends of the mature mRNA encoding the protein to be produced contain **untranslated regions (UTRs).** The UTRs influence the stability of the mRNA and the efficiency of translation to protein. These regions have been shown to play an important role in regulating the proteins involved in iron metabolism in developing erythrocytes (∞ Chapter 9).

Sometimes large genes with multiple exons can be "read" in a variety of ways, resulting in different proteins based on alternative transcriptions of the gene. The human genome is estimated to contain ~35,000 genes; however, alternate splicing allows for greater genetic complexity than the number of genes would suggest.

Different individuals do not have identical DNA sequences. When a cell replicates its DNA during S phase of the cell cycle (discussed later), the process does not occur without error. It has been estimated that ~0.01% of the 6 billion base pairs are copied incorrectly during each S-phase.[2] The process of DNA replication is coupled with DNA repair systems to make sure that errors in copying are corrected. If these errors cannot be corrected, the cell may activate its internal apoptotic mechanism (discussed later), resulting in cell death. Errors in DNA replication that cannot be corrected and that subsequently result in activation of apoptosis are believed to be the underlying basis for the large degree of ineffective erythropoiesis in megaloblastic anemias (∞ Chapter 12). In addition to correcting copying errors, DNA repair mechanisms correct other damage to DNA that could have occurred. Failure of these DNA repair mechanisms often contribute to the development of a malignancy.

If the miscopied base pair is not corrected, a mutation (or new polymorphism) may occur. Variations of the genetic sequence of a gene that may be seen in different individuals are called *alleles*. **Polymorphism** is the term used to describe the presence of alternate copies (alleles) of a gene. Not every alteration in DNA produces an abnormality. For instance, many of the alternate alleles identified for human globin chains do not result in any abnormality of function (∞ Chapter 10). Generally, if the change in DNA sequence does not result in an abnormality of function, the change is called a *polymorphism*. Often the word **mutation** is used only to describe a deleterious change in a gene (e.g., the β^S globin mutation in sickle cell anemia; ∞ Chapter 10).

A region of DNA that differs in only a single DNA nucleotide is called a **single nucleotide polymorphism (SNP).** SNPs are found at approximately 1 in every 1000 base pairs in the human genome (resulting in ~2.5 million SNPs in the entire genome). To be considered a true polymorphism, an SNP must occur with a frequency of >1% in the population. If the alteration is known to be the cause of a disease, the nucleotide change is considered a mutation rather than an SNP.

CONTROL OF GENE EXPRESSION

Control of gene expression is a complex process. It must be regulated in both time (i.e., developmentally) and location (i.e., tissue-specific gene expression). Most genes have a promoter region upstream of the coding region of the gene. **Transcription factors (TFs)** are proteins that bind to the

DNA of the promoter region of a target gene and regulate expression of that gene. TFs may function to either activate or repress the target gene (some TFs do both, depending on the specific targeted gene). Often TFs are tissue specific, such as GATA-1, a known erythroid specific TF that regulates expression of glycophorin and globin chains in developing cells of the erythroid lineage.[3]

In addition to the basic on/off function of the promoter region, there are additional layers of control of gene expression. Some genes have enhancer elements or silencer elements, which are nucleotide sequences that can amplify or suppress gene expression, respectively.[2] These response elements influence gene expression by binding specific regulatory proteins (activators, repressors).

Many signals that regulate genes come from outside the cell (e.g., cytokine control of hematopoiesis; ∞ Chapter 3). The external molecule (cytokine) or ligand binds to its specific receptor on the surface of the cell. The binding of ligand to receptor activates the receptor and initiates a cell-signaling pathway that conveys the activation signal from the receptor to the nucleus. The end result is an interaction with DNA (e.g., TF binding to one or more gene promoter regions) that either activates or represses the target gene(s).

PROTEIN SYNTHESIS AND PROCESSING

Synthesis of proteins (polypeptides) occurs on ribosomes. The newly formed polyeptides are transported to their eventual destination through a sorting mechanism within the cytoplasm.[4] If the polypeptide lacks a "signal sequence," translation is completed in the cytosol, and the protein either stays in the cytosol or is incorporated into the nucleus, mitochondria, or peroxisomes. If the polypeptide contains a signal sequence, the polypeptide is extruded into the lumen of the endoplasmic reticulum (which ultimately gives rise to the more distal structures of the secretory apparatus—the Golgi, endosomes, lysosomes, and plasma membrane).

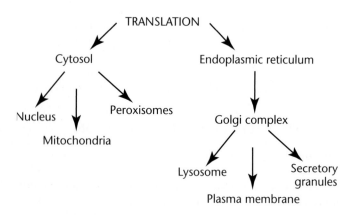

Following import into the ER, proteins undergo appropriate folding and may undergo **post-translational modifications.** These are modifications in protein structure that occur after the protein is produced by translation on the ribosome. These changes include the addition of nonprotein groups (such as sugars or lipids), modification of existing amino acids (such as the γ-carboxylation of certain coagulation proteins; ∞ Chapter 30), or cleavage of the initial polypeptide product resulting in a multichain molecule. As the proteins exit the ER, they may be accompanied by molecules that facilitate their transfer from the ER to the Golgi apparatus. A mutation in one of these transfer molecules, ERGIC-53, is the cause of the hemostatic disorder combined F-V-VIII deficiency (∞ Chapter 32). During transport through the Golgi, additional processing of the proteins occurs.

The primary structure of a protein is defined by its amino acid sequence (see Web Table 2-1 ✪ for review of the amino acids and their shorthand notations). A protein emerges from the ribosome in an extended, linear conformation. Subsequently, local regions are folded into specific conformations, the protein's secondary structure, determined by the primary amino acid sequence. The two major secondary protein structures are α-helices and β-pleated sheets. Most proteins are made up of combinations of α-helices and β-sheets connected by regions of a less regular structure termed *loops*. *Molecular chaperones* are cytoplasmic proteins that assist the polypeptide in this folding process. The tertiary structure of a protein refers to its unique three-dimensional shape determined by the folding of secondary structures. Sometimes appropriately folded protein monomers are assembled with other proteins to form multisubunit complexes (also facilitated by chaperones). The *quaternary structure of a protein* refers to the assembly of independently synthesized polypeptide chains into a multimeric protein (e.g., the $\alpha_2\beta_2$ tetramer, which constitutes hemoglobin A; ∞ Chapter 6).

Proteins are often described as being made up of *domains*. Frequently, a domain is encoded in a single exon and represents a region of the polypeptide chain that can fold into a stable tertiary structure. The domains of a protein are often used to designate the location of a particular functional or structural attribute.

A mutation that alters a protein's amino acid sequence can result in failure to function. Failure to function can result from a mutation of a critical functional residue or from the amino acid alteration preventing the protein from folding into its proper three-dimensional structure. Improperly folded proteins are marked for destruction and degraded (via the ubiquitin system).

✓ **Checkpoint! 3**

What is the difference between a polymorphism and a mutation?

THE UBIQUITIN SYSTEM

The ubiquitin system is responsible for disposing of damaged or misfolded proteins.[4] In addition, it regulates numerous cellular processes (e.g., cell-cycle progression, cellular differentiation) by the timed destruction of key regulatory proteins (e.g., cyclins, membrane receptors, transcription factors). It is a nonlysosomal, proteolytic mechanism in the cytoplasm of most cells.

Molecules destined for destruction are tagged with a small (76 amino acid) polypeptide called **ubiquitin** (Figure 2-2 ■). Appropriately labeled molecules are then transferred to an ATP-dependent protease complex (the proteosome) for destruction. Generally, proteins bearing a single ubiquitin molecule are marked for endocytosis and degradation in lysosomes. Multi-ubiquitinated proteins are marked for destruction by the proteosome, which is assembled into a cylinder through which proteins are channeled for destruction.

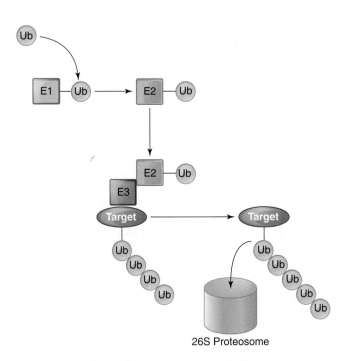

26S Proteosome

■ FIGURE 2-2   Ubiquitin-Proteosome system. E1 = ubiquitin activating enzyme; E2 = ubiquitin conjugating enzyme; E3 = ubiquitin ligase; Ub = ubiquitin; E1 activates Ub, which is then transferred to the E2 enzyme; E3 functions in target substrate recognition; it brings together the target and E2-Ub and then catalyzes the transfer of Ub from E2-Ub to the target. Once a target has become multi-ubiquitinated, it is directed to the 26S proteosome for degradation.

▶ TISSUE HOMEOSTASIS: PROLIFERATION, DIFFERENTIATION, AND APOPTOSIS

Tissue homeostasis refers to the maintenance of an adequate number of cells to carry out the functions of the organism. In the human body, somatic cells (including blood cells) generally undergo one of three possible fates: They (1) proliferate by mitotic cell division, (2) differentiate and acquire specialized functions, or (3) die and are eliminated from the body. Cell proliferation is required for the replacement of cells lost to terminal differentiation, cell death, or cell loss. Differentiation provides a variety of cells, each of which is capable of executing specific and specialized functions. Recently, it has become apparent that cell death is also an active process (**apoptosis**) that the cell itself can initiate. Apoptosis is physiologically as important as cell proliferation and differentiation in controlling the overall homeostasis of various tissues. When the regulation of any of these three cellular processes malfunctions or the processes become unbalanced, the consequence may be tissue atrophy, functional insufficiency, or neoplasia (cancer). The following sections present an overview of the physiologic processes first followed by a discussion of the molecular regulation of each. Not all readers may be interested in the molecular aspects of regulation, but it is included in this book for those who want to gain a foundation for understanding the development of hematologic malignancies (∞ Chapters 21–26).

THE CELL CYCLE

Cell division is a fundamental process that is required throughout the life of all eukaryotes. Although it has been known for many years that cells have the ability to grow and replicate, the actual mechanisms involved were discovered relatively recently.[5] When a cell is stimulated to divide, it goes through a series of well-defined (biochemical and morphological) stages called the **cell cycle,** which is divided into four phases: G_1 (Gap-1), S (DNA synthesis), G_2 (Gap-2), and M (mitosis) (Figure 2-3 ■).

Stages of the Cell Cycle

The physical process of cell division is preceded by a series of morphologically recognizable stages referred to as *mitosis* (*M phase*) (Web Figure 2-2 ■). During mitosis, chromosomes condense (*prophase*), align on a microtubular spindle (*metaphase*), and sister chromatids segregate to opposite poles of the cell (*anaphase* and *telophase*). The interval between successive mitoses (known as *interphase*) shows little morphologic variation except that cells grow in volume. During interphase, the cell synthesizes molecules and duplicates its components in preparation for the next mitosis. However, DNA synthesis occurs only during a narrow window of time of interphase. In *S phase,* DNA synthesis takes place and is separated from M phase (mitosis) by two gap periods: G_1,

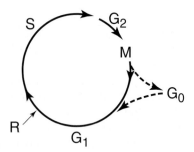

■ **FIGURE 2-3**   The four phases of the cell cycle: G_1, S, G_2, and M. G_0 represents the state of quiescence when a cell is withdrawn from the cell cycle. R represents the restriction point—the point in the cell cycle after which the cell no longer depends on extracellular signals but can complete the cycle in the absence of mitogenic stimuli. (Reprinted with permission from *Recombinant DNA*, 2nd ed., New York: W. H. Freeman; 1992.)

the time between the end of mitosis and the onset of the next round of DNA replication, and G_2, the time between the completion of S and the onset of mitosis.

Not all of the cells in the body are actively dividing (i.e., actively engaged in the cell cycle). Cells may exit the cell cycle at G_1 and enter a nonproliferative phase called G_0, or **quiescence** (Figure 2-3). To proliferate, a cell must re-enter the cell cycle. In response to specific mitogenic stimuli, quiescent cells can exit G_0 and re-enter the cell cycle at the level of early G_1. In unicellular organisms such as bacteria, cell division depends only on an adequate supply of nutrients. In mammalian cells, all cell division cycles are initiated by specific growth factors, or mitogens, that drive the cell from G_0 to G_1 ($G_0 \rightarrow G_1$). Some cells, such as terminally differentiated neutrophils, have irreversibly exited the cell cycle during differentiation and are in G_0. Other cells, such as hematopoietic stem cells or antigen-specific memory lymphocytes, primarily reside in G_0 but can be induced to return to G_1 and begin cycling with appropriate cytokine or antigen stimulation.

G_1 is characterized by a period of cell growth and synthesis of components necessary for replication. If conditions are unsuitable for proliferation (insufficient nutrients or mitogens), cells will arrest in G_1. As cells transit through the G_1 phase of the cell cycle, they pass through what has been called the **restriction point (R)** in late G_1. R defines a point in the cell cycle after which the cell no longer depends on extracellular signals but is committed to completing that cell cycle *independent* of further mitogenic stimuli (i.e., cell-cycle completion becomes autonomous).[6] Cells then transit across the G_1/S boundary into the S phase of the cycle where DNA synthesis occurs followed by the G_2 phase and finally mitosis (where nuclear division [*karyokinesis*] and cytoplasmic separation [*cytokinesis*] occur).

Molecular Regulation of the Cell Cycle

The fundamental task of the cell cycle is to faithfully replicate DNA once during S phase and to distribute identical chromosome copies equally to both daughter cells during M

phase. Organized progression through the cell cycle normally ensures that this takes place, so most cells never initiate mitosis before DNA duplication is completed, never attempt to segregate sister chromatids until all pairs are aligned on the mitotic spindle at metaphase, and never reduplicate their chromosomes (reinitiate S phase) before the paired chromatids have been separated at the previous mitosis. Cells must ensure that chromosome duplication and segregation occur in the correct order (i.e., $S \rightarrow M \rightarrow S \rightarrow M$). They must also see that the next event in the cycle begins *only*[7] when the previous events have been successfully completed (i.e., chromosome duplication is complete before the chromosomes are segregated into the two daughter cells). Entry into and exit from each phase of the cell cycle are tightly regulated. Failure to regulate this process results in aneuploidy (abnormal chromosome number) seen in many malignancies. Research over the past 20 years has begun to reveal how cells guarantee the orderliness of this process.[5]

Cyclins and Cyclin-Dependent Kinases

Enzymatic activities of specific kinases (phosphorylating enzymes) regulate the transition between the various phases of the cell cycle. These kinase proteins (**Cdks**, or cyclin-dependent kinases) phosphorylate target molecules important for cell cycle control. To be active, the kinase (Cdk) must be complexed with a regulatory protein named **cyclin** (hence, the name, **c**yclin-**d**ependent **k**inase). Numerous cyclins and Cdks exist in the cell. Different complexes with differing cyclin and Cdk components drive the cell from one cell cycle stage to the next. The sequential activation of successive cyclin/kinase complexes, each of which in turn phosphorylates key substrates, facilitates or regulates the movement of the cell through the cycle (Figure 2-4a ■). Cdk inhibitors that function to inhibit the active kinase activity by binding to the Cdks or the Cdk/cyclin complexes also exist.

At least 14 cyclins and at least 9 different Cdks have been discovered so far, although not all of them have been shown to play an essential role in regulating the cell cycle. The concentration of the different cyclin proteins rises and falls at specific times during the cell cycle (hence, they are *cycling* proteins). Different cyclin/Cdk complexes are functional at different phases of the cell cycle as summarized in Table 2-2 ✪.

A mammalian cell must receive external signals (growth factors and/or hormones) that trigger the cell to proliferate.[7] These external signals result in an increase of one (or more) of the D cyclins (of which there are three: D1, D2, and D3). Cyclin D complexes with Cdk4 or Cdk6 and phosphorylates target molecules required for $G_1 \rightarrow S$ progression. The D cyclins are unique in that they are synthesized in response to growth factor stimulation and remain active in the cell as long as the mitotic stimulus is present. Toward mid to late G_1, levels of cyclin E increase and bind with Cdk2. The cyclin E/Cdk2 complex is required for the

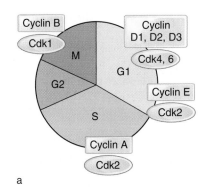

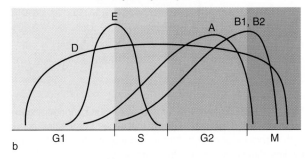

Cell cycle cyclin patterns

a

b

■ FIGURE 2-4   **a.** The phases of the cell cycle with the major regulatory cyclin/Cdk complexes depicted for each. **b.** The levels of the various cyclin proteins during the cell cycle. The cyclins rise and fall in a periodic fashion, thus controlling the cyclin-dependent kinases and their activities.

G_1 to S transition. Once the cell enters S phase, cyclin E degrades rapidly, and cyclin A takes over the activation of Cdk2. Cyclin A/Cdk2 is required for the onset of DNA synthesis, progression through S phase, and entry into mitosis. Toward the end of S phase, cyclin A starts to activate another kinase, Cdk1 (previously called cdc2), which signals the completion of S phase and the onset of G_2. Cyclin B takes over from cyclin A as the activating partner of Cdk1, and Cyclin B/Cdk1 controls the onset, sequence of events, and the completion of mitosis. Cyclin B must be destroyed for the cell to exit mitosis and for cytokinesis to take place (Figure 2-4b ■).

❂ TABLE 2-2

Cell Cycle Regulatory Proteins

Cell Cycle Phase	Cyclin	Partner Cdk
G_1	D1, D2, D3	Cdk4, Cdk6
G_1/S	E	Cdk2
S	A	Cdk2
M	A	Cdk1 (Cdc2)
	B	Cdk1 (Cdc2)

Regulation of Cell-Cycle Kinase Activity

Control of cell-cycle kinase activity is somewhat unique in that protein levels of the enzyme (kinase) subunit remain constant throughout the cell cycle and do not require activation from a proenzyme precursor form (unlike the activation of the serine proteases of the blood coagulation cascade; ∞ Chapter 30). Regulation is achieved by varying the availability of the regulatory cofactor (the cyclins) through periodic (and cell-cycle phase-specific) synthesis and degradation (by the ubiquitin system) of the appropriate cyclin partners (Figure 2-4b).[8] The periodic accumulation of different cyclins determines the sequential rise and fall of kinase activities, which in turn regulates the events of the cell cycle.

Multiple mechanisms regulate cell-cycle kinase activity. In addition to the requirement for the appropriate cyclin partner (controlled by cell-cycle specific synthesis and degradation of the different cyclins), the kinase subunit (Cdk) must be phosphorylated and/or dephosphorylated at specific amino acid residues.[9] Full kinase activity requires the phosphorylation of threonine (Thr) 161 (using the amino acid numbering of Cdk1). The kinase responsible for this activating phosphorylation is called CAK (Cdk-activating kinase) and is itself a Cdk (Cdk7 complexed with cyclin H). CAK is responsible for the activating phosphorylation of *all* the kinases important for mammalian cell cycle control including Cdks 1, 2, 4, and 6. On the other hand, phosphorylation of Thr 14 and tyrosine (Tyr) 15 suppresses kinase activity, and these phosphates must be removed by the phosphatase called *CDC25* in order to have a fully active cyclin/Cdk complex (Web Figure 2-3 ■).

The final level of regulation involves two groups of proteins that function as inhibitors of Cdks and cyclin/Cdk complexes (Figure 2-5 ■).[10] The first Cdk inhibitor identified was p21; other Cdk inhibitors with structural and functional similarities to p21 include p27 and p57. (This nomenclature indicates they are **p**roteins of the indicated molecular mass in kilodaltons, e.g., p21 is a protein of molecular weight of 21,000.) These three inhibitors bind multiple cyclin/Cdk complexes of various phases of the cell cycle (cyclin D/Cdk4/6, cyclin E/Cdk2, and cyclin A/Cdk2). The second group of inhibitors is a family of structurally related proteins that include p15, p16, p18, and p19. These inhibitors are more restricted in their inhibitory activity, inhibit only Cdk4 and Cdk6, and can induce cell cycle arrest in G_1.

Cell-Cycle Checkpoints

Cell proliferation and differentiation depend on the accurate duplication and transfer of genetic information, which requires the precise ordering of cell-cycle events. Cells achieve this coordination by using **cell-cycle checkpoints** to monitor events at critical points in the cycle and, if necessary, halt progression of the cycle.[11,12,13] The main functions of checkpoints are to detect malfunctions within the system and to assess whether certain events are properly completed before the cell is allowed to proceed through the cycle.

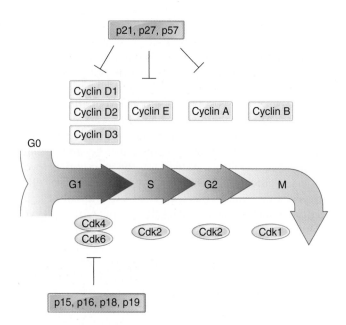

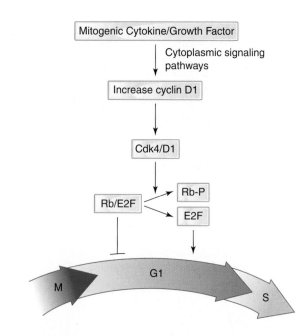

■ FIGURE 2-5   Cdk inhibitors. There are two families of Cyclin-dependent kinase inhibitors. The first group, including p15, p16, p18, and p19, inhibits only D-type cyclin/Cdk4 or Cdk6 complexes. The second group of inhibitors, including p21, p27, and p57, possesses a greater spectrum of inhibitory activity, inhibiting the G_1 as well as S-phase cyclin/Cdk complexes (Cyclin D/Cdk4/6, Cyclin E/Cdk2 and Cyclin A/Cdk2). ⊥ indicates inhibition of the pathway.

■ FIGURE 2-6   Role of the retinoblastoma susceptibility gene product (Rb) in regulation of the cell cycle. Stimulation of a cell with mitogens or growth factors induces synthesis of the D-type cyclins. Activation of G_1 phase kinase activity (Cyclin D/Cdk4/6) phosphorylates a number of intracellular substrates including the Rb protein. In the hypophosphorylated (active) state, Rb binds and sequesters transcription factors known as E2F, rendering them inactive. When Cyclin D/Cdk4 or Cdk6 phosphorylates Rb, it releases the E2F transcription factors, which then move to the nucleus, and initiate transcription of genes required for cell-cycle progression (including the genes for Cyclin E and Cyclin A). ↓ indicates stimulation of the pathway; ⊥ indicates inhibition of the pathway.

When problems are detected, check point mechanisms interrupt cell cycling to allow correction of the problem or elimination of the defective cell.

Several major cell-cycle checkpoints have been described. The G_1 *checkpoint* checks for DNA damage and prevents progression into S-phase if the integrity of the genome is compromised. The *S-phase checkpoint* monitors the accuracy of DNA replication. The G_2/M *checkpoint* also monitors the accuracy of DNA replication during S-phase. It checks for damaged or unreplicated DNA and can block mitosis if any is found. The *metaphase checkpoint* (also called the *mitotic-spindle checkpoint*) functions to ensure that all chromosomes are properly aligned on the spindle apparatus prior to initiating chromosomal separation and segregation at anaphase. If defects are detected at any of these checkpoints, the cell cycle is stopped by inhibiting the cyclin/Cdk kinase complexes. Activation of repair pathways may be initiated, or if the damage is severe, apoptosis may be triggered (discussed later).

Two proteins critical for effective function of the G_1 checkpoint are p53 and Rb. Rb is the protein product of the retinoblastoma susceptibility gene, which predisposes individuals to retinoblastomas and other tumors when only one functional copy is present. Rb is present throughout the cell cycle, although its phosphorylation state changes markedly in different phases of the cell cycle (Figure 2-6 ■).[14,15] In its *hypo*phosphorylated (active) state, Rb has antiproliferative

effects, inhibiting cell cycling. It does so by binding transcription factors (the E2F proteins) required for the transcription of genes needed for cell proliferation, rendering them nonfunctional. When growth factors induce activation of cyclin D/Cdk4/6, the Rb protein is one of the targets of this kinase activity. As cells progress through G_1, *hyper*phosphorylation of Rb by cyclin D/Cdk4/6 kinase results in inactivation of Rb and release of the active E2F transcription factors, resulting in the activation and expression of genes required for cell-cycle progression. Rb hyperphosphorylation is subsequently maintained through the cell cycle by cyclin E/Cdk2 and cyclin A/Cdk2. *RB* functions as a tumor suppressor gene. Cells lacking functional Rb protein show deregulated cell-cycle genes and cell proliferation, sometimes resulting in malignancy.

Although p53 is not required for normal cell function (i.e., it is not required for cell-cycle progression), it serves an important function as a molecular policeman, monitoring the integrity of the genome;[16] p53 is a transcription factor that can both activate and inhibit gene expression (depending on the target gene). It is induced in response to DNA damage and puts the brakes on cell growth and division, allowing time for DNA repair, or triggering apoptosis if repair is not possible.

Elevated levels of p53 result in upregulation of the Cdk inhibitor p21 and inhibition of the CDC25 phosphatase (blocking kinase function), induction of proapoptotic Bax and inhibition of anti-apoptotic Bcl-2. p53 is an important component of both the G_1 and the G_2/M checkpoints. Like Rb, p53 functions as a tumor suppressor gene and is the most commonly mutated gene in human tumors.

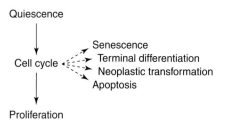

■ **FIGURE 2-7** Alternative fates for a cell induced to enter the cell cycle.

✓ **Checkpoint! 4**

A cell undergoing mitosis fails to attach one of its duplicated chromosomes to the microtubules of the spindle apparatus during metaphase. The cell's metaphase checkpoint malfunctions and does not detect the error. What is the effect (if any) on the daughter cells produced?

APOPTOSIS

Cells stimulated to enter the cell cycle may experience outcomes other than proliferation (Figure 2-7 ■). Cells can undergo senescence in which they are permanently growth arrested and no longer respond to mitogenic stimuli. Cells entering the cell cycle can also become terminally differentiated (committed) into specialized cell types. Uncontrolled cell cycling is a characteristic feature of malignant cells. Finally, cells can exit at any phase of the cell cycle by undergoing programmed cell death (apoptosis).

Cells can die by either of two major mechanisms: **necrosis** or **apoptosis**. The criteria for determining whether a cell is undergoing apoptosis or necrosis originally relied on distinct morphologic changes in the appearance of the cell (Table 2-3 ✪).[17] Necrotic death is induced by lethal chemical, biological, or physical events (extracellular assault). Such a death is analogous to "cell murder." In contrast, apoptosis, or "programmed cell death," is a self-induced death program regulated by the genetic material of the cell ("cell suicide").

Apoptosis is now recognized to play an essential role in the development and homeostasis of all multicellular organisms.[18] Apoptosis is essential to maintain a constant organ size in tissues that undergo continuous renewal by balancing cell proliferation and cell death. It also occurs at defined times and locations during development.

Apoptosis plays a major role in sculpting the developing organism (embryogenesis/organogenesis): It is responsible for the morphogenesis of the hands and feet (removal of interdigital webs), the formation of hollow tubes in the body (including the blood vessels, gastrointestinal tract, and heart), and the development of the immune system (the selection of appropriate T and B lymphocyte clones).

In adults, apoptosis is important in tissue homeostasis; homeostasis generally balances generation of new cells with the loss of terminally differentiated cells. Apoptosis is responsible for the elimination of excess cells (such as expanded clones of T or B lymphocytes following immune stimulation or excess PMNs following a bacterial challenge).

✪ TABLE 2-3

Cardinal Features of Apoptosis and Necrosis

Feature	Necrosis	Apoptosis
Stimuli	Toxins, severe hypoxia, massive insult, conditions of ATP depletion	Physiologic and pathologic conditions without ATP depletion
Energy requirement	None	ATP dependent
Histology	Cellular swelling; disruption of organelles; death of patches of tissue	Cellular shrinkage; chromatin condensation; fragmentation into apoptotic bodies; death of single isolated cells
DNA breakdown pattern	Randomly sized fragments	Ladder of fragments in internucleosomal multiples of 185 base pairs
Plasma membrane	Lysed	Intact, blebbed with molecular alterations (loss of phospholipid asymmetry)
Phagocytosis of dead cells	Immigrant phagocytes	Neighboring cells
Tissue reaction	Inflammation	No inflammation

✪ TABLE 2-4

Diseases Associated with Increased and Decreased Apoptosis

Increased Apoptosis	Decreased Apoptosis
AIDS	Cancer
Neurodegenerative disorders	• Follicular lymphomas
• Alzheimer's disease	• Other leukemias/lymphomas
• Parkinson's disease	• Carcinomas with p53 mutations
• Amyotrophic lateral sclerosis	• Hormone-dependent tumors (breast, prostate, ovarian)
• Retinitis pigmentosa	Autoimmune disorders
Myelodysplastic syndromes	• Systemic lupus erythematosus
Aplastic anemia	• Other autoimmune diseases
Ischemic injury	Viral infections
• Myocardial infarction	• Herpes viruses
• Stroke	• Poxviruses
• Reperfusion injury	• Adenoviruses
Toxin-induced liver disease	

As a defense mechanism, apoptosis is used to remove unwanted and potentially dangerous cells such as self-reactive lymphocytes, cells infected by viruses, and tumor cells. Diverse forms of cellular damage can trigger apoptotic death including DNA damage or errors of DNA replication, which prevents the cell with abnormal DNA from proliferating. Similarly, intracellular protein aggregates or misfolded proteins can stimulate apoptosis (e.g., the ineffective erythropoiesis and intramedullary apoptotic death of erythroblasts in β-thalassemia major triggered by aggregates of α globin chains [∞ Chapter 11]). In addition to the beneficial effects of programmed cell death, the inappropriate activation of apoptosis may cause or contribute to a variety of diseases (Table 2-4 ✪).[19,20]

Apoptosis is initiated by three major types of stimuli (see Table 2-5 ✪):

1. Deprivation of survival factors (growth factor withdrawal or loss of attachment to extracellular matrix)
2. Signals by "death" cytokines through apoptotic "death" receptors (tumor necrosis factor-TNF, Fas Ligand)
3. Cell-damaging stress

✪ TABLE 2-5

Inhibitors and Initiators/Inducers of Apoptosis

Inhibitors	Initiators/Inducers
Presence of survival factors	Deprivation of survival factors
• Growth factors	• Growth factor withdrawal
• Extracellular matrix	• Loss of matrix attachment
• Interleukins	Death cytokines
• Estrogens, androgens	• TNF
Viral products that block apoptosis	• Fas ligand
• Cowpox virus CrmA	Cell damaging stress
• Epstein Barr virus BHRF-1	• Bacterial toxins
Pharmacologic inhibitors	• Viral infections
Oncogene and tumor suppressor gene products (Bcl-2, Bcl-x$_L$, Mcl-1, Rb, c-Abl)	• Oxidants
	• Glucocorticoids
	• Cytotoxic drugs
	• Radiation therapy
	Oncogene and tumor suppressor gene products (c-myc, p53, Bax, Bad, Bcl-x$_S$, c-Fos, c-Jun)

Conversely, apoptosis is inhibited by growth-promoting cytokines and interaction with appropriate extracellular environmental stimuli. The disruption of cell physiology as a result of viral infections can cause an infected cell to undergo apoptosis. The suicide of an infected cell may be viewed as a cellular defense mechanism to prevent viral propagation. To circumvent these host defenses, a number of viruses have developed mechanisms to disrupt the normal regulation of apoptosis within the infected cell. Finally, a number of oncogenes and tumor suppressor genes have been described that may either stimulate or inhibit apoptosis.

Necrosis vs Apoptosis

When a cell is damaged, the plasma membrane loses its ability to regulate cation fluxes, resulting in the accumulation of Na^+, Ca^{++}, and water (Table 2-3, and Figure 2-8■). Consequently, the necrotic cell exhibits a swollen morphology. The organelles also accumulate cations and water, swell, and ultimately lyse. The rupture of the cytoplasmic membrane and organelles releases cytoplasmic components (including proteases and lysozymes) into the surrounding tissue, triggering an inflammatory response. In contrast, apoptosis is characterized by cellular shrinking rather than swelling with condensation of both the cytoplasm and the nucleus. Apoptotic cells do not lyse, but portions of the cell pinch off as apoptotic bodies that are phagocytosed by neighboring cells or macrophages. Thus, apoptosis is a very efficient process by which the body can remove a population of cells at a given time or in response to a given stimulus *without* the activation of an inflammatory response. Necrosis is a passive event elicited by the external injurious agent and generally leads to the destruction of a large group of cells in the same area. In contrast, apoptosis is an energy-dependent process orchestrated by the cell itself and generally affects only single, individual cells. In addition, apoptosis is characterized by a particular type of DNA fragmentation. DNA in an apoptotic cell is enzymatically cleaved by a specific endonuclease into oligonucleotides whose sizes are multiples of ~185 base pairs (corresponding to nucleosomal fragments). When electrophoresed on agarose gel, these nucleotide fragments make a discrete "ladder pattern" that is considered the hallmark of apoptosis. This is in contrast to the "smudge" pattern seen in cells undergoing necrosis, which indicates the presence of randomly and fully degraded DNA.

Molecular Regulation of Apoptosis

Caspases and the Initiation of Apoptosis   The cellular events responsible for apoptotic cell death are directed by a group of proteins called **caspases.**[21,22] Caspases are a family of **c**ysteine proteases that cleave after **asp**artic acid amino acids in a peptide substrate and are responsible for the orderly dismantling of the cell undergoing apoptosis. A number of similarities exist between the configuration and function of the apoptotic system (caspases) and the blood coagulation system (serine proteases) (∞ Chapter 30).

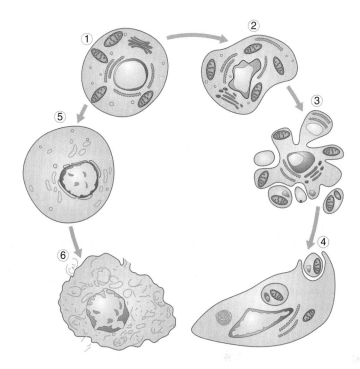

■ FIGURE 2-8   Diagram illustrating the sequential ultrastructural changes in apoptosis (clockwise arrows) and necrosis (counterclockwise arrows). A normal cell is shown (1). The onset of apoptosis (2) is heralded by compaction and segregation of chromatin into sharply delineated masses that lie against the nuclear envelope, condensation of the cytoplasm, and mild convolution of the nuclear and cellular outlines. Rapid progression of the process over the next few minutes (3) is associated with nuclear fragmentation and marked convolution of the cellular surface with the development of protuberances. The latter then separate to produce membrane-bound apoptotic bodies, which are phagocytosed and digested by adjacent cells (4). Signs of early necrosis in an irreversibly injured cell (5) include clumping of chromatin into ill-defined masses, gross swelling of organelles, and the appearance of flocculent densities in the matrix of mitochondria. At a later stage (6), membranes break down and the cell disintegrates. (With permission from Definition and incidence of apoptosis: An historical perspective. In: *Apoptosis: The molecular basis of cell death.* Eds: Kerr, JRF, Harmon, BV. New York: Cold Spring Harbor Laboratory Press; 1991.)

At least 14 caspase enzymes (caspase 1–14) have been identified in humans, although not all play a significant role in apoptosis. Those that are involved in apoptosis form the effector arm of the apoptotic machinery that, once activated, carries out the proteolysis necessary for apoptosis to occur. Caspases are found in healthy cells as zymogens (inactive form) and express their protease activity following either proteolytic cleavage or autocatalytic activation at high concentrations. A hierarchical relationship similar to that described for the blood coagulation proteins exists among the various apoptotic caspases. Early acting, initiator caspases (caspase-2, -8, -9, -10) are recruited in response to apoptotic stimuli and are activated. They then initiate the apoptotic cascade by proteolytically activating downstream, effector caspases (caspase-3, -6, -7), which in turn orchestrate the ordered dismantling of the cell resulting in cell death (Figure 2-9 ■).[22,23] Activation of caspases in apoptosis does not lead to indiscriminate proteolytic degradation but to specific cleavage of key substrates including proteins involved in cell structure, cell cycle regulation, DNA repair, RNA splicing, and the activation of a key endonuclease (CAD/caspase activated DNAse) responsible for the characteristic DNA fragmentation (Web Table 2-2 ✪).

Two major cell death pathways (Web Figure 2-4 ■) are initiated by a variety of events. Similar to the coagulation cascade (∞ Chapter 30) are an "extrinsic pathway" and an "intrinsic pathway." The extrinsic pathway is triggered by extracellular signals ("death cytokines") and transmitted through "death receptors" on the surface of the cell. The intrinsic pathway is a mitochondria-dependent pathway, initiated by intracellular signals in response to stress, exposure to cytotoxic agents, or radiation.

Eight death receptors have been described in mammalian cells to date.[24,25,26] The two best-known death cytokines and death receptors (DR) are tumor necrosis factor (TNF) and the TNF receptor, and Fas Ligand and CD95 (Fas receptor). DRs and initiator caspases do not bind each other directly but interact through adapter molecules containing "docking sites" for each protein (Web Figure 2-5 ■). Once the death cytokine, death receptor, adapter molecules, and initiator caspases are assembled in a complex, the caspase is activated by the process of autocatalysis.

The sequence of events triggering apoptosis via the internal pathway is less understood. It involves the assembly of a second caspase-activating complex called the *apoptosome* (Web Figure 2-5). DNA damage, cell-cycle check point defects, or loss of survival factors increase expression of pro-apoptotic Bcl family members (discussed later) and trigger mitochondrial release of cytochrome-c which serves as a cofactor for caspase activation. Cytochrome-c assembles with a different adapter protein and initiator caspase, again triggering autocatalysis. The activated initiator caspase from both pathways converge on the proteolytic activation of the effector caspase, caspase-3, and the activation of apoptosis.

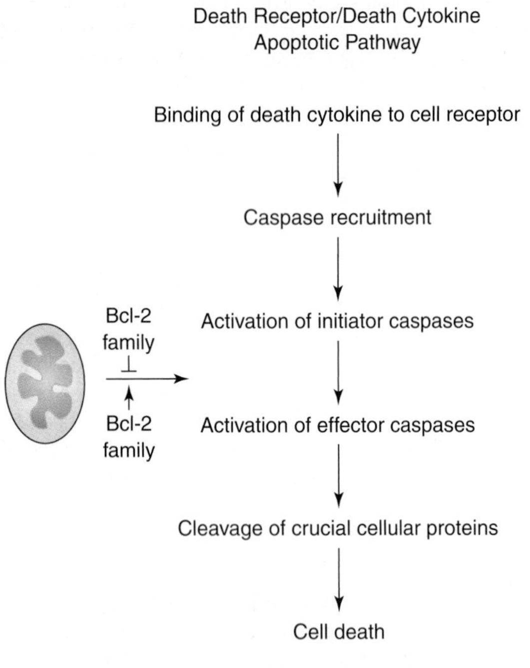

Role of Bcl-2 Protein   Apoptosis is a closely regulated physiologic process in which the Bcl-2 family of proteins plays an important role. The Bcl-2 family of proteins includes both pro-apoptotic and anti-apoptotic members and constitutes a critical intracellular checkpoint of apoptosis.[27,28] The founding member, Bcl-2, was a protein originally cloned from B-cell lymphomas with the characteristic t(14;18) chromosomal translocation (∞ Chapter 26). Since that initial discovery, several additional related proteins have been identified, some of which promote and others oppose apoptosis. At present, there are at least six known apoptosis-inhibitory proteins (survival factors) including the originally described Bcl-2 and at least 12 proapoptotic family members.[26] The Bcl-2 family of proteins is localized at or near the mitochondrial membranes and constitutes a critical intracellular checkpoint of apoptosis, determining whether early activation of initiator caspases will proceed to full activation of effector caspases (see Figure 2-9).[29,30]

The relative levels of anti-apoptotic and pro-apoptotic Bcl-2 members constitute a *rheostat* for apoptosis. This rheostat is regulated by different associations between survival and pro-death Bcl proteins. They all share similar structural regions that allow them to form dimers or higher oligomers (either homo- or hetero-oligomers). Bax (the first proapoptotic member discovered) can associate with itself (Figure 2-10 ■), and Bax:Bax homo-oligomers promote apoptosis. They induce permeabilization of the mitochondrial membrane, release of proteins including cytochrome-c, and activate the caspase cascade. With elevated levels of Bcl-2, Bax:Bcl-2 hetero-oligomers that repress apoptosis are formed. Actually, it is the overall ratio of death agonists (Bax and related proteins) to death antagonists (Bcl-2 and related proteins) and their interactions with each other that determine the susceptibility of a cell to a death stimulus (Figure 2-11 ■). Thus, the

Death Receptor/Death Cytokine
Apoptotic Pathway

Binding of death cytokine to cell receptor

↓

Caspase recruitment

↓

Bcl-2
family
⊥ →   Activation of initiator caspases
↑
Bcl-2
family

↓

Activation of effector caspases

↓

Cleavage of crucial cellular proteins

↓

Cell death

■ FIGURE 2-9   The apoptotic pathway triggered by death cytokine binding to death receptors. Activation of a death receptor by binding of death cytokine results in the recruitment of specific adapter proteins and activation of initiator caspases. Activated initiator caspases can then proceed to activate downstream effector caspases that mediate the cleavage of various cellular proteins during apoptosis. The contribution of the Bcl-2 family of proapoptotic and antiapoptotic proteins in determining whether activation of initiator caspases will proceed through to activation of effector caspases is depicted. ↓ indicates stimulation of the pathway; ⊥ indicates inhibition of the pathway.

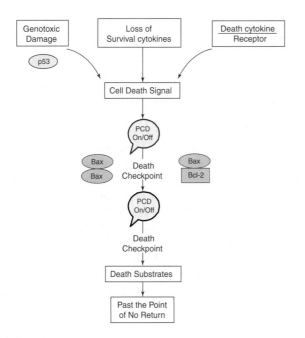

cell receives and processes *death signals* from a variety of sources. They converge on this rheostat, which determines whether the cell will activate effector caspases and subsequently whether there will be cleavage of the *death substrates* necessary for apoptosis.[28]

Cells utilize a variety of safeguards to prevent inappropriate apoptosis. Cells possess a number of proteins that modulate cell death by binding to activated caspases and interfering with their activity, the so-called inhibitors of apoptosis proteins (IAPs).[21,22] Some viruses contain viral proteins that perform the same function (e.g., cowpox viral protein CrmA, Adenovirus E1B, and Baculovirus p35). These viral proteins block the apoptosis-activating defense of the host cell against viral replication (i.e., block apoptosis).

Apoptosis and the Hematopoietic System

Apoptosis is important in the hematopoietic system (Table 2-6 ✪). The default cellular status of hematopoietic precursor cells is *cell death* (∞ Chapter 3). Cytokines and components of the extracellular matrix function to suppress apoptosis, allowing survival of hematopoietic cells when appropriate cytokines are present. Apoptosis plays an essential role in the selection of appropriate recognition repertoires of T and B lymphocytes, eliminating those with nonfunctional or autoreactive antigen receptors. Apoptosis helps regulate the overall number of mature cells by inducing elimination (cell death) of excess cells when expanded numbers of mature cells are no longer needed (i.e., expanded T and B cell clones, following elimination of foreign antigen; elimination

■ **FIGURE 2-10** Model of cell death checkpoints. Following delivery of a cell death signal (genotoxic damage, loss of survival cytokines, or presence of death cytokines), the ratio of proapoptotic components (Bax and related molecules) vs. antiapoptotic components (Bcl-2 and related molecules) determines whether or not the death program will continue to completion. A preponderance of Bax:Bax homodimers promotes continuation of the process while Bax–Bcl-2 heterodimers will shut it down. PCD = programmed cell death (apoptosis). (Adapted, with permission, from: Chao DT, Korsmeyer SJ: Bcl-2 family: Regulators of cell death. *Ann Rev Immunol.* 1998; 16:395.)

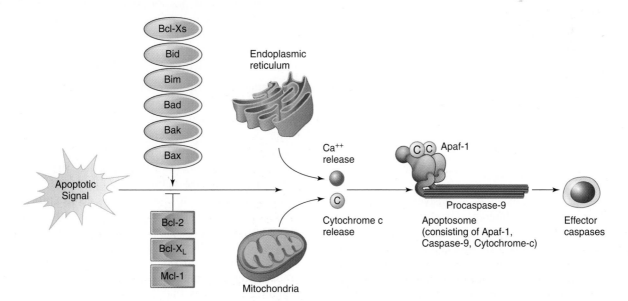

■ **FIGURE 2-11** Bcl-2-related proteins and control of apoptosis. Pro-apoptotic (blue ovals) and anti-apoptotic (pink rectangles) Bcl-2 related proteins interact in response to an apoptotic signal. If the pro-apoptotic signals prevail, cytochrome-c (yellow circle) is released from the mitochondria, binds to an adapter protein (Apaf-1) and recruits an initiator caspase (procaspase-9); the resulting caspase-activating assembly, the apoptosome, is associated with the intrinsic pathway of apoptosis.

✪ TABLE 2-6

The Role of Apoptosis in the Hematopoietic and Lymphoid Systems

I. Default cellular status for hematopoietic stem cells and progenitor cells

    Apoptosis regulated by cytokines and extracellular matrix

II. Lymphoid homeostasis

    Selection of recognition repertoires of T and B cells

    Elimination of autoreactive lymphocytes

    Down regulation of immune response following antigen stimulation

    Cytotoxic killing by CTL* and NK* cells

III. Elimination of eosinophils, monocytes, and neutrophils following infection/inflammatory response

IV. Developmental pathways for erythropoiesis and thrombopoiesis

*CTL = cytotoxic T lymphocytes; NK = natural killer cells

of PMNs, eosinophils, and monocytes following an infection/inflammatory response). Apoptosis is the mechanism employed in cytotoxic killing by cytotoxic T lymphocytes (CTL) and natural killer (NK) cells. Finally, activation of apoptotic caspases is involved in platelet production and release from mature megakaryocytes and in the final stages of erythrocyte maturation (chromatin condensation and organelle removal).[31,32]

Dysregulation of apoptosis also contributes to hematologic disorders. Apoptosis is increased in the myelodysplastic syndromes and tends to be decreased in the acute leukemias, perhaps partly explaining the pancytopenias and leukocytosis, respectively, seen in those disorders (∞ Chapters 23–25).

✓ Checkpoint! 5

What would be the effect on the hematopoietic system homeostasis if the expanded clone of antigen-activated B lymphocytes failed to undergo apoptosis after the antigenic challenge was removed?

▶ ABNORMAL TISSUE HOMEOSTASIS AND CANCER

In recent years, there has been an explosive growth in our knowledge of cancer cell biology. Of significance is the recognition that scattered throughout our own genome are genes that have the potential to cause cancer (**proto-oncogenes**)[33,34] and other genes that have the power to block it (**anti-oncogenes** or **tumor suppressor genes**).[35] As researchers have worked to understand the function of these oncogenes and tumor suppressor genes, they have found that many of them are molecules that regulate normal cell growth and differentiation and/or apoptosis.[36,37]

Cancer is a genetic disease: Most tumors are clonally derived from a single cancer "stem cell" that divides incessantly to generate a tumor of "identical" sibling cells. The cancer cell genotype is generally maintained (stably inherited) during cell division. This implies that the tumor cell DNA determines the disease phenotype. Researchers have found that certain viruses, when inoculated into animals, are capable of causing tumors. In an effort to discover the particular viral genes capable of inducing malignant transformation, it has been shown that tumor viruses carry discrete genetic elements, **oncogenes,** responsible for their ability to transform cells. The proteins encoded by these oncogenes play important roles in the cell cycle, such as initiation of DNA replication and transcriptional control of genes. Importantly, many viral oncogenes have normal counterparts in the human genome, now called *cellular proto-oncogenes.* The identification of cellular proto-oncogenes verified that the human genome carries genes with the potential to dramatically alter cell growth and to cause malignancy.

ONCOGENES

One of the defining features of cancer cells is their ability to proliferate under conditions in which normal cells do not.[38] The proteins encoded by proto-oncogenes function in the signaling pathways by which cells receive and execute growth instructions. The mutations that convert these proto-oncogenes to active oncogenes are usually either structural mutations resulting in the constitutive (formed continuously) activity of a protein without an incoming signal or regulatory mutations that lead to the production of the protein at the wrong place or time. The result in either case is a persistent internal growth signal uncoupled from environmental controls. It is possible that any gene playing a key role in cellular growth can become an oncogene if mutated in an appropriate way.

Generally, the proto-oncogenes that have been identified serve one of the following functions in normal growth control:

- Some encode growth factors (the molecules that are themselves the signals to grow) that when activated to an "oncogene" result in an autocrine growth stimulation.
- Other proto-oncogenes encode growth factor receptors; when activated to an oncogene, the mutated receptors are capable of triggering growth-promoting signals even in the absence of ligand (cytokine) binding.
- The largest class of proto-oncogenes encodes proteins that associate with growth factor receptors within the cytoplasm and function to pass receptor signals to downstream targets. Many of these proto-oncogenes encode protein-tyrosine kinases found on the inner surface of the membrane. Often the oncogenic form of these genes produces signaling molecules that exist in a constantly activated state in the absence of growth factor/receptor interaction and signaling.
- Some proto-oncogenes are transcription factors, proteins that bind DNA and function to control the expression of cellular genes required for proliferation.

Thus, proto-oncogenes are genes that regulate the initiation of DNA replication, cell division, and/or the commitment to cellular differentiation. As such, they are obvious targets for processes that damage the growth-control apparatus of the cell. Damage to these regulatory genes, referred to as *activation of the proto-oncogene* (resulting in the creation of an oncogene), occurs by one of three mechanisms: genetic mutation, genetic rearrangement, or genetic amplification. The result is either (1) a *qualitative* change in function of the protein product of the gene, resulting in enhanced activity, (2) a protein that is no longer subject to the control of regulatory factors, or (3) a *quantitative* change (increased production) of an otherwise normal oncogene protein.

TUMOR SUPPRESSOR GENES

It is now widely accepted that cancer is a multihit phenomenon, resulting from several independent genetic alterations occuring sequentially within a single cell. Specific tumor suppressor genes, or anti-oncogenes, in normal cells function to inhibit cell growth. Thus, in addition to mutations of oncogenes resulting in a growth-promoting activity, tumor cells often have inactivating mutations of growth-suppressing genes that may also contribute to tumor development. Mutations in tumor suppressor genes behave differently from oncogene mutations (Table 2-7 ✪). Oncogene mutations tend to be activating mutations, which functionally are dominant to wild-type (nonmutated) gene products; they produce proliferation signals even when a single copy of the oncogene is present. Tumor suppressor mutations, on the other hand, are recessive, loss-of-function mutations. Mutation in one gene copy usually has no effect, as long as a reasonable amount of normally functioning wild-type protein remains.

Understanding the function of tumor suppressor genes has been greatly aided by studies of rare cancers that run in families. Members of affected families appear to inherit susceptibility to cancer and develop certain kinds of tumors at rates much higher than the normal population. The first of these to be explained at the molecular level was the inherited susceptibility to retinoblastoma (a tumor of the eye) seen in certain families.[39,40] Although retinoblastoma can occur sporadically, about one-third of the cases occurs in related siblings, suggesting an inherited susceptibility to the disease. The development of retinoblastoma requires two mutations resulting in the inactivation of both of the *RB* loci on each of the chromosomes #13. In the familial form of the disease, the affected children inherit one mutant *RB* allele and one normal allele. Retinoblastoma (or other malignancies) develops when acquired mutations eliminate the function of the remaining normal (wild-type) allele (Web Figure 2-6 ■). Thus, the *RB* gene acts as a tumor suppressor gene (anti-oncogene) that normally functions to arrest excessive growth of cells. As is typically true of tumor suppressor genes, even one copy is sufficient to keep growth in check. However, loss of both copies of *RB* eliminates the block and a tumor develops. As discussed above, the protein product of the *RB* gene (Rb protein) is not specific to retinal tissue but serves as a universal cell-cycle brake in most cells. Acquired mutations of *RB* (i.e., nonfamilial) are found in about 25% of sporadic cancers.

Inactivation of the *p53* gene, also a tumor suppressor anti-oncogene, is seen in more than half of all human cancers, making it the most common genetic defect detectable in human tumors.[41,42] Interestingly, a damaged *p53* gene, the Li-Fraumeini syndrome, can also be inherited resulting (like familial retinoblastoma) in an inherited susceptibility to a variety of cancers.[43,44] In affected individuals, 50% develop cancer by age 30 and 90% by age 70. The function of p53 in cell-cycle regulation is to block cell-cycle progression in the event of damaged DNA or to trigger apoptosis if the damaged DNA cannot be repaired. The p53 protein is a major component of the body's antitumor army, serving as a "molecular policeman" monitoring the integrity of the genome. Loss of function of the *p53* gene facilitates tumor formation by allowing damaged cells to proceed through the cell cycle and continue to replicate.

Although all of the Cdk inhibitors could potentially act as tumor suppressors,[45] the one that seems to have the strongest link to malignancy is *p16*.[46] Loss-of-function mutations of *p16* have been described in a wide variety of human cancers. To date, there is much less information on the involvement of other Cdk inhibitors, although it is likely that they also function as tumor suppressors and thus play a role in tumorigenesis. In addition, there are tumor suppressor genes that tend to show tissue preference in terms of site of malignancy. These include the *WT-1* gene, mutated in Wilms' tumor; the *APC* gene, mutated in adenomatous

---

✪ TABLE 2-7

Properties of Oncogenes and Tumor Suppressor Genes

Property	Oncogenes	Tumor suppressor gene
Nature of mutation	Dominant	Recessive
	Gain of function	Loss of function
Inherited mutant allele	Never observed	Common—basis for inherited predisposition in cancers
Somatic mutations in cancers	Yes	Yes

polyposis; the *DCC* gene, deleted in colon carcinomas; and *BRCA-1* and *BRCA-2,* mutated in breast cancers.

CELL-CYCLE CHECKPOINTS AND CANCER

A common feature of many cancer cells is the loss of regulation of cell-cycle checkpoints, either by overexpression of positive regulators (for example, cyclins and Cdks) or the loss of function of negative regulators (the Cdk inhibitors, p53, or Rb).[47,48] Cyclin D, cyclin E, and cyclin A are overexpressed in a variety of human cancers and function as oncogenes in their mutated configuration. Often specific chromosomal translocations activate the expression of the cyclin gene by placing it under the influence of other transcriptional control elements. For example, the t[11;14] translocation seen in some B-lymphocyte malignancies places the cyclin D gene under the control of the immunoglobulin heavy chain locus, resulting in activation of cyclin D expression. Thus, the Bcl-1 oncogene defined by the t(11;14) translocation is now known to represent a translocated cyclin D locus (∞ Chapter 25). Mutations (overexpression) of *Cdk4* also have been reported in a number of human tumors, contributing to the excessive growth characteristics of those diseases. The p16-cyclin D-Rb pathway, which controls the G_1 checkpoint in cell-cycle regulation, is believed to play a pivotal role in tumorigenesis (Figure 2-12■). Some investigators

have proposed that a mutation involving at least one member of this checkpoint must occur in order for a malignant phenotype to be established.[49]

APOPTOSIS AND CANCER

The accumulation of excess numbers of cells characteristic of malignancies may be due to increased cell proliferation (see previous discussion of cell cycle checkpoints and cancer) and/or to decreased cell death (apoptosis).[50] Thus, mutations of genes important in regulating apoptosis have also been identified as oncogenes and tumor suppressor genes. These include loss-of-function mutations of initiators of apoptosis such as p53, Bax, and other proapoptotic Bcl-2 family members, as well as overexpression of Bcl-2 and other Bcl-2 family members that function to inhibit apoptosis. Bcl-2 is overexpressed in most cases of B-cell follicular lymphoma, many cases of B-cell chronic lymphocytic leukemia (CLL), and some cases of acute myelocytic leukemia (AML) (∞ Chapters 24, 25, 26). Mutations of Bax (resulting in loss of proapoptotic function) have been reported in about 20% of leukemic cell lines. The result is production of cells with an extended life span, increased proliferation capacity, and diminished cell death.

EPIGENETICS

In addition to mutations (changes in the nucleotide sequence of the gene) of various oncogenes or tumor suppressor genes that have been described in association with malignancy, there is a second group of alterations, the so-called *epigenetic alterations*. **Epigenetics** (meaning literally "on top of genetics") refers to stable changes in gene function that are transferred through mitosis and passed from one cell to its progeny. Epigenetic changes play an important role in normal development and differentiation and are associated with "silencing" genes and chromatin condensation into heterochromatin.

One of the most common epigenetic changes found in the human genome involves the methylation of certain cytosine nucleotides (C^M) within genes and/or their promoter regions. Cytosine nucleotides particularly susceptible to methylation are those found adjacent to a guanine nucleotide, the so-called CpG dinucleotide.

$$CGATCGATCGAT \rightarrow C^MGATC^MGATC^MGAT$$

These methylations or epigenetic changes become incorporated into the heritable genetic/epigenetic regulatory mechanisms of the cell and play a significant role in differentiation and development. The methylation of CpG dinucleotides is a potentially reversible process, and approximately 70–75% of CpG dinucleotides in the human genome are methylated. In addition, CpG dinucleotides are often clustered in *CpG islands,* many of which are in and around the promoter regions of genes. The unmethylated state of the promoter region of a gene favors a *transcription-ready status* or accompanies active transcription. Typically, methyla-

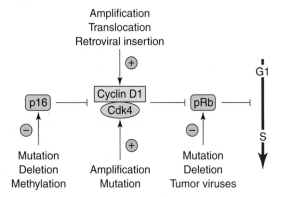

■ FIGURE 2-12 Alterations of the G_1 checkpoint that can lead to malignancy. Loss-of-function alterations of negative regulators of the cell cycle (i.e., Cdk inhibitor p16 or cell-cycle inhibitor Rb protein) may contribute to uncontrolled proliferation. Similarly, gain-of-function mutations of positive regulators of proliferation (i.e., Cyclin D, Cdk4) may contribute to uncontrolled proliferation. Inhibitory regulatory proteins with the potential to influence malignant transformation are called *tumor suppressor genes*, and positive regulatory proteins are called *proto-oncogenes*. ↓ indicates stimulation of the pathway; ⊥ indicates inhibition of the pathway. (+) indicates a mutation that increases activity of the indicated proteins; (−) indicates a mutation that decreases activity of the indicated proteins.

tion of the promoter regions is associated with gene silencing and is part of the normal terminal differentiation process seen in many diverse tissue types.

Cancer is a complex disorder that may involve DNA methylation. One may see demethylation of the genome in regions where it should be methylated, or methylation of regions of the genome that are typically unmethylated. There is a growing list of genes that acquire hypermethylation of CpGs in their promoter regions and contribute to tumorigenesis. This change is associated with transcriptional silencing of these genes and is the explanation for one of the most common causes of loss of function of key tumor suppressor genes.

Extensive information also can be encoded in the protein component of the chromatin in what is now being called the *histone code*. Modifications of the histone proteins include lysine acetylation, serine phosphorylation, lysine, and arginine methylation. These modifications can be stably passed from one cell generation to the next as well. These modifications of histones also play an important role in the complex system responsible for regulating euchromatin to heterochromatin transitions. Hypo-acetylated histones bind tightly to the phosphate backbone of DNA and help maintain chromatin in an inactive, silent state. Various types of malignant cells utilize enzymes called *histone deacetylases* (*HDACs*) to deacetylate key lysine aminoacids, resulting in silencing of key genes, which favors cell growth over differentiation.

Many of the newer approaches to treating cancer patients involve *demethylating agents* or *HDAC inhibitors* with the goal of reversing epigenetic changes associated with certain types of cancer.

 Checkpoint! 6

Mutations of proto-oncogenes predisposing to malignancy are said to be dominant mutations while mutations of antioncogenes are said to behave as recessive mutations, requiring loss of both alleles. Explain this difference in behavior of the gene products.

SUMMARY

The cell is an intricate, complex structure bound by a membrane. The membrane is a phospholipid bilayer with integral proteins throughout and containing receptors that bind extracellular molecules and transmit messages to the cell's nucleus. Within the cell is the cytoplasm with numerous organelles and the nucleus. The cellular organelles include ribosomes, endoplasmic reticulum, the Golgi apparatus, lysosomes, mitochondria, microfilaments, and microtubules. The nucleus contains the genetic material, DNA, which regulates all cell functions.

The cell cycle is a highly ordered process that results in the accurate duplication and transmission of genetic information from one cell generation to the next. The cell cycle is divided into four stages: M phase (in which cell division or mitosis takes place), S phase (during which DNA synthesis occurs), and two gap phases, G_1 and G_2. G_0 refers to quiescent cells that are temporarily or permanently out of cycle. The normal cell depends on external stimuli (growth factors) to move it out of G_0 and through G_1. The cell cycle is regulated by a series of protein kinases (Cdks), whose activity is controlled by complexing with a regulatory partner (cyclin). Different cyclins with their associated (and activated) Cdks function at specific stages of the cell cycle. Kinase activity is further modulated by both activating and inactivating phosphorylation of kinase subunits and by specific cell-cycle kinase (Cdk) inhibitors. A series of checkpoint controls or surveillance systems functions to ensure the integrity of the process.

To maintain tissue homeostasis, cells utilize the process of programmed cell death, or apoptosis, as well as proliferation. Apoptosis is a unique form of cell death that can be morphologically and biochemically distinguished from necrosis. Apoptosis plays important roles in the development of the organism, in controlling the number of various types of cells, and as a defense mechanism to eliminate unwanted and potentially dangerous cells. Apoptosis is an active process initiated by the cell and resulting in the orderly dismantling of cellular constituents. It is directed by cysteine proteases called *caspases*. Proapoptotic and antiapoptotic proteins (Bcl-2 family members) and specific protein inhibitors (IAPs, or inhibitors of apoptosis) regulate this process. Apoptosis is triggered by loss of survival factors (survival cytokines or extracellular matrix components), presence of death cytokines, or cell-damaging stress.

The various processes that govern tissue homeostasis—proliferation, differentiation, cytokine regulation, and apoptosis—are highly ordered and tightly regulated. When the regulation of these processes malfunctions, the result can be deregulated cell production and malignant transformation. Oncogenes and tumor suppressor genes are genes whose normal transcription products regulate the processes that govern tissue homeostasis. Mutations or epigenetic changes that alter the structure or function of these genes may result in uncontrolled cell growth and malignancy.

REVIEW QUESTIONS

LEVEL I

1. Selective cellular permeability and structural stability are provided by: (Objective 1)
   a. membrane lipids
   b. membrane proteins
   c. ribosomes
   d. the nucleus

2. Rough endoplasmic reticulum is important in: (Objective 1)
   a. synthesizing lipid
   b. synthesizing hormones
   c. synthesizing and assembling proteins
   d. phagocytosis

3. The fundamental subunit of chromatin composed of ~180 base pairs of DNA wrapped around a histone protein is called: (Objective 1)
   a. nucleolus
   b. genome
   c. heterochromatin
   d. nucleosome

4. Condensation of chromosomes occurs during which phase of mitosis? (Objective 3)
   a. anaphase
   b. telophase
   c. prophase
   d. metaphase

5. Cells that have exited the cell cycle and entered a nonproliferative phase are said to be in: (Objective 3)
   a. quiescence
   b. interphase
   c. G_1
   d. G_2

6. The regulatory subunit of the active enzyme complex responsible for regulating passage through the various phases of the cell cycle is: (Objective 3)
   a. cyclin
   b. Cdk
   c. Cdk inhibitor
   d. p21

7. The point in the cell cycle at which cell proliferation (cycling) no longer depends on extracellular signals is: (Objective 4)
   a. G_1
   b. R
   c. G_2
   d. M

8. Programmed cell death (cell suicide) is also known as: (Objective 5)
   a. necrosis
   b. senescence
   c. apoptosis
   d. terminal differentiation

LEVEL II

1. UTRs are regions of mRNA: (Objective 1)
   a. representing the introns of the gene
   b. representing the exons of the gene
   c. representing the splice sites for mRNA processing
   d. representing regions at either end of the mRNA that are not part of the coding sequence

2. The main function of the ubiquitin-proteosome system is to: (Objective 2)
   a. assist in the three-dimensional folding of polypeptides into their tertiary structure
   b. degrade unwanted or damaged polypeptides
   c. facilitate transfer of polypeptides from the endoplasmic reticulum to the Golgi
   d. direct post-translational modifications of proteins

3. The kinase complex responsible for passage through and exit from mitosis is composed of: (Objective 3)
   a. cyclin A/Cdk2
   b. cyclin D/Cdk4
   c. cyclin B/Cdk1
   d. cyclin E/Cdk2

4. CAK, the kinase activity responsible for the activating phosphorylations of Cdks, consists of: (Objective 4)
   a. cyclin A/Cdk1
   b. cyclin H/Cdk7
   c. cyclin F/Cdk6
   d. cyclin C/Cdk2

5. Overexpression of the p21 protein would have what effect on the cell cycle of proliferating cells? (Objective 4)
   a. decrease cell cycle progression
   b. increase cell cycle progression
   c. trigger apoptosis
   d. have no effect

6. The protein responsible for binding the transcription factors E2F blocking cell cycle progression beyond the restriction point (R) is: (Objective 6)
   a. p53
   b. p15
   c. p21
   d. Rb

7. Apoptotic cell death is characterized by all of the following *except:* (Objective 14)
   a. triggering an inflammatory response
   b. condensation of the nucleus
   c. cleavage of chromatin into discrete fragments (multiples of 185 base pairs)
   d. condensation of the cytoplasm and cell shrinkage

REVIEW QUESTIONS *(continued)*

LEVEL I

9. All of the following are considered initiators of apoptosis *except:* (Objective 6)
   a. estrogens
   b. death cytokines
   c. loss of matrix attachment
   d. cell-damaging stress

10. Which of the following events in hematopoiesis is regulated by apoptosis? (Objective 7)
    a. removal of excess neutrophils following cessation of bacterial challenge
    b. removal of excess B lymphocytes following immune stimulation
    c. removal of excess platelets following hemostatic challenge
    d. a and b

LEVEL II

8. The components of apoptosis directly responsible for dismantling the cell during the programmed cell death process are: (Objective 8)
   a. Bcl-2 family members
   b. IAPs
   c. initiator caspases
   d. effector caspases

9. A predominance of Bax-Bax homodimers has what effect on apoptosis? (Objective 11)
   a. inhibits initiator caspases
   b. promotes activation of effector caspases
   c. activates death receptors on the cell surface
   d. neutralizes IAPs

10. All of the following are considered characteristics of tumor suppressor genes *except:* (Objective 13)
    a. function normally as negative regulators of the cell cycle
    b. undergo gain-of-function mutations resulting in malignant transformation
    c. have mutated forms of the genes often found in inherited predispositions to malignancy
    d. have characteristic mutations that are recessive in expression patterns.

www.pearsonhighered.com/mckenzie

Use this address to access the interactive Companion Website created for this textbook. Find additional information, tables and figures. Evaluate your command of the chapter information using case studies and critical thinking and multiple choice questions.

REFERENCES

1. Singer SJ, Nicholson GL. The fluid mosaic model of the structure of cell membranes. *Science.* 1972;175:720–31.

2. Wagner AJ, Berliner N, Benz EJ. Anatomy and physiology of the gene. In: R Hoffman, EJ Benz, SJ Shattil, B Furie, HJ Cohen, LE Silberstein, P McGlave, eds. *Hematology: Basic principles and procedures.* 4th ed. New York: Churchill Livingstone; 2005:2–16.

3. Papayannopoulou T, D'Andrea AD, Abkowitz JL, Migliaccio AR. Biology of erythropoiesis, erythroid differentiation, and maturation. In: R Hoffman, EJ Benz, SJ Shattil, B Furie, HJ Cohen, LE Silberstein, P McGlave, eds. *Hematology: Basic principles and procedures.* 4th ed. New York: Churchill Livingstone; 2005:267–88.

4. Toby GG, Wiest DL. Protein synthesis, processing, and degradation. In: R Hoffman, EJ Benz, SJ Shattil, B Furie, HJ Cohen, LE Silberstein, P McGlave, eds. *Hematology: Basic Principles and Procedures,* 4th ed. New York: Churchill Livingstone; 2005:27–38.

5. Nasmyth K. Viewpoint. Putting the cell cycle in order. *Science.* 1996;274:1643–45.

6. Pardee AB. G_1 events and regulation of cell proliferation. *Science.* 1989;246:603–8.

7. Sherr CJ. G_1 phase progression: Cycling on cue. *Cell.* 1994;79:551–55.

8. King RW, Deshaies RJ, Peters JM, Kirschner MW. How proteolysis drives the cell cycle. *Science.* 1996;274:1652–59.

9. Morgan DO. Principles of Cdk regulation. *Nature.* 1995;374:131–34.

10. Sherr CJ, Roberts JM. Inhibitors of mammalian G-1 cyclin dependent kinases. *Genes Develop.* 1995;9:1149–63.

11. Murray AW. Creative blocks: Cell cycle checkpoints and feedback controls. *Nature.* 1992;359:599–604.

12. Gorbsky GJ. Cell cycle checkpoints: Arresting progress in mitosis. *BioEssays.* 1997;19:193–97.

13. Nurse P. Checkpoint pathways come of age. *Cell.* 1997;91:865–67.

14. Weinberg RA. The retinoblastoma protein and cell cycle control. *Cell.* 1995;81:323–30.

15. Herwig S, Strauss M. The retinoblastoma protein: A master regulator of cell cycle, differentiation, and apoptosis. *Eur J Biochem.* 1997; 246:581–601.

16. Sidransky D, Hollstein M. Clinical implications of the p53 gene. *Ann Rev Med.* 1996;47:285–301.

17. Kerr JFR, Harmon BV. Definition and incidence of apoptosis: An historical perspective. In: *Apoptosis: The molecular basis of cell death.* New York: Cold Spring Harbor Laboratory Press; 1991:5–25.

18. Steller H. Mechanisms and genes of cellular suicide. *Science.* 1995; 267:1445–49.

19. Thompson CB. Apoptosis in the pathogenesis and treatment of disease. *Science.* 1995;267:1456–62.

20. Hetts SW. To die or not to die: An overview of apoptosis and its role in disease. *JAMA.* 1998;279:300–7.

21. Thornberry NA, Lazebik Y. Caspases: Enemies within. *Science.* 1998;281:1312–16.

22. Earnshaw WC, Martins LM, Kaufmann SH. Mammalian caspases: Structure, activation, substrates, and functions during apoptosis. *Ann Rev Biochem.* 1999;68:383–424.

23. Salvesen GS, Dixit VM. Caspase activation: The induced proximity model. *Proc Natl Acad Sci USA.* 1999;96:10:964–67.

24. Nagata S, Golstein P. The Fas death factor. *Science.* 1995;267:1449–56.

25. Ashkenazi A, Dixit VM. Death receptors: Signaling and modulation. *Science.* 1998;281:1305–8.

26. Hockenbery DM, Korsmeyer SJ. Cell Death. In: *Hematology: Basic Principles and Procedures,* 4th ed. Edited by R Hoffman, EJ Benz, SJ Shattil, B Furie, HJ Cohen, LE Silberstein, P McGlave. New York: Churchill Livingstone; 2005:83–92.

27. Adams JM, Cory S. The Bcl-2 protein family: Arbiters of cell survival. *Science.* 1998;281:1322–26.

28. Chao DT, Korsmeyer SJ. Bcl-2 family: Regulators of cell death. *Ann Rev Immunol.* 1998;16:395–419.

29. Susin SA, Zamzami N, Kroemer G. Mitochondria as regulators of apoptosis: Doubt no more. *Biochem Biophys Acta.* 1998;1366:151–65.

30. Green DR, Reed JC. Mitochondria and apoptosis. *Science.* 1998; 281:1309–12.

31. Kaluzhny Y, Ravid, K. Role of apoptotic processes in platelet biogenesis. *Acta Haematol.* 2004;111:67–77.

32. Kolbus A, Pilat S, Huszk A. et al. Raf-1 antagonizes erythroid differentiation by restraining caspase activation, *J Exp Med.* 2002;196: 1347–53.

33. Prochownik E. Protooncogenes and cell differentiation. *Trans Med Rev.* 1989;3:24–38.

34. Studzinski GP. Oncogenes, growth, and the cell cycle: An overview. *Cell Tissue Kinet.* 1989;22:405–24.

35. Carbone DP, Minna JD. Antioncogenes and human cancer. *Ann Rev Med.* 1993;44:451–64.

36. Marx J. How cells cycle toward cancer. *Science.* 1994;263:319–21.

37. Marx J. Learning how to suppress cancer. *Science.* 1993;261:1385–87.

38. Sherr CJ. Cancer cell cycles. *Science.* 1996;274:1672–77.

39. Benedict WF, Xu HJ, Hu SX, Takahashi R. Role of the retinoblastoma gene in the initiation and progression of human cancer. *J Clin Invest.* 1990;85:988–93.

40. Bartek J, Bartkova J, Lukas J. The retinoblastoma protein pathway in cell cycle control and cancer. *Exp Cell Res.* 1997;237:1–6.

41. Levine AJ, Momand J, Finlay CA. The p53 tumour suppressor gene. *Nature.* 1991;351:453–56.

42. Greenblatt MS, Bennett WP, Hollstein M, Harris CC. Mutations in the p53 tumor suppressor gene: Clues to cancer etiology and molecular pathogenesis. *Cancer Res.* 1994;54:4855–78.

43. Srivastava S, Zou ZQ, Pirollo K, et al. Germ-line transmission of a mutated p53 gene in a cancer-prone family with Li-Fraumeini syndrome. *Nature.* 1990;348:747–79.

44. Malkin D, Li FP, Strong LC, Fraumeini JF, et al. Germline p53 mutations in a familial syndrome of breast cancer, sarcomas and other neoplasms. *Science.* 1990;250:1233–38.

45. Tsihlias J, Kapusta L, Slingerland J. The prognostic significance of altered cyclin-dependent kinase inhibitors in human cancer. *Ann Rev Med.* 1999;50:401–23.

46. Nobori T, Miura K, Wu DJ et al. Deletions of the cyclin-dependent kinase-4 inhibitor gene in multiple human cancers. *Nature.* 1994; 368:753–56.

47. Hall M, Peters G. Genetic alterations of cyclins, cyclin-dependent kinases, and Cdk inhibitors in human cancer. *Adv Cancer Res.* 1996; 68:67–108.

48. Bartek J, Lukas J, Bartkove J. Perspective: Defects in cell cycle control and cancer. *J Pathol.* 1999;187:95–99.

49. Rosenberg N, Krantiris RG. Molecular basis of neoplasia. In: *Hematology: Basic principles and procedures,* 3rd ed. Edited by R Hoffman, EJ Benz, SJ Shattil, B Furie, HJ Cohen, LE Silberstein, P McGlave. New York: Churchill Livingstone; 2000:870–84.

50. Rinkenberger JL, Korsmeyer SJ. Errors of homeostasis and deregulated apoptosis. *Curr Opin Genet Dev.* 1997;7:589–96.

3

Hematopoiesis

J. Lynne Williams, Ph.D.

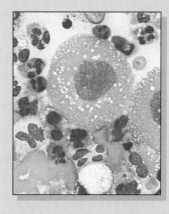

■ OBJECTIVES—LEVEL I

At the end of this unit of study, the student should be able to:

1. Describe the basic concepts of cell differentiation and maturation.
2. Compare and contrast the categories of hematopoietic precursor cells: hematopoietic stem cells, hematopoietic progenitor cells, and maturing cells, including proliferation and differentiation potential, morphology, and population size.
3. Describe the hierarchy of hematopoietic precursor cells and the relationships of the various blood cell lineages to each other (including the concept of colony-forming units/CFUs).
4. Discuss the general characteristics of growth factors and identify the major examples of early acting (multilineage), later acting (lineage restricted), and indirect acting growth factors.
5. Differentiate between paracrine, autocrine, and juxtacrine regulation.
6. List examples of negative regulators of hematopoiesis.
7. Define *hematopoietic microenvironment*.

■ OBJECTIVES—LEVEL II

At the end of this unit of study, the student should be able to:

1. Identify the phenotypic characteristics differentiating the hematopoietic stem cells and progenitor cells.
2. Identify the key cytokines required for lineage-specific regulation.
3. Describe the structure and role of growth factor receptors.
4. Summarize the concept of signal transduction pathways.
5. Discuss the roles of transcription factors in the regulation of hematopoiesis and differentiation.
6. Outline current clinical uses of cytokines.
7. Describe the cellular and extracellular components of the hematopoietic microenvironment.
8. Discuss the proposed mechanisms used to regulate hematopoietic stem/progenitor cell proliferation/differentiation.

KEY TERMS

Autocrine
Commitment
Cytokine
Differentiation
Extracellular matrix (ECM)
Hematopoiesis
Hematopoietic microenvironment (HM)
Hematopoietic progenitor cells
Hematopoietic stem cells
JAK/STAT signaling pathway
Juxtacrine
Maturation
Maturing cell
Paracrine
Progenitor cell
Stromal cells
Transcription factors (TF)

BACKGROUND BASICS

The information in this chapter will build on the concepts learned in previous chapters. To maximize your learning experience you should review these concepts before starting this unit of study.

Level I and Level II

▶ Identify the component parts of a cell, including the structure and function of cellular organelles (Chapter 2).

▶ Describe the *cell cycle* and the molecules that regulate it (Chapter 2).

▶ Describe *apoptosis*, the two activation pathways, and the roles of caspases and the Bcl-2 family of proteins in the process (Chapter 2).

▶ OVERVIEW

This chapter begins with an introduction to the concepts of commitment and differentiation in the hematopoietic system. It discusses the defining characteristics of the hematopoietic precursor cells and then the cytokines that regulate the development of these precursor cells. The structure and function of the cytokine receptors are presented with a summary of the signaling pathways and transcription factors activated by receptor-cytokine binding. Finally, the hematopoietic microenvironment is described and its role in hematopoiesis summarized.

▶ INTRODUCTION

The maintenance of an adequate number of cells to carry out the functions of the organism is referred to as *tissue homeostasis,* and depends on a careful balance between

cellular proliferation, cellular differentiation, and cell death (apoptosis). The hematopoietic system presents a challenge when considering the homeostasis of the circulating blood because the majority of circulating cells are postmitotic cells that are relatively short lived. Thus, circulating blood cells are intrinsically incapable of providing their replacements when they reach the end of their life spans. **Hematopoiesis** is the process responsible for the replacement of circulating blood cells and depends on the proliferation of precursor cells that still retain mitotic capability. This process is governed by a multitude of cytokines (both stimulating and inhibitory growth factors) and takes place in a specialized microenvironment uniquely suited to regulate the process.

▶ HEMATOPOIESIS

Whereas cell proliferation and programmed cell death (apoptosis) work together to provide an adequate number of cells (∞ Chapter 2), **differentiation** is the process responsible for generating the diverse cell populations that provide the specialized functions needed by the organism. Differentiation has been defined as the appearance of different properties in cells that were initially equivalent. Because all cells of an organism have the same genetic information, differentiation (or the appearance of specific characteristics) occurs by the progressive restriction of other potentialities of the cell.[1] **Commitment** is the term used to define the instance when two cells derived from the same precursor take a separate route of development.[1] Commitment "assigns the program," and the maturation process executes it (**maturation** encompasses the totality of phenomena that begins with commitment and ends when the cell has all its characteristics).[1]

Hematopoiesis (the development of all the different cell lineages of the blood) has two striking characteristics: the variety of distinct blood cell types produced and the relatively brief life span of the individual cells. The cells circulating in the peripheral blood are mature blood cells and, with the exception of lymphocytes, are generally incapable of mitosis. Also they have a limited life span from days for granulocytes and platelets to ~4 months for erythrocytes. As a result, they are described as *terminally differentiated*. This constant death of mature, functional blood cells (by apoptosis) means that new cells must be produced to replace those that are removed either as a consequence of performing their biologic functions (e.g., platelets, granulocytes) or through cellular senescence or "old age" (erythrocytes). The replacement of circulating, terminally differentiated cells depends on the function of less differentiated hematopoietic precursor cells that still retain significant proliferative capabilities. These hematopoietic precursor cells, located primarily in the bone marrow in adults, consist of a hierarchy of cells with enormous proliferation potential. They maintain a daily production of approximately 2×10^{11} red blood cells (RBC) and 1×10^{11} (each) white blood cells (WBC) and platelets for the lifetime of the individual.[2] In addition, acute stress (blood loss or infection) can result in a rapid, efficient, and specific increase in production over baseline of the particular cell lineage needed. For example, acute blood loss results in a specific increased production of erythrocytes while a bacterial infection results in an increased production of phagocytic cells (granulocytes and monocytes).

HEMATOPOIETIC PRECURSOR CELLS

The pioneering work of Till and McCulloch began to define the hierarchical organization of hematopoietic precursor cells using in vivo clonal assays.[3] However, it was not until the development of clonal in vitro assays that the current model of blood cell production began to evolve.[3,4,5,6,7] Hematopoietic precursor cells can be divided into three cellular compartments defined by relative maturity: **hematopoietic stem cells, progenitor cells,** and **maturing cells** (Table 3-1 ✪). The nomenclature used to define these various compartments over the past 20 years has lacked uniformity. Although there is now general agreement on the designations *stem cells* and *progenitor cells,* various authors have called the third category precursor cells,[8] maturing cells,[9] or morphologically recognizable precursor cells.[10] In this textbook, we use the term *precursor* to include all cells antecedent to the mature cells in each lineage and the term *maturing cells* to include those precursor cells within each lineage that are morphologically identifiable under the microscope.

Stem Cells

All hematopoiesis derives from a pool of undifferentiated cells, hematopoietic stem cells (HSC), which give rise to all of the bone marrow cells by the processes of proliferation and differentiation.[11] The stem cell compartment is the smallest of the hematopoietic precursor compartments, constituting of only ~0.5% of the total marrow nucleated cells. However, these rare cells are capable of regenerating the entire hematopoietic system. Thus, they are defined as multipotential precursors (i.e., they maintain the capacity to give rise to *all* lineages of blood cells). The other defining characteristic of stem cells is their high self-renewal capacity (i.e., they give rise to daughter stem cells that are exact replicas of the parent cell). Despite their responsibility for generating the entire hematopoietic system, the majority of stem cells are not dividing at any one time ($< 5\%$) with the majority being withdrawn from the cell cycle or quiescent (G_0 phase of the cell cycle).

Stem cells are not morphologically distinguishable. Primitive stem cells, isolated by fluorescent-activated cell sorting, appear morphologically very similar to small lymphocytes. Because stem cells are not morphologically identifiable, they have been defined functionally by their ability to reconstitute both lymphoid and myeloid hematopoiesis when transplanted into a recipient. In mice, the existence of the true HSC has been unequivocally demonstrated by occasional successful transplants with single purified stem cells, providing direct proof that single cells capable of sustaining lifelong hematopoiesis do exist.[12] There are no practical and quantitative assays for human HSC. Despite the difficulties (both practical and ethical) surrounding an effective assay for human stem cells, a number of characteristics have been used to define their phenotype, and these can be used in cell-separation protocols resulting in a high degree of purity. The currently proposed phenotype of a human HSC is:

$$CD34^+Thy\text{-}1^{lo}CD38^-Lin^-HLA\text{-}DR^-Rh123^{Dull}$$

In addition, HSCs are positive for the receptor for stem cell factor (SCF-R or c-kit, CD-117) and the thrombopoietin receptor (TPO-R, CD-110). CD-34, SCF-R, and TPO-R are not found exclusively on HSCs but also on cells that have begun to differentiate.

CD34 is a 110 kDa glycoprotein expressed by human hematopoietic stem cells and early progenitor cells.[13] Expression of CD34 is lost as cells mature beyond the progenitor cell compartment. Thy-1 is a membrane glycoprotein that participates in T-lymphocyte adhesion to stromal cells. CD38 is a 45 kDa glycoprotein considered to be an early myeloid differentiation antigen. *Lin⁻* refers to the absence of known differentiation markers or antigens present on more

---

✪ TABLE 3-1

Comparison of Hematopoietic Precursor Cells

Stem Cells	Progenitor Cells	Maturing Cells
~0.5% of total hematopoietic precursor cells	3 percent of total hematopoietic precursor cells	>95% of total hematopoietic precursor cells
Multilineage differentiation potential	Restricted developmental potential (multipotential → unipotential)	Committed (unipotential) transit population
Quiescent cell population—population size stable	Population amplified by proliferation	Population amplified by proliferation
Population maintained by self-renewal	Transit population without true self-renewal	Proliferative sequence complete before full maturation
Not morphologically recognizable	Not morphologically recognizable	Morphologically recognizable
Measured by functional clonal assays in vivo and in vitro	Measured by clonal assays in vitro	Measured by morphologic analysis; cell counting differentials

⊗ TABLE 3-2

Lineage-Specific Markers Used in Purification of HSC

Erythrocytes	Glycophorin A
Megakaryocytes	Glycoprotein (GP) IIb/IIIa
Neutrophils	CD13, CD15, CD33
Monocytes and macrophages	CD11b, CD14
B lymphocytes	CD10, CD19, CD20
T lymphocytes	CD3, CD4, CD5, CD8, CD38, HLA-DR

lineage-restricted progenitors (Table 3-2 ⊗). The HLA-DR antigens are a component of the human major histocompatibility complex antigens. Rhodamine[123] is a fluorescent supravital dye that is taken up by cells.[14] HSCs have high levels of pumps capable of effluxing dyes (and drugs). They transport the dye out of the cells and are functionally Rho123^{Dull}. Thus, the long-term reconstituting multipotential stem cells are found in the population of cells that contain no lineage-specific antigens, CD38, or HLA-DR antigens but express CD34, SCF-R, and TPO-R and are largely quiescent.

The process of self-renewal, which is a *nondifferentiating cell division,* ensures that the stem cell population is sustained throughout the individual's the lifespan. It is estimated that humans have only ~2 × 10^4 HSCs.[15] This small group of cells is able to maintain tremendous hematopoietic cell supplies through the division of only a tiny fraction of its members, keeping the remainder of the stem cells in reserve. The size of the stem cell compartment is relatively stable under homeostatic conditions. In a stem cell compartment that remains stable in size but supplies differentiating cells, a cell must be added to the compartment by proliferation within the compartment (self-renewal) for each cell that leaves by the process of differentiation. Thus, the stem cell pool must carefully balance the simultaneous processes of expansion (self-renewal) and differentiation. For an individual stem cell undergoing mitosis, these two processes are mutually exclusive.

The regulation of cell-fate decisions of the HSC—whether to remain quiescent, self-renew, or initiate differentiation—is complex and not fully understood. It is thought to involve the interplay of cytokine-receptor interactions and transcription factor activation (see discussion that follows). Quiescence is maintained through interaction with stromal cells and molecules in the hematopoietic microenvironment and interaction with cytokines that have an inhibitory effect on hematopoiesis (see discussion that follows). As an example, TGF-β, a negative regulator of hematopoiesis, upregulates the cell cycle inhibitor p21 (∞ Chapter 2) to help maintain the quiescent status of HSC.[16]

It has been suggested that HSCs reside in unique "stem cell niches" in the bone marrow, which regulate and balance the processes of self-renewal and differentiation. Actually, HSC have a third option available: apoptosis or programmed cell death (which may be triggered if the appropriate cytokines or

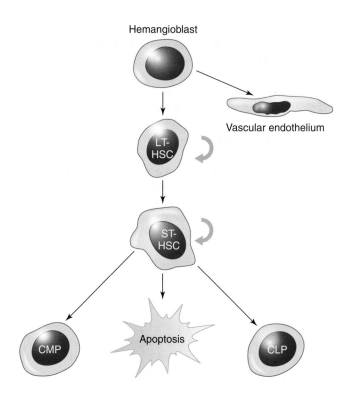

■ **FIGURE 3-1** Derivation and fates of hematopoietic stem cells (HSC). Hemangioblasts are precursor cells giving rise to both HSC and vascular endothelium during embryonic development. LT (long-term) HSC and ST (short-term) HSC refer to the length of time these subpopulations of HSC take to repopulate depleted hematopoietic tissue with LT cells being developmentally more primitive than ST cells. HSCs have three possible fates: self-renewal, commitment to differentiation (becoming common lymphoid progenitors [CLP] or common myeloid progenitors (CMP]), or apoptosis. This cell-fate decision is highly regulated and involves specific transcription factors. (Adapted from Zhu J, Emerson SG. Hematopoietic cytokines, transcription factors and lineage commitment. *Oncogene.* 2002;21:3295–3313.)

microenvironment are not available to sustain the HSC) (Figure 3-1■). Figure 3-1 also depicts the hemangioblast, which is a multipotential precursor capable of producing both HSC and vascular endothelium.[16] Not all HSCs are identical; there is an "age" hierarchy that has been described based on the time it takes for transplanted marrow cells to repopulate a lethally irradiated animal. Thus, the terms *long-term repopulating cells* and *short-term repopulating cells* are used, the short-term repopulating cells are further along the hematopoietic developmental pathway[2] (Figure 3-1).

Progenitor Cells

To meet the cell demands imposed on the hematopoietic system, some stem cells ultimately undergo differentiation. The molecular mechanisms that HSCs utilize to control whether they will self-renew or differentiate upon mitosis remain a mystery. The transition from an HSC to a committed progenitor correlates with the down-regulation of HSC-associated genes via gene silencing and the up-regulation or activation of lineage-specific genes.[17] Evidence suggests that pluripotential stem and progenitor cells simultaneously express low levels of many different genes characteristic of multiple different, discreet lineages (e.g., transcriptions factors, cytokine receptors).[18] This so-called "promiscuous" gene expression is actually characteristic of most multipotent cells. The process of down-regulating HSC-associated genes reduces the promiscuous gene expression so that genes of

the lineage to which the cell has committed are upregulated while the expression of genes associated with alternate lineages are silenced. Lineage-specific transcription factors are thought to play essential roles in this process (see below).

Upon commitment to development, the stem cell enters the next compartment, the progenitor cell (PC) compartment. Initially, the daughter cells arising from undifferentiated stem cells retain the potential to generate cells of all hematopoietic lineages (multipotential progenitor cells/MPP, see Figure 3-2 ■). After additional divisions, however, the

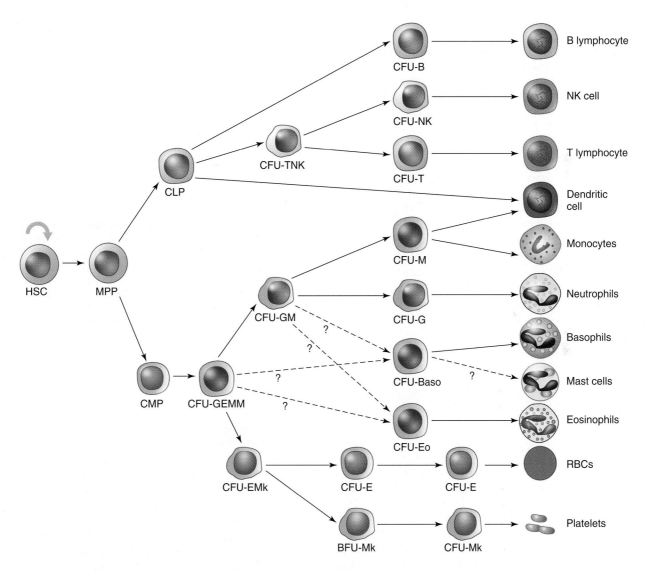

■ FIGURE 3-2   The differentiation of blood cells from a pluripotential stem cell. The pluripotential hematopoietic stem cell (HSC), multipotential progenitor cell (MPP), common myeloid progenitor (CMP), and the colony-forming unit (CFU)-granulocyte, erythrocyte, macrophage, and megakaryocyte (CFU-GEMM) have the potential to differentiate into one of several cell lines and are therefore multilineage precursor cells. The CFU-GM (granulocyte, monocyte) CFU-EMk (erythrocyte, megakaryocyte) and CFU-TNK (T-lymphocyte, natural killer cell) are bipotential progenitors. The committed (unilineage) progenitors—CFU-G (granulocyte), CFU-M (monocyte), CFU-Eo (eosinophil), CFU-Baso (basophil), BFU (burst-forming unit)-E and CFU-E (erythrocyte), and BFU-Mk and CFU-Mk (megakaryocyte),—differentiate into only one cell line. The BFUs are more immature than the CFUs. The mature blood cells are those found in the peripheral blood. The common lymphoid progenitor cell (CLP) may differentiate into T- or B-lymphocytes, natural killer cells, or lymphoid dendritic cells.

progeny of daughter cells lose their ability to generate cells of progressively more lineages and gradually become restricted in differentiation potential to a single cell lineage (unilineage or committed progenitor cells). The progenitor cell compartment thus includes all precursor cells developmentally located between stem cells and the morphologically recognizable precursor cells.

The PC compartment is larger than the HSC compartment, constituting ~3% of the total nucleated hematopoietic cells. PCs do not possess self-renewal ability; in general, their process of cell division is obligatorily linked to differentiation. They are, in essence, transit cells said to be on a suicide maturation pathway (because full maturation and differentiation result in a *terminally differentiated* cell with a finite life span). Like the HSC, PCs are not morphologically identifiable but are functionally defined based on the mature progeny that they produce. Both multipotential and unipotential PCs can be assayed by their ability to form colonies of cells in semisolid media in vitro and are described as *colony-forming units* (CFU) with the appropriate lineage(s) appended. For example, a CFU-GEMM would be a progenitor cell capable of giving rise to a mixture of all myeloid lineages: **g**ranulocytic, **e**rythrocytic, **m**onocytic, and **m**egakaryocytic while a CFU-GM would be a bipotential PC with both granulocytic and monocytic differentiation potential, and a CFU-Mk would be a unilineage progenitor giving rise exclusively to cells of the megakaryocytic series. PCs are mitotically more active than stem cells and are capable of expanding the size of the PC compartment by proliferation in response to increased needs of the body. Thus, the PC compartment consists of a potentially *amplifying* population of cells as opposed to the stable size of the stem cell compartment.

Lineage commitment is a fundamental but poorly understood step in normal hematopoiesis. The factors that regulate this process remain unknown. It is clear, however, that differentiation is accompanied by the increased expression of certain lineage-specific genes and the silencing of genes associated with differentiation along alternate lineages by epigenetic alterations of the chromatin structure (∞ Chapter 2). A number of growth-regulatory glycoproteins, or cytokines (see cytokine section), influence the survival and differentiation of hematopoietic precursor cells.

Maturing Cells

After a series of amplifying cell divisions, the committed precursor undergoes a further change when the cell takes on the morphologic characteristics of its lineage. Maturing cells constitute the majority of hematopoietic precursor cells; proliferation and amplification boost these cells to more than 95% of the total precursor cell pool. In general, the capacity to proliferate is lost before full maturation of these cells is complete. They exhibit recognizable nuclear and cytoplasmic morphologic characteristics that can be used to classify their lineage and stage of development. Because these cells can be morphologically categorized, different nomenclature

is used. Generally, the earliest morphologically recognizable cell of each lineage is identified by the suffix *-blast,* with the lineage indicated (i.e., lymphoblast [lymphocytes], myeloblast [granulocytes], or megakaryoblast [megakaryocytes/platelets]). In some lineages, additional differentiation stages are indicated by prefixes or qualifying adjectives (i.e., proerythroblast, basophilic erythroblast). A complete discussion of the stages of maturing cells of each lineage can be found in the appropriate chapters (∞ Chapter 5, erythrocytic; ∞ Chapter 7, granulocytic and lymphocytic).

✓ Checkpoint! 1

Hematopoietic stem cells that have initiated a differentiation program are sometimes described as undergoing death by differentiation. Explain.

Hematopoietic Precursor Cell Model

The head of the hierarchy of hematopoietic cells is the *pluripotent hematopoietic stem cell (HSC).* These are the cells that have full self-renewal abilities and that give rise to all other hematopoietic elements (Figure 3-2). The progeny of HSCs gradually loses one or more developmental potentials and eventually becomes committed to a single lineage.

The earliest differentiating daughters of the HSC are slightly more restricted in differentiation potential. One group of daughter cells is a precursor capable of giving rise to all cells of the lymphoid system: the *common lymphoid progenitor cell (CLP).*[19] The other group is composed of daughter cells restricted to producing cells of the myeloid system (the cell lineages of the bone marrow): the *common myeloid progenitor cell (CMP).*[20] These cells, although multipotential, have no self-renewal ability and are ultimately destined to differentiate. The phenotypes for the various levels of PC can be seen in Table 3-3 .

TABLE 3-3	
Phenotype of Hematopoietic Precursor Cells	
HSC	CD34$^+$, Thy-1^{Lo}, CD38$^-$, Lin$^-$, HLA-DR$^-$, Rh123^{Dull}, SCF-R$^+$, TPO-R$^+$
CLP	CD34$^+$, Lin$^-$, IL7R$^+$, Thy-1$^-$, SCFR^{lo}
CMP	CD34$^+$, Lin$^-$, IL7R$^-$, SCFR$^+$
CFU-GM	CD34$^+$, SCFR$^+$, FcRγ^{Hi}, CD33$^+$, CD13$^+$
CFU-EMk	CD34$^-$, SCFR$^+$, FcRγ^{Lo}, CD33$^-$, CD13$^-$

HSC = hematopoietic stem cell; Lin$^-$ = lineage markers negative; Rh123^{Dull} = negative for supravital dye Rhodamine123; SCF-R = receptor for stem cell factor; TPO-R = receptor for thrombopoietin; CLP = common lymphoid progenitor; IL7R = receptor for IL7; CMP = common myeloid progenitor; CFU-GM = granulocyte, monocyte colony forming unit; CFU-EMk = erythroid, megakaryocytic colony forming unit; FcRγ = receptor for Fc component of IgG γ chain

Following additional differentiation steps (Figure 3-2), the CLP gives rise to T and B lymphocytes, NK (natural killer) cells and lymphoid dendritic cells, while the CMP gives rise to at least six different lines of cellular differentiation, ultimately producing mature neutrophils, monocytes, eosinophils, basophils, erythrocytes, and megakaryocytes/platelets. One of the first precursor cells defined as arising from the CMP was the CFU-GEMM, a cell capable of producing colonies in culture consisting of granulocytic, eosinophilic, erythrocytic, and megakaryocytic elements. However, it soon was shown that there are layers of functionally defined cells between the true CMP and the CFU-GEMM. Various authors have assigned names to these intermediate cells, including CFU-Blast,[21] HPP-CFC[22] (high proliferative potential, colony-forming cell), CFU-D12[23] (colony-forming unit, day 12), and LT-CIC[24] (long-term culture initiating cell). Whether these represent distinct subpopulations of early progenitor cells or overlapping subpopulations is unclear. In general, they require two to seven growth factors for optimal growth, are characterized by their capacity to produce large colonies of cells (>50,000 cells per colony) after prolonged growth periods in culture, and represent cell populations more primitive than the CFU-GEMM.[25]

The sequence of events during the differentiation of a myeloid or lymphoid multipotential progenitor cell to a unilineage, committed progenitor cell is still being resolved. Neutrophils and monocytes are derived from a common committed bipotential progenitor cell, the CFU-GM, which ultimately gives rise to lineage restricted and morphologically recognizable precursor cells (myeloblasts and monoblasts).[20] Similarly, erythrocytes and megakaryocytes appear to be derived from a common bipotential progenitor cell, the CFU-EMk,[20,26] and T lymphocytes and natural killer cells share a common precursor, the CFU-TNK.[27] The developmental pathway for eosinophils and basophils/mast cells remains uncertain. Some authors describe the CFU-Eo and CFU-B developing from the CFU-GM[2] while others depict them deriving from the CFU-GEMM.[28]

Each of the unilineage or committed progenitor cells is named for the cell lineage to which it is committed (e.g., CFU-Mk for megakaryocytes, CFU-E for erythrocytes, CFU-M for monocytes, CFU-G for neutrophils, CFU-Eo for eosinophils, and CFU-B for basophils). Within some lineages are designated subpopulations of committed progenitor cells. Committed erythroid progenitors are designated as erythroid burst-forming units (BFU-E) and erythroid colony forming units (CFU-E) with the BFU-E being the more primitive precursor cell antecedent to the CFU-E. A similar BFU-Mk/CFU-Mk hierarchy has been described for the megakaryocyte lineage.[29] Each committed progenitor cell differentiates into morphologically identifiable precursors of their respective lineage (e.g., CFU-E → Proerythroblast; CFU-G → myeloblast).

Under normal steady-state physiological conditions, the majority of hematopoietic precursor cells (SC and PC) are retained in the bone marrow. A small population of SC and PC can, however, be found circulating in the peripheral blood.

The number of circulating SC/PC can be further increased by the infusion of various cytokines, enabling the collection of "mobilized" peripheral blood SC/PC for transplantation purposes rather than from a direct bone marrow harvest.

✓ Checkpoint! 2

Explain the difference in the nomenclature used to label progenitor cells from that used to label maturing cells within the hematopoietic hierarchy of cells.

► CYTOKINES AND THE CONTROL OF HEMATOPOIESIS

The regulation of hematopoietic stem/progenitor cell differentiation and expansion is critical because it determines the concentration of various lineages in the marrow and eventually in the peripheral blood. Hematopoietic precursor cell survival, self-renewal, proliferation, and differentiation are governed by specific glycoproteins called *hematopoietic growth factors,* or **cytokines** (Figure 3-3 ■). Growth factor control of hematopoiesis is an extraordinarily complex and highly efficient intercellular molecular communication system that allows the coordinated increases in the production and functional activity of appropriate hematopoietic cell types without expansion of the irrelevant ones. The first identified growth factors (GF) were described as *colony-stimulating factors* (CSFs) because they sustained the growth of hematopoietic colonies in in vitro cultures. Subsequently, as additional cytokines were discovered, the system of nomenclature was changed to that of *interleukins*. When a new cytokine is discovered, the initial description is based on its biologic properties; when the amino acid sequence has been defined, an interleukin number is assigned. The system has some exceptions and inconsistencies, however. For historic reasons, some cytokines retain their original names (e.g., GM-CSF, G-CSF, M-CSF, EPO, and TPO). The initial research into the biologic activities of other cytokines focused on activities outside hematopoietic regulation, and their original names have been retained (e.g., kit-ligand/SCF, Flt3 ligand/FL). More than 30 interleukins have been isolated and characterized to date.

The growth of hematopoietic precursor cells requires the continuous presence of GFs. If the relevant GFs are withdrawn, the cells die within hours by the active process of self-destruction or apoptosis. Thus, the first effect of GFs is to promote cell survival by suppressing apoptosis (programmed cell death). Second, GFs promote proliferation. Hematopoietic cells are intrinsically incapable of unstimulated cell division. All cell division or proliferation depends on stimulation by appropriate regulatory cytokines. Additionally, GFs control and regulate the process of differentiation, which ultimately produces the mature functional cells from their multipotential progenitor cell precursors (Figure 3-3). Finally, GFs that induce proliferation of precursor cells

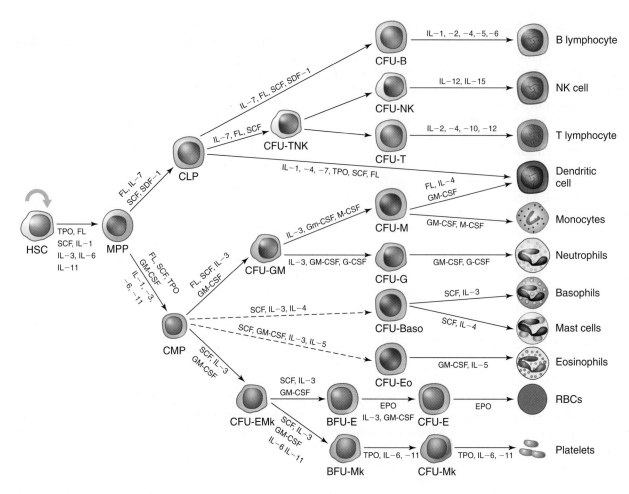

FIGURE 3-3 The pluripotential hematopoietic stem cell (HSC) gives rise to erythrocytes, platelets, monocytes, macrophages, granulocytes, and lymphoid cells. Under stimulation from selective growth factors, stem cell factor (SCF), Flt ligand (FL), and interleukins (IL), the HSC in quiescence (G_0) enters the cell cycle (G_1) and differentiates to the common myeloid progenitor cell (CMP) and, subsequently, to the colony-forming unit-granulocyte, erythroid, macrophage, and megakaryocyte (CFU-GEMM). The CFU-GEMM then differentiates into granulocytes, erythrocytes, monocytes, and megakaryocytes under the influence of specific growth factors, erythropoietin (EPO), thrombopoietin (TPO), granulocyte-monocyte colony-stimulating factor (GM-CSF), granulocyte colony stimulating factor (G-CSF), macrophage colony-stimulating factor (M-CSF), and interleukin-5 (IL-5). Different combinations of hematopoietic cytokines regulate the differentiation of HSC into the common lymphoid progenitor cell (CLP) and subsequently into B and T lymphocytes, natural killer (NK) cells, and lymphoid dendritic cells. (SDF-1 = stromal cell derived factor-1.)

sometimes have the capacity to enhance the functional activity of the terminally differentiated progeny of these precursor cells.

CHARACTERISTICS OF GROWTH FACTORS

Although many different cytokines have been identified as hematopoietic growth factors, many of them share a number of characteristics (Table 3-4 ✪). Most GFs are produced by a number of different cells, including monocytes, macrophages, activated T lymphocytes, fibroblasts, endothelial cells, osteoblasts, and adipocytes (bone marrow stromal cells). With the notable exception of erythropoietin (EPO), most GFs are produced by stromal cells in the hematopoietic microenviron-

---

✪ TABLE 3-4

Characteristics of Hematopoietic Growth Factors

- GFs are produced by stromal cells in the hematopoietic microenvironment.
- Individual GFs have multiple biologic activities (pleiotrophy).
- Many different GFs have similar or identical activities (redundancy).
- By themselves individual GFs are poor stimulators of colony growth; control of hematopoiesis generally involves the interplay of at least several GFs.
- GFs interact with membrane receptors restricted to cells of appropriate lineage.
- GF requirements change during the differentiation process.
- GFs can affect hematopoiesis directly or indirectly.
- Regulatory cytokines are organized in a complex, interdependent network and exhibit many signal amplification circuits.
- GFs commonly act synergistically with other cytokines.

ment. EPO production is atypical of the lymphohematopoietic GFs in that it is produced mainly in the kidney, released into the peripheral blood, and carried to the bone marrow where it regulates red blood cell production. As such, it is the only true hormone (endocrine cytokine), whereas the majority of the other cytokines exert their effects on cells in the local environment where they are produced. Often a single stromal cell source may produce multiple cytokines.

The majority of GFs are not lineage specific; each GF has multiple functions, and most of the GFs act on more than one cell type (i.e., they are *pleiotrophic*) (Table 3-5 ✪). Cytokines must be bound to surface receptors on their target cells to express their activity. They interact with membrane receptors restricted to cells of the appropriate lineage. Be-

cause many precursor cells respond to more than one GF, they obviously express receptors for multiple GFs. Some GFs influence hematopoiesis directly by binding to receptors on precursor cells and inducing the appropriate response (survival, proliferation, differentiation). Other GFs influence the process indirectly by binding to receptors on accessory cells, which in turn respond by releasing other direct-acting cytokines. Some GFs trigger cell division while others support survival without inducing proliferation.

Hematopoietic regulatory cytokines interact in a highly ordered, interdependent network creating a complex cell-to-cell communication system. Individual GFs by themselves are poor stimulators of colony growth; the control of hematopoiesis generally involves the interplay of at least several GFs. Some

✪ TABLE 3-5

Hematopoietic Growth Factors (GFs)

GF	Mol. Wt.	Chromosome	Source	Major Target Cells
EPO	34–39,000	7	Kidney (liver)	Erythroid
GM-CSF	18–30,000	5	T cells, EC, fibroblasts, mast cells	Granulocytes, monos, eos, erythroid, megs, progenitor cells
IL-3	14–28,000	5	Activ T cells, mast cells	Granulocytes, monos, eos, erythroid, megs basos, progenitor cells
G-CSF	18,888	17	Monos, macros, fibroblasts, EC	Granulocytes, early progenitor cells
M-CSF	70–90,000	1	Monos, macros, fibroblasts, EC	Monos, macros, osteoclasts
IL-1	17,000	2	Monos, macros, dendritic cells	Monos, EC, fibroblasts, lymphs, PMN, early progenitor cells
IL-2	23,000	4	Activ T_H1 cells	Prolif and activ of T, B, and NK cells
IL-4	18,000	5	Activ T_H2 cells	Stim T_H2, suppress T_H1; B cells, mast cells basos, fibroblasts
IL-5	50–60,000	5	Activ T_H2 cells	Eos, B cells, cytotoxic T cells
IL-6	21–26,000	7	Fibroblasts, EC, macros, T_H2 cells	Early progenitor cells, B and T cells; megs; myeloid; myeloma cells
IL-7	17,000	8	Stromal cells (BM and thymus)	Pre-T, pre-B cells, NK cells, T_S differentiation
IL-8	8,000	4	Monos, macros, EC, fibroblasts	Chemotaxis of granulocytes (chemokine)
IL-9	40,000	5	Activ T_H cells	T cells, early erythroid cells, mast cells
IL-10	18,000	1	T_H2 cells, monos, macros, activated B cells	B cells, mast cells, T_H2 cells, inhib T_H1 cells
IL-11	24,000	19	Stromal cells, fibroblasts	B cells, megs, early progenitor cells
IL-12	75,000	3,5	Monos, macros, B cells	T_H1 cells, NK cells
IL-13	18,000	5	T cells, basos	Isotype switching of B cells; inhib cytotoxic and inflamm functions of monos and macros
IL-14	53–65,000	16	T cells	Activ B cells
IL-15	14–18,000	4	Monos, macros, E.C., fibroblasts	T cells (CTL), NK cells (LAK), co-stim for B cells
IL-16	16–18,000	15	T cells, Eos, mast cells	Chemotactic for $CD4^+$ T cells, monos, eos
IL-17	22,000	2	Activ T cells	Induces cytokine production by stromal cells
IL-18	18,000	7	Macros, keratinocytes	Induces IFN production by lymphocytes
SCF/KL	28–36,000	12	Fibroblasts, EC, stromal cells	Stem cells, progenitor cells, mast cells
FL	18,000	19	Stromal cells, monos, macros, T cells	Stem cells, progenitor cells, B cells, dendritic cells
TPO	65–85,000	3	Stromal cells, hepatocytes, kidney	Megs, early progenitor and stem cells

Abbreviations used: T cell, B cell = T or B lymphocytes; NK = natural killer cells; EC = endothelial cells; monos = monocytes; macros = macrophages; basos = basophils; eos = eosinophils; megs = megakaryocytes; PMN = neutrophils; activ = activates; inhib = inhibits; inflamm = inflammation; activ T cells = T lymphocytes activated by antigens, mitogens, or cytokines; CTL = cytotoxic T lymphocytes; LAK = lymphokine activated killer cells; prolif = proliferation; stim = stimulation

GFs act synergistically with other cytokines (synergism occurs when the net effect of two or more events is greater than the sum of the individual effects). Many cytokines have overlapping activities (redundancy). The cytokine network often exhibits signal amplification circuits including autocrine, paracrine, and juxtacrine mechanisms of stimulation/amplification (Figure 3-4■). **Autocrine** signals are produced by and act on the same cell. **Paracrine** signals are produced by one cell and act on an adjacent cell, typically over short distances. **Juxtacrine** signals represent a specialized type of paracrine signaling in which the cytokine is not secreted by the cell that produced it but remains membrane bound, necessitating direct producer cell-target cell contact to achieve the desired effect. In contrast, endocrine signals (classic hormones) typically act over fairly long distances. The majority of cytokines regulating hematopoiesis exert their effects via paracrine or juxtacrine interactions.

GF requirements change during the differentiation process so that the cytokines/GFs needed by the HSC and early multipotential PC differ from the GF requirements of the later, lineage-restricted progenitors and the maturing precursor cells. These are described as early-acting (multilineage) GFs and later-acting (lineage-restricted) GFs, respectively. GFs and their receptors share a number of structural features, perhaps explaining some of observed functional redundancies. Most of the GFs have been cloned and characterized, and recombinant proteins are available; certain of these GFs have been shown to have important clinical applications.

Early-Acting (Multilineage) Growth Factors

Several GFs have direct effects on multipotential precursor cells and thus are capable of inducing cell production within several lineages. Early-acting cytokines primarily affect proliferation of these noncommitted progenitor cells. These include SCF, FL, IL-3, GM-CSF, IL-6, and IL-11. Although these factors can initiate proliferation in several cell lineages, in many instances additional factors are necessary for the production of mature cells in these lineages (Figure 3-3).

Stem Cell Factor and Flt3 Ligand (FL) Stem cell factor (SCF) [also known as steel factor (SF), kit ligand (KL), or mast cell growth factor (MCGF)] promotes the proliferation and differentiation of stem cells and primitive multilineage progenitor cells as well as committed progenitor cells (CFU-GEMM, CFU-GM, CFU-Mk, BFU-E). SCF also promotes the survival, proliferation, and differentiation of mast cell precursors and has functional activity outside the hematopoietic system; it plays a role in normal melanocyte development and gametogenesis. Hematopoietic cells responsive to FL appear to be more primitive than SCF-responsive cells. FL increases recruitment of primitive SC/PC into cell cycle and inhibits apoptosis.[30] In contrast to SCF, FL has little effect on unilineage BFU-E/CFU-E, CFU-mast cell, or CFU-Eo but is a potent stimulator of granulo/monocytic, B cell, and dendritic cell proliferation and differentiation. FL and SCF have similar protein structures and share some common characteristics. Both cytokines may be found as either membrane-bound or soluble forms, although the membrane-bound form appears more important physiologically; thus, the cytokines operate primarily through juxtacrine interactions.[31] Neither cytokine has independent in vitro colony-stimulating activity, but both act synergistically with IL-3, GM-CSF, G-CSF, and other cytokines to promote early progenitor cell proliferation.

Interleukin 3 and GM-CSF Interleukin 3 (IL-3) is one of the earliest recognized multipotential growth factors that directly affects multilineage progenitor cells and early committed progenitors such as BFU-E. IL-3 also has indirect actions and can induce the expression of other cytokines. GM-CSF is also a multipotential GF that stimulates clonal growth of all lineages except basophils. GM-CSF also activates the functional activity of most mature phagocytes including neutrophils, macrophages, and eosinophils.

Interleukin 6 and Interleukin 11 Interleukin 6 (IL-6) and Interleukin 11 (IL-11) are pleiotropic cytokines with overlapping growth stimulatory effects on myeloid and lymphoid cells as well as on primitive multilineage cells.[32,33] Each cytokine rarely acts alone but functions synergistically with IL-3, SCF, and other cytokines in supporting hematopoiesis. Both cytokines have significant effects on megakaryocytopoiesis and platelet production.[34] Both mediate the acute phase response of hepatocytes and are major pyrogens in vivo.

Later-Acting (Lineage-Restricted) Growth Factors

The growth factors included here tend to have a narrower spectrum of influence and function primarily to induce mat-

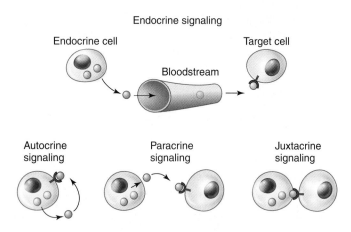

Endocrine signaling

Endocrine cell

Target cell

Bloodstream

Autocrine signaling

Paracrine signaling

Juxtacrine signaling

■ FIGURE 3-4 Mechanisms of cytokine regulation. Autocrine signals are produced by and act on the same cell. Paracrine signals are produced by one cell and act on an adjacent cell, typically over short distances. A juxtacrine signal is a specialized type of paracrine signaling in which the cytokine is not secreted by the producing cell but remains membrane bound, necessitating direct cell-cell contact to achieve the desired effect. In contrast, endocrine signals (classic hormones) typically act over fairly long distances.

uration along a specific lineage. However, most are *not* lineage specific but instead demonstrate a predominant effect on the committed progenitor cell of a single lineage, inducing differentiation of these more mature cells. These growth factors (cytokines) include granulocyte colony-stimulating factor/G-CSF (granulocytes), monocyte colony-stimulating factor/M-CSF (monocytes), erythropoietin/EPO (erythrocytes), thrombopoietin/TPO (megakaryocytes and platelets), interleukin-5/IL-5 (eosinophils), and the interleukins important in lymphopoiesis (ILs-2, -4, -7, -10, -12, -13, -14, -15).

EPO is the only cytokine to function as a true hormone as it is produced at a distant site and travels via the circulation to the bone marrow to influence erythrocyte production. It is expressed largely by cells in the liver in embryonic life and by cells of the kidney (and to a lesser extent, liver) in adult life. Its release is regulated by the body's oxygen needs and is induced by hypoxia (∞ Chapter 5). EPO stimulates survival, growth, and differentiation of erythroid progenitor cells (with its major effect on CFU-E). It also stimulates proliferation, and RNA and protein synthesis in erythroid-maturing cells. Reticulocytes and mature erythrocytes do not have receptors for EPO and thus are not influenced by this cytokine.

G-CSF, M-CSF, and IL-5 stimulate the proliferation of granulocyte, monocyte/macrophage, and eosinophil progenitor cells, respectively. All three also influence the function of mature cells of their respective lineages, increasing migration, phagocytosis, metabolic activities and augmenting prolongation of their life spans. M-CSF also regulates the genesis of osteoclasts, and IL-5 stimulates lymphocyte development.

TPO, also known as *mpl-ligand* or *megakaryocyte growth and development factor* (MGDF), is the major physiologic regulator of megakaryocyte proliferation and platelet production. In vitro, TPO primes mature platelets to respond to aggregation-inducing stimuli and increases the platelet release reaction.[35] TPO also synergizes with a variety of other GFs (SCF, IL-3, FL) to stimulate the maintenance and growth of primitive progenitor cells.

Indirect-Acting Growth Factors

Some cytokines that regulate hematopoiesis do so indirectly by inducing accessory cells to release direct-acting factors. An example is IL-1, which has no colony-stimulating activity itself. However, when administered in vivo, it induces neutrophilic leukocytosis by promoting the release of other direct-acting cytokines from accessory cells.

LINEAGE-SPECIFIC CYTOKINE REGULATION

Erythropoiesis

In the erythroid lineage, progenitor cells give rise to two distinct types of erythroid colonies in culture (∞ Chapter 5). A primitive progenitor cell, the BFU-E, is relatively insensitive to EPO and forms large colonies after 14 days in the form of bursts. Production of BFU-E colonies was originally described

as being supported by *burst-promoting activity,* or BPA, now known to be IL-3 or GM-CSF. CFU-E colonies grow to maximal size in 7 to 8 days and depend primarily on EPO. The CFU-E are the descendants of BFU-E and subsequently give rise to the first recognizable erythrocyte precursor, the pronormoblast. Other cytokines reported to influence production of red cells include IL-9, IL-11, and SCF. However, EPO is the pivotal humoral factor that functions to prevent apoptosis and induce proliferation/differentiation of the most committed erythroid progenitor cells and their progeny.

Granulopoiesis and Monopoiesis

Granulocytes and monocytes are derived from a common bipotential progenitor cell, the CFU-GM, derived from CFU-GEMM. Specific GFs for granulocytes and monocytes, acting synergistically with GM-CSF and/or IL-3, support the differentiation pathway of each lineage. M-CSF supports monocyte differentiation while G-CSF induces neutrophilic granulocyte differentiation. Eosinophils and basophils also are derived from the CFU-GEMM under the influence of growth factors IL-5 and IL-3/IL-4, respectively.

Megakaryocytopoiesis/Thrombopoiesis

Platelets are derived from megakaryocytes, which are progeny of the CFU-EMk. CFU-Mk are induced to proliferate and differentiate into megakaryocytes by several cytokines. However, the cytokines that induce the greatest increase in platelet production are IL-11 and TPO.

Lymphopoiesis

The growth and development of lymphoid cells from the common lymphoid progenitor cell occurs in multiple anatomic locations including the bone marrow, thymus, lymph nodes, and spleen (∞ Chapter 7). Multiple GFs play a role in T and B lymphocyte growth and development, most of which act synergistically (Figure 3-3).

> ✓ **Checkpoint! 3**
>
> *Cytokine control of hematopoiesis is said to be characterized by redundancy and pleiotrophy. What does this mean?*

NEGATIVE REGULATORS OF HEMATOPOIESIS

In addition to the well-studied cytokines that function as positive regulators of hematopoiesis, there exists a second group of polypeptides that inhibit cellular proliferation (Table 3-6). The proliferation of hematopoietic precursor cells can be limited by either decreasing production of stimulating factors or increasing factors that inhibit cell growth. There appears to be a homeostatic network of counteracting growth inhibitors secreted in response to GFs, which normally limit cell proliferation after growth stimuli. These negative regulators of hematopoiesis (e.g., TGF$_\beta$) may be

✪ TABLE 3-6

Negative Regulators of Hematopoiesis

- Interferons
- TGF-β
- TNF-α
- PGEs
- Acidic isoferritins
- Lactoferrin
- Di-OH vitamin D_3
- T_s and NK cells
- SCI (MIP-1α)

responsible for the quiescent state with respect to DNA synthesis of stem cells and early progenitor cells.[18] Several negative regulators have been shown to upregulate some cell cycle inhibitors such as p16 and p21. Alternatively, they may oppose the actions of positive regulators that act on these same cells. Whether or not precursor cells synthesize DNA and proliferate depends on a balance between these opposing influences.

The interferons and transforming growth factor-β (TGF-β) suppress hematopoietic progenitor cells, largely by inhibiting proliferation or inducing programmed cell death. Tumor necrosis factor (TNF-α) directly suppresses colony growth of CFU-GEMM, CFU-GM, and BFU-E while prostaglandins of the E series (PGEs) suppress granulopoiesis and monopoiesis by inhibiting CFU-GM, CFU-G, and CFU-M. Acidic ferritins and lactoferrin are products of mature neutrophils that inhibit hematopoiesis via feedback regulation. Di-hydroxyvitamin D_3 (Di-OH Vitamin D3), classically associated with the stimulation of bone formation, also functions to inhibit myelopoiesis. Additionally, there are cellular components of the immune system, including T-suppressor (Ts) cells and NK cells, which function as negative regulators of hematopoiesis.

Stem cell inhibitor (SCI), also known as *macrophage inflammatory protein*-1α (*MIP*-1α), is believed to be a primary negative regulator of stem cell proliferation.[36] It is believed to be a local-acting regulatory cytokine present in the stromal microenvironment, that controls the steady-state quiescence of stem cells. SCI functions largely via juxtacrine interactions between stromal cells and stem cells (see below) to maintain stem cells in the G_0 phase of the cell cycle.

▶ CYTOKINE RECEPTORS, SIGNALING PATHWAYS, AND TRANSCRIPTION FACTORS

Cytokines must bind to surface receptors on their target cells to express their activity. They interact with membrane receptors restricted to cells of the appropriate lineage. Cells also need a mechanism to transfer signals from extracellular stimuli (cytokines) into appropriate cellular responses intracellularly. Binding of a cytokine (ligand) to its specific receptor transduces an intracellular signal through which the par-

ticular survival, proliferation, or differentiation responses are initiated. The intracellular portion of the receptor binds to associated intracellular molecules that activate signaling pathways. These signaling molecules translocate to the nucleus, recruit appropriate transcription factors, and activate or silence gene transcription (Figure 3-5 ■). Ultimately, changes in protein synthesis lead to alterations in cell proliferation or other modifications of cellular response induced by the cytokine involved. Many of these receptors have been characterized, and they can be grouped according to certain structural characteristics.[37] Some cytokine receptors including the receptors for Epo, G-CSF, and TPO are homodimers (i.e., they consist of two identical subunits). Other receptors are heterodimers or heterotrimers, consisting of different polypeptide subunits (the receptors for most of the other hematopoietic cytokines).

RECEPTORS WITH CYTOPLASMIC TYROSINE KINASE DOMAINS

These receptors are transmembrane proteins with cytoplasmic "tails" that contain a tyrosine kinase catalytic site or domain. When GF binds to the receptor, the receptor chains dimerize enhancing the catalytic activity of the kinase do-

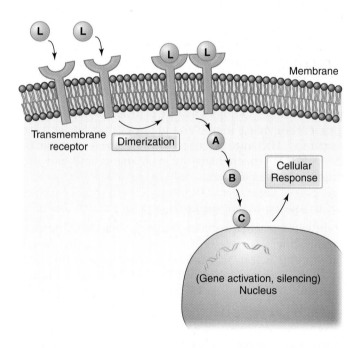

■ FIGURE 3-5   A model for the transfer of signals from extracellular stimuli (cytokines) into appropriate intracellular responses. The binding of a cytokine or ligand (L) to its cognate receptor generally induces receptor dimerization, the activation of a cascade of downstream signaling molecules (A, B, C-signal transduction pathways), converging on the nucleus to induce or repress cytokine-specific genes. The result is an alteration of transcription, RNA processing, translation, or the cellular metabolic machinery.

main and activating intracellular signaling pathways directly. Included in this group are the receptors for M-CSF, SCF, and FL.

HEMATOPOIETIC GROWTH FACTOR RECEPTOR SUPERFAMILY

The receptors for the majority of hematopoietic GFs do not possess intrinsic kinase activity. However, ligand binding and receptor activation leads to phosphorylation of cellular substrates by the activated receptor, which serves as a docking site for adaptor molecules that do have kinase activity. All of these receptors are multichain transmembrane proteins that demonstrate enhanced binding and/or signal transduction (phosphorylation of cellular proteins) when configured as a heterodimer or homodimer. The receptors for many of the GF receptors in this large group share peptide subunits with other receptors[37] (Web Figure 3-1). There are three major subgroups:

1. IL-3, IL-5, and GM-CSF receptors have unique ligand-specific α chains but share a common signal-transducing β chain (the βc family).

2. IL-6 and IL-11 similarly have ligand-specific α chains and share a common signal-transducing β chain called GP 130.

3. The receptors for IL-2, IL-4, IL-7, IL-9, and IL-15 have unique, ligand-specific α chains and share a common signaling γ chain. IL-2 and IL-15 are actually trimeric structures and share a common β subunit as well. Inherited abnormalities of the γ chain gene are responsible for the X-linked form of severe combined immunodeficiency (SCID) (∞ Chapter 20).

It has been suggested that the functional *redundancy* seen in the cytokine regulation of hematopoiesis (i.e., the fact that multiple GFs often have overlapping activities) may be at least partly explained by the sharing of common receptor signaling subunits. For example, IL-3 and GM-CSF have very similar spectra of biologic activities and share a common β subunit.

RECEPTOR FUNCTIONAL DOMAINS

Most receptors have discrete functional domains in the cytoplasmic region of one or more of the receptor chains. Thus, mutations disrupting a discrete domain of the receptor may disrupt part, but not all, of the functions of that receptor. Kostmann's syndrome (congenital agranulocytosis) is a rare disorder characterized by a profound absolute neutropenia with a maturation arrest of precursor cells at the promyelocyte/myelocyte stage. Erythropoiesis and thrombopoiesis are normal. In some patients, molecular studies have revealed a mutation of the G-CSF receptor that disrupts a terminal *maturation-inducing* domain but leaves intact a subterminal *proliferation-inducing* domain.[38] These patients sustain prolif-

eration of neutrophilic progenitor and early maturing cells but fail to complete final maturation of cells in this lineage. Similarly, some individuals with previously unexplained primary erythrocytosis (i.e., *not* secondary to smoking, high altitude, or increased EPO levels) have been shown to have a mutation affecting their EPO-receptors.[39] The EPO-R has been shown to have two separate domains in the cytoplasmic region of the receptor: The domain closest to the membrane constitutes a positive control domain promoting proliferation, and the terminal, negative control domain slows down the intracellular signaling from the receptor. In some patients with familial erythrocytosis, a mutation results in the generation of a truncated protein receptor that lacks the terminal negative control domain. The loss of this negative control region results in enhanced responsiveness of target cells (BFU-E and CFU-E) to the growth stimulatory effects of EPO, resulting in a (benign) erythrocytosis.

✓ Checkpoint! 4

Individuals with congenital defects of the γ chain of the IL-2 receptor suffer from profound defects of lymphopoiesis for greater than individuals with congenital defects of the α chain of the IL-2 receptor. Why?

SIGNALING PATHWAYS

To transfer signals from the receptor into an appropriate response, cells use a variety of "signal transduction pathways" that are initiated by a ligand binding to its specific receptor followed by the activation of "downstream signaling molecules." The downstream signals often result in a cascade of activation steps, ultimately converging on the nucleus to modulate transcription, RNA processing, the protein synthetic machinery (translation), the cellular metabolic machinery, or cytoskeletal-dependent functions[40] (Figure 3-5). Protein phosphorylation is often an important part of the signaling response from cell surface receptors involved in hematopoiesis. These receptors either contain a kinase domain as an integral component of the receptor itself or activate a cytoplasmic kinase as part of the signaling pathway. The signaling cascades that are activated can involve the formation of multiprotein complexes, proteolytic cascades, and phosphorylation/dephosphorylation reactions.

Receptors that contain intrinsic kinase (or phosphatase) activity are identified by the target amino acid to be modified as receptor tyrosine kinases (RTKs), receptor serine kinases (RSKs), or receptor protein tyrosine phosphatases (PTPs).[40] Ligands generally activate these receptors by promoting receptor oligomerization resulting in juxtaposition and activation of their cytoplasmic kinase domains. The result is cross-phosphorylation of the associated subunit kinases.

Receptors that do not have intrinsic enzymatic activity recruit cytoplasmic proteins to their intracellular "tails" and induce the association and assembly of multisubunit protein complexes that generate the enzymatic activity. The recruited proteins are termed *protein tyrosine kinases (PTKs)*. Most hematopoietic receptors signal through the Janus family of PTKs, called *JAKs*. Once activated, the JAK kinases recruit signal relay molecules, often including members of the STAT family of transcription factors (**S**ignal **T**ransducers and **A**ctivators of **T**ranscription), referred to as the **JAK-STAT signaling pathway.** Four different JAK kinases and ~10 different STAT proteins have been identified. Once STAT proteins are phosphorylated by activated JAK kinases, they dimerize, translocate to the nucleus, bind to cytokine-specific DNA sequences, and activate (or inhibit) specific gene expression[40,41] (Figure 3-6■). Abnormalities of the erythrocyte JAK-STAT signaling pathway are the major cause of polycythemia vera (∞ Chapter 22).

TRANSCRIPTION FACTORS

The growth factors that maintain hematopoiesis are *not* thought to be "instructive" for the pathway of differentiation but to be "permissive" for cell viability and proliferation.[42] The components that actually establish the patterns of gene expression associated with lineage differentiation are the nuclear **transcription factors (TF).** Cell-fate decisions are regulated by the integrated effects of internal transcription factors and signaling pathways initiated by external regulatory cytokines.[16]

Different transcription factors are restricted in their expression to particular lineages and to particular differentiation stages within one or more lineages (Web Table 3-1 ✪, Web Figures 3-2■, 3-3a■, 3-3b■). The effect of a particular TF may be either gene expression or gene suppression, depending on the additional molecules (co-activators or co-repressors) recruited to the gene promoter region upon TF binding. TFs associated with activation of lineage-specific differentiation programs often simultaneously inhibit alternate lineage-specific transcription factors.[43] Interestingly, more than half of the hematopoietic transcription factors identified have been shown to be involved in chromosomal translocations associated with leukemias (∞ Chapters 21–26). Thus, the impaired differentiation seen in leukemias is likely due to the perturbation of critical, discrete pathways of transcriptional control.

Although certain TFs are often associated with lineage-specific differentiation pathways, most are also expressed, usually at much lower levels, in hematopoietic progenitor cells that are not yet committed to a specific differentiation pathway. It is thought that this simultaneous expression of TFs for different lineages is associated with the progenitor cell's potential for multilineage development.[16] Once a differentiation decision has been reached (commitment), there is upregulation of TFs for one lineage and down-regulation or antagonism of the others.

CLINICAL USE OF HEMATOPOIETIC GROWTH FACTORS

The cloning and characterization of genes encoding the hematopoietic GFs have allowed scientists to produce these cytokines in large quantity using recombinant DNA technology. As a result, GFs can be used in therapeutic regimens for hematopoietic disorders (Table 3-7 ✪). Some cytokines approved by the Food and Drug Administration (FDA) for clini-

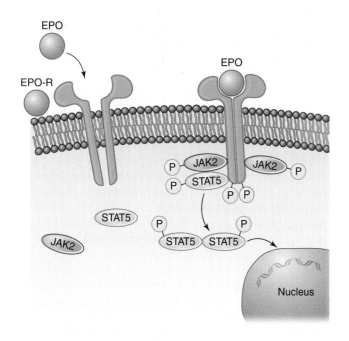

■ FIGURE 3-6 Cytokine receptor-JAK-STAT model of signal transduction. Cytokine (e.g., EPO) interaction with its specific receptor leads to receptor dimerization and activation of JAK kinases associated with the activated receptor. Activated JAK kinases mediate autophosphosphorylation as well as phosphorylation of the receptor, which then serves as a docking site for STATs (signal transducers and activators of transcription). These STATs are phosphorylated, dissociate from the receptor, dimerize, and translocate to the nucleus where they activate gene transcription.

✪ TABLE 3-7
Clinical Applications of Hematopoietic Growth Factors

- Stimulation of erythropoiesis in renal disease (EPO)
- Recovery from treatment-induced myelosuppression (G-CSF and GM-CSF)
- Therapy of myelodysplastic syndromes (IL-3, GM-CSF, EPO)
- Enhanced killing of malignant cells (IL-2, etc.)
- Priming of bone marrow for donation (IL-3, G-CSF, GM-CSF, FL)
- Stimulation of malignant cells to differentiate (various)
- Enhancement of the acute phase response (IL-1, IL-6)
- Enhancement of the immune system (IL-2, IL-15, etc.)
- Stimulation of marrow recovery in BM transplantation (G-CSF, GM-CSF, EPO, IL-11)
- Treatment in bone marrow failure (IL-3, G-CSF, GM-CSF)

cal use include G-CSF and GM-CSF (used primarily to accelerate recovery from granulocytopenia), EPO (for treatment of anemia of various etiologies), IL-11 (for treatment of thrombocytopenia), the interferons (IFNα, IFNβ, and IFNγ used to treat a number of malignant and nonmalignant disorders), and IL-2 (for treatment of metastatic renal cell cancer and melanoma). In vitro studies show that cytokines used in combination often show synergy in terms of their biologic effects. Consequently, the use of combinations of growth factors is being evaluated clinically as well, often with dramatic results. For a more thorough discussion of the biologic therapies currently in clinical use or undergoing clinical evaluations, see Gordon and Sosman.[44]

► HEMATOPOIETIC MICROENVIRONMENT

Hematopoiesis is normally confined to certain organs and tissues (∞ Chapter 4). The proliferation and maturation of hematopoietic precursor cells take place within a microenvironment that provides the appropriate milieu for these events.[45] Patients undergoing bone marrow transplants receive donor cells by intravenous infusion; the cells "home" to and initiate significant hematopoiesis only in the recipient's bone marrow. No biologically significant hematopoietic activity occurs in nonhematopoietic organs. For successful engraftment, the HSCs require an appropriate microenvironment, which presumably has specific properties that make it a unique site for stem cell renewal, growth, and differentiation.

The term **hematopoietic microenvironment (HM)** refers to this localized environment in the hematopoietic organs that is crucial for the development of hematopoietic cells and maintaining the hematopoietic system throughout the individuals lifetime. The HM includes cellular elements and extracellular components including matrix proteins and regulatory cytokines (Table 3-8 ✪). The HM provides homing and adhesive interactions important for the co-localization of stem cells, progenitor cells, and growth regulatory proteins within the marrow cavity.

Stromal Cells

The cellular elements of the HM are referred to as hematopoietic **stromal cells.** They include adipocytes (fat cells), endothelial cells, fibroblasts (referred to by some authors as reticular cells), T lymphocytes, and macrophages. Although the last two cell types are actually hematopoietic cells, they are included in the discussion of stromal cells because they are important sources of cytokine production. The stromal cells' capacity to support hematopoiesis derives from a number of characteristics: They are thought to express homing receptors although the exact mechanisms involved in mediating homing of hematopoietic cells are unclear; they produce and secrete a number of soluble growth and differentiation factors as well as a number of membrane-bound cytokines that function as juxtacrine regulators of hematopoiesis (such as SCF and FL); and finally, they produce the various components constituting the extracellular matrix of the HM.

Extracellular Matrix

The **extracellular matrix (ECM)** produced and secreted by the stromal cells provides the adhesive interactions important for the co-localization of stem cells (SC), progenitor cells (PC), and the growth regulatory proteins. The ECM is composed of collagens, glycoproteins, and glycosaminoglycans. Variations in the type and relative amounts of these components produce the characteristic properties of ECMs in different tissues. Collagen provides the structural support for the other components. Glycosaminoglycans (heparan-sulfate, chondroitin-sulfate, dermatan-sulfate) play a role in cell-cell interactions, helping to mediate progenitor-cell binding to the stroma. They also serve to bind and localize cytokines in the vicinity of the hematopoietic cells.

Within the hematopoietic bone marrow, precursor cells of different lineages and at different stages of differentiation can be found in distinct areas throughout the marrow space. Precursor cells at different stages of differentiation can interact with certain, but not all, ECM components and can be induced to proliferate or differentiate by some but not all cytokines. It has been proposed that at specific stages of

✪ TABLE 3-8

Hematopoietic Microenvironment

Cellular (Stroma)		Extracellular	
Components	Function	Components	Function
Adipocytes, endothelial cells, fibroblasts, T-cells, macrophages	Expression of homing receptors Production of soluble growth and differentiation factors Production of integral membrane proteins that function as juxtacrine regulators (SCF, FL) Production of ECM components	Soluble factors (cytokines and growth factors) Extracellular matrix (ECM) Collagen Glycosaminoglycans (heparan, chondroitin, dermatan-sulfate) Cytoadhesion molecules	Regulation of hematopoietic stem/progenitor cell differentiation and expansion Structural support Cell-to-cell interactions; localization of growth factors Adhesion of hematopoietic precursors to ECM proteins

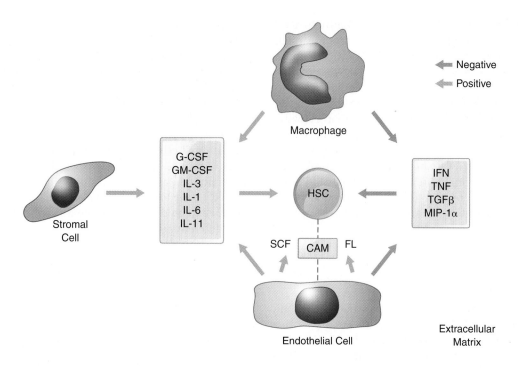

■ FIGURE 3-7   A model for regulation of hematopoietic precursor cells in the bone marrow microenvironment. The hematopoietic stem cell (HSC) attaches to bone marrow stromal cells via specific receptors and ligands. The HSC is then influenced by both positive and negative regulatory growth factors. (CAM: cell adhesion molecule; SCF: stem cell factor; FL: Flt3-ligand; IFN: interferon; TNF: tumor necrosis factor; TGFβ transforming growth factor β; MIP-1α: macrophage inflammatory protein-1α [stem cell inhibitor]; G-CSF: granulocyte-colony stimulating factor; GM-CSF: granulocyte-monocyte CSF; IL-: interleukin-).

differentiation, specialized stromal cells produce extracellular matrix components and hematopoietic supportive cytokines that are conducive for the commitment and/or differentiation of precursor cells of a specific hematopoietic lineage. These interactions could explain the observed tight regulation of precursor cell differentiation and proliferation.[46]

One of the important molecular determinants of the geographic localization of hematopoiesis appears to be the presence of membrane receptors on hematopoietic precursors for ECM proteins. Fibronectin (Fn) is a large, adhesive glycoprotein that can bind cells, growth factors, and ECM components. SC/PC and developing erythroblasts have Fn receptors on their surface membrane. As developing erythroblasts mature to the reticulocyte stage, they lose their Fn receptor; loss of attachment via Fn facilitates the egress of reticulocytes and erythrocytes from the erythroblastic islands in the bone marrow. Likewise, hemonectin (Hn) is an adhesive glycoprotein found in the HM that interacts with Hn receptors on SC, PC, and granulocytes and is important for the attachment of these cells to the marrow. Loss of Hn receptors by developing granulocytes and loss of adhesion to ECM mediates release of mature granulocytes to the circulation. Adhesive interactions between the SC, PC, and the ECM function to help hold the hematopoietic precursor cells in microenvironmental niches, bringing cells into close proximity with

growth regulatory cytokines that are also bound and held by the ECM.[46]

It has been suggested that the quiescent state of stem cells is controlled by their localization in niches that block their responsiveness to differentiation-inducing signals (Figure 3-7 ■). Stromal cells produce cell-surface–associated (juxtacrine) factors that restrain SC differentiation (TGF-β, MIP-1α). Any manipulation that removed SC from their niche would result in a cascade of differentiation events. A major role of stromal tissue in the regulation of hematopoiesis may be to safeguard and ensure stem cell maintenance. This may explain the observation that bone marrow cells removed from their marrow environment do not retain their "stemness" for more than a few weeks when cultured in the absence of stromal cells. Inevitably, they differentiate into progenitor cells and mature cells of the various lineages and thus undergo death by differentiation.

SUMMARY

Hematopoiesis is the production of the various types or lineages of blood cells. Mature, terminally differentiated blood cells are derived from mitotically active precursor cells found primarily in the bone marrow in adults. Hematopoietic precursor cells include pluripotential hematopoietic stem cells, hematopoietic progenitor cells (multilineage and unilineage), and maturing (morphologically recognizable) cells.

Hematopoietic precursor cells are stimulated to proliferate and differentiate by hematopoietic growth factors or cytokines (colony-stimulating factors and interleukins). Cytokine control of hematopoiesis is characterized by redundancy (more than one cytokine is capable of exerting the same effect on the system) and pleiotrophy (a given cytokine usually exerts more than one biologic effect). These cytokines interact with their target cell by means of unique transmembrane receptors responsible for generating the intracellular signals that govern proliferation and differentiation. Hematopoiesis takes place in a unique microenvironment in the marrow consisting of stromal cells and extracellular matrix, which plays a vital role in controlling hematopoiesis.

REVIEW QUESTIONS

LEVEL I

1. Self-renewal and pluripotential differentiation potential are characteristics of: (Objective 2)
   a. mature cells
   b. stem cells
   c. progenitor cells
   d. maturing cells

2. Precursor cells that are morphologically recognizable are found in the: (Objective 2)
   a. stem cell compartment
   b. progenitor cell compartment
   c. maturing cell compartment
   d. differentiating cell compartment

3. The CFU-EMk gives rise to: (Objective 3)
   a. eosinophils and megakaryocytes
   b. erythrocytes and monocytes
   c. eosinophils and megakaryocytes
   d. erythrocytes and megakaryocytes

4. All hematopoietic cells are derived from the CFU-GEMM except: (Objective 3)
   a. lymphocytes
   b. platelets
   c. eosinophils
   d. erythrocytes

5. The following cell is most sensitive to erythropoietin: (Objective 4)
   a. reticulocyte
   b. CFU-GEMM
   c. BFU-E
   d. CFU-E

6. All of the following are considered "early acting, multilineage" cytokines except: (Objective 4)
   a. IL-5
   b. GM-CSF
   c. SCF
   d. IL-3

7. Pleiotrophy refers to: (Objective 4)
   a. multiple different cells that can produce the same cytokine
   b. a cytokine with multiple biologic activities
   c. multiple cytokines that can induce the same cellular effect
   d. a cytokine that can be produced by multiple different tissues

LEVEL II

1. Hematopoietic stem cells are characterized by all of the following markers except: (Objective 1)
   a. CD34$^+$
   b. Lin$^-$
   c. HLA-DR$^+$
   d. Rhodamine^{Dull}

2. The major molecular marker that differentiates CLP from CMP is: (Objective 1)
   a. IL7-R
   b. FcRγ
   c. CD33
   d. CD13

3. All of the following are important regulators of granulopoiesis except: (Objective 2)
   a. GM-CSF
   b. FL
   c. IL-2
   d. IL-3

4. The major cytokine important for eosinophil differentiation is: (Objective 2)
   a. IL-3
   b. IL-5
   c. IL-7
   d. IL-11

5. Which of the following growth factor receptors share a common β chain? (Objective 3)
   a. IL-3 and GM-CSF
   b. TPO and EPO
   c. IL-2 and IL-3
   d. G-CSF and GM-CSF

6. Cytokine receptors that lack an intrinsic kinase domain generally signal through: (Objective 4)
   a. an intrinsic phosphatase domain
   b. recruiting membrane-embedded kinases
   c. an intrinsic protease domain
   d. recruiting cytoplasmic kinases

REVIEW QUESTIONS *(continued)*

LEVEL I

8. Cytokine regulation in which the cytokine is not secreted by the producing cell but remains membrane bound, necessitating direct cell-cell contact to achieve the desired effect is: (Objective 5)
   a. paracrine
   b. endocrine
   c. juxtacrine
   d. autocrine

9. All of the following are thought to be negative regulators of hematopoiesis *except:* (Objective 6)
   a. TGFβ
   b. SCF
   c. TNF
   d. MIP-1α

10. The hematopoietic microenvironment is composed of: (Objective 7)
   a. hepatocytes and extrahepatic matrix
   b. osteoblasts and osteoclasts
   c. marrow stromal cells and extracellular matrix
   d. hepatocytes and splenic macrophages

LEVEL II

7. The function of the JAK-STAT pathway in hematopoiesis is to: (Objective 4)
   a. localize cytokines in the hematopoietic microenvironment
   b. generate homing receptors for stem and progenitor cells
   c. produce cytoadhesion molecules to retain precursor cells in the marrow
   d. function as a signal transduction pathway for cytokine-activated receptors

8. The stromal elements of the hematopoietic microenvironment include all of the following *except:* (Objective 7)
   a. B-lymphocytes
   b. adipocytes
   c. fibroblasts
   d. macrophages

9. Which of the following cytoadhesion molecules plays an important role in retaining erythroid-developing cells in the bone marrow microenvironment? (Objective 7)
   a. hemonectin
   b. fibronectin
   c. thrombospondin
   d. glycosaminoglycans

10. The role of stem cell "niche" in the bone marrow is thought to be to: (Objective 7)
   a. protect hematopoietic precursor cells from the lytic action of osteoclasts
   b. provide nourishment (oxygen, nutrients) to developing precursor cells
   c. regulate the quiescent state of stem cells blocking differentiation-inducing signals
   d. produce cytoadhesion molecules important for homing to the marrow

www.pearsonhighered.com/mckenzie
Use this address to access the interactive Companion Website created for this textbook. Find additional information, tables and figures. Evaluate your command of the chapter information using case studies and critical thinking and multiple choice questions.

REFERENCES

1. Bessis M. *Blood smears reinterpreted.* Berlin-Heidelberg-New York: Springer-Verlag; 1977:17. Trans. G Brecher.

2. Kaushansky K. Hematopoietic stem cells, progenitors, and cytokines. In MA Lichtman, E Beutler, TJ Kipps, U Seligsohn, K Kaushansky, JT Prchal, eds. *Williams hematology,* 7th ed. New York: McGraw-Hill; 2006:201–20.

3. Till JE, McCulloch CE. A direct measurement of the radiation sensitivity of normal mouse bone marrow cells. *Radiat Res.* 1961;14: 213–22.

4. Bradley TR, Metcalf D. The growth of mouse bone marrow cells in vitro. *Aust J Exp Biol Med Sci.* 1966;44:287–99.

5. Silver RK, Erslev AJ. The action of erythropoietin on erythroid cells in vitro. *Scand J Haematol.* 1974;13:338–51.

6. Metcalf D, MacDonald HR, Odartchenko N et al. Growth of mouse megakaryocyte colonies in vitro. *Proc Natl Acad Sci USA.* 1975;72: 1744–48.

7. Vainchenker W, Bouguet J, Guichard J et al. Megakaryocyte colony formation from human bone marrow precursors. *Blood.* 1979;54:940–45.

8. Williams DA. Stem cell model of hematopoiesis. In: R Hoffman, EJ Benz, SJ Shattil, B Furie, HJ Cohen, LE Silberstein, P McGlave, eds. *Hematology: Basic principles and procedures,* 3rd ed. New York: Churchill Livingstone; 2000:126–38.

9. Lord BI, Testa NG. The hemopoietic system: Structure and regulation. In: NG Testa and RP Gale, eds. *Hematopoiesis: Long-Term effects of chemotherapy and radiation.* New York: Marcel Dekker; 1988:1–25.

10. Bagby GC Jr. Hematopoiesis. In: G Stamatoyannopoulos, AW Nienhuis, PW Majerus, H Varmus, eds. *The molecular basis of blood diseases,* 2nd ed. Philadelphia: W B Saunders; 1994.

11. Prchal JT et al. A common progenitor for human myeloid and lymphoid cells. *Nature.* 1978;197:590–91.

12. Bhatia M, Wang JCY, Kapp U, Bonnet D, Dick JE. Purification of primitive human hematopoietic cells capable of repopulating immune-deficient mice. *Proc Natl Acad Sci USA.* 1997;94:5320–125.

13. Berenson RJ, Andrews RG, Bensinger WI, Kalamasz D, Knitter G, Buckner CD, Bernstein ID. Antigen CD34+ marrow cells engraft lethally irradiated baboons. *J Clin Invest.* 1988;81:951–55.

14. Leung AYH, Verfaillie CM. Stem cell model of hematopoiesis. In: R Hoffman, EJ Benz, SJ Shattil, B Furie, HJ Cohen, LE Silberstein, P McGlave, eds. *Hematology: Basic principles and procedures,* 4th ed. New York: Churchill Livingstone; 2005:200–13.

15. Abkowitz JL, Catlin SN, McCallie MT et al. Evidence that the number of hematopoietic stem cells per animal is conserved in mammals. *Blood.* 2002;100:2665–67.

16. Zhu J, Emerson SG. Hematopoietic cytokines, transcription factors and lineage commitment. *Oncogene.* 2002;21:3295–3313.

17. Terskikh AV, Miyamoto T, Chang C et al. Gene expression analysis of purified hematopoietic stem cells. *Blood.* 2003;103:94–101.

18. Krause DS. Regulation of hematopoietic stem cell fate. *Oncogene.* 2002;21:3262–69.

19. Galy A, Travis M, Cen D et al: Human T, B, natural killer, and dendritic cells arise from a common bone marrow progenitor cell subset. *Immunity.* 1995;3:459.

20. Akashi K, Traver D, Miyamoto T et al: A clonogenic common myeloid progenitor that gives rise to all myeloid lineaeges. *Nature.* 2000;404:193.

21. Nakahata T, Ogawa M. Identification in culture of a new class of hemopoietic colony forming units with extensive ability to self-renew and generate multipotential colonies. *Proc Natl Acad Sci USA.* 1982;79:3843–47.

22. Bradley TR, Hodgson GS. Detection of primitive macrophage progenitor cells in mouse bone marrow. *Blood.* 1979;54:1446–50.

23. Magli MC, Iscove NN, Odartchenko V. Transient nature of early haematopoietic spleen colonies. *Nature.* 1982;295:527–29.

24. Sutherland HJ, Lannsdorp PM, Henkelman DH et al. Functional characterization of individual human haematopoietic stem cells cultured at limiting dilution on supportive marrow stromal layers. *Proc Natl Acad Sci USA.* 1990;87:3584–88.

25. Quesenberry PJ. Hemopoietic stem cells, progenitor cells and cytokines. In: E Beutler, MA Lichtman, BS Coller, TJ Kipps, eds. *Williams hematology,* 5th ed. New York: McGraw-Hill; 1995:211–28.

26. McDonald TP, Sullivan PS. Megakaryocytic and erythrocytic cell lines share a common precursor cell. *Exp Hematol.* 1993;21:1316.

27. Ikawa T, Kawamoto H, Fujimoto S et al. Commitment of common T/Natural killer (NK) progenitors to unipotent T and NK progenitors in the murine fetal thymus revealed by a single progenitor assay. *J Exp Med.* 1999;190:1617.

28. Khanna-Gupta A, Berliner N. Granulocytopoiesis and monocytopoiesis. In: R Hoffman, EJ Benz, SJ Shattil, B Furie, HJ Cohen, LE Silberstein, P McGlave, eds. *Hematology: Basic principles and procedures,* 4th ed. New York: Churchill Livingstone; 2005:289–301.

29. Long MW, Gragowski LL, Heffner CH et al. Phorbol diesters stimulate the development of an early murine progenitor cell: The burst forming unit-megakaryocyte. *J Clin Invest.* 1985;76:431–38.

30. Veiby OP, Jacobsen FW, Cui L et al. The Flt3 ligand promotes the survival of primitive hemopoietic progenitor cells with myeloid as well as B lymphoid potential: Suppression of apoptosis and counteraction by TNF-alpha and TGF-beta. *J Immunol.* 1996;157:2953–60.

31. Flanagan JG, Chan DC, Leder P. Transmembrane form of the kit ligand growth factor is determined by alternative splicing and is missing in the Sld mutant. *Cell.* 1991;64:1025–35.

32. Kopf M, Ramsay A, Brombacher F et al. Pleiotropic defects of IL-6 deficient mice including early hematopoiesis, T and B cell function, and acute-phase responses. *Ann NY Acad Sci.* 1995;762:308–18.

33. Musashi M, Clark SC, Sudo T et al. Synergistic interactions between interleukin-11 and interleukin-4 in support of proliferation of primitive hematopoietic progenitors of mice. *Blood.* 1991;778:1448–51.

34. Du XX, Neven T, Goldman S, Williams DA. Effects of recombinant human interleukin-11 on hematopoietic reconstitution in transplant mice: Acceleration of recovery of peripheral blood neutrophils and platelets. *Blood.* 1993;81:27–34.

35. Toombs CF, Young CH, Glaspy JA, Varnum BC. Megakaryocyte growth and development factor (MGDF) moderately enhances in-vitro platelet aggregation. *Thromb Res.* 1995;80:23–33.

36. Graham GJ, Wright EG, Hewick R et al. Identification and characterization of an inhibitor of haemopoietic stem cell proliferation. *Nature.* 1990;344:442–44.

37. Shaheen M, Broxmeyer HE. The humoral regulation of hematopoiesis. In: R Hoffman, EJ Benz, SJ Shattil, B Furie, HJ Cohen, LE Silberstein, P McGlave, ed. *Hematology: Basic principles and procedures,* 4th ed. New York: Churchill Livingstone; 2005:233–65.

38. Dong F, Hoefsloot LH, Schelen AM et al. Identification of a nonsense mutation in the granulocyte-colony-stimulating factor receptor in severe congenital neutropenia. *Proc Natl Acad Sci USA.* 1994;91:4480–84.

39. de la Chapelle H, Traskelin AL, Jubonen E. Truncated erythropoietin receptor causes dominantly inherited benign human erythrocytosis. *Proc Natl Acad Sci USA.* 1993;90:4495–99.

40. Carpenter CL, Neel BG. Regulation of cellular response. In: R Hoffman, EJ Benz, SJ Shattil, B Furie, HJ Cohen, LE Silberstein, P McGlave, eds. *Hematology: Basic principles and procedures,* 4th ed. New York: Churchill Livingstone; 2005:47–59.

41. Rane SG, Reddy EP. JAKs, STATs and Src kinases in hematopoiesis. *Oncogene.* 2002;21:3334–58.

42. Orkin SH. Diversification of haematopoietic stem cells to specific lineages. *Nature Reviews.* 2000;1:57–64.

43. Cantor AB, Orkin SH. Transcriptional regulation of erythropoiesis: An affair involving multiple partners. *Oncogene.* 2002;21:3368–76.

44. Gordon MS, Sosman JA. Clinical application of cytokines and biologic response modifiers. In: R Hoffman, EJ Benz, SJ Shattil, B Furie, HJ Cohen, LE Silberstein, P McGlave, eds. *Hematology: Basic principles and procedures,* 3rd ed. New York: Churchill Livingstone; 2000:939–78.

45. Verfaillie CM. Anatomy and physiology of hematopoiesis. In: R Hoffman, EJ Benz, SJ Shattil, B Furie, HJ Cohen, LE Silberstein, P McGlave, eds. *Hematology: Basic principles and procedures,* 3rd ed. New York: Churchill Livingstone; 2000:139–53.

46. Quesenberry PF, Crittenden RB, Lowry P et al. In vitro and in vivo studies of stromal niches. *Blood Cells.* 1994;2:97–104.

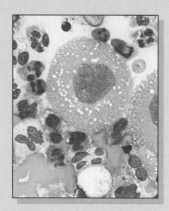

SECTION TWO
THE HEMATOPOIETIC SYSTEM

4

Structure and Function of Hematopoietic Organs

Annette J. Schlueter, M.D., Ph.D.

■ OBJECTIVES—LEVEL I

At the end of this unit of study, the student should be able to:

1. Identify the sites of hematopoiesis during embryonic and fetal development as well as in childhood and adulthood.
2. Identify organ/tissue sites in which each hematopoietic cell type differentiates.
3. Explain the difference between primary and secondary lymphoid tissue.
4. Describe the function of bone marrow, spleen, lymph nodes, and thymus.

■ OBJECTIVES—LEVEL II

At the end of this unit of study, the student should be able to:

1. Associate physical findings (hypersplenism, lymphadenopathy) with the presence of hematologic disease.
2. Describe the pathophysiologic changes that lead to bone marrow hyperplasia or extramedullary hematopoiesis.
3. Identify sites of extramedullary hematopoiesis.
4. Describe the structure of bone marrow, spleen, lymph nodes, and thymus.

KEY TERMS

- Adipocyte
- Culling
- Endosteum
- Erythroblastic island
- Extramedullary hematopoiesis
- Germinal center
- Hyperplasia
- Lymphoid follicle
- Medullary hematopoiesis
- Osteoblast
- Osteoclast
- Pitting
- Reticular cell
- Stroma
- Trabecula

BACKGROUND BASICS

The information in this chapter builds on the concepts learned in the first three chapters. A basic anatomy and physiology course could also be helpful. To maximize your learning experience, you should review these concepts before starting this unit of study:

Level I

- ▶ Define *microenvironment* as related to hematopoietic cell development (Chapter 3).
- ▶ Summarize the process of cell maturation in the bone marrow (Chapter 3).

Level II

- ▶ Summarize the mechanisms of positive and negative regulators of hematopoietic cell development (Chapter 3).
- ▶ Describe the details of hematopoiesis and the role of cytokines/growth factors in blood cell development (Chapter 3).

 CASE STUDY

We will refer to this case throughout this chapter.
Francine, a 40-year-old female, saw her physician for complaints of fatigue and shortness of breath. Physical examination revealed splenomegaly and lymphadenopathy. A complete blood count was ordered with the following results: Hb 8g/dL; WBC 6.5 × 10⁹/L; Platelets 21 × 10⁹/L.

1. Refer to the tables on the front inside cover of the book and determine which blood cell parameters if any, are abnormal.

▶ OVERVIEW

This chapter includes a description of the tissues involved in the production and maturation of blood cells. It begins with a sequential look at blood cell production from the embryo to the adult. The histologic structure of each tissue and its function in hematopoiesis are discussed. Abnormalities in hematopoiesis that are associated with histologic and functional changes in these tissues are briefly described.

▶ INTRODUCTION

Cellular proliferation, differentiation, and maturation of blood cells take place in the hematopoietic tissue, which in the adult consists primarily of bone marrow although some lymphocyte development also takes place in spleen and thymus. Mature cells are released to the peripheral blood and can live out their lifespan in the blood or take up residence primarily in the spleen or a lymph node. In pathologic conditions, mature cells can also reside in other tissues of the body. The link between the bone marrow and blood cell production was not established until it was recognized that blood formation was a continuous process. Before 1850, it was believed that blood cells formed in the fetus were viable until the host's death and that there was no need for a continuous source of new elements.

▶ DEVELOPMENT OF HEMATOPOIESIS

Hematopoiesis begins as early as the eighteenth day after fertilization in an extraembryonic location, the yolk sac of the human embryo.[1] The cells made in the yolk sac include erythrocytes and a few macrophages.[2] The ability to make erythrocytes is important because the embryo must be able to transport oxygen to developing tissue early in gestation. Shortly thereafter, intraembryonic hematopoiesis begins in the aorta-gonads-mesonephros (AGM) region located along the developing aorta. This region has the ability to make a wider range of hematopoietic cells including lymphocytes.[3] Cell production at this time is called *primitive erythropoiesis* because the hemoglobin is not typical of that seen in later developing erythroblasts. The primitive embryonic erythroblasts in the yolk sac arise from clusters of cells in the mesenchyme called *blood islands* and are closely related to development of endothelium, the cells lining blood vessels.[4] Embryonic red cells have a megaloblastic appearance with coarse clumped chromatin (∞ Chapter 12). The hemoglobin in these cells consists of the embryonic varieties, Gower 1, Gower 2, and Portland (∞ Chapter 6).[5]

At about the third month of fetal life, the liver becomes the chief site of blood cell production, and the yolk sac and

AGM discontinue their role in hematopoiesis. The liver continues to produce a high proportion of erythroid cells, but myeloid and lymphoid cells begin to appear in greater numbers.[6] This is the beginning of a transition to adult patterns of hematopoiesis in which myeloid differentiation predominates over erythroid differentiation.

As fetal development progresses, hematopoiesis also begins to a lesser degree in the spleen, kidney, thymus, and lymph nodes. Erythroid and myeloid cell production as well as early B cell (lymphocyte) development gradually shifts from these sites to bone marrow during late fetal and neonatal life as the hollow cavities within the bones begin to form. The bone marrow becomes the primary site of hematopoiesis at about the sixth month of gestation and continues as the primary source of blood production after birth and throughout adult life (Figure 4-1 ■). Granulocytic and megakaryocytic production shifts to the bone marrow before erythropoiesis, which does not transition until the end of gestation. The thymus becomes the major site of T cell (lymphocyte) production during fetal development and continues to be active throughout the neonatal period and childhood. As is true for erythrocytes in the yolk sac, the first T cells to develop are different than their adult counterparts. They use a different set of genes to make the T cell receptor, which the T cell uses to recognize and react to foreign substances[7] (∞ Chapter 7). Lymph nodes and spleen continue as an important site of late B cell differentiation throughout life.

▶ HEMATOPOIETIC TISSUE

The adult hematopoietic system includes tissues and organs involved in the proliferation, maturation, and destruction of blood cells. These organs and tissues include the bone marrow, thymus, spleen, and lymph nodes. Bone marrow is the site of myeloid, erythroid, and megakaryocytic as well as lymphoid cell development. Thymus, spleen, and lymph nodes are primarily sites of lymphoid cell development. Tissues in which lymphoid cell development occurs are divided into primary and secondary lymphoid tissue. Primary lymphoid tissues (bone marrow and thymus) are those in which T and B cells develop from nonfunctional precursors into cells that are capable of responding to foreign antigens (immunocompetent cells). Secondary lymphoid tissues (spleen and lymph nodes) are those in which immunocompetent T and B cells further differentiate and divide in response to antigens.

BONE MARROW

Blood-forming tissue located between the **trabeculae** of spongy bone is known as *bone marrow*. (*Trabecula* refers to a projection of calcified bone extending from cortical bone into the marrow space; it provides support for marrow cells.) This major hematopoietic organ is a cellular, highly vascularized, loose connective tissue. It is composed of two major compartments: the vascular compartment and the hematopoietic compartment. The vascular compartment is composed of the nutrient artery, periosteal arteries, central longitudinal vein, arterioles, and sinuses. The hematopoietic compartment is the site of formation and maturation of blood cells (Figure 4-2 ■). This compartment includes both hematopoietic cells and stromal cells.

Vasculature

The vascular supply of bone marrow is served by two arterial sources, a nutrient artery and a periosteal artery that enter the bone through small holes, the bone foramina. Blood is drained from the marrow via the central vein (Figure 4-3 ■). The nutrient artery branches around the central sinus that spans the marrow cavity. Arterioles radiate outward from the nutrient artery to the **endosteum** (the inner lining of the cortical bone), giving rise to capillaries that merge with capillaries from periostial arteries to form venous sinuses within the marrow. The sinuses, lined by single endothelial cells

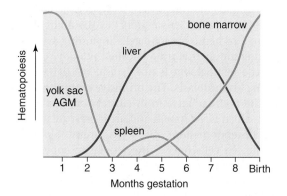

■ FIGURE 4-1   Location of hematopoiesis during fetal development. At birth most blood cell production is limited to the marrow.

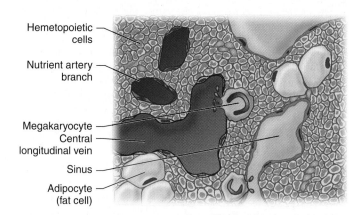

■ FIGURE 4-2   Schematic drawing of a section of bone marrow.

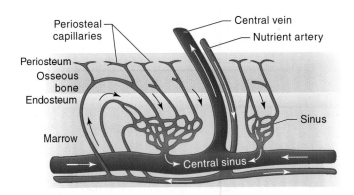

■ **FIGURE 4-3**   Diagram of the microcirculation of bone marrow. The major arterial supply to the marrow is from periosteal capillaries and from capillary branches of the nutrient artery, which have traversed the bony enclosure of the marrow through the bone foramina. The capillaries join with the venous sinuses as they reenter the marrow. The sinuses gather into wider collecting sinuses that then open into the central longitudinal vein (central sinus). (Adapted with permission from: DeBruyn PPH: Structural substrates of bone marrow function. *Semin Hematol.* 1981;18:179.)

and supported on the abluminal side by adventitial **reticular cells,** ultimately gather into wider collecting sinuses, which open into the central longitudinal vein.[8] The central longitudinal vein continues through the length of the marrow and exits through the foramina where the nutrient artery entered.

Stroma

The bone marrow **stroma** (supporting tissue) forms a favorable microenvironment for sustained proliferation of hematopoietic cells.[9] It forms a meshwork that provides a three-dimensional scaffolding for hematopoietic cells. Stromal components also provide cytokines that regulate hematopoiesis. The stroma is composed of three major cell types: macrophages, reticular cells (fibroblasts), and **adipocytes.**

Macrophages serve two major functions in the bone marrow: phagocytosis and secretion of hematopoietic cytokines. Macrophages phagocytose the extruded nuclei of maturing erythrocytes and abnormal cells such as B cells that have not differentiated properly. Some macrophages serve as the center of the erythroblastic islands as discussed below. It has been believed that these cells supply the developing erythroblasts with iron and cytokines; more recent studies suggest, however, that the majority of the iron is supplied by transferrin delivery from the plasma. Macrophages also provide many colony-stimulating factors needed for the development of myeloid lineage cells. Macrophages stain acid phosphatase positive.

Reticular cells are located on the abluminal surfce of the vascular sinuses and send long cytoplasmic processes into the stroma. These cells also produce reticular fibers, which contribute to the three-dimensional supporting network that holds the vascular sinuses and hematopoietic elements.

The fibers can be visualized with light microscopy and after silver staining. Reticular cells are alkaline phosphatase positive.

Adipocytes are cells whose cytoplasm is largely replaced with a single fat vacuole. They most likely develop from reticular cells that synthesize fat. These cells mechanically control the volume of bone marrow in which active hematopoiesis takes place. They also provide steroids that influence erythropoiesis and maintain osseous bone integrity.[10,11]

The proportion of bone marrow composed of adipocytes changes with age. For the first four years of life, nearly all marrow cavities are composed of hematopoietic cells, or red marrow. After four years of age, the red marrow in the shafts of long bones is gradually replaced by adipocytes, or yellow marrow. By the age of 25 years, hematopoiesis is limited to the marrow of the skull, ribs, sternum, scapulae, clavicles, vertebrae, pelvis, upper half of the sacrum, and proximal ends of the long bones. The distribution of red:yellow marrow in these bones is about 1:1. The fraction of red marrow in these areas may decrease after age 70.

Osteoblasts and osteoclasts are found in the endosteum (internal surface of calcified bone). These cells can be dislodged during bone marrow biopsy and can be found in the specimen with hematopoietic cells. Osteoblasts differentiate from a common precursor with hematopoietic cells.[12] They are involved in the formation of calcified bone and provide a niche for resting hematopoietic stem cells.[13] They are large cells (up to 30 μm in diameter) that resemble plasma cells except that the perinuclear halo (Golgi apparatus) is detached from the nuclear membrane and, in Wright-stained specimens, appears as a light area away from the nucleus (Figure 4-4■). In addition, the cytoplasm may be less basophilic, and the nucleus has a finer chromatin pattern than plasma cells. Osteoblasts are normally found in groups. These cells are more commonly seen in children and in metabolic bone diseases. The cells are alkaline phosphatase positive.

Osteoclasts are cells related to macrophages that are involved in resorption and remodeling of calcified bone. They are even larger than osteoblasts and can reach up to 100 μm in diameter. The cells are multinucleated and have granular cytoplasm that can be either acidophilic or basophilic. They resemble megakaryocytes except that the nuclei are usually discrete (whereas the megakaryocyte has a single, large multilobulated nucleus) and often contain nucleoli (Figure 4-4).

Hematopoietic Compartment

Hematopoietic cells are arranged in distinct niches within the marrow cavity. Erythroblasts constitute 25–30% of the marrow cells and are produced near the sinuses. They develop in **erythroblastic islands** composed of a single macrophage surrounded by erythroblasts in varying states of maturation. The macrophage cytoplasm extends out to surround the erythroblasts. During this close association, the macrophages regulate erythropoiesis by secreting various

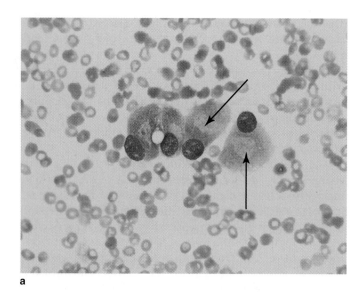

a

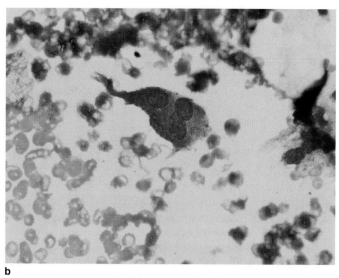

b

■ FIGURE 4-4   **a.** Osteoblast; arrows point to the Golgi apparatus (perinuclear halo) **b.** Osteoclast in bone marrow aspirate. (Wright-Giemsa stain; 1000× magnification)

cytokines.[14] The least mature cells are closest to the center of the island, and the more mature cells are at the periphery.

The location of leukocyte development differs depending on its type. Granulocytes are produced in nests close to the trabeculae and arterioles and are relatively distant from the venous sinuses. These nests are not quite as apparent morphologically as are erythroblastic islands. Megakaryocytes are very large, polyploid cells that produce platelets from their cytoplasm. They are located adjacent to the vascular sinus.[15] Cytoplasmic processes of the megakaryocyte form long proplatelet processes that pinch off to form platelets (Figure 4-5 ■). Lymphocytes are normally produced in lymphoid aggregates located near arterioles. Lymphoid progenitor cells can leave the bone marrow and travel to the thymus where they mature into T lymphocytes. Some remain in the bone marrow where they mature into B lymphocytes. Some B cells return to the bone marrow after being activated in the spleen or lymph node. Activated B cells transform into plasma cells, which can reside in the bone marrow and produce antibody.

✓ Checkpoint! 1

Describe the bone marrow stromal location of erythrocyte, granulocyte, platelet, and lymphocyte differentiation.

Bone forms a rigid compartment for the marrow. Thus, any change in volume of the hematopoietic elements as occurs in many anemias and leukemias must be compensated for by a change in the space-occupying adipocytes. Normal red marrow can respond to stimuli and increase its activity to several times the normal rate. As a result, the red marrow becomes hyperplastic and replaces portions of the fatty marrow. Bone marrow **hyperplasia** (an excessive proliferation

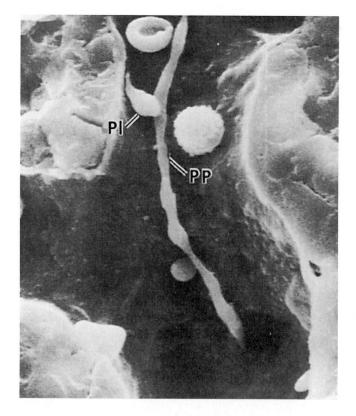

■ FIGURE 4-5   Scanning electron micrograph of the luminal face of the myeloid sinus wall with an intraluminal segment of a pro-platelet process (PP) showing periodic constriction along its length. Pl: platelet displaying tear-drop shape. (Reprinted with permission from: DeBruyn PPH: Structural substrates of bone marrow function. *Semin Hematol.* 1981;18:179.)

of normal cells) accompanies all conditions with increased or ineffective hematopoiesis. The degree of hyperplasia is related to the severity and duration of the pathologic state. Acute blood loss can cause erythropoietic tissue to temporarily replace fatty tissue whereas severe chronic anemia can cause erythropoiesis to be so intense that it not only replaces fatty marrow but also erodes the bone's internal surface. In malignant diseases that invade or originate in the bone marrow such as leukemia, proliferating abnormal cells can replace both normal hematopoietic tissue and fat.

In contrast, the hematopoietic tissue can become inactive or hypoplastic. Fat cells then increase, providing a cushion for the marrow. Environmental factors such as chemicals and toxins can suppress hematopoiesis whereas other types of hypoplasia can be genetically determined (∞ Chapter 13). Myeloproliferative disease, which begins as a hypercellular disease, frequently terminates in a state of aplasia in which hematopoietic tissue is replaced by fibrous tissue (∞ Chapter 22).

CASE STUDY (continued from page 51)

Microscopic examination of a stained blood smear from Francine revealed a predominance of very young blood cells (blasts) in the peripheral blood. These cells are normally found only in the bone marrow. Subsequently, she had a bone marrow aspirated for examination. This revealed 100% cellularity (red marrow) with a predominance of the same type of blasts as those found in the peripheral blood.

2. Describe Francine's bone marrow as normal, hyperplastic, or hypoplastic.
3. What conditions can cause this bone marrow finding?

Blood Cell Egress

Special properties of the maturing hematopoietic cell as well as of the venous sinus wall are important in migration of blood cells from the bone marrow.[16] These cells must migrate between reticular cells but through endothelial cells to reach the circulation. As cell traffic across the sinus increases, the reticular cells contract creating a less continuous layer over the abluminal sinus wall. This provides the mature hematopoietic cells more interaction sites on the sinus endothelial surface. In areas in which the reticular cell layer contracts, it creates compartments between the reticular cell layer and the endothelial layer where mature cells accumulate.

The new blood cell interacts with the abluminal endothelial membrane by a receptor-mediated process, forcing the abluminal membrane into contact with the luminal endothelial membrane. The two membranes fuse, and then under pressure from the passing cell, they separate, creating a pore through which the remainder of the hematopoietic cell enters the lumen of the sinus. These pores are only

2–3 µm in diameter. Because of the small size of the endothelial cell pores, blood cells must have the ability to deform so that they can pass through the sinusoidal lining. Progressive increases in deformability and motility have been noted as granulocytes mature from the myeloblast to the segmented granulocyte stage. This facilitates the movement of cells into the sinus lumen.

Many soluble factors are important in facilitating the release of blood cells from bone marrow. Among these are G-CSF, GM-CSF, and a large number of chemokines.[17,18] Some of these molecules are used clinically to increase circulating granulocytes or hematopoietic stem cells into the circulation to obtain granulocytes for transfusion or stem cells for transplantation.

✓ Checkpoint! 2

Describe the process by which a blood cell moves from the marrow to the vascular space.

Extramedullary Hematopoiesis

Hematopoiesis in the bone marrow is called **medullary hematopoiesis**. **Extramedullary hematopoiesis** denotes blood cell production in hematopoietic tissue other than bone marrow. In certain hematologic disorders when hyperplasia of the marrow cannot meet the physiologic blood needs of the tissues, extramedullary hematopoiesis can occur in the hematopoietic organs that were active in the fetus, principally the liver and spleen. Organomegaly frequently accompanies significant hematopoietic activity at these sites. This extramedullary hematopoiesis in postnatal life reflects the ability of inert hematopoietic cells to become active, functional cells if the need arises.

THYMUS

The thymus is a lymphopoietic organ located in the upper part of the anterior mediastinum. It is a bilobular organ demarcated into an outer cortex and central medulla. The cortex is densely packed with small lymphocytes (thymocytes), cortical epithelial cells, and a few macrophages. The medulla is less cellular and contains more mature thymocytes mixed with medullary epithelial cells, dendritic cells, and macrophages (Figure 4-6).

The primary purpose of the thymus is to serve as a compartment for maturation of T lymphocytes.[19] Precursor T cells leave the bone marrow and enter the thymus through arterioles in the cortex. As they travel through the cortex and the medulla, they interact with epithelial cells and dendritic cells, which provide signals to ensure that T cells can recognize foreign antigen but not self-antigen. They also undergo rapid proliferation. Only about 3% of the cells generated in the thymus exit the medulla as mature T cells. The rest die by apoptosis and are removed by thymic macrophages. The thymus is responsible for supplying the T-dependent areas of lymph nodes, spleen, and other peripheral lymphoid tissue with immunocompetent T lymphocytes.

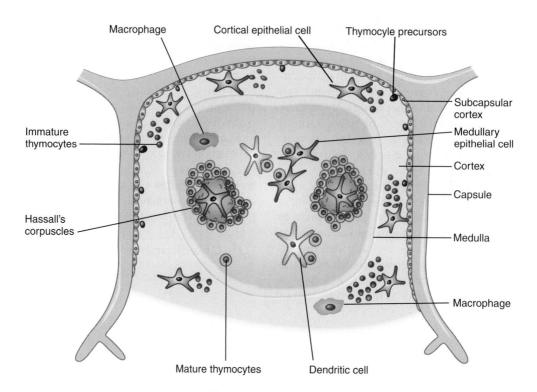

Macrophage   Cortical epithelial cell   Thymocyte precursors

Subcapsular cortex

Medullary epithelial cell

Cortex

Capsule

Medulla

Macrophage

Immature thymocytes

Hassall's corpuscles

Mature thymocytes   Dendritic cell

■ FIGURE 4-6   A schematic drawing of the thymus. See text for the role of the various cell types. Hassall's corpuscles are collections of epithelial cells that may be involved in the development of certain (regulatory) T cell subsets in the thymus.

The thymus is a well-developed organ at birth and continues to increase in size until puberty. After puberty, however, it begins to atrophy until in old age it becomes barely recognizable. This atrophy could be driven by increased steroid levels beginning in puberty and decreased growth factor levels in adults.[20,21] The atrophied thymus is still capable of producing new T cells if the peripheral pool becomes depleted as occurs after the lymphoid irradiation that accompanies bone marrow transplantation.[22]

SPLEEN

The spleen is located in the upper left quadrant of the abdomen beneath the diaphragm and to the left of the stomach. After several emergency splenectomies were performed without causing permanent harm to the patients, it was recognized that the spleen was not essential to life. However, it does play a role in filtration of foreign substances and old erythrocytes from the circulation, storage of platelets, and immune defense.

Architecture

The spleen, enclosed by a capsule of connective tissue, contains the largest collection of lymphocytes and macrophages in the body (Figure 4-7 ■). These cells together with a reticular meshwork are concentrated in different areas of the spleen and contribute to the formation of three zones of tissue: white pulp, red pulp, and the marginal zone.

The white pulp, a visible grayish white zone, is composed of lymphocytes and located around a central artery. The area closest to the artery, which contains many T cells as well as macrophages and dendritic cells, is termed the *periarterial lymphatic sheath.* Peripheral to this area are B cells arranged into follicles (a sphere of B cells within lymphatic tissue). Activated B cells are found in specialized follicular areas called **germinal centers.** Germinal centers appear as lightly stained areas in the center of a **lymphoid follicle.** They consist of a mixture of B lymphocytes, follicular dendritic cells, and phagocytic macrophages. The immune response is initiated in the white pulp. In some cases of heightened immunologic activity, the white pulp can increase to occupy half the volume of the spleen (it is normally 20% or less).

White pulp is surrounded by the marginal zone, a reticular meshwork containing blood vessels, macrophages, and specialized B cells. This zone lies at the junction of the white pulp and red pulp and is important in initiating certain types of immune responses as well as performing functions similar to that of the red pulp (see below).

The red pulp contains sinuses and cords. The sinuses are dilated vascular spaces for venous blood. The red color of the pulp is caused by the presence of erythrocytes in the sinuses. The cords are composed of masses of reticular tissue and macrophages that lie between the sinuses. The cords of the red pulp provide zones for platelet storage and destruction of damaged blood cells.

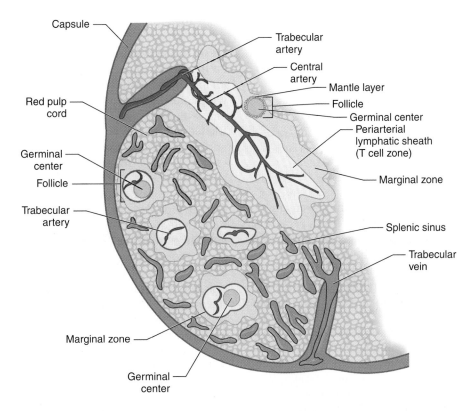

■ FIGURE 4-7   A schematic drawing of splenic tissue. See text for an explanation of the splenic tissue architecture. The periarterial lymphatic sheath contains many T cells, macrophages and dendritic cells. B cells are arranged into follicles. Activated B cells are in the germinal centers. (Adapted from *Seminars in Hematology*, V7(4), Weiss L et al: Anatomical hazards to the passage of erthrocytes through the spleen, p. 373, 1970, with permission from Elsevier.)

Blood Flow

The spleen is richly supplied with blood. It receives 5% of the total cardiac output, a blood volume of 300 mL/minute. Blood enters the spleen through the splenic artery, which branches into many vessels in the trabeculae. Vessel branches can terminate in the white pulp, red pulp, or marginal zone. Blood entering the spleen can follow either the rapid transit pathway (closed circulation) or the slow transit pathway (open circulation). The rapid transit pathway is a relatively unobstructed route by which blood enters the sinuses in red pulp from arteries and passes directly to the venous collecting system. In contrast, blood entering the slow transit pathway moves sluggishly through a circuitous route of macrophage-lined cords before it gains access to the sinuses. Plasma in the cords freely enters the sinuses, but erythrocytes meet resistance at the sinus wall where they squeeze through the tiny openings. This skimming of the plasma from blood cells in the cords to the sinuses sharply increases the hematocrit in the cords. Sluggish blood flow and continued erythrocyte metabolic activity in cords results in a splenic environment that is hypoxic, acidic, and hypoglycemic. Hypoxia and hypoglycemia occur as erythrocytes utilize available oxygen and glucose. Metabolic byproducts create the acidic environment.

Functions

Blood that empties into the cords of the red pulp and of the white pulp and marginal zone takes the slow transit pathway, which is very important to splenic function including culling, pitting, immune defense, and storage. The discriminatory filtering and destruction of senescent or damaged red cells by the spleen is termed **culling.** Cells entering the spleen through the slow transit pathway become concentrated in the hypoglycemic, hypoxic cords of the red pulp, a hazardous environment for aged or damaged erythrocytes. Slow passage through a macrophage-rich route allows the phagocytic cells to remove these old or damaged, less deformable erythrocytes before or during their squeeze through the 3 μm pores to cords and sinuses. Normal erythrocytes withstand this adverse environment and eventually reenter the circulation.

Pitting refers to the spleen's ability to "pluck out" particles from intact erythrocytes without destroying them. Blood cells coated with antibody are susceptible to pitting by macrophages. The macrophage removes the antigen-antibody complex and the attached membrane. The pinched off cell membrane can reseal itself, but the cell cannot synthesize lipids and proteins for new membrane due to its lack of cellular organelles. Therefore, extensive pitting causes a reduced surface-area-to-volume ratio, resulting in the formation of spherocytes (erythrocytes that have no central area of pallor on stained blood smears). The presence of spherocytes on a blood film is evidence that the erythrocyte has undergone membrane assault in the spleen.

 Checkpoint! 3

Describe how old or damaged erythrocytes are removed from the circulation by the spleen.

The white pulp and marginal zones of the spleen are important lines of defense in blood-borne infections because of their rich supply of lymphocytes and phagocytic cells as well as the slow transit circulation through these areas. Blood-borne antigens are forced into close contact with phagocytes (antigen-presenting cells) and lymphocytes allowing for recognition of the antigen as foreign and leading to phagocytosis and antibody formation.

The immunologic function of the spleen is probably less important in the well-developed immune system of the adult than in the less-developed immune system of the child. Young children who undergo splenectomy may develop overwhelming, often fatal, infections with encapsulated organisms such as *S. pneumoniae* and *H. influenzae*. This can also be a rare complication of splenectomy in adults. The loss of the marginal zone can be especially important in this regard.[23]

Sequestering approximately one-third of the platelet mass, the red pulp cords of the spleen act as a reservoir for platelets. Massive splenomegaly can result in a pooling of 80–90% of the platelets, producing peripheral blood thrombocytopenia. Removal of the spleen results in a transient thrombocytosis with a return to normal platelet concentrations in about 10 days.

Hypersplenism

In a number of conditions, the spleen may become enlarged and, through exaggeration of its normal activities of filtering and phagocytosing, cause anemia, leukopenia, thrombocytopenia, or combinations of cytopenias. A diagnosis of hypersplenism is made when three conditions are met: (1) the presence of anemia, leukopenia, or thrombocytopenia in the peripheral blood, (2) the existence of a cellular or hyperplastic bone marrow corresponding to the peripheral blood cytopenias, and (3) the occurrence of splenomegaly. The correction of cytopenias following splenectomy confirms the diagnosis.

Hypersplenism has been categorized into two types: primary and secondary. The primary type is said to occur when no underlying disease can be identified. The spleen functions abnormally and causes the disease. This type of hypersplenism is very rare.

Secondary hypersplenism occurs in those cases in which an underlying disorder causes the splenic abnormalities. The causes of secondary hypersplenism are many and varied. Hypersplenism can occur secondary to compensatory (or workload) hypertrophy of this organ. Inflammatory and infectious diseases are thought to cause splenomegaly by an increase in the defensive functions of the spleen. For example, an increase in the clearing of particulate matter can lead to an increase in the number of macrophages, or hyperplasia of lymphoid cells can result from prolonged infection. Several blood disorders can cause splenomegaly. In these disorders, the blood cells can be intrinsically abnormal or coated with antibody and are removed from circulation in large numbers (e.g., hereditary spherocytosis, immune thrombocytopenic purpura).

Infiltration of the spleen with additional cells or metabolic byproducts can also cause hypersplenism. Such conditions include disorders in which the macrophages accumulate large quantities of undigestible substances; some of these disorders, such as Gaucher's disease, will be discussed later (∞ Chapter 19). Neoplasms in which the malignant cells occupy much of the splenic volume can cause splenomegaly. If the tumor cells incapacitate the spleen, the peripheral blood shows the evidence of hyposplenism (similar to the findings after splenectomy). An outstanding feature of myelofibrosis, a disorder in which the bone marrow is progressively replaced with fibrous tissue, is splenomegaly. In these cases, the spleen contains foci of extramedullary hematopoiesis. Congestive splenomegaly can occur following liver cirrhosis with portal hypertension or congestive heart failure when blood that does not flow easily through the liver is rerouted through the spleen.

 Checkpoint! 4

List three causes each of workload and infiltrative splenic hypertrophy.

Splenectomy

The effects of hypersplenism can be relieved by splenectomy; however, this procedure is not always advisable, especially when the spleen is performing a constructive role such as antibody production or filtering protozoa or bacteria. Splenectomy appears to be most beneficial in patients with hereditary or acquired conditions in which erythrocytes or platelets undergo increased destruction, such as hemolytic disorders or idiopathic thrombocytopenic purpura. The blood cells are still abnormal after splenectomy, but the major site of their destruction is removed. Consequently, the cells have a more normal life span. Splenectomy results in characteristic erythrocyte abnormalities easily noted on blood smears by experienced clinical laboratory professionals. After splenectomy, the erythrocytes often contain inclusions (e.g., Howell Jolly bodies, Pappenheimer bodies). Abnormal shapes may also be seen (∞ Chapter 8).

The lifespan of healthy erythrocytes is not increased after splenectomy. Other organs, primarily the liver assume the culling function. Blood flow through the liver also is slowed by passage through sinusoids, which are lined with specialized macrophages called *Kupffer cells*. These macrophages can perform functions similar to the phagocytes in the splenic cords and marginal zone. Even when a spleen is present, the liver, because of its larger blood flow, is responsible for removing most of the particulate matter of the blood. The liver, however, is not as effective as the spleen in filtering abnormal erythrocytes. This is probably because of the relatively rapid flow of blood past hepatic macrophages.

Acquired hyposplenism is a complication of sickle cell anemia. The acidic, hypoxic, hypoglycemic environment of the spleen leads to sickling of the erythrocytes in the spleen. This leads to blockage of the blood vessels and infarcts of the surrounding tissue. The tissue damage is progressive and leads to functional splenectomy (also referred to as *autosplenectomy*) (∞ Chapter 10).

CASE STUDY *(continued from page 55)*

Francine was diagnosed as having leukemia.

4. What do you think is the cause of the splenomegaly?
5. Why might the peripheral blood reveal changes associated with hyposplenism when the spleen is enlarged?

▶ LYMPH NODES

The lymphatic system is composed of lymph nodes and lymphatic vessels that drain into the left and right lymphatic ducts. The vessels, which originate in connective tissue spaces throughout the body, carry lymph toward the ducts near the neck where lymph enters the blood. Lymph is formed from blood fluid that escapes into connective tissue. The bean-shaped lymph nodes occur in groups or chains along the larger lymphatic vessels. Lymph nodes contain an outer area called the *cortex* and an inner area called the *medulla* (Figure 4-8 ■). Fibrous trabeculae extend inward from the capsule to form irregular communicating compartments within the parenchyma. The cortex contains B cell follicles surrounded by T lymphocytes and macrophages. Similar to the spleen, follicles contain areas of activated B cells known as *germinal centers*. A stimulated node can have many germinal centers whereas a resting node contains follicles with small resting lymphocytes and macrophages. The medulla, which surrounds the efferent lymphatics, consists of cords of plasma cells that lie between sinusoids.

Lymph nodes act as filters removing foreign particles from lymph by dendritic cells and macrophages. Dendritic cells in turn stimulate T and B cells. Stimulated B cells move from the germinal centers to the medulla where they reside as plasma cells and secrete antibody. Thus, lymph nodes provide immune defense against pathogens in virtually all tissues.

MUCOSA-ASSOCIATED LYMPHOID TISSUE (MALT)

MALT is a collection of loosely organized aggregates of lymphocytes found throughout the body in association with mucosal surfaces.[24] Its basic organization is similar to that of

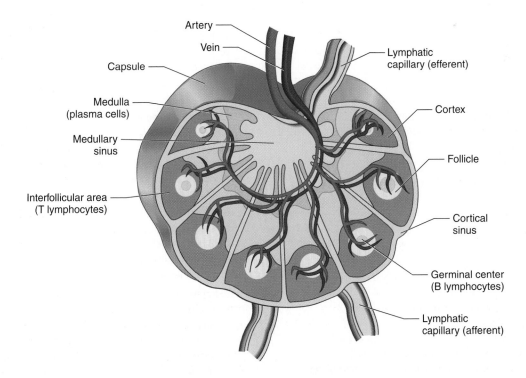

■ **FIGURE 4-8**   A schematic drawing of a lymph node. Note the location of T and B lymphocyte populations.

lymph nodes in that T- and B-cell-rich areas can be identified, but they are not as clearly demarcated as in lymph nodes. The medulla is not present as a separate structure, and no fibrous capsule can be identified. In the intestine, some of these aggregates are known as *Peyer's patches*. Tonsils and the appendix also are part of MALT. The function of MALT is to trap antigens that are crossing mucosal surfaces and initiate immune responses rapidly.

LYMPHADENOPATHY

Lymph nodes can become enlarged by expansion of the tissue within the node due to inflammation, prolonged immune response to infectious agents, or malignant transformation of lymphocytes or macrophages. Alternatively, lymph node enlargement can occur because of metastatic tumors that originate in extranodal sites.

 CASE STUDY *(continued from page 59)*

Francine had lymphadenopathy. The leukemia was diagnosed as a leukemia of the lymphocytic cells.

6. What might explain the lymphadenopathy?

SUMMARY

Hematopoiesis occurs in several different locations during human development. The major locations include the yolk sac, aorta-gonads-mesonephros (AGM) region, liver, bone marrow, and thymus. Further differentiation of lymphocytes also occurs in the spleen and lymph nodes. In the adult, the bone marrow is the location of the most primitive stem cells and thus is ultimately responsible for initiating all hematopoiesis. Myeloid cells, platelets, and erythrocytes essentially complete their differentiation in the bone marrow. T cells finish most of their differentiation in the thymus. B cells are able to respond to antigens by the time they leave the bone marrow but differentiate further into antibody-secreting plasma cells in the spleen and lymph nodes. The spleen removes senescent or abnormal erythrocytes and removes particulate matter from erythrocytes. Hypersplenism may occur and is most commonly secondary to another disorder. This leads to exaggeration of its normal activity. Lymph nodes are important in immune defense, initiating immune responses to foreign particles found in lymph.

REVIEW QUESTIONS

LEVEL I

1. B cells develop or differentiate in all of the following tissues *except*: (Objective 2)
   a. thymus
   b. bone marrow
   c. spleen
   d. lymph nodes

2. Lack of a spleen results in: (Objective 4)
   a. younger circulating erythrocytes
   b. granular inclusions in erythrocytes
   c. pitting of erythrocytes
   d. spherocytes

3. Peyer's patches are most closely related to the: (Objective 3)
   a. lymph node
   b. spleen
   c. thymus
   d. liver

4. All of the following are functions of bone marrow stroma *except* that it: (Objective 4)
   a. controls the volume of marrow available for hematopoiesis
   b. provides structural support for marrow elements
   c. secretes growth factors for hematopoiesis
   d. provides an exit route from marrow for mature blood cells

LEVEL II

1. A common site of adult extramedullary hematopoiesis is the: (Objective 3)
   a. liver
   b. thymus
   c. lymph node
   d. yolk sac

2. Which of the following is a criterion for a diagnosis of hypersplenism? (Objective 1)
   a. presence of a low WBC count in the blood
   b. low cell counts in the bone marrow
   c. circulating antibody-coated platelets
   d. splenic macrophages containing undigestible substances

3. Hypersplenism can result from increased: (Objective 1)
   a. splenic macrophages
   b. B cell proliferation
   c. abnormal erythrocytes
   d. all of the above

4. Extramedullary hematopoiesis in the adult is often accompanied by: (Objectives 1, 2, 3)
   a. splenomegaly
   b. liver atrophy
   c. leukocytosis
   d. hyposplenism

REVIEW QUESTIONS *(continued)*

LEVEL I

5. Which site of early hematopoiesis is extraembryonic? (Objective 1)
   a. yolk sac
   b. liver
   c. AGM
   d. spleen

LEVEL II

5. Hypersplenism associated with compensatory hypertrophy of the spleen can be found: (Objectives 1, 4)
   a. in neoplasms when malignant cells occupy much of the splenic space
   b. when there are intrinsically abnormal erythrocytes
   c. in liver cirrhosis with portal hypertension
   d. when splenic macrophages accumulate large amounts of undigestible substances

www.pearsonhighered.com/mckenzie

Use this address to access the interactive Companion Website created for this textbook. Find additional information, tables and figures. Evaluate your command of the chapter information using case studies and critical thinking and multiple choice questions.

REFERENCES

1. Palis J, Yoder MC. Yolk-sac hematopoiesis: The first blood cells of mouse and man. *Exp Hematol.* 2001;29:927–36.

2. Gordon S, Fraser I, Nath D, Hughes D, Clarke S. Macrophages in tissues and in vitro. *Curr Opin Immunol.* 1992;4:25–32.

3. Marcos MA, Godin I, Cumano A, Morales S, Garc a-Porrero JA, Dieterlen-Livre F et al. Developmental events from hemopoietic stem cells to B-cell populations and Ig repertoires. *Immunol Rev.* 1994; 137:155–71.

4. Pardanaud L, Luton D, Prigent M, Bourcheix LM, Catala M, Dieterlen-Livre F. Two distinct endothelial lineages in ontogeny, one of them related to hemopoiesis. *Development.* 1996;122:1363–71.

5. Farace MG, Brown BA, Raschella G, Alexander J, Gambari R, Fantoni A et al. The mouse beta h1 gene codes for the z chain of embryonic hemoglobin. *J Biol Chem.* 1984;259:7123–28.

6. Chang Y, Paige CJ, Wu GE. Enumeration and characterization of DJH structures in mouse fetal liver. *EMBO J.* 1992;11:1891–99.

7. Elliott JF, Rock EP, Patten PA, Davis MM, Chien YH. The adult T-cell receptor delta-chain is diverse and distinct from that of fetal thymocytes. *Nature.* 1988;331:627–31.

8. Iversen PO. Blood flow to the haemopoietic bone marrow. *Acta Physiol Scand.* 1997;159:269–76.

9. Mayani H, Guilbert LJ, Janowska-Wieczorek A. Biology of the hemopoietic microenvironment. *Eur J Haematol.* 1992;49:225–33.

10. Rickard DJ, Subramaniam M, Spelsberg TC. Molecular and cellular mechanisms of estrogen action on the skeleton. *J Cell Biochem.* 1999;Suppl 32–33:123–32.

11. Moriyama Y, Fisher JW. Effects of testosterone and erythropoietin on erythroid colony formation in human bone marrow cultures. *Blood.* 1975;45:665–70.

12. Dominici M, Pritchard C, Garlits JE Hofmann Tj, Persons DA, Horwitz EM. Hematopoietic cells and osteoblasts are derived from a common marrow progenitor after bone marrow transplantation. *Proc Natl Acad Sci USA.* 2004;101:11761–66.

13. Yin T, Li, L. The stem cell niches in bone. *J Clin Invest.* 2006; 116:1195–1201.

14. Sadahira Y, Mori M. Role of the macrophage in erythropoiesis. *Pathol Int.* 1999;49(10):841–48.

15. Lichtman MA, Chamberlain JK, Simon W, Santillo PA. Parasinusoidal location of megakaryocytes in marrow: A determinant of platelet release. *Am J Hematol.* 1978;4:303–12.

16. Lichtman MA, Packman CH, Costine LS. Molecular and cellular traffic across the marrow sinus wall. In: M. Tavassol, ed. *Blood cell formation: The role of the hematopoietic microenvironment.* Clifton, NJ: Humana Press; 1989.

17. Yong, K. Granulocyte colony-stimulating factor (G-CSF) increases neutrophil migration across vascular endothelium independent of an effect on adhesion: Comparison with granulocyte macrophage colony stimulating factor (GM-CSF). *Br J Haematol.* 1996;94:40–47.

18. Laurence ADJ. Location, movement and survival: The role of chemokines in haematopoiesis and malignancy. *Br J Haematol.* 2005;132:255–67.

19. Shortman K, Egerton M, Spangrude GJ, Scollay R. The generation and fate of thymocytes. *Semin Immunol.* 1990;2:3–12.

20. Zoller AL, Kersh GJ. Estrogen induces thymic atrophy by eliminating early thymic progenitors and inhibiting proliferation of beta-selected thymocytes. *J Immunol.* 2006;176:7371–78.

21. Garcia-Suarez O, Perez-Perez M, Germana A, Esteban I, Germana G. Involvement of growth factors in thymic involution. *Microsc Res Tech.* 2003;62:524–23.

22. Douek DC, Koup RA. Evidence for thymic function in the elderly. *Vaccine.* 2000;18(16):1638–41.

23. Kraal G. Cells in the marginal zone of the spleen. *Int Rev Cytol.* 1992;132:31–74.

24. MacDonald TT. The mucosal immune system. *Parasite Immunol.* 2003;25:235–46.

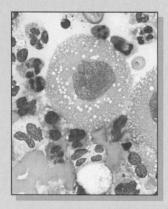

5

The Erythrocyte

Joel Hubbard, Ph.D.

CHAPTER OUTLINE

■ OBJECTIVES—LEVEL I

At the end of this unit of study, the student should be able to:

1. List and describe the stages of erythrocyte maturation in the marrow from youngest to most mature cells.
2. Explain the maturation process of reticulocytes and the cellular changes that take place.
3. Identify the normal range for reticulocytes.
4. Explain the function of erythropoietin; include the origin of production, bone marrow effects, and normal values.
5. Describe the function of the erythrocyte membrane.
6. Name the energy substrate of the erythrocyte.
7. Diagram the mechanism of extravascular erythrocyte destruction and hemoglobin catabolism.
8. Diagram the mechanism of intravascular erythrocyte destruction and hemoglobin catabolism.
9. State the average dimensions and life span of the normal erythrocyte.
10. Describe the function of 2,3-BPG and its relationship to the erythrocyte.

■ OBJECTIVES—LEVEL II

At the end of this unit of study, the student should be able to:

1. Summarize the mechanisms involved in the regulation of erythrocyte production.
2. Describe the structure of the erythrocyte membrane, including general dimensions and features; assess the function of the major membrane components.
3. Explain the mechanisms used by the erythrocyte to regulate permeability to cations, anions, glucose, and water.
4. Compare and contrast three pathways of erythrocyte metabolism and identify key intermediates as well as the relationship of each to erythrocyte survival and longevity.
5. Generalize the metabolic and catabolic changes within the erythrocyte that occur with time that "label" the erythrocyte for removal by the spleen.
6. Compare and contrast erythrocyte extravascular destruction with intravascular destruction and identify which process is dominant given laboratory results.
7. Predict the effects of increased and decreased erythropoietin levels in the blood.

KEY TERMS

- Acanthocytes
- BFU-E
- Bilirubin
- CFU-E
- Cyanosis
- Erythroblasts
- Erythron
- Erythropoiesis
- Erythropoietin
- Glycolysis
- Haptoglobin
- Heinz bodies
- Hemopexin
- Hemosiderin
- Hemosiderinuria
- Hypoxic
- Integral proteins
- Normoblast
- Peripheral proteins
- Polychromatophilic erythrocyte
- Reticulocyte
- Spectrin

BACKGROUND BASICS

The information in this chapter builds on the concepts learned in previous chapters. To maximize your learning experience, you should review these concepts before starting this unit of study.

Level I

- ▶ Describe the process of cell differentiation and maturation, regulation, and the function of growth factors; describe cell organelles and their function (Chapter 2 and 3).
- ▶ Give the functional description of the erythroid marrow (Chapter 4).

Level II

- ▶ List and describe the function of specific growth factors important in erythrocyte development (Chapter 3).
- ▶ Describe the structure and function of the spleen and bone marrow (Chapter 4).

CASE STUDY

We will address this case study throughout the chapter.

Stephen, a 28-year-old Caucasian male of Italian descent, became progressively ill following a safari vacation to West Africa. The patient arrived at the ER for evaluation following several days of fever, chills, and malaise. The advent of hemoglobinuria prompted the patient to seek emergency aid. A clinical history and physical examination supported a diagnosis of anemia. Because Stephen had recently returned from a malarial endemic area, the physician first suspected malaria although the patient had been on primaquine preventive drug therapy while traveling abroad. Blood smears examined for malaria, however, resulted in a negative diagnosis. Consider additional laboratory tests that could help identify the cause of Stephen's anemia.

▶ OVERVIEW

This chapter is a study of the erythrocyte. It begins with a description of erythrocyte production and maturation. This is followed by an account of the erythrocyte membrane composition and function, cell metabolism, and kinetics of cell production. The chapter concludes with a description of the destruction of the senescent cell.

▶ INTRODUCTION

The erythrocyte (red blood cell, RBC) was one of the first microscopic elements recognized and described after the discovery of the microscope. For centuries, these corpuscles were considered inert particles with no function. In 1817, Francois Magendie diluted blood with water, found no microscopic corpuscles, and erroneously surmised that the red blood cells seen by others were probably air bubbles.[1] We now know that erythrocytes suspended in water will burst, which explains Magendie's negative findings. Magendie eventually recognized his mistake and later provided a morphologic description of the erythrocyte. Not until 1865, however, when Felix Hoppe-Seyler discovered the oxygen-carrying capacity of the red pigment (hemoglobin) within the red blood cells, did the function of these "globules" begin to be understood. Today, we recognize the erythrocyte as being one of the most highly specialized cells in the body.

▶ ERYTHROPOIESIS AND RED BLOOD CELL MATURATION

Erythron refers to the totality of all stages of erythrocytes, including precursor cells in the marrow and mature cells in the peripheral blood and within vascular areas of specific organs such as the spleen. **Erythropoiesis,** or the production of erythrocytes, is normally an orderly process through which the peripheral concentration of erythrocytes is maintained at a steady state. The life cycle of erythrocytes includes stimulation of lineage commitment and maturation of precursor cells in the marrow by **erythropoietin;** a circulating life span for mature cells of approximately 120 days +/- 10 days, and the destruction of senescent cells by mononuclear cells in the liver, spleen, and bone marrow.

ERYTHROID PROGENITOR CELLS

Red cell production begins with the hematopoietic stem cell (HSC) (∞ Chapter 3). Stem cell differentiation is induced by certain microenvironmental influences to produce a committed erythroid progenitor cell. The committed (unipotential) erythroid progenitor cell compartment consists of two populations of cells, neither identifiable microscopically but defined by their behavior in cell culture systems: the burst-forming unit-erythroid **(BFU-E)** and colony-forming unit-erythroid **(CFU-E).**[2] The

BFU-E progenitor cells proliferate under the influence of what was originally called "burst-promoting activity" (BPA), now known to be IL-3 or GM-CSF, released by local microenvironmental stromal cells. BFU-Es have a low concentration of erythropoietin (EPO) receptors and thus are relatively insensitive to EPO except in high concentrations. The BFU-Es are defined as progenitor cells that give rise to a "burst" or multifocal colony of cells in an in vitro colony assay in 10 to 14 days. The colony consists of several hundred to several thousand cells recognizable as hemoglobin-containing RBC precursors. Maturation of the BFU-E gives rise to the CFU-E progenitor cell. An individual CFU-E, which undergoes only a few cell divisions, gives rise to a single, discrete colony of 8 to 60 identifiable cells after 2–5 days of culture.[2] CFU-Es have a high concentration of EPO membrane receptors; hence, they respond to lower EPO concentrations than do BFU-Es. The CFU-E is the immediate precursor of the earliest morphologically recognizable erythroid precursor, the pronormoblast. The graph below shows the relationship of the various hematopoietic progenitor cells to the cytokines that affect their maturation.

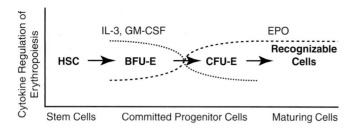

BFU-Es are CD34$^+$ and have a high proliferative potential but a low rate of cycling. As they mature to the CFU-E stage, they lose CD34$^+$ expression but begin to express surface proteins characteristic of the erythroid lineage including gly-

cophorin A, Rh antigens, and in a subset of CFU-E, the ABH and Ii antigens.[2]

Additional cytokines shown to have a positive effect on erythrocyte precursor proliferation include stem cell factor (SCF), thrombopoietin, and IL-11 while tumor necrosis factor-α, transforming growth factor-β, and interferon-γ have a negative effect on erythropoiesis.

ERYTHROID-MATURING CELLS

Erythroid-maturing cells include those precursor cells in the bone marrow that are morphologically identifiable. Nucleated erythrocyte precursors in the bone marrow are collectively called **erythroblasts.** If the maturation sequence is "normal," the cells are often called **normoblasts.** Young erythrocytes with residual RNA but without a nucleus are referred to as **reticulocytes** (polychromatophilic erythrocytes). Bone marrow normoblast maturation occurs in an orderly and well-defined sequence under normal conditions encompassing six morphologically defined stages. The process involves a gradual decrease in cell size together with progressive condensation of the nuclear chromatin and eventual expulsion of the pyknotic nucleus. The cytoplasm in the younger normoblasts stains deeply basophilic due to the predominance of RNA (Figure 5-1 ■). As the cell matures, there is an increase in hemoglobin production, which is acidophilic, and the cytoplasm takes on a gray to pink or salmon color (Figures 5-1 and 5-2■). Two terminology systems are used to describe erythrocyte precursors. One uses the word *normoblast* and the other *rubriblast.* This text uses the normoblast terminology. The stages in order from most immature to mature cell are pronormoblast (rubriblast), basophilic normoblast (prorubricyte), polychromatophilic normoblast (rubricyte), orthochromatic normoblast (metarubricyte), reticulocyte, and erythrocyte (Table 5-1 ✪).

■ FIGURE 5-1   Pronormoblast in the center. Note the large N:C ratio, presence of nucleoli, and lacy chromatin. The cytoplasm is deep blue with a lighter pinkish area next to the nucleus. Also note above at about one o'clock the polychromatophilic normoblast (arrow). (Bone marrow; Wright-Giemsa stain, 1000× magnification)

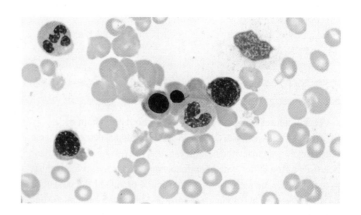

■ FIGURE 5-2   Developing normoblasts. At nine o'clock there is an early polychromatophilic normoblast; in the center from left to right are an early orthochromic normoblast, late orthochromic normoblast, band neutrophil, and a basophilic normoblast. (Bone marrow; Wright-Giemsa stain, 1000× magnification)

✪ TABLE 5-1

Morphologic Characteristics of Erythroid Precursors

Cell Type (% of nucleated cells in BM)	Image (Wright stain)	Size	N/C Ratio	Cytoplasmic Characteristics	Nuclear Characteristics
Pronormoblast (rubriblast) (1%)		20–25 μm	High (8:1)	Small to moderate amount of deep blue cytoplasm; pale area next to nucleus might be seen	1–3 faint nucleoli; reddish purple color; homogeneous, lacy chromatin
Basophilic normoblast (prorubricyte) (1–3%)		16–18 μm	Moderate (6:1)	Deep blue-purple color; occasionally small patches of pink; irregular cell borders may be present; perinuclear halo might be apparent	Indistinct nucleoli; coarsening chromatin; deep purplish-blue color
Polychromatophilic normoblast (rubricyte) (13–30%)		12–15 μm	Low (4:1)	Abundant; gray-blue color	Chromatin irregular and coarsely clumped, eccentric
Orthochromic normoblast (metarubricyte) (1–4%)		10–15 μm	Low (1:2)	Pink-salmon color; may have varying degrees of basophilia	Small; dense; pyknotic; round or bizarre shape; eccentric
Reticulocyte (new methylene blue stain)		7–10 μm	—	Punctuate purplish-blue inclusions	No nucleus
(Wright's stain)				Polychromatophilic (diffusely basophilic)	
Mature RBC		7–8 μm	—	Salmon color	No nucleus

The normoblasts generally spend from 5 to 7 days in the proliferating and maturing compartment of the bone marrow. After reaching the reticulocyte stage, there is an additional 2–3 days of maturation, the first 1–2 days of which are spent in the marrow before the cell is released to the peripheral blood. The mature circulating erthrocyte has a life span of 100–120 days. This lengthy life span accounts for the relatively small number of erythroid precursors in the marrow in comparison to the large circulating erythrocyte mass.

Erythropoietin (EPO) is the only cytokine important in regulating the final stages of erythroid maturation (the maturing cells). A number of hormones are known to have some erythropoietic effect, however. The most notable is the erythropoietic effect of androgens, which was exploited for the treatment of various anemias before the development of recombinant EPO. Androgens appear to both stimulate EPO secretion and directly affect the erythropoietic marrow, which partially explains the difference in hemoglobin concentrations according to sex and age. Other hormones, which have varying (although minor) effects on erythropoiesis, include thyroid hormones, adrenal cortical hormones, and growth hormone.[3] Anemic patients with hypopituitarism, hypothyroidism, and adrenocortical insufficiency show an increase in erythrocyte concentration when the appropriate deficient hormone is administered. The reduction of EPO in hypothyroidism may partially be the result of the reduced demand for cellular oxygen by metabolically hypoactive tissue.

 Checkpoint! 1

What is meant by the term erythron?

CHARACTERISTICS OF CELL MATURATION

Although the stages of erythrocyte maturation are usually described in steplike fashion, the actual maturation is a gradual and continuous process (Table 5-1). Some normoblasts may not conform to all criteria for a particular stage, and a judgment must be made when identifying those cells. The more experience one has in examining the blood and bone marrow, the easier it becomes to make these judgments.

Pronormoblast

This is the earliest morphologically recognizable erythrocyte precursor. Each pronormoblast produces between 8 and 32 mature erythrocytes (a total of 3 to 5 cell divisions during the maturation sequence). The cell is the largest of the normoblast series, from 20–25 μm in diameter with a high nuclear:cytoplasmic (N:C) ratio. The nucleus occupies 80% or more of the cell. This cell is rather rare in the bone marrow.

Cytoplasm The cytoplasm contains a large number of ribosomes and stains deeply basophilic. A pale area next to the nucleus is sometimes apparent. This represents the Golgi apparatus, which does not take up the dyes of the Romanowsky stain. Small amounts of hemoglobin are present but are not visible by light microscopy.

Nucleus The nucleus is large, taking up most of the cell volume, and stains bluish-purple. The chromatin is in a fine linear network often described as lacy. The pronormoblast chromatin has a coarser appearance and stains darker than the chromatin of a white cell blast. The nucleus contains from 1 to 3 faint nucleoli.

Basophilic Normoblast

This cell is similar to the pronormoblast except that it is usually smaller (16–18 μm in diameter) and has a slightly decreased N:C ratio. The nucleus occupies approximately three-fourths of the cell volume. Because these cells are actively dividing, it is posible to find a basophilic normoblast (in G2, prior to mitosis) that is larger than the pronormoblast (in G1).

Cytoplasm The cytoplasm is still deeply basophilic, often more so than that of the previous stage due to the increased number of ribosomes. However, in late basophilic normoblasts, the presence of varying amounts of hemoglobin can cause the cell to take on a lighter blue hue or show scattered pink areas. A pale area surrounding the nucleus, the perinuclear halo, is sometimes seen. This halo corresponds to the mitochondria, which also do not stain with Romanowsky stains.

Nucleus The chromatin is coarser than that of the pronormoblast. The dark violet heterochromatin interspersed with the lighter-staining euchromatin can give the chromatin a wheel-spoke appearance. A few small masses of clumped chromatin may be seen along the rim of the nuclear membrane. Nucleoli usually are not apparant.

Polychromatophilic Normoblast

The cell is about 12–15 μm in diameter with a decreased N:C ratio due to continued condensation of the nuclear chromatin. This is the last stage capable of mitosis.

Cytoplasm The most characteristic change in the cell at this stage is the presence of abundant gray-blue cytoplasm. The staining properties of the cytoplasm are due to the synthesis of large amounts of hemoglobin and decreasing numbers of ribosomes. The cell derives its name, polychromatophilic, from this characteristic cytoplasmic feature.

Nucleus The nuclear chromatin is irregular and coarsely clumped due to increased aggregation of nuclear heterochromatin.

Orthochromic Normoblast

This cell is about 10–15 µm in diameter with a low N:C ratio.

Cytoplasm   After the final mitotic division of the erythropoietic precursors, the concentration of hemoglobin increases within the erythroblast. The cytoplasm is predominantly pink or salmon color but retains a tinge of blue due to residual ribosomes.

Nucleus   The nuclear chromatin is heavily condensed. In late stages, the nucleus is structureless (pyknotic) or fragmented. The nucleus is often eccentric or even partially extruded. Using phase-contrast microscopy, these cells demonstrate motility with protraction and retraction of cytoplasmic projections.[4] These movements are in preparation for ejection of the nucleus, which usually occurs while the erythroblast is still part of the erythroblastic island (see below). Alternatively, the nucleus may be lost as the cell passes through the wall of a marrow sinus. The expelled nucleus is engulfed by a marrow macrophage.

Reticulocyte

After the nucleus is extruded, the cell is known as a *reticulocyte.* When the nucleus is first extruded, the cell has an irregular lobulated or puckered shape. The cell is remodeled, eliminating excess membrane and gradually acquiring its final biconcave shape while it completes its maturation program. The reticulocyte matures over a span of 2–3 days, the first half of which is spent in the bone marrow and the latter half in the circulating blood.

The reticulocyte has residual RNA and mitochondria in the cytoplasm, which give the young cell a bluish tinge with Romanowsky stains; thus, the cell is appropriately described as a diffusely basophilic erythrocyte or **polychromatophilic erythrocyte.** About 80% of the cell's hemoglobin is made during the normoblast stages with the remaining 20% made during the reticulocyte stage. The reticulocyte is slightly larger, 7–10 µm, than a mature erythrocyte. After 1 1/2 to 2 days in the bone marrow, the reticulocyte is released into the vascular sinuses of the marrow. From there, it gains access to the peripheral blood. Reticulocyte maturation continues in the peripheral blood for another day or two. These cells can be identified in vitro by reaction with supravital stains, new methylene blue N, or brilliant cresyl blue, which cause precipitation of the RNA and mitochondria. This supravital staining method identifies the reticulocytes by the presence of punctate purplish blue inclusions (∞ Chapter 34). Normally, reticulocytes compose 0.5–2.5% (absolute concentration 18–158 × 10^9/L) of peripheral blood erythrocytes in a nonanemic adult. The actual reference interval varies among laboratories. The absolute concentration of reticulocytes is calculated by multiplying the percent of reticulocytes by the RBC count. When reticulocytes are increased, an increased number of polychromatophilic erythrocytes (polychromasia) may be seen on the Romanowsky-stained peripheral blood smear.

Reticulocytes may contain small amounts of iron dispersed throughout the cytoplasm, which can be identified with Perl's Prussian blue stain. Erythrocytes with identified iron are called *siderocytes.* Nucleated RBC precursors that stain with Prussian blue are called *sideroblasts.* The spleen is responsible for removal of these iron-containing granules and the normal mature circulating cell is devoid of granular inclusions.

 Checkpoint! 2

What is the first stage of red cell maturation that has visible cytoplasmic evidence of hemoglobin production on a Romanowsky-stained smear?

 CASE STUDY *(continued from 63)*

In addition to malaria screening, the ER physician also ordered a CBC with the following results:

		Differential	
WBC	14 × 10^9/L		
RBC	3.10 × 10^{12}/L	Segs	70%
HGB	9.2 gm/dL	Bands	11%
HCT	28%	Metas	2%
MCV	93 fL	Lymphs	13%
MCH	30.6 pg/dL	Monos	2%
MCHC	32.5 gm/dL	Eos	2%
PLT	230 × 10^9/L	NRBCs/100 WBCs	18
		RBC Morphology	
		Anisocytosis	3+
		Poikilocytosis	2+
		Spherocytosis	1+
		Schistocytes	1+
		Polychromasia	2+

1. Predict Stephen's reticulocyte count: low, normal, or increased.

Erythrocyte

The mature erythrocyte is a biconcave disc about 7–8 µm in diameter and 80–100 fL in volume. It stains pink to orange because of its content of the intracellular acidophilic protein, hemoglobin (28–34 pg/cell). The cell has lost its residual RNA and mitochondria as well as important enzymes; therefore, it is incapable of synthesizing new protein or lipid.

ERYTHROBLASTIC ISLANDS

Erythropoiesis occurs in distinctive histologic configurations called *erythroblastic islands* (EI) that consist of concentric circles of developing erythroblasts clustered around a central macrophage. The central macrophage sends out slender cytoplasmic processes that maintain direct contact with each erythroblast. Erythroblasts adhere to the central macrophage by a variety of cytoadhesion molecules including fibronectin (Fn) and thrombospondin (Tsp). As the erythroblast matures, it moves along a cytoplasmic extension of the macrophage. As the cell becomes sufficiently mature for nuclear expulsion, cytoadhesion molecule receptors (FnR, Tsp-R, and others) are no longer expressed on the cell membrane. As a result, the cell detaches from the EI, passes through a pore in the cytoplasm of endothelial cells lining the marrow sinuses, and enters the circulation.[4] The central macrophage phagocytizes the nucleus, which is extruded from the orthochromatic erythroblasts before the cell leaves the bone marrow. Any defective erythroblasts produced during the process of erythropoiesis ("ineffective erythropoiesis") also are phagocytized by the macrophage.

Surrounding the EI are fibroblasts, macrophages, and endothelial cells, which provide the optimal microenvironment for terminal erythroid maturation. The EI is a fragile structure and is usually disrupted by the process of marrow aspiration. However, maturing erythroblasts with adherent macrophage cytoplasmic fragments may be seen on marrow aspirate smears. Intact erythroblastic islands can occasionally be seen in marrow core biopsies.[4]

► ERYTHROCYTE MEMBRANE

Around the beginning of the twentieth century, investigations began that established the complexity of the erythrocyte membrane. Steven Hedin performed experiments that demonstrated the osmotic properties and selective permeability of the erythrocyte.[5] He found that erythrocyte volume increased in hypotonic solutions (these having a lower osmotic pressure than the erythrocyte) and solutions such as urea or glycerol. Other solutions, however, caused the cell to shrink. Antigenic properties of the membrane were recognized several years later by Karl Landsteiner, who observed that human sera caused clumping of the erythrocytes in different individuals. He originally divided these individuals into three groups, A, B, and C, according to their erythrocyte agglutination patterns with human sera.[6] Today we identify these blood types as groups A, B, and O. Hundreds of other erythrocyte antigens have since been identified.

The red cell membrane is essential for erythrocyte development and function. Developing erythroblasts have membrane receptors for EPO and transferrin (iron), which are required during erythropoiesis. The erythrocyte membrane selectively sequesters vital components (e.g., organic phosphates such as 2,3-BPG) and lets metabolic waste products (lactate, pyruvate) escape. The membrane helps regulate metabolism by reversibly binding and inactivating many glycolytic enzymes. It carefully balances exchange of bicarbonate and chloride ions, which aid in the transfer of carbon dioxide from tissues to lungs and balance cation and water concentrations to maintain erythrocyte ionic composition.

Finally, in association with the "membrane skeleton," the erythrocyte membrane provides the red cell with the dual characteristics of strength and flexibility needed to survive its 120-day life span in the circulation.

MEMBRANE COMPOSITION

The erythrocyte membrane is a phospholipid bilayer-protein complex composed of ~52% protein, 40% lipid, and 8% carbohydrate (Table 5-2).[7] The chemical structure and composition control the membrane functions (e.g., transport, durability/strength, flexibility) and determine the membrane's antigenic properties. Any defect in structure or alteration in chemical composition can alter erythrocyte membrane functions and lead to the cell's premature death (∞ Chapter 15). Mature erythrocytes lack the cellular organelles (nucleus, ribosomes, and mitochondria) and enzymes necessary to synthesize new lipid and protein. Thus, extensive damage to the membrane cannot be repaired, and the damaged cell will be culled from the circulation by the spleen.

✓ Checkpoint! 3

How would an increase in RBC membrane permeability affect intracellular sodium balance?

✪ TABLE 5-2

Erythrocyte Membrane Composition

Lipids and glycolipids (~45%)	Unesterified cholesterol
	Phospholipids
	Phosphatidylionsitol/PI
	Phosphatidylethanolamine/PE
	Phosphatidylserine/PS
	Phosphatidylcholine/PC (lecithin)
	Sphingomyelin/SM
	Lysophospholipids (Lysophosphatidylcholine/LPC, Lysophosphatidylethanolamine/LPE)
	Glycolipids
Proteins and glycoproteins (~55%)	Integral proteins
	Glycophorins A, B, C, D, E (carry antigens on exterior of membrane)
	Band 3 (attaches skeletal lattice to membrane lipid bilayer; anion exchange channel)
	Peripheral proteins (form membrane skeletal lattice and attach it to membrane)
	Spectrin (α and β polypeptides)
	Actin (band 5)
	Ankyrin (band 2.1)
	Band 4.2
	Band 4.1
	Adducin (band 2.9)
	Band 4.9 (dematin)
	Tropomyosin (band 7)
	Tropomodulin (band 5)

Lipid Composition

Approximately 95% of the lipid content of the membrane consists of equal amounts of unesterified cholesterol and phospholipids. The remaining lipids are free fatty acids (FA) and glycolipids (e.g., globoside). Mature erythrocytes are unable to synthesize fatty acids, phospholipids, or cholesterol. Consequently, they depend on lipid exchange with the plasma and fatty acid acylation for phospholipid repair and renewal during their 120-day lifespan.

The overall structure of the membrane is that of a phospholipid bilayer with the phospholipid molecules arranged with polar heads exposed at each membrane surface and their hydrophobic fatty acid sidechains directed to the interior of the bilayer. The major phospholipids are phosphatidylcholine (PC), phosphatidylethanolamine (PE), phosphatidylserine (PS), and sphingomyelin (SM). Small amounts of phosphatidylinositol (PI), phosphatidic acid (PA), and lysophospholipids are also present.[8] The phospholipids are asymmetrically distributed within the membrane bilayer. The choline phospholipids (PC, SM) are concentrated in the outer half of the bilayer, and the amino phospholipids (PE, PS, PI) are largely confined to the inner half. Although there is transmembrane diffusion of the phospholipids from areas of higher concentration to the bilayer leaflet of lower concentration, the asymmetry is maintained by an ATP-dependent transport system, the aminophospholipid translocase (also nicknamed "flippase").[9] Considerable evidence that the mobility of phospholipids within the membrane contributes to membrane fluidity exists. Exchange between phospholipids of the membrane and plasma can occur, especially with the phospholipids of the outer bilayer leaflet.

Cholesterol and glycolipids are intercalated between the phospholipids in the membrane bilayer.[8] Cholesterol is present in approximately equal proportions on both sides of the lipid bilayer. Cholesterol affects the surface area of the cell and membrane permeability. Membrane cholesterol exists in free equilibrium with unesterified cholesterol of plasma lipoproteins. Once in the plasma, cholesterol is partially converted to esterified cholesterol by the action of lecithin-cholesterol acyl transferase (LCAT). Once esterified, cholesterol cannot return to the red cell membrane; thus, LCAT catalyzes a unidirection pathway of cholesterol transfer that tends to deplete the red cell membrane of cholesterol. It is not surprising that when LCAT is absent (congenital LCAT deficiency or hepatocellular disease), free plasma cholesterol increases, resulting in accumulation of cholesterol within erythrocyte membranes, and RBC membrane surface area expands. An excess of cell membrane due to proportional increases in cholesterol and phospholipids, maintaining the normal ratio, results in the formation of macrocodocytes (large target cells). An increase in the cholesterol-to-phospholipid ratio, however, increases the membrane's microviscosity (decreased fluidity). An increase in membrane lipids due to a disproportionate increase in cholesterol results in

the formation of **acanthocytes** (∞ Chapter 8), which have reduced survival as compared to normal RBCs.

The shape of the red cell can also be altered by expansions of the separate lipid bilayers relative to each other. Processes that expand the bilayer's outer leaflet (or contract the inner) result in the formation of membrane spicules, producing echinocytes (see Figure 5-3 ■). Conversely, expansion of the inner leaflet of the bilayer leads to invagination of the membrane and the formation of stomatocytes (cup-shaped cells) (Figure 5-3).

Reticulocytes normally contain more membrane lipid and cholesterol than do older erythrocytes. This excess lipid material is removed from the reticulocytes during the final stages of maturation in the circulation by the spleenic macrophages. Splenectomized patients can have cells with an abnormal accumulation of cholesterol and/or other lipids in the membrane, which will present as target cells, acanthocytes, and/or echinocytes on the blood smear. (Alterations of red cell shape are described in ∞ Chapter 8.)

A small portion of membrane lipids consists of glycolipids in the form of glycosphingolipid. Red cell glycolipids are located entirely in the external half of the lipid bilayer with their carbohydrate portions extending into the plasma. Glycolipids are responsible for some important antigenic properties of the red cell membrane; they carry the ABH, Lewis, and P blood group antigens.

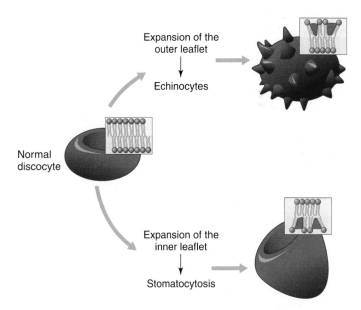

■ FIGURE 5-3 Model of discocyte-echinocyte and discocyte-stomatocyte transformation. RBC shape is determined by the ratio of the surface areas of the two hemileaflets of the lipid bilayer. Preferential accumulation of compounds in the outer leaflet of the lipid bilayer cause expansion and results in RBC crenation and echinocytosis; expansion of the inner leaflet of the bilayer results in stomatocytosis. (Palek J, Jarolim P. Clinical expression and laboratory detection of red cell membrane protein mutations. *Semin Hematol.* 1993;30:249–83, with permission).

Checkpoint! 4

Compare and contrast the placement of lipids in the erythrocyte membrane and their functions.

Protein Composition

Erythrocyte membrane proteins are of two types: integral and peripheral (Figure 5-4 ■). Integral proteins penetrate or traverse the lipid bilayer and interact with the hydrophobic lipid core of the membrane. In contrast, peripheral proteins do not penetrate into the lipid bilayer but interact with integral proteins or lipids at the membrane surface. In the red cell, the major peripheral proteins are on the cytoplasmic side of the membrane attached to membrane lipids or integral proteins by ionic and hydrogen bonds. Both types of membrane proteins are synthesized during erythroblast development. The proteins of the red cell have been studied by first lysing the cell by hypotonic hemolysis, extracting the proteins, and analyzing them by polyacrylamide gel electrophoresis in sodium dodecyl sulfate (SDS-PAGE). The proteins, separated according to molecular weight, were initially identified by number according to their migration during electrophoresis with the larger proteins (which migrated the shortest distance) beginning the numbering sequence.

Integral proteins include transport proteins and the glycophorins. The three major glycophorins—A, B, and C (GPA, GPB, GPC)—are made up of three domains: the cytoplasmic domain, the hydrophobic domain, which spans the bilayer,

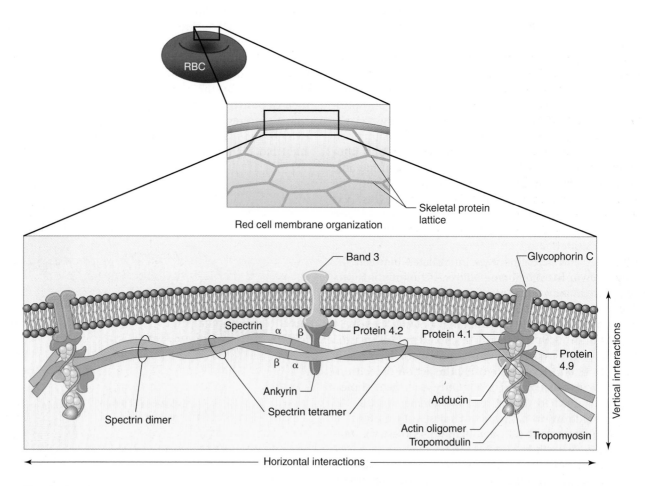

■ FIGURE 5-4   Model of the organization of the erythrocyte membrane showing the peripheral and integral proteins and lipids. Spectrin is the predominant protein of the skeletal protein lattice. Spectrin dimers join head to head to form spectrin tetramers. At the tail end, spectrin tetramers come together at the junctional complex. This complex is composed of actin oligomer and stabilized by tropomyosin, which sits in the groove of the actin filaments. The actin oligomer is capped on one end by tropomodulin and on the other by adducin. Band 4.9 protein (dematin) binds to actin and bundles actin filaments. Spectrin is attached to actin by protein 4.1, which also attaches the skeletal lattice to the lipid membrane via its interaction with glycophorin C (minor attachment site). Ankyrin links the skeletal protein network to the inner side of the lipid bilayer via band 3. Protein 4.2 interacts with ankyrin and band 3 (major attachment site).

and the extracellular domain on the exterior surface of the membrane.[7] The extracellular domain is heavily glycosylated and is responsible for most of the negative surface charge (zeta potential) that keeps red cells from sticking to each other and to the vessel wall. They also carry various red cell antigens. Genetic polymorphisms at the GPA locus are responsible for the MN blood group antigens; GPB carries the S, s, and U antigens, and GPC carries the Gerbich antigens.[8] Glycophorin C also plays a role in attaching the skeletal protein network located on the cytoplasmic side of the membrane to the bilipid layer. The glycophorins are synthesized early in erythroid differentiation (GPC is found in BFU-E) and thus serve as lineage-specific markers for erythrocytic differentiation.

Band 3, also known as the *anion exchange protein 1* (AE1), is the major integral protein of the red cell with more than 1 million copies per cell. Band 3/AE1 is the transport channel for the chloride-bicarbonate exchange, which occurs during the transport of CO_2 from the tissues back to the lungs (∞ Chapter 6). Like most transport channels, Band 3 spans the membrane multiple times (12–14). Anion exchange is thought to occur by a "ping-pong" mechanism. An intracellular anion enters the transport channel and is translocated outward and released. The channel remains in the outward conformation until an extracellular anion enters and triggers the reverse cycle.[8]

In addition to its role as an anion exchanger, band 3 is a major binding site for a variety of enzymes and cytoplasmic membrane components.[8] The N-terminal, cytoplasmic domain of band 3, binds glycolytic enzymes, regulating their activity and serving as a regulator of red cell glycolysis. Band 3 also binds hemoglobin at its cytoplasmic domain with intact hemoglobin binding weakly but partially denatured hemoglobin (Heinz bodies) binding more avidly. Binding of hemoglobin to band 3 is thought to play a role in erythrocyte senescence. Band 3 is also important in attaching the skeletal protein network to the lipid bilayer by binding to the skeletal proteins ankyrin and band 4.2. The Ii blood group antigens are carried on the carbohydrate component of the red cell band 3 protein.[10,11]

The red cell membrane contains more than 100 additional integral proteins.[8] These include all of the various transporter proteins (glucose transporter, urea transporter, Na^+/K^+-ATPase, Ca^{2+}-ATPase, Mg^{2+}-ATPase), the Rh protein, the Kell antigen protein, various receptors (transferrin, insulin, insulinlike growth factor, etc.) and decay-accelerating factor (DAF; ∞ Chapter 15).

Peripheral proteins are found primarily on the cytoplasmic face of the erythrocyte membrane and include enzymes and structural proteins. The structural proteins are organized into a two-dimensional lattice network directly laminating the inner side of the membrane lipid bilayer called the *red cell membrane skeleton*.[12] The horizontal interactions of this lattice are parallel to the plane of the membrane and serve as a skeletal support for the membrane lipid layer. The vertical interactions of the lattice are perpendicular to the

plane of the membrane and serve to attach the skeletal lattice network to the lipid layer of the membrane. The skeletal proteins give red cell membranes their viscoelastic properties and contribute to cell shape, deformability, and membrane stability. The red cell skeleton proteins include spectrin, actin, ankyrin (band 2.1), band 4.2, band 4.1, adducin, band 4.9 (dematin), tropomyosin, and tropomodulin. Defects in this erythrocyte cytoskeleton are associated with abnormal cell shape, decreased stability, and hemolytic anemia (∞ Chapter 15).

Spectrin, the predominant skeletal protein, exists as a heterodimer of two large chains (α and β). The two chains associate in a side-by-side, antiparallel arrangement (N-terminal of α chain associated with C-terminal of β chain). The $\alpha\beta$ heterodimers form a slender, twisted, highly flexible molecule ~100 nm in length. Spectrin heterodimers in turn self-associate head to head to form tetramers and some larger oligomers.[8] Spectrin is described as functioning as a kind of spring. In the red cell, spectrin tetramers (which would have an extended length of ~200 nm) are tightly coiled in vivo with an end-to-end distance of only ~76 nm.[13] These coiled tetramers can extend reversibly when the membrane is stretched but cannot exceed their maximum extended length (200 nm) without rupturing.

Ankyrin is a large protein that serves as the high-affinity binding site for the attachment of spectrin to the inner membrane surface. It binds spectrin near the region involved in dimer-tetramer associations. In turn, ankyrin is bound with high affinity to the cytoplasmic portion of band 3 (the actual anchor for the membrane skeleton).[14] *Band 4.2* binds to ankyrin and band 3, strengthening their interaction and helping to bind the skeleton to the lipid bilayer at its major attachment point.[15]

Red cell *actin* is functionally similar to actin in other cells. However, unlike its organization in muscle cells, red cell actin is organized into short, double-helical protofilaments of 12–14 actin monomers. These short filaments are stabilized by their interactions with other proteins of the red cell skeleton including *tropomodulin, adducin, tropomyosin,* and *band 4.9.* Spectrin dimers bind to actin filaments near the tail end of the spectrin dimer. *Protein 4.1* interacts with spectrin and actin and with GPC in the overlying lipid bilayer. It serves to stabilize the otherwise weak interaction between spectrin and actin and is necessary for normal membrane stability.[8] This complex of spectrin, actin, tropomodulin, tropomyosin, adducin, band 4.9, and band 4.1 serves as the secondary attachment point for the red cell skeleton, binding to GPC of the membrane.

The skeletal proteins are not static but are in a continuous disassociation–association equilibrium with each other (e.g., spectrin dimer-tetramer interconversions) and with their attachment sites. This equilibrium occurs in response to various physical and chemical stimuli that affect the erythrocytes as they journey throughout the body. Calcium also influences the red cell cytoskeleton. Most intracellular calcium (80%) is found in association with the erythrocyte membrane. Calcium is normally maintained at a low intracellular concentration by the activity of an ATP-fueled Ca^{2+} pump (Ca^{2+}-ATPase). Elevated Ca^{2+} levels induce membrane protein cross-linking.[16] This cross-linking essentially acts as a fixative, stabilizing red cell shape and reducing the cell's deformability. The abnormal erythrocyte shape of irreversibly sickled cells (∞ Chapter 10) can be produced by calcium-induced irreversible cross-linking and alteration of the cyoskeletal proteins.

The erythrocyte membrane together with the membrane skeleton is responsible for the dual cellular characteristics of structural integrity as well as deformability. The 7 μm erythrocyte must be sufficiently flexible to squeeze through the tiny capillary openings, particularly in the splenic vasculature (~3 μm); this requires significant deformations of the cell. At the same time, cells must be able to withstand the rigors of the turbulent circulation as they travel throughout the body for 120 days. Deformability of the red cell is due to three unique cellular characteristics[17]:

- its biconcave shape (large surface area-to-volume ratio)
- the viscosity of its internal contents (the "solution" of hemoglobin)
- the unique viscoelastic properties of the erythrocyte membrane

Red cells have an "elastic extension" capability (primarily due to the elasticity of coiled spectrin tetramers and association–dissociation of skeletal proteins) whereby the cells can resume a normal shape after being distorted by an external applied force. However, application of large or prolonged forces can be associated with reorganization of the cytoskeletal proteins, producing a permanent deformation or, if the force is excessive, fragmentation.[17] In addition to being a major component of erythrocyte deformability, the membrane skeleton is the principal determinant of erythrocyte stability. The proportion of spectrin dimers versus tetramers (or higher oligomers) is a key factor influencing membrane stability.[18] Higher proportions of dimers result in increased fragility while higher proportions of tetramers and oligomers result in stabilization. Also, interaction of the cytoskeleton with the lipid bilayer and integral membrane proteins stabilizes the cell membrane. If the bilayer uncouples from the skeleton, portions of lipid-rich membrane will be released in the form of microvesicles, resulting in a decrease in the surface area-to-volume ratio and the formation of spherocytes.[19]

 Checkpoint! 5

Compare placement in the membrane and function of peripheral and integral erythrocyte membrane proteins.

MEMBRANE PERMEABILITY

The red cell membrane is freely permeable to water (exchanged by a water channel protein[20]) and to anions (ex-

TABLE 5-3

Concentration of Cations in the Erythrocyte versus Plasma

Cation	Erythrocyte (mmoles/L)	Plasma (mmoles/L)
Sodium (Na$^+$)	5.4–7.0	135–145
Potassium (K$^+$)	98–106	3.6–5.0
Calcium (Ca$^+$)	0.0059–0.019	2.1–2.6
Magnesium (Mg^{++})	3.06	0.65–1.05

changed by the anion transport protein, band 3). In contrast, the red cell membrane is nearly impermeable to monovalent and divalent cations. Glucose is taken up by a glucose transporter in a process that does not require ATP.[21]

The cations, Na$^+$, K$^+$, Ca^{2+}, and Mg^{2+} are maintained in the erythrocyte at levels much different than those in plasma (Table 5-3 ✪). Erythrocyte osmotic equilibrium is normally maintained by both the selective (low) permeability of the membrane to cations and cation pumps located in the cell membrane. To maintain low intracellular Na$^+$ and Ca^{2+} and high K$^+$ concentrations (relative to plasma concentrations), the red cell utilizes two cation pumps, both of which use intracellular ATP as an energy source.

The Na$^+$/K$^+$ cation pump hydrolyzes one mole of ATP in the expulsion of 3Na$^+$ and the uptake of 2K$^+$. This normally balances exactly the passive "leaks" of each cation along its respective concentration gradient between plasma and cytoplasm. This Na$^+$/K$^+$-ATPase is activated by intracellular Na$^+$ and extracellular K$^+$, although physiologic regulation of Na$^+$ and K$^+$ transport is primarily due to increased intracellular Na$^+$.[8] Calcium plays a role in maintaining low membrane permeability to Na$^+$ and K$^+$. An increase in intracellular Ca^{2+} allows Na$^+$ and K$^+$ to move in the direction of their concentration gradients.[8] Additionally, increased intracellular Ca^{2+} activates the Gárdos channel, which causes selective loss of K$^+$ and, consequently, water, resulting in dehydration. Low intracellular Ca^{2+} is maintained by a Ca^{2+}-ATPase pump. The Ca^{2+} pump depends on magnesium to maintain its transport function. Although Mg^{2+} is necessary for active extrusion of Ca^{2+} from the cell, Mg^{++} is not moved out of the cell in the process.

If erythrocyte membrane permeability to cations increases or the cation pumps fail (either due to decreased glucose for generation of ATP via glycolysis or decreased ATP), Na$^+$ accumulates in the cells in excess of K$^+$ loss. The result is an increase in intracellular monovalent cations and water, cell swelling, and, ultimately, osmotic hemolysis.

▶ ERYTHROCYTE METABOLISM

The metabolism of the erythrocyte is limited because of the absence of a nucleus, mitochondria, and other subcellular organelles. Although the binding, transport, and release of

O_2 and CO_2 are passive processes not requiring energy, various energy-dependent metabolic processes that are essential to cell viability occur. Energy is required by the erythrocyte to:

1. maintain the cation pumps, moving cations against electrochemical gradients
2. maintain hemoglobin iron in the reduced state
3. maintain reduced sulfhydryl groups in hemoglobin and other proteins
4. maintain red cell membrane integrity and deformability

The most important metabolic pathways in the mature erythrocyte are linked to glucose metabolism. These pathways include: (Table 5-4 ❂)

1. glycolysis (glycolytic pathway, formerly known as Embden-Meyerhof pathway)
2. hexose-monophosphate shunt
3. methemoglobin reductase pathway
4. Rapoport-Luebering shunt

Because the red cell lacks a citric acid cycle (due to the lack of mitochondria), it is limited to obtaining energy (ATP) solely by anaerobic glycolysis. Glucose enters the red cell through a membrane-associated glucose carrier, which transports glucose into the cell in a process that does not require ATP. Transport of glucose into the RBC is independent of insulin.

GLYCOLYTIC PATHWAY

The erythrocyte obtains its energy in the form of ATP from glucose breakdown in the glycolytic pathway, formerly known as the Embden-Meyerhof pathway (Figure 5-5 ■). About 90–95% of the cell's glucose consumption is metabolized by this pathway. Normal erythrocytes have no glycogen deposits and depend entirely on environmental glucose for **glycolysis.** Glucose is metabolized by this pathway to lactate or pyruvate, producing a net gain of 2 moles of ATP per mole of glucose. If NADH is available in the cell, pyruvate is reduced to lactate. The lactate or pyruvate formed is transported from the cell to the plasma and metabolized elsewhere in the body.

Adequate amounts of ATP are necessary to maintain erythrocyte shape, flexibility, and membrane integrity by regulating intracellular cation concentration (see previous discussion of membrane permeability). ATP is needed to maintain normal levels of intracellular cations against their concentration gradients. Increased osmotic fragility is noted in cells with abnormally permeable membranes and/or decreased ATP production. Upon the exhaustion of glucose, ATP for the cation pumps is no longer available, and cells cannot maintain normal intracellular cation concentrations. The cells become sodium and calcium logged and potassium depleted. The cell accumulates water and changes from a biconcave disc to a sphere and is removed from the circulation.

HEXOSE MONOPHOSPHATE (HMP) SHUNT

Not all of the glucose metabolized by the red cell goes through the direct glycolytic pathway. Five to 10% of cellular glucose enters the oxidative HMP shunt, an ancillary system for producing reducing substances (Figure 5-5). Glucose-6-phosphate is oxidized by the enzyme glucose-6-phosphate dehydrogenase (G6PD) in the first step of the HMP. In the process, $NADP^+$ is reduced to NADPH.

Glutathione is highly concentrated in the erythrocyte and is important in protecting the cell from oxidant damage by reactive oxygen species (ROS), which are produced during oxygen transport and by other oxidants such as chemicals

❂ TABLE 5-4

Role of Metabolic Pathways in the Erythrocyte

Metabolic Pathway	Key Enzymes	Function	Hemopathology
Glycolytic pathway	Phosphofructokinase Pyruvate kinase (PK)	Produces ATP accounting for 90% of glucose consumption in RBC	Hemolytic anemia Hereditary PK deficiency
Hexose-monophosphate shunt	Glutathione reductase Glucose-6-phosphate dehydrogenase (G6PD)	Provides NADPH and glutathione to reduce oxidants that would shift the balance of oxyhemoglobin to methemoglobin	Hemolytic anemia Hereditary G6PD deficiency Glutathione reductase deficiency Hemoglobinopathies
Rapoport-Leubering	BPG-Synthetase	Controls the amount of 2,3-BPG produced, which in turn affects the oxygen affinity of hemoglobin	Hypoxia
Methemoglobin reductase	Methemoglobin reductase	Protects hemoglobin from oxidation via NADH (from glycolytic pathway) and methemoglobin reductase	Hemolytic anemia Hypoxia

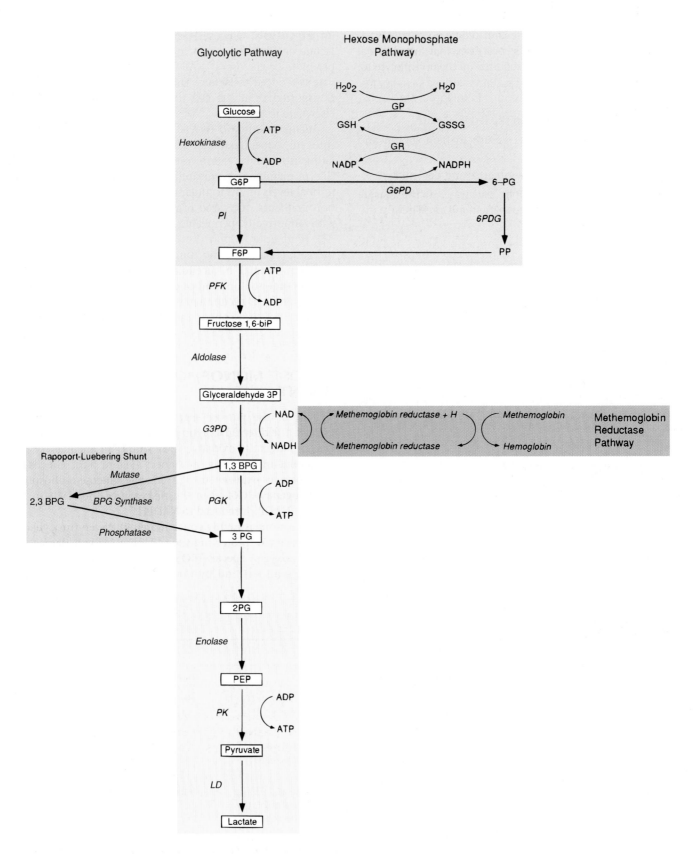

■ FIGURE 5-5   Erythrocyte metabolic pathways. The glycolytic pathway is the major source of energy for the erythrocyte through production of ATP. The hexose-monophosphate pathway is important for reducing oxidants by coupling oxidative metabolism with pyridine nucleotide (NADP) and glutathione (GSSG) reduction. The methemoglobin reductase pathway supports methemoglobin reduction. The Rapoport-Luebering shunt produces 2,3-BPG, which alters hemoglobin-oxygen affinity.

and drugs. In the process of reducing oxidants, glutathione itself is oxidized. (The reduced glutathione is referred to as GSH while the oxidized form is referred to as GSSG.) NADPH produced by the HMP converts GSSG back to GSH, the form necessary to maintain hemoglobin in the reduced funcitonal state. The erythrocyte normally maintains a large ratio of NADPH to $NADP^+$. When the HMP is defective, hemoglobin sulfhydryl groups (-SH) are oxidized, which leads to denaturation and precipitation of hemoglobin in the form of **Heinz bodies.** Heinz bodies attach to the inner surface of the cell membrane, decreasing cell flexibility. Heinz bodies are removed from the cell with a portion of the membrane by macrophages in the spleen. These bodies can be visualized with supravital stains (∞ Chapter 34). If large portions of the membrane are damaged in this manner, the whole cell may be removed. This commonly occurs in patients with G6PD deficiency (∞ Chapter 16).

Reduced GSH also is responsible for maintaining reduced -SH groups of membrane proteins. Decreased GSH leads to oxidative injury of membrane protein -SH groups, compromising protein function and resulting in "leaky" cell membranes. Cellular depletion of ATP can then occur due to increased consumption of energy by the cation pumps.

Ascorbic acid, or vitamin C, is also an important antioxidant in the erythrocyte where it consumes oxygen free radicals and helps preserve alpha-tocopherol (vitamin E, another important antioxidant) in membrane lipoproteins.[22]

METHEMOGLOBIN REDUCTASE PATHWAY

The methemoglobin reductase pathway, an offshoot of the glycolytic pathway, is essential to maintain heme iron in the reduced (ferrous) state, Fe^{++} (Figure 5-5). Methemoglobin (hemoglobin with iron in the oxidized ferric state, Fe^{+++}) is generated simultaneously with the oxidative compounds discussed above as O_2 dissociates from the heme iron. Methemoglobin cannot bind oxygen. The enzyme methemoglobin reductase (also known as NADH diaphorase, or cytochrome b_5) with NADH produced by the glycolytic pathway functions to reduce the ferric iron in methemoglobin, converting it back to ferrous hemoglobin. In the absence of this system, the 2% of methemoglobin formed daily eventually builds up to 20–40%, severely limiting the bloods oxygen-carrying capacity. Challenges by oxidant drugs can interfere with methemoglobin reductase and cause even higher levels of methemoglobin. This results in **cyanosis** (a bluish discoloration of the skin due to an increased concentration of deoxyhemoglobin in the blood).

Checkpoint! 6

Uncontrolled oxidation of hemoglobin results in what RBC intracellular inclusion?

RAPOPORT-LEUBERING SHUNT

The Rapoport-Leubering shunt is a part of the glycolytic pathway (Figure 5-5). This pathway bypasses the formation of 3-phosphoglycerate and ATP from 1,3-bisphosphoglycerate (1,3 BPG). Instead, 1,3-BPG forms 2,3-BPG (also known as *2,3-diphosphoglycerate, 2,3-DPG*) catalyzed by BPG mutase. Therefore, the erythrocyte sacrifices one of its two ATP-producing steps in order to form 2,3-BPG. When hemoglobin binds 2,3-BPG, oxygen release is facilitated (i.e., binding 2,3-BPG causes a decrease in hemoglobin affinity for oxygen). Thus, 2,3-BPG plays an important role in regulating oxygen delivery to the tissues (∞ Chapter 6).

CASE STUDY *(continued from page 67)*

Stephen was admitted for identification and treatment of the anemia. More lab tests were ordered with the following results:

	Patient	Reference Interval
Total bilirubin	4.8 mg/dL	0.1–1.2
Direct bilirubin	1.6 mg/dL	0.1–1.0
Haptoglobin	25 mg/dL	35–165
Hemoglobin electrophoresis		
HbA	98%	>95%
Hb-F	1%	<2%
Hb-A2	1%	1.5–3.7%
Heinz body stain	Positive	Negative
Fluorescent spot test for G6PD deficiency	Positive	

2. What cellular mechanism results in hemolysis due to a deficiency in G6PD?

3. Explain how Heinz body inclusions cause damage to the erythrocyte membrane.

✓ Checkpoint! 7

Which erythrocyte metabolic pathway is responsible for providing the majority of cellular energy? For regulating oxygen affinity? For maintaining hemoglobin iron in the reduced state?

▶ ERYTHROCYTE KINETICS

In the middle of the nineteenth century, Dr. Dennis Jourdanet, a French physician practicing in the highlands of Mexico, noted that patients with altitude sickness exhibited symptoms similar to those of patients with anemia at sea level.[23] Those with altitude sickness, however, had no decrease in red corpuscles as was typical of anemic patients at sea level. He also noted that his "healthy" patients in the highlands had more than the normal number of red corpuscles and that their blood flowed more slowly than normal. He believed that the increased number of red corpuscles in an individual at high altitude compensated for the reduced atmospheric pressure of oxygen. Not until 1890, however, was the increase in erythrocytes accepted as an acquired adjustment to high altitude.[23]

Over the following decades, it was discovered that the stimulation of erythropoiesis in the bone marrow in response to decreased oxygen pressure was the result of a hormone, erythropoietin (EPO) that is released into the peripheral blood by renal tissue in response to hypoxia. Hormonal control of red blood cell mass is closely regulated and is normally maintained in a steady state within narrow limits.

ERYTHROCYTE CONCENTRATION

The normal erythrocyte concentration varies with sex, age, and geographic location. A high erythrocyte count (5.2×10^{12}/L) and hemoglobin concentration (19 g/dL) at birth are followed by a gradual decrease that continues until about the second or third month of extrauterine life. At this time, red blood cell and hemoglobin values fall to $\sim3.5 \times 10^{12}$/L and 10–11 g/dL, respectively.[24] This erythrocyte decrease in infancy is sometimes called *physiologic anemia* of the newborn; its most likely cause is a temporary cessation of bone marrow erythropoiesis after birth due to a low concentration of erythropoietin. EPO levels are high in the fetus due to the relatively **hypoxic** environment in utero and the high oxygen affinity of hemoglobin F (fetal hemoglobin). After birth, however, when the lungs replace the placenta as a means of providing oxygen, the arterial blood oxygen saturation rises from 45% to 95%. EPO cannot be detected in the infant's plasma from about the first week of extrauterine life until the second or third month. Reticulocytes reflect the bone marrow activity during this time. At birth and for the next few days, the mean reticulocyte count is high (4–7%). Within a week, the count drops and remains low (<1%) until about the second month of life, at which time EPO levels rise again (when the hemoglobin levels fall to ~12 g/dL). This corresponds to the recovery from "physiologic anemia of the newborn."

Males have a higher erythrocyte concentration than females after the age of puberty due to the presence of testosterone. Before puberty, and after "male menopause," males and females have comparable erythrocyte levels.[25,26] Testosterone stimulates renal and extrarenal EPO production and directly enhances differentiation of marrow stem and progenitor cells.[27]

Individuals living at high altitudes have a higher mean erythrocyte concentration than those living at sea level. Decreases in the partial pressure of atmospheric oxygen at high altitudes result in a physiologic increase in erythrocytes in the body's attempt to provide adequate tissue oxygenation.

Checkpoint! 8

Why are there different reference ranges for hemoglobin concentration in male and female adults but not in male and female children?

REGULATION OF ERYTHROCYTE PRODUCTION

The body can regulate the number of circulating erythrocytes by changing the rate of cell production in the marrow and/or the rate of cell release from the marrow. Delivery of erythrocytes to the circulation is normally well balanced to match the rate of erythrocyte destruction, which does not vary significantly under steady-state conditions. Impaired oxygen delivery to the tissues and low intracellular oxygen tension (PO_2) trigger increased EPO release and increased erythrocyte production by the marrow. Conditions that stimulate erythropoiesis include anemia, cardiac or pulmonary disorders, abnormal hemoglobins, and high altitude. Erythropoiesis is influenced by a number of cytokines including SCF, IL-3, GM-CSF, and EPO (∞ Chapter 3). However, EPO is the principal cytokine essential for terminal erythrocyte maturation.

Erythropoietin (EPO) is a thermostable renal glycoprotein hormone with a MW of about 34,000 daltons. Renal cortical interstitial cells[28] secrete EPO in response to cellular hypoxia. This feedback control of erythropoiesis is the mechanism by which the body maintains optimal erythrocyte mass for tissue oxygenation. Plasma levels of EPO are constant when the hemoglobin concentration is within the normal range but increase steeply when the hemoglobin decreases below 12 g/dL.[29] EPO is also produced by extrarenal sources, including marrow macrophages and stromal cells, which likely contributes to steady-state erythropoiesis.[2] However, under conditions of tissue hypoxia, oxygen sensors in the kidneys trigger the release of renal EPO, resulting in an increased stimulus for erythropoiesis.

EPO has been defined in biologic terms to have an activity of ~130,000 IU/mg of protein.[30] Normal plasma contains from 5 to 25 U of EPO per L of plasma. EPO can also be found in the urine at concentrations proportional to that found in the plasma (Table 5-5 ☻).[31] In anemia, plasma levels of EPO are related to both hemoglobin concentration and the pathophysiology of the anemia. For example, patients with pure erythrocyte aplasia (∞ Chapter 13) have plasma EPO levels significantly higher than patients with iron deficiency anemia or megaloblastic anemia even though hemoglobin concentration in all three types of anemia can be similar. Plasma EPO levels are significant because they reflect

TABLE 5-5

Characteristics of Erythropoietin

General Characteristics

Composition	Glycoprotein
Stimulus for synthesis	Cellular hypoxia
Origin	Kidneys 80–90%
	Liver <15%
Normal range	Plasma 2–25 IU/L

Functions

Stimulates BFU-E and CFU-E to divide and mature
Increases rate of mRNA and protein (hemoglobin) synthesis
Decreases normoblast maturation time
Increases rate of enucleation (extrusion of nucleus)
Stimulates early release of bone marrow reticulocytes (shift)

Response to Anemia

Generally increased except in anemia of renal disease

not only EPO production but also its disappearance from the blood or utilization by the bone marrow.

Patients with renal disease and nephrectomized patients are usually severely anemic, but they continue to make some erythrocytes and produce limited amounts of EPO in response to hypoxia. Anephric individuals have detectable but low plasma EPO concentrations. In addition to the production of EPO by marrow macrophages and stromal cells, hepatocytes act as an extrarenal source of EPO, accounting for <15% of the total EPO production in humans.[32] In addition, the adult liver appears to require a more severe hypoxic stimulus for EPO production than the kidney. The liver is the major site of EPO production during fetal development. At birth, a gradual and irreversible switch from hepatic to renal production of EPO occurs.[33]

Increased EPO production is due to synthesis of EPO rather than release of preformed stores. The hypoxia-induced increase of EPO is due to both increased gene transcription and stabilization of EPO mRNA.[34] Regulation of EPO production is mediated by the transcription factor hypoxia-inducible factor-1 (HIF-1).[35] Under hypoxic conditions, HIF-1 binds to DNA regulatory sequences (hypoxia-responsive element/HRE) in the EPO gene, activating transcription of EPO. Under conditions of normal oxygen concentration, HIF-1 is degraded by a hydroxylase enzyme that requires oxygen for activity; as levels of HIF-1 decrease, HIF-1 cannot bind DNA or activate transcription of EPO.[32]

EPO exerts its action by binding to specific receptors (EPO-R) on erythropoietin-responsive cells. EPOs major action is stimulation of committed progenitor cells, primarily the CFU-E to survive, proliferate, and differentiate (see discussion of erythropoiesis earlier in this chapter). A small subset of BFU-E has EPO-R but in low number, and BFU-E are largely unresponsive to the effects of EPO. Thus, under conditions of EPO stimulation, the primary elements of the

erythroid precursor cells to respond are the CFU-Es and early normoblasts. However, acute demands for erythropoiesis with extremely high EPO levels can induce influx from the pre-CFU-E pool (the BFU-E). When this occurs, the characteristics of the resulting erythrocytes include an increase in mean corpuscular volume (MCV) and an increase in i antigen and HbF concentration.[2] EPO-Rs on the cell membrane increase as the BFU-E matures to the CFU-E and gradually decrease as the normoblasts mature. The EPO-R is absent on reticulocytes. Other effects of EPO include decreasing normoblast maturation time, increasing rate of mRNA and protein (hemoglobin) synthesis, increasing rate of enucleation (extrusion of the nucleus), and stimulating early release of bone marrow reticulocytes (stress or shift reticulocytes).

The primary way by which EPO stimulates erythropoiesis is by preventing apoptosis. Erythropoiesis is maintained by a finely tuned balance between the positive signals generated by EPO and negative signals from death receptor ligands and inhibitory cytokines (∞ Chapter 2). Erythroid progenitors differ in their sensitivity to EPO; some progenitors require much less EPO than others to survive and mature to reticulocytes.[36] Progenitors with increased sensitivity to EPO are thought to provide RBC production when EPO levels are normal or decreased. Progenitors that require high concentrations of EPO die of apoptosis under these conditions. Progenitors requiring high concentrations of EPO, however, could be rescued from apoptosis when EPO concentrations are elevated as occurs in anemia, thus providing increased erythrocytes under these conditions.

The EPO-R exists in the membrane as a homodimer and lacks intrinsic kinase activity. However, the cytoplasmic tail of the receptor recruits and binds cytoplasmic kinases, Janus kinases 2 (JAK-2), which are activated when EPO binds to the EPO-R (see Figure 3-6). At least four different signaling pathways are activated by this EPO/EPO-R/JAK-2 interaction. Abnormal interactions and/or function of these components have been linked to familial forms of erythrocytosis and certain myeloproliferative disorders (∞ Chapter 22).

The normal bone marrow can increase erythropoiesis 5- to 10-fold in response to increased EPO stimulation if sufficient iron is available. Erythropoiesis is affected (and limited) by serum iron levels and by transferrin saturation (∞ Chapter 6).[37] In hemolytic anemia, there is a readily available supply of iron recycled from erythrocytes destroyed in vivo that results in a sustained ~6-fold increase in erythropoiesis. The rate of erythropoiesis in blood loss anemia during which iron is lost from the body, however may be dependent on preexisting iron stores. In this case, the rate of erythropoiesis usually does not exceed 2.5 times normal unless large parenteral or oral doses of iron are administered.

A number of tumors have been reported to cause an increase in erythropoietin production. Stimulation of the hypothalmus can cause an increase in release of EPO from the kidneys, explaining the association of polycythemia and cerebellar tumors. The serum EPO level increases dramatically in patients undergoing chemotherapy for leukemia as well as other cancers in response to marrow suppression by chemotherapeutic agents.[37]

The production of synthetic hematopoietic growth factors using recombinant DNA technology has revolutionized the management of patients with some anemias. Several recombinant forms of human EPO (rHuEPO) are available and are commonly used for treatment of the anemia associated with end-stage renal disease and chemotherapy as well as HIV-related anemia.[30,38]

CASE STUDY *(continued from page 75)*

4. Would you predict Stephen's serum erythropoietin levels to be low, normal, or increased? Why?

Checkpoint! 9

What would the predicted serum EPO levels be in a patient with an anemia due to end-stage kidney disease?

▶ ERTHROCYTE DESTRUCTION

Red blood cell destruction is normally the result of senescence. Erythrocyte aging is characterized by a decline in certain cellular enzyme systems. It has been suggested that declines in enzymes in the glycolytic pathway, which in turn would lead to decreased ATP production and loss of adequate reducing systems, would result in a loss of the ability to maintain cell shape and deformability as well as membrane integrity. Although many of these enzymes are higher in reticulocytes than in mature erythrocytes, it is unclear whether the activities of these enzymes continue to decline during the aging of the erythrocyte.[39,40,41]

The exposure of phosphatidylserine (PS) on the outer leaflet of the erythrocyte membrane is one of the signals that allows macrophages to recognize senescent erythrocytes.[42] This is the only major difference between senescent and nonsenescent erythrocytes that has been clearly documented.[43] The chromatin condensation and mitochondrial destruction that play a role in erythrocyte production parallel changes seen in apoptotic cells as does the PS externalization seen in erythrocyte senescence. The parallels with apoptosis has led some researchers to speculate that erythrocyte maturation and senescence represent "apoptosis in slow motion."[44]

About 90% of aged erythrocyte destruction is extravascular, taking place in the mononuclear phagocytic cells of the spleen, liver, and bone marrow. The remaining 10% is catabolized intravascularly, whereby the erythrocyteslyse and release hemoglobin directly into the bloodstream.

EXTRAVASCULAR DESTRUCTION

Erythrocyte removal by the spleen, bone marrow, and liver is referred to as extravascular destruction. This pathway, which is the most efficient method of cell removal, conserves and recycles essential erythrocyte components such as amino acids and iron (Figure 5-6 ■). Most extravascular destruction of erythrocytes takes place in the macrophages of the spleen. The exact signal(s) that marks erythrocytes for destruction remains unknown. However, the architecture of the spleen with its torturous circulation, sluggish blood flow, and relative hypoxic and hypoglycemic environment, makes it well suited for culling aged erythrocytes.

Several theories have been proposed to explain the underlying pathology of senescent red cells. Erythrocytes accumulate surface membrane damage during their 120-day lifespan in the circulation at least in part from oxidative damage as well as circulatory "wear and tear."[41] These damaged regions of the membranes are removed by macrophages in the spleen. The biconcave disk shape of the RBC, essential for its deformability, requires a high surface area to volume ratio. Progressive loss of membrane should cause the erythrocyte to assume a more rigid spherical shape with less deformability and reduced ability to pass through the spleen's small apertures. To whatever extent RBCs progressively lose some of the critical enzymes needed for ATP production and antioxidant protection, they can suffer oxidation of critical membrane proteins, lipids, and hemoglobin. This may cause protein denaturation, distortion, and rigidity of the membrane and contribute to the cell's removal. Oxidative damage also causes clustering of band 3 molecules, which can be a "senescence"-identifying feature. The glucose supply in the spleen is low, limiting the energy-producing process of glycolysis within the erythrocyte. Aged erythrocytes can quickly deplete their cellular level of ATP, resulting in limited ability to maintain osmotic equilibrium via the energy-dependent cation pumps. Any combination of these events could contribute to the trapping of erythrocytes in the vasculature of the spleen and their removal by splenic macrophages.

Hemoglobin is composed of a porphyrin ring (heme) complexed with iron and bound to protein chains called *globin* (∞ Chapter 6). Within the macrophage, the hemoglobin molecule is broken down into heme, iron, and globin. Iron and globin (a polypeptide) are conserved and reused for new hemoglobin or other protein synthesis. Heme iron can be stored as ferritin or hemosiderin within the macrophage or released to the transport protein, transferrin, for delivery to developing normoblasts in the bone marrow. This endogenous iron exchange is responsible for about 80% of the iron passing through the transferrin pool. Thus, iron from the normal erythrocyte aging process is conserved and reutilized. The globin portion of the hemoglobin molecule is broken down and recycled into the amino acid pool.

Heme is further catabolized by the macrophage and eventually excreted in the feces. The α-methane bridge of the

EXTRAVASCULAR HEMOGLOBIN DEGRADATION

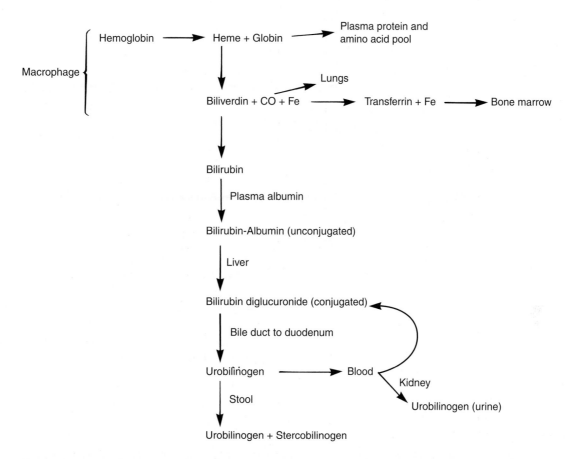

■ **FIGURE 5-6**   Most hemoglobin degradation occurs within the macrophages of the spleen. The globin and iron portions are conserved and reutilized. Heme is reduced to bilirubin, eventually degraded to urobilinogen, and excreted in the feces. Thus, indirect indicators of erythrocyte destruction include the blood bilirubin level and urobilinogen concentration in the urine.

porphyrin ring is cleaved, producing a molecule of carbon monoxide and the linear tetrapyrrole biliverdin. Carbon monoxide is released to the blood stream, carried to the lungs, and expired. The biliverdin is rapidly reduced within the cell to bilirubin. **Bilirubin**, released from the macrophage, is bound by plasma albumin and carried to the liver (unconjugated or "indirect" bilirubin). Upon uptake by the liver, bilirubin is conjugated with two molecules of bilirubin glucuronide by the enzyme bilirubin UDP-glucuronyltransferase present in the endoplasmic reticulum of the hepatocyte. Once conjugated, bilirubin becomes polar and lipid insoluble. Bilirubin diglucuronide (conjugated or "direct" bilirubin) is excreted into the bile, eventually reaching the intestinal tract where it is converted into urobilinogen by intestinal bacterial flora. Most urobilinogen is excreted in the feces where it is quickly oxidized to urobilin or stercobilin. Ten to 20% of urobilinogen is reabsorbed from the gut back to the plasma. The reabsorbed urobilinogen is either excreted in urine or returned to the gut via an entero-

hepatic cycle. In liver disease, the enterohepatic cycle is impaired and an increased amount of urobilinogen is excreted in the urine.

INTRAVASCULAR DESTRUCTION

The small amount of hemoglobin released into the peripheral blood circulation through intravascular erythrocyte breakdown undergoes dissociation into $\alpha-\beta$ dimers, which are quickly bound to the plasma glycoprotein **haptoglobin** (Hp) in a 1:1 ratio (Figure 5-7 ■). Haptoglobin is an $\alpha2$-globulin present in plasma at a concentration of 35-164 mg/d (males) or 40-175 mg/dl (females). The haptoglobin-hemoglobin (HpHb) complex is too large to be filtered by the kidney, so haptoglobin carries hemoglobin dimers to the liver. Hepatocytes, which have haptoglobin receptors, take up the HpHb and process it in a manner similar to that of hemoglobin released by extravascular destruction (∞ Chapter 14).

INTRAVASCULAR HEMOGLOBIN DEGRADATION

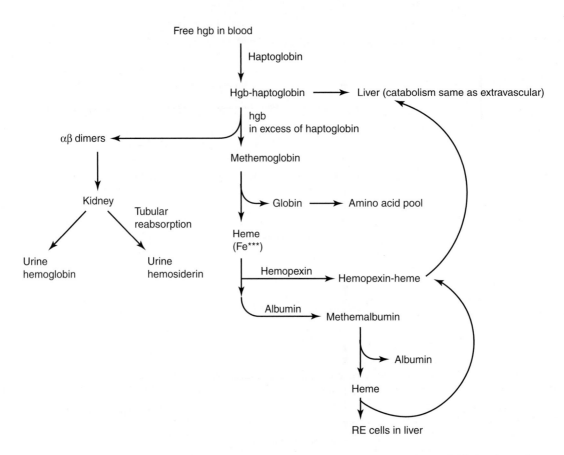

■ FIGURE 5-7   When the erythrocyte is destroyed within the vascular system, hemoglobin is released directly into the blood. Normally, the free hemoglobin quickly complexes with haptoglobin, and the complex is degraded in the liver. In severe hemolytic states, haptoglobin can become depleted, and free hemoglobin dimers are filtered by the kidney. Additionally, with haptoglobin depletion, some hemoglobin is quickly oxidized to methemoglobin and bound to either hemopexin or albumin for eventual degradation in the liver.

The HpHb complex is cleared very rapidly from the bloodstream with a $T_{1/2}$ disappearance rate of 10–30 minutes. The haptoglobin concentration can be depleted very rapidly in acute hemolytic states because the liver is unable to maintain plasma haptoglobin levels. Haptoglobin, however, is an acute-phase reactant, and increased concentrations can be found in inflammatory, infectious, or neoplastic conditions. Therefore, patients with hemolytic anemia accompanied by an underlying infectious or inflammatory process may have normal haptoglobin levels.

When haptoglobin is depleted, as in severe hemolysis, free $\alpha-\beta$ dimers can be filtered by the kidney and reabsorbed by the proximal tubular cells. $\alpha-\beta$ dimers passing through the kidney in excess of the reabsorption capabilities of the tubular cells appear in the urine as free hemoglobin. Dimers reabsorbed by the tubular cells are catabolized to bilirubin and iron, both of which may reenter the plasma pool. However, some iron remains in the tubular cell and is complexed to storage proteins forming ferritin and **hemosiderin**.

Eventually, tubular cells loaded with iron are sloughed off and excreted in the urine (**hemosiderinuria**). The iron inclusions can be visualized with the Prussian blue stain (∞ Chapter 34). Thus, the presence hemosiderinuria is a sign of recent increased intravascular hemolysis.

Hemoglobin not excreted by the kidney or bound to haptoglobin is either cleared directly by hepatic uptake or oxidized to methemoglobin. Heme dissociates from methemoglobin and avidly binds to a β-globulin glycoprotein, **hemopexin**. Hemopexin is synthesized in the liver and combines with heme in a 1:1 ratio. The hemopexin–heme complex is cleared from the plasma slowly with a $T_{1/2}$ disappearance of 7–8 hours. When hemopexin becomes depleted, the dissociated oxidized heme combines with plasma albumin in a 1:1 ratio to form methemalbumin. Methemalbumin clearance by the liver is also very slow. In fact, methemalbumin could only be a temporary carrier for heme until more hemopexin or haptoglobin becomes available. Heme is transferred from methemalbumin to hemopexin for clearance by the liver as it becomes available. When present in large quantity, methemalbumin and hemopexin-heme complexes impart a brownish color to the plasma. Schumm's test is designed to detect these abnormal compounds spectrophotometrically.

 Checkpoint! 10

What lab tests would diagnose an increase in RBC destruction (i.e., hemolysis), and what would be the expected results?

 CASE STUDY *(continued from page 78)*

5. Stephen's haptoglobin level is 25 mg/dL. Explain why he has a low haptoglobin value.

SUMMARY

Erythrocytes are derived from the unipotent committed progenitor cells BFU-E and CFU-E. Morphologic developmental stages of the erythroid cell include (in order of increasing maturity) the pronormoblast, basophilic normoblast, polychromatophilic normoblast, orthochromatic normoblast, reticulocyte, and erythrocyte. Erythropoietin, a hormone produced in renal tissues, stimulates erythropoiesis and is responsible for maintaining a steady-state erythrocyte mass. Erythropoietin stimulates survival and differentiation of erythroid progenitor cells, increases the rate of erythropoiesis, and effects an early release of reticulocytes from the marrow.

The erythrocyte concentration varies with sex, age, and geographic location. Higher concentrations are found in males (post-puberty) and newborns and at high altitudes. Decreases below the reference range result in a condition called *anemia*.

The erythrocyte membrane is a lipid-protein bilayer complex that is important for maintaining cellular deformability and selective permeability. As the cell ages, the membrane is reduced in surface area relative to cell volume and becomes more rigid, and the cell is culled in the spleen. The normal erythrocyte life span is 100–120 days.

The erythrocyte derives its energy and reducing power from glycolysis and ancillary pathways. The glycolytic pathway provides ATP to help the cell maintain erythrocyte shape, flexibility, and membrane integrity through regulation of intracellular cation permeability. The HMP shunt provides reducing power to protect the cell from permanent oxidative injury. The methemoglobin reductase pathway helps reduce heme from the ferric (Fe^{3+}) back to the ferrous (Fe^{2+}) state. The Rapoport-Leubering shunt facilitates oxygen delivery to the tissue by producing 2,3-BPG.

Destruction of aged erythrocytes occurs primarily in the macrophages of the spleen and liver through processes known as *extravascular* and *intravascular destruction*. Extravascular destruction of the erythrocyte is the physiologically preferred pathway for aged or abnormal erythrocyte removal (splenic and hepatic macrophages). Hemoglobin is broken down into heme, globin and iron. Iron and globin are conserved and reused. Heme is catabolized to bilirubin and excreted. Intravascular destruction of erythrocytes results in release of hemoglobin into the peripheral blood circulation. Hemoglobin or its derivatives combine with albumin, haptoglobin, and/or hemopexin and are transported to the liver where it is catabolized. Free hemoglobin can be filtered by the kidney and some reabsorbed by renal tubular cells. Free hemoglobin in the urine is a sign of acute intravascular hemolysis.

REVIEW QUESTIONS

LEVEL I

1. The earliest recognizable erythroid precursor on a Wright-stained smear of the bone marrow is: (Objective 1)
   a. pronormoblast
   b. basophilic normoblast
   c. CFU-E
   d. BFU-E

2. This renal hormone stimulates erythropoiesis in the bone marrow: (Objective 4)
   a. IL-1
   b. erythropoietin
   c. granulopoietin
   d. thrombopoietin

3. Haptoglobin can become depleted in: (Objective 8)
   a. inflammatory conditions
   b. intravascular hemolysis
   c. infectious diseases
   d. kidney disease

LEVEL II

1. The last stage of erythrocyte maturation that can undergo mitosis is: (Objective 1)
   a. basophilic normoblast
   b. orthochromic normoblast
   c. pronormoblast
   d. polychromatophilic normoblast

2. Spherocytes are erythrocytes with an increase in cell hemoglobin concentration. This could result in: (Objective 3)
   a. increased membrane permeability
   b. increased cell elasticity
   c. absence of the MN antigens
   d. decreased cell deformability

3. As a person ascends to high altitudes, the increased activity of the Rapoport-Leubering pathway: (Objective 4)
   a. causes precipitation of hemoglobin as Heinz bodies
   b. has no effect on oxygen delivery to tissues
   c. causes increased release of oxygen to tissues
   d. causes decreased release of oxygen to tissues

REVIEW QUESTIONS (continued)

LEVEL I

4. The erythrocyte life span is most directly determined by: (Objective 5)
   a. spleen size
   b. serum haptoglobin level
   c. membrane deformability
   d. cell size and shape

5. Which of the following depicts the normal sequence of erythroid maturation? (Objective 1)
   a. pronormoblast → basophilic normoblast → polychromatic normoblast → orthochromic normoblast → reticulocyte
   b. pronormoblast → polychromatic normoblast → orthochromic normoblast → basophilic normoblast → reticulocyte
   c. basophilic normoblast → polychromatic normoblast → reticulocyte → orthochromic normoblast → pronormoblast
   d. orthochromic normoblast → basophilic normoblast → reticulocyte → polychromatic normoblast → pronormoblast

6. The primary effector (cause) of increased erythrocyte production, or erythropoiesis, is: (Objective 4)
   a. supply of iron
   b. rate of bilirubin production
   c. tissue hypoxia
   d. rate of EPO secretion

7. An increase in the reticulocyte count should be accompanied by: (Objective 2)
   a. a shift to the left in the Hb-O_2 dissociation curve
   b. abnormal maturation of normoblasts in the bone marrow
   c. an increase in total and direct serum bilirubin
   d. polychromasia on the Wright's stained blood smear

8. What property of the normal erythrocyte membrane allows the 7-μm cell to squeeze through 3-μm fenestrations in the spleen? (Objective 5)
   a. fluidity
   b. elasticity
   c. permeability
   d. deformability

9. An increase of erythrocyte membrane rigidity would be predicted to have what effect? (Objective 5)
   a. increase in erythropoietin production
   b. increase in cell volume
   c. decrease in cell life span
   d. decrease in reticulocytosis

10. A patient with an anemia due to increased intravascular hemolysis would likely present with which of the following lab results? (Objective 8)
    a. increased haptoglobin
    b. hemoglobinuria
    c. normal hemoglobin and hematocrit
    d. decreased serum bilirubin

LEVEL II

4. A newborn has a hemoglobin level of 16.0 g/dL at birth. Two months later a CBC indicates a hemoglobin concentration of 11.0 g/dL. The difference in hemoglobin concentration is most likely due to: (Objective 1)
   a. chronic blood loss
   b. inherited anemia
   c. increased intravascular hemolysis
   d. physiologic anemia of the newborn

5. Compared to sea level, at high altitudes an individual's erythrocytes are: (Objective 1)
   a. produced at a lower rate
   b. larger than normal
   c. destroyed at an increased rate
   d. at a higher concentration

6. Which of the following is necessary to maintain reduced levels of methemoglobin in the erythrocyte? (Objective 4)
   a. vitamin B_6
   b. NADH
   c. 2,3-BPG
   d. lactate

7. A patient lost about 1500 mL of blood during surgery but was not given blood transfusions. His hemoglobin before surgery was in the reference range. What would be the most likely finding 3 days later. (Objective 1, 6)
   a. increase in total bilirubin
   b. increase in indirect bilirubin
   c. increase in erythropoietin
   d. increased haptoglobin

8. An anemic patient has hemosiderinuria, increased serum bilirubin, and decreased haptoglobin. This is an indication that there is: (Objective 6)
   a. increased intravascular hemolysis
   b. decreased extravascular hemolysis
   c. hemolysis accompanied by renal disease
   d. a defect in the Rapoport-Leubering pathway

9. A laboratory professional finds evidence of Heinz bodies in the erythrocytes of a 30-year-old male. This is evidence of: (Objective 4)
   a. increased oxidant concentration in the cell
   b. decreased hemoglobin-oxygen affinity
   c. decreased production of ATP
   d. decreased stability of the cell membrane

10. A 65-year-old female presents with an anemia of 3 weeks' duration. In addition to a decrease in her hemoglobin and hematocrit, she has an increased serum bilirubin, a decrease in serum haptoglobin, and 3^+ polychromasia on her blood smear. Based on these preliminary findings, what serum erythropoietin result is expected? (Objective 6, 7)
    a. decreased
    b. normal
    c. increased
    d. no correlation

www.pearsonhighered.com/mckenzie
Use this address to access the free, interactive Companion Website created for this textbook. Find additional information, tables and figures. Evaluate your command of the chapter information using case studies and critical thinking and multiple choice questions.

REFERENCES

1. Beutler E. The red cell: A tiny dynamo. In: Wintrobe, MM ed. *Blood, pure and eloquent.* New York: McGraw-Hill; 1980:141–68.

2. Papayannopoulou T, D'Andrea AD, Abkowitz JL, Migliaccio AR. Biology of erythropoiesis, erythroid differentiation and maturation. In: Hoffman R, Benz EJ Jr, Shattil SJ, Furie B, Cohen HJ, Silberstein LE, McGlave P, eds. *Hematology: Basic principles and practice,* 4th ed. Philadelphia: Elsevier Churchill Livingstone; 2005:267–88.

3. Gregg XT, Prchal JT. Anemia of endocrine disorders. In: Lichtman MA, Beutler E, Kipps TJ, Seligsohn U, Kaushansky K, Prchal JT, eds. *Williams hematology,* 7th ed. New York: McGraw-Hill; 2006;459–62.

4. Bull BS. Morphology of the erythron. In: Lichtman MA, Beutler E, Kipps TJ, Seligsohn U, Kaushansky K, Prchal JT, eds. *Williams hematology,* 7th ed. New York: McGraw-Hill; 2006;369–85.

5. Hedin SG. Uber die Permeabilitaet der Blutkorperchen. *Pflugers Arch.* 1897;68:229–338.

6. Landsteiner K. Uber Agglutinationserscheinungen normalen menschlichen Blutes. *Wien Klin Wochenschr.* 1902;14:1132–34.

7. Mohandas N. The red cell membrane. In: Hoffman R, Benz Jr. EJ, Shattil SF, Furie B, Cohen HJ, eds. *Hematology: Basic principles and practice.* Philadelphia: Elsevier Churchill Livingstone; 1995:264–69.

8. Lux SE, Palek J. Disorders of the red cell membrane. In: Handin RI, Lux SE, Stossel TP, eds. *Blood principles and practice of hematology.* Philadelphia: JB Lippincott; 1995:1701–1818.

9. Devaux PF. Protein involvement in transmembrane lipid asymmetry. *Annu Rev Biophys Biomol Struct.* 1992;21:417–39.

10. Fukuda M, Dell A, Fukuda MN. Structure of fetal lactosaminoglycan: The carbohydrate moiety of band 3 isolated from human umbilical cord erythrocytes. *J Biol Chem.* 1984;259:4782–91.

11. Fukuda M, Dell A, Oates JE, Fukuda MN. Structure of branched lactosaminoglycan, the carbohydrate moiety of band 3 isolated from adult erythrocytes. *J Biol Chem.* 1984;259:8260–73.

12. Platt OS. Inherited disorders of red cell membrane proteins. In: Nagel RL, ed. *Genetically abnormal red cells.* Boca Raton, FL: CRC Press; 1988.

13. Vertessy BG, Steck TL. Elasticity of the human red cell membrane skeleton: Effects of temperature and denaturants. *Biophys J.* 1989; 55:255–62.

14. Bennett V, Stenbuck PJ. The membrane attachment protein for spectrin is associated with band 3 in human erythrocyte membranes. *Nature.* 1979;280:468–73.

15. Cohen CM, Dotimas E, Korsgren C. Human erythrocyte membrane proein band 4.2 (pallidin). *Semin Hematol.* 1993;30:119–37.

16. Lorand L, Siefring GE Jr, Lowe-Krentz L. Enzymatic basis of membrane stiffening in human erythrocytes. *Semin Hematol.* 1979;16: 65–74.

17. Mohandas N, Chasis JA. Red cell deformability, membrane material properties, and shape: Regulation by transmembrane, skeletal, and cytosolic proteins and lipids. *Semin Hematol.* 1993;30:171–92.

18. Liu S-C, Pallek J. Spectrin tetramer-dimer equilibrium and the stability of erythrocyte membrane skeletons. *Nature.* 1980;285: 586–188.

19. Liu S-C, Derick LH. Molecular anatomy of the red blood cell membrane skeleton: Structure-function relationships. *Semin Hematol.* 1992;29:231–43.

20. Zeidel ML, Ambudkar SV, Smith BL, Agre P. Reconstitution of functional water channels in liposomes containing purified red cell CHIP28 protein. *Biochemistry.* 1992;31:7436–40.

21. Mueckler M, Caruso C, Baldwin SA et al. Sequence and structure of a human glucose transporter. *Science.* 1983;229:941–45.

22. May JM. Ascorbate function and metabolism in the human erythrocyte. *Frontiers in Bio.* 1998;3(1):1–10.

23. Viault F. Sur l'augmentation considerable du nombre des globules ranges dans le sang chez les habitants des haute plateaux de l'amerique du sud. *CR Acad Sci* (Paris). 1890;119:917–18.

24. Bao W et. al. Normative distribution of complete blood count from early childhood through adolescence: The Bogalusa Heart Study. *Prev Med.* 1993;22:825–37.

25. Cavalieri TA, Chopra A, Bryman PN. When outside the norm is normal: Interpreting lab data in the aged. *Geriat.* 1992;47:66–70.

26. Kosower NS. Altered properties of erythrocytes in the aged. *Am J Hematol.* 1993;42:241–47.

27. Besa EC. Hematologic effects of androgens revisted: An alternative therapy in various hematologic conditions. *Semin Hematol.* 1994;31: 134–45.

28. Bachmann S, Le Hir M, Eckardt KU. Co-localization of erythropoietin mRNA and ecto-5'-nucleotidase immuno-reactivity in peritubular cells of rat renal cortex indicates that fibroblasts produce erythropoietin. *J Histochem Cytochem.* 1993;41:335–41.

29. Gabrilove J. Overview: Erythropoiesis, anemia, and the impact of erythropoietin. *Sem Hematol.* 2000;suppl37(4):1–3.

30. Jelkmann W. Erythropoietin after a century of research: Younger than ever. *Eur J Haematol.* 2007;78:183–205.

31. Marsden JT. Erythropoietin measurement and clinical application. *Ann Clin Biochem.* 2006;43:97–104.

32. Hodges VM, Rainey S, Lappin TR, Maxwell AP. Pathophysiology of anemia and erythrocytosis. *Crit Rev Oncol Hematol.* 2007;64:139–58.

33. Zanjani ED, Ascensao JL, McGlave PB, Banisadre M, and Ash RC. Studies on the liver to kidney switch of erythropoietin production. *J Clin Invest.* 1981;67:1183–88.

34. Nangaku M. Eckardt KU. Hypoxia and the HIF system in kidney disease. *J Mol Med.* 2007;85:1325–30.

35. Wang GL, Semenza GL. A nuclear factor induced by hypoxia via de novo protein synthesis binds to the human erythropoietin gene enhancer at a site required for transcriptional activation. *Mol Cell Biol.* 1992;12:5447–54.

36. Kelley LL, Koury MJ, Bondurant MC et al. Survival or death of individual proerythroblasts results from differing erythropoietin sensitivities: A mechanism for controlled rates of erythrocyte production. *Blood.* 1993;82:2340–52.

37. Swabe Y, Takiguchi Y, Kikuno K et. al. Changes in levels of serum erythropoietin, serum iron, and unsaturated iron binding capacity during chemotherapy for lung cancer. *J Clin Onc.* 1998;28(3):182–86.

38. Kimmel PL, Greer JW, Milam RA, Thamer M. Trends in erythropoietin therapy in the U.S. dialysis population. *Semin Nephrol.* 2000; 20(4):335–44.

39. Suzuki T, Dale GI. Senescent erythrocytes. Isolation of in vivo aged cells and their biochemical characteristics. *Proc Natl Acad Sci USA.* 1998;85:1647–51.

40. Zimran A, Forman L, Suzuki T et al. In vivo aging of red cell enzymes. Study of biotinylated red cells in rabbits. *Am J Haematol.* 1990;33:249–54.

41. Steinberg MH, Benz EJ Jr., Adewoye HA, Ebert B. Pathobiology of the human erythrocyte and its hemoglobins. In: Hoffman R, Benz EJ Jr, Shattil SJ, Furie B, Cohen HJ, Silberstein LE, McGlave P, eds. *Hematology: Basic principles and practice,* 4th ed. Philadelphia: Elsevier Churchill Livingstone; 2005:442–54.

42. Boas FE, Forman L, Beutler E. Phosphatidylserine exposure and red cell viability in red cell aging and in hemolytic anemia. *Proc Natl Acad Sci USA.* 1998;95:3077–81.

43. Beutler E. Destruction of erythrocytes. In: Lichtman MA, Beutler E, Kipps TJ, Seligsohn U, Kaushansky K, Prchal JT, eds. *Williams hematology,* 7th ed. New York: McGraw-Hill; 2006;405–10.

44. Gottlieb RA. Apoptosis. In: Lichtman MA, Beutler E, Kipps TJ, Seligsohn U, Kaushansky K, Prchal JT, eds. *Williams hematology,* 7th ed. New York: McGraw-Hill; 2006;151–7.

6

Hemoglobin

Shirlyn B. McKenzie, Ph.D.

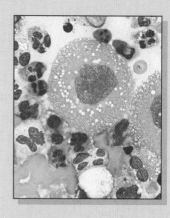

CHAPTER OUTLINE

■ OBJECTIVES—LEVEL I

At the end of this unit of study, the student should be able to:

1. Diagram the quaternary structure of a molecule of hemoglobin identifying the heme ring, globin chains, and iron.

2. Assemble fetal and adult hemoglobin molecules with appropriate globin chains.

3. Explain how pH, temperature, 2,3-BPG, and PO_2 affect the oxygen dissociation curve (ODC).

4. List the types of hemoglobin normally found in adults and newborns and give their approximate concentration.

5. Summarize hemoglobin's function in gaseous transport.

6. Define *normal hemoglobin values.*

7. Explain how the fine balance of hemoglobin concentration is maintained.

8. Compare HbA with HbA1c and explain what an increased concentration of HbA1c means.

OBJECTIVES—LEVEL II

At the end of this unit of study, the student should be able to:

1. Construct a diagram to show the synthesis of a hemoglobin molecule.

2. Describe the ontogeny of hemoglobin types; contrast differences in oxygen affinity of HbF and HbA, and relate them to the structure of the molecule.

3. Explain the molecular control of heme synthesis.

4. Given information on pH, 2,3-BPG, CO_2, temperature, and HbF concentration, interpret the ODC and translate it into the physiologic effect on oxygen delivery.

5. Contrast the structures and functions of relaxed and tense hemoglobin and propose how these structures affect gaseous transport.

6. Describe how abnormal hemoglobins are acquired, and select a method by which they can be detected in the laboratory.

7. Assess the oxygen affinity of abnormal, acquired hemoglobins and reason as to how this affects oxygen transport.

8. Compare and contrast the exchange of O_2, CO_2, H^+, and Cl^- at the level of capillaries and the lungs.

KEY TERMS

Artificial oxygen carriers (AOCs)
Bohr effect
Carboxyhemoglobin
Chloride shift
Cyanosis
Deoxyhemoglobin
Glycosylated hemoglobin
Heme
Hypoxia
Iron regulatory element (IRE)
Iron regulatory protein (IRP)
Oxygen affinity
Oxyhemoglobin
Methemoglobin
(R) structure
Sulfhemoglobin
(T) structure

BACKGROUND BASICS

The information in this chapter builds on the concepts learned in previous chapters. To maximize your learning experience, you should review these concepts before starting this unit of study.

Level I

▶ List and describe the stages of erythrocyte maturation (Chapter 5).
▶ Summarize the role of erythropoietin in erythropoiesis (Chapter 5).
▶ Describe the site of erythropoiesis (Chapter 4).

Level II

▶ Describe the metabolic pathways present in the mature erythrocyte, and explain their role in maintaining viability of the erythrocyte (Chapter 5).
▶ Describe the appearance of the bone marrow when erythropoiesis is decreased or increased (Chapter 5).
▶ Summarize the development of hematopoiesis from the embryonic stage to the adult (Chapter 4).

CASE STUDY

We will address this case study throughout the chapter.

Jerry, a 44-year-old male, arrived in the emergency room by ambulance after a bicycle accident. Examination revealed multiple fractures of the femur. He was otherwise healthy. The next day, he was taken to surgery to repair the fractures. After surgery, his hemoglobin was 7 gm/dL. He refused blood transfusions and was discharged 6 days later. Jerry called his doctor within days of being discharged and told him that he had difficulty walking around the house on crutches because of shortness of breath and lack of stamina. Consider why Jerry's hemoglobin was decreased after surgery and how this could be related to his current symptoms.

▶ OVERVIEW

This chapter describes the synthesis and structure of hemoglobin and factors that regulate its production. The different types of hemoglobin produced according to developmental stage are compared. The function of hemoglobin in gaseous exchange is considered, and factors that affect this function are analyzed. Structure, formation, and laboratory detection of abnormal hemoglobins are also discussed.

▶ INTRODUCTION

Hemoglobin is a highly specialized intracellular erythrocyte protein responsible for transporting oxygen from the lungs to tissue and facilitating carbon dioxide transport from the tissue to the lungs. Each gram of hemoglobin can carry 1.34 mL of oxygen.

Hemoglobin occupies approximately 33% of the volume of the erythrocyte and accounts for 90% of the cell's dry weight. Each cell contains between 28 and 34 pg of hemoglobin. This concentration is measured by cell analyzers and reported as mean corpuscular hemoglobin (MCH). In anemic states, the erythrocyte may contain less hemoglobin (decreased MCH) and/or have fewer erythrocytes present, which results in a decrease of the blood's oxygen-carrying capacity.

The erythrocyte's membrane and its metabolic pathways are responsible for protecting and maintaining the hemoglobin molecule in its functional state. Abnormalities in the membrane that alter its permeability or alterations of the cell's enzyme systems can lead to changes in the structure and/or function of the hemoglobin molecule and affect the capacity of this protein to deliver oxygen.

Although a small amount of hemoglobin is synthesized as early as the pronormoblast stage, most hemoglobin synthesized in the developing normoblasts occurs at the polychromatophilic normoblast stage. All together, 75–80% of the cell's hemoglobin is made before the extrusion of the nucleus. Because the reticulocyte does not have a nucleus, it cannot make new RNA for protein synthesis. However, residual RNA and mitochondria in the reticulocyte enable the cell to make the remaining 20–25% of the cell's hemoglobin. The mature erythrocyte contains no nucleus, ribosomes, or mitochondria and is unable to synthesize new protein.

Hemoglobin concentration in the body is the result of a fine balance between production and destruction of erythrocytes. The normal hemoglobin concentration in an adult male is about 15 g/dL with a total blood volume of about 5000 mL. Therefore, the total body mass of hemoglobin is approximately 750 g:

$$15 \text{ g/dL} \times 5000 \text{ mL} \times 1 \text{ dL}/100 \text{ mL} = 750 \text{ g}$$

Because the normal erythrocyte life span is ~120 days, $\frac{1}{120}$ of the total amount of hemoglobin is lost each day through removal of senescent erythrocytes. Thus, an equivalent amount must be synthesized each day to maintain a steady-state concentration. This amounts to approximately 6 g of new hemoglobin per day:

$$\frac{750 \text{ g}}{120 \text{ days}} = 6.25 \text{ g/day (amount of hemoglobin lost and synthesized each day)}$$

If we divide the total amount of hemoglobin synthesized each day (6.25 g) by the mean amount of hemoglobin in a red cell (MCH, ~ 30 pg), we can determine the daily production of new red blood cells:

$$\frac{6.25 \text{ g/day}}{30 \text{ pg/cell}} \times 10^{12} \text{ pg/g} = 2 \times 10^{11} \text{ cells/day}$$

► HEMOGLOBIN STRUCTURE

Hemoglobin is a large tetrameric molecule, molecular weight 66,700 daltons, composed of four globular protein subunits (Figure 6-1 ■). Each of the four subunits contains a heme group and a globin chain. Heme, the prosthetic group of hemoglobin, is a tetrapyrrole ring with a ferrous iron located in the center of the ring. Hemoglobin structure is described in Table 6-1 ✪ (Figure 6-2 ■). Each heme subunit can carry one molecule of oxygen bound to the central ferrous iron; thus, each hemoglobin molecule can carry four molecules of oxygen.

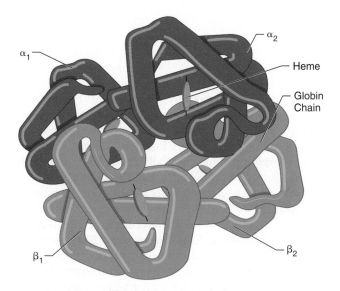

■ FIGURE 6-1   Hemoglobin is a molecule composed of four polypeptide subunits. Each subunit has a globin chain with a heme nestled in a hydrophobic crevice that protects the iron from being oxidized. Four different types of globin chains—α, β, δ, γ—occur in pairs. The types of globin chains present determine the type of hemoglobin. Depicted here is hemoglobin A, consisting of 2 α and 2 β chains. The contacts between the α, β-chains in a dimer (i.e., $\alpha_1\beta_1$) are extensive and allow little movement. The contacts between the dimer pairs (i.e., $\alpha_1\beta_2$ and $\alpha_2\beta_1$), however, are smaller and allow conformational change of the molecule as it goes from oxyhemoglobin to deoxyhemoglobin.

✪ TABLE 6-1

The Structure of Hemoglobin

Structure	Conformational Description
Primary	Sequence of individual amino acids held together by peptide bonds in the globin chains; is critical to stability and function of molecule; determines the overall structure
Secondary	Arrangement of the amino acids resulting from hydrogen bonding between the peptide bonds of the amino acids next to or near each other (75% α-helix; consists of 8 α-helical segments, labeled A → H, separated by nonhelical segments)
Tertiary	Folding superimposed on the helical and pleated domains; forms the heme hydrophobic pocket within globin chains; this tertiary structure changes upon ligand binding
Quaternary	Relationship of the four protein subunits to one another; quaternary structural changes seen upon ligand binding result from the tertiary changes

The composition of the globin chains is responsible for the different functional and physical properties of hemoglobin. Two types of globin chains are produced: alphalike (alpha [α], zeta [ζ]), and nonalpha (epsilon [ε], beta [β], delta [δ], and gamma [γ]). The tetrameric hemoglobin molecule consists of two pairs of unlike chains: two identical α-like and two identical non-α-chains. A pair of α-like chains (α or ζ) combines with a pair of non-α-chains (ε, β, δ, or γ) to form the various types of hemoglobin (Table 6-2 ✪). The arrangement of each globin chain is similar. Each α- and ζ-chain has 141 amino acids while each ε, β-, δ-, and γ-chain has 146 amino acids. Each chain is wound up into eight spiral or α-helical segments separated by seven short, nonhelical segments. The helical segments are lettered A–H, starting at the amino end of the chain. The amino acids of the globin chains are identified by their helix location and amino acid number (i.e., F8 is the eighth amino acid in the F helix). Amino acids between helices are identified by amino acid number and the letters of the two helices (i.e., EF3). The nonhelical segments allow the chains to fold upon themselves.

The four subunits of hemoglobin, each consisting of a heme group surrounded by a globin chain, are held together by salt bonds, hydrophobic contacts, and hydrogen bonds in a tetrahedral formation giving the hemoglobin molecule a nearly spherical shape. When ligands, such as oxygen, bind to hemoglobin, the number and strigency of intersubunit contacts change. Mutations in the globin chains can affect subunit or dimer pair interactions and thus alter hemoglobin-oxygen affinity or the molecule's stability.

✓ Checkpoint! 1

Describe the quaternary structure of a molecule of hemoglobin. How can a mutation in one of the globin chains at the subunit interaction site, $\alpha_1\beta_2$, affect hemoglobin function?

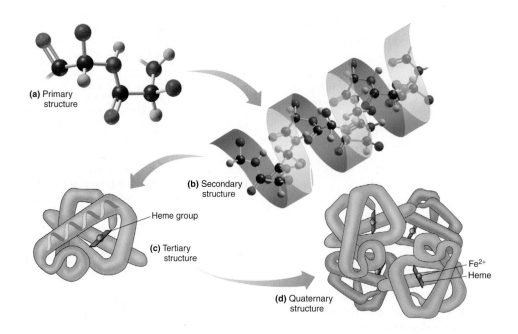

■ FIGURE 6-2   The structure of hemoglobin: Primary structure is the sequence of amino acids; secondary structure is the coiled α helix and B-pleated sheet formed by hydrogen bonding between the peptide bonds in the chain; tertiary structure is the folding of the molecule into a three-dimensional structure; quarternary structure is the combination of the four polypeptide subunits, each of which contains a heme group, into a larger protein. (Timberlake, Karen C.; Timberlake, William. *Basic Chemistry*, 2nd, © N/A. 2008. Electronically reproduced by permission of Pearson Education, Inc., Upper Saddle River, New Jersey.)

✪ TABLE 6-2

Normal Types of Hemoglobin According to Developmental Stage

Developmental Stage	Type	Globin Chains	Reference Interval
Embryonic	Gower I	$\zeta_2\varepsilon_2$	—
	Gower II	$\alpha_2\varepsilon_2$	—
	Portland	$\zeta_2\gamma_2$	—
Fetal	HbF	$\alpha_2\gamma_2$	90–95% before birth
			50–85% at birth
	HbA	$\alpha_2\beta_2$	10–40% at birth
	HbA$_2$	$\alpha_2\delta_2$	<1% at birth
>1 year old	HbF	$\alpha_2\gamma_2$	<2%
	HbA	$\alpha_2\beta_2$	>95%
	HbA$_2$	$\alpha_2\delta_2$	<3.5%
Adult	HbA	$\alpha_2\beta_2$	>95%
	HbA$_2$	$\alpha_2\delta_2$	1.5–3.7%
	HbF	$\alpha_2\gamma_2$	<2%

▶ HEMOGLOBIN SYNTHESIS

HEME

Heme is an iron-chelated porphyrin ring that functions as a prosthetic group (nonamino acid component) of a protein. The porphyrin ring, protoporphyrin IX, is composed of a flat tetrapyrrole ring with ferrous iron (Fe^{++}) inserted into the center. (Porphyrins are metabolically active only when chelated.) Ferrous ions have six electron pairs per atom. In heme, four of these electron pairs are coordinately bound to the N atoms of each of the four pyrrole rings. In hemoglobin, one (fifth) of the two remaining electron pairs is coordinately bound with the N of the proximal histidine (F8) of the globin chain, and the other pair (sixth) is the binding site for molecular oxygen. In the deoxygenated state, the sixth electron pair is occupied by a water molecule.[1] Iron must be in the ferrous (Fe^{++}) state for oxygen binding to occur. Ferric iron (Fe^{+++}), which has lost an electron, cannot serve as an oxygen carrier because the sixth potential binding site (electron pair) for oxygen is no longer available.

Heme synthesis begins in the mitochondria with the condensation of glycine and succinyl coenzyme A (CoA) to form 5-aminolevulinic acid (ALA). This reaction occurs in the presence of the cofactor pyridoxal phosphate, succinyl CoA synthase, and the enzyme 5-aminolevulinate synthase (ALAS). This first reaction is the rate-limiting step in the synthesis of heme and occurs only when the cell has an adequate supply of iron (∞ Chapter 9). Synthesis continues through a series of steps in the cytoplasm, eventually forming coproporphyrinogen. Coproporphyrinogen then reenters the mitochondria and is further modified to form the protoporphyrin IX ring (Figure 6-3■). The final step, also occuring in the mitochondria, is the chelation of iron with protoporphyrin IX catalyzed by ferrochelatase to form heme (Figure 6-4■). Heme then leaves the mitochondria to combine with a globin chain in the cytoplasm. See Web Figure 6-1■ for detailed molecular structures of intermediates in heme synthesis.

GLOBIN

Globin chain synthesis is directed by eight genetic loci (Figure 6-5■). These genes produce the seven different types of globin chains: zeta, alpha, epsilon, gamma-A, gamma-G, delta, and beta (α, ζ, ε, γ^A, γ^G, δ, β). Two are found only in embryonic hemoglobins (ζ, ε). The genes for the ζ-chain (the fetal equivalent of the α-chain) and α-chain are located on chromosome 16 (the α gene cluster). The ζ-chain is synthesized very early in embryonic development. After 8–12 weeks, ζ-chain synthesis is replaced by α-chain synthesis. There are two α-loci (α-1 and α-2), both of which transcribe mRNA for α-chain synthesis. The protein product from each locus is identical. The non-α-globin genes are arranged in linear fashion in order of activation on chromosome 11 (the non-α-gene cluster). The non-α-globin chains show a high degree of homology.

The ε-gene is located toward the 5' end of chromosome 11; during embryonic development, ε-chain synthesis is switched off, and the two γ-genes are activated. One γ-gene directs the production of a γ-chain with glycine at amino acid position 136, γ^G while the other directs the production of a γ-chain with alanine at position 136, γ^A. The γ^G-chain synthesis predominates before birth (3:l), but γ^G- and γ^A-chain syntheses are equal (l:l) in adults. The next two genes on chromosome 11, δ and β, are switched on to a small degree when the γ-genes are activated, but they are not fully activated until γ-chain synthesis diminishes at about 35 weeks of gestation. The rate of synthesis of the δ-chain is only $\frac{1}{140}$ that of the β-chain. After birth, most cells produce predominantly α and β chains for the formation of HbA, the major adult hemoglobin.

The synthesis of globin peptide chains occurs on polyribosomes in the cytoplasm of developing erythroblasts (Figure 6-6■). Globin chains are released from the polyribosomes and combine with heme molecules released from the mitochondria. The globin chains are folded to create a hydrophobic pocket near the exterior surface of the chain between the E and F helices. Heme is inserted into this hydrophobic pocket where it is readily accessible to oxygen. A newly formed α-chain-heme subunit and a non–α-chain-heme subunit combine spontaneously, facilitated by electrostatic attraction, to form a dimer (e.g., $\alpha\beta$). Two dimers then combine to form the tetrameric hemoglobin molecule (e.g., $\alpha_2\beta_2$). The heme is positioned between two

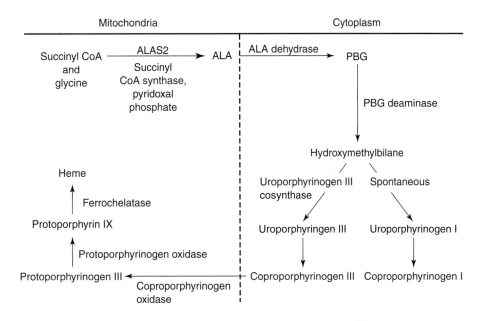

■ FIGURE 6-3   Synthesis of heme: It begins in the mitochondria with the condensation of glycine and succinyl CoA. The product, 5-aminolevulinate (ALA), leaves the mitochondria to form the pyrrole ring, porphobilinogen (PBG). The combination of four pyrroles to form a linear tetrapyrrole (hydroxymethylbilane), the cyclizing of the linear form to uroporphyrinogen, and the decarboxylation of the side chains to form coproporphyrinogen occur in the cytoplasm. The final reactions, the formation of protoporphyrin IX, and the insertion of iron into the protoporphyrin ring occur in the mitochondria.

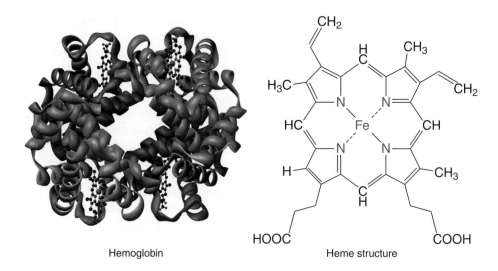

Hemoglobin   Heme structure

■ FIGURE 6-4   The hemoglobin molecule on the left reveals the quartenary structure of hemoglobin with four protein chains folded around a heme molecule. On the right is a heme molecule. Heme is composed of a flat tetrapyrrole ligand (porphyrin) and iron. The iron has six coordinate sites. Nitrogen atoms of porphyrin occupy four coordination sites in a square planar arrangement around the iron. Iron, which is in the ferrous state, has two other coordinate sites, one of which is occupied by the N of the proximal histidine (F8) of globin and one with molecular oxygen or H_2O. (Tro, Nivaldo Jose. *Chemistry: A Molecular Approach* 1st, © 2008. Electronically reproduced by permission of Pearson Education, Inc., Upper Saddle River, New Jersey.)

histidines of the globin chain called the *proximal* (F8) and *distal* (E7) *histidines.* The proximal histidine (F8) is bonded with the heme iron. The iron is protected in the reduced ferrous state in this hydrophobic pocket. The exterior of the chain is hydrophilic, which makes the molecule soluble.

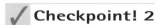 **Checkpoint! 2**

What globin chains are synthesized in the adult?

▶ REGULATION OF HEMOGLOBIN SYNTHESIS

Normally, the production of α subunits, non-α subunits, and heme are nearly equal. This indicates that tight regulatory mechanisms exist, controlling the production of hemoglobin. Hemoglobin synthesis is regulated by several mechanisms including:

• Activity of the erythroid enzyme 5-aminolevulinate synthase (ALAS2)
• Activity of porphobilinogen deaminase (PBGD)

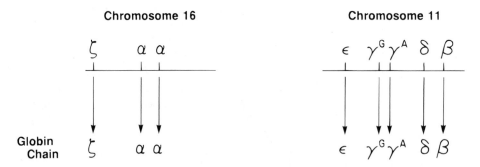

■ FIGURE 6-5   The genes for the globin chains are located on chromosomes 11 and 16. The ζ-chain appears to be the embryonic equivalent of the α-chain, both of which are located on chromosome 16. Note that the α-gene is duplicated. The other globin genes are located on chromosome 11.

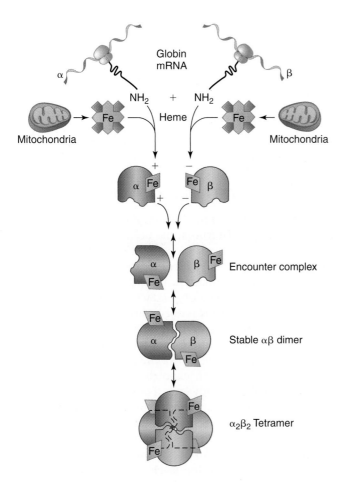

FIGURE 6-6 Assembly of hemoglobin. The α and β globin polypeptides are translated on their respective mRNAs. On binding of heme, the protein folds into its native three-dimensional structure. The binding of α and β hemoglobin subunits to each other is facilitated by electrostatic attraction. An unstable intermediate encounter complex can rearrange to form the stable $\alpha\beta$ dimer. Two dimers combine to form the functional $\alpha_2\beta_2$ tetramer. (Adapted, with permission, from Bunn HF: Subunit assembly of hemoglobin: An important determinant of hematologic phenotype. *Blood.* 1987; 69:1.)

- Concentration of iron
- Regulation of globin chain synthesis

The first enzyme in the heme synthetic pathway, ALAS, catalyzes the initial reaction of condensation of glycine and succinyl-CoA to form 5-ALA, the rate-limiting step in heme synthesis. As mentioned previously, this reaction takes place in the mitochondria. Because ALAS is synthesized on ribosomes in the cytosol, it must be imported into the mitochondria to catalyze the reaction. This mitochondrial import can be inhibited by high concentrations of heme.[2] When iron is scarce, the synthesis of ALAS is decreased.

Iron entering the developing erythroblast can be in either the pool available for metabolic *processes* (heme synthesis) or the storage pool (ferritin and hemosiderin). An **iron regulatory protein** (**IRP**), previously referred to as **iron respon-**

sive element-binding protein (IRE-BP), is the primary physiologic iron sensor.[3] It plays an important role in regulating the available iron in each of these pools by affecting heme synthesis, synthesis of proteins involved in iron metabolism and the formation of ferritin and transferrin receptors.[2,3,4,5,6] When iron is scarce, translation of ALAS is prevented, the synthesis of ferritin and hemosiderin decreases, and the synthesis of transferrin receptors increases. Iron metabolism is discussed in detail in ∞ Chapter 9.

The rate of globin synthesis is governed primarily by the rate at which the DNA code is transcribed to mRNA, but it is also modified by the processing of globin pre-mRNA to mRNA, the translation of mRNA to protein, and the stability of globin mRNA. The individual globin genes have separate promoter regions that are available for activation at variable times during embryonic and fetal development. In addition, the β-gene cluster has a locus control region (LCR), located upstream (5′) of the genes, which plays an important role in regulating the entire gene cluster. The α-gene cluster has a similar control region, the HS40, which is thought to have a similar function. Heme plays an important role in controlling the synthesis of globin chains. It stimulates globin synthesis by inactivating an inhibitor of translation.

CASE STUDY *(continued from page 86)*

Jerry's doctor gave him iron supplements to take every day.
1. If Jerry is iron deficient, what is the effect of this deficient state on the synthesis of ALAS, transferrin receptor, and ferritin?
2. What was the rationale for giving Jerry the iron?

▶ ONTOGENY OF HEMOGLOBIN

The type of hemoglobin is determined by its composition of globin chains (Table 6-2). Individual globin chains are expressed at different levels in developing erythroblasts of the human embryo, fetus, and adult. Some hemoglobins (Gower I, Gower II, and Portland) occur only in the embryonic stage of development. HbF is the predominant hemoglobin in the fetus and newborn, and hemoglobin A is the predominant hemoglobin after 1 year of age.

Studies have suggested that the synthesis of different globin chains occurs in sequence depending on the developmental stage. This is due to the sequential activation and then inactivation (i.e., "switching") among the α- and non-α-globin gene clusters. In vitro cultures of burst forming unit—Erythrocyte (BFU-E, ∞ Chapter 3) from fetal liver, neonatal (umbilical cord) blood, and adult blood show HbF production from these three sources to decrease in concentration from fetal to neonatal to adult. The switch from fetal to adult hemoglobin synthesis is closely related to gestational age and is unaffected by the time of birth: Premature infants do not switch over to adult hemoglobin synthesis any earlier than they would if they had been carried full term. The perinatal switch from HbF to HbA synthesis is probably time controlled by a developmental clock.[7,8] The stem cells are gradually reprogrammed during the perinatal period leading to a switching from γ-chain production to predominantly β-chain production.

EMBRYONIC HEMOGLOBINS

Intrauterine erythropoiesis is associated with the production of the embryonic hemoglobins Gower 1, Gower 2, and Portland in the first trimester of gestation. The embryonic hemoglobins are made from the combination of pairs of embryonic globin chains, ζ and ε in pairs ($\zeta_2 \varepsilon_2$) or embryonic chains in combination with α- and γ-chains ($\alpha_2 \varepsilon_2$; $\zeta_2 \gamma_2$). These primitive hemoglobins are detectable during early hematopoiesis in the yolk sac and liver and are not usually detectable after the third month of gestation.

FETAL HEMOGLOBIN

Hemoglobin F (HbF; $\alpha_2 \gamma_2$) is the predominant hemoglobin formed during liver and bone marrow erythropoiesis in the fetus. HbF composes 90–95% of the total hemoglobin production in the fetus until ~34–36 weeks of gestation. At birth, the infant has 50–85% HbF.

ADULT HEMOGLOBINS

In adults, hemoglobin A (HbA; $\alpha_2 \beta_2$) is the major hemoglobin. It is formed in during erythropoiesis in the bone marrow. Although HbA is found as early as 9 weeks gestation, β-chain synthesis continues at a low level and does not exceed γ-chain synthesis until after birth. At ~36 weeks gestation, β-chain synthesis significantly increases while γ-chain synthesis declines so that at birth, approximately equal amounts of γ- and β-chains are being produced. After birth, the percentage of HbA continues to increase with the infant's age until normal adult levels (>95%) are reached by the end of the first year of life.

HbF production constitutes less than 2% of the total hemoglobin of adults. In normal adults, most if not all HbF is restricted to a few erythrocytes, referred to as *F cells*. F cells constitute less than 8% of adult RBC, and from 13% to 25% of the hemoglobin in each F cell is HbF. The switch from HbF to HbA after birth is incomplete and in part reversible. For example, patients with hemoglobinopathies or severe anemia can have increased levels of HbF, often proportionate to the decrease in HbA. In bone marrow recovering from suppression and in some neoplastic hematologic diseases, HbF levels often rise.

HbA2 ($\alpha_2 \delta_2$) appears late in fetal life, composes less than 1% of the total hemoglobin at birth, and reaches normal adult values (1.5–3.7%) after one year. The δ-gene locus is transcribed very inefficiently compared to the β-locus. This low level of transcription is thought to be due to changes in the region of the gene that recognizes erythroid-specific transcription factors (e.g., GATA-1). HbA2 has a slightly higher oxygen affinity than HbA; otherwise, the two hemoglobins have similar or identical ligand binding curves, Bohr effect, and response to 2,3-BPG.

 Checkpoint! 3

What are the names and globin composition of the embryonic, fetal, and adult hemoglobins?

GLYCOSYLATED HEMOGLOBIN

HbA1 on chromatography is a minor component of normal adult hemoglobin (HbA) that has been modified posttranslationally (HbA3 on starch block electrophoresis). A component usually has been added to the N terminus of the β-chain. The most important subgroup of HbA1 is HbA1C, which has glucose irreversibly attached. This hemoglobin is referred to as **glycosylated hemoglobin**. HbA1C is produced throughout the erythrocyte's life, its synthesis dependent on the concentration of blood glucose. Older erythrocytes typically contain more HbA1C than younger erythrocytes having been exposed to plasma glucose for a longer period of time. However, if young cells are exposed to extremely high concentrations of glucose (>400 mg/dL) for several hours, the concentration of HbA1C increases with both concentration and time of exposure.

Measurement of HbA1C is routinely used as an indicator of control of blood glucose levels in diabetics because it is proportional to the average blood glucose level over the previous two to three months. Average levels of HbA1C are 7.5% in diabetics and 3.5% in normal individuals.

 Checkpoint! 4

A patient has an anemia caused by a shortened RBC life span (hemolysis); how would this affect the HbA1C measurement?

▶ HEMOGLOBIN FUNCTION

The function of hemoglobin is to transport and exchange respiratory gases. The air we breathe is a mixture of nitrogen (78.6%), oxygen (20.8%), water, and carbon dioxide (CO_2). The sea level atmospheric pressure is 760 torr. Each of the gases in the air contributes to this pressure in proportion to its concentration. The partial pressure each gas exerts is referred to as P. Thus, the partial pressure of oxygen in the atmosphere is $20.8\% \times 760 = 159$ torr.

The partial pressure gradient of a gas (in this case, oxygen) determines the rate of diffusion of that gas across the alveolar-capillary membrane. When air is inspired, water vapor is added to the incoming gas to bring its relative humidity up to 100% at body temperature. This amounts to a relatively constant water vapor pressure of 47 torr. Therefore, the PO2 of inspired air is $(760-47) \times 20.8\% = 148$ torr. As the inspired air mixes with alveolar gas, the PO_2 is diluted further by the presence of carbon dioxide given off at the lungs as a byproduct of metabolism. The now arterialized blood leaves the lungs with a PO_2 of 100 torr and a PCO_2 of 40 torr. In comparison, the PO_2 of interstitial fluid in tissues is about 40 torr and the PCO_2 is about 45 torr. Thus, when blood reaches the tissues, oxygen diffuses out of the blood (because the PO_2 in blood is higher than in tissues), and CO_2 diffuses into the blood (because the PCO_2 is higher in tissues than in blood). The amount of dissolved O_2 and CO_2 the plasma can carry is limited. Most O_2 and CO_2 diffuse into the erythrocyte to be transported to tissue or lungs.

OXYGEN TRANSPORT

Hemoglobin with bound oxygen is called **oxyhemoglobin**; hemoglobin without oxygen is called **deoxyhemoglobin**. The amount of oxygen bound to hemoglobin and released to tissues depends not only on the PO_2 and PCO_2 but also on the affinity of Hb for O_2. The ease with which hemoglobin binds and releases oxygen is known as **oxygen affinity**. Hemoglobin affinity for oxygen determines the proportion of oxygen released to the tissues or loaded onto the cell at a given oxygen pressure (PO_2). Increased oxygen affinity

means that the hemoglobin has a high affinity for oxygen, will bind oxygen more avidly, and does not readily give it up whereas decreased oxygen affinity means the hemoglobin has a low affinity for oxygen and releases its oxygen more readily.

Oxyhemoglobin and deoxyhemoglobin have different three-dimensional configurations. In the unliganded or deoxy state, the tetramer is stabilized by intersubunit salt bridges and is described as being in the tense **(T) structure** or state. In oxyhemoglobin, the salt bridges are broken, and the molecule is described as being in the **relaxed (R) structure** state. The change in conformation of hemoglobin (from T to R) occurs as a result of a coordinated series of changes in the quaternary structure of the tetramer as the subunits bind oxygen (see below). The T configuration is a low oxygen-affinity conformation, and the R state is a high oxygen-affinity conformation.

Oxygen affinity of hemoglobin is usually expressed as the PO_2 at which 50% of the hemoglobin is saturated with oxygen (P_{50}). The P_{50} in humans is normally about 26 torr. If hemoglobin-oxygen saturation is plotted versus the partial pressure of oxygen (PO_2), a sigmoid-shaped (S-shaped) curve results. This is referred to as the *oxygen dissociation curve* (*ODC*) (Figure 6-7 ■). The shape of the curve reflects subunit

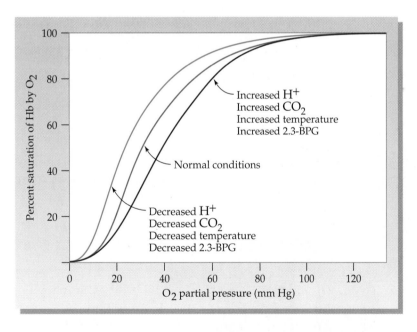

■ FIGURE 6-7   The oxygen affinity of hemoglobin is depicted by the oxygen dissociaton curve (ODC). The fractional saturation of hemoglobin (*Y* axis) is plotted against the concentration of oxygen measured as the PO_2 (*X* axis). At a pH of 7.4 and an oxygen tension (PO_2) of 26 torr hemoglobin is 50% saturated with oxygen (red line). The curve shifts in response to temperature, CO_2, O_2, 2,3-BPG concentration and pH. When the curve shifts left (blue line), there is increased affinity of Hb for O_2. When the curve shifts right (black line), there is decreased affinity of Hb for O_2. (McMurry, John; Castellion, Mary E.; Ballantine, David S., *Fundamentals of General, Organic, and Biological Chemistry*, 5th ed., © 2007. Electronically reproduced by permission of Pearson Education, Inc., Upper Saddle River, New Jersey.)

interactions between the four subunits of hemoglobin (heme-heme interaction or cooperativity). Monomeric molecules such as myoglobin have a hyperbolic ODC. The sigmoid-shaped curve indicates that more than one molecule of O_2 is binding to a molecule of hemoglobin and that binding of one molecule of O_2 to hemoglobin facilitates the binding of additional O_2.

The shape of the curve has certain physiologic advantages. The "flattened" top of the S reflects the fact that >90% saturation of hemoglobin still occurs over a fairly broad range of pO_2. This enables us to survive and function in conditions of lower oxygen availability, such as living (or skiing) at high altitudes. Note that the steepest part of the curve occurs at oxygen tensions found in tissues. This allows the release of large amounts of oxygen from hemoglobin during the small physiologic changes in PO_2 encountered in the capillary beds of tissues. This is physiologically of great importance, for it allows the overall transfer of oxygen from the lungs to the tissues with relatively small changes in PO_2. The ODC shows that the oxygen saturation of hemoglobin drops from ~100% in the arteries where the PO_2 is about 100 torr to ~75% in the veins where the PO_2 is about 40 torr. This indicates that hemoglobin gives up about 25% of

its oxygen to the tissues. When the curve is shifted to the right, the P_{50} is increased, indicating that the oxygen affinity has decreased. This results in the release of more oxygen to the tissues. When the curve is shifted to the left, the P_{50} is decreased, indicating that oxygen affinity has increased. In this case, less oxygen is released to the tissues.

CASE STUDY (continued from page 91)

Jerry was lethargic and pale. He was having problems with activities of daily living.

3. Explain why Jerry could have these symptoms.

The Allosteric Property of Hemoglobin

The sigmoid shape of the ODC is primarily due to heme-heme interactions described below. While the sigmoid shape of the ODC is due to heme-heme subunit interactions, the relative position of the curve (shifted right or left) is due to other variables.

Hemoglobin is an allosteric protein. This means that hemoglobin's structure (conformation) and function are affected by other molecules, primarily 2,3-bisphosphoglycer-

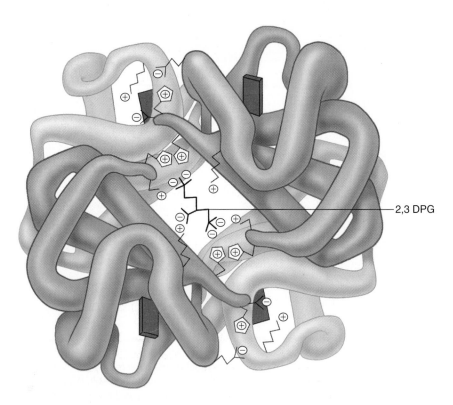

2,3 DPG

■ FIGURE 6-8   2,3 BPG binds in the central cavity of deoxyhemoglobin. This cavity is lined with positively charged groups on the beta chains that interact electrostatically with the negative charges on 2,3-BPG. The α-globin chains are in pink, the β-chains are in blue and the heme prosthetic groups in red. (Horton, Robert; Moran, Laurence A.; Scrimgeour, Gary; Perry, Mark; Rawn, David, *Principles of Biochemistry,* 4th ed., © 2006. Electronically reproduced by permission of Pearson Education, Inc., Upper Saddle River, New Jersey.)

ate (2,3-BPG; also referred to as diphosphoglycerate [2,3-DPG]) known as the *allosteric regulator*. A byproduct of the glycolytic pathway, 2,3-BPG, is present at almost equimolar quantities with hemoglobin in erythrocytes. In the presence of physiologic concentrations of 2,3-BPG, the P_{50} of hemoglobin is about 26 torr. In the absence of 2,3-BPG, the P_{50} of hemoglobin is 10 torr, a very high oxygen affinity. Thus, in the absence of 2,3-BPG, little oxygen is released to the tissues.

Protons (H^+), CO_2, and organic phosphates (2,3-BPG) are all allosteric effectors of hemoglobin, which preferentially bind to deoxyhemoglobin, forming salt bridges within and between chains and stabilizing the deoxyhemoglobin (T) structure. 2,3-BPG binds to deoxyhemoglobin in a 1:1 ratio. The binding site for 2,3-BPG is in a central cavity of the hemoglobin tetramer structure between the β-globin chains. It binds to the positive charges on both β-chains, thereby crosslinking the chains and stabilizing the quaternary structure of T/deoxyhemoglobin. (Figure 6-8 ■)

Hemoglobin also binds oxygen allosterically. Oxygen binds to hemoglobin in a 4:1 ratio because one molecule of O_2 binds to each of the 4 heme portions of the tetramer. The binding of oxygen by a hemoglobin molecule depends on the interaction of the four heme groups, referred to as *heme-heme interaction*. The interaction of the heme groups is the result of movements within the tetramer triggered by the uptake of a molecule of oxygen by one of the heme groups.

In the deoxygenated state, the heme iron is 0.4–0.6Å out of the plane of the porphyrin ring because the iron atom is too large to align within the plane. The iron is displaced toward the proximal histidine of the globin chain to which it is linked by a coordinate bond. Fully deoxygenated hemoglobin (T state) has a low oxygen affinity, and loading of the first oxygen onto the tetramer does not occur easily. On binding of oxygen, the atomic diameter of iron becomes smaller due to changes in the distribution of electrons, and the iron moves into the plane of the porphyrin ring, pulling the histidine of the globin chain with it (Figure 6-9 ■). These small changes in the tertiary structure of the molecule near the heme group result in a large shift in the quaternary structure, altering the bonds and contacts between chains and weakening the intersubunit salt bridges. Likewise, loading of a second O_2 onto the tetramer while it is still in the T conformation does not occur easily. However, the iron atom of the second heme is likewise shifted, further destabilizing the salt bridges. During the course of loading the third O_2 onto

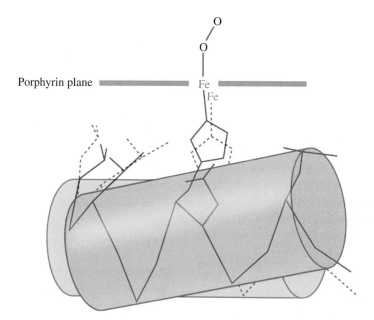

■ **FIGURE 6-9** Changes in the conformation of hemoglobin occur when the molecule takes up O_2. In the deoxyhemoglobin state, the heme iron of a hemoglobin subunit is below the porphyrin plane (blue). On uptake of an O_2 molecule, the iron decreases in diameter and moves into the plane of the porphyrin ring, pulling the proximal histidine with it (red). The helix containing the histidine also shifts disrupting ion pairs that link the subunits. 2,3-BPG is expelled, and the remaining subunits are able to combine with O_2 more readily. (Horton, Robert; Moran, Laurence A.; Scrimgeour, Gary; Perry, Marc; Rawn, David. *Principles of Biochemistry*, 4th ed., © 2006. Electronically reproduced by permission of Pearson Education, Inc., Upper Saddle River, New Jersey.)

hemoglobin, the salt bridges are broken, and the hemoglobin molecule shifts from the T to the R configuration, pulling the β-chains together. Consequently, the size of the central cavity between the β-chains decreases, and 2,3-BPG is expelled. In the high oxygen–affinity R configuration, the third and fourth O_2 are added easily. The structural changes within successive heme subunits facilitate the binding of oxygen by the remaining heme subunits because fewer subunit crosslinks need to be broken to bind subsequent oxygen molecules.

Oxygen interacts weakly with heme iron, and the two can dissociate easily. As O_2 is released by hemoglobin in the tissues, the heme pockets narrow and restrict entry of O_2 while the space between the β-chains widens and 2,3-BPG binds again in the central cavity. Thus, as 2,3-BPG concentration increases, the T configuration of hemoglobin is favored and the oxygen affinity decreases.

This cooperative binding of oxygen makes hemoglobin a very efficient oxygen transporter. Cooperativity ensures that once a hemoglobin tetramer begins to accept oxygen, it promptly is fully oxygenated. In the process of oxygen release to the tissues, the same general principle is followed. Individual hemoglobin molecules are either fully deoxygenated or fully oxygenated. Only a small portion of the molecules exists in a partially oxygenated state.

Adjustments in Hemoglobin-Oxygen Affinity

Variations in environmental conditions or physiological demand for oxygen result in changes in erythrocyte and plasma parameters that directly affect hemoglobin-oxygen affinity. In particular, PO_2, pH (H^+), PCO_2, 2,3-BPG, and temperature affect hemoglobin-oxygen affinity (Table 6-3 ⚙).

Several physiologic mechanisms of oxygen delivery can be explained by the hemoglobin–2,3-BPG interaction. When a person goes from sea level to high altitudes, the body adapts to the decreased atmospheric pressure of oxygen by releasing more oxygen to the tissues. This adaptation is mediated by increases of 2,3-BPG in the erythrocyte, usually noted within 36 hours of ascent. EPO and erythrocyte mass also increase as a part of the adaptive mechanism to decreased PO_2, but this adaptation can take several days to improve tissue oxygenation.[9]

Fetal hemoglobin (HbF) has a higher oxygen affinity compared to adult hemoglobin, HbA. Fetal blood's higher oxygen affinity is primarily due to the fact that hemoglobin F does not readily bind 2,3-BPG. The more efficient binding of 2,3-BPG to HbA facilitates the transfer of oxygen from the maternal (HbA) to the fetal (HbF) circulation.

Rapidly metabolizing tissue as occurs during exercise produces CO_2 and acid (H^+) as well as heat. These factors decrease oxygen affinity and promote the release of oxygen from hemoglobin to the tissue. However, in the alveolar capillaries of the lungs, the high PO_2 and low PCO_2 drives off the CO_2 in the blood and reduces H^+ concentration, promoting the uptake of O_2 by hemoglobin (increasing oxygen affinity). Thus, PO_2, PCO_2, and H^+ facilitate the transport and exchange of respiratory gases.

The effect of pH on hemoglobin-oxygen affinity is known as the **Bohr effect**, an example of the acid-base equilibrium of hemoglobin that is one of the most important buffer systems of the body. A molecule of hemoglobin can accept H^+ when it releases a molecule of oxygen. Deoxyhemoglobin accepts and holds the H^+ better than oxyhemoglobin. In the tissues, the H^+ concentration is higher because of the presence of lactic acid and CO_2. When blood reaches the tissues, the affinity of hemoglobin for oxygen is decreased by the high H^+ concentration, thereby permitting the more efficient unloading of oxygen at these sites.

$$Hb(O_2) + H^+ \rightarrow HHb + O_2$$

Thus, proton binding facilitates O_2 release and helps minimize changes in the hydrogen ion concentration of the blood when tissue metabolism is releasing CO_2 and lactic acid. Up to 75% of the hemoglobin oxygen can be released if needed (as in strenuous exercise) as the erythrocytes pass through the capillaries.

✓ Checkpoint! 5

What factors influence an increase in the amount of oxygen delivered to tissue during an aerobic workout?

CARBON DIOXIDE TRANSPORT

After diffusing into the blood from the tissues, carbon dioxide is carried to the lungs by three separate mechanisms: dissolution in the plasma, formation of bicarbonic acid, and binding to the N-terminus groups of hemoglobin (carbaminohemoglobin) (Table 6-4 ⚙; Figure 6-10).

Plasma Transport

A small amount of carbon dioxide is dissolved in the plasma and carried to the lungs. There it diffuses out of the plasma and is expired.

Bicarbonic Acid

Most of the carbon dioxide transported by the blood is in the form of bicarbonic acid, which is produced when carbon dioxide diffuses from the plasma into the erythrocyte. In the

---

⚙ TABLE 6-3

Factors That Affect Oxygen-Hemoglobin Affinity	
Increase Affinity	Decrease Affinity
↑ O_2	↑ CO_2
↓ CO_2	↑ H^+
↓ H^+	↑ Temperature
↓ Temperature	↑ 2,3-BPG
↓ 2,3-BPG	

Key: ↑ = increased

⊛ TABLE 6-4

Carbon Dioxide Transport in Blood

Mechanism	Percent of Transportation
Dissolved in plasma	7
Formation of carbonic acid, H_2CO_3	70
Bound to Hb	23

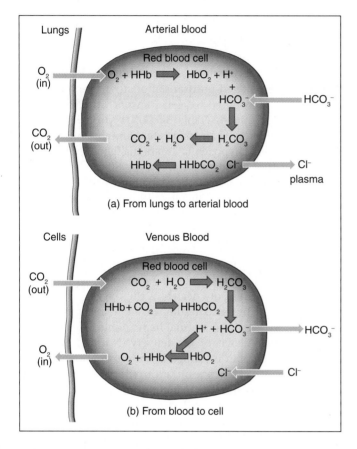

(a) From lungs to arterial blood

(b) From blood to cell

■ **FIGURE 6-10** Transport of oxygen and carbon dioxide in the erythrocyte is depicted. Lower figure: CO_2 diffuses from the tissue into the venous blood and then into the erythrocyte. Within the erythrocyte, CO_2 reacts with water to form bicarbonic acid, H_2CO_3. The bicarbonic acid dissociates into bicarbonate (HCO_3^-) and a proton (H^+). The HCO_3^- leaves the cell and enters the blood. In exchange, chloride (Cl^-) from the blood enters the erythrocyte (chloride shift). The proton is accepted by oxyhemoglobin (HbO_2), which facilitates through the Bohr effect the dissociation of oxygen into the tissues. Upper figure: In the lungs, O_2 and HCO_3^- enter the red cell. O_2 combines with Hb, releasing H^+. HCO_3^- combines with H^+ to form H_2CO_3, which dissociates into H_2O and CO_2, and are expired. To maintain electrolyte balance, at the same time that the HCO_3^- flows into the RBCs, the Cl^- flows out (the reverse chloride shift). The cell membrane anion-exchange protein controls this ion exchange. (Sackheim, George I.; Lehman, Dennis D. *Chemistry for the Health Sciences,* 8th ed., © 1998. Electronically reproduced by permission of Pearson Education, Inc., Upper Saddle River, New Jersey.)

presence of the erythrocyte enzyme, carbonic anhydrase (CA), CO_2 reacts with water to form bicarbonic acid:

$$H_2O + CO_2 \xleftarrow{} CA \xrightarrow{} H_2CO_3$$

Subsequently, hydrogen ion and bicarbonate are liberated from carbonic acid and the H^+ is accepted by deoxyhemoglobin:

$$H_2CO_3 \xleftarrow{} CA \xrightarrow{} H^+ + HCO_3^-$$

These bicarbonate ions do not remain in the RBC because the cell can hold only a small amount of bicarbonate. Thus, the free bicarbonate diffuses out of the erythrocyte into the plasma. The cell cannot tolerate a loss in negative ions, so in exchange for the loss of bicarbonate, Cl^- diffuses into the cell from the plasma, a phenomenon called the **chloride shift**. This occurs via the anion exchange channel (band 3). The bicarbonate combines with Na^+ ($NaHCO_3$) in the plasma and is carried to the lungs where the PCO_2 is low. There the bicarbonate diffuses back into the erythrocyte, is rapidly converted back into CO_2 and H_2O, and expired.

Hemoglobin Binding

Approximately 23% of the total CO_2 exchanged by the erythrocyte in respiration is through carbaminohemoglobin. Deoxyhemoglobin directly binds 0.4 moles of CO_2 per mole of hemoglobin. Carbon dioxide reacts with uncharged N-terminal amino groups of the four globin chains to form carbaminohemoglobin. At the lungs, the plasma PCO_2 decreases, and the CO_2 bound to hemoglobin is released and diffuses out of the erythrocyte to the plasma. It then is expired as it enters the alveolar air space.

ⓔ CASE STUDY *(continued from page 94)*

After a week at home, Jerry called his doctor, who sent him back to the hospital where he was given 2 units of packed red cells. Within a day, he had more energy.

4. Explain why Jerry could have had more energy after the transfusions.

NITRIC OXIDE AND HEMOGLOBIN

Nitric oxide (NO) is produced in the endothelium by the action of NO synthase. NO derives its name as the endothelium-derived relaxing factor (EDRF) due to its ability to relax smooth muscle and dilate blood vessels.[10] It is important in other aspects of normal vessel physiology as well as inhibition of platelet activation. Some NO diffuses into the blood from the endothelium where it reacts with hemoglobin and other plasma molecules. Reaction of oxyhemoglobin with NO destroys the NO and forms methemoglobin and nitrate. This is referred to as *dioxygenation.*

$$HbO_2 + NO \rightarrow MetHb + NO_3^-$$

This reaction is responsible for complications such as vasoconstriction and increase of blood pressure due to loss of NO that are encountered when using artificial hemoglobin-based oxygen carriers in solution.

NO also reacts with deoxyhemoglobin to form iron-nitrosyl hemoglobin (HbNO) and with the cysteine at position 93 of the β-chain to form S-nitroso hemoglobin. It has been proposed that these later two reactions could serve to preserve NO by acting as a carrier of NO in the circulation and later reversing the reaction, releasing NO.[10,11] The rate of reaction of NO with hemoglobin within the erythrocyte is decreased by a factor of at least 1000 from the rate of reaction with free hemoglobin because of the slow diffusion of NO through the RBC membrane and the laminar blood flow that pushes the erythrocytes inward away from the vessel endothelium where the NO is concentrated.[11]

ARTIFICIAL OXYGEN CARRIERS

Efforts to reduce allogeneic blood transfusions and improve oxygen delivery to tissues have resulted in development of **artificial oxygen carriers** (AOCs). Two groups of AOCs include hemoglobin-based oxygen carriers (HBOCs) in solution and perfluorocarbons (PFCs). The HBOCs consist of purified human or bovine hemoglobin and recombinant hemoglobin. The hemoglobin is altered chemically or genetically or is microencapsulated to decrease oxygen affinity and to prevent its breakdown into dimers that have significant nephrotic toxicity.[12] The oxygen dissociation curve of HBOCs is similar to that of native human blood. Side effects of these AOCs are Hb-induced vasoconstriction and resulting hypertension. These side effects are related to NO scavenging by the free hemoglobin as well as endothelin release and sensitization of peripheral adrenergic receptors.[13] Because hemoglobin in solution imparts color to plasma, it might not be possible to perform laboratory tests based on colorimetric analysis of patients receiving this product because measurements could give erroneous results.

PFCs are fluorinated hydrocarbons with high gas-dissolving capacity. They do not mix in aqueous solution and must be emulsified. In contrast to HBOCs, a linear relationship between pO_2 and oxygen content in PFCs exists. This means that relatively high O_2 partial pressure is required to maximize delivery of O_2 by PFCs. The PFC droplets are taken up by the mononuclear-phagocyte (MNP) system, broken down, bound to blood lipids, transported to the lungs, and exhaled.[13]

AOCs are not approved for use in the United States although HBOCs are approved for compassionate use.[13] Phase III trials are complete or in progress for HBOCs, but no trials are in place for PFCs.

► ACQUIRED NONFUNCTIONAL HEMOGLOBINS

The acquired, nonfunctional hemoglobins are hemoglobins that have been altered posttranslationally to produce molecules with compromised oxygen transport, thereby causing *hypoxia* and/or *cyanosis* (Table 6-5 ✪). **Hypoxia** is a condition in which there is an inadequate amount of oxygen at the tissue level. (Hypoxemia is an inadequate amount of oxygen in the blood, arterial $PO_2 < 80$ torr.) **Cyanosis** refers to a bluish color of the skin due to the presence of more than 5 g/dL of deoxyhemoglobin in the blood.

METHEMOGLOBIN

Methemoglobin is hemoglobin with iron in the ferric (Fe^{+++}) state. It is incapable of combining with oxygen. Methemoglobin not only decreases the oxygen-carrying capacity of blood but also results in an increase in oxygen affinity of the remaining normal hemoglobin. This results in an even higher deficit of O_2 delivery. Normally less than 1.5% methemoglobin is formed by auto-oxidation of hemoglobin per day. At this concentration, the abnormal pigment is not harmful because the reduction in oxygen-carrying capacity of the blood is insignificant. Several reducing systems hold the accumulation of higher concentrations in control (Table 6-6 ✪). Of these reducing systems, the most important, accounting for more than 60% of the reduction of methemoglobin, is NADH methemoglobin reductase.

Increased levels of methemoglobin are formed when an individual is exposed to certain oxidizing chemicals or drugs. Even small amounts of these chemicals and drugs can

✪ TABLE 6-5

Abnormal Acquired Hemoglobins

Hemoglobin	Acquired Change	Abnormal Function	Lab Detection
Methemoglobin	Hb iron in ferric state	Cannot combine with oxygen	Demonstration of maximal absorption band at wavelength of 630 nm; chocolate color blood
Sulfhemoglobin	Sulfur combined with hemoglobin	$\frac{1}{100}$ oxygen affinity of HbA	Absorption band at 620 nm
Carboxyhemoglobin	Carbon monoxide combined with hemoglobin	Affinity for carbon monoxide is 200 times higher than for oxygen	Absorption band at 541 nm

TABLE 6-6

Erythrocyte Systems Responsible for Methemoglobin Reduction

Rank in Order of Decreasing Methemoglobin Reduction	System
First	NADH methemoglobin reductase (also known as *cytochrome b5 methemoglobin reductase, diaphorase I, DPNH-diaphorase, DPNH dehydrogenase I, NADH dehydrogenase, NADH methemoglobin-ferrocyanide reductase*)
Second	Ascorbic acid
Third	Glutathione
Fourth	NADPH methemoglobin reductase

cause oxidation of large amounts of hemoglobin. If the offending agent is removed, methemoglobinemia disappears within 24–48 hours.

Infants are more susceptible to methemoglobin production than adults because HbF is more readily converted to methemoglobin and because infants' erythrocytes are deficient in reducing enzymes. Exposure to certain drugs or chemicals that increase oxidation of hemoglobin or water high in nitrates can cause methemoglobinemia in the infant segment of the population. Color crayons containing aniline can cause methemoglobinemia if ingested.

Cyanosis develops when methemoglobin levels exceed 10% (more than 1.5 g/dL) while hypoxia is produced at levels exceeding 30–40%. Methemoglobin can be reduced by medical treatment with methylene blue or ascorbic acid, which speeds up reduction by NADPH-reducing enzymes. In some cases of severe methemoglobinemia, exchange transfusions are helpful.

Methemoglobinemia can also result from congenital defects in the reducing systems mentioned above or from an inherited hemoglobin variant, HbM (Table 6-7 ☺). A deficiency or abnormality of NADH methemoglobin reductase causes the most severe methemoglobinemia. In this condition, cyanosis is observed from birth, and methemoglobin levels reach 10–20%. The oxygen affinity of normal hemo-

globin is increased in these children, resulting in increased erythropoiesis and subsequently higher than normal hemoglobin levels. The hereditary structural hemoglobin variant, HbM, also results in methemoglobinemia. HbM is characterized by amino acid substitutions in the globin chains near the heme pocket that stabilize the iron in the oxidized, Fe^{+++}, state. Methemoglobinemia caused by these hereditary defects cannot be reduced by treatment with methylene blue or ascorbic acid. However, even in the homozygous state, individuals with HbM or defects in the reducing systems rarely have methemoglobin levels of more than 30% and are usually asymptomatic.

Laboratory diagnosis of methemoglobinemia involves demonstration of a maximum absorbance band at a wavelength of 630 nm at pH 7.0–7.4. The blood sample can be chocolate brown in color when compared to a normal blood specimen. Differentiation of acquired types from hereditary types of methemoglobin requires assay of NADH methemoglobin reductase and hemoglobin electrophoresis (Table 6-7). Enzyme activity is reduced only in hereditary NADH-methemoglobin reductase deficiency, and hemoglobin electrophoresis is abnormal only in HbM disease. The acquired types of methemoglobinemia show normal enzyme activity and a normal electrophoresis pattern.

In the presence of methemoglobinemia, oxygen saturation obtained by a cutaneous pulse oximeter (fractional oxyhemoglobin, $FhbO_2$) can be lower than the oxygen saturation reported from a blood–gas analysis. This is so because $FhbO_2$ is calculated as the amount of oxyhemoglobin compared to the total hemoglobin (oxyhemoglobin, deoxyhemoglobin, methemoglobin, and other inactive hemoglobin forms) whereas oxygen saturation in a blood–gas analysis is the amount of oxyhemoglobin compared to the total amount of hemoglobin able to combine with oxygen (oxyhemoglobin plus deoxyhemoglobin). $FhbO_2$ and oxygen saturation are the same if no abnormal hemoglobin is present.[14]

Sulfhemoglobin

Sulfhemoglobin is a stable compound formed when a sulfur atom combines with the heme group of hemoglobin. The sulfur atom binds to a pyrrole carbon at the periphery of the porphyrin ring. Sulfuration of heme groups results in a drastically right-shifted oxygenation dissociation curve,

TABLE 6-7

Differentiation of Types of Methemoglobinemia

Cause of Methemoglobinemia	Inherited/Acquired	Enzyme Activity	Hb Electrophoresis
Exposure to oxidants	Acquired	Normal	Normal
Decreased enzyme activity	Inherited	Decreased	Normal
Presence of hemoglobin M	Inherited	Normal	Abnormal

which renders the heme groups ineffective for oxygen transport. This effect appears to be due to the fact that even half-sulfurated, half-oxygen–liganded tetramers exist in the T configuration (the low oxygen-affinity form) of hemoglobin. Although the heme iron is in the ferrous state, sulfhemoglobin binds to oxygen with an affinity only one-hundredth that of normal hemoglobin. Thus, oxygen delivery to the tissues can be compromised if there is an increase in this abnormal hemoglobin. The bright green sulfhemoglobin compound is so stable that the erythrocyte carries it until the cell is removed from circulation. Ascorbic acid or methylene blue cannot reduce it; however, sulfhemoglobin can combine with carbon monoxide to form carboxysulfhemoglobin. Normal levels of sulfhemoglobin do not exceed 2.2%. Cyanosis is produced at levels exceeding 3–4%.

Sulfhemoglobin has been associated with occupational exposure to sulfur compounds, environmental exposure to polluted air, and exposure to certain drugs. Sulfhemoglobinemia is formed during the oxidative denaturation of hemoglobin and can accompany methemoglobinemia, especially in certain drug- or chemical-induced hemoglobinopathies. Sulfhemoglobin is formed on exposure of blood to trinitroluene, acetanilid, phenacetin, and sulfonamides. It also is found to be elevated in severe constipation and in bacteremia with *Clostridium welchii*. Diagnosis of sulfhemoglobinemia is made spectrophotometrically by demonstrating an absorption band at 620 nm. Confirmation testing is done by isoelectric focusing. This is the only abnormal hemoglobin pigment not measured by the cyanmethemoglobin method, which is used to measure hemoglobin concentration.

Carboxyhemoglobin

Carboxyhemoglobin is formed when hemoglobin is exposed to carbon monoxide. Hemoglobin's affinity for carbon monoxide is more than 200 times higher than its affinity for oxygen. Carboxyhemoglobin is incapable of transporting oxygen because CO occupies the same ligand-binding position as O_2. As is the case with methemoglobinemia, carboxyhemoglobin has a great impact on oxygen delivery because it destroys the molecule's cooperativity. CO also has a pronounced effect on the oxygen dissociation curve, shifting it to the left, resulting in increased affinity and a decreased release of O_2 by remaining normal hemoglobin molecules. High levels of carboxyhemoglobin impart a cherry red color to the blood and skin. However, high levels of carboxyhemoglobin with high levels of deoxyhemoglobin can give blood a purple pink color.

Blood normally carries small amounts of carboxyhemoglobin formed from the carbon monoxide produced during heme catabolism. The normal level of carboxyhemoglobin varies depending on individuals' smoking habits and their environment. City dwellers have higher levels than country dwellers due to the carbon monoxide produced from automobiles and industrial pollutants in cities.

Acute carboxyhemoglobinemia causes irreversible tissue damage and death from anoxia. Chronic carboxyhemoglobinemia is accompanied by increased oxygen affinity and polycythemia. In severe cases of carbon monoxide poisoning, patients can be treated in hyperbaric oxygen chambers.

Carboxyhemoglobin is commonly measured in whole blood by a spectrophotometric method. Sodium hydrosulfite reduces hemoglobin to deoxyhemoglobin, and the absorbances of the hemolysate are measured at 555 nm and 541 nm. Carboxyhemoglobin has a greater absorbance at 541 nm.

 Checkpoint! 6

A 2-year-old child was found to have 15% methemoglobin by spectral absorbance at 630 nm. What tests would you suggest to help differentiate whether this is an inherited or acquired methemoglobinemia, and what results would you expect with each diagnosis?

SUMMARY

Hemoglobin is the intracellular protein of erythrocytes responsible for transport of oxygen from the lungs to the tissues. A fine balance between production and destruction of erythrocytes serves to maintain a steady-state concentration.

Hemoglobin is a globular protein composed of four subunits. Each subunit contains a porphyrin ring with an iron molecule (heme) and a globin chain. The four globin chains are arranged in identical pairs, each composed of two different globin chains. Hemoglobin synthesis is controlled by iron concentration within the cell, activity and synthesis of the first enzyme in the heme synthetic pathway, ALAS, activity of PBGD and globin chain synthesis.

The oxygen affinity of hemoglobin depends on PO_2, pH, PCO_2, 2,3-BPG, and temperature. Hemoglobin-oxygen affinity can be graphically depicted by the ODC. When the curve shifts to the right, oxygen affinity decreases; when it shifts to the left, oxygen affinity increases. Increased CO_2, heat, and acid decrease oxygen affinity; high O_2 concentrations increase oxygen affinity.

Hemoglobin is an allosteric protein, which means that hemoglobin structure and function are affected by other molecules. In particular, the uptake of 2,3-BPG or oxygen can cause conformational changes in the molecule. The structure of deoxyhemoglobin is known as the T structure and that of oxyhemoglobin is known as the R structure.

When hemoglobin is exposed to oxidants or other compounds, the molecule can be altered, which compromises its ability to carry oxygen. High concentrations of these abnormal hemoglobins can cause hypoxia and cyanosis, which can be detected by spectrophotometric methods.

REVIEW QUESTIONS

LEVEL I

1. Which of the following types of hemoglobin is the major component of adult hemoglobin? (Objective 4)
   a. HbA
   b. HbF
   c. HbA_2
   d. Hb Portland

2. One of the most important buffer systems of the body is the: (Objective 5)
   a. chloride shift
   b. Bohr effect
   c. heme-heme interaction
   d. ODC

3. When iron is depleted from the developing erythrocyte, the: (Objective 7)
   a. synthesis of heme is increased
   b. activity of ALAS is decreased
   c. formation of globin chains stops
   d. heme synthesis is not affected

4. When the H^+ concentration in blood increases, the oxygen affinity of hemoglobin: (Objective 3)
   a. increases
   b. is unaffected
   c. decreases
   d. cannot be measured

5. Which of the following is the correct molecular structure of hemoglobin? (Objective 1)
   a. four heme groups, two iron, two globin chains
   b. two heme groups, two iron, four globin chains
   c. two heme groups, four iron, four globin chains
   d. four heme groups, four iron, four globin chains

6. 2,3-BPG combines with which type of hemoglobin? (Objectives 3, 5)
   a. oxyhemoglobin
   b. relaxed structure of hemoglobin
   c. deoxyhemoglobin
   d. $\alpha\beta$ dimer

7. During exercise, the oxygen affinity of hemoglobin is: (Objective 3)
   a. increased in males but not females
   b. decreased due to production of heat and lactic acid
   c. unaffected in those who are physically fit
   d. affected only if the duration is more than 1 hour

8. Which of the following hemoglobins is *not* normally found in adults? (Objective 4)
   a. hemoglobin A
   b. hemoglobin A_2
   c. hemoglobin F
   d. hemoglobin Portland

LEVEL II

1. Which of the following hemoglobins is *not* found in the normal adult? (Objective 2)
   a. $\alpha_2\beta_2$
   b. $\alpha_2\gamma_2$
   c. $\alpha_2\delta_2$
   d. $\alpha_2\varepsilon_2$

2. Which of the following is the major hemoglobin in the newborn? (Objective 2)
   a. $\alpha_2\beta_2$
   b. $\alpha_2\gamma_2$
   c. $\alpha_2\delta_2$
   d. $\alpha_2\varepsilon_2$

3. A 2-year-old child was found to have 15% methemoglobin by spectral absorbance at 630 nm. What test would you suggest to help differentiate whether this is an inherited or acquired state? (Objective 6)
   a. hemoglobin electrophoresis and NADPH reductase determination
   b. bone marrow aspiration and examination
   c. haptoglobin and sulfhemoglobin determination
   d. glycosylated hemoglobin measurement by column chromatography

4. A 25-year-old male was found unconscious in a car with the motor running. Blood was drawn and sent to the chemistry lab for spectral analysis. The blood was cherry red in color. What hemoglobin should be tested for? (Objective 6)
   a. sulfhemoglobin
   b. methemoglobin
   c. carboxyhemoglobin
   d. oxyhemoglobin

5. The oxygen dissociation curve in a case of chronic carboxyhemoglobin poisoning would show: (Objective 7)
   a. a shift to the right
   b. a shift to the left
   c. a normal curve
   d. decreased oxygen affinity

6. A college student from Louisiana vacationed in Colorado for spring break. He arrived at Keystone Resort area on the first day. The second day he was nauseated and had a headache. He went to the medical clinic at the resort and was told he had altitude sickness. The doctor told him to rest for another 24 hours before participating in any activities. What is the most likely reason he will overcome this condition in the next 24 hours? (Objective 4)
   a. His level of HbF will increase to help release more oxygen to the tissues.
   b. The amount of carboxyhemoglobin will decrease to normal levels.
   c. The levels of ATP in his blood will reach maximal levels.
   d. The level of 2,3-BPG will increase and, in turn, decrease oxygen affinity.

REVIEW QUESTIONS *(continued)*

LEVEL I

9. Which of the following is considered a normal hemoglobin concentration in an adult male? (Objective 6)
   a. 11.0 g/dL
   b. 21.0 g/dL
   c. 15.0 g/dL
   d. 9.0 g/dL

10. Which of the following plays an important role in hemoglobin-oxygen affinity? (Objective 3)
    a. 2,3-BPG
    b. NADPH reductase
    c. $NaHCO_3$
    d. Cl^-

LEVEL II

7. When iron in the cell is replete, the translation of ferritin mRNA is: (Objective 3)
   a. decreased
   b. increased
   c. unaffected
   d. variable

8. An aerobics instructor just finished an hour of instruction. Blood is drawn from her for a research study and the oxygen dissociation is measured. What would you expect to find? (Objective 4)
   a. a shift to the left
   b. a shift to the right
   c. no shift
   d. an increased oxygen affinity

9. In the lungs, a hemoglobin molecule takes up two oxygen molecules. What effect will this have on the hemoglobin molecule? (Objectives 5, 8)
   a. It will increase oxygen affinity.
   b. It will narrow the heme pockets blocking entry of additional oxygen.
   c. The hemoglobin molecule will take on the tense structure.
   d. The center cavity will expand, and 2,3-BPG will enter.

10. A patient with emphysema would be expected to have (Objective 4):
    a. increased blood pH
    b. decreased blood pH
    c. increased oxygen affinity
    d. decreased 2,3-BPG level

www.pearsonhighered.com/mckenzie

Use this address to access the interactive Companion Website created for this textbook. Find additional information, tables and figures. Evaluate your command of the chapter information using case studies and critical thinking and multiple choice questions.

REFERENCES

1. Horton HR, Moran LA, Scrimgeour KG, Perry MD, Rawn JD. Proteins: Three-dimensional structure and function. In: *Principles of Biochemistry*, 4th ed. New Jersey: Prentice-Hall; 2006:84–128.

2. Ferreira GC, Gong J. 5-aminolevulinate synthase and the first step of heme biosynthesis. *J Bioenerg Biomembr*. 1995;27:151–59.

3. Rouault TA. The role of iron regulatory proteins in mammalian iron homeostasis and disease. *Nature Chem Biol*. 2006;2(8):406–14.

4. Klausner RD, Rouault TA, Harford JB. Regulating the fate of mRNA: The control of cellular iron metabolism. *Cell*. 1993;72:19–28.

5. Kawasaki N, Morimoto K, Tanimoto T, Hayakawa T. Control of hemoglobin synthesis in erythroid differentiating K562 cells. I. Role of iron in erythroid cell heme synthesis. *Arch Biochem Biophys*. 1996;328:289–94.

6. Kawasaki N, Morimoto K, Hayakawa T. Control of hemoglobin synthesis in erythroid differentiating K562 cells. II. Studies of iron mo-

bilization in erythroid cells by high-performance liquid chromatography-electrochemical detection. *J Chromatogr B Biomed Sci Appl*. 1998;705:193–201.

7. Peschle C, Migliaccio AR, Migliaccio G, Lettieri F, Maguire YP, Condorelli M et al. Regulation of Hb synthesis in ontogenesis and erythropoietic differentiation: In vitro studies on fetal liver, cord blood, normal adult blood or marrow, and blood from HPFH patients. In: Stamatoyannopoulos G, Nienhuis AW, eds. *Hemoglobins in Development and Differentiation*. New York: Alan R. Liss; 1980: 359–71.

8. Papayannopoulou T, Nakamoto B, Agostinelli F, Manna M, Lucarelli G, Stamatoyannopoulos G et al. Fetal to adult hemopoietic cell transplantation in humans: Insights into hemoglobin switching. *Blood*. 1986;67:99–104.

9. Boning D, Maassen N, Jochum F, Steinacker J, Halder A, Thomas A et al. Aftereffects of a high altitude expedition on blood. *Int J Sports Med.* 1997;18:179–85.

10. Schechter AN, Gladwin MT. Hemoglobin and the paracrine and endocrine functions of nitric oxide. *N Engl J Med.* 2003;348(15): 1483–85.

11. Kim-Shapiro DB, Schechter AN, Gladwin MT. Unraveling the reactions of nitric oxide, nitrite, and hemoglobin in physiology and therapeutics. *Arterioscler Thromb Vasc Biol.* 2006;26:697–705.

12. Henkel-Hanke T, Oleck M. Artificial oxygen carriers: A current view. *AANA Journal.* 2007;75(3):205–11.

13. Spahn DR. Blood substitutes artificial oxygen carriers: Perfluorocarbon emulsions. *Crit Care.* 1999;3:R93–97.

14. Wentworth P, Roy M, Wilson B, Padusenko J, Smeaton A, Burchell N. Clinical pathology rounds: Toxic methemoglobinemia in a 2-year-old child. *Lab Med.* 1999;30:311–15.

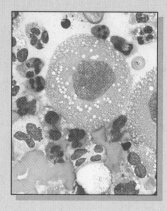

CHAPTER OUTLINE

7

The Leukocyte

Rebecca J. Laudicina, Ph.D.
Yasmen Simonian, Ph.D.

■ OBJECTIVES—LEVEL I

At the end of this unit of study, the student should be able to:

1. Identify terms associated with increases and decreases in leukocytes.
2. Differentiate morphologically the leukocyte precursors found in the proliferative compartment of the bone marrow.
3. Compare and contrast the development including distinguishing maturation and cell features of the granulocytic, monocytic-macrophage, and lymphocytic cell lineages.
4. Compare and contrast the morphologic and other distinguishing cell features of each of the leukocytes found in the peripheral blood.
5. Compare and contrast the function of each of the leukocytes found in the peripheral blood.
6. Summarize the process of neutrophil migration and phagocytosis.
7. List the adult reference ranges for the leukocytes found in the peripheral blood.
8. Calculate absolute cell counts from data provided.
9. Differentiate absolute values and relative values of cell count data.
10. List causes/conditions that increase or decrease absolute numbers of individual leukocytes found in the peripheral blood.
11. Compare and contrast pediatric and newborn reference ranges and adult reference ranges.
12. Explain immunoglobulin diversity.

■ OBJECTIVES—LEVEL II

At the end of this unit of study, the student should be able to:

1. Summarize the kinetics of the granulocytic, monocytic-macrophage, and lymphocytic cell lineages.
2. Describe the processes that permit neutrophils to leave the peripheral blood circulation and move to a site of infection and propose how defects in these processes affect the body's defense mechanism.
3. Compare and contrast the immunologic features and functions of each of the leukocytes found in the peripheral blood.
4. Summarize lymphocyte membrane characteristics and molecular changes used to differentiate subtypes.
5. Differentiate between polyclonal and monoclonal antibodies and discuss each type in relationship to a patient's clinical condition.

■ OBJECTIVES—LEVEL II *(continued)*

6. Compare and discriminate morphological features of Russell bodies, Mott cells, and flame cells.

7. Design systems to evaluate laboratory data of leukocytes for error detection.

8. Formulate pathways to correlate laboratory data of leukocytes with clinical knowledge of the patient.

KEY TERMS

Adaptive immune response
Agranulocytosis
Antigen-presenting cells (APC)
Azurophilic granules
Barr body (drumstick)
B cell receptor (BCR)
Charcot-Leyden crystals
Cell-mediated immunity
Chemokines
Chemotaxis
Degranulation
Diapedesis
Drumstick (Barr body)
Dutcher bodies
Erythrophagocytosis
Flame cell
Granulocytosis
Humoral immunity
Immune response (IR)
Immunoblast
Immunoglobulin
Innate immune response
Large granular lymphocyte (LGL)
Leukocytosis
Leukopenia
Memory cell
Monoclonal gammopathies
Monocyte-macrophage system
Mononuclear phagocyte (MNP) system
Mott cell
Natural killer (NK) cell
Neutrophilia
Neutropenia
Pathogen-associated molecular pattern (PAMP)
Pattern recognition receptors (PRR)
Phagocytosis
Plasma cell
Plasmacytoid lymphocyte
Reactive lymphocyte
Russell bodies
T cell receptor (TCR)

BACKGROUND BASICS

In addition to the basics from previous chapters, it is helpful to have a basic understanding of immunology (immune system and function), biochemistry (proteins, carbohydrates, and lipids), algebra, the use of percentages, ratios and proportions, and the metric system.

To maximize your learning experience, you should review these concepts from previous chapters before starting this unit of study:

Level I

▶ Identify components of the cell and describe their function. (Chapter 2)

▶ Summarize the function of growth factors and the hierarchy of hematopoiesis. (Chapter 3)

▶ Describe the structure and function of the hematopoietic organs. (Chapter 4)

Level II

▶ List the growth factors and identify their function in leukocyte differentiation and maturation. (Chapter 3)

CASE STUDY

We will refer to this case study throughout the chapter.

Harry, a 30-year-old male in good physical condition, had a routine physical examination as a requirement for purchasing a life insurance policy. A CBC was ordered with the following results: Hb 15.5 g/dL (155 g/L); hct 47% (0.47 L/L); RBC count 5.2×10^{12}/L; platelet count 175×10^9/L; and WBC count 12×10^9/L. Consider how you could explain these results in a healthy male.

▶ OVERVIEW

Leukocytes develop from the pluripotential hematopoietic stem cell in the bone marrow. They are involved in the defense against foreign pathogens or antigens. In the presence of infection or inflammation, the number of these cells can increase and can show morphologic changes. Thus, an important screening test for a wide variety of conditions is the leukocyte (WBC) count. This chapter is a study of the normal differentiation and maturation of leukocytes. Each type of leukocyte is discussed including cell morphology, concentration, and function. Because of the length of the chapter, it is divided into two parts: Part I includes the granulocytes and monocytes, and Part II covers lymphocytes. The lymphocyte section is divided into T, B, and NK cell development and function. The synthesis and structure of immunoglobulins, lymphocyte receptors, and cell antigens are described with attention to the use of these markers in identifying lymphocyte types.

▶ INTRODUCTION

Leukocytes (white blood cells, WBC) are essential cellular components of the peripheral blood. With the exception of T lymphocytes, leukocyte precursors differentiate, proliferate, and mature in the bone marrow. Mature leukocytes are released into the peripheral blood where they circulate briefly until they move into the tissues in response to stimulation. They perform their function of host defense primarily in the tissues. The neutrophil, band neutrophil, eosinophil, basophil, monocyte, and lymphocyte are the leukocytes normally found in the peripheral blood of children and adults.

The era of morphologic hematology began in 1877 with Paul Ehrlich's discovery of a triacidic stain.[1] The stain allowed differentiation of leukocytes on fixed blood smears by different staining properties of the components of the cells. Wright stain, a Romanowsky-type stain, is used to stain the cellular components of blood and bone marrow that are smeared on glass slides. Methylene blue and eosin are the major components of the Wright stain. Basic cellular elements react with the acidic dye, eosin, and acidic cellular elements react with the basic dye, methylene blue. The eosinophil contains large amounts of basic protein in its granules, which react with the eosin dye, hence, the name *eosinophil*. The basophil has granules that are acidic and react with the basic dye, methylene blue, hence, the name *basophil*. The neutrophil granules react with both acid and basic components of the stain, giving the cell cytoplasm a neutral to pinkish appearance. The nuclear DNA and cytoplasmic RNA of cells are acidic and pick up the basic stain, methylene blue. Hemoglobin is a basic cellular component of red blood cells and reacts with the acid dye, eosin, and stains orange red to salmon pink. The eosinophil, basophil, and neutrophil are polymorphonuclear and contain many granules and thus are classified as granulocytes. Monocytes and lymphocytes are mononuclear cells and contain small numbers of fine granules or no granules. The monocyte cytoplasm is a bluish gray, and the lymphocyte cytoplasm is sky blue.

Leukocytes were first observed by William Hewson, the father of hematology, in the eighteenth century. In the nineteenth century, the studies of inflammation and bacterial infection intensified interest in leukocytes.[2] Many researchers studied the similarity of pus cells in areas of inflammation and the leukocytes of the blood. Ilya Metchnikov observed the presence of nucleated blood cells surrounding a thorn introduced beneath the skin of a larval starfish.[1]

Many of Ehrlich's observations and Metchnikov's experiments provided the groundwork for understanding the leukocytes as defenders against infection. Ehrlich recognized that variations in numbers of leukocytes accompanied specific pathologic conditions, such as eosinophilia in allergies, parasitic infections, and dermatitis as well as neutrophilia in bacterial infections.

It is now recognized that the leukocyte function of fighting infection includes two separate but interrelated events: phagocytosis (innate immune response) and the development of the adaptive immune response. Granulocytes and monocytes are responsible for phagocytosis while monocytes and lymphocytes interact to produce an effective adaptive immune response. Eosinophils and basophils interact in mediating allergic and hypersensitivity reactions.

▶ LEUKOCYTE CONCENTRATION IN THE PERIPHERAL BLOOD

Leukocytes develop from pluripotential hematopoietic stem cells (HSC) in the bone marrow. On specific hematopoietic growth factor stimulation, the stem cell proliferates and differentiates into the various types of leukocytes: granulocytes (neutrophils, eosinophils, basophils), monocytes, and lymphocytes. On maturation, these cells can be released into the peripheral blood or remain in the bone marrow storage pool until needed.

The total peripheral blood leukocyte count is high at birth, 9–$30 \times 10^9/L$. A few immature granulocytic cells (myelocytes, metamyelocytes) can be seen in the circulation the first few days of life; however, immature leukocytes are not present in the peripheral blood after this age except in certain diseases. Within the first week, the leukocyte count drops to 5–$21 \times 10^9/L$. A gradual decline continues until the age of 8 years at which time the leukocyte concentration averages $8 \times 10^9/L$. The Bogalusa Heart Study found that in children between the ages of 5 and 17, females had, on the average, leukocyte counts $0.5 \times 10^9/L$ higher than males.[3] Adult values average from 4.5 to $11.0 \times 10^9/L$. Although reports on the reference interval for older adults have been conflicting, it is now generally accepted that total leukocyte counts in adults do not decline with age. The concentration of neutrophils and lymphocytes remains constant in the adult years.[4]

Various physiologic and pathological events affect the concentrations of leukocytes. Pregnancy, time of day, and activity level affect the WBC concentration. Infections and immune-regulated responses cause significant changes in leukocytes. Many other pathologic disorders also can cause quantitative and/or qualitative changes in white cells. Considerable heterogeneity in leukocyte concentration has been found among racial, ethnic, and sex subgroups, suggesting the need for unique reference intervals for specific populations.[5]

Thus, when evaluating cell count data, knowing the patient's age, sex, and possibly race/ethnicity as well as previous cell counts on the same patient is helpful. It also is helpful to assess the accuracy of cell counts by correlating them with the patient's clinical history. Additional testing can be done as a result of abnormalities in the WBC count. Changes associated with diseases and disorders will be discussed in subsequent chapters on leukocytes.

 CASE STUDY *(continued from page 105)*

The CBC results on Harry were Hb 15.5 g/dL; Hct 0.47 L/L; RBC count 5.2 × 10^{12}/L; platelet count 175 × 10^9/L; and WBC count 12 × 10^9/L.

1. Are any of these results outside the reference range? If so, which one(s)?

2. If this were a newborn, would you change your evaluation? Why?

An increase or decrease in the total number of leukocytes can be caused by an altered concentration of all leukocyte types or, more commonly, by an alteration in one specific type of leukocyte. For this reason, an abnormal total WBC count should be followed by a leukocyte differential count. A manual leukocyte differential count enumerates each leukocyte type within a total of 100 leukocytes. The differential results are reported as the percentage of each type counted. To accurately interpret whether an increase or decrease in cell types exists, however, it is necessary to calculate the absolute concentration using the results of the WBC count and the differential (relative concentration) in the following manner:

Differential count (in decimal form) × WBC count × (10^9/L) = Absolute cell count × (10^9/L)

The usefulness of this calculation is emphasized in the following example. Each of two different blood specimens had a relative lymphocyte concentration of 60%. The total leukocyte count of one was 3 × 10^9/L and of the other was 9 × 10^9/L. The relative lymphocyte concentration on both specimens appears elevated (reference range is 25%–35%); however, calculation of the absolute concentration (reference range 1.0 to 4.8 × 10^9/L) shows that only one specimen has an absolute increase in lymphocytes; the other is within the reference range:

$$0.6 \times (3 \times 10^9/L) = 1.8 \times 10^9/L \text{ (within reference range)}$$
$$0.6 \times (9 \times 10^9/L) = 5.4 \times 10^9/L \text{ (increased)}$$

The neutrophil is the most numerous leukocyte in the adult peripheral blood, composing 40–80% of total leukocytes (1.8–7 × 10^9/L). At birth, the neutrophil concentration is about 50–60%; this level drops to ~30% by 4–6 months of age. After 4 years of life, the concentration of neutrophils gradually increases until adult values are reached at ~6 years of age. Most peripheral blood neutrophils are mature segmented forms; however, a few nonsegmented forms (bands) (up to 5%) can be seen in normal specimens. Most variations in the total leukocyte count are due to an increase or decrease in neutrophils.

Peripheral blood eosinophil concentrations are maintained at 0–5% (up to 0.4 × 10^9/L) throughout life. It is possible that no eosinophils are seen on a 100-cell differential; however, careful scanning of the entire smear should reveal an occasional eosinophil.

Basophils are the least plentiful cells in the peripheral blood, 0–1% (up to 0.2 × 10^9/L). It is common to find no basophils on a 100-cell differential; the finding of an absolute basophilia, however, is very important because it can indicate the presence of a hematologic malignancy.

Monocytes usually compose 2–10% (0.1–0.8 × 10^9/L) of circulating leukocytes. Occasionally, reactive lymphocytes resemble monocytes, possibly giving even the experienced clinical laboratory scientist difficulty in performing the differential.

The lymphocyte concentration varies with the age of the individual. About 30% of the leukocytes at birth are lymphocytes. This increases to ~60% at about 4–6 months of age and remains at this level until ~4 years of age. Then a gradual decline occurs until a mean level of ~34% at age 21 is reached. The concentration in adults ranges from 25% to 35% (1.0–4.8 × 10^9/L).

► LEUKOCYTE SURFACE MARKERS

Leukocytes as well as other cells express a variety of molecules on their surface. These surface molecules can be used as markers to help identify the lineage of a cell as well as subsets within the lineage. These markers can be identified by reactions with specific monoclonal antibodies. A nomenclature system was developed to identify antibodies with similar characteristics using cluster of differentiation (CD) and a number. The CD designation is now used to identify the molecule recognized by the monoclonal antibody. In addition to using CD markers to identify cell lineage, some surface markers are used to identify stages of maturation as they are transiently expressed at a specific stage of development. Other markers are expressed only after the cell has been stimulated and thus can be used as a marker of cell activation. Cell markers are very helpful in differentiating neoplastic hematologic disorders (∞ Chapter 21). Surface markers can be identified by flow cytometry or cytochemical stains (∞ Chapters 34, 37).

CASE STUDY *(continued from page 107)*

A leukocyte differential was performed with the following results:

Neutrophils	58%
Lymphocytes	32%
Monocytes	6%
Eosinophils	3%
Basophils	1%

3. Are any of the WBC concentrations outside the reference interval (relative or absolute)?

▶ LEUKOCYTE FUNCTION

The leukocytes' primary function is to protect the host from infectious agents or pathogens. The innate system (natural) with the acquired (adaptive) or specific immune system is the body's major defense system. The **innate immune response** (innate IR) is the body's first response to common classes of invading pathogens. When a pathogen enters the body, it must be recognized as foreign (nonself) by soluble proteins (e.g., antibody or complement) and leukocyte cell-surface receptors (FcγR, CR1, CR3) before specific effector mechanisms can eliminate it. The leukocyte receptors that participate in the innate IR are always available and do not require cell activation to be expressed. Other leukocyte receptors recognize structures that are shared by different pathogens or common alterations that the pathogen makes to the body's cells (known as **pathogen-associated molecular patterns [PAMP]**). Examples of PAMP include bacterial lipopolysaccharide, viral RNA and bacterial DNA. Receptors for PAMP are sometimes referred to as **pattern recognition receptors (PRR)**.[6] Once a pathogen has been recognized, effector cells can attack, engulf, and kill it. Neutrophils, monocytes, and macrophages play a major role in the innate immune system. The innate IR is rapid but limited.

The **adaptive immune response** (adaptive IR) is initiated in lymphoid tissue where pathogens encounter lymphocytes, the major cells involved in this response. The lymphocytes recognize antigens on the pathogens (or antigens presented by antigen-presenting cells [APC]) and become activated. During lymphopoiesis, lymphocyte precursor cells are capable of rearranging their antigen receptor genes (immunoglobulin light and heavy chain loci in B cells and T cell receptor polypeptides [αβ- or δγ-loci] in T cells). This results in a subset of mature T and B lymphocytes (effector cells) that express receptors for the specific antigens of various pathogens. Thus, the effector cells mount a highly specialized defense. The successful adaptive IR eliminates the pathogen. This IR is slower to develop than the innate IR, but it provides long-lasting immunity (memory) against the pathogen with which it interacts.

PART I

GRANULOCYTES AND MONOCYTES

▶ NEUTROPHILS

Neutrophils are the most numerous leukocyte in the peripheral blood. They are easily identified on Romanowsky-stained peripheral blood smears as cells with a segmented nucleus and fine pinkish granules.

DIFFERENTIATION, MATURATION, AND MORPHOLOGY

Leukocytes develop from HSC in the bone marrow. The common myeloid progenitor (CMP) cell gives rise to the committed precursor cells for the neutrophilic, eosinophilic, basophilic, and monocytic lineages. The common lymphoid progenitor (CLP) cell gives rise to committed precursor cells for T, B, and natural killer (NK) lymphocytes[7] (∞ Chapter 3). When lineage commitment has occurred, maturation begins. Myeloid, monocytic, and lymphoid elements go through unique maturation processes. The myeloid elements include the granulocytes and their precursors' colony-forming unit—granulocyte monocyte (CFU-GM), colony-forming unit-granulocyte (CFU-G), the monocytic elements including monocytes and their precursors (CFU-GM, colony-forming unit-monocyte [CFU-M]), and the lymphoid elements including the lymphocytes and their precursors (CFU-T/NK, CFU-T, and CFU-B).

Normally, the life span of the neutrophil is spent in three compartments: the bone marrow (site of differentiation, proliferation, and maturation), the peripheral blood (where they circulate for a few hours), and the tissues (where they perform their function of host defense). Neutrophilic production is primarily regulated by three cytokines, interleukin-3, granulocyte monocyte-colony–stimulating factor, and granulocyte-colony–stimulating factor (IL-3, GM-CSF, G-CSF). GM-CSF and G-CSF also regulate survival and functional activity of mature neutrophils. The neutrophil undergoes six morphologically identifiable stages in the process of maturation. The stages from the first morphologically identifiable cell to the mature segmented neutrophil include (1) myeloblast, (2) promyelocyte, (3) myelocyte, (4) metamyelocyte, (5) band or unsegmented neutrophil, and (6) segmented neutrophil or polymorphonuclear neutrophil (PMN).

During the maturation process, obvious progressive changes occur in the nucleus. The nucleoli disappear, the chromatin condenses, and the once round nuclear mass indents and eventually segments. These nuclear changes are accompanied by distinct cytoplasmic changes. The scanty, agranular, basophilic cytoplasm of the earliest stage is gradually replaced by pink-to- neutral-staining granular cytoplasm in the mature differentiated stage (Figures 7-1 ■ and 7-2 ■, Table 7-1 ✪). There

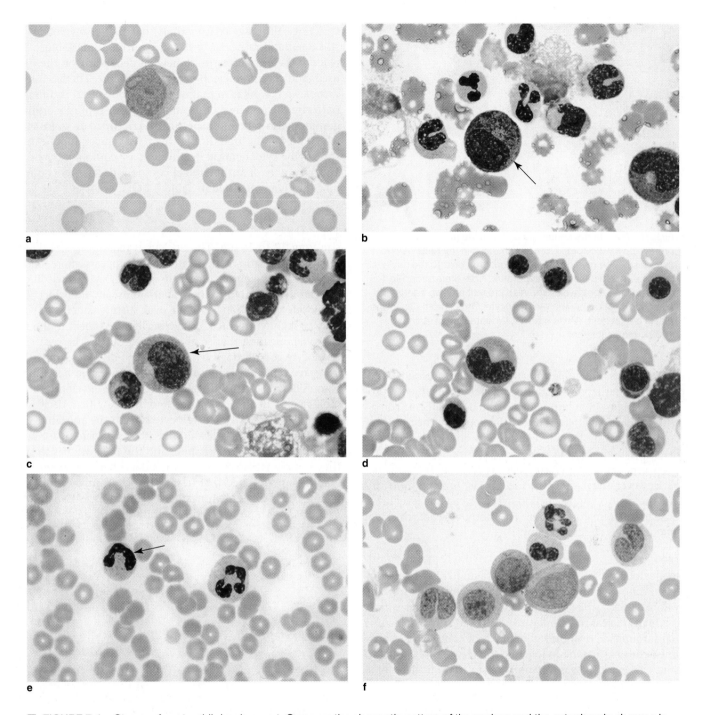

■ FIGURE 7-1   Stages of neutrophil development. Compare the chromatin pattern of the nucleus and the cytoplasmic changes in the various stages. **a.** myeloblast: nucleus has fine chromatin and nucleoli; cytoplasm is agranular; **b.** promyelocyte: nucleus has coarser chromatin, nucleoli are still visible, and there are primary granules in the cytoplasm; **c.** myelocyte: nuclear chromatin is condensed and nucleoli are not visible; secondary granules give the cytoplasm a pinkish color; **d.** metamyelocyte: nucleus is kidney shaped and cytoplasm is pinkish; **e.** band (arrow) and segmented neutrophil: the nuclear chromatin is condensed and the cytoplasm is pinkish; **f.** compare the nuclear and cytoplasmic features of these maturing neutrophilic cells. From left are a very early band, myelocyte, promyelocyte, myeloblast, and very early band; above the myeloblast are 2 segmented neutrophils. (Bone marrow; Wright-Giemsa stain; 1000× magnification)

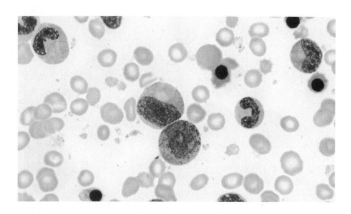

■ FIGURE 7-2   In the center are a myelocyte (top) and a promyelocyte (bottom). Note the changes in the nucleus and cytoplasm. The myelocyte has a clear area next to the nucleus, which represents the Golgi apparatus. Note the azurophilic granules in the promyelocyte. Also present are two bands and in the top right corner a metamyelocyte. Orthochromatic normoblasts are present. (Bone marrow, Wright-Giemsa stain, 1000× magnification)

are four subsets of granules/organelles (primary, secondary, secretory, and tertiary) containing different constituents produced at various times during neutrophil development. The diversity of granule content is due to differences in the timing of biosynthesis of the granule constituents and is regulated by different transcription factors. Leukopoiesis is an amazing process generating $1–5 \times 10^9$ cells per hour or 10^{11} cells per day.[7] However, the marrow has the capacity to significantly increase the neutrophil production over this baseline level in response to inflammatory stimuli. The morphology of the stages of maturation is discussed below.

Myeloblast

The myeloblast (Table 7-1, Figures 7-1a and 7-3 ■) is the earliest morphologically recognizable neutrophil precursor. The myeloblast size varies from 14 to 20 μm in diameter, and it has a high nuclear to cytoplasmic (N:C) ratio. The nucleus is usually round or oval and contains a delicate, lacy, evenly stained chromatin. One to five nucleoli are visible. The small amount of cytoplasm is agranular, staining from deep blue to a lighter blue. A distinct unstained area adjacent to the nucleus representing the Golgi apparatus can be seen. These cells can stain faintly positive for peroxidase and esterase enzymes and for lipids (Sudan black B) although granules are not evident by light microscopy. Staining reactions with peroxidase and esterase help differentiate myeloblasts from monoblasts and lymphoblasts. CD markers also aid in identifying the lineage of blasts. Myeloblast CD markers include CD34, CD33, CD13, CD38, and CD45RA.[8]

Promyelocyte

The promyelocyte/progranulocyte (Table 7-1, Figures 7-1b and 7-2) varies in size from 15 to 21 μm. The nucleus is still quite large, and the N:C ratio is high. The nuclear chromatin

structure, although coarser than that of the myeloblast, is still open and rather lacy, staining purple to dark blue. The color of the nucleus varies somewhat depending on the stain used, and several nucleoli can still be visible. The basophilic cytoplasm is similar to that of the myeloblast but is differentiated by the presence of prominent, reddish-purple primary granules, also called nonspecific or **azurophilic granules**, which are synthesized during this stage. The granules can be shown by cytochemical techniques to contain peroxidase and a number of antimicrobial compounds. Contents of primary granules are listed in Table 7-2 ✪.

Myelocyte

The myelocyte (Table 7-1, Figures 7-1c, 7-2, and 7-3) varies in size from 12 to 18 μm. The nucleus is reduced in size due to nuclear chromatin condensation and appears more darkly stained than the chromatin of the promyelocyte. Nucleoli can be seen in the early myelocyte but are usually indistinct. The myelocyte nucleus can be round, oval, slightly flattened on one side, or slightly indented.[9] The clear light area next to the nucleus, representing the Golgi apparatus, can still be seen. The myelocyte goes through two to three cell divisions; this is the last stage capable of mitosis. The early myelocyte has a more basophilic cytoplasm; the later more mature myelocyte has a more neutral to pink cytoplasm, and the N:C ratio is decreased.

The hallmark for the myelocyte stage is the appearance of specific or secondary granules. Synthesis of peroxidase-positive primary granules is halted, and the cell switches to synthesis of peroxidase-negative secondary granules. Secondary granules are detected first near the nucleus in the Golgi apparatus. This has sometimes been referred to as the *dawn of neutrophilia*. These neutrophilic granules are small, sandlike

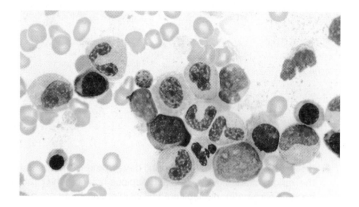

■ FIGURE 7-3   At about nine o'clock in the central group of cells is a pronormoblast. At about five o'clock is a myeloblast. Note that the myeloblast has a more lacy, lighter-staining chromatin with distinct nucleoli and bluish cytoplasm. The normoblast chromatin is more smudged with indistinct nucleoli and very deep blue-purple cytoplasm. Also pictured are bands, metamyelocyte, myelocytes, basophilic normoblast, polychromatophilic normoblast, and orthochromatic normoblast. (Bone marrow, Wright-Giemsa stain, 1000× magnification)

✪ TABLE 7-1

Characteristics of Cells in the Maturation Stages of the Neutrophil

Cell Stage (% in bone marrow)	Size (μm)	Nucleus	Cytoplasm	N:C ratio	Granules	CD Markers	Maturation Transit Time
Myeloblast (0.2–1.5) (see Fig. 7–1a)	14–20	Round or oval; delicate, lacy chromatin; nucleoli	Deep blue	High	Absent	CD13, CD33, CD34, CD38	~1 day
Promyelocyte (2–4) (see Fig. 7–1b)	15–21	Round or oval, chromatin lacy but more condensed than blast; nucleoli present	Deep blue	High but less than myeloblast	Large, reddish-purple (azurophilic) primary or nonspecific granules	CD33, CD38	1–3 days
Myelocyte (8–16) (see Fig. 7–1c)	12–18	Round to oval; chromatin more condensed; nucleoli usually absent	Light pink; can have patches of blue	Decreased from promyelocyte	Small pinkish-red specific granules; azurophilic granules; secretory vesicles		1–5 days
Metamyelocyte (9–25) (see Fig. 7–1d)	10–18	Chromatin condensed; stains dark purple; kidney bean shape to oval	Pink	Decreased	Predominance of small pinkish red specific granules; some azurophilic granules present; secretory vesicles		0.5–4 days
Band (nonsegmented) (9–15) (see Fig. 7–1e)	9–15	Chromatin condensed at ends of horseshoe shaped nucleus; stains dark purple	Pink	Decreased	Abundant small, pinkish-red specific granules; some azurophilic granules present; secretory vesicles; tertiary granules		0.5–4 days
Polymorphonuclear (segmented) (6–12) (see Fig. 7–1f)	9–15	Nucleus segmented into 2–4 lobes; chromatin condensed; stains dark purple	Pink	Decreased	As in band	CD15, CD16, CD11b/CD18	1–5 days

granules with a pink-red to pink-violet tint. Like the primary granules, the secondary granules are surrounded by a phospholipid membrane that stains with Sudan black B. Large primary azurophilic granules can still be apparent, but their concentration decreases with each successive cell division because their synthesis has ceased. Their ability to pick up stain also decreases with successive mitotic divisions. A partial list of secondary granule contents is found in Table 7-2.[9]

Secretory vesicles are scattered throughout the cytoplasm of myelocytes, metamyelocytes, band neutrophils, and segmented neutrophils (Table 7-2).[10] Secretory vesicles are specialized vesicles formed by endocytosis in the later stages of neutrophil maturation; they contain plasma proteins including albumin. The secretory vesicles fuse with the plasma membrane on neutrophil stimulation, increasing the neutrophil surface membrane and expression of adhesion and chemotactic receptors. Tertiary or gelatinase-containing granules are synthesized mainly during the metamyelocyte and band neutrophil stages.[9]

Metamyelocyte

The metamyelocyte (Table 7-1, Figures 7-1d and 7-3) varies in size from 10 to 18 μm in diameter. Traditionally, the characteristic most apparently differentiating it from the myelocyte was nuclear indentation, giving the nucleus a kidney bean shape. More recent research suggests that nuclear shape is variable and is not the most reliable identifying feature. Care should be taken to review other cellular features such as the degree of the chromatin clumping, color of the cytoplasm, predominant granules present, and the cell size. The nuclear chromatin is coarse and clumped and stains dark purple. Nucleoli are not visible. The cytoplasm is a neutral pink color with a predominance of secondary and secretory granules. The ratio of secondary to primary granules is ~2:1. The metamyelocyte's cytoplasm resembles the color of the cytoplasm of a fully mature neutrophil.[9]

Band Neutrophil

The band neutrophil, also called *nonsegmented neutrophil*, is slightly smaller in diameter, 9–15 μm, than the metamyelocyte. The metamyelocyte becomes a band when the indentation of the nucleus is more than half the diameter of the hypothetical round nucleus (Table 7-1, Figure 7-1e). The indentation gives the nucleus a horseshoe shape. The chromatin displays increased condensation at either end of the nucleus. The cytoplasm appears pinkish, resembling both the previous stage and the fully mature segmented forms. The band neutrophil is the first stage that normally is found in the peripheral blood. All four types of granules (primary, secondary, secretory, and tertiary) can be found at this stage,

but primary granules are not usually differentiated with Wright's stain in bands

Segmented Neutrophil

Although similar in size to the band form, 9–15 μm, the PMN is recognized, as its name implies, by a segmented nucleus with two or more lobes connected by a thin nuclear filament (Table 7-1, Figures 7-1e, f). The chromatin is condensed and stains a deep purple black. Most neutrophils have three or four nuclear lobes, but a range of two to five lobes is possible. Fewer than three lobes are considered hyposegmented. A cell with more than five lobes is considered abnormal and referred to as a *hypersegmented neutrophil*. Observing three or more five-lobed neutrophils in a 100-cell differential is also considered hypersegmentation. Nuclear lobes are often touching or superimposed on one another, sometimes making it difficult to differentiate the cell as a band or PMN.

Individual laboratories and agencies such as the Clinical and Laboratory Standards Institute (CLSI) have outlined criteria for differentiating bands from PMNs in manual differentials.[11] A *band* is defined as having a nucleus with a connecting strip or isthmus with parallel sides and having width enough to reveal two distinct margins with nuclear chromatin material visible between the margins. If a margin of a given lobe can be traced as a definite and continuing line from one side across the isthmus to the other side, a filament is assumed to be present although it is not visible. If a clinical laboratory scientist is not sure whether a neutrophil is a band form or a segmented form, it is arbitrarily classified as a segmented neutrophil. From a traditional clinical viewpoint, determining whether young forms of neutrophils (band forms and younger) are increased has been useful.[9] However, differentials performed by automated hematology instruments do not differentiate between band and segmented neutrophils. Band neutrophils are fully functional phagocytes and often are included with the total neutrophil count.[11]

The cytoplasm of the mature PMN stains a pinkish to clear color. It contains many secondary granules, tertiary granules, and secretory vesicles. Primary granules are pres-

⊙ TABLE 7-2

Neutrophil Granule Contents

Primary Granules	Secondary Granules	Secretory Vesicles	Tertiary Granules
Myeloperoxidase	Lactoferrin	Alkaline phosphatase	Gelatinase
Lysozyme	Lysozyme	Complement receptor 1	Lysozyme
Cathespin G, B, and D	Histaminase	Cytochrome b_{558}	
Defensins (group of cationic proteins)	Collagenase		
Bactericidal permeability increasing protein (BPI)	Gelatinase		
Esterase N	Heparinase		
Elastase			

ent, but because of their loss of staining quality, might not be readily evident. The ratio of secondary to primary granules remains ~2:1.

In addition to protein material found in neutrophilic granules, lipids and carbohydrates also can be found. About one-third of the lipids in neutrophils consists of phospholipids. Much of the phospholipid is present in the plasma membrane or membranes of the various granules. Cholesterol and triglycerides constitute most of the nonphospholipid neutrophil lipid. Cytoplasmic nonmembrane lipid bodies can also be found in neutrophils; their role in cell function is unclear. Lipid material is likewise found in neutrophilic precursors. A cytochemical stain for lipids, Sudan black B, is used to differentiate myeloid precursors from lymphoid precursors (∞ Chapter 21). Glycogen is also found in both neutrophils and some myeloid precursors. Neutrophils sometimes function in hypoxic conditions as at an abscess site and obtain energy by glycolysis, utilizing glycogen. The periodic acid-Schiff (PAS) stain is used to detect glycogen in cells. CD markers on the neutrophil include CD15, CD16, and CD11b/CD18.[8]

In females with two X chromosomes or males with XXY chromosomes (Klinefelter syndrome), one X chromosome is randomly inactivated in each somatic cell of the embryo and remains inactive in all daughter cells produced from that cell. The inactive X chromosome appears as an appendage of the neutrophil nucleus and is called a **drumstick** or an *X chromatin body* (**Barr body**) (Figure 7-4■). The number of chromatin bodies detected in the neutrophil is one less than the number of X chromosomes present; however, chromatin bodies are not visible in every neutrophil. The X chromatin bodies can be identified in 2–3% of the circulating PMNs of 46, XX females, and Klinefelter males.[9]

> ✓ **Checkpoint! 1**
>
> *An adult patient's peripheral blood smear revealed many myelocytes, metamyelocytes, and band forms of neutrophils. Is this a normal finding?*

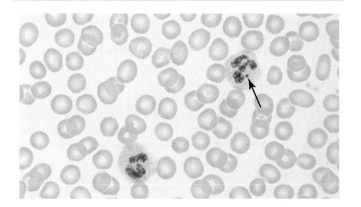

■ **FIGURE 7-4**   The segmented neutrophil on the right has an X chromatin body (arrow). (Peripheral blood, Wright-Giemsa stain, 1000× magnification)

DISTRIBUTION, CONCENTRATION, AND KINETICS

The kinetics of a group of cells—their production, distribution, and destruction—also is described as the *cell turnover rate*. For the neutrophil, kinetics follows the movement of the cell through a series of interconnected compartments (the marrow, blood, and tissues).

Bone Marrow

Neutrophils in the bone marrow can be divided into two pools: the mitotic pool and the postmitotic pool (Figure 7-5■). The *mitotic pool*, also called the *proliferating pool*, includes cells capable of DNA synthesis: myeloblasts, promyelocytes, and myelocytes. Cells spend about 3–6 days in this proliferating pool undergoing four to five cell divisions. Two to three of these divisions occur in the myelocyte stage, but the number of cell divisions at each stage is variable. The postmitotic pool, also known as the *maturation and storage pool*, includes metamyelocytes, bands, and segmented neutrophils. Cells spend about 5–7 days in this compartment before they are released to the peripheral blood. However, during infections, the myelocyte-to-blood transit time can be as short as 2 days. The postmitotic storage pool is almost three times the size of the mitotic pool.[10]

The largest compartment of PMNs is found within the bone marrow and is referred to as the *mature neutrophil reserve*. The blood compartment is about one-third the size of the bone marrow compartment, and only one-half of the blood compartment PMNs are circulating. The other half are attached to the vascular endothelium.[10]

Once precursor cells have matured in the bone marrow, they are released into the peripheral blood (∞ Chapter 3). Normally, input of neutrophils from the bone marrow to the peripheral blood equals output of neutrophils from the blood to the tissues, maintaining a relative steady-state blood concentration. However, when the demand for neutrophils is increased as in infectious states, the neutrophil concentration in the peripheral blood can increase quickly as neutrophils from the bone marrow storage (reserve) pool are released. Depending on the strength and duration of the stimulus, the marrow myeloid precursor cells (CFU-GM, CFU-G) also can be induced to proliferate and differentiate to form additional neutrophils. The transit time between development in the bone marrow and release to the peripheral blood can be decreased as a result of several mechanisms: (1) acceleration of maturation, (2) skipped cellular divisions, and (3) early release of cells from the marrow.

The mechanism regulating the production and release of neutrophils from the bone marrow to the peripheral blood is not completely understood but likely includes a feedback loop between the circulating neutrophils and the bone marrow. G-CSF is probably the primary humoral feedback mediator in normal steady-state conditions. The major sources of G-CSF are marrow stromal cells and macrophages. Inflammatory cytokines such as IL-1 and tumor necrosis factor

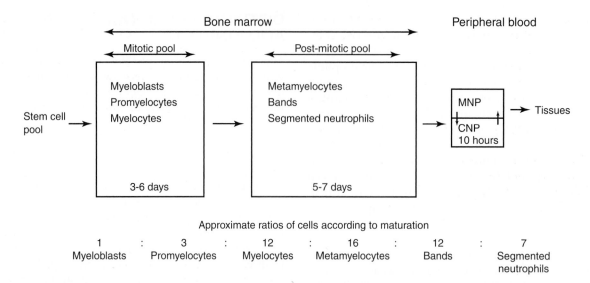

■ FIGURE 7-5   Neutrophils are produced from stem cells in the bone marrow and spend about 1–2 weeks in this maturation compartment. Most neutrophils are released to the peripheral blood as segmented forms. When the demand for these cells is increased, more immature forms can be released. One-half of the neutrophils in the perpheral blood is in the marginating pool (MNP); the other half is in the circulating pool (CNP). Neutrophils spend <10 hours in the blood before marginating and exiting randomly to tissue. (Adapted from Boggs DR, Winkelstein A. *White Cell Manual,* 4th ed. Philadelphia: FA Davis Co.; 1983.)

(TNF) are important in causing an increase in the neutrophil concentration in pathologic conditions. These cytokines induce the macrophage to release G-CSF and GM-CSF. The vascular endothelial cell that forms the inner lining of blood vessels also generates cytokines that govern activation and recruitment of leukocytes. Endothelial cells can be important in recruiting neutrophils in the earliest phases of inflammation and injury.

The release mechanism of the bone marrow storage pool is selective in normal, steady-state kinetics, releasing only segmented neutrophils and a few band neutrophils. The mechanisms controlling this regulated release are not fully understood. The release is partially regulated by the small pore size in the vascular endothelium of bone marrow sinusoids and by the mature segmented neutrophil's ability to deform enough to squeeze through the narrow opening. Immature cells are larger and less deformable and cannot penetrate the small pores; however, when an increased demand for neutrophils exists, a higher proportion of less mature neutrophils is released into the peripheral blood. Glucocorticoids, endotoxin (bacterial lipopolysaccharide), and G-CSF can increase neutrophil release from the marrow.

Peripheral Blood

Neutrophils are released from the bone marrow to the peripheral blood, but not all neutrophils are circulating freely at the same time. About half the *total blood neutrophil pool* (TBNP) is temporarily marginated along the vessel walls (*marginating pool*/MNP) while the other half is freely circulating (*circulating pool*/CNP). Thus, if all marginated neutrophils were to circulate freely, the total neutrophil count would double. Marginating neutrophils roll on the endothelial surface at a slow rate caused by a loose binding interaction between selectin adhesion proteins on neutrophils (L-selectin) and the L-selectin ligand on endothelial cells. The two pools are in equilibrium and rapidly and freely exchange neutrophils. Stimulants such as strenuous exercise, epinephrine, or stress can induce a shift from the MNP to the CNP, temporarily increasing the neutrophil count.

The average neutrophil circulates ~7.5 hours in the blood before diapedesing (transendothelial migration) to the tissues, although a few die of senescence (apoptosis) while in the circulation. These are occasionally seen as "necrobiotic neutrophils" on the peripheral blood smear.

Tissues

Most neutrophils move into the tissues from the marginated pool in response to chemotactic stimulation (see below). In the tissues, the neutrophil is either destroyed by trauma (cell necrosis) or lives until programmed cell death, apoptosis, occurs (∞ Chapter 2). PMNs that do not receive activation signals generally die within 1–2 days. However, elevated levels of GM-CSF or G-CSF associated with an infection or inflammatory process can prolong the neutrophil life span to 3–5 days by blocking apoptosis. Senescent (apoptotic) neutrophils are phagocytosed by macrophages.[9]

Neutrophil Kinetics

Neutrophils constitute the majority of circulating leukocytes. The absolute concentration varies between 1.8 and 7.0×10^9/L. A number of physiologic and pathologic variations affect the concentration of circulating leukocytes.

Pathologic causes of changes in leukocyte numbers are discussed in subsequent chapters on white cell disorders including ∞ Chapters 19–26.

Alteration in the concentration of peripheral blood leukocytes is often the first sign of an underlying pathology. A normal leukocyte count does not rule out the presence of disease, but **leukocytosis** (an increase in leukocytes) or **leukopenia** (a decrease in leukocytes) is an important clue to disease processes and deserves further investigation including a leukocyte differential count to identify the concentration of the different types of leukocytes. Granulocytopenia (granulocytes $<2 \times 10^9$/L) defines a decrease in all types of granulocytes (i.e., eosinophils, basophils, and neutrophils). **Neutropenia** is a more specific term denoting a decrease in only neutrophils. Neutropenia in adults exists if the absolute neutrophil count falls below 1.8×10^9/L. The condition of absence of granulocytes is called **agranulocytosis,** and the patient is at high risk of developing an infection. **Granulocytosis** is a term used to denote an increase in all granulocytes. **Neutrophilia** is a more specific term indicating an increase in neutrophils. Neutrophilia in adults occurs when the absolute concentration of neutrophils exceeds 7×10^9/L. This condition is most often the result of the body's reactive response to bacterial infection, metabolic intoxication, drug intoxication, or tissue necrosis.

Although the WBC count and absolute neutrophil count are used to evaluate neutrophil production, they reflect a transient moment in overall neutrophil kinetics and do not provide accurate, quantitative information on the rate of production or destruction, status of marrow reserves, or abnormalities in cell distribution in the tissues.

✓ Checkpoint! 2

An adult patient's WBC count is 10×10^9/L, and there are 90% neutrophils. What is the absolute number of neutrophils? Is this in the reference range for neutrophils? If not, what term would be used to describe it?

FUNCTION

To be effective in its role in host defense, the neutrophil must move to the site of the foreign agent, engulf it, and destroy it. Thus, neutrophils function primarily in the tissues where microbial invasion typically occurs. Monocytes-macrophages help in this process but are slower to arrive at the site. The four steps in the innate immune response can be described as adherence, migration (chemotaxis), phagocytosis, and bacterial killing.

Adherence

Neutrophils flow freely along the vascular endothelium when neither the neutrophil nor vascular endothelial cell (VEC) is activated. Neutrophil adherence and migration to the site of infection begin with a series of interactions between the neutrophils and VEC when these cells are activated by a variety of inflammatory mediators (cytokines).

Several different families of cytoadhesion molecules (CAM) and their ligands play a major role in the adherance process. Adhesion molecules include: (Table 7-3 ⚙)

- Selectins and their ligands
- Intercellular adhesion molecules (ICAMs)
- β_2 (CD18) family of leukocyte integrins and their ligands (Immunoglobulin-like CAM)

Adhesion molecules and their ligands located on the leukocytes and VEC act together to induce activation-dependent adhesion events. They are critical for every step of cell recruitment to sites of tissue injury including margination along vessel walls, **diapedesis,** and **chemotaxis.** Adhesion molecules are transmembrane proteins with three domain types: extracellular, transmembrane, and intracellular. A ligand's binding to the extracellular domain sends a signal across the membrane to the cell's interior, which activates secondary messengers within the cell. These secondary messengers affect calcium flux, NADPH oxidase activity, cytoskeleton assembly, and phagocytosis.

Neutrophils and endothelial cells are transformed from a basal state to an activated state by inflammatory mediators (cytokines and chemokines). The initial result is activation of all three classes of CAMs. Springer has proposed a model of the neutrophil-endothelial cell adhesion process[12] that can be divided into four stages: (1) activation of VEC, (2) activation of neutrophils, (3) binding of neutrophils to inner vessel linings, and (4) transendothelial migration (Figure 7-6 ■).

Stage one involves the activation of VEC, which mediates a loose association of VECs with neutrophils. Inflammatory cytokines (IL-1, tumor necrosis factor-α [TNF-α], or interferon-γ [IFN-γ]) activate VEC to express E- and P-selectins as well as L-selectin ligands. E-selectin is newly synthesized by the activated VEC; P-selectin is mobilized and translocated from storage sites in the Weibel-Palade bodies to the surface of the VEC. E- and P-selectin molecules on the VEC surface interact with their ligands on the neutrophil. Additionally L-selectin, which is constitutively present in the neutrophil membrane, interacts with its ligands that are upregulated on the activated VEC. These interactions induce the neutrophil to transiently associate and dissociate with the VEC, causing the neutrophil to "roll" on the VEC surface. The rolling neutrophils are thus situated to respond to additional signals from chemoattractants (chemotactic substances—chemical messengers that cause directional migration of cells along a concentration gradient) generated by infectious agents or an inflammatory response.[10]

Stage two is the activation of neutrophils. **Chemokines** (cytokines with chemotactic activity) or other chemoattractants released by tissue cells, microorganisms, and activated VEC bind to the endothelial cell surface. There they interact with the loosely bound leukocytes, resulting in activation of leukocyte integrins. Chemoattractants include specific and

✪ TABLE 7-3

Adhesion Molecules Important in Leukocyte-Endothelial Cell Interactions

Molecules	CD Designation	Expressed By	Counter-Receptor/Ligand
1. β_2-integrins/Neutrophils $\alpha_L\beta_2$ (LFA-1)	CD11a-CD18	Activated leukocytes	ICAM-1 on VEC (CD54) ICAM-2 on VEC (CD102) ICAM-3 (CD50)
$\alpha_M\beta_2$ (Mac-1)	CD11b-CD18	Activated leukocytes	ICAM-1 on EC iC3b, fibrinogen, factor X
$\alpha_x\beta_2$ (p150,95)	CD11c-CD18	Activated leukocytes	iC3b, fibrinogen
2. Selectins			
L-selectin	CD62L	Leukocytes	Sialylated carbohydrates; PSGL-1
E-selectin	CD62E	Activated VEC	Sialylated carbohydrates (SLe^x) and L-selectin on activated leukocytes
P-selectin	CD62P	Activated VEC and platelets	PSGL-1; sialylated carbohydrates
3. Immunoglobulin supergene family			
ICAM-1	CD54	VEC	LFA-1 (CD11a-CD18)
ICAM-2	CD102	VEC	LFA-1 (CD11a-CD18)
ICAM-3	CD50	Neutrophils	VEC
PECAM-1	CD31	VEC	CD31, $\alpha_v\beta_3$
LFA-2	CD2	T lymphocytes	LFA-3 (CD58) on EC
LFA-3	CD58	VEC	CD2 on T lymphocytes
VCAM-1	CD106	VEC	VLA-4(CD49d) on monocytes, lymphocytes, eosinophils, basophils
T cell receptor	CD3	T lymphocytes	Antigen
CD4	CD4	T$_H$ lymphocytes	MHC Class II
CD8	—	T$_S$ lymphocytes	MHC Class I
MHC Class II	—	B lymphocytes Activated T lymphocytes Monocytes	
MHC Class I	—	Nucleated cells	CD8 on T$_S$ lymphocytes

LFA = leukocyte function-related antigen, CD = cluster of differentiation, EC = endothelial cell, ICAM = intercellular adhesion molecules, PSGL-1 = P selectin glycoprotein ligand-1.

nonspecific proinflammatory mediators such as C5a (complement activation peptide), bacterial products, lipid mediators (e.g., platelet-activating factor [PAF]), and chemokines. The neutrophil activation-dependent adhesion receptors include the β_2 integrin molecules. Leukocyte plasma membranes have at least three β_2-integrins: CD11a/CD18 (LFA-1/leukocyte function associated antigen-1), CD11b/CD18 (Mac-1, also known as the *CR3 complement receptor*), and CD11c/CD18. Each has an α subunit (CD11a, CD11b, and CD11c) noncovalently linked to a β subunit (CD18).[10] The neutrophil L-selectin molecule is downregulated at this time.

An autosomal recessive disorder, leukocyte adhesion deficiency type-I (LAD-I), has partial or total absence of expression of the β_2 integrins on leukocyte membranes, often due to a mutation of the CD18 gene. This results in absence of leukocyte adhesion to the VEC as well as lack of mobility or migration and can result in life-threatening bacterial infections. An inability to synthesize the E- and L-selectin ligand SLe^x is seen in leukocyte adhesion deficiency type 2 (LAD-2) and results in reoccurring infections.[13] (∞ Chapter 19)

Stage three involves arrest of neutrophil rolling because activated neutrophils are more tightly bound to inner vessel linings. Expression of the neutrophils' activation-dependent β_2 integrin adhesion receptors mediates firm adherence of neutrophils to ICAMs expressed by activated VEC near the site of infection or inflammation. The integrin receptors' intracellular domains react with the neutrophil's cytoskeleton, triggering a rapid cytoskeletal rearrangement in the neutrophil on ligand interaction. This induces a cytoskeletal and morphologic change in the leukocyte required for cellular migration. Stage three ends with a strong, sustained attachment of the leukocyte to the VEC. At this time, leukocyte NADPH oxidase membrane complexes are assembled and activated (discussed later).

Stage four involves the transendothelial migration phase that occurs when neutrophils move through the vessel wall by the process of diapedesis, occurring predominantly at the borders of VECs. Passing out of the vessel to the tissue requires modification of the VEC cell-to-cell adherent junctions. The neutrophils use pseudopods to squeeze between endothelial cells, leaving the vascular space and passing through the subendothelial basement membranes and peri-

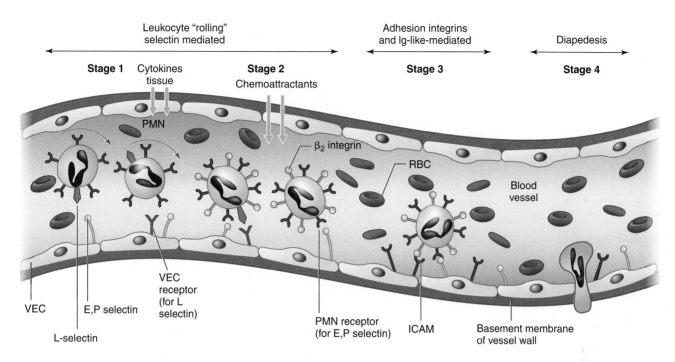

■ **FIGURE 7-6**   Adhesion of neutrophils to the vascular endothelium and eventual migration of neutrophils into the tissue occur as a result of activation of endothelial cells (EC) and neutrophils by exposure to chemoattractants. When the cells are activated, they are induced to express adhesion molecules. These transmembrane molecules send a signal across the membrane to the interior of the cell when they attach to their receptor. The process occurs in 4 stages: In stage 1, E,P-selectin and L-selectin (VEC) receptor are expressed on activated EC. The neutrophil's L-selectin and receptors for E,P-selectin cause the neutrophil to attach loosely to the EC and roll along the endothelium. Neutrophils in stage 2 are activated by the presence of chemoattractants in the local environment and express the $\beta 2$-integrins. These chemoattractants also activate the ECs. The neutrophils in stage 3 attach to the activated ECs via the attachment of their $\beta 2$-integrins to ICAMs of the EC, resulting in a firmer attachment than in stage 1 and halting the rolling of the neutrophil. The neutrophil in stage 4 migrates through the endothelium and basement membrane (diapedesis) to the area of inflammation. They move in the direction of the chemoattractants (chemotaxis).

endothelial cells. Subendothelial basement membranes are eroded, presumably by secretion of neutrophil gelatinase B and elastase from neutrophil granules. Migration is enhanced when the VEC is activated by IL-1 and/or TNF.[10]

Migration

Once in the tissues, neutrophil migration (*chemotaxis*) is guided by chemoattractant gradients. Neutrophils continue their migration through the extravascular tissue, moving by directed ameboid motion toward the infected site. Locomotion of neutrophils (and other leukocytes) is a process of "crawling," not "swimming." During locomotion along a chemotactic gradient, the neutrophils acquire a characteristic asymmetric shape, a process made possible by the alterations of the cytoskeleton triggered by neutrophil activation. There is an extension of a broad pseudopodium (protopod) at the anterior of the cell (containing the nucleus and organelles) and a narrow knoblike tail (uropod) at the rear of the cell. Neutrophil migration through the tissues requires β_1 and β_2 integrins with the continuous formation of new adhesive contacts at the cell front and detachment from the adhesive substrate at the rear of the cell. Chemotaxis is induced by a variety of chemoattractant molecules including bacterial formyl

peptides (fMLP), $C5_a$, LTB_4, IL-8, and PAF, many of the same molecules which activated the PMN during stage two.[12]

✓ **Checkpoint! 3**

A patient with life-threatening recurrent infections is found to have a chromosomal mutation that results in a loss of active integrin molecules on the neutrophil surface. Why would this result in life-threatening infections?

Phagocytosis

After arriving at the site of infection, phagocytosis by neutrophils can begin. Monocytes and macrophages also arrive at the site of injury and continue to accumulate and contribute to the inflammatory process. Phagocytes must recognize the pathogen as foreign before attachment occurs and phagocytosis begins (Figure 7-7 ■). Recognition is followed by ingestion of the particle, fusion of the neutrophil granules with the phagosome (degranulation), and finally the process of bacterial killing and digestion. **Phagocytosis** is an active process that requires a large expenditure of energy by the cells. The required energy can be provided by anaerobic glycolysis or aerobic processes.

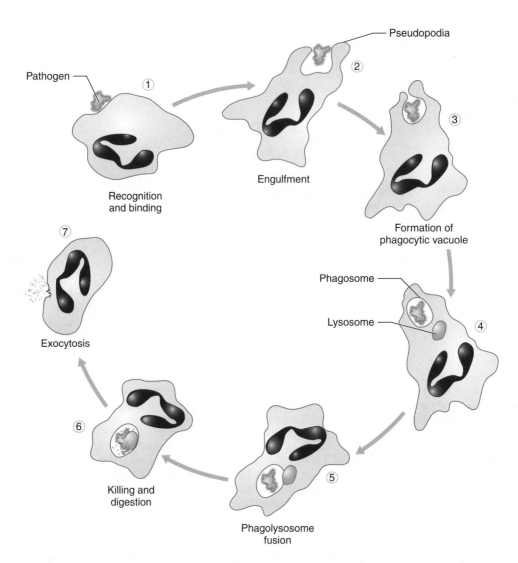

■ **FIGURE 7-7**   Phagocytosis begins with recognition and attachment of the pathogen to the neutrophil (or macrophage). The pathogen is then internalized, forming a phagocytic vacuole. Next the granule fuses with the vacuole, forming a phagolysosome, and releases its contents into the vacuole to help kill and digest the microbe (degranulation). This is followed by extrusion of undigested vacuole contents from the neutrophil (exocytosis).

The principal factor in determining whether or not phagocytosis can occur is the physical nature of the surfaces of both the foreign particle and the phagocytic cell. Phagocytes recognize unique molecular characteristics of the pathogen's surface (PAMP) and bind to the invading organism via specific PRR (see leukocyte function, discussed previously). Some pathogens can be recognized by the process of opsonization (the coating of a particle with a soluble factor). Enhancement of phagocytosis through the process of opsonization speeds the ingestion of particles. Two well-characterized opsonins are immunoglobulin G (IgG) and complement component C3b (see lymphocyte section for description of structure of IgG). The antibody, IgG, binds to the microorganism/particle by means of its Fab region while the Fc region of the antibody attaches to Fc receptors on the neutrophil membrane (FcγRI/CD64, FcγRII/CD32, FcγRIII/CD16). Thus, the antibody forms a connecting link between the microorganism/particle and the neutrophil. The neutrophil also has receptors for activated complement component C3b (CR1/CD35, CR3/CD11b/CD18, CR4/CD11c/CD18). Some bacteria with polysaccharide capsules avoid recognition, thus reducing the effectiveness of phagocytosis.

Following recognition and attachment, the particle is surrounded by neutrophil cytoplasmic extensions or pseudopods (Figure 7-7). As the pseudopods touch, they fuse, encompassing the particle within a phagosome that is bound by the cytoplasmic membrane turned "inside out." A plasma membrane-bound oxidase is activated during ingestion, which plays an important role in microbactericidal activities.

Bacterial Killing and/or Digestion

Bacterial killing and/or digestion follows ingestion of particles. After formation of the phagosome, neutrophil granules migrate toward and fuse with the phagosome membrane, discharging their granule contents into the phagocytic vesicle, forming a phagolysosome (**degranulation**). The bactericidal and digestive proteins contained within both primary and secondary granules are thus normally sequestered from the cytoplasm of the neutrophil, selectively released, and activated within a membrane-enclosed system.

Microbicidal mechanisms that follow ingestion can be divided into oxygen-dependent/oxidative or oxygen-independent/nonoxidative activities (Table 7-4 ✪). Oxygen-dependent microbicidal activity is most important physiologically. Phagocytosis is accompanied by an energy-dependent "respiratory burst" that generates oxidizing compounds produced from partial oxygen reduction. The respiratory burst is described as including a significant increase in glycolysis, a 2–3-fold increase in oxygen consumption, a 2–10-fold increase in hexose monophosphate shunt (HMS) activity and generation of NADPH, and the production of a series of reactive oxygen species (ROS).[14] The oxidizing compounds—ROS—are important agents in killing ingested organisms. The enzyme activity needed to generate ROS is provided by NADPH oxidase, also known as *respiratory burst oxidase* (*RBO*). In resting cells, NADPH oxidase is found as separate components of the plasma membrane (gp^{91phox}, p^{22phox}, and Rap^1) and intracellular stores (p^{47phox} and p^{67phox}). When phagocytosis takes place, the plasma membrane is internalized as the wall of the phagocytic vessicle with the outer plasma membrane surface now facing the interior of the phagosome. When the resting cell is exposed to any of a wide variety of activating stimuli, activated NADPH oxidase is assembled from the cytoplasmic and membrane-associated subunits at the phagosome membrane. From this location, the NADPH oxidase generates and pours ROS into the phagosome.

Once assembled, the oxidase produces superoxide anion, (O_2^-) and $NADP^+$. The $NADP^+$ activates the hexose monophosphate (HMP) shunt (∞ Chapter 5), generating more NADPH. O_2^- is further metabolized to produce additional ROS (H_2O_2, OH^-, $^1O_2$) with increasing bactericidal potency.

$$\overset{\text{NADPH oxidase}}{2\ NADPH + 2\ O_2 \rightarrow 2\ NADP^+ + 2\ O_2^- + 2\ H^+}$$

$$\overset{\text{Superoxide oxidase}}{2\ H^+ + O_2^- + O_2^- \rightarrow H_2O_2 + O_2}$$

$$H_2O_2 + O_2^- \rightarrow 2\ OH^- + {}^1O_2$$

The activated oxidase can be detected in the laboratory by a nitroblue tetrazolium (NBT) test, cytochrome reduction, or chemiluminescence test.

The second oxygen-dependent microbicidal system involves the primary granule enzyme myeloperoxidase (MPO). Myeloperoxidase catalyzes the interaction of hydrogen peroxide produced during the respiratory bust with halide ions (e.g., chloride/Cl^-) giving rise to oxidized halogens (e.g., hypochlorous acid/HOCl), which increase bacterial killing.[14]

$$H_2O_2 + Cl^- \overset{\text{MPO}}{\rightarrow} OCl^- + H_2O$$

The oxidants generated by the respiratory burst have potent microbicidal activity against a wide variety of microorganisms such as bacteria, fungi, and multicellular and unicellular parasites. However, the phagocyte and surrounding tissues are also susceptible to damage. Phagocytes use a variety of mechanisms to detoxify the oxidant radicals, such as the superoxide dismutase, catalase, and a variety of other antioxidants.

Oxygen-independent granular proteins present in primary, gelatinase, and specific granules of neutrophils can successfully kill and degrade many strains of both gram-negative and gram-positive bacteria. The most important nonoxygen-dependent antimicrobial proteins of PMNs are listed in Table 7-4. Initially, the pH within the phagolysosome decreases, which inhibits bacterial growth, but this alone is insufficient to kill most microbes. Acidic conditions, however, can enhance the activity of some granular proteins such as hydrolases and lactoferrin, which perform optimally at low pH. In the extracellular environment, microorganisms that escape phagocytosis are also subject to killing by reactive oxygen metabolites such as H_2O_2 that forms from the O_2^- secreted by active plasma membrane NADPH complexes into the tissue matrices. Neutrophils themselves are not resistant to the toxic effects of the oxidants they secrete and

✪ TABLE 7-4

Neutrophil Antimicrobial Systems

Oxygen Dependent	Oxygen Independent
Myeloperoxidase independent	Acid pH of phagosome: antibacterial; enhances some oxygen-dependent antimicrobial mechanisms and other enzymes
Hydrogen peroxide (H_2O_2)	Lysozyme (primary and secondary granules): hydrolyzes cell wall of some bacteria; digests killed microbes
Superoxide anion (O_2^-)	Lactoferrin (secondary granules): binds iron necessary for bacterial growth; also directly bactericidal
Hydroxyl radicals (OH^-)	BPI—Bactericidal permeability inducing protein (primary granules); coat microbes; alters cell permeability
Singlet oxygen ($^1O_2$)	Defensins—small cationic peptides; broad spectrum of bactericidal activity
Myeloperoxidase dependent	Collagenase (secondary granules): degrades microbe macromolecules
(forms oxidized halogens)	Hydrolases (primary granules): digests microbe

thus have high mortality during any sustained inflammatory response.[15]

In patients with chronic granulomatous disease, neutrophils are missing one of the components of the NADPH oxidase complex and therefore fail to produce the respiratory burst. They are still capable of eliminating infection caused by strains of bacteria susceptible to killing by oxygen-independent mechanisms, but this antimicrobial system is not very effective alone. Often these patients eventually die of multiple infections with bacteria resistant to the killing actions of these granular proteins (∞ Chapter 19).

In addition to their primary functions of phagocytosis and killing of microorganisms, neutrophils interact in other physiologic processes. Neutrophils stimulate coagulation by releasing a substance that activates prekallikrein to kallikrein, which then cleaves kinins from high-molecular-weight kininogen. Kinins are responsible for vascular dilation and increased vessel permeability. Kinins, which are also chemotactic for neutrophils, attract them to sites of inflammation. Neutrophils initially activate kinin production, but as the cells accumulate, they break down kinins. Neutrophils also secrete pyrogen, a substance that acts on the hypothalamus to produce fever. This endogenous pyrogen is now known to be interleukin-1 (IL-1).

✓ Checkpoint! 4

A patient has a compromised ability to utilize the oxygen-dependent pathway in neutrophils. What two important microbial killing mechanisms could be affected?

▶ EOSINOPHILS

The eosinophil originates from the IL-5–responsive CD34⁺ myeloid progenitor cells. Cytokines that influence the proliferation and the differentiation of the eosinophil lineage include GM-CSF, IL-3, and IL-5. However, it is now recognized that IL-5, released by T_{H2} lymphocytes, has relative lineage specificity for eosinophils and is the major cytokine required for eosinophil production and terminal differentiation.[16]

DIFFERENTIATION, MATURATION, AND MORPHOLOGY

The eosinophil undergoes a morphologic maturation similar to the neutrophil with the same six stages of maturation identified. It is not possible to morphologically differentiate eosinophilic precursors from neutrophilic precursors with the light microscope until the myelocyte stage, however, when the typical acidophilic crystalloid granules of the eosinophil appear. Granule formation begins in the promyelocyte with small coreless granules. The first two stages (eosinophilic myeloblast and promyelocyte) will not be described because they are morphologically identical to the neutrophilic myeloblast and promyelocyte.

Eosinophilic Myelocyte to Mature Eosinophil

The eosinophilic myelocyte contains large, eosin-staining, crystalloid granules. Maturation from the myelocyte to the metamyelocyte, band, and segmented eosinophil stage is similar to that described for the neutrophils with gradual nuclear indentation and segmentation. No appreciable change occurs in the cytoplasm in these latter stages of development. The reddish orange spherical granules are larger than neutrophilic granules, are uniform in size, and are evenly distributed throughout the cell. Because of the low percentage of eosinophils in the bone marrow, differentiating the eosinophil into its maturational stages (e.g., eosinophilic myelocyte) serves no useful purpose when the count is normal. Bone marrow maturation and storage time are about 9 days.

The mature eosinophil (Figure 7-8 ■) is 12 to 15 μm in diameter. The nucleus usually has no more than two or three lobes, and the cytoplasm is completely filled with granules. The eosinophil contains three types of granules: primary granules, granules called *small granules* (which contain the enzymes acid phosphatase and aryl-sulphatase), and the eosinophil-specific, or crystalloid, granules that are bound by a phospholipid membrane and have a central crystalloid core surrounded by a matrix. The eosinophil-specific granules contain four major proteins: major basic protein (MBP), eosinophil cationic protein (ECP), eosinophil peroxidase (EPO), and eosinophil-derived neurotoxin (EDN), also known as *protein x* (*EPX*) (Table 7-5 ✪). The MBP is located in the crystalloid core; the other three proteins are found in the granule matrix. The crystalloid core also appears to store a number of proinflammatory cytokines such as IL-2, IL-4, and GM-CSF, and the matrix contains IL-5 and TNF-α. The eosinophil has the capacity to synthesize and elaborate a number of other cytokines as well. The eosinophil's capacity to produce cytokines has led to increased interest and re-

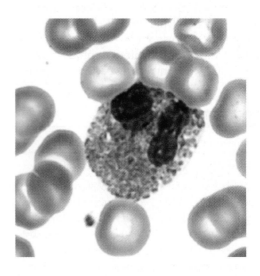

■ FIGURE 7-8   Eosinophil (Peripheral blood, Wright-Giemsa stain, 1000× magnification)

⊗ TABLE 7-5

Major Constituents of Eosinophil Granules

Protein (Abbreviation)	Characteristics
Major basic protein (MBP)	Is cytotoxic for protozoans and helminth parasites Stimulates release of histamine from mast cells and basophils Neutralizes mast cell and basophil heparin
Eosinophil cationic protein (ECP)	Is capable of killing mammalian and nonmammalian cells Stimulates release of histamine from mast cells and basophils Inhibits T lymphocyte proliferation Activates plasminogen Enhances mucus production in the bronchi Stimulates glycosaminoglycan production by fibroblasts
Eosinophil-derived neurotoxin (EDN)	Can provoke cerebral and cerebellar dysfunction in animals Inhibits T cell responses
Eosinophil peroxidase (EPO)	Combines with H_2O_2 and halide ions to produce a potent bactericidal and helminthicidal action Is cytotoxic for tumor and host cells Stimulates histamine release and degranulation of mast cells Diminishes roles of other inflammatory cells by inactivating leukotrienes
Lysophospholipase	Forms Charcot-Leyden crystals
Miscellaneous enzymes	Phospholipase D: inactivates mast cell PAF (platelet activating factor) Arylsulphatase: inactivates mast cell LT-D_4 (leukotriene D4) Histaminase: neutralizes mast cell histamine Acid phosphatase, catalase, nonspecific esterases
Lipid-derived mediators	LT-C_4: promotes smooth muscle contraction and mucus secretion PG-E_1 and E_2: inhibits mast cell degranulation PAF TXB_2 (thromboxand B2)

search into the eosinophil's role as an effector cell in allergic inflammation. The eosinophil, like the neutrophil, contains a number of lipid bodies that increase during eosinophil activation in vitro.[16,17] Eosinophils express the CD9, CD11a, and CD13 molecules.

Tissue Eosinophils

Smears of bone marrow can contain large cells with a well-defined reticular chromatin pattern in the nucleus, nucleoli, an irregular cytoplasmic outline, and cytoplasmic granules similar to the reddish orange granules of blood eosinophils. It is thought that these cells are tissue variants of the more motile eosinophils of the peripheral blood. Tissue eosinophils can be found in tissue other than bone marrow (see section below). Some evidence indicates that tissue eosinophils can develop and mature in extramedulary sites in response to locally produced cytokines.[16]

DISTRIBUTION, CONCENTRATION, AND KINETICS

Eosinophils in adults have a concentration in the peripheral blood $\leq 0.40 \times 10^9$/L. The cell shows a diurnal variation with highest concentration in the morning and the lowest concentration in the evening.[16]

Eosinophilia in adults is defined as $>0.40 \times 10^9$/L; it is associated with allergic diseases, parasitic infections, toxic reactions, gastrointestinal diseases, respiratory tract disorders, neoplastic disorders, and other conditions. (See ∞ Chapter 19 for a complete list.) Eosinophilia is T cell dependent; T cells are the predominant source of IL-5. Persistant eosinophilia is seen in hypereosinophilic syndrome, a myeloproliferative disorder (∞ Chapter 22).

Very little is known about the kinetics of eosinophils. Most of the body's eosinophil population lies in connective tissue below the epithelial layer in tissues that are exposed to the external environment such as the nasal passages, lung, skin, gastrointestinal tract, and urinary tract. These cells spend ~18 hours in the peripheral blood before migrating to the tissues where they can live for several weeks. Once in the tissues, eosinophils do not reenter the circulation.[16]

FUNCTION

Eosinophils have multiple biologic functions and contribute to a variety of immune defense mechanisms. Eosinophil production and function are influenced by the cellular arm of the immune system (T cells). Eosinophils are associated with allergic diseases, parasitic infections, and chronic inflammation. Their major role is host defense against helminth parasites via a complex interaction of the eosinophils, adaptive immune system, and parasite. The eosinophil adheres to the organism and releases its granule contents onto the surface of the parasite via exocytosis. A number of eosinophil proteins are highly toxic for larval parasites, including MBP, ECP, and EPO. Eosinophils also are capable of phagocytosing bacteria (although less efficiently than neutrophils and macrophages) and have been shown to function as antigen-presenting cells.[18]

The eosinophils are proinflammatory cells that are capable of either protecting or damaging the host depending on the situation. Eosinophils respond weakly to IL-3, IL-5, and GM-CSF as chemotaxins, but IL-5 synthesized by T lymphocytes has been shown to prime eosinophils for a better chemotactic response to PAF, LTB$_4$, or IL-8. Products released from basophils and mast cells (eosinophil chemotactic factor/ECF), lymphokines from sensitized lymphocytes, and allergy-related antigen/antibody complexes are strongly chemotactic for eosinophils. Eosinophils express Fc receptors for IgE, which is prevalent in the response to parasitic infections and mediates activation of eosinophil killing mechanisms. The cytokines IL-3, IL-5, and GM-CSF promote the adherence of eosinophils; transendothelial migration is 10 times higher in the presence of these cytokines. These cytokines also prolong the survival of eosinophils in culture.

Eosinophils have a β_2 integrin-independent mechanism for recruitment into the tissues. This was first suggested when eosinophils and mononuclear leukocytes—but not neutrophils—were found at sites of infection in children with congenital β_2-integrin deficiency (LAD-1). Eosinophil recruitment appears to be modulated by the eosinophil adhesion receptor, VLA-4, and its ligand on VEC and VCAM-1. VCAM-1 has been shown to be expressed on VEC when the vascular endothelium is activated by IL-1, TNF, or IL-4. Changes in eosinophil adhesion molecule expression occur during eosinophil migration. This implies that dynamic changes in cell adhesion molecules are involved in cell recruitment to areas of inflammation.

The eosinophil liberates substances that can neutralize mast cell and basophil products, thereby down modulating the allergic response (Table 7-5). Increasing evidence suggests a direct correlation between the degree of eosinophilia and severity of inflammatory diseases such as asthma. In these conditions, the cytotoxic potential of eosinophils is turned against the host's own tissue.[19]

Charcot-Leyden crystals are bipyramidal crystals commonly found in fluids or tissues in association with eosinophilic inflammatory reactions. They are composed primarily of lysophospholipase, an eosinophil component found in eosinophil primary granules as opposed to the crystal-containing secondary or specific granules.

▶ BASOPHILS

Basophils (Figure 7-9 ■) originate from the CD34$^+$ myeloid progenitors in the bone marrow. IL-3 is the main cytokine involved in human basophil growth and differentiation, but it is believed that GM-CSF, SCF, IL-4, and IL-5 also have a role.[20,21]

DIFFERENTIATION, MATURATION, AND MORPHOLOGY

Basophils undergo a maturation process similar to that described for the neutrophil. The first recognizable stage is the promyelocyte, although this stage is very difficult to differentiate from the promyelocyte of the neutrophil or eosinophil. As with eosinophils and neutrophils, the various stages of the maturing basophil are characterized by a gradual indentation and segmentation of the nucleus.

Basophilic Myelocyte to Mature Basophil

The basophilic myelocyte, metamyelocyte, band, and segmented form are easily differentiated from other granulocytes by the presence of the large purple-black granules unevenly distributed throughout the cytoplasm. The granules are described as metachromatic and contain histamine, heparin, cathepsin G, major basic protein, and lysophospholipase.[20] The mature basophil ranges in size from 10 to 15 μm and has a segmented nucleus and many purple granules obscuring both the background of the cytoplasm and the nu-

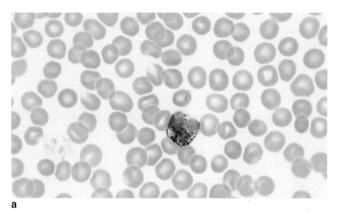

a

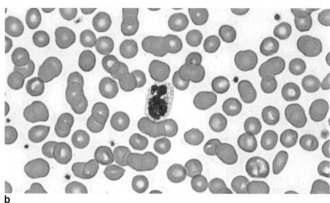

b

■ FIGURE 7-9   **a.** Basophil. (Peripheral blood, Wright-Giemsa stain, 1000× magnification). **b.** Basophil with washed out granules (staining artifact).

cleus. Basophil granules contain peroxidase and are positive with the PAS reaction. Basophil granules are water soluble and can dissolve on a well-rinsed Wright-stained smear, resulting in clear areas within the cytoplasm. Usually a few deep-purple–staining granules remain to aid in the identification of the cell. Basophils express the CD9, CD11a, and CD13 molecules.

Mast Cell (Tissue Basophil)

The relationship between basophils and mast cells continues to be investigated. Research shows that mast cells and basophils represent distinct, terminally differentiated cells derived from the CD34+ common myeloid progenitor cell. Distinct committed progenitor cells (CFU-B and CFU-MC) have been identified for each lineage.[22] Mast cells are found in the bone marrow and tissues but are not found in peripheral blood. Mast cells have proliferative potential and live for several weeks to months. At times, differentiating the mast cell and the basophil precursors in the bone marrow is difficult although some differences exist (Table 7-6). The mast cell nucleus is round and surrounded by a dense population of granules. The mast cell granules contain acid phosphatase, protease, and alkaline phosphatase. Mast cells have an antigen profile similar to that of macrophages.

CONCENTRATION, DISTRIBUTION, AND DESTRUCTION

Basophils' maturation in the bone marrow requires 2.5–7 days before they are released into circulation. In the peripheral blood, they number less than 0.2×10^9/L (<1% of the total leukocytes). Basophilia in adults is defined as $>0.2 \times 10^9$/L in the peripheral blood. Basophils are end-stage cells incapable of proliferation and spend only hours in the peripheral blood.

FUNCTION

The basophil and mast cell function as mediators of inflammatory responses, especially those of immediate hypersensitivity reactions such as asthma, urticaria, allergic rhinitis, and anaphylaxis. These cells have membrane receptors for IgE (FcεR). When IgE attaches to the receptor, the cell is activated and degranulation is initiated. Degranulation releases enzymes that are vasoactive, bronchoconstrictive, and chemotactic (especially for eosinophils). This release of mediators initiates the classic clinical signs of immediate hypersensitivity. These cells can synthesize more granules after degranulation occurs. Basophils and mast cells express CD40L, the ligand for CD40, an antigen on B lymphocytes. The interaction of B lymphocyte CD40 and basophil CD40L, in conjunction with IL-4, can induce IgE synthesis by B lymphocytes. Thus, basophils can play an important role in inducing and maintaining allergic reactions.[21]

✓ Checkpoint! 5

Indicate which of the granulocytes will be increased in the following conditions: a bacterial infection, an immediate hypersensitivity reaction, and an asthmatic reaction.

▶ MONOCYTES

The monocyte is produced in the bone marrow from a bipotential progenitor cell (CFU-GM) that is capable of maturing into either a monocyte or a granulocyte. The differentiation and proliferation of CFU-GM into monocytes depend on the action of GM-CSF, IL-3, and M-CSF (monocyte-stimulating factor). Monocytes continue to differentiate, transforming to macrophages in the tissues. Monocytes and macrophages can be stimulated by T lymphocytes and endotoxin to liberate

---

✪ TABLE 7-6

Comparison of the Characteristics of Basophils and Mast Cells

Characteristics	Basophils	Mast Cells
Origin	Hematopoietic stem cell	Hematopoietic stem cell
Site of maturation	Bone marrow	Connective or mucosal tissue
Proliferative potential	No	Yes
Life span	Days	Weeks to months
Size	Small	Large
Nucleus	Segmented	Round
Granules	Few, small (peroxidase positive)	Many, large (acid phosphatase, alkaline phosphatase positive)
Key cytokine regulating development	IL-3	Stem cell factor (SCF)
Surface receptors		
IL-3-R	Present	Absent
c-kit (SCF-R)	Absent	Present
IgE receptor (FcεR)	Present	Present

M-CSF, which can be one mechanism for the monocytosis associated with some infections. M-CSF also activates the secretory and phagocytic activity of monocytes and macrophages.[23] Monocytes and macrophages make up the **monocyte-macrophage system**. More recently, it has been proposed to call this continuum of cells the **mononuclear phagocyte system** (**MNP**).

DIFFERENTIATION, MATURATION, AND MORPHOLOGY

The morphologically recognizable monocyte precursors in the bone marrow are the monoblast and the promonocyte. These cells are present in very low concentration in the normal bone marrow and are found in abundance only in leukemic processes involving the MNP system. The monoblast of the marrow cannot be morphologically distinguished from the myeloblast by light microscopy unless proliferation of the monocytic series is marked as occurs in monocytic leukemia. Cytochemical stains and immunophenotyping frequently are used to help differentiate myeloblasts and monoblasts in suspected cases of leukemia.

The promonocyte is usually the first stage to develop morphologic characteristics that allow it to be clearly differentiated as a monocyte precursor by light microscopy. The identification of early monocyte precursors is aided by observing folds or indentations in the nucleus and by their association with mature monocytes.

Monoblast

The monoblast's (Figure 7-10a ■) nucleus is most often ovoid or round but can be folded or indented. Monoblasts are large, from 12–20 μm in diameter. The pale blue-purple nuclear chromatin is finely dispersed (lacy), and several nucleoli are easily identified. The monoblast has abundant agranular blue-gray cytoplasm. Differentiation of the monoblast from the myeloblast may be possible with special cytochemical stains (∞ Chapter 21). The monoblast has nonspecific esterase activity demonstrated by reaction with the substrates α-naphthyl butyrate or naphthol AS-D acetate (NASDA). Sodium fluoride inhibits NASDA activity. The myeloblast has both specific esterase activity (demonstrated by reaction with the substrate naphthol AS-D chloroacetate) and nonspecific esterase activity, but the nonspecific esterases are not inhibited by sodium fluoride. Immunophenotyping is

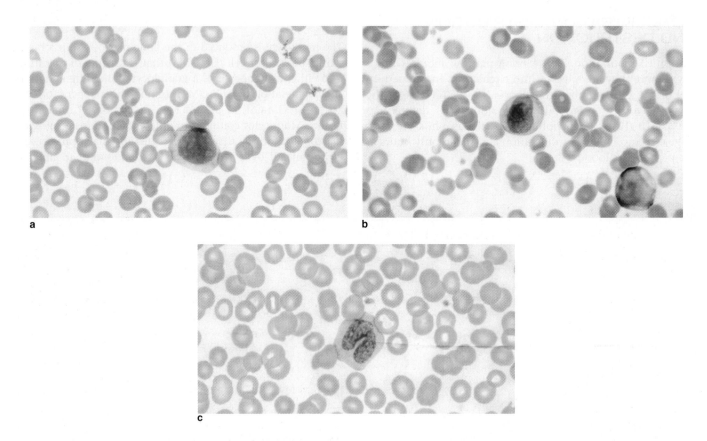

a

b

c

■ FIGURE 7-10 Stages of monocyte maturation: **a.** monoblast: Note lacy chromatin, nucleoli, and high N:C ratio; **b.** promonocyte: The chromatin is somewhat more coarse and the amount of cytoplasm is increased; **c.** monocyte: The nucleus is more lacy than that of a neutrophil or lymphocyte and is irregular in shape. (a, b: Bone marrow, Wright-Giemsa stain, 1000× magnification; c: Peripheral blood, Wright-Giemsa stain, 1000× magnification) also used to differentiate myeloblasts and monoblasts (∞ Chapter 24).

Promonocyte

The promonocyte (Figure 7-10b ■) is an intermediate form between the monoblast and the monocyte. The cell is large, 12–20 μm in diameter. The nucleus is most often irregular and indented with a fine chromatin network. Nuclear chromatin is coarser than the monoblast, and nucleoli can be present. The promonocyte's cytoplasm is abundant with a blue-gray color; azurophilic granules can be present. Cytochemical stains for nonspecific esterase, peroxidase, acid phosphatase, and arylsulfatase are positive.

Monocyte

Mature monocytes (Figure 7-10c ■) range in size from 12 to 20 μm with an average size of 18 μm, making them the largest mature cells in peripheral blood. The nucleus is frequently horseshoe- or bean-shaped and possesses numerous folds, giving it the appearance of brainlike convolutions. The chromatin is loose and linear, forming a lacy pattern in comparison to the clumped dense chromatin of mature lymphocytes or granulocytes. Monocytes, however, are sometimes difficult to distinguish from large lymphocytes, especially in reactive states when there are many reactive lymphocytes. The monocyte cytoplasm has variable morphologic characteristics depending on its activity. The cell adheres to glass and "spreads" or sends out numerous pseudopods resulting in a wide variation of size and shape on blood smears. The blue-gray cytoplasm is evenly dispersed with fine, dustlike membrane-bound granules, which give the cell cytoplasm the appearance of ground glass. Vacuoles are frequently observed in the cytoplasm.

Electron-microscopic cytochemistry reveals two types of granules present in monocytes. One type contains peroxidase, acid phosphatase, and arylsulfatase, suggesting that these granules are similar to the lysosomes (azurophilic granules) of neutrophils. Less is known about the content of the other type of granule except that it does not contain alkaline phosphatase. The lipid membrane of the granules stains faintly with Sudan black B. Many CD markers including CD11b/CD18, CD13, CD14, and CD15 are found on monocytes.

Macrophage

The monocyte leaves the blood and enters the tissues where it matures into a macrophage (Figure 7-11 ■). The transition from monocyte to macrophage is characterized by progressive cellular enlargement, reaching a 15–80 μm size. The nucleus becomes round with a reticular (netlike) appearance, nucleoli appear, and the cytoplasm appears blue-gray with ragged edges and many vacuoles present. As it matures, the macrophage loses peroxidase, but increases are seen in the amount of endoplasmic reticulum (ER), lysosomes, and mitochondria. Also, distinct granules are noted in the maturing macrophage. Macrophages acquire the expression of CD68, a glycoprotein that can be important in lipid metabolism. These cells can live for months in the tissues. Macrophages do not normally reen-

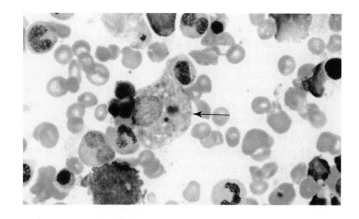

■ FIGURE 7-11   A macrophage. Note the numerous vacuoles and cellular debris. (Bone marrow, Wright-Giemsa stain, 1000× magnification)

ter the blood, but in areas of inflammation, some can gain access to the lymph, eventually entering the circulating blood.

Tissue macrophages, also known as *histiocytes,* develop different cytochemical and morphologic characteristics that depend on the site of maturation and habitation in tissue. These cells are widely distributed in the body and have been given specific names depending on their anatomic location. For example, macrophages in the liver are known as *Kupffer cells,* those in the lung as *alveolar macrophages,* those in the skin as *Langerhans cells,* and those in the brain as *microglial cells.*

Macrophages can proliferate in the tissue, especially in areas of inflammation, thereby increasing the number of cells at these sites. Occasionally, two or more macrophages fuse to produce giant multinucleated cells. This occurs in chronic inflammatory states and granulomatous lesions where many macrophages are tightly packed together. Fusion also occurs when particulate matter is too large for one cell to ingest or when two cells simultaneously ingest a particle.

DISTRIBUTION, CONCENTRATION, AND KINETICS

Before maturing into monocytes, the promonocyte undergoes two or three divisions. Bone marrow transit time is about 54 hours. In contrast to the large neutrophil storage pool, there is no significant reserve pool of monocytes in the bone marrow; most are released within a day after their derivation from promonocytes. Monocytes diapedese into the tissue from the peripheral blood in a random manner after an average transit time in the vascular system of ~8 hours.[23]

The total vascular monocyte pool consists of a marginated pool and a circulating pool; the marginating pool is about three times the size of the circulating pool. Monocytes in the circulating peripheral blood number about $0.1–0.8 \times 10^9$/L in the normal adult, or ~2%–10% of the total leukocytes. Children have a slightly higher concentration. Monocytosis (increase in monocytes) in adults occurs when the absolute monocyte count is $>0.8 \times 10^9$/L.

FUNCTION

Monocytes and macrophages are active in both the innate and adaptive IR. In addition to their phagocytic function, they secrete a variety of substances that affect the function of other cells, especially lymphocytes. Lymphocytes in turn secrete soluble products—lymphokines—that modulate monocytic functions.

Monocytes and macrophages ingest and kill microorganisms. They are particularly important in inhibiting the growth of intracellular microorganisms. This inhibition requires cellular activation (enhancement of function) of monocytes by soluble products of T lymphocytes. Killing by activated monocytes is nonspecific (i.e., the secretions from *Listeria*-sensitized T cells activate a killing mechanism in monocytes not only to *Listeria* but also to other microorganisms). Activation also can occur as the result of the actions of other substances on monocytes such as endotoxins and naturally occurring opsonins. Activation results in the production of many large granules, enhanced phagocytosis, and an increase in the activity of the HMP shunt.

Monocytes/macrophages have some ability to bind directly to microorganisms via PAMP and PRR (see leukocyte function), but binding is enhanced if the microorganism has been opsonized by complement or immunoglobulin (Web Figure 7-1 ■). Macrophages possess receptors for the Fc component of IgG and for the complement component C3b. Following attachment, the opsonized organism is ingested in a manner similar to that of neutrophils (see Figure 7-7). Primary lysosomes fuse with the phagosome, releasing hydrolytic enzymes and other microbicidal substances. The most powerful microbicidal substances of monocytes and macrophages are products of oxygen metabolism—superoxide (O_2^-), hydroxy radical (OH^-), singlet oxygen ($^1O_2$), and hydrogen peroxide (H_2O_2)—generated in a reaction analogous to the neutrophil respiratory burst.

Activated macrophages attach to tumor cells and kill them by a direct cytotoxic effect. If the tumor cell has immunoglobulin attached, the macrophage Fc receptor attaches to the Fc portion of the immunoglobulin and exerts a lytic effect on the tumor cell.

Macrophages are important scavengers, phagocytosing cellular debris, effete cells, and other particulate matter. Monocytes in the blood ingest activated clotting factors, thus limiting the coagulation process. They also ingest denatured protein and antigen–antibody complexes. Macrophages lining the blood vessels remove toxic substances from the blood, preventing their escape into tissues. The macrophages of the spleen are important in removing aged erythrocytes from the blood; they conserve the iron of hemoglobin by either storing it for future use or releasing it to transferrin for use by developing normoblasts in the marrow. By virtue of their Fc receptor, the splenic macrophages also remove cells sensitized with antibody. In autoimmune hemolytic anemias or in autoimmune thrombocytopenia, the spleen is sometimes removed to prevent premature destruction of these an-

tibody-coated cells in an attempt to alleviate the resulting cytopenias.

For unknown reasons, erythrocytes in some pathologic conditions are randomly phagocytosed and destroyed by monocytes and macrophages in the blood and bone marrow (erythrophagocytosis) (Figure 7-12 ■). **Erythrophagocytosis** is readily identified when the ingested erythrocytes still contain hemoglobin. At times, erythrocyte digestion can be inferred by finding ghost spheres within the macrophage.

In addition to its role in pathogen control and tissue homeostasis, the MNP plays a major role in initiating and regulating the adaptive IR.[23] Macrophages phagocytize and degrade both soluble and particulate substances that are foreign to the host. Through unknown mechanisms, they spare critical portions of these antigens known as *antigenic determinants* or *epitopes*. These antigenic determinants are bound by MHC molecules on the macrophage membrane and are presented to antigen-dependent T lymphocytes. Thus, monocytes and macrophages can function as **antigen-presenting cells** (APC). In addition to antigen presentation, the macrophage produces a number of cytokines that regulate the adaptive IR as well as the inflammatory response. Antigen-specific T lymphocyte proliferation requires antigen presentation in context with cell surface MHC antigens and stimulation with soluble mediators such as IL-1 and IL-2. T lymphocytes respond to foreign antigens only when the antigens are displayed on APCs that have the same MHC phenotype as the lymphocyte itself.

Macrophages stimulate the proliferation and differentiation of lymphocytes through secretion of cytokines. They secrete IL-1, which stimulates T lymphocytes to secrete interleukin-2 (IL-2), a growth factor that stimulates the proliferation of other T lymphocytes. In addition, IL-2 acts in synergy with interferon (IFN) to activate macrophages. When released from macrophages, arachidonic metabolites (e.g., leukotrienes, prostaglandins) inhibit the function of activated lymphocytes. Activated lymphocytes in turn secrete lymphokines that regulate the function of macrophages. For these interdependent reactions to occur between the macrophage and lymphocyte, the two cell populations must express compatible MHC antigens.

In addition to IL-1, macrophages release a variety of substances that are involved in host defense or that can affect

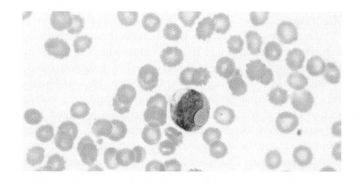

■ FIGURE 7-12 Erythrophagocytosis by a monocyte. (Peripheral blood, Wright-Giemsa stain, 1000× magnification)

the function of other cells. Other secretory products involved in host defense include lysozymes, complement components, and IFN (an antiviral compound). Secreted substances that modulate other cells include hematopoietic growth factors (e.g., G-CSF, M-CSF, GM-CSF), substances which stimulate the growth of new capillaries (angiogenic cytokines), factors that stimulate and suppress the activity of lymphocytes, chemotactic substances for neutrophils, and a substance that stimulates the hepatocyte to secrete fibrinogen. After death, activated macrophages also release enzymes such as collagenase, elastase, and neutral proteinase that hydrolyze tissue components.

 Checkpoint! 6

An adult patient's neutrophil count and monocyte count are extremely low ($<0.50 \times 10^9$/L and $<0.050 \times 10^9$/L, respectively). What body defense mechanism is at risk?

PART II

LYMPHOCYTES

For many years after its discovery, the lymphocyte was considered an insignificant component of blood and lymph. Since 1960, major advances in immunology have targeted lymphocytes as the effector cells of the adaptive immune response. The lymphocyte's primary functions are to: recognize and react with antigens; work with monocytes to eliminate pathogens; and provide long-lasting immunity to previously encountered pathogens.

▶ LYMPHOCYTES

COMMITMENT AND DIFFERENTIATION

The lymphoid lineage arises from the pluripotential HSC found in the bone marrow. This stem cell gives rise to committed progenitor cells: the CLP and the CMP (∞ Chapter 3). The lymphoid progenitor cell differentiates and matures under the inductive influence of selective microenvironments into three types of morphologically identical but immunologically and functionally diverse lymphocytes. T lymphocytes and B lymphocytes are the major cells of the adaptive immune response. A third type of lymphocyte, the natural killer (NK) cell, has characteristics distinctly different from those of T and B lymphocytes and is an effector cell of innate immunity against infectious agents and transformed cells that have altered expression of histocompatibility antigens (see section on NK cells).

T and B lymphopoiesis can be divided into two distinct phases: antigen-independent lymphopoiesis and antigen-dependent lymphopoiesis (Figure 7-13■). Antigen-independent lymphopoiesis takes place within the primary lymphoid tissue

(bone marrow, thymus, fetal liver). Antigen-independent lymphopoiesis begins with the committed lymphoid progenitor cell and results in the formation of immunocompetent T and B lymphocytes (referred to as *virgin* or *naïve lymphocytes* because they have not yet reacted with antigens). These cells exit the primary lymphoid tissue and migrate to secondary lymphoid tissue (spleen, lymph nodes, gut-associated lymphoid tissue) where the secondary phase of lymphopoiesis continues. Antigen-dependent lymphopoiesis begins with recognition of and interaction with antigens by specific antigen receptors on the surface of the immunocompetent T and B lymphocytes (T cell receptors [TCR] and B cell receptors [BCR]). Interaction with antigen results in the formation of effector T and B lymphocytes. These effector cells mediate the adaptive immune response.

Effector T cells are responsible for cell-mediated cytotoxic reactions (T_c), suppressor functions (T_S), and delayed hypersensitivity responses (T_{DHS}). They also produce cytokines that regulate immune responses (T regulatory cells, T_{reg}) and provide helper activity for B cells (T_H). B lymphocytes can concentrate and present antigens to T cells and are the precursors of immunoglobulin-secreting plasma cells. Each B lymphocyte can be programmed to make a specific antibody targeted against a specific triggering antigen by rearrangement of its immunoglobulin genes. The NK cells are a form of cytotoxic lymphocyte that composes a major component of the innate immune system. NK cells play a key role in the cytolysis of both tumor- and pathogen-infected cells. They do not rearrange or express T-cell receptor genes or B-cell immunoglobulin genes and thus do not express antigen-specific receptors.

Morphologic criteria cannot be used to differentiate between T, B, and NK lymphocytes. When there is a need to distinguish between them, monoclonal antibodies and flow cytometry for subset-specific CD molecules are most often used.

DIFFERENTIATION: MORPHOLOGY OF IMMATURE LYMPHOCYTES

Three morphologic stages of lymphoid maturation are recognized: lymphoblast, prolymphocyte, and lymphocyte. The morphologic changes that occur during differentiation or activation are shared by the major lymphocyte subgroups. T, B, and NK lymphocytes and their precursors are indistinguishable by morphologic criteria.

Lymphoblast

The lymphoblast (Figure 7-14a■) is about 10–18 μm in diameter with a high N:C ratio. The nuclear chromatin is lacy and fine, but it appears more smudged or heavy than that of myeloblasts. One or two well-defined pale blue nucleoli are visible. The nuclear membrane is dense, and a perinuclear clear zone can be seen; it has less basophilic agranular cytoplasm than other white cell blasts. Subtle morphologic differences exist, but lymphoblasts are usually indistinguishable from myeloblasts. Cytochemical stains can be used to help identify their lymphoid origin (∞ Chapter 21). Unlike myeloblasts, lymphoblasts stain negative for peroxidase, lipid,

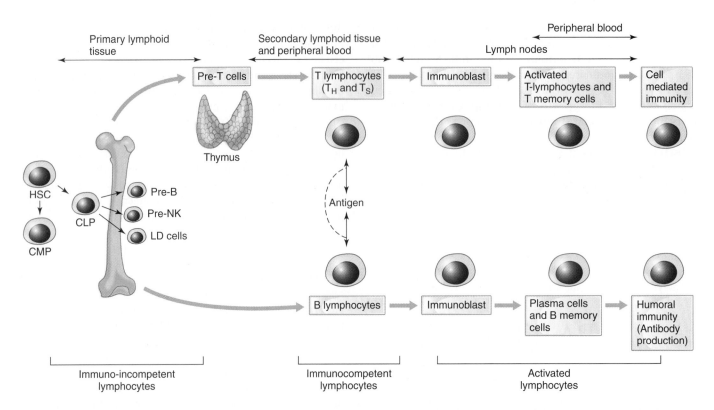

■ FIGURE 7-13   Lymphocytes originate from the common lymphoid progenitor cell/CLP (derived from the pluripotential hematopoietic stem cell/HSC) in the bone marrow. Lymphocyte progenitors that mature in the thymus become T lymphocytes, and those that mature in the bone marrow become B lymphocytes, natural killer cells (NK), or lymphoid-derived dendritic cells (LD). Three *morphologic* stages can be identified in this development to T- and B-cells: lymphoblast, prolymphocyte, and lymphocyte. On encounter with antigen, these immunocompetent T and B lymphocytes undergo blast transformation, usually in the lymph nodes, to form effector lymphocytes. The B lymphocytes eventually emerge as plasma cells. Effector T lymphocytes, however, are often morphologically indistinguishable from the original T lymphocytes. The recognizable morphologic stages of blast transformation include reactive lymphocytes, immunoblasts, plasmacytoid lymphocytes (B-cells), and plasma cells (B-cells). Flow cytometry indicates that some morphologic stages could represent several stages of immunologic maturation.

and esterase but contain acid phosphatase and sometimes deposits of glycogen (PAS+). Both T and B lymphoblasts contain a DNA polymerase, terminal deoxynucleotidyl transferase (TdT), present in immature lymphoid cells intermediate between the CLP and differentiated T and B cells.

Prolymphocyte

The prolymphocyte is difficult to distinguish in normal bone marrow specimens (Figure 7-14b■). The prolymphocyte is slightly smaller than the lymphoblast with a lower N:C ratio. The nuclear chromatin is clumped but more finely dispersed than that of the lymphocyte. Nucleoli are usually present, and the cytoplasm is light blue and agranular.

Lymphocyte

The mature lymphocyte has extreme size variability, 7–16 μm when flattened on a glass slide, which is primarily dependent on the amount of cytoplasm present (Figure 7-14c■). Small lymphocytes range in size from 7–10 μm. In these cells, the nucleus is about the size of an erythrocyte and occupies about 90% of the cell area. The chromatin is deeply con-

densed, staining a dark purple. Nucleoli, although always present, are rarely visible with the light microscope as small, light areas within the nucleus. The nucleus is surrounded by a narrow rim of sky blue cytoplasm. A few azurophilic granules and vacuoles can be present. Lymphocytes are motile and can show a peculiar hand-mirror shape on stained blood smears with the nucleus in the rounded anterior portion (protopod) trailed by an elongated section of cytoplasm known as the *uropod*. Small lymphocytes include a diversity of functional subsets including resting, immunocompetent, differentiated effector, and memory T and B lymphocytes.

Large lymphocytes are heterogeneous and range in size from 11 to 16 μm in diameter. The nucleus can be slightly larger than in the small lymphocyte, but the difference in cell size is mainly attributable to a larger amount of cytoplasm. The cytoplasm can be lighter blue with peripheral basophilia or darker than the cytoplasm of small lymphocytes. Azurophilic granules can be present; if prominent, the cell is described as a large granular lymphocyte. These granules differ from those of the myelocytic cells in that they are peroxidase negative. The nuclear chromatin can appear similar to that of the small lym-

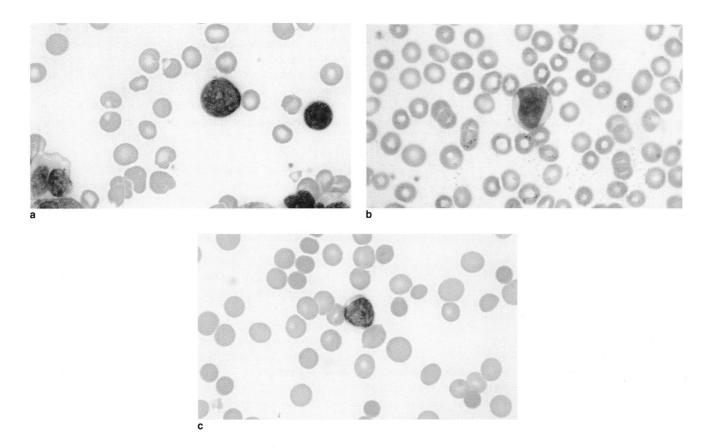

■ FIGURE 7-14 Morphologic stages of lymphocyte maturation. **a.** lymphoblast: Note the lacy chromatin and high N:C ratio; **b.** prolymphocyte: Note the increased amount of cytoplasm; **c.** lymphocyte: The nuclear chromatin is coarse and smudged. (a, b: Bone marrow, Wright-Giemsa stain, 1000× magnification; c: Peripheral blood, Wright-Giemsa stain, 1000× magnification)

phocyte or more dispersed, and the nucleus can be slightly indented. These large cells, like small lymphocytes, probably represent a diversity of functional subsets.

Normally ~3% of blood lymphocytes are described as **large granular lymphocytes (LGL)**, so named because of the presence of large granules in their cytoplasm. These cells consist of a mixed population of both NK cells and some mature CD8+ (cytotoxic) T cells (T_C). These cells have a round or indented nucleus and abundant pale blue cytoplasm containing coarse pink granules (Figure 7-15 ■). The granules, thought to be related to the cells' cytolytic capacity, contain the pore-forming proteolytic enzyme perforin and granzymes (serine proteases with pro-apoptotic activity).

ACTIVATION: MORPHOLOGY OF ACTIVATED LYMPHOCYTES

During development into immunocompetent T and B lymphocytes (cells with the ability to respond to stimulation by an antigen), the cells acquire specific receptors for a particular antigen, which commits them to an antigen specificity. During the antigen-dependent phase of lymphocyte development, contact and binding of this specific antigen to receptors on immunocompetent T and B lymphocytes begin a

complex sequence of cellular events known as *blast transformation* (*blastogenesis*). The end result is a clonal amplification of cells responsible for the overt expression of immunity to the specific antigen. Usually occurring within the lymph node, this series of events includes cell enlargement, an increase in the rough endoplasmic reticulum (RER), enlargement of the nucleolus, dispersal of chromatin and an increase in DNA synthesis, and mitosis. These transformed cells, called *immunoblasts,* have the option to differentiate into terminally differentiated effector cells capable of mediating the immune response or long-lived memory cells. The morphologically identifiable forms of antigen-stimulated lymphocytes include the reactive lymphocyte, reactive immunoblast, plasmacytoid lymphocyte, and plasma cell.

Reactive lymphocytes and immunoblasts can be either T or B lymphocytes, which can be determined only by cell marker studies (flow cytometry). In the past, reactive lymphocytes and immunoblasts were referred to as *Downey cells* (a term usually used to describe the cells seen in infectious mononucleosis) and were classified as Types I, II, or III, depending on various morphologic criteria. This classification is obsolete because the various types of Downey cells are simply morphologic variations accompanying the process of blast transformation.

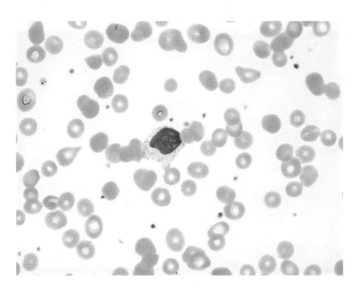

■ FIGURE 7-15   Large granular lymphocyte. (Peripheral blood, Wright-Giemsa stain, 1000× magnification)

Reactive Lymphocyte

The **reactive lymphocyte** (Figure 7-16a■) exhibits a variety of morphologic features, including one or more of the following. It can increase in size (16–30 μm) and have a decreased N:C ratio. The nucleus can be round but is more frequently elongated, stretched, or irregular. The chromatin becomes more dispersed, staining lighter than the chromatin of a resting lymphocyte, and nucleoli can be seen. There usually is an increase in diffuse or localized basophilia of the cytoplasm, and azurophilic granules and/or vacuoles can be present. The cytoplasmic membrane can be indented by surrounded erythrocytes, which sometimes gives the cell a scalloped edge.

The reactive lymphocyte is also referred to as a *stimulated, transformed, atypical, activated,* or *variant lymphocyte.* However, the word *atypical* carries the connotation of abnormal or malignant, and some hematologists therefore prefer not to use the term to describe normal lymphocytes in various stages of reaction to antigenic stimulation.

A few reactive lymphocytes can be seen in the blood of healthy individuals, but they are found in increased numbers in viral infections. For this reason, the reactive lymphocyte has also been called a *virocyte.*

Immunoblast

The **immunoblast** (Figure 7-16b■) is the next stage in blast transformation. The cell is large, 12–25 μm in size. The cell is characterized by prominent nucleoli and a fine nuclear chromatin pattern (but coarser than that of other leukocyte blasts). The large nucleus is usually central and stains a purple-blue color. The abundant cytoplasm stains an intense blue color due to the high density of polyribosomes. These are cells preparing for or engaged in mitosis. The immunoblast proliferates, increasing the pool of cells programmed to respond to the initial stimulating antigen.

These programmed daughter cells (effector lymphocytes) mature into cells that mediate the effector arm of the immune response.

The daughter cells of B immunoblasts, which mediate **humoral immunity,** are plasmacytoid lymphocytes (Figure 7-16c■) and plasma cells (Figure 7-16d■). Humoral immunity is the production of antibodies by activated B lymphocytes stimulated by antigen. The plasmacytoid lymphocyte (also referred to as lymphocytoid plasma cell) is believed to be an intermediate cell between the B lymphocyte and the plasma cell. It gains its descriptive name from its morphologic similarity to the lymphocyte but has marked cytoplasmic basophila similar to that of plasma cells.

In contrast to the progeny of the B immunoblast, effector cells produced from the T immunoblast, T cytotoxic cells (T_C), T suppressor cells (T_S), or T helper cells (T_H) are morphologically indistinguishable from the original unsensitized lymphocytes or appear as LGL.

Plasmacytoid Lymphocyte

The **plasmacytoid lymphocyte** ranges in size from 15 to 20 μm. The nuclear chromatin is less clumped (more immature) than that of a plasma cell, and it can have a single visible nucleolus. The nucleus is central or slightly eccentric, and the cytoplasm is deeply basophilic. The cell has some cytoplasmic immunoglobulin (cIg) as well as surface membrane immunoglobulin (sIg). This cell is occasionally seen in the peripheral blood of patients with viral infections.

Plasma Cells

Plasma cells are round or slightly oval with a 9–20 μm diameter. The nucleus is eccentrically placed and contains coarse blocklike radial masses of chromatin, often referred to as the *cartwheel* or *spoke wheel arrangement.* Nucleoli are not present. The paranuclear Golgi complex is obvious and surrounded by deeply basophilic cytoplasm. The cytoplasm stains red with pyronine (pyroninophilic) because of the high RNA content. The RER is well developed, and the cytoplasm enlarges because of the production of large amounts of immunoglobulin. As cytoplasmic immunoglobulin increases, the cell's secretory capacity increases. Membrane sIg is usually absent, but azurophilic granules and rodlike crystal inclusions can be present.

Memory Cells

A number of the T and B immunoblast daughter cells alternatively form T and B memory cells. **Memory cells** are morphologically similar to the resting small lymphocytes, retain the ability to react with the stimulating antigen, and are capable of eliciting a rapid secondary immune response when challenged again by the same antigen.

The reactive lymphocyte is commonly found in the blood during viral infection; the immunoblast, plasmacytoid lymphocyte, and plasma cell usually are found only in lymph nodes and other secondary lymphoid tissue. During intense stimulation of the immune system, however, these trans-

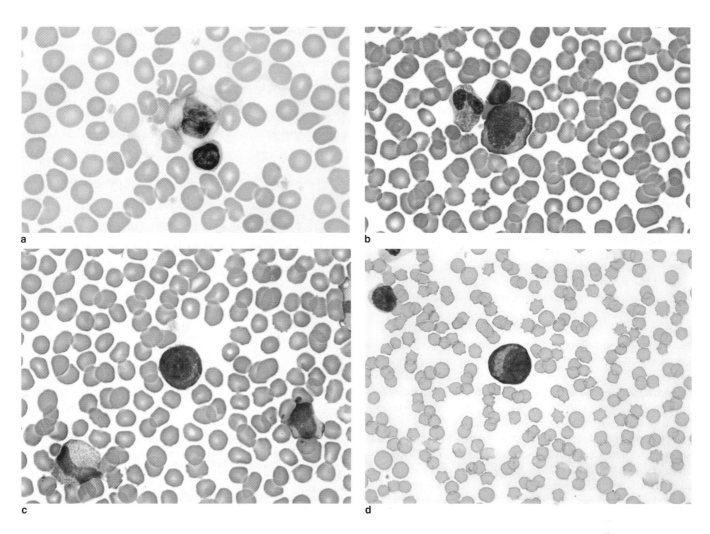

■ FIGURE 7-16   Stages of lymphocyte activation. **a.** Reactive lymphocyte: The cell is large with an increased amount of basophilic cytoplasm. Note the normal lymphocyte below the reactive lymphocyte; **b.** Immunoblast: The N:C ratio is high. The nucleus has a lacy chromatin pattern, and the cytoplasm is deep blue; a small lymphocyte is above the immunoblast **c.** Plasmacytoid lymphocyte: The nuclear chromatin is coarse, and there is a moderate amount of deep blue cytoplasm; there is a reactive lymphocyte to the lower right. **d.** Plasma cell: The fully differentiated B cell has an eccentric nucleus and there is a large amount of basophilic cytoplasm. (Peripheral blood, Wright-Giemsa stain, 1000× magnification)

formed cells can be found in the peripheral blood due to lymphocyte recirculation.

 Checkpoint! 7

How would you morphologically differentiate a reactive lymphocyte from a plasma cell on a peripheral blood smear?

LYMPHOID LINEAGE DIFFERENTIATION

The phenotypic features of lymphocytes that allow them to be identified as T lymphocytes or B lymphocytes include cytochemical staining properties, CD surface markers, and membrane antigens. This differentiation is possible throughout antigen-independent and antigen-dependent lympho-poiesis. Examples of markers for B cell precursors include CD10, CD19, CD21, CD22, and CD24. Markers for T cell precursors include CD1, CD2, CD3, CD5, and CD7. T lymphoblasts contain nonspecific esterase, β-glucuronidase, and N-acetyl β-glucosamidase, as well as a punctuate pattern of acid phosphatase positivity. The esterase and acid phosphatase stains for B lymphoblasts are either negative or have a scattered granular pattern of positivity. B lymphoblasts can contain small amounts of immunoglobulin or the μ immunoglobulin heavy chain, which can be detected by using immunofluorescent techniques.

T Lymphocytes
Bone marrow lymphoid precursor cells migrate to the thymus (primary lymphoid organ) where they proliferate and

differentiate to acquire cellular characteristics of T lymphocytes. It is unclear which specific precursor cell migrates, the HSC, CLP, CFU-T/NK, or CFU-T (∞ Chapter 3). Lymphopoiesis at this stage correlates to the antigen-independent stage of lymphoid development.

The hormone thymosin, synthesized and secreted by epithelial cells in the thymus, is believed to influence T lymphocyte maturation. Intrathymic proliferation and death for potential T lymphocytes is high with about 95% of the cells produced undergoing apoptosis. Consequently, only a small portion of T-precursor cells leave the thymus as immunocompetent, naïve T lymphocytes.

The historic viewpoint has been that the thymus functions in T lymphopoiesis primarily during fetal life and the first few years after birth, and the T lymphoid system was considered to be nearly fully developed at birth. Surgical removal of the thymus after birth does not severely impair immunologic defense; however, lack of thymus development in the fetus (DiGeorge syndrome) results in the absence of T lymphocytes and severe impairment of cell mediated immunity. However, more recent studies utilizing polymerase chain reaction–based assays to detect excised products of the TCR gene rearrangement (described below) have demonstrated that while thymic function declines significantly (by 5-fold at age 35 years), the T cell pool continues to be replenished by a functioning thymus throughout life.[24]

Cell-mediated immunity is the basis of the immune response mediated by T lymphocytes and requires interaction between histocompatible T lymphocytes, macrophages, and antigens. Several important T lymphocyte subsets are involved. T cells diversify late in thymic maturation into either T helper/effector (T_H, T_{Reg} CD4$^+$, or T_4) lymphocytes or T cytotoxic/suppressor (T_C/T_S, CD8$^+$, or T_8) lymphocytes. When activated, these cells proliferate, produce lymphokines, and a mount a diverse set of effector functions. These subsets are phenotypically and functionally distinct but morphologically indistinguishable

T lymphocytes confer protection against antigens that have the ability to avoid contact with antibodies by residing and replicating within the cells of the host. Thus, serious infection with intracellular parasites (bacteria, fungi, and viruses) can occur if T lymphocytes are deficient.

T Lymphocyte Membrane Markers   Lymphocyte subpopulations were first identified by virtue of unique surface receptors, which have a binding affinity for certain ligands. Binding of sheep red blood cells (SRBC) by T lymphocytes via the E (erythrocyte) receptor traditionally has been a marker for identifying T cells. The E receptor, now known as *CD2* or *lymphocyte function antigen-3* (*LFA-3*), binds SRBC, forming a rosette. The T lymphocyte is the center of the rosette, and the SRBCs form the petals.

T lymphocytes also possess receptors for the Fc portion of IgM and IgG (CD16). T lymphocytes can change the specificity of their Fc receptor upon antigenic stimulation. Additionally, CD surface markers (including CD4 and CD8, discussed above)

and/or other antigens are used to differentiate developmental stages of T precursor cells. CD4 and CD8 are members of the immunoglobulin supergene family of adhesion molecules.

T Lymphocyte Antigen Receptor   The T lymphocyte has an antigen receptor on its surface (**T cell receptor,** [TCR]), responsible for initiating the cellular immune response. The TCR is a heterodimer of two peptide chains linked by a disulfide bond (Figure 7-17 ■). This receptor is a member of the immunoglobulin supergene family of adhesion molecules. Two subsets of T cells are defined by expression of distinct TCR polypeptides: TCR with gamma and delta chains ($\gamma\delta$ T cells) and TCR with alpha and beta chains ($\alpha\beta$ T cells). More than 90% of T lymphocytes are $\alpha\beta$ T cells.[25,26] The organization of the TCR chains is similar to

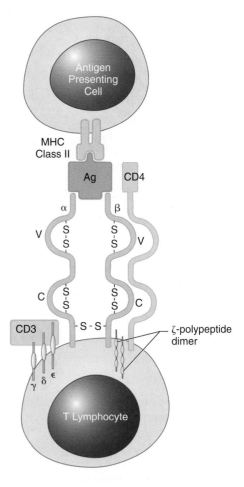

■ **FIGURE 7-17**   The T lymphocyte has an antigen receptor (TCR) on its surface that is composed of two peptide chains linked by a disulfide bond. This receptor is expressed in a complex with CD3 (γ, δ, ε polypeptides) and a ζ-polypeptide dimer. This TCR is in close proximity to an MHC-restricted receptor (CD4 or CD8) that recognizes the appropriate molecule on antigen presenting cells (APCs). The helper T lymphocyte receptor (CD4), shown here, recognizes Class II MHC molecules, and the suppressor T lymphocytes receptor (CD8) recognizes Class I MHC molecules.

that of the immunoglobulin chains. Each TCR chain is composed of a variable region that binds an antigen and a constant region that anchors the TCR to the cell membrane. The variable (V) region is made from three DNA segments—variable (V), diversity (D), and joining (J)—in the beta and delta chains but only two segments, V and J, in the alpha and gamma chains. A complete V region (i.e., VDJ) is translocated to a constant (C) segment to form the individual TCR chains. Random rearrangement and recombination of various V, D, and J segments and subsequent joining with a C segment provide the antigenic diversity of T cell receptors. This diversity allows the T lymphocyte to recognize many different antigens.

The $\alpha\beta$ and $\gamma\delta$ TCR are expressed as a molecular complex with several other transmembrane polypeptide chains (CD3γ, CD3δ, and CD3ε) in the cell membrane. These chains form δ:ε and γ:ε heterodimers in the cell membrane producing the CD3 complex. Also included in the TCR is a ζ-chain homodimer (CD247). These auxiliary molecules (CD3 and CD247) with the $\gamma\delta$TCR or $\alpha\beta$TCR mediate intracellular signal transduction when antigen binds to the TCR antigen-receptor.[27] Antigenic stimulation of T lymphocytes requires presentation of antigen bound to major histocompatibility (MHC) molecules of antigen-presenting cells (APC). T cell response is "MHC restricted," that is, T lymphocytes respond only to foreign antigens displayed by APCs having the same MHC phenotype as the T cell. APCs include dendritic cells, macrophages, and B lymphocytes.

Dendritic cells are derived from the HSC and are present in all tissues. There are two pathways of development for dendritic cells: one group originates from the CMP (myeloid-derived) and the other group originates from the CLP (lymphoid-derived). Their function is to process the antigen and present it in a recognizable form to T lymphocytes.

The different subsets of T lymphocytes recognize different classes of MHC molecules with the CD4 and CD8 molecules of the T cell serving as "coreceptors" in the interaction. In cytotoxic or suppressor T cells, the CD8 molecule recognizes and interacts with Class I MHC molecules, but in T helper cells, the CD4 molecule recognizes and interacts with Class II MHC molecules.

T Lymphocyte Developmental Stages Differentiation of the various developmental stages for both T and B lymphocytes is based on the appearance of specific molecular changes as well as membrane molecules. It is possible to define distinct stages of intrathymic differentiation of T lymphocytes using monoclonal probes to identify the presence of CD antigens on the cell surface as well as molecular evidence of TCR gene rearrangement. Some antigenic determinants appear at a very early developmental stage of the cell and disappear with maturity; other unique determinants appear on more mature cells (Figure 7-18 ■).[28]

Commitment to the T cell lineage depends on cytokines produced by the thymic stroma including IL-1α and tumor necrosis factor-α (TNF-α). The exact lymphoid progenitor

cell that migrates to the thymus is unclear; however, acquisition of cell surface CD1 identifies a precursor cell committed to T lineage differentiation.[29,30] The stages of T cell development are most reliably defined based on changes in rearrangement of the gene loci for the TCR polypeptides and the presence of the TCR coreceptors, CD4 and CD8. The major developmental stages are termed pro-T cell, pre-T cell, double positive (DP) and single positive (SP) thymocyte, and T cell (Figure 7-18).

The earliest committed T-cell precursor, a *pro-T cell*, is CD34+ and contains germline configuration of the TCR α-, β-, γ-, and δ-loci. These cells are also CD25+ (IL-2 receptor) and CD44+ (thymic homing receptor) but CD4−CD8− ("double negative" cells). They contain TdT (terminal deoxynucleotidyl transferase). During transition from pro-T to pre-T cell, rearrangement of the β-chain locus occurs. If the rearrangement is successful, the β-chain is expressed in the cytoplasm (cβ) toward the end of the pro-T stage.

At the next developmental stage, pre-T cell, the TCR β-chain appears on the cell surface complexed with a surrogate α-chain (preTα) and the CD3 polypeptides as a pre-TCR (pre-Tα/ TCRβ). Expression of the pre-TCR signals expression of both CD4 and CD8, forming *double positive (DP) thymocytes* (late pre-T cell). During the pre-T cell stage, the α-chain undergoes rearrangement.

When a functional α-chain has been produced, it pairs with the β-chain to form the $\alpha\beta$TCR. This appears on the surface of the cell with the CD3 complex (DP, $\alpha\beta$TCR:CD3). In the next step, the DP thymocyte undergoes selection and differentiation into either SP CD4+CD8− (T$_H$) or CD4−CD8+ (T$_{S/C}$)T cells. At this point, the cells are immunocompetent but naïve T cells. SP T$_H$ or T$_{S/C}$ cells leave the thymus and enter the circulation to complete final maturation. In the periphery, encounters with the antigen specifically recognized by the unique variable region of the TCR result in activation and generation of appropriate effector cells and memory T cells (antigen-dependent phase of lymphopoiesis).

Thus, early thymocytes have markers of both helper (CD4+) and suppressor (CD8+) cells (DP thymocytes); later mature (though naïve) T cells express one or the other (CD4+ T$_H$ cells or CD8+ T$_{S/C}$ cells). About 60–80% of peripheral blood T lymphocytes are CD4 cells (T$_4$). They are also the predominant T lymphocytes of the lymph nodes. CD8 cells (T$_8$) make up only 35% of peripheral blood T lymphocytes but are the predominant T lymphocyte found in the bone marrow. The normal T$_4$:T$_8$ ratio in circulating blood is thus ~2:1. The balance between T$_4$ and T$_8$ must be maintained for normal activity of the immune system. This ratio can be depressed in viral infections, immune deficiency states, and acquired immune deficiency syndrome (AIDS) and can be increased in disorders such as acute graft versus host disease, scleroderma, and multiple sclerosis.

There are two subtypes of CD4+ cells: T$_{H1}$ and T$_{H2}$. They differ as to the cytokines they produce, the cells they affect, and the pathogens with which they react. T$_{H1}$ cells participate in cell-mediated immunity against intracellular

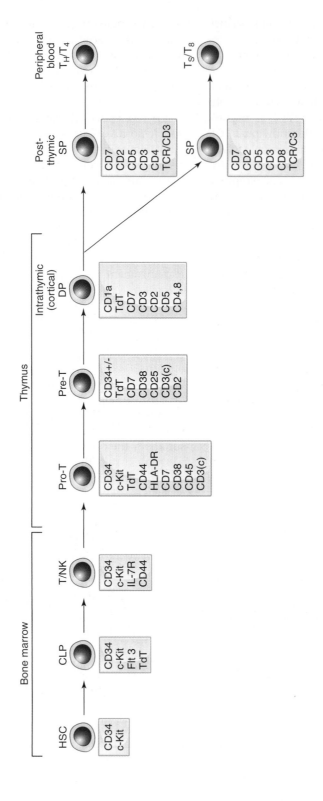

■ FIGURE 7-18 Immunologic maturation of the T lymphocyte from the common lymphoid progenitor cell (CLP) to the peripheral blood T helper (T$_H$) and T suppressor/cytotoxic (T$_S$/T$_C$) lymphocytes. Monoclonal antibodies and molecular studies for TCR gene rearrangements have identified at least four intrathymic stages of maturation before the cells are released to the peripheral blood as mature T lymphocytes. These include pro-T cell, pre-T cell, double positive (DP), and single positive (SP). Differentiation into either helper or suppressor lymphocytes occurs at the last intrathymic stage of maturation. (CD = cluster of differentiation; TCR = T cell receptor; TdT = terminyldeoxynucleotidyl transferase; IL-7R = interleukin 7 receptor; c-Kit = stem cell factor receptor, also called CD117)

pathogens and activate macrophages. T_{H2} cells provide help to the B cells and are essential for antibody-mediated immunity. Table 7-7 ✪ summarizes the T helper cell functions.

B Lymphocytes

B lymphocyte precursors derived from the CLP undergo the antigen-independent phase of B cell maturation in the bone marrow. The immunocompetent (naïve) mature B lymphocytes then enter the blood and migrate to the germinal centers (follicles) and medullary cords of lymph nodes, the germinal centers of the spleen, and other secondary lymphoid tissue. If B cells fail either to enter a lymphoid follicle or to encounter and be stimulated by specific antigens, the cells die (by apoptosis) within several days to several weeks. Upon encounter with specific antigen, the B cells finish their differentiation program. Antigenic stimulation causes the B lymphocytes to undergo proliferation and differentiation into plasmacytoid lymphocytes and finally into immunoglobulin antibody-secreting plasma cells. The immunoglobulin recognizes and binds to foreign antigen. B lymphocytes compose 15–30% of peripheral blood lymphocytes.

B Lymphocyte Membrane Markers B lymphocytes can be identified and differentiated from T lymphocytes by virtue of complement receptors and surface membrane immunoglobulin as well as CD antigens/markers. B lymphocytes form rosettes with mice erythrocytes as well as sheep erythrocytes that are coated with antibody and complement (EAC). EACs attach to B lymphocytes by means of B lymphocyte complement receptors. Surface membrane immunoglobulin can be detected by fluorescein-conjugated antisera to the different classes of immunoglobulins.

Membrane markers are present at various stages in B lymphocyte development. B lymphocytes are identified using flow cytometry and a panel of antibodies to surface antigens that corresponds to the stage of the cell's differentiation (Figure 7-19 ■). CD markers expressed by B lymphocytes and their precursors include CD10, CD19, CD20, CD21, CD22, CD24, and CD38. The CD19 antigen is considered a "pan-B" antigen because it is found on the earliest B lymphocyte and is retained until the latest stages of activation. The CD10 antigen, the common acute lymphoblastic leukemia antigen (CALLA), was originally believed to be a specific marker of leukemia cells in acute lymphoblastic leukemia. It is now known that CALLA is present on a small percentage (<3%) of normal bone marrow cells and is found on only early B lymphocyte precursors, disappearing as cell maturation occurs. B cells also express Fc receptors capable of binding the Fc portion of IgG, IgM, IgA and IgE on their membranes.[31,32]

B Lymphocyte Antigen Receptor

Like T cells, B cells recognize and interact with specific antigens via an antigen-specific **B cell receptor (BCR).** The antigen-binding component of the BCR consists of an immunoglobulin (Ig) molecule identical to that produced by the mature B lymphocyte/plasma cell. The complete BCR consists of the immunoglobulin molecule with two accessory molecules, Igα and Igβ, which function as signaling molecules in B cell activation.

Immunoglobulin A unique molecule produced by B lymphocytes and plasma cells, **immunoglobulin** (antibody) consists of two pairs of polypeptide chains: two heavy and two light chains linked together by disulfide bonds (Figure 7-20 ■). The number and arrangement of these bonds are specific for the various immunoglobulin classes and subclasses. The five types of heavy chains (HC) are α, δ, ε, γ, and μ, which determine the class of the antibody (IgA, IgD, IgE, IgG, and IgM, respectively). Although each B cell precursor has two sets of HC genes (one on each chromosome 14), only one encodes the HC protein in any given cell. Thus, within a given immunoglobulin molecule, the two heavy chains are always identical. The two classes of light chains, κ and λ, have many subclasses. As with the heavy chains, the two light chains within an immunoglobulin molecule are always identical. Either -κ or λ-chain can be found in association with any of the various heavy chains. Each of the classes and subclasses of immunoglobulin has distinct physical and biologic properties (Web Table 7-1 ✪).

Each heavy and light immunoglobulin chain consists of a variable region and a constant region. The constant region is the same for all antibodies within a given class or subclass, but the variable region in each immunoglobulin molecule is different. The constant region mediates effector functions such as complement fixation. Together, the variable regions of the light (V_L) and heavy (V_H) chains determine the antibody-combining site. Rearrangement of gene segments of the heavy chain variable regions (see below) allows a diverse repertoire of immunoglobulin specificity for foreign antigens.

✪ TABLE 7-7

Helper T Cell Functions

Type	Stimulating Cytokine	Effector Cytokines	Functions	Detrimental Effects
T_{H1}	IL-12	INF-γ, IL-2, TNF$_\alpha$, TGF$_\beta$	Targets intracellular pathogens, mediates DTH and cytotoxicity, promotes secretion of IgG$_2$	Arthritis, autoimmunity, organ transplant rejection
T_{H2}	IL-4	IL-4, IL-5, IL-6, IL-10, IL-13, TGF-β	Targets extracellular pathogens, activates eosinophils and mast cells, promotes IgG, activates B lymphocytes by secreting lymphokines	IgE mediated allergies and asthma

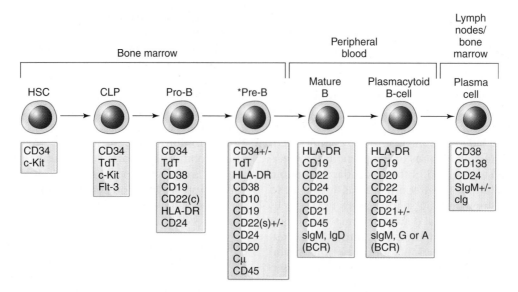

FIGURE 7-19 Immunologic maturation of the B lymphocyte from the pluripotential hematopoietic stem cell (HSC) to the plasma cell. Each stage of maturation can be defined by specific antigens (CD) that appear sequentially on the developing cell. Stem cells, pro-B lymphocytes, and pre-B lymphocytes are normally found in the bone marrow. The mature B lymphocyte is found in the peripheral blood. When stimulated by antigens, the B lymphocytes undergo maturation to plasma cells in the lymph nodes or bone marrow. In this figure, the pre-B cell stage includes the pre-pre-B cell, also referred to as the intermediate pre-B cell. (Cµ = cytoplasmic µ chains; sIg = surface membrane immunoglobulin; cIg = cytoplasmic immunoglobulin; CD = cluster of differentiation; BCR = B-cell receptor; c-Kit = stem cell factor receptor, also called CD117.)

The rate-limiting step in antibody production is the synthesis of heavy chain. A balance between production of heavy and light chains normally ensures no excess of one or the other. Neoplastic diseases of plasma cells, however, upset the balance; excesses of light chains or heavy chains can then be found in both serum and urine.

Immunoglobulin Gene Rearrangement During B lymphocyte development, a rearrangement of the gene loci coding for immunoglobulin heavy and light chains in the B progenitor cells similar to that for the TCR components occurs. This is one of the earliest features allowing the cell to be recognized as a B cell precursor. HC and LC gene rearrangement occurs at different stages of B cell development (see below). The gene rearrangement of the HC locus involves random selection of coding sequences from menus of three serially arranged DNA segments (V, D, and J) and recombination to form a variety of unique coding sequences and antibody specificities. This is described and diagrammed in ∞ Chapter 39 (see Figure 39-10). The κ and λ LC also rearrange gene segments to provide additional immunoglobulin diversity. Light chain-variable gene segments include the V and J regions but no D region.

B Lymphocyte Developmental Stages Early antigen-independent stages of B lymphopoiesis occur in the bone marrow. The earliest committed B cell precursor is the pro-B cell (Figure 7-19).[31] The *pro-B cell* is characterized by the presence of CD34 (an early hematopoietic cell antigen) and CD19 (pan-B antigen) and TdT. During the pro-B stage, HC rearrangement (DJ and VDJ) of the µ heavy chain of IgM takes place.

When a successful µ HC rearrangement has been completed, free cytoplasmic µ chains (Cµ) can be seen and the cell becomes an early (large) pre-B cell. *Pre-B cells* are characterized by the loss of CD34, persistence of CD19, and the appearance of CD10 (CALLA), CD20, and CD24. Similar to the parallel stage in T cell development, pre-B cells produce a "pre-BCR" complex on the cell surface consisting of the µ HC complexed with a surrogate light chain (ψLC). The µ/ψLC associates with the accessory molecules Igα and Igβ to form the pre-BCR. Toward the end of the pre-B cell stage, LC gene rearrangement occurs; it is characterized by loss of TdT and persistence of CD-19, -20, and -24.

When successful rearrangement of the LC locus is complete and the cell expresses either a µκ or a µλ IgM, the molecule is transported to the cell surface to form a functional BCR (sIgM). The cell is now a *mature B cell*; it is positive for CD-19, -20, -21, -22, and -24. The immunocompetent but naïve mature B cell is characterized by the dual expression of both µ (IgM) and δ (IgD) BCR on the cell surface.

As with T cells, during antigen-independent lymphopoiesis in the marrow, proliferation and apoptotic cell death are significant. This eliminates those cells with nonfunctional immunoglobulin gene rearrangement as well as those that produce autoreactive antigen receptors.

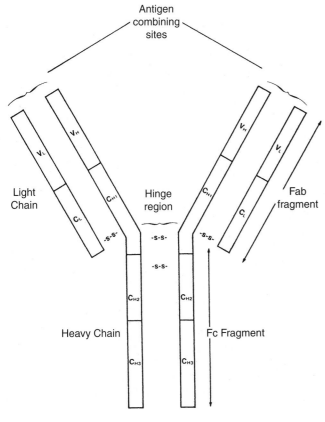

Antigen combining sites

Light Chain

Hinge region

Fab fragment

Heavy Chain

Fc Fragment

Basic structure of Immunoglobulin

■ FIGURE 7-20   Schematic drawing of an IgG molecule. The four peptide chains include two light and two heavy chains. Disulfide bonds between the chains are indicated by—s-s-. The variable domains are indicated by V, and the constant regions by C. The variable regions have variable amino acid sequences depending on the antibody specificity, and the constant regions have a constant sequence among immunoglobulins of the same class. The two heavy chains (H) determine the class of immunoglobulin, in this case for IgG. The two light chains can be either kappa or lambda.

B lymphocytes are not capable of reacting with antigens until they develop both IgM and IgD on their surface (i.e., mature B cell stage). At this stage, the immunocompetent but naïve cells leave the marrow and travel to the secondary lymphoid tissue (primarily lymph nodes) where the antigen-dependent phase of B cell development continues.

These naïve B cells recirculate through the blood and enter the peripheral lymph nodes and spleen. In these tissues, the B cells can undergo further differentiation into effector cells in response to antigenic challenge. After encountering the antigen recognized by the specific BCR, some activated B cells undergo isotype switching of the constant region of the HC gene, converting to IgG, IgA, or IgE BCR. Most mature B lymphocytes possess only one class of immunoglobulin on their membrane, although a small percentage can express IgG or IgA with IgM and IgD. Surface-bound immunoglobulin serves as the receptor for a particular antigen.

There are two subclasses of mature B lymphocytes. B-1 lymphocytes are also known as CD5$^+$ B cells because they express CD5 (normally considered a T cell marker). These cells are produced early in embryonic development and are found primarily in pleural and peritoneal cavities where they are thought to provide defense against environmental flora. B-2 lymphocytes are produced primarily after birth, are CD5$^-$, and are found primarily in the circulation and secondary lymphoid tissues. CD5$^+$ B-1 lymphocytes are the cells most commonly associated with autoimmune diseases and chronic lymphocytic leukemia (CLL).

Plasma Cell Development   When stimulated by antigens, mature B lymphocytes undergo proliferation and transformation into plasma cells (the antigen-dependent phase of B-lymphopoiesis). Antigen activation of B lymphocytes results in the transformation from reactive lymphocytes to immunoblasts, to plasmacytoid lymphocytes, and finally to plasma cells in the lymph nodes. Plasma cells are the fully activated terminal form of the B lymphocyte lineage. Their primary function is formation and secretion of immunoglobulin that recognizes a particular antigen. Each plasma cell is committed to secreting large amounts of specific immunoglobulin of the same isotype (Ig class) and idiotype (antigen specificity) as the BCR of its precursor B cell. Plasma cells have large quantities of cytoplasmic immunoglobulin (cIg$^+$) but contain little or no surface immunoglobulin (sIg). On the other hand, B cells from which plasma cells are derived are sIg$^+$, but cIg$^-$.

Plasma cells are not normally present in the peripheral blood or lymph and constitute less than 4% of the cells in the bone marrow. Most plasma cells are found in the medullary cores of lymph nodes although intense stimulation of the immune system can cause them to be found in the peripheral blood. Plasma cells are sometimes found in the blood in rubeola, infectious mononucleosis, toxoplasmosis, syphilis, tuberculosis, and multiple myeloma.

Normal plasma cell morphology was included with the discussion of lymphocyte morphology. Morphologic variations of plasma cells include *flame cells* and *Mott cells*. **Flame cells** are named for their reddish-purple cytoplasm (Figure 7-21 ■). The red tinge is caused by a glycoprotein produced in the RER, and the purple tinge is caused by the presence of ribosomes. These cells contain more immunoglobulin than do normal plasma cells. At one time, flame cells were believed to be associated with IgA multiple myeloma, but it is now recognized that these cells can be seen in a variety of pathologies and occasionally in normal bone marrow.

Mott cells, also called *grape cells,* are plasma cells filled with globules containing immunoglobulin (Russell bodies) (Figure 7-22 ■). **Russell bodies** normally stain blue-violet or pink, but in the staining process, the globulin can dissolve and the cell then appears to be filled with colorless vacuoles. The globules form as a result of the accumulation of material in the RER, smooth endoplasmic reticulum (SER), and the

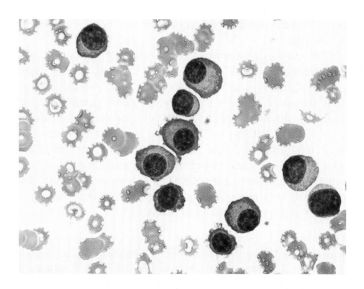

■ FIGURE 7-21   Flame cells. Note the reddish tinge of cyto-plasm. The color is especially apparent at the periphery of the cytoplasm. These are variants of plasma cells. (Bone marrow, Wright-Giemsa stain, 1000× magnification).

Golgi complex caused by an obstruction of secretion. This pathologic plasma cell is associated with chronic plasmocyte hyperplasia, parasitic infection, and malignant tumors.

Intranuclear membrane-bound inclusion bodies known as **Dutcher bodies,** have been described in plasma cells from patients with dysproteinemias. These inclusions stain with PAS, indicating that they contain glycogen or glycoprotein. Dutcher bodies are most often found in neoplastic plasma cells.

Alterations in immunoglobulin production can be classi-fied as hypogammaglobulinemia, polyclonal gammopathy, and monoclonal gammopathy. These conditions are most commonly detected by serum protein electrophoresis be-

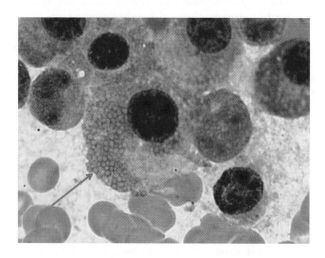

■ FIGURE 7-22   Mott cell (grape cell). Note the large globules in the cytoplasm. This is a variant of a plasma cell. (Bone marrow, Wright-Giemsa stain, 1000× magnification)

cause each class of immunoglobulin has a specific electrical charge that permits migration in an electrical field. Hy-pogammaglobulinemia is a decrease in the total concentra-tion of immunoglobulins (∞ Chapter 20). Polyclonal gam-mopathies result in an increase in immunoglobulin in more than one class (polyclonal antibodies) and are frequently seen in viral or bacterial infections. **Monoclonal gam-mopathies** arising from one clone of cells (a monoclonal antibody) are characterized by an increase in one specific class of immunoglobulin with identical heavy and light chains. This type of alteration is usually the result of unregu-lated proliferation (neoplastic) of one clone of plasma cells (∞ Chapter 26).

Natural Killer Cells

The third population of lymphoid cells, **natural killer cells (NK)**, have the capacity for spontaneous cytotoxicity for vari-ous target cells. Unlike Tc cells whose cytotoxic activity is "MHC restricted," NK cells are effector cells whose cytotoxic-ity is non-MHC restricted (they do not require interaction with appropriate MHC molecules on the target cell).[33] Their CD markers are not characteristic of either T or B cells. NK cells do not rearrange either the BCR (immunoglobulin) or TCR (α-, β-, γ-, δ-) gene loci. NK cells possess CD16 (the FcγIII receptor for IgG) and CD56. The CD16 marker is shared with neutrophils and some macrophages. NK cells have some T cell antigens on their cell membranes (up to 50% of NK cells can have weak expression of CD8 and CD2) but not CD3.[34]

NK cells originate in the bone marrow from the CLP (Figure 7-23 ■). NK cells and T cells have a close develop-mental relationship with evidence that the immediate pre-cursor of an NK-committed progenitor is a bipotential CFU-T/NK.[29] IL-15 is the major cytokine regulating NK cell differentiation and development (Figure 7-23). NK cells con-stitute about 15% of the circulating lymphocytes in the pe-ripheral blood. Most NK cells are short lived with life spans from a few days to a few weeks.[34]

Most (but not all) NK cells have an LGL morphology, but not all LGLs are NK cells. Under normal circumstances, most LGLs are CD3−. CD3+ LGLs are thought to be activated cyto-toxic T cells that recognize specific epitopes of foreign pro-tein such as those of viruses and are non-MHC restricted.[35] The separation between the two cell types is not absolute. There may be an intermediate cell population whose rela-tionship with these two cell populations has not been deter-mined.[25,36]

NK cells mediate two cytolytic activities. They recognize and kill tumor cells and those infected with a virus (natural killing). They also can recognize and attack antigens with at-tached IgG via their IgG receptor (CD16) referred to as *antibody-dependent cellular cytotoxicity* (ADCC). NK cells are activated by IL-2 to express nonspecific cytotoxic functions. Together with a small population of T$_C$ cells (that have the LGL morphology and are activated by IL-2), they are called *lymphokine-activated killer (LAK)* cells. NK cells also can be ac-

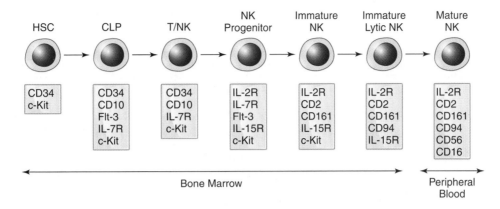

■ FIGURE 7-23 Natural killer (NK) cell maturation pathway. Immunologic maturation of NK cells from the pluripotential hematopoietic stem cell (HSC) and common lymphoid progenitor cell (CLP) to the mature NK cell. Each stage of maturation can be defined by specific antigens (CD) and/or presence of cytokine receptors that appear on the developing cell. NK progenitors and immature cells are found in the bone marrow, and mature NK cells are found in the peripheral blood. (CD = cluster of differentiation; IL-7R = IL-7 receptor; c-Kit = stem cell factor receptor, also referred to as CD117)

tivated by IL-12, a cytokine produced by macrophages. The activated Tc and NK cells rely primarily on the perforin/granzyme system to kill their targets.[33] On contact with their target, perforin released from the granules introduces a hole in the target cell membrane, allowing activated granzymes and other granule contents to enter. Granzymes activate the target cell apoptotic pathway, inducing target cell death. Fas Ligand or other apoptosis-inducing cytokines on NK cell membranes can also contribute to cytotoxicity through death-receptors on target cells (∞ Chapter 2). In addition, NK cells appear to be involved in regulation of hematopoiesis with a suppressive effect on hematopoietic cell proliferation.[34]

NK cells have a "fail-safe" mechanism to guard against an inappropriate response against self.[35] The NK cells have killer-cell immunoglobulin-like receptors (KIR) that include both activating and inhibiting subgroups of receptors. Ligands for these receptors include both cell surface proteins that are altered when a cell is infected and MHC class I molecules. The inhibiting receptors bind to the MHC class I molecules of autologous cells and allogeneic cells of similar HLA-C type. This interaction between the "target" cell MHC molecules and the inhibitory KIR receptors blocks NK cell activation and protects healthy self-cells and allogeneic cells with similar HLA-C phenotypes from NK attack. The NK cell is said to be tolerant of these cells. Allogeneic cells that lack similar MHC class I molecules, or autologous cells that are infected and lose expression or alter conformation of the MHC class I molecules, fail to bind to the NK cell's inhibitory KIR receptors. These uninhibited NK cells become activated via their activating receptors and can mount an attack on the altered or allogeneic cell and kill it. Thus, the NK cell attacks cells when a self-MHC Class I determinant is missing. The alloreactive NK cell is said to recognize "miss-

ing-self."[37] KIR-mediated inhibition can block activation that is triggered by engaging a single activating receptor.[37] On the other hand, if several activating receptors are activated at once, KIR inhibition can be overcome and the resting NK cell is activated. This suggests that for a potential target cell to activate the NK cell, it must be able to upregulate an array of activating NK receptors; activating just one would not necessarily trigger an NK response.

The activity of NK cells is firmly regulated and is activated by signals from a variety of sources, which are listed in Table 7-8 ✪.

LYMPHOCYTE FUNCTION

The T lymphocyte, B lymphocyte, and macrophage interact in a series of events that allows the body to attack and eliminate foreign antigens. This series is known collectively as the adaptive immune response (IR). The body's ability to mount an IR against a particular foreign antigen is controlled by IR genes located in the major histocompatibility complex (MHC) loci on chromosome 6. These genes code for histocompatible antigens found on the surface of essentially all nucleated cells.

The MHC gene cluster in humans is called the *human leukocyte antigen (HLA) region* (Table 7-9 ✪). The HLA genes are located in specific regions within the complex known as HLA-A, HLA-B, HLA-C, and HLA-D (HLA-DP, HLA-DQ, and HLA-DR). The regions are classified according to their structure and specific role in the IR. Class I MHC include HLA-A, HLA-B, and HLA-C genes, which code for cell surface recognition proteins found on essentially all nucleated cells. These proteins are utilized by T_C and NK cells to distinguish self from nonself. HLA-D genes code for MHC Class II antigens on B lymphocytes, dendritic cells, a subpopulation of macrophages,

⊘ TABLE 7-8

Regulation of NK Activity

Source of Activating Signal	Activating Signal	Mode of Action
Cytokines	IFNα/β IL-12	Stress molecules serve to signal NK cells in the presence of viral pathogens Produced by macrophages for NK cell stimulation
Fc Receptor	Activating molecule that binds Fc portion of antibody	Allows NK cells to target cells against which a humoral response has been mounted and lyse the cells by antibody-dependant cellular cytotoxicity (ADCC)
Activating and Inhibitory Receptors	Variety of receptors that bind ligands on both endogenous and exogenous target cells *Activating* NKG2D, NKp46, CD2 or DNAM *Inhibiting* KIR, Ly49, CD94/NKG2A	Either activate or suppress NK cell cytolytic activity

and activated T lymphocytes. The Class II antigens, also known as *Ia antigens,* determine the ability of immune cells to cooperate and interact in the IR. The D region is arranged into at least three subregions: DP, DQ, and DR. The Class III genes code for components of the complement system.

The B lymphocytes are responsible for the part of the IR known as *humoral immunity* (i.e., the production of antibodies). To accomplish effective humoral immunity, the peripheral B lymphocyte must be activated and must differentiate to a plasma cell. The antibodies circulate in body fluids and can bind directly to the pathogen, which makes it a target for phagocytosis by cells that have receptors for the antibody (FcγR-I, -II, -III).

The T lymphocytes are responsible for part of the IR known as *cell-mediated immunity* (*CMI*), which requires interaction among histocompatible macrophages, T lymphocytes, and antigens. CMI is independent of antibody production by B lymphocytes. At least three important functional subsets of T lymphocytes are involved in the IR: helper T lymphocytes (T_H), suppressor T lymphocytes (T_S), and cytotoxic T lymphocytes (T_C). When these cells become activated in the IR, they proliferate, produce lymphokines, and perform a variety of other effector functions.

Lymphokines are cytokines released primarily from T lymphocytes that influence the function of other lymphocytes, macrophages, and other body cells (Table 7-10 ⊘). B lympho-

⊘ TABLE 7-9

Major Histocompatibility Complex Antigens

Class I	Class II (Ia antigens)	Class III
HLA-A	HLA-DP	Complement components
HLA-B	HLA-DQ	
HLA-C	HLA-DR	

⊘ TABLE 7-10

Some Soluble Mediators Released from T Lymphocytes and Their Effects on Other Cells

Lymphokine	Action
Macrophage inhibition factor (MIF)	Prevents migration of macrophages from site of inflammation
INFγ	Inhibits intracellular viral multiplication, inhibits proliferation of T_{H2} cells, activates macrophages
IL-2	Induces proliferation and activation of other lymphocytes
IL-3	Is multilineage colony-stimulating factor; acts in synergy with other cytokines to stimulate growth of hematopoietic colonies, has a negative effect on lymphoid progenitors
IL-4	Stimulates proliferation of B lymphocytes
IL-5	Stimulates proliferation/differentiation of B lymphocytes and eosinophils
IL-6	Stimulates proliferation/differentiation of B lymphocytes
IL-9	Enhances T cell survival, activates mast cells
IL-10	Inhibits production of IFNγ by T_{H1} cells, suppresses macrophage function
IL-13	B cell growth and differentiation, inhibits production of proinflammatory cytokines
IL-14	Stimulates proliferation of activated B-cells
IL-16	Serves as a chemoattractant of CD4$^+$ lymphocytes
IL-17	Has an indirect effect on hematopoiesis by inducing other cytokines, releases IL-6, G-CSF, PGE2; enhances ICAM-1
IFN α and IFN β	Activates macrophages, granulocytes, T_c lymphocytes
MIP-1α	Is responsible for chemotaxis, respiratory burst

cytes and NK cells also can secrete lymphokines. Under the influence of lymphokines, monocytes can produce monocyte-derived cytokines. Most cytokines work synergistically in inducing their physiologic response (∞ Chapter 3).

T cells do not react directly with the pathogen but with short peptides derived from the breakdown of pathogens or their protein products by antigen-presenting cells (e.g., macrophages or dendritic cells). The processed peptide is bound by an MHC molecule on the APC, forming a peptide:MHC complex. The T cell receptor (TCR) binds to the complex on the infected cell and "kills" it or activates the APC. Recognition of and binding to a target cell requires the TCR to bind with the antigen/MHC complex and the T cell co-receptor (CD4 or CD8) to bind to appropriate MHC molecules (class I or II). MHC class I molecules form a complex with antigens that are derived from intracellular pathogens. MHC class I molecules in the infected cell bind processed viral proteins and transport the complex to the cell surface. These MHC:protein complexes bind and activate $CD8^+$ T cells. Class II MHC molecules complex with peptides derived from extracellular pathogens; this complex binds to $CD4^+$ T cells.

Macrophages phagocytize and degrade extracellular pathogens. The peptide fragments complex with MHC class II molecules, and the complex is transported to the cell surface where it is recognized by lymphocytes with the CD4 receptor (T-helper cells, T_H). The T_H cell activates the macrophage through direct cell contact and secretion of cytokines. B lymphocytes can bind pathogens by their surface immunoglobulin. The pathogen is engulfed and degraded, and its peptides are complexed with class II MHC molecules. As in the macrophage, the complex is transported to the cell surface where T_H cells recognize it. B cells are activated by contact with the T_H cell and secretion of cytokines.

Adhesion Molecules of the Adaptive Immune Response

Adhesion receptors are important in the congregation of lymphoid cells at sites of infection (Table 7-11 ✪). The TCR/CD3 complex recognizes antigens bound to monocytes/macrophages. LFA-1 (leukocyte function-related antigen) on activated leukocytes and LFA-3 on VEC are important in the antigen-independent adhesion of activated T lymphocytes, localizing these cells in sites of antigen accumulation. LFA-1 on T lymphocytes is required for the lymphocytes' interaction with other cells, most likely by promoting adherence. The ligand for LFA-1 is the intercellular adhesion molecule on VEC, ICAM-1, which modulates inflammatory responses by up-regulation (promoting lymphocyte adherence) or down-regulation of expression. Inflammatory mediators such as lipopolysaccharide (LPS, endotoxin), IL-1, and TNF cause strong expression of ICAM-1 in tissues, increasing adherence of lymphocytes and monocytes expressing LFA-1 in areas of inflammation. LFA-3 is expressed on endothelial cells and is the ligand for CD2 on T lymphocytes. Reaction of CD2 with its VEC ligand generates an activation signal in the T lymphocyte.

The B_1 integrin subfamily of very late activation (VLA) molecules appears on lymphocytes several weeks after antigen stimulation. The six VLA molecules—VLA-1–VLA-6—are recognized as CD49a through CD49f, respectively. VLA-4 binds to the VCAM-1 receptor on VEC, a member of the immunoglobulin superfamily. The VCAM-1 receptor is induced on the endothelium by inflammatory mediators. Other B_1

✪ TABLE 7-11

Adhesion Molecules Involved in the Interaction of Lymphocytes with Other Cells in the Immune Response

Adhesion Molecule	CD Designation	Expressed By	Ligand	Function
LFA-1	CD11a/CD18	Activated leukocytes	ICAM-1, ICAM-2 on endothelial cells	Mediates interaction of lymphocytes with other cells, possibly by promoting adherence to target cells at site of antigen
CD2	CD2	T lymphocytes Monocytes	LFA-3 (CD58) on EC	Promotes adherence of the monocytes and T lymphocytes to EC, mediates activation of T lymphocytes
CD4	CD4	T_H lymphocytes	Class II MHC	Enhances adhesion of T_H lymphocytes to other cells, mediates activation of T_H lymphocytes
CD8	CD8	T_S lymphocytes	Class 1 MHC	Enhances adhesion and activation of T_S lymphocytes, promotes avidity of cytotoxic T lymphocytes and target cells
VLA1, VLA2, VLA3 VLA4, VLA5, VLA6	CD49a, CD49b, CD49c, CD49d, CD49e, CD49f	Lymphocytes (VLA-4 also on monocytes)	VLA4 ligand VCAM-1 on EC	Increases adhesion of cells in area of inflammation

EC = endothelial cell, CD = cluster of differentiation, LFA = leukocyte function-related antigen, ICAM = intercellular cytoadhesion molecule, MHC = major histocompatibility complex antigens, VLA = very late activation

integrin molecules bind to extracellular matrix components such as collagen and are expressed on many leukocytes and other nonhematopoietic cells.

Aging and Lymphocyte Function

Although many immune functions are well conserved throughout life, some investigators believe that a derangement of some immune responses occurs in the elderly, possibly contributing to an increased risk of morbidity and mortality in this age group. Although there is a decrease in absolute numbers of lymphocytes, there is an increase in activated NK cells and T lymphocytes that mediate non-MHC-restricted spontaneous cytotoxicity.

Lymphocyte Metabolism

Lymphocytes contain all enzymes of the glycolytic and tricarboxylic acid cycle. Glucose enters the cell through facilitated diffusion and is catabolized to produce ATP through oxidative phosphorylation. The ATP is used for recirculation and locomotion as well as replacement of lipids and proteins and maintenance of ionic equilibrium. The HMP shunt provides only a fraction of the needed energy, but it is important for purine and pyrimidine synthesis required for DNA replication and mitosis as well as provision of reducing energy by production of NADPH.

DISTRIBUTION, CONCENTRATION, AND KINETICS

Lymphocytes have a peripheral blood concentration in adults ranging from 1.0 to 4.8×10^9/L. At birth, the mean lymphocyte count is 5.5×10^9/L. This value rises to a mean of 7×10^9/L in the next 6 months and remains at that level until ~age 4. A gradual decrease in lymphocytes is noted from 4 years of age until reaching adult reference range values in the second decade of life. *Lymphocytosis,* an increase in lymphocytes, occurs in adults when the absolute number of lymphocytes exceeds 4.8×10^9/L. Lymphocytopenia, a decrease in lymphocytes, occurs in adults when the absolute number of lymphocytes is $<1.0 \times 10^9$/L.

Although lymphocytes are the second most numerous intravascular leukocyte in adults, peripheral blood lymphocytes comprise only ~5% of the total body lymphocyte concentration. Ninety-five percent of the lymphocytes are located in extravascular tissue of the lymph nodes and spleen. Movement of lymphocytes between the intravascular and extravascular compartments is continuous. Lymphocytes from lymph nodes enter the lymphatic channels and gain entry to the blood as the lymph drains into the right lymphatic duct and the thoracic duct. When blood lymphocytes are stimulated by an antigen, they migrate to specific areas of lymphoid tissue where they undergo proliferation and transformation into effector cells. These cells also can pass directly through the cytoplasm of postcapillary or high endothelial venule cells (emperipolesis) as they recirculate between intravascular and extravascular compartments.

Lymphocytes leave and reenter the blood (recirculate) many times during their life spans. About 80% of lymphocytes in the peripheral blood are "long lived" with a life span ranging from a few months to many years. These cells spend most of their lives in a prolonged, intermitotic, G_0 phase. The remaining 20% of the lymphocytes live from a few hours to ~5 days. The majority of these short-lived, rapidly turning over lymphocytes are immunocompetent, naïve B lymphocytes.

 Checkpoint! 8

A young adult patient's blood smear reveals 70% reactive lymphocytes and 10% nonreactive lymphocytes (80% total lymphocytes) in a 10×10^9/L WBC count. What is the absolute concentration of total lymphocytes and reactive lymphocytes? What is a probable cause of these findings?

 CASE STUDY *(continued from page 108)*

4. Is there a need for reflex testing on Harry? Explain your answer.

SUMMARY

Leukocytes include five morphologically and functionally distinct types of nucleated blood cells: neutrophils, eosinophils, basophils, monocytes, and lymphocytes. The leukocytes develop from the pluripotential hematopoietic stem cells in the bone marrow. Under the influence of hematopoietic growth factors, the stem cell matures into terminally differentiated cells. These cells circulate only a matter of hours in the peripheral blood before diapedesing into the tissues.

The leukocytes serve as the defenders of the body against foreign invaders and noninfectious challenges by participating in phagocytosis and the immune response. The leukocytes are attracted to sites of inflammation, infection, or tissue injury by chemoattractants and leave the circulation using special adhesion molecules and ligands located on the leukocytes and endothelial cells of the vessel walls. Neutrophils and monocytes are active in phagocytosis, and eosinophils function in defending the body against parasites. Eosinophils are involved in allergic reactions and chronic inflammation. Basophils are also involved in allergic reactions by releasing histamine and heparin when activated via the binding of IgE to membrane Fc receptors.

Monocytes function as phagocytes and secrete a variety of cytokines that affect the function of other cells, especially that of lymphocytes. Monocytes, also referred to as *antigen-processing* (or *presenting*) *cells* (APC), play a major role in initiating and regulating the immune response.

The three types of lymphocytes are T, B, and NK cells. T and B lymphocytes have antigen-independent and antigen-dependent phases of maturation. In the antigen-independent maturation process, B lymphocytes mature in the bone marrow and T lymphocytes mature in the thymus. There are at least three different major types of T lymphocytes: CD4$^+$ helper T lymphocytes (T$_H$), CD8$^+$

suppressor T lymphocytes (T_S), and CD8$^+$ cytotoxic lymphocytes (T_C). The lymphoid precursor cell from the bone marrow matures and acquires cellular molecular characteristics of a T or B lymphocyte. In the antigen-dependent maturation process, these lymphocytes mature, and immunocompetent T and B lymphocytes undergo a series of cellular events in response to encounters with antigens known as *blast transformation.* The end result is a clonal amplification of lymphocytes responsible for immunity to the specific antigen that stimulated transformation. Reactive lymphocytes are the most common form of antigen-stimulated lymphocyte found in the peripheral blood. NK cells, also known as *large granular lymphocytes* (*LGL*), are a form of cytotoxic lymphocyte. LGLs have two distinct populations categorized by the presence or absence of CD3. Natural killer cells are thought to be CD3$^-$ (NK-LGL), and activated cytotoxic T-cells are thought to be CD3$^+$ (T-LGL) with the possibility of existing intermediate forms. The cytotoxicity of NK cells is not MHC restricted.

T and B lymphocytes have separate but related functions in the immune response. Monocytes/macrophages and dendritic cells phagocytize antigens, preserving critical immunologic determinants that are presented to the T lymphocytes. The T lymphocytes bind to the antigens and the MHC molecules on the surface of the macrophage by means of the TCR and either CD4 or CD8. Cytokines released by the macrophage and the T lymphocyte activate the lymphocyte. T_S lymphocytes also are activated by the released cytokines and serve to suppress the immune response. The B lymphocyte's functional activity includes the synthesis and secretion of antibodies. Surface immunoglobulin serves as the B lymphocyte receptor for the processed antigen that is bound to the macrophage and T_H lymphocyte. The B lymphocyte can also bind to the MHC receptors on the T_H lymphocyte. As a result of this interaction, the B lymphocyte transforms to an antibody-secreting plasma cell.

NK-LGLs function in the first line (innate) defense mechanism. They can target virus-infected cells or tumor cells for killing. T-LGLs are thought to be activated cytotoxic T-cells that recognize specific epitopes of foreign protein such as viruses.

REVIEW QUESTIONS

LEVEL I

1. Leukocytosis can be defined as an increase in: (Objective 1)
   a. neutrophils, monocytes, and macrophages
   b. neutrophils, eosinophils, erythrocytes, and basophils
   c. neutrophils, eosinophils, basophils, monocytes, lymphocytes
   d. neutrophils, eosinophils, basophils, monocytes, lymphocytes, megakaryocytes

2. The hallmark of differentiating myelocytes from promyelocytes morphologically is the visual identification of what in the myelocytes? (Objective 2)
   a. primary granules
   b. secondary granules
   c. loss of nucleoli
   d. pink cytoplasm

3. The granulocytic maturation process differs from the lymphocytic and monocytic-macrophage maturation process in that: (Objective 3)
   a. granules never develop in cells in the monocytic-macrophage cell line
   b. the nucleus in the granulocytic cell line eventually segments
   c. the scanty cytoplasm in the lymphocytic cell line eventually becomes abundant and very granular
   d. the nucleoli disappear in only the granulocytic line

4. Primary granules first appear in the: (Objective 2)
   a. myeloblast
   b. promyelocyte
   c. myelocyte
   d. band

LEVEL II

1. The average cell turnover rate for granulocytes and monocytes in the peripheral blood is: (Objective 1)
   a. <12 hours
   b. 24 hours
   c. 8–10 days
   d. 10 years

2. The following cells are found in the granulocytic proliferating pool (mitotic pool) of the marrow: (Objective 1)
   a. pluripotential stem cells
   b. unipotential progenitor cells
   c. monoblasts, myeloblasts, and macrophages
   d. myeloblasts, promyelocytes, and myelocytes

3. The most likely explanation for a patient who has a WBC count of 16×10^9/L with many reactive lymphocytes and a few immunoblasts present is: (Objective 3)
   a. a heightened immune response
   b. early leukemia or lymphoma
   c. the presence of immunodeficiency
   d. qualitatively abnormal lymphocytes

4. A patient has lymphocytic leukemia with 60% lymphoblasts in the peripheral blood. The best way for the clinical laboratory scientist to determine whether these are T or B lymphoblasts is to: (Objective 4)
   a. do a TdT stain on the blood
   b. determine the CD surface markers on the blasts
   c. do a molecular analysis to find oncogenes
   d. send the peripheral blood specimen to cytogenetics

REVIEW QUESTIONS (continued)

LEVEL I

5. The first heavy immunoglobulin chain produced in the maturing B lymphocyte is: (Objective 12)
   a. alpha
   b. beta
   c. mu
   d. gamma

6. Lymphocytes can be differentiated from monocytes because monocytes have a: (Objective 4)
   a. large variation in cell size
   b. more lobular nucleus and fine granular grey cytoplasm
   c. low N:C ratio with intense basophilia on the cytoplasmic edges
   d. round dense chromatin nuclear pattern and sky blue cytoplasm

7. The eosinophil's primary function is to: (Objective 5)
   a. protect the host from helminth parasites
   b. protect the host from autoimmune destruction
   c. secrete cytokines to attract monocytes to the site of infection
   d. secrete cytokines to attract lymphocytes to the site of infection

8. Leukocyte migration to the tissues is regulated by leukocyte-endothelial cell recognition which requires: (Objective 6)
   a. interaction of adhesion molecules and their receptors
   b. activation of membrane oxidase
   c. leukocyte degranulation
   d. hematopoietic growth factors

9. The adult reference range for lymphocytes found in the peripheral blood is: (Objective 7)
   a. $0.2–0.8 \times 10^9$/L
   b. $1.0–4.8 \times 10^9$/L
   c. $2.0–7.0 \times 10^9$/L
   d. $3.9–10.6 \times 10^9$/L

10. An 80% lymphocyte count with a total WBC count of 4.4×10^9/L on an adult would indicate a: (Objectives 1, 8, 9)
   a. relative and absolute decrease in lymphocytes
   b. relative decrease in lymphocytes but an absolute number in the reference range
   c. relative increase in lymphocytes but an absolute number in the reference range
   d. relative and absolute increase in lymphocytes

LEVEL II

5. The largest compartment of neutrophils is found in the: (Objective 1)
   a. granulocyte proliferating/mitotic compartment
   b. granulocyte maturation/postmitotic compartment
   c. peripheral blood compartment
   d. tissues

6. Which of the following is felt to have a controlling influence on the release of neutrophils from the bone marrow? (Objective 2)
   a. pore diameter of histiocytes lining the vessel
   b. morphologic age of endothelial cells
   c. size of postmitotic storage pool
   d. morphologic age of cells and growth factors

7. A 30-year-old healthy male needed a CBC as part of his physical examination for purchasing a life insurance policy. He decided to combine his daily 5-mile run with his appointment to get his blood drawn. He ran 3 miles to the laboratory, had his blood drawn, and returned home. His WBC count was increased to 15×10^9/L, but all other CBC parameters were normal. What is the most likely explanation for the increased WBC count? (Objectives 1, 8)
   a. He has a bacterial or viral infection.
   b. He has a leukemia with leukemic cells present.
   c. Nucleated RBCs have entered the peripheral blood.
   d. The marginating neutrophil pool entered the circulating pool.

8. The adhesion molecules that play a role in neutrophil adhesion include: (Objective 2)
   a. selectins, superoxides, integrins
   b. ICAMs, integrins, superoxides
   c. NADPH, superoxides, myeloperoxidase
   d. selectins, ICAMs, integrins

9. A patient with a strep throat would most likely produce: (Objective 5)
   a. monoclonal antibody
   b. paraprotein
   c. polyclonal antibody
   d. M protein

10. A patient who is immunosuppressed would most likely have: (Objective 3)
   a. an increase in CD4$^+$ lymphocytes
   b. lymphocytosis and eosinophilia
   c. a decrease in CD4$^+$ lymphs
   d. an increase in T_H to T_s ratio

www.pearsonhighered.com/mckenzie
Use this address to access the interactive Companion Website created for this textbook. Find additional information, tables and figures. Evaluate your command of the chapter information using case studies and critical thinking and multiple choice questions.

REFERENCES

1. Wintrobe MM. *Blood, Pure and Eloquent.* New York: McGraw-Hill; 1980:19–22, 428–31.

2. Weaver AD. The development of the knowledge of the leukocyte. *Bull NY Acad Med.* 1954;30:988–92.

3. Bao W, Dalferes ER Jr, Srinivasan SR, Webber LS, Berenson GS. Normative distribution of complete blood count from early childhood through adolescence: The Bogalusa Heart Study. *Prev Med.* 1993; 22:825–37.

4. Berger NA, Rosenblum D. Geriatric hematology. In: Young NS, Gerson SL, High KA, eds. *Clinical Hematology.* Philadelphia: Mosby Elsevier; 2006:944–55.

5. Saxena S, Wong ET. Heterogeneity of common hematologic parameters among racial, ethnic, and gender subgroups. *Arch Pathol Lab Med.* 1990:114(7):715–19.

6. Beutler B. Innate Immunity. In: Lightman MA, Beutler E, Kipps TJ, Seligsohn U, Kaushansky K, Prchal JT, eds. *Williams Hematology,* 7th ed. New York: McGraw-Hill; 2006:233–38.

7. Williams DA. Stem cell model of hematopoiesis. In: Hoffman R, Benz EJ, Shattil SJ, Furie B, Cohen HJ, Silberstein LE, McGlave P, eds. *Hematology: Basic Principles and Practice,* 3rd ed. New York: Churchill Livingstone; 2000:126–38.

8. Khanna-Gupta A, Berliner N. Granulopoiesis and monocytopoiesis. In: Hoffman R, Benz EJ Jr, Shattil SJ, Furie B, Cohen HJ, Silberstein LE, McGlave P, eds. *Hematology: Basic Principles and Practice,* 4th ed. Philadelphia: Elsevier Churchill Livingstone; 2005:289–301.

9. Skubitz KM. Neutrophilic leukocytes. In: Greer JP, Foerster J, Lukens J, Rodgers GM, Paraskevas F, Glader B, eds. *Wintrobe's Clinical Hematology,* 11th ed. Philadelphia: Lippincott Williams & Wilkins; 2004: 267–310.

10. Baehner RL. Normal phagocyte structure and function. In: Hoffman R, Benz EJ Jr, Shattil SJ, Furie B, Cohen HJ, Silberstein LE, McGlave P, eds. *Hematology: Basic Principles and Practice,* 4th ed. Philadelphia: Elsevier Churchill Livingstone; 2005:737–62.

11. Clinical and Laboratory Standards Institute. Reference leukocyte (WBC) differential count (proportional) and evaluation of instrumental methods. *Approved Standard,* 2nd ed. CLSI document H-20-A2. Villanova, PA: CLSI; 2007:27(1).

12. Springer TA. Traffic signals for lymphocyte recirculation and leukocyte emigration: The multistep paradigm. *Cell.* 1994;76:301–14.

13. Malech HL, Nauseef WM. Primary inherited defects in neutrophil function: Etiology and treatment. *Semin Hematol.* 1997;34: 279–90.

14. Paraskevas F. Phagocytosis. In: Greer JP, Foerster J, Lukens J, Rodgers GM, Paraskevas F, Glader B, eds. *Wintrobe's Clinical Hematology,* 11th ed. Philadelphia: Lippincott Williams & Wilkins; 2004:387–407.

15. Wilson JM, Ziemba SE. Neutrophils fight infectious disease but may promote other human pathologies. *Lab Med.* 1999; 30:123–28.

16. Lacy P, Becker AB, Moqbel R. The human eosinophil. In: Greer JP, Foerster J, Lukens J, Rodgers GM, Paraskevas F, Glader B, eds. *Wintrobe's Clinical Hematology,* 11th ed. Philadelphia: Lippincott Williams & Wilkins; 2004:311–33.

17. Gleich GJ, Adolphson CR, Leiferman KM. The biology of the eosinophilic leukocyte. *Ann Rev Med.* 1993;44:85–101.

18. Shi HZ. Eosinophils function as antigen-presenting cells. *J Leuk Biol.* 2004;76:520–27.

19. Gleich GJ. Mechanisms of eosinophil-associated inflammation. *J Allergy Clin Immunol.* 2000;105:651–63.

20. Parker RI, Metcalfe DD. Basophils, mast cells, and systemic mastocytosis. In: Hoffman R, Benz EJ Jr, Shattil SJ, Furie B, Cohen HJ, Silberstein LE, McGlave P, eds. *Hematology: Basic Principles and Practice,* 4th ed. Philadelphia: Elsevier Churchill Livingstone; 2005:911–925.

21. Befus AD, Denburg JA. Basophilic leukocytes: Mast cells and basophils. In: Greer JP, Foerster J, Lukens J, Rodgers GM, Paraskevas F, Glader B, eds. *Wintrobe's Clinical Hematology,* 11th ed. Philadelphia: Lippincott Williams & Wilkins; 2004:335–48.

22. Rodewald HR, Dessing M, Dvorak AM et al. Identification of a committed precursor for the mast cell lineage. *Science.* 1996;271:818–22.

23. Weinberg JB. Mononuclear phagocytes. In: Greer JP, Foerster J, Lukens J, Rodgers GM, Paraskevas F, Glader B, eds. *Wintrobe's Clinical Hematology,* 11th ed. Philadelphia: Lippincott Williams & Wilkins; 2004:349–86.

24. Douek DC, McFarland RD, Keiser PH et al. Changes in thymic function with age and during treatment of HIV infection. *Nature.* 1998;396:690–95.

25. Powell LD, Baum LG. Overview and compartmentalization of the immune system. In: Hoffman R, Benz EJ Jr, Shattil SJ, Furie B, Cohen HJ, Silberstein LE, McGlave P, eds. *Hematology: Basic Principles and Practice,* 4th ed. Philadelphia: Elsevier Churchill Livingstone; 2005:108–117.

26. McCoy KL. Programmed B and T cell development. *Nutr Rev.* 1998; 56(1 Pt 2):S19–S26.

27. Kipps TJ. Functions of T lymphocytes: T cell receptors for antigen. In: Lightman MA, Beutler E, Kipps TJ, Seligsohn U, Kaushansky K, Prchal JT, eds. *Williams Hematology,* 7th ed. New York: McGraw-Hill; 2006;1065–75.

28. Paraskevas F. Clusters of differentiation. In: Greer JP, Foerster J, Lukens J, Rodgers GM, Paraskevas F, Glader B, eds. *Wintrobe's Clinical Hematology,* 11th ed. Philadelphia: Lippincott Williams & Wilkins; 2004:27–98.

29. Sanchez M-J, Muench MO, Roncarolo MG et al. Identification of a common T/NK cell progenitor in human fetal thymus. *J Exp Med.* 1994;180:569–76.

30. Spits H. Development of alphabeta T cells in the human thymus. *Nat Rev Immunol.* 2002;2:760–72.

31. Dorshkind K, Rawlings DJ. B-cell development. In: Hoffman R, Benz EJ Jr, Shattil SJ, Furie B, Cohen HJ, Silberstein LE, McGlave P, eds. *Hematology: Basic Principles and Practice,* 4th ed. Philadelphia: Elsevier Churchill Livingstone; 2005:119–33.

32. Paraskevas F. B lymphocytes. In: Greer JP, Foerster J, Lukens J, Rodgers GM, Paraskevas F, Glader B, eds. *Wintrobe's Clinical Hematology,* 11th ed. Philadelphia: Lippincott Williams & Wilkins; 2004: 439–73.

33. Shresta S, Pham CT, Thomas DA et al. How do cytotoxic lymphocytes kill their targets? *Curr Opin Immunol.* 1998;10:581–87.

34. Trinchieri G, Lanier LL. Functions of natural killer cells. In: Lightman MA, Beutler E, Kipps TJ, Seligsohn U, Kaushansky K, Prchal JT, eds. *Williams Hematology,* 7th ed. New York: McGraw-Hill; 2006; 1077–82.

35. Lanier L. Lewis. Natural killer cells: Roundup. *Immunological Reviews.* 2006;214:5–8.

36. Paraskevas F. T lymphocytes and natural killer cells. In: Greer JP, Foerster J, Lukens J, Rodgers GM, Paraskevas F, Glader B, eds. *Wintrobe's Clinical Hematology,* 11th ed. Philadelphia: Lippincott Williams & Wilkins; 2004:475–526.

37. Parham P. *The immune system,* 2nd ed. New York: Garland Science Publishing; 2005, 254–255.

38. Loughran TP. Large granular lymphocytic leukemia: An overview. *Hosp Prac* (off. ed). 1998; 33:133–38.

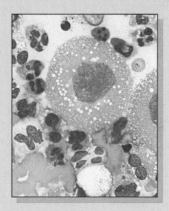

Introduction to Anemia

Shirlyn B. McKenzie, Ph.D.
Catherine N. Otto, Ph.D., M.B.A.

CHAPTER OUTLINE

■ OBJECTIVES—LEVEL I

Upon completion of this chapter, the student should be able to:

1. Describe and identify specific anisocytes and poikilocytes.
2. Classify and describe erythrocytes based on erythrocyte indices.
3. Calculate absolute reticulocyte count, corrected reticulocyte count and reticulocyte production index from reticulocyte results, hematocrit, and RBC count.
4. Describe and identify erythrocyte inclusions including staining characteristics.
5. Describe and recognize abnormal variation in erythrocyte distribution on stained smears.
6. Identify laboratory tests to evaluate erythrocyte destruction.
7. Given CBC and RPI results, categorize an anemia according to morphologic classification.
8. Correlate polychromatophilia on a blood smear with other laboratory results of erythrocyte production and destruction.

■ OBJECTIVES—LEVEL II

Upon completion of this chapter, the student should be able to:

1. Relate adaptations to anemia with patient symptoms.
2. Correlate patient history and clinical symptoms with laboratory results in anemia.
3. Interpret RDW results.
4. Assess bone marrow response to anemia given CBC and reticulocyte results.
5. Correlate poikilocytes with the mechanism of formation and assess their clinical significance.
6. Correlate CBC results with findings on a blood smear and troubleshoot discrepancies.
7. Determine the clinical significance of erythrocyte inclusions and select methods to differentiate the inclusions.
8. Evaluate the distribution of erythrocytes on stained smears and determine its clinical significance.
9. Assess and interpret bone marrow findings in the presence of anemia.
10. Compare the sensitivity and specificity of tests used to screen and confirm a differential diagnosis of anemia.
11. Compare the morphologic and functional classification of anemia.
12. Given laboratory results, classify an anemia in terms of morphology and pathophysiologic mechanism (function).
13. Choose appropriate follow-up tests to determine anemia classification and evaluate the results.

KEY TERMS

Acanthocyte
Anisocytosis
Basophilic stippling
Cabot ring
Codocyte
Echinocyte
Elliptocyte
Heinz body
Helmet cell
Howell-Jolly body
Immature reticulocyte fraction (IRF)
Knizocyte
Leptocyte
Macrocyte
Megaloblastic
Microcyte
Pancytopenia
Pappenheimer body
Poikilocytosis
Reticulocyte production index (RPI)
Schistocyte
Sickle cell
Spherocyte
Stomatocyte
Target cell
Teardrop/dacryocyte

BACKGROUND BASICS

The information in this chapter builds on the concepts learned in previous chapters. To maximize your learning experience, you should review these concepts before starting this unit of study.

Level I

▶ Describe the production, maturation, and destruction of blood cells and explain how the balance between erythrocyte production and destruction is maintained; describe the normal concentration and appearance of an erythrocyte. (Chapters 3, 5)

▶ Summarize the role of hemoglobin in gaseous transport; explain how 2,3-BPG, and H^+ affect oxygen affinity. (Chapter 6)

▶ Discuss the appearance of a normal bone marrow and list reasons why a bone marrow examination could be necessary. (Chapter 35)

▶ Discuss the principle and normal results of the following tests: hemoglobin, hematocrit, reticulocyte count, erythrocyte count, and erythrocyte indices; calculate indices. (Chapter 34)

Level II

▶ Identify the helpful stains in assessing bone marrow; correlate peripheral blood findings with bone marrow appearance. (Chapter 35)

▶ Correlate CBC results with findings on the peripheral blood smear and other laboratory test results; determine the validity and accuracy of CBC results and suggest corrective action when necessary. (Chapter 34)

℮ CASE STUDY

We will address this case study throughout the chapter.

George, a 50-year-old male, visited his doctor when he noted the whites of his eyes appeared yellow and that he had dark urine. His CBC revealed a hemoglobin of 31 g/L. Given this clinical description, consider what laboratory tests should be ordered to assist in diagnosis.

▶ OVERVIEW

This chapter is a general introduction to anemia. It begins with a description of how anemia develops and the body's adaptations to a decrease in hemoglobin. The emphasis of the chapter is on the laboratory investigation of anemia. This includes discussion of screening tests used to diagnose anemia and other more specific tests used to identify the etiology and pathophysiology of the anemia. Identification of abnormal erythrocyte morphology and its association with anemia is discussed in depth. The chapter concludes with a description of the morphologic and functional classification schemes of anemia and the use of laboratory tests to correctly classify an anemia.

▶ INTRODUCTION

Anemia is functionally defined as a decrease in the competence of blood to carry oxygen to tissues, thereby causing tissue hypoxia. In clinical medicine, it refers to a decrease in the normal concentration of hemoglobin or erythrocytes. It is one of the most common problems encountered in clinical medicine. However, anemia is not a disease but the expression of an underlying disorder or disease; it is an important clinical marker of a disorder that could be basic or sometimes more complex. Therefore, once the diagnosis of anemia is made, the physician must determine its exact cause.

Treating anemia without identifying its cause could not only be ineffective but also could lead to more serious problems. For example, if a patient experiencing iron deficiency anemia due to chronic blood loss were given iron or a blood transfusion, the hemoglobin level might temporarily rise; however, if the cause of the deficiency is not isolated and treated, serious complications of the primary disease may develop, and the anemia would probably return after cessation of treatment. Thus, it is necessary to identify and understand the etiology and pathogenesis of an anemia to institute correct treatment.

▶ HOW DOES ANEMIA DEVELOP?

To understand how anemia develops, it is necessary to understand normal erythrocyte kinetics. Total erythrocyte mass (M) in the steady state is equal to the number of new erythrocytes produced per day (P) times the erythrocyte life span (S), which is normally about 100–120 days.

$$M \quad = \quad P \quad \times \quad S$$

Mass   Production   Survival

Thus, the average 70 kg man with 2 liters of erythrocytes must produce 20 mL of new erythrocytes each day to replace the 20 mL normally lost due to cell senescence.[1]

$$\frac{2,000 \text{ mL (M)}}{100 \text{ days (S)}} = 20 \text{ mL/day (P)}$$

From this formula, it is clear that if the survival time of the erythrocyte is decreased by one-half as can occur in hemolysis or hemorrhage, the bone marrow must double production to maintain mass at 2,000 mL.

$$\frac{2,000 \text{ mL (M)}}{50 \text{ days (S)}} = 40 \text{ mL/day (P)}$$

New erythrocytes are released as reticulocytes. Thus, the increased production of cells is reflected by an increase in the absolute reticulocyte count in the peripheral blood. The marrow can compensate for decreased survival in this manner until production is increased to a level 5–10 times normal, which is the maximal functional capacity of the marrow. Thus, if all necessary raw products for cell synthesis are readily available, erythrocyte life span can decrease to about 18 days before marrow compensation is inadequate and anemia develops. If, however, bone marrow production of erythrocytes does not adequately increase when the erythrocyte survival is decreased, the erythrocyte mass cannot be maintained and anemia develops. There is no mechanism for increasing erythrocyte life span to help accommodate an inadequate bone marrow response.

Thus, anemia can develop if (1) erythrocyte loss or destruction exceeds the maximal capacity of bone marrow erythrocyte production or (2) the bone marrow erythrocyte production is impaired. Anemia can be classified according to these principles (functional classification) based on laboratory test results, which aid the physician in diagnosis. The functional classification includes survival defects, proliferation defects, and maturation defects (which have a high degree of ineffective erythropoiesis). A morphologic classification is also possible based on the erythrocyte indices and reticulocyte count. These classifications are discussed later in this chapter.

▶ INTERPRETATION OF ABNORMAL HEMOGLOBIN CONCENTRATIONS

Diagnosis of anemia is usually made after the discovery of a decreased hemoglobin concentration. Hemoglobin is the carrier protein of oxygen; thus, it is expected that a decrease

in its concentration is accompanied by a decrease in oxygen delivery to tissues (functional anemia).

Screening for anemia generally relies on the relative hemoglobin and hematocrit. However, the hemoglobin or hematocrit concentration can be misleading in a few instances (Table 8-1 ✪).

- In *hypervolemia*, the total blood volume increases. This is primarily caused by a plasma volume increase while the erythrocyte mass remains stable. In this case, the relative hemoglobin/hematocrit concentration appears falsely decreased.
- In *hypovolemia*, such as occurs in dehydration, a relative decrease in plasma volume occurs, resulting in a falsely elevated hemoglobin/hematocrit.

Diagnosis of anemia requires an upward adjustment of hemoglobin and hematocrit values dependent on the altitude.[2] The hemoglobin reference interval at high altitudes is higher than the reference interval at lower altitude. Therefore, signs of anemia at high altitudes can occur at higher hemoglobin concentrations than at sea level. Cigarette smoking has a similar effect. The hemoglobin reference interval for cigarette smokers is higher than in nonsmokers.[3]

✪ TABLE 8-1

Conditions in which the Hemoglobin or Hematocrit Can Be Misleading and Require Further Investigation or Interpretation in Light of Other Factors

Hematocrit disproportionately low (relative increase in plasma volume):
- Hydremia of pregnancy
- Overhydration in oliguric renal failure
- Congestive heart failure
- Congestive splenomegaly
- Chronic diseases
- Hypoalbuminemia
- Recumbency

Hematocrit disproportionately high relative to red cell mass (relative decrease in plasma volume):
- Dehydration
- Protracted diarrhea (especially in infants), cholera
- Stress erythrocytosis
- Intestinal malfunction (pyloric destruction, etc.)
- Abdominal paracentesis with fluid restriction
- Peritoneal dialysis with hypertonic solution
- Diabetic acidosis
- Diabetes insipidus with restricted fluid

Higher reference interval:
- High altitudes
- Smokers

Presence of abnormal hemoglobins with altered oxygen affinity

Decrease in both plasma volume and RBC mass (hematocrit normal, RBC low):
- Acute blood loss
- Cancer
- Myxedema, Addison disease, panhypopituitarism

(Adapted, with permission from *Wintrob's Clinical Hematology*, 10th ed. Edited by GR Lee, J Foerster, J Lukens, F Paraskevas, GP Greer, GM Rodgers. Baltimore: Williams & Wilkins. 1999.)

In most cases, the physician integrates the patient's clinical findings with laboratory test results to correctly diagnose the illness. The examples mentioned serve to emphasize the fact that when making a diagnosis of anemia, the physician cannot depend solely on laboratory test results but also must consider patient history, physical examination, and symptoms.

▶ ADAPTATIONS TO ANEMIA

Signs and symptoms of anemia range from slight fatigue or barely noticeable physiologic changes to life-threatening reactions depending on:

- Rate of onset
- Severity of blood loss
- Ability of the body to adapt

With rapid loss of blood as occurs in acute hemorrhage, clinical manifestations are related to hypovolemia and vary with the amount of blood lost. A normal person may lose up to 1,000 mL or 20% of total blood volume and not exhibit clinical signs of the loss at rest, but with mild exercise, tachycardia is common.[4] Severe blood loss of 1,500–2,000 mL or 30–40% of total blood volume leads to circulatory collapse and shock. Death is imminent if the acute loss reaches 50% of total blood volume (2,500 mL).

Slowly developing anemias can show an equally severe drop in hemoglobin as is seen in acute blood loss, but the threat of shock or death is not usually present. The reason for this apparent discrepancy is that in slowly developing anemias, the body has several adaptive mechanisms that allow organs to function at hemoglobin levels of up to 50% less than normal. The adaptive mechanisms are of two types: an increase in the oxygenated blood flow to the tissues and an increase in oxygen utilization by the tissues (Table 8-2 ✪).

INCREASE IN OXYGENATED BLOOD FLOW

Oxygenated blood flow to the tissues can be increased by increasing the cardiac rate, cardiac output, and circulation rate. Oxygen uptake by hemoglobin in the alveoli of the lungs is increased by deepening the amount of inspiration and increasing the respiration rate. In anemia, decreased blood viscosity due to the decrease in erythrocytes and decrease in peripheral resistance help to increase the circulation rate, delivering oxygen to tissues at an increased rate. Blood flow to the vital organs, the heart and brain, can preferentially increase while flow to tissues with low oxygen requirements and normally high blood supply such as skin and the kidneys is decreased.

INCREASE IN OXYGEN UTILIZATION BY TISSUE

An important compensatory mechanism at the cellular level that allows the tissue to extract more oxygen from hemoglobin involves an increase in 2,3-BPG (2,3-bisphosphoglycerate—also known as *2,3-diphosphoglycerate/2,3-DPG*) within the erythrocytes (∞ Chapter 6). An increase in erythrocyte 2,3-BPG permits the tissues to extract more oxygen from the blood even though the PO_2 remains constant and shifts the oxygen dissociation curve to the right. It is not clear exactly how anemia stimulates this increase in cellular 2,3-BPG.

Another adaptive mechanism at the cellular level involves the Bohr effect. The scarcity of oxygen causes anaerobic glycolysis by muscles and other tissue, which produces a buildup of lactic acid. Additionally, H^+ are generated from bicarbonic acid (H_2CO_3) formed during the transport of CO_2 from the tissues to the lungs (∞ Chapter 6). This acidosis decreases hemoglobin's affinity for oxygen in the capillaries, thus causing release of more oxygen to the tissues.

Even with these physiologic adaptations, different anemic patients respond differently to similar changes in hemoglobin levels. The extent of the physiologic adaptations is influenced by:

1. Severity of the anemia
2. Competency of the cardiovascular and respiratory systems
3. Oxygen requirements of the individual (physical and metabolic activity)
4. Duration of the anemia
5. Disease or condition that caused the anemia
6. Presence and severity of coexisting disease

▶ DIAGNOSIS OF ANEMIA

Anemia can impair an individual's ability to carry on activities of daily living and decrease the individual's quality of life (QOL). Thus, accurate diagnosis and treatment are essential to improve patient outcomes. The diagnosis of anemia and determination of its cause are made by using a combination of information received from the patient history, the physical examination, and the laboratory investigation (Table 8-3 ✪).

✪ TABLE 8-2
Adaptations to Anemia
Increase in oxygenated blood flow • Increase in cardiac rate • Increase in cardiac output • Increase in circulation rate • Preferential increase in blood flow to vital organs Increase in oxygen utilization by tissues • Increase in 2,3-BPG in erythrocytes • Decreased oxygen affinity of hemoglobin in tissues due to Bohr effect

⊛ TABLE 8-3

Important Information for Evaluating a Patient for Anemia

Diagnosis of anemia and determination of its cause requires information obtained from the patient history, physical examination, and laboratory data

I. Patient history
   A. Dietary habits
   B. Medications
   C. Exposure to chemicals and toxins
   D. Symptoms and their duration
      1. Fatigue
      2. Muscle weakness
      3. Headache
      4. Vertigo
      5. Syncope
      6. Dyspnea
      7. Palpitations
   E. Previous record of abnormal blood examination
   F. Family history of abnormal blood examination

II. Signs of anemia obtained by physical examination
   A. Skin pallor
   B. Pale conjunctiva
   C. Koilonychia
   D. Hypotension
   E. Jaundice
   F. Smooth tongue
   G. Neurological dysfunction
   H. Hepatomegaly
   I. Splenomegaly
   J. Bone deformities in congenital anemias

III. Laboratory investigation
   A. Erythrocyte count
   B. Hemoglobin
   C. Hematocrit
   D. Erythrocyte indices: MCV, MCH, MCHC
   E. Reticulocyte count and reticulocyte production index
   F. Blood smear examination
   G. Leukocyte and platelet quantitative and qualitative examination
   H. Tests to measure erythrocyte destruction depending on other information available: serum bilirubin, haptoglobin, lactate dehydrogenase (LD), methemalbumin, urine hemosiderin
   I. Bone marrow examination (depending upon results of other laboratory tests and patient clinical data)

HISTORY

The patient's history including symptoms can reveal some important clues as to the cause of the anemia. Information solicited by the physician should include dietary habits, medication taken, possible exposure to chemicals or toxins, and description and duration of the symptoms. The most common complaint is tiredness. Muscle weakness and fatigue develop when there is not enough oxygen available to burn fuel for the production of energy.

Severe drops in hemoglobin can lead to a variety of additional symptoms. When oxygen to the brain is decreased, headache, vertigo, and syncope can occur. Dyspnea and palpitations from exertion, or occasionally while at rest, are not uncommon complaints. The patient should be questioned as to any overt signs of blood loss, such as hematuria, hematemesis, and bloody or black stools. Family history can help define the rarer hereditary types of hematologic disorders. For example, sickle cell anemia and thalassemia are frequently manifested to some degree in several members of the immediate family.

PHYSICAL EXAMINATION

Physical examination of the patient helps the physician detect the adverse effects of a long-standing anemia (Table 8-3).

- Changes in epithelial tissue from oxygen deprivation is noted in some patients. Skin pallor is easily noted in most Caucasian patients, but because of variability in natural skin tone, pale conjunctiva is a more reliable indicator of anemia. The presence of pallor, particularly conjunctival pallor, has been shown to be a cost effective and feasible method to screen for anemia in a variety of settings.[5,6]
- Hypotension can accompany significant decreases in blood volume.
- Heart abnormalities can occur as a result of the increased cardiac workload associated with the physiologic adaptations to anemia. Cardiac problems usually occur only with chronic or severe anemias (hemoglobin <7 g/dL).
- Organomegaly of the spleen and liver are of primary importance in establishing the extent of involvement of the hematopoietic system in the production and destruction of erythrocytes. Massive splenomegaly is characteristic of some hereditary chronic anemias. The spleen can also become enlarged in some autoimmune hemolytic anemias when it is the primary site of destruction of antibody-sensitized erythrocytes.
- Anemia can also occur secondarily to a defect in hemostasis. The presence of bruises, ecchymoses, and petechiae indicates that the platelets can be involved in the disorder that is producing the anemia.

In addition to these general physical findings associated with anemia, there can be findings associated with a particular type of anemia. These include koilonychia in iron deficiency, a smooth tongue in megaloblastic anemia, jaundice in hemolytic anemias, bone deformities and extramedullary hematopoietic tissue masses in the hereditary hemoglobinopathies, and neurological dysfunction in pernicious anemia.

In addition to determining the extent of anemic manifestations, physical examination helps to establish the underlying disease process causing the anemia. Some disorders associated with anemia include chronic diseases such as rheumatoid arthritis as well as malignancies, gastrointestinal lesions, kidney disease, parasitic infection, and liver dysfunction.

LABORATORY INVESTIGATION

After the physical examination and patient history, a physician who suspects the patient has anemia orders laboratory tests. Initially, screening tests are performed to determine whether anemia is present and to evaluate erythrocyte production and destruction/loss. The initial screening test is the complete blood count (CBC), which includes red blood cell (RBC) count, hemoglobin, hematocrit, RBC indices, white blood cell (WBC) count, and platelet count. Depending on these test results, additional tests such as the reticulocyte count, bilirubin, and review of the blood smear can be suggested. In addition, the urine and stool can be examined for the presence of blood. When combined with the information from the history and physical examination of the patient, results of these tests can give insight to the cause of the anemia. These routine tests can be followed by a protocol of specific diagnostic tests that help establish the etiology and pathophysiology of the anemia. These specific tests will be discussed in the appropriate chapters on anemia.

Erythrocyte Count, Hematocrit, and Hemoglobin

The erythrocyte count, hematocrit, and hemoglobin are determined using routine laboratory tests used to screen for the presence of anemia. Generally, concentrations for these parameters parallel each other. A diurnal variation in hemoglobin, hematocrit, and erythrocyte values occurs with highest values in the morning and lowest values in the evening.

Erythrocyte counts are usually performed only if automated instruments are available. Thus, in a clinic or physician's office with limited resources, screening can be limited to either the hematocrit or hemoglobin. If one of the three screening tests is abnormal, it is helpful to have the results of the other two so that the red cell indices can be calculated.

A decreased concentration in one or more of these parameters based on the individual's age and sex should be followed by other laboratory tests to help establish criteria for diagnosis. The Centers for Disease Control (CDC) recommended cutoff values for a diagnosis of anemia according to age and sex are provided in Table 8-4 ✪. Upward adjustments for these cutoff values should be utilized for individuals living at high altitudes and for those who smoke. There is a direct dose–response relationship between the amount smoked and the hemoglobin level.[3] The CDC recommended adjustments are included in Tables 8-5 ✪ and 8-6 ✪. Hemoglobin and hematocrit values also vary in pregnancy with a gradual decrease in the first two trimesters and a rise during the third trimester (Table 8-7 ✪).

The highest normal hemoglobin, hematocrit, and erythrocyte counts are seen at birth. In the neonate, erythrocytes are macrocytic, and the reticulocyte count is 2–6%. From 3 to 10 nucleated erythrocytes per 100 leukocytes can be observed in the peripheral blood during the first week of

✪ TABLE 8-4

Hemoglobin (Hb) and Hematocrit (Hct) Cutoffs for a Diagnosis of Anemia in Children, Nonpregnant Females, and Males

Age (yrs)/Sex	Hb (g/dL)	Hct (%)
Both sexes		
1–1.9	11.0	33.0
2–4.9	11.2	34.0
5–7.9	11.4	34.5
8–11.9	11.6	35.0
Female		
12–14.9	11.8	35.5
15–17.9	12.0	36.0
≥18	12.0	36.0
Male		
12–14.9	12.3	37.0
15–17.9	12.6	38.0
≥18	13.6	41.0

*Based on fifth percentile values from the Second National Health and Nutrition Examination survey conducted after excluding persons with a higher likelihood of iron deficiency.
From Centers for Disease Control. *MMWR*. 1989, June 8; 38 [22].

✪ TABLE 8-5

Altitude Adjustments for Hemoglobin (Hb) and Hematocrit (Hct) Cutoffs for a Diagnosis of Anemia

Altitude (ft)	Hb (g/dL)	Hct (%)
<3000	—	—
3000–3999	+0.2	+0.5
4000–4999	+0.3	+1.0
5000–5999	+0.5	+1.5
6000–6999	+0.7	+2.0
7000–7999	+1.0	+3.0
8000–8999	+1.3	+4.0
9000–9999	+1.6	+5.0
>10,000	+2.0	+6.0

From Centers for Disease Control. *MMWR*. 1989, June 8; 38 [22].

✪ TABLE 8-6

Adjustments for Hemoglobin (Hb) and Hematocrit (Hct) Cutoffs for a Diagnosis of Anemia in Smokers

Characteristic	Hb (g/dL)	Hct (%)
Nonsmoker	—	—
Smoker (all)	+0.3	+1.0
1/2–1 pack/day	+0.3	+1.0
1–2 packs/day	+0.5	+1.5
>2 packs/day	+0.7	+2.0

From Centers for Disease Control. *MMWR*. 1989, June 8; 38 [22].

☼ TABLE 8-7

Hemoglobin Cutoffs for a Diagnosis of Anemia in Pregnancy by Month and Trimester*

Gestation (wks)/Trimester	12/1[†]	16/2	20/2[†]	24/2	28/3	32/3[†]	36/3	40/Term
Mean Hb (g/dL)	12.2	11.8	11.6	11.6	11.8	12.1	12.5	12.9
5th percentile Hb values (g/dL)	11.0	10.6	10.5	10.5	10.7	11.0	11.4	11.9
Equivalent 5th percentile Hct values (%)[‡]	33.0	32.0	32.0	32.0	32.0	33.0	34.0	36.0

*Based on pooled data from four European surveys of healthy women taking iron supplements
[†]Hb values adapted for the trimester-specific cutoffs
[‡]Hematocrit
From Centers for Disease Control. *MMWR.* 1989, June 8; 38 [22].

life. A gradual decrease in these parameters occurs for 2 months after birth. This decline is followed by a gradual increase until normal adult values are reached at about 14 years of age. A difference in erythrocyte values between sexes is noted at puberty, females having lower values than males.

Although anemia in the elderly is prevalent, it should not be considered a normal part of aging. Hematologic values change very little in normal older adults and increase slightly after menopause.[7] In men over 70 years of age, the hemoglobin decreases about 1 g/dL partly due to a decrease in androgens. A slight decline in the hemoglobin of about 0.2 g/dL occurs in women over 70.[8,9] The third National Health and Nutrition Examination Survey (NHANES III, 1988–94) studied a group of noninstitutionalized older individuals and found that after age 65, the prevalence of anemia rose to 11% in men and 10.2% in women.[10,11] The highest prevalence of anemia is in those over 85 years of age (26% of men and 20% of women). In this anemic group, one-third had a nutritional deficiency, one-third had anemia of chronic disease or inflammation, and one-third were unexplained.

Variations in hemoglobin are also reported to occur as a result of blood-drawing techniques. Hemoglobin values are about 0.7 g/dL higher if the patient's blood is obtained while the individual is in an upright position rather than supine. Prolonged vasoconstriction by the tourniquet can cause hemoconcentration of the sample and elevate the hemoglobin value.

Erythrocyte Indices

The erythrocyte indices help classify the erythrocytes as to their size and hemoglobin content (∞ Chapter 34). Hemoglobin, hematocrit, and erythrocyte count values are used to calculate the three indices: mean corpuscular volume (MCV), mean corpuscular hemoglobin (MCH), and mean corpuscular hemoglobin concentration (MCHC). (The conversion factors in the formulas for the indices vary depending on the use of conventional units or Systeme International Units [SI] for the hemoglobin and hematocrit. Chapter 34 gives both conversion factors.) The indices give a clue as to what the erythrocytes should look like on the stained blood film. Because abnormal erythrocyte morphology is characteristic of distinct types of anemia, the indices are useful for classification of anemic states. Indices may be falsely increased or decreased depending upon a number of factors (see ∞ Table 41-7). The laboratory scientist should always correlate the indices with the Hb, Hct, RBC count, and other indices to ensure that technical problems are identified when they occur.

Mean Cell Volume   The MCV indicates the average volume of individual erythrocytes expressed in femtoliters (fL), (10^{-15} L). It is measured directly on automated cell counters and also can be manually calculated from the hematocrit and RBC count. The reference interval is 80.0–100.0 fL. The mean MCV is slightly increased in nonanemic individuals over the age of 65 (about 90.0 fL versus 87.0 fL).[8]

$$MCV(fL) = \frac{hct(L/L) \times 1000}{RBC\ count\ (\times 10^{12}/L)}$$

(Multiply by 10 if hct is expressed in %).

Example   A patient has a hematocrit of 0.45 L/L and an RBC count of 5.0×10^{12}/L.

$$MCV(fL) = \frac{0.45\ L/L\ (hct) \times 1000}{5 \times 10^{12}/L\ (RBC\ count)} = 90.0\ fL$$

The value 90.0 fL means the cell has a normal volume and therefore is normocytic.

The MCV is used to classify cells as normocytic, microcytic, or macrocytic (Table 8-8 ☼). Abnormalities in the MCV are clues to disease processes of the hematopoietic system;

☼ TABLE 8-8

Classification of Erythrocytes Based on MCV

Normocytic	80.0–100.0 fL
Microcytic	<80.0 fL
Macrocytic	>100.0 fL

they are useful in preliminary assessment of anemia pathophysiology.

This index usually correlates with the appearance of cells on stained blood smears (i.e., cells with an increased MCV appear larger [macrocytes], and cells with a decreased MCV appear smaller [microcytes]). However, it must be remembered that MCV is a measurement of volume whereas estimation of flattened cells on a blood smear is a measurement of cell diameter. Cell diameter and cell volume are not the same. Spherocytes usually have a normal or only slightly decreased volume (MCV), but on a stained smear, they are unable to flatten as much as normal erythrocytes because of a decreased surface area and increased rigidity. Spherocytes, therefore, often appear to have a smaller diameter than normal cells. On the other hand, target cells can appear larger due to an increased diameter, but the MCV is often normal.

On instruments using hydrodynamic focusing technology, the MCV can change by up to 4.0 fL if the blood specimen is left uncapped for 4 hours or more due to oxygenation of the blood.[12] The MCV also can increase significantly if blood is stored for 24 hours at room temperature.

Mean Corpuscular Hemoglobin The MCH is a measurement of the average weight of hemoglobin in individual erythrocytes. The MCH is calculated from the hemoglobin and erythrocyte count. The reference interval of MCH for normocytic cells is 28.0–34.0 pg.

$$MCH(pg) = \frac{Hb\ (g/dL) \times 10}{RBC\ count\ (\times 10^{12}/L)}$$

Example A patient has a hemoglobin concentration of 15 g/dL and an RBC count of $5 \times 10^{12}/L$.

$$MCH(pg) = \frac{15\ g/dL\ (Hb) \times 10}{5 \times 10^{12}/L\ (RBC\ count)} = 30.0\ pg$$

(If hemoglobin is expressed in g/L, do not multiply by 10.)

The value 30.0 pg means the cell contains an average weight of hemoglobin that is within the reference range (28–34 pg).

The MCH does not take into account the size of a cell; it should not be interpreted without taking into consideration the MCV. It varies in a direct linear relationship with MCV. Smaller cells normally contain less hemoglobin, and larger cells normally contain more hemoglobin. In some anemias, a decrease or increase in cell size (MCV) is associated with a proportional decrease or increase in the amount of hemoglobin within the cell (MCH), resulting in a normochromic cell (normal MCHC). In other anemias, however, the decrease in the amount of hemoglobin within the cell (MCH) is substantially more than the decrease in cell size, and the cell appears hypochromic (decreased MCHC). It is important to understand this concept because microcytic cells with an MCH <28.0 pg are not necessarily hypochromic, and macrocytes with a MCH >34.0 pg are usually normochromic.

Mean Corpuscular Hemoglobin Concentration

The MCHC is the ratio of hemoglobin mass to volume in which it is contained (i.e., average concentration of hemoglobin in a deciliter of erythrocytes expressed in g/dL). The MCHC is calculated from the hemoglobin and hematocrit. The reference interval of MCHC is 32.0–36.0 g/dL.

$$MCHC(g/dL) = \frac{Hb(g/dL)}{Hct\ (L/L)}$$

Example A patient has a hemoglobin concentration of 15.0 g/dL and a hematocrit of 0.45 L/L.

$$MCHC(g/dL) = \frac{15\ g/dL\ (Hb)}{.45\ L/L\ (hct)} = 33.3\ g/dL$$

(If hematocrit is expressed in percent, multiply by 100.)

The value, 33.3 g/dL, reveals that the cells contain a normal concentration of hemoglobin and are therefore normochromic.

This index indicates whether the general cell population is normochromic or hypochromic (Table 8-9 ✪). The word *hyperchromic* should be used sparingly. The only erythrocyte that is hyperchromic with an MCHC more than 36.0 g/dL is the spherocyte. Spherocytes have a decreased surface-to-volume ratio due to a loss of membrane but have not lost an appreciable amount of their hemoglobin. The MCHC can be increased in some cases of sickle cell anemia and hemoglobin C disease when the hemoglobin concentration in the cell is close to the solubility value of hemoglobin.[10] The MCHC can be falsely increased with hemolysis, cold agglutinins, and/or insufficient blood in relation to EDTA in the collection tube. The erythrocyte's deformability and its viscosity affect the MCV and MCHC measurements using different automated technologies. The MCHC rarely changes using impedance analyzers and, therefore, its usefulness in classifying anemias can be limited.[12] The MCHC from analyzers using hydrodynamic focusing can be more clinically useful.

In certain conditions, the indices MCV, MCH, and MCHC can be falsely elevated. These are discussed in ∞ Chapters 34 and 41.

Developmental Changes in Erythrocyte Indices

The MCV is increased to a mean of 108 fL at birth but decreases to a mean of 77 fL between the ages of 6 months and 2 years (Figure 8-1 ■).[13] It increases to a mean of 80.0 fL by

✪ TABLE 8-9	
Classification of Erythrocytes Based on MCHC	
Normochromic	32.0–36.0 g/dL
Hypochromic	<32.0 g/dL
Hyperchromic	>36.0 g/dL

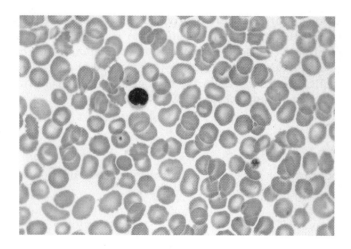

■ FIGURE 8-1 Peripheral blood from a newborn; note the macrocytic erythrocytes. (Wright-Giemsa stain; 1000× magnification)

5 years of age but does not reach the adult mean of 90 fL until about 18 years of age. The MCH changes in parallel to the MCV throughout infancy and childhood. The MCHC, however, remains constant within the adult reference interval. Between the ages of 12 and 17 years, males have a higher MCHC and lower MCH and MCV than females.[14]

✓ Checkpoint! 1

Calculate the indices and describe the erythrocytes given the following information: Hb 7.1 g/dL, Hct 0.23L/L; RBC count 3.59 × 10^{12}/L.

Red Cell Distribution Width Because the MCV represents an average of erythrocyte volume, it is less reliable in describing the erythrocyte population when considerable variation in erythrocyte size (anisocytosis occurs). The RDW (red cell distribution width), the coefficient of variation of MCV, is a calculated index provided by hematology analyzers to help identify anisocytosis. It is calculated as follows:

$$\frac{\text{Standard deviation of MCV} \times 100}{\text{Mean MCV}} = \text{RDW}$$

The reference interval for RDW is 11.5–14.5%. All abnormalities found to this time have been on the high side, indicating an increase in the heterogeneity of erythrocyte size.

Caution must be used in interpreting the RDW because it reflects the ratio of the standard deviation of cell size and the mean MCV. An increased standard deviation (heterogeneous cell population) with a high MCV can give a normal RDW. Conversely, a normal standard deviation (homogeneous cell population) with a low MCV can give an increased RDW. Examination of the erythrocyte histogram/cytogram and stained blood smear gives clues as to the accuracy of the RDW in these cases. When the standard deviation is increased, indicating a true variability in cell size, the base of the erythrocyte histogram is broader than usual.

ⓒ CASE STUDY *(continued from page 147)*

George's only complaint was dark urine and the yellow color of his eyes. His CBC results were hemoglobin 3.1 g/dL; hematocrit 0.08 L/L; RBC count 0.71 × 10^{12}/L; RDW 21.6; reticulocytes 22%. Calculate the erythrocyte indices.

1. Does the information given suggest acute or chronic blood loss? What is the significance of the RDW?

✓ Checkpoint! 2

A patient has an MCV of 130 fL and an RDW of 14.5. Review of the blood smear reveals anisocytosis. Explain the discrepancy between the blood smear finding and RDW.

Reticulocyte Count

Immature, anuclear erythrocytes containing organelles and residual ribosomes for hemoglobin synthesis are known as reticulocytes (∞ Chapter 5). Reticulocytes usually spend 2–3 days in the bone marrow and an additional day in the peripheral blood before losing their RNA and becoming mature erythrocytes. The peripheral blood reticulocyte count indicates the degree of effective bone marrow activity and is one of the most useful and cost-effective laboratory tests in monitoring anemia and response to therapy (∞ Chapter 34). It is also helpful in classifying the pathophysiology of anemia. Reticulocytes can sometimes be identified as *polychromatophilic* erythrocytes (erythrocytes with a bluish tinge) on Romanowsky-stained smears. The polychromatophilia is due to the presence of basophilic ribosomes (RNA) mixed with acidophilic hemoglobin (Figure 8-2 ■).

Methods for Counting Reticulocytes The reticulocyte count is one of the few remaining common hematology tests to be performed manually (Figure 8-3 ■). Although au-

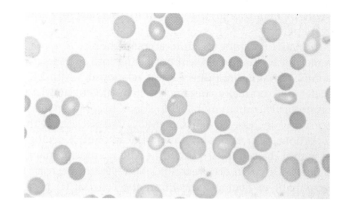

■ FIGURE 8-2 The large erythrocytes with a bluish tinge are polychromatophilic erythrocytes, which are larger than the more mature erythrocytes. Note also the spherocytes. (Peripheral blood; Wright-Giemsa stain; 1000× magnification)

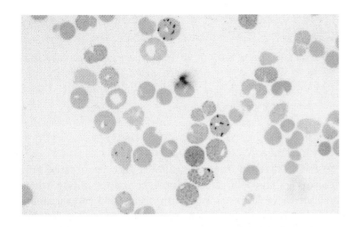

■ **FIGURE 8-3** The erythrocytes with the particulate inclusions are reticulocytes. The inclusions represent reticulum that stains with the supravital stain brilliant cresyl blue. (Peripheral blood; 1000× magnification)

tomated methods are available on hematology analyzers, more than half of the laboratories still use the manual method[15] (∞ Chapter 36). Test results are expressed as a percentage of reticulocytes in relation to total RBC count or can be expressed as the absolute number (see next section). The reference interval varies among laboratories and the procedure used, but it is about 0.5–2.5% or 18–158 × 10^9/L. In the automated method, more than 30,000 RBCs are assessed, so the method is more precise than the manual method (which assesses 1000 RBCs) and is more accurate when the reticulocyte count is very low.

In the healthy aged, there appears to be a decrease in the lifespan of the erythrocyte.[16] This is compensated for by an active bone marrow so that the hemoglobin and hematocrit remain in the reference interval of other adults. There is, however, a slight reticulocytosis, reflecting the increased production of erythrocytes.

Absolute Reticulocyte Count   In anemia, a more informative index of erythropoietic activity than the relative reticulocyte count is needed. When reported in percentage, the reticulocyte count does not indicate the relationship between the peripheral blood erythrocyte mass and the number of reticulocytes being produced. The percentage can be increased due to either an increase in the number of reticulocytes in the circulation or a decrease in the number of total RBCs. Therefore, it is recommended that in addition to the percentage of reticulocytes, labs report the absolute reticulocyte count to provide a more useful estimate of reticulocyte production. The absolute count is provided by automated analyzers and can be calculated when using manual methods for reticulocytes:

Absolute reticulocyte ($\times 10^9$/L) =
RBC count ($\times 10^{12}$/L) × Reticulocyte count (%)

For example, in a patient with an RBC count of 3.5×10^{12}/L and a 10% reticulocyte count, the absolute

reticulocyte count is $(3.5 \times 10^{12}/\text{L}) \times 10\% = 350 \times 10^9/\text{L}$. The mean normal value is $90 \times 10^9/\text{L}$.

The corrected reticulocyte count is another means to adjust the reticulocyte count in proportion to the severity of anemia. In this procedure, the percentage of reticulocytes is multiplied by the ratio of the patient's hematocrit to an average age and sex appropriate normal hematocrit:

$$\text{Corrected reticulocyte count} = \frac{\text{Patient hematocrit}}{\text{Normal hematocrit}} \times \% \text{ reticulocyte}$$

Corrected reticulocyte counts less than 2% are associated with hypoproliferative anemias. For practical purposes, the corrected reticulocyte count or preferably absolute reticulocyte count is used to assess the degree of erythropoiesis in anemic patients.[15,17]

✓ **Checkpoint! 3**

Is it possible to have an increased relative reticulocyte count but an absolute reticulocyte count in the normal interval? Explain.

Quantitation of Reticulocyte Immaturity   Under normal physiologic conditions when there is no anemia, the reticulocytes are released into the peripheral blood where they spend another day maturing to the erythrocyte. When the need for erythrocytes in the circulation increases, the bone marrow releases reticulocytes earlier than normal. These more immature reticulocytes are called *stress reticulocytes* or *shift reticulocytes*. They appear as large polychromatophilic cells on the Romanowsky-stained blood smear. It takes longer for these reticulocytes to mature in the peripheral blood because the remainder of the bone marrow maturation time is added to the peripheral blood maturation time (Table 8-10 ✪). The more severe the anemia, the earlier the reticulocyte is released. In a stimulated marrow, hematocrit levels of 0.35L/L, 0.25 L/L, and 0.15 L/L are associated with early reticulocyte release and a prolongation of the reticulocyte maturation in peripheral blood to approximately 1.5, 2.0, and 2.5 days, respectively. This is similar to the left shift in granulocytes seen in peripheral blood when the need for granulocytes is increased. To correct for the prolongation of maturation of these circulating shift reticulocytes and

✪ **TABLE 8-10**

Correlation of the Hematocrit with Reticulocyte Maturation Time in the Peripheral Blood	
Hematocrit (L/L)	Reticulocyte Maturation Time (Days)
.35	1.5
.25	2.0
.15	2.5

anemia, the **reticulocyte production index (RPI)** is calculated. The following formula is used:

$$\frac{\text{Patient's hematocrit}}{0.45 \text{ L/L}} \times \frac{\text{Reticulocyte count (\%)}}{\text{Reticulocyte maturation time (days)}}$$

For example, if a patient with a 0.25 L/L hematocrit had a 15% reticulocyte count, the RPI would be:

$$\frac{.25 \text{ L/L}}{.45 \text{ L/L}} \times \frac{15\%}{2.0} = 3.3 \text{ RPI}$$

The RPI is a good indicator of the adequacy of the bone marrow response in anemia. Generally speaking, an RPI > 2 indicates an appropriate bone marrow response, whereas an RPI < 2 indicates an inadequate compensatory bone marrow response (hypoproliferation) or an ineffective bone marrow response. When utilized in this way, the reticulocyte count provides a direction for the course of investigation concerning anemia etiology and pathophysiology.

Reticulocyte maturity level also can be classified based on semi quantitative assessment of RNA concentration within the maturing erythrocyte. Younger reticulocytes contain more RNA than more mature reticulocytes. Some automated hematology instruments not only provide a relative and absolute reticulocyte count but they also assess reticulocytes for maturity level based on RNA content level (assessed by intensity of staining) and report an index of maturity. The term used for this index varies by instrument manufacturer, but it is recommended that it be called the **immature reticulocyte fraction (IRF)**.

The Miles H.3/Advia 120 System by Bayer Diagnostics uses a different method to classify reticulocyte maturity. It reports a reticulocyte hemoglobin content (CHr) and mean reticulocyte cell hemoglobin concentration (CHCMr) for reticulocyte maturity level.

The IRF can be helpful in evaluating bone marrow erythropoietic response to anemia, monitoring anemia, and evaluating response to therapy. In anemia, an increased IRF generally indicates an adequate erythropoietic response while a normal or subnormal IRF reflects an inadequate or no response to the anemia.[18] (The normal reference interval using the Cell-Dyn 3500 and 3700 systems with impedance technology is 0.29 +/− 0.6.)[12] When the bone marrow increases production of erythrocytes, an observable increase in the IRF occurs *before* an increase in the reticulocyte count or an increase in hemoglobin, hematocrit, or RBC count occurs. After bone marrow transplantation, it is the first sign of a successful engraftment. In patients receiving human recombinant erythropoietin (rHuEPO) or iron therapy for anemia, an increased IRF predicts a successful outcome.

The Clinical Laboratory Standards Institute (CLSI), recommends that the IRF index replace the reticulocyte production index (RPI).[15] Laboratories that do not have instruments that measure this parameter may use the RPI.

 CASE STUDY *(continued from page 154)*

George's RBC count is 0.7×10^{12}/L and his reticulocyte count is 22%.

2. Calculate his absolute reticulocyte count. Is this count increased, decreased, or normal?

Blood Smear Examination

The erythrocyte is sometimes called a *discocyte* because of its biconcave shape. On a Romanowsky-stained blood smear, the erythrocyte appears as a 7 μm disc with a central area of pallor surrounded by a rim of pink-staining hemoglobin. The area of pallor is caused by the closeness occurring between the two concave portions of the membrane when the cell becomes flattened on a glass slide. Normally the area of pallor occupies about one-third the diameter of the cell. The area of pallor is not seen in erythrocytes suspended in saline or plasma and viewed with the light microscope.

Although doing so is not always necessary, reviewing the stained blood smear assists in diagnosing the type of anemia in 25% of the cases.[19] The normal morphology of the erythrocyte can be altered by various pathological conditions intrinsic or extrinsic to the cell. Careful examination of a stained blood smear reveals these morphologic aberrations. **Anisocytosis** denotes a nonspecific variation in the size of the cells. Some variation in size is normal because of the variation in age of the erythrocytes, younger cells being larger and older cells smaller (Figures 8-4a■ and 8-4b■). **Poikilocytosis** is the general term used to describe a nonspecific variation in the shape of erythrocytes (Figures 8-5a■ and 8-5b■). Some shapes and sizes, however, are particularly characteristic of specific underlying hematologic disorders or malignancies. These include nucleated erythrocytes (except in newborns), schistocytes, teardrop erythrocytes, spherocytes, acanthocytes, and marked erythrocyte shape abnormalities in normocytic anemia without evidence of hemolysis. It is important to keep in mind that some abnormal morphology can be artifactual because of poorly made or improperly stained smears. If artifactual morphology is suspected, the erythrocytes should be examined in a wet preparation. If the abnormal morphology is present in this preparation, the possibility of artifacts can be eliminated.

Anisocytosis   Anisocytosis, variation in cell size, can be detected by examining the blood smear and/or by reviewing the MCV and RDW. Normal erythrocytes have a diameter of about 7–8 μm and an MCV of 80–100 fL. If the majority of cells are larger than normal, the cells are macrocytic; if smaller than normal, they are microcytic (Table 8-11✪). If there is a significant variation in size with microcytic, normocytic, and macrocytic cells present, the MCV can be normal because it is an average of cell size. In this case, the RDW is helpful. An RDW more than 14.5 suggests that the erythrocytes are heterogeneous in size, which makes

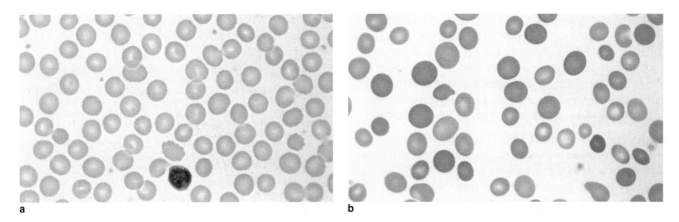

■ FIGURE 8-4   **a.** Normocytic, normochromic erythrocytes. Compare the size of the cells to the nucleus of the lymphocytes. **b.** These erythrocytes show marked anisocytosis. Note the spherocytes. (MCV 104 fL; RDW 30.2) (Peripheral blood; Wright-Giemsa stain; 1000× magnification)

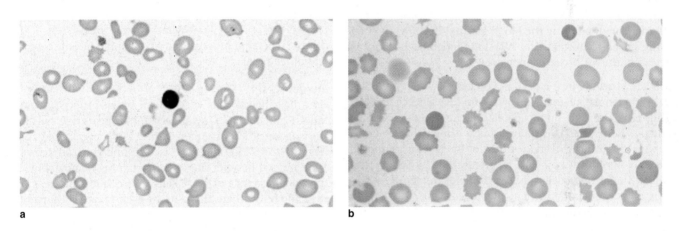

■ FIGURE 8-5   **a.** Erythrocytes with marked anisocytosis and poikilocytosis. (Peripheral blood; Wright-Giemsa stain; 400× magnification). **b.** Poikilocytosis with acanthocytes, helmet cell, elliptocytes, echinocytes, schistocytes, and spherocytes. There is also anisocytosis with microcytes and macrocytes. At least two of the macrocytes are polychromatophilic, indicating that they are reticulocytes. (Peripheral blood; 1000× magnification Wright-Giemsa stain)

✪ TABLE 8-11

Abnormalities in Erythrocyte Size

Terminology	Description	Associated Disease States
Anisocytosis	Increased variation in the range of red cell sizes	See disease states associated with microcytes and macrocytes below
Microcytosis	Red cells with a reduced volume (<80 fL)	Iron deficiency anemia; thalassemia; sideroblastic anemia
Macrocytosis	Red cells with an increased volume (>100 fL)	Megaloblastic anemias; hemolytic anemia; recovery from acute hemorrhage; liver disease; asplenia; aplastic anemia; myelodysplasia; endocrinopathies

the MCV less reliable.[18] Microscopic examination of the cells is especially helpful when the RDW is elevated. To evaluate erythrocyte size microscopically, the cells are compared with the nucleus of a normal small lymphocyte. Normocytic erythrocytes are about the same size as the lymphocyte nucleus (Figure 8-4a). Figures 8-4b and 8-5a show erythrocytes with a marked degree of anisocytosis.

Microcytes   Microcytes are erythrocytes with a diameter less than 7.0 μm and an MCV less than 80 fL. The cell is usually hypochromic but can be normochromic (Figure 8-6 ■). Microcytes in the shape of spheres (microspherocytes) can appear hyperchromic. Microcytes are usually associated with defective hemoglobin formation (Table 8-11).

Macrocytes   Macrocytes are larger than normal erythrocytes, having a diameter more than 8.0 μm and an MCV of more than 100 fL. The cell usually contains an adequate amount of hemoglobin resulting in a normal MCHC and normal to increased MCH. Macrocytes are associated with impaired DNA synthesis as occurs in Vitamin B_{12}, or folate, deficiency as well as other diseases (Table 8-11). Young erythrocytes are normally larger than mature erythrocytes, but within a day of entering the blood stream, they are groomed by the spleen to normal size. When the reticulocyte count is increased, the MCV can be increased.

Poikilocytosis   In the past, poikilocytosis was reported as slight, moderate, or marked (or 1+ to 4+). This practice is being replaced, and many laboratories report only significant poikilocytosis. The stained smear should be reviewed keeping in mind the overall context of the laboratory results and the significance of the reported findings. Using the 40X–50X objective, review at least 10 fields to identify variations in size, shape, and hemoglobin content. To evaluate abnormalities including inclusions, review with the 100X objective. When determining significance and deciding whether to report poikilocytes, the following should be considered:

1. Will it assist in differential diagnosis of the anemia?
2. Will it make a difference in the management of the patient?
3. Is the dominant poikilocyte significant in this setting?
4. Is the specific constellation of findings indicative of a particular pathologic state?

Figure 8-4a illustrates normal erythrocytes, and Figure 8-5a and 8-5b illustrate poikilocytosis. Following is a description of specific types of poikilocytes, their physiologic significance, and disorders with which they are associated (Table 8-12 ✪).

Acanthocytes   Acanthocytes, or spur cells, are small spherical cells with irregular thornlike projections (Figures 8-5b and 8-7e ■). Often the projections have small bulblike tips. Acanthocytes do not have a central area of pallor. These cells have membranes with altered lipid content. Acanthocytes have a normal life span with a normal to slightly decreased osmotic fragility. Acanthocytes can be seen in liver disease, abetalipoproteinemia (congenital acanthocytosis), and other diseases (Table 8-12).

Target Cells   Target cells, also called codocytes, are thin, bell-shaped cells with an increased surface-to-volume ratio (Figure 8-7f ■). On stained blood smears, the cells have the appearance of a target with a bull's eye in the center (Figure 8-8 ■). The bull's eye is surrounded by an achromic zone and a thin outer ring of pink-staining hemoglobin. The typical appearance of these cells is discernible in the area of the slide only where the cells are well separated but not in the extreme outer feather edge where all cells are flattened. Target cells can appear as artifacts when smears are made in a high-humidity environment or when a wet smear is blown dry rather than fan dried. Target cells have decreased osmotic fragility due to the increased surface-to-volume ratio of the cell.

Target cells can be seen in disorders in which there is an increase in membrane lipids, such as liver disease. Increased surface-to-volume ratio can also occur as a result of diminution of corpuscular hemoglobin as in iron deficiency anemia and thalassemia. Target cells can occur in some hemoglobinopathies, especially hemoglobin S and hemoglobin C disease (Table 8-12).

Teardrops   Teardrops, also called dacryocytes, are erythrocytes that are elongated at one end to form a teardrop or pear-shaped cell (Figures 8-7g ■ and 8-9 ■). Some teardrops can form after erythrocytes containing cellular inclusions have transversed the spleen. Erythrocytes with inclusions are more rigid in the area of the inclusion, and this portion of the cell has more difficulty passing through the splenic filter than the rest of the cell. As splenic macrophages attempt to

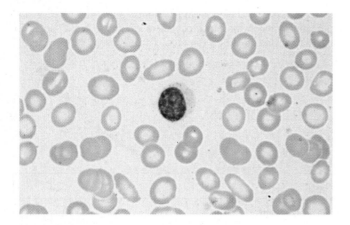

■ FIGURE 8-6   Microcytic, hypochromic erythrocytes. Compare the size of the erythrocytes with the nucleus of the lymphocyte. Normocytic cells are about the same size as the nucleus. There is only a thin rim of hemoglobin around the periphery of the cells indicating they are hypochromic. Note the elliptocytes. (Peripheral blood; Wright-Giemsa stain; 1000× magnification)

⭐ TABLE 8-12

Abnormalities in the Shape of Erythrocytes

Terminology	Synonyms	Description	Associated Disease States
Poikilocytosis	—	Increased variation in the shape of red cells	See disease states associated with specific poikilocytes on this table
Acanthocyte (spike)	Spur cell	Red cells with spicules of varying length irregularly distributed over the surface	Abetalipoproteinemia; alcoholic liver disease; disorders of lipid metabolism; post splenectomy; fat malabsorption; retinitis pigmentosa
Codocyte (bell)	Target cell	Thin bell-shaped cells with an increased surface-to-volume ratio; on stained blood smears, they assume the appearance of a target with a bull's eye in the center surrounded by an achromic zone and outer ring of hemoglobin; osmotic fragility is decreased	Hemoglobinopathies; thalassemias; obstructive liver disease; iron deficiency anemia; splenectomy; renal disease; LCAT deficiency
Dacryocyte (tear)	Teardrop; tennis racquet cell	Round cell with a single elongated or pointed extremity; often microcytic and/or hypochromic	Myelophthisic anemias; thalassemias
Drepanocyte (sickle)	Sickle cell	Red cells containing polymerized HbS showing various shapes: sickle, crescent, or boat shaped	Sickle cell disorders
Echinocyte (sea urchin)	Burr cells; crenated cell	Spiculated red cells with short equally spaced projections over the entire surface	Liver disease; uremia; pyruvate kinase deficiency; peptic ulcers; cancer of stomach; heparin therapy
Elliptocyte (oval)	Ovalocyte; pencil cell; cigar cell	Oval to elongated ellipsoid cell with central area of pallor and hemoglobin at both ends	Hereditary elliptocytosis; iron deficiency anemia; thalassemia; anemia associated with leukemia
Keratocyte (horn)	Helmet cells; horn-shaped cells	Red cells with one or several notches with projections that look like horns on either end	Microangiopathic hemolytic anemias; heart-valve hemolysis; Heinz-body hemolytic anemia; glomerulonephritis; cavernous hemangiomas
Knizocyte	—	Red cells with more than two concavities; on stained blood smears has a dark band of hemoglobin across the center with a pale area on either side	Conditions in which spherocytes are found
Leptocyte (thin)	Thin cell	Thin, flat cell with hemoglobin at periphery; usually cup shaped, MCV is decreased but diameter of cell is normal	Thalassemia; iron deficiency anemia; hemoglobinopathies; liver disease
Schistocyte (cut)	Schistocyte; fragmented cell	Fragments of red cells; variety of shapes including triangles, comma shaped; microcytic	Microangiopathic hemolytic anemias; heart-valve hemolysis; DIC; severe burns; uremia
Spherocyte	—	Spherocytic red cells with dense hemoglobin content (hyperchromatic); lack an area of central pallor; osmotic fragility increased	Hereditary spherocytosis; immune hemolytic anemias; severe burns; ABO incompatibility; Heinz-body hemolytic anemias
Stomatocyte (mouth)	Mouth cell; cup form; mushroom cap	Uniconcave red cells with the shape of a very thick cup; on stained blood smears cells have an oval or slitlike area of central pallor	Hereditary stomatocytosis; spherocytosis; alcoholic cirrhosis; anemia associated with Rh null disease; lead intoxication; neoplasms
Xerocytes	—	Dense, irregularly contracted cells; hemoglobin can be concentrated at periphery of the cell	Familial xerocytosis

remove this rigid inclusion, the cell is stretched into an abnormal shape. The teardrop cannot return to its original shape because the cell either has been stretched beyond the limits of deformability of the membrane or has been in the abnormal shape for too long a time. This is most likely the mechanism of formation of teardrops observed in thalassemia when Heinz bodies are present. Teardrops are also observed in myelofibrosis with myeloid metaplasia and metastatic cancer to the bone marrow. The mechanism of formation of dacryocytes in these pathologic states is unclear (Table 8-12).

Sickle Cells Sickle cells, also called *drepanocytes,* are elongated, crescent-shaped erythrocytes with pointed ends (Figure 8-7h ■). Some forms have more rounded ends with a flat rather than concave side (Table 8-12). These modified forms of sickle shape can be capable of reversing to the normal discocyte. Sickle cell formation can be observed in wet preparations or in stained blood smears from patients with sickle cell anemia. The hemoglobin within the cell is abnormal and polymerizes into rods at decreased oxygen tension or decreased pH. The cell first transforms into a holly leaf shape (Figure 8-7i ■). Then, as the hemoglobin polymerization

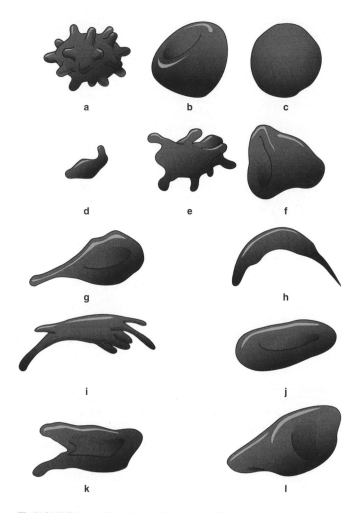

continues, it transforms into a sickle-shaped cell. Some holly-leaf forms may be observed on stained blood smears in addition to the typical sickle shape. The sickle cell has decreased osmotic fragility but increased mechanical fragility. The irregular shape of the cell decreases the erythrocyte sedimentation rate by inhibiting rouleaux formation.

Echinocytes Echinocytes, also called *burr cells*, are usually smaller than normal erythrocytes with regular, spinelike projections on their surface (Figures 8-5b, 8-7a■, and 8-9). For true "in vivo" echinocytes, the characteristic appearance is not related to tonicity of the medium in which the cells are suspended. The shape change is instead thought to be the result of an increase in the area of the outer leaflet of the lipid bilayer as compared to the inner layer. Echinocyte formation is reversible (i.e., the cell can revert to a discocyte). Echinocytes can eventually assume the shape of a spherocyte, presumably because of grooming (removal) of the membrane spines by the spleen; in this circumstance, the cell cannot revert to a normal shape.

Normal discocytes can be transformed into echinocytes under certain in vitro conditions. Echinocytes are a common artifact in stained blood smears because of the "glass effect" of the slide. The glass releases certain basic substances, raising the pH of the medium surrounding the cell and inducing echinocyte formation. Plasma provides a buffering effect on the cells, and for this reason, blood films made from whole blood may show only certain areas of echinocyte transformation. To determine the in vivo or in vitro nature of echinocytes, it can be necessary to enclose a drop of blood between two plastic cover slips (wet preparation) and observe the unstained individual erythrocytes. If no echinocytes are in the wet preparation but were noted on the stained blood smears, the cell abnormality occurred as an in vitro artifact.

■ FIGURE 8-7 Drawings of various poikilocytes: **a.** Echinocyte, **b.** Stomatocyte, **c.** Spherocyte, **d.** Schistocyte, **e.** Acanthocyte, **f.** Codocyte (target cell), **g.** Dacryocyte (teardrop), **h.** Drepanocyte, (sickle cell), **i.** Drepanocyte (holly leaf), **j.** Elliptocyte, **k.** Keratocyte (helmet cell), **l.** Knizocyte.

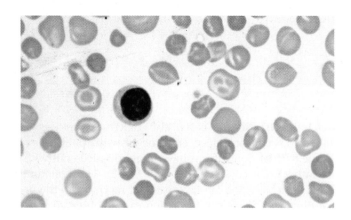

■ FIGURE 8-8   Target cells. (Peripheral blood; Wright-Giemsa stain; 1000× magnification)

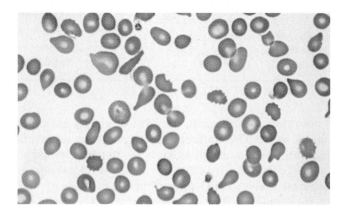

■ FIGURE 8-9   Note the presence of teardrops. Note also the echinocytes, acanthocytes, and spherocytes. (Peripheral blood; Wright-Giemsa stain; 1000× magnification)

Echinocytes have been reported to occur in vivo in a variety of conditions (Table 8-12). Echinocytes appear within several days in blood stored at 4°C. Consequently, blood from patients receiving transfusions can show the presence of echinocytes if blood is taken from the patient immediately after transfusion; however, after a few minutes, the buffering action of patient's plasma causes the transfused echinocyte to resume a normal discoid shape.

Elliptocytes   Elliptocytes, also called *pencil cells* and *cigar cells*, vary from elongated oval shapes (ovalocytes) to elongated rodlike cells (Figures 8-7j■ and 8-6). Elliptocytes have a central area of biconcavity with hemoglobin concentrated at both ends. Elliptocytes are formed after the erythrocyte matures and leaves the bone marrow because reticulocytes and young erythrocytes in patients with elliptocytosis are normal in shape. The mechanism of formation is not known but is assumed to involve alterations of the erythrocyte membrane skeleton (∞ Chapter 5). The osmotic fragility of elliptocytes is normal except in hemolytic hereditary elliptocytosis when osmotic fragility is increased. Autohemolysis at 48 hours is increased but is corrected by the addition of both glucose and ATP, suggesting that elliptocytes have abnormal membrane permeability. Rouleaux formation is normal. Elliptocytes are the predominant shape of erythrocytes in hereditary elliptocytosis. These abnormal shapes also can occur in other diseases (Table 8-12). Megaloblastic anemia is associated with abnormally large oval erythrocytes called *macroovalocytes*.

Helmet Cells   Helmet cells, also called *keratocytes*, have a concavity on one side and two hornlike protrusions on either end (Figures 8-7k■ and 8-5b). They are produced by impalement on a fibrin strand. The two halves of the erythrocyte hang over the strand as saddlebags; the membranes of the touching sides fuse, producing a vacuole-like inclusion on one side. This cell with an eccentric vacuole is called a *blister cell*. The vacuole bursts, leaving a notch with two spicules on the ends. It has also been suggested that these cells could result from repeated collisions in abnormalities of the circulation. Helmet cells are associated with microangiopathic hemolytic anemia (Table 8-12).

Knizocytes   Knizocytes are cells with more than two concavities (Figure 8-7l■). The appearance of this cell on stained blood smears can vary depending upon how the cell comes to rest on the flat surface; however, most knizocytes have a dark-staining band across the center with a pale area on either side surrounded by a rim of pink-staining hemoglobin. The mechanism of formation is unknown. Knizocytes are associated with spherocytosis (Table 8-12).

Leptocytes   Leptocytes are thin, flat, cells with normal or larger than normal diameter. Although the diameter of the cell is normal or increased, the MCV is usually decreased. The cells have an increased surface-to-volume ratio either as a result of decreased hemoglobin content or increased surface area. The leptocyte is usually cup shaped like stomatocytes, but the cup has little depth. Target cells can be formed from leptocytes on dried blood smears when the depth of the cup increases. Leptocytes are seen in liver disease and in anemias characterized by hypochromic erythrocytes (Table 8-12).

Schistocytes   Schistocytes are erythrocyte fragments caused by mechanical damage to the cell (Figures 8-5a, 8-5b, and 8-7d■, Table 8-12). They appear in a variety of shapes: triangular, comma shaped, helmet shaped, and others. Because schistocytes are fragments of erythrocytes, they are usually microcytic. They maintain normal deformability, but their survival in the peripheral blood is reduced. The fragments can assume a spherical shape and hemolyze or can be removed in the spleen.

Schistocytes are found whenever blood vessel pathology is present. Erythrocyte fragmentation is particularly associated with intravascular fibrin formation. Erythrocytes become hung up on fibrin strands in the vessels (termed the *clothesline effect*). The force of blood flow can release the distressed cell intact, or the cell can be fragmented by the fibrin strand, producing schistocytes. This mechanism of erythrocyte damage predominates in microangiopathic hemolytic anemias. Schistocytes can also be seen in valvular lesions, uremia, and march hemoglobinurea. Seen in severe burn victims, spheroschistocytes are the result of heat damage to the spectrin in the membrane cytoskeleton.

Spherocytes   Spherocytes (Figures 8-4b and 8-7c■) are erythrocytes that have lost their biconcavity due to a decreased surface-to-volume ratio. On stained blood smears, the spherocyte appears as a densely stained sphere lacking a central area of pallor. Although the cell often appears microcytic on stained blood smears, the volume (MCV) is usually normal. The spherocyte is the only erythrocyte that can be called hyperchromic because of an increased MCHC. Spherocytes have increased osmotic fragility with hemolysis beginning in NaCl concentrations of about 0.6% and complete at about 0.4%. Autohemolysis (in vitro suspension of patients' cells and serum) is increased. Spherocytes, which are less deformable than discocytes, have a decreased life span and are removed in the spleen. Spherocytes are seen in hereditary spherocytosis and a variety of other disorders (Table 8-12). They represent a significant finding when associated with hemolytic anemia because it is an indication of immune hemolytic anemia.

Stomatocytes   In wet preparations, stomatocytes appear as small cup-shaped uniconcave discs (Figures 8-7b■ and 8-10■). Upon staining, these cells exhibit a slitlike (mouthlike) area of pallor. Normal discocytes can be transformed under certain conditions to stomatocytes and, eventually, to spherostomatocytes. The stomatocyte shape is

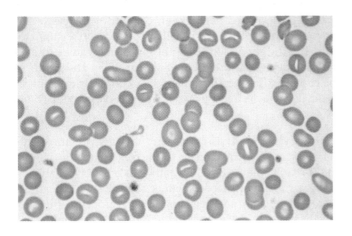

■ FIGURE 8-10   Stomatocytes. Note the slitlike area of pallor. (Peripheral blood; Wright-Giemsa stain; 1000× magnification)

reversible, but the spherostomatocyte is not. Cationic drugs and low pH cause a gradual loss of biconcavity leading to the stomatocyte and eventually formation of a sphere. Stomatocytosis is the opposite of echinocytosis; the shape change in stomatocytosis is thought to be the result of an increase in the lipid content or area of the inner leaflet of the membrane lipid bilayer.

Stomatocytes also can appear as an artifact on stained blood smears and, thus, care should be used in identifying them. Stomatocytes in vivo are characteristic of a rare autosomal dominant hemolytic anemia called *hereditary stomatocytosis*. Stomatocytes are also associated with a variety of other diseases (Table 8-12).

 CASE STUDY *(continued from page 156)*

George's blood smear revealed marked spherocytosis.

3. Explain the importance of this finding.

4. Explain George's abnormal indices.

Variation in Hemoglobin (Color)   Normal erythrocytes have an MCH of approximately 30 pg. On stained smears, the erythrocyte has a central area of pallor approximately one-third the diameter of the cell. In certain conditions, the cells contain less hemoglobin than normal. The only erythrocyte that contains more hemoglobin than normal in relation to its volume is the spherocyte. Spherocytes lack a central area of pallor and stain uniformly dense.

Hypochromic Cells   Hypochromic cells are poorly hemoglobinized erythrocytes with an exaggerated area of pallor (>1/3 the diameter of the cell) on Romanowsky-stained blood smears. Hypochromic cells, although occasionally normocytic, are usually microcytic (Figure 8-6). Hypochromic cells are the result of decreased or impaired hemoglobin synthesis (Table 8-13 ✪).

Polychromatophilic Erythrocytes   Polychromatophilic erythrocytes (reticulocytes) are usually larger than normal cells with a bluish tinge on Romanowsky-stained blood smears (Figure 8-2). The bluish tinge is caused by the presence of residual RNA in the cytoplasm. Large numbers of these cells are associated with decreased erythrocyte survival or hemorrhage and an erythroid hyperplastic marrow (Table 8-13).

Erythrocyte Inclusions   Erythrocytes do not normally contain any particulate inclusions. When present, inclusions can help direct further investigation because they are associated with certain disease states. Diseases/conditions associated with these inclusions are listed in Table 8-14 ✪. The erythrocyte inclusions are described here as they appear on Romanowsky-stained blood smears unless otherwise stated.

Basophilic Stippling   Erythrocytes with **basophilic stippling** are cells with bluish-black granular inclusions distributed across their entire cell area (Figure 8-11a ■). The granules may vary in size and distribution from small diffuse to coarse and punctate. The granules, which are composed of aggregated ribosomes, are sometimes associated with mitochondria and siderosomes. It is believed that basophilic stippling is not present in living cells; instead, stippling probably is produced during preparation of the blood smear or during the staining process. Electron microscopy has not shown an intracellular structure similar to basophilic stippling. Cells dried slowly or stained rapidly can demonstrate fine, diffuse stippling as an artifact. Pathologic basophilic stippling is more coarse and punctate.

✪ TABLE 8-13

Variations in Erythrocyte Color		
Terminology	Description	Associated Disease or Physiologic States
Hypochromia	Decreased concentration of hemoglobin in the red cell; red cells have an increased area of central pallor (>1/3 diameter of cell)	Iron deficiency anemia; thalassemia; other anemias associated with a defect in hemoglobin production
Polychromasia	Young red cells containing residual RNA; stain a pinkish-gray to pinkish-blue color on Wright's stained blood smears; usually appear slightly larger than mature red cells	Hemolytic anemias; newborns; recovery from acute hemorrhage

⊘ TABLE 8-14

Abnormal Erythrocyte Inclusions

Terminology	Description	Associated Disease States
Basophilic stippling	Round or irregularly shaped granules of variable number and size distributed throughout the red cell; composed of aggregates of ribosomes (RNA); stain bluish black with Wright's stain	Lead poisoning; anemias associated with abnormal hemoglobin synthesis; thalassemia
Cabot rings	Appear as a figure-8, ring, or incomplete ring; thought to be composed of the microtubules of the mitotic spindle; stain reddish violet with Wright's stain	Severe anemias; dyserythropoiesis
Howell-Jolly bodies	Small, round bodies composed of DNA usually located eccentrically in the red cell; usually occurs singly, rarely more than 2 per cell; stains dark purple with Wright's stain	Post-splenectomy; megaloblastic anemias; some hemolytic anemias; functional asplenia; severe anemia
Pappenheimer bodies	Clusters of granules containing iron that are usually found at the periphery of the cell; visible with Prussian blue stain and Wright's stain	Sideroblastic anemia; thalassemia; other severe anemias
Heinz bodies	Bodies composed of denatured or precipitated hemoglobin; not visible on Wright's stained blood smears; with supravital stain appear as purple, round-shaped bodies of varying size, usually close to the cell membrane; can also be observed with phase microscopy on wet preparations	G6PD deficiency; unstable hemoglobin disorders; oxidizing drugs or toxins; post-splenectomy
Reticulofilamentous substance	Artifactual aggregation of ribosomes; not visible on Wright's stained smears; supravital stain must be used (new methylene blue), appears as deep blue reticular network	Normal reticulocytes

Cabot Rings Cabot rings are reddish-violet erythrocytic inclusions usually occurring in the formation of a figure eight or oval ring. Cabot rings are thought to be remnants of spindle fibers, which form during mitosis. They occur in severe anemias and in dyserythropoiesis (Figure 8-11f ■).

Howell-Jolly Bodies Howell-Jolly bodies are dark purple or violet spherical granules in the erythrocyte (Figure 8-11b ■). These inclusions are nuclear (DNA) fragments usually occurring singly in cells, rarely more than two per cell. Howell-Jolly bodies are associated with nuclear maturation abnormalities. They are thought to occur as a result of an individual chromosome failing to attach to the spindle apparatus during mitosis, and, thus, it is not included in the reformed nucleus. When the nucleus is extruded, the Howell-Jolly body is left behind (until removed by splenic macrophages).

Pappenheimer Bodies Pappenheimer bodies are secondary lysosomes variable in their composition of iron and protein, or mitochondria with iron micelles (Figure 8-11d ■). This type of inclusion appears as clusters of small granules in erythrocytes and normoblasts and stains with both Romanowsky and Perl's Prussian blue stains. Romanowsky stains visualize Pappenheimer bodies by staining the protein matrix of the granules whereas Perl's Prussian blue is responsible for staining the iron portion of the granules. Pappenheimer bodies occur only in pathologic states.

Heinz Bodies Heinz bodies do not stain with Romanowsky stains but can be visualized with supravital stains or with phase microscopy of the living cell. They appear as 2–3 μm round masses lying just under or attached to the cell membrane. Heinz bodies are composed of aggregated denatured hemoglobin.

Sideroblasts Sideroblasts are nucleated erythrocytes that contain stainable iron granules whereas siderocytes are nonnucleated erythrocytes containing stainable iron granules (Figures 8-11c ■ and 8-11e ■). Sideroblasts and siderocytes can be identified with Perl's Prussian blue iron stain, which stains iron aggregates blue. Finely dispersed ferritin cannot be visualized by this technique. It is hypothesized that when ferritin is not used rapidly by cells, it aggregates and is proteolyzed within lysosomes, forming hemosiderin (a nonspecific complex of iron and partially degraded proteins and lipids). Thus, hemosiderin represents an abundant supply of iron or an abnormality in iron use by the cell. It is usually found in cells heavily loaded with iron, such as macrophages. About 50–70% of all erythroblasts in the marrow contain iron, which can be visualized with Perl's Prussian blue stain. This number decreases in some pathologic states and can be markedly increased in others. Reticulocytes and erythrocytes in the peripheral blood do not normally contain ferritin aggregates.

Variation in Erythrocyte Distribution on Stained Smears On a well-made blood smear, the erythrocytes are evenly distributed and well separated on the feather edge of the smear. Stacking or aggregating of cells is associated with certain pathologic states (Table 8-15 ⊘).

Agglutination In the presence of IgM antibodies (cold agglutinins) directed against erythrocyte antigens, erythrocytes can agglutinate forming irregular clusters of varying sizes (Figure 8-12 ■). These clusters are readily differentiated

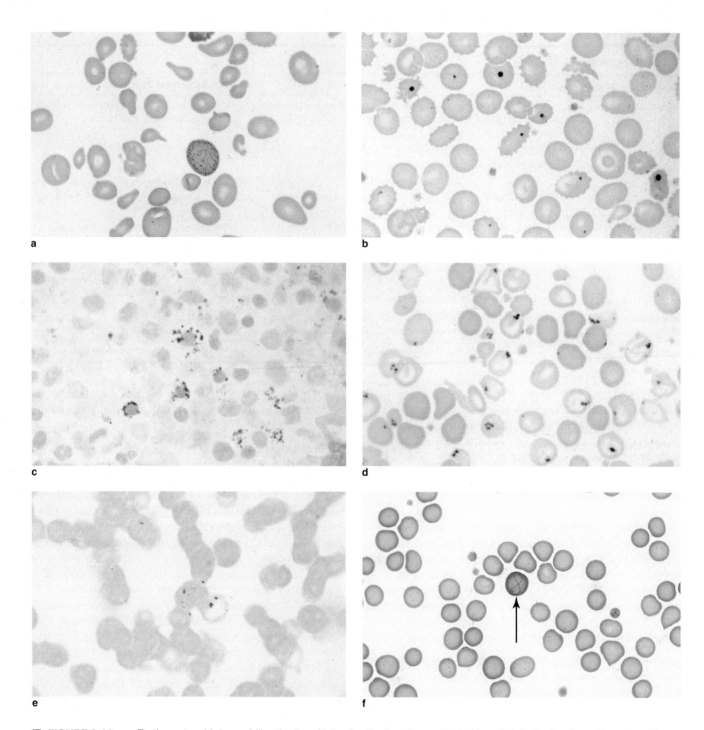

■ FIGURE 8-11   **a.** Erythrocyte with basophilic stippling. Note also the teardrop cells. **b.** Howell-Jolly bodies in erythrocytes. These bodies are the single round purple inclusions. Note echinocytes, acanthocytes, target cells, and spherocytes. **c.** The erythroblasts with blue inclusions (iron granules) are referred to as sideroblasts. These granules do not stain with Romanowsky stains. **d.** These erythrocytes contain iron granules called *Pappenheimer bodies*, which will stain with both Romanowsky and Perl's Prussian blue stains. **e.** Siderocytes. **f.** Cabot ring (a, b, d, f. Peripheral blood, Wright-Giemsa stain, 1000× magnification; c. Bone marrow, Perl's Prussian blue stain, 1000× magnification; e. Peripheral blood, Perl's Prussian blue stain, 1000× magnification)

⊛ TABLE 8-15

Abnormalities in Erythrocyte Arrangement

Terminology	Description	Associated Disease States
Agglutination	Irregular clumps of red blood cells from antigen–antibody reaction	Cold agglutinins; autoimmune hemolytic anemias
Rouleaux	Red blood cells arranged in rolls or stacks; usually associated with abnormal or increased plasma proteins; red blood cells can be dispersed by mixing cells with saline	Multiple myeloma and other gammopathies

from rouleaux by their irregular conformations (grape-like clusters). On automated cell counters, a blood count with a grossly elevated MCV and low RBC count but a normal hemoglobin suggests the presence of cold-reacting erythrocyte agglutinins. The effect of cold agglutinins is overcome by keeping the blood at 37°C. When performing blood counts, the diluting fluid must also be kept at 37°C.

Rouleaux *Rouleaux* is an alignment of erythrocytes one on top of another resembling a stack of coins (Figure 8-13 ■). This phenomenon occurs normally when blood is collected and allowed to stand in tubes. It can also be seen in the thick portion of blood smears. In certain pathologic states that are accompanied by an increase in fibrinogen or globulins, rouleaux become marked and are readily seen in the feather edge of blood smears. When the erythrocyte assumes abnormal shapes, such as sickled forms, rouleaux formation is inhibited. Rouleaux is also inhibited when erythrocytes are suspended in saline.

Leukocyte and Platelet Abnormalities

Some nutritional deficiencies, stem cell disorders, and bone marrow abnormalities affect the production, function, and/or morphology of all hematopoietic cells; thus, evaluation of the quantity and morphology of leukocytes and platelets can supply additional important data as to the cause of anemia.

Bone Marrow Examination

Bone marrow evaluation usually is not necessary to determine the cause of an anemia. However, it can provide supplemental diagnostic information in anemic patients when other laboratory tests are not conclusive. For example, in hypoproliferative anemias, bone marrow evaluation can reveal myelodysplasia or infiltration of the marrow with malignant cells or granulomas.

Microcytic, Hypochromic Anemia Serum iron studies and occasionally hemoglobin electrophoresis are usually adequate to differentiate the causes of a microcytic, hypochromic anemia (∞ Chapters 9, 11). When iron studies are not definitive, a bone marrow exam can be helpful. However, measurement of serum ferritin levels have largely negated the need for bone marrow iron assessment. Low or absent bone marrow iron or serum ferritin confirms iron deficiency anemia. In patients with sideroblastic anemia, the diagnostic bone marrow finding is the presence of sideroblasts with iron deposits circling the nucleus. These ringed sideroblasts represent iron-laden mitochondria.

Macrocytic Anemias Macrocytic anemias can be due to hemolytic anemias, megaloblastic anemia, or nonmegaloblastic anemia. Diagnostic features of megaloblastic anemia

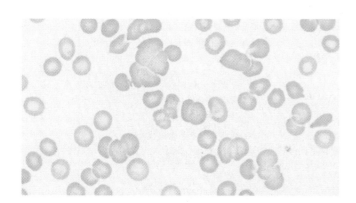

■ **FIGURE 8-12** This blood smear is from a patient with cold agglutinin disease. Notice the clumping of the erythrocytes. (Peripheral blood; Wright-Giemsa stain; 1000× magnification)

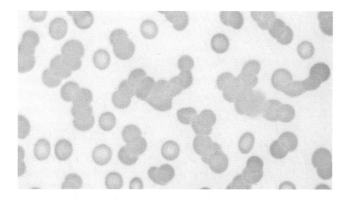

■ **FIGURE 8-13** Rouleaux. The erythrocytes are stacked on one another like a stack of coins. This blood smear is from a patient with multiple myeloma, a malignant plasma cell disorder. The background of the slide has a bluish hue due to the large amount of protein in the plasma. (Peripheral blood; Wright-Giemsa stain; 1000× magnification)

such as hypersegmented granulocytes can be found on peripheral blood smears and supported by low vitamin B_{12} or folic acid levels (∞ Chapter 12). However, if vitamin B_{12} and folic acid levels are normal, a bone marrow examination is suggested to rule out myelodysplastic syndrome (∞ Chapter 23). Hemolytic anemias with an increased MCV due to reticulocytosis can usually be diagnosed by other laboratory tests and review of the blood smear (∞ Chapter 14). Nonmegaloblastic anemias have various causes, but clinical symptoms, history, and other laboratory tests are usually sufficient to arrive at a diagnosis. However, if aplastic anemia (often macrocytic but not megaloblastic) is suspected, a bone marrow examination is indicated (∞ Chapter 13).

Normocytic, Normochromic Anemia   If a diagnosis of aplastic anemia or pure red cell aplasia is suspected, a bone marrow examination is essential to demonstrate hypoplasia and an increase in fat and/or fibrosis.

Tests for Erythrocyte Destruction

Tests of erythrocyte destruction are important in evaluating erythrocyte survival. If the hemoglobin concentration is stable over at least several days in an anemic patient, then the measurements of erythrocyte production including marrow cellularity and RPI are indirect measurements of erythrocyte destruction. Serum unconjugated bilirubin is primarily derived from hemoglobin catabolism; its concentration in the absence of hepatobiliary disease can yield further information concerning erythrokinetics. Increased unconjugated bilirubin indicates increased hemoglobin catabolism, either intravascular or extravascular. Conversely, anemia due to chronic and acute blood loss as well as hypoproliferative anemias are associated with normal or decreased serum bilirubin because the number of erythrocytes catabolized is decreased. Cytoplasmic maturation abnormalities can also be accompanied by normal to decreased serum bilirubin even though there is an increase in erythrocyte destruction. This happens because when insufficient heme is being synthesized (hypochromic cells), less heme is being catabolized. Thus, the bilirubin level should always be interpreted with the degree of anemia. It has been suggested that too many variables affect serum bilirubin levels to make it a reliable measurement of RBC destruction.

Other laboratory tests are used to evaluate erythrocyte turnover or blood loss. Hemosiderin in urine, decreased plasma haptoglobin, and increased methemalbumin are associated with increased intravascular hemolysis. Certain biochemical constituents that are concentrated in blood cells are released to the peripheral blood as the cell lyses, and these constituents are indicators of the degree of cellular destruction. In anemias associated with ineffective erythropoiesis or hemolysis, these products will be increased in the blood. The most commonly measured constituents include uric acid, the main end product of purine metabolism, and lactate dehydrogenase (LD), an enzyme that is present in the cell cytoplasm.

The choice of laboratory tests for the differential diagnosis of anemia should depend on the test's specificity and sensitivity. A highly sensitive test is one that will likely be positive when the disorder is present. A highly specific test is one that will be negative when the disorder is not present. Highly sensitive tests are good for screening for the disorder, and highly specific tests are good for confirming the diagnosis of the disorder. Table 8-16 ✪ shows a variety of tests used

---

✪ TABLE 8-16

Operating Characteristics of Discriminating Tests Used in Diagnosing Anemia

Test	Sensitivity (%)	Specificity (%)	Disease
RDW >15	87–100	66	Iron deficiency anemia
Ferritin <12	65–97	99	Iron deficiency anemia
Transferrin saturation <16	95	70–95	Iron deficiency anemia
Reticulocyte count	62–90	99(>10%)	Hemolysis
Coombs' test	90	95	Autoimmune hemolytic anemia
MCHC >36	100	100*	Hereditary spherocytosis
Splenomegaly	100	?	Hereditary spherocytosis
MCV >105	11	95	Vitamin B_{12} or folic acid deficiency
MCV <100	100	40–50	Iron deficiency anemia
MCV <80	100	?	Thalassemia
Hemosiderin (urine)	100	?	Paroxysmal nocturnal hemoglobinuria

*Provided that artifacts are excluded

MCHC, mean corpuscular hemoglobin concentration; MCV, mean corpuscular volume; RDW, red cell distribution width

(From Djulbegovic B, Hadley T, Pasic R. A. new algorithm for diagnosis of anemia. *Postgrad Med* 85(5):119–30, 1989.)

in diagnosing anemia together with their rates of sensitivity and specificity.

 Checkpoint! 4

What laboratory test is the least invasive and most cost efficient to evaluate erythrocyte production in the presence of anemia?

▶ CLASSIFICATION OF ANEMIA

The purpose of the classification of anemias is to assist the physician in identifying the cause by using laboratory test results in addition to other clinical data. The classification also is useful to laboratory professionals when correlating various test results for accuracy and when making suggestions for additional follow-up tests. Although specific diagnosis is the ultimate goal of any anemia classification system, it must be kept in mind that anemia frequently develops from more than one mechanism, complicating correlation and interpretation of laboratory test results. In addition, complicating factors can alter the typical findings of a specific anemia. For example, preexisting iron deficiency can inhibit the reticulocytosis that normally accompanies acute blood loss or mask the macrocytic features of folic acid deficiency. In these cases, laboratory test results can depend on which mechanism predominates. Anemias can be classified by either morphology or pathophysiology (function).

MORPHOLOGIC CLASSIFICATION

Anemias can be initially classified morphologically according to the average size and hemoglobin concentration of the erythrocytes as indicated by the erythrocyte indices. This morphologic classification is helpful because MCV, MCH, and MCHC are determined when anemia is diagnosed, and certain causes of anemia are characteristically associated with specific erythrocyte size (large, small, or normal) and hemoglobin content (normal or abnormal). The general categories of a morphologic classification include macrocytic, normochromic; normocytic, normochromic; and microcytic, hypochromic.

It must again be stressed that, although an anemia initially seems to belong in one of these categories, the morphologic expression can be the result of a combination of factors. For example, a combined deficiency of iron and folate can result in a normal MCV even though iron deficiency is normally microcytic and folate deficiency is normally macrocytic. These complicated cases usually can be detected by examining the blood smear for specifics of erythrocyte morphology.

A morphologic assessment of anemia, however, is not sufficient; determining the etiology of anemia through additional laboratory tests yields even more meaningful information. Patient history and physical examination are essential for a differential diagnosis within given classifications.

FUNCTIONAL CLASSIFICATION

Considering that the normal bone marrow compensatory response to decreased peripheral blood hemoglobin levels is an increase in erythrocyte production, persistent anemia can be expected as the result of three pathophysiologic mechanisms: (1) a proliferation defect (decreased production), (2) a maturation defect, or (3) a survival defect (increased destruction). These are considered to be the three functional classifications of anemia. The functional classification uses the absolute reticulocyte count, corrected reticulocyte count, IRF or RPI, and/or serum iron studies to categorize an anemia. Proliferation and maturation defects usually have a normal or decreased IRF and/or RPI < 2 and corrected reticulocyte count < 2%; survival defects are characterized by an increased IRF and/or RPI > 2 and corrected reticulocyte count > 2%. Serum iron studies are most helpful in identifying the pathophysiology of microcytic anemias because the IRF or RPI is variable in these cases.

Although some anemias can be the result of several mechanisms, one mechanism is usually dominant. The initial step in approaching an anemic patient is the identification of this dominant mechanism. If the functional and morphologic classifications of anemia are combined, the result is a classification using the corrected reticulocyte count, IRF or RPI, iron studies, and morphology of the erythrocyte (Figure 8-14■). If an anemia does not fit into any of these categories, it is probably multifactorial.

Proliferative Defects

Proliferative defects are characterized by decreased proliferation, maturation, and release rates of erythrocytes in response to anemia (Figure 8-15■). The most characteristic laboratory findings of proliferation defects are normocytic, normochromic erythrocytes, decreased absolute reticulocyte count, corrected reticulocyte count, and IRF, and RPI <2, signifying a marrow output of reticulocytes inadequate for the degree of anemia. Serum bilirubin levels are normal or decreased because of the decrease in cell production. The bone marrow is hypocellular with normal or increased iron stores. Decreased proliferation can be caused by inappropriate erythropoietin production or production of cytokines that inhibit erythropoiesis. This trophic basis is responsible for the anemias associated with malignancies, chronic renal disease, and certain endocrinopathies.

Conversely, erythropoietic stimulating mechanisms can be normal, but the bone marrow can fail to respond to the stimulus appropriately. This occurs when the bone marrow is infiltrated with fibrous, neoplastic, or granulomatous tissue or when the marrow is damaged by chemicals, drugs, or radiation. It is possible to differentiate these causes of hypoproliferation by observing whether all cell lineages are affected or only the erythrocytes are involved. If the proliferation defect is due to inappropriate erythropoietin production, decreased proliferation is limited to the erythrocytic lineage. In contrast, marrow damage or infiltration is

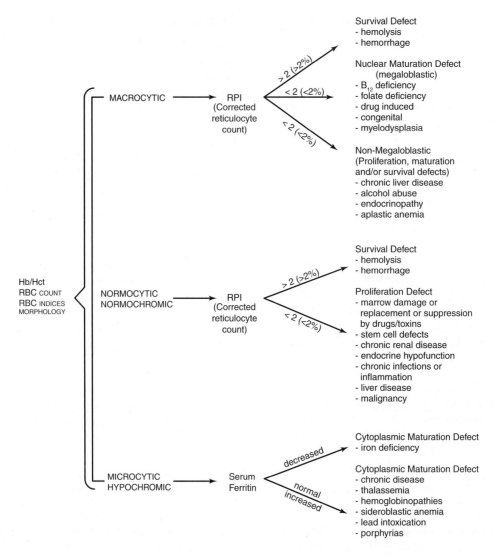

■ FIGURE 8-14 Classification of anemias using function and morphology. (Corrected reticulocyte count is in parentheses.)

characterized by hypoplasia of all normal hematopoietic cells in the bone marrow, producing **pancytopenia** (decrease in all blood cells) in the peripheral blood. In addition, marrow infiltration is usually accompanied by poikilocytosis and a leukoerythroblastic peripheral blood picture, presumably caused by damage of the normal sinusoidal barrier.

Many proliferative defects also are associated with decreased erythrocyte lifespan; however, survival is only moderately decreased and could easily be compensated for by a normal functioning marrow or a normal cytokine stimulus. Rarely is hypoproliferation caused by an abnormality in the hematopoietic stem cells.

Maturation Defects

Maturation defects disrupt the orderly process of either nuclear or cytoplasmic development producing qualitatively abnormal cells (Figure 8-15). The erythrocytes are macro-

cytic in nuclear defects and microcytic in cytoplasmic defects. Despite the abnormal maturation process, the marrow attempts to increase production of erythrocytes, resulting in bone marrow erythroid hyperplasia. However, because these cells are often intrinsically abnormal, many are destroyed before they can be released to the peripheral blood (ineffective erythropoiesis). Because many of the abnormal erythrocytes are not released to the peripheral blood, the corrected reticulocyte count, the absolute reticulocyte concentration and IRF are decreased, and the RPI <2. Poikilocytes indicative of abnormal erythropoiesis are frequently present in direct proportion to the severity of the anemia.

Cytoplasmic maturation defects are caused by abnormal hemoglobin production. Therefore, the defect is limited to the erythroid lineage. Hemoglobin production can be impaired due to one or more of the following: limited iron supply, defective iron utilization, decreased globin synthesis,

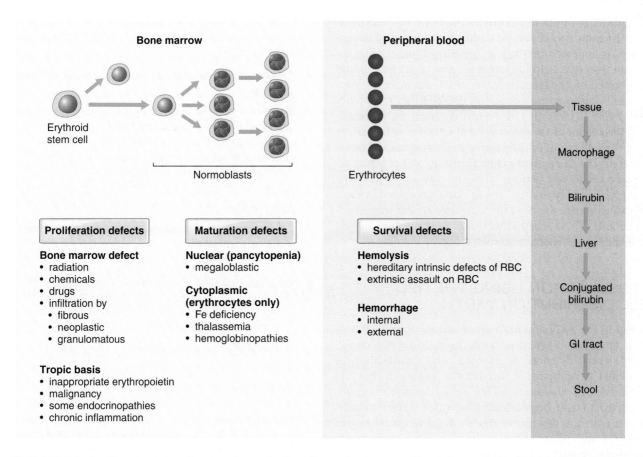

Bone marrow

Erythroid
stem cell

Normoblasts

Peripheral blood

Erythrocytes

Tissue

Macrophage

Bilirubin

Liver

Conjugated
bilirubin

GI tract

Stool

Proliferation defects

Bone marrow defect
• radiation
• chemicals
• drugs
• infiltration by
  • fibrous
  • neoplastic
  • granulomatous

Tropic basis
• inappropriate erythropoietin
• malignancy
• some endocrinopathies
• chronic inflammation

Maturation defects

Nuclear (pancytopenia)
• megaloblastic

**Cytoplasmic
(erythrocytes only)**
• Fe deficiency
• thalassemia
• hemoglobinopathies

Survival defects

Hemolysis
• hereditary intrinsic defects of RBC
• extrinsic assault on RBC

Hemorrhage
• internal
• external

■ **FIGURE 8-15** Functional classification of anemia. Anemia may be due to proliferation, maturation, and/or survival defects. Proliferation and maturation defects are due to defective erythropoiesis in the bone marrow. Survival defects are caused by increased destruction of erythrocytes. This destruction may occur in the bone marrow if the cells are intrinsically abnormal and/or in the peripheral circulation. If cells are destroyed in the bone marrow, it is called ineffective erythropoiesis. In some cases an anemia may be due to several causes such as in megaloblastic anemia. Although this anemia is classified as a maturation defect, it also is characterized by ineffective erythropoiesis in which the abnormal cells are destroyed before they reach the peripheral blood. Thus, there also is a survival defect.

and defective porphyrin (heme) synthesis. Most erythrocytes produced in association with cytoplasmic maturation defects are microcytic and hypochromic with a variable degree of poikilocytosis. These anemias are best differentiated using iron studies (∞ Chapter 9).

Because all developing hematopoietic cells have nuclei, nuclear maturation defects affect all hematopoietic cell lineages and probably other body cells as well. As a result, the peripheral blood could reflect not only anemia but also pancytopenia with characteristic morphologic changes apparent in all cell lines. The distinctive morphologic changes in cells are collectively termed **megaloblastic** (delayed nuclear development in comparison to cytoplasmic development).

Survival Defects

Survival defects are the result of premature loss of circulating erythrocytes either by hemorrhage or hemolysis (Figure 8-15). In this type of defect, bone marrow proliferation increases and maturation is orderly. The absolute reticulocyte concentration and IRF are increased, the corrected reticulocyte count is >2% and the RPI is typically >2. The blood film reflects this increased erythropoietic activity by the presence of polychromatophilic macrocytes. If anemia persists despite increased erythrocyte production, the patient has persistent blood loss or active hemolytic disease.

In contrast to poikilocytes that are formed in the bone marrow as a result of dyserythropoiesis typical of proliferation and maturation defects, poikilocytes of a survival defect are formed after the cell leaves the marrow. The most common poikilocytes are schistocytes and spherocytes. The schistocyte is the result of intravascular mechanical trauma to the cell, such as a shearing by fibrin strands or damage by passage through abnormal capillaries. Spherocytes indicate extravascular erythrocyte membrane damage. Generally, the erythrocyte population is normocytic and normochromic. It is possible, however, that macrocytosis can prevail depending on the degree of reticulocytosis or that microcytosis can predominate depending on the number of schistocytes or microspherocytes.

Other indications of decreased erythrocyte survival can include increased serum bilirubin, decreased haptoglobin, and increased methemalbumin, hemosiderinuria, hemoglobinuria, hemoglobinemia, exhaled CO, and urine or fecal urobilinogen.

A knowledge of the functional and morphologic classification of anemias is necessary to design a cost-effective laboratory testing approach that aids in specific diagnosis. Only appropriate tests that help identify the cause of anemia should be performed on the laboratory workup. Guidelines for reimbursement of laboratory tests within ICD codes by third-party payers make it clear that test ordering must be rationally based. Web Figure 8-1 ■ shows general schemas of laboratory testing that are useful in diagnosing anemias. It should be remembered that the patient's clinical history and physical examination are always performed by the physician before beginning a laboratory workup. The information gained in these areas can eliminate the need for some tests and/or suggest additional tests. These schemas will gain more meaning as you read the following chapters on each group of anemias.

CLASSIFICATION USING THE RED CELL DISTRIBUTION WIDTH

Changes in the MCV and RDW are relatively reproducible in certain anemias. When used with the reticulocytes count, the differential diagnosis is narrowed and classification of the anemia is facilitated.[20] (It has been suggested that the classification of anemias use the terms *heterogeneous* (increased RDW) and *homogeneous* (decreased RDW) in conjunction with the descriptive morphologic terms *microcytic*, *normocytic*, and *macrocytic* (e.g., homogeneous macrocytic, heterogeneous macrocytic) (Table 8-17 ✪).

Studies of anemic individuals provided the following information regarding the relation between categories of anemia and RDW.[9,20]

1. Hypoproliferative anemias have a normal RDW regardless of the MCV.
2. Maturational defect anemias (excluding the rare hereditary types) have an increased RDW regardless of the MCV or the degree of anemia. The RDW is increased in these individuals before anemia develops or before abnormal cells can be identified on the smear.
3. The RDW is normal after acute hemorrhage if iron supplies are adequate.
4. Uncompensated hemolytic anemias have a high RDW while compensated hemolytic states have a normal RDW.

⊙ **CASE STUDY** *(continued from page 162)*

5. Classify George's anemia morphologically and functionally.

SUMMARY

Anemia is a decrease in the competence of blood to carry oxygen to the tissue due to a decrease in the concentration of hemoglobin. Diagnosis of anemia is made with a combination of information from the patient history, physical examination, and laboratory investigation. Initially, routine laboratory tests are performed to determine the presence of anemia and to evaluate erythrocyte production and destruction. These tests include erythrocyte count, hemoglobin, hematocrit, erythrocyte indices, reticulocyte count, blood smear examination, and serum bilirubin. More specific tests can be performed based on the results of these routine tests.

The erythrocyte indices can be used to determine the size and hemoglobin content of erythrocytes. Because some anemias are characterized by specific erythrocyte morphology, the indices are helpful in initially classifying the anemia.

The manual reticulocyte count is routinely reported in relative terms: the number of reticulocytes per erythrocytes in percent. Automated reticulocyte counts are reported in both relative and absolute terms. More information is available from the absolute count, corrected reticulocyte count, estimate of IRF, and RPI. Generally, the reticulocyte count in an anemic patient should be increased if the bone marrow is increasing production of erythrocytes.

Examination of the blood film is helpful in assessing anisocytosis and poikilocytosis. Anisocytosis is a variation in erythrocyte size. It is also calculated and expressed as the red cell distribution width (RDW) on some automated cell counters. Macrocytes are erythrocytes with a volume of more than 100 fL while microcytes have a cell volume of less than 80 fL. It is not uncommon to find a variety of cell sizes in some anemias. Poikilocytosis is a variation in cell shape. Specific shapes give clues to the cause of anemia. When present, erythrocyte inclusions also are helpful in determining the cause of anemia. Pappenheimer bodies indicate faulty iron

---

✪ **TABLE 8-17**

Classification of Anemias by MCV and RDW

	Normal RDW	Increased RDW
Normocytic	Acute hemorrhage Splenic pooling Chronic disease Chronic leukemia	Immune hemolytic anemia Early iron, B_{12}, or folate deficiency Sideroblastic anemia Myelofibrosis Sickle cell anemia/trait Chronic liver disease Myelodysplastic syndrome
Microcytic	Heterozygous thalassemia Chronic disease Hemoglobin E trait	Iron deficiency Homozygous thalassemia Hb S/B^{thal} Hb H disease Hemolytic anemia with schistocytes
Macrocytic	Chronic liver disease Aplastic anemia Chemotherapy Alcohol ingestions Antiviral medications	Immune hemolytic anemia with marked reticulocytosis B_{12} or folate deficiency CLL with high lymph count Cytotoxic chemotherapy Chronic liver disease Myelodysplastic syndrome

metabolism, and Howell-Jolly bodies are found in megaloblastic anemia after splenectomy and in some hemolytic anemias.

Bone marrow examination is indicated if laboratory tests give inconclusive results. Bone marrow is examined for cellularity, cellular structure, M:E ratio, and iron stores.

Anemias are generally classified by a functional or morphologic scheme or by a combination of the two. The morphologic classification includes three general categories based on erythrocyte indices: normocytic, normochromic; macrocytic, normochromic; and microcytic, hypochromic. The functional classification uses the IRF or RPI and serum iron studies to classify the anemias according to pathophysiology: proliferation defect, maturation defect, and survival defect. These classifications help the laboratory scientist and physician design a cost-effective approach to laboratory testing to reach a specific diagnosis.

REVIEW QUESTIONS

LEVEL I

1. Which erythrocyte inclusions are composed of aggregated, denatured hemoglobin and stain with supravital stains but not with Romanowsky stains? (Objective 4)
   a. Howell-Jolly bodies
   b. Pappenheimer bodies
   c. sideroblasts
   d. Heinz bodies

2. A patient with anemia has an RPI of 2.3 with an MCV of 103 fL. How would you classify this anemia? (Objective 7)
   a. macrocytic
   b. normocytic
   c. microcytic
   d. maturation defect

3. A blood smear reveals uneven distribution of blood cells, and the cells appear to be stacked together like a stack of coins. How would you describe this distribution? (Objective 5)
   a. agglutination
   b. rouleaux
   c. anisocytosis
   d. poikilocytosis

4. Which of the following tests will give information about rate of erythrocyte destruction? (Objective 6)
   a. RPI
   b. serum bilirubin
   c. serum ferritin
   d. MCV

5. A patient has the following results: RBC count, 2.5×10^{12}/L and hemoglobin 5.3 g/dL, hematocrit 0.17 L/L, reticulocyte count 1%. What are the absolute reticulocyte count and RPI? (Objective 3)
   a. absolute count, 25×10^9/L; RPI, 0.15
   b. absolute count, 250×10^9/L; RPI, 0.15
   c. absolute count, 170×10^9/L; RPI, 0.38
   d. absolute count, 100×10^9/L; RPI, 1.5

LEVEL II

1. What follow-up test is most appropriate to determine the cause of anemia in a patient with the following results: RBC count, 2.5×10^{12}/L, and hemoglobin 5.3 g/dL, hematocrit 0.17 L/L, reticulocyte count 1% (Objective 13)
   a. LDH
   b. vitamin B_{12}
   c. serum ferritin
   d. IRF

2. What is the functional classification of the anemia in the preceding question? (Objective 12)
   a. proliferation defect
   b. survival defect
   c. nuclear maturation defect
   d. cytoplasmic maturation defect

3. Why might the serum bilirubin results be misleading as an indicator of erythrocyte destruction in the patient in question 1? (Objective 2)
   a. The cells are not being destroyed at an increased rate, and the liver is not excreting the bilirubin due to liver failure.
   b. The cells are being produced in the bone marrow and released as fast as they are being destroyed, so the bilirubin will be normal.
   c. The cells could be destroyed at an increased rate, but the hypochromic cells do not release much hemoglobin, and, hence, less bilirubin is formed.
   d. The cells are not destroyed as fast in anemic individuals as in normal individuals, and the bilirubin will be falsely decreased.

4. Which of the following laboratory tests is most specific for an anemia due to vitamin B_{12} or folic acid deficiency? (Objective 10)
   a. low ferritin
   b. high RDW
   c. Coomb's test
   d. MCV > 105 fL

REVIEW QUESTIONS (continued)

LEVEL I

6. How would you classify the cell population with the following indices: MCV 70 fL, MCH 25 pg, MCHC 32 g/dL? (Objective 2)
   a. normocytic, normochromic
   b. macrocytic, normochromic
   c. microcytic, normochromic
   d. microcytic, hypochromic

7. If the cell population in question 6 were homogeneous (absence of anisocytosis), what might the RDW show? (Objective 2)
   a. false increase
   b. false decrease
   c. normal reference interval
   d. true increase

8. A peripheral blood smear that has an erythrocyte mixture of macrocytes, microcytes, and normocytes present can best be described by which term? (Objective 1)
   a. poikilocytosis
   b. polychromatophilia
   c. megaloblastosis
   d. anisocytosis

9. Which of the following erythrocyte inclusions cannot be stained and visualized with Romanowsky stains? (Objective 4)
   a. Pappenheimer bodies
   b. Howell-Jolly bodies
   c. Heinz bodies
   d. basophilic stippling

10. If there is an increase in macrocytic polychromatophilic erythrocytes on the Romanowsky-stained blood smear, with what laboratory test result should you correlate this? (Objective 8)
    a. serum bilirubin
    b. reticulocyte count
    c. leukocyte count
    d. MCHC

LEVEL II

5. In anemia caused by hemorrhage, what would you expect to find in your laboratory investigation? (Objective 2)
   a. presence of polychromatophilic macrocytes on the peripheral blood smear
   b. hypoplastic bone marrow with nuclear maturation abnormalities
   c. megaloblastosis in the bone marrow and pancytopenia in the peripheral blood
   d. decreased IRF and RPI

6. Bone marrow examination in a patient with a hemoglobin of 80 g/L reveals erythrocytic hyperplasia with normal appearing erythrocytic precursors. This is an indication that the anemia is due to a: (Objective 9)
   a. proliferation defect
   b. nuclear maturation defect
   c. survival defect
   d. cytoplasmic maturation defect

7. Which of the following is an adaptation to anemia that tends to increase blood flow to tissues? (Objective 1)
   a. decrease in 2,3-DPG
   b. shallow inspiration
   c. decreased respiratory rate
   d. increased heart rate

8. A 53-year-old patient had a hemoglobin of 70 g/L. The reticulocyte count is 15%. Which of the following would you expect on the blood smear? (Objective 6)
   a. poikilocytes
   b. polychromatophilia
   c. agglutination
   d. Howell-Jolly bodies

9. In the patient in question 8, numerous schistocytes were identified on the blood smear. How could this finding affect the RDW? (Objective 3)
   a. increase it
   b. decrease it
   c. have no effect
   d. invalidate it

10. A patient has a hemoglobin of 90 g/L and a reticulocyte count of 20%. A bone marrow revealed an M:E ratio of 1:2 and 70% cellularity. How would you describe this marrow? (Objective 4)
    a. aplasia
    b. erythrocytic hypoplasia
    c. dysplasia
    d. erythrocytic hyperplasia

www.pearsonhighered.com/mckenzie
Use this address to access the interactive Companion Website created for this textbook. Find additional information, tables and figures. Evaluate your command of the chapter information using case studies and critical thinking and multiple choice questions.

REFERENCES

1. Crosby WH. Reticulocyte counts. *Arch Intern Med.* 1981;141: 1747–48.

2. Centers for Disease Control. CDC criteria for anemia in children and childbearing-aged women. *MMWR.* 1989 Jun 9; 38:400–4.

3. Nordenberg D, Yip R, Binkin NJ. The effect of cigarette smoking on hemoglobin levels and anemia screening. *JAMA.* 1990;264:1556–59.

4. Hillman RS. Hershko, C. Acute blood loss anemia. In:, Lichtman MA, Beutler E, Kipps TJ, Seligsohn U, Kaushansky K, Prchal JT, eds. *Hematology,* 7th ed. New York: McGraw-Hill; 2007:Chapter 54.

5. Sheth TN, Choudhry NK, Bowes M, Detsky AS. The relation of conjunctival pallor to the presence of anemia. *J Gen Intern Med.* 1997; 12(2):102–6.

6. Stoltzfus RJ, Edward-Raj A, Dreyfuss ML, Albonico M, Montresor A, Dhoj Thapa M, et al. Clinical pallor is useful to detect severe anemia in populations where anemia is prevalent and severe. *J Nutrit.* 1999;129(9):1675–81.

7. Scott RB. Common blood disorders: A primary care approach. *Geriatrics.* 1993;48:72–76, 79–80.

8. Freedman, M.L. Anemias in the elderly: Physiologic or pathologic. *Hosp. Pract.* 1982;17(5):121.

9. Mark PW, Glader B. Approach to anemia in the adult and child. In: Hoffman R, Benz EJ, Shattil SJ, Furie B, Cohen HJ, Silberstein LE, McGlave P, eds. *Hematology Basic Principles and Practice.* Philadelphia: Elsevier; Churchill Livingstone 2004:455–63.

10. Guralnik JM, Eisenstaedt RS, Ferrucci L, Klein HG, Woodman RC. Prevalence of anemia in persons 65 years and older in the United States: Evidence for a high rate of unexplained anemia. *Blood.* 2004; 104:2263–68.

11. Steensma DP, Tefferi A. Anemia in the elderly: How should we define it, when does it matter, and what can be done. *Mayo Clin Proc.* 2007;82(2):958-66.

12. Van Hove L, Schisano T, Brace L. Anemia diagnosis, classification, and monitoring using Cell-Dyn technology reviewed for the new millennium. *Lab Hematol.* 2000;6:93–108.

13. Perkins SL. Examination of the blood and bone marrow. In: Lee GR, Foerster J, Lukens J, Paraskevas JPG, Rodgers GM, eds. *Wintrobe's Clinical Hematology,* 10th ed. Baltimore: Williams and Wilkins; 1999:9–35.

14. Weihang B, Dalfares ER, Srinivasan AR, Webber LS, Berensen GS. Normative distribution of complete blood count from early childhood through adolescence. The Bogalusa Heart Study. *Prev Med.* 1993;22:825–37.

15. NCCLS. Methods for reticulocyte counting (flow cytometry and supravital dyes): Approved guideline. *NCCLS Document H44-A.* 1997;17(15).

16. Kosower NS. Altered properties of erythrocytes in the aged. *Am J Hematol.* 1993;42:241–47.

17. Koepke JA. Update on reticulocyte counting. *Lab Med.* 1999; 30(5): 339–43.

18. Chang CC, Kass L. Clinical significance of immature reticulocyte fraction determined by automated reticulocyte counting. *Am J Clin Pathol.* 1997;108(1):69–73.

19. Djulbegovic B. Red blood cell problems. In: Djulbegovic B, ed. *Reasoning and Decision Making in Hematology.* Edinburgh, UK: Churchill Livingstone; 1992:13.

20. Bessman JD, Gilmer PR, Gardner FH. Improved classification of anemias by MCV and RDW. *Am J Clin Pathol.* 1983;80:322–26.

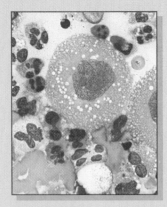

CHAPTER OUTLINE

9

Anemias of Disordered Iron Metabolism and Heme Synthesis

Shirlyn B. McKenzie, Ph. D.

■ OBJECTIVES—LEVEL I

At the end of this unit of study, the student should be able to:

1. Define *sideropenic* and *sideroachrestic* as they relate to anemias.
2. Diagram the transport of iron from ingestion to incorporation into heme.
3. Define the following terms and explain their role in iron metabolism: *transferrin, hemosiderin, ferritin, TIBC*.
4. Describe physiologic factors that affect the amount of iron needed by the body.
5. Compare and contrast the typical blood features and iron studies associated with iron deficiency anemia (IDA), anemia of chronic disease (ACD), lead poisoning, and sideroblastic anemia.
6. Explain the etiology and pathophysiology of iron deficiency anemia, anemia of chronic disease, and sideroblastic anemia.
7. Define *hemosiderosis*.
8. Calculate transferrin saturation and UIBC.

■ OBJECTIVES—LEVEL II

At the end of this unit of study, the student should be able to:

1. List the three stages of iron deficiency and define characteristic RBC morphology of each stage.
2. Compare and contrast iron stores, hemoglobin, serum iron, TIBC, saturation, serum ferritin, and RBC morphology in the three stages of iron deficiency.
3. Describe the function of the proteins involved in iron metabolism including hepcidin, HFE, transferrin receptor, hemojuvelin, divalent metal transporter 1, duodenal cytochrome–B reductase, hephaestin, and ferroportin.
4. Explain the molecular control of total body iron and cellular iron.
5. Describe how genetic defects in the iron metabolism proteins can affect the body's iron homeostasis.
6. Contrast the basic defects in iron deficiency anemia, sideroblastic anemia, and anemia of chronic disease, and describe how these defects affect hemoglobin synthesis.
7. Recognize the clinical features associated with iron deficiency.

■ OBJECTIVES—LEVEL II (continued)

8. Correlate the following laboratory features with iron deficiency anemia and sideroblastic anemia: erythrocyte morphology and protoporphyrin studies, iron studies, and bone marrow.

9. Select laboratory tests and discuss test results that help differentiate iron deficiency anemia, anemia of chronic disease, and sideroblastic anemia.

10. Summarize the results of bone marrow analysis in sideroblastic anemia and anemia of chronic disease, and contrast them with those found in iron deficiency anemia.

11. Outline the classification of sideroblastic anemias and describe the differentiating feature of the hereditary type.

12. Describe the relationship of the anemias associated with alcoholism and malignant disease to sideroblastic anemia.

13. Describe the role of molecular diagnostics in hereditary sideroblastic anemia.

14. Explain the significance of finding microcytic anemia in the presence of lead poisoning, and suggest reflex testing that would help define an accurate diagnosis.

15. Explain how lead poisoning and alcohol affect erythropoiesis and their relationship to sideroblastic anemia, and recognize the abnormal peripheral blood and clinical features that can be associated with these disorders.

16. Discuss the treatment for iron deficiency, sideroblastic anemia, and anemia of chronic disease and expected laboratory findings associated with successful therapy.

17. Differentiate primary (hereditary) and secondary hemochromatosis and summarize typical results of iron studies in this disease.

18. Describe the genetic abnormality associated with hereditary hemochromatosis and identify the screening and diagnostic tests for this disease.

19. Describe the basic defect in porphyria and its effect on the blood.

20. Develop a reflex-testing pathway for an effective and cost-efficient diagnosis when microcytic and/or hypochromic cells are present.

21. Evaluate laboratory test results and use them to identify the etiology and pathophysiology of the anemias that have a defective heme synthesis component.

KEY TERMS

Anemia of chronic disease (ACD)
Anemia of inflammation (AI)
Apoferritin
DcytB
DMT1
Ferritin
Ferroportin 1
Hemochromatosis
Hemojuvelin (HJV)
Hemosiderin
Hepcidin
Hephaestin
HFE

Pappenheimer bodies
Pica
Plumbism
Porphyrias
Rhopheocytosis
Sideroacrestic anemia
Sideroblastic anemia
Sideropenic anemia
Total iron-binding capacity (TIBC)
Transferrin
Transferrin saturation
Unsaturated iron-binding capacity (UIBC)

BACKGROUND BASICS

The information in this chapter builds on the concepts learned in previous chapters. To maximize your learning experience, you should review these concepts before starting this unit of study.

Level I

▸ Diagnosis of anemia: List the laboratory tests used to diagnose and classify anemias and identify abnormal values. (Chapter 8)

▸ Classification of anemia: Outline the morphologic and functional classification of anemias. (Chapter 8)

Level II

▸ Function, structure, and synthesis of hemoglobin: Diagram the synthesis of heme and explain the role of iron in hemoglobin synthesis. (Chapter 6)

▸ Erythrocyte destruction: Diagram degradation of hemoglobin when the erythrocyte is destroyed and interpret laboratory tests associated with increased erythrocyte destruction. (Chapter 5)

CASE STUDY

We will address this case study throughout the chapter.
Jose, an 83-year-old anemic male, was admitted to a local hospital with recurrent urinary tract bleeding and an infection associated with prostatitis. Consider how these conditions can affect the hematopoietic system.

▸ OVERVIEW

This chapter includes a discussion of a group of anemias associated with defective hemoglobin synthesis due to faulty iron metabolism or porphyrin biosynthesis. The discussion begins with a detailed description of iron metabolism and laboratory tests used to assess the body's iron concentration. This is followed by a description of the specific anemias included in this group—iron deficiency anemia, anemia of chronic disease, and sideroblastic anemia. Hemochromatosis is also discussed even though it is not characterized by anemia. In this disease, iron metabolism is abnormal, and results of iron studies must be differentiated from those found in sideroblastic anemia. The rare porphyrias are briefly discussed because porphyrin is an integral component in the synthesis of heme.

▸ INTRODUCTION

Defective hemoglobin production can be due to disturbances in either heme or globin synthesis (Table 9-1 ✪). The result of these disturbances is a cytoplasmic maturation defect reflected by a microcytic, hypochromic anemia. Defective heme synthesis is caused by abnormalities of iron homeostasis (deficiency and/or metabolism) or rarely by defective porphyrin metabolism (Figure 9-1 ■). Defective globin synthesis is caused by a deletion or mutation of globin genes. These globin deletions and mutations are the result of a hereditary condition known as *thalassemia*. Thalassemias are discussed in ∞ Chapter 11.

Anemia characterized by deficient iron for hemoglobin synthesis is known as **sideropenic anemia**, commonly referred to as *iron deficiency anemia* (IDA). Iron deficiency primarily affects the erythrocyte and developing central nervous system. Sideropenic anemia caused by inadequate iron intake or absorption or increased blood loss responds to iron therapy given either orally or less commonly, parenterally.

Defective heme synthesis also can result from defective iron metabolism. **Sideroachrestic anemias** are characterized by adequate or excess stores of iron but defective utilization in the synthesis of hemoglobin. The **anemia of chronic disease (ACD)**, also referred to as the **anemia of inflammation (AI)**, is characterized by iron retention in the macrophages, thus making iron unavailable to the erythrocyte for heme synthesis.

Defects in porphyrin synthesis involve the enzymes required for heme synthesis. The defect can affect the insertion of iron into the porphyrin ring to form heme. These conditions include primary and secondary **sideroblastic anemias**. For convenience, the **porphyrias** are included in this chapter, although the porphyrias except for the erythropoietic porphyria type are not generally characterized by the presence of anemia.

✪ TABLE 9-1

Causes of Defective Hemoglobin Production That May Result in a Microcytic Hypochromic Anemia

Defects in heme synthesis
- Abnormal iron metabolism
  - Iron deficiency
  - Defective iron utilization
- Defective porphyrin metabolism

Defects in globin synthesis (thalassemias): deletions or mutations of globin genes

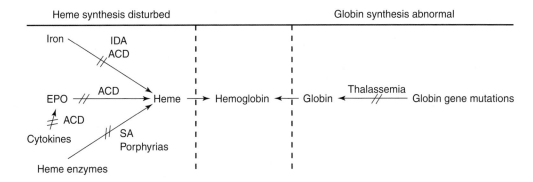

■ FIGURE 9-1   Sites of defective hemoglobin synthesis that can result in anemia. Some of these anemias are hereditary or congenital and others are acquired. (ACD = anemia of chronic disease; IDA = iron deficiency anemia; SA = sideroblastic anemia; EPO = erythropoietin; ─//➤ = defective or disturbed)

► IRON METABOLISM

Iron is required by every cell in the body. It has vital roles in oxidative metabolism, cellular growth and proliferation, and oxygen transport and storage.[1] Iron must be bound to protein compounds to fulfill these functions. Iron in inorganic compounds or in an ionized form is potentially dangerous. If the amount of iron exceeds the body's capacity for transport and storage in the protein-bound form, iron toxicity can develop, causing damage to cells and a potentially lethal condition. Conversely, if too little iron is available, the synthesis of physiologically active iron compounds is limited and critical metabolic processes are inhibited.

Important advances in our understanding of iron metabolism are the result of the discovery of genes and proteins that participate in the regulation of iron homeostasis. As the roles of these proteins are explained, the pathophysiology of disorders involving iron metabolism is revealed. Proteins that play a role in iron metabolism include hepcidin, HFE (hemochromatosis), transferrin receptor (TfR), hemojuvelin, divalent metal transporter 1 (DMT1), duodenal cytochrome–B reductase (DcytB), and ferroportin, also known as IREG1. The role of these proteins is described in the following sections.

DISTRIBUTION

Iron-containing compounds in the body are one of two types: (1) functional compounds that serve in metabolic (hemoglobin, myoglobin, iron-responsive element-binding protein) or enzymatic (cytochromes, cytochrome oxygenase, catalase, peroxidase) functions and (2) compounds that serve as transport (transferrin, transferrin receptor) or storage forms (ferritin and hemosiderin) for iron (Table 9-2 ✪). A poorly understood iron compartment is the intracellular "labile pool." Iron leaves the plasma and enters the intracellular fluid compartment for a brief time before it is incorporated into cellular components (heme or enzymes) or storage

compounds. This labile pool is believed to be the chelatable iron pool (see Therapy, Hemochromatosis). The total iron concentration in the body is 40–50 mg of iron/kg of body weight. Men have higher amounts than women.

Iron is found primarily in erythrocytes, macrophages, hepatocytes, and enterocytes (absorptive cells at the luminal [apical] surface of the duodenum). Hemoglobin constitutes the major fraction of body iron (functional iron) with a concentration of 1 gm iron/kg of erythrocytes, or about 1 mg iron/mL erythrocytes. Iron in hemoglobin remains in the erythrocyte until the cell is removed from the circulation. Hemoglobin released from the erythrocyte is then degraded in the macrophages of the spleen and liver, releasing iron. Approximately 85% of this iron from degraded hemoglobin is promptly recycled from the macrophage to the plasma where it is bound to the transport protein, transferrin, and delivered to developing normoblasts in the bone marrow for heme synthesis. The macrophages recycle 10 to 20 times more iron than is absorbed in the gut.[2] This iron recycling provides most of the marrow's daily iron requirement for erythropoiesis (∞ Chapter 5).

Iron in hepatocytes and intestinal enterocytes is stored and utilized as needed to maintain iron homeostasis. The hepatocytes store iron that can be released and utilized when the amount of iron in the plasma is not sufficient to support erythropoiesis. Enterocytes that absorb dietary iron can either export it to the plasma or store it. Iron stored in enterocytes is lost when the cells are sloughed into the intestine.

ABSORPTION

Total body iron homeostasis depends on balancing and linking the absorption of iron by the enterocytes of the duodenum with total body requirements. No significant mechanism regulates iron loss. Factors influencing iron absorption are listed in Table 9-3 ✪.

Dietary iron exists in two forms: nonheme iron (ionic or ferric form) present in vegetables and whole grains and

⊕ TABLE 9-2

Composition and Distribution of Iron in Adults

Compound	Iron Content, Male (mg Iron/ Kg Body Weight)	Iron Content, Female (mg Iron/ Kg Body Weight)	Percent of Total Iron
Functional iron			
Hemoglobin	31	28	60–75
Myoglobin	5	4	3.5
Other tissue iron	<1	<1	0.2
Heme enzymes (cytochromes, catalases, peroxidases)			
Nonheme enzymes (iron-sulfur proteins, metalloflavoproteins, ribonucleotide reductase)			
Transport			
Transferrin	<1	<1	0.1
Storage			
Ferritin	~8	4	10–20
Hemosiderin	~4	2	5–10
Labile pool	~1	~1	2
Total iron	50	40	

heme iron (ferrous form) present primarily in red meats in the form of hemoglobin. Nonheme iron is the most common form ingested worldwide, but heme iron is more common in Western countries. The ferric complexes from nonheme sources are not easily absorbed. Gastric acid solubilizes this form of iron and provides an acidic environment around the apical brush border of the enterocytes. This low pH facilitates the transport of iron across the enterocyte membrane. The ferric iron is reduced to the ferrous state at the enterocyte brush border through the action of the enzyme, **DcytB**, a ferric reductase. The ferrous iron is then

⊕ TABLE 9-3

Factors Affecting Iron Absorption in the GI Tract

- Bioavailability of iron: from the diet and from macrophage recycling
- Condition of mucosal cells in the GI tract
- Intraluminal factors: parasites, toxins, intestinal motility; increased motility or decreased absorptive surface area can decrease absorption
- Hematopoietic activity of bone marrow: rate of erythropoietic activity directly related to the amount absorbed
- Tissue iron stores: Amount of storage iron inversely related to the amount absorbed
- Oxygen content of the blood: hypoxia associated with increased absorption
- Systemic inflammation or infection: decreases absorption
- Blood hemoglobin concentration: anemia associated with increased absorption

transported across the apical enterocyte plasma membrane by **DMT1**, an integral membrane protein. DMT1 also transports the divalent forms of manganese, lead, zinc, cobalt, and copper across the enterocyte membrane[3] (Figure 9-2 ■).

Heme iron is more readily absorbed than nonheme iron, but the mechanism of absorption is less well understood. Heme is split from the globin portion of hemoglobin in the intestine, and is then assimilated directly by the enterocytes. Once inside the cell, iron is released from heme by heme oxygenase. The iron then enters the same iron pool as the nonheme iron. A heme carrier protein (HCP1) found in the duodenal enterocyte was recently described, but its contribution to iron absorption has not been documented.[4]

In the enterocyte, the iron can be stored as ferritin or transported across the basolateral membrane into the plasma. The iron stored as ferritin is lost when the enterocyte is sloughed off into the intestinal tract. Iron transport across the basolateral membrane is via a basolateral transporter protein known as **ferroportin 1** (also known as IREG1). Ferroportin 1, an integral membrane protein, transports ferrous ions and is the only known cellular exporter of iron. Export is facilitated by the ferroxidase, **hephaestin** (a homologue of the plasma protein ceruloplasmin). Hephaestin oxidizes the Fe^{2+} to Fe^{3+}, the form of iron required for binding to apotransferrin in the blood. Hephaestin is a copper-containing ferroxidase that requires adequate amounts of copper for its function. Thus, it is not surprising that copper deficiency is associated with abnormal iron metabolism. Export of iron from nonintestinal cells requires

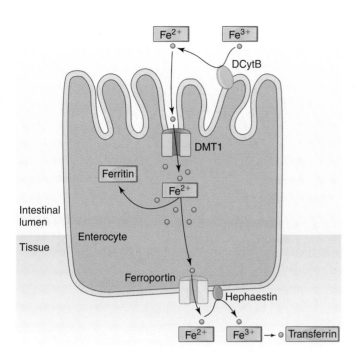

FIGURE 9-2 The absorption of nonheme iron in the intestine. Most nonheme iron in the diet is in the ferric iron form (Fe^{+3}). When the Fe^{+3} reaches the intestine and comes into contact with the cells lining the gut (enterocytes), the iron is reduced to the ferrous form (Fe^{+2}) by a reductase, DCytB, located at the apical enterocyte membrane. The Fe^{+2} then can be transported across the membrane by DMT1. Ferroportin transports the iron across the enterocyte basolateral membrane, a process thought to be facilitated by hephaestin. Hephaestin is an oxidase that oxidizes the iron to Fe^{+3}, the form that combines with transferrin. Some iron can remain in the cell as ferritin, depending on the systemic iron balance.

ceruloplasmin, which also converts Fe^{2+} to Fe^{3+} for binding to transferrin.

There appears to be a predetermined set point of iron stores that results in a negative correlation between the amount of iron absorbed and the amount of iron stored.[5] The efficiency of intestinal absorption of iron increases in response to accelerated erythropoietic activity and depletion of body iron stores. Thus, bleeding, hypoxia, or hemolysis results in accelerated erythrocyte production and enhanced absorption of iron. However, increased iron uptake in extravascular hemolytic anemias and anemias associated with a high degree of ineffective erythropoiesis can lead to an excess of iron in various organs because the body does not lose the iron from erythrocytes hemolyzed in vivo. Conversely, diminished erythropoiesis as occurs in starvation decreases the absorption of iron.

IDA due to a lack of dietary iron is usually treated with daily oral doses of ferrous salts. The efficiency of absorption of this therapeutic iron is greatest during the initial treatment period when body stores are depleted. Increased absorption occurs up to 6 months after hemoglobin values return to normal or until iron stores are replenished. Absorption also increases 10–20% in early stages of developing ID.

TRANSPORT

Transferrin is a plasma transport protein that mediates iron exchange between tissues (Table 9-4 ✪; Figure 9-3 ■). It is not lost in delivering iron to the cells but returns to the plasma and is reused. Transferrin is a single polypeptide chain composed of two homologous lobes, each of which contains a single iron-binding site. The binding of a ferric iron to either site is random. If only one transferrin lobe binds an iron molecule, it is termed *monoferric transferrin*; if both sites are occupied, it is *diferric transferrin*. Transferrin without iron is called *apotransferrin*.

Each gram of transferrin binds 1.4 mg of iron. Enough transferrin is present in plasma to bind 253–435 μg of iron per deciliter of plasma. This is referred to as the **total iron-binding capacity (TIBC)**.

The serum iron concentration is about 70–201 μg/dL and almost all (95%) of this iron is complexed with transferrin; thus, transferrin is about one-third saturated with iron (serum iron/TIBC × 100 = % **transferrin saturation**). The reserve iron-binding capacity of transferrin (transferrin without bound iron) is referred to as the serum **unsaturated iron-binding capacity (UIBC)** (TIBC − Serum iron = UIBC).

The majority of transferrin-bound iron is delivered to the developing bone marrow normoblasts where the iron is released for use in hemoglobin synthesis. Iron in excess of physiologic requirements is deposited in tissues (primarily the liver) for storage.

Only a small amount of transferrin-bound iron is derived from iron absorbed by enterocytes. Most of the iron bound to transferrin is recycled iron derived from the monocyte-macrophage system. The major flow of iron in the body is from transferrin to erythroid marrow, then to erythrocytes, and finally to macrophages when the senescent erythrocyte is removed and degraded by liver, bone marrow, and splenic macrophages. Recovered iron from hemoglobin catabolism in the monocyte-macrophage system enters the plasma and is again bound to transferrin for transfer back to the bone marrow (Figure 9-4 ■). In disorders associated with

✪ TABLE 9-4
Characteristics of Transferrin
• Function: responsible for transporting iron • B_1-globulin • MW 79,570 D • Half-life: 18 days • Synthesized in the liver

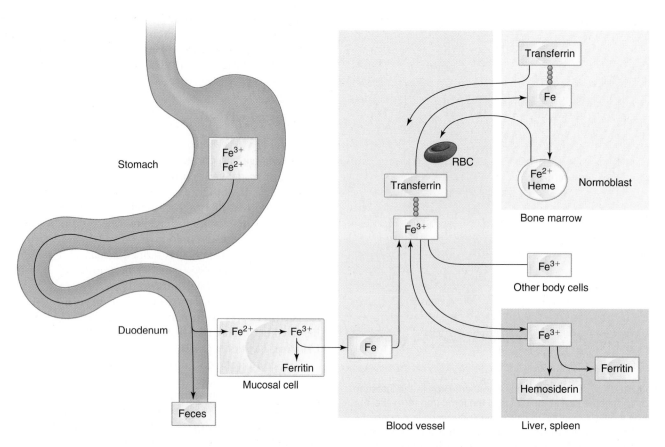

■ **FIGURE 9-3**   Iron is absorbed by the mucosal cells in the gut as ferrous iron. It can be stored in the mucosal cell as ferritin or it can leave the cell as oxidized ferric iron and be transported in the blood by transferrin. Transferrin can deliver iron to developing normoblasts in the bone marrow, other body cells or macrophanges in the liver or spleen. Transferrin is reutilized after it delivers iron to the cells.

intravascular hemolysis, plasma hemoglobin combines with haptoglobin. The haptoglobin-hemoglobin complex is taken into the macrophage via the cell's hemoglobin scavenger receptor, CD163.[6]

In contrast to serum ferritin, transferrin is a negative acute phase reactant (levels decrease during the acute phase response). Increased levels are found in pregnancy and in estrogen therapy.

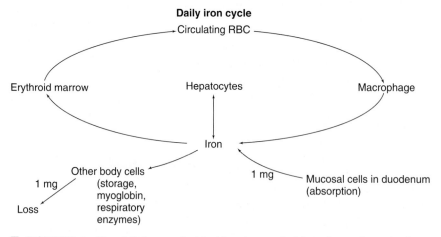

■ **FIGURE 9-4**   The daily iron cycle. Most iron is recycled from the erythrocytes to the bone marrow. Only a small amount of iron is lost from the body through loss of iron containing cells. To maintain iron balance, a similar amount of iron is absorbed from the duodenum.

Lactoferrin also functions as an iron transport protein but is found primarily in tissue fluid and cells. It has antimicrobial properties and is important in protecting the body from infection.

Transferrin releases iron at specific receptor sites on the developing cell, referred to as the *transferrin receptor1* (*TfR*1). These receptors are expressed on virtually all cells, but the number per cell is a function of cellular iron requirements. Cells with high iron requirements have high numbers of TfR1. Erythroid precursors, especially intermediate normoblasts that are rapidly synthesizing hemoglobin, have high numbers of transferrin receptors, about 800,000 per cell. The TfR1 is a transmembrane glycoprotein dimer with two identical subunits, each of which can bind a molecule of transferrin. A homologous protein, TfR2, is more limited in expression. It is found on hepatocytes, duodenal crypt cells, and erythroid cells.

Iron enters the cell in an energy- and temperature-dependent process. After transferrin binds to its receptor, the transferrin-TfR complex clusters with other transferrin-TfR complexes on the cell membrane, and the membrane invaginates and seals, forming an endosome with the complex inside (endocytosis) (Figure 9-5 ■). In the acidic endosome, iron is released from transferrin and transported into the cy-toplasm via DMT1 transport proteins present in the endosomal membrane. The endosome with the apotransferrin and TfR is transported back to the cell surface. The apotransferrin is released, making both it and the receptor available for recycling. Ferritin molecules are also endocytosed on erythroblasts in a process called **rhopheocytosis** (a form of micropinocytosis). However, ferritin iron incorporated into the cell this way does not appear to be utilized for hemoglobin synthesis.

Cells release the extracellular portion of their transferrin receptors through proteolytic cleavage as they mature. These cleaved receptors referred to as *serum* or *soluble transferrin receptors* (*sTfR*) are found in the blood. With increased erythropoiesis, soluble transferrin receptors in the plasma increase.

STORAGE

The primary iron storage depot is the liver. The largest nonheme iron stores in the body are hemosiderin and ferritin (Table 9-5 ✪). Storage iron provides a readily available iron supply in the event of increased iron loss through bleeding. Depletion of these storage compounds reflects an excess iron loss over what is absorbed.

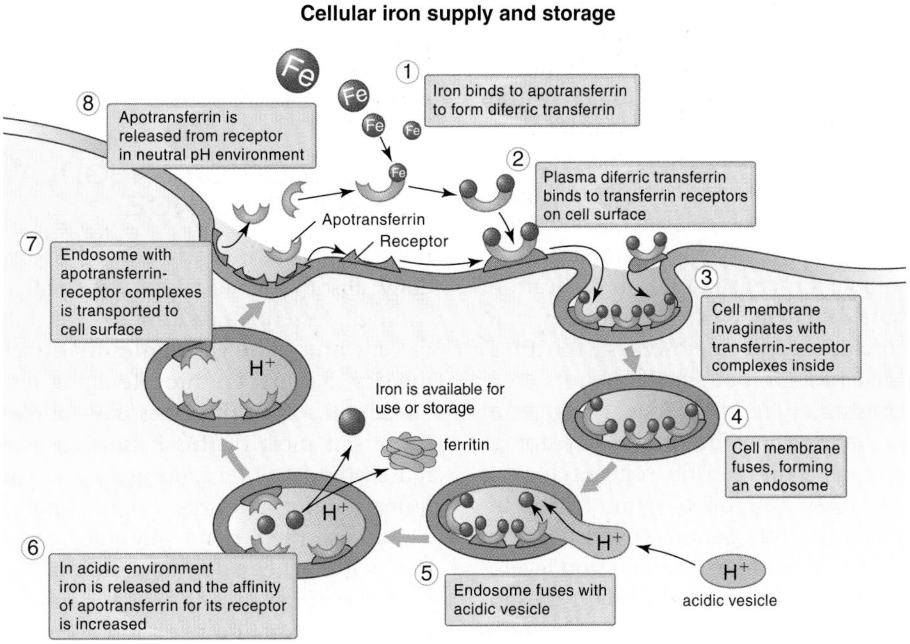

Cellular iron supply and storage

⑧ Apotransferrin is released from receptor in neutral pH environment

① Iron binds to apotransferrin to form diferric transferrin

② Plasma diferric transferrin binds to transferrin receptors on cell surface

⑦ Endosome with apotransferrin-receptor complexes is transported to cell surface

③ Cell membrane invaginates with transferrin-receptor complexes inside

④ Cell membrane fuses, forming an endosome

⑥ In acidic environment iron is released and the affinity of apotransferrin for its receptor is increased

⑤ Endosome fuses with acidic vesicle

Apotransferrin Receptor

Iron is available for use or storage

ferritin

acidic vesicle

■ **FIGURE 9-5** Iron binds to apotransferrin in the plasma forming monoferric or diferric transferrin. Transferrin binds to transferrin receptors on the cell surface. The transferrin-receptor complex enters the cell where the iron is released. The apotransferrin-receptor complex is transported to the cell surface where the apotransferrin is released to the plasma for reutilization. (Adapted from: Hoffman R, Benz EJ, Shattil SJ, Furie B, Cohen HJ, eds. *Hematology: Basic Principles and Procedures.* New York: Churchill Livingstone; 1991.)

⊘ TABLE 9-5

Storage Forms of Iron

Iron Form	Role	Laboratory Analysis	Reference Interval
Ferritin	Primary storage form of soluble iron; readily released for heme synthesis	Serum ferritin levels Prussian blue staining	20–300 µg/L males 12–200 µg/L females
Hemosiderin	Partially degraded storage form of iron; slow release	Bone marrow estimation using Prussian blue stain	40–60% sideroblasts in bone marrow

Ferritin

Ferritin consists of a spherical protein shell that can store up to 4500 iron atoms. Ferritin is 17–33% iron by weight. Ferritin without iron in its shell is called **apoferritin**.

Ferritin is a multimer composed of 24 subunits arranged to form a hollow sphere. There are two types of subunit polypeptides, heavy (H) and light (L). The H polypeptide has ferroxidase activity, but the L form does not. Although ferritin contains 24 subunits, the proportion of H and L subunits varies by cell type. Ferritins in the heart, placenta, and erythrocytes are rich in the H subunit, and ferritins in the iron storage sites, such as the liver and spleen, are rich in the L subunits.

Ferritin acts as the primary storage compound for the body's iron needs and is readily available for erythropoiesis. It controls the amount of iron released for cellular activity and by binding the iron, protects the cellular constituents from oxidative damage catalyzed by free ferrous ions. Ferritin is found in the bone marrow, liver, and spleen, usually within membrane-bound vesicles called *siderosomes*. Normally from 30% to 60% of the normoblasts contain iron aggregates (ferritin). Mature erythrocytes usually do not contain iron aggregates because any excess iron in the cell after hemoglobin synthesis is complete is removed by splenic macrophages.

Ferritin is a water-soluble form of storage iron that cannot be visualized by unstained light microscopy but does stain with iron stains (when clustered in siderosomes). Ferritin is primarily an intracellular protein, but small amounts enter the blood through active secretion or cell lysis. The amount of circulating ferritin parallels the concentration of storage iron in the body. Therefore, serum ferritin concentration is used as an index of iron stores: 1 ng/mL of serum ferritin indicates about 8 mg of storage iron. Serum ferritin does not exhibit diurnal variations as are seen with serum iron levels.

The patient's comorbidities must be considered when interpreting serum ferritin levels. Ferritin is not a reliable indicator of iron stores in the presence of inflammation or tissue damage because it is an acute phase reactant. However, if serum ferritin is decreased, it invariably means that iron stores are low or depleted.

Hemosiderin

Hemosiderin is a heterogeneous aggregate of carbohydrate, lipid, protein, and iron; up to 50% of its weight is iron. Hemosiderin is found primarily in macrophages and is formed by the partial degradation of ferritin. At high levels of cellular iron, ferritin forms aggregates, which are taken up by lysosomes and degraded, forming hemosiderin. The ratio of ferritin to hemosiderin varies with the total body iron concentration. At lower cellular iron concentrations, the ferritin form predominates, but at higher concentrations, the majority of storage iron exists as hemosiderin. Iron from hemosiderin is released slowly and is not readily available for cellular metabolism. Binding in the form of hemosiderin probably keeps iron from harming cellular constituents.

Storage iron in the form of hemosiderin can be estimated on bone marrow tissue sections. Bone marrow macrophages contain hemosiderin if body iron stores are normal or increased. Hemosiderin appears as yellow to brown refractile pigment on unstained marrow or liver specimens. On Prussian blue-stained specimens, the iron appears as blue intracellular particles. Stores can be graded from 0 to 4+ or as markedly reduced, normal, or increased (∞ Chapter 35).

PHYSIOLOGICAL REGULATION OF IRON BALANCE

Body iron is stringently conserved by reutilization so that daily absorption and loss are small. Total body iron lost through secretions of urine, sweat, bile, and desquamation of cells lining the gastrointestinal tract amounts to about 1 mg/day. Normal erythrocyte aging results in destruction of 20–25 mL of erythrocytes/day (releasing about 20–25 mg iron), but most of this hemoglobin iron is scavenged and reused by developing normoblasts. Thus, the total daily requirement for new iron is about 1 mg (∞ Chapter 5).

Because there is no physiological route for excretion of excess iron, the major regulation of total body iron depends on accurate sensing of systemic iron and the adjustment of iron absorption and retention according to needs. Iron deficiency can occur if dietary intake of iron is not adequate, if absorption is impaired, or if there is increased loss of iron through bleeding. Iron overload can occur if absorption abnormally increases or if the individual receives transfusions or iron injections (Table 9-6 ⊘).

Iron Balance at the Tissue Level

Iron homeostasis is accomplished by the interaction of iron with proteins that aide in its absorption, retention, export,

---

⊛ TABLE 9-6

Causes of Iron Deficiency and Iron Overload

Causes of Iron Deficiency	Causes of Iron Overload
Increased requirement/demand due to blood loss, rapid growth, treatment with EPO	Increased absorption of iron
	Multiple transfusions
	Iron injections
Inadequate diet	
Malabsorption	

---

and transport. These proteins include hepcidin, DcytB, DMT1, ferroportin, HFE, TfR, and hemojuvelin (Table 9-7 ⊛). The liver is the primary storage depot for iron and plays a central role in the regulation of total body iron homeostasis by synthesizing hepcidin in response to multiple signals.[2] Thus, the liver has been called the *command central* of iron homeostasis. The proteins involved in iron absorption can be upregulated or downregulated depending on total body iron status.

Hepcidin   **Hepcidin** (also referred to as *HAMP*) is the master iron-regulating hormone that acts by inhibiting expression or activity of genes involved in intestinal iron transport. It decreases absorption and/or transfer of iron from enterocytes to plasma transferrin when iron stores are adequate. Hepcidin also blocks the export of iron stored in macrophages. Downregulation of hepcidin permits increased

---

⊛ TABLE 9-7

Proteins Involved in Iron Homeostasis

Protein	Metabolic Role
Hepcidin	Master iron-regulating protein; regulates iron recycling/balance via interaction with ferroportin1; is negative regulator of intestinal iron absorption
DMT1	Transports iron across the enterocyte apical plasma membrane
DCytB	Reduces Fe^{3+} iron to Fe^{2+} at enterocyte border
Ferroportin1	Transports iron across the basolateral membrane of enterocyte
Hephaestin	Facilitates cellular export of iron; oxidizes Fe^{++} iron to Fe^{+++} for binding to apotransferrin
Transferrin receptor (TfR)	Binds transferrin to cell for internalization of iron
HFE	Interacts with TfR to regulate the receptor's affinity for transferrin
Transferrin (Tf)	Transports iron found in blood
Hemojuvelin (HJV)	Regulates hepcidin expression

---

iron absorption when total body iron is low. Hepcidin synthesis is induced by an excess of iron and inhibited by lack of iron. Thus, it is a negative regulator of iron absorption and/or transfer. Hepcidin synthesis also is controlled by anemia and hypoxia.[7] The body's response to insufficient oxygen delivery is an increase in erythropoiesis. An increase in erythropoietic activity results in a decrease in hepcidin secretion, which allows absorption of more iron in the intestine and increased availability of iron from iron stores. The specific mediator that conveys this signal from the bone marrow to the hepatic sites of hepcidin synthesis is not yet known.

Hepcidin synthesis is affected by not only iron status and erythropoietic activity but also infection and inflammation. Bacteria-activated macrophages and neutrophils synthesize hepcidin but at lower levels than the hepatocytes. In the presence of inflammation, the cytokine interleukin-6 (IL-6) induces synthesis of hepcidin resulting in hypoferremia (decreased serum iron). Other cytokines can be involved in this process but have not been specifically identified. Because hepcidin induces iron retention in the macrophages (traps intracellular iron) and most iron used in erythropoiesis comes from recycled iron from the macrophage, hypoferremia can develop rapidly in the presence of inflammation or infection even though total body iron can be normal or even increased. This appears to be the pathologic basis for the anemia of chronic disease (ACD, see below).

Hepcidin decreases iron absorption by inhibiting the expression of genes involved in the uptake or transfer of iron (e.g., DMT1, DcytB) and by binding to the iron exporter ferroportin. When there is dietary iron deficiency, hepcidin release is blocked, and DMT1, DcytB and ferroportin are upregulated.[8] When hepcidin binds ferroportin, ferroportin is internalized within the cell and degraded. Since ferroportin determines if iron is delivered to the plasma or remains within the enterocyte and is shed, its presence or absence plays a vital role in iron homeostasis. Hepcidin's interaction with ferroportin is thought to be the major mechanism that controls systemic iron homeostasis while DMT1 and DcytB are strongly regulated by local iron concentration in the enterocytes.[9]

HFE   **HFE** is a transmembrane protein that associates with beta2-microglobulin (Beta2M). HFE binds to the transferrin receptor (TfR) on cells and regulates the receptor's interaction with transferrin. When bound to TfR, HFE reduces the affinity of the receptor for iron-bound transferrin (Tf-Fe) by 5- to 10-fold. Thus, HFE is involved in regulating iron absorption and uptake. Mutations of HFE are associated with hereditary hemochromatosis (a condition of total body iron overload).

TfR2 can bind transferrin but less efficiently than TfR, and it does not complex with HFE. It appears that TfR2 influences the synthesis or release of hepcidin. In TfR2 knockout mice (mice that do not express TfR2), hepcidin expression is decreased and hepatocytes are overloaded with iron, resulting in hemochromatosis.[10] On the other hand, the interaction of Tf-Fe with hepatocyte TfR2 results in an increase in hepcidin secretion into the circulation. Thus, it appears that TfR2 may be the iron sensor of hepatocytes. The expression of TfR2 is not controlled by the IRE/IRE-BP complex (discussed in the next section).

Hemojuvelin Hemojuvelin (HJV), a glycosylphosphatidylinositol-anchored protein, has been shown to regulate hepcidin expression in mice.[11] When the HJV gene is mutated, the mice fail to express hepcidin in response to dietary or injected iron, resulting in increased absorption of iron. In humans, HJV mutations are associated with severe iron overload.

Thus, it appears that although hepcidin is the major iron-regulating protein, additional proteins are involved in iron homeostasis by their influence on hepcidin synthesis or function.

Iron Balance at the Cellular Level

Control of iron balance at the cellular level occurs by regulation of transcription and translation of proteins involved in iron metabolism. Transcriptional control has not yet been explained, but regulation at the translational level has been described. Several proteins of iron metabolism have mRNA with similar RNA stem-loop-stem structures in either the 5′ or 3′ noncoding regions, referred to as the iron responsive element (IRE). These regions are recognized and bound by an iron-binding protein (IRE-BP; also known as *iron-regulatory protein*/IRP). The binding affinity of IRP for the IRE is determined by the amount of cellular iron. The IRP binds to the IRE region when iron is scarce and dissociates when iron is plentiful.

When bound to the IRE of mRNA, the IRP modulates the translation of the mRNA.[12] The IRP regulates translation in one of two ways, depending on the location of the IRE (stem-loop-stem structure) in the mRNA. If the IRE is in the 5′ untranslated region (UTR) of the mRNA, binding of the IRP results in the disruption of translation by preventing the assembly of initiation factors at the initiator site (Figure 9-6 ■). Because binding occurs when iron is scarce, translation of these proteins is decreased in the absence of iron.[13–16] The mRNAs of ferritin, ferroportin, and ALA synthase2 (ALAS2) fall into this group. If the IRE is in the 3′ UTR of the mRNA, binding of the IRP stabilizes the mRNA that would otherwise be digested/degraded (Figure 9-7 ■). Thus, translation increases when iron is scarce. The mRNAs of TfR and DMT1 fall into this second group.

Thus, IRP regulates cellular iron by coordinating synthesis of ferritin and TfR in opposite directions. The level of TfR expression reflects the need of the cell for iron and is an important factor in hemoglobin synthesis. When the cell needs more iron, TfRs increase to maximize the amount of iron incorporated into the cell and formation of ferritin decreases. When cells have adequate or excess iron, the ferritin levels

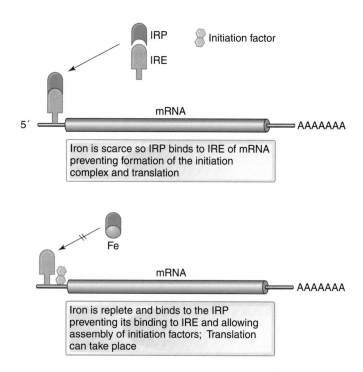

■ **FIGURE 9-6** Regulation of iron at the cellular level. A stem-loop-stem structure in the 5′ noncoding region, referred to as the *iron responsive element* (*IRE*), is present in some mRNA. Binding of iron regulatory protein (IRP) to the IRE prevents initiation of translation. When the level of cellular iron is replete, the iron binds to IRP, preventing IRP binding to the IRE and allowing assembly of initiation factors at the initiation site which allows translation to take place. The translation of mRNAs of ferritin, ferroportin, and ALAS2 is regulated in this fashion.

rise and transferrin receptors decrease. Regulation of the ALAS2 gene serves to coordinate the synthesis of porphyrin (heme) with iron availability.

Iron Metabolism in the Mitochondria

Most iron entering the erythroid cells is routed to the mitochondria for hemoglobin synthesis and Fe-S cluster biogenesis. Key mitochondrial proteins thought to be involved in this iron metabolism include frataxin, ATP-binding cassette protein B7 (ABC7), and mitochondrial ferritin.

The mitochondria contain a variety of Fe-S cluster (iron-containing functional group) proteins including ferrochelatase and aconitase. The ABC7 protein is thought to function in the export of the Fe-S assembled clusters from the mitochondria to the cytosol. Mutations in this protein are characterized by anemia, neurological symptoms, and erythroid cells containing iron aggregates in the mitochondria. ABC7 also interacts with ferrochelatase in heme synthesis.[6]

Mitochondrial ferritin serves as an iron storage molecule and is highly expressed in tissue with numerous mitochondria. It is encoded by a gene on chromosome 5 (5q23). It is highly expressed also in the sideroblasts of patients with

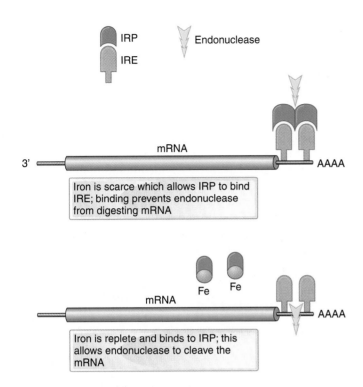

■ **FIGURE 9-7** Regulation of iron at the cellular level. A stem-loop-stem structure in the 3' noncoding region, referred to as the *iron-responsive element* (*IRE*), is present in some mRNA. Binding of iron regulatory protein (IRP) to the IRE stabilizes the mRNA. When cellular iron is replete, the iron binds to the IRP and prevents its binding to the IRE. This results in degradation of the mRNA by endonuclease. The translation of the mRNAs of TfR and DMT1 is regulated in this fashion.

X-linked sideroblastic anemia, a disease in which iron accumulates in the mitochondria to form ringed sideroblasts. Frataxin is a protein in the mitochondrial matrix that is thought to play a role in mitochondrial iron export and storage.[17]

IRON REQUIREMENTS

Normally, humans maintain a relatively constant body concentration of iron throughout the life span. This is accomplished by maintaining a positive iron balance during growing years and establishing an equilibrium between loss and absorption in adult life. Humans are unable to excrete iron to achieve this balance. Therefore, the rate of absorption and loss of iron must be matched to avoid iron deficiency or excess.

Factors That Increase Fe Requirements

Normal physiologic factors that increase the daily requirement for iron include menstruation, pregnancy, and growth. Pathologic factors that increase the need for iron include blood loss, malabsorption, and human recombinant erythropoietin (rHuEPO) therapy in hemodialysis patients with ane-

mia. The pathologic factors are discussed in the next section on iron deficiency anemia.

Menstruation   The average daily iron loss in menstruating females is twice that of their male counterparts. To maintain total body iron balance, menstruating females must absorb about 2 mg of iron daily. National statistics from the third National Health and Nutrition Examination Survey from 1988 to 1994 (NHANES III) reveal that 9–11% of adolescent and young adult females are in an iron deficient state and 2–5% have IDA.[18] In women of childbearing age, ID is more prevalent in minority, low-income, and multiparous women.

Pregnancy   The daily iron requirement during pregnancy is about 3.4 mg; if spread out as a daily average over the three trimesters, it would be about 1,000 mg per pregnancy. The fetus accumulates ~250 mg of iron from maternal stores via the placenta; added to this is the iron requirement for increased maternal blood volume and iron loss at delivery due to bleeding. Thus, a single pregnancy without supplemental iron could exhaust iron stores.

Infancy/Children   In infancy, rapid growth of body size and hemoglobin mass requires more iron in proportion to food intake than at any other time of life. During the first six months of life, an infant synthesizes ~50 g of new hemoglobin. In addition, iron is needed for tissue growth. At birth, normal iron stores of 30 mg are adequate to see the infant through the first 4 to 5 months of life but can be depleted quickly in an infant on an iron-deficient, milk-only diet. Premature infants are at an even higher risk of rapid iron depletion because much of the placental transfer of iron occurs in the last trimester of pregnancy, and they have a faster rate of postnatal growth than full-term infants.[17] It is recommended that full-term infants begin iron supplements no later than 4 months of age and that low-birth-weight infants begin no later than two months of age.[19]

Iron requirements are also high in childhood, especially in 1–3 year olds. Data from NHANES III revealed that in 1-year-olds, the prevalence of ID is 13%,[18] yet 1–3 year olds, especially those from low income families, have the lowest daily iron intake of any age group.[20] A recent study of 1–3-year-old children from urban lower- and middle-class socioeconomic groups showed that 35% had evidence of iron insufficiency in various stages. Of these, 10% had overt IDA.[21]

▶ LABORATORY ASSESSMENT OF IRON

Laboratory testing to determine iron status includes measurement of serum iron, total iron-binding capacity (TIBC), calculation of percent saturation of transferrin, serum ferritin, and serum transferrin receptor (sTfR) (Table G, back cover). An indirect assessment of iron availability is provided by the zinc protoporphyrin (ZPP).

IRON STUDIES

Transferrin can be measured as a protein by immunochemical methods, but because the percent saturation (with iron) is helpful in the differential diagnosis of anemia, it is usually measured functionally as the maximum amount of iron able to be bound in the serum (TIBC). The measured serum iron and TIBC are used to calculate the percent saturation.

As a general rule, changes in the quantity of total body storage iron are accompanied by fluctuations in the serum iron and TIBC. As storage iron increases, serum iron increases and TIBC decreases; conversely, if storage iron decreases or is absent, serum iron decreases and TIBC increases. A transferrin saturation below 16% is an indicator of iron deficiency (ID) while a saturation above 55% is diagnostic for iron overload or hemochromatosis.

Ferritin can be measured in the serum where its concentration is directly proportional to the amount of storage iron in the body. Generally, serum ferritin levels less than 12 µg/L indicate depletion of iron stores while levels >1000 µg/L indicate iron overload. Decreased serum ferritin levels can be the first indication of developing IDA. Serum ferritin levels decrease before the exhaustion of mobilizable iron stores whereas abnormalities in the TIBC and serum iron may become detectable only when iron stores are depleted. Care should be used in interpreting serum ferritin levels, however, because ferritin is an acute phase reactant. Nonspecific increases can be seen in malignancy, infections, and liver disease as well as in inflammatory responses even though storage iron can be decreased. Thus, concommitant ID can be masked in these conditions if other tests of iron status are not considered. Table 9-8 ✪ shows the variations in tissue iron in various disease states.

Small concentrations of TfR can be identified in serum by sensitive immunoassay techniques. TfR in serum (sTfR) is a truncated form of the intact protein found on the cell membrane and circulates bound to Tf. The level of circulating sTfR mirrors the amount of cellular receptor. The sTfR is thus inversely proportional to the amount of body iron because cellular receptor synthesis increases when cells lack iron. The level of sTfR is not affected by concurrent disease states (i.e., inflammation, infection) as is serum ferritin. Circulating sTfR increases in iron-deficiency anemia but not anemia of chronic disease.

When iron is not available for incorporation into the protoporphyrin ring to form heme or the heme synthesis is disturbed, zinc is an alternate protoporphyrin ligand and can be incorporated instead, forming zinc protoporphyrin (ZPP). As a result, excess protoporphyrin in the form of ZPP can accumulate in the cell. This can be detected by measuring fluorescence in the blood.

✓ Checkpoint! 1

A patient's iron studies revealed serum iron 100 µg/dL and TIBC 360 µg/dL. Calculate % saturation and UIBC. Are these values normal or abnormal?

FERROKINETICS

Quantitative measurement of internal iron exchange (ferrokinetics) is useful in understanding the pathophysiology of certain erythropoietic disorders. Ferrokinetic studies monitor the movement of radioactively labelled iron (^{59}Fe) from the plasma to the bone marrow and its subsequent uptake into circulating erythrocytes. Plasma iron is labeled by intravenous injection of a tracer amount of radioiron. The labeled iron binds to transferrin for transport. Its clearance from the plasma can be followed by counting the radioactiv-

---

 TABLE 9-8

Effects of Disease on Tissue Iron

Disease	Percent Transferrin Saturation	Ferritin	Bone Marrow Iron
Iron-deficiency anemia	Low	Low	Absent
Anemia of chronic disease	Normal/low	Normal/high	Abundant
Anemia of chronic renal disease	Normal/high	Normal/high	Abundant
Anemia of chronic liver disease	High	High	Abundant
Anemia of hypothyroidism	Normal	Normal	Normal
Sideroblastic anemias	High	High	Abundant with ringed sideroblasts
Hypoplastic/aplastic anemias	High	High	Abundant
Polycythemia vera	Low	Low	Low or absent
Hemolytic anemia	Normal	Normal	Normal
Megaloblastic anemia	High	High	Abundant
Thalassemia minor	Normal	Normal	Normal

(*Hospital Practice.* 1986;21(3A):115. © 1986 The McGraw Hill Companies, Inc.)

ity that remains in the plasma at intervals up to 90 minutes. The rate at which iron leaves the plasma is called the *plasma iron turnover (PIT)* rate. Tissue need is the primary determinant of PIT. The PIT is a good indicator of total erythropoiesis and correlates well with the erythroid cellularity of bone marrow.

The amount of iron used for effective hemoglobin synthesis can also be measured by determining the amount of labeled iron incorporated into circulating erythrocytes over time. Normal erythrocyte utilization is 70–90% by day 10 to 14. This is termed the *erythrocyte iron turnover* (EIT) rate. The EIT is a good measure of effective erythropoiesis and correlates with the reticulocyte production index.

The normal discrepancy between the rate at which iron leaves the plasma (PIT = 0.7 mg/day/dL) and the rate at which it moves from marrow to circulating erythrocytes (EIT = 0.56 mg/day/dL) suggests that the red cell utilization (RCU) of iron is <100%. Some of the labeled iron can enter the liver or bone marrow macrophages. In addition, 5–10% of bone marrow iron is involved in ineffective erythropoiesis, causing a loss of the labeled iron by intramedullary destruction of abnormal erythrocytes.

A rapid or increased PIT coupled with a normal or increased RCU indicates increased erythropoiesis. A normal to increased PIT coupled with a decreased RCU indicates ineffective erythropoiesis, and a decreased PIT with corresponding decreased RCU indicates decreased erythropoiesis.

Ferrokinetic studies can be of value in locating sites of medullary and extramedullary erythropoiesis by counting surface radioactivity over the liver, spleen, and sacrum.

▶ IRON-DEFICIENCY ANEMIA

Iron deficiency (ID) is the most common nutritional deficiency in the world. It is prevalent in countries where grain is the mainstay of the diet or meat is scarce. Unfortunately, these are also countries where hookworm infestation is endemic. The combination of decreased availability of dietary iron and chronic blood loss from parasitic infection increases the risk of developing IDA. Malnutrition is associated not only with decreased iron intake but also with decreased intake of other essential nutrients including folate. Thus, causes of anemia associated with malnutrition may be multifactorial.

HISTORICAL ASPECTS

In America between 1870 and 1920, *chlorosis,* a word used to describe the condition of ID, was so common in young women it was believed that every female had some form of the disease during puberty.[22] The word *chlorosis* was coined because of the greenish tinge of the skin in these patients; however, often the greenish hue was not apparent but pallor (paleness of the skin) was pronounced. Other classic clinical signs and symptoms of anemia were present including shortness of breath on exertion, lethargy, and heart palpitations. These chlorotic girls were found to have decreased numbers of red cells and an increase in the proportion of serum to cells. Some of the chlorotic girls were also noted to have perverted appetites, craving substances such as chalk, cinders, charcoal, and bugs. As therapy for these patients, doctors prescribed iron salts even though the exact nature of the disease had not been identified. Some physicians linked chlorosis to dietary habits; others implicated menstruation as a possible cause of the disease because chlorosis affected girls in puberty but not boys.

ETIOLOGY

ID can occur due to normal or pathologic conditions that result in an increased demand for iron, malabsorption, or poor diet. In malabsorption or with an iron deficient diet, iron stores can become depleted over a period of years. With an increase in the demand for iron, iron depletion can occur more rapidly, sometimes over a period of months.

Dietary Deficiency

In most developed countries, inadequate dietary intake of iron is rarely the cause of anemia (except in infancy, pregnancy, and adolescence). Diet and socioeconomic status, however, are factors in the development of iron deficiency in children.

Blood Loss

The average adult male in the United States ingests many times more iron than is required. It would take an adult male about eight years to develop IDA if he absorbed no iron during those years. ID in adult males is almost always due to chronic blood loss from the gastrointestinal or genitourinary tracts. For each milliliter of blood lost, there is a loss of about 0.5 mg of iron. Gastrointestinal lesions leading to blood loss include peptic ulcers, hiatus hernia, malignancies, alcoholic gastritis, excessive salicylate ingestion, hookworm infestation, and hemorrhoids. The correlation of ID and GI lesions in elderly patients is high.[23] Genitourinary tract blood loss occurs less frequently; it can result from lesions within the genitourinary system.

Less often, blood loss is the result of intravascular hemolysis. If haptoglobin becomes depleted, the free circulating hemoglobin dissociates into dimers, is filtered by the kidneys, and appears in the urine (hemoglobinuria). This results in a loss of iron, the amount of which is proportional to the amount of hemoglobin in the urine. Some of the hemoglobin is reabsorbed by the renal tubules, resulting in the deposition of iron as hemosiderin in renal tubular cells and eventual sloughing of these cells into the urine (hemosiderinuria). Such is the case with paroxysmal nocturnal hemoglobinuria (PNH) or malfunctioning prosthetic heart valves.

Hemodialysis

Anemia is a common finding in patients with kidney disease. The causes are varied, but the most important factor is a loss or decrease in erythropoietin (EPO) production by the diseased kidneys. Thus, hemodialysis patients are often given recombinant human EPO (rHuEPO), also referred to as *epoetin alfa*, to increase erythropoiesis. However, sufficient iron cannot be mobilized from storage sites rapidly enough to meet the need for a 2- to 4-fold increase in the rate of erythropoiesis that can result from this therapy. The result can be a functional iron deficiency.[24] Lack of an adequate response to EPO therapy is primarily due to functional ID.[25] However, if the patient is given intravenous iron injections with rHuEPO, the hematopoietic response is enhanced.

Malabsorption

Malabsorption is an uncommon cause of ID except in malabsorption syndromes (such as sprue), after gastrectomy, in atrophic gastritis, and in achlorhydria. Gastrectomy results in impaired iron absorption due to the absence of gastric juice, which helps to solubilize and reduce dietary iron into the more easily absorbed ferrous form. In addition, with the loss of the reservoir function of the stomach, nutrients can transit rapidly through the duodenum, allowing insufficient time for iron absorption.

IDA is frequently accompanied by atrophic gastritis and achlorhydria, but it is unknown whether achlorhydria and gastritis are causes of iron malabsorption or the ID is a cause of atrophic gastritis and hence achlorhydria. In patients with gastritis and achlorhydria, therapy with oral iron can be ineffective due to poor iron absorption.

 Checkpoint! 2

A 30-year-old female and a 25-year-old male both had a bleeding ulcer. Assume that each acquired the ulcer at the same time, was losing about the same amount of blood, had equal amounts of storage iron to begin with, and was taking in about 15 mg of dietary iron each day. Would you expect that the woman and man would develop ID at the same time? Explain.

PATHOPHYSIOLOGY

Defined as a diminished total body iron content, ID develops in sequential stages over a period of negative iron balance (losing more iron than is absorbed in the gut). These stages are commonly referred to as:

- Iron depletion
- Iron deficient erythropoiesis
- Iron deficiency anemia (IDA)

Thus, ID can range in severity from reduced iron stores with no functional effect (Stages 1 and 2) to severe anemia with deficiencies of tissue iron-containing enzymes (Stage 3). Laboratory evaluation of iron status is helpful in defining these three stages (Table 9-9 ✪).

- *Stage 1*   During the iron depletion stage, iron stores are exhausted as indicated by a decrease in serum ferritin. There is no anemia, and erythrocyte morphology is normal, but the red cell distribution width (RDW) is frequently elevated. The abnormal RDW can be the first hematologic indication of a developing ID in the nonanemic patient.

  In hospitalized patients, the RDW is not as specific and the ferritin not as sensitive in detecting ID.[26] Hospitalized patients have a high incidence of other diseases that can affect these parameters.

- *Stage 2*   The second stage of ID is characterized by iron-deficient erythropoiesis. There is insufficient iron to insert into the protoporphyrin ring to form heme. As a result, the protoporphyrin accumulates in the cell and complexes with zinc to form zinc protoporphyrin (ZPP). Bone marrow sideroblasts are absent.

  Anemia and hypochromia are still not detectable, but the erythrocytes can become slightly microcytic. The reticulocyte index, reticulocyte hemoglobin content (CHr; Technicon H*3), however, can decrease even in the absence of anemia[27] (∞ Chapter 8). The CHr measures the functional availability of iron during hemoglobin synthesis in the erythrocyte. This index is not available on all hematology analyzers.

- *Stage 3*   A long-standing negative iron flow eventually leads to the last stage of iron deficiency: IDA. Blood loss can significantly shorten the time for this stage to develop. All laboratory tests for iron status become markedly abnormal. The most significant finding is the classic microcytic hypochromic anemia.

  It is apparent then, that when microcytic hypochromic anemia is present, the situation represents the advanced stage of severely deficient total body iron.

CLINICAL FEATURES

The onset of IDA is insidious, usually occuring over a period of months to years. Early stages of ID usually show no clinical manifestations, but as anemia develops, clinical symptoms appear. In addition to symptoms of anemia, a variety of other abnormalities may occur due to a decrease or absence of iron-containing enzymes in various tissues. These include koilonychia (concavity of nails), glossitis, pharyngeal webs, muscle dysfunction, inability to regulate body temperature when cold or stressed, and gastritis.

A curious manifestation of ID is the *pica* syndrome. **Pica** is an unusual craving for ingesting unnatural items. The most common dysphagias described in patients with ID include ice-eating (phagophagia), dirt/clay-eating (geophagia), and starch-eating (amylophagia).[28,29] In one study of 55 patients with IDA, 58% had pica, and of these, 88% had phagophagia.[28]

Iron-deficient infants perform worse in tests of mental and motor development than do nonanemic infants.[30] There is speculation that untreated ID at this stage of human develop-

✪ TABLE 9-9

Laboratory Test Profile of Fe Status

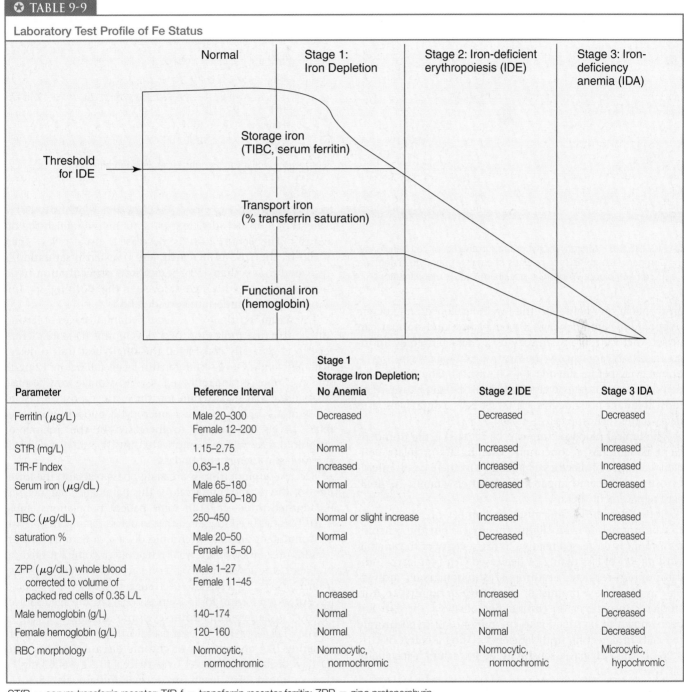

Parameter	Reference Interval	Stage 1 Storage Iron Depletion; No Anemia	Stage 2 IDE	Stage 3 IDA
Ferritin (μg/L)	Male 20–300 Female 12–200	Decreased	Decreased	Decreased
STfR (mg/L)	1.15–2.75	Normal	Increased	Increased
TfR-F Index	0.63–1.8	Increased	Increased	Increased
Serum iron (μg/dL)	Male 65–180 Female 50–180	Normal	Decreased	Decreased
TIBC (μg/dL)	250–450	Normal or slight increase	Increased	Increased
saturation %	Male 20–50 Female 15–50	Normal	Decreased	Decreased
ZPP (μg/dL) whole blood corrected to volume of packed red cells of 0.35 L/L	Male 1–27 Female 11–45	Increased	Increased	Increased
Male hemoglobin (g/L)	140–174	Normal	Normal	Decreased
Female hemoglobin (g/L)	120–160	Normal	Normal	Decreased
RBC morphology	Normocytic, normochromic	Normocytic, normochromic	Normocytic, normochromic	Microcytic, hypochromic

STfR = serum transferrin receptor; TfR-f = transferrin receptor-ferritin; ZPP = zinc protoporphyrin

ment has long-lasting effects on the central nervous system.[31] Symptoms reported to occur in iron deficient children include irritability, loss of memory, and difficulties in learning. Deficiencies of the immune system have been attributed to iron-related impairment of host defense mechanisms.

In the absence of iron in the gut, other metals are absorbed in increased amounts. This can be significant when an iron deficient person is exposed to toxic metals such as lead, cadmium, and plutonium.

LABORATORY FEATURES

Laboratory tests are essential for an accurate diagnosis of ID and in evaluation of therapy.

Peripheral Blood

The blood picture in well-developed ID is microcytic (MCV 55–74 fL) and hypochromic (MCHC 22–31 g/dL, MCH 14–26 pg) (Figure 9-8■). Because ID develops progressively,

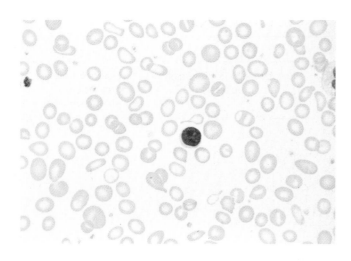

■ FIGURE 9-8   Microcytic, hypochromic anemia of iron deficiency. Compare size of RBCs to nucleus of small lymphocyte in center. (Peripheral blood; Wright-Giemsa stain; 1000× magnification)

any gradation between the well-developed microcytic hypochromic iron-deficient blood picture and normal can occur. Microcytosis and anisocytosis, characterized by an increased RDW, are usually the first morphologic signs, developing even before anemia (∞ Chapter 8). The blood film demonstrates progressively abnormal poikilocytosis. The most frequent poikilocytes are target cells, elliptocytes, and dacryocytes (teardrop cells).

The typical blood picture can be masked if the iron-deficient patient has a concurrent vitamin B_{12} or folate deficiency (causes of macrocytic anemia). In these cases, microcytosis can become apparent only after vitamin B_{12}/folic acid replacement therapy.

Both the relative and absolute number of reticulocytes can be normal or even slightly increased, but the reticulocyte count is decreased relative to the severity of the anemia with an RPI of less than 2. A decreased CHr is an early indicator of iron-restricted erythropoiesis in nonanemic individuals and can be a promising alternative or adjunct to iron studies.[27] In patients on chronic hemodialysis, the CHr has been shown to be superior to the presence of hypochromic red cells in detecting iron deficiency. Using a cutoff of CHr <26 pg, the CHr has a sensitivity of 100% and a specificity of 73%.[32]

The leukocyte count is usually normal but can increase due to chronic marrow stimulation in long-standing cases or after hemorrhage. With concomitant hookworm infestation, eosinophilia can be present.

Platelets can be normal, increased, or decreased. Thrombocytosis frequently accompanies ID. It has been proposed that thrombocytosis is related to ID caused by chronic blood loss. Thrombocytopenia can occur in patients with severe or long-standing anemia, especially if accompanied by folate deficiency. Numeric changes seen in platelets are corrected with treatment that replenishes iron stores.

ⓒ CASE STUDY (continued from page 176)

Jose, the 83-year-old patient, had a CBC upon admission. The results were:

RBC	4.15×10^{12}/L
Hb	81 g/L
Hct	0.26 L/L
Platelets	174×10^9/L
WBC	2.8×10^9/L

1. How would you describe his anemia morphologically?

Iron Studies

Iron studies on iron-deficient patients help establish the diagnosis. The serum iron is decreased, usually less than 30 μg/dL, the TIBC is increased, and transferrin saturation is decreased to less than 15%. Serum iron concentration has a diurnal variation with highest levels in the morning, so sampling time is an important consideration.

The serum ferritin level is decreased in all stages of ID and can be the first indication of a developing ID state. Serum ferritin is generally considered the single best test to detect iron deficiency. Once serum ferritin levels fall below 12 μg/L, the levels may no longer correlate with storage iron because stores are exhausted. Serum ferritin is an important test to differentiate IDA from other microcytic hypochromic anemias. Levels are normal to increased in the anemia of chronic disease unless complicated by ID and increased in sideroblastic anemia and thalassemia.

Because serum ferritin is an acute phase reactant, the lower limit of the reference interval for this parameter may need to be adjusted to detect ID in some patient populations (Table 9-10 ❁). It has been suggested that to detect ID in patients with concommitant anemia of chronic disease, inflammation, infection, pregnancy, and a wide range of concomitant medical problems, the lower limit of serum ferritin should be raised from 12 g/L.[25,33-36] It has also been suggested that the threshold level of serum ferritin for a diagnosis of ID in the aged subject be raised because serum ferritin levels rise with age.[37]

The sTfR assay has proved useful in detecting and differentiating IDA and anemia of chronic disease. Patients with ID have a mean sTfR level over twice (13.91 + 4.63 mg/L) that of mean sTfR levels in normal individuals (5.36 + 0.82 mg/L). Conversely, patients with chronic disease and acute infection (ACD) have mean levels almost identical to those of normal individuals (Table 9-11 ❁). Receptor levels also parallel the reticulocyte count, suggesting that the receptor level can reflect the turnover of transferrin receptors as cells mature. Thus, the sTfR level can provide an index of erythrocyte production in the marrow.

A combination of sTfR and serum ferritin can be used to calculate the TfR-F index:

$$\text{TfR-F Index} = \text{sTfR/log ferritin}$$

✪ TABLE 9-10

Serum Ferritin Cutoff Levels for Detecting Iron Deficiency in Patients with Other Diseases and Conditions

Disease	Upper Serum Ferritin Cutoff Levels for a Diagnosis of ID
Chronic renal disease (absolute ID)	100 µg/L
Chronic renal disease on EPO therapy* (functional ID)	100–800 µg/L
Anemia of chronic disease	50 µg/L
Rheumatoid arthritis	70 µg/L
Other medical problems	100 µg/L
Pregnancy	30 µg/L

Reference interval:
  Males
  Females
	
	20–300 µg/L
	12–200 µg/L

*Functional iron deficiency is present when iron saturation is 20–50%, serum ferritin 100–800 µg/L, and the patient responds to intravenous iron therapy with an increase in hemoglobin and/or a decrease in requirement for EPO.

This index can improve detection of subclinical iron-deficient states in healthy individuals.[38,39] An index of >1.8 indicates depletion of iron stores.

Combinations of serum ferritin, MCV, TIBC, percent saturation, and sTfR can eliminate the need for costly, inconvenient, and painful bone marrow examination to assess iron stores in patients with inflammation or chronic disease and in early stages of ID.[33,40,41]

CASE STUDY *(continued from page 190)*

Reflex testing for anemia on Jose followed based on the CBC results. The following test results were obtained:

Reticulocyte count	2.6%
Serum iron	18 µg/dL
TIBC	425 µg/dL

2. Calculate % saturation.
3. Is this value normal, decreased, or increased?
4. What disease, if any, is suggested by this value?

Erythrocyte Protoporphyrin (EP) Studies

Using ZPP measurement, the evaluation of EP is useful when attempting to identify the etiology of microcytic hypochromic anemia. The concentration of ZPP increases in iron-deficient erythropoiesis and in anemias in which heme synthesis is disturbed. Because ZPP persists throughout the cell's life span, a measure of ZPP utilizing a hematofluorimeter provides a retrospective indicator of iron availability at the time of cell maturation. The ZPP measurement correlates inversely with serum ferritin concentration but is more cost effective.[42] It can detect iron depletion even before anemia develops and thus is a good screening tool for the early stages of ID. Because there is a significant number of nonanemic toddlers with iron depletion and ID has a detrimental effect on development in children, ZPP should be considered as a more sensitive test of ID than the hematocrit.[43] ZPP is also more diagnostically efficient than serum iron or serum

✪ TABLE 9-11

Comparison of Iron Status Parameters Between Groups of Patients with Various Diseases

Patient Group	Hemoglobin (gm/L)*	MCV (fL)*	Serum Iron (µg/dL)*	TIBC (µg/dL)*	Saturation (%)*	Ferritin (µg/L)†	Transferrin Receptor (mg/L)
Normal controls (n = 17)	143 ± 12	93 ± 3	75 ± 28	377 ± 67	20 ± 8	43 (23–80)	5.36 ± 0.82
Iron-deficiency anemia (n = 17)	95 ± 12	74 ± 8	21 ± 15	428 ± 76	5 ± 4	7 (4–12)	13.91 ± 4.63
Acute infection (n = 15)	139 ± 12	88 ± 5	32 ± 23	302 ± 120	14 ± 15	252 (103–613)	5.11 ± 1.42
Anemia of chronic disease (n = 41)	102 ± 12	84 ± 7	35 ± 25	257 ± 87	14 ± 11	220 (86–559)	5.65 ± 1.91
Acute hepatitis (n = 5)	144 ± 8	94 ± 4	121 ± 72	400 ± 70	33 ± 24	2438 (1071–5552)	4.80 ± 1.19
Chronic liver disease with anemia (n = 10)	111 ± 13	97 ± 9	52 ± 32	193 ± 80	28 ± 19	280 (116–677)	5.98 ± 2.06

*Data expressed as mean ± standard deviation
†Data expressed as geometric mean ± standard deviation
MCV = mean cell volume; TIBC = total iron binding capacity
(With permission from: Ferguson BJ et al. Serum transferrin receptor distinguishes the anemia of chronic disease from iron deficiency anemia. *Journal of Laboratory and Clinical Medicine* 119:385, 1992.)

ferritin in screening for ID in the presence of infection or inflammation and in hospitalized patients with microcytic anemia.[42,44] Thus, ZPP can be a valuable screening assay for these populations.

The level of ZPP is useful also as a screening test to differentiate ID and thalassemia, the two most common causes of microcytic hypochromic anemia. ZPP can be elevated in thalassemia, but the increase in ID is 3 to 4 times higher than in thalasssemia.[45] When laboratory analysis reveals a high ZPP combined with a high RDW, ID is strongly suggested.[46] The RDW is typically normal or only slightly elevated in thalassemia trait. Table 9-12 ✪ lists other conditions associated with increased EP levels.

In patients with concurrent lead poisoning, the ZPP cannot be used to distinguish ID and thalassemia because lead inhibits ferrochelatase, the enzyme needed to incorporate iron into the protoporphyrin ring. Consequently, the free erythrocyte porphyrin complexes with zinc, and ZPP is increased in lead poisoning whether or not iron is available.

Bone Marrow

The bone marrow shows mild to moderate erythroid hyperplasia with a decreased M:E ratio. Total cellularity is often moderately increased. This increase in marrow erythropoietic activity without a corresponding increase in peripheral blood reticulocytes suggests an ineffective erthropoietic component. With appropriate iron therapy, the erythroid hyperplasia initially increases and then returns to normal. A common finding (not exclusive to IDA) is the presence of poorly hemoglobinized erythroblasts with scanty irregular (ragged) cytoplasm. This change is most evident at the polychromatophilic stage. Erythroid nuclear abnormalities are sometimes present and can resemble the changes found in dyserythropoietic anemia. These changes include budding, karyorrhexis, nuclear fragmentation, and multinuclearity. Stains for iron reveal an absence of hemosiderin in the macrophages, an invariable characteristic of ID. Sideroblasts are markedly reduced or absent.

Evaluation of iron stores using serum iron studies eliminates the need for bone marrow examination in almost all cases.

✪ TABLE 9-12

Conditions Associated with Increased Erythrocyte Protoporphyrin (EP)

- Anemia of chronic disease
- Iron-deficiency anemia
- Lead poisoning
- Erythropoietic protoporphyria
- Some sideroblastic anemias
- Conditions with markedly increased levels of erythropoiesis
- Thalassemia

THERAPY

Once the cause of the anemia has been established, the principles of treatment are to treat the underlying disorder (e.g., bleeding ulcer), administer iron, and observe the response. The anemia is usually corrected by the oral administration of ferrous sulfate. Parenteral iron therapy, which is more dangerous and expensive than oral iron therapy, is indicated only rarely for unusual circumstances. Intravenous iron dextran is often required in patients with chronic renal disease who are receiving therapy with recombinant human EPO (rHuEPO).[47] To maintain a twofold to threefold increase in the rate of erythrocyte production in patients treated with epoetin alfa, enough iron should be given to maintain serum iron concentrations at 80–100 µg/dL.[48]

Iron-deficient patients treated with iron experience a return of strength, appetite, and a feeling of well-being within 3–5 days whereas the anemia is not alleviated for weeks. The dysphagias also are corrected before the anemia is relieved.

A response to iron therapy is defined as an increase of 1 gm/hemoglobin in one month. Because reticulocytes are new red cells just released from the bone marrow, reticulocyte counts and the CHr or IRF give a snapshot of recent red cell production. Reticulocyte response to iron therapy begins at about the 3rd day after the start of therapy, peaks at about the 9th to 10th day (4–10% reticulocytes), and declines thereafter. Increases in reticulocyte hemoglobin content (CHr) or the immature reticulocyte fraction (IRF) (∞ Chapter 8) are early indicators of a response to iron therapy and begin to increase well in advance of an increase in reticulocytes and hemoglobin.[32,49] If therapy is successful, the hemoglobin should rise until levels within normal limits are established, usually within 6–10 weeks. To restore iron stores, extended therapy with small amounts of iron salts could be required (usually for 6 months) after the hemoglobin has returned to normal.

Due to the high prevalence of ID in toddlers, screening all 1-year-olds for iron deficiency and/or anemia is a well-accepted practice. It has been suggested that if the hemoglobin concentration is decreased, a therapeutic trial of iron be initiated in this population. If anemia persists after one month of therapy, further evaluation is necessary[50] (Web Figure 9-1 ■).

▶ ANEMIA OF CHRONIC DISEASE

The anemia of chronic disease (ACD), also called anemia of inflammation or infection (AI) is usually defined as the anemia that occurs in patients with chronic infections, chronic inflammatory disorders, trauma, organ failure, or neoplastic disorders not due to bleeding, hemolysis, or marrow involvement. ACD is characterized by low serum iron but normal iron stores (Table 9-13 ✪). The anemia appears to be a specific entity and does not relate to any nutritional deficiency. Anemias associated with renal, endocrine, or hepatic insufficiency are usually excluded from ACD.

TABLE 9-13

Conditions Associated with Anemia of Chronic Disorders

Category	Conditions
Chronic infections (after 1–2 months of sustained infection)	Pulmonary infections Subacute bacterial endocarditis Pelvic inflammatory disease Osteomyelitis Chronic urinary tract infection Chronic fungal disease Tuberculosis
Chronic, noninfectious inflammation	Rheumatoid arthritis Rheumatic fever Systemic lupus erythematosus Sterile abscess Regional enteritis Ulcerative colitis
Other	Malignant diseases Alcoholic liver disease Congestive heart failure Thrombophlebitis Ischemic heart disease Severe tissue trauma Thermal injury Fractures

Anemia of chronic disease is the most common anemia other than IDA due to blood loss. It accounts for the anemia in more than one-third of anemic hospitalized patients without blood loss. Anemia is present in up to 50% of patients with malignant solid tumors and is often the clue that leads to a diagnosis of cancer. The most common anemia in these patients is ACD.

PATHOPHYSIOLOGY

ACD is characterized by hypoferremia, decreased transferrin (decreased TIBC), increased serum ferritin, and increased iron in bone marrow macrophages. This suggests a block in the mobilization of iron from macrophages for recycling to the bone marrow normoblasts. Because macrophages recycle 10–20 times more iron than is absorbed by enterocytes, any changes in iron flux through the macrophages affect iron balance more rapidly than changes in iron absorption and transport by enterocytes. Studies reveal that this block in iron release from macrophages is mediated by hepcidin, which is produced in response to interleukin 6 (IL-6) and other inflammatory cytokines (Web Figure 9-2 ■). These cytokines are produced as a result of the immune response and/or inflammatory response and are increased in patients with ACD. Hepcidin plays a role in the body's innate immune system, which is designed to sequester iron from pathogens and thus restrict their growth. The severity of ACD is roughly correlated to the activity of the associated

disease. Absorption of iron in the intestine also is decreased leading to iron deficiency over time.

Other contributing factors to this anemia are decreased erythropoietin (EPO) production and direct suppression of erythropoiesis by cytokines[51,52] (Table 9-14 ❂). In general, the EPO levels in patients with anemia of chronic disease are lower than in anemic patients with similar hemoglobin levels but without chronic disease.[53,54] This finding suggests a blunted EPO response to anemia in ACD. Pharmacologic doses of EPO overcome this inhibitory effect and correct the anemia in some patients.[55]

ACD is also associated with shortened erythrocyte survival as a result of extracorpuscular factors. The reason for the decreased erythrocyte life span is unknown, but several mechanisms have been suggested including nonspecific macrophage activation, hemolytic factors elaborated by tumors, vascular factors, and the presence of bacterial toxins capable of hemolyzing erythrocytes.

Of all mechanisms described, the block in release of iron from macrophages is the most significant.

CLINICAL FEATURES

The signs and symptoms of ACD are usually those associated with the underlying disorder. Rarely severe, the degree of the anemia roughly correlates with the activity of the underlying disease.

LABORATORY FEATURES

Many of the laboratory test results are nonspecific in ACD, but with clinical signs and primary diagnosis, they help to establish that the anemia is ACD. This is important because ACD does not usually require therapy for the anemia.

Peripheral Blood

A mild anemia with a hemoglobin of not less than 90 g/L and hematocrit of not less than 0.27 L/L is characteristic. Erythrocytes are usually normocytic (MCV>85 fL) and normochromic but can present as normocytic, hypochromic, or, in long-standing cases, microcytic and hypochromic (Figure 9-9 ■). The reticulocyte production index is <2. The white blood cell count and platelet count are normal unless they are changed due to the primary disease state.

TABLE 9-14

Mechanisms of Anemia in ACD

- Block in release of iron from macrophages due to increased hepcidin
- Cytokine inhibition of EPO production
- Direct cytokine inhibition of erythropoiesis
- Shortened erythrocyte survival

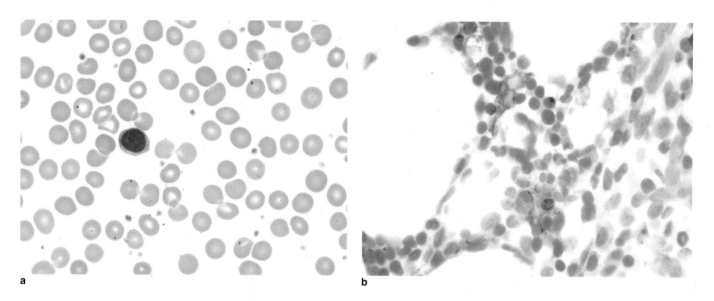

a

b

■ FIGURE 9-9   **a.** Blood film from a patient with anemia of chronic disease. Hb 9.6 g/dL; MCV 76;MCH 24 pg;MCHC 30.6 g/dL. The erythrocytes appear microcytic. (Peripheral blood; Wright-Giemsa stain; 1000× magnification) **b.** Bone marrow from same patient in (a) stained with Prussian blue. Note the macrophages with abundant blue staining iron. (Bone marrow; Prussian blue stain; 1000× magnification)

✓ **Checkpoint! 3**

How does the peripheral blood picture in ACD differ from that seen in IDA?

Iron studies show decreased serum iron (10–70 µg/dL), decreased or normal TIBC (100–300 µg/dL), normal to low transferrin saturation (10–25%), and normal or increased serum ferritin. Serum ferritin can be helpful in distinguishing this anemia from IDA. Although serum iron is low in both anemias, serum ferritin, which reflects body iron stores, is normal or increased in ACD and low in IDA. Because ACD is partially due to iron-deficient erythropoiesis, the ZPP levels are increased.

It is important to keep in mind that ferritin is an acute phase reactant and is very often increased in inflammatory conditions. Therefore, in ACD, serum ferritin can be normal even if concurrent ID exists. If serum ferritin falls in the interval of 20–100 µg/L in ACD, another means of assessing iron should be considered, such as sTfR assay or bone marrow examination.[56] Serum TfR is high in IDA but normal in uncomplicated ACD.

CASE STUDY *(continued from page 191)*

5. How do the patient's iron study results help in differentiating the diagnosis of iron defiency from ACD?

6. What additional iron test that was not done would be most helpful in this case?

Bone Marrow   The bone marrow usually shows an increased M:E ratio because of a decrease in erythrocyte precursors. The proportion of younger erythroblasts is increased. Poor hemoglobin production is apparent, especially in the polychromatophilic erythroblasts. The proportion of sideroblasts decreases to less than 30%; however, the macrophages appear to have increased amounts of hemosiderin in the form of coarse iron aggregates (Figure 9-9b). This finding helps to distinguish the anemia of chronic disease from IDA. In IDA, macrophage iron and sideroblasts are absent.

Bone marrow examination is usually not necessary for distinguishing ACD from IDA. An algorithm using the MCV, serum ferritin, and iron saturation can correctly differentiate and classify most cases of ACD and IDA[45] (Web Figure 9-3 ■). Additional tests, such as sTfR and calculation of the sTfR-F index, can provide additional diagnostic information in some cases.

THERAPY

Anemia can be alleviated by successful treatment of the underlying disease. Anemia is usually mild and nonprogressive; thus, transfusion is rarely warranted except in older patients with vascular disease and circulatory insufficiency.

▶ ANEMIAS ASSOCIATED WITH ABNORMAL HEME SYNTHESIS

These anemias are associated with defects in enzymes of the heme biosynthetic pathway leading to abnormal heme synthesis. Iron incorporation into the protoporphyrin ring to form heme can be blocked. In contrast to IDA, the positive iron balance in these anemias can lead to an increase in iron stores predominantly in the spleen, liver, and bone marrow. Serum ferritin levels above 250 µg/L in the male and above 200 µg/L in the female indicate increased iron stores.

The conditions discussed in this section include sideroblastic anemia and the porphyrias. Lead poisoning also is included because of its pathophysiologic relationship to these anemias through a block in heme synthesis.

SIDEROBLASTIC ANEMIAS

Mutations that affect the first enzymatic step in heme synthesis, the formation of ALA, result in sideroblastic anemia. Mutations in the subsequent steps of heme synthesis result in metabolic disorders called *porphyrias*. Sideroblastic anemia (SA) is the result of diverse clinical and biochemical manifestations that reflect multiple underlying hereditary, congenital, or acquired pathogenic mechanisms. However, all types are characterized by (1) an increase in total body iron, (2) the presence of ringed sideroblasts in the bone marrow, and (3) hypochromic anemia.

Classification

The classification of sideroblastic anemia is arbitrary at best, and many different schemes of classification exist. The classification in Table 9-15 ✪ is one of the most descriptive. The two major groups are those that are inherited and those that are acquired.

Hereditary Form   The most common form of hereditary sideroblastic anemia is due to a defective sex-linked recessive gene. Although carrier females often show a dimorphic population of morphologically abnormal and normal erythrocytes, they rarely have anemia. Affected males demonstrate the typical findings of sideroblastic anemia. In rare instances, both sexes are equally affected implying the presence of another hereditary form that is transmitted in an autosomal recessive manner. In the hereditary forms, anemia can become apparent in infancy but most commonly appears in young adulthood. Symptoms rarely do not occur until age 60.

Acquired Form   The acquired forms of sideroblastic anemia are more common than the hereditary forms. The acquired forms are classified according to whether the basis of

the anemia is unknown (idiopathic) or is secondary to an underlying disease or toxin (secondary type). The idiopathic form, *refractory anemia with ringed sideroblasts (RARS)*, can affect either sex in adult life. It is included in a group of acquired stem cell disorders called *myelodysplastic syndromes* (∞ Chapter 23) that have a tendency to terminate in acute leukemia.

The acquired secondary type sideroblastic anemias are associated with malignancy, drugs, or other toxic substances. In this type, once the underlying disorder is effectively treated or the toxin removed, the anemia abates.

Pathophysiology

Studies of patients with sideroblastic anemia have shown disturbances of the enzymes regulating heme synthesis. Ringed sideroblasts are specific findings for these heme enzyme abnormalities. Ringed sideroblasts are formed from an accumulation of nonferritin iron in the mitochondria that encircle the erythroblast nucleus. The mitochondria eventually rupture as they become iron laden. When stained with Prussian blue, the iron appears as blue punctate deposits circling the nucleus (ringed sideroblasts). Iron within the erythroblasts is normally deposited diffusely throughout the cytoplasm.

Hereditary Sideroblastic Anemia   Defective heme synthesis appears to be involved in the pathogenesis of the hereditary form of sideroblastic anemia. The most common form of SA in this group is sex linked and due to an abnormal δ-aminolevulinate synthase enzyme (ALAS).

Two different forms of ALAS are the nonerythroid or hepatic form (ALAS1) and the erythroid form (ALAS2). The nonerythroid form, also known as the *housekeeping form,* is coded for by a gene expressed in all tissues and has been assigned to the chromosomal region 3p21. The erythroid form is coded for by a gene that has been assigned to the Xp21-q21 chromosomal region. ALAS2 is the first and rate-limiting enzyme in heme synthesis.

Sex-linked SA (XLSA) is due to an abnormal ALAS2 enzyme that is the result of heterogeneous point mutations in the catalytic domain of the ALAS2 gene.[57] More than 22 different mutations have been described in this gene.[58] The mutations are located in exons 5–11 and all but one are missense (single-base change) leading to substitution of a single amino acid in the protein.

Evidence indicates that the activity of ALAS2 depends totally on the presence of the cofactor, pyridoxal phosphate. This cofactor binds to the enzyme and is crucial for its stability, for the maintenance of a conformation optimal for substrate binding and product release, and for its catalytic activity. In 17 of the 22 ALAS2 mutations, there is a partial to complete clinical response to pharmacologic doses of pyridoxine. Excess pyridoxine possibly enhances the abnormal ALAS enzyme activity by stabilizing it after synthesis.[58] In the pyridoxine-refractory sex-linked SA, it appears that the gene mutation affects the processing of ALAS2 precursor, which terminates ALAS2 translation prematurely or abolishes its function.[58,59]

✪ TABLE 9-15	
Classification of Sideroblastic Anemia	
Hereditary	**Acquired**
Sex linked	Idiopathic refractory sideroblastic anemia
Autosomal recessive	(IRSA) or refractory anemia with ringed
	sideroblasts (RARS)
	Secondary to drugs, toxins, lead
	Associated with malignancy

Significant ineffective erythropoiesis is characterized by bone marrow erythroid hyperplasia. This increased erythropoietic activity results in increased iron absorption in the gut. Iron overload can be significant and can lead to complications such as cardiac failure and diabetes.

Other hereditary forms of sideroblastic anemia have been described but are less common than the sex-linked type.[60]

Acquired Sideroblastic Anemia   The acquired SA can be categorized as refractory anemia with ringed sideroblasts (RARS) and those secondary to drugs or toxins.

RARS.   This form of SA is considered to be the result of an acquired stem cell disorder. It is discussed in the chapter on myelodysplastic syndromes (∞ Chapter 23).

Secondary to Drugs or Toxins.   Acquired sideroblastic anemia secondary to drugs or toxins is the result of the interference of the drugs or toxins with the activity of heme enzymes. Lead and alcohol are the most common causes of this form of SA.

Lead Poisoning. Lead poisoning (**plumbism**) has been recognized for centuries. In children, it generally results from ingestion of flaked lead-based paint from painted items. Lead was removed from paint after 1978. Children from lower socioeconomic backgrounds are at increased risk; those between 1 and 3 years of age are at greatest risk. Clinically, lead toxicity in children is associated with hyperactivity, low IQ, concentration disorders, hearing loss, and impaired growth and development. In adults, lead poisoning is primarily the result of inhalation of lead or lead compounds from industrial processes. It is the most common disease of toxic environmental origin in the United States.[61]

Many states require laboratories and physicians to report elevated blood lead levels to the state health department, which can report to the Centers for Disease Control (CDC). Thirty-seven states reported elevated blood levels to the CDC in 2004. Although average blood lead levels have dropped by 80% since the late 1970s, about 10,000 adults had blood lead levels >25 μg/dL in 2004.[62] Hundreds of thousands of children under age six still have increased blood lead levels.

Lead serves no physiological purpose. Although lead poisoning consistently shortens the erythrocyte life span, the anemia accompanying plumbism is not primarily the result of hemolysis but of a marked abnormality in heme synthesis. Once ingested, lead passes through the blood to the bone marrow, where it accumulates in the mitochondria of erythroblasts and inhibits cellular enzymes involved in heme synthesis. The heme enzymes most sensitive to lead inhibition are δ-aminolevulinic acid dehydrase (δ-ALA-D) and ferrocheletase (heme synthase) (∞ Chapter 6). The effect of lead on ferrochelatase is competitive inhibition with iron. Other enzymes can be affected at higher lead concentrations. Thus, the synthesis of heme is primarily disturbed at the conversion of δ-ALA to porphobilinogen (which uses the enzyme δ-ALA-D), and at the incorporation of iron into protoporphyrin to form heme (which uses the enzyme fer-

rochelatase). As a result, urine excretion of δ-ALA increases. The erythrocyte protoporphyrin (in the form of ZPP) is also strikingly increased. Iron accumulates in the cell.

Studies have revealed that microcytic, hypochromic anemia is not characteristic of elevated lead levels in children. Evidence suggests that the presence of a microcytic anemia in plumbism is most likely due to complications of ID or to the coexistence of alpha-thalassemia trait.[63–65] One study found that 33% of African American children with lead poisoning and microcytosis had alpha-thalassemia trait.[63]

Coexistent ID and lead poisoning put children at a higher risk for developing even more serious lead poisoning because children absorb larger portions of lead in iron-deficient states and the competitive inhibition of ferrochelatase by lead is even greater in the absence of iron. Thus, it is critical to make a diagnosis of ID when it coexists with lead poisoning.

In 1991, the Centers for Disease Control and Prevention (CDC) set a new acceptable blood lead level at 10 μg/dL or less, down from the 30 μg/dL level set in the mid-1970s. The CDC also recommended five decision levels for evaluation and treatment depending on the lead level (Web Table 9-1 ✪).

Although the zinc protoporphyrin (ZPP) measurement has been utilized to screen for lead in the past, it is no longer recommended as an appropriate screening tool because ZPP is unaffected until lead levels reach approximately 20 μg/dL.[66] It is now apparent that lead levels <20 μg/dL can impair neuropsychologic development. Thus, ZPP can be useful as a screening tool in children with very high lead levels, but screening generally should be done by direct lead measurements. ZPP cannot be used to differentiate IDA and thalassemia in the presence of lead poisoning because of the increase in erythrocyte protoporphyrin caused by lead.

Alcoholism. Anemia is a common finding (up to 62%) in hospitalized chronic alcoholics.[26] Megaloblastic and sideroblastic anemia occur in the majority, but anemia in this population has many other causes including ACD, IDA, acute blood loss and chronic hemolysis[67] (Table 9-16 ✪). Less than one-half have an isolated cause for the anemia (Table 9-17 ✪). Studies show that sideroblastic anemia is particularly common among alcoholics with a poor diet and can be

---

✪ TABLE 9-16

Mechanisms of Anemia in Chronic Alcoholism

- Megaloblastosis associated with folate deficiency
- Iron-deficiency anemia from chronic or acute blood loss
- Sideroblastic anemia from toxic effects of alcohol on enzymes needed for heme synthesis
- Hemolytic anemia

    Chronic hemolysis due to splenic sequestration

    Spur cell anemia occurring in the setting of severe liver disease, splenomegaly, and jaundice

    Transient hemolytic anemia associated with portal hypertension and acute congestive splenomegaly

TABLE 9-17

Incidence and Causes of Anemia in Study
of 121 Hospitalized Alcoholics[67]

Number of Causes of Anemia	Proportion	Associated Causes as Defined by Laboratory Findings	Percentage
One	45%	ACD	81%
Two	37%	Megaloblastic changes in BM	34
Three	18%	Ringed sideroblasts	23
		Iron deficiency	13

ACD = Anemia of Chronic Disease

associated with a concommitant decrease in folic acid and megaloblastosis (∞ Chapter 12). The presence of a dimorphic erythrocyte population and siderocytes in the peripheral blood is a clue to a diagnosis of SA. Alcohol is believed to interfere with some enzymes of hemoglobin synthesis including inhibition of the synthesis of pyridoxal phosphate and of activity of uroporphyrinogen decarboxylase and ferrochelatase but enhancement of activity of δ-aminolevulinic acid synthase. Alcoholics with a poor diet can also have an inadequate intake of pyridoxine. Alcohol is directly toxic to hematologic cells as evidenced by the frequent presence of vacuoles in bone marrow precursor cells, thrombocytopenia, and granulocytopenia.

Interpreting laboratory tests in alcoholism is difficult because the alcohol has effects on multiple parameters. Even in the absence of megaloblastosis and anemia, the cells are frequently macrocytic (MCV 100–110 fL). Alcohol has a direct effect on folate metabolism, interfering with absorption, storage, and release. Serum iron levels are increased during drinking episodes but return to normal after cessation.

Secondary to Malignancy   Ringed sideroblasts can be found in diseases other than sideroblastic anemia (Table 9-18 ✪). For example, ringed sideroblasts are often associated with hematologic malignancies (e.g., leukemia, malignant histiocytosis, multiple myeloma, lymphoma). Some investigators believe that the presence of ringed sideroblasts in these disorders suggests that the malignancy can result from

TABLE 9-18

Diseases Associated with the Presence
of Ringed Sideroblasts

- Sideroblastic anemia
- Myelodysplastic syndromes: refractory anemia with ringed sideroblasts
- Megaloblastic anemia
- Primary bone marrow disorders
- Chemotherapy

an abnormal clone of pluripotential stem cells that affects the erythrocyte as well as other cell lineages. Occasionally, ringed sideroblasts appear in the bone marrow following treatment of malignant disease (e.g., multiple myeloma, Hodgkin's disease). The appearance of ringed sideroblasts after treatment is a very poor prognostic sign, as these cases almost always terminate in acute leukemia.

Clinical Features
In patients with acquired sideroblastic anemias secondary to drugs or malignancy, the manifestations of the underlying disorder dominate. Patients with hereditary sideroblastic anemia or RARS, however, generally show primary signs and symptoms of anemia. In hereditary sideroblastic anemias, most patients also exhibit signs associated with iron overload including hepatomegaly, splenomegaly, and diabetes. In the latter stages of the disease, cardiac function may be affected.

Laboratory Features
See Table 9-19 ✪ for laboratory findings in sideroblastic anemia.

Peripheral Blood   The anemia is usually moderate to severe. A dimorphic picture of normochromic and hypochromic cells is characteristically seen in inherited and acquired secondary forms of sideroblastic anemia (Figure 9-10■). Dual

TABLE 9-19

Laboratory Findings in Sideroblastic Anemia

- Dual population of hypochromic and normochromic erythrocytes
- Pappenheimer bodies in erythrocytes
- Normal or increased platelets
- Increased serum iron, serum ferritin, and percent saturation
- Ringed sideroblasts in the bone marrow

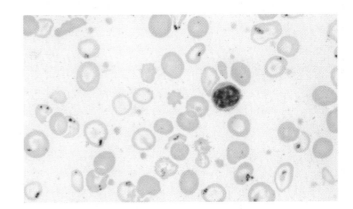

■ FIGURE 9-10   Blood film from a patient with sideroblastic anemia. Two populations of erythrocytes are present: hypochromic and normochromic. This is the dimorphic blood picture typical of sideroblastic anemia. Note also the numerous inclusions (Pappenheimer bodies). (Peripheral blood; Wright-Giemsa stain; 1000× magnification)

populations of macrocytes and microcytes or normocytes can also be found. Hypochromic macrocytes are especially prevalent in RARS whereas hypochromic microcytes are common in the hereditary form of SA. Macrocytes are common in SA associated with alcoholism.

If a dimorphic erythrocyte population is present, the MCV, MCH, and MCHC can be normal because these parameters represent an average of all erythrocytes, thus emphasizing the need for careful examination of CBC parameters and the blood smear. The RDW and erythrocyte histogram/cytogram are useful in detecting these dual populations. The RDW is increased, and the RBC histogram/cytogram shows two peaks representing the dual population.

Other abnormalities of erythrocytes are often seen. Poikilocytosis and target cells can be present. Erythrocytes can contain **Pappenheimer bodies** (iron deposits) (∞ Chapter 35). When Pappenheimer bodies are present, reticulocyte counts must be performed carefully because both RNA and Pappenheimer bodies take up supravital stains. On the other hand, Pappenheimer bodies stain with both Romanowsky stains and Prussian blue stain, whereas reticulated RNA does not stain with either. (Polychromatophilic erythrocytes, which are young red cells with RNA, do stain with Romanowsky stain. These cells stain as reticulocytes with supravital stains.) Nucleated erythrocytes are rarely present.

Basophilic stippling can be seen in any of the sideroblastic anemias. However, coarse, punctate, basophilic stippling resulting from aggregated ribosomes and degenerating mitochrondria is a particularly characteristic feature of lead poisoning (Figure 9-11 ■). The punctate stippling occurs in the reticulocyte and is found in developing erythroblasts. It has been shown that the granules in these stippled erythroblasts contain free ionized iron and that the hemoglobin

production in the cells is grossly deficient. Many stippled cells in peripheral blood in lead poisoning are actually siderocytes.

Other laboratory test results can be abnormal. Even though the bone marrow is usually hyperplastic, the reticulocyte production index is <2, indicating that the anemia has an ineffective erythropoietic component. Other indications of ineffective erythropoiesis including a slightly increased serum bilirubin (usually <2.0 mg/dL), decreased haptoglobin, and increased lactate dehydrogenase (LD) are usually present. Iron studies show increased serum iron, normal or decreased TIBC with increased saturation levels (sometimes reaching 100%), and increased serum ferritin. Leukocyte and platelet counts are usually normal but can be decreased. Thrombocytosis is found in about a one-third of patients.

In alcoholics, the direct and indirect effects of alcohol complicate the interpretation of laboratory tests used to diagnose anemia including MCV, serum iron, TIBC, serum ferritin, and red cell and serum folate (Figure 9-12 ■).

CASE STUDY *(continued from page 194)*

7. Do the iron studies in Jose (serum iron 18 μg/dL, TIBC 425 μg/dL) suggest sideroblastic anemia?

Bone Marrow   Bone marrow changes include erythroid hyperplasia often accompanied by various degrees of megaloblastosis. The megaloblastosis is sometimes responsive to folate, which indicates the presence of a complicating folate deficiency. Erythroblasts appear poorly hemoglobinized with scanty, irregular cytoplasm. Macrophages contain increased amounts of storage iron. Ringed sideroblasts constitute more than 40% of the erythroblasts (Figure 9-13 ■). Ringed sideroblasts are erythroblasts with iron granules that encircle one-third or more of the nucleus. The siderotic granules are

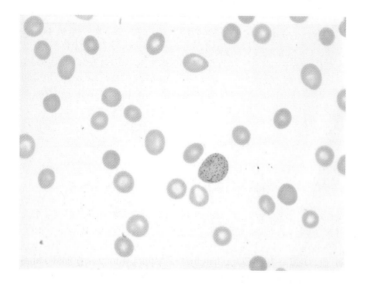

■ FIGURE 9-11   Peripheral blood smear from a patient with lead poisoning. Note the heavy basophilic stippling in erythrocyte. (Peripheral blood; Wright-Giemsa stain; 1000× magnification)

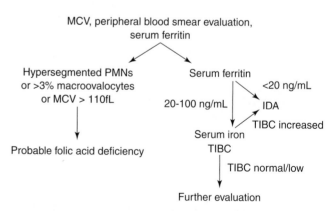

■ FIGURE 9-12   An algorithm for diagnosis of anemia in alcoholics

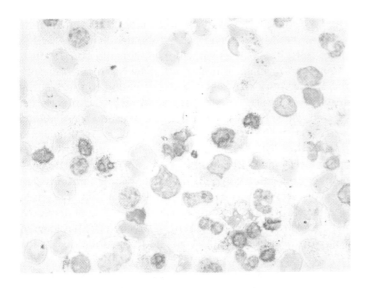

■ **FIGURE 9-13**   Ringed sideroblasts. (Bone marrow; Prussian blue stain; 1000× magnification)

larger than those found in normal sideroblasts. In the hereditary forms of sideroblastic anemia, the abnormal granules occur primarily in the later stages of erythroblast development and the polychromatophilic and orthochromatic erythroblast stages. In the idiopathic and secondary forms, the abnormal granules occur beginning at the earlier erythroblast stages.

The ringed sideroblasts must be present for the diagnosis of sideroblastic anemia; however, it is important to recognize that other disease entities may have ringed sideroblasts present without involving a diagnosis of sideroblastic anemia.

Molecular Studies   If hereditary sex-linked sideroblastic anemia is suspected based on erythrocyte morphology and iron studies, the patient should be tested for the presence of ALAS2 gene mutations. This can be done by studying genomic DNA or cDNA (from RNA) of reticulocytes[58] (∞ Chapter 39). If a mutation is found, other family members should be tested. Even if anemia is not present in family members, there is a risk of iron overload. Molecular studies also allow a distinction to be made between hereditary sideroblastic anemia and RARS.

 CASE STUDY *(continued from page 198)*

8. Do Jose's laboratory test results and clinical history indicate that a bone marrow examination is necessary?

Therapy
Pyridoxine therapy is generally tried on patients with the hereditary form of sideroblastic anemia; less than one-half experience a return to normal hemoglobin levels with this form of therapy, although some have a partial response. In some patients, iron overload decreases responsiveness to pyridoxine, but when the iron load is reduced by phlebotomy, hemoglobin concentration increases.[68] Folic acid is administered to those with megaloblastic features. Although the anemia can be treated, iron overload is the primary complication of this anemia. Sometimes the risk of hemochromatosis is lessened by removal of excess body iron through phlebotomy or chelation therapy. Iron overload is monitored by iron studies (percent saturation of transferrin). Female carriers should also be monitored. Some patients live for many years tolerating their anemia well; others die because of complications of iron overload, infections, or bone marrow failure.

Secondary sideroblastic anemia resulting from a disease, toxin, or drug may be corrected by successful treatment of the disease or by elimination of the toxin/drug.

▶ **HEMOCHROMATOSIS**

Hemochromatosis is a term used to describe the clinical disorder that results in parenchymal tissue damage from progressive iron overload. Hemochromatosis typically is not associated with anemia but is included in this chapter because iron studies are markedly abnormal in patients with the disorder. Due to its prevalence, hemochromatosis should be considered when symptoms are present, when there is a family history of the disorder, or when iron studies suggest iron overload. Iron overload is said to exist when serum ferritin is higher than 200 µg/L in premenopausal women or higher than 300 µg/L in men and postmenopausal women. The danger of hemochromatosis lies in the fact that excess iron deposits are stored not only in macrophages but also in hepatocytes, cardiac cells, endocrine cells, and other parenchymal tissue. Iron interferes with the normal function of these cells. This situation has potentially fatal consequences, especially in relation to cardiac and hepatic tissue.

Hemochromatosis is classified as hereditary or secondary. The hereditary form is caused by genetic mutations. The secondary type is associated with other hematologic diseases and a variety of other conditions. (Table 9-20 ✪)

HEREDITARY HEMOCHROMATOSIS

Etiology and Pathophysiology
Hereditary hemochromatosis (HH) is characterized by increased iron absorption in the gut and progressive iron overload. It is a genetic disorder with a prevalence of 1 in 200–250 persons. One in 10 Caucasians in the United States is a carrier. It is the most common genetic abnormality in those with a European ancestry. At least five genes have been implicated in causing HH including hepcidin, *HFE*, *TfR2*, ferroportin, and *HJV* genes. Mutations in *HFE*, *TfR2* and *HJV* appear to cause aberrant regulation of hepcidin (Table 9-21 ✪).

✪ TABLE 9-20

Causes of Iron Overload

Hereditary
- Classical hemochromatosis: HFE mutations (type I)
- Juvenile hemochromatosis (type 2)
- Hemojuvelin (HJV) mutations
- Hepcidin mutations
- Transferrin-receptor 2 deficiency (type 3)
- Ferroportin deficiency (type 4)
- DMT1 mutations and congenital atransferrinemia

Secondary
- Anemias with ineffective erythropoiesis (i.e., Sickle cell anemia, thalassemia, refractory anemias with erythroid hypercellular bone marrow, X-linked sideroblastic anemia)
- Chronic transfusions
- Chronic liver disease
- Viral hepatitis
- Dietary iron overload
- Overload from injections or ingestion of iron supplements
- Alcoholism

The most common form of HH in populations of European origin is due to mutations in the *HFE* gene, identified in 1996.[69] Mutations result in an autosomal recessive disorder of low penetrance with adult onset. Clinical disease is more common in males than females. The *HFE* gene is mapped to chromosome 6(6q21,3). The most common mutation is cys282 → tyrosine: C282Y. Less common are the mutations his63 → asp: H63D and ser65 → cys: S65C. Clinical signs of the disease may be found in homozygous C282Y and compound heterozygosity for C282Y and H63D. The penetrance of C282Y is low with only half of homozygotes developing iron overload (increased serum Tf saturation and serum ferritin levels) and ~1% with clinical features of hemosiderosis. This suggests that modifier genes and epigenetic or environmental factors affect the severity of the HH phenotype. Genetic mutations in at least two genes have been proposed to affect the phenotypic expression of homozygous *C282Y*: *HJV* and hepcidin.[70,71]

The normal HFE protein is a cell surface transmembrane protein found in the crypt cells of the duodenum as well as other cells. It associates with B_2-microglobulin and TfR. It is thought to regulate iron absorption by its interaction with the TfR in those cells.[72] When HFE is bound to the TfR, the affinity of the TfR for the iron-transferrin complex is decreased. Thus, the ability of the mucosal cell to sense plasma iron and regulate iron absorption depends on the interaction of HFE with TfR. The mechanism of how mutations in the HFE protein may affect iron metabolism is unclear but may involve interactions of HFE with proteins in addition to TfR as it has been shown that HFE can regulate iron concentration in cells without binding to TfR. The finding of decreased hepatic expression of hepcidin in *HFE* related HH has focused attention on the role of HFE in the liver. Mutations in the *HFE* gene result in inappropriately low hepcidin expression, suggesting that the *HFE* gene is involved in the normal regulation of synthesis of hepcidin and that the effect of the mutated *HFE* gene is due to hepcidin deficiency. About 3–4 mg of iron a day is absorbed from the GI tract as compared to 1–2 mg normally. Because the body has no mechanism to excrete excess iron, it accumulates at about 0.5–1.0 gm/year. Cells' capacity to store iron by complexing with apoferritin is exceeded and "free" intracellular iron accumulates. This free iron facilitates the buildup of reactive oxygen species that cause cell injury and cell death and leads to organ failure. Most of the excess iron is deposited in the liver.

Other less common forms of HH are due to mutations in other genes involved in iron sensing and regulation but all appear to result in deregulation of hepcidin expression. Mutations of the TfR2 gene results in a disease that is clinically indistinguishable from HFE-associated HH.

Genetic mutations in the ferroportin gene are expressed in an autosomal dominant fashion. Mutations that affect ferroportin's ability to export iron cause iron overload in reticuloendothelial cells ("ferroportin disease"), and mutations that cause hyporesponsiveness of ferroportin to hepcidin result in increased absorption of iron and iron overload in parenchymal cells of the liver and other organs.

✪ TABLE 9-21

Role of Iron-Regulating Proteins in the Pathogenesis of Disorders of Iron Metabolism

Disorder	Defect/Mutation	Fe Absorption	Fe in Macrophages	Plasma Iron	Ferritin
ACD	IL-6 increases hepcidin, which binds ferroportin	Decreased	Increased	Decreased	Increased
Hereditary hemochromatosis (autosomal recessive)	*HFE* gene; *TfR2* gene	Increased	Decreased	Increased	Increased
Hereditary hemochromatosis (juvenile; autosomal recessive)	*HJV* gene Hepcidin gene	Increased	Decreased	Increased	Increased
Hereditary hemochromatosis (autosomal dominant)	Ferroportin gene	Increased	Increased	Normal until late in disease	Increased
Iron-loading anemias (ineffective erythropoiesis)	Erythropoietic drive-suppresses hepcidin synthesis	Increased	Increased (due to hemolysis)	Increased	Increased

Mutations in the hemojuvelin (*HJV*) gene cause a severe autosomal dominant type of HH. This type affects young men and women usually in the second decade of life. A marked decrease in hepcidin occurs, resulting in severe iron overload. A subgroup of patients with juvenile hemochromatosis have a null mutation in the hepcidin gene. The consequence is a complete absence of hepcidin-mediated control of intestinal iron absorption and severe iron overload.

Rare mutations in the transferrin gene and ceruloplasmin gene produce autosomal recessive disorders affecting iron metabolism. Congenital hypotransferrinemia is characterized by increased iron absorption but the unbound iron circulates in plasma without a mechanism for uptake into developing erythroblasts. There is severe hypochromic, microcytic anemia. The circulating nontransferrin-bound iron is deposited in the parenchymal cells of the liver, heart, and pancreas. Ceruloplasmin serves an essential role in catalyzing the oxidation of Fe^{++} to Fe^{+++}, which is the form necessary for binding to apotransferrin. Although excess iron is deposited in tissues, liver injury does not occur. A mild normochromic, normocytic anemia is characteristically found.

Clinical Findings

Clinical penetrance of the most common form of HH is incomplete and only 1 in 5,000 have clinical symptoms. About 81% of symptomatic patients have the C282Y/C282Y genotype. Asymptomatic patients who have the C282Y/C282Y genotype or the H63D/C282Y genotype should have their serum iron and ferritin levels monitored for they are at risk for developing iron storage disease. Clinical findings include chronic fatigue, arthralgia, infertility, impotence, cardiac disease, diabetes, and/or cirrhosis.[73] Hyperpigmentation of the skin is also found.

Laboratory Findings

Screening tests for hemochromatosis usually include percent saturation of transferrin and serum ferritin. The criterion for a diagnosis of hemochromatosis is usually >50% transferrin saturation in females and >60% saturation in males. Saturation often approaches 100%. Adding serum ferritin analysis increases specificity for HH. Iron overload is suggested when the serum ferritin is elevated. Although an increase in transferrin saturation is sensitive for hemochromatosis, DNA testing to identify the mutated gene is necessary to definitively diagnose hereditary hemochromatosis (HH). Biopsy of the liver and/or bone marrow usually are not needed. Liver enzymes are usually elevated. Anemia is not present unless complicating conditions exist.

Screening for HH is controversial. Some have recommended population screening with transferrin saturation and suggest that laboratories include transferrin saturation in their routine lab panels.[74] Genetic screening is still very costly for population screening, and unresolved ethical issues including patient privacy, counseling, and insurance concerns exist. With the recognition of the low penetrance of clinical disease (<1%), interest in large-scale screening has largely disappeared. It is recommended, however, that both symptomatic and asymptomatic first-degree relatives of those with HH be tested because transferrin saturation will not detect carriers.[75] The goal in screening and identifying the disease early is to allow treatment with phlebotomy before the onset of clinical disease.

SECONDARY HEMOCHROMATOSIS

Secondary hemochromatosis is associated with a number of conditions including anemias that have an ineffective erythropoietic component and increased iron absorption. These include β-thalassemia, congenital dyserythropoietic anemia, X-linked sideroblastic anemia, and anemias associated with DMT1 mutations. Iron overload often develops in patients who have transfusion-dependent anemias such as sickle cell disease. Iron overload is also found in chronic liver disease and congenital atransfrerrinemia. Serum iron studies are also abnormal in 40–50% of patients with chronic viral hepatitis, alcoholic liver disease, and nonalcoholic steatohepatitis. Alcohol disrupts normal iron metabolism and results in excess iron deposition in the liver in about one-third of alcoholics.[76]

TREATMENT

Phlebotomy is usually the treatment for HH. Each unit of blood removes about 250 mg of iron from the body. It is suggested that following initial venesection therapy to deplete iron stores, iron status be monitored annually by serum ferritin levels.[77]

Treatment of secondary hemochromatosis sometimes includes the infusion of iron chelators (e.g., deferoxamine) to bind iron and enable urinary excretion. Only a very small amount of iron is available for chelation (from the labile pool) at one time; thus, continuous infusion of the chelator over a long period of time is required to remove this iron. Chelation therapy is the primary form of treatment for transfusion-induced hemochromatosis.

 Checkpoint! 4

What is the risk of population genetic screening for HH? What is the benefit of population genetic screening for HH?

▶ PORPHYRIAS

Heme is an iron-chelated porphyrin ring. Its biosynthesis occurs in most cells, but the major sites of synthesis are in the erythroid cells of the bone marrow and hepatocytes. Thus, the activity of the enzymes catalyzing porphyrin metabolism is highest in these cells.

The porphyrias represent a group of inherited disorders characterized by a block in porphyrin synthesis. Abnormal porphyrin metabolism is due to a defect in one or more of the enzymes in the heme synthesis pathway. As a result of these enzyme deficiencies, the porphyrin heme precursors behind the bottleneck accumulate in tissues, and large amounts are excreted in the urine and/or feces. These excess porphyrin deposits cause most of the symptoms and clinical findings associated with porphyria. The most common findings include photosensitivity, abdominal pain, and neuropathy (motor dysfunction, sensory loss, and mental disturbances). However, usually adequate production of heme for hemoglobin synthesis occurs.

Although rare, the porphyrias have received wide recognition and stimulated interest because the disease affected the royal families of England and Scotland, especially those descended from Mary, Queen of Scots. Historians have described George III as suffering from a mental and physical disorder thought to have been porphyria. Princess Charlotte, the granddaughter of George III and heir to the throne, died in childbirth; her death was attributed to an acute porphyria attack at the time of delivery.

Two forms of porphyria (erythropoietic and hepatic) are expressed, depending on the primary site (bone marrow or liver) of defective porphyrin metabolism (Table 9-22 ✪). Only the erythropoietic porphyrias affect the erythrocytes. Therefore, these porphyrias are discussed here.

PATHOPHYSIOLOGY

The erythropoietic prophyrias result from an abnormality of the enzymes in the heme biosynthetic pathway within the erythroblasts of the bone marrow. At least two types exist: congenital erythropoietic porphyria (CEP) and erythropoietic protoporphyria (EPP). These two types are classified according to the particular enzyme defect and the excessive porphyrin intermediates produced. Although CEP is associated with hemolytic anemia, anemia in EPP is rare.

Porphyrins are functionless products produced by the irreversible oxidation of type I and type III porphyrinogens.

✪ TABLE 9-22

Classification and Characteristics of the Porphyrias

| Porphyria | Mode of Inheritance | Enzymatic Defect | Metabolites in Excess | | | Tissue Source |
			Urine	Feces	Erythroid Cells	
Erythropoietic						
Congenital erythropoietic porphyria (CEP)	Autosomal recessive	Uroporphyrinogen III cosynthase	Uroporphyrin I, Coproporphyrin I	Coproporphyrin I, uroporphyrin I	Uroporphyrin I, coproporphyrin I	Erythropoietic
Congenital erythropoietic protoporphyria (EPP)	Autosomal dominant	Ferrocheletase (Heme synthase)	Normal	Protoporphyrin	Protoporphyrin	Erythropoietic and occasionally hepatic
Hepatic and erythropoietic						
Hepatoerythropoietic porphyria (HEP)	Recessive	Uroporphyrinogen decarboxylase	Uroporphyrin	Uroporphyrin	ZPP	Hepatic and erythropoietic
Hepatic						
Acute intermittent porphyria (AIP)	Autosomal dominant	Porphobilinogen deaminase	δ-ALA, Porphobilinogen	Sometimes coproporphyrin and protoporphyrin	Normal	Hepatic
Hereditary coproporphyria (HCP)	Autosomal dominant	Coproporphyrinogen oxidase	Coproporphyrin III; Uroporphyrin (in attack)	Coproporphyrin III	Normal	Hepatic
Variegate porphyria (PV)	Autosomal dominant	Protoporphyrinogen oxidase	Porphobilinogen, δ-ALA, Uroporphyrin, Coproporphyrin	Protoporphyrin Coproporphyrin	Normal	Hepatic
Porphyria cutanea tarda (PCT)	Autosomal dominant	Uroporphyrinogen decarboxylase	Uroporphyrin I Uroporphyrin III, Coproporphyrin (slight)	Protoporphyrin Coproporphyrin	Normal	Hepatic
ALA dehydratase deficiency porphyria (ADP)	Autosomal recessive	ALA dehydratase	δ-ALA, Coproporphyrin III		Normal	Hepatic

Porphyrinogens of the type III series are the precursors of heme whereas the type I isomers do not produce any useful metabolites and cannot be used in heme synthesis (∞ Chapter 6). In normal heme synthesis, both type I and III isomers are formed but in a 1:10,000 ratio. Normally, most porphyrinogens are readily converted during heme synthesis to heme, and very small amounts of the porphyrin intermediates are formed. If, for some reason, excessive amounts of porphyrinogen are produced, the oxidized porphyrin compounds also increase. Porphyrins are tetrapyrroles and resonating compounds (contain alternating single and double bonds); erythrocytes that contain these substances show red fluorescence with UV light.

Congenital Erythropoietic Porphyria

CEP (Gunther's disease) is characterized by the presence of excessive amounts of type I porphyrins: uroporphyrin I (UroI) and coproporphyrin I (CoproI). A defect in uroporphyrinogen III cosynthase results from point mutations in the gene, which channels the porphobilinogen into the functionless UroI isomer (Figure 9-14■). However, enough Uro III is produced to generate adequate amounts of heme. This suggests that a deficiency of cosynthetase is not the only abnormality. Another possibility for the excessive amounts of UroI isomer is hyperactivity of the uroporphyrin I synthetase. Validation of either of these hypotheses requires purification, characterization, and accurate measurement of these enzymes.

The excess porphyrins are deposited in body tissues and excreted in urine and feces. Intense fluorescence with ultraviolet light can verify their presence. The cause of the hemolytic anemia that accompanies CEP is unknown but is thought to be closely associated with the excessive porphyrin deposits within erythrocytes. The finding that normal erythrocytes infused into CEP patients have a normal life span supports this. The erythrocytes in CEP can be subject to photohemolysis as they pass through the dermal capillaries exposed to UV light. The erythrocytes show increased photohemolysis in vitro, but whether this is also an in vivo phenomenon is uncertain.

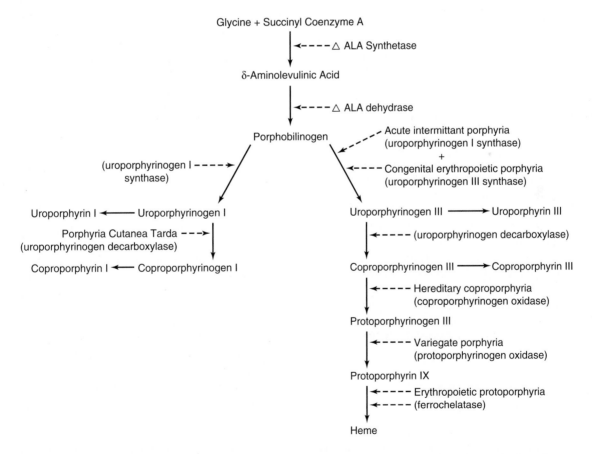

■ FIGURE 9-14   The formation of heme from glycine and succinyl-coenzyme A involves the production of porphyrinogen intermediates. Normally, only very small amounts of the series I isomers are formed. However, in the hereditary condition erythropoietic porphyria, there is an abnormality in this pathway, and large amounts of the functionless series I isomers are formed. These isomers are oxidized to porphyrin and accumulate in the tissues. Another form of porphyria, erythropoietic protoporphyria, is characterized by excessive production of protoporphyrin.

Erythropoietic Protoporphyria

EPP is characterized by an overproduction of protoporphyrin, the immediate precursor of heme, and is associated with a defect in ferrochelatase (Figure 9-10). Adequate amounts of heme are produced, however, and no anemia is present. Excess protoporphyrin IX builds up in the cell, can leak into skin dermal capillaries and can be found in the skin, liver, blood, and feces. Due to its insolubility in water, protoporphyrin is not present in the urine. This porphyria is thought to be of both erythropoietic and hepatic origin.[78]

CLINICAL FEATURES

CEP is a rare autosomal recessive disease with ~130 cases reported. EPP is inherited as an autosomal dominant trait, but recessive inheritance is possible.[79] About 300 cases of EPP have been reported, but the actual rate of occurence is probably masked due to the subtlety of the clinical signs and the absence of colored porphyrins in the urine.

The first signs of CEP occur in infancy. The urine is colored pink to reddish brown, depending on the amount of uroporphyrin excreted. This is usually first noted as a pink stain on the infant's diaper. The excess porphyrins in the skin create an extreme photosensitivity to sunlight. Vesicular or bullous eruptions appear on bared areas shortly after exposure to sunlight. The lesions heal slowly and can become infected. Repeated eruptions and skin injury cause scarring and can lead to severe mutilation of the face, ears, and hands. The excess porphyrin stains the teeth a dirty brown. Under UV light, the teeth fluoresce bright red. Hypertrichosis affects the entire body but is especially present in exposed areas. The hair can be blond and downy or dark and coarse. Splenomegaly is a consistent finding and is usually progressive with the disease. A mild to severe hemolytic anemia is present with erythrocyte life span decreased to as little as 18 days. Patients with CEP never exhibit the abdominal pain or neurologic and psychotic signs associated with hepatic porphyrias.

Clinical signs of EPP are more subtle, and its course is relatively mild in comparison to CEP. Photosensitivity is not severe, and scarring is usually absent. Sunlight exposure leads to erythema and urticaria. Protoporphyrin accumulates in the erythrocytes, which causes them to fluoresce intensely, but there is no hemolytic anemia. Occasionally hepatic damage occurs.

LABORATORY FEATURES

CEP

The peripheral blood in CEP exhibits a mild to severe normocytic anemia with anisocytosis and poikilocytosis. The blood smear reveals significant polychromatophilia and nucleated erythrocytes. Reticulocytes are increased. The erythrocytes fluoresce with UV light.

The bone marrow in CEP shows erythroid hyperplasia. A large portion of the erythroblasts demonstrate intense fluorescence with UV light. The fluorescence is localized principally in the nuclei. The fact that not all erythroblasts fluoresce suggests that two populations of erythrocytes exist, and one of which is normal.

Serum iron and storage iron are usually normal. Haptoglobin is absent and unconjugated bilirubin, urinary, and fecal urobilinogen are increased.

Large amounts of uroporphyrin I and coproporphyrin I are excreted in the urine and feces. These isomers are also found in the plasma and in erythrocytes.

EPP

The blood and bone marrow in EPP usually reveal no abnormalities on routine examination; however, under UV light, the cytoplasm of erythroblasts fluoresces intensely. The erythrocytes, plasma, and feces contain large amounts of protoporphyrin. The protoporphyrins are not found in the urine. The protophophyrin in erythrocytes is free (FEP), not bound to zinc as in IDA and lead poisoning. The FEP is higher than in other disorders associated with an increase in erythrocyte protoporphyrin levels. This block in heme synthesis, which occurrs in the reaction just prior to insertion of iron into the porphyrin ring, would be expected to cause an accumulation of iron within the erythroblasts. The fact that this iron buildup does not occur cannot be explained.

PROGNOSIS AND THERAPY

Individuals with CEP do not usually survive beyond the fifth decade of life. Attempts to decrease the excess porphyrins have been unsuccessful, but the quality of life for CEP patients has improved by minimizing the scarring and mutilation with effective dermatologic treatment. Avoidance of exposure to sunlight is critical. Splenectomy has sometimes resulted in a decrease of porphyrin production and helped ameliorate the hemolytic anemia. Evidence for long-term success with splenectomy, however, is questionable. Blood transfusion in conjunction with administration of chelators to reduce iron overload suppresses erythropoiesis and decreases or eliminates symptoms. Bone marrow transplantation is suggested in severe phenotypes because the predominant site of prophyrin production is the bone marrow.

Treatment of EPP is aimed at protecting the skin from sunlight and minimizing the toxic effects of protoporphyrin on the liver. In most patients with EPP, high doses of β-carotene improves tolerance to sunlight. Blood transfusions and hematin can be utilized to suppress erythropoiesis. Splenectomy can be helpful if hemolysis and splenomegaly are prominent. Cholestyramine can promote excretion of liver protoporphyrin.[80]

Genes of the heme biosynthetic pathway have been cloned, and mutations associated with porphyrias have been identified. Gene therapy will likely be an option for porphyrias in the future.[78] In this type of therapy, a functional gene would be transferred to specific hematopoietic or hepatic stem cells of the patient, restoring normal heme synthesis pathways.

SUMMARY

Hemoglobin synthesis requires adequate production of heme and globin. Inadequate amounts of either can result in anemia—usually microcytic, hypochromic anemia. Defects in heme synthesis could be due to faulty iron or porphyrin metabolism (Table 9-23 ☻).

Many proteins that play a role in iron homeostasis have been identified. These include hepcidin, ferroportin1, hephaestin, DMT1, DCytB, HFE, transferrin receptor and transferrin. The anemias with a faulty iron metabolic component include IDA and ACD. IDA is due to inadequate amounts of iron for heme synthesis. This ID usually occurs because of blood loss or a nutritional deficiency of iron. ACD has several pathophysiologic mechanisms related to cytokines produced as a result of inflammation or infection. The major mechanism is a block in reutilization of macrophage iron. The erythrocytes are normocytic, normochromic, but in long-standing anemia, they can be microcytic, hypochromic.

Abnormal porphyrin metabolism results in SA and porphyrias. Defects in globin synthesis are due to genetic defects that affect production of the globin chains. These globin defects are known as thalassemias.

Sideroblastic anemia (SA) is due to defective porphyrin synthesis and a block in the insertion of iron into the poryphyrin ring to form heme. The erythrocyte population in SA characteristically contains cells that are normochromic and hypochromic (dual population). The bone marrow has ringed sideroblasts. Hereditary SA is due to defective ALAS2, the enzyme in the first step of heme synthesis. SA can also occur because of the effects of drugs or toxins on enzymes involved in heme synthesis.

Iron studies are helpful in differentiating these disorders. Serum iron is decreased in IDA and ACD; it is normal to increased in SA. The serum transferrin is increased and saturation decreased if total body iron is decreased, whereas if storage iron is normal or increased, the serum transferrin is normal or decreased with normal or increased saturation. Serum ferritin is a reliable indicator of iron stores except in the presence of inflammation when it is falsely increased. It is decreased in ID and normal or increased in SA, ACD, and hemochromatosis. The serum transferrin receptor assay is

☻ TABLE 9-23

Summary of Conditions Associated with Abnormal Heme Synthesis and/or Iron Metabolism/Utilization

Condition	Etiology	CBC	Iron Studies	Other
Iron deficiency anemia	Inadequate iron due to deficient dietary intake; decreased absorption; increased loss	Microcytic, hypochromic, anisocytosis, poikilocytosis	Decreased serum iron, serum ferritin, and percent saturation of transferrin; increased TIBC and sTfR	Increased ZPP (do not use to evaluate if possibility of concurrent lead poisoning); decreased CHr
Anemia of chronic disease	Impaired release of iron from macrophages due to increased hepcidin induced by cytokines; inhibition of EPO production and impaired erythropoiesis; shortened erythrocyte survival	Normocytic, normochromic; in long-standing cases can be microcytic, hypochromic	Decreased serum iron and low to normal TIBC; low/normal transferrin saturation; serum ferritin normal or increased; sTfR normal	Increased ZPP
Sideroblastic anemia	Defect in enzymes needed for heme synthesis; can be hereditary or acquired (secondary to drugs/toxins)	Dual population of normochromic and hypochromic erythrocytes	Increased serum iron and transferrin saturation; normal or decreased TIBC; increased serum ferritin	Bone marrow shows ringed sideroblasts; peripheral blood erythrocytes may contain Pappenheimer bodies
Hemochromatosis (no anemia)	Hereditary: genetic mutation (C282Y and/or H63D); acquired: transfusion, iron injections, chronic liver disease	No anemia or characteristic peripheral blood cell morphology	Increased serum iron, transferrin saturation, and serum ferritin	Molecular testing to identify mutated gene is suggested if transferrin saturation is >55%
Porphyrias (anemia not characteristic)	Block in porphyrin synthesis due to defect in enzymes for heme synthesis; CEP and EPP affect erythrocytes	CEP: normocytic hemolytic anemia; anisocytosis and poikilocytosis; polychromatophilia; NRBC EPP: no abnormalities	Storage iron and serum iron normal	CEP: increased uroporphyrin I and coproporphyrin I excreted in urine and feces, plasma, and erythrocytes; series III isomers also increased CEP, EPP: normoblasts demonstrate intense fluorescence with UV light

useful in differentiating ID and ACD. Levels are increased in ID and normal in ACD.

Hemochromatosis is a disorder characterized by total body iron excess. Anemia is not a characteristic of this disorder, but it is included in this chapter to help the reader compare and differentiate iron study results with those associated with defective heme synthesis. Hemochromatosis can be caused by a genetic defect or chronic transfusion. The most common hereditary form of hemochromatosis (HH) is due to a mutation of the *HFE* gene. Mutations in several other genes associated with iron metabolism can also cause HH. These mutations are believed to affect the synthesis of hepcidin. Serum iron studies reflect the excessive iron overload with increased serum ferritin and a very high saturation of transferrin.

The porphyrias are a heterogeneous group of hereditary disorders that are due to a block in porphyrin synthesis. The defect is in a critical enzyme in the porphyrin metabolic pathway. Two forms have an erythropoietic component, CEP and EPP. Erythrocytes have very high levels of free erythrocyte protoporphyrin, and excess prophyrins are deposited in tissues and excreted in feces/urine.

REVIEW QUESTIONS

LEVEL I

1. What is the iron transport protein? (Objective 3)
   a. ferritin
   b. transferrin
   c. hemosiderin
   d. albumin

2. The term *sideropenic* is most closely associated with which of the following anemias? (Objective 1)
   a. iron deficiency
   b. sideroblastic
   c. lead poisoning
   d. anemia of chronic disease

3. Microcytic, hypochromic erythrocytes are most characteristic of which of the following anemias? (Objective 5)
   a. megaloblastic
   b. lead poisoning
   c. iron deficiency
   d. anemia of chronic disease

4. Which of the following individuals is most likely to require an increased intake of iron? (Objective 4)
   a. adult male
   b. menopausal female
   c. mother of 3 preschool children
   d. 75-year-old male

5. The basic defect in sideroblastic anemia is: (Objective 6)
   a. inadequate iron intake
   b. inadequate absorption of iron in the gut
   c. cytokine inhibition of erythropoiesis
   d. faulty enzymes regulating heme synthesis

6. Anemia(s) characterized by defective heme synthesis include: (Objective 6)
   a. hemochromatosis
   b. megaloblastic anemia
   c. thalassemia
   d. sideroblastic anemia

7. The most common cause of ID in middle-aged men is: (Objective 6)
   a. inadequate iron in the diet
   b. cancer
   c. prescription drugs
   d. chronic bleeding

LEVEL II

Use this history for questions 1–4.

A 75-year-old male experiencing mental confusion and fatigue was seen by his physician. Laboratory tests were ordered:

RBC	3.3×10^{12}/L
Hb	9.3 g/dL
Hct	0.29 L/L
PLT	168×10^9/L
WBC	4.0×10^9/L
Differential	
Segmented neutrophils	60%
Band neutrophils	9%
Lymphocytes	25%
Monocytes	3%
Eosinophils	3%

RBC morphology: Anisocytosis with microcytic, hypochromic RBCs, and normocytic, normochromic RBCs present
Laboratory data for anemia workup:

Reticulocyte count	1.0%
Serum iron	274 µg/dL
Total iron-binding capacity (TIBC)	285 µg/dL

1. Which anemia of defective heme synthesis is associated with this type of red cell morphology? (Objective 8)
   a. sideroblastic anemia
   b. anemia of chronic disease
   c. IDA
   d. erythropoietic porphyria

2. Which laboratory result(s) is (are) most useful in distinguishing this patient's anemia from IDA? (Objective 9)
   a. bone marrow
   b. MCV
   c. hemoglobin
   d. iron studies

LEVEL I

8. Which of the following is most often associated with microcytic, hypochromic anemia? (Objective 5)
   a. lead poisoning
   b. ID
   c. sideroblastic anemia
   d. anemia of chronic disease

9. Which of the following best describes hemosiderosis? (Objective 7)
   a. decrease in serum iron
   b. increase in serum iron
   c. increase in macrophage iron
   d. increase in total body iron

10. A patient with anemia of chronic disease would be expected to have which set of laboratory test results? (Objective 5)
    a. MCV decreased, serum iron increased, serum ferritin increased, TIBC and % saturation increased
    b. MCV normal, serum iron increased, serum ferritin decreased, TIBC and % saturation decreased
    c. MCV normal, serum iron decreased, serum ferritin increased, TIBC and % saturation decreased
    d. MCV decreased, serum iron decreased, serum ferritin decreased, TIBC and % saturation decreased

LEVEL II

3. From the results of these laboratory studies, how would you describe the patient's red blood cells? (Objective 8)
   a. microcytic, hypochromic
   b. dual population of microcytes and normocytes
   c. macrocytic, normochromic
   d. normocytic, normochromic

4. A bone marrow was performed and sections were stained with Prussian blue. Numerous sideroblasts were present with a large number of ringed sideroblasts. What is the most probable cause of this anemia? (Objectives 6, 8, 10)
   a. poor diet
   b. chronic blood loss
   c. abnormality of ALAS2
   d. increased iron requirement

5. A hematocrit is not recommended to screen for iron deficiency in children because: (Objectives 1, 2, 8, 9)
   a. It is not sensitive enough to pick up anemia in children.
   b. Iron deficiency can be present without the presence of anemia.
   c. High levels of lead will affect the hematocrit accuracy.
   d. Serum ferritin is more cost effective.

6. If a child with lead poisoning also had a significant microcytic, hypochromic anemia, what complicating pathology/pathologies should be considered? (Objective 14)
   a. iron deficiency
   b. thalassemia
   c. iron deficiency and thalassemia
   d. thalassemia and sideroblastic anemia

7. What laboratory test is best for screening for iron deficiency in a population of 1- to 3-year-old children who have a high incidence of elevated blood lead levels? (Objective 14)
   a. hematocrit
   b. serum ferritin
   c. serum iron
   d. ZPP

8. A 2-year-old child was tested for blood lead level. The result was 25 µg/dL. He also had microcytic, hypochromic anemia. The child's parents were questioned, and it was determined that the source of lead was a painted crib in his day care center. The child was enrolled in another day care center. Follow-up testing revealed that the blood lead level was within normal limits but the microcytic, hypochromic anemia was still present. Which follow-up test(s) would you recommend to help identify the etiology of this anemia? (Objectives 9,14,15)
   a. serum iron, serum ferritin, TIBC, % saturation
   b. hemoglobin electrophoresis
   c. molecular diagnostic testing for sideroblastic anemia
   d. molecular diagnostic testing for hemosiderosis

REVIEW QUESTIONS (continued)

LEVEL I

LEVEL II

9. A health maintenance organization (HMO) has a contract for laboratory testing services with your laboratory. The HMO has decided to screen its members for hereditary hemochromatosis. Which laboratory test will you recommend for this screening? (Objective 18)
   a. serum iron
   b. % transferrin saturation
   c. serum ferritin
   d. molecular test for mutated HFE gene

10. In regard to question 9, what test should you recommend to be done reflexively on patients with an abnormal screening test? (Objective 18)
    a. molecular test for HFE gene
    b. serum iron
    c. serum ferritin
    d. % saturation

11. Which protein regulates iron absorption in the gut and transport of iron from cells to the plasma? (Objective 3)
    a. DcytB
    b. DMT1
    c. hepcidin
    d. hephaestin

12. What effect would a high degree of ineffective erythropoiesis have on iron metabolism? (Objective 4)
    a. Decreased amount of iron released from enterocytes
    b. Increased absorption of iron in the intestine
    c. Decreased hepcidin synthesis
    d. Increased serum transferrin saturation

www.pearsonhighered.com/mckenzie
Use this address to access the interactive Companion Website created for this textbook. Find additional information, tables and figures. Evaluate your command of the chapter information using case studies and critical thinking and multiple choice questions.

REFERENCES

1. Brittenham GM. Disorders of iron metabolism: Iron deficiency and overload. In: Hoffman R, Benz Jr. EJ, Shattil SJ, Furie B, Cohen HJ, eds. *Hematology: Basic Principles and Practice.* New York: Churchill Livingstone; 1991:327–49.

2. Roy CN, Andrews NC. Anemia of inflammation: The hepcidin link. *Cur Opi Hemat.* 2005;12(2):107–11.

3. Guschin H, Mackenzie B, Berger UV et al. Cloning and characterization of a mammalian proton-coupled metal-iron transporter. *Nature.* 1997;388:482–88.

4. Shayeghi M, Latunde-Dada GO, Oakhill JS et al. Identification of an intestinal heme transporter. *Cell.* 2005;122:789–801.

5. Gavin MW, McCarthy DM, Garry PJ. Evidence that iron stores regulate iron absorption: A setpoint theory. *Am J Clin Nutr* 1994;59:1376–80.

6. Hentze MW, Muckenthaler MU, Andrews NC. Balancing Acts: Molecular control of mammalian iron metabolism. *Cell.* 2004;117:285–97.

7. Nicolas G, Chauvet C, Viatte L et al. The gene encoding the iron regulatory peptide hepcidin is regulated by anaemia, hypoxia, and inflammation. *J Clin Invest.* 2002;110:1037–44.

8. Latunde-Dad GO, Van der Westhuizen J, Vulpe CD, Anderson GJ, Simpson RJ, McKie AT. Molecular and functional roles of duodenal Cytochrome B (Dcytb) in iron metabolism. *Blood Cells Mol Dis.* 2002;29(3):356–60.

9. Frazer DM, Wilkins SJ, Becker EM et al. A rapid decrease in the expression of DMT1 and DCytb but not Ireg1 or hephaestin explains the mucosal block phenomenon of iron absorption. *Gut.* 2003;52 (3):340–46.

10. Kawabata H, Fleming RE, Rui D et al. Expression of hepcidin is down-regulated in TfR2 mutant mice manifesting a phenotype of hereditary hemochromatosis. *Blood.* 2004;105:378–81.

11. Niederkofler V, Salie R, Arber S. Hemojuvelin is essential for dietary iron sensing, and its mutation leads to severe iron overload. *J Clin Invest.* 2005;115(8):2180–86.

12. Ferreira GC, Gong J. 5-aminolevulinate synthase and the first step of heme biosynthesis. *J Bioenerg Biomembr.* 1995;27:151–59.

13. Klausner RD, Rouault TA, Harford JB. Regulating the fate of mRNA: The control of cellular iron metabolism. *Cell.* 1993;72:19–28.

14. Kawasaki N, Morimoto K, Tanimoto T, Hayakawa T. Control of hemoglobin synthesis in erythroid differentiating K562 cells. I. Role of iron in erythroid cell heme synthesis. *Arch Biochem Biophys.* 1996; 328:289–94.

15. Kawasaki N, Morimoto K, Hayakawa T. Control of hemoglobin synthesis in erythroid differentiating K562 cells. II. Studies of iron mobilization in erythroid cells by high-performance liquid chromatography-electrochemical detection. *J Chromatogr B Biomed Sci Appl.* 1998;705:193–201.

16. Rouault TA, Klausner RD. Iron-sulfur clusters as biosensors of oxidants and iron. *Trends Biochem Sci.* 1996;21:174–77.

17. Muhlenhoff U, Gerber J, Richhardt N, Lill R. Components involved in assembly and dislocation of iron-sulfur clusters on the scaffold protein Isu1p. *EMBO J.* 2003;22:4815–25.

18. Looker AC, Dallman PR, Carroll MD, Gunter EW, Johnson CL. Prevalence of iron deficiency in the United States. *JAMA.* 1997;277 (12):973–76.

19. Oski FA. Iron deficiency in infancy and childhood. *NEJM.* 1993; 329(3):190–93.

20. Kazal LA Jr. Failure of hematocrit to detect iron deficiency in infants. *J Fam Pract.* 1996;42(3):237–40.

21. Eden AN, Mier MA. Iron deficiency in 1- to 3-year-old children: A pediatric failure? *Arch Ped Adoles Med.* 1997;151(10):986–88.

22. Brumberg, JJ. Chlorotic girls, 1870–1920: A historical perspective on female adolescence. *Child Dev.* 1982;53:1468–77.

23. Joosten E, Ghesquiere B, Linthoudt H et al. Upper and lower gastrointestinal evaluation of elderly inpatients who are iron deficient. *Amer J Med.* 1999;107(1):24–29.

24. Major A, Mathez-Loic F, Rohling R, Gautschi K, Brugnara C. The effect of intravenous iron on the reticulocyte response to recombinant human erythropoietin. *Br J Haematol.* 1997;98(2):292–94.

25. Fernandez-Rodriquez AM, Guindeo-Casasus MC, Molero-Labarta T et al. Diagnosis of iron deficiency in chronic renal disease. *Amer J Kidney Dis.* 1999;34(3):508–13.

26. Thompson WG, Meola T, Lipkin M Jr., Freedman ML. Red cell distribution width, mean corpuscular volume, and transferrin saturation in the diagnosis of iron deficiency. *Arch Intern Med.* 1988;148: 2128–30.

27. Braugnara C, Zurakowski D, Dicanzio J, Boyd T, Platt O. Reticulocyte hemoglobin content to diagnose iron deficiency in children. *JAMA.* 1999;281:2247–48.

28. Rector WG Jr.: Pica: Its frequency and significance in patients with iron-deficiency anemia due to chronic gastrointestinal blood loss. *J Gen Intern Med.* 1989;4:512–13.

29. Geissler PW, Shulman CE, Prince RJ et al. Geophage, iron status, and anaemia among pregnant women on the coast of Kenya. *Transac Royal Soc Trop Med Hyg.* 1998;92(5):549–53.

30. Idjradinata P, Pollitt E. Reversal of developmental delays in iron-deficient anaemic infants treated with iron. *Lancet.* 1993;341:1–4.

31. Roncagliolo M, Garrido M, Walter T, Peirano P, Lozoff B. Evidence of altered central nervous system development in infants with iron deficiency anemia at 6 months: Delayed maturation of auditory brainstem responses. *Am J Clin Nutri.* 1998; 68(3):683–90.

32. Cullen P, Soffker J, Hopfl M, Bremer C et al. Hypochromic red cells and reticulocyte hemoglobin content as markers of iron-deficient-erythropoiesis in patients undergoing chronic haemodialysis. *Nephrol Dial Transplant.* 1999;14(3):659–65.

33. Vreugdenhil G, Baltus CA, van Eijk HG, Swaak AJ. Anaemia of chronic disease: Diagnostic significance of erythrocyte and serological parameters in iron deficient rheumatoid arthritis patients. *Br J Rheumatol.* 1990;29:105–10.

34. Coenen JL et al. Measurements of serum ferritin used to predict concentrations of iron in bone marrow in anemia of chronic disease. *Clin. Chem.* 1991;37:560–63.

35. Kis AM, Carnes M. Detecting iron deficiency in anemic patients with concomitant medical problems. *J Gen Intern Med.* 1998;13(7): 455–61.

36. Van den Broek NR, Letsky EA, White SA, Shenkin A. Iron status in pregnant women: Which measurements are valid? *Br J Haematol.* 1998;103(3):817–24.

37. McKay R, Scott BB. Iron deficiency anemia: How far to investigate? *Gut.* 1993;34:1427–28.

38. Wong SS, Qutishat AS, Lange J, Gornet TG, Buja LM. Detection of iron-deficiency anemia in hospitalized patients by zinc protoporphyrin. *Clin Chim Acta.* 1996;244(1):91–101.

39. Rettmer Rl, Carlson TH, Origenes ML, Jack RM, Laab RF. Zinc protoporphyrin/heme ratio for diagnosis of preanemic iron deficiency. *Pediatrics.* 1999;104(3):e37.

40. Lowenstein W et al. Free erythrocyte protoporphyrin assay in the diagnosis of iron deficiency in the anemic aged subject: A prospective study of 103 anemic patients. *Ann Med Intern.* 1991;142: 13–16.

41. Harthoorn-Lasthuizen EJ, Lindemans J, Langenhuipen MM. Combined use of erythrocyte zinc protoporphyrin and mean corpuscular volume in differentiation of thalassemia from iron deficiency anemia. *Europ J Haematol.* 1998;60(4):245–51.

42. Junca J, Flores A, Roy C, Alberti R, Milla F. Red cell distribution width, free erythrocyte protoporphyrin, and England-Fraser index in the differential diagnosis of microcytosis due to iron deficiency or beta-thalassemia trait: A study of 200 cases of microcytic anemia. *Hematol Pathol.* 1991;5:33–36.

43. Suominen P, Punnonen K, Ragamaki A, Irjala K. Serum transferrin receptor and transferrin receptor-ferritin index identify healthy subjects with subclinical iron deficits. *Blood.* 1998;92(8):2934–39.

44. Punnonen K, Irjala K, Rajamaki A. Serum transferrin receptor and its ratio to serum ferritin in the diagnosis of iron deficiency. *Blood.* 1997;89(3):1052–57.

45. Mulherin D, Skelly M, Saunders A et al. The diagnosis of iron deficiency in patients with rheumatoid arthritis and anemia: An algorithm using simple laboratory measures. *J Rheum.* 1996;23(2): 237–40.

46. Ahluwalia N. Diagnostic utility of serum transferrin receptors measurement in assessing iron status. *Nutri Rev.* 1998;56(5 Pt1):133–41.

47. Case G. Maintaining iron balance with total-dose infusion of intravenous iron dextran. *Anna J.* 1998;25(1):65–68.

48. Adamson J. Erythropoietin, iron metabolism, and red blood cell production. *Sem Hematol.* 1996;33:5–9.

49. Chang CC, Kass L. Clinical significance of immature reticulocyte fraction determined by automated reticulocyte counting. *Am J Clin Pathol.* 1997;108(1):69–73.

50. Dallman PR, Reeves JD, Driggers DA, Lo YET. Diagnosis of iron deficiency: The limitations of laboratory tests in predicting response to iron treatment in 1-year-old infants. *J Pediatr.* 1981;99(3):376–81.

51. Krantz SB: Pathogenesis and treatment of the anemia of chronic disease. *Am J Med Sci.* 1994;307:353–59.

52. Means RT. Clinical application of recombinant erythropoietin in the anemia of chronic disease. *Hematol Oncol Clin No Amer.* 1994;8 (5):933–44.

53. Miller CB et al. Decreased erythropoietin response in patients with the anemia of cancer. *N Engl J Med.* 1990;322:1689–92.

54. Baer AN, Dessypris EN, Goldwasser E, and Krantz SB. Blunted erythropoietin response to anemia in rheumatoid arthritis. *Br J Haematol.* 1987;66:559–64.

55. Means RT Jr., Krantz SB. Progress in understanding the pathogenesis of the anemia of chronic disease. *Blood.* 1992;80:1639–47.

56. Ferguson BJ et al. Serum transferrin receptor distinguishes the anemia of chronic disease from iron deficiency anemia. *J Lab Clin Med.* 1992;19:385–90.

57. Bottomley SS, May BK, Cox TC, Cotter PD, Bishop DF. Molecular defects of erythroid 5-aminolevulinate synthase in s-linked sideroblastic anemia. *J Bioenerg Biomembr.* 1995;27(2):161–68.

58. May A, Bishop DF. The molecular biology and pyridoxine responsiveness of x-linked sideroblastic anemia. *Haematologica.* 1998;83: 56–70.

59. Furuyama K, Fujita H, Nagi T et al. Pyridoxine refractory x-linked sideroblastic anemia caused by a point mutation in the erythroid 5-aminolevulinate synthase gene. *Blood.* 1997;90 (2):822–30.

60. Koc S, Harris JW. Sideroblastic anemias: Variations on imprecision in diagnostic criteria; Proposal for an extended classification of siderblastic anemias. *Am J Hematol.* 1998;57:1–6.

61. Landrigan PJ, Todd AC. Lead Poisoning. *West J Med.* 1994;161: 153–59.

62. CDC. Blood lead level data on adults reported from 2002 through 2004 by the states in CDC, NIOSH's adult blood lead epidemiology and surveillance (ABLES) Program. http://origin.cdc.gov/niosh/topics/ABLES/pdfs/2002-2005%20lead-data.pdf.Accessed 11/11/08.

63. Bhambhani K, Aronow R. Lead poisoning and thalassemia trait or iron deficiency: The value of the red blood cell distribution width. *Am J Dis Child.* 1990;144:1231–33.

64. Carraccio CL, Bergman GE, Daley BP. Combined iron deficiency and lead poisoning in children: Effect on FEP levels. *Clin Pediatr.* 1987;26:644–47.

65. Clark M, Royal J, Seeler, R. Interaction of iron deficiency and lead and the hematologic findings in children with severe lead poisoning. *Pediatrics.* 1988;81:247–54.

66. Rainey PM. Lead: A heavy burden for small children. *Clin Chem News.* 1992;18 (6):37.

67. Savage D, Lindenbaum J. Anemia in alcoholics. *Medicine.* 1986;5: 322–39.

68. Cotter PD, May A, Li L, al-Sabah AI, Fitzsimons EJ, Cazzola M, Bishop DF. Four new mutations in the erythroid-specific 5-aminolevulinate synthase (ALSA2) gene causing x-linked sideroblastic anemia: Increased pyridoxine responsiveness after removal of iron overload by phlebotomy and coinheritance of hereditary hemochromatosis. *Blood.* 1999;93(5):1757–69.

69. Feder JN, Gnirke A, Thomas W. A novel class-I like gene is mutated in patients with hereditary hemochromatosis. *Nature Genet.* 1996; 13:399–408.

70. Jacolot S, LeGac G, Scotet V, Quere I, Mura C, Ferec C. *HAMP* as a modifier gene that increase the phenotypic expression of the *HFE* p.C282Y homozygous genotype. *Blood.* 2004;103:2835–40.

71. Le Gac G, Scotet V, Ka C, Gourlaouen I, Bryckaert L, Jacolot S, Mura C, Ferec C. The recently identified type 2A juvenile haemochromatosis gene (HJV), a second candidate modifier of the C282Y homozygous phenotype. *Human Mol Genet.* 2004;13(17):1913–18.

72. Lebron JA, Bjorkman PJ. The transferrin receptor binding site on HFE: The class I MCH-related protein mutated in hereditary hemochromatosis. *J Mole Biol.* 1999;289:1109–18.

73. Swinkles DW, Marx JJ. Diagnosis and treatment of primary hemochromatosis. *Nederlands Tijdschrift voor Geneeskunde.* 1999;143: 1404–8.

74. Cogswell ME, Burke W, McDonnell SM, Franks AL. Screening for hemochromatosis: A public health perspective. *Am J Prev Med.* 1999; 16(2):134–40.

75. Olynyk JK. Hereditary haemochromatosis: Diagnosis and management in the gene era. *Liver.* 1999;19:73–80.

76. Fletcher LM, Halliday JW, Powell LW. Interrelationships of alcohol and iron in liver disease with particular reference to the iron-binding proteins, ferritin, and transferrin. *J Gastroentero Hepat.* 1999;14: 202–14.

77. Adams PC, Kertesz AE, Valberg LS. Rate of iron reaccumulation following iron depletion in hereditary hemochromatosis: Implications for venesection therapy. *J Clin Gastroenterol.* 1993;16(3):207–10.

78. DeVerneuil H, Ged C, Bouleihfar S, Moreau-Gaudry F. Porphyrias: Animal models and prospects for cellular and gene therapy. *J Bioenerg Biomembr.* 1995;27(2):239–48.

79. Mascaro JM. Porphyrias in children. *Pediatr Dermatol.* 1992;9: 371–72.

80. Desnick RJ, Anderson KE. Heme biosynthesis and its disorders: The porphyrias and sideroblastic anemias. In: R. Hoffman R, Benz Jr. EJ, Shattil SJ, Furie B, Cohen HJ, eds. *Hematology: Basic principles and practice.* New York: Churchill Livingstone; 1991:350–67.

10

Hemoglobinopathies: Qualitative Defects

Rebecca J. Laudicina, Ph.D.

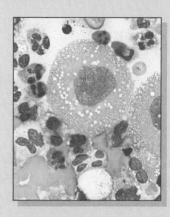

■ OBJECTIVES—LEVEL I

At the end of this unit of study, the student should be able to:

1. Define *hemoglobinopathy*.
2. Explain the basis of defects resulting in the production of abnormal hemoglobins.
3. Explain the basis of the hemoglobin electrophoresis method in identifying abnormal hemoglobins.
4. Describe the epidemiology of sickle cell anemia (SCA) and other hemoglobinopathies.
5. Identify the globin chain defects causing SCA and hemoglobin C disease.
6. Associate laboratory analyses with their use in detecting and identifying hemoglobinopathies.
7. Recognize and identify abnormal laboratory test results, including peripheral blood findings and screening and confirmatory tests, typically associated with homozygous and heterozygous conditions involving HbS, HbC, HbD, HbE, and compound heterozygous conditions involving hemoglobin S and other abnormal hemoglobins.
8. List major clinical findings typically associated with the hemoglobinopathies listed in Objective 7.

■ OBJECTIVES—LEVEL II

At the end of this unit of study, the student should be able to:

1. Compare the synthesis and concentration of abnormal hemoglobins in homozygous and heterozygous conditions.
2. Compare the prevalence of hemoglobins S, C, D, and E.
3. Compare and contrast the pathophysiology of hemoglobin variants in terms of altered solubility, function, and stability.
4. Analyze the structure of the hemoglobin molecule in sickle cell anemia (SCA) and relate it to the pathophysiology of the disease.
5. Contrast clinical findings in persons who are homozygous and heterozygous for hemoglobins S, C, D, and E and in those who have compound heterozygotes for these abnormal hemoglobins.
6. Identify and explain current therapies for SCA.
7. Evaluate and interpret mobility patterns obtained on cellulose acetate and citrate agar gel hemoglobin electrophoresis when structurally abnormal hemoglobins are present.

■ OBJECTIVES—LEVEL II (continued)

8. Select, evaluate, and interpret tests used in detecting and identifying abnormal hemoglobins.

9. Design a laboratory testing algorithm for optimizing tests used in detecting and identifying abnormal hemoglobins.

10. Evaluate laboratory test results and medical history of a clinical case for a patient with a hemoglobinopathy and suggest a possible diagnosis.

11. Explain the physiologic abnormality resulting in unstable hemoglobins, methemoglobinemia, and hemoglobin variants with increased or decreased oxygen affinity.

12. Interpret laboratory findings associated with the disorders in Objective 11.

KEY TERMS

Aplastic crisis
Autosplenectomy
Compound heterozygote
Congenital Heinz body hemolytic anemia
Hemoglobin electrophoresis
Hemoglobinopathy
Irreversibly sickled cells
Methemoglobinemia
Sequestration crisis
Thalassemia
Vaso-occlusive crisis

BACKGROUND BASICS

The information in this chapter builds on the concepts learned in previous chapters. To maximize your learning experience, you should review these concepts before starting this unit of study.

Level I

▶ Describe erythrocyte metabolism and erythrocyte destruction. (Chapter 5)

▶ Describe the structure and function of hemoglobin; list abnormal hemoglobins. (Chapter 6)

▶ Name and describe basic laboratory procedures used to screen for and assess anemia. (Chapters 8, 34)

▶ Recognize abnormal values and results for basic hematologic procedures. (Chapter 34)

▶ Describe the classification systems of anemias. (Chapter 8)

Level II

▶ Describe bone marrow structure and explain laboratory examination of bone marrow aspirates and biopsy. (Chapters 4, 35)

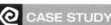 CASE STUDY

We will refer to this case throughout the chapter.
Shane, a 16-year-old African American male with a previously diagnosed hemoglobinopathy, was admitted to the hospital complaining of severe pain in his knees and back. Two of his four siblings have the same disorder. He has been admitted to the hospital on numerous occasions throughout his life for complications of his disease. Physical examination reveals a thin male in acute distress, complaining of severe pain. HEENT (head, eyes, ears, nose, and throat) exam is positive for corkscrew vessels of the schlerae, schleral icterus, and small, ill-defined, mobile (shotty) cervical lymph nodes. Abdominal exam revealed no splenomegaly, hepatomegaly, tenderness, or masses. Vital signs included temperature 37.8°C, blood pressure 95/70, and pulse 82. Blood was drawn for laboratory tests, and a chest radiograph and MRI of the head were ordered. Consider whether the patient's current condition is likely to be related to his previous diagnosis and what the laboratory's role is at this time.

▶ OVERVIEW

When the hemoglobin's molecular structure is altered, the molecule's function, stability, and/or solubility can be altered, often resulting in anemia. Laboratory screening tests are based on the altered characteristics of the hemoglobin molecule. If screening tests are abnormal, reflex tests are required to confirm the presence of an abnormal hemoglobin. This chapter discusses the most common abnormal hemoglobins including epidemiology, pathophysiology, clinical findings, laboratory findings, and treatment. Emphasis is on the correlation of clinical history and symptoms with laboratory tests and interpretation of test results.

▶ INTRODUCTION

Clinical diseases that result from a genetically determined abnormality of the structure or synthesis of the hemoglobin molecule are called **hemoglobinopathies.** The abnormality is associated with the globin chains; the heme portion of the molecule is normal. The globin abnormality can be either a qualitative defect in the globin chain (structural abnormality) or a quantitative defect in globin synthesis.

Qualitatively abnormal hemoglobin molecules result from genetic mutations in the coding region of a globin gene, resulting in amino acid deletions or substitutions in the globin protein chain. These mutations cause structural variation in one of the globin chain classes (structural hemoglobin variants). The nomenclature of these disorders is discussed in a later section. The most common clinical disorder of this type of mutation is sickle cell anemia.

The quantitative globin disorders result from various genetic defects that reduce synthesis of structurally normal globin chains. The quantitative disorders are known collectively as the **thalassemias.**

As a result of the globin chain defects, hemoglobinopathies can be associated with a chronic hemolytic anemia or can be asymptomatic. Clinical expression of the hemoglobinopathy varies depending on the class of globin chain involved (α, β, δ, or γ), the severity of hemolysis, and the compensatory production of other normal globin chains. Some of the hemoglobinopathies produce no clinical signs or symptoms of disease and are identified only through population studies specifically designed to reveal "silent" carriers. As discovery of silent carriers increases, the incidence of these genetic disorders is proving to be much higher than originally thought. Hemoglobinopathies are believed to be the most common lethal hereditary diseases in humans.[1]

Hemoglobinopathies are found worldwide but occur most commonly in African blacks and ethnic groups from the Mediterranean basin and Southeast Asia. The geographic locations where the quantitative and qualitative hemoglobin disorders are found frequently overlap; thus, it is not uncommon for individuals to have both a structural hemoglobin variant and a form of thalassemia. This could partly explain the extreme variation in clinical findings associated with hemoglobinopathies.

This chapter discusses the structural hemoglobin variants and (∞ Chapter 11) discusses the thalassemias.

▶ STRUCTURAL HEMOGLOBIN VARIANTS

The largest group of hemoglobinopathies results from an inherited structural change in one of the globin chains; however, synthesis of the abnormal chain usually is not significantly impaired. Any of the globin chain classes, α, β, δ, or γ, can be affected.

Sickle cell anemia, the most common structural hemoglobin variant, was reported by James Herrick of Chicago in 1910.[2] He described the typical crescent-shaped sickled erythrocytes in a young black student from the West Indies. Following this initial report, additional cases of the disease

were described, and the clinical pattern of sickle cell anemia was established. The pathophysiologic aspects of the disease, however, remained a mystery until Linus Pauling in 1949 discovered the altered electrophoretic mobility of the hemoglobin in patients with sickle cell disease.[3] The molecule's altered electrical charge was ascribed to a molecular abnormality of the globin chain.

More than 900 abnormal hemoglobins have since been discovered. A molecular data base can be accessed at globin.cse.psu.edu/globin/hbvar/menu.html. The number of identified β-chain mutations exceeds the number identified for α-, δ-, or γ-chains (Table 10-1 ✪). Part of the explanation for this distribution likely resides in the genetics and phenotypic expression of the globin gene loci. Hemoglobin F (γ-chain) is expressed to a significant extent only during fetal development; therefore, variant F hemoglobins are unlikely to be detectable after 3–6 months of age. Mutations affecting the γ-chain locus with the potential to produce a clinically significant abnormality would likely either cause fetal death or be insignificant at birth. At birth, as β-chain synthesis becomes predominant, the residual abnormal Hb F is likely masked by the increasing concentration of HbA.

Because HbA$_2$ (δ-chain) is usually a minor hemoglobin with a concentration of <4% of the total hemoglobin in adults, HbA$_2$ variants are also unlikely to cause clinical complications and are discovered "accidentally" during laboratory evaluation for other purposes.

The α-chain gene is duplicated on each of the 16 chromosomes. Thus, a mutation of a single α-locus resulting in a variant α-chain containing hemoglobin produces only a small amount of the abnormal hemoglobin and is less likely to cause clinical complications.

The β-gene, which is found in a single copy on each of the 11 chromosomes, is most likely to be associated with a clinical phenotype when mutated as the β-globin chain is a component of HbA, the major adult hemoglobin.

IDENTIFICATION OF HEMOGLOBIN VARIANTS

Most structural hemoglobin variants result from a single amino acid substitution or deletion in the globin polypeptide

✪ TABLE 10-1

Globin Structural Variants*

Globin Polypeptide	Number of Variants
α1- and/or α2-globin gene(s)	338
β-globin gene	518
δ-globin gene	53
Aγ-globin gene	34
Gγ-globin gene	48

*globin.cse.psu.edu/globin/hbvar/menu.html (accessed April 2008)

chain. Most structural variants result in no clinical or hematologic abnormality and have been discovered only by population studies or family studies. Mutations result in clinical manifestations only when the function (oxygen affinity) and/or the stability/solubility of the hemoglobin molecule are altered. These phenotypic variants produce both clinical and hematologic abnormalities of varying severity, depending on the nature and site of the mutation. Laboratory tests designed to detect hemoglobin variants are based on the molecule's altered structure or function.

METHODS OF ANALYSIS

Hemoglobin carries an electrical charge resulting from the presence of ionized carboxyl (COO^-) and protonated (H^+) amino (NH_3^+) groups. The type (net positive, net negative) and strength of the charge depend on both the amino acid sequence hemoglobin molecule and the pH of the surrounding medium. Many amino acid substitutions alter the molecule's electrophoretic charge, enabling detection of a structural hemoglobin variant by **hemoglobin electrophoresis.** However, different substitutions can cause identical changes in the net charge of the molecule; thus, two different mutant hemoglobins can have identical electrophoretic mobility. By varying the medium and pH of the procedure, many clinically significant hemoglobins can be identified. Methods for performing hemoglobin electrophoresis, examples of electrophoretic patterns, and more complete discussions of the tests that follow are included in ∞ Chapter 34.

The most common clinically symptomatic hemoglobinopathies involve abnormalities of the β-globin chain, resulting in a decrease or absence of HbA ($\alpha_2\beta_2$) and an increase in HbF ($\alpha_2\gamma_2$) and/or HbA$_2$ ($\alpha_2\delta_2$). Typically, an elevation in HbF and/or HbA$_2$ is the clue to the presence of a hemoglobinopathy, although HbF is frequently elevated in other hematologic disorders as well. HbF concentrations >10% can be measured by electrophoresis and densitometry. Smaller but significant increases in HbF can be measured more accurately by alkali denaturation. Hb F distribution among the erythrocyte population, however, is evaluated by the acid elution test. These tests are based on the fact that HbF is more resistant to alkali and acid treatment than other hemoglobins.

Various laboratory tests provide essential information when a hemoglobinopathy is suspected. The CBC indicates whether anemia is present, and RDW and erythrocyte indices should be evaluated to help distinguish hemoglobinopathies from thalassemia (which is usually a microcytic, hypochromic anemia). An important next step is to detect hemoglobin variants and quantify hemoglobins A$_2$ and F.[4] Several options, ranging from traditional to newer methods are available; many laboratories use a combination of both. Some laboratories are using advanced testing methods such as isoelectric focusing (IEF) and high-performance liquid

chromatography (HPLC). These laboratory methods are suitable for testing large numbers of individuals for hemoglobinopathies. They offer improved resolution and identification of certain hemoglobin variants over results obtained with alkaline electrophoresis.[5] HPLC also has the advantage over electrophoresis of quantifying low concentrations of Hb A$_2$ and Hb F and is emerging as the method of choice for this purpose.[4] Most states have instituted newborn screening programs for sickle cell disease,[6] often using HPLC or mass spectrometry methods that are appropriate for high-volume testing.

Other traditional tests for abnormal hemoglobins are based on altered physical properties of the structural variants. These include solubility tests, heat precipitation tests, and tests for Heinz bodies. The uses of these methods are included in the following discussion of the corresponding specific structural variants. Procedures are included in ∞ Chapter 34.

Techniques are also available to identify the specific molecular defect of hemoglobin disorders.[7] These techniques are discussed in ∞ Chapter 39. The polymerase chain reaction (PCR) has been incorporated into diagnostic procedures for identifying point mutations because it enhances sensitivity and reduces the amount of DNA and time required for analysis. Prenatal diagnosis can be carried out in the first trimester of pregnancy using DNA obtained from chorionic villus sampling. In cases of hemoglobinopathies caused by known common mutations, such as sickle cell anemia, the fetal DNA can be analyzed directly. If prenatal diagnosis is desired in cases in which the exact mutation is not known, the parents' DNA could be analyzed first (e.g., RFLP—restriction fragment length polymorphism) to help identify the mutation (∞ Chapter 39).

 Checkpoint! 1

Why can't all structural hemoglobin variants be identified by hemoglobin electrophoresis?

 CASE STUDY *(continued from page 212)*

1. Identify a laboratory test needed to determine Shane's hemoglobinopathy.

NOMENCLATURE

The first abnormal hemoglobin discovered was called *hemoglobin S (HbS)* because it was associated with crescent (sickle)-shaped erythrocytes (S for sickle). Subsequently, other hemoglobin variants were discovered and were given successive letters of the alphabet according to electrophoretic mobility beginning with the letter C. The letter *A* was already in use to describe the normal adult hemoglobin, HbA. The letter *B* was not used to avoid confusion with the ABO blood group system. The letter *F* had been designated to describe fetal hemoglobin, HbF. The letter *M* was given to those hemoglobins that tended to form methemoglobin (HbM).

As more and more variants were discovered, it was recognized that the alphabetical system was not sufficient and a different nomenclature system was needed. Thus, subsequent hemoglobins were given common names according to the geographic area in which they were discovered (e.g., Hb Ft. Worth). It also became apparent that some variants with the same letter designation (same electrophoretic mobility) had different structural variations. If the hemoglobin has the electrophoretic mobility of a previously lettered hemoglobin, that letter is used in addition to the geographic area (e.g., HbG Honolulu).

A standardized hemoglobin nomenclature has been recommended for use when possible. All variants should be given a scientific designation as well as a common name. The scientific designation includes the following: (1) the mutated chain, (2) the position of the affected amino acid, (3) the helical position of the mutation, and (4) the amino acid substitution. (If the mutation affects amino acids between helices, the number of the amino acid and the letters of the two bracketing helices are used.) For example, HbS would be designated $\beta6$ (A3) Glu $\rightarrow$ Val. The mutation is in the β-chain affecting the amino acid in the sixth position of the chain located in the A3 helix position. The amino acid valine is substituted for glutamic acid. Hemoglobins with amino acid deletions include the word *missing* after the amino acid and helix designation (e.g., $\beta56$-59 [D7-E3] missing). The advantage of the helical designation is that amino acid substitutions in the same helix can lead to similar functional and structural alterations of the hemoglobin molecule, allowing a better understanding of the clinical manifestations of each.

Not all globin chain mutations cause symptoms of disease; thus, many go undetected. Only those that cause clinical symptoms are likely to be brought to a physician's attention. If an individual is homozygous for the gene coding for a structural β-globin mutant, no HbA is produced, and the term *disease* or *anemia* is used to describe the specific disorder (e.g., sickle cell anemia). If, however, one of the genes coding for the β-chain is normal and the other β-gene codes for a structural variant, both HbA and the abnormal hemoglobin are produced, and the word *trait* is used to describe the heterozygous disorder (e.g., sickle cell trait).

With the most common β-chain hemoglobin variants (HbS, HbC), the abnormal hemoglobin usually accounts for less than 50% of the total hemoglobin in the trait form whereas in the homozygous state of disease, the abnormal hemoglobin usually constitutes 90–95% of the total hemoglobin. This is explained by the effect of the abnormal globin chain on the formation of the hemoglobin tetramers. The normal α-chain has a net positive charge; the normal β-chain(β^A) has a negative charge, and $\alpha\beta$ dimers form ini-

tially through positive-negative electrostatic interactions. β-chain mutants with a lesser negative charge than β^A form $\alpha\beta$ dimers more slowly than do β^A (and, conversely mutations that increased the negative charge of the β-globin chain would form $\alpha\beta$ dimers more rapidly). Both β^S and β^C mutations cause a net reduction of the β-chain negative charge and form $\alpha\beta^S$ or $\alpha\beta^C$ dimers more slowly than $\alpha\beta^A$ dimers. As a result, heterozygotes have ~60% HbA and ~35–40% HbS or HbC. If HbS or HbC constitutes more than 50% of the total hemoglobin in a heterozygote, the patient could have inherited two different abnormal hemoglobin genes (**compound heterozygote**) or a form of thalassemia with the hemoglobin variant.

 Checkpoint! 2

What does the term silent carrier mean when referring to a hemoglobinopathy?

 CASE STUDY *(continued from page 214)*

Results of hemoglobin electrophoresis were 90% HbS, 9% HbF, and 1% HbA$_2$.

2. What is the abnormal hemoglobin causing Shane's disease?

3. Is Shane heterozygous or homozygous for the disorder?

4. What is this disorder called?

PATHOPHYSIOLOGY

The structural hemoglobin variants cause symptoms if the amino acid substitution occurs at a critical site within the molecule. Most mutations cause clinical signs of disease because the mutation affects the solubility, function (oxygen-affinity), and/or stability of the hemoglobin molecule.

Altered Solubility

If a nonpolar amino acid is substituted for a polar residue near the molecule's surface, the solubility of the hemoglobin molecule can be affected. Hemoglobin S and hemoglobin C are examples of this type of substitution. In the deoxygenated state, the HbS molecule polymerizes into insoluble, rigid aggregates. The majority of surface substitutions, however, do not affect the tertiary structure, heme function, or subunit interactions and are therefore innocuous.

Altered Function

Some amino acid substitutions can affect the oxygen affinity of hemoglobin by stabilizing heme iron in the ferric state, producing methemoglobin, which cannot combine with oxygen (∞ Chapter 6). Hemoglobins M and Chesapeake are examples. Mutations within the subunit interface, $\alpha_1\beta_2$, can affect the allosteric properties of the molecule leading to increased or decreased oxygen affinity. Considerable movement occurs at the $\alpha_1\beta_2$ contact region on oxygenation, which triggers these allosteric interactions (∞ Chapter 6). High oxygen-affinity hemoglobin variants produce congenital erythrocytosis whereas decreased oxygen-affinity variants produce pseudoanemia and cyanosis.

Altered Stability

Amino acid substitutions that reduce the stability of the hemoglobin tetramer result in *unstable hemoglobins*. The mutations usually disrupt hydrogen bonding or hydrophobic interactions that retain the heme component within the heme-binding pocket of the globin chain or that hold the tetramer together. The result is a weakening of the binding of heme to globin and detachment of the heme or the disruption of the integrity of hemoglobin's tetrameric structure. Consequently, hemoglobin denatures, aggregates, and precipitates as Heinz bodies. Clinically, the unstable variants are known as **congenital Heinz body hemolytic anemias.** In addition to altering the molecule's stability, disruption of normal conformation also can affect the molecule's function.

✓ **Checkpoint! 3**

The mutation in HbJ-Capetown, $\alpha92$, Arg $\rightarrow$ Gln, stabilizes hemoglobin in the R state (∞ Chapter 6). What functional effect does this have on the hemoglobin molecule?

▶ **SICKLE CELL ANEMIA**

Worldwide, sickle cell anemia is the most common symptomatic hemoglobinopathy with greatest prevalence in tropical Africa (Table 10-2 ✪). Gene frequency in equatorial Africa can exceed 20%. The sickle cell gene is also common in areas around the Mediterranean, the Middle East, India, Nepal, and in geographic regions in which there has been migration from endemic areas, such as North, Central, and South America.[8] Sickle cell disease occurs in 0.3–1.3%, and sickle cell trait occurs in 8–10% of African Americans.

It is interesting to note that geographic areas with the highest frequency of sickle cell genes are also areas where infection with *Plasmodium falciparum* is common. This correlation strongly suggests that HbS in heterozygotes confers a selective advantage against fatal malarial infections, resulting in an increase in the gene frequency. Children with sickle cell trait are readily infected with the malarial parasite, but the parasite counts remain low. It has been suggested that resistance to malaria occurs because parasitized cells sickle more readily, leading to sequestration and phagocytosis of the infected cell by the spleen. Other, as yet undefined, factors can also contribute to reduced malarial susceptibility in individuals with HbS.[9] Epidemiological data also suggest there could be similar selective advantages to HbE and HbC.[8] Molecular evidence indicates that the identical sickle mutation arose in these geographic areas independently at least five times.

PATHOPHYSIOLOGY

Hemoglobin S is the mutant hemoglobin produced when nonpolar valine is substituted for polar glutamic acid at the seventh position in the A3 helix of the β-chain ($\beta7$ [A3] Glu $\rightarrow$ Val). (Older literature refers to the mutation at the sixth position because of confusion about numbering.) This substitution is on the surface of the molecule, producing a net decrease in negative charge; hence, it changes the molecule's electrophoretic mobility. The solubility of HbS in the deoxygenated state is markedly reduced, producing a tendency for deoxyhemoglobin S molecules to polymerize into rigid aggregates. Following polymerization, the cells assume a crescent shape. Polymerization is reversible on reoxygenation.

Polymerization is time dependent. A time delay occurs between deoxygenation and the formation of a significant amount of HbS polymers. It takes ~2–4 minutes for the development of significant polymerization and red cell distortion. The delay time for polymerization is important in considering the overall clinical consequences of HbS. Even though most red cells contain some sickle hemoglobin poly-

---

 TABLE 10-2

Summary of the Most Common Hemoglobin Variants

Hb	Peripheral Blood	Electrophoresis	Mutation	Geographic Distribution
HbS	Normocytic, normochromic anemia; reticulocytosis; poikilocytosis with sickled and boat-shaped cells	Homozygous: HbS, F, A$_2$ Heterozygous: HbA, S, F, A$_2$	$\beta7$(A3)Glu $\rightarrow$ Val	Tropical Africa and Mediterranean areas, Middle East, India, Nepal
HbE	Microcytic, hypochromic anemia; target cells	Homozygous: HbE, F, A$_2$ Heterozygous: HbA, E, F, A$_2$	$\beta26$(B8)Glu $\rightarrow$ Lys	Burma, Thailand, Cambodia, Malaysia, Indonesia
HbC	Normocytic, normochromic anemia with reticulocytosis; poikilocytosis with folded, irregularly contracted cells; target cells	Homozygous: HbC, F, A$_2$ Heterozygous: HbA, C, F, A$_2$	$\beta6$(A3)Glu $\rightarrow$ Lys	West Africa

mer at the oxygen concentration in venous blood, the majority of the cells do not sickle during their journey through the circulation because they reach the lungs and are reoxygenated before significant polymerization and cell distortion occurs. The length of delay depends highly on temperature, pH, ionic strength, and oxygen tension in the cell's environment. Hypoxia, acidosis, hypertonicity, and temperatures higher than 37°C promote deoxygenation and the formation of HbS polymers. The spleen, kidney, retina, and bone marrow provide a sufficiently hypoxic, acidotic, and hypertonic microenvironment to promote HbS polymerization and sickling.

Sickling (delay time) also depends on intracellular hemoglobin composition (the proportion of HbA, HbS, HbA$_2$, and HbF present) as well as total hemoglobin concentration (MCHC). Non-S hemoglobins increase the delay time for polymerization, presumably by interfering with the HbS polymerization process. The delay time is also inversely related to the total hemoglobin concentration. The more concentrated the hemoglobin solution within the cell (the higher the MCHC), the shorter is the delay time and the greater is the potential for HbS aggregates to form. Using this concept, attempts are made to treat the disease by hydrating the cells, which would decrease the MCHC and prevent sickling.

Polymerization of deoxyhemoglobin S begins when the oxygen saturation of hemoglobin falls below 85% and is generally complete at about 38% oxygen saturation. The HbS aggregates cause the erythrocyte to become rigid and less deformable. With repeated cycles of deoxygenation, polymerization, and sickling, disruption of cation homeostasis occurs, resulting in an increase in intracellular Ca^{2+} and loss of K$^+$ and water from the cell. This cellular dehydration increases the MCHC (predisposing the cell to sickling on subsequent deoxygenation). In addition, the increased MCHC is associated with an increase in cytoplasmic viscosity and a decrease in cell deformability. HbS is also prone to oxidation. Oxidation of membrane proteins and lipids weakens critical skeletal associations. In addition, repeated sickling tends to decouple the lipid bilayer from the membrane skeleton, and loss of membrane phospholipid asymmetry occurs. The aggregates also damage the erythrocyte membrane directly, and with the weakened cytoskeleton, the cell's fragility increases.

Irreversibly Sickled Cells

The sickled erythrocyte can return to a normal biconcave shape upon reoxygenation of the hemoglobin; however, as described above, with repeated cycles of sickling, the erythrocyte membrane undergoes changes that cause it to become leaky and rigid. After repeated sickling episodes, the cells become **irreversibly sickled cells** (ISC), which are locked in a sickle shape whether oxygenated or deoxygenated (i.e., regardless of polymerization state of the hemoglobin molecules). This is due to abnormal interactions of red cell skeletal proteins, most likely caused by oxidative damage and increased Ca^{2+} concentrations. The ISC is the

result of permanent alterations of the submembrane skeletal lattice.[10] From 5 to 50% of the circulating erythrocytes in sickle cell anemia are ISC. This varies from person to person but is relatively constant for a given individual. The ISC have a very high MCHC and a low MCV. They are ovoid or boat shaped with a smooth outline and lack the spicules characteristic of deoxygenated sickled cells.

The ISC are removed by mononuclear phagocytes in the spleen, liver, or bone marrow. ISC account for most, if not all, of the sickle forms on a peripheral blood smear (most reversible sickle cells regain a discocyte shape when the blood is exposed to air while making the slide). The ISC can also initiate or increase the severity of vaso-occlusive crises because of impaired cell deformability and increased cell adherence to vascular endothelium. The mechanism for this interaction between sickled cells and the endothelium is unclear but could be related to changes in the surface properties of sickled cells and endothelial cells as well as plasma factors.[11,12]

Oxygen Affinity of HbS

The oxygen affinity of HbS differs from that of HbA, resulting in important physiologic changes in vivo. HbS has decreased oxygen affinity, and the 2,3-BPG level of homozygotes is increased. This decreased oxygen affinity, depicted by a shift to the right in the oxygen dissociation curve, facilitates the release of more oxygen to the tissues. However, this phenomenon increases the concentration of deoxyhemoglobin S, promoting the formation of sickle cells.

RBC Destruction

The primary cause of anemia in sickle cell anemia is extravascular hemolysis. Erythrocyte survival depends on intracellular HbF concentration and degree of membrane damage.[13] Changes in the erythrocyte membrane resulting in increased fragility coupled with Heinz body formation from denatured HbS lead to increased membrane shedding (vesiculation), a decreased cell surface area, and the removal of the cell by the mononuclear phagocyte system.[14] The life span of circulating HbS erythrocytes can decrease to as few as 14 days. The sluggish blood flow and the hypoglycemic, hypoxic environment of the spleen promotes HbS polymerization and sickling, further slowing blood circulation in the splenic cords and enhancing phagocytosis of erythrocytes containing HbS. Eventually, however, the spleen loses its functional capacity as repeated ischemic crises (see below) lead to splenic tissue necrosis and atrophy. With splenic atrophy, other cells of the mononuclear phagocyte system in the liver and bone marrow take over the destruction of these abnormal cells.

CLINICAL FINDINGS

The first clinical signs of sickle cell anemia appear at about 6 months of age when the concentration of HbS predominates over HbF. Clinical manifestations result from chronic hemolytic anemia, vaso-occlusion of the microvasculature, overwhelming infections, and acute splenic sequestration.

Anemia

A moderate to severe chronic anemia as the result of extravascular hemolysis is characteristic of the disease. Gallstones, a complication of any chronic hemolytic disorder, are a common finding due to cholestasis and increased bilirubin turnover. Folate deficiency due to increased erythrocyte turnover can further exacerbate the anemia, producing megaloblastosis (∞ Chapter 12).

Hemodynamic changes occur in an attempt to compensate for the tissue oxygen deficit; as a result, symptoms of cardiac overload including cardiac hypertrophy, cardiac enlargement, and eventually congestive heart failure are frequent complications of the disease.

The hyperplastic bone marrow, secondary to chronic hemolysis, is accompanied by bone changes, such as thinning of cortices and a "hair-on-end" appearance in x-rays of the skull. Hyperplasia results from a futile attempt by the marrow to compensate for premature erythrocyte destruction. Conversely, **aplastic crises** can accompany or follow viral, bacterial, and mycoplasmal infections. This temporary cessation of erythropoiesis in the face of chronic hemolysis leads to an acute worsening of the anemia. The aplasia can last from a few days to a week and because of the significantly decreased red cell life span can induce a catastrophic fall in the hemoglobin concentration. Increasing evidence suggests that many cases of aplasia occur as a result of infection with human parvovirus B19. Parvovirus also causes a cessation of erythropoiesis in normal individuals, but with a normal RBC life span, normal blood cell production in these individuals is restored before any clinically significant changes in erythrocyte concentration take place.

Vaso-Occlusive Crisis

HbS cells are poorly deformable. Sickled cells have difficulty squeezing through small capillaries, and consequently, the rigid cells tend to aggregate in the microvasculature, increasing vascular stasis. Erythrocytes behind the blockage release their oxygen to the surrounding hypoxic tissue, deoxygenate, polymerize, and sickle, increasing the plug's size (Figure 10-1 ■). Erythrocytes from nearby capillaries are forced to give up more oxygen than they normally would to feed the oxygen-deprived tissue around the blockage. These cells then form rigid aggregates of deoxyhemoglobin S, expanding the blockaded region. If severe, lack of oxygen can cause local tissue necrosis. Vaso-occlusion occurs more often in tissues prone to vascular stasis (spleen, marrow, retina, kidney).

The blockage of the microvasculature by rigid sickled cells accounts for the majority of the clinical signs of sickle cell anemia. The occlusions do not occur continuously but sporadically, causing acute signs of distress. These episodes are called **vaso-occlusive crises** and are the most frequent

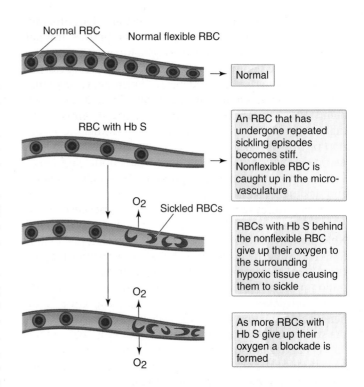

■ FIGURE 10-1   How sickle cells block a vessel and precipitate a vaso-occlusive crisis.

causes of hospitalization. The crises can be triggered by infection, decreased atmospheric oxygen pressure, dehydration, or slow blood flow, but frequently they occur without any known cause. The occlusions are accompanied by pain, low-grade fever, organ dysfunction, and tissue necrosis. The episodes generally last for 4 to 5 days and subside spontaneously.

Recurrent occlusive episodes can lead to infarctions of tissue of the genitourinary tract, liver, bone, lung, and spleen. The chronic organ damage is accompanied by organ dysfunction. Although splenomegaly is present in early childhood, repeated splenic infarctions eventually result in splenic fibrosis and calcifications (usually by age 4 or 5). This organ damage, secondary to infarction, is known as **autosplenectomy.** As a result, splenomegaly is rare in adults with this disease. Aseptic necrosis of the head of the femur is common. Dactylitis, a painful symmetrical swelling of the hands and feet (hand-foot syndrome) caused by infarction of the metacarpals and metatarsals, is often the first sign of the disease in infants. Recurrent priapism is a characteristic, painful complication that occasionally requires surgical intervention.

The slow flow of blood in occlusive areas can lead to thrombosis. Thrombosis of the cerebral arteries resulting in stroke is common. Magnetic resonance imaging shows evidence of subclinical cerebral infarction in 20–30% of children with sickle cell anemia. If the arterioles of the eye are affected, blindness can occur. Chronic leg ulcers, found also in other hemolytic anemias, can occur at any age. The ulcers appear without any known injury. These painful sores do not readily respond to treatment and can take months to heal.

Placental infarctions in pregnant women with sickle cell disease can be a hazard to the fetus. Maternal anemia often becomes more severe during pregnancy. In addition, other clinical findings can be exacerbated during pregnancy, endangering the life of both the mother and the fetus.

Bacterial Infection

Overwhelming bacterial infection is a common cause of death in young patients. The risk of septicemia from encapsulated microorganisms, such as *Streptococcus pneumoniae* and *Hemophilus influenzae,* is extremely high. Bacterial pneumonia is the most common infection, but meningitis is also prevalent. The reasons for this increased susceptibility to infection are not fully understood but could be related to functional asplenia, impaired opsonization, and abnormal complement activation.[15] The spleen is particularly important to host defense in the young. Significant impairment of in vivo neutrophil adherence to vascular endothelium in HbS disease also occurs. This could prevent neutrophils from rapidly relocating to areas of inflammation.[15] Prophylactic penicillin is given to children with sickle cell anemia to reduce morbidity and mortality from infection, but compliance with therapy may not be optimal. The pneumococcal and *H. influenzae* type B vaccines protect patients from infections with *S. pneumoniae* and *H. influenzae,* reducing the incidence of infection in children with sickle cell disease. Children with sickle cell disease are also routinely immunized for hepatitis B.

 Checkpoint! 4

Why do newborns with sickle cell anemia not experience episodes of vaso-occlusive crisis?

Acute Splenic Sequestration

In young children, sudden splenic pooling of sickled erythrocytes can cause a massive decrease in erythrocyte mass within a few hours (**sequestration crisis**). Thrombocytopenia can also occur. Hypovolemia and shock follow. At one time, this was the leading cause of death in infants with sickle cell anemia. Early diagnosis, instruction of parents in detecting an enlarging spleen, and rapid intervention with transfusion have decreased morbidity and mortality associated with splenic sequestration.

Acute Chest Syndrome

This illness resembling pneumonia is the most common cause of death in children with sickle cell disease and the second most common cause of hospitalization.[16] Clinical findings include cough, fever, chest pain, dyspnea, chills, wheezing, and pulmonary infiltrates. Hemoglobin concentration and oxygen saturation decrease.[17] The etiology of acute chest syndrome is not clear. In children, an infectious agent can often be identified. Other possible causes include pulmonary edema from overhydration, fat embolism from infarcted bone marrow, and hypoventilation due to pain from rib infarcts or from narcotic analgesics used to combat pain. The long-term effects of recurrent episodes of acute chest syndrome are unknown.

 CASE STUDY *(continued from page 215)*

The chest radiograph showed consolidation in the left lower lobe, indicating that Shane has pneumonia.

5. What physiological conditions does Shane have that could lead to sickling of his erythrocytes?

6. What is the cause of Shane's pain and acute distress?

7. Why might Shane be more susceptible to pneumonia than an individual without sickle cell disease?

LABORATORY FINDINGS

Peripheral Blood

A normocytic, normochromic anemia is characteristic of sickle cell anemia; however, with marked reticulocytosis, the anemia can appear macrocytic (Figure 10-2 ■). Reticulocytosis from 10–20% is typical. The hemoglobin ranges from 60 to 100 g/L and the hematocrit from 0.18 to 0.30 L/L. A calculated hematocrit from an electronic cell counter is more reliable than a centrifuged microhematocrit because excessive plasma trapped by sickled cells in centrifuged specimens falsely elevates the manual hematocrit.

The Cooperative Study of Sickle Cell Disease revealed that individuals homozygous for HbS have higher steady-state leukocyte counts than do normal individuals, especially children less than 10 years of age.[18] Platelet counts are also frequently higher than normal. After the age of 40, the hemoglobin concentration, reticulocyte count, leukocyte count, and platelet count decrease.[19]

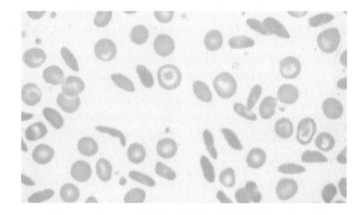

■ FIGURE 10-2   Hemoglobin S disease (sickle cell anemia). Note abnormal boat-shaped, sickled, and ovoid erythrocytes. (Peripheral blood; Wright-Giemsa stain; 1000× magnification)

The blood smear shows variable anisocytosis with polychromatophilic macrocytes and variable poikilocytosis with the presence of sickled cells and target cells. Nucleated erythrocytes can usually be found. The RDW is increased. During and following a hemolytic crisis, the RDW increases linearly with increases in reticulocytes.[20] If the patient is not experiencing a crisis, sickled cells might not be present.

In older children and adults, signs of splenic hypofunction are apparent on the peripheral blood smear with the presence of basophilic stippling, Howell-Jolly bodies, siderocytes, and poikilocytes.

 CASE STUDY *(continued from page 219)*

Admission laboratory data on Shane included:

WBC	16.4×10^9/L
RBC	2.5×10^{12}/L
HGB	78 g/L
Hct	0.24 L/L
PLT	467×10^9/L

Differential: Segs 76%, bands 10%, lymphs 9%, monos 3%, eos 1%, basos 1%

RBC morphology: Sickle cells 3+, target cells 1+, ovalocytes 1+, polychromasia, 3 NRBC/100 WBCs, Howell-Jolly bodies

8. Which of Shane's hematologic test results are consistent with a diagnosis of sickle cell anemia?

9. What does the presence of polychromatophilic erythrocytes signify?

10. Why is the absolute neutrophil count elevated?

11. What is the significance of ovalocytes on the blood smear?

12. What is the significance of Howell-Jolly bodies on the smear?

Bone Marrow

Bone marrow aspiration shows erythroid hyperplasia, reflecting the attempt of the bone marrow to compensate for chronic hemolysis. Erythrocyte production increases to 4–5 times normal. If the patient is deficient in folic acid, megaloblastosis can be seen. Iron stores are most often increased but can be diminished if hematuria is excessive. Bone marrow examination is not usually performed because it yields no definitive diagnostic information.

Hemoglobin Electrophoresis

The presence of HbS is confirmed by hemoglobin electrophoresis. Electrophoresis on cellulose acetate at pH 8.4 shows 85–100% HbS. HbF is usually not more than 15%. Higher levels of HbF (25–35%) can indicate compound heterozygosity for HbS and hereditary persistence of fetal hemoglobin (∞ Chapter 11). HbA_2 is normal. Newborns have 60–80% HbF with the remainder HbS. In infants less than 3 months of age with small amounts of HbS, electrophoresis

on citrate agar gel at pH 6.2 permits more reliable separation of HbF from both HbA and HbS. Citrate agar gel electrophoresis is also useful in separating HbD and HbG from HbS. Both of these nonsickling hemoglobins migrate with HbS on alkaline electrophoresis with paper or starch gel but migrate with HbA on agar gel electrophoresis at acid pH.

Solubility Test

The solubility test is a rapid test for detecting HbS in the heterozygous or homozygous state. In severe anemia, the amount of HbS can be too low to be accurately detected, and the procedure may need to be altered. This test should not be used as a screening test for newborns because of the low concentration of HbS in this age group. Unstable hemoglobins can give a false positive test if many Heinz bodies are present. Other rare hemoglobin variants (e.g., HbC Harlem, HbI) can also give positive tests. False positive tests can also occur with elevated plasma proteins and lipids.

Sickling Test

Another confirmatory test that is performed less often is the sodium metabisulfite slide test for sickling. This test is positive in both sickle cell anemia and sickle cell trait.

Other Diagnostic Tests

IEF in agar gels and HPLC can be used to identify abnormal hemoglobins such as HbS. Preferred methods for prenatal screening and diagnosis use DNA-based analysis (polymerase chain reaction) to detect point mutations in globin gene sequences.[7] This DNA testing provides a genotype diagnosis and eliminates the need for later neonatal testing when the phenotype results can be inconclusive. The molecular techniques are discussed in ∞ Chapter 39.

Other Laboratory Findings

Other laboratory findings are less specific. The hemolytic nature of the disease causes indirect bilirubin to increase, haptoglobin to decrease, and uric acid and serum lactic dehydrogenase (LD) to increase. Osmotic fragility can be decreased due to the presence of target cells. These tests offer no diagnostic information on sickle cell anemia but can be performed to evaluate complicating conditions.

 CASE STUDY *(continued from page 220)*

The LD level was reported as 1260 U/L. (Reference interval 75–200 U/L)

13. What is the significance of Shane's elevated LD?

THERAPY

Preventive therapy is aimed at eliminating conditions known to precipitate vaso-occlusion, such as dehydration and infection. Transfusion of packed erythrocytes or whole blood can be required in aplastic crises or splenic sequestration. Preoperative transfusion is helpful in preventing the complications of anesthesia-induced sickling. Long-term transfusion therapy can be useful in preventing complications of sickle cell anemia but is usually not required. This therapy is aimed at suppressing the formation of new HbS-containing RBC by the patient's bone marrow. Complications of chronic transfusion therapy include transmission of blood-borne diseases, alloimmunization, expense, inconvenience, and iron overload.

Various pharmacologic agents have been used to reduce intracellular sickling by increasing the level of HbF including hydroxyurea (HU), 5-azacytidine, and 5-aza 2'-deoxycitidine. Of these, HU has been tested most extensively and elevates HbF in most HbS-containing erythrocytes. Children and adults respond well to HU, experiencing fewer vaso-occlusive crises and hospitalizations. The most frequent side effects are neutropenia, reticulocytopenia, and thrombocytopenia. HU is a potential teratogen, so contraceptive precautions are recommended. HU does not seem to produce serious irreversible toxicity; however, long-term effects are unknown.[6]

Hematopoietic stem cell transplantation (SCT) affords the potential cure of sickle cell disease. Results of multicenter case series show disease-free survival rates ranging from 80 to 85% with the best outcomes obtained when children received stem cells from HLA-identical siblings. Risk of complications, including graft versus host disease and neurological problems, is high for patients with sickle cell disease undergoing SCT. Because of a wide range of heterogeneity in clinical severity of sickle cell disease, it is difficult to predict which patients will benefit from SCT. Furthermore, SCT is extremely expensive and can be beyond the financial means of many patients. Gene therapy, in which normal genes are inserted into a patient's defective stem cells and returned to the patient, also holds a promise of cure but is not feasible at this time. Progress toward finding a stable gene vector capable of expressing therapeutic levels of normal β-globin chains over time has been slow.[21,22]

Checkpoint! 5

Outline the treatment options for a patient with HbS disease, pneumonia, and vaso-occlusive crisis. Discuss how each would affect the patient's clinical condition.

SICKLE CELL TRAIT

Sickle cell trait is the heterozygous β^S state, and typically the patient has one normal β-gene and one β^S-gene ($\beta^A\beta^S$). Sickle cell trait is not as severe a disorder as sickle cell anemia because the presence of HbA or other non-S hemoglobins interferes with the process of HbS polymerization, preventing sickling under most physiologic conditions. However, sickle cell trait cells can sickle under very low oxygen tension (~15 torr). Although some hemoglobins other than HbS (especially HbC, HbD, and HbE) can be incorporated into the polymer of deoxyhemoglobin S, the presence of molecules of these hemoglobins intermixed with the molecules of HbS creates a weakened structure and decreases the degree of polymerization. Because HbA constitutes more than 50% of the total hemoglobin in these individuals, sickle cell trait has no clinical symptoms, and results of physical examination appear normal. However, sickle cell trait is important to diagnose because, statistically, one of four children born to parents each of whom has the trait will have sickle cell anemia and two of four will have the trait.

Complications of splenic infarction and renal papillary necrosis have occasionally been reported in affected individuals subjected to extreme and prolonged hypoxia such as after flying at high altitude in unpressurized aircraft or following general anesthesia.

Hematologic parameters are normal. No anemia or sickled cells are found in routine blood counts and differentials. Sickling can be induced with the sodium metabisulfite test, however, and the solubility test is also positive. Hemoglobin electrophoresis results show 50–65% HbA, 35–45% HbS, normal HbF, and normal or slightly increased HbA_2. If HbA constitutes less than 50% of the total hemoglobin in sickle cell trait, the patient is probably heterozygous for another hemoglobinopathy such as thalassemia.

Checkpoint! 6

A child's parents both have sickle cell trait. The physician orders a hemoglobin electrophoresis on the child. Results of electrophoresis on cellulose acetate at pH 8.4 show 65% HbS, 30% HbA, 3% HbF, 2% HbA_2. Explain these results and suggest further testing that could help in diagnosis.

▶ HEMOGLOBIN C DISEASE

Hemoglobin C, the second hemoglobinopathy to be recognized, is the third most prevalent hemoglobin variant worldwide.[8] The first cases of HbC were discovered in the heterozygous state with HbS; this is not surprising because both hemoglobinopathies are prevalent in the same geographic area. Hemoglobin C is found predominantly in West African blacks in whom the incidence of the trait can reach 17–28% of the population. From 2–3% of African Americans carry the trait, and 0.02% have the disease.

Hemoglobin C is produced when lysine is substituted for glutamic acid at the sixth position (A3) in the β-chain (β6 [A3] Glu → Lys). Because the nonpolar lysine amino acid substitution is in the same β-chain position as the substitution for HbS, a decrease in hemoglobin solubility can be expected. Intraerythrocytic crystals of oxygenated HbC can be found in the red cells, especially in splenectomized individuals. HbF inhibits the formation of crystals. Crystal formation is enhanced when cells are dehydrated or in hypertonic solutions. Erythrocytes with crystals become rigid and are trapped and destroyed in the spleen. Erythrocyte life span is decreased to 30–55 days.

Hemoglobin C disease (β^C/β^C) is usually asymptomatic, but patients occasionally experience joint and abdominal pain. In contrast to sickle cell anemia, the spleen is most often enlarged. Variable hemolysis results in a mild to moderate anemia.

The hemoglobin ranges from 80 to 120 g/L and the hematocrit from 0.25 to 0.35 L/L. The anemia is accompanied by a slight to moderate increase in reticulocytes. The stained blood smear contains small cells that appear to be folded and irregularly contracted as well as many target cells (Figure 10-3 ■). Intracellular hemoglobin crystals can be found if the smear has been dried slowly. Microspherocytes are occasionally present. Osmotic fragility can be decreased, especially in the presence of large numbers of target cells.

Hemoglobin electrophoresis on citrate agar gel at acid pH demonstrates more than 90% HbC with a slight increase in HbF (not more than 7%). On cellulose acetate at an alkaline pH, HbC migrates with HbA_2, HbE, and HbO-Arab. HbC can be separated from these other hemoglobins by agar gel electrophoresis at an acid pH.

Hemoglobin C trait (β^C/β^A) is asymptomatic. No hematologic abnormalities are produced except that target cells are noted on blood smears. Mild hypochromia can be present. About 60–70% of the hemoglobin is HbA and 30–40% is HbC. Higher levels of HbC and microcytosis are found when HbC is associated with β-thalassemia (β^C/β^{thal}) (Figure 10-4 ■).

Considerable heterogeneity occurs in the clinical and hematological features of HbC/β^{thal}, depending on the particular β-thalassemia gene interacting with HbC. HbC/β^+ thalassemia is characterized by mild anemia similar to that found in heterozygous β-thalassemia. (β^+-thalassemia is characterized by a decrease in β-chain synthesis.) There is 65–80% HbC, 2–5% HbF, and the remainder is HbA. HbC/B^0 thalassemia is characterized by more severe anemia and an absence of HbA (β^0-thalassemia is characterized by an absence of β-chain synthesis). Hemoglobin electrophoresis reveals only HbC, HbA_2, and HbF with HbF ranging from 3–10%.

▶ HEMOGLOBIN S/C DISEASE

In hemoglobin S/C disease, both β-chains are abnormal. One β-gene codes for β^S-chains, and the other gene codes for β^C-chains ($\beta^S\beta^C$), thus, HbA is absent. This double heterozygous state for HbS and HbC results in a disease less severe then homozygous HbS but more severe than homozygous HbC. The concentration of hemoglobin in individual erythrocytes (MCHC) is increased, and the concentration of HbS is more than in sickle cell trait (the percent of HbS is higher than that of HbC because the β^C-globin has a less negative charge than β^S-globin, thus, the cell does not form $\alpha\beta^C$-dimers as readily as $\alpha\beta^S$-dimers). The presence of HbC makes the HbS/C cells more prone to sickling than cells that contain HbA/HbS because HbC molecules participate in the polymerization process with HbS molecules more easily than do HbA molecules. Increased erythrocyte rigidity is noted at oxygen tensions less than 50 mm Hg. Additionally, cells containing HbS/C have formation of aggregates of intracellular HbC crystals.[23] Thus, in HbS/C disease, both sickling and crystal formation contribute to the pathophysiology of the disease.

The clinical signs and symptoms of the disease are similar to those of mild sickle cell anemia. Because of the poorly deformable red cells, patients can develop vaso-occlusive crises leading to the complications associated with this pathology. A notable difference from sickle cell anemia, however, is that in HbS/C disease, splenomegaly is prominent.

Mild to moderate normocytic, normochromic anemia is present. The hematocrit is usually above 0.25 L/L, and the hemoglobin concentration is between 100 and 140 g/L. The

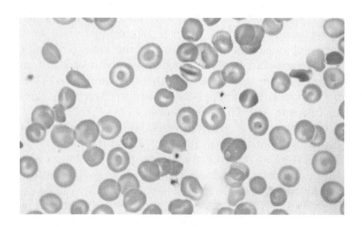

■ FIGURE 10-3 Hemoglobin C disease. Note the cell in the center with HbC crystal, target cells, and folded cells. (Peripheral blood; Wright-Giemsa stain; 1000× magnification)

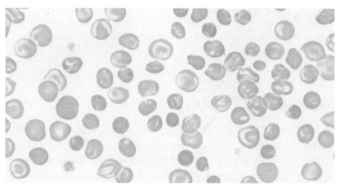

■ FIGURE 10-4 Hemoglobin C/β-thalassemia. Note the microspherocytes and target cells. This patient had 94% HbC and 6% HbF. (Peripheral blood; Wright-Giemsa stain; 1000× magnification)

higher hemoglobin concentration does not necessarily mean that hemolysis is less severe than in sickle cell anemia; it could be that the higher oxygen affinity of HbS/C cells stimulates higher erythropoietin levels. Peripheral blood smears reveal a large number of target cells (up to 85%), folded cells, and boat-shaped cells but rarely sickled forms (Figure 10-5 ■). Typical HbC crystals are rarely found. Some erythrocytes contain a single eccentrically located, densely stained, round mass of hemoglobin that makes part of the cell appear empty. These cells have been referred to as *billiard-ball cells*.[23] Anisocytosis and poikilocytosis range from mild to severe. Small, dense, misshapen cells, some with crystals of various shapes jutting out at angles, have been referred to as *HbSC poikilocytes*.[24] Hemoglobin electrophoresis shows a higher concentration of HbS than HbC. HbF can be increased up to 7%. No HbA is found due to the absence of normal β-chains.

 Checkpoint! 7

What is the functional abnormality of HbC and HbS? Why do these two abnormal hemoglobins have the same altered functions?

▶ HEMOGLOBIN D

Hemoglobin D is due to several molecular variants of which the identical variants HbD Punjab and HbD Los Angeles ($\beta121$ [GH4] Glu → Gln) are the most common in African Americans (<0.02%). HbD migrates with HbS on hemoglobin electrophoresis at alkaline pH. However, the HbD molecules do not sickle and have normal solubility properties. The heterozygous and homozygous states are both asymptomatic. Although there are no hematologic abnormalities, the homozygous state occasionally has an increase in target cells and a decrease in osmotic fragility. Although rare, the compound heterozygous state of HbD with HbS exists. HbD molecules can interact with HbS molecules, producing aggregates of deoxyhemoglobin (Figure 10-6 ■). This produces a relatively mild form of sickle cell anemia.

In homozygous HbD, electrophoresis on cellulose acetate at pH 8.4 demonstrates 95% HbD with the same electrophoretic mobility as HbS. Electrophoresis on citrate agar at pH 6.0 allows separation of HbS and HbD. At acid pH, HbD migrates with HbA.

✓ **Checkpoint! 8**

A 13-year-old black female had a routine physical. Her CBC was normal, but the differential revealed many target cells. Hemoglobin electrophoresis revealed a band that migrated like HbS on cellulose acetate at pH 8.4. Her hemoglobin solubility test was negative. Explain the results and suggest a follow-up test to determine a diagnosis.

▶ HEMOGLOBIN E

Hemoglobin E is the second most prevalent hemoglobinopathy worldwide.[8] It is most often encountered in individuals from southeast Asia. The trait has reached frequencies of almost 50% in areas of Thailand. It is estimated that 15–30% of immigrants from southeast Asia in North America have HbE with the highest frequencies occurring in those from Cambodia and Laos. Although found mainly in Asians, the HbE trait can also occur in blacks.

Hemoglobin E is the result of a substitution of lysine for glutamic acid in the β-chain ($\beta26$ [B8] Glu → Lys). The hemoglobin is slightly unstable when subjected to oxidant stress. Also, the nucleotide substitution creates a potential new splicing sequence so that some of the mRNA can be improperly processed. As a result, synthesis of the abnormal

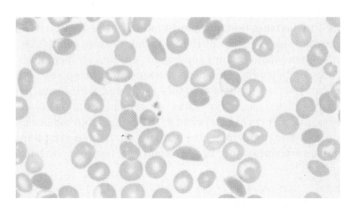

■ **FIGURE 10-5**   Hemoglobin S/C disease. Notice the elongated cells and boat-shaped cells. The small contracted cells are typical of those seen in hemoglobin C disease. (Peripheral blood; Wright-Giemsa stain; 1000× magnification)

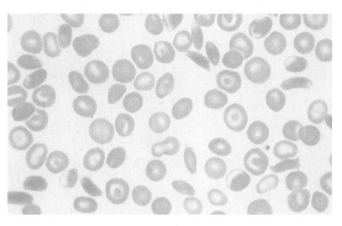

■ **FIGURE 10-6**   A blood film from a patient with hemoglobin D/S. Homozygous HbD does not usually cause anemia, but when combined with HbS, it potentiates the aggregating of deoxyhemoglobin and sickling of erythrocytes, producing a mild sickle cell anemia. Notice the boat-shaped cells and target cells. (Peripheral blood; Wright-Giemsa stain; 1000× magnification)

β-chain is decreased and HbE trait and disease have some thalassemia-like characteristics including an increased ratio of α:non-α-chain synthesis and α-chain excess (∞ Chapter 11). The oxygen dissociation curve is shifted to the right, indicating that HbE has decreased oxygen affinity.

Homozygous HbE is characterized by the presence of a mild, asymptomatic, microcytic hypochromic anemia (similar to thalassemia) with decreased erythrocyte survival (Figure 10-7 ■). Target cells are prominent and osmotic fragility is decreased. Electrophoresis demonstrates mostly HbE (90% or more) with the remainder HbA_2 and HbF. On alkaline electrophoresis, HbE migrates with HbA_2, HbC, and HbO-Arab. On agar gel at an acid pH, HbE migrates with HbA.

HbE trait is asymptomatic, and hematologic parameters are normal except for slight microcytosis. Hemoglobin electrophoresis at alkaline pH shows about 35–45% HbE. The remainder is HbA with normal HbA_2 and HbF.

▶ HEMOGLOBIN E/THALASSEMIA

Compound heterozygosity for HbE and β-thalassemia causes a moderate to severe anemia similar to thalassemia. This is a common combination in people from southeast Asia in whom both genes have a high frequency. The most severe type (β^E/β^0-thalassemia) reveals only HbE and HbF. The amount of HbE, however, is less than that expected for homozygous HbE, and the HbF is increased proportionately. A more moderate anemia can result if the β^+-thalassemia gene is inherited with HbE. In this form of the disease, there are HbE, HbA, HbF, and HbA_2. The HbA, however, is less than would be expected in HbE trait, but the anemia is more severe. When the β-thalassemia gene is inherited with the β^E gene, the result is microcytic, hypochromic anemia with significant poikilocytosis and nucleated erythrocytes.

Hemoglobin E can also be found in combination with α-thalassemia (Figure 10-8 ■). This combination produces a

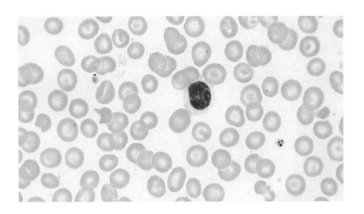

■ FIGURE 10-7   A blood film from a patient with homozygous hemoglobin E (HbEE). Note the microcytosis and prominent target cells. (Peripheral blood; Wright-Giemsa stain; 1000× magnification)

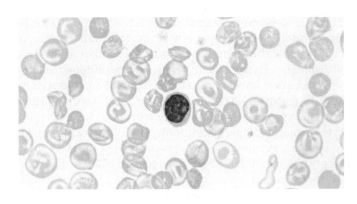

■ FIGURE 10-8   A blood film from a splenectomized patient with homozygous hemoglobin E and α-thalassemia. The erythrocytes are microcytic, hypochromic with many target cells and poikilocytosis. The patient was from southeast Asia and had a lifelong history of anemia. (Peripheral blood; Wright-Giemsa stain; 1000× magnification)

more severe anemia than does HbE alone. The amount of HbE depends on whether the patient is heterozygous or homozygous for HbE and which α-thalassemia genotype is inherited (∞ Chapter 11).

✔ **Checkpoint! 9**

The red cell morphology in HbE disease and β-thalassemia are similar: microcytic, hypochromic anemia with target cells. What laboratory test(s) could differentiate these two conditions?

▶ UNSTABLE HEMOGLOBIN VARIANTS

Unstable hemoglobins can result from structurally abnormal globin chains, and more than 130 unstable variants have been described. The abnormal chains contain amino acid mutations at critical internal portions of the chains, which affect the molecular stability.[25] The disorders are characterized by denaturation and precipitation of the abnormal hemoglobin in the form of Heinz bodies, causing cell rigidity, membrane damage, and subsequent erythrocyte hemolysis. Although hemoglobin denaturation and hemolysis can occur spontaneously, symptoms associated with acute hemolysis often occur only after drug administration, infection, or other events that change the hemoglobin molecule's normal environment. Those variants that cause symptoms are known collectively as *congenital Heinz body hemolytic anemias*.

PATHOPHYSIOLOGY

Most affected individuals with unstable hemoglobins are heterozygous. Most unstable hemoglobins are inherited as autosomal-dominant disorders, but a large number arise from spontaneous mutations with no evidence of hemoglobin instability in parents or other family members.

Unstable hemoglobin variants can result from a variety of globin chain amino acid substitutions or deletions that disrupt the stability of the globin subunit or hemoglobin tetramer or the binding of heme to globin. Such mutations resulting in unstable hemoglobin variants include:

1. Mutation of a globin amino acid that is involved in contact with the heme group or that results in a tendency to dissociate heme from the abnormal globin chains

2. Replacement of nonpolar by polar amino acids at the interior of the molecule resulting in a distortion of the folding of the globin chain

3. Deletion or insertion of additional amino acids, particularly in the helical regions of the molecule, creating instability

4. Mutations of amino acids at intersubunit contacts (especially the α_1-β_1 contact points), creating instability and a tendency to dissociate into monomers

5. Replacement of a hydrophobic residue with a more hydrophilic amino acid in the hydrophobic pocket, disrupting the conformation of the hydrophobic heme cleft

Unstable hemoglobin denatures and precipitates as Heinz bodies, which attach to the inner surface of the membrane, thereby decreasing cell deformability. The inclusions are pitted by macrophages in the spleen, leaving the cell with less hemoglobin and decreased membrane. This process leads to rigid cells and their premature destruction in the spleen.

In addition to altering the molecule's stability, disruption of the normal conformation also can affect the molecule's function. Many of the unstable hemoglobins also have altered oxygen affinity. If the amino acid substitution is strategically located to affect the oxygen-binding site, oxygen affinity can be increased or decreased. In addition, some unstable hemoglobin variants have a tendency to spontaneously oxidize to methemoglobin.

CLINICAL FINDINGS

Congenital hemolytic anemia indicative of an unstable hemoglobin disorder requires further investigation to establish a definitive diagnosis. Family history is extremely important in defining the hereditary nature of the disease. Patient history can also provide information about the nature of events such as infection or drug administration, that precipitate acute hemolytic episodes. The severity of the disorder can range from asymptomatic to a chronic severe hemolytic anemia.

The severity of the anemia depends on the degree of instability of the hemoglobin tetramer and the change, if any, in oxygen affinity. For example, Hb Köln is an unstable hemoglobin (β-chain mutation) that also demonstrates increased oxygen affinity. Hemoglobins with increased oxygen affinity (hemoglobin-oxygen dissociation curve is shifted

left) release less oxygen to the tissues which result in relatively higher levels of tissue hypoxia and of erythropoietin as well as higher hematocrits than expected relative to the severity of hemolysis. Conversely, unstable hemoglobins with decreased oxygen affinity (e.g., Hb Hammersmith) have a hemoglobin-oxygen dissociation curve that is shifted right, increasing the oxygen delivery to the tissues and allowing patients to function at a lower hematocrit. When the oxygen affinity of an unstable hemoglobin is decreased, the reticulocyte count is not increased as much as would be expected for the degree of anemia relative to an uncomplicated hemolytic anemia.

Most clinical findings occur as the result of increased erythrocyte hemolysis. Jaundice and splenomegaly are common when there is chronic extravascular hemolysis. Cyanosis can result from the formation of sulfhemoglobin and methemoglobin that accompanies hemoglobin denaturation. Weakness and jaundice frequently follow the administration of oxidant drugs, which increase the hemoglobin's instability. Acute hemolysis can also be accompanied by the excretion of dark urine due to the presence of dipyrroles in the urine.

LABORATORY FINDINGS

Peripheral Blood

The anemia of congenital Heinz body hemolytic anemia is usually normocytic and normochromic and occasionally has a slightly decreased MCH and MCHC because of the removal of Heinz bodies from erythrocytes and loss of hemoglobin in the spleen. The reticulocyte count is typically increased. The blood film can show basophilic stippling, pitted cells (bite cells), and small contracted cells. Osmotic fragility is usually abnormal after 24 hours of incubation.

If splenic function is efficient, Heinz bodies are not detectable in peripheral blood cells. Heinz bodies can be found in the peripheral blood following splenectomy; however, this finding is not specific for unstable hemoglobin disorders. Heinz bodies can also be seen in erythrocyte enzyme abnormalities that permit oxidation of hemoglobin, in thalassemia, and after administration of oxidant drugs in normal individuals. Heinz bodies of unstable hemoglobins can be generated in vitro by incubation of the erythrocytes with brilliant cresyl blue or other redox agents. These intracellular inclusions cannot be observed on smears stained with Wright's stain.

Other Laboratory Findings

Many unstable hemoglobins identified to date have the same charge and electrophoretic mobility as normal hemoglobin. Only about 45% can be diagnosed by electrophoresis. Hemoglobin A_2 and HbF are sometimes increased, which could provide a clue to the presence of an abnormal hemoglobin when it is not detected by its electrophoretic pattern.

Diagnosis usually depends on the demonstration of the presence of an unstable hemoglobin (i.e., one that precipitates more readily than normal hemoglobin). The heat instability test (heating a hemoglobin solution to 50°C) is always positive in unstable hemoglobin disorders. The unstable hemoglobin is also precipitated within 20 minutes in the isopropanol (17% by volume) precipitation test. Normal hemoglobin remains in solution 30–40 minutes.

Checkpoint! 10

a. Explain why patients with an unstable hemoglobin variant usually experience acute hemolysis only after administration of certain drugs or with infections.

b. A patient is suspected of having a congenital Heinz body hemolytic anemia but hemoglobin electrophoresis is normal. Why is it necessary to perform additional tests?

THERAPY

Many patients with these disorders do not require any therapy. Splenectomy can be performed if hemolysis is severe. Patients are advised to avoid oxidizing drugs, which can precipitate a hemolytic episode.

▶ HEMOGLOBIN VARIANTS WITH ALTERED OXYGEN AFFINITY

Amino acid substitutions in the globin chains close to the heme pocket can affect the hemoglobin's ability to carry oxygen by preventing heme from binding to the globin chain or by stabilizing iron in the oxidized ferric state. Other substitutions that affect oxygen affinity include substitutions near the $\alpha_1\beta_2$ contacts, substitutions at the C terminal end of the β-chain, and substitutions near the 2,3-BPG binding site. These are critical sites involved in the allosteric properties of hemoglobin and/or in the physiologic regulation of hemoglobin affinity for oxygen. Either the α- or β-chain can be affected, but most substitutions are associated with the β-chain. Hemoglobinopathies causing perma-

nent methemoglobin formation are associated with psuedocyanosis while cyanosis characterizes hemoglobins with decreased oxygen affinity. Increased oxygen affinity results in congenital erythrocytosis, a compensatory mechanism for the reduced release of oxygen to the tissues.

METHEMOGLOBINEMIAS

Methemoglobin is hemoglobin with iron oxidized to the ferric state, which cannot carry oxygen. The amount of methemoglobin produced under normal physiologic conditions is maintained at concentrations less than 1% through the NADH-dependent enzyme, methemoglobin reductase. This system is capable of reducing methemoglobin to deoxyhemoglobin at a rate 250 times the rate at which heme is normally oxidized.

Methemoglobinemia is a clinical condition that occurs when methemoglobin encompasses more than 1% of the hemoglobin. This condition can occur when the methemoglobin reductase system is overwhelmed (acquired) or deficient (congenital) and when a structurally abnormal globin chain results in increased formation of methemoglobin by rendering the molecule relatively resistant to reduction by methemoglobin reductase (congenital) (Table 10-3 ✪).

Acquired methemoglobinemia can occur in normal individuals when drugs or other toxic substances oxidize hemoglobin in circulation at a rate that exceeds the reducing capacity of the methemoglobin reductase system (∞ Chapter 6).

Congenital methemoglobinemia can be inherited as a dominant or recessive characteristic. Recessive inheritance is usually associated with a defect in the methemoglobin reduction system, NADH diphorase (NADH reductase, dehydrogenase) deficiency rather than with an alteration in the structure of the hemoglobin molecule. With defects in the methemoglobin reduction system, the small amount of methemoglobin formed daily cannot be reduced and consequently accumulates within the cell. Dominant inheritance of methemoglobinemia is usually ascribed to the presence of a structural variant of hemoglobin called *hemoglobin M*

✪ TABLE 10-3

Causes and Characteristics of Methemoglobinemia

Type	Cause	Electrophoretic Pattern	NADH-Diaphorase Activity	Reduction with Methylene Blue
Acquired	Hb oxidized at a rate exceeding capacity of methemoglobin reductase system	Normal	Normal	Yes
Congenital				
Recessive	Defect in methemoglobin reductase system (recessive)	Normal	Decreased	Yes
Dominant	Structural abnormality of hemoglobin (HbM) (dominant)	HbM variant	Normal	No

(*HbM*). Nine variants of HbM have been described; however, all variants have been found only in the heterozygous state.

Most HbM variants are produced by a tyrosine substitution for the proximal or distal histidine in the heme pocket of the α- or β-chains. Tyrosine forms a covalent link with heme iron, stabilizing the iron in the ferric state. The stabilized, oxidized iron is relatively resistant to reduction by the methemoglobin reductase pathway. If the substitution occurs in the α-chain, cyanosis (or actually pseudocyanosis) is present from birth because the α-chain is a component of HbF ($\alpha_2\gamma_2$), the major hemoglobin at birth. If the substitution occurs in the β-chain, cyanosis does not occur until about the sixth month after birth when HbA ($\alpha_2\beta_2$) becomes the major hemoglobin. The presence of methemoglobin imparts a brownish color to the blood. Except for this abnormal color, no other hematologic abnormality is present because methemoglobin levels are rarely higher than 30%. Patients with methemoglobinemia appear to be cyanotic, but unlike truly cyanotic people, arterial blood pO$_2$ levels are usually normal (i.e., pseudocyanosis).

Hemoglobin M will not always separate from HbA at an alkaline pH. Hemoglobin electrophoresis on agar gel at pH 7.1 of a blood sample containing HbM reveals a brown band (HbM) running anodal to a red band (HbA). The pattern can appear sharper with gel electrofocusing. Oxidizing the erythrocyte hemolysate with ferricyanide before electrophoresis reveals a sharp separation of congenital HbM and methemoglobin formed from HbA. Methemoglobin formed from HbA by oxidation of iron has no change in molecular charge and therefore has the same electrophoretic mobility as HbA.

Although HbM can be detected by spectral abnormalities of the hemoglobin (absorption peaks at ~630 and 502 nm), methemoglobin formed in NADH-diaphorase deficiency has a normal absorption spectrum. In addition, methemoglobin formed as the result of NADH-diaphorase deficiency can be readily reduced by incubation of blood with methylene blue whereas methemoglobin caused by a structural hemoglobin variant such as HbM does not reduce with the methylene blue. To confirm NADH-diaphorase deficiency, a quantitative assay of the enzyme activity is necessary.

Congenital methemoglobinemia resulting from NADH-diaphorase deficiency and acquired toxic methemoglobinemia can be treated by administering ascorbic acid or methylene blue. Conversely, no treatment for the HbM structural variants exists because the abnormal hemoglobin resists reduction. However, most patients are asymptomatic and require no management. Most patients have methemoglobin levels <30%, below the level at which symptoms of oxygen deprivation occur.

DECREASED OXYGEN AFFINITY

Low oxygen-affinity hemoglobins result from mutations that stabilize or favor the deoxygenated (T) conformation of the hemoglobin molecule or destabilize the oxygenated (R) form. These mutations impair oxygen binding or reduce heme-heme subunit interactions (cooperativity). Low oxygen affinity hemoglobins are often associated with mutations involving the $\alpha_1\beta_2$ contact points, which are involved in intramolecular movement as hemoglobin goes from the oxy (R) to the deoxy (T) state. The low-affinity variants result in a right-shifted oxygen dissociation curve.

Most low oxygen-affinity hemoglobins possess enough oxygen affinity to become fully saturated in the lungs but at the capillary PO$_2$ in the peripheral tissues deliver higher than normal amounts of oxygen (i.e., become more unsaturated). Two physiologic effects result:

* Because oxygen delivery is so efficient, oxygen requirements of the tissues can be met by lower than normal hematocrits, producing a pseudoanemia (hematocrits lower than "normal").
* The amount of deoxygenated hemoglobin in the capillaries and veins is increased, resulting in a cyanosis. However, no adverse clinical effect is associated with this cyanosis. Patients are asymptomatic and require no treatment. Diagnosis requires determining the P$_{50}$ (the PO$_2$ at which hemoglobin is 50% saturated).

INCREASED OXYGEN AFFINITY

High-affinity hemoglobins are inherited as autosomal dominant traits. All such hemoglobins discovered have been in the heterozygous state. The variants also result from amino acid substitutions that involve the $\alpha_1\beta_2$ contacts. Mutations alter the quaternary structure of hemoglobin to favor the R (oxy) state by either stabilizing this conformation or destabilizing the T (deoxy) state. Other substitutions affect the C-terminal end of the β-chain, which is important in maintaining the stability of the T form. A few substitutions affect the 2,3-BPG binding sites, which alter oxygen affinity when bound to hemoglobin.

The high-affinity hemoglobins bind oxygen more readily than normal and retain more oxygen at lower PO$_2$ levels, which results in a shift to the left of the oxygen dissociation curve. The P$_{50}$ of the hemoglobin is decreased to 12–18 mm Hg, meaning less oxygen is released to tissues at the tissue PO$_2$ of ~26 mm Hg. The resulting tissue hypoxia stimulates erythropoietin release and, subsequently, formation of a compensatory increased erythrocyte mass. In addition to the primary effect of increasing oxygen affinity, secondary effects of the mutations can also occur, including hemoglobin instability, reduced Bohr effect, and reduced cooperativity of the oxygen binding.[26]

Erythrocyte counts and hematocrit levels are increased, and hemoglobin levels are increased to about 200 g/L. Other hematologic parameters are normal. About half of the hemoglobin variants have an altered electrophoretic mobility-enabling diagnosis by starch gel or cellulose acetate electrophoresis. Diagnosis is established by measuring oxygen affinity (determining the P$_{50}$ of the patient's hemoglobin).

Individuals with these hemoglobin variants are asymptomatic. A ruddy complexion is occasionally apparent as a result of the erythrocytosis. The importance of identifying the presence of a high-affinity hemoglobin is for the differential diagnosis of other causes of erythrocytosis and the avoidance of unnecessary and expensive diagnostic and therapeutic interventions.

 Checkpoint! 11

Why should red cell enzyme assays and hemoglobin electrophoresis both be performed on a patient with congenital cyanosis?

SUMMARY

The hemoglobinopathies are a group of chronic hemolytic anemias caused by either qualitative or quantitative defects in the globin chains of hemoglobin. Quantitative defects in globin chains, or thalassemias, are included in ∞ Chapter 11.

Qualitative defects are due to genetic mutations that cause a structural change in the globin chain. Although the mutation can affect any of the globin chain classes, most clinically significant mutations affect the β-chain. The mutation can affect the hemoglobin molecule's solubility, stability, or oxygen affinity. Hemoglobin electrophoresis can be used to detect those mutants in which amino acid mutations cause a change in the hemoglobin molecule's electrophoretic mobility. However, not all variants can be detected by electrophoresis. Other tests detect alterations in hemoglobin solubility and/or stability or oxygen affinity. Molecular techniques are available to help definitively diagnose hemoglobinopathies but are not always necessary for routine diagnostic purposes.

In the United States, the most common structural variants are HbS and HbC. Both are characterized by decreased hemoglobin solubility and can be detected electrophoretically. Hemoglobin S has decreased solubility when deoxygenated, forming rigid aggregates and reduced erythrocyte deformability. The rigid cells aggregate in the microvasculature, resulting in tissue hypoxia. In HbC disease, the erythrocytes become trapped and destroyed in the spleen when intracellular crystals of HbC form. Generally, these variants produce a normocytic, normochromic anemia with anisocytosis and poikilocytosis characteristic for the specific hemoglobinopathy. The blood smear in HbS disease can show sickled forms and target cells. In HbC disease, there are numerous target cells and irregularly contracted cells and the erythrocytes occasionally contain HbC crystals. In the United States, both HbS and HbC are found in highest frequency among African Americans. Hemoglobin E is especially prevalent in people from southeast Asia and is characterized by a mild, asymptomatic microcytic anemia in the homozygous form.

Unstable hemoglobin variants are known as *congenital Heinz body hemolytic anemias.* The hemoglobin denatures in the form of Heinz bodies, decreasing cell deformability and resulting in membrane damage and premature destruction. Hemoglobin variants with increased or decreased oxygen affinity can result in erythrocytosis or cyanosis, respectively. Hemoglobin variants resulting in methemoglobin formation are associated with pseudocyanosis.

REVIEW QUESTIONS

LEVEL I

1. Which ethnic group has the lowest incidence of hemoglobinopathies? (Objective 4)
   a. African Americans
   b. Caucasian Americans
   c. immigrants from southeast Asia
   d. immigrants from the Mediterranean basin

2. The most common clinical disorder resulting from an amino acid substitution in the globin chain is: (Objectives 4, 5)
   a. sickle cell disease
   b. hemoglobin C disease
   c. thalassemia
   d. hemoglobin E disease

3. Hemoglobinopathies are clinical diseases that result from genetically determined abnormalities of the hemoglobin molecule and include those involving: (Objective 1)
   1. heme structure
   2. decreased heme synthesis
   3. globin chain structure
   4. reduced globin chain synthesis
      a. 1 and 3 only
      b. 1 and 2 only
      c. 3 and 4 only
      d. all of the above

LEVEL II

1. Rank the following hemoglobinopathies on the basis of quantity of HbS starting with the lowest amount. (Objective 1)
   1. adult with sickle cell disease
   2. adult with sickle cell trait
   3. neonate with sickle cell disease
      a. 3, 2, 1
      b. 2, 3, 1
      c. 1, 2, 3
      d. 2, 1, 3

2. Rank the following hemoglobinopathies in terms of worldwide prevalence, starting with the most common. (Objective 2)
   1. HbE
   2. HbS
   3. HbC
      a. 3, 1, 2
      b. 1, 2, 3
      c. 2, 3, 1
      d. 2, 1, 3

3. HbS is an example of a hemoglobin with a globin chain mutation that alters hemoglobin: (Objective 3)
   a. function
   b. solubility
   c. stability
   d. oxygen binding

REVIEW QUESTIONS (continued)

LEVEL I

4. Amino acid substitutions on globin chains often alter the hemoglobin molecule's charge and mobility. This is the principle of which test for identifying hemoglobins? (Objective 3)
   a. HbA$_2$ quantitation
   b. HbF quantitation
   c. hemoglobin electrophoresis
   d. solubility test

5. The defect resulting in production of HbC is: (Objective 5)
   a. β6 (A3) Glu → Val
   b. β6 (A3) Glu → Lys
   c. β121 (GH4) Glu → Gly
   d. β26 (B8) Glu → Lys

6. Tests that quantitate HbF and HbA$_2$ are useful in detecting hemoglobinopathies because: (Objective 6)
   a. they are the only valid tests available for this purpose
   b. they are routinely performed in most laboratories
   c. HbF and HbA$_2$ are typically decreased in hemoglobinopathies
   d. HbF and HbA$_2$ are typically increased in hemoglobinopathies

7. The presence of many sickled erythrocytes on a peripheral blood smear is most likely to be found in a person who is: (Objective 7)
   a. heterozygous for HbC
   b. homozygous for HbC
   c. heterozygous for HbS
   d. homozygous for HbS

8. Clinical findings for persons with sickle cell trait typically include: (Objective 8)
   a. mild to moderate anemia
   b. rare complications after exposure to prolonged hypoxia
   c. increased susceptibility to infection
   d. aplastic crisis

9. Synthesis of abnormal hemoglobins is the result of: (Objective 2)
   a. genetic defects that result in amino acid substitutions in globin chains
   b. genetic defects in genes that code for erythrocyte enzymes
   c. presence of toxins (i.e., lead) during hemoglobin synthesis
   d. genetic defects that result in abnormal synthesis of heme

10. A hemoglobin electrophoresis showed 45% HbS, 46% HbC, 6% HbF, and 3% HbA$_2$. These results are consistent with a diagnosis of: (Objective 7)
    a. sickle cell anemia
    b. sickle cell trait
    c. hemoglobin S/C disease
    d. hemoglobin C trait

LEVEL II

4. Anemia develops in persons with sickle cell disease because: (Objective 4)
   a. the production of erythroid precursors is impaired.
   b. antibodies coat the erythrocyte membrane leading to cell lysis.
   c. erythrocytes have a greatly shortened life span.
   d. marrow stem cells are inhibited or crowded out.

5. Cells containing large amounts of HbS sickle when the following conditions occur: (Objective 4)
   a. high oxygen tension and acidosis
   b. hypoxia and alkalosis
   c. temperatures less than 37°C and alkalosis
   d. temperatures greater than 37°C and hypoxia

6. Infants with sickle cell disease typically do not become symptomatic until 6 months of age. How can this be explained? (Objective 4)
   a. Environmental conditions conducive to sickling are not experienced by infants.
   b. Physical examinations are not sufficiently sensitive with infants.
   c. The immature infant spleen is incapable of extravascular hemolysis.
   d. The concentration of HbF predominates over HbS.

7. Hydroxyurea therapy for sickle cell disease is used to: (Objective 6)
   a. increase the level of HbF within erythrocytes
   b. decrease the production of mutated globin chains
   c. increase the pH of the blood
   d. decrease the risk of bacterial infection

8. A hemoglobin electrophoresis on cellulose acetate at pH 8.5 is performed on a 2-year-old African American patient with severe anemia. An abnormal band appears halfway between the HbA and HbA$_2$ positions on the strip. The HbF level is 10%, and the HbA$_2$ level is normal. No HbA is present. What is the most likely identity of the abnormal hemoglobin? (Objective 7)
   a. HbC
   b. HbS
   c. HbD
   d. HbE

9. The presence of HbE disease in an adult is best confirmed using which routine laboratory test? (Objective 8)
   a. hemoglobin electrophoresis
   b. the CBC and peripheral blood smear
   c. solubility test
   d. PCR for molecular defect

REVIEW QUESTIONS *(continued)*

LEVEL I

LEVEL II

10. When amino acid substitutions or deletions disrupt the stability of the globin subunit or hemoglobin tetramer, a likely consequence is production of a hemoglobin: (Objective 11)
    a. with altered solubility
    b. that tends to form crystals
    c. that can result in the formation of Heinz bodies
    d. that is composed of only alpha globin chains

www.pearsonhighered.com/mckenzie
Use this address to access the interactive Companion Website created for this textbook. Find additional information, tables and figures. Evaluate your command of the chapter information using case studies and critical thinking and multiple choice questions.

REFERENCES

1. Weatherall DJ, Clegg JB. Genetic disorders of hemoglobin. *Semin Hematol.* 1999;36 (4 Suppl 7):24–37.

2. Herrick JB. Peculiar elongated and sickle-shaped red blood corpuscles in a case of severe anemia. *Trans Assoc Am Physicians.* 1910;25:553–61.

3. Pauling L, Itano HA, Singer SJ, Wells IC. Sickle cell anemia: A molecular disease. *Science.* 1949;ll0:543–48.

4. Clarke GM, Higgins TN. Laboratory investigation of hemoglobinopathies and thalassemias: Review and update. *Clin Chem.* 2000;46:1284–90.

5. Houtovsky A, Hadzi-Nesic J, Nardi MA. HPLC retention time as a diagnostic tool for hemoglobin variants and hemoglobinopathies: A study of 60000 samples in a clinical diagnostics laboratory. *Clin Chem.* 2004:50:1736–47.

6. Thompson AA. Advances in the management of sickle cell disease. *Pediatr Blood Cancer.* 2005;46:533–39.

7. Old JM. Screening and genetic diagnosis of haemoglobin disorder. *Blood Rev.* 2003;17:43–53.

8. Flint J, Harding RM, Boyce AJ, Clegg JB. The population genetics of the haemoglobinopathies. *Baillieres Clin Haematol.* 1998;11:1–51.

9. Bunyaratvej A, Butthep P, Sae-Ung N, Fucharoen S, Yuthavong Y. Reduced deformability of thalassemic erythrocytes and erythrocytes with abnormal hemoglobins and relation with susceptibility to *Plasmodium falciparum* invasion. *Blood.* 1992;79:2460–63.

10. Liu SC, Derick LH, Palek J. Dependence of the permanent deformation of red blood cell membranes on spectrin dimer-tetramer equilibrium: Implication for permanent membrane deformation of irreversibly sickled cells. *Blood.* 1993;81:522–28.

11. Ballas SK, Smith ED. Red blood cell changes during the evolution of the sickle cell painful crisis. *Blood.* 1992;79:2154–63.

12. Mackie LH, Hochmuth RM. The influence of oxygen tension, temperature, and hemoglobin concentration on the rheologic properties of sickle erythrocytes. *Blood.* 1990;76:1256–61.

13. Steinberg MH. Pathophysiology of sickle cell disease. *Baillieres Clin Haematol.* 1998;11:163–84.

14. Liu SC, Yi SJ, Mehta JR, Nichols PE, Ballas SK, Yacono PW et al. Red cell membrane remodeling in sickle cell anemia. *J Clin Invest.* 1996;97:29–36.

15. Boghossian SH, Nash G, Dormandy J, Bevan DH. Abnormal neutrophil adhesion in sickle cell anaemia and crisis: Relationship to blood rheology. *Br J Haematol.* 1991;78:437–41.

16. Ballas SK. Sickle cell disease: Clinical management. *Baillieres Clin Haematol.* 1998;11:185–14.

17. Quinn CT, Buchanan GR. The acute chest syndrome of sickle cell disease. *J Pediatr.* 1999;135:416–22.

18. West MS, Wethers D, Smith J, Steinberg M. Laboratory profile of sickle cell disease: A cross-sectional analysis. The Cooperative Study of Sickle Cell Disease. *J Clin Epidemiol.* 1992;45:893–909.

19. Morris J, Dunn D, Beckford M, Grandison Y, Mason K, Higgs D et al. The haematology of homozygous sickle cell disease after the age of 40 years. *Br J Haematol.* 1991;77:382–85.

20. el Sayed HL, Tawfik ZM. Red cell profile in normal and sickle cell diseased children. *J Egypt Soc Parasitol.* 1994;24:147–54.

21. Walters MC. Stem cell therapy for sickle cell disease: Transplantation and gene therapy. *Hematology Am Soc Hematol Educ Program.* 2005:66–73

22. Persons DA, Nienhuis AW. Gene therapy for the hemoglobin disorders: Past, present, and future. *Proc Natl Acad Sci USA.* 2000;97(10):5022–24.

23. Lawrence C, Fabry ME, Nagel RL. The unique red cell heterogeneity of SC disease: Crystal formation, dense reticulocytes, and unusual morphology. *Blood.* 1991;78:2104–12.

24. Bain BJ. Blood film features of sickle cell–haemoglobin C disease. *Br J Haematol.* 1993;83:516–18.

25. Williamson D. The unstable haemoglobins. *Blood Reviews.* 1993;7:146–63.

26. Benz Jr. EJ. Hemoglobin variants associated with hemolytic anemia, altered oxygen affinity, and methemoglobinemias. In: Hoffman R, Benz EJ Jr, Shattil SJ, Furie B, Cohen HJ, eds. *Hematology: Basic Principles and Practice.* Philadelphia: Elsevier Churchill Livingstone; 2005.

11

Thalassemia

Tim R. Randolph, Ph.D.

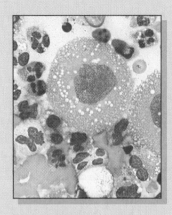

■ OBJECTIVES—LEVEL I

At the end of this unit of study, the student should be able to:

1. Define *thalassemia*.
2. Differentiate thalassemias from hemoglobinopathies based on definition and basic pathophysiology.
3. Describe the typical peripheral blood morphology associated with thalassemia.
4. Compare and contrast the etiology of α- and β-thalassemia.
5. For each of the four genotypes of α-thalassemia describe the:
   a. Number of affected alleles
   b. Individuals affected
   c. Basic pathophysiology
   d. Symptoms
   e. Laboratory results including blood cell morphology and hemoglobin electrophoresis
6. For each of the six genotypes of β-thalassemia describe the:
   a. Individuals affected
   b. Basic pathophysiology
   c. Symptoms
   d. Laboratory results including blood cell morphology and hemoglobin electrophoresis

■ OBJECTIVES—LEVEL II

At the end of this unit of study, the student should be able to:

1. List and describe five genetic defects found in thalassemias.
2. Compare and contrast α- and β-thalassemia
3. Correlate the outcomes in hemoglobin synthesis resulting from the five genetic defects in thalassemia.
4. For all four genotypes of α-thalassemia:
   a. Correlate all three nomenclature systems: genotype, genotype description, and phenotype.
   b. Explain advanced pathophysiology.
   c. Describe treatment and prognosis.

■ OBJECTIVES—LEVEL II *(continued)*

5. For all four phenotypes of β-thalassemia

   a. List expected genotypes.

   b. Explain advanced pathophysiology.

   c. Describe treatment and prognosis.

6. Correlate clinical severities of both α- and β-thalassemia with their respective genotypes.

7. Compare and contrast other thalassemia and thalassemia-like conditions to include:

   a. $\delta\beta$-thalassemia

   b. $\gamma\delta\beta$-thalassemia

   c. Hemoglobin Constant Spring

   d. Hereditary persistence of fetal hemoglobin (HPFH)

   e. Hemoglobin Lepore

   f. Thalassemia/hemoglobinopathy combination disorders

8. Differentiate iron deficiency anemia and HPFH from thalassemia based on results of laboratory tests and clinical findings.

KEY TERMS

Allele

Compression syndrome

Congenital

Crossover

Diploid

Double heterozygous

Extramedullary erythropoiesis

Functional hyposplenism

Gene cluster

Genotype

Haplotypes

Heterozygous

Homozygous

Ineffective erythropoiesis

P_{50} value

Phenotype

Zygosity

BACKGROUND BASICS

The information in this chapter builds on concepts presented in previous chapters. To maximize your learning experience, you should review the following concepts before beginning this unit of study.

Level I

► Describe the pathophysiology of hemoglobinopathies. (Chapter 10).

► Describe the morphologic and functional classification of anemias and the associated lab tests. (Chapter 8)

► Interpret routine laboratory tests, such as CBC and differential, and apply both normal and abnormal results in the diagnosis of anemias. (Chapters 8, 34)

► Describe the basic structure and function of hemoglobin and identify the globin chain composition of normal hemoglobin types. (Chapter 6)

► Describe the extravascular destruction of erythrocytes. (Chapter 5)

Level II

► Summarize the synthesis and molecular structure of hemoglobin and correlate alterations in structure with function; describe globin chain synthesis in utero and throughout life. (Chapters 4, 6)

► Interpret hemoglobin migration patterns on electrophoresis, acid elution of fetal hemoglobins, hemoglobin solubility tests, and iron panels to distinguish iron metabolism disorders and hemoglobinopathies from thalassemias. (Chapter 34)

CASE STUDY

We will refer to this case throughout the chapter.
John is a 4-year-old boy who frequently complains of weakness, fatigue, and dyspnea. The family moved to the United States from Greece before the child's birth. Both parents experienced fatigue from time to time but never consulted a physician. Consider the types of anemia most often found at this age and the laboratory tests that could help establish a diagnosis. What is the significance, if any, of knowing the parents' background and medical history?

▶ OVERVIEW

This chapter discusses a group of hereditary anemias collectively called *thalassemias*. It begins with a general description of thalassemias including the genetic defects and types, pathophysiology, and clinical and laboratory findings. Subsequently, each type is discussed in the following format: pathophysiology, clinical findings, laboratory findings, treatment, and prognosis. Other thalassemia-like conditions are described and compared and contrasted with thalassemia. The chapter concludes by describing the laboratory differential diagnosis of types of thalassemia and other disorders that have similar peripheral blood morphology.

▶ INTRODUCTION

Thalassemia constitutes a family of **congenital** disorders in which mutations in one or more of the globin genes of hemoglobin cause decreased or absent synthesis of the corresponding globin chains. Almost 400 unique mutations have been described among this diverse group of disorders.[1] Consequences of the mutation depend on the particular chain affected and the amount of globin chain produced. Limited availability of globin chains results in a reduction in the assembly of hemoglobin. Patients with mild genetic defects are generally asymptomatic. Patients with more severe defects present with symptoms that result from one or more of the following: decreased production of normal hemoglobin, synthesis of abnormal hemoglobins, **ineffective erythropoiesis**, and disproportionate production of unaffected globin chains. Symptoms include anemia, hepatosplenomegaly, infections, gallstones, and bone deformities that alter facial features and result in pathologic fractures.

The most important thalassemias are alpha- (α) and beta- (β). α-thalassemia results from a decreased or absent production of α-globin chains, and β-thalassemia is caused by a reduction or absence of β-globin chains. Reduction in the quantity of α- and β-chains can cause anemia because approximately 97% of normal adult hemoglobin (HbA) is composed of α- and β-globin chains.

Thomas Cooley offered the first clinical description of thalassemia in Detroit in 1925.[2] At that time, thalassemia was thought to be a rare disorder restricted to the Mediterranean ethnicities. Dr. Cooley's work broadened our understanding of the nationalities that potentially could be affected by thalassemia and suggested that the disease was hemolytic in nature. By 1960, it was apparent that the thalassemias composed a heterogeneous group of genetic disorders. With the advent of molecular biology, many groups of researchers have widely studied thalassemias. Methods developed in the last 25 years have enabled researchers to measure the number of globin chains synthesized and identify specific genetic mutations.

Thalassemia is now recognized as one of the most common genetic disorders affecting the world's population. It is estimated that between 100,000 and 200,000 individuals worldwide are born each year with severe forms of thalassemia. In North America, about 20% of immigrants from Southeast Asia and 6–11% of African Americans have detectable α-thalassemia. Many more are silent carriers. About 6% of individuals with Mediterranean ancestry, 5% of Southeast Asians, and 0.8% of African Americans have β-thalassemia.

Thalassemia is a major health problem in countries where these disorders are prevalent. Prevention is seen as an essential part in the management of the problem. Thus, many of these countries now have large screening and education programs to detect carriers. This has drastically reduced the number of individuals born with both homozygous and heterozygous forms of the disease.

THALASSEMIA VERSUS HEMOGLOBINOPATHY

The system of categorizing thalassemias and hemoglobinopathies differs among hematologists. Some use hemoglobinopathy as a disease category that includes structural variants of hemoglobin, such as sickle cell anemia and thalassemias. Others categorize only structural variants as hemoglobinopathies and describe thalassemias as a separate disease entity. In this text, we refer to the two diseases separately.

In the preceding chapter, hemoglobinopathies were defined as qualitative defects in the structure of globin chains resulting in production of abnormal hemoglobin molecules. Thalassemias, on the other hand, are typically quantitative disorders of hemoglobin synthesis that produce reduced amounts of normal hemoglobin.

The different outcomes of hemoglobinopathies and thalassemia are a direct result of the types of mutations encountered in these disease states. Most hemoglobinopathies result predominantly from a point mutation in the β-globin gene that is translated into a β-globin chain containing a single amino acid substitution. Hemoglobin types containing a point mutation in the β-chains may be produced at normal levels but are structurally abnormal. In contrast, thalassemias result from both deletional and nondeletional

✪ TABLE 11-1

Comparison of Hemoglobinopathies and Thalassemias

Disease	RBC Count	Indices	Erythrocyte Morphology	Abnormal Hb	Hb Solubility Test	Ancestry	Reticulocyte Count
Hemoglobinopathy	↓	Normocytic, normochromic	Target cells, sickle cells (in HbS), HbC crystals (in HbC), others	HbS, HbC, HbE, etc.	+ in HbS, Hb Bart's, and HbC^{Harlem}	African, Mediterranean, Middle Eastern, Southeast Asian	↑↑
Thalassemia	↑ Compared to what is expected for the Hb level	Microcytic, hypochromic	Target cells, basophilic stippling	HbH (β^4), Hb Bart's (γ^4)	Negative	Mediterranean, Southeast Asian, African	↑

↓ = slight decrease, ↑ = slight increase, ↑↑ = moderate increase, Hb = hemoglobin, RBC = red blood cell, + = positive

mutations in globin genes that reduce or eliminate the synthesis of the corresponding globin chain. This results in the assembly of inadequate amounts of normal hemoglobin and a reduced oxygen-carrying capacity of the blood. Unlike hemoglobinopathies, the amino acid sequence of the chain, if produced, is normal and is assembled into the appropriate hemoglobin as usual, albeit in reduced amounts. In some of the less common thalassemias, the globin chains can be lengthened or truncated (Table 11-1 ✪).

 Checkpoint! 1

Differentiate the etiology of thalassemias and hemoglobinopathies.

GENETIC DEFECTS IN THALASSEMIA

Nearly all thalassemic mutations fall into one of five categories of genetic lesions: gene deletion, promoter mutation, nonsense mutation, mutated termination (stop) codon, and splice site mutation (Table 11-2 ✪). Regardless of the type of mutation encountered, the results are the same: The globin chain corresponding to the mutated globin gene is absent, reduced in concentration, or occasionally somewhat longer or shorter than normal.

If all globin genes of a single type of globin chain are deleted, the corresponding hemoglobin is absent. Deleted genes are most common in α-thalassemia. Reduction in globin chain production from nondeletional mutations is more common in the β-thalassemias. The degree of reduction in globin chain production is a direct reflection of the type of

✪ TABLE 11-2

Five Common Genetic Defects in Thalassemia

Mutation Type	Thalassemia Encountered	Effect on Gene	Effect on Globin Chain
Deletion (large)	Predominantly α-thalassemia, some β-thalassemia	Loss of gene	Absence of production
Promoter	Predominantly β-thalassemia	Impaired transcription	Reduced or absent production
Nonsense	Predominantly β-thalassemia	In frame substitution	Amino acid change
		Frame shift	Amino acid changes distal to shift
			Longer or shorter globin chains
Stop codon	Predominantly β-thalassemia	Convert stop codons to amino acid codons	Slightly lengthened globin chain (retained)
			Significantly lengthened globin chain (degraded)
Splice site	Predominantly β-thalassemia	Create new splice sites	Slightly shortened globin chain (retained)
			Significantly shortened globin chain (degraded)
		Loss of splice sites	Slightly lengthened globin chain (retained)
			Significantly lengthened globin chain (degraded)
			Unaltered globin chain

mutation encountered and parallels the severity of the clinical disorder (Table 11-2).

 Checkpoint! 2:

What are the most common genetic mutations associated with α-thalassemia?

TYPES OF THALASSEMIA

Because six different normal globin genes (α, β, γ, δ, ε, ζ) exist, at least six versions of thalassemia are possible. In addition, deletions can occur to entire **gene clusters** concurrently affecting more than one globin chain. Of the six normal globin genes, epsilon and zeta (ε, ζ) are normally synthesized only in utero, and gamma (γ) is produced in high amounts from approximately the third trimester of pregnancy until birth. After birth, γ-chain synthesis begins to decrease but can still be detected in low amounts in adult life. The three remaining globin chains (α, β, and δ) and the γ-chains are considered normal adult globin chains and combine to form hemoglobin A ($\alpha_2\beta_2$), hemoglobin A$_2$ ($\alpha_2\delta_2$), and hemoglobin F ($\alpha_2\gamma_2$), respectively. Because approximately 97% of normal adult hemoglobin is HbA, a deficiency of either α- or β-chains affects hemoglobin A assembly, reducing HbA concentration and thus affecting the blood's oxygen-carrying capacity.

Two major types of classical thalassemia, α-thalassemia and β-thalassemia, have been described. When synthesis of the α-chain is impaired, the disease is α-thalassemia. When synthesis of the β-chain is affected, the disease is β-thalassemia. A third type of thalassemia, δ-thalassemia, has been reported, but its occurrence is rare and it is not clinically significant because the δ-chain is a component of the minor hemoglobin HbA$_2$, which composes only ~2.5% of total hemoglobin. Combinations of gene deletions like $\delta\beta$-thalassemia or $\gamma\delta\beta$-thalassemia occur but are rare. The affected chains are all synthesized at a reduced rate.

Occasionally, synthesis of a structural hemoglobin variant decreases hemoglobin concentration, giving the clinical picture of thalassemia. These structural variants include those hemoglobins with abnormally long or short globin chains (hemoglobin Constant Spring) as well as variants with a point mutation (hemoglobin E). Hemoglobin Lepore is a hemoglobin variant in which the non–α-globin chains are not only structurally abnormal but also ineffectively synthesized. Because of their clinical similarity to thalassemias, these particular structural variants are discussed in this section.

A variant of β-thalassemia known as *hereditary persistence of fetal hemoglobin* (HPFH) is characterized by continued production of HbF throughout life. This disorder is characterized by a failure in the switch of γ-chain production to β-chain production after birth. In the homozygotes, 100% of circulating hemoglobin is HbF.

PATHOPHYSIOLOGY

Normally equal amounts of α- and β-chains are synthesized by the maturing erythrocyte, resulting in a β-chain to α-chain ratio of 1.0. In α- and β-thalassemia, synthesis of one of these chains is decreased or absent, resulting in an excess of the other chain. If the α-chain is affected, there is an excess of β-chains, and if the β-chain is affected, there is an excess of α-chains. This imbalanced synthesis of chains has several effects, all of which contribute to anemia: (1) a decrease in total erythrocyte hemoglobin production, (2) ineffective erythropoiesis, and (3) chronic hemolysis.

Excess α-chains are unstable and precipitate within the cell. The precipitates bind to the cell membrane, causing membrane damage and decreased erythrocyte deformability. Macrophages may destroy the precipitate-filled erythrocytes in the bone marrow, resulting in a large degree of ineffective erythropoiesis. Circulating erythrocytes with precipitates are pitted and/or removed by the spleen, causing chronic extravascular hemolysis.

Excess β-chains can combine to form hemoglobin molecules with four β-chains, hemoglobin H (HbH). This hemoglobin has a high oxygen affinity and is also unstable. Thus, it is a poor transporter of oxygen. In the infant, when α-chains are decreased, excess γ-chains can combine to form hemoglobin molecules with four γ-chains, hemoglobin Bart's (Hb Bart's). This hemoglobin also has a very high oxygen affinity.

In addition to α- and β-thalassemia, other thalassemias and thalassemia-like conditions can occur. Structural hemoglobin variants can result in decreased synthesis of globin chains, giving the clinical picture of thalassemia (e.g., Hemoglobin E).

CLINICAL FINDINGS

Clinical findings are related to anemia, chronic hemolysis, and ineffective erythropoiesis (Table 11-3 ☺). The combination of reduced HbA synthesis, ineffective erythropoiesis, and hemolysis results in anemia. The severity of anemia varies widely depending on the specific genetic mutation and number of genes affected. Hypoxia from anemia is exacerbated in some cases by the presence of abnormal hemoglobins that have a high oxygen affinity (HbH and Hb Bart's). These hemoglobins do not release oxygen readily to the tissues.

Chronic hemolysis has several adverse effects. Splenomegaly is frequently present because the spleen is a major site of extravascular hemolysis. Occasionally, the spleen can become overburdened by the process of erythrocyte destruction resulting in **functional hyposplenism**. In this case, the spleen's function as a secondary lymphoid tissue is compromised, leading to an increase in infections (∞ Chapter 4). Chronic hemolysis can also result in the formation of gallstones.

The chronic demand for erythrocytes also has adverse effects. The bone marrow responds by increasing erythropoiesis,

❂ TABLE 11-3

Clinical and Laboratory Findings Associated with Thalassemia

Clinical Finding	Pathophysiology	Laboratory Finding
Anemia/hypoxia	Decreased hemoglobin production/erythropoiesis	↓ –N RBC count, ↓ hemoglobin, ↓ hematocrit
	Ineffective erythropoiesis	Microcytic/hypochromic RBCs
	Presence of high-affinity hemoglobins (HbH and Hb Bart's)	↓MCV, ↓MCH, ↓MCHC
	Increased extravascular hemolysis	↑ Reticulocyte count
		Anisocytosis and poikilocytosis
		Target cells, basophilic stippling, nucleated RBCs
		BM erythroid hyperplasia
		↑ RDW
		Abnormal hemoglobin electrophoresis
Splenomegaly/hemolysis	Splenic removal of abnormal erythrocytes	↑ Bilirubin
	Ineffective erythropoiesis	↓ Haptoglobin
Gallstones	Increased intravascular and extravascular hemolysis	↑ Bilirubin
Skeletal abnormalities	Expansion of bone marrow	BM erythroid hyperplasia
Pathologic fractures	Thinning of calcified bone	
Iron toxicity	Iron overload	
	Multiple transfusions	↑ Prussian blue staining in BM
	Increased iron absorption	↑ Serum iron/ferritin and ↓ TIBC

resulting in erythroid hyperplasia and in some of the more severe thalassemias, in bone marrow expansion and thinning of calcified bone. Consequently, patients develop skeletal abnormalities and pathologic fractures. The increased iron demand needed to support the erythropoietic activity stimulates the absorption of more iron. This additional iron is not effectively incorporated into hemoglobin, so it accumulates in macrophages in the bone marrow, liver, and spleen. As this process continues, iron eventually accumulates in parenchymal cells of various organs and adversely affects organ function. Iron toxicity commonly affects such organs as the liver, pituitary, heart, and bone, resulting in dysfunctions such as cirrhosis, hypogonadism and growth failure, arrhythmias and cardiomyopathies, and pathologic fractures, respectively.[3] Ineffective erythropoiesis in the bone marrow can be accompanied by **extramedullary erythropoiesis** in the liver and spleen. Extramedullary erythropoiesis can produce masses large enough to cause **compression syndromes** (Table 11-3).

Pregnant women with thalassemia have physiological demands that impact the developing baby to a greater extent than the mother. Developing infants can experience diminished growth, premature birth, and even intrauterine death if the woman's oxygen concentration falls below 70 mmHg. Pregnant women who present with a hemoglobin level of between 9 and 10 g/dL around the time of delivery are often given a blood transfusion to improve oxygen delivery. To avoid iron overload caused primarily by the combination of transfusion therapy and increased iron absorption, pregnant women can be given deferoxamine during and after the transfusion.[4]

 Checkpoint! 3

Why do α- and β-thalassemia result in more clinically severe disease than other types of thalassemia?

LABORATORY FINDINGS

Peripheral blood findings provide clues to the disease (Table 11-3). Thalassemias are characterized by microcytic, hypochromic anemia with a decrease in MCV, MCH, and usually MCHC. The erythrocyte count is often normal or slightly decreased but increased for the degree of anemia. The RDW can be increased although often is not. Target cells and microcytosis usually are present even in cases without anemia or symptoms of anemia. Basophilic stippling and nucleated erythrocytes can be present. Anisocytosis and poikilocytosis are common. Precipitates of excess chains or unstable hemoglobin can be visualized with supravital stains. Reticulocytes and bilirubin are usually increased due to the chronic hemolysis. Haptoglobin, a protein that transports free plasma hemoglobin to the liver, can be decreased depending on the degree of intravascular hemolysis.

Hemoglobin electrophoresis is always indicated if thalassemia is suspected. HbA is usually decreased. HbF and

HbA_2 are increased in β-thalassemia but decreased in α-thalassemia. Hemoglobin Bart's and HbH can also be present in α-thalassemia.

Bone marrow studies are not necessary for diagnosis but when performed show marked erythroid hyperplasia. Erythroblasts appear abnormal with very little cytoplasm, uneven cytoplasmic membranes, and striking basophilic stippling. Prussian blue stain reveals an abundance of iron and occasionally a few ringed sideroblasts. Phagocytic "foam" cells similar to Gaucher cells have been reported in the more severe forms of the disease. The foam probably results from partially digested red cell membrane lipids associated with intense ineffective erythropoiesis.

Because the emphasis is now on screening programs to detect thalassemia carriers in areas of high prevalence and in certain populations, laboratory professionals must look for assays that are uncomplicated, time efficient, and accurate. The reverse dot-blot procedure, a molecular technique, seems to be the most popular for this purpose because it is rapid and accurate. It allows for the screening of several mutations with a single hybridization reaction. In this procedure, probes for the mutated genes are fixed on a membrane. Because hundreds of different globin gene mutants lead to thalassemia, the probes selected are those commonly found in a particular geographic region. The patient's DNA is PCR-amplified, labeled, and added to the membrane with the probes. The patient's DNA hybridizes only to probes complementary to its sequence. The pattern of hybridization of the patient's DNA with the probes determines whether a particular mutation is present. Molecular techniques can also be performed on a fetus in utero within the first or second trimester of pregnancy by using fetal blood sampling or chorionic villous sampling followed by similar PCR-based methods of DNA analysis.[4]

▶ α-THALASSEMIA

GENERAL CONSIDERATIONS

Alpha-thalassemia is a group of four disorders characterized by decreased synthesis of α-chains. Although each is discussed separately, several features common to each type are presented here.

Etiology

In the human genome, two α-genes are located on each of the two chromosome 16 structures, totaling four α-genes in the **diploid** state (Figure 11-1 ■). Mutations can affect one or more of the α-genes resulting in four discrete clinical severities that have been described. A patient in whom all four α-genes are deleted produces no α-chains, a condition referred to as *hydrops fetalis*. When three of the four α-genes are deleted, the disorder is known as *hemoglobin H (HbH) disease*. The deletion of two α-genes is known as *α-thalassemia minor*, and the deletion of a single α-gene is known as *silent carrier*. Though less common, nondeletional mutations and muta-

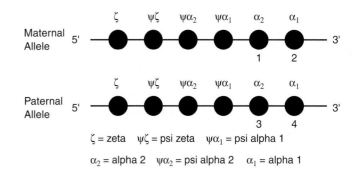

■ FIGURE 11-1   A short section of chromosome 16 showing the 5' to 3' orientation of three functional genes ζ, α_2, and α_1 along with three pseudogenes $\psi\zeta$, $\psi\alpha_2$, and $\psi\alpha_1$. Pseudogenes are the result of partial gene duplications but are not expressed. There are two α-genes on each chromosome; the α_2-gene expresses 2 to 3 times as much protein product as the α_1-gene.

tions that produce unstable α-chains are also found in α-thalassemia. The outcome is usually the same as a deletion mutation, a reduction in α-chains and in the corresponding α-containing hemoglobins.

Affected Alleles

The amount of α-chains synthesized is somewhat proportional to the number of affected **alleles**. In general, erythrocytes produce higher concentrations of α-chains than the number of affected alleles predict. There are two main reasons for this phenomenon. First, the four α-genes can be described as two pairs of genes designated as α_1 and α_2. Each chromosome 16 contains an α_1- and an α_2-gene oriented with the α_2-gene positioned upstream (5') from the α_1-gene (Figure 11-1). It has been shown that the α_2-gene produces two to three times the amount of mRNA as the α_1-gene.[5] Therefore, a deletion of the α_2-gene would reduce α-chain production to a greater degree than would a deletion of the α_1-gene. Second, the erythropoietic system has an internal mechanism designed to stimulate increased production of α-chains from the unaffected genes to compensate for deletions, thus minimizing the reduction of α-chains.

Affected Individuals

Alpha-thalassemia is concentrated in people of Mediterranean, Asian, and African ancestry. In particular, it is commonly seen in blacks, Indians, Chinese, and Middle Eastern people, with blacks expressing a milder version of the disease. The reason patients of African descent tend to present with a milder version of α-thalassemia is because the deletion in this ethnic group usually involves the α_1-gene.

Genotypes

Three nomenclature systems—genotypic, genotypic description, and phenotypic—have been developed to classify the α-thalassemias into five discrete categories. The addition of the normal **genotype** produces a total of six possibilities.

The genotypic system designates deleted genes as $(-)$ and unaffected genes as (α). The genotypic description system combines the **zygosity** state, **homozygous** or **heterozygous**, with either a gene symbol (α^0 or α^+) or a nominal descriptor (thal-1 or thal-2) to designate the number of deleted α-genes on each chromosome. Both thal-1 and α^0 indicate the deletion of both α-genes on the same chromosome $(-,-)$. Likewise, thal-2 and α^+ refer to one deleted and one unaffected α-gene on a given chromosome $(-, \alpha)$. The phenotypic system describes four clinical types, hydrops fetalis, hemoglobin H disease, α-thalassemia minor, and silent carrier with the α-thalassemia minor type exhibiting two clinical severities (Table 11-4 ✪).[5] Patients occasionally bear a nondeletional mutation of the α-thalassemia gene, designated as α^T, that functions to reduce but not eliminate α-chain production from that gene.

α-THALASSEMIA MAJOR (α^0-THAL-1/α^0-THAL-1; HYDROPS FETALIS)

The most severe form of α-thalassemia, α-thalassemia major, involves the deletion of all four α-genes $(--/--)$. Both parents of the thalassemia patient must have α-thalassemia to have a child with hydrops fetalis because both α-genes on each parental chromosome inherited by the child are deleted.

Pathophysiology

Because all four α-genes are deleted in hydrops fetalis, no normal adult hemoglobins can be synthesized. Therefore, this disorder is incompatible with life, and infants are either stillborn or die within hours of birth. In the absence of α-chains, erythrocytes assemble hemoglobin using the γ-, δ-, and β-chains available. Therefore, abnormal hemoglobin tetramers involving γ-chains (Hb Bart's, γ_4) and β-chains (HbH, β_4) are produced. Hb Bart's has a very high oxygen affinity and no Bohr effect (∞ Chapter 6). Therefore, this hemoglobin cannot supply tissues with sufficient oxygen to sustain life, and the developing infant dies of hypoxia and congestive heart failure. Hemoglobin Portland, although normally absent following the first trimester, continues to be synthesized until birth in α-thalassemia because it does not contain α-chains.

Clinical Findings

Infants who survive until birth exhibit significant physical abnormalities upon routine exam. The babies are underweight and edematous with a distended abdomen. The liver and often the spleen are enlarged due to extramedullary hematopoiesis. There is massive bone marrow hyperplasia. Hemolysis in the fetus is probably severe because there is extensive deposition of hemosiderin.

✪ TABLE 11-4

Characteristics of α-thalassemia

Genotype	Genotypic Description	Phenotype	Hematologic Findings	Severity	Hemoglobins Present
$(--/--)$	Homozygous α^0-thalassemia-1	Hydrops fetalis	Marked anemia Microcytic/hypochromic RBCs ↑↑↑ anisopoikilocytosis ↑ NRBC	Fatal	Hb Bart's (80–90%) Hb Portland (10–20%)
$(--/-\alpha)$	Heterozygous α^0-thalassemia-1/ α^+-thalassemia-2	Hemoglobin H disease	Moderate to marked anemia Microcytic/hypochromic RBCs Target cells Basophilic stippling Poikilocytosis	Chronic, moderately severe hemolytic anemia	Birth=Hb Bart's; Adult=HbH
$(--/\alpha\alpha)$	Heterozygous α^0-thalassemia-1	α-thalassemia-minor	Slight anemia Microcytic/hypochromic RBCs Target cells Basophilic stippling Poikilocytosis	Mild to moderate	Birth=Hb Bart's; Adult=normal
$(-\alpha/-\alpha)$	Homozygous α^+-thalassemia-2	α-thalassemia-minor	Slight anemia Microcytic/hypochromic RBCs Target cells Basophilic stippling Poikilocytosis	Mild	Birth=Hb Bart's; Adult=normal
$(-\alpha/\alpha\alpha)$	Heterozygous α^+-thalassemia-2	Silent carrier	Normocytic or slightly microcytic RBCs	Normal	Normal
$(\alpha\alpha/\alpha\alpha)$	Normal	None	Normal	Normal	Normal

↑↑↑ = marked increase, ↑ = slight increase

α-thalassemia Major Laboratory Results

Laboratory results can confirm the diagnosis. There is severe anemia with hemoglobin values ranging from 3 to 10 g/dL. Hemoglobin electrophoresis on cellulose acetate agarose at alkaline pH shows 80–90% Hb Bart's and 10–20% Hb Portland with HbH sometimes detectable. HbA, HbA$_2$, and HbF are absent due to the lack of α-chain production (Figure 11-2 ■).

 ### Checkpoint! 4

Which of the three normal adult hemoglobins would be affected in hydrops fetalis?

HEMOGLOBIN H DISEASE (α^0-THAL-1/α^+-THAL-2)

HbH disease, a symptomatic but nonfatal type of α-thalassemia, was the first type to be described, in 1956. It occurs when three of the four α-genes are deleted. African Americans seldom present with HbH disease because they rarely express a deletion of two α-genes on the same chromosome.[6]

This disorder usually results when two heterozygous parents, one with α^0-thal-1 $(--/\alpha\alpha)$ and the other expressing the α^+-thal-2 $(-\alpha/\alpha\alpha)$ genotype, bear children.[5] All children from a patient with HbH disease will have one of the four types of α-thalassemia, the severity of which depends on the other parent's genotype.

Pathophysiology

The dramatic reduction in α-chain synthesis results in a decrease in the assembly of HbA, HbA$_2$, and HbF. In addition, a decrease in α-chains creates a relative excess of β-chains, which unite to form tetrads of four β-chains called *HbH*. γ-chains are also produced in excess of α-chains, especially at birth, and combine to form Hb Bart's.

HbH is thermolabile, unstable, and tends to precipitate inside erythrocytes triggering chronic hemolytic anemia. Its oxygen affinity is 10 times that of HbA, reducing oxygen delivery to the tissues. Its high oxygen affinity is attributed to the lack of heme-heme interaction and absence of the Bohr effect (∞ Chapter 6). This increased oxygen affinity is reflected in the lower **P$_{50}$ value** of HbH relative to HbA and myoglobin (Figure 11-3 ■).

Hemoglobin H also occurs as an acquired defect in erythroleukemia and other myeloproliferative disorders. However, the clinical manifestations and hematological abnormalities of these acquired disorders make it possible to distinguish them from HbH disease. Acquired HbH is probably due to a defect that prohibits the transcription of the α-gene.

 ### Checkpoint! 5

Compare oxygen binding characteristics of HbH relative to HbA and myoglobin.

	CA	CS	A2	COE Lepore	F	A	Portland	Barts	H
Hydrops fetalis	I						I	■	
Hgb H (neonate)	I		I		I	I		■	
Hgb H (adult)	I		I		I	■			I
Hgb H/ CS	I	I	I		I	■			I
α-Thal minor	I		I		I	■		I (neonates only)	
Silent carrier	I		I		I	■			

CA = Carbonic anhydrase
CS = Constant spring

■ **FIGURE 11-2** Hemoglobin electrophoresis on cellulose acetate at pH 8.4 is helpful in distinguishing the type of thalassemia and in differentiating thalassemias from hemoglobinopathies. In α-thalassemias, there is a reduction in α-containing hemoglobins (HbA, HbA$_2$, and HbF) proportional to the number of deleted α-genes and in the more severe cases, the emergence of non–α-containing hemoglobins (HbH and Hb Bart's).

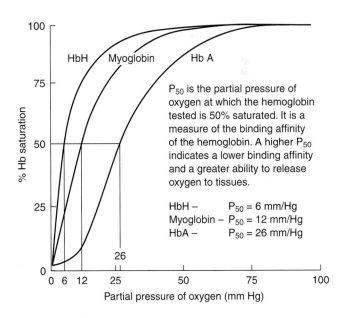

P$_{50}$ is the partial pressure of oxygen at which the hemoglobin tested is 50% saturated. It is a measure of the binding affinity of the hemoglobin. A higher P$_{50}$ indicates a lower binding affinity and a greater ability to release oxygen to tissues.

HbH – P$_{50}$ = 6 mm/Hg
Myoglobin – P$_{50}$ = 12 mm/Hg
HbA – P$_{50}$ = 26 mm/Hg

■ **FIGURE 11-3** The Hb dissociation curve illustrates the relative binding affinities of HbA, HbH, and myoglobin using the P$_{50}$ value. The monomeric myoglobin molecule lacks heme-heme interactions, causing it to bind oxygen tightly, decreasing the P$_{50}$ value relative to HbA. The P$_{50}$ value is even lower for HbH, indicating an even stronger affinity for oxygen estimated to be 10 times more than the oxygen affinity of HbA.

Clinical Findings

Symptoms are related to anemia and chronic hemolysis. Hemoglobin H disease shows a wide variation from mild to severe in the degree of anemia, which worsens during pregnancy, in infectious states, and during administration of oxidant drugs. Splenomegaly and, less often, hepatomegaly are present. Less than half of affected patients exhibit skeletal changes similar to those found in β-thalassemia major.

Laboratory Results

Hemoglobin H disease is characterized by a microcytic, hypochromic anemia with hemoglobin levels usually ranging from 8 to 10 g/dL. Reticulocytes are moderately increased from 5 to 10%, and nucleated red blood cells are observed on the peripheral blood smear (Figure 11-4a ■).

Hemoglobin electrophoresis of affected neonates shows about 25% Hb Bart's with decreased levels of HbA, HbA$_2$, and HbF. After birth, β-chains begin to replace γ-chains, and HbH eventually replaces Hb Bart's. Hemoglobin H, a fast-migrating hemoglobin at alkaline pH, makes up from 2 to 40% of the hemoglobin in adults with HbH disease. HbA$_2$ is decreased to a mean of 1.5%, but HbF is normal. A trace of Hb Bart's can be demonstrated in approximately 10% of affected adults with remaining hemoglobin being HbA (Figure 11-2). Other laboratory tests are available to assess patients with HbH disease. Hemoglobin H inclusions are easily found upon incubation of blood with brilliant cresyl blue (Figure 11-4b ■). These inclusions tend to cover the inside of the plasma membrane, giving the appearance of a golf ball.

Treatment and Prognosis for Hemoglobin H Disease

Treatment for patients with HbH disease is variable but when indicated involves long-term transfusion therapy and splenectomy. Regular transfusions minimize the stunting of growth and the other consequences of chronic severe anemia. Iron chelation therapy with deferoxamine avoids iron overload and the effects of iron toxicity. Deferipone is an oral chelator that is an alternative to deferoxamine but has significant dose-related sequelae like neutropenia, arthropathy, and agranulocytosis. The increased and ineffective erythropoiesis places high demands on the bone marrow requiring folate supplementation to avoid a deficiency.[3] Early treatment is necessary to prevent the typical clinical manifestations of thalassemia. With supportive and behavioral interventions, patients with HbH disease experience a normal life expectancy. For patients in whom transfusion and chelation therapy are not efficacious, a bone marrow transplant could be indicated.[3]

α-THALASSEMIA MINOR (α^+-THAL-2/ α^+- THAL-2, OR α^0-THAL-1/NORMAL)

The α-thalassemia trait (homozygous α^+-thal-2 or α^0-thal-1 trait) occurs when two of the four α-genes, either on the same or opposite chromosomes, are missing. The condition is found in all geographic locations.[7] In African Americans, the homozygous α^+-thal-2 form is the most common presentation. Genetic testing has identified at least nine **haplotypes**, representing different mutations, all of which result in the deletion of both α-genes on the same chromosome, which is more common in patients of Southeast Asian or Mediterranean descent.[8]

Pathophysiology

Although a measurable decrease in the production of α-containing hemoglobins occurs, the unaffected globin genes are able to direct synthesis of α-globin chains to a greater than normal degree and therefore compensate for the affected genes. Only minor changes occur in the erythrocyte count, indices, hemoglobin electrophoresis patterns, and red cell morphology.

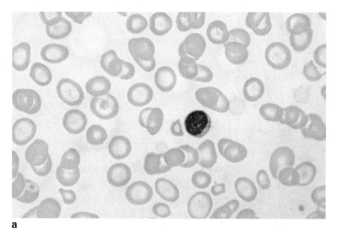

a

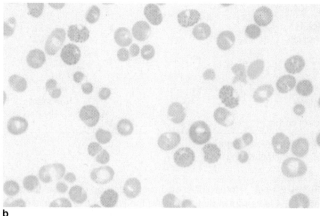

b

■ FIGURE 11-4   a. This peripheral blood smear is from a patient with HbH disease. Note the microcytic, hypochromic anemia with target cells. b. Peripheral blood from patient in Figure 11-4a after incubation with brilliant cresyl blue. Notice the cells that have dimples and look like golf balls. These are the cells with precipitated HbH. (a. Brilliant cresyl blue stain; 1000× magnification)

Clinical Findings

Patients with α-thalassemia trait are asymptomatic with a mild anemia and are often diagnosed incidentally or when being evaluated for family studies. This mild **phenotype** is the reason this form is called *thalassemia minor*.

Laboratory Results

The most demonstrable laboratory abnormalities are observed in the newborn. The presence of 5–6% Hb Bart's in neonates can be helpful in diagnosing this condition.[9] Three months after birth, Hb Bart's decreases to undetectable levels and hemoglobin electrophoresis becomes normal. The only persistent hematological abnormality thereafter is a variable microcytic, hypochromic anemia.

In adult patients, hemoglobin levels are above 10 g/dL and the erythrocyte count is above 5×10^{12}/L. The peripheral blood film usually demonstrates significant microcytosis with an MCV of 60–70 fL with few target cells (Figure 11-5 ■). Occasional cells can exhibit HbH inclusions after incubation with brilliant cresyl blue.

In some cases, α-thalassemia is masked by iron-deficiency anemia. Persistence of microcytes following successful treatment of iron deficiency is suggestive of thalassemia, but further investigation is suggested.

Treatment and Prognosis

These patients have a normal life span and do not require medical intervention for their thalassemia.

SILENT CARRIER (α^+-THAL-2/NORMAL)

The silent carrier version of α-thalassemia (α^+-thal-2 trait) is missing only one of four functioning α-genes. More than 25% of African Americans have been shown to express a deletion of one α-gene.[10–12]

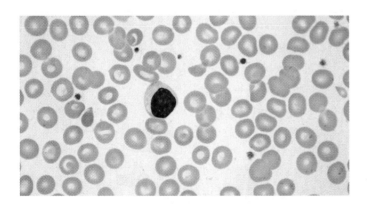

■ FIGURE 11-5 This is a peripheral blood smear from a patient with α-thalassemia trait. The hemoglobin is 15 g/dL, RBC 6.4 $\times$ 10^{12}/L, MCV 69.4 fL. The high RBC count with microcytosis is typical of thalassemia minor or trait. (Peripheral blood; Wright-Giemsa stain; 1000$\times$ magnification)

Pathogenesis/Clinical Findings/Laboratory Results

In silent carrier disease, the three remaining α-genes direct the synthesis of an adequate number of α-chains for normal hemoglobin synthesis. This carrier state is asymptomatic and totally benign, but adults often present with a borderline normal MCV of around 78–80 fL.[8] In affected infants, 1–2% Hb Bart's is found at birth but cannot be detected after three months of age. The only definitive diagnostic test for thalassemias in adults with one or two gene deletions is globin gene analysis.

Treatment and Prognosis

Patients with silent carrier disease require no treatment and have a normal life span.

CASE STUDY (continued from page 233)

Following are the CBC and differential results for John, the 4-year-old Grecian patient.

CBC		Differential	
WBC	11.4×10^9/L	Segs	55%
RBC	1.7×10^{12}/L	Bands	1%
Hb	8.3 g/dL	Lymphs	36%
Hct	0.24L/L	Mono	7%
MCV	69 fL	Eos	1%
MCH	21 pg	Moderate poikilocytosis,	
MCHC	29.2 g/dL	polychromasia, and tar-	
Plt	172×10^9/L	get cells; few teardrop	
		cells	

1. Based on the indices, classify the anemia morphologically.
2. Name the dominant poikilocyte observed in this peripheral blood smear.
3. Name three disorders that frequently present with the same poikilocyte that dominates in this peripheral blood smear.
4. List two additional lab tests that would help to confirm the diagnosis and predict the results of each.

▶ β-THALASSEMIA

GENERAL CONSIDERATIONS

As with α-thalassemias, some features of β-thalassemias are common to all forms of the disease. The genetics of β-thalassemia and the individuals affected with the disorder are presented before the discussion of its various forms.

Genetics

Whereas a total of four α-globin genes result in four major genotypes of α-thalassemia, there are only two β-globin

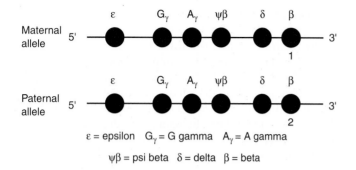

ε = epsilon   G$_γ$ = G gamma   A$_γ$ = A gamma

ψβ = psi beta   δ = delta   β = beta

■ **FIGURE 11-6**   Chromosome 11 is the location of four types of globin genes (ε, γ, δ, β). The 5′ to 3′ orientation of the genes is depicted. There is a gene for ε, δ, and β and two γ-genes. A β-pseudogene (ψβ) has been identified but does not express protein product.

genes, one located on each chromosome 11 (Figure 11-6■). If the prominent type of mutation found in β-thalassemia were also deletional, one would expect two severities, the severe homozygote and the mild heterozygote. However, in β-thalassemia, most mutations are non-deletional, resulting in a near continuum of clinical severities. In an attempt to gain some control over nomenclature of this diverse group of diseases, two classification systems are currently used. The genotypic system classifies β-thalassemia patients into six genotypes based on zygosity and the degree of alteration of the β-genes, and the phenotypic system divides patients into four categories based on the severity of clinical symptoms.

In the genotypic system, all β-gene mutations are categorized into two groups based on the impact of the mutation on β-globin production. The two gene varieties are termed $β^+$ and $β^0$. The $β^+$-gene mutation causes a partial block in β-chain synthesis, and the $β^0$-gene mutation results in a complete absence of β-chain synthesis from that allele. In addition, a minimally affected β-allele called *silent carrier* has been identified. It is found only in the most benign version of β-thalassemia. When the two gene designations ($β^0$ and $β^+$) are combined with the normal allele (β) and the two possible zygosity patterns (homozygous and heterozygous), six possible genotypes ($β^0/β^0$, $β^0/β^+$, $β^+/β^+$, $β^0/β$, $β^+/β$, $β/β$) emerge. When the silent carrier mutation is added, a total of seven β-genotypes can be described (Table 11-5 ✪).

β-thalassemia is the result of several different types of molecular defects. More than 180 mutations that result in partial to complete absence of β-gene expression have been described, but only 20 mutations account for 80% of the diagnosed β-thalassemias.[1,6] β-thalassemia is rarely due to deletion of the structural gene as is the case in the α-thalassemias. Most defects in β-thalassemia are point mutations in regions of the DNA that control β-gene expression. These types of mutations can affect gene expression ranging from minor reductions in β-globin production to complete absence of synthesis. Mutations can affect any step in the pathway of globin gene expression including gene transcription, RNA processing, m-RNA translation, and post-translational integrity of the protein.[13,14] Within a given population, a few genetic lesions account for most of the β-thalassemia mutations. For instance, in Greece, five mutations account for 87% of the gene defects.[14]

The phenotypic system recognizes four groups of patients categorized by the severity of symptoms, medical interventions, and prognoses. The four groups, listed in order from most severe to least severe, are β-thalassemia major, β-thalassemia intermedia, β-thalassemia minor, and β-thalassemia minima (Table 11-5).

One reason some prefer to organize β-thalassemias into a genotypic system is that phenotypic terms do not accurately

✪ TABLE 11-5

Characteristics of β-Thalassemia

Genotype	Zygosity	Phenotype	RBC Count	RBC Morphology	Hb Electrophoresis	Severity
$β^0/β^0$	Homozygous	Major	Relative ↑	↑↑↑ Target cells	No A, ↑A$_2$, ↑↑F	Severe
$β^0/β^+$	Double heterozygous	Major	Relative ↑	↑↑↑ Target cells	↓A, ↑A$_2$, ↑↑F	Severe
		Intermedia		↑↑ Target cells	↓A, ↑A$_2$, ↑↑F	Moderate
$β^+/β^+$	Homozygous	Major	Relative ↑	↑↑↑ Target cells	↓A, ↑A$_2$, ↑↑F	Severe
		Intermedia		↑↑ Target cells	↓A, ↑A$_2$, ↑↑F	Moderate
$β^0/β$	Heterozygous	Intermedia	Relative ↑	↑↑ Target cells	↓A, ↑A$_2$, ↑F	Moderate
		Minor		↑ Target cells	↓A, ↑A$_2$, ↑F	Mild
$β^+/β$	Heterozygous	Minor	Relative ↑	↑ Target cells	↓A, ↑A$_2$, ↑F	Mild
$β^{SC}/β$	Heterozygous	Minima	Normal	± Target cells	Normal	Normal
$β/β$	Homozygous	Normal	Normal	Normal	Normal	Normal

↑ = slight increase, ↑↑ = moderate increase, ↑↑↑ = marked increase, +/− = occasionally seen, ↓ = slight decrease, A = HbA, A$_2$ = HbA$_2$, F = HbF, $β^{sc}$ = silent carrier

reflect the genetic description of the disease. However, a disadvantage to the genotypic system is that patients with identical genotype designations can express β-thalassemia that is phenotypically diverse. For instance, a severe form of β^+/β^+-thalassemia (Mediterranean form) is characterized by an increase in HbF (50–90%) and a normal or only slightly elevated HbA$_2$ whereas a milder form of β^+/β^+-thalassemia (black form) has 20–40% HbF with normal or elevated HbA$_2$ and the remainder HbA. For this reason, some clinicians prefer the phenotypic system that more closely parallels symptoms and better predicts clinical interventions necessary for appropriate management of the patient.

This section combines the genotypic and phenotypic systems with an emphasis on the phenotypic system. The two more recognized phenotypic groups, β-thalassemia major and minor, are discussed first followed by intermedia and minima (Table 11-5).

Affected Individuals

The most severe mutation (β^0) occurs more frequently in the Mediterranean regions—specifically in northern Italy, Greece, Algeria, Saudi Arabia—and Southeast Asia. Two severities of the β^+ mutation tend to originate in different ethnic populations. The more severe version is observed in the Mediterranean region, the Middle East, the Indian subcontinent, and Southeast Asia, the milder version is localized to patients of African descent.[7]

β-THALASSEMIA MAJOR (β^0/β^0, β^0/β^+, $\beta^+\beta^+$)

Expected Genotypes

Beta-thalassemia major, also referred to as *Cooley's anemia*, is caused by a homozygous (β^0/β^0, $\beta^+\beta^+$), or **double heterozygous** (β^0/β^+), inheritance of abnormal β-genes resulting in marked reduction or absence of β-chain synthesis. As can be seen in Table 11-5, two of these three genotypes (β^0/β^+, β^+/β^+) can also present as the milder β-thalassemia intermedia phenotype that will be discussed later.

Pathophysiology

The dramatic reduction or absence of β-chain synthesis affects the production of HbA. The symptoms that result from β-thalassemia major begin to manifest in infants approximately six months after birth. Other non–β-containing hemoglobins, HbA$_2$ and HbF, are increased in partial compensation for the decreased HbA levels.

The pathophysiologic mechanisms that result from a lack of β-chain production can be classified into four categories (Figure 11-7 ■):

* reduced HbA
* compensatory production of abnormal hemoglobins
* ineffective erythropoiesis with hemolysis
* erythroid hyperplasia

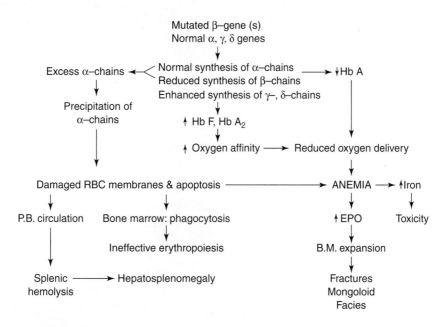

■ FIGURE 11-7   In β-thalassemia major, the decreased synthesis of β-chains reduces the production of HbA and increases the production of non-β-chain containing hemoglobins (HbA$_2$ and HbF). Excess α-chains form insoluble precipitates inside erythrocytes, damaging the membranes and reducing RBC lifespan through splenic sequestration and ineffective erythropoiesis. All of these factors contribute to a reduced oxygen delivery to the tissues resulting in anemia and hypoxia. The compensatory erythroid hyperplasia in the bone marrow expands the marrow cavity, resulting in pathologic fractures and mongoloid facial features.

A dramatic reduction in HbA compromises the blood's oxygen-carrying capacity. Other non-β-containing hemoglobins, HbF and HbA$_2$, are increased. HbF has a higher affinity for oxygen than HbA (∞ Chapter 6). The result is to exacerbate the already compromised oxygen delivery to tissues.

In β-thalassemia major, reduced synthesis of β-chains results in an excess of free α-chains and a β-to-α chain ratio of less than 0.25. The free excess α-chains cannot form hemoglobin tetramers, so they precipitate within the cell, damaging the cell membrane, leading to chronic hemolysis.[15] The accumulating α-chains contain free iron and hemichromes that generate reactive oxygen species (ROS). The ROS damage hemoglobin as well as the membrane's proteins and lipids, decreasing membrane stability.[16,17] Oxidation of membrane band 3 produces clustering of the proteins, creating new antigens on the cell surface that bind IgG and complement.[18] Many IgG- and complement-sensitized erythrocytes in the bone marrow are destroyed by binding to marrow macrophages via F$_c$ receptors, resulting in phagocytosis and a large degree of hemolysis.

The majority of the hemolysis occurs within the bone marrow primarily at the polychromatophilic normoblast stage of erythroid development, resulting in ineffective erythropoiesis.[19] The ineffective erythropoiesis is due to activation of apoptotic mechanisms by the precipitated α-globin chains and damaged cellular components.[20,21] If the patient has inherited α-thalassemia with β-thalassemia, the symptoms associated with hemolysis can be reduced because the relative excess of α-chains is reduced by the α-thalassemia.

The combination of reduced HbA, increased HbF, ineffective erythropoiesis, and chronic hemolysis results in significant anemia. The body attempts to compensate by stimulating erythropoiesis. The resulting erythroid hyperplasia causes bone marrow expansion and thinning of calcified bone. Increased erythropoietic activity also stimulates the absorption of more iron in the gut, leading to iron toxicity. Ineffective erythropoiesis in the bone marrow can be accompanied by extramedullary hematopoiesis in the liver and spleen, often producing hepatosplenomegaly (Figure 11-7).

 Checkpoint! 6

Why do the symptoms of β-thalassemia major delay until approximately the sixth month of life?

CLINICAL FINDINGS

Early symptoms of β-thalassemia first observed in infants include irritability, pallor, and a failure to thrive and gain weight. Diarrhea, fever, and an enlarged abdomen are also common findings. If therapy does not begin during early childhood, the clinical picture of thalassemia develops within a few years.

Severe anemia is the clinical condition responsible for many of the problems experienced by these children. The anemia places a tremendous burden on the cardiovascular system as it attempts to maintain tissue perfusion. Constant high output of blood usually results in cardiac failure in the first decade of life and is the major cause of death in untreated children. Growth is retarded, and a bronze pigmentation of the skin is notable. Chronic hemolysis often produces gallstones, gout, and icterus.

Bone changes accompany the hyperplastic marrow. Marrow cavities enlarge in every bone, expanding the bone and producing characteristic bossing of the skull, facial deformities, and "hair-on-end" appearance of the skull on x-ray (Figure 11-8 ■). The thinning cortical bone in long bones can lead to pathologic fractures.

Extramedullary hematopoiesis can be found in the liver and spleen and occasionally elsewhere in the body. The spleen can become massively enlarged and congested with abnormal erythrocytes.

Other clinical findings are associated with the body's attempt to increase erythrocyte production. Features that suggest an increased metabolic rate include fever, lethargy, weakened musculature, decreased body fat, and decreased appetite. Infection is a common cause of death. Folic acid deficiency can develop as a consequence of increased utilization by the hyperplastic marrow.

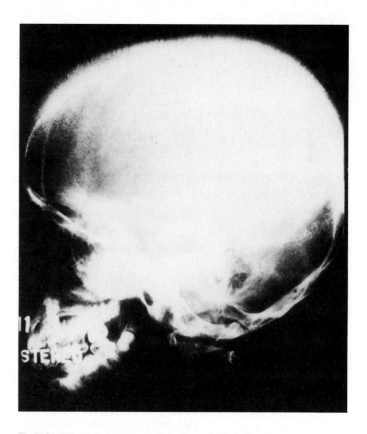

■ FIGURE 11-8 Increased erythropoiesis in the bone marrow of patients with β-thalassemia major expands the marrow cavity producing the typical "hair-on-end" appearance as seen on this radiograph of the skull of a boy with β-thalassemia.

Laboratory Results

The hemoglobin level can be as low as 2 or 3 g/dL in the more severe forms of the disease. The anemia is markedly microcytic and hypochromic with an MCV of less than 67 fL[22] and a markedly reduced MCH and MCHC. The peripheral blood smear shows marked anisocytosis and poikilocytosis (Figure 11-9 ■). Precipitates of α-chains can be visualized with methyl violet stain. Variable basophilic stippling and polychromasia are noted. Reticulocytes are not increased to the degree expected for the severity of the anemia because of the high degree of ineffective erythropoiesis. Nucleated erythrocytes are almost always found, and the RDW can be increased.[23] Secondary leukopenia and thrombocytopenia are produced because these components also become trapped in the enlarged spleen. Chronic hemolysis is reflected by increased unconjugated bilirubin. Urine can appear dark brown from the presence of dipyrroles.

Bone marrow studies are not usually necessary for diagnosis but when performed show marked erythroid hyperplasia with an M:E ratio of 0.1 or less.

Hemoglobin electrophoresis performed on cord blood samples provides evidence of deficient β-chain production at birth. Although normal cord blood contains about 20% HbA, cord blood from infants with β-thalassemia major has less than 2% HbA.[13] In adults, hemoglobin electrophoresis shows variable results depending on the thalassemia genes inherited. Absence of HbA, 90% HbF, and low, normal, or increased HbA₂ is characteristic of β^0/β^0-thalassemia.[24] The other genotypes, β^0/β^+ and β^+/β^+, show some HbA, but the majority of the hemoglobin is HbF with normal to increased HbA₂[25] (Figure 11-10 ■). The increased HbF in thalassemia is thought to be due to the expansion of a subpopulation of erythrocytes that have the ability to synthesize γ-chains. The distribution of HbF among erythrocytes is heterogeneous.

Definitive diagnosis of β-thalassemia can be made by demonstration of a β-to-α-chain ratio of less than 0.25. Molecular techniques demonstrating specific genetic mutations can also define the presence of thalassemia.

	CA	CS	COE A2	GDS Lepore	F	A	Portland	Bart's	H
Beta-thal major	|		|		■				
Beta-thal major (med)	|		|		■	|			
Beta-thal intermediate	|		|		|	■			
Beta-thal minor	|		|		|	■			
Beta-thal minima	|		|			■			

CA = Carbonic anhydrase
CS = Constant spring
med = Mediterranean

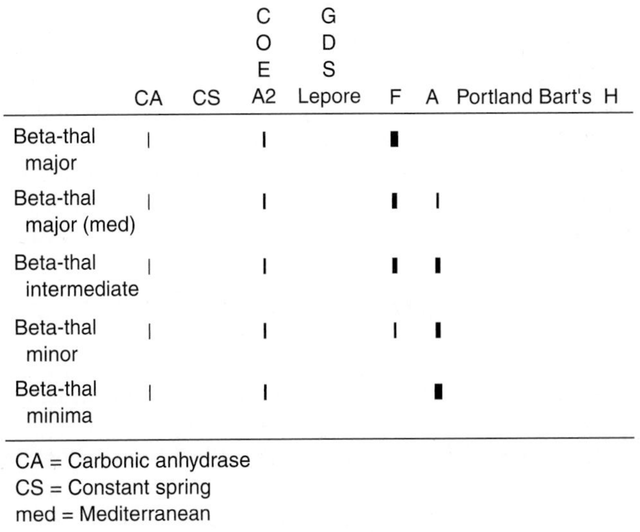

■ **FIGURE 11-10** Hemoglobin electrophoresis pattern from patients with β-thalassemia shows a reduction in β-containing HbA and an increase in non–β-containing HbA₂ and HbF.

TREATMENT

Most children with β-thalassemia major participate in a regular transfusion program, which prolongs life into the second or third decade and allows normal developmental and growth patterns. Initial treatment protocols were mainly palliative and designed to maintain the hemoglobin level ~7–8 g/dL; however, evidence of erythroid expansion and increased iron absorption persisted. Clinical evidence suggests that the more aggressive hypertransfusion programs (maintaining a hemoglobin level between 9 and 10.5 g/dL) offer the highest quality of life without significant sequelae.[26] The objectives of hypertransfusion programs are to minimize the anemia, reduce excess iron absorption, and suppress ineffective erythropoiesis. The large doses of iron received with these transfusions, however, lead to tissue damage from iron overload similar to that seen in hereditary hemochromatosis. Iron-chelating agents such as deferoxamine are given to decrease the deposition of iron in the tissues. Splenectomy can be performed in an attempt to decrease hemolysis and prolong red cell survival; however, it is usually reserved for patients over 5 years of age.

Within the last several years, bone marrow transplants have been attempted in an effort to provide the individual with stem cells capable of producing normal erythrocytes. Although bone marrow transplantation is an option for thalassemia patients with a suitable donor, this technology is not widely used at this time.[27] Clinical efficacy is questionable with the highest risk factor being lack of engraftment.

Drugs to treat leukemia are being used to induce the reexpression of latent γ-genes that would combine with the excess α-chains and produce HbF. The two major risk factors for this treatment approach include lack of γ-chain stimulation and induction of malignancy from the antileukemic drugs.[28,29] Correction of the molecular defect with gene therapy may be achievable in the future.[30]

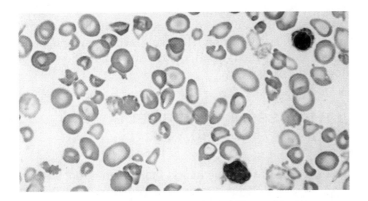

■ **FIGURE 11-9** Peripheral blood smear from a patient with β-thalassemia major showing marked anisopoikilocytosis. Target cells, schistocytes, teardrops, and ovalocytes are the major poikilocytes observed. An NRBC is also present. (1000× magnification; Wright-Giemsa stain)

Prognosis

Untreated patients generally expire during the first or second decade of life. Patients enrolled in a hypertransfusion program with chelation therapy can extend their life expectancy by at least a decade.[31] Usually in the second decade of life, endocrine disorders (e.g., diabetes) and hepatic and cardiac disturbances develop from excessive deposits of iron in these tissues if chelation therapy has not been successful.

β-THALASSEMIA MINOR (β^0/β OR β^+/β)

Expected Genotypes

Beta-thalassemia minor results from the heterozygous inheritance of either a β^+- or β^0-gene with one normal β-gene (Table 11-5). Evidence is mounting that there is no major clinical difference in the expression between the two thalassemia genes in the heterozygous state due primarily to the enhanced output of β-chains from the normal β-allele. About 1% of African Americans are heterozygous for β-thalassemia.

Pathophysiology

The normal β-gene directs synthesis of sufficient amounts of β-chains to synthesize enough HbA for near normal oxygen delivery and erythrocyte survival. In the case of a heterozygous β^+ patient, the thalassemic gene can also contribute to β-chain production.

Clinical Findings

The heterozygote appears to be asymptomatic except in periods of stress as can occur during pregnancy and with infections and folic acid deficiency. Under such conditions, a moderate microcytic anemia can develop.

Laboratory Results

The anemia in β-thalassemia minor is mild with hemoglobin values ranging from 9 to 14 g/dL with the mean value for women being 10.9 g/dL and for men 12.9 g/dL.[32-34] The erythrocyte count is increased ($> 5 \times 10^{12}$/L) for what is expected at the given hemoglobin concentration. The condition is usually discovered incidentally during testing for unrelated symptoms or during family study workups.

The erythrocytes are microcytic (MCV=55–70 fL) and hypochromic (MCHC=29–33 g/dL) or sometimes normochromic with an MCH that is usually less than 22 pg (Figure 11-11 ■). The degree of microcytosis, as indicated by the MCV, is directly related to the anemia's severity.[22] Although the anemia is mild, the peripheral blood smear shows variable anisocytosis and poikilocytosis with target cells and basophilic stippling. Nucleated red blood cells are not usually found, but anemic patients can have a slightly elevated reticulocyte count. Bone marrow shows slight erythroid hyperplasia and normoblasts poorly filled with hemoglobin.

Hemoglobin electrophoresis demonstrates an increase in HbA$_2$ from 3.5 to 7% with a mean of 5.5%. Newborns have a

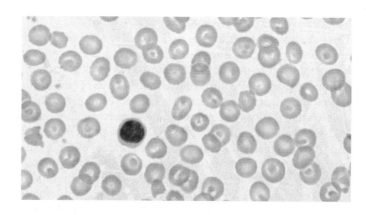

■ FIGURE 11-11   Patients with β-thalassemia minor show minimal morphologic abnormalities to include microcytosis with target cells. The CBC in this patient showed the following results: Hb 11.1 g/dL; RBC count 5.2 $\times$ 10^{12}/L; MCV 61 fL; MCH 20.2 pg; MCHC 33 g/L. (Wright-Giemsa stain; 1000$\times$ magnification)

normal HbA$_2$ concentration of 0.27 $\pm$ 0.02%.[24] HbF is normal in approximately half of the patients and increased in the other half (Figure 11-10).[35,36] If HbF exceeds 5%, however, the individual has probably inherited an HPFH gene (discussed later) in addition to the β-thalassemia gene. Vital stains to detect Heinz bodies are usually negative.

DNA-probing techniques can be performed to identify the type of mutation present and validate the heterozygous inheritance pattern but are of limited diagnostic value. Such information, however, can be helpful in counseling prospective parents with β-thalassemia minor.

✓ Checkpoint! 7

In β-thalassemia, what erythrocyte parameter on the CBC differs significantly from that found in iron deficiency?

Treatment and Prognosis

Patients generally do not require treatment if they maintain good health and nutrition. They are generally asymptomatic except during periods of physiologic stress, and they have a normal life expectancy.

β-THALASSEMIA INTERMEDIA (β^+/β^+, β^0/β^+, β^0/β)

Expected Genotypes

All three patterns of inheritance—homozygous, double heterozygous, and heterozygous—can produce β-thalassemia intermedia (Table 11-5). The homozygous and double heterozygous forms represent a mutation in both β-alleles resulting in a moderate reduction in β-chain synthesis. Patients who inherit a mutation of one β-gene in conjunction with a normal β-gene occasionally exhibit clinical symptoms significant enough to be classified as β-thalassemia intermedia rather than β-thalassemia minor.

Patients with β-thalassemia intermedia who coexpress α-thalassemia or HPFH can actually experience milder symptoms as compared to those with pure β-thalassemia. In both cases, α-chain accumulation and precipitation is decreased, reducing the ineffective erythropoiesis and extravascular hemolysis responsible for much of the pathology. In the case of concomitant β-thalassemia intermedia and HPFH, the overexpressed γ-chains combine with the excessive α-chains to produce HbF, which reduces α-chain precipitation.

Clinical Findings

Patients with β-thalassemia intermedia can present with symptoms of intermediate hematologic severity between severe β-thalassemia major and mild β-thalassemia minor. The β^0/β^+-genotype produces the greatest reduction in β-chain synthesis but has a variable clinical presentation; some patients have symptoms that can rival β-thalassemia major, and other patients have a much milder clinical phenotype. Patients expressing the β^0/β-genotype generally express mild symptoms. The generally accepted criterion for β-thalassemia intermedia is the ability to maintain a hemoglobin level associated with a comfortable survival without requiring regular transfusions.[26] The need for transfusions is defined by the quality of life, not the hemoglobin level per se. Some patients with a hemoglobin level of 7 g/dL can be relatively symptom free, but other patients with a hemoglobin of 9 g/dL can have clinical symptoms related to ineffective erythropoiesis. Clinical symptoms often intensify during periods of physiological stress as with pregnancy and infection and can require short-term transfusion therapy. Even in the absence of regular transfusions, some patients develop progressive iron overload and require iron-chelation therapy.

Laboratory Results

The CBC reflects a moderate microcytic hypochromic anemia with a hemoglobin value ranging from 7 to 10 g/dL. In the milder versions, patients express only a slight reduction in hemoglobin values. The red blood cell count is disproportionately higher than the hemoglobin values that often approach normal.

Target cells are the predominant poikilocytes observed. Basophilic stippling and nucleated red blood cells are also present. The bone marrow shows hypochromic normoblasts in the context of erythroid hyperplasia. However, bone marrow examination is not needed for diagnosis.

Hemoglobin electrophoresis patterns in patients with the more severe forms of β-thalassemia intermedia ($\beta^0\beta^+$ and $\beta^+\beta^+$) are nearly indistinguishable from those observed in the milder forms of β-thalassemia major ($\beta^+\beta^+$). Patients express elevated HbA$_2$ (5–10%) and HbF (30–75%) with the re-

mainder being HbA. Milder versions of β-thalassemia intermedia produce lower HbA$_2$ (>3.2%) and HbF levels (1.5–12.0%) (Figure 11-10). Although hemoglobin electrophoresis is helpful in the diagnosis of β-thalassemia intermedia, differentiation from β-thalassemia major and minor is a clinical decision.

Treatment and Prognosis

Splenomegaly is common. Functional hyposplenism leads to infections requiring regular interventions with antibiotic therapy. Chelation therapy is generally warranted to combat iron overload, which tends to develop later than in patients with β-thalassemia major. Most patients have a normal life span.

β-THALASSEMIA MINIMA (β^{SC}/β)

Beta-thalassemia minima is a form of asymptomatic β-thalassemia and exhibits no major laboratory abnormalities. The disorder is usually discovered serendipitously during family studies. The gene has been given the designation β^{SC} for silent carrier. The genotype used to describe a patient with β-thalassemia minima is β^{SC}/β.[37]

CASE STUDY *(continued from page 241)*

Additional tests were performed on John's blood to determine the cause of his anemia.

Hemoglobin Electrophoresis		Iron Panel	
HbA	66%	Serum iron	92 µg/dL
HbA$_2$	1.0%	TIBC	310 µg/dL
HbF	1.0%	Serum ferritin	88 ng/mL
Hb Bart's	8%	Iron saturation	33%
HbH	24%		

5. Is the hemoglobin electrophoresis normal or abnormal?

6. If abnormal, list hemoglobins that are elevated, decreased, or abnormally present.

7. If abnormal, which globin chain(s) is (are) decreased?

8. If abnormal, which globin chains are produced in excess?

9. Is the iron panel normal or abnormal?

10. If the iron tests are abnormal, list those outside the normal range and indicate whether they are elevated or decreased.

11. If the iron tests are abnormal, state the disorder(s) consistent with the abnormal iron panel.

12. Given all the data supplied, what is the definitive diagnosis of John's anemia?

► OTHER THALASSEMIAS AND THALASSEMIA-LIKE CONDITIONS

In theory, any globin gene can be mutated, resulting in a reduction in the synthesis of globin chains and the corresponding hemoglobin. Patients have been observed with deficiencies in each of the normal adult globin chains. However, the thalassemias that involve globin chains other than α and β are relatively benign in their clinical course because they are not constituents of the major adult hemoglobin, HbA. Thalassemias have been observed involving more than one globin gene and in combination with structural hemoglobin disorders such as sickle cell anemia and HbC disease (Table 11-6 ✪).

$\delta\beta$-THALASSEMIA

Delta, beta-thalassemia is a rare thalassemia observed primarily in patients of Greek, African, Italian, and Arabian ancestry in which production of both β- and δ-chains is affected. The $\delta\beta$-mutation can be categorized into two genotypes, $\delta\beta^0$ and $\delta\beta^+$. The $\delta\beta^0$ designation indicates a complete lack of synthesis of both β- and δ-chains from a given chromosome, whereas the $\delta\beta^+$-genotype suggests a reduction in β- and δ-chain synthesis. The absence of β- and δ-chains is most often due to deletion of the structural β- and δ-gene complex. One or both of the γ-genes remain, resulting in 100% HbF in homozygous $\delta\beta^0/\delta\beta^0$.[30] However, increased γ-chain production fails to fully compensate for the loss of β-chain

✪ TABLE 11-6

Characteristics of Other Thalassemias and Thalassemia-Like Conditions

Disorder	Defect	Ancestry	CBC/diff	Hb Electrophoresis	Other
$\delta\beta$ thalassemia homozygous ($\delta\beta^0/\delta\beta^0$)	Deletion of $\delta\beta$-gene complex	Greek, African, Italian, Arabian	Micro/hypo RBCs Hb 10–12 g/dL	$\downarrow\downarrow$HbA, $\downarrow\downarrow$HbA$_2$, $\uparrow\uparrow$HbF	Thalassemia intermedia
heterozygous ($\delta\beta^0/\beta$)		Same as heterozygous	No anemia	$\downarrow$HbA, N-$\downarrow$HbA$_2$, $\uparrow$HbF	Thalassemia minor
$\gamma\delta\beta$ thalassemia heterozygous ($\gamma\delta\beta^0/\beta$)	Deletion or inactivation of β-gene complex	Mediterranean regions	Birth: Marked anemia; Adult: Slight anemia	$\downarrow$HbA, $\downarrow$HbA$_2$, $\downarrow$HbF	Thalassemia minor
homozygous ($\gamma\delta\beta^0/\gamma\delta\beta^0$)		Same as heterozygous	Unable to observe	No adult Hb	Fatal
Constant Spring homozygous ($\alpha\alpha^{CS}/\alpha\alpha^{CS}$)	Long α-chain, mutated stop codon, reduced synthesis	Thailand	Micro/hypo RBCs, Hb 9–11 g/dL, $\uparrow$ Reticulocytes	Hb Bart's at birth, $\uparrow\uparrow$HbCS, $\downarrow$HbA, N-HbA$_2$ and HbF	
heterozygous ($\alpha\alpha^{CS}/\alpha\alpha$)		Same as homozygous	Normal	$\uparrow$ HbCS	Can be seen with α-thal2 trait
HPFH homozygous ($\delta\beta^0/\delta\beta^0$)	Deletion or inactivation of $\delta\beta$-gene complex	Greek, Swiss, black	Mild micro/hypo RBCs, no anemia, $\uparrow\uparrow$ RBC, Hb 14–18 g/dL	100% HbF	2 variants— pancellular, heterocellular Asymptomatic
heterozygous ($\delta\beta^0/\beta$)		Same as homozygous	Near normal	$\uparrow$ HbF, $\downarrow$ HbA, $\downarrow$ HbA$_2$	Asymptomatic
Hb Lepore homozygous ($\delta\beta^{Lepore}/\delta\beta^{Lepore}$)	$\delta\beta$-hybrid chain	European	Marked micro/hypo RBCs, Hb 4–11 g/dL, $\uparrow\uparrow\uparrow$ anisopoikilocytosis	No HbA, No HbA$_2$, $\uparrow\uparrow$ Hb Lepore, $\uparrow\uparrow$ HbF	Thalassemia major or intermedia
heterozygous ($\delta\beta^{Lepore}/\beta$)		Same as homozygous	Slight micro/hypo RBCs, Hb 12 g/dL	$\downarrow$ HbA, $\downarrow$ HbA$_2$, $\uparrow$ Hb Lepore	Thalassemia minor

$\uparrow\uparrow\uparrow$ = marked increase; $\uparrow\uparrow$ = moderate increase; $\uparrow$ = slight increase; $\downarrow\downarrow$ moderate decrease; $\downarrow$ = slight decrease; N = normal production, resulting in a thalassemic phenotype and anemia.

It appears that in $\delta\beta$-thalassemia, the compensation of γ-chain synthesis is less than in HPFH but more than in homozygous β^0-thalassemia. Clinically, the disease is classified as thalassemia intermedia and rarely requires blood transfusions except in cases of physiological stress such as in pregnancy or infection. Thus, most patients with $\delta\beta$-thalassemia have a mild hypochromic, microcytic anemia. Patients have slight hepatosplenomegaly and some bone changes associated with chronic erythroid hyperplasia. Hemolysis probably contributes to the anemia because both reticulocytes and bilirubin are elevated.

The heterozygous form of $\delta\beta$-thalassemia ($\delta\beta^0/\beta$) is not identified with any specific clinical finding. There is no anemia or splenomegaly. The hematological picture, however, is similar to that of β-thalassemia minor with microcytic, hypochromic erythrocytes. Hemoglobin A_2 is normal or slightly decreased while HbF is increased to 5–20%. HbA is usually less than 90% (Table 11-6).

$\gamma\delta\beta$-Thalassemia

This rare form of thalassemia has several variants and is characterized by deletion or inactivation of the entire β-gene complex.[25] Deletion of the γ-, δ-, and β-genes would result in the absence of all normal adult hemoglobin production from that chromosome. Therefore, only the heterozygous state has been encountered, presumably because a homozygous condition would be incompatible with life. Although neonates have severe hemolytic anemia, as the child grows, the disease evolves to a mild form of β-thalassemia.

HEMOGLOBIN CONSTANT SPRING

Hemoglobin Constant Spring (HbCS) is a hemoglobin tetramer formed from the combination of two structurally abnormal α-chains, each elongated by 31 amino acids at the carboxy-terminal end, and two normal β-chains. This genetic mutation is common in Thailand. The chromosome with the α^{CS} gene carries one normal α-gene (remember that each chromosome 16 has 2 α-genes for a total of 4 α-genes); thus, the homozygous HbCS individual has two normal α-genes, one on each chromosome, and the heterozygous HbCS carrier has three normal α-genes.

The elongated α-chains of HbCS are thought to result from a mutation of the α-chain termination codon by a single base substitution.[38] The abnormal α-chains are synthesized at very low levels (~1% of the output compared to a normal α gene) due to reduced stability of the mRNA. The result is an overall deficiency of α-chain synthesis producing an α-thalassemia-like phenotype.

Clinical Findings

The homozygous state is phenotypically similar to α-thalassemia minor. A slight anemia accompanied by mild jaundice and splenomegaly is typical. Heterozygotes show no clinical abnormalities.

Laboratory Results

In homozygotes, clinical findings are similar to a relatively mild form of HbH disease with a mild microcytic hypochromic anemia. Hemoglobin electrophoresis demonstrates the presence of Hb Bart's at birth. In homozygous adults, HbCS makes up 5–7% of the hemoglobin and HbA_2 and HbF remain normal. The remainder of hemoglobin is HbA (Figure 11-2).

Heterozygotes show no hematological abnormalities, but a small amount of HbCS (0.2–1.7%) can be found on electrophoresis. HbA_2 and HbF are normal with the remainder being HbA (Figure 11-2).

In some areas, the coexistence of HbCS with α-thalassemia trait ($--/\alpha\alpha^{CS}$) is a rather common finding. The clinical findings are similar to those of HbH disease. Hemoglobin electrophoresis characteristically shows HbA, HbH, Hb Bart's, HbA_2, and 1.5–2.5% HbCS[39] (Figure 11-2) (Table 11-6).

 Checkpoint! 8

Why is $\gamma\delta\beta$-thalassemia more severe than $\delta\beta$-thalassemia and CS-thalassemia?

HEREDITARY PERSISTENCE OF FETAL HEMOGLOBIN (HPFH)

Hereditary persistence of fetal hemoglobin (HPFH) is actually a group of heterogeneous disorders in which the absence of δ- and β-chain synthesis is compensated for by increased γ-chain production into adult life. In homozygotes, the result is an absence of HbA and HbA_2 with 100% of hemoglobin production being HbF. Hemoglobin F production continues at high levels throughout life, preventing the clinical symptoms and hematological abnormalities associated with thalassemia. The condition occurs in 0.1% of African Americans.

Genetics

HPFH is characterized by either deletion or inactivation of the β- and δ-structural gene complex. Most α-chains combine with the available γ-chains to produce HbF. Consequently, no accumulation and no precipitation of excess α-chains occur. In HPFH, increased production of γ-chains with the corresponding elevations of HbF compensates for the reduction in HbA and A_2 synthesis and differentiates it from $\delta\beta$-thalassemia, in which only modest elevations in HbF are observed.

Variants

HPFH can be categorized into two major groups, pancellular and heterocellular, based on the distribution of HbF in erythrocytes. The HbF distribution patterns can be visualized using the acid elution stain developed by Kleihauer and Betke. Pancellular refers to the observance of HbF in most of the erythrocytes; in the heterocellular version, HbF is concentrated in a small subset of erythrocytes.

Several different types of HPFH have been described: the black, Greek, and Swiss types. In the black and Swiss types, both $^G\gamma$- and $^A\gamma$-chains are produced in approximately equal amounts. The Greek form is characterized by production of both $^G\gamma$- and $^A\gamma$-chains, but most HbF is made up of the $^A\gamma$-chains. Both the black and Greek types have the characteristic pancellular distribution pattern of HbF in erythrocytes. However, the Swiss form exhibits a heterocellular distribution of HbF. This heterocellular distribution results from a hereditary increase (3%) in the number of fetal (F) cells.[13,14] (Table 11-7 ✪).

When present, the pancellular distribution of HbF in erythrocytes helps to distinguish this disorder from other disorders associated with an increase in HbF. Most other disorders with elevated HbF levels present with the heterocellular distribution pattern.

It has been suggested that the various categories of HPFH actually represent a continuum of a spectrum of β-thalassemias with homozygous β^0-thalassemia at one end where the lack of β-chain synthesis is poorly compensated for by γ-chain production and with pancellular HPFH at the other end where the lack of β-chain synthesis is almost completely compensated for by γ-chain production.

Homozygotes

Homozygous HPFH is asymptomatic including no evidence of abnormal growth patterns or splenomegaly. The abundant γ-chains combine with the normal α-chains to produce HbF.

Erythrocytosis ranging from 6×10^{12}/L to 7×10^{12}/L occurs as the result of the higher oxygen affinity of HbF as compared to HbA. Correspondingly, high hemoglobin levels from 14.8 to 18.2 g/dL are also typical in HPFH. Erythrocytes are microcytic and slightly hypochromic with a mean MCV of 75 fL and a mean MCH of 25.0 pg. There is a mild degree of anisocytosis and poikilocytosis. The reticulocyte count

ranges from 1 to 2%. It is doubtful that this disorder has any significant degree of hemolysis because the reticulocyte count, bilirubin, and haptoglobin levels are normal. Electrophoresis demonstrates 100% HbF.

Heterozygotes

Heterozygous HPFH is usually found incidentally through family studies. Patients present with a slightly elevated erythrocyte count with the corresponding elevation of the hematocrit and a slightly decreased MCH (27 pg). HbF increases to 10 to 30%. Hemoglobin A_2 is decreased to 1–2% and the remainder is HbA. In the presence of iron deficiency, HbF levels are lower (Table 11-6).

HEMOGLOBIN LEPORE

Incidence and Affected Individuals

Hemoglobin Lepore was first described in 1958 as a structural hemoglobin variant with hematological changes and clinical manifestations resembling those of thalassemia.[40] The disorder is widely distributed throughout the world but is especially common in Middle and Eastern Europe.

Genetics

In Hb Lepore, the non-α-chain is a δ/β-globin hybrid in which the N-terminal end of a δ-chain is fused to the C-terminal end of a β-chain. The variant hybrid genes are thought to occur during meiosis from an aberrant **crossover** event resulting in recombination of misaligned δ- and β-genes on separate chromosomes. The result of the unequal crossover event is two fusion genes, the δ/β-Lepore and the β/δ-anti-Lepore fusion genes. The δ/β-Lepore fusion gene is transcribed and translated into the δ/β-fusion globin chain, two of which combine with two α-chains to form Hb Lepore. The chromosome containing the β/δ-anti-Lepore fusion gene still contains intact β- and δ-genes that are synthesized normally to form HbA and A_2, respectively. Progeny bear genes from the involved chromosome that are neither fully paternal nor fully maternal. Because the recombination event occurred in the germ cells, the newly formed chromosomes become a permanent part of the family's gene pool. Hb Lepore is stable and has normal functional properties except for a slight increase in oxygen affinity.

Pathophysiology

The pathophysiology of hemoglobin Lepore is similar to that of β-thalassemia. No intact β-gene is present, so β-chain synthesis is absent. The Hb Lepore gene is under the influence of the δ-gene promoter, which limits synthesis of the Lepore hybrid chain to approximately 2.5% of normal β-chain production. Thus, the abnormal Lepore chains are inadequately synthesized, leading to an excess of α-chains. In the homozygous state, no normal β-chains or δ-chains would be synthesized to combine with the α-chains being produced, thus no HbA or HbA$_2$. The more severely affected children can

✪ TABLE 11-7

Characteristics of HPFH Variants

HPFH Type	Types of γ-chains Produced	Distribution of HbF in Erythrocytes
Black	$^G\gamma$- and $^A\gamma$-	Pancellular
Swiss	$^G\gamma$- and $^A\gamma$-	Heterocellular
Greek	Primarily $^A\gamma$-	Pancellular

become transfusion dependent and develop complications of hemosiderosis. The combination of ineffective erythropoiesis, decreased HbA, increased oxygen affinity of HbF, and chronic extravascular hemolysis produces a microcytic hypochromic anemia that is classified as β-thalassemia major in the more severe cases and as β-thalassemia intermedia in the remaining cases. As with β-thalassemia major, symptoms emerge within the first few years of life.

Patients with heterozygous Hb Lepore are asymptomatic and classified as β-thalassemia minor. The blood picture is similar to that seen in β-thalassemia minor.

Laboratory Results

In the homozygous state, hematologic findings are similar to β-thalassemia major. There is no detectable HbA or A_2 on hemoglobin electrophoresis, Hb Lepore ranges from 8–30%, and the remainder consists of HbF. Hemoglobin electrophoresis must be interpreted with caution because Hb Lepore comigrates with HbS on cellulose acetate agarose at an alkaline pH and with HbA on citrate agar at an acid pH.

In the heterozygous state, hematologic findings are similar to thalassemia minor (Figure 11-12 ■): Hemoglobin electrophoresis reveals a mean Hb Lepore concentration of 10%; HbA_2 is decreased with a mean of 2%; HbF is usually slightly elevated to 2–3%; and HbA makes up the remainder (Table 11-6).

The severely anemic cases of Hb Lepore require a regular transfusion protocol from early childhood. Splenectomy is also performed in an attempt to lessen the degree of anemia.

COMBINATION DISORDERS

Occasionally an individual is doubly heterozygous for a structural hemoglobin variant and thalassemia, inheriting one of the two abnormalities from each parent. The most common structural hemoglobin variants involved in combination disorders are HbS, HbC, and HbE. When a structural variant is inherited with a β-thalassemia gene, the severity of the combination disorder depends on the type of α- or β-gene mutation. Patients expressing the β^0-gene produce no HbA and experience moderate to severe symptoms. The β^+-gene produces some β-chains resulting in HbA synthesis and fewer to no symptoms. The most common example is HbS/β-thalassemia accounting for 1 in 1,667 births among African Americans.[41] This has also been reported in patients of Greek, Turkish, Indian, North American, Mediterranean, and Rumanian ancestry.[42] Three clinical severities have been identified: HbS/β^0-Type 1 (severe), HbS/β^+-Type 1 (moderate), and HbS/β^+-Type 2 (asymptomatic). Differentiating this combination disorder from sickle cell disease (HbSS) and trait (HbAS) is sometimes difficult, but a comparison of β/α ratio can be helpful (Web Table 11-1 ✪). In sickle cell disorders, the β/α ratio is approximately 1/1, whereas it is closer to 0.5/1 in HbS/β-thalassemia.[43]

Combination disorders are more complex when the structural hemoglobin gene mutation is on the β-gene and the thalassemia mutation involves the α-gene because different chromosomes are involved. These patients can be either homozygous or heterozygous for the structural hemoglobin variant and coexpress any of the possible α-gene combinations.

The severity of the combination disorder is directly proportional to the total number of affected genes and ranges from moderate to asymptomatic.[44-46] Coexistent α-thalassemia decreases synthesis of α-chains resulting in fewer α-globin chains available to combine with the structurally abnormal β-chain. Thus, the concentration of the structural variant is usually decreased because the limited number of α chains preferentially combine with the normal β or δ (or γ) chains. The percentage of HbA, HbF, and HbA_2 increases relative to a typical heterozygote, reducing the abnormal pathophysiology associated with the particular structural hemoglobin variant inherited.

In the case of a homozogous $\beta^S\beta^S$ individual with an α-thalassemia syndrome, the clinical severity of sickling is often reduced because of a net decrease in MCHC, which reduces the tendency of HbS to polymerize. Thus, cell hemolysis and the clinical symptoms associated with occlusion of the microvasculature decrease (∞ Chapter 10). HbF has also been shown to decrease the sickling process.[7] The wide variety of clinical severities seen in sickle cell anemia can be related to the high incidence of α-thalassemia in the same population (Figure 11-13 ■).

Laboratory diagnosis is accomplished by applying the techniques used to identify each of the disorders individually. Patients present with a mild microcytic, hypochromic anemia with target cells and the poikilocytes associated with the structural hemoglobin variant inherited. Patients who inherit HbS can have sickle cells, and those with HbC sometimes show HbC crystals. Hemoglobin electrophoresis is helpful in resolving the structural hemoglobin variant and shows the quantitative changes in normal and abnormal hemoglobins associated with α- and β-thalassemias. In HbS/α-thalassemia, the concentration of HbS is inversely

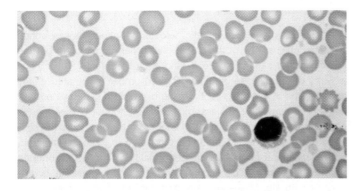

■ **FIGURE 11-12** Peripheral blood smear from a patient with hemoglobin Lepore. Note the anisocytosis, poikilocytosis, and microcytosis. (Wright-Giemsa stain; 1000× magnification)

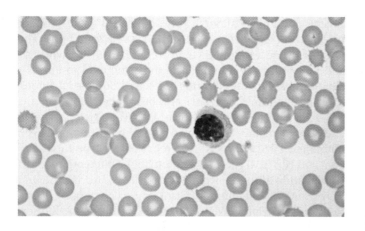

■ FIGURE 11-13   Peripheral blood smear from a patient with hemoglobin S and α-thalassemia. The cells are microcytic. There are acanthocytes and cells with pointed ends present. (Wright-Giemsa stain; 1000× magnification)

proportional to the number α-gene deletions. HbS concentration is ~35% with one α-gene deletion, ~28% with two α-deletions, and ~20% with three α-genes deletions.[47]

When less common structural variants (HbE, HbO, HbD, etc.) are coexpressed with thalassemias, more testing can be necessary because they comigrate with HbS or HbC on hemoglobin electrophoresis (Figure 11-2). Molecular techniques including automated sequencing, dot-blot analysis, or allele-specific amplification can be used in these cases.[48]

The incidence of double heterozygotes expressing both HbE and β-thalassemia is increasing in Southeast Asia, and many patients are presenting with symptoms that rival β-thalassemia major in severity.[49] Approximately 3,000 of these people with double heterozygotes are born each year in Thailand, and many others are diagnosed in other parts of Southeast Asia, India, and Burma. In Thailand, Laos, and Cambodia, HbE penetrance is approximately 50%. HbE heterozygotes usually have relatively mild disease; HbE/β-thal double heterozygotes might be expected to have a moderately severe disease.[50] However, the HbE mutation at the 26th position of the β-globin gene activates a cryptic splice site at codon 25, resulting in significantly reduced β-chain production. Therefore, in double heterozygotes of HbE and β^0-thal, few to no β^E or β^A-chains are produced. This results in the accumulation of α-chains that precipitate within the erythrocytes, producing hemolysis as in β-thalassemia major.[50,51]

Double heterozygotes for sickle cell and HPFH (deletion variant) exhibit a mild form of sickle cell trait with no occurrence of crises or anemia. It has been suggested that the surprisingly favorable clinical picture is related to the distribution of HbF in erythrocytes. The peripheral blood smear shows anisocytosis and target cells, and the sodium metabisulfite and solubility tests are positive. Hemoglobin electrophoresis produces a pattern that is easily confused with that of sickle cell anemia. Only HbS, HbF, and HbA_2 are present with HbF levels ranging from 15 to 35%. Hemoglo-

bin A_2 is normal or reduced. Family studies are helpful in identifying double heterozygous states.

Due to the significant variations in clinical expression of the various hemoglobin structural variants and β-thalassemia alleles, it is suggested that identification of these conditions should go beyond hematologic analysis and hemoglobin electrophoresis.[48] A diagnosis defined at the molecular level to identify the genetic mutation can lead to better clinical management of the disease. A summary of the differentiating characteristics of combination thalassemia and hemoglobinopathy disorders can be found in Web Table 11-1.

✓ Checkpoint! 9

In combination disorders of structural Hb variants and thalassemia, why is the severity less when α-thalassemia is inherited with sickle cell trait than when β-thalassemia is coexpressed with sickle cell trait?

▶ DIFFERENTIAL DIAGNOSIS OF THALASSEMIA

Clinical signs, symptoms, and CBC results are strikingly similar in microcytic hypochromic anemias regardless of the etiology of the anemia, making the clinical diagnosis difficult. Differentiating the various thalassemias is even more difficult because they are all inherited and occur in similar nationalities. Additional laboratory tests are therefore crucial in making the differential diagnosis.[52,53] Web Table 11-2 summarizes the tests used to differentiate thalassemia from other anemias.

✓ Checkpoint! 10

Which laboratory tests should be done first to differentiate thalassemia and iron deficiency?

SUMMARY

Thalassemias result from genetic defects that affect the production of globin chains. Any of the globin chains can be affected, but the most clinically significant are α- and β-chain defects. The clinical severity of the disease is related to the number of mutated genes and the type of genetic defect. The human diploid genome normally has four α-genes. In α-thalassemia, from one to four of the α-genes can be deleted. If only one gene is affected, the condition is not clinically or hematologically apparent, but if two or three are affected, both clinical and hematological abnormalities of mild or moderate severity, respectively, occur. Deletion of all four α-genes is incompatable with life. There are two β-alleles and two β-thalassemia gene defects; one causes a complete absence of β-chain production (β^0-thalassemia), and the other causes decreased synthesis of β-chain production (β^+-thalassemia). This results in five potential

β-thalassemia genotypes ($\beta^0\beta^0$, $\beta^0\beta^+$, $\beta^+\beta^+$, $\beta^0\beta$, $\beta^+\beta$) that are categorized into four clinical severities (β-thalassemia major, intermedia, minor, and silent carrier) ranging from severe to asymptomatic.

The thalassemias generally produce a microcytic, hypochromic anemia with changes in the concentrations of HbF, HbA$_2$, and HbA. HbF and HbA$_2$ are elevated in β-thalassemia and decreased in α-thalassemia with decreased concentrations of HbA in both. In the more severe α-thalassemias, HbH (β^4) and Hb Bart's (γ^4) can be detected. Erythrocyte morphology is similar in both major forms of thalassemia and in iron deficiency anemia; however, hemoglobin electrophoresis and iron studies assist in differentiating these two entities. Some structural hemoglobin variants are synthesized in decreased quantities (i.e., Hb Lepore, Hb Constant Spring, HbE) and have morphologic similarities to thalassemias. Molecular techniques are now available to identify the genetic mutation in the globin gene but are not always necessary for diagnostic purposes.

Current therapies are improving, and medical access in underdeveloped countries is expanding. As a result of these advances, the general health and quality of life are improving for patients with thalassemia.

REVIEW QUESTIONS

LEVEL I

1. Select the statement that best defines thalassemia. (Objective 1)
   a. a qualitative disorder of hemoglobin synthesis derived primarily from a genetic point mutation in one or more globin genes
   b. a disorder of inappropriate iron metabolism due to abnormal transferrin
   c. a quantitative disorder of hemoglobin synthesis resulting from deletional and nondeletional mutations of globin genes
   d. a single amino acid substitution in a globin chain affecting the function of hemoglobin

2. Which of the following statements is *false* for a patient with thalassemia but *true* in certain hemoglobinopathies? (Objective 2)
   a. Abnormal hemoglobin will polymerize inside erythrocytes, altering red cell shape.
   b. Novel hemoglobins composed of abnormal combinations of normal globin chains can be detected on hemoglobin electrophoresis.
   c. Elevations in embryonic and fetal hemoglobins can be observed.
   d. The amino acid sequence of the globin chains of the abnormal hemoglobins is normal.

3. What is the typical morphologic classification of erythrocytes in thalassemia? (Objective 3)
   a. macrocytic, normochromic
   b. normocytic, normochromic
   c. microcytic, hyperchromic
   d. microcytic, hypochromic

4. Select the disorder that is an α-thalassemia. (Objectives 5a, 5b)
   a. HbH disease
   b. Cooley's anemia
   c. HPFH
   d. Hb Lepore

LEVEL II

1. Alpha-thalassemia most commonly results from which of the following genetic lesions? (Objective 1)
   a. gene deletion
   b. promoter mutation
   c. termination codon mutation
   d. splice site mutation

2. Why is hydrops fetalis incompatible with life? (Objective 4b)
   a. Life cannot exist without HbA.
   b. Lack of embryonic hemoglobins precludes fetal development.
   c. All three normal adult hemoglobins contain α-chains.
   d. Fetal hemoglobin is essential to sustain life after birth.

3. Which pathophysiologic event is involved in the pathogenesis of HbH disease? (Objective 4b)
   a. HbH has a higher affinity for oxygen that hampers oxygen release.
   b. HbH is an embryonic hemoglobin that is not present at birth.
   c. HbH cannot bind and transport oxygen.
   d. Polymerization of abnormal hemoglobin alters erythrocyte shape.

4. The genetic designation heterozygous α^0-thal-1/normal refers to: (Objective 4a)
   a. α-thalassemia minor
   b. Cooley's anemia
   c. HbH disease
   d. silent carrier

5. The single best laboratory test to distinguish β-thalassemia minor from α-thalassemia, iron-deficiency anemia, HPFH, and hemoglobinopathies is: (Objective 8)
   a. hemoglobin solubility
   b. serum iron
   c. Heinz body stain
   d. HbA$_2$ level

REVIEW QUESTIONS *(continued)*

LEVEL I

5. Alpha-thalassemia is characterized by: (Objective 5c)
   a. deletion of β-genes
   b. amino acid substitutions in the α-chain
   c. excess α-chain production
   d. deletion of α-genes

6. Which nationality is *most* likely to be affected by thalassemia? (Objectives 5b, 6a)
   a. Chinese
   b. South American Indians
   c. Southeast Asians
   d. Europeans

7. Which of the following laboratory results would be expected in a patient with α-thalassemia? (Objective 5e)
   a. MCH=32 pg
   b. MCV=70 fL
   c. stomatocytes
   d. increased HbA

8. The pathogenesis of β-thalassemia includes: (Objective 6b)
   a. decreased production of β-chains
   b. abnormal structure of α-chains
   c. bone marrow hypoproliferation
   d. decreased synthesis of erythropoietin

9. In β-thalassemia major, hemoglobin electrophoresis will show: (Objective 6d)
   a. reduced HbF
   b. reduced HbA_2
   c. reduced HbA
   d. increased HbH

10. Select the thalassemia type in which the patient survives and presents with an abnormal hemoglobin that is sensitive to oxidation and precipitates in red cells after incubation with brilliant cresyl blue. (Objective 6d)
    a. hydrops fetalis
    b. HbH disease
    c. β-thalassemia minor
    d. silent carrier

LEVEL II

6. Hemoglobin constant spring can best be described as: (Objective 7c)
   a. deletion of three α-genes
   b. two normal β-chains and two elongated α-chains
   c. two normal α-chains and two β/γ-fusion chains
   d. continued synthesis of γ-chains throughout adult life

7. Select the statement that best describes hereditary persistence of fetal hemoglobin. (Objective 7d)
   a. The homozygous state is incompatible with life.
   b. HbF is elevated in adults.
   c. It results from the deletion of the γ-gene.
   d. It is a form of β-thalassemia.

8. A 4-year-old male patient has a microcytic, hypochromic anemia. Hemoglobin electrophoresis shows 46% HbS, 49%HbA, 3.5% HbA_2, 1.5% HbF. His parents have no symptoms of anemia. What are his parents' most likely phenotypes? (Objectives 5, 7)
   a. sickle cell trait and β-thalassemia major
   b. sickle cell anemia and α-thalassemia
   c. sickle cell anemia and heterozygous β-thalassemia
   d. sickle cell trait and normal

9. Which combination disorder would exhibit more severe symptoms? (Objective 7f)
   a. HbS and β-thalassemia minor
   b. HbC trait and α-thalassemia minor
   c. HPFH and β-thalassemia minor
   d. HbS and HPFH

10. A 28-year-old female from Laos who had a hemoglobin of 11.2 g/dL was diagnosed with iron deficiency anemia. She was given iron supplements. Her reticulocyte count increased from 4% to 5% after 6 days of treatment. Six months later, she returned for a follow-up CBC. Her hemoglobin was 11.5 g/dL, and the red cells were microcytic (75 fL), normochromic. What reflex test should be done? (Objective 8)
    a. hemoglobin electrophoresis
    b. serum iron
    c. bone marrow
    d. serum ferritin

www.pearsonhighered.com/mckenzie
Use this address to access the interactive Companion Website created for this textbook. Find additional information, tables and figures. Evaluate your command of the chapter information using case studies and critical thinking and multiple choice questions.

REFERENCES

1. http://globin.bx.psu.edu/cgi-bin/hbvar/counter (Accessed 3/9/09).

2. Cooley TB, Lee P. A series of cases of splenomegaly in children with anemia and peculiar bone changes. *Trans Am Pediatr Soc.* 1925;37:29.

3. Sarnaik, SA. Thalassemia and related hemoglobinopathies. *Indian J Pediatr.* 2005;72:319–24.

4. Poole JH. Thalassemia and pregnancy. *J Perinat Neonatal Nurs.* 2003; 17(3):196–208.

5. Williams JL. Anemias of abnormal globin development. In: Steine-Martin EA, Lotspeich-Steininger CA, Koepke JA, eds. *Clinical Hematology: Principles, Procedures, Correlations,* 2nd ed. Philadelphia: Lippincott-Raven; 1998:217–40.

6. LeCrone CN, Detter JC. Screening for hemoglobinopathies and thalassemia. *J Med Technol.* 1985;2:389–95.

7. Harrison CR. Hemolytic anemias: Intracorpuscular defects. In: Harmening DM, ed. *Clinical Hematology and Fundamentals of Hemostasis,* 3rd ed. Philadelphia: F.A. Davis; 1997:193–210.

8. Na-Nakorn S, Wasi P. Alpha-thalassemia in Northern Thailand. *Am J Hum Genet.* 1970;22:645–51.

9. Lehmann H, Carrell RW. Nomenclature of the alpha-thalassaemias. *Lancet.* 1984;1(8376):552–53.

10. Dozy AM, Kan YW, Embury SH, Mentzer WC, Wang WC, Lubin B et al. Alpha-globin gene organisation in blacks precludes the severe form of alpha-thalassemia. *Nature.* 1979;280:605–7.

11. Graham EA. The changing face of anemia in infancy. *Ped Rev.* 1994; 15:175–83.

12. Huisman THJ, Carver MFH, Baysal E. *A syllabus of thalassemia mutations.* Augusta, GA: The Sickle Cell Anemia Foundation; 1997.

13. Schwartz E, Benz EJ Jr, Forget BG. Thalassemia syndromes. In: Hoffman R, Benz EJ Jr, Shattil SJ, Furie B, Cohen HJ, Silberstein LE, eds. *Hematology: Basic Principles and Practice,* 2nd ed. Philadelphia: Churchill Livingstone; 1995:586–610.

14. Kattamis C, Hu H, Cheng G, Reese AL, Gonzalez-Redondo JM, Kutlar A et al. Molecular characterization of beta-thalassaemia in 174 Greek patients with thalassaemia major. *Br J Haematol.* 1990;74: 342–46.

15. Scott MD, Rouyer-Fessard P, Ba MS, Lubin BH, Beuzard Y. Alpha- and beta-haemoglobin chain induced changes in normal erythrocyte deformability: Comparison to beta thalassaemia intermedia and HbH disease. *Br J Haematol.* 1992;80:519–26.

16. Shinar E, Rachmilewitz EA, Lux SE. Differing erythrocyte membrane skeletal protein defects in alpha and beta thalassemia. *J Clin Invest.* 1989;83:404–10.

17. Advani R, Sorenson S, Shinar E et al. Characterization and comparison of the RBC membrane damage in severe human alpha and beta thalassemia. *Blood.* 1992;79:1058–63.

18. Yuan J, Kannan R, Shinar E et al. Isolation, characterization, and immunoprecipitation studies of immune complexes from membranes of [beta]-thalassemia erythrocytes. *Blood.* 1992;79:3007–13.

19. Mathias LA, Fisher TC, Zeng L et al. Ineffective erythropoiesis in beta-thalassemia major is due to apoptosis at the polychromatophilic normoblast stage. *Exp Hematol.* 2000;28:1343–53.

20. Schrier SL. Thalassemia: Pathophysiology of red cell changes. *Ann Rev Med.* 1994;45:211–18.

21. Schrier SL. Pathophysiology of thalassemia. *Curr Opin Hematol.* 2002;9(2):123–26.

22. Rund D, Filon D, Strauss N, Rachmilewitz EA, Oppenheim A. Mean corpuscular volume of heterozygotes for beta-thalassemia correlates with the severity of mutations. *Blood.* 1992;79:238–43.

23. Bagar MS, Khurshid M, Molla A. Does red blood cell distribution width (RDW) improve evaluation of microcytic anaemias? *JPMA J Pak Med Assoc.* 1993;43:149–51.

24. Steinberg MH, Coleman MB, Adams JG III. Beta-thalassemia with exceptionally high hemoglobin A2: Differential expression of the delta-globin gene in the presence of beta-thalassemia. *J Lab Clin Med.* 1982;100:548–57.

25. Fearon ER, Kazazian HH Jr, Waber PG, Lee JI, Antonarakis SE, Orkin SH et al. The entire beta-globin gene cluster is deleted in a form of gamma delta beta-thalassemia. *Blood.* 1983;61:1269–74.

26. Forget BG, Cohen AR. Thalassemia syndromes. In: R Hoffman, EJ Benz, SJ Shattil, B Furie, HJ Cohen, LE Silberstein, P McGlave, eds. *Hematology: Basic Principles and Procedures,* 4th ed. Philadelphia: Churchill Livingstone; 2005:557–89.

27. Lucarelli G, Weatherall DJ. For debate: Bone marrow transplantation for severe thalassaemia. *Br J Haematol.* 1991;78:300–3.

28. Ley TJ, DeSimone J, Anagnou NP, Keller GH, Humphries RK, Turner PH et al. 5-azacytidine selectively increases gamma-globin synthesis in a patient with beta-thalassemia. *N Engl J Med.* 1982;307: 1469–75.

29. Veith R, Galanello R, Papayannopoulou T, Stamatoyannopoulos G. Stimulation of F-cell production in patients with sickle-cell anemia treated with cytarabine or hydroxyurea. *N Engl J Med.* 1985;313: 1571–75.

30. Thomas ED. Marrow transplantation for nonmalignant disorders. *N Engl J Med.* 1985;312:46–48.

31. Weatherall DJ. The thalassemias. In: Stamatoyannopoulos G, Nienhaus AW, Leder P, Majerus PW, eds. *The Molecular Basis of Blood Diseases,* 2nd ed. Philadelphia: WB Saunders; 1994:157–206.

32. Malamos B, Fessas P, Stamatoyannopoulos G. Types of thalassemia-trait carriers as revealed by a study of their incidence in Greece. *Br J Haematol.* 1962;8:5–14.

33. Mazza U, Saglio G, Cappio FC, Camaschella C, Neretto G, Gallo E. Clinical and haematological data in 254 cases of beta-thalassaemia trait in Italy. *Br J Haematol.* 1976;33:91–99.

34. Pootrakul P, Wasi P, Na-Nakorn S. Haematological data in 312 cases of β-thalassaemia trait in Thailand. *Br J Haematol.* 1973;24:703–12.

35. Fairbanks VF. *Hemoglobinopathies and Thalassemias: Laboratory Methods and Case Studies.* New York: BC Decker;1980.

36. Metaxotou-Mavromati AD, Antonopoulou HK, Laskari SS, Tsiarta HK, Ladis VA, Kattamis CA et al. Developmental changes in hemoglobin F levels during the first two years of life in normal and heterozygous beta-thalassemia infants. *Pediatr.* 1982;69:734–38.

37. Weatherall DJ. The thalassemias. In: *Methods in Hematology, vol 6.* Philadelphia: Churchill Livingstone; 1983.

38. Clegg JB, Weatherall DJ, Milner PF. Haemoglobin Constant Spring: A chain termination mutant? *Nature.* 1971;234:337–40.

39. Weatherall DJ, Clegg JB. α thalassaemia in association with structural haemoglobin variants and disorders of δ and β chain production. *The Thalassaemia Syndromes,* 3rd ed. Oxford: Blackwell Scientific Publications; 1981:613–44.

40. Gerald PS, Diamond LK. The diagnosis of thalassemia trait by starch block electrophoresis of the hemoglobin. *Blood.* 1958;13:61–69.

41. Motulsky AG. Frequency of sickling disorders in U.S. blacks. *N Engl J Med.* 1973;288:31–33.

42. Wood WG, Weatherall DJ, Hart GH, Bennett M, Marsh GW. Hematologic changes and hemoglobin analysis in beta thalassemia heterozygotes during the first year of life. *Pediatr Res.* 1982;16:286–89.

43. Bunn HF, Forget BG. Sickle cell disease: Clinical and epidemiological aspects. *Hemoglobin: Molecular, Genetic, and Clinical Aspects.* Philadelphia: WB Saunders; 1986:502–64.

44. Embury SH, Clark MR, Monroy G, Mohandas N. Concurrent sickle cell anemia and alpha-thalassemia: Effect on pathological properties of sickle erythrocytes. *J Clin Invest.* 1984;73:116–23.

45. de Ceulaer K, Higgs DR, Weatherall DJ, Hayes RJ, Serjeant BE, Serjeant GR. Alpha-thalassemia reduces the hemolytic rate in homozygous sickle-cell disease. *N Engl J Med.* 1983;309:189–90.

46. Higgs DR, Aldridge BE, Lamb J, Clegg JB, Weatherall DJ, Hayes RJ et al. The interaction of alpha-thalassemia and homozygous sickle-cell disease. *N Engl J Med.* 1982;306(24):1441–46.

47. Embury SH, Dozy AM, Miller J, Davis JR Jr, Kleman KM, Preisler H et al. Concurrent sickle-cell anemia and alpha-thalassemia: Effect on severity of anemia. *N Engl J Med.* 1982;306:270–74.

48. Huisman, TH. Combinations of beta-chain abnormal hemoglobins with each other or with beta-thalassemia determinants with known mutations: Influence on phenotype. *Clin Chem.* 1997;43:1850–56.

49. Weatherall DJ. Introduction to the problem of hemoglobin E-beta thalassemia. *J Pediatr Hematol Oncol* 2000;22:551.

50. Winichogoon P, Fucharoen S, Chen P et al. Genetic factors affecting clinical severity of beta-thalassemia syndromes. *J Pediatr Hematol Oncol.* 2000;22:573–80.

51. Fucharoen S, Ketvichit P, Pootrakul P et al. Clinical manifestations of beta-thalassemia/hemoglobin E disease. *J Pediatr Hematol Oncol.* 2000;552–57.

52. Johnson CS, Tegos C, Beutler E. Thalassemia minor: Routine erythrocyte measurements and differentiation from iron deficiency. *Am J Clin Path.* 1983;80:31–36.

53. Steinberg MH, Dreiling BJ. Microcytosis: Its significance and evaluation. *JAMA.* 1983;249:85–87.

12

Megaloblastic and Nonmegaloblastic Macrocytic Anemias

Joel Hubbard, Ph.D.

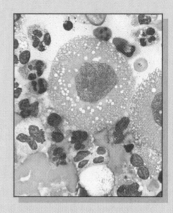

■ OBJECTIVES—LEVEL I

At the end of this unit of study, the student should be able to:

1. Explain the cause and process of megaloblastic maturation in the bone marrow.
2. Describe the body's requirements for vitamin B_{12} and folate and their physiologic role.
3. List the laboratory tests used to confirm a diagnosis of vitamin B_{12} deficiency and give expected results.
4. List the laboratory tests used to confirm a diagnosis of folic acid deficiency and give expected results.
5. Recognize the six most common disorders that result in a macrocytic anemia.
6. Name four causes of a vitamin B_{12} deficiency and give two distinguishing clinical or laboratory characteristics of each.
7. Describe the etiology and pathophysiology of pernicious anemia, clinical symptoms, and clinical subtypes.
8. Name three causes of a folate deficiency and give two distinguishing clinical or laboratory characteristics of each.
9. Differentiate the pathophysiology and peripheral blood findings of nonmegaloblastic anemia from those of megaloblastic anemias.
10. Summarize the common or typical blood picture seen with a folate or vitamin B_{12} deficiency.

■ OBJECTIVES—LEVEL II

At the end of this unit of study, the student should be able to:

1. Summarize the process of vitamin B_{12} and folic acid metabolism and explain how a deficiency can result in megaloblastosis.
2. Compare macrocytosis associated with a normoblastic marrow and macrocytosis associated with a megaloblastic marrow on the basis of physiological defect or cause, and differentiate based on the laboratory blood picture.
3. Summarize the mechanism of maturation defects that lead to megaloblastosis and recognize the morphologic blood cell abnormalities.

■ OBJECTIVES—LEVEL II *(continued)*

4. Compare and contrast the various clinical forms and causes of a vitamin B_{12} and folate deficiency on the basis of clinical symptoms and laboratory results.

5. Categorize the causes and clinical variations of pernicious anemia.

6. Compare and contrast the various clinical forms and causes of a folic acid deficiency.

7. Demonstrate how a folate or vitamin B_{12} deficiency results in megaloblastic maturation.

8. Choose and briefly explain four laboratory tests used to identify the cause of a macrocytic anemia; give the expected results of these four tests in a patient with an autoantibody directed against intrinsic factor.

9. Assess Schilling's test results and provide a differential diagnosis.

10. Compare and contrast the causes of macrocytosis with a normoblastic marrow.

11. Construct an algorithm of laboratory testing to distinguish between a megaloblastic anemia and a macrocytic, normoblastic anemia.

12. Evaluate a case study from a patient with anemia. Determine the most probable diagnosis from the medical history and laboratory results.

KEY TERMS

Achlorhydria
Cobalamin
Demyelination
Dyspepsia
Glossitis
Intrinsic factor (IF)
Megaloblastic
Nuclear-cytoplasmic asynchrony
Pernicious anemia (PA)
Schilling test

BACKGROUND BASICS

The information in this chapter builds on the concepts learned in previous chapters. To maximize your learning experience, you should review these concepts before starting this unit of study.

Level I

▶ Describe the maturation process of erythrocytes in the marrow. (Chapter 5)

▶ Outline the functional and morphologic classification of anemia and list the basic laboratory tests to diagnose anemia. (Chapter 8)

Level II

▶ Summarize the concepts of cell development, regulation, and the process of cell division. (Chapter 2)

▶ List and describe the laboratory tests used in differential diagnosis of anemia. (Chapter 8)

CASE STUDY

We will refer to this case study throughout the chapter.
Kathy, a 36-year-old female, experienced a recent 35-pound weight loss. Her tongue was red and fissured. She also complained of chronic fatigue and shortness of breath upon exertion. Physical examination suggested signs of jaundice and increased numbness and a tingling sensation of fingers and toes. She was hospitalized with the general diagnosis of moderate anemia, jaundice, and neurological symptoms. Her admitting CBC demonstrated the following laboratory results:

WBC	4.5×10^9/L	Differential	
RBC	2.50×10^{12}/L	Lymphs %	36.0
HGB	10.0 g/dL	Monos %	3.8
HCT	0.31 L/L	Neutrophils %	59.4
MCV	124.0 fL	Eosinophils %	1.0
MCH	40.5 pg/dL	Basophils %	0.0
MCHC	32.7 gm/dL	NRBCs/100WBCs	5
RDW	21.2	Moderate hyper-	
PLT	155×10^9/L	segmented	
		neutrophils	

The following abnormal erythrocyte morphology was reported:

Macrocytes:	2+
Anisocytosis:	3+
Poikilocytosis:	2+
Ovalocytes:	1+
Basophilic stippling:	1+
Occasional Howell-Jolly bodies	

Consider the reflex tests that might be important in identifying the etiology of this anemia.

▶ OVERVIEW

This chapter is a study of the macrocytic anemias, which can be megaloblastic or nonmegaloblastic. The first part of the chapter discusses the megaloblastic anemias beginning with a description of the clinical and laboratory findings. Because megaloblastic anemia is most often due to deficiencies or abnormal metabolism of folate or vitamin B_{12}, the metabolism of these vitamins is discussed in detail. The latter part of the chapter reviews the causes of nonmegaloblastic macrocytic anemia and compares the laboratory test results in nonmegaloblastic and megaloblastic anemia. The experienced laboratory professional can often identify diagnostic clues on review of a blood smear.

▶ INTRODUCTION

Macrocytic anemias are characterized by large erythrocytes (mean MCV >l00 fL) with an increased MCH and a normal hemoglobin content (MCHC). This is an important group of anemias because macrocytosis is frequently a sign of a disease process that can result in significant morbidity if left untreated.

Macrocytosis is found in 2.5–4% of adults who have a routine complete blood count.[1] In up to 60% of cases, macrocytosis is not accompanied by anemia,[2] but isolated macrocytosis should always be investigated. Macrocytosis without anemia can indicate early folate or **cobalamin** (vitamin B_{12}) deficiency because macrocytosis precedes the development of anemia.

Macrocytosis detected by automated cell counters is not always apparent microscopically on stained blood smears. In some cases, the erythrocyte size on automated counters is falsely elevated due to hyperglycemia, cold agglutinins, and extreme leukocytosis. These causes of false macrocytosis need to be differentiated from true macrocytosis.

The most common cause of true macrocytosis is alcoholism. Other causes include folate and cobalamin deficiencies, drugs including chemotherapy, reticulocytosis due to hemolysis or bleeding, myelodysplasia, liver disease, and hypothyroidism.[2]

Macrocytic anemias are generally classified as **megaloblastic** or nonmegaloblastic (normoblastic) depending on morphologic characteristics of erythroid precursors in the bone marrow (Table 12-1 ✪). The megaloblastic anemias are the result of abnormal DNA synthesis (a nuclear maturation defect), most often due to vitamin B_{12} or folate deficiencies. As a result, delayed nuclear development prevents cell division. RNA synthesis and cytoplasmic maturation are not affected. The result is production of large cells with **nuclear-cytoplasmic asynchrony**. The basis for the nonmegaloblastic anemias is not always as well defined but can be related to an increase in membrane lipids. The macrocytes in nonmegaloblastic macrocytic anemia often are

✪ TABLE 12-1

Conditions Associated with Megaloblastic and Nonmegaloblastic Macrocytic (Normoblastic) Anemias

Megaloblastic	Normoblastic
Folate deficiency	Alcoholism
Nutritional deficiency	Liver disease
Increased requirement (i.e., pregnancy)	Shift reticulocytosis in hemo-
Intestinal malabsorption	lytic anemia or hemorrhage
Drug inhibition	Hypothroidism
B_{12} deficiency	Aplastic anemia
Pernicious anemia	Obstructive jaundice
Small bowel resection	Splenectomy
Gastrectomy	Pregnancy
Intestinal malabsorption	Artifactual: hyperglycemia,
Nutritional deficiency	cold agglutinins, leukocytosis
Increased requirement (i.e., pregnancy)	
Transcobalamin II deficiency	
Nitrous oxide abuse	
Other causes	
Chemotherapy with metabolic inhibitors	
Orotic aciduria	
CDA	

round but in megaloblastic anemia are oval. A flow chart for laboratory analysis to help distinguish causes of macrocytic anemia is shown in Figure 12-1 .

✓ Checkpoint! 1

Explain why patients with B_{12} or folate deficiency have megaloblastic maturation.

▶ MEGALOBLASTIC ANEMIA

Although very little was known about the function or origin of blood cells before the twentieth century, some perceptive individuals began to make associations between anemia and other clinical patient signs. In 1822, J. S. Coombe, a Scottish physician, made the initial clinical description of a patient who appeared to have megaloblastic anemia. He was the first to suggest that this anemia might be related to **dyspepsia**.[3] In 1855, Thomas Addison reported his description of a macrocytic anemia, but he made no reference to the typical microscopic blood findings.[4] The discovery and description of the abnormal erythroid precursors in the bone marrow associated with this anemia were made possible by the advent of triacid stains. Paul Ehrlich is credited with coining the term *megaloblast* in 1891 to describe the large abnormal precursors in megaloblastic anemia.[5]

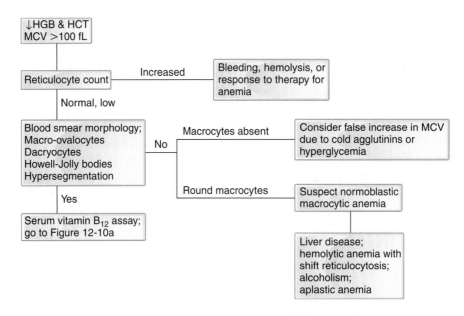

Megaloblastic anemia is classified as a nuclear maturation defect. Anemia is attributed primarily to a large degree of ineffective erythropoiesis resulting from disrupted DNA synthesis. The anemia was called *megaloblastic* in an attempt to describe the giant, abnormal-appearing erythroid precursors (megaloblasts) in the bone marrow. The generic word *megaloblast* describes any maturation stage of the megaloblastic erythroid series (i.e., polychromatic megaloblast). Other nucleated cells of the marrow are also typically abnormal.

About 95% of megaloblastic anemias are caused by deficiencies of either vitamin B_{12} or folic acid, vitamins necessary as coenzymes for nucleic acid synthesis. In the majority of cases, vitamin B_{12} deficiency is secondary to a deficiency of the **intrinsic factor (IF)**, a factor necessary for absorption of vitamin B_{12} rather than to a nutritional deficiency of the vitamin. Folic acid deficiency, on the other hand, is most often due to an inadequate dietary intake. Inherited disorders affecting DNA synthesis or vitamin metabolism are rare causes of megaloblastosis.

CLINICAL FINDINGS

The onset of megaloblastic anemia is usually insidious; because the anemia develops slowly, it produces few symptoms until the hemoglobin and hematocrit are significantly depressed. Patients can present with typical anemic symptoms of lethargy, weakness, and a yellow or waxy pallor. Dyspeptic symptoms are common. **Glossitis** with a beefy red tongue or, more commonly, a smooth pale tongue is characteristic. Loss of weight and loss of appetite are common complaints.

In pernicious anemia (see below), atrophy of the gastric parietal cells causes decreased secretion of intrinsic factor and hydrochloric acid. Bouts of diarrhea can result from epithelial changes in the gastrointestinal tract.

Neurological disturbances occur only in vitamin B_{12} deficiency, not in folic acid deficiency. They are the most serious and dangerous clinical signs because neurological damage can be permanent if the deficiency is not treated promptly. The patient's initial complaints occasionally are related to neurological dysfunction rather than to anemia. Neurological damage has been reported to occur even before anemia or macrocytosis in some cases. The bone marrow, however, usually reveals megaloblastic changes even in the absence of anemia. Tingling, numbness, and weakness of the extremities reflect peripheral neuropathy. Loss of vibratory and position (proprioceptive) sensibilities in the lower extremities can cause the patient to have an abnormal gait. Mental disturbances such as loss of memory, depression, and irritability are sometimes noted by the patient's relatives. *Megaloblastic madness* is a term used to describe severe psychotic manifestations of vitamin B_{12} deficiency. A patient with severe anemia occasionally is asymptomatic, which is probably a reflection of a very slowly developing anemia.

> ## ✓ Checkpoint! 2
>
> *Patients with megaloblastic anemia often present with a yellow or waxy pallor. What is the diagnostic significance of this clinical symptom?*

LABORATORY FINDINGS

Laboratory tests are critical to a diagnosis of megaloblastic anemia. The routine CBC with a review of the blood smear gives important diagnostic clues and helps in selecting reflex tests.

Peripheral Blood

Megaloblastic anemia is typically a macrocytic, normochromic anemia. The MCV is usually higher than 100 fL and can reach a volume of 140 fL. However, an increased MCV is not specific for megaloblastic anemia. The MCH is increased because of the large cell volume, but the MCHC is normal. In vitamin B_{12} deficiency, a macrocytosis can precede the development of anemia by months to years.[6-8] On the other hand, the MCV can remain in the reference range. Epithelial changes in the gastrointestinal tract can cause iron absorption to be impaired. If an iron deficiency—which characteristically produces a microcytic, hypochromic anemia—coexists with megaloblastic anemia, macrocytosis can be masked and the MCV can be in the normal range.[9] Other conditions that have been shown to coexist with megaloblastic anemia in the absence of an increased MCV include thalassemia, chronic renal insufficiency, and chronic inflammation or infection.[8] Sometimes these coexisting causes of anemia are not recognized until after the megaloblastic anemia has been treated. It has been suggested that if coexisting iron deficiency, thalassemia, or chronic disease is suspected, patient medical history, racial background, and previous MCV should be considered.[10]

Hematologic parameters vary considerably (Table 12-2 ✪). The hemoglobin and erythrocyte count range from normal to very low. The erythrocyte count is occasionally less than 1×10^{12}/L. However, anemia is not always evident. In one study of 100 patients with confirmed B_{12} deficiency, only 29% had a hemoglobin of less than 12 g/dL.[11] This is significant because neurologic symptoms can be present even if the MCV and/or hematocrit are normal.[12] Because the abnormality is a nuclear maturation defect, the megaloblastic anemias affect all three blood cell lineages: erythrocytes, leukocytes, and platelets. This is unlike other anemias that typically involve only erythrocytes. The leukocyte count can be decreased due to an absolute neutropenia. Platelets can also be decreased but do not usually fall below 100×10^9/L. The relative reticulocyte count (percentage) is usually normal; however, because of the severe anemia, the corrected reticulocyte count is <2% and RPI is less than 2 (∞ Chapter 8).

The distinguishing features of megaloblastic anemia on the stained blood smear include the triad of oval macrocytes (macroovalocytes), Howell-Jolly bodies, and hypersegmented neutrophils (Figure 12-2 ■). Anisocytosis is moderate to severe with normocytes and a few microcytes in addition to the macrocytes. Poikilocytosis can be striking and is usually more severe when the anemia is severe. Polychromatophilia

✪ TABLE 12-2

Comparison of Common Laboratory Values in Megaloblastic and Nonmegaloblastic Macrocytosis

Laboratory Value	Megaloblastic Macrocytosis	Nonmegaloblastic Macrocytosis
WBC count	Decreased	Normal
Platelet count	Decreased	Normal
RBC count	Decreased	Decreased
Hemoglobin	Decreased	Decreased
Hematocrit	Decreased	Decreased
MCV	Usually >110 fL	>100 fL
RBC morphology	Ovalocytes, Howell-Jolly bodies, polychromasia	Polychromasia, target cells, and stomatocytes (liver disease), schistocytes (hemolytic anemias)
Hypersegmentation of neutrophils	Present	Absent
Reticulocyte count	Normal to decreased	Normal, decreased, or increased
Serum B_{12}	Decreased in B_{12} deficiency	Usually normal
Serum folate	Decreased in folate deficiency	Normal (except in alcoholism where it may be decreased)
FIGLU	Increased in folate deficiency	Normal
MMA	Increased in B_{12} deficiency	Normal
Homocysteine	Increased	Normal
Serum bilirubin	Increased	Normal to increased
LD	Increased	Normal to increased

MCV = mean corpuscular volume; FIGLU = formiminoglutamic acid; MMA = methylmalonic acid; LD = lactic dehydrogenase

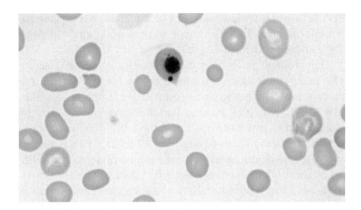

■ FIGURE 12-2   Peripheral blood film from a patient with pernicious anemia. Note the anisocytosis with oval macrocytes and the nucleated red blood cell with a Howell-Jolly body. (Wright-Giemsa stain; 1000× magnification)

and megaloblastic erythroblasts can be seen, especially when the anemia is severe, indicating the futile attempt of the bone marrow to increase peripheral erythrocyte mass. Erythrocytes can contain Cabot rings.

Granulocytes and platelets can also show changes evident of abnormal hematopoiesis. Hypersegmented neutrophils (>5 nuclear lobes) can be found in megaloblastic anemia even in the absence of macrocytosis (Figure 12-3). Finding 5% or more PMNs with 5 lobes or one PMN with six or more lobes is considered hypersegmentation of neutrophils. This finding of hypersegmented neutrophils is considered highly sensitive and specific for megaloblastic anemia. Therefore, hypersegmented neutrophils can be an important clue to megaloblastic anemia in the face of a coexisting disease that tends to keep erythrocyte volume below 100 fL. One study showed that in patients with renal disease, iron deficiency, or chronic disease with a normal or decreased MCV and 1% hypersegmented neutrophils, 94% had vitamin B_{12} or folic acid deficiency.[8] If 5% hypersegmented neutrophils

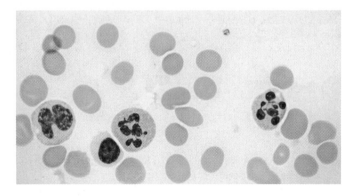

■ FIGURE 12-3   Hypersegmented neutrophils from the peripheral blood of a patient with pernicious anemia. (Wright-Giemsa stain; 1000× magnification)

were counted, the incidence of the vitamin B_{12} or folic acid deficiency increased to 98%. Hypersegmented neutrophils tend to be larger than normal neutrophils. A mild shift to the left with large hypogranular bands can also be noted. Platelets can be large, especially when the platelet count is decreased.

✓ **Checkpoint! 3**

Why are abnormalities of leukocytes and platelets present in megaloblastic anemia?

CASE STUDY *(continued from page 258)*

Based on the initial CBC results, further testing was ordered with the following results:

B_{12}	50 pg/mL	Low
Folate	10.3 ng/mL	Normal
Total Bilirubin	2.5 mg/dL	High
Direct Bilirubin	0.8 mg/dL	Normal
AST	35 U/mL	Normal
ALT	30 U/mL	Normal

Examination of a bone marrow aspirate revealed an erythroblastic hyperplasia with megaloblastic erythroblasts.

1. What is the morphologic classification of the patient's anemia?

2. Based on the information obtained so far, what is the most likely defect?

3. What is the significance of the AST/ALT results?

4. What further testing can be done to obtain a definitive diagnosis?

Bone Marrow

If physical examination, patient history, and peripheral blood findings suggest megaloblastic anemia, a bone marrow examination helps establish a definitive diagnosis. In megaloblastic states, the bone marrow is hypercellular with megaloblastic erythroid precursors and a decreased M:E ratio. In a long-standing anemia, red marrow can expand into the long bones. About half the erythroid precursors show megaloblastic changes. Megaloblasts are large nucleated erythroid precursors with nuclear maturation lagging behind cytoplasmic maturation (Figure 12-4). The nucleus of the megaloblast contains loose, open chromatin that stains poorly; cytoplasmic development continues in normal fashion. At each stage of development, the cells contain more cytoplasm with a more mature appearance relative to the size and maturity of the nucleus (resulting in a decreased nuclear:cytoplasmic [N:C] ratio). Thus, the term *nuclear-cytoplasmic asynchrony* is used to describe these cells.

The megaloblastic features are more easily noted in later stages of erythroid development, especially at the polychro-

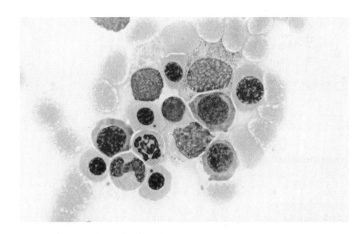

■ FIGURE 12-4   Basophilic and orthochromatic megaloblasts in the bone marrow from a patient with pernicious anemia. Note the large size of the cells, the open chromatin network in the nuclei, and the presence of Howell-Jolly bodies in the orthochromatic megaloblasts. There is also a large band neutrophil and segmented neutrophil with five nuclear lobes. (Wright-Giemsa stain; 1000× magnification)

matophilic stage in which the presence of hemoglobin mixed with RNA gives the cytoplasm the gray-blue color typical of this erythroid precursor. The megaloblast nucleus, however, still has an open (lacy) chromatin pattern more typical of a younger stage of development.

Leukocytes and platelets also show typical features of a nuclear maturation defect as well as ineffective leukopoiesis and thrombopoiesis. Giant metamyelocytes and bands with loose, open chromatin in the nuclei are diagnostic (Figure 12-5 ■). The myelocytes can show poor granulation as do more mature stages. Megakaryocytes can be decreased, nor-

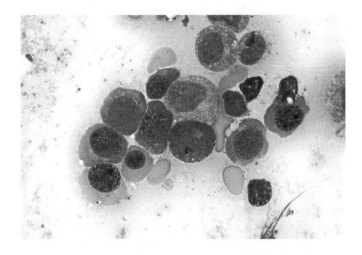

■ FIGURE 12-5   Nuclear-cytoplasmic asynchrony in the bone marrow. There are basophilic (arrow on right), polychromatophilic (arrow on left), and orthochromatic megaloblasts with the typical immature looking nuclei. Note the large size of the cells. (Bone marrow; Wright stain; 1000× magnification)

mal, or increased. Maturation, however, is distinctly abnormal. Some larger than normal forms can be found with separation of nuclear lobes and nuclear fragments.

Other Laboratory Findings

Vitamin B_{12} and serum or red cell folate are commonly measured to diagnose megaloblastosis. Measurement of erythrocyte folate is not influenced as much by recent dietary changes as is serum folate and gives an accurate estimate of the average folate levels over the preceding several months.[14] Automated ligand binding measurements are the easiest to perform and are commonly used. These tests, however, are not the most sensitive indicators of megaloblastosis.

Early megaloblastic changes can be detected by testing for methylmalonic acid (MMA) and homocysteine levels in the blood. These components are intermediaries in folate and vitamin B_{12} metabolism and are elevated early in functional vitamin deficiencies. By performing tests for both MMA and homocysteine, it is possible to differentiate between vitamin B_{12} deficiency and folate deficiency. MMA is usually normal in folate deficiency and elevated in vitamin B_{12} deficiency. Homocysteine is increased in both vitamin B_{12} and folate deficiency. Clinical information is important to help distinguish vitamin B_{12} deficiency from a combined vitamin B_{12} and folate deficiency. A block in the metabolism of histidine to glutamic acid in folic acid deficiency causes urinary excretion of formiminoglutamic acid (FIGLU), an intermediate metabolite, to increase after the administration of histidine.

The large degree of ineffective erythropoiesis results in hemolysis in the marrow and an increase in plasma iron turnover, serum iron, indirect bilirubin, and urobilinogen. The characteristic marked increase in fractions 1 and 2 of serum lactic dehydrogenase (LD) is partially caused by the destruction of megaloblasts rich in LD. The increase is roughly proportional to the degree of anemia. Haptoglobin, uric acid, and alkaline phosphatase are decreased. These and additional tests are discussed in the following sections.

✓ Checkpoint! 4

What abnormal morphological findings on a stained blood smear compose the triad in megaloblastic anemia?

FOLIC ACID

A folic acid deficiency must be considered in the differential diagnosis of macrocytosis due to megaloblastic anemia. Folate deficiency can generally occur as the result of decreased dietary intake, an increased physiological requirement, malabsorption in the small intestine, or drug inhibition.

Structure and Function

Folic acid is the parent substance of a large group of compounds known as *folates*. Chemically, folate is known as

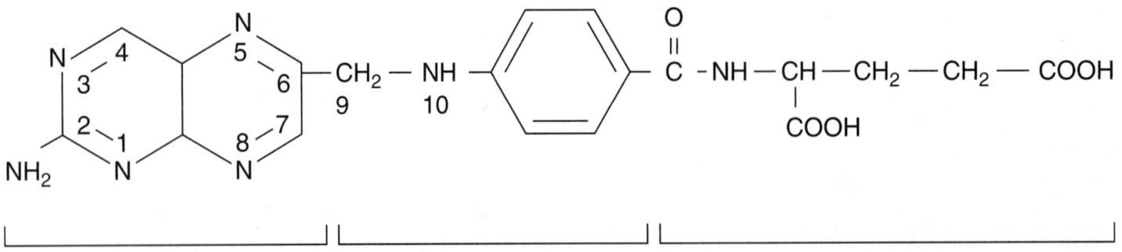

■ FIGURE 12-6   Molecular structure of the folic acid molecule.

pteroylglutamic acid. Structurally, folate is composed of three parts: (1) pteridine, a nitrogen-containing ring, (2) a ring of p-amino-benzoic acid, and (3) a chain of glutamic acid residues. This structure composes the inert form of folate (F) (Figure 12-6 ■). Tetrahydrofolate (THF or FH_4), the active form, is produced by a four-hydrogen reduction of the pteridine ring. Dihydrofolate (DHF or FH_2) is an intermediate in this reaction. The enzyme, DHF reductase, catalyzes both $F \rightarrow FH_2$ and $FH_2 \rightarrow FH_4$.

The function of THF is to transfer one-carbon compounds from donor molecules to acceptor molecules in intermediary metabolism. A variety of one-carbon substituents can be carried by THF, including formyl ($-CH=O$), forminimo ($-CH= NH_2$), hydroxymethyl ($-CH_2OH$), methenyl ($=CH-$), methylene ($=CH_2$), and methyl ($-CH_3$). In this capacity, folate serves a vital role in the metabolism of nucleotides and amino acids:

1. The carbon transfer reaction most important in the development of megaloblastosis is initiated when the carbon side chain of serine is transferred to THF to form N^5,N^{10}-methylene THF (Figure 12-7a ■). This reaction requires the cofactor pyridoxal-5-phosphate (PLP), a derivative of vitamin B_6. The carbon of N^5,N^{10}-methylene-THF is then transferred to deoxyuridilate (dUMP) to form deoxythymidylate (dTMP), a pyrimidine of DNA. In this reaction, THF is oxidized to DHF. The DHF is reduced back to THF by DHF reductase and then to N^5,N^{10}-methylene THF by the serine reaction discussed above. Folates also transport formate (as N^{10}-formyl THF) for purine synthesis. Thus, folate is necessary for the de novo synthesis of DNA (Table 12-3 ✪).

2. The metabolism of histidine to glutamic acid requires THF (Figure 12-7b ■, Table 12-3). The intermediate metabolite of this reaction is formiminoglutamic acid (FIGLU), which requires THF for conversion to glutamic acid. A deficiency of folate blocks this reaction, resulting in an increase in FIGLU excretion.

3. The synthesis of methionine from homocysteine requires the donation of a methyl group from N^5-methyl THF and the action of vitamin B_{12} as a cofactor, resulting in methionine and THF (Figure 12-7a). A deficiency of either folate or B_{12} blocks this reaction, resulting in an increase in homocysteine levels.

Metabolism

Folic acid is present in food and also is synthesized by microorganisms. Most folic acid in food is in the conjugated polyglutamate form. It is deconjugated in the intestine to a monoglutamate prior to absorption. Absorption can take place throughout the small intestine but is especially significant in the proximal jejunum. Once taken up by the intestinal epithelial cell, the folate is reduced to N^5-methyl THF, the primary circulating form of THF in the blood. N^5-methyl THF is distributed throughout the body via the blood and attaches to cells by means of specific receptors. Once inside the cell, N^5-methyl THF must be demethylated and reconjugated by the addition of seven or eight glutamic acid residues to keep it from leaking out again. Demethylation is a reaction that requires vitamin B_{12} and methionine synthase (Figure 12-7a). Thus, a deficiency of vitamin B_{12} traps folate in its methylated form and blocks the formation of other forms of THF. (This is commonly referred to as the *folate trap.*) Although free THF is easily conjugated within cells, methyl-THF is not; consequently, much of the methyl-THF taken up by a B_{12}-deficient cell leaks out before additional glutamates can be added.[13] Consequently, the cells in vitamin B_{12} deficiency are unable to retain their folate, leading to tissue folate depletion. In the demethylation of N^5-methyl THF by vitamin B_{12}, homocysteine is methylated to methionine, a precursor of S-adenosylmethionine (SAM). This reaction requires methionine synthase and vitamin B_{12}. SAM is thought to be critical to nervous system function.

Requirements

Folic acid is present in most foods including eggs, milk, yeast, mushrooms, and liver but is especially abundant in green leafy vegetables (from which it gets its name). It is also synthesized by microorganisms. The vitamin is destroyed by heat; thus, when food is overcooked, much of the folate is destroyed. Ascorbate protects folate from oxidation and, when present, can protect folate to some extent from heat degradation. The recommended daily dietary allowance of food folic acid for adults is ~400 µg of which about 50–80% is absorbed in the intestine. This is adequate to provide the minimum daily requirement of ~50 µg/day needed to sustain normal metabolism. The liver stores from 5 to 10 mg of

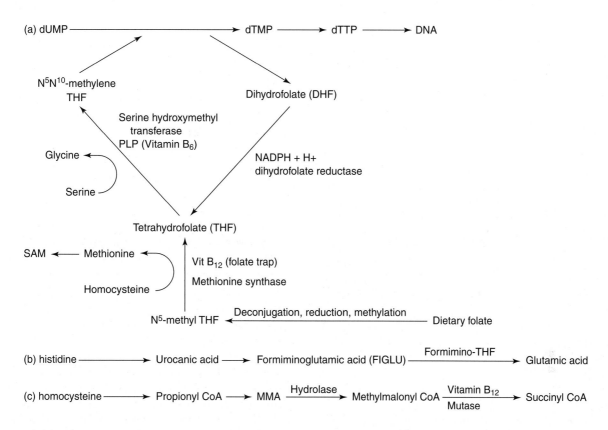

FIGURE 12-7 Biochemical reactions using folic acid, vitamin B_{12}, and derivatives. **a.** The role of folate and vitamin B_{12} in the synthesis of DNA. A deficiency of methylcobalamin causes a failure of methylation of homocysteine, which leads to a reduction in tetrahydrofolate (THF) and the trapping of the folate as N^5-methyl THF. This causes a deficiency of N^{5-10}-methylene THF, a coenzyme needed in the synthesis of dTTP, a nucleotide of DNA. **b.** The role of folate in the catabolism of histidine. **c.** The role of vitamin B_{12} (adenosyl-cobalamin form) in the conversion of methylmalonic acid (MMA) to succinyl CoA. Tests to detect vitamin B_{12} deficiency include direct measurement of vitamin B_{12} and tests to detect increased MMA and homocysteine, intermediaries that require vitamin B_{12} for metabolism. Tests to detect folic acid deficiency include direct measurement of folate or measurement of homocysteine and FIGLU, intermediaries that require folate for metabolism. With deficiencies of vitamin B_{12} and/or folate, the intermediaries MMA, homocysteine, and FIGLU are trapped and increase in concentration.

folate, which is sufficient to provide the daily requirement for three to six months if folic acid is omitted from the diet.

Folate plays an important role in normal embryogenesis. Observations reveal a high incidence of low folate levels in women who give birth to babies with neural tube defects (NTD) compared to women who give birth to normal babies. Several studies have shown that supplementation of folate during pregnancy can reduce the rate of neural tube closure birth defects by as much as one-half. The basis for this protective effect is not clear, but it has been suggested that the effect may be confined to a subset of women who have defective folate metabolism. In an effort to reduce NTDs, the United States government required the fortifications of grain products with folic acid beginning in the fall of 1997.[15] The goal was to increase the daily dietary folate to 100 µg per person. It has been suggested that pregnant women need an intake of about 800 µg/day.

Folic acid can become depleted quickly in conditions with rapid cell turnover such as sickle cell anemia and other hemolytic anemias, during growth and in pregnancy and lactation. Thus, the daily requirement in patients with these conditions is increased.

⊙ **TABLE 12-3**

Metabolic Reactions Requiring Folic Acid Coenzymes

System	Reaction
Serine ↔ Glycine	Ser + THF ↔ N^5,N^{10}-methylene THF + Gly
Thymidylate synthesis	dUMP + N^5,N^{10}-methylene THF → DHF + dTMP
Histidine catabolism	Formininoglutamate + THF → N^5-formimino THF + glutamic acid
Methionine synthesis	Homocysteine + N^5-methyl THF → THF + Methionine

✓ **Checkpoint! 5**

Hal had small bowel resection due to carcinoma. Explain why he is at high risk for folate deficiency.

Pathophysiology of Folic Acid Deficiency

Folate deficiency results in decreased synthesis of N^5, N^{10}-methylene THF, which is needed as a cofactor in DNA synthesis. Consequently, there is a marked slowing of DNA synthesis and the S phase is prolonged. The impairment of DNA synthesis is due to the inability to convert deoxyuridine monophosphate (dUMP) to deoxythymidine monophosphate (dTMP) (see below). The dUMP is subsequently phosphorylated to the triphosphate form (dUTP). DNA polymerase does not effectively distinguish dUTP from dTTP (which is synthesized from dTMP), and dUTP is erroneously incorporated into the DNA of folate-deficient cells. The DNA "proof-reading" function of the cells recognizes the mistake and tries to repair the DNA by replacing uridine with thymidine, but the repair attempt fails due to the lack of available dTTP. The result is ultimately DNA fragmentation and cell death by apoptosis.[13] Increased apoptosis of the blood cell precursors (ineffective erythropoiesis) leads to increased heme catabolism and iron turnover and leads to signs of hemolysis and jaundice. Extramedullary hemolysis also occurs, and circulating red cell survival can be decreased by 30–50%. The intermediaries requiring folic acid as a cofactor for metabolism (homocysteine and FIGLU) accumulate. Mildly elevated levels of homocysteine are considered a major risk factor for atherosclerosis and venous thrombosis (∞ Chapter 33).

All rapidly dividing cells—including erythrocytes, leukocytes, platelets, and intestinal epithelium—are affected by a folate deficiency. Hematopoietic cells show characteristic megaloblastic changes. The bone marrow can exhibit a 3-fold increase in erythropoiesis, but the peripheral blood reticulocyte count is low, indicating a large degree of ineffective erythropoiesis. Survival of the erythrocytes in the peripheral blood also decreases significantly.

The clinical findings of folate deficiency develop sequentially. Serum folate decreases within 1 to 2 weeks of a folic acid deficiency. Hypersegmented neutrophils are the first morphologic change and occur at about 2 weeks. The urinary excretion of FIGLU increases next at about 13 weeks, and anemia appears last at about 19–20 weeks.

Causes of Folate Deficiency

Folate deficiency can occur as the result of an inadequate dietary intake, an increased requirement, malabsorption in the small intestine, or drug inhibition (Table 12-4 ✪).

Inadequate Diet   The most common cause of folate deficiency is an inadequate dietary intake of folic acid. This is seen most often in poor and elderly people who fail to obtain enough of the appropriate foods to maintain adequate folic acid intake due to financial reasons, lack of motivation,

✪ TABLE 12-4

Causes of Folate Deficiency

Cause	Examples
Inadequate diet	Low income, elderly people with limited function/income, people who are alcoholics
Increased requirement	Diseases associated with rapid cell turnover (sickle cell anemia, thalassemia, leukemias, other malignancies, pregnancy, infancy)
Malabsorption	Ileitis, tropical sprue, nontropical sprue, blind loop syndrome
Drug inhibition	Oral contraceptives, long-term anticoagulant therapy, phenobarbital, primidome, phenytoin, antimetabolite chemotherapy
Biologic competition	Bacterial overgrowth in small intestine

physical disabilities, or lack of knowledge concerning nutrition. People who are alcoholics whose diet consists mainly of large quantities of ethanol have a deficiency of many vitamins in addition to folic acid. Complicating the folate deficiency in alcoholic individuals, the ethanol appears to impair release of folate from the liver and can be toxic to erythroid precursors. (Erythroid precursors in alcoholism are frequently vacuolated.) In alcoholic individuals who have liver disease but have an adequate diet, the anemia is macrocytic but not megaloblastic.

Increased Requirement   In individuals with increased cell replication, the normal daily intake of folic acid is perhaps not sufficient to maintain normal DNA synthesis. Without folate supplements, folate stores can be rapidly depleted. This occurs in hemolytic anemias such as sickle cell anemia and thalassemia, in myeloproliferative diseases such as leukemia, in pregnancy, and in metastatic cancers. Anemia in pregnancy is common and can be caused by deficiencies of iron and/or folic acid. The deficiency of folic acid is related to the limited reserves of this nutrient and a 5–10 time increased demand for its use created by the growing fetus. Prophylactic folic acid supplements are usually prescribed to prevent anemia during pregnancy. Supplements are also recommended preconception in an effort to decrease neural tube defects in the fetus.[16]

Malabsorption   Intestinal diseases affecting the upper small intestine, which interfere with the absorption of nutrients, can cause a folate deficiency. The most common conditions of this type include ileitis, tropical sprue, and nontropical sprue. The blind loop syndrome associated with an overgrowth of bacteria can cause a folate deficiency because the bacteria preferentially utilize the folate.

Drug Inhibition   Megaloblastic anemia has also been associated with certain drugs including oral contraceptives, long-term anticoagulant drugs, phenobarbital, primidone, and phenytoin. Anemia occasionally is not present even though serum and erythrocyte folate are depressed.

✓ Checkpoint! 6

What is the most common cause of folate deficiency and in what groups of individuals is it usually found?

Laboratory Analysis of Folate Deficiency

Both serum and erythrocyte folate levels must be decreased to diagnose folate deficiency. Serum folate reflects the folic acid intake over the last several days, whereas erythrocyte folate reflects the folate available when the red cell was maturing in the bone marrow and reflects the net folate level over the preceding several months. Serum folate can be falsely increased with even slight hemolysis of the sample. Erythrocyte folate, then, is a better indication of folate stores. Low serum folate can indicate an imminent folic acid deficiency and precedes erythrocyte folate deficiency.[14]

Neither serum nor erythrocyte folate is a good indicator of folate stores in the presence of vitamin B_{12} deficiency. A deficiency of vitamin B_{12} impairs methionine synthesis and leads to the accumulation of methyl-THF as the donation of the methyl group to homocysteine, and the generation of free THF is impaired. In addition, vitamin B_{12} is required for normal transfer of methyl-THF to the cells and for keeping the folate in the cell as conjugated folate (methyl-THF is not easily conjugated and leaks out of the cell). Thus, serum folate can be falsely increased and erythrocyte folate falsely decreased in vitamin B_{12} deficiency. In about two-thirds of vitamin B_{12}-deficient patients, erythrocyte folate is decreased.[17] In addition, epithelial changes in the GI tract that accompany vitamin B_{12} deficiency can lead to malabsorption of folic acid in which case both serum and erythrocyte folate are decreased. Care must be taken in interpreting the folate results because both serum and erythrocyte folate can be falsely increased or decreased in a variety of conditions (Table 12-5 ✪).

VITAMIN B_{12} (COBALAMIN)

By the early 1900s, megaloblastic anemia was recognized as a unique anemia of adults with typical symptoms and clinical findings. The disease was called *pernicious anemia* because of the certainty of a fatal outcome. The average survival after the onset of the disease was from 1 to 3 years. It is now recognized that pernicious anemia is a specific form of megaloblastic anemia characterized by a deficiency of vitamin B_{12} that is secondary to an absence of intrinsic factor.

Structure and Function

Vitamin B_{12} is a commonly used generic term for a family of cobalamin vitamins in which ligands can be chelated to cobalt. The more accurate terminology when referring to this family of vitamins is *cobalamin*. Vitamin B_{12} refers specifically to the therapeutic form of cobalamin that contains the ligand, cyanide (cyanocobalamin), a form not naturally found in the body but is the crystalline form used for treating cobalamin deficiency. In hematology literature, the terms *cobalamin* and *vitamin B_{12}* are often used interchangably. However, in the following discussion, for sake of consistency with clinical testing, the term vitamin B_{12} is used.

Vitamin B_{12} (cobalamin) is structurally classified as a corrinoid, a family of compounds with a corrin ring. The molecule has three portions: (1) a corrin ring composed of four reduced pyrrole groups with a cobalt at the center (cobalamin gets it name from the central cobalt), (2) a nucleotide (5,6-dimethylbenzimidazole) that lies almost perpendicular to the ring attached to the cobalt, and (3) various ligands (a β-group) attached to the cobalt on the opposite side of the ring from the nucleotide (Figure 12-8 ■). The β-group in tissue cobalamins is either cyanide, methyl, adenosyl, or hydroxyl. Adenosylcobalamin (AdoCbl) and methylcobalamin (MeCbl) act as coenzymes in biological reactions. Hydroxycobalamin (OHCbl) and cyanocobalamin (CnCbl) are not metabolically active forms of cobalamin but can be converted to the active methyl and adenosyl forms by tissue enzymes.

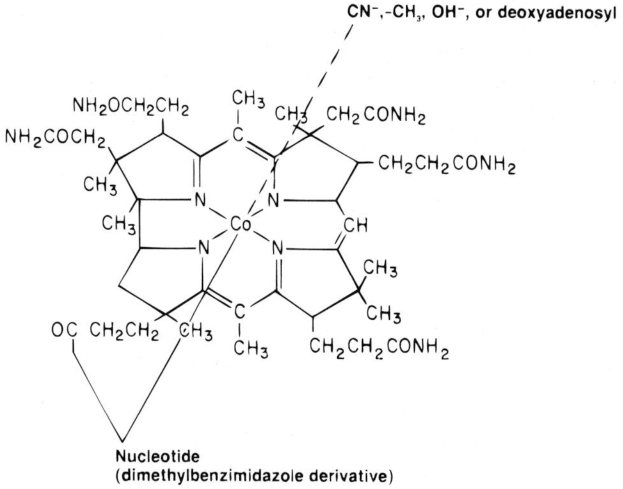

✪ TABLE 12-5

Causes of False Increases and Decreases in Folate Levels

	Erythrocyte Folate	Serum Folate
False increase	Early folate deficiency	Recent increase in dietary folate
	Reticulocytosis	Hemolysis of blood sample
	Recent RBC transfusion	Coexisting vitamin B_{12} deficiency
False decrease	B_{12} deficiency	Recent low dietary intake
	Recent alcohol consumption	Gallium or technetium administration

■ FIGURE 12-8   Molecular structure of the cobalamin molecule.

As mentioned previously, methionine is formed from homocysteine when a methyl group is transferred from N^5-methyl THF to homocysteine in a vitamin B_{12}-dependent reaction catalyzed by methionine synthase (Figure 12-7a). For this reaction, the vitamin must be in the MeCbl form. The significance of the reaction is that THF is formed from the demethylation of N^5-methyl THF, which is then converted to N^5N^{10}-methylene THF, the folate form necessary for thymidylate synthesis that is needed for DNA synthesis. A vitamin B_{12} deficiency traps newly acquired folate in the N^5-methyl THF form (in which it is acquired from the plasma), which is not efficiently conjugated with glutamic acids and thus leaks back out of cells (see discussion of folate metabolism). The result is an intracellular functional deficiency of folate and a block of DNA synthesis. Methionine is the precursor of SAM, a metabolite thought to be critical to the normal functioning of the nervous system.

AdoCbl is required for only one mammalian reaction: the conversion of methylmalonyl CoA to succinyl CoA (Figure 12-7c ■). AdoCbl acts as a coenzyme with methylmalonyl CoA mutase in this reaction. Increased urinary excretion of methylmalonic acid (MMA), a precursor of methylmalonyl-CoA, is a diagnostic aid in vitamin B_{12} deficiency.

 Checkpoint! 7

A patient has the following results: vitamin B_{12} 50 pg/mL, serum folate 4 ng/dL, RBC folate 100 ng/mL. Interpret these results.

Metabolism

Defects in any of the steps of vitamin B_{12} metabolism can lead to a vitamin B_{12} deficiency and megaloblastic anemia. The laboratory plays a critical role in both assessing the level of the vitamin and determining the cause of low levels. Thus, it is important to understand the metabolism of this important nutrient.

Absorption   Vitamin B_{12} is present in most foods of animal origin including milk, eggs, and meat. The vitamin complex is released from food by peptic digestion at a low pH in the stomach and binds to an R-protein, a vitamin B_{12} binding protein secreted in the saliva and in the stomach. R-protein, named because of its rapid electrophoretic mobility compared with the intrinsic factor, is the preferred binding protein for vitamin B_{12} released from food at the acid pH of the stomach. In the duodenum, pancreatic proteases degrade the R-proteins, releasing vitamin B_{12}. The released vitamin B_{12} quickly binds to the intrinsic factor (IF), which is resistant to pancreatic degradation. The intrinsic factor is a glycoprotein secreted by parietal cells of the gastric mucosa in response to the presence of food, vagal stimulation, histamine, and gastrin. The IF binds vitamin B_{12} in a 1:1 stoichiometry and is required for the absorption of vitamin B_{12}. The IF-B_{12} complex resists digestion and passes through the jejunum into the ileum where it binds the specific IF receptor (cubulin) on the microvilli of ileal mucosal cells[13] (Figure 12-9 ■). Because the ileal receptors are specific for IF, not R-proteins, a lack of pancreatic protease ties up the vitamin B_{12} in a form that cannot be absorbed (R-protein:cobalamin) and results in vitamin B_{12} deficiency. Following attachment of the IF-B_{12} complex to the receptor, the vitamin is taken into the mucosal cell. The entire IF-B12 complex appears to be taken into the cell where the B_{12} is released while the IF is degraded.[13]

Transport   Vitamin B_{12} leaves the mucosal cell and is transported in the blood by a group of transport proteins. These transport proteins include transcobalamin I (TCI), transcobalamin II (TCII), and transcobalamin III (TCIII). TCI and TCIII are R-proteins, but TCII is not.

The release of the vitamin from each of these transcobalamins is different. TCII is an α-globulin produced in the liver and the ileum and by macrophages. Although TCII carries only a small fraction of the total vitamin in the plasma, it is the primary plasma protein that mediates transfer of vitamin B_{12} into the tissues. The vitamin B_{12}:TCII complex is thought to be formed within the ileal mucosal cells and released to the blood.[13] TCII binds 90% of the newly absorbed vitamin B_{12}. This transport complex disappears rapidly from blood (T 1/2 of 6–9 minutes) as it is taken up by cells in the liver, bone marrow, and other dividing cells that have spe-

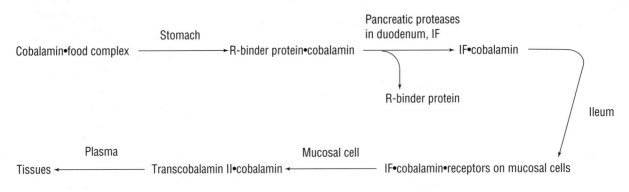

■ FIGURE 12-9   Assimilation of vitamin B_{12}.

cific receptors for TCII. The B_{12}-TCII complex is internalized, and once inside the cell, vitamin B_{12} is released and utilized, and the TC is degraded. Congenital deficiency of TCII produces a severe megaloblastic anemia in infancy. However, serum vitamin B_{12} concentration in this condition is normal.

The functions of the R-proteins TCI and TCIII are less well understood. TCI has an electrophoretic mobility of α_1-globulin and is produced in part by granulocytes. TCI is the main R-protein of plasma and carries 75% of the recycled endogenous vitamin B_{12} in the body. TCI is only about 50% saturated, its turnover is slow (T l/2 of 10 days), and its function is unknown. It has been suggested that TCI serves to carry cobalamins to hepatocytes where they are excreted in the bile, thus serving to clear the body of nonphysiologic cobalamins. An alternative theory suggests that TCI is a storage protein for cobalamins.[13] Lack of TCI produces no megaloblastosis or anemia but results in a decreased serum vitamin B_{12} level.

TCIII has an electrophoretic mobility of the α_2-globulins and is found in plasma and in granulocytes. It appears to be released from granulocytes during the clotting process and does not bind significant portions of cobalamin. Both TCI and III are increased in myeloproliferative disorders, presumably due to proliferation of granulocytes that produce the protein. Other vitamin B_{12} binder proteins are present in plasma, saliva, gastric juice, pancreatic juice, amniotic fluid, and milk.

Requirements

About 3–5 μg of vitamin B_{12} per day is needed to maintain normal biochemical functions. It is estimated that only about 70% of vitamin B_{12} intake is absorbed, which suggests that the diet should include from 5 to 7 μg of the vitamin per day. This amount is available in a regular mixed ("balanced") diet but a strict vegetarian diet does not. Vitamin B_{12} stores (~5000 μg) are sufficient to provide the normal daily requirement for about 1000 days. Therefore, it takes several years to develop a deficiency if no vitamin B_{12} is absorbed from the diet. About half of this storage vitamin is in the liver.[18] The rest is located in the heart and kidneys.

 Checkpoint! 8

Explain why there is a megaloblastic anemia in transcobalamin II deficiency when the serum vitamin B_{12} concentration is normal.

Pathophysiology of Vitamin B_{12} Deficiency

Deficiency of vitamin B_{12} is reflected by (1) impaired DNA synthesis (megaloblastic anemia) and (2) defective fatty acid degradation (neurologic symptoms).

Impaired DNA Synthesis   A deficiency in either vitamin B_{12} or folic acid results in impaired production of methylene-THF, a defect in thymidylate synthesis, and ultimately a defect in DNA synthesis. This produces megaloblastic ane-

mia and epithelial cell abnormalities. All dividing cells including the hematopoietic cells in the bone marrow are affected.

$$\text{Homocysteine + Methyltetrahydrofolate} \longrightarrow$$
$$\uparrow \qquad\qquad\qquad \uparrow$$
$$\text{Dietary Folate} \qquad \text{MeCbl}$$
$$\text{Methionine + Tetrahydrofolate} \longrightarrow \quad \text{DNA Synthesis}$$

Defective Fatty Acid Degradation   AdoCbl is a cofactor in the conversion of methylmalonyl CoA to succinyl CoA. In vitamin B_{12} deficiency, there is a defect in degradation of propionyl CoA to methylmalonyl CoA and, finally, to succinyl CoA. As propionyl CoA accumulates, it is used as a primer for fatty acid synthesis, replacing the usual primer acetyl CoA. This results in fatty acids with an odd number of carbons. These odd-chain fatty acids are incorporated into neuronal membranes causing disruption of membrane function. It is probable that **demyelination** (destruction, removal, or loss of the lipid substance that forms a myelin sheath around the axons of nerve fibers), a characteristic finding in vitamin B_{12} deficiency is a result of this erroneous fatty acid synthesis.

A critical feature of demyelination in vitamin B_{12} deficiency is neurological disease. Peripheral nerves are most often affected, presenting initially as motor and sensory neuropathy. The brain and spinal cord can also be affected leading to dementia, spastic paralysis, and other serious neurological disturbances. Demyelination has been known to occur occasionally without any sign of anemia or macrocytosis, making accurate diagnosis difficult but critical. The bone marrow, however, always shows megaloblastic hematopoiesis.[19] Neurological disease might not be totally reversible but, if treated early, can be partially resolved. Neurological disease does not occur in folic acid deficiency. Administration of synthetic folic acid corrects the anemia of vitamin B_{12} deficiency but does not halt or reverse neurological disease because synthetic folic acid, unlike dietary folic acid, is reduced directly to THF without the requirement of vitamin B_{12} as a cofactor.[20] The THF can correct the megaloblastosis, but because there is a bypass of the vitamin B_{12}-dependent reaction of conversion of homocysteine to methionine, SAM—a metabolite considered critical to nervous system function—is not formed. Thus, it is essential to differentiate between folate deficiency and vitamin B_{12} deficiency so that appropriate treatment can be given.

Gastritis and abnormalities of the gastrointestinal epithelium secondary to vitamin B_{12} deficiency can interfere with the absorption of folic acid and iron, complicating the anemia.

 Checkpoint! 9

Explain why severe B_{12} deficiency sometimes presents with neurological disease.

Causes of Vitamin B$_{12}$ Deficiency

Vitamin B$_{12}$ deficiency has many causes including lack of intrinsic factor (pernicious anemia), malabsorption, nutritional deficiency, and impaired utilization by tissues due to defective or absent transport proteins or enzyme deficiencies (Table 12-6 ✪).

Pernicious Anemia   **Pernicious anemia (PA)** is a specific term used to define the megaloblastic anemia caused by an absence of IF secondary to gastric atrophy. An absence of IF leads to vitamin B$_{12}$ deficiency because the vitamin cannot be absorbed without it. PA is the most common cause of vitamin B$_{12}$ deficiency, accounting for 85% of all deficiencies. Total atrophy of gastric parietal cells is demonstrated by finding **achlorhydria** of gastric juice after histamine stimulation (these cells also produce HCl). It is generally a disease of older adults, usually occurring after 40 years of age. This anemia is seen more commonly among people of Northern European background, especially Great Britain and Scandinavia, but can be found in all racial groups. More women than men are affected. Although no particular genetic abnormality has been identified, some patients have prematurely graying or whitening hair. A positive family history of PA increases the

risk of developing it by 20 times. The incidence of gastric carcinoma in these patients is also increased.[21]

PA is an autoimmune disease. The gastric atrophy is thought to result from immune destruction of the acid-secreting portion of the gastric mucosa.[13] Up to 90% of PA patients have antibodies against parietal cells.[23] However, these antibodies are not specific for pernicious anemia patients and are also found in patients with gastritis, thyroid disease, and Addison's disease. On the other hand, serum antibodies against intrinsic factor are found in ~75% of PA patients and are highly specific for PA. These IF antibodies are of two types: blocking and binding. Type I, or blocking, antibodies are antibodies to IF and prevent formation of the IF-vitamin B$_{12}$ complex. Type II, or binding, antibodies are directed against the IF-B$_{12}$ complex and prevent the IF-B$_{12}$ complex from binding to ileal receptors. Binding antibodies are found in about half the sera that contain blocking antibody. A number of findings suggest that the immune destruction of the gastric mucosa is not antibody mediated but more likely T cell mediated. Patients with agammaglobulinemia have a higher than expected incidence of PA. Also, lymphocytes from PA patients have been shown to be hyperresponsive to gastric antigens.[13]

Pernicious anemia frequently occurs with other autoimmune diseases such as Graves' disease and Hashimoto's thyroiditis, type I diabetes, and Addison's disease. In addition, a predisposition to PA can be inherited. Relatives of patients with PA have a higher incidence of antiparietal cell antibodies and anti-intrinsic factor antibodies than the general population.[13]

Juvenile pernicious anemia is rare in children. It can occur secondary to a variety of conditions, including a congenital deficiency or abnormality of IF (the more common type with lack of IF but otherwise normal gastric secretion), or more rarely, true PA of childhood. In true PA of childhood, there is absence of intrinsic factor and gastric atrophy, decreased gastric secretion, and antibodies against IF and parietal cells. Megaloblastic anemia in childhood due to malabsorption of vitamin B$_{12}$ can also be due to a congenital deficiency of TCII, a congenital R-protein deficiency, or selective malabsorption of vitamin B$_{12}$ (Imerslund-Gräsbeck disease). The latter can be due to abnormal vitamin B$_{12}$-IF receptors in the ileum.

Laboratory diagnosis of pernicious anemia and/or vitamin B$_{12}$ deficiency usually involves gastric analysis and/or the Schilling test, serum vitamin B$_{12}$ assay, and methylmalonic acid (MMA) assay. The serum vitamin B$_{12}$ and MMA assays establish the fact that a deficiency exists but does not provide a distinction of PA from other causes of vitamin B$_{12}$ deficiency. Gastric analysis and the Schilling test are more useful in establishing the specific diagnosis of PA but are rarely performed anymore.

Gastric Analysis   Because atrophy of the parietal cells is a universal feature of PA, an absence of free HCl in gastric

✪ TABLE 12-6

Causes of Vitamin B$_{12}$ Deficiency and Associated Conditions

Cause	Associated Conditions
Malabsorption	Pernicious anemia (lack of IF)
	Gastrectomy or gastric bypass
	Crohn's disease
	Tropical sprue
	Celiac disease
	Surgical resection of the ileum
	Imerslund-Gräsbeck disease
	Pancreatic insufficiency
	Drugs (colchicine, neomycin, p-aminosalicylic acid, or omeprazole)
	Blind loop syndrome
	Diverticulitis
	Intestinal parasite—*Diphyllobothrium latum*
Biologic competition	Intestinal parasite (i.e., *Diphyllobothrium latum*)
	Leishmaniasis[22]
	Bacterial overgrowth
Nutritional deficiency	Strict vegetarian diets
	Pregnant women on a poor diet
	Malnutrition
Impaired utilization	Transcobalamin II deficiency
	Nitrous oxide inhalation

juice after histamine stimulation is indicative of PA. Because parietal cells secrete both HCl and intrinsic factor, an absence of HCl is indirect evidence for lack of IF. After histamine stimulation in patients with pernicious anemia, the pH fails to fall below 3.5, and gastric volume, pepsin, and rennin are decreased. Approximately 80% of cases of PA have increased gastrin. Testing for anti-intrinsic factor antibodies, serum gastrin, and serum pepsinogin A and C together as a group provides a sensitive indication of gastric atrophy and pernicious anemia.[24]

Schilling Test   The **Schilling test** is a definitive test useful in distinguishing vitamin B_{12} deficiency due to malabsorption, dietary deficiency, or absence of IF. The test measures the amount of an oral dose of radioactively labeled crystalline B_{12} that is absorbed in the gut and excreted in the urine. The patient is given 0.5–1.0 µg dose of ^{57}Co-labeled B_{12} orally. This is given with or followed within two hours by an intramuscular injection of 1000 µg of unlabeled vitamin B_{12}. The injection is termed the *flushing dose*; its purpose is to saturate all vitamin B_{12} receptors in the tissues. Thus, any of the labeled oral dose absorbed in the gut and passing into the blood will be in excess of available uptake receptors. The excess is filtered by the kidney and appears in the urine. Urine is collected for 24 hours, and its radioactivity is determined. If more than 7.5% of the standard oral dose is excreted, absorption is said to be normal. In PA and in malabsorption, excretion is less than 7.5% because the labeled oral vitamin B_{12} is not absorbed.

If excretion is less than 7.5%, part II of the Schilling test is performed to distinguish between PA and other causes of malabsorption. In part II, the oral dose of labeled B_{12} is accompanied by a dose of intrinsic factor. The rest of the test is the same as in part I. If part II shows more than 7.5% excretion, absorption is considered normal with the lack of absorption in part I simply due to the lack of IF. The diagnosis is PA. If part II is abnormal, the patient can have another malabsorption defect such as sprue (Table 12-7 ☺).

Several points must be considered when interpreting the results of a Schilling test. First, the test results are not valid with the presence of renal disease. The patient could have been able to absorb the vitamin but cannot filter the excess vitamin efficiently because of abnormal kidney function. Second, incomplete collection of urine invalidates the results. Incontinence or inability to empty the bladder gives false low values even when absorption was normal. Spuriously low urinary excretion in part II can also be due to the inability to absorb IF-B_{12} because of megaloblastoid epithelial changes in the gut.

The Schilling test is seldom used now in this country because of the difficulties in using radioisotopes and the inconvenience of the test for the patient. An additional problem is that the absorption of crystalline vitamin B_{12} used in the oral dose can differ from the absorption of vitamin B_{12} in

TABLE 12-7

Conditions Associated with Abnormal Schilling Test Results

Corrected by Intrinsic Factor in Part II	Not Corrected by Intrinsic Factor in Part II
Pernicious anemia	Crohn's disease
Abnormal intrinsic factor molecule	Tropical sprue
	Celiac disease
Hereditary intrinsic factor deficiency	Surgical resection of the ileum
	Imerslund-Gräsbeck disease
Gastrectomy	Pancreatic insufficiency
	Drugs
	Blind loop syndrome
	Diverticulitis
	Intestinal parasite—*Diphyllobothrium latum*
	Transcobalamin II deficiency

food.[14,25] For these reasons, MMA and homocysteine are emerging as better markers for early detection of PA or vitamin B_{12} deficiency.

On the other hand, there are advantages of the Schilling test. First, the test results can suggest what further testing (i.e., stool analysis for *D. latum*) should be done. Second, results can help identify how to treat the clinical condition and the duration of treatment.[26]

Other Causes of Malabsorption   Pernicious anemia is only one specific cause of vitamin B_{12} malabsorption, which also can be caused by a loss of IF secondary to gastrectomy or secondary to diseases that prevent binding of the IF-B_{12} complex in the ileum. An iron deficiency usually precedes vitamin B_{12} deficiency in patients who have had a gastrectomy. Diseases that can affect the absorption of the IF-B_{12} complex in the ileum include Crohn's disease, tropical sprue, celiac disease, and surgical resection of the ileum. In Imerslund-Gräsbeck disease, the IF receptors are missing or abnormal, causing a form of juvenile megaloblastic anemia. In patients with severe pancreatic insufficiency, there is a lack of absorption of the vitamin B_{12} because the vitamin cannot be released from the R-proteins and transferred to IF. Normally, pancreatic proteases are responsible for degrading the R-proteins. Certain medications can interfere with intestinal absorption. In addition, conditions that allow a buildup of bacteria in the small bowel can cause a vitamin B_{12} deficiency. The bacteria preferentially take up the vitamin before it reaches the ileum. This situation occurs in the blind loop syndrome and in diverticulitis. Infestation with the fish tapeworm *Diphyllobothrium latum* can cause a deficiency as the worm accumulates the vitamin avidly.

CASE STUDY *(continued from page 262)*

A Schilling test and antibody testing were done, with the following results:

Schilling test	Part I, before intrinsic factor, 1%
	Part II, after intrinsic factor, 8%
Intrinsic-factor-blocking antibodies	Positive to a titer of 1:6400

5. What is this patient's definitive diagnosis?

Nutritional Deficiency Dietary deficiency of vitamin B_{12} is rare in the United States. Food from animal sources, especially liver, is rich in vitamin B_{12}. Strict vegetarian diets, however, do not supply vitamin B_{12}, and these individuals can develop a deficiency over a period of years. Occasionally, pregnant women with a poor diet can develop a deficiency presumably due to an increased demand by the developing fetus. However, folic acid deficiency is a more common cause of megaloblastic anemia in pregnancy due to the lower stores of this nutrient.

Other Causes TCII deficiency is the only transcobalamin deficiency that produces megaloblastic anemia because it is the major transport protein responsible for delivering the vitamin to the tissues. In TCII deficiency, vitamin B_{12} is absorbed normally and serum vitamin B_{12} is normal because of the relatively high levels bound to TCI. Tissue vitamin B_{12} deficiency develops, however, including megaloblastic anemia, because the cellular receptors recognize only TCII, not the R-proteins (TCI and TCIII).[13]

Nitrous oxide, N_2O ("laughing gas"), abuse has been reported to result in a B_{12} deficiency and megaloblastic anemias. N_2O rapidly inactivates methionine synthetase of which cobalamin is a coenzyme. Vitamin B_{12} cleaves N_2O and at the same time is oxidized to an inert form. This leads to a rapid deficiency.

 Checkpoint! 10

Explain why some believe that pernicious anemia is an autoimmune disorder.

Laboratory Analysis of Vitamin B_{12} Deficiency

Vitamin B_{12} in serum is a reflection of vitamin stores. The normal range of serum vitamin B_{12} varies from newborn to adult, in men, the concentration depends significantly on age.[27] Serum vitamin B_{12} can appear falsely decreased (no actual vitamin B_{12} deficiency) in folic acid deficiency, in pregnancy, with oral contraceptive use, with antibiotic therapy (using the microbiologic assay), and in multiple myeloma

TABLE 12-8

Causes of False Decrease and False Normal/Increase in Serum Vitamin B_{12} Levels

False Decrease	False Normal/Increase
Folate deficiency	B_{12} treatment
Pregnancy (last trimester)	Liver disease
Oral contraceptive use	Nitrous oxide inhalation
Multiple myeloma	Chronic myelogenous leukemia
Elderly	Polycythemia vera
Transcobalamin I deficiency	Transcobalamin II deficiency

(Table 12-8 ✪). Vitamin B_{12} deficiency can be masked by folate therapy.

A specific test that measures the increased excretion of methylmalonic acid (MMA) in the urine indirectly indicates decreases in vitamin B_{12} concentration. Up to 40% of patients may have increased MMA levels in the urine but normal serum B_{12} levels.[20] These patients, however, show laboratory and clinical evidence of vitamin B_{12} deficiency. The only condition in which methylmalonic acid is increased in addition to vitamin B_{12} deficiency is in congenital methylmalonic aciduria. The congenital condition, however, has no megaloblastic anemia. Thus, determination of MMA concentration is useful in distinguishing a vitamin B_{12} deficiency from folate deficiency.

Homocysteine is increased in the plasma of patients with vitamin B_{12}, or folate deficiency.[28] Monitoring serum levels can serve as an early detector of vitamin B_{12} deficiency. Many recent studies have concluded that MMA and homocysteine are the most sensitive and specific indicators of vitamin B_{12} deficiency.[27–30] Some studies have shown that besides being a good indicator of vitamin B_{12} deficiency, increased homocysteine levels could also predict a 3-fold increase risk in myocardial infarction as well as venous thrombosis.[29] Increased concentrations of both analytes can be found in many patients with normal serum vitamin B_{12} concentrations.[29] Some clinicians now recommend initial testing for serum vitamin B_{12} levels and following up low or borderline normal results with MMA and homocysteine measurements.[30] By contrast, some have found that MMA and homocysteine measurements are more sensitive tests of early pernicious anemia preceding hematologic abnormalities and decreased serum vitamin B_{12} levels and recommend them as a superior testing regimen (Figure 12-10 ■).

Homocysteine and MMA tests are also helpful in determining a patient's response to treatment with vitamin B_{12} and folate. The serum MMA level remains increased in vitamin B_{12}-deficient patients treated inappropriately with folate. Folate-deficient patients treated inappropriately with cobalamin have increased serum homocysteine level.

A new technology, electrospray tandem mass spectrometry, could make testing for serum levels of MMA and homocysteine easier and more practical.[31] The procedure does not require expensive immunodiagnostic reagents and chromatographic columns and can be performed in under five minutes.

 ### ✓ **Checkpoint! 11**

What two lab tests are the most specific indicators of B₁₂ deficiency?

THERAPY

Therapeutic trials in megaloblastic anemia using *physiologic* doses of either vitamin B₁₂ or folic acid produce a reticulocyte response only if the specific vitamin that is deficient is being administered. For instance, small doses (1 µg) of vitamin B₁₂ given daily produce a reticulocyte response in vitamin B₁₂ deficiency but not in folic acid deficiency. On the other hand, large therapeutic doses of vitamin B₁₂ or folic acid can induce a partial response to the other vitamin deficiency, as well as the specific deficiency.

Generally, it is best to determine which deficiency exists and treat the patient with the specific deficient vitamin. Large doses of folic acid are proven to correct the anemia in vitamin B₁₂ deficiency but do not correct or halt demyelination and neurologic disease. This makes diagnosis and specific therapy critical in vitamin B₁₂ deficiency. Specific therapy causes a rise in the reticulocyte count after the 4th day of therapy. Reticulocytosis peaks at about 5 to 8 days and returns to normal after 2 weeks. The degree of reticulocytosis is proportional to the severity of the anemia with more striking reticulocytosis in patients with severe anemia. The hemoglobin rises about 2–3 g/dL every 2 weeks until normal levels are reached. The marrow responds quickly to therapy as evidenced by pronormoblasts (normal) appearing within 4–6 hours and nearly complete recovery of erythroid abnormalities within 2–4 days. Granulocyte abnormalities disappear more slowly. Hypersegmented neutrophils can usually be found for 12–14 days after therapy is begun.[18]

Specific therapy can reverse the peripheral neuropathy of vitamin B₁₂ deficiency, but spinal cord damage is usually irreversible. Pernicious anemia must be treated with lifelong monthly parenteral doses of hydroxycobalamin (OHCbl) because of these patients' inability to absorb oral vitamin B₁₂. Recently it was reported that large doses of vitamin B₁₂ therapy (usually 1000 to 2000 µg/day) administered orally could be feasible if the patient is followed carefully.[23] The oral treatment can be better tolerated and less expensive.[32] The rationale behind oral therapy using large doses of vitamin is that a small amount (from 1 to 3%) of the vitamin is absorbed by mass action without IF.

CASE STUDY (continued from page 272)

6. How would the diagnosis change if the special testing results were as follows?

Schilling test	Part I, before intrinsic factor, 1%
	Part II, after intrinsic factor, 3%
Intrinsic-factor-blocking antibodies	Negative

7. What would you predict this patient's reticulocyte count to be?

OTHER MEGALOBLASTIC ANEMIAS

A megaloblastic anemia occasionally is associated drugs, congenital enzyme deficiencies, or other hematopoietic diseases.

Drugs

A large number of drugs that act as metabolic inhibitors can cause megaloblastosis (Table 12-9 ✪). Some of these drugs are used in chemotherapy for malignancy. Although aimed at eliminating rapidly proliferating malignant cells, these drugs are not selective for malignant cells. Any normal proliferating cell including hematopoietic cells, is also affected.

Enzyme Deficiencies

Methionine synthase reductase (MSR) deficiency is a rare autosomal recessive disorder. A deficiency of this enzyme leads to a dysfunction of folate/cobalamin metabolism and results in hyperhomocysteinemia, hypomethioninemia, and megaloblastic anemia.[33] MSR is necessary for the reductive activation of methionine synthase and the resultant folate/vitamin B₁₂ dependent conversion of homocysteine to methionine.

Congenital Deficiencies

A congenital deficiency is a physiological aberration present at birth. The following congenital deficiencies result in megaloblastosis.

Orotic Aciduria   Inborn defects in enzymes required for pyrimidine synthesis or folate metabolism can result in megaloblastic anemia. Orotic aciduria is a rare autosomal recessive disorder in which there is a failure to convert orotic acid to uridylic acid. The result is excessive excretion of orotic acid. Children with this disorder also fail to grow and develop normally. The condition responds to treatment with oral uridine.

Congenital Dyserythropoietic Anemia   Congenital dyserythropoietic anemia (CDA) is actually a heterogeneous group of refractory, congenital anemias characterized by

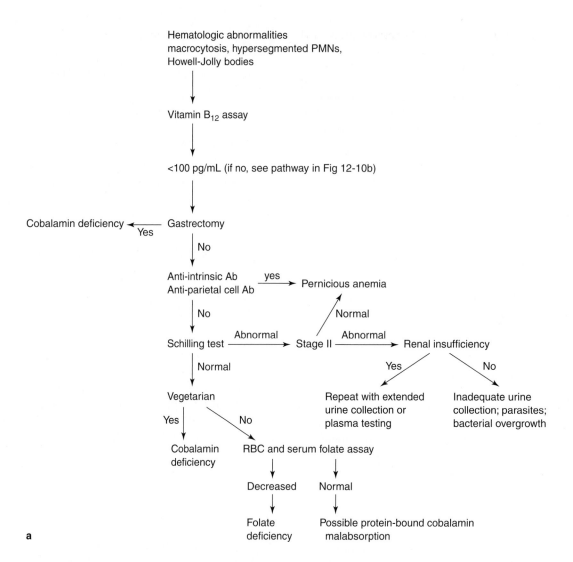

a

■ FIGURE 12-10   Algorithm of diagnosis of vitamin B$_{12}$ and folic acid deficiency using laboratory tests. The algorithm above (a) is followed if the serum vitamin B$_{12}$ level is <100 pg/mL. If higher, follow the algorithm to the right (b) Use this figure with Figure 12-1 to determine whether macrocytosis is megaloblastic or nonmegaloblastic. (Adapted, with permission, from: Snow CF. Laboratory diagnosis of vitamin B$_{12}$ and folate deficiency. *Arch Intern Med.* 1999;159:1289–98.)

✪ TABLE 12-9			
Drugs That Can Cause Megaloblastosis			
DNA Base Inhibitors			
Pyrimidine	Purine	Antimetabolites	Other
Azauridine	Acyclovir	Cytosine arabinoside	Azacytidine
	Adenosine arabinoside	Fluorocytidine	Cyclophosphamide
	Azathioprine	Fluorouracil	Zidovudine
	Gancyclovir	Hydroxyurea	
	Mercaptopurine	Methotrexate	
	Thioguanine		
	Vidarabine		

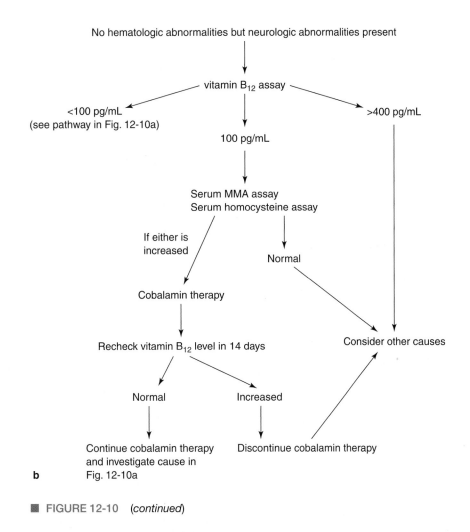

No hematologic abnormalities but neurologic abnormalities present

↓

vitamin B_{12} assay

<100 pg/mL
(see pathway in Fig. 12-10a)

100 pg/mL

>400 pg/mL

Serum MMA assay
Serum homocysteine assay

If either is
increased

Normal

Cobalamin therapy

Recheck vitamin B_{12} level in 14 days

Consider other causes

Normal

Increased

Continue cobalamin therapy
and investigate cause in
Fig. 12-10a

Discontinue cobalamin therapy

b

■ FIGURE 12-10   (*continued*)

both abnormal erythropoiesis and ineffective erythropoiesis (Table 12-10 ✪). There are three types: CDA I, CDA II, and CDA III. Types I and II are inherited as autosomal recessive disorders, and Type III is inherited in an autosomal dominant fashion. Red cell multinuclearity in the bone marrow and secondary siderosis are recognized in all types; however, megaloblastic erythroid precursors are present only in Type I and Type III.

- **CDA I.** Bone marrow erythroblasts are megaloblastic and often binucleate with incomplete division of nuclear segments. The incomplete nuclear division is characterized by internuclear chromatin bridges.
- **CDA II.** Bone marrow precursors are not megaloblastic but are typically multinucleated with up to seven nuclei (Figure 12-11 ■). Type II is distinguished by a positive acidified serum test (Ham test) but a negative sucrose

✪ TABLE 12-10

Comparison of Congenital Dyserythropoietic Anemia (CDA) Types

Characteristics	CDA I	CDA II	CDA III
Inheritance	Autosomal recessive	Autosomal recessive	Autosomal dominant
RBC multinuclearity	Present	Present	Present
Number of nuclear lobes	2	Up to 7	Up to 16
Siderosis	Present	Present	Present
Megaloblastosis	Present	Absent	Present
Other characteristics	Incomplete nuclear division	Positive Ham test (HEMPAS)	RBC agglutination by anti-I and anti-i antibodies

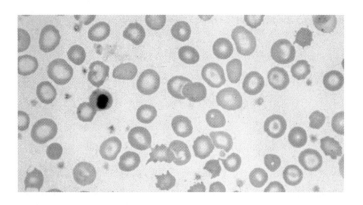

■ FIGURE 12-11   Peripheral blood of a case of congenital dyserythropoietic anemia type II (CDA-II). There is anisocytosis with microcytic, hypochromic cells as well as macrocytes and normocytes. Cabot's rings are visible. The nucleated cell is an orthochromic normoblast showing lobulation of the nucleus. (Wright-Giemsa stain; 1000× magnification).

hemolysis test. In the Ham test, only about 30% of normal sera are effective in lysing CDA II cells. This type has also been termed *hereditary erythroblastic multinuclearity* with positive acidified serum test (HEMPAS). CDA II is the most common of the three types of CDA.

- **CDA III.**   This type of CDA is morphologically distinct from Types I and II because of the presence of giant erythroblasts (up to 50 μm) containing up to l6 nuclei. Sometimes the erythrocytes are agglutinated by anti-I and anti-i antibodies.

Other Hematopoietic Diseases

The myelodysplastic syndromes are a group of stem cell disorders characterized by peripheral cytopenias and dyshematopoiesis. Erythroid precursors in the bone marrow frequently exhibit megaloblasticlike changes. There is occasionally a nonmegaloblastic macrocytic anemia. These diseases will be discussed in ∞ Chapter 23.

 Checkpoint! 12

Which clinical type of CDA gives a positive HAM test result and presents with a normoblastic marrow?

▶ MACROCYTIC ANEMIA WITHOUT MEGALOBLASTOSIS

The typical findings of megaloblastic anemia are not evident in other macrocytic anemias. The macrocytes in macrocytic anemias without megaloblastosis are not usually as pronounced as the macrocytes in megaloblastic anemia. In addition, these macrocytes are usually round rather than oval as seen in megaloblastic anemia. Hypersegmented neutrophils are not present, and leukocytes and platelets are quantita-

tively normal. Jaundice, glossitis, and neuropathy, the typical clinical findings in megaloblastosis are absent. The cause of the macrocytosis without megaloblastosis is unknown in many cases. It has been suggested that macrocytes could be due to an increase in membrane lipids or to a delay in blast maturation. Some diseases associated with nonmegaloblastic macrocytic anemia are listed in Table 12-11 ✪. Three of the most common are discussed in this section: alcoholism, liver disease, and reticulocytosis (stimulated erythropoiesis).

ALCOHOLISM

Alcohol abuse is one of the most common causes of nonanemic macrocytosis. It has been suggested that all patients with macrocytosis should be questioned about their alcohol consumption.[34] The macrocytosis associated with alcoholism is usually multifactorial and can be megaloblastic. Macrocytosis is probably the result of one or more of four causes: (1) folate deficiency due to decreased dietary intake, (2) reticulocytosis associated with hemolysis or gastrointestinal bleeding, (3) associated liver disease, and (4) alcohol toxicity.

Folate deficiency associated with a megaloblastic anemia is the most common cause of the macrocytosis found in hospitalized alcoholic patients. The deficiency probably results from poor dietary habits, although ethanol also appears to interfere with folate metabolism.

The reduced erythrocyte survival with a corresponding reticulocytosis has been associated with chronic gastrointestinal bleeding secondary to hepatic dysfunction (de-

✪ TABLE 12-11	
Conditions Associated with Nonmegaloblastic Macrocytosis	
Condition	**Cause of Macrocytosis**
Alcoholism	Direct toxic effect of alcohol on erythroid precursors
	Reticulocytosis associated with hemolysis or GI bleeding
	Liver disease: abnormal RBC membrane lipid composition
	Can also be megaloblastic from folate deficiency
Liver disease	Reticulocytosis associated with stimulated erythropoiesis; increased RBC membrane lipids
Hemolysis or post-hemorrhagic anemia	Reticulocytosis associated with stimulated erythropoiesis
Hypothroidism	Unknown
Aplastic anemia	Unknown
Artifactual	Cold agglutinin disease
	Severe hyperglycemia
	RBC clumping
	Swelling of RBCs

creased coagulation proteins) or thrombocytopenia, hypersplenism from increased portal and splenic vein pressure, pooling of cells in splenomegaly, and altered erythrocyte membranes caused by abnormal blood lipid content in liver disease (∞ Chapter 15). Stomatocytes are associated with acute alcoholism, but there appear to be no significant cation leaks, and hemolysis of these cells is not significant.

Liver disease is common in alcoholic individuals; typical hematologic findings associated with this disease are discussed in the following section. Even when anemia is absent, most alcoholic individuals have a mild macrocytosis (100–110 fL) unrelated to liver disease or folate deficiency. This can be caused by a direct toxic effect of the ethanol on developing erythroblasts. Vacuolization of red cell precursors, similar to that seen in patients taking chloramphenicol, is a common finding after prolonged alcohol ingestion. If alcohol intake is eliminated, the cells gradually assume their normal size, and the bone marrow changes disappear. The association of a sideroblastic anemia and alcoholism is discussed in ∞ Chapter 9.

The multiple pathologies of this type of anemia result in the possibility of a variety of abnormal hematologic findings. Thus, it is possible to have a blood picture resembling that of megaloblastic anemia, chronic hemolysis, chronic or acute blood loss, liver disease, or (more than likely) a combination of these conditions. Alcohol can also cause disordered heme synthesis as discussed in ∞ Chapter 9.

LIVER DISEASE

The most common disease associated with a nonmegaloblastic macrocytic anemia is liver disease (including alcoholic cirrhosis). The causes of this anemia are multifactorial and include hemolysis, impaired bone marrow response, folate deficiency, and blood loss (Table 12-12 ✪). Although macrocytic anemia is the most common form of anemia in liver disease, occurring in more than 50% of the patients, normocytic or microcytic anemia can also be found depending on the predominant pathologic mechanism.

Erythrocyte survival appears to be significantly shortened in alcoholic liver disease, infectious hepatitis, biliary cirrhosis, and obstructive jaundice. The reason for this is unknown. Cross-transfusion studies in which patient cells are infused into normal individuals demonstrate an increase in patient cell survival. These studies suggest an extracorpuscular factor is probably responsible for cell hemolysis. The spleen is thought to play an important role in sequestration and hemolysis in individuals with splenomegaly or hypersplenism. In some cases, hemolysis is well compensated for by an increase in erythropoiesis and there is no anemia. In some patients with alcoholic liver disease, a heavy drinking spree produces a brisk but transient hemolysis. These patients also show abnormal liver function and have markedly increased levels of plasma triglycerides.

Abnormalities in erythrocyte membrane lipid composition are common in hepatitis, cirrhosis, and obstructive jaundice. Both cholesterol and phospholipid are increased, resulting in cells with an increased surface-to-volume ratio. This abnormality is not thought to cause decreased cell survival. In contrast, in severe hepatocellular disease, erythrocyte membranes have an excessive amount of cholesterol relative to phospholipid, which decreases the erythrocyte deformability. This is associated with the formation of spur cells in which the erythrocyte exhibits spikelike projections. These cells have a pronounced shortened life span leading to an anemia termed *spur cell* (∞ Chapter 15).

Kinetic iron studies have revealed that the bone marrow response in liver disease can be impaired. It has been proposed that liver disease can affect the production of erythropoietin because this organ has been shown to be an important extrarenal source of the hormone in rats.[35] In alcoholic cirrhosis, the alcohol can have a direct suppressive effect on the bone marrow.

Clinical findings and symptoms in liver disease are secondary to the abnormalities in liver function. The liver is involved in many essential metabolic reactions and in the synthesis of many proteins and lipids. Therefore, the anemia is only a minor finding among the abnormalities associated with this organ's dysfunction.

The anemia is usually mild with an average hemoglobin concentration around 12 g/dL. With complications, the anemia can be severe. The erythrocytes can appear normocytic, macrocytic (usually not more than 115 fL MCV), or microcytic. A discrepancy between the MCV and the appearance of the cells microscopically often occurs. In these cases, thin, round macrocytes (as determined by diameter) with target cell formation are found on the blood smear, but the MCV is within normal limits. The reticulocyte count can be increased, but the RPI is usually less than 2 unless hemolysis is a significant factor. Thrombocytopenia is a frequent finding, and platelet function can be abnormal. Various nonspecific leukocyte abnormalities have been described including neutropenia, neutrophilia, and lymphopenia. The bone marrow is either normocellular or hypercellular, often with erythroid hyperplasia. The precursors are qualitatively normal unless folic acid deficiency is present. In this case, megaloblastosis is apparent with the typical associated blood abnormalities.

Other laboratory tests of liver function are variably abnormal including increased serum bilirubin and increased hepatic enzymes. Tests for carbohydrate and lipid metabolites are frequently abnormal depending on the degree of liver disease.

 Checkpoint! 13

What is the main cause of nonanemic macrocytosis?

STIMULATED ERYTHROPOIESIS

Increased erythropoietin (stimulation) in the presence of an adequate iron supply (e.g., autoimmune hemolytic anemia) can result in the release of shift reticulocytes from the bone

TABLE 12-12

Causes and Characteristics of Anemia in Liver Disease

Causes	Anemia Type	Characteristics
Abnormal liver function	Macrocytic	MCV normal to increased
		Increased RBC membrane cholesterol resulting in target cells and acanthocytes
		Normal to slightly increased reticulocytes
Folic acid deficiency	Macrocytic	MCV increased
		Pancytopenia
		Ovalocytes and teardrop cells
		Normal to decreased reticulocytes
		Functional folate deficiency
Stimulated erythropoiesis	Macrocytic	MCV increased
		Slightly increased WBC count
		Normal platelet count
		Shift reticulocytosis
Hemolysis	Normocytic or macrocytic	MCV normal to increased
		Spur cells and schistocytes
		Increased reticulocytes
Hypersplenism	Normocytic	MCV normal
		Pancytopenia
		Increased reticulocytes
		Portal hypertension
Marrow hypoproliferation	Normocytic	MCV normal
		Pancytopenia
		Decreased reticulocytes
		Associated with renal disease or alcohol suppression
Chronic blood loss	Microcytic	MCV decreased
		Iron deficiency
		Leukocyte and platelet counts slightly increased
		Reticulocytes increased
		Commonly associated with gastrointestinal bleeding

marrow. These cells are larger than normal with an MCV as high as 130 fL. A reticulocyte count and examination of the blood smear allow distinction of this macrocytic entity from megaloblastic anemia. In the presence of large numbers of shift reticulocytes, polychromasia has a marked increase. In addition, the oval macrocytes typical of megaloblastic anemia are not present in conditions associated with increased erythropoietin stimulation.

HYPOTHYROIDISM

Anemia of hypothyroidism presents as a mild to moderate anemia with a normal reticulocyte count. Thyroid hormone regulates cellular metabolic rate, and therefore tissue oxygen requirement. With a decrease in thyroid hormone (i.e., hy-

pothyroidism), tissue oxygen requirement is smaller, which is interpreted by the kidneys as a more than adequate oxygen tension. The net result is a decrease in the production of EPO and, correspondingly, erythrocytes. This type of anemia often presents as a macrocytic, normochromic anemia but can also be a normocytic, normochromic anemia. The anemia can be complicated by iron, folic acid, or B_{12} deficiencies, and the blood picture can reflect these forms of anemia.

 Checkpoint! 14

What are three clinical or laboratory findings (besides assessing the bone marrow) that can distinguish a nonmegaloblastic macrocytic anemia from a megaloblastic anemia?

SUMMARY

Macrocytosis due to megaloblastic anemia must be differentiated from macrocytosis with a normoblastic marrow. The laboratory test profile of a patient with megaloblastic anemia commonly indicates pancytopenia. The blood smear reveals macrocytes (i.e., large ovalocytes), poikilocytosis, teardrop cells, Howell-Jolly bodies, and neutrophil hypersegmentation. The marrow is characterized by megaloblastosis of precursor cells due to a block in thymidine production. Because thymidine is one of the four DNA bases, the deficiency leads to a diminished capacity for DNA synthesis and a block in mitosis. The marrow is hypercellular, but erythropoiesis is ineffective. Causes of megaloblastosis are nearly always due to vitamin B_{12} or folic acid deficiencies.

Folate is primarily acquired from the diet. Liver tissue is the main storage site of folic acid. Folate deficiency results in decreased synthesis of N^5,N^{10}-methylene THF, a cofactor in DNA synthesis. Consequently, DNA synthesis slows. Clinically, symptoms from inadequate dietary folate can occur within months as compared to years for a B_{12} deficiency.

Vitamin B_{12} (i.e., cyanocobalamin) absorption occurs in the small intestine. Dietary vitamin B_{12} is released from digestion of animal proteins in meats and bound by gastric R-proteins, and subsequently intrinsic factor (IF). Once absorbed, vitamin B_{12} is bound to specific plasma proteins known as *transcobalamin I, II,* or *III*. Normal serum vitamin B_{12} values are highly variable on age and sex. B_{12} function is related to DNA synthesis because vitamin B_{12} is a vital cofactor in the conversion of methyl tetrahydrofolate (i.e., folic acid) to tetrahydrofolate. This product is an important cofactor needed for the production of DNA thymidine.

Defective production of intrinsic factor is the most common cause of vitamin B_{12} deficiency (pernicious anemia—PA), which is caused by failure of the gastric mucosa to secrete IF. PA most commonly occurs in people after 40 years of age. Central nervous system symptoms such as numbness and tingling of the extremities, difficulty with balance and gait, loss of vibration sensation, weakness, spasticity, and personality changes can be present in advanced cases. The Schilling test is a definitive test useful in the diagnosis of intrinsic factor deficiency but is rarely used. Other causes of vitamin B_{12} deficiency include gastrectomy, malabsorption diseases such as Crohn's disease, and drugs. Megaloblastic anemia rarely results from chemotherapeutic drugs or congenital enzyme deficiencies or with other hematopoietic diseases such as congenital dyserythropoietic anemia.

Serum and RBC folate can be measured to diagnose folate deficiency, but the tests do not reliably indicate folate stores in the presence of vitamin B_{12} deficiency. Vitamin B_{12} levels can be directly assessed by measuring serum vitamin B_{12} or indirectly by measuring MMA in the urine/serum/plasma or homocysteine in plasma.

Macrocytosis due to megaloblastic anemia must be differentiated from macrocytosis with a normoblastic marrow. Normoblastic, macrocytic anemias can result from acute blood loss or hemolysis due to shift reticulocytosis from the marrow. Alcohol abuse is one of the most common causes of normoblastic macrocytosis. Liver disease, often resulting from alcohol abuse, is also commonly associated with macrocytosis without a megaloblastic marrow.

REVIEW QUESTIONS

LEVEL I

1. The most common cause of macrocytosis is: (Objective 5)
   a. folate deficiency
   b. alcoholism
   c. liver disease
   d. pernicious anemia

2. In the majority of cases, B_{12} deficiency is due to a deficiency of: (Objective 6)
   a. intrinsic factor
   b. vitamin B_6
   c. folate
   d. methylmalonic acid

3. Which of the following is the best clue in diagnosing megaloblastic anemia? (Objective 3)
   a. decreased hemoglobin and hematocrit
   b. leukocytosis
   c. hypersegmented neutrophils
   d. poikilocytosis

LEVEL II

1. If a patient presents with anemia, macrocytosis, pancytopenia, and malnutrition, which of the following should be investigated first as a possible cause of the anemia? (Objectives 4, 12)
   a. pernicious anemia
   b. folic acid deficiency
   c. B_{12} deficiency
   d. celiac disease

2. Which laboratory tests are most sensitive to decreased levels of vitamin B_{12}? (Objectives 8, 11)
   a. red cell and serum folate
   b. serum vitamin B_{12} and red cell folate
   c. transcobalamin II and III assays
   d. MMA and homocysteine

REVIEW QUESTIONS (continued)

LEVEL I

4. Increases in urinary excretion of formiminoglutamic acid (FIGLU) most likely indicates which of the following? (Objective 4)
   a. vitamin B_{12} deficiency
   b. autoantibodies to intrinsic factor
   c. folic acid deficiency
   d. hemolysis

5. The liver stores enough folate to meet daily requirement needs for how long? (Objective 2)
   a. 1 month
   b. 6–8 weeks
   c. 2 years
   d. 3–6 months

6. Which of the following conditions increases the daily requirement for vitamin B_{12}? (Objective 2)
   a. pregnancy
   b. aplastic anemia
   c. hypothyroidism
   d. splenectomy

7. A deficiency of vitamin B_{12} leads to impaired: (Objective 1)
   a. folic acid synthesis
   b. DNA synthesis
   c. intrinsic factor secretion
   d. absorption of folate

8. Laboratory diagnosis of pernicious anemia may include which of the following? (Objective 3)
   a. urinary FIGLU
   b. WBC count
   c. Gastric analysis
   d. LDH

9. Alcoholic individuals commonly develop a macrocytic anemia due to: (Objective 8)
   a. folate deficiency
   b. increased blood cholesterol levels
   c. development of autoantibodies against intrinsic factor
   d. intestinal malabsorption of B_{12}

10. Anemia due to liver disease is often associated with which of the following RBC morphological forms? (Objective 9)
    a. ovalocytes
    b. microcytes
    c. spur cells
    d. teardrop cells

LEVEL II

3. Which of the following can be found in a patient with megaloblastic anemia? (Objectives 2, 8, 11)
   a. giant metamyelocytes and hypolobated neutrophils
   b. Howell-Jolly bodies and Pappenheimer bodies
   c. hypersegmented neutrophils and oval macrocytes
   d. hypochromic macrocytes and thrombocytosis

4. The metabolic function of tetrahydrofolate is to: (Objective 1)
   a. synthesize methionine
   b. transfer carbon units from donors to receptors
   c. serve as a cofactor with cobalamin in the synthesis of thymidylate
   d. synthesize intrinsic factor

5. Folic acid deficiency can be caused by: (Objective 6)
   a. alcoholism
   b. chronic blood loss
   c. strict vegetarian diet
   d. vitamin B_6 deficiency

6. A lack of intrinsic factor could be due to: (Objective 7)
   a. gastrectomy
   b. vitamin B_{12} deficiency
   c. folate deficiency
   d. large bowel resection

7. Which of the following is more typical of nonmegaloblastic than megaloblastic anemia? (Objectives 2, 3)
   a. oval macrocytes
   b. round macrocytes
   c. Howell-Jolly bodies
   d. hypersegmented PMN

8. If a patient excretes less than 7.5% of a radioactively tagged crystalline B_{12} dose after 24 hours both before and after administration of a dose of oral intrinsic factor, which of the following is a possible diagnosis? (Objective 9)
   a. pernicious anemia
   b. liver disease
   c. gastrectomy
   d. celiac disease

9. Which type of congenital dyserythropoietic anemia (CDA) presents with giant multinucleated erythrocytes in the marrow? (Objective 10)
   a. CDA I
   b. CDA II
   c. CDA III
   d. CDA IV

REVIEW QUESTIONS (continued)

LEVEL I

LEVEL II

10. A 48-year-old Caucasian female experiencing fatigue, loss of appetite, and weight loss over a period of three months was seen by her physician. A medical history revealed she had a history of alcohol abuse. An initial laboratory workup demonstrated that she was anemic, had a leukocyte count of 3×10^9/L, and had an MCV of 119 fL. Macroovalocytes and neutrophil hypersegmentation was noted on her blood smear evaluation. Based on the initial laboratory test results, her physician obtained a serum vitamin B_{12} and folate workup. Results were as follows:

Serum vitamin B_{12}	550 pg/mL
Serum folate	4.0 ng/mL
RBC folate	105 ng/mL

Based on her clinical history and laboratory results, the best possible diagnosis is which of the following? (Objective 12)
a. pernicious anemia
b. folate deficiency
c. primary B_{12} deficiency
d. anemia of liver disease

www.pearsonhighered.com/mckenzie

Use this address to access the interactive Companion Website created for this textbook. Find additional information, tables and figures. Evaluate your command of the chapter information using case studies and critical thinking and multiple choice questions.

REFERENCES

1. Hoggarth K. Macrocytic anaemias. *Practitioner.* 1993;237(1525): 331–32, 335.

2. Colon-Otero G, Menke D, Hook CC. A practical approach to the differential diagnosis and evaluation of the adult patient with macrocytic anemia. *Med Clin North Am.* 1992;76:581–97.

3. Kass L. Pernicious anemia. In: Smith LH Jr, ed. *Major Problems in Internal Medicine, vol. 7.* Philadelphia: W.B. Saunders, Co; 1976:1–62.

4. Addison T. *On the Constitutional and Local Effects of Disease of the Suprarenal Capsules.* London, England: Sam Highley; 1855:43.

5. Ehrlich P. *Farbenanalytische Untersuchungen zur Histologie und Klinik des Blutes.* Berlin, Germany: A. Hirschwald; 1891:137.

6. Carmel R. Macrocytosis, mild anemia, and delay in the diagnosis of pernicious anemia. *Arch Intern Med.* 1979;139:47–50.

7. Hall CA. Vitamin B_{12} deficiency and early rise in mean corpuscular volume. *JAMA.* 1981;245:1144–46.

8. Spivak JL. Masked megaloblastic anemia. *Arch Intern Med.* 1982;142: 2111–14.

9. Carmel R, Weiner JM, Johnson CS. Iron deficiency occurs frequently in patients with pernicious anemia. *JAMA.* 1987;257:1081–83.

10. Chan CW et al. Diagnostic clues to megaloblastic anemia without macrocytosis. *Intern J Lab Hematol.* 2007;29(3):163–171.

11. Pruthi RK, Tafferi A. Pernicious anemia revisited. *Mayo Clin Pro.* 1994;69:144–50.

12. Lindenbaum J, Healton EB, Savage DG et al. Neuropsychiatric disorders caused by cobalamin deficiency in the absence of anemia or macrocytosis. *N Engl J Med.* 1988;318:1720–28.

13. Babior BM. Folate, cobalamin, and megaloblastic anemias. In: MA Lichtman, E Beutler, TJ Kipps, U Seligsohn, K Kaushansky, JT Prchal, eds. In *Williams Hematology*, 7th ed. New York: McGraw-Hill; 2006; 477–509.

14. Klee GG. Cobalamin and folate evaluation: Measurement of methylmalonic acid and homocysteine vs vitamin B_{12} and folate. *Clin Chem.* 2000;46(8 Pt 2):1277–83.

15. Jacques PF, Selhub J, Bostom AG, Wilson PWF, Rosenberg IH. The effect of folic acid fortification on plasma folate and total homocysteine concentrations. *N Engl J Med.* 1999;340:1449–54.

16. MRC Vitamin Study Research Group. Prevention of neural tube defects: Results of the Medical Research Council Vitamin Study. *Lancet.* 1991;338(8760):131–37.

17. Minot GR, Murphy W. Observations on patients with pernicious anemia partaking of a special diet. A. Clinical aspects. *Trans Assoc Am Physicians.* 1926;41:72–75.

18. Chanarin I. Megaloblastic anaemia, cobalamin, and folate. *J Clin Pathol.* 1987;40:978–84.

19. Hsing AW et al. Pernicious anemia and subsequent cancer: A population-based cohort study. *Cancer.* 1993;71:745–50.

20. Elin RJ, Winter WE. Methylmalonic acid: A test whose time has come. *Arc Path & Lab Med.* 2001;125(6):824–27.

21. Carson-Dewitt RS. Pernicious anemia. In *Gale Encyclopedia of Medicine.* Farmington Hills, MI: The Thomson Corp.; 2002;2224.

22. Sinha AK, Rijal S, Majhi S. Incidence of megaloblastic anemia and its correction in leishmaniasis—a prospective study at BPKIHS Hospital Hepal. *Ind J Path Micro.* 2006;49:528–31.

23. Oh R, Brown OL. Vitamin B12 deficiency. *Am Fam Phys.* 2003; 67(5):979–92.

24. Kumar V. Pernicious anemia. *MLO.* 2007;39(2):28–30.

25. Norman EJ, Morrison JA. Screening elderly populations for cobalamin (vitamin B_{12}) deficiency using the urinary methylmalonic acid assay by gas chromatography mass spectrometry. *Am J Med.* 1993;94:589–94.

26. Antony AC. Megaloblastic anemias. In R Hoffman et al., eds. *Hematology Basic Principles and Practice.* Philadelphia: Churchill Livingstone; 2005;519.

27. Welch GN, Loscalzo J. Homocysteine and atherothrombosis. *N Engl J Med.* 1998;338:1042–1050.

28. Carmel R, Melnyk S, James SJ. Cobalamin deficiency with and without neurologic abnormalities: Differences in homocysteine and methionine metabolism. *Blood.* 2003;101(8)3302–08.

29. Ridker PM, Hennekens CH, Selhub J, Miletich JP, Malinow MR, Stampfer MF. Interrelation of hyperhomocyst(e)inemia, factor V Leiden, and risk of future venous thromboembolism. *Circulation.* 1997;95:1777–82.

30. Holleland G, Schneede J, Ueland PM, Lund PK, Refsum H, Sandberg S. Cobalamin deficiency in general practice: Assessment of the diagnostic utility and cost-benefit analysis of methylmalonic acid determination in relation to current diagnostic strategies. *Clin Chem.* 1999;45:189–98.

31. Magera MF, Lacey JM, Casetta B, Rinaldo P. Method for the determination of total homocysteine in plasma and urine by stable isotope dilution and electrospray tandem mass spectrometry. *Clin Chem.* 1999;45:1517–22.

32. Balaman Z et al. Oral versus intramuscular cobalamin treatment in megaloblastic anemia: A single-center, prospective, randomized open-label study. *Clin Ther.* 2004;26(6):936.

33. Wilson A, Leclerc D, Rosenblatt DS, Gravel RA. Molecular basis for methionine synthase reductase deficiency in patients belonging to the cblE complementation group of disorders in folate/cobalamin metabolism. *Hu Mol Gene.* 1999;8:2009–16.

34. Seppa K, Sillanaukee P, Saarni M. Blood count and hematologic morphology in nonanemic macrocytosis: Differences between alcohol abuse and pernicious anemia. *Alcohol.* 1993;10:343–47.

35. Katz R et al. Studies on the site of production of erythropoietin. *Ann NY Acad Sci.* 1968;149:120–27.

13

Hypoproliferative Anemias

Rebecca Laudicina, Ph.D.

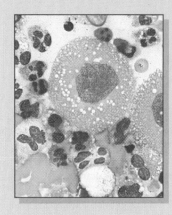

■ OBJECTIVES—LEVEL I

At the end of this unit of study, the student should be able to:

1. Define *hypoproliferative anemia*.
2. Cite the diagnostic criteria for aplastic anemia.
3. Describe the epidemiology and etiology of aplastic anemia.
4. Explain the pathophysiology of aplastic anemia.
5. Explain the difference between acquired and constitutional aplastic anemia.
6. List the major clinical and laboratory characteristics of aplastic anemia.
7. Identify environmental factors associated with the development of aplastic anemia.
8. Describe the etiology, bone marrow, and peripheral blood in pure red cell aplasia.
9. Identify peripheral blood findings associated with the following: aplastic anemia, pure red cell aplasia, and anemia due to renal disease.

■ OBJECTIVES—LEVEL II

At the end of this unit of study, the student should be able to:

1. List and explain possible causes of aplastic anemia.
2. Discuss prognosis in aplastic anemia.
3. Compare methods of treatment and management of patients with aplastic anemia.
4. Contrast aplastic anemia with other causes of pancytopenia on the basis of clinical findings and peripheral blood and bone marrow findings.
5. Compare and contrast pure red cell aplasia with aplastic anemia and other causes of erythroid hypoproliferation.
6. Compare and contrast major characteristics of Diamond-Blackfan syndrome and transient erythroblastopenia of childhood.
7. Explain the pathophysiology of anemia due to renal disease.
8. Evaluate laboratory test results and medical history of a clinical case for a patient with hypoproliferative anemia and suggest a possible diagnosis.

KEY TERMS

Aplasia
Aplastic anemia
Diamond-Blackfan anemia (DBA)
Dyshematopoiesis
Fanconi anemia (FA)
Hypocellularity
Hypoplasia
Hypoproliferative
Idiopathic
Myelophthisic anemia
Pancytopenia
Pure red cell aplasia

BACKGROUND BASICS

The information in this chapter builds on the concepts learned in previous chapters. To maximize your learning experience, you should review these concepts before starting this unit of study.

Level I

▶ Describe basic laboratory procedures used to screen for and assess anemia. (Chapter 34)
▶ Identify abnormal values and results for basic hematologic laboratory procedures. (Chapter 34)
▶ Outline the classification of anemias. (Chapter 8)
▶ Explain the process of hematopoiesis. (Chapter 3)

Level II

▶ Explain the concepts of stem cell renewal and differentiation. (Chapter 3)
▶ Describe the normal bone marrow structure and cellularity and the process of bone marrow examination. (Chapter 35)

ⓒ CASE STUDY

We will address this case study throughout the chapter.
Rachael, a 13-year-old female, was admitted to the hospital with complaints of progressive weakness and shortness of breath with minimal physical effort. She has experienced recurrent fevers reaching 102°F. Physical examination reveals a well-developed adolescent with good nutritional status and in no acute distress. There is no lymphadenopathy or organomegaly. Many petechial hemorrhages cover her chest and legs. Several bruises are found on her legs and thighs. Laboratory tests were ordered upon admission. Consider the diagnostic possiblilities in this case and how laboratory tests can be used to assist in differential diagnosis.

▶ OVERVIEW

The finding of cytopenias in the peripheral blood is a cause for concern. Although there are a variety of causes, bone marrow hypoproliferation is one of the most serious. This chapter discusses the acquired and constitutional anemias that are associated with bone marrow hypoproliferation. The first section describes the classification of hypoproliferative anemias followed by a discussion of aplastic anemia and pure red cell aplasia. These anemias are contrasted to other causes of cytopenia.

▶ INTRODUCTION

The **hypoproliferative** anemias are a heterogeneous group of acquired and constitutional disorders in which there is a normocytic or macrocytic, normochromic anemia associated with chronic bone marrow **hypocellularity**. Much of the area in the bone marrow normally occupied by hematopoietic tissue is replaced by fat. The terms *aplastic*, **aplasia**, and *hypoplastic* refer to a bone marrow with an overall decrease in hematopoietic cellularity. If there is **hypoplasia** of only one of the cellular elements, the terms *erythroid, myeloid,* or *megakaryocytic hypoplasia* should be used to define the specific entity.

The hematopoietic defect is due to depletion, damage, or inhibition of stem and/or progenitor cells. Either the unipotent erythroid progenitor cell or a multilineage hematopoietic precursor cell can be affected. The peripheral blood findings provide important clues to help identify the bone marrow abnormality. If only the erythroid progenitor cells are affected (BFU-E, CFU-E), platelets and leukocytes remain normal, and the diagnosis is **pure red cell aplasia.** More commonly, the multilineage hematopoietic precursor cells are affected (HSC, MPP, CMP, CFU-GEMM, etc.), resulting in **pancytopenia** (decrease of all three cell lineages), and the diagnosis is **aplastic anemia.**

▶ APLASTIC ANEMIA

The mature blood cells produced in aplastic anemia usually appear normal. Aplasia of the bone marrow is only one of several possible causes of peripheral blood pancytopenia. The term *aplastic anemia* should be reserved to describe the pancytopenia that is associated with a hypocellular bone marrow. Diagnostic criteria for aplastic anemia include:

- Bone marrow cellularity <25% plus at least two of the following:
  - Granulocyte count $<0.5 \times 10^9$/L
  - Platelet count $<20 \times 10^9$/L
  - Anemia with corrected reticulocyte count <1% (absolute count $<40 \times 10^9$/L))

Additional diagnostic criteria are based on disease severity.[1] With progression, all three cell lines eventually become decreased. This reflects an impaired proliferative capacity of the marrow stem cells, which loose their ability for normal cellular renewal.

 CASE STUDY *(continued from page 284)*

1. Select laboratory tests appropriate for screening for aplastic anemia.
2. Justify the selection of laboratory screening tests based on Rachael's clinical signs and symptoms.

 Checkpoint! 1

An anemic patient has a (corrected) reticulocyte count of 1.5%, hemoglobin of 100 g/L, hematocrit of 0.30 L/L, total neutrophil count of 0.4 × 10⁹/L, and a platelet count of 30 × 10⁹/L. Is it likely that this patient has aplastic anemia?

EPIDEMIOLOGY

These anemias are rare but are encountered more frequently now than at the beginning of the twentieth century. Aplastic anemia is most commonly seen in three age groups: 2–5 year olds, 15–25 year olds, and adults over 60. The occurrence of aplastic anemia in children is mostly due to inherited forms, but the occurrence in adults is due to acquired forms, although there are exceptions.[1,2] A geographic variation in incidence occurs with more cases in Asia than in western countries. It is believed that this variation is related to environmental and occupational factors.[3] Individual susceptibility can also play a role.

PATHOPHYSIOLOGY

Recent attention has been focused on immunologic suppression of hematopoiesis as a cause of acquired aplastic anemia. Response of marrow failure to immunosuppressive therapy has led to the characterization of most cases of acquired aplastic anemia as an autoimmune disease.[4] The immune mechanism responsible is thought to involve the suppression of stem cell growth and differentiation by abnormal T lymphocytes. This is supported by finding that treatment of patients with immunosuppressive drugs including antilymphocyte globulin (ALG), antithymocyte globulin (ATG), and cyclosporine results in improvement in the majority.[5]

Immunosuppressive therapy presumably eliminates an abnormal population of activated T lymphocytes that produce interferon-γ (IFN-γ) and tumor necrosis factor (TNF), substances known to inhibit hematopoiesis.[4,6] One mechanism of inhibition is likely cell killing through induction of apoptosis. Both IFN-γ and TNF induce overexpression of Fas

(a cell membrane receptor) by progenitor cells. When the Fas receptor is activated by binding with its ligand, apoptosis is initiated (∞ Chapter 2). It is estimated that stem cell concentration in severe acquired aplastic anemia is decreased to <1% of normal. Experimental studies using lymphocytes from patients with acquired aplastic anemia also tend to support the immunosuppression hypothesis. Flow cytometric analysis of lymphocyte subpopulations in acquired aplastic anemia has revealed a marked increase in activated CD8⁺ lymphocytes.

In Epstein-Barr viral infections as well as other viral infections, the virus can infect the hematopoietic stem cell, triggering an immune response. Cytotoxic lymphocytes then destroy the stem cell. Other mechanisms of stem cell damage in viral infections have been postulated, including direct cytotoxicity of the virus and inhibition of cellular proliferation and differentiation.[4]

The success of hematopoietic stem cell transplants (SCT) in many patients with aplastic anemia suggests that the bone marrow deficit can be corrected by repopulation of the marrow with normal stem cells. Thus, defective or deficient stem cells are apparently a common cause of this type of anemia rather than a defective marrow hematopoietic microenvironment. This is also supported by the results of long-term bone marrow culture assays in which marrow cells from patients with aplastic anemia exhibit defective hematopoiesis when grown on normal bone marrow stroma.[7,8] Aplastic anemia bone marrow cells grow significantly lower numbers of colonies compared to normal marrow. Likewise, deficiency of hematopoietic cytokine stimulation does not appear to be causative because most patients have normal or even elevated levels of growth factors. The stem cell abnormality can either be acquired or hereditary in nature.

CLASSIFICATION AND ETIOLOGY

Aplastic anemia can be classified into two groups: acquired and constitutional (Table 13-1 ⊙). Historically, much attention has focused on association between acquired aplastic anemia and environmental exposures. Drugs, chemicals, radiation, infectious agents, and other factors have been linked to the development of acquired aplastic anemia, which can be temporary or persistent. In most cases, no environmental link can be identified, and the cause is said to be **idiopathic**. The immune pathophysiologic model (discussed in previous section) provides a unifying basis for understanding the disorder regardless of the presence or absence of environmental factors. Although acquired aplastic anemia is more common in adults, it is also a cause of aplasia in children.

Constitutional aplastic anemia is a chronic failure of the bone marrow due to an inherited abnormality; it may or may not be present at birth. A congenital condition is one that is manifest early in life, often at birth, but that is not necessarily inherited or constitutional; it can be caused by acquired factors (e.g., maternal exposure to an environmental toxin

TABLE 13-1

Classification of Hypoproliferative Anemias

Aplastic Anemia	Pure Red Cell Aplasia	Other Hypoproliferative Anemias
Acquired	Transitory infections	Anemia of chronic renal disease
Idiopathic	Acquired pure red cell aplasia	Anemia associated with endocrine abnormalities
Drugs: chloramphenicol, phenylbutazone, old compounds, sulfa drugs, antihistamines, antithyroid, tetracyclines, penicillin, methylphenylethylhydantoin	Acute: infections, transient erythroblastopenia of childhood (TEC), drugs	
Chemical agents: benzene, insecticides, hair dye, carbon tetrachloride, chemotherapeutics (vincristine, busulfan, etc.), arsenic	Chronic: thymoma, autoimmune disorders	
Ioninzing radiation	Constitutional: Diamond-Blackfan anemia	
Biological agents: parovirus, infectious mononucleosis, infectious hepatitis, measles, influenza, errors of amino acid metabolism, starvation		
Pregnancy		
Paroxysmal nocturnal hemoglobinuria		
Constitutional		
Fanconi anemia		
Familial aplastic anemia		

while pregnant). Constitutional aplastic anemia can be associated with other congenital anomalies. This form is rare and less understood than acquired aplastic anemia. The defect can be a quantitative or qualitative abnormality of stem cells.

CASE STUDY *(continued from page 285)*

3. Evaluate the relationship between Rachael's age and the likelihood that she has aplastic anemia.

4. If aplastic anemia is present, would you expect her to have an idiopathic or secondary form? Explain your answer.

Acquired Forms of Aplastic Anemia

Idiopathic Approximately 50–70% of cases of aplastic anemia cannot be linked to an environmental factor; however, some unrecognized previous agent or event could be responsible for stimulation of the immune system.

Drugs About 30% of acquired forms of aplastic anemia are associated with drug exposure. It has been proposed that some drugs are not easily metabolized by the individual; as a result, the drug accumulates, causing injury to stem cells.[9] It is also possible that drugs can induce an antibody-mediated suppression of the marrow. With drug injury, neutropenia usually develops before anemia or thrombocytopenia be-

cause of the relatively short life span of the neutrophil. Within 7 days after stem cell injury or suppression, the neutrophil bone marrow reserve is exhausted and neutropenia develops. The longer life span of erythrocytes and platelets provides a buffer for a limited time until stem cell differentiation can resume if it does.

Chloramphenicol, a broad spectrum antibiotic, is a well-known drug associated with aplastic anemia. Because of concerns about bone marrow toxicity, the drug is rarely prescribed in the United States.[10]

Because aplasia develops in some individuals after exposure to certain drugs and chemicals while in others it does not, there is probably a genetic or acquired defect in drug elimination or detoxification. Also perhaps some individuals have stem cells that are more vulnerable to damage or inhibition by drugs and chemicals than others.

Chemical Agents The widespread use of toxic chemical agents in industry and agriculture is probably responsible for the increased incidence of toxic bone marrow aplasia.[9] Benzene derivatives are well established as a cause of bone marrow depression. Most cases develop within a few weeks after exposure, but some occur months or years after chronic exposure. Although stem cells can be damaged, the main toxic effect of benzene is usually expressed on transient stages of committed proliferating blood cells.

Most of the chemicals used in chemotherapy of malignant diseases kill rapidly proliferating cells. However, the chemicals do not distinguish between malignant and normal cells. Therefore, all proliferating cells are damaged, including normal cells of the hematopoietic compartment. Although quiescent (G_0) stem cells are spared, repeated doses of the chemical over a long period of time can eventually deplete the remaining stem cells as they enter the proliferating pool.

Ionizing Radiation   Aplastic anemia due to x-irradiation has been encountered in persons exposed in industrial accidents, military nuclear tests, and therapeutic regimens for malignancy. The effects of irradiation are dose dependent. Small doses affect all cells but are especially destructive to rapidly dividing cells. The bone marrow can recover from sublethal doses of irradiation because quiescent stem cells become active after exposure-induced depletion of more differented progeny. In high doses, more than 4000 rads, bone marrow aplasia and peripheral blood pancytopenia are usually permanent. The aplasia appears to be caused by damage of the supporting marrow matrix. Thus, bone marrow transplantation is usually unsuccessful in alleviating pancytopenia in these cases.

Infectious Agents   Viral and bacterial infections can be followed by a transient cytopenia. The aplasia can be limited to the erythroid elements or can include all three cell lineages. Aplasia has been described in patients after recovery from infectious mononucleosis, tuberculosis, and hepatitis. Hepatitis-associated aplastic anemia does not appear to be caused by any of the known hepatitis viruses and is often fatal if untreated.[11,12] In patients with hereditary hemolytic anemias, aplastic crisis is commonly associated with human parvovirus infection. This aplasia, however, is limited to the erythroid lineage.

Metabolic   The rare inborn errors of amino acid metabolism, which result in accumulation of ketones and glycine, have been associated with aplastic anemia.

Starvation or protein deficiency results in hypoproliferative anemia after about three months of deprivation. Starvation that is not self-induced usually occurs in areas where other endemic pathologies are also present, such as parasitic infection and blood loss. Thus, the causes of this anemia can be multifactorial.

Decreased hormonal stimulation of hematopoietic stem cells is important primarily as a factor in erythroid hypoplasia. Renal disease and endocrine diseases are examples of hypoproliferation caused by a decrease in erythropoietin.

Rarely, a life-threatening pancytopenia occurs during pregnancy. The condition usually remits after delivery or abortion. It has been suggested that the aplasia can be related to estrogen inhibition of stem cell proliferation.[13]

Paroxysmal Nocturnal Hemoglobinuria   Paroxysmal nocturnal hemoglobinuria (PNH) is an acquired stem cell disease in which a blood cell membrane abnormality makes the cells susceptible to in vivo complement hemolysis. The defect is the absence of a membrane glycolipid that serves to attach and anchor proteins to the cell. Although considerable variation in clinical manifestations occurs, the typical picture in severe cases is pancytopenia and marrow hypoplasia. Between 10–25% of patients with an initial diagnosis of aplastic anemia develop an abnormal erythrocyte population typical of that seen in PNH, but they do not usually develop the full clinical manifestations (intravascular hemolysis and venous thrombosis) of PNH. PNH is a prominent, later complication in aplastic anemia patients who have received immunosuppressive ALG therapy.[14] PNH will be discussed in detail in ∞ Chapter 15.

Other Diseases   Aplastic anemia also is associated with myelodysplastic syndromes (∞ Chapter 23), leukemia, and solid tumors. Some evidence suggests that the high frequency of these neoplastic, clonal disorders in patients treated for aplastic anemia can be inherent in the disease, not simply secondary to treatment.[14]

 CASE STUDY *(continued from page 286)*

For the past three months, Rachael's family physician has been following her recovery from viral hepatitis. Her recovery was uneventful; her liver enzyme levels returned to normal within two months. She has no other past medical history. There is no family history of hematologic disorders.

5. What aspect of this patient's history could be associated with the occurrence of aplastic anemia?

Constitutional Aplastic Anemia

This group of anemias has a congenital predisposition. Included are Fanconi anemia and other causes of constitutional aplastic anemia.

Fanconi Anemia   **Fanconi anemia (FA)** is an autosomal recessive disorder resulting from a heterogeneous molecular defect and is characterized by abnormal chromosomal fragility. It has a prevalence of about 1 in 350,000 live births in North America with a heterozygote frequency of ~1 in 300. Patients can have a complex assortment of congenital anomalies in addition to a progressive bone marrow hypoplasia. The congenital defects include dysplasia of bones, renal abnormalities, and other organ malformations as well as mental retardation, dwarfism, microcephaly, hypogonadism, and skin hyperpigmentation. Some patients lack congenital defects and may not be diagnosed until aplastic anemia develops, which may not occur until adulthood.[15]

Aplastic anemia eventually develops in ~90% of FA patients. The hematological manifestations are slowly progressive from birth and need to be monitored closely. Usually clinical signs of pancytopenia appear between the ages of 5 and 10 years with the median age of 7 at diagnosis. Anemia is usually macrocytic (although it can be normocytic) with macrocytosis often preceding anemia. Erythrocytes often show increased levels of Hemoglobin F and the "i" antigen (reflecting hematologic stress and the development of erythrocytes from earlier erythroid progenitor cells). Leukopenia primarily involves the granulocytes. Thrombocytopenia often precedes anemia and leukopenia. Androgen therapy can reverse the pancytopenia for several years (in about 50% of FA patients). Cytokine therapy can help increase neutophil counts.

SCT offers the only possible curative treatment for bone marrow failure in FA patients. In patients with HLA-matched sibling donors, 5-year survival is close to 75%. Stem cells from HLA-matched unrelated donors have also been used. Because FA patients are acutely sensitive to chemotherapeutic agents and radiation, pretransplant conditioning protocols must be altered to reduce toxicity.

The risk for developing cancer in FA is 20%.[16] Acute non-lymphocytic leukemia and solid tumors are common complications. Leukemia is difficult to treat and survival is poor. The median survival for FA patients is now about 30 years of age.[1]

Karyotyping of FA cells shows increased spontaneous chromosomal breakage, gaps, rearrangements, exchanges, and duplications. Diagnosis of FA has involved exposing blood lymphocytes or skin fibroblasts to crosslinking agents such as mitomycin C, diepoxybutane, or cisplatin that amplify chromosomal breakage.[1,16] Molecular techniques are or will soon be available to identify the various FA molecular subtypes. Testing is performed when warranted based on clinical findings and/or abnormal blood counts.

Research to identify the genes involved in FA has revealed that the molecular defect is heterogeneous. Eleven FA genes have been identified (*FANCA, B, C, D1, D2, E, F, G, I, J,* and *L*), but the biologic role has not been determined for all of them.[17] Interestingly, the breast cancer susceptibility gene, *BRCA2*, has been identified as the abnormal gene in *FANCB* and perhaps *FANCD1*. Six of the Fanconi proteins (A, B, C, E, F, and G) function in a common cellular pathway, activated in response to DNA damage, which in turn activates DNA repair proteins, including *BRCA1* and *FANCD1/BRCA2*. Defective FA proteins are thus responsible for the genetic instability and increased apoptosis of hematopoietic stem cells, resulting in aplastic anemia.[1,17] In addition to the genetic defects leading to defective DNA repair and DNA instability, TNFα is elevated in most patients. Also the telomeres of the hematopoietic stem and progenitor cells are shortened, suggesting an abnormally high proliferative rate, ultimately leading to their premature senescence.

Other Causes of Constitutional Aplastic Anemia.
Several other, rare disorders have a predisposition to developing aplastic anemia. Congenital amegakaryocytic thrombocytopenia (CAT) presents in infancy with isolated thrombocytopenia due to reduced or absent marrow megakaryocytes. Aplastic anemia subsequently develops in ~45% of the pa-

tients, usually in the first years of life. The defect is a mutation in the gene for the thrombopoietin (TPO) receptor *MPL* with the loss of the antiapoptotic effect of TPO on hematopoietic stem cells (∞ Chapter 3).

Patients with Shwachman-Diamond Syndrome can present with some of the same congenital anomalies including aplastic anemia as is seen in FA patients. However, they also have exocrine pancreatic dysfunction and do not display increased chromosomal fragility and defective DNA repair processes. This disorder is due to mutations of the *SBDS* gene, although the exact pathogenesis of the disorder is still unknown.

Dyskeratosis congenita (DC) is also an inherited bone marrow failure syndrome, resulting in aplastic anemia in ~50% of cases. Types of physical abnormalities and mutations differ for patients with DC and FA. Mutations in two genes have been associated with DC: *DKC1* and *TERC*. Mutations in these two genes result in markedly reduced telomerase activity, telomere shortening, early progenitor senescence, and a reduced stem cell compartment. Because not all persons carrying these mutations develop aplastic anemia, it may be that an additional acquired factor(s) (e.g., viral infection) is needed for bone marrow failure to develop.[1]

 CASE STUDY *(continued from page 287)*

6. Is it likely that Rachael has a constitutional form of aplastic anemia? Explain your answer.

CLINICAL FINDINGS

The onset of symptoms in aplastic anemia is usually insidious and related to the cytopenias. The most common initial sign is bleeding accompanied by petechial and fundal hemorrhages. Anemia and infection can occur separately or in combination with the bleeding. Hepatosplenomegaly and lymphadenopathy are absent. Splenomegaly has occasionally been noted in later stages of the disease, but if found in the early stages, the diagnosis of aplastic anemia should be questioned.

LABORATORY FINDINGS

Laboratory studies of peripheral blood and bone marrow are always indicated if a diagnosis of aplastic anemia is suspected.

Peripheral Blood
Pancytopenia is typical. Although the degree of severity can vary, it is good practice to question the diagnosis of aplastic anemia unless the leukocyte count, erythrocyte count, and platelet count are all below the reference intervals. Hemoglobin is usually < 70 g/L. Erythrocytes appear normocytic and

normochromic, or they can be slightly macrocytic. Mild to moderate anisocytosis and poikilocytosis occur. The presence of nucleated erythrocytes and teardrops is not typical of aplastic anemia but suggests marrow replacement (myelophthisic anemia). The relative reticulocyte count (%) alone can be misleading due to the severe anemia. Therefore, the reticulocyte count should always be determined in absolute numbers or be corrected for the anemia before interpretation. The absolute reticulocyte count is usually $< 25 \times 10^9$/L. The corrected reticulocyte count is less than 1%. Most often, thrombocytopenia is present at the time of diagnosis. Neutropenia precedes leukopenia; initially, lymphocyte and monocyte counts are normal. Because of the neutropenia, the differential count reflects a relative lymphocytosis. When the leukocyte count is below 1.5×10^9/L, an absolute lymphocytopenia is also present. The band to segmented neutrophil ratio increases, and occasionally more immature forms are found. Neutrophil granules are frequently larger than normal and stain a dark red; these granules should be distinguished from toxic granules, which are bluish black.

CASE STUDY (continued from page 288)

7. Correlate Rachael's clinical findings of weakness and shortness of breath, as well as petechial hemorrhages and bruises, with her laboratory screening results, which follow.

   Admission laboratory data for patient:

RBC	2.42×10^{12}/L
Hb	71 g/L
Hct	0.24 L/L
PLT	8.0×10^9/L
WBC	1.2×10^9/L
Differential	
Segmented neutrophils	2%
Lymphocytes	94%
Monocytes	4%
Uncorrected reticulocyte count	0.7%

8. Evaluate each of the patient's laboratory results by comparing them to reference ranges.
9. Which of the patient's routine laboratory results are consistent with those expected for aplastic anemia?
10. Classify the morphologic type of anemia.
11. Calculate the absolute lymphocyte count. Are her lymphocytes truly elevated as suggested by the relative lymphocyte count?
12. Correct the reticulocyte count. Why is this step important?
13. Calculate the absolute reticulocyte count.

Bone Marrow

Examination of the bone marrow is necessary to differentiate aplastic anemia from other diseases accompanied by pancytopenia. In aplastic anemia, the bone marrow is hypocellular with more than 70% fat (Figure 13-1 ■). This sometimes makes aspiration difficult. Bone marrow infiltration with granulomas or cancer cells can lead to fibrosis, also resulting in a hypocellular dry tap on aspiration. Thus, both aspiration and biopsy are needed for a correct diagnosis. It is recommended that several different sites be aspirated because spot sampling of an organ as large as the marrow can be misleading. Some areas of acellular stroma and fat can be infiltrated with clusters of lymphocytes, plasma cells, and reticulum cells. Areas of focal hyperplasia termed *hot spots* are found predominantly in early remission but can also be found in severe refractory cases. Iron stain reveals many iron granules in macrophages but granules are rarely seen in normoblasts.

CASE STUDY (continued)

Rachael was referred to a hematologist who ordered a bone marrow examination. The aspirate obtained was inadequate for evaluation due to lack of marrow spicules. Only a single site was aspirated. Touch preps made from the biopsy showed a markedly hypocellular marrow with very few hematopoietic cells. Cells present consisted of lymphocytes, plasma cells, and stromal cells. There were no malignant cells present.

14. Compare these results with those expected for a person with aplastic anemia.
15. Interpret the significance of the lack of malignant cells and hematopoietic blasts.
16. Suggest a way to improve the validity of bone marrow examination results for this patient.

Other Laboratory Findings

Other abnormal findings are not specific for aplastic anemia but are frequently found associated with the disease. Hemoglobin F can be increased, especially in children.

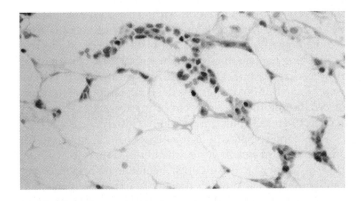

■ FIGURE 13-1   Bone marrow preparation from a patient with aplastic anemia shows marked hypocellularity (10%). The patches of cells remaining are primarily lymphocytes. (Wright-Giemsa stain; 100× magnification)

Erythropoietin is often increased, particularly when compared to the erythropoietin levels in patients with similar degrees of anemia. Serum iron is increased with > 50% saturation of transferrin, reflecting erythroid suppression. The clearance rate of iron (Fe^{59}) from the plasma is decreased because of the decrease in iron utilization by a hypoactive marrow. Coagulation tests that reflect platelet activity are abnormal in relation to the degree of thrombocytopenia.

PROGNOSIS AND THERAPY

Recent advances in treatment have tempered the previously grim prognosis of patients diagnosed with aplastic anemia. Bone marrow transplantation and immunosuppression have improved survival. Presently the 2-year survival rate is 60–90%.[18]

The first aim in management of acquired aplastic anemia is removal of a putative causative agent. This can involve withdrawal of drugs or removal of the patient from a hazardous environment. The immediate mode of treatment is often supportive. Patients can require multiple transfusions of erythrocytes, platelets, and leukocytes.

Stem cell transplants using cells collected from bone marrow or peripheral blood have become a relatively common procedure and are curative in most patients with aplastic anemia. Treatment complications and posttransplant mortality remain high; therefore, the probability for long-term cure must be weighed against the inherent risks of complications, including graft-versus-host disease and early and late toxicities of the conditioning regimen.[19] Survival rates range from 91% (identical-twin donor) to 37% (mismatched donors).[20] Although replacement of needed stem cells is successful in most cases, some transplants, even some performed between identical twins, do not induce remission. These unsuccessful transplants suggest that stem cell growth is immunosuppressed, or damage to the hematopoietic microenvironment may occur, preventing successful engraftment.[19] (See ∞ Chapter 27 on hematopoietic SCT.)

Immunosuppressive therapy (IST) using ATG or ALG, either solely or in combination with cyclosporine A, has become standard treatment for the majority of patients with acquired aplastic anemia.[5] IST with ALG or ATG is effective in restoring hematopoiesis in between 40–70% of patients.[21] However, at least 15–20% of patients treated with IST develop some form of clonal disease. Long-term complications of IST include the development of marrow clonal disorders such as PNH, leukemia, and myelodysplasia.[15,21]

Hematopoietic growth factors (HGF), G-CSF and GM-CSF, are also used in treatment (∞ Chapter 3). When used alone, HGF do not result in sustained hematologic responses but can be useful as an adjunct therapy to immunosuppression. Serious side effects and the potential for development of clonal disorders raise questions about HGF use in treating aplastic anemia. The use of HGF in combination with IST requires further study.[22]

CASE STUDY *(continued from page 289)*

17. Appraise the prognosis for Rachael.
18. Predict a treatment regimen.

DIFFERENTIATION OF APLASTIC ANEMIA FROM OTHER CAUSES OF PANCYTOPENIA

Pancytopenia can be associated with anemias other than aplastic anemia, but these anemias differ from aplastic anemia in that the pancytopenia is not the result of a defect in stem cell proliferation. Rather, the bone marrow is normocellular, hypercellular, or infiltrated with abnormal cellular elements. These anemias are mentioned here to help the health care professional differentiate them from the true hypoproliferative anemias.

Myelophthisic Anemia

Myelophthisic signifies marrow replacement or infiltration by fibrotic, granulomatous, or neoplastic cells (∞ Chapter 22). The abnormal replacement cells reduce normal hematopoiesis and disrupt the normal bone marrow architecture, allowing the release of immature cells into the peripheral blood. Anemia can be accompanied by normal, increased, or decreased leukocyte and platelet counts. The most characteristic findings are a leukoerythroblastic reaction and a moderate to marked poikilocytosis. Dacryocytes are common, as are large bizarre platelets. By contrast, nucleated erythrocytes and significant morphologic changes are almost never found in the peripheral blood in aplastic anemia. **Myelophthisic anemia** is associated with diffuse cancer of the prostate, breast, and stomach. It is also typical of myelofibrosis and lipid storage disorders.

Myelodysplastic Syndromes

Myelodysplastic syndromes (MDS) are a group of hematological disorders that have a propensity to terminate in acute leukemia (∞ Chapter 23). The principal peripheral blood findings are pancytopenia, bicytopenia, or isolated cytopenias with reticulocytopenia. A macrocytic anemia is common. The bone marrow, however, is usually normocellular or hypercellular with various degrees of qualitative abnormalities of one or more cell lines (**dyshematopoiesis**). Signs of dyshematopoiesis are also reflected in morphologic abnormalities of one or more cell lineages in the peripheral blood. These qualitative abnormalities of peripheral blood cells are useful in differentiating cytopenias due to true hypoproliferation of stem cells (aplastic anemia) from cytopenias due to dyshematopoiesis (ineffective erythropoiesis).

On the other hand, a subgroup of patients with an MDS diagnosis has a hypocellular marrow. This condition is referred to as *hypoplastic MDS (HMDS)*. In these cases, differentiation of MDS and aplastic anemia can be complicated if there are few bone marrow cells from a biopsy or aspirate to examine. If granulocytic and megakaryocytic dysplasia are seen and/or if an abnormal karyotype consistent with MDS is present, HMDS can be diagnosed. However, if only erythroid dysplasia is present, the evidence is insufficient to differentiate HMDS and aplastic anemia because erythroid dysplasia can be found in some cases of aplastic anemia.[23]

Congenital Dyserythropoietic Anemia

Congenital dyserythropoietic anemia (CDA) is a very rare familial refractory anemia characterized by both abnormal erythropoiesis and ineffective erythropoiesis. The bone marrow is normocellular or hypercellular, but the peripheral blood is pancytopenic. In contrast to the normal erythroid precursors found in aplastic anemia, erythrocyte precursors in the bone marrow of CDA patients exhibit multinuclearity, and myeloblasts and promyelocytes are increased. The anemia can be normocytic, but most often it is macrocytic. The three types of CDA are discussed in ∞ Chapter 12.

Hypersplenism

Hypersplenism from a variety of causes can result in a lack of one or more cellular elements of the blood as these elements become pooled and sequestered in the spleen. In this condition, the bone marrow is hyperplastic, corresponding to the peripheral blood cytopenia. Anemia is accompanied by a reticulocytosis as opposed to the reticulocytopenia found in the true hypoproliferative anemias. Granulocytopenia can be accompanied by a shift to the left in these cells. From a clinical standpoint, splenomegaly and other findings of the underlying disease are important in diagnosing this disorder. Splenectomy, although not always advisable, corrects the cytopenias.

Other

Deficiency of cobalamin or folic acid can be accompanied by pancytopenia (∞ Chapter 12). The bone marrow in these cases, however, reveals normocellularity or hypercellularity with megaloblastic changes. In the peripheral blood, hypersegmented neutrophils and Howell-Jolly bodies are typical but are not found in pancytopenia of aplastic anemia.

CASE STUDY *(continued from page 290)*

19. What other hematologic conditions must be ruled out for this patient?

20. What laboratory test is most beneficial in differentiating aplastic anemia from these other disorders? Compare the expected results of aplastic anemia with those of the other disorders.

▶ PURE RED CELL APLASIA

Pure red cell aplasia is characterized by a selective decrease in erythroid precursor cells in the marrow and by peripheral blood anemia. The disease is thought to occur due to selective hypoproliferation of the committed erythroid progenitor cell. The term *aplastic anemia* should be avoided in describing this disease because there is no disturbance of granulopoiesis or thrombopoiesis. Reticulocytes can be present but are less than 1% when corrected for the degree of anemia. Pure red cell aplasia can be acquired (acute or chronic) or inherited. Acquired pure red cell aplasia is seen in thymoma with administration of certain drugs, in autoimmune disorders, and in infection. Transient erythroblastopenia of childhood (TEC) is an acquired, self-limiting form of erythroid hypoplasia found in children. Results of laboratory tests in pure red cell aplasia are shown in Table 13-2 ☉.

ACQUIRED ACUTE PURE RED CELL APLASIA

Viral (parvovirus, Epstein-Barr virus, and viral hepatitis) and/or bacterial infections can be associated with a temporary depression of erythropoiesis. Transient erythroblastopenia of childhood is a form of acquired acute pure red cell aplasia, but because of the importance of distinguishing this pediatric anemia from Diamond-Blackfan anemia (DBA), it will be discussed with DBA in a following section.

In individuals who have a normal erythrocyte life span and hemoglobin level, temporary erythroid hypoproliferation is not noticed. However, if the erythrocyte life span is decreased, the complication of erythroid hypoproliferation

---

☉ TABLE 13-2

Laboratory Findings in Pure Red Cell Aplasia

Test	Findings
Erythrocyte count, hematocrit, and hemoglobin	Decreased
Reticulocyte count	Severely decreased
Leukocyte count	Normal or possibly increased
Platelet count	Normal or possibly increased
Bilirubin	Low or normal
Bone marrow	Absence of erythroid cells if examined early in disease; if examined later in disease progression, increase in young erythroid cells, which can be mistaken for an erythroid maturation arrest. If the patient is followed, however, these cells show normal maturation and differentiation. There is normal myelopoiesis and granulopoiesis.

can be life threatening (aplastic crises). These aplastic crises are most frequently noted in hemolytic anemias including sickle cell anemia, paroxysmal nocturnal hemoglobinuria, and autoimmune hemolytic anemias.

The aplastic crisis cases brought to the attention of a physician probably represent only a minor fraction of the actual occurrence of temporary erythroid aplasia. The aplastic crises are often preceded by fever with upper respiratory and intestinal complaints. Several members of the same family are frequently affected with the illness. Patients with concurrent hemolytic anemia have a rapid onset of lethargy and pallor. Patients without hemolytic anemia may seek medical attention because of the primary illness, and anemia is only an incidental finding.

If the anemia is severe, supportive therapy of packed erythrocyte transfusions can be necessary until spontaneous recovery occurs. Pure red cell aplasia associated with viral hepatitis has a poor prognosis.

Acute erythroid hypoplasia also occurs with the administration of some drugs and chemicals. After removal of the inciting agent, normal erythropoiesis usually resumes.

ACQUIRED CHRONIC PURE RED CELL APLASIA

An acquired selective depression of erythroid precursors is a rare disorder encountered in middle-aged adults. This disease usually occurs in association with thymoma, autoimmune hemolytic anemia, systemic lupus erythematosus, rheumatoid arthritis, and hematologic neoplasms (CLL, Hodgkin Disease). The high incidence of autoimmune disorders in this anemia suggests that an immunologic mechanism may be responsible for the red cell aplasia. Cytotoxic antibodies to erythropoietin-sensitive cells in the marrow and to erythropoietin have been demonstrated in some cases. More commonly, the mechanism appears to be a T cell-mediated immunosuppression of erythropoiesis.

Clinical findings are nonspecific. Pallor is usually the only physical finding. Therapies include transfusion with packed erythrocytes, thymectomy if the thymus is enlarged, and immunosuppression. Various treatments including prednisone, cyclosporine, cytotoxic agents, antithymocyte globulin, and monoclonal antibodies against B lymphocytes (rituximab/anti-CD20, alemtuzumab/anti-CD52) have been used to suppress the immune response. Androgens or erythropoietin to stimulate erythrocyte production is rarely used. In drug-induced red cell aplasia, withdrawal of the drug is indicated. Approximately 80% of patients with acquired pure red cell aplasia have a spontaneous remission or remission induced by immunosuppression. About half will relapse, but with additional immunosuppression, 80% will enter a second remission. By retreating relapsing patients or continuing maintenance immunosuppression, many can be maintained transfusion free for years.[24] Stem cell transplants are rarely indicated for pure red cell aplasia.

DIAMOND-BLACKFAN SYNDROME

Diamond-Blackfan anemia (DBA) is a rare congenital progressive erythrocyte aplasia that occurs in very young children. In 90% of cases, symptoms of the anemia are apparent in the first year of life. Unlike Fanconi anemia, there is no leukopenia or thrombocytopenia.

DBA is actually a diverse family of diseases with a common hematologic phenotype. There is evidence for both autosomal dominant and autosomal recessive modes of inheritance. About 25% of cases have a mutation of the *RPS19* gene (which encodes a protein involved in ribosome assembly). Other genes related to DBA have been identified. A wide range of congenital defects can be observed in 47% of DBA patients, and patients are predisposed to occurrences of cancer.[1] Many cases have no familial pattern, suggesting spontaneous mutations or acquired disease.

The disease is not due to a deficiency of erythropoietin (EPO) because EPO levels are consistently increased and higher than expected for the degree of anemia. The EPO is active, and no antibodies are directed against this hormone, nor are there apparent mutations in either EPO or the EPO receptor. The most probable defect in DBA is an intrinsic defect of erythroid progenitor cells. BFU-E and CFU-E are decreased, but early erythropoietin-independent erythropoiesis is relatively normal in cell culture systems.

Physical findings and symptoms are those associated with anemia or related to congenital defects. Anemia is severe with erythroid hypoplasia in an otherwise normocellular bone marrow.

Diagnostic criteria for all cases of DBA are included in Table 13-3 ✪ [24] Testing for *RPS19* mutations is helpful in only about 25% of cases.[1] Testing for the chromosomal breakage associated with FA is negative. Vitamin B_{12} and folate levels are normal. Fetal-like erythrocytes are present, hemoglobin F is increased from 5 to 25%, and the i antigen is increased. The presence of fetal-like erythrocytes is not particularly useful, however, in diagnosing DBA in children younger than 1 year of age because children in this age group normally possess erythrocytes with fetal characteristics. Serum iron and serum ferritin are increased, and transferrin is 100% saturated.

✪ TABLE 13-3

Diagnostic Criteria for Diamond-Blackfan Anemia

- Macrocytic (or normocytic) normochromic anemia in first year of life
- Reticulocytopenia
- Normocellular marrow with marked erythroid hypoplasia
- Increased serum erythropoietin (EPO)
- Normal or slightly decreased leukocyte count
- Normal or increased platelet count

⊙ TABLE 13-4

Comparison of the Features of Diamond-Blackfan Anemia and Transient Erythroblastopenia of Childhood (TEC)

Feature	Diamond-Blackfan	TEC
PRCA	Present	Present
Fetal erythrocyte characteristics (i antigen, HbF increased)	Present	Absent (if child is >1 year old)
Etiology	Inherited	Follows viral infection (mechanism unkown)
MCV	Can be increased	Normal
Age at onset	Birth to 1 year	Up to 4 years
Therapy	Corticosteroids, transfusions	None, spontaneous recovery

PRCA = pure red cell aplasia

Therapy includes erythrocyte transfusions and administration of adrenal corticosteroids.[25] Up to half of patients develop prolonged remission, but most eventually require additional therapy. Transfusion dependence requires the initiation of iron-chelation therapy (desferroximine). Most deaths are due to complications of therapy such as hemosiderosis.

Diamond-Blackfan anemia must be distinguished from transient erythroblastopenia of childhood (TEC), a temporary suppression of erythropoiesis that frequently occurs after a viral infection in otherwise normal children (Table 13-4 ⊙). The age of onset of TEC ranges from 1 month to 10 years. Progressive pallor in a previously healthy child is the primary clinical finding. Fetal characteristics of erythrocytes (HbF, i antigen) seen in DBA are not found in TEC. The pathophysiology of TEC is thought to be either a virus-associated, antibody-mediated, or a T cell-mediated suppression/inhibition of erythroid precursors. Although a preceding viral infection is associated with TEC, parvovirus B19 is not the etiologic agent. Transient aplastic crisis is a similar disorder of temporary failure of erythropoiesis, usually seen in young children with an underlying hemolytic disease (sickle cell anemia, hereditary spherocytosis). It is associated with acute B19 parvovirus infection, a virus that infects erythroid progenitor cells, lysing the target cell and blocking erythropoiesis. Infection, as well as the block to erythropoiesis, is terminated by the production of neutralizing antibodies to the virus.

It is important that the distinction be made between DBA and TEC because DBA requires treatment that is unnecessary and potentially harmful to children with TEC.[26] Patients with TEC recover within 2 months of diagnosis. Therapy involves only supportive care.

▶ OTHER HYPOPROLIFERATIVE ANEMIAS

Other hypoproliferative anemias due primarily to defective hormonal stimulation of erythroid progenitor cells include the anemia associated with chronic renal disease and the anemias associated with endocrine disorders. In most cases, these anemias can be traced to a decrease in erythropoietin production.

RENAL DISEASE

Chronic renal disease is a common cause of anemia. Anemia, however, is only an incidental finding; the patient primarily seeks medical attention for symptoms related to renal failure. The hemoglobin begins to decrease when the blood urea nitrogen level increases to more than 30 mg/dL. Anemia is slow developing, and most patients tolerate the low hemoglobin levels well.

Pathophysiology

Due to the complexity of the clinical settings in uremia, anemia is frequently the result of several different pathophysiologies (Table 13-5 ⊙):

1. The most important and consistent factor is bone marrow erythroid hypoproliferation attributed to a decrease in erythropoietin (EPO) production by the diseased kidney.

2. In some cases, the EPO level is normal, but the bone marrow does not respond. The unresponsiveness can be caused by the presence of a low molecular weight dialyzable inhibitor of erythropoiesis present in the serum of uremic patients. Improvement in hemoglobin levels is seen after dialysis.

⊙ TABLE 13-5

Possible Causes of Anemia in Chronic Renal Disease

- Decreased erythropoietin production
- Presence of an inhibitor of erythropoiesis
- Decreased erythrocyte survival
- Blood loss
- Iron deficiency
- Folate deficiency

3. In addition to hypoproliferation, decreased erythrocyte survival compounds the anemia. One factor responsible for the shortened survival is related to an unknown extracorpuscular cause, perhaps an unfavorable metabolic environment or mechanical trauma. Another cause of hemolysis can be related to an acquired abnormality in erythrocyte metabolism that involves the pentose phosphate shunt. This abnormality causes impaired generation of NADPH and reduced glutathione.[27] Thus, when exposed to oxidants, the erythrocytes develop Heinz bodies, inducing acute hemolysis. Hemolysis can also be related to a reversible defect in erythrocyte membrane sodium-potassium ATPase.

4. The anemia can be related to blood loss from the gastrointestinal tract because of a decrease in platelets and/or platelet dysfunction. Blood is also lost during priming for dialysis. Patients receiving dialysis lose about 5–6 mg of iron daily. Thus, an anemia associated with iron deficiency is common (∞ Chapter 9).

5. Patients on dialysis can become folate deficient because folate is dialyzable. Without folate supplements, the patient can develop a megaloblastic anemia.

Laboratory Findings

A normocytic and normochromic anemia is typical in renal disease except when the patient is deficient in folate or iron; then a macrocytic anemia or microcytic anemia prevails. Moderate anisocytosis with some degree of microcytosis can be present. Hemoglobin levels are reduced to 50–80 g/L, and the reticulocyte production index is approximately 1. There is moderate to severe poikilocytosis with echinocytes and schistocytes. The number of echinocytes correlates roughly with the severity of azotemia. Spherocytes are associated with hypersplenism. Nucleated erythrocytes are noted in the peripheral blood. Leukocytes and platelets are usually normal. The bone marrow reveals erythroid hypoproliferation, especially when compared to the degree of anemia.

Other laboratory findings vary depending on the severity of renal impairment. Blood urea nitrogen is >30 mg/dL, serum creatinine is increased, and electrolytes are abnormal. Hemostatic abnormalities can be present. Serum ferritin levels are higher than normal in chronic renal failure even if iron deficiency is present. Therefore, it has been suggested that if the serum ferritin level is below 40 ng/mL, iron deficiency should be considered. Increased iron-binding capacity can be a useful predictor of iron deficiency in these cases.

Therapy

Therapy for chronic renal disease includes renal transplantation, hemodialysis, and continuous ambulatory peritoneal dialysis. All treatments tend to ameliorate the anemia, but hemodialysis exposes the patient to additional causes of anemia including blood loss, iron and folate deficiency, and hemolysis. Thus, iron and folic acid supplements are frequently given in conjunction with hemodialysis. Intermittent doses of EPO three times a week cause improvement in 1–2 weeks. In some cases, a normal hemoglobin is achieved, and in all cases, the patients remain transfusion independent.

ENDOCRINE ABNORMALITIES

Endocrine deficiencies are sometimes associated with a decrease in EPO. The resulting anemia is usually normocytic, normochromic with normal erythrocyte morphology. The bone marrow findings suggest erythroid hypoproliferation.

A slowly developing normocytic, normochromic anemia is characteristic of hypothyroidism. Erythrocyte survival is normal, and reticulocytosis is absent. The anemia is most likely a physiologic response to a decrease in tissue demands for oxygen. With hormone replacement therapy, the anemia slowly remits.

Hypopituitarism is associated with an anemia more severe than that of hypothyroidism, and the leukocyte count can be decreased. However, anemia is a minor component of the other manifestations of hypopituitarism. The pituitary has an effect on multiple endocrine glands including the thyroid and adrenals. In males, a decrease in androgens (gonadal dysfunction) can be partly responsible for the anemia because they stimulate erythropoiesis. In addition, a decrease in the growth hormone can have a trophic effect on the bone marrow. Mild anemia has also been associated with hyperparathyroidism.

SUMMARY

The hypoproliferative anemias include a group of acquired and constitutional disorders in which a chronic marrow failure of erythropoiesis occurs. If only the erythrocytes are affected, the term *pure red cell aplasia* is appropriate. More commonly, a hypocellularity affects all cell lineages, and the diagnosis is aplastic anemia.

Immune suppression has been shown to underlie the hypocellularity in acquired aplastic anemia. Acquired aplastic anemia can be idiopathic or secondary to drugs, chemical agents, ionizing radiation, or infectious agents. Constitutional aplastic anemia has a congenital cause and can be associated with other congenital anomalies. Fanconi anemia is a form of constitutional anemia with progressive bone marrow hypoplasia and other congenital defects. The disorder is characterized by chromosomal instability and fragility, secondary to defective DNA repair mechanisms.

The laboratory findings in aplastic anemia reveal pancytopenia. The erythrocytes are usually normocytic, normochromic but can be macrocytic. The reticulocyte count is low and the corrected reticulocyte count is less than 1%. The bone marrow is less than 25% cellular.

Pure red cell aplasia is characterized by a selective decrease in erythroid cells. This disorder can be acquired or inherited. The acquired forms are seen in thymoma with administration of certain drugs, autoimmune disorders, and infection, especially viral infections. Diamond-Blackfan anemia is a constitutional progressive erythrocyte aplasia occurring in young children. This inherited form of aplasia must be differentiated from TEC, a temporary aplasia occurring after viral infection.

Other hypoproliferative anemias are due primarily to defective hormonal stimulation of erythroid stem cells. These include anemia associated with renal disease and with endocrinopathies. The laboratory findings reflect not only anemia but also pathologies of the primary disorder.

Immunosuppressive therapy using antithymocyte globulin, antilymphocyte globulin, cyclosporine A, or monoclonal antibodies against B cell antigens is the treatment of choice for the majority of older patients who are not candidates for hematopoietic stem cell transplants (SCT). SCT is potentially curative but not without risks. Transplantation still remains unavailable for many patients due to the inability to find matched donors.

REVIEW QUESTIONS

LEVEL I

1. What is the typical morphologic classification of erythrocytes in aplastic anemia? (Objective 8)
   a. hypochromic, microcytic
   b. normochromic, normocytic
   c. normochromic, microcytic
   d. hypochromic, macrocytic

2. The bone marrow in aplastic anemia is typically: (Objective 8)
   a. hypocellular
   b. hypercellular
   c. dysplastic
   d. normal

3. Which of the following is (are) considered a cause of hypoproliferation in aplastic anemia? (Objective 3)
   1. damage to stem cells
   2. depletion of stem cells
   3. inhibition of stem cells
      a. 1 only
      b. 1 and 2 only
      c. 2 and 3 only
      d. 1, 2, and 3

4. What term best describes the peripheral blood findings of a person with aplastic anemia? (Objective 8)
   a. pancytopenia
   b. bicytopenia
   c. granulocytopenia only
   d. anemia only

5. Diagnostic criteria for aplastic anemia include: (Objective 2)
   a. corrected reticulocyte count of more than 1%
   b. platelet count less than 100×10^9/L
   c. granulocyte count less than 0.5×10^9/L
   d. bone marrow less than 50% cellular

6. Which age group is *least* likely to have a high incidence of aplastic anemia? (Objective 3)
   a. 2–5 years old
   b. 20–25 years old
   c. 40–50 years old
   d. adults over 60

LEVEL II

1. What confirmatory test should be performed in suspected cases of aplastic anemia? (Objective 4)
   a. serum iron and TIBC
   b. hemoglobin electrophoresis
   c. bone marrow examination
   d. direct antiglobulin test

2. A 3-year-old patient presents with severe normocytic, normochromic anemia. Platelet counts and leukocyte counts are normal. The mother reported that the child has been healthy since birth but recently had a cold. Which of the following laboratory test results would support a diagosis of TEC? (Objectives 1, 5, 6)
   a. decreased numbers of erythrocyte precursors on bone marrow examination
   b. normal hemoglobin F level on hemoglobin electrophoresis
   c. abnormal karyotype
   d. i antigen on the patient's erythrocytes

3. A bone marrow from an anemic patient that demonstrates a marked erythroid hypoplasia but normal numbers of other cell lines is most consistent with a diagnosis of: (Objective 5)
   a. Fanconi anemia
   b. aplastic anemia
   c. pure red cell aplasia
   d. myelophthisic anemia

4. A male patient with previously diagnosed infectious mononucleosis infection has become suddenly anemic. A possible cause of the anemia is: (Objective 1)
   a. iron deficiency
   b. folic acid deficiency
   c. anemia of chronic disease
   d. aplastic anemia

5. What is the standard treatment for patients with acquired aplastic anemia? (Objective 3)
   a. immunosuppressive therapy
   b. bone marrow transplant
   c. administration of growth factors
   d. none; treatment typically not needed

REVIEW QUESTIONS *(continued)*

LEVEL I

7. Exposure to drugs, radiation, or infectious agents can result in which type of aplastic anemia? (Objective 7)
   a. idiopathic
   b. congenital
   c. constitutional
   d. acquired

8. If a patient with anemia had a decrease in only the red cells in the bone marrow, this might indicate: (Objective 8)
   a. pure red cell aplasia
   b. acquired aplastic anemia
   c. megaloblastic anemia
   d. constitutional aplastic anemia

9. Which of the following is most characteristic of the peripheral blood picture in pure red cell aplasia? (Objective 8)
   a. pancytopenia
   b. granulocytopenia and thrombocytopenia
   c. leukocytosis
   d. decreased hemoglobin and hematocrit

10. Peripheral blood findings in patients with chronic renal disease include: (Objective 9)
    a. mild anemia with hemoglobin levels around 10 g/dL
    b. poikilocytosis with echinocytes and schistocytes
    c. normally shaped erythrocytes
    d. decreased leukocytes and platelets

LEVEL II

6. The peripheral blood finding that helps differentiate aplastic anemia from myelophthisic anemia is: (Objective 5)
   a. leukoerythroblastic reaction in aplastic anemia
   b. fetal-like erythrocytes in aplastic anemia
   c. poikilocytosis in myelophthisic anemia
   d. microcytic anemia in myelophthisic anemia

7. Which patient with aplastic anemia could have the best prognosis for recovery? (Objective 2)
   a. one with a parvovirus infection
   b. one with idiopathic aplastic anemia
   c. one who has severe bone marrow hypoplasia
   d. one who has severe pancytopenia

8. A bone marrow biopsy is performed on an infant with severe congenital abnormalities and severe anemia. Results of the biopsy demonstrate marked hypoplasia of all cell lines. These findings are most consistent with a diagnosis of: (Objective 4)
   a. transient erythroblastopenia of childhood
   b. familial aplastic anemia
   c. Diamond-Blackfan anemia
   d. Fanconi anemia

9. Clinical signs and symptoms of aplastic anemia include: (Objective 4)
   a. hepatomegaly
   b. bleeding
   c. splenomegaly
   d. lymphadenopathy

10. A 75-year-old male was diagnosed with aplastic anemia. He has no known living blood relatives. What treatment would most likely be initiated? (Objective 3)
    a. none
    b. bone marrow transplant
    c. immunosuppressive therapy
    d. chemotherapy

www.pearsonhighered.com/mckenzie
Use this address to access the interactive Companion Website created for this textbook. Find additional information, tables and figures. Evaluate your command of the chapter information using case studies and critical thinking and multiple choice questions.

REFERENCES

1. Bagby GC, Lipton JM, Sloand EM, Schiffer CA. Marrow failure. *Hematology* 2004;1:318–43

2. Shimamura, A, Guinan, EA. Acquired aplastic anemia. In: Nathan, DG, Orkin, SH, eds. *Hematology of Infancy and Childhood*. Philadelphia: WB Saunders; 2003, 256.

3. Issaragrisil S, Leaverton PE, Chansung K, Thamprasit T, Porapakham Y, Vannasaeng S et al. Regional patterns in the incidence of aplastic anemia in Thailand. The Aplastic Anemia Study Group. *Am J Hematol.* 1999;61:164–68.

4. Young NS. Hematopoietic cell destruction by immune mechanisms in acquired aplastic anemia. *Semin Hematol.* 2000;37:3–14.

5. Marsh JC. Results of immunosuppression in aplastic anaemia. *Acta Haematol.* 2000;103:26–32.

6. Stewart FM. Hypoplastic/aplastic anemia: Role of bone marrow transplantation. *Med Clin North Am.* 1992;76:683–97.

7. Marsh JC, Chang J, Testa NG, Hows JM, Dexter TM. The hematopoietic defect in aplastic anemia assessed by long-term marrow culture. *Blood.* 1990;76:1748–57.

8. Marsh JC, Chang J, Testa NG, Hows JM, Dexter TM. In vitro assessment of marrow "stem cell" and stromal cell function in aplastic anaemia. *Br J Haematol.* 1991;78:258–67.

9. Levere RD, Ibraham NG. The bone marrow as a metabolic organ. *Am J Med.* 1982;73:615–16.

10. Kasten MJ. Clindamycin, metronidazole, and chloramphenicol. *Mayo Clin Proc.* 1999;74:825–33.

11. Brown KE, Tisdale J, Barrett AJ, Dunbar CE, Young NS. Hepatitis-associated aplastic anemia. *N Engl J Med.* 1997;336(15):1059–64.

12. Tisdale JF, Dunn DE, Maciejewski J. Cyclophosphamide and other new agents for the treatment of severe aplastic anemia. *Semin Hematol.* 2000;37:102–9.

13. Baker RI, Manoharan A, de Luca E, Begley CG. Pure red cell aplasia of pregnancy: A distinct clinical entity. *Br J Haematol.* 1993;85: 619–22.

14. Socie G, Rosenfeld S, Frickhofen N, Gluckman E, Tichelli A. Late clonal diseases of treated aplastic anemia. *Semin Hematol.* 2000;37: 91–101.

15. Alter BP. Bone marrow failure: A child is not just a small adult but an adult can have a childhood disease. *Hematology.* 2005;2005: 96–103

16. Garcia-Higuera I, Kuang Y, D'Andrea AD. The molecular and cellular biology of Fanconi anemia. *Curr Opin Hematol.* 1999;6:83–88.

17. Segel GB, Lichtman MA. Aplastic anemia. In: Lichtman MA, Beutler E, Kipps TJ, Seligsohn U, Kaushansky K, Prchal JT, eds. *Williams Hematology,* 7th ed. New York: McGraw-Hill; 2006;419–36.

18. Socie G, Gluckman E. Cure from severe aplastic anemia in vivo and late effects. *Acta Haematol.* 2000;103:49–54.

19. Horowitz MM. Current status of allogeneic bone marrow transplantation in acquired aplastic anemia. *Semin Hematol.* 2000;37:30–42.

20. Bacigalupo A, Oneto R, Bruno B, Socie G, Passweg J, Locasciulli A et al. Current results of bone marrow transplantation in patients with acquired severe aplastic anemia: Report of the European Group for Blood and Marrow Transplantation, on behalf of the Working Party on Severe Aplastic Anemia of the European Group for Blood and Marrow Transplantation. *Acta Haematol.* 2000;103:19–25.

21. Frickhofen N, Rosenfeld SJ. Immunosuppressive treatment of aplastic anemia with antithymocyte globulin and cyclosporine. *Semin Hematol.* 2000;37:56–68.

22. Marsh JC. Hematopoietic growth factors in the pathogenesis and for the treatment of aplastic anemia. *Semin Hematol.* 2000;37:81–90.

23. Barrett J, Saunthararajah Y, Molldrem J. Myelodysplastic syndrome and aplastic anemia: Distinct entities or diseases linked by a common pathophysiology. *Semin Hematol.* 2000;37:15–29.

24. Freedman MH. Pure red cell aplasia in childhood and adolescence: Pathogenesis and approaches to diagnosis. *Br J Haematol.* 1993;85: 246–53.

25. Krijanovski OI, Sieff CA. Diamond-Blackfan anemia. *Hematol Oncol Clin North Am.* 1997;11:1061–77.

26. Miller R, Berman B. Transient erythroblastopenia of childhood in infants <6 months of age. *Am J Ped Hematol Oncol.* 1994;16:246–48.

27. Hocking WG. Hematologic abnormalities in patients with renal diseases. *Hematol Oncol Clin North Am.* 1987;1:229–60.

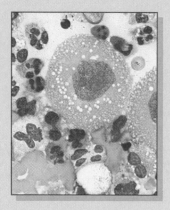

14

Introduction
to Hemolytic Anemia

Shirlyn B. McKenzie, Ph.D.

CHAPTER OUTLINE

■ OBJECTIVES—LEVEL I

At the end of this unit of study, the student should be able to:

1. List the laboratory tests that can be used to assess a hemolytic anemia and give expected results.
2. Define *hemolysis* and reconcile a normal hemoglobin in compensated hemolytic disease.
3. Assess laboratory results in intravascular and extravascular hemolysis.
4. Summarize the clinical findings associated with a hemolytic anemia.
5. Explain the difference between intrinsic and extrinsic erythrocyte defects and give an example of each.

■ OBJECTIVES—LEVEL II

At the end of this unit of study, the student should be able to:

1. Evaluate clinical findings of hemolytic anemia and differentiate those associated with acute and chronic disease.
2. Compare and contrast the processes of intravascular and extravascular hemolysis and explain how laboratory results can be used to differentiate.
3. Interpret laboratory and clinical findings in hemolytic anemia and determine the type of hematologic defect present.
4. Recommend follow-up tests that could be necessary for a diagnosis of hemolytic disease.

KEY TERMS

Compensated hemolytic disease
Hemoglobinemia
Hemoglobinuria
Hemolysis
Hemosiderinuria

BACKGROUND BASICS

The information in this chapter builds on the concepts learned in previous chapters. To maximize your learning experience, you should review these concepts before starting this unit of study.

Level I

▶ Diagram the process of intravascular and extravascular hemolysis. (Chapter 5)
▶ Identify and define types of poikilocytes. (Chapter 8)
▶ Explain the morphologic and functional classification of anemia. (Chapter 8)
▶ Identify laboratory tests used to assess anemia. (Chapters 5, 8)

Level II

▶ Classify an anemia based on laboratory findings. (Chapter 8)
▶ Interpret results of laboratory tests and clinical findings based on type of hemolysis and functional defect. (Chapters 5, 8)
▶ Review the erythrocyte membrane structure. (Chapter 5)

CASE STUDY

We will address this case study throughout the chapter.

Sashi is a 58-year-old female. Her amylase and lipase values were markedly increased. Her hemoglobin was 15.5 g/dL. Two months later she had surgery for a pancreatic pseudocyst. She received 3 units of packed red blood cells. Three days after surgery, her hemoglobin was 5.2 g/dL, RBC 1.5×10^{12}/L, hematocrit 0.148 L/L. The physician is concerned about the possibility of internal bleeding. Consider what other laboratory tests could be helpful in defining the source of blood loss in this patient.

▶ OVERVIEW

The laboratory plays an important role in differentiating the etiology of hemolytic disease. This chapter introduces the next four chapters on hemolytic anemia. It describes the classification schemes of hemolytic disease and gives the general laboratory and clinical findings characteristic of this group of anemias. The use of laboratory tests in differentiating the intravascular or extravascular sites of erythrocyte destruction and in defining the source of defect (intrinsic or extrinsic to the red cell) is discussed.

▶ INTRODUCTION

The hemolytic anemias are a heterogeneous group of normocytic, normochromic anemias in which the erythrocyte is prematurely destroyed. This premature destruction is referred to as **hemolysis.** Hemolytic anemia can be classified according to the source of the defect causing the hemolysis (intrinsic or extrinsic to the erythrocyte), mode of onset (inherited or acquired), and location of hemolysis (intravascular or extravascular) (Table 14-1 ✪). Intrinsic abnormalities are generally genetically determined, extrinsic abnormalities are acquired. There are exceptions to these classifications. For example, paroxysmal nocturnal hemoglobinuria (PNH) is an intrinsic erthrocytic defect that is acquired, and abetalipoproteinemia and LCAT deficiency are inherited extrinsic defects. Depending on the type and extent of injury, hemolysis can be intravascular or extravascular.

These anemias can also be classified by type of poikilocyte present on the blood smear: schistocytes or spherocytes (Figure 14-1 ■). Schistocytes indicate physical/mechanical trauma to the erythrocyte. Hemolysis can be either extravascular or intravascular hemolysis, depending on the severity of cell damage. Spherocytes indicate that part of the cell's membrane has been removed by phagocytes or shed from the cell in the form of microvesicles. Membrane can be removed by phagocytes in the spleen because of antigen/antibody complexes on the membrane, a defective membrane, or abnormal inclusions in the cell. Spherocytes are hemolyzed extravascularly.

The ultimate aim of any classification is to help identify the etiology of the anemia so that the appropriate treatment

✪ TABLE 14-1

Possible Classifications of Hemolytic Anemia Based on Pathophysiology, Etiology, and/or Laboratory Findings

Source of Defect	Mode of Onset	Site of Hemolysis	Predominant Poikilocyte
Intrinsic to red cell (intracorpuscular)	Inherited	Intravascular	Spherocyte
Extrinsic to red cell (extracorpuscular)	Acquired	Extravascular	Schistocyte (fragmented erythrocyte)/spherocyte

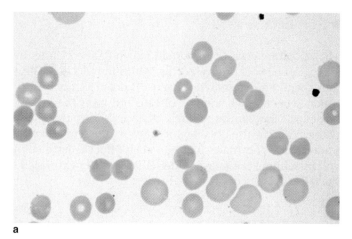
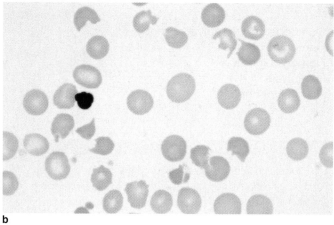

a

b

■ FIGURE 14-1   **a.** Peripheral blood smear from a patient with autoimmune hemolytic anemia. There is marked anisocytosis with numerous spherocytes and large polychromatophilic erythrocytes. **b.** Peripheral blood smear from a patient with thrombotic, thrombocytopenic purpura, a microangiopathic hemolytic anemia. Many schistocytes are present as are spherocytes, but the predominant poikilocyte is the schistocyte. (both: 1000× magnification; Wright-Giemsa stain)

can be given and prognosis determined. Laboratory tests are a very important part of this process.

Reticulocytosis is a constant feature of all hemolytic anemias reflecting the increased activity of the bone marrow as it attempts to maintain erythrocyte mass in the peripheral blood. If the bone marrow is able to increase erythropoiesis enough to compensate for the decreased erythrocyte life span, anemia does not develop. In this case, cells are being produced at the same or nearly the same rate as they are hemolyzed. This condition is called **compensated hemolytic disease.** Compensated hemolytic disease can rapidly develop into anemia if one of the following occurs: (1) erythrocyte destruction accelerates beyond the compensatory capacity of the marrow (hemolytic crises) or (2) the marrow suddenly stops producing erythrocytes (aplastic crisis).

It has been shown that in individuals scheduled for surgery who undergo aggressive autologous blood donation (two 450-ml units per week), the bone marrow can increase its production rate twofold to fourfold over the basal rate if sufficient iron is mobilized.[1] Thus, it is possible that the erythrocyte life span can drop to one-fourth of normal, or about 30 days, without anemia developing. If the life span decreases to less than 30 days, however, anemia can develop. The increase in erythropoiesis is limited by the amount of iron that can be mobilized for hemoglobin synthesis. The term *functional iron deficiency* is used when total body iron is adequate but iron stores cannot be mobilized fast enough for the increase in erythropoiesis. Patients with chronic hemolytic anemia can increase erythropoiesis sixfold if adequate iron is available. Individuals with hemochromatosis have very high serum iron and transferrin saturation levels, and it has been shown that they can increase erythropoiesis up to eightfold.[2]

▶ **LABORATORY FINDINGS**

Hematologic characteristics of hemolytic anemia reflect the increased activity of the bone marrow and the increased erythrocyte destruction (Table 14-2✿). Erythroid hyperplasia of the bone marrow with decreased amounts of fat is more pronounced in hemolytic anemias than in any of the nonhemolytic anemias. Consequently, the myeloid-to-erythroid ratio (M:E) is decreased. Increased plasma iron turnover reflects the increased erythrocyte destruction and increased utilization of iron by erythroid precursors in the bone marrow.

Peripheral blood reticulocytosis, increased immature reticulocyte fraction (IRF), marked polychromasia, and nucleated erythrocytes in the peripheral blood are clues to the presence of increased erythropoietic activity in the bone marrow. (∞ Chapter 8) The hemolytic anemias are the only anemias with a reticulocyte production index (RPI) of more than 2 (except in acute hemorrhage). Thus, the RPI is useful in differentiating hemolytic anemias from other normocytic, normochromic anemias in which the bone marrow is not increasing effective erythropoiesis. The degree of reticulocytosis occasionally is great enough to cause an increased MCV in which case the anemia is classified as macrocytic, normochromic. (Reticulocytes are larger than mature erythrocytes.)

Results of laboratory tests that are used to evaluate heme catabolism are usually abnormal. Unconjugated/indirect bilirubin is often increased, but the conjugated/direct fraction is usually normal unless hepatic or biliary dysfunction is present. (Reference intervals: total bilirubin = 0.2–1 mg/dL; unconjugated bilirubin = 0–0.2 mg/dL) However, a significant number of patients with hemolytic disease have normal serum bilirubin levels, suggesting that serum bilirubin is not

✪ TABLE 14-2

Common Laboratory Findings Reflecting Increased Production and Destruction of Erythrocytes in Hemolytic Anemias

Increased Bone Marrow Production of Erythrocytes	Increased Erythrocyte Destruction
Reticulocytosis (RPI >2)	Anemia
Increased IRF	Presence of spherocytes, schisto-cytes, and/or other poikilocytes
Leukocytosis	
Nucleated erythrocytes in the peripheral blood	Positive direct antihuman globulin test (DAT)
Polychromasia of erythrocytes on Romanowsky-stained blood smears	Decreased haptoglobin and hemo-pexin
	Decreased glycosylated hemoglobin
Normoblastic erythroid hyper-plasia in the bone marrow	Increased fecal and urine urobilinogen
	Increased bilirubin (unconjugated)
	Hemoglobinemia*
	Hemoglobinuria*
	Hemosiderinuria*
	Methemoglobinemia*
	Increased serum LD
	Increased expired CO

*Associated only with intravascular hemolysis. IRF = immature reticulocyte fraction; LD = lactic dehydrogenase; RPI = reticulocyte production index; CO = carbon monoxide

a reliable index of erythrocyte destruction. Bilirubin levels of more than 5 mg/dL are unusual in hemolytic disease except in neonates and in those with coexisting liver dysfunction. Urine and fecal urobilinogen is elevated.

The heme-binding plasma proteins, haptoglobin and hemopexin, are often decreased as a result of increased consumption. Haptoglobin levels less than 25 mg/dL are highly specific for hemolytic anemia.

Review of the peripheral blood smear is helpful in directing the course of laboratory investigation. Poikilocytes other than spherocytes suggest mechanical damage to the cell whereas spherocytes suggest membrane grooming (loss) by phagocytes in the spleen.

⊘ CASE STUDY *(continued from page 299)*

Sashi's reticulocyte count is 19%, total serum bilirubin 9.8 mg/dL, and haptoglobin <13 mg/dL. The peripheral blood smear revealed many spherocytes.

1. What type of anemia do the laboratory results and clinical history suggest?

✓ Checkpoint! 1

A patient is suspected of having a hemolytic disease. The reticulocyte count is increased, but the hemoglobin, serum bilirubin, and haptoglobin are within the normal range. Explain.

▶ CLINICAL FINDINGS

Clinical signs of hemolytic anemia are associated with increases in both heme catabolism (erythrocyte destruction) and erythropoiesis (Table 14-3 ✪). Jaundice reflects an increase in bilirubin production. Gallstones consisting primarily of bilirubin are common in congenital and other chronic hemolytic anemias. Dark or red urine due to excretion of plasma hemoglobin can be noted in intravascular hemolysis.

Chronic severe hemolytic anemias stimulate the expansion of bone marrow, consequently thinning cortical bone and widening the spaces between inner and outer tables of bone. In children, this expansion is evident in skeletal abnormalities. These bone changes can result in spontaneous fractures and a type of arthritis termed *osteoarthropathy.*[3] Extramedullary hematopoietic masses can be found. Some of these masses are believed to represent extrusions of the marrow cavity through thinned bone cortex. Small colonies of erythrocytes also can be found in the spleen, liver, lymph nodes, and perinephric tissue. The hematopoietic masses can cause pressure symptoms on adjacent organs.[3] In extravascular hemolysis, splenic hypertrophy is a constant finding.

Other clinical findings and the primary symptoms are those associated with anemia including pallor, fatigue, and cardiac symptoms.

▶ SITES OF DESTRUCTION

Hemolysis can occur within the circulation (intravascular) or within the macrophages of the spleen, liver, or bone marrow (extravascular). In some cases, depending on the degree of

✪ TABLE 14-3

Clinical Findings Associated with Hemolytic Anemia

- Jaundice
- Gallstones
- Dark or red urine (intravascular hemolysis)
- Symptoms of anemia
- Thinning of cortical bone (in chronic hemolytic anemia)
- Extramedullary hematopoietic masses (in chronic hemolytic anemia)
- Splenomegaly

damage to the cell, destruction occurs both intravascularly and extravascularly. The results of laboratory tests can provide important clues to the hemolytic process.[4] To correlate laboratory results with the etiology and pathophysiology of the anemia, an understanding of intravascular and extravascular hemolysis is essential (∞ Chapter 5).

INTRAVASCULAR HEMOLYSIS

In intravascular hemolysis, the erythrocyte is destroyed within the blood vessels. When the erythrocyte is hemolyzed, free hemoglobin is released into the plasma. The hemoglobin is bound to the plasma protein haptoglobin, transported as a complex to the liver where it is metabolized to bilirubin, and excreted to the intestinal tract via the bile duct. Normally the concentration of hemoglobin in plasma is less than 5 mg/dL. In severe intravascular hemolysis, synthesis of haptoglobin might not be sufficient to replace that being used, and free hemoglobin accumulates in the plasma. It should be remembered, however, that haptoglobin is an acute phase reactant and can be normal or even increased in individuals with concomitant infections, inflammation, or malignant disease despite an increase in intravascular hemolysis. Levels also can be decreased in liver disease due to decreased synthesis of the protein and in hereditary deficiency of haptoglobin. Although haptoglobin functions as an intravascular heme-binding protein, it also can be decreased in association with extravascular hemolytic diseases. Thus, by itself, the haptoglobin level cannot be used to differentiate intravascular and extravascular hemolysis.

Another plasma protein, hemopexin, complexes with heme when haptoglobin is depleted. This complex can also be cleared from the plasma by the liver faster than hemopexin can be synthesized and is quickly depleted. A decrease in hemopexin is secondary to a reduction in haptoglobin.

Hemoglobin bound to haptoglobin or hemopexin forms complexes that are too large to pass through the glomerulus of the kidney. When these two transport proteins are depleted, free hemoglobin circulates in the plasma (**hemoglobinemia**). The liver directly removes some of this hemoglobin, but some dissociates into dimers small enough to be filtered by the glomerulus. Filtered hemoglobin can be reabsorbed in the proximal renal tubules, but when the rate of filtration exceeds the tubular reabsorption capabilities, free hemoglobin appears in the urine (**hemoglobinuria**). The presence of free hemoglobin in the urine is a sign of rapid and severe intravascular hemolysis.[5] Depending on the degree of hemolysis, the urine can be pink, red, or brownish black.

Some renal tubular cells can become laden with hemoglobin iron. When these tubular cells are sloughed off into the urine, hemosiderin granules can be visualized by staining the urine sediment with an iron stain and examining it microscopically. Hemosiderin in the urine (**hemosiderinuria**) is a sign that the kidney has filtered a significant amount of hemoglobin.[3] In chronic intravascular hemolysis, hemosiderin granules can appear in the urine even in the absence of hemoglobinuria.

Free hemoglobin not bound to either of the two transport proteins or not excreted by the kidney is quickly oxidized to methemoglobin. Methemoglobin dissociates into hemin (oxidized form of heme) and globin. Hemin can bind to hemopexin if it is available or to albumin, forming methemalbumin. Methemalbumin is not excreted in the urine but circulates in the blood can be detected in the plasma by Schumm's test.

As described above laboratory findings of intravascular hemolysis include hemoglobinemia, hemoglobinuria, hemosiderinuria, methemoglobinemia, decreased haptoglobin, and decreased hemopexin. In addition, the serum lactic dehydrogenase (LD) can increase to as much as 800 IU/L (upper limit of reference range is 207 IU/L). LD, an enzyme present in high concentration in erythrocytes, is released from the erythrocyte into the plasma in intravascular hemolysis, and it is cleared from plasma even more slowly than hemoglobin. It can be an early and sensitive indicator of intravascular hemolysis.[6]

Erythrocytes must be severely damaged to undergo intravascular destruction because phagocytes in the spleen or liver remove minimally or moderately damaged erythrocytes. Intravascular hemolysis can be caused by the (1) activation of complement on the erythrocyte membrane, (2) physical or mechanical trauma to the erythrocyte, or (3) the presence of soluble toxic substances in the erythrocyte's environment (Table 14-4 ✪).

EXTRAVASCULAR HEMOLYSIS

If premature erythrocyte destruction is the result of extravascular hemolysis, the erythrocytes are removed from circulation by phagocytes in the tissues. This type of hemolysis is more common than intravascular hemolysis. There is no hemoglobinemia, hemoglobinuria, or hemosiderinuria because hemoglobin is not released directly into the plasma. Instead, the hemoglobin is degraded within the phagocyte to heme and globin. The heme is further catabolized to iron, biliverdin, and carbon monoxide. The biliverdin then enters the plasma as bilirubin, binds to albumin, and is excreted by the liver.

Significant laboratory findings in hemolytic anemias associated with extravascular hemolysis are measurements of the products of heme catabolism. These findings include increases in expired carbon monoxide, carboxyhemoglobin, serum bilirubin (especially the unconjugated fraction), and both urine and fecal urobilinogen. In severe or chronic extravascular hemolysis, haptoglobin and hemopexin levels also can be decreased.

✪ TABLE 14-4

Anemias Characterized by Intravascular Hemolysis

Activation of Complement on the Erythrocyte Membrane	Physical or Mechanical Trauma to the Erythrocyte	Toxic Microenvironment of the Erythrocyte
Paroxysmal nocturnal hemoglobinuria	Microangiopathic hemolytic anemia	Bacterial infections
Paroxysmal cold hemoglobinuria	Abnormalities of the heart and great vessels	*Plasmodium falciparum* infection
Some transfusion reactions	Disseminated intravascular coagulation	Venoms
Some autoimmune hemolytic anemias		Arsine poisoning
		Acute drug reaction in G6PD deficiency
		Intravenous administration of distilled water
		Thermal injury

G6PD = glucose-6-phosphate dehydrogenase

Extravascular hemolysis can occur in phagocytes of the spleen, liver, or bone marrow. The type and degree of erythrocyte damage determines the primary site of erythrocyte destruction. The spleen is more efficient at removing slightly damaged erythrocytes because of the unique circulation pattern in the splenic cords. In this relatively static environment, erythrocytes are susceptible to fine scrutiny by splenic macrophages. The liver blood flow exceeds blood flow in the spleen and is an important site for the removal and phagocytosis of extensively damaged erythrocytes. The bone marrow can remove intrinsically abnormal erythrocytes before they are released to the peripheral circulation (ineffective erythropoiesis).

Antibodies directed against the erythrocyte commonly cause hemolytic anemia associated with extravascular hemolysis. Antibody and complement attached to the cell membrane make the erythrocyte a target for removal from the circulation by phagocytes. The sites and extent of extravascular hemolysis depend on the class of antibody attached to the erythrocyte as well as on whether complement is present. Thus, in immune mediated hemolytic anemia, determining the specific class of antibody present is sometimes helpful. The antihuman globulin (AHG) test (or direct antiglobulin test, DAT) is helpful in identifying erythrocytes sensitized with antibodies and/or complement. This test will be discussed in ∞ Chapter 17.

Erythrocytes sensitized with both complement and IgM are readily removed in the liver by hepatic macrophages, which have receptors for the complement component, C3b. However, if the terminal complement components are activated on the cell membrane, hemolysis is intravascular. Cells sensitized with IgM but without attached complement components appear to survive normally because macrophages lack Fc receptors for IgM. Clearance of IgM sensitized cells thus depends completely on activation of complement.

Erythrocytes sensitized with IgG may or may not activate complement because it takes multiple molecules of IgG on the erythrocyte membrane to bind one molecule of complement. However, cells sensitized with IgG can be removed by macrophages even in the absence of complement. IgG-sensitized erythrocytes are cleared primarily in the spleen by macrophages that have Fc receptors for IgG (FcγR) in addition to C3b receptors (CR3). The clearance of erythrocytes sensitized by both IgG and complement is accelerated because phagocytosis is mediated by two receptors.

Bone marrow macrophages are responsible for the removal of maturing precursor cells that are intrinsically abnormal. Cytoplasmic or nuclear maturation abnormalities (iron deficiency and megaloblastic anemia) are associated with this type of extravascular hemolysis resulting in a high degree of ineffective erythropoiesis. Many of the abnormal cells never enter the peripheral blood. Many hemolytic anemias that are associated with inherited defects of the erythrocyte membrane, hemoglobin, and intracellular enzymes have some degree of ineffective erythropoiesis. (This is a major factor in the clinical complications found in thalassemia [∞ Chapter 11], a disease with a large degree of ineffective erythropoiesis.) In most cases, however, a significant number of the defective cells gain access to the peripheral blood. These cells are not physiologically equipped to withstand the assaults of the peripheral circulation and are damaged. The damaged cells are then removed by liver or splenic macrophages. Anemias associated with extravascular hemolysis are listed in Table 14-5 ✪.

 CASE STUDY *(continued from page 301)*

Hemoglobinuria and hemoglobinemia are not present in Sashi, but haptoglobin is decreased.

2. Do the laboratory test results indicate intravascular or extravascular hemolysis? Explain.

✪ TABLE 14-5

Anemias Characterized by Extravascular Hemolysis

Origin	Anemias
Inherited erythrocyte defects	Thalassemia
	Hemoglobinopathies
	Enzyme deficiencies
	Membrane disorders
Acquired erythrocyte defects	Megaloblastic anemia
	Spur cell anemia
	Vitamin E deficiency in newborns
Immunohemolytic anemias	Autoimmune
	Drug induced
	Some transfusion reactions

✓ Checkpoint! 2

Explain why it is helpful for the clinical laboratory professional to know whether a particular hemolytic anemia is characterized by intravascular or extravascular hemolysis.

ERYTHROCYTE SURVIVAL STUDIES

Erythrocyte survival studies are helpful in defining a hemolytic process in which erythrocyte survival is only mildly decreased. In mild hemolysis, laboratory findings typical of extravascular or intravascular hemolysis can be absent. Survival studies give insight into the rate and mechanism of hemolysis.

To study erythrocyte survival, a sample of the patient's blood is removed and labeled in vitro with tracer amounts of radionuclide. The most common random label for erythrocytes and that recommended by the International Committee for Standardization in Hematology is radioactive chromium (^{51}Cr). The chromium penetrates the erythrocyte and remains trapped there. This labeled sample is injected intravenously into the patient. To determine the erythrocyte survival pattern, small samples of the patient's blood are assayed at specified time intervals for radioactivity levels. The erythrocyte life span is expressed as the time it takes for blood radioactivity to decrease by one-half (T 1/2 ^{51}Cr) starting 24 hours after injection. About 1% of the ^{51}Cr is normally eluted from surviving cells daily. In addition, only 1% of the labeled cells can be expected to have a life span of 100–120 days, because only 1% of the total erythrocyte mass is replaced each day. The remaining labeled cells have expected life spans from 0 to 100 days. Taking these facts into consideration, the normal T 1/2 with this method has been determined to be 25–32 days. A steady state is necessary for accurate interpretation of erythrocyte survival studies because blood loss or transfusions can alter the data significantly. Labeled erythrocytes in this method are also useful in

determining the sites of erythrocyte destruction. The amount of radioactivity taken up by an organ can be measured by scanning the body for ^{51}Cr deposition and is proportional to the number of erythrocytes destroyed there.

▶ SOURCE OF DEFECT

Hemolytic anemias can be classified as intrinsic or extrinsic according to the cause of the shortened erythrocyte survival (Table 14-6 ✪). *Intrinsic* refers to an abnormality of the erythrocyte itself. The abnormality can be in the membrane, cell enzymes, or hemoglobin molecule. *Extrinsic* refers to an antagonist in the cell's environment that causes injury to the erythrocyte. Contrary to intrinsic defects, the erythrocyte in extrinsic defects is normal.

INTRINSIC DEFECTS

With a few exceptions, intrinsic defects are hereditary. The site of hemolysis in intrinsic defects is usually extravascular. In some cases, intrinsic defects render the cell more susceptible than normal cells to damage by environmental (extracorpuscular) factors. Although extracorpuscular factors can be involved, the initiating event in hemolysis is considered to be the intrinsic abnormality. For example, a patient with a deficiency of glucose-6-phosphate dehydrogenase (G6PD; an enzyme in the erythrocyte that is necessary to reduce oxidants via production of glutathione) might not be able to produce enough glutathione to handle the oxidation products that occur when certain drugs are administered. Consequently, the erythrocytes suffer oxidant injury precipitated by the drug, which leads to hemolysis. Intrinsic defects causing hemolysis are discussed next.

Defects of the Erythrocyte Membrane
Structural defects of the erythrocyte membrane can cause the membrane to become abnormally permeable, rigid, or unstable and easily fragmented. In most cases, the defect is in one or more of the cytoskeletal proteins under the membrane lipid bilayer, causing abnormal interaction between the lipid bilayer and the cytoskeleton. In other cases, the membrane is abnormally permeable to cations because of defects in integral proteins and/or lipids.

In paroxysmal nocturnal hemoglobinuria, the erythrocyte membrane lacks a protein that serves a critical role in controlling complement attachment and activation on the cell membrane. As a result, the cell is abnormally sensitive to complement hemolysis. The defective membrane is an acquired abnormality.

Defects of Hemoglobin Structure or Production
Structurally abnormal hemoglobins that result in hemoglobin insolubility or instability can cause erythrocyte rigidity

✪ TABLE 14-6

Classification of Hemolytic Anemias Based on Underlying Defect

Classification	Underlying Defect	Examples
Intrinsic (inherited)	Membrane defects	Hereditary spherocytosis
		Hereditary elliptocytosis
		Hereditary pyropoikilocytosis
		Hereditary stomatocytosis
		Hereditary xerocytosis
		Paroxysmal nocturnal hemoglobinuria (acquired)
	Enzyme disorders	Glycolytic pathway enzyme deficiencies
		Hexose-monophosphate shunt enzyme deficiencies
	Abnormal hemoglobins	Thalassemia
		Structural hemoglobin variants (i.e., sickle cell anemia)
Extrinsic (acquired)	Antagonistic plasma factors	Chemicals, drugs
		Animal venoms
		Infectious agents
		Plasma lipid abnormalities
		Intracellular parasites
		Splenomegaly
	Traumatic physical cell injury	Microcirculation lesions
		Thermal injury
		March hemoglobinuria
	Immune mediated cell destruction	Autoimmune
		Alloimmune
		Drug induced

and, ultimately, hemolysis. In thalassemia, precipitates of excess globin chains (Heinz bodies) damage the erythrocyte membrane and cause erythrocytes to become rigid, and a severe hemolytic anemia develops.

Defects of Erythrocyte Enzymes

Deficiencies of erythrocyte enzymes necessary for maintaining hemoglobin and membrane sulfhydryl groups in the reduced state or for maintaining adequate levels of adenosine triphosphate (ATP) for cation exchange can result in hemolytic anemia. The enzyme disorders can be divided into two groups: (1) deficiencies in enzymes of the glycolytic pathway and (2) deficiencies in enzymes of the hexose-monophosphate shunt.

EXTRINSIC DEFECTS

Extrinsic defects are usually acquired. The erythrocytes, as innocent bystanders, are damaged by chemical, mechanical, or physical agents. Hemolysis can be either intravascular or extravascular. Discussion of the external factors causing hemolysis follows.

Antagonistic Plasma or Soluble Factors in the Erythrocyte's Environment

These factors include substances in the circulation that are toxic to the cell, cause direct cell hemolysis, or in the case of lipid abnormalities, alter the cell membrane and lead to removal of the cell in the spleen. Many drugs and chemicals are known to cause hemolysis. The European Union (EU) recognizes that prolonged exposure to a variety of chemical substances can result in hemolytic anemia.[7] They propose criteria that can be used to classify these chemicals as dangerous.[7]

Physical or Mechanical Trauma

Trauma to the erythrocyte in the peripheral circulation can cause the erythrocyte to fragment, producing striking abnormalities on the blood smear (schistocytes). In addition, splenomegaly can cause anemia by hypersequestration of erythrocytes.

Immune Mediated Cell Destruction

Antibodies or complement attached to the erythrocyte membrane sensitize the cell, and it is prematurely removed by macrophages in the spleen or liver. This can be an autoimmune or alloimmune process or can be drug induced.

 CASE STUDY *(continued from page 303)*

3. The indirect AHG test (used to detect antibodies in patient's serum) on Sashi is positive. Her serum was tested with panel cells that revealed anti-Jk^b and anti-S alloantibodies and possible anti-K (antibodies against red cell antigens). Is this anemia due to an intrinsic or extrinsic erythrocyte defect?

 Checkpoint! 3

Why is it helpful for the clinical laboratory professional to know the clinical history and suspected cause of a hemolytic anemia?

The next three chapters discuss these various kinds of hemolytic anemia. Note that many anemias, although not primarily hemolytic, have a hemolytic component. These include the hemoglobinopathies, thalassemia, iron-deficiency anemia, and megaloblastic anemia discussed in ∞ Chapters 11–14.

SUMMARY

Hemolytic anemias are characterized by decreased erythrocyte survival. Hemolysis can be caused by an intrinsic erythrocyte abnormality or an abnormality extrinsic to the cell. Intrinsic abnormalities are generally inherited and include defects in the cell's membrane, hemoglobin, or enzymes. Extrinsic abnormalities are generally acquired. These include hemolysis due to factors in the erythrocyte environment such as drugs, toxins, antibodies, complement, and physical or mechanical trauma to the erythrocyte.

Laboratory findings in hemolytic anemia reflect increased bone marrow production as well as increased erythrocyte destruction. Reticulocytosis, increased IRF, erythroid hyperplasia of the bone marrow, and increased iron turnover, all signs of increased bone marrow activity, can be present. Findings associated with increased erythrocyte destruction include decreased haptoglobin, hemosiderinuria, hemoglobinuria, increased unconjugated serum bilirubin, increased LD, and increased urine and fecal urobilinogen. Schistocytes are signs of intravascular erythrocyte trauma whereas spherocytes are indications that part of the cell's membrane has been removed by phagocytes. Hemolysis is usually extravascular but also can occur intravascularly. Laboratory test results can be used to help differentiate sites of hemolysis.

REVIEW QUESTIONS

LEVEL I

1. Which of the following is characteristic of severe intravascular hemolysis? (Objective 3)
   a. decreased bilirubin
   b. increased hemopexin
   c. decreased urobilinogen
   d. decreased haptoglobin

2. Hemolytic anemias caused by intrinsic erythrocyte abnormalities include: (Objective 5)
   a. immune hemolytic anemia
   b. hereditary spherocytosis
   c. microangiopathic hemolytic anemia
   d. thermal injury anemia

3. Which of the following indicates that compensated hemolytic disease is present in a patient with hereditary spherocytosis? (Objective 2)
   a. increased carboxyhemoglobin
   b. normal hemoglobin
   c. increased hemoglobin
   d. decreased hemoglobin

4. Which of the following is helpful in defining the presence of a hemolytic process? (Objective 1)
   a. RPI >2
   b. decreased IRF
   c. reticulocytopenia
   d. increased M:E ratio in bone marrow

LEVEL II

1. A 2-year-old child was seen by his physician for pallor and an enlarged abdomen. Results of laboratory tests showed a severe anemia. Family history revealed a mother and maternal uncle who had lifelong anemia. Further testing revealed the child had thalassemia. This anemia is an example of an: (Objective 3)
   a. extrinsic erythrocyte defect
   b. erythrocyte enzyme defect
   c. intrinsic erythrocyte defect
   d. acquired hemolytic anemia

2. Which of the following findings are characteristic of the bone marrow in a hemolytic anemia? (Objective 3)
   a. erythroid hyperplasia
   b. increased M:E ratio
   c. increased amount of fat
   d. hypoplasia

3. A patient is suspected of having an autoimmune hemolytic anemia. Many spherocytes are present on the blood smear, and the reticulocyte count is 20%. What test should be done to determine whether this is an autoimmune process? (Objective 4)
   a. serum bilirubin
   b. serum LD
   c. urinalysis
   d. AHG (DAT) test

REVIEW QUESTIONS *(continued)*

LEVEL I

5. This clinical finding is common in a patient with hemolytic anemia. (Objective 4)
   a. pica
   b. kidney stones
   c. jaundice
   d. lymph node enlargement

LEVEL II

4. A 4-year-old boy has thalassemia. His x-rays reveal thinning cortical bone, and he had splenomegaly. This diagnosis and clinical symptoms indicate: (Objective 1)
   a. a chronic hemolytic process
   b. an acute hemolytic anemia
   c. intravascular hemolysis
   d. extravascular hemolysis

5. A 50-year-old male has a hemoglobin of 8 g/dL. The serum bilirubin is elevated, and schistocytes are on the blood smear. Microangiopathic hemolytic anemia is suspected. What laboratory test would assist in determining whether intravascular hemolysis is present? (Objective 2)
   a. serum bilirubin
   b. haptoglobin level
   c. reticulocyte count
   d. amount of CO exhaled

www.pearsonhighered.com/mckenzie

Use this address to access the interactive Companion Website created for this textbook. Find additional information, tables and figures. Evaluate your command of the chapter information using case studies and critical thinking and multiple choice questions.

REFERENCES

1. Goodnough LT. Erythropoietin and iron-restricted erythropoiesis. *Exp Hemat.* 2007;35(4, Supplement 1):167–72.

2. Crosby WH. Treatment of haemochromatosis by energetic phlebotomy. One patient's response to the letting of 55 liters of blood in 11 months. *Br J Haematol.* 1958;4:82–88.

3. Tabbara, IA. Hemolytic anemias: Diagnosis and management. *Med Clin N Amer.* 1992;76:649–68.

4. Beutler E, Luzzatto L. Hemolytic anemia. *Sem Hematol.* 1999;36(4, Suppl 7):38–34.

5. Schreiber, AD. Autoimmune hemolytic anemia. *Pediatr Clin N Amer.* 1980;27(2):253–67.

6. Cunha BA, Nausheen S, Szalda D. Pulmonary complications of babesiosis: Case report and literature review. *Cur J Clin Microbiol Infec Dis.* 2007;26:505–08.

7. Muller A, Jacobsen H, Healy E, McMickan S, Istace F, Blaude MN et al. Classification of chemicals inducing haemolytic anaemia: An EU regulatory perspective. *Reg Toxi Pharmacol* 2006;45(3):229–41.

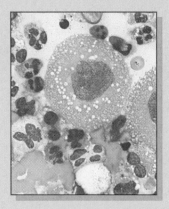

CHAPTER OUTLINE

15

Hemolytic Anemia: Membrane Defects

Diana Cochran-Black, Ph.D.

■ OBJECTIVES—LEVEL I

At the end of this unit of study, the student should be able to:

1. List the hereditary membrane disorders involved with erythrocyte skeletal protein abnormalities.

2. List the hereditary erythrocyte membrane disorders involved with abnormal membrane permeability.

3. Describe the pathophysiology and recognize laboratory features associated with hereditary spherocytosis, hereditary elliptocytosis, and hereditary pyropoikilocytosis.

4. Discuss the principle of the osmotic fragility test and interpret the results.

5. Describe the etiology, pathophysiology, and laboratory features of paroxysmal nocturnal hemoglobinuria (PNH).

6. Explain the principle of the sugar water (sucrose hemolysis) test and interpret its results.

■ OBJECTIVES—LEVEL II

At the end of this unit of study, the student should be able to:

1. Differentiate the protein defects associated with each hereditary membrane defect discussed in the chapter.

2. Create a flow chart using laboratory tests to differentiate hereditary spherocytosis, elliptocytosis, pyropoikilocytosis, stomatocytosis syndromes, and paroxysmal nocturnal hemoglobinuria.

3. Explain the role of decay-accelerating factor (DAF) and membrane inhibitor of reactive lysis (MIRL) in PNH.

4. Explain the results of the sucrose hemolysis test and immunophenotyping to determine a diagnosis of paroxysmal nocturnal hemoglobinuria (PNH).

5. Evaluate a clinical case study and determine the type of membrane disorder present by correlating clinical history and laboratory features.

KEY TERMS

- Cholecystitis
- Cholelithiasis
- Decay-accelerating factor (DAF)
- Exchange transfusion
- Hereditary elliptocytosis (HE)
- Hereditary pyropoikilocytosis (HPP)
- Hereditary spherocytosis (HS)
- Dehydrated hereditary stomatocytosis (DHS)
- Overhydrated hereditary stomatocytosis (OHS)
- Horizontal interactions
- Paroxysmal nocturnal hemoglobinuria (PNH)
- Rh null disease
- Spur cell anemia
- Vertical interactions

BACKGROUND BASICS

The information in this chapter builds on concepts learned in previous chapters. To maximize your learning experience, you should review these concepts before starting this unit of study.

Level I

▶ Describe the function, composition, and metabolism of the erythrocyte membrane. (Chapter 5)

▶ Identify the differences between extravascular and intravascular erythrocyte destruction. (Chapters 5, 14)

▶ Describe the general clinical and laboratory features associated with hemolytic anemias. (Chapter 14)

▶ Calculate erythrocyte indices, recognize abnormal erythrocyte morphology, and list reference ranges for common hematology parameters. (Chapters 8, 34)

Level II

▶ List the erythrocyte membrane proteins associated with cell deformability and permeability, and describe their involvement in horizontal and vertical interactions. (Chapter 5)

CASE STUDY

We will refer to this case study throughout the chapter.
Jack, a 12-year-old male, was brought to his family physician for evaluation of right-upper-quadrant pain. He has a lifelong history of hemolytic and aplastic crises. Consider why this patient history is important in selecting and evaluating laboratory tests.

▶ OVERVIEW

This chapter is a study of a group of hemolytic anemias that result from defects in the erythrocyte membrane. These defects include hereditary spherocytosis, hereditary elliptocy-tosis, hereditary pyropoikilocytosis, overhydrated and dehydrated hereditary stomatocytosis, membrane lipid disorders, and paroxysmal nocturnal hemoglobinuria. The format for presentation of each of these disorders is pathophysiology, clinical features, laboratory findings, and therapy. Because these anemias are due to defects in the erythrocyte membrane, the reader should have a good understanding of the normal erythrocyte membrane structure (∞ Chapter 5) before beginning.

▶ INTRODUCTION

Erythrocyte life span can be significantly shortened if the cell is intrinsically defective (intracorpuscular defect). Hemolytic anemia has been associated with defective erythrocyte membranes, structurally abnormal hemoglobins (hemoglobinopathies), defective globin synthesis (thalassemias), and deficiencies of erythrocyte enzymes. Almost all of these defects are hereditary. The hemoglobinopathies and thalassemias, which have a significant hemolytic component, have been discussed previously (∞ Chapters 10 and 11). This chapter includes the hemolytic anemias due to membrane defects.

An erythrocyte membrane that is normal in both structure and function is essential to the survival of the cell (∞ Chapter 5). Composed of proteins and lipids, the membrane is responsible for maintaining stability and the normal discoid shape of the cell, preserving cell deformability, and retaining selective permeability.

▶ MEMBRANE DEFECTS

Hemolytic anemia can result from abnormalities in constituent membrane proteins or lipids, both of which can alter the membrane's stability, shape, deformability, and/or permeability. The abnormal cells are particularly susceptible to entrapment in the splenic cords. Anemia results when the rate of hemolysis is increased to the point at which the bone marrow cannot adequately compensate. Most hemolysis associated with abnormal membranes is extravascular, occurring primarily in the splenic cords.

SKELETAL PROTEIN ABNORMALITIES

The membrane protein and lipid interactions associated with abnormal erythrocyte membranes can be divided into two categories, vertical and horizontal[1] (Figure 15-1 ■; Table 15-1 ✪).

Vertical Interactions

Vertical interactions are perpendicular to the plane of the erythrocyte membrane and include interactions between

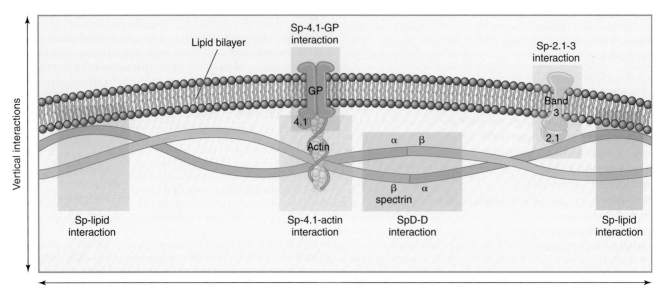

FIGURE 15-1   Pathobiology of the red cell lesions in hereditary red blood cell membrane defects. Vertical interactions of membrane lipids and proteins are perpendicular to the plane of the membrane. These interactions stabilize the lipid bilayer. Deficiencies of spectrin, ankyrin (2.1), or band 3 protein causes decoupling of the lipid bilayer from the underlying skeletal lattice and subsequent membrane loss in the form of microvesicles. This leads to the formation of spherocytes (hereditary spherocytosis). Horizontal interactions are parallel to the plane of the membrane. These interactions provide mechanical stability to the membrane. Horizontal defects include abnormal spectrin heterodimer association to form tetramers and defective skeletal protein interactions of junctional complexes at the end of the spectrin tetramers (spectrin, actin, protein 4.1) Horizontal defects result in fragmentation of the red blood cell. (Hereditary elliptocytosis, hereditary pyropoikilocytosis). Sp = spectrin; GP = glycophorin; SpD-D = spectrin dimer dimer. (This figure was published in *Seminars in Hematology, vol 30*, Palek J, Jarolim P, Clinical expression and laboratory detection of red blood cell membrane protein mutations, p. 249–83. Copyright Elsevier. 1993. Used with permission.)

the skeletal lattice on the cytoplasmic side of the membrane and its attachment to the integral proteins and lipids of the membrane. These interactions stabilize the lipid bilayer membrane. Defects in vertical contacts between the skeletal lattice proteins and the membrane's integral proteins and

lipids cause uncoupling of the lipid bilayer from the underlying skeletal lattice, causing a selective loss of portions of the lipid bilayer. The net loss of cell membrane results in a decrease in the surface area-to-volume ratio, the formation of a spherocyte, and the eventual hemolysis of the cell. The skeletal lattice, however, is not disrupted, and the cell is mechanically stable. The genetic defects associated with the vertical protein interaction of the red cell membrane are listed in Table 15-1.

Horizontal Interactions

Horizontal interactions are parallel to the plane of the membrane and are important in the formation of the stress-supporting skeletal protein lattice. This lattice provides mechanical stability to the membrane. Horizontal interactions include spectrin heterodimer head-to-head association to form tetramers as well as skeletal protein interactions in the junctional complexes at the distal ends of spectrin tetramers (spectrin, actin, protein 4.1, glycophorin C, and adducin contacts). Horizontal defects characterized by defects of the skeletal protein interactions beneath the lipid bilayer lead to disruption of the skeletal lattice and, consequently, membrane destabilization. This causes cell fragmentation with formation of poikilocytes.

✪ TABLE 15-1	
Protein Mutations in the Erythrocyte Membrane That Result in Vertical or Horizontal Interaction Defects and Cause Hemolytic Anemia	
Interaction Defect	**Causes**
Vertical	Ankyrin
	Band 3
	Protein 4.2
	α-spectrin
	β-spectrin
Horizontal	Protein 4.1
	Glycophorin C
	α-spectrin
	β-spectrin

LIPID COMPOSITION ABNORMALITIES

Disorders that affect the composition of the membrane lipid bilayer lead to the formation of acanthocytes. The erythrocyte membrane normally contains equal amounts of free cholesterol and phospholipids. Excess free plasma cholesterol in patients accumulates in the outer bilayer of the erythrocyte. It has been hypothesized that preferential expansion of the outer face of the lipid bilayer in comparison to the inner face leads to formation of acanthocytes as the spleen attempts to remodel the cell.[2] Acanthocytes are more spheroidal cells with sharp irregular projections and an absence of central pallor. These cells are poorly deformable and readily trapped in the spleen. A variety of conditions can lead to acanthocytosis.

Hemolytic anemias associated with the various membrane defects are listed in Table 15-2 ✪. In general, vertical interaction defects are characterized by the presence of spherocytes; horizontal defects are characterized by the presence of other types of poikilocytes; and lipid composition defects are characterized by the presence of acanthocytes.

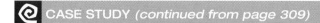

CASE STUDY (continued from page 309)

A CBC was ordered on the patient and the results follow:

WBC	8.0×10^9/L
RBC	4.0×10^{12}/L
Hgb	108 g/L
Hct	0.292 L/L
Platelets	504×10^9/L

1. Calculate the erythrocyte indices.
2. Based on the calculated indices, describe the patient's red blood cells.

► HEREDITARY SPHEROCYTOSIS

Hereditary spherocytosis (HS) is a common inherited membrane disorder that affects 1 in 2000 northern Europeans. In about two-thirds of patients, the disease is inherited in an autosomal-dominant fashion.[3] De novo mutations

✪ TABLE 15-2

Hemolytic Anemias Associated with Erythrocyte Membrane Defects

Disorder	Inheritance Pattern	Membrane Defect	Abnormal Membrane Function	Erythrocyte Morphology
Hereditary spherocytosis (HS)	Usually autosomal dominant; autosomal recessive; de novo mutations	Ankyrin and spectrin deficiency or deficiencies of band 3 and protein 4.2	Defective vertical protein interaction between RBC skeleton and membrane; loss of lipid bilayer and subsequent formation of a spherocyte with decreased deformability; abnormal permeability to Na^+	Spherocytes
Hereditary elliptocytosis (HE)	Autosomal dominant or rare de novo mutation; Melanesian variant is autosomal recessive	Defective spectrin Deficiency or defect in band 4.1 Abnormal integral proteins	Defect in horizontal protein interactions resulting in membrane instability; also can be a defect in permeability	Elliptocytes
Hereditary pyropoikilocytosis (HPP)	Autosomal recessive	Two defects: Partial spectrin deficiency and presence of a mutant spectrin	Defect in horizontal protein interactions resulting in membrane instability	Schistocytes, elliptocytes, and microspherocytes
Overhydrated hereditary stomatocytosis	Autosomal dominant	Unknown	Abnormally permeable to Na^+ and K^+; overhydration and swelling; decreased deformability	Stomatocytes
Dehydrated hereditary stomatocytosis	Autosomal dominant	Unknown	Abnormally permeable resulting in loss of K^+; water loss; decreased deformability	Target cells
Acanthocytosis (abetalipoproteinemia)	Autosomal recessive	Increased sphingomyelin, which can be secondary to abnormal plasma lipid composition	Expansion of outer lipid layer causes abnormal shape; increased membrane viscosity and decreased fluidity/deformability	Acanthocytes
Paroxysmal nocturnal hemoglobinuria (PNH)	Acquired	Deficiency of DAF and MIRL	Increased sensitivity to complement lysis	Normocytic or macrocytic; microcytic, hypochromic if iron deficient

DAF = decay-accelerating factor; MIRL = membrane inhibitor of reactive lysis

account for about one-half of sporadic cases[4] with the rest assumed to be caused by a recessive gene.

PATHOPHYSIOLOGY

Hereditary spherocytosis is a clinically heterogeneous disorder characterized by mild to moderate hemolysis. The erythrocytes in this disorder are deficient in spectrin and are abnormally permeable to Na^+. These features lead to erythrocytes that have problems with both deformability and permeability.

The membrane defect in hereditary spherocytosis is a disorder of vertical protein interactions most often characterized by a combined deficiency of spectrin and ankyrin, although there is considerable genetic heterogeneity at the molecular level.[5,6] The spectrin deficiency can be a primary deficiency of spectrin or a secondary deficiency due to defective attachment of the skeleton to the lipid bilayer. Defective attachment can occur as a result of mutations of ankyrin, α- or β-spectrin, protein 4.2, or band 3 protein.[7-9]

These defects in spectrin and ankyrin and their interactions with other skeletal proteins result in a weakening of the vertical connections between the skeletal proteins and lipid bilayer membrane. The uncoupling between the inner membrane skeleton and outer lipid bilayer leads to the shedding of the lipid bilayer in the form of microvesicles.[3] Secondary to membrane loss, the cell has a decreased surface-area-to-volume ratio, changing the morphology of the cell from a discocyte to a spherocyte. The most spheroidal cells have a greatly increased cytoplasmic viscosity. The spheroidal shape and increased viscosity result in reduced cellular flexibility. Reticulocytes in HS are normal in shape, emphasizing the fact that erythrocytes lose their membrane fragments after encountering the stress of the circulation.

In addition to the abnormal cytoskeleton of HS erythrocytes, other membrane abnormalities may be present. The total lipids in the HS erythrocyte membrane is decreased both before and after splenectomy. Although the organization of lipids in the membrane is known to affect membrane fluidity, an association between abnormal fluidity and HS erythrocytes has not been established. The HS erythrocytes also are abnormally permeable to sodium, causing an influx of Na^+ at 10 times the normal rate.[10] An increase in the activity of the cation pump can compensate for the leak if adequate glucose is available for ATP production. The increased permeability is probably related to a functional abnormality of the membrane proteins.

The spherocytic shape, increased cytoplasmic viscosity, and increased membrane permeability account for the eventual destruction of HS cells in the spleen. Spherocytes lack the flexibility of normal cells, causing them to become trapped in the splenic cords. In this environment of very low glucose concentrations, the cell quickly runs out of the ATP needed to pump out excess Na^+. As energy production ceases, splenic macrophages destroy the metabolically stressed cells.

CLINICAL FINDINGS

The clinical severity of HS varies among families and even among patients in the same family. About 25% of the patients have compensated hemolytic disease, no anemia, little or no jaundice, and only slight splenomegaly. In contrast, the disease can be lethal for some patients, especially in those homozygous for dominant HS. Most patients, however, develop a partially compensated hemolytic anemia in childhood and appear asymptomatic. HS in some asymptomatic individuals can be detected only when family studies are done on patients with more severe forms of the disease. Intermittent jaundice can occur. The jaundice is especially apparent during viral infections. Splenomegaly is present in about 50% of affected infants increasing to 75–95% in older children and adults. Aplastic crisis is a life-threatening complication that can occur in childhood during or following a viral infection. Untreated older patients commonly develop pigment bile stones from excess bilirubin catabolism (**cholelithiasis**). These patients also are predisposed to **cholecystitis**.

LABORATORY FINDINGS

Hemoglobin levels in patients with HS can be normal or decreased, varying directly with the age of the individual upon presentation of symptoms. Infants have the lowest values, 8–11 g/dL. Older children usually have concentrations above 10 g/dL. The reticulocyte count is usually more than 8%. The diagnosis of hereditary spherocytosis is suspected with the finding of many densely stained spherocytic cells with a decreased diameter and increased polychromasia on the blood smear (Figure 15-2 ■). Small, dense microspherocytes with a decreased MCV and increased MCHC also can be found. The number of microspherocytes varies considerably, and microspherocytes might not be prominent in 20–25% of

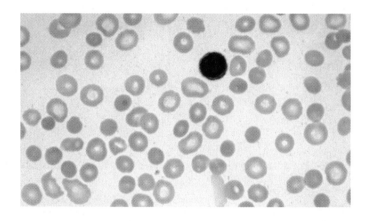

■ FIGURE 15-2   Peripheral blood from a patient with hereditary spherocytosis shows the presence of many densely staining spherocytes. (Peripheral blood; Wright-Giemsa stain; 1000× magnification)

patients. In mild forms of HS, the changes in erythrocyte morphology can be too subtle to detect even by experienced hematologists. Nucleated erythrocytes can be found in children with severe anemia.

When the inheritance pattern of HS cannot be established, HS must be distinguished from other conditions causing spherocytosis. Spherocytes also can be found in acquired immune hemolytic anemia (AIHA), but in HS, the spherocytes are more uniform in size and shape than in AIHA.

Erythrocyte indices are helpful in the diagnosis of HS. The MCV usually is normal or only slightly decreased (77–87 fL). If reticulocytosis is marked, the MCV can be increased. The MCH is normal, but the MCHC is generally more than 36 g/dL.[11] Spherocytes are the only erythrocytes with an increased MCHC. Modern generation blood analyzers utilizing laser or aperture impedance methodology are extremely sensitive in detecting erythrocytes with an MCHC of more than 41 g/dL (hyperhemoglobin).[12] These erythrocytes are typically spherocytes. This technology can detect even the mild forms of HS. It is important to remember that the indices can vary depending on iron and folate stores. Folate frequently becomes depleted in chronic hemolytic states.

As in other hemolytic states, the bone marrow demonstrates normoblastic erythroid hyperplasia with an increase in storage iron.

✓ Checkpoint! 1

List various factors related to changes in the erythrocyte that can lead to a decrease or increase in the MCV in hereditary spherocytosis.

Osmotic Fragility Test

The principal confirmation test in the diagnosis of HS, the osmotic fragility test, measures the erythrocyte's resistance to hemolysis by osmotic stress, which depends primarily on the volume of the cell, the surface area, and its membrane function. Erythrocytes are incubated in varying concentrations of hypotonic sodium chloride (NaCl) solution. Because of their decreased surface-area-to-volume ratio, spherocytes are unable to expand as much as normal discoid shaped cells can. Very little fluid needs to be absorbed before the cells hemolyze. The spherocytes also may have increased membrane permeability, contributing to their increased fragility. Lysis of HS erythrocytes, therefore, begins at higher NaCl concentrations than normal cells. These HS cells are said to exhibit increased osmotic fragility.

The osmotic fragility test is not abnormal unless spherocytes constitute at least 1–2% of the erythrocyte population; thus, patients with mild HS can have a normal osmotic fragility. These cells, however, show marked abnormal hemolysis if the blood is incubated overnight (24 hours) at 37°C before it is added to the NaCl solution. Incubation increases the loss of erythrocyte surface area. Because of its increased sensitivity, this incubated osmotic

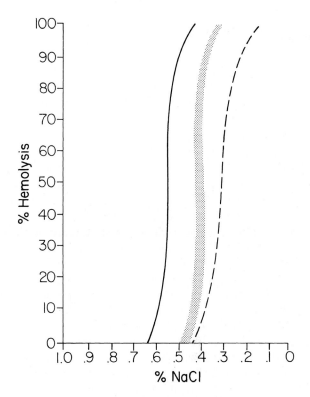

FIGURE 15-3 Graph depicting the osmotic fragility of normal cells, spherocytes, and cells from a patient with thalassemia. Spherocytes show an increased fragility with a shift to the left in the osmotic fragility curve, and the thalassemia cells show a decreased fragility with a shift to the right in the osmotic fragility curve. The decreased fragility in thalassemia is caused primarily by the presence of target cells.

fragility test is the most reliable diagnostic test for hereditary spherocytosis.

In most laboratories, the osmotic fragility test results are graphed to depict the degree of fragility in comparison to the normal state (Figure 15-3 ■). A shift to the left of normal in the curve indicates increased osmotic fragility, whereas a shift to the right indicates decreased osmotic fragility (Table 15-3 ✪). Decreased osmotic fragility occurs in thalassemia, sickle cell anemia, and conditions associated with target cells.

✪ TABLE 15-3

Example of Increased Osmotic Fragility

	Patient	Normal Control
Initial hemolysis	0.65% NaCl	0.45% NaCl
Complete hemolysis	0.45% NaCl	0.30% NaCl

✓ Checkpoint! 2

Interpret the results of the following osmotic fragility test:

	Patient	Control
Initial hemolysis	*0.35% NaCl*	*0.45% NaCl*
Complete hemolysis	*0.25% NaCl*	*0.30% NaCl*

Autohemolysis Test

The autohemolysis test also is used in the diagnosis of HS but does not have an advantage over the osmotic fragility test. It is of more value in differentiating various types of congenital, nonspherocytic hemolytic anemias. This test measures the degree of spontaneous hemolysis of blood incubated at 37°C. The degree of hemolysis depends on the integrity of the cell membrane and the adequacy of cell enzymes involved in glycolysis. Incubation of blood in vitro probably causes the alteration of membrane lipids. This alteration leads to a change in cell permeability and an increase in the utilization of both glucose and ATP.

In HS, autohemolysis is increased to between 5 and 25% at 24 hours (normal is 0.2–2.0%) and can increase to 75% at 48 hours. If glucose is added to the blood before incubation, hemolysis is significantly decreased. If large numbers of microspherocytes are present, hemolysis might not be corrected with glucose. Autohemolysis also is increased in the immune spherocytic anemias, but glucose does not usually affect the test results.

Other Lab Tests

Other laboratory tests including increased indirect serum bilirubin, and increased fecal urobilinogen reflect the usual findings of increased extravascular hemolysis. Lactic dehydrogenase (LD) can be increased, and haptoglobin levels are often decreased. The antihuman globulin (AHG) test is negative, a finding helpful in distinguishing HS from immune hemolytic anemias in which large numbers of spherocytes also are found (∞ Chapter 17). The AHG test detects antibodies or complement bound to erythrocytes in vivo (direct antiglobulin test, DAT) or free antibodies in the serum (indirect antiglobulin test, IAT). Immune hemolytic anemias are usually associated with a positive DAT.

IDENTIFICATION OF DEFICIENT MEMBRANE PROTEIN

To determine which erythrocyte membrane protein is deficient, initial studies usually include sodium dodecyl sulfate polyacrylamide gel electrophoresis (SDS-PAGE) followed by densitometric quantitation and enzyme linked immunosorbent assay (ELISA) techniques.[11] Genetic linkage analysis using PCR-based techniques can be used to determine a patient's precise molecular defect[2] (∞ Chapter 39). A test utilizing flow cytometry technology that can detect band 3 binding by the dye eosin-5-maleimide (EMA) has recently been introduced. This test is highly specific and sensitive for HS.[13]

THERAPY

Mild forms of HS do not require therapeutic intervention. Total or partial splenectomy is the standard treatment in patients with symptomatic hemolysis.[14,15] This therapy corrects the anemia and hemolysis, but the basic membrane defect, however, remains, and spherocytes can still be found in the peripheral blood. Fragments of the unstable membrane are probably removed in the liver.

@ CASE STUDY *(continued from page 311)*

The patient's peripheral smear revealed numerous elliptocytes, spherocytes, teardrop cells, and micropoikilocytes.

3. What additional lab tests should be ordered?

▶ HEREDITARY ELLIPTOCYTOSIS

Hereditary elliptocytosis (HE) is inherited as an autosomal-dominant trait except for a rare Melanesian type that is inherited as a recessive trait. Worldwide, the incidence is 1 case per 2000–4000 individuals, although the true incidence is unknown because many patients with HE are asymptomatic.[3] The disease is heterogeneous in the degree of hemolysis and in clinical severity. As its name indicates, the most prominent peripheral blood finding is an increase in oval and elongated erythrocytes (elliptocytes).

Three classifications of HE can be distinguished based on erythrocyte morphology:[9] (1) common HE, (2) spherocytic HE (hemolytic ovalocytosis), and (3) stomatocytic HE, Melanesian ovalocytosis, or Southeast Asian ovalocytosis (SAO) (Table 15-4).

PATHOPHYSIOLOGY

The abnormal erythrocyte shape in hereditary elliptocytosis is the result of a defect in one of the skeletal proteins. It is interesting to note that similar to HS, reticulocytes and nucle-

✪ TABLE 15-4

Classification of Hereditary Elliptocytosis (HE) Based on Erythrocyte Morphology

Type of HE	Hemolysis	Erythrocyte Shape
Common HE	Variable; minimal to severe	Elliptocytes
Spherocytic HE (hemolytic ovalocytosis)	Present	Spherocytes and fat elliptocytes
Southeast Asian ovalocytosis (SAO) (stomatocytic HE; Melanesian ovalocytosis)	Mild or absent	Roundish elliptocytes that are also stomatocytic

ated erythrocytes in this disorder are normal in shape; therefore, the elliptical erythrocyte form is acquired in the circulation. In the microcirculation, erythrocytes are subjected to shear stress and normally acquire an elliptical shape. Normal erythrocytes, however, revert to a biconcave shape in the absence of the circulatory stress while HE erythrocytes remain in the elliptical shape. It is possible that the stress in the microcirculation causes disruption of the skeletal protein contacts in the membrane of HE erythrocytes that leads to the formation of new protein contacts that prevent HE erythrocytes from resuming the normal biconcave shape.

The principal defect involves horizontal membrane protein interactions. Evidence indicates that several different membrane protein defects can be linked to this disease:[16,17]

1. decreased association of spectrin dimers to form tetramers due to defective spectrin chains

2. a deficiency or defect in band 4.1 that aids in binding spectrin to actin

3. abnormalities of the integral proteins including deficiency of glycophorin C and abnormal anion transport protein (band 3) with increased affinity to ankyrin (vertical interaction defect).

Each of these defects can lead to skeletal disruptions that can cause the cell to become elliptical in shape and/or fragment under the stresses of the circulation, depending on the extent of the defect. Mildly dysfunctional proteins cause only elliptocytosis whereas severely dysfunctional proteins cause membrane fragmentation in addition to elliptocytosis. Alteration in shape only does not appear to affect cell deformability, and the cells have a nearly normal life span. Elliptocytosis with membrane fragmentation, however, causes a decrease in cell surface area and reduced cell deformability. The life span of these cells is severely shortened.

In addition to membrane instability, HE erythrocytes are abnormally permeable to Na^+. This altered permeability demands an increase in ATP to run the cation pump and maintain osmotic equilibrium. Cells detained in the spleen can quickly deplete their ATP and become osmotically fragile.

The defect in the SAO variant of HE is an abnormal band 3 protein rather than a defect in the cytoskeletal proteins under the lipid bilayer. There is a deletion of nine amino acids near the boundary of the membrane and cytoplasmic domains of the protein. This is associated with a tighter binding of band 3 to ankyrin, a lack of transport of sulfate anions, and a restriction in the lateral and rotational mobility of band 3 protein within the membrane. As a result, these erythrocytes are very rigid.[9]

CLINICAL FINDINGS

Ninety percent of patients with HE show no overt signs of hemolysis. Although erythrocyte survival can be decreased, the hemolysis is usually mild and well compensated for by the bone marrow (compensated hemolytic disease). Anemia is not characteristic.

Common HE is rare in the Western population but more common in blacks, particularly in equatorial Africa. The severity ranges from asymptomatic to severe clinical disease. There can be minimal hemolysis and only mild elliptocytosis (15%) or severe hemolysis with cell fragmentation and formation of poikilocytes.

A variant of common HE noted in black infants is associated with a moderately severe anemia at birth and neonatal jaundice. The peripheral blood smear exhibits erythrocytes similar to those seen in hereditary pyropoikilocytosis with budding and fragile bizarre poikilocytes. Variable numbers of elliptocytes are noted. Between 6 and 12 months of age, the hemolysis decreases, and the number of elliptocytes increases. One of the parents of affected infants has mild hereditary elliptocytosis.

The spherocytic HE variant constitutes a relatively rare form of HE characterized by the presence of hemolysis despite minimal changes in erythrocyte morphology. The erythrocytes have characteristics of both HS and HE cells: Some are spherocytic and others are fat elliptocytes.

The Southeast Asian variant of HE (SAO, stomatocytic HE) is characterized by a mild or absent hemolytic component. Erythrocyte cation permeability appears to be increased, and the expression of blood group antigens is muted. The elliptocytes are roundish and stomatocytic with one or two transverse bars or a longitudinal slit. Evidence indicates these cells can have more stable cytoskeletons than normal.[16]

The high prevalence of the SAO variety of HE in some parts of the world is related to the resistance of the HE erythrocytes to invasion by malarial parasites. The resistance can result from the abnormal rigidity of the erythrocyte membrane. This protection against malaria has led to natural selection of individuals with HE in areas of the world where malaria is endemic and, thus, the incidence of HE increases.[18,19]

HE cells are poorly agglutinable with antisera against erythrocyte antigens. This is presumably the result of defective lateral movement and clustering of surface antigens associated with the abnormal band 3 protein. The laboratory scientist should be aware of this problem because it can interfere with testing of patients' cells in the blood bank.

LABORATORY FINDINGS

The most consistent and characteristic laboratory finding in all variants is prominent elliptocytosis (Figure 15-4 ■). Elliptocytes also can be found in association with other diseases, but elliptocytes in these conditions usually constitute less than 25% of the erythrocytes. Acquired elliptocytosis is seen in megaloblastic anemias and iron-deficiency anemia. In contrast, the elliptocytes in HE make up more than 25% of the erythrocytes and usually more than 60%. In the asymptomatic variety of HE, elliptocytes can be the only morphologic clue to the disease. Hemoglobin levels are usually higher than 12 g/dL. Reticulocytes are mildly elevated, up to about 4%.

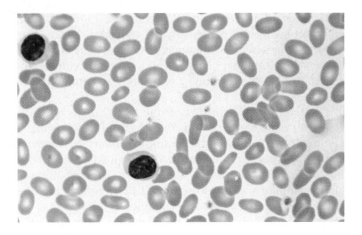

■ FIGURE 15-4   Peripheral blood from a patient with non-hemolytic HE reveals almost 100% elliptocytes. (Peripheral blood; Wright-Giemsa stain; 1000× original magnification)

In the hemolytic HE variants, hemoglobin concentration is 9–10 g/dL, and reticulocytes are elevated to as high as 20%. Microelliptocytes, bizarre poikilocytes, schistocytes, and spherocytes are usually evident (Figure 15-5 ■). The bone marrow shows erythroid hyperplasia with normal maturation.

The incubated and unincubated osmotic fragility tests and autohemolysis tests are usually abnormally increased in the overt hemolytic variants. However, the obvious blood picture suggests that there is no need to perform these tests.

THERAPY

The hemolytic variants of HE respond well to splenectomy. As in HS, splenectomy prevents hemolysis and protects the patient from complications of chronic hemolysis. The membrane defect, however, remains, and elliptocytes are still present. The asymptomatic variants require no therapy.

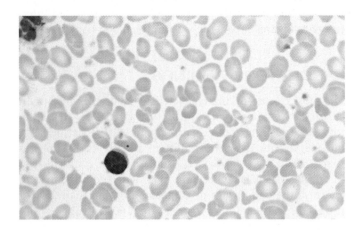

■ FIGURE 15-5   Blood smear from a patient with the hemolytic hereditary elliptocytosis. Schistocytes as well as elliptocytes are present. (Wright-Giemsa stain; 1000× original magnification)

✓ **Checkpoint! 3**

Why do the elliptocytes in HE demonstrate normal osmotic fragility?

ⓔ **CASE STUDY** *(continued from page 314)*

Jack's osmotic fragility test revealed the following:

	Patient	Control
Initial hemolysis	.65% NaCl	.45% NaCl
Complete hemolysis	.40% NaCl	.30% NaCl

4. Interpret the results of the osmotic fragility test.

▶ HEREDITARY PYROPOIKILOCYTOSIS (HPP)

Hereditary pyropoikilocytosis (HPP), a rare autosomal recessive disorder, is closely related to HE. Based on recent genetic and biochemical data, it has now been established that HPP is a severe subtype of HE.[17] It occurs primarily in blacks, although it also has been diagnosed in Arabs and Caucasians.[3] The disease presents in infancy or early childhood as a severe hemolytic anemia with extreme poikilocytosis. The morphological similarities of erythrocytes in HPP and that of erythrocytes associated with thermal injury led investigators to examine the thermal stability of HPP cells. In contrast to normal erythrocytes that fragment at 49–50°C, HPP cell membranes fragment when heated to 45–46°C. In addition, pyropoikilocytes disintegrate when incubated at 37°C for more than 6 hours.

PATHOPHYSIOLOGY

The HPP cells have two defects with one inherited from each parent. One is related to a deficiency of α-spectrin and the other to the presence of a mutant spectrin that prevents self-association of heterodimers to tetramers.[16] The parent carrying the mutant spectrin trait either has mild HE or is asymptomatic. The other parent, with the deficiency of spectrin trait, is hematologically normal. The HPP phenotype also is found in patients who are homozygous or doubly heterozygous for one or two spectrin mutations characteristically found in HE trait.[16] The defects lead to a disruption of the membrane skeletal lattice and cell destabilization followed by erythrocyte fragmentation and poikilocytosis.[9] Poikilocytes are removed in the spleen.

CLINICAL FINDINGS

Clinical features consistent with a hemolytic anemia are present at birth. Hyperbilirubinemia requiring **exchange transfusion** (a procedure involving simultaneous withdrawal of blood and infusion with compatible blood) or

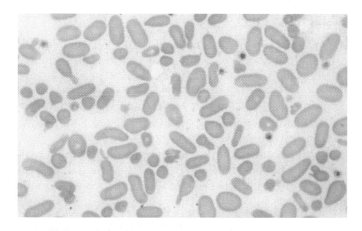

■ FIGURE 15-6 Peripheral blood from a patient with hereditary pyropoikilocytosis. (Peripheral blood; Wright-Giemsa stain; 1000× original magnification)

phototherapy (therapeutic exposure to sunlight or artificial light) is present.[16] Laboratory serologic studies for hemolytic disease of the newborn, however, are negative.

LABORATORY FINDINGS

Stained blood smears exhibit striking erythrocyte morphologic abnormalities including budding, fragments, microspherocytes (2–4 fL), elliptocytes, triangulocytes (fragmented erythrocytes that are triangle shaped), and other bizarre erythrocyte shapes (Figure 15-6■). The MCV is decreased (25–55 fL), most likely as a result of the many erythrocyte fragments. The osmotic fragility is abnormal, especially after incubation, and the thermal sensitivity test demonstrates an increase in erythrocyte fragmentation (Figure 15-7■). Autohemolysis is increased and the hemolysis is not corrected with glucose.

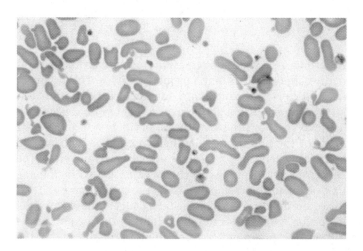

■ FIGURE 15-7 Peripheral blood from a patient with hereditary pyropoikilocytosis (in Figure 15-6). Smear made after incubation of blood for 10 minutes at 46°C. (Peripheral blood; Wright-Giemsa stain; 1000× original magnification)

THERAPY

Patients show improvement after splenectomy, but the membrane defect remains, and fragmented erythrocytes are still present.

CASE STUDY (continued from page 316)

A thermal sensitivity test demonstrated that Jack's erythrocytes fragment when incubated for 10 minutes at 46°C.

5. What do the results of the thermal sensitivity test reveal about the patient's red blood cells?

✓ Checkpoint! 4

Interpret the results of the following thermal sensitivity test:

Patient's erythrocytes	*Marked erythrocyte fragmentation after 10-minute incubation at 46°C*
Normal control	*No significant change in erythrocyte morphology after 10-minute incubation at 46°C*

▶ HEREDITARY STOMATOCYTOSIS SYNDROMES

The hereditary stomatocytosis syndromes are rare autosomal dominant hemolytic anemias in which the erythrocyte membrane exhibits abnormalities in cation permeability.[1] These syndromes include **overhydrated hereditary stomatocytosis (OHS)** and **dehydrated hereditary stomatocytosis (DHS)** (formally known as hereditary xerocytosis). The red cell membrane in OHS is abnormally permeable to both Na^+ and K^+. The net gain of Na^+ ions is more than the net loss of K^+ ions because the capacity of the cation pump (fueled by ATP derived from glycolysis) to maintain normal intracellular osmolality is exceeded. As a result, the intracellular concentration of cations increases, water enters the cell, and the overhydrated cells take on the appearance of stomatocytes. Stomatocytes (hydrocytes) on dried, stained blood films are erythrocytes with a slitlike (mouthlike) area of pallor (Figure 15-8■). These cells are uniconcave and appear bowl shaped on wet preparations.

The primary defect in DHS is a net loss of intracellular K^+ that exceeds the passive Na^+ influx and thus net intracellular cation and water content are decreased. Consequently, the cell dehydrates and the cells appear targeted or contracted and spiculated.[12]

PATHOPHYSIOLOGY

The specific membrane defect for OHS and DHS has not been identified. Patients with OHS demonstrate a deficiency of stomatin, an intregal red cell membrane protein, which is secondary to an unknown protein mutation.[1,20]

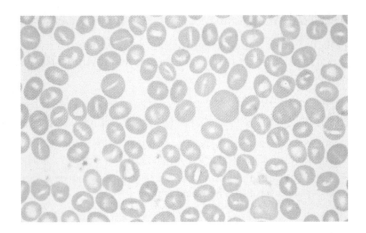

■ FIGURE 15-8   This peripheral blood picture from a patient with hereditary overhydrated stomatocytosis reveals erythrocytes with slitlike or mouthlike (stoma = mouth) areas of pallor. (Peripheral blood; Wright-Giemsa stain; 1000× magnification)

Abnormalities of erythrocyte lipids have been demonstrated to induce stomatocytosis with impaired sodium transport. However, stomatocytosis also occurs when membrane lipids are normal. In these cases, membrane proteins can be abnormal. Although membrane proteins are usually electrophoretically normal, there can be an alteration in their conformation. A deficiency in band 7 proteins has been described.

From the variability of clinical findings, laboratory results, and response to splenectomy, these disorders appear to be caused by several different membrane defects. Some patients have marked stomatocytosis but no abnormal sodium transport. Up to one-third of patients with stomatocytosis do not have overt hemolysis.[21,22] **Rh null disease** (a disorder associated with the lack of Rh antigen on erythrocytes) also is associated with the presence of stomatocytes.[23] The association between a lack of the Rh complex and the membrane abnormality has not been explained.

The stomatocytic cells in OHS are osmotically fragile and less deformable than normal cells, and, as a result, the cells are sequestered in the spleen where glucose supplies are readily exhausted. As the ATP levels fall, the cation pump is unable to maintain osmotic equilibrium, causing cell lysis or phagocytosis.

OHS must be differentiated from acquired stomatocytosis. Stomatocytes are seen as an acquired defect in acute alcoholism, liver disease, and cardiovascular disease. However, these acquired conditions, have no cation leaks, and little hemolysis is present.

The cells are dehydrated in DHS, which is reflected by an increased MCHC. As the MCHC of the cell increases beyond 37 g/dl, the cytoplasmic viscosity increases, and cellular deformability decreases. The rigid cells become trapped in the spleen.

LABORATORY FINDINGS

Anemia is usually mild to moderate with a hemoglobin concentration of 8–10 g/dL. Bilirubin is increased and reticulocytosis is moderate. The MCHC of the stomatocytes seen in OHS is decreased, and the MCV can be increased. The blood smear is remarkable for 10–50% stomatocytes. Osmotic fragility and autohemolysis are increased, and autohemolysis is partially corrected with glucose and ATP.

Target cells and erythrocytes that have hemoglobin puddled at the periphery are observed in DHS. The cells demonstrate a slightly increased MCV and decreased osmotic fragility.

THERAPY

Splenectomy is not a required therapeutic measure for OHS and DHS. In fact, this procedure is usually contraindicated because some patients have experienced catastrophic thrombotic episodes after splenectomy.[1,24] Most patients are able to maintain an adequate hemoglobin level without this procedure.

 Checkpoint! 5

Determine the type of erythrocyte membrane disorder present based on the following lab results: retic count: 4%; osmotic fragility: increased; autohemolysis: increased; bilirubin: increased; peripheral smear: 30% stomatocytes present.

 Checkpoint! 6

Explain why the osmotic fragility is decreased in DHS.

► **ABNORMAL MEMBRANE LIPID COMPOSITION: ACANTHOCYTOSIS**

Acanthocytosis is most often associated with acquired or inherited abnormalities of the membrane lipids. This occurs in liver disease and in a rare inherited condition, *abetalipoproteinemia*. Although the mature cell has no capacity for de novo synthesis (new synthesis) of lipids or proteins, the lipids of the membrane continually exchange with plasma lipids. Thus, erythrocytes can acquire excess lipids when the concentration of plasma lipids increases. Excess membrane lipids expand the membrane surface area and cause the cell to acquire abnormal shapes, including target cells (codocytes), leptocytes, or acanthocytes. If portions of the membrane are lost due to "grooming" of excess lipids in the spleen or if the membrane's lipid viscosity increases, the cells lose their ability to deform and are sequestered in the spleen. On the other hand, a significant decrease in one or more lipids in the cell membrane can also lead to increased destruction. The rare hereditary forms of acanthocytosis also can result from abnormal proteins.

SPUR CELL ANEMIA

Spur cell anemia is an acquired hemolytic condition associated with severe hepatocellular disease such as cirrhosis in which serum lipoproteins increase, leading to an excess of erythrocyte membrane cholesterol. The total phospholipid content of the membrane, however, is normal. As the membrane ratio of cholesterol to phospholipid increases, the cell becomes flattened (leptocyte) with a scalloped edge. The increased cholesterol to phospholipid ratio also causes a decrease in membrane fluidity and an associated decrease in cell deformability. During repeated splenic passage or conditioning, membrane fragments are lost, and the cell acquires irregular spikelike projections typical of acanthocytes (spur cells). Eventually, the cell is hemolyzed. In patients with cirrhosis, this hemolysis is enhanced by congestive splenomegaly.

The peripheral blood shows a moderate to severe normocytic, normochromic anemia with a hemoglobin concentration of 5–10 g/dL. Reticulocytes are increased to 5–15%. Approximately 20–80% of the erythrocytes are acanthocytes (Figure 15-9 ■). On the peripheral blood smear, acanthocytes must be distinguished from echinocytes (burr cells) and keratocytes. (Echinocytes have regular, small, spiny projections throughout the cell membrane; keratocytes have just a few large surface projections.) Spherocytes and echinocytes can also be found. An increase in indirect bilirubin and liver enzymes and a decrease in serum albumin reflect evidence of liver disease.

Studies with transfused cells have shown that spur cells acquire their shape as innocent by-standers and that when normal cells are transfused into the patient, they acquire the abnormal shape and are hemolyzed at the same rate as the patient's cells, suggesting that the diseased liver can contribute to the transformation of normal red cells into spur cells.[25]

Biliary obstruction is often associated with the presence of normocytic or slightly macrocytic target cells that result from an acquired excess of lipids on the cell membrane. However, in contrast to the acanthocytes found in severe hepatocellular disease, the excess lipid on target cells associated with biliary obstruction includes an increase in both cholesterol and phospholipids in a ratio similar to that of normal cells. As a result, lipid viscosity and membrane deformability are normal. These target cells have a normal survival.

ABETALIPOPROTEINEMIA (HEREDITARY ACANTHOCYTOSIS)

This rare autosomal recessive disorder is characterized by the absence of serum β-lipoprotein, low serum cholesterol, low triglyceride, and low phospholipid and an increase in the ratio of cholesterol to phospholipid.[26,27] The primary abnormality is the defective synthesis of apoprotein B, a microsomal triglyceride transfer protein. Mutations in band 3 protein of the erythrocyte membrane that alters band 3 conformation have also been described in hereditary acanthocytosis.[28,29] Acanthocytes are typically found, but hemolysis is minimal with little or no anemia. Reticulocytes are usually normal but can be slightly increased. The acanthocytes have normal cholesterol levels, but lecithin decreases and sphingomyelin increases. This is in contrast to spur cells found in severe liver disease, which have increased membrane cholesterol. Membrane fluidity is decreased, presumably because of the increase in sphingomyelin, which is less fluid than other phospholipids. The degree of distortion of erythrocytes increases with cell age. The acanthocytes have normal membrane permeability, normal glucose metabolism, and normal osmotic fragility. Autohemolysis at 48 hours is increased and only partially corrected by glucose. In addition to hypolipidemia, the disorder is characterized by steatorrhea, retinitis pigmentosa, and neurological abnormalities. Transport of fat soluble vitamins (A, D, E, K) is impaired, and prothrombin time can be increased due to decreased vitamin K stores (∞ Chapters 30 and 40).

LECITHIN-CHOLESTEROL ACYL TRANSFERASE (LCAT) DEFICIENCY

This rare autosomal recessive disorder affects metabolism of high-density lipoproteins. Onset is usually during young adulthood. The disorder is characterized by a deficiency of LCAT, the enzyme that catalyzes the formation of cholesterol esters from cholesterol. As a result, patients with this deficiency demonstrate low levels of high-density

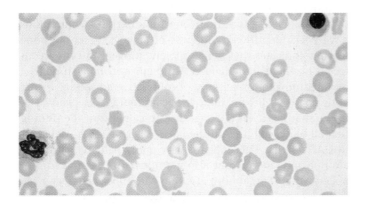

■ FIGURE 15-9   Spur cell anemia in a patient with alcoholic cirrhosis. Note the echinocytes and acanthocytes (spur cells). Spherocytes are also present. (Peripheral blood; Wright-Giemsa stain; 1000× magnification)

lipoprotein (HDL) and low-density lipoprotein (LDL) and elevated levels of very low-density lipoproteins (VLDL) and lipoprotein X.[30] Because erythrocyte membrane cholesterol is in a comparatively rapid equilibrium with unesterified plasma cholesterol, the activity of LCAT indirectly regulates the amount of free cholesterol in the cell. The most characteristic hematologic findings include a mild hemolytic anemia marked by the presence of numerous target cells. The target cells are loaded with cholesterol. LCAT activity is decreased in most patients with spur cells and target cells, but the relationship to lipid abnormalities of the membrane is not known.

RARE FORMS

The rare forms of acanthocytosis associated with abnormalities of membrane proteins include the McLeod phenotype with a deficiency of Kx substance and the K antigen, chorea-acanthocytosis syndrome, and acanthocytosis with band 3 protein abnormalities.

 Checkpoint! 7

Compare the membrane lipid abnormalities seen in LCAT deficiency, spur cell anemia, and abetalipoproteinemia, and explain how they result in hemolysis of the cell.

▶ PAROXYSMAL NOCTURNAL HEMOGLOBINURIA (PNH)

All erythrocyte membrane disorders discussed so far are hereditary in nature except spur cell anemia. **Paroxysmal nocturnal hemoglobinuria (PNH)** is a rare acquired disorder of the erythrocyte membrane. The membrane defect makes the cell abnormally sensitive to lysis by complement. The disease derives its name from the classic pattern of intermittent bouts of intravascular hemolysis and nocturnal hemoglobinuria. The condition is exacerbated during sleep and remits during the day. However, many patients have chronic hemolysis that is not associated with sleep and with no obvious hemoglobinuria.

PATHOPHYSIOLOGY

An intrinsic erythrocyte disorder, PNH results from an acquired stem cell somatic mutation that leads to an abnormal clone of differentiated hematopoietic cells. The abnormal stem cell clone produces erythrocytes, platelets, and neutrophils that bind abnormally large amounts of complement and that are abnormally sensitive to complement lysis (∞ Chapter 17). Complement is composed of at least 20 proteins responsible for a variety of biologic activities. These proteins are abbreviated as C1, C2, C3, etc. They normally circulate in an inactive form. Under some circumstances, complement components are activated. If the components attach to the erythrocyte membrane and are activated, the cell can be hemolyzed.

The susceptibility of PNH cells to complement-induced lysis is related to deficient regulation of complement activation. At least two regulatory proteins found on normal cell membranes are responsible for preventing amplification of complement activation. The first, **decay-accelerating factor (DAF)** (CD55), a complement regulatory protein that amplifies the decay of C3 convertase, accelerates decay (dissociation) of membrane-bound C3bBb, and thus prevents amplification of C3 convertase and activation of other complement components. Membrane inhibitor of reactive lysis (MIRL) (CD59) is the second regulatory protein that is deficient on PNH erythrocytes.[31] Its major role is to prevent the interaction between C8 and C9, and it thus interferes with the formation of membrane attack complex (MAC) (the final steps of complement activation). These regulating factors help normal cells avoid lysis by autologous complement. Lack of DAF and MIRL on PNH cells is causally related to excessive sensitivity of these cells to complement.[31]

Evidence suggests that deficiency of DAF and MIRL in PNH is not due to lack of production of these proteins but to the absence of a membrane glycolipid that serves as an anchor that attaches these proteins to the cell membrane. Other proteins anchored to the cell membrane in a similar manner also are deficient on hematopoietic cells in PNH. It appears that the common link to these membrane protein deficiencies is the lack of the glycolipid anchoring structure. This anchor has been identified as glycosyl-phosphatidyl inositol (GPI), a molecule embedded in the cell membrane that is important for the covalent linkage of a wide variety of proteins to the cell membrane. These GPI-linked proteins vary in structure and function. They include adhesion molecules, hydrolases, and receptors[31] (∞ Chapter 28).

The GPI-anchoring deficiency is due to a somatic mutation of the *PIGA* gene,[32] which encodes an enzyme (phosphatidyl inositol glycan Class A) essential for synthesis of the GPI anchor. More than one hundred PIG-A mutations have been identified.[33] Analysis of stem cells in the bone marrow indicates that hematopoietic progenitor cells are affected by the genetic defect. Although not understood, the mutated progenitor cell has a proliferative advantage in the bone marrow. Before the genetic mutation discovery, evidence that PNH was a clonal disease came from the finding that all blood cell lines in the patient with PNH are deficient in DAF activity. This explains why many patients with PNH are not only anemic but also granulocytopenic and thrombocytopenic. The abnormal clone can appear after damage to the marrow or spontaneously (idiopathic). A significant number of patients with PNH have or eventually develop another clonal blood disorder such as acute nonlymphocytic leukemia (∞ Chapter 24), chronic lymphocytic leukemia (∞ Chapter 26), myeloproliferative disorder (∞ Chapter 22), or myelodysplastic syndrome (∞ Chapter 23).[34]

The increased sensitivity of PNH cells to complement can be demonstrated to occur in vitro whether the complement is activated by the classic or the alternate pathway. In vivo, however, activation is probably by the alternate pathway.

CLINICAL FINDINGS

PNH occurs most often in adults but is occasionally found in children. The four basic disease mechanisms are hyperhemolysis, venous thrombosis, infection, and bone marrow hypoplasia.[35] The disease begins insidiously with irregular brisk episodes of acute intravascular hemolysis accompanied by hemoglobinuria. The patient usually seeks medical attention when reddish-brown urine is noted. In some patients, the irregular exacerbations of hemolysis are associated with sleep, hence the name *paroxysmal nocturnal hemoglobinuria*. In other patients, these hemolytic episodes can follow infections, transfusions, vaccinations, surgery, or ingestion of iron salts. In a large number of patients, hemolysis is unrelated to any specific event. Iron-deficiency anemia can occur due to the chronic blood loss through the kidneys. Renal functions can become abnormal as the result of chronic iron deposition. Folic acid deficiency can occur because of increased demand for this nutrient. Abdominal and lower back pain, eye pain, and headaches can occur during hemolytic episodes.

Even with moderate thrombocytopenia, venous thrombosis is a prominent and severe complication. Thrombosis is a common cause of death. Thrombotic events may be related to abnormal platelet or neutrophil function due to lack of GPI-anchored proteins.

When leukopenia is present, infections are common. Propensity for infection also can be related to the absence of granulocyte glycoproteins and altered response of granulocytes. Immunological abnormalities may be present.

LABORATORY FINDINGS

Most patients with PNH experience anemia with a hemoglobin concentration of 8–10 g/dL. The erythrocytes are normocytic or macrocytic but can appear microcytic and hypochromic if iron deficiency develops. Reticulocytes are increased (5–10%) but not to the extent expected for a hemolytic anemia. Nucleated red blood cells can be found on the blood smear. Isolated development of leukopenia and/or thrombocytopenia often occurs during the course of the disease. Neutrophil alkaline phosphatase and erythrocyte acetylcholinesterase are decreased (∞ Chapter 21). Although hemoglobinuria can be intermittent or even mild, hemosiderinuria is a constant finding, indicating chronic intravascular hemolysis.

The bone marrow usually exhibits normoblastic hyperplasia but can be hypocellular. In some cases, marrow failure develops during the course of the disease. Interestingly, aplastic anemia can be the initial diagnosis with an abnormal clone of PNH cells developing during the course of the disease (in up to 50% of patients with aplastic anemia). PNH rarely precedes aplastic anemia and should be considered as a diagnosis when hypoplastic anemia is found in association with hemolysis.[35] Bone marrow iron is decreased or absent.

The osmotic fragility is normal. Autohemolysis is increased after 48 hours, and when glucose is added, the hemolysis can increase even more. The DAT is negative for immunoglobulin (Ig) but can be positive for complement given the fact that PNH cells have a propensity to bind C3b.

The screening sucrose hemolysis (sugar-water) test is useful in identifying erythrocytes that are abnormally sensitive to complement lysis. The patient's blood is incubated in a sucrose solution. The sucrose provides a low-ionic-strength medium that promotes the binding of complement to the erythrocytes. PNH cells show hemolysis in this medium.

The Ham (acid-serum lysis) test is a more specific test for PNH cells (∞ Chapter 34), but laboratories have replaced it with immunophenotyping for confirmation of PNH (∞ Chapter 37). Immunophenotyping uses monoclonal antibodies directed against the GPI anchored molecules. When the GPI link is missing, these molecules are also missing. This technology can detect three types of cells in PNH related to the degree of deficiency of GPI-linked proteins on cell membranes:

- Type I   Little or no hemolysis by complement; nearly normal GPI expression
- Type II   Moderately sensitive to complement lysis; intermediate GPI expression
- Type III Highly sensitive to complement lysis; no expression of GPI

Because different hematopoietic cells display different kinds of GPI-anchored proteins, it is recommended that at least two different antibodies be used for a diagnosis of PNH (CD55, CD59, CD14). CD55 (DAF) and CD59 (MIRL) antibodies are used most frequently and are most attractive because they are involved in the complement pathway that leads to the hemolysis in PNH. PNH cells show low-intensity staining for these molecules. CD55 and CD59 are both normally found on neutrophils, and CD59 also is present on normal erythrocytes. CD14 is normally on monocytes, and some use it to verify PNH. Analyzing molecules that can be expressed on the membrane in a GPI-anchor form as well as a transmembrane form is not so useful because it can give false normal results.

The most accurate measurement of the PNH defect with immunophenotyping is performed using nucleated cells rather than erythrocytes because the patient with PNH often receives red blood cell transfusions. In addition, test results on erythrocytes might not be accurate because PNH type III erythrocytes have a shorter life span than do type I or II, thus underestimating type III erythrocyte concentration.

Recently a fluorochrome that binds to the GPI anchor itself, not to an attached protein, was developed.[36] This is a more direct technique to detect GPI deficient cells and is more sensitive in detecting abnormal granulocyte populations.

 Checkpoint! 8

Explain why immunophenotyping with CD14, CD55, and CD59 is used to establish a diagnosis of PNH.

THERAPY

Treatment is primarily supportive in the form of transfusions, antibiotics, and anticoagulants. A humanized monoclonal antibody has shown to relieve the hemoglobinuria in PNH patients by inhibiting the formation of the membrane attack complex (MAC).[37] In patients with PNH-induced marrow aplasia, bone marrow transplantation may be indicated.

 CASE STUDY *(continued from page 317)*

This case study depicts a young man who presented with right-upper-quadrant pain. The complete blood count disclosed anemia with a decreased MCV and and increased MCHC. The peripheral blood smear revealed numerous elliptocytes, teardrop cells, and micropoikilocytes. The patient's erythrocytes demonstrated increased osmotic fragility and thermal sensitivity.

6. What disorder is suggested by the patient's lab findings?

SUMMARY

The erythrocyte life span can be significantly shortened if the erythrocyte has intrinsic defects such as an abnormal membrane, structurally abnormal hemoglobin, defective globin synthesis, or deficient erythrocyte enzymes. These abnormalities are almost always inherited defects. When the bone marrow is unable to compensate, hemolytic anemia results.

Erythrocyte membrane defects can be caused by abnormalities of membrane proteins or lipids, which can affect cell deformability, stability, shape, and/or permeability. The abnormal erythrocytes become trapped in splenic cords and are removed from the circulation. Interactions between the skeletal lattice proteins and integral proteins and lipids of the membrane are vertical interactions that when disrupted cause a reduced density of spectrin and uncoupling of the lipid bilayer. This causes selective loss of lipid bilayer and formation of spherocytes. Skeletal lattice proteins interact horizontally to form the stress-supporting skeletal protein lattice. Defects in these proteins result in the cell's mechanical instability and fragmentation. Inherited defects in membrane proteins produce the hereditary hemolytic anemias including hereditary spherocytosis, hereditary elliptocytosis, and hereditary pyropoikilocytosis. Abnormally permeable membranes can cause hereditary overhydrated and dehydrated stomatocytosis, but the specific abnormality of the membrane in these two disorders has not been definitively identified. Abnormalities in the lipid portion of the membrane can be inherited or acquired. These disorders result in the formation of acanthocytes.

Paroxysmal nocturnal hemoglobinuria (PNH), a stem cell disorder, is an acquired membrane abnormality in which complement-mediated destruction of the cell occurs. The defect is due to a lack of decay-accelerating factor (DAF) and membrane inhibitor of reactive lysis (MIRL) on the erythrocytes, secondary to the absence of a membrane glycolipid, glycosyl-phosphatidyl inositol (GPI) to anchor these proteins to the cell membrane. Hemolysis is intravascular, resulting in hemoglobinuria and decreased haptoglobin. Leukopenia and thrombocytopenia are common because these cells also are susceptible to complement destruction. The sucrose hemolysis test is a screening test for PNH. Although the Ham test was used in the past, immunophenotyping is now the standard technology for confirming a diagnosis of PNH.

REVIEW QUESTIONS

LEVEL I

1. What is the most common type of erythrocyte found in hereditary spherocytosis? (Objectives 1, 3)
   a. spherocyte
   b. acanthocyte
   c. schistocyte
   d. elliptocyte

2. What erythrocyte membrane disorder has erythrocytes that are thermally unstable and fragment when heated to 45–46°C? (Objectives 1, 3)
   a. hereditary spherocytosis
   b. hereditary elliptocytosis
   c. hereditary pyropoikilocytosis
   d. PNH

LEVEL II

1. Which of the following is the red blood cell membrane protein defect associated with hereditary pyropoikilocytosis? (Objective 1)
   a. deficiency of band 3
   b. defective ankyrin protein
   c. mutant spectrin
   d. excess cholesterol

REVIEW QUESTIONS *(continued)*

LEVEL I

3. Choose the principal confirmation test for a diagnosis of hereditary spherocytosis. (Objective 3)
   a. autohemolysis test
   b. sucrose hemolysis test
   c. thermal stability test
   d. osmotic fragility test

4. Erythrocyte membrane disorders associated with known skeletal protein mutations include all of the following *except:* (Objective 1)
   a. hereditary spherocytosis
   b. hereditary overhydrated stomatocytosis
   c. hereditary elliptocytosis
   d. hereditary pyropoikilocytosis

5. Which of the following erythrocyte disorders is associated with abnormal membrane permeability? (Objective 2)
   a. hereditary elliptocytosis
   b. hereditary dehydrated stomatocytosis
   c. PNH
   d. HPP

6. Laboratory features associated with hereditary spherocytosis include: (Objective 3)
   a. spherocytes on the peripheral smear
   b. MCHC more than 36%
   c. increased osmotic fragility
   d. all of the above

7. The red blood cells in paroxysmal nocturnal hemoglobinuria (PNH) demonstrate a(n) _____ osmotic fragility test. (Objectives 4, 5)
   a. decreased
   b. increased
   c. normal
   d. unpredictable

8. Which of the following statements describes the basic principle behind the sucrose hemolysis test? (Objective 6)
   a. This test determines whether a patient's erythrocytes incubated in their own serum will demonstrate increased hemolysis.
   b. This test determines whether a patient's erythrocytes are sensitive to complement lysis when exposed to acidified serum.
   c. This test determines whether the patient's erythrocytes incubated in a low ionic medium such as sucrose will demonstrate increased hemolysis.
   d. This test determines whether the patient's erythrocytes will resist acid elution.

9. The laboratory features associated with asymptomatic common hereditary elliptocytosis include: (Objective 3)
   a. fragmented erythrocytes on the peripheral smear
   b. increased osmotic fragility
   c. positive autohemolysis test
   d. mild reticulocytosis

LEVEL II

2. Which of the following erythrocyte disorders will demonstrate an increased osmotic fragility pattern? (Objective 2)
   a. hereditary elliptocytosis and paroxysmal nocturnal hemoglobinuria
   b. hereditary overhydrated stomatocytosis and hereditary spherocytosis
   c. paroxysmal noctural hemoglobinuria and hereditary xerocytosis
   d. sickle cell anemia and thalassemia

Use this case study to answer questions 3 and 4.

A 5-year-old white male was admitted with the diagnosis of a fractured tibia following a playground accident. His admission laboratory results follow:

WBC: 12.5×10^9/L	*Differential*
RBC: 3.6×10^{12}/L	Segmented neutrophils: 70%
Hgb: 10.2 g/dL	Lymphocytes: 22%
Hct: 27%	Monocytes: 5%
MCV: 96.3 fL	Eosinophils 2%
MCH: 28.3 fL	Basophils 1%
MCHC: 38 g/dL	

RBC morphology: Slight polychromasia and spherocytes present

Osmotic fragility test: Initial hemolysis: .65% NaCl
Complete hemolysis: .45% NaCl

3. Which erythrocyte index differentiates this membrane disorder from most of the other erythrocyte membrane disorders discussed in this chapter? (Objectives 2, 5)
   a. MCV
   b. MCH
   c. MCHC
   d. both the MCV and MCH

4. The patient's osmotic fragility test demonstrates that his erythrocytes have what type of osmotic fragility. (Objectives 2, 5)
   a. increased
   b. decreased
   c. normal
   d. questionable

5. Immunophenotyping for a diagnosis of PNH uses the following monoclonal antibodies: (Objective 4)
   a. CD 55 and CD59
   b. CD11b/CD18
   c. CD 33 and CD34
   d. CD56 and CD10

6. The RBC membrane permeability in hereditary overhydrated stomatocytosis is _____, and the cells have a(n) _____ osmotic fragility. (Objective 2)
   a. increased, decreased
   b. decreased, increased
   c. increased, increased
   d. decreased, decreased

REVIEW QUESTIONS *(continued)*

LEVEL I

10. The osmotic fragility test determines whether a patient's erythrocytes are osmotically fragile by: (Objective 4)
    a. measuring the amount of hemolysis that occurs after a patient's erythrocytes have been incubated for 24 hours in acidified serum
    b. measuring the amount of hemolysis that occurs when a patient's erythrocytes are incubated in various concentrations of hypotonic saline
    c. measuring the amount of hemolysis that occurs when the patient's erythrocytes are incubated in a sucrose solution
    d. measuring the amount of hemolysis that occurs when the patient's erythrocytes are incubated in their own serum for 48 hours

LEVEL II

7. The following results were obtained on an osmotic fragility test.

	Normal Control	Patient
Initial hemolysis	0.50%	0.65% NaCl
Complete hemolysis	0.30%	0.45% NaCl

    These results most closely relate to which of the following statements? (Objective 2)
    a. The patient's peripheral smear will reveal spherocytes.
    b. The patient's peripheral smear will reveal target cells.
    c. The patient's peripheral smear will reveal sickle cells.
    d. The test is out of control and should be repeated.

8. A decrease in the level of which erythrocyte enzyme is seen in PNH? (Objective 3)
    a. leukocyte alkaline phosphatase (LAP)
    b. acid phosphatase
    c. C5 convertase
    d. acetylcholinesterase

9. Which of the following statements best describes the role of the decay-accelerating factor (DAF)? (Objective 3)
    a. This regulatory protein enhances the amplification of complement lysis.
    b. This complement regulatory protein stimulates erythrocyte lysis.
    c. This regulatory protein prevents the amplification of C3/C5 convertase activity.
    d. None of the above adequately describes the role of decay-accelerating factor.

10. The function of the membrane inhibitor of reactive lysis (MIRL) is to: (Objective 3)
    a. induce erythrocyte aggregation
    b. interfere with the end stages of complement activation
    c. prevent production of an autoantibody
    d. all of the above

www.pearsonhighered.com/mckenzie
Use this address to access the interactive Companion Website created for this textbook. Find additional information, tables and figures. Evaluate your command of the chapter information using case studies and critical thinking and multiple choice questions.

REFERENCES

1. Delauney, J. The molecular basis of hereditary red cell membrane disorders. *Blood Rev.* 2004;21:1–20.

2. Gallagher PG, Jarolim P. Red blood cell membrane disorders. In R Hoffman, EJ Benz, Jr, SJ Shattil, B Furie, HJ Cohen, LE Silberstein, P McGlave, eds. *Hematology: Basic Principles and Practice*, 4th ed. Philadelphia: Elsevier Churchill Livingstone; 2005.

3. Gallagher, PG. Update on the clinical spectrum and genetics of red blood cell membrane disorders. *Curr Hematol Rep.* 2004;3:85–91.

4. Miraglia del Giudice E, Lombardi C, Francese M et al. Frequent de novo monallelic expression of β-spectrin gene (SPTB) in children

with hereditary spherocytosis and isolated spectrin deficiency. *Br J Haematol.* 1998;101:251–54.

5. Gallagher, PG. Hematologically important mutations: Ankyrin variants in hereditary spherocytosis. *Blood Cells Mol Dis.* 2005;35:345–47.

6. Gallagher PG. Erythrocyte ankyrin promoter mutations associated with recessive hereditary spherocytosis cause significant abnormalities in ankyrin expression. *J Biol Chem.* 2001;276:41683–89.

7. Lanciotti M, Perutelli P, Valetto A, DiMartino D, Mori PG. Ankyrin deficiency is the most common defect in dominant and nondominant hereditary spherocytosis. *Haematologica.* 1997;82:460–62.

8. Basseres DS, Vincentim DL, Costa FF, Saad STO, Hassoun H. Beta-spectrin Promiss-ao: A translation initiation codon mutation of the beta-spectrin gene (ATG → GTG) associated with hereditary spherocytosis and spectrin deficiency in a Brazilian family. *Blood.* 1998; 91:368–69.

9. Tsx WT, Lux SE. Red blood cell membrane disorders. *Br J Haematol.* 1999;104:2–13.

10. DeFranceschi L, Olivieri O, Miraglia del Giudice E et al. Membrane cation and anion transport activities in erythrocytes of hereditary spherocytosis: Effects of different membrane protein defects. *Am J Hematol.* 1997;55:121–28.

11. Eber S, Lux SE. Hereditary spherocytosis—Defects in proteins that connect the membrane skeleton to the lipid bilayer. *Semin Hematol.* 2004;41:118–41.

12. Michaels LA, Cohen AR, Zhao H. Screening for hereditary spherocytosis by use of automated erythrocyte indexes. *J Pediatr.* 1997;130: 957–60.

13. King MJ, Behrens J, Rogers C et al. Rapid flow cytometric tests for the diagnosis of membrane cytoskeleton-associated haemolytic anaemia. *Br J Haematol.* 2000;111:924–33.

14. Rice HE, Oldham KT, Hillery CA et al. Clinical benefits and hematologic benefits of partial splenectomy for congenital hemolytic anemia in children. *Ann Surg.* 2003;237:281–288.

15. deBuys Roessingh AS, de Lagausie P, Rohrlich P et al. Follow-up of partial splenectomy in children with hereditary spherocytosis. *J Pediatr Surg.* 2002;37:1459–63.

16. Gallagher PG. Hereditary elliptocytosis: spectrin and protein 4.1R. *Semin Hematol.* 2004;41;142–64.

17. McMullin MF. The molecular basis of disorders of the red cell membrane. *J Clin Pathol.* 1999;52:245–48.

18. O'Donnell A, Allen SJ, Mgone CS et al. Red cell morphology and malaria anaemia in children with Southeast-Asian ovalocytosis band 3 in Papua New Guinea. *Br J Haematol.* 1998;101:407–12.

19. Allen SJ, O'Donnel A, Alexander ND et al. Prevention of cerebral malaria in children in Papua New Guinea by Southeast Asian ovalocytosis band 3. *Am J Trop Med Hyg.* 1999;60:1056–60.

20. Fricke B, Argent AC, Chetty MC et al. The "stomatin" gene and protein in overhydrated hereditary stomatocytosis. *Blood.* 2003;102: 2268–77.

21. Coles SE, Stewart GW. Temperature effects on cation transport in hereditary stomatocytosis and allied disorders. *Int J Exp Pathol.* 1999;80:251–58.

22. Haines PG, Jarvis HG, King S et al. Two further British families with the "cryodrocytosis" form of hereditary stomatocytosis. *Br J Haematol.* 2001;113:932–37.

23. Reid ME, Mohandas N. Red blood cell blood group antigens: Structure and function. *Semin Hematol.* 2004;41:93–117.

24. Gallagher PG. Red cell membrane disorders. *Hematology Am Soc Hematol Educ.* 2005;1:13–18.

25. Chitale AA, Sterling RK, Post AB et al. Resolution of spur cell anemia with liver transplantation: A case report and review of literature. *Transplant.* 1998;65:993–95.

26. Rader DJ, Brewer HB. Abetalipoproteinemia. New insights into lipoprotein assembly and vitamin E metabolism from a rare genetic disease. *JAMA.* 1993;270:865–69.

27. Gregg RE, Wetterau JR. The molecular basis of abetlipoproteinemia. *Curr. Opin. Lipidol.* 1994;5:81–86.

28. Jarolim P. Sequencing of antigens of the Diego blood group system helps to characterize ectoplasmic loops of erythroid band 3 protein. *Br J Haematol.* 1998;102:12.

29. Wong, P. A basis of the acanthocytosis in inherited and acquired disorders. *Med Hypotheses.* 2004;62:966–69.

30. Nishiwaki, M, Ikewaki, K, Bader G et al. Human lecithin cholesterol acyltransferase deficiency in vivo kinetics of low-density lipoprotein and lipoprotein X. *Arterioscler Thromb Vasc Biol.* 2006;26: 1370–75.

31. Parker C, Ormine M, Richard S et al. Diagnosis and management of paroxysmal nocturnal hemoglobinuria. *Blood.* 2005;106:3699–709.

32. Takeda J, Miyata T, Kawagoe K et al. Deficiency of the GPI anchor caused by a somatic mutation of the PIG-A gene in paroxysmal nocturnal hemoglobinuria. *Cell.* 1993;73:703–11.

33. Luzzatto L. Somatic mutation in paroxysmal nocturnal hemoglobinuria. *Hosp Pract (Off Ed).* 1997;32:125–31, 135–36, 139–40.

34. Brodsky RA. Paroxysmal nocturnal hemoglobinuria. In Hoffman R, Benz EJ, Shattil SJ, Furie B, Cohen HJ, Silberstein LE, McGlave P, eds. *Hematology: Basic Principles and Practice,* 3rd ed. New York: Churchill Livingstone; 2005:331–42.

35. Fieni S, Bonfanti L, Gramelli D, Benassi L, Delsignore, R. Clinical management of paroxysmal nocturnal hemoglobinuria in pregnancy: A case report and updated review. *Obstet Gynecol Surv.* 2006; 61:593–601.

36. Brodsky RA, Mukhina GL, Li S et al. Improved detection and characterization of paroxysmal nocturnal hemoglobinuria using fluorescent aerolysin. *AJCP.* 2000;114(3):459–66.

37. Hillmen P, Young NS, Schubert J et al. The complement inhibitor eculizumab in paroxysmal nocturnal hemoglobinuria. *N Engl J Med.* 2006;355:1233–43.

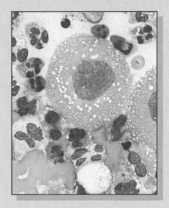

CHAPTER OUTLINE

16

Hemolytic Anemia: Enzyme Deficiencies

Martha Lake, Ed.D.
Dan Bessmer, M.S.

■ OBJECTIVES—LEVEL I

At the end of this unit of study, the student should be able to:

1. Identify the two main pathways by which erythrocytes catabolize glucose.

2. Explain the role of erythrocyte enzymes in maintaining the cell's integrity, and describe how deficiencies in these enzymes lead to anemia.

3. Identify the most common erythrocyte enzyme deficiency.

4. Describe the inheritance pattern for glucose-6-phosphate dehydrogenase (G6PD).

5. Explain how the diagnosis of G6PD deficiency is made.

6. List the tests used to detect G6PD deficiency and describe their principles.

7. Recognize the erythrocyte morphology in a Romanowsky-stained blood smear associated with G6PD deficiency.

8. Identify common compounds that induce anemia in G6PD deficiency.

■ OBJECTIVES—LEVEL II

At the end of this unit of study, the student should be able to:

1. Recommend appropriate laboratory testing and interpret results for suspected G6PD deficiency following a hemolytic episode.

2. Explain the function of glutathione in maintaining cellular integrity.

3. Associate the mechanisms of hemolysis with defects in the glycolytic and hexose-monophosphate shunt pathways.

4. Correlate clinical and laboratory findings with the common G6PD isoenzyme variants.

5. Diagram the reaction catalyzed by pyruvate kinase, and explain how a defect of this enzyme can cause hemolysis.

6. Recognize erythrocyte morphology associated with pyruvate kinase deficiency.

7. Review and interpret laboratory findings in a case study presentation of G6PD deficiency.

KEY TERMS

Bite cells
Blister cells
Chronic nonspherocytic hemolytic anemia
Favism
Hypoxia
Lyonization

BACKGROUND BASICS

The information in this chapter builds on concepts learned in previous chapters. To maximize your learning experience, you should review the following concepts from previous chapters.

Level I and Level II

▶ Describe the normal erythrocyte metabolic processes. (Chapter 5)

▶ Recognize RBC morphology as it relates to hemolytic disease processes. (Chapter 14)

▶ Understand basic enzymology and techniques to measure enzyme activity.

CASE STUDY

We will address this case study throughout the chapter.

The patient, Henry, is a 25-year-old African American male soldier who was in the process of being deployed to West Africa for a 3-month temporary duty. Because of the high prevalence of malaria in the area, he was started on antimalarial prophylaxis (primaquine) 3 days prior to leaving to join his command. Twenty-four hours after starting the medication, he developed fever, chills, and general malaise. He subsequently reported to the emergency department and was admitted to the hospital for observation and additional testing.

The physical exam revealed a normal appearing, well-nourished adult male in no acute distress. His family history was noncontributory, and he had no known drug allergies. Laboratory analysis yielded the following.

CBC		
White blood cells	12 × 10⁹/L	
Hemoglobin	9.1 g/dL (91 g/L)	
Hematocrit	27% (0.27 L/L)	
MCV	90 fL	
Platelet count	423 × 10⁹/L	
Total bilirubin	5.0 mg/dL	
Conjugated	0.2 mg/dL	
Unconjugated	4.8 mg/dL	
Haptoglobin	39 mg/dL	

Based on the clinical history and these laboratory results, consider what could have precipitated this patient's condition.

▶ OVERVIEW

Intrinsic defects in the erythrocyte membrane, hemoglobin, or enzymes can lead to hemolysis. This chapter discusses defects of enzymes within the erythrocyte that lead to hemolytic anemia. The most common enzyme deficiencies are those associated with the hexose monophosphate shunt and the glycolytic pathway. Thus, the chapter begins with a description of the role of these two pathways in erythrocyte metabolism and a general overview of the clinical and laboratory findings in enzyme deficiencies associated with the pathways. The two most common enzyme deficiencies, glucose-6-phosphate dehydrogenase and pyruvate kinase, are discussed in detail in the format of pathophysiology, clinical and laboratory findings, and therapy.

▶ INTRODUCTION

The erythrocyte life span can be significantly shortened if the cell is intrinsically abnormal. Although the enzymes in the erythrocyte are limited, those involved in processes that protect the cell from oxidant damage and provide the cell with energy through glycolysis are essential for cell survival. As reticulocytes mature, they lose their nucleus, mitochondria, and microsomes. Consequently, reticulocytes also lose their ability to synthesize protein and undergo oxidative phosphorylation for ATP production. Thus, the mature erythrocyte depends entirely on anaerobic glucose metabolism for its energy needs. Maturation of the reticulocyte is associated with a decline in the activity of some enzymes, but the activity is usually stable in the mature erythrocyte.[1] The erythrocyte cannot synthesize new enzymes. An inherited deficiency in one of the erythrocyte enzymes can compromise the integrity of the cell membrane or hemoglobin and cause hemolysis. The more common hereditary enzyme deficiencies known to cause hemolytic anemia are listed in Table 16-1 ✪. Most are associated with the two erythrocyte metabolic pathways: hexose monophosphate (HMP) shunt and the glycolytic (Embden-Meyerhof, EM) pathway. To understand how defects in these two pathways can result in hemolysis, they will be reviewed next. (For a more thorough discussion of each, review Chapter 5.)

HEXOSE MONOPHOSPHATE SHUNT

Glucose, the cell's primary metabolic substrate, enters the cell in a carrier-mediated, energy-free transport process and is catabolized via the glycolytic pathway or the HMP shunt. The HMP shunt catabolizes approximately 10% of the glucose, which is essential for maintaining adequate concentrations of reduced glutathione (GSH). GSH levels are maintained by conversion of NADPH to NADP; NADP is reduced back to NADPH in a reaction catalyzed by glucose-6-

✪ TABLE 16-1

Erythrocyte Enzyme Deficiencies Associated with Congenital (Chronic) Nonspherocytic Hemolytic Anemia

Metabolic Pathway	Enzyme Deficiency
Glycolytic (Embden-Meyerhof)	Pyruvate kinase (PK)
	Glucose phosphate isomerase (GPI)
	Hexokinase (HK)
	Phosphoglyceratekinase (PGK)
	Phosphofructokinase (PFK)
	Triosephosphate isomerase (TPI)
Hexose-monophosphate	Glucose-6-phosphate dehydrogenase (G6PD)
	Glutathione synthetase
	Glutamylcysteine synthetase
Nucleotide	Pyrimidine 5'-nucleotidase (P5N)

phosphate dehydrogenase (G6PD) (Figure 16-1 ■). GSH protects the erythrocyte from oxidant damage; it maintains hemoglobin in the reduced functional state and preserves vital cellular enzymes from oxidant damage. When the cell is exposed to an oxidizing agent, the metabolism of NADPH increases. NADPH is consumed as part of the cell's protective mechanism and subsequently reduced back to NADPH via

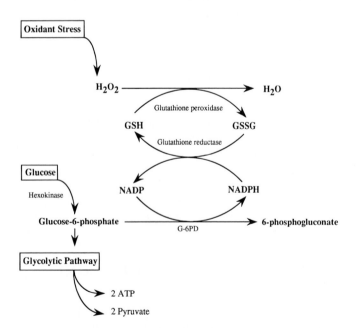

■ FIGURE 16-1   G6PD is needed for maintaining adequate quantities of gultathione (GSH), an important buffer to oxidants within the erythrocyte. As GSH reduces H_2O_2 to H_2O, it is oxidized (GSSG). G6PD generates NADPH in the conversion of glucose-6-phosphate to 6-phosphogluconate. NADPH, in turn, regenerates reduced glutathione from oxidized glutathione.

G6PD. If enzymes in the HMP shunt are deficient, the cell's reducing power is compromised, and oxidized hemoglobin accumulates, subsequently denaturing in the form of Heinz bodies. Heinz bodies aggregate at the cell membrane, causing membrane damage. As the cells pass through the spleen, the macrophages attempt to remove the Heinz bodies, leading to premature extravascular hemolysis. The most common enzyme deficiency of the HMP shunt is G6PD deficiency.

GLYCOLYTIC PATHWAY

Most of the cell's energy is produced via glycolysis in the glycolytic pathway. About 90% of the glucose is utilized by this pathway as 1 mole of glucose is catabolized to lactic acid with a net production of 2 moles of ATP. ATP is needed for active cation transport of Na^+, K^+, and Ca^{++}, maintaining membrane deformability (membrane's ability to temporarily change shape in response to multiple forces in the cell's environment); and maintaining normal erythrocyte biconcave disc shape in the resting or steady state.[1] The erythrocyte's ability to deform is an important determinant of its survival. Deficiencies in enzymes of the glycolytic pathway decrease ATP production and lead to hemolysis. Heinz bodies are not formed because the cell's reducing power is primarily linked to the HMP shunt. The mechanism of hemolysis is related to decreased ATP leading to impaired cation pumping. Membrane integrity is compromised, and increased osmotic fragility results. The osmotically fragile cells are trapped in the hostile splenic environment and phagocytosed.

The Rapoport-Luebering shunt of the glycolytic pathway provides the erythrocyte with 2,3-bisphosphoglycerate (2,3-BPG). If this shunt is used, there is no net gain of ATP from glycolysis. The activity of this shunt is stimulated during **hypoxia**, a state of decreased oxygen tension and delivery to tissues. This is sometimes evidenced by a blue appearance of normally pink tissues, such as the fingernail beds. When 2,3-BPG combines with hemoglobin, the hemoglobin's oxygen affinity decreases, making more oxygen available to the tissues.

CLINICAL AND LABORATORY FINDINGS IN ERYTHROCYTE ENZYME DEFICIENCIES

Most erythrocyte enzyme deficiencies are inherited as autosomal recessive traits. However, the most common enzyme deficiency, G6PD, is inherited as an X-linked recessive (sex-linked) disorder. Patients with the homozygous autosomal recessive enzyme deficiencies and males with X-linked G6PD deficiency generally have chronic normocytic, normochromic anemia, reticulocytosis, hyperbilirubinemia, and neonatal jaundice. The direct antiglobulin test (DAT) is negative, indicating an absence of antibodies coating the erythrocytes, and no evidence suggests a defect in either the erythrocyte membrane or hemoglobin. Sometimes no anemia is present or hemolysis is sporadic, depending on the specific allele(s) inherited. These anemias associated with inherited defects of erythrocyte metabolism are often collectively referred to as **chronic** (hereditary or congenital) **nonspherocytic hemolytic anemias.** The preferred term is *hereditary nonspherocytic hemolytic* anemia, for this heterogeneous group of anemias does not have significant poikilocytosis. Although the anemias are not life threatening, they can be disabling and lead to debilitating complications.[2]

DIAGNOSIS

Definitive diagnosis of enzyme deficiencies requires spectrophotometric measurement of the suspected deficient enzyme. The time of testing and interpreting the results is important for accurate diagnosis. Sometimes the abnormal cells are selectively removed from circulation in vivo, and the enzyme activity of the remaining circulating cells is normal. Some abnormal enzymes have normal activity in the reticulocytes, but enzyme activity decreases as the cell ages (G6PD-A⁻). Thus, depending on the degree of reticulocytosis, the enzyme content can appear normal. For these reasons, it is important not to test the patient immediately after a hemolytic attack when most of the enzyme deficient cells have been hemolyzed and there is a compensatory reticulocytosis. It has been reported that diagnosis during or shortly after a hemolytic attack can be made if the blood is centrigured and the older dense erythrocytes at the bottom of the column of blood are tested.[2,3] If a patient has been transfused, testing should be delayed until the transfused cells have outlived their life span.[1]

✓ Checkpoint! 1

Transfusion of red blood cells in a patient with chronic nonspherocytic, hemolytic anemia due to an erythrocyte enzyme deficiency does not reverse or prevent the recipient's condition. However, a transfusion does help to raise the patient's hemoglobin. If tests are performed to quantitate the enzyme after a transfusion, the results can be within the normal reference intervals. Explain.

▶ GLUCOSE-6-PHOSPHATE DEHYDROGENASE DEFICIENCY

G6PD deficiency is the most common erythrocyte enzyme disorder. It was first recognized during the Korean War when 10% of African American soldiers who were given the antimalarial drug primaquine developed a self-limited hemolytic anemia. G6PD deficiency is found worldwide in Caucasians, blacks, and Asians. It occurs most frequently in the Mediterranean area, Africa, and China. The geographic distribution coincides with that of malaria, suggesting that G6PD-defi-

cient cells may be more resistant to malarial parasites than normal cells and/or are more readily phagocytosed.[4,5]

The disease is a sex-linked disorder carried by a gene on the X chromosome (band Xq28) and therefore fully expressed in males with the genetic mutation or in females homozygous for the mutation. Heterozygote females appear to have two populations of cells, one deficient in G6PD and one normal. This occurs because of **lyonization** (random inactivation of one set of X-linked genes in each cell) of an X chromosome. The degree to which females are affected depends on the relative amount of deficient cells present. Web Figure 16-1 ■ illustrates the expected progeny from G6PD deficient males or females.

The disease is heterogenous with differences in severity among races and sexes. The majority of people with G6PD deficiency have no clinical expression of the deficiency unless they have neonatal jaundice, are exposed to oxidative chemicals or drugs, or have severe infections. Compounds that have been associated with hemolytic anemia in G6PD deficiency are listed in Table 16-2 ✪.

✪ TABLE 16-2	
Compounds Associated with Hemolysis in G6PD Deficiency	
Antimalarials	primaquine
	pamaquine
	pentaquine
	quinacrine (Atabrine)
Sulfonamides	sulfanilamide
	sulfacetamide
	sulfapyridine
	sulfamethoxazole (Gantonol)
	sulfasalazine (Azulfidine)
Sulfones	thiazosulfone
	diaphenylsulfone (DDS, Dapsone)
	sulfoxone (Diasone)
Nitrofurans	nitrofurantoin (Furadantin)
Analgesics	acetanilid
Miscellaneous	fava beans
	hydroxylamines
	methylene blue
	naphthalene (moth balls)
	naxidlic acid
	niridazole
	phenylhydrazine
	toluidine blue
	trinitrotoluene (TNT)

✓ Checkpoint! 2

Oxidant compounds are harmful because they result in the production of harmful peroxides or other oxygen radicals that overwhelm the body's natural mechanisms to scavenge them. Why is the mechanism of protection against oxidants easily compromised in G6PD deficiency?

PATHOPHYSIOLOGY

G6PD is necessary for maintaining adequate levels of GSH for reducing cellular oxidants (Figure 16-1). In G6PD deficiency, the generation of NADPH, and subsequently GSH, is impaired and cellular oxidants accumulate. The buildup of cellular oxidants leads to erythrocyte injury and hemolysis. Hemoglobin is oxidized to methemoglobin, which precipitates in the form of Heinz bodies. Heinz bodies attach to the erythrocyte membrane causing increased membrane permeability to cations, osmotic fragility, and cell rigidity. Heinz bodies are removed from the erthrocytes by splenic macrophages, producing "bite" cells and **blister cells.** With progressive membrane loss, spherocytes can be formed. Spherocytes are less deformable than normal and become trapped and hemolyzed in the spleen (extravascular hemolysis). Heinz bodies require a supravital stain to be visualized because they are not evident on Romanowsky-stained blood smear stains. Oxidant stress also can oxidize membrane lipids and proteins. This disruption of the membrane structural integrity results in removal of the cell from circulation by splenic macrophages. Cell membrane damage can be severe enough for the cell to hemolyze in the circulation. This intravascular hemolysis can be acute and accompanied by hemoglobinemia and hemoglobinurea.

Normally, G6PD activity is highest in young cells and decreases as the cell ages. Normal erythrocytes have been shown to use only 0.1% of their maximum G6PD enzyme capacity.[6] Thus, even older cells normally retain enough G6PD activity to maintain adequate GSH levels. This also explains why even G6PD-deficient cells can maintain normal function and hemolysis is sporadic. It is in situations that create excessive oxidant stress that the G6PD activity usually is inadequate to maintain normal metabolic function. Those cells that are most deficient undergo oxidant damage and are rapidly removed from circulation. This accounts for the sporadic hemolysis that accompanies oxidant stress in G6PD deficiency. In most G6PD variants, hemolysis is self-limited (referring to the fact that hemolysis stops after a time even if the oxidant stress continues). Self-limited hemolysis occurs because the older, most G6PD-deficient erythrocytes initially are destroyed, but the younger cells remain because they have sufficient enzyme activity to avoid hemolysis. The reticulocytes released from the bone marrow in response to the hemolytic episode also have enough enzyme activity to maintain metabolic activity even under oxidant stress. However, it is important to recognize that under the stress of severe oxidants (drugs, chemicals), even normal cells can experience oxidant damage and hemolyze.

✓ Checkpoint! 3

Erythrocyte morphology should always be examined carefully. The ability to pick up subtle clues as to the cause of a disease process can be acquired from a comprehensive evaluation of abnormal erythrocyte morphology. How is this likely to aid the diagnosis of G6PD deficiency?

G6PD VARIANTS

More than 400 variants (isoenzymes) of the G6PD enzyme have been identified.[1] Many of them differ in activity, stability, and electrophoretic mobility. The mutant enzymes have been categorized into four classes according to the degree of deficiency and hemolysis (Table 16-3). Most variants have normal enzyme activity. Deficient enzyme variants tend to have mutations clustered in domains responsible for stable dimerization of the protein or the NADP binding site.[7] Variants except G6PD-B, G6PD-A+, and G6PD-A− are given geographic names or other types of names.

✪ TABLE 16-3

Classes of Mutant G6PD Isoenzymes

Class	G6PD Activity	Hemolysis	Important Variants
I	Severely deficient	Chronic (nonspherocytic hemolytic anemia); not self-limited	Minnesota; Iowa
II	Severely deficient (<10%)	Acute, episodic; can be chronic and not self-limited	G6PD-Mediterranean
III	Moderately to mildly deficient (10–60%)	Acute, episodic	G6PD-A−; G6PD-Canton
IV	Normal (60–150%)	Absent	G6PD-B, G6PD-A+

FEMALES WITH G6PD DEFICIENCY

Female heterozygotes for G6PD deficiency always contain two populations of cells, one normal and one with G6PD deficiency. In contrast, all cells in affected males are G6PD deficient. The dual population in females is caused by random inactivation of one X chromosome in a given stem cell. Depending on the proportion of abnormal erythrocytes, females may have no clinical expression of the deficiency or may be affected as severely as males. Although rare, there are case reports of homozygous-deficient females.[8]

CLINICAL FINDINGS

A spectrum of clinical presentations is associated with this disorder: acute, acquired hemolytic anemia (episodic) including favism; congenital nonspherocytic hemolytic anemia (chronic); and neonatal hyperbilirubinemia with jaundice. Homozygotes and heterozygotes can be symptomatic depending on the severity of the deficiency. G6PD deficiency is most common in those of African, Asian, Mediterranean, and Middle-Eastern descent.

Acute, Acquired Hemolytic Anemia

Most persons with G6PD deficiency have no clinical symptoms, and they are not anemic. Diagnosis usually occurs during or after infectious illnesses or following exposure to certain drugs because these conditions commonly precipitate hemolytic attacks. Hemolysis is variable and depends on the degree of oxidant stress, the G6PD isoenzyme, and sex of the patient. The symptoms are those of acute intravascular hemolytic anemia (∞ Chapter 14). Drug-induced hemolysis usually occurs within 1 to 3 days after exposure to the drug. Sudden anemia develops with a 3–4 g/dL drop in hemoglobin. Jaundice is not prominent. The patient may experience abdominal and low back pain, as well as dark or black urine due to hemoglobinuria. In one study of 35 G6PD-deficient children in India, the most common significant complication, occuring in more than 50% of the cases, was renal failure.[9] Hemoglobinemia is prominent. Often, however, hemolysis is less striking and is not accompanied by hemoglobinuria or conspicuous symptoms.

Favism refers to the sudden severe hemolytic episode that develops in some individuals with G6PD deficiency after the ingestion of fava beans (broad beans). Hemolytic episodes occur in much the same way as drug-induced hemolytic episodes. The most likely components of the bean responsible for the sensitivity are isouramil and divicine. This complication is often thought to be associated with severe G6PD deficiency, especially the G6PD Mediterranean variant. It is now clear, however, that other forms of G6PD deficiency are also associated with favism, including G6PD-A⁻ and G6PD Aures, a type identified in Algerian subjects.[10]

The hemolysis is similar to the acute hemolytic episodes that occur after primaquine administration in individuals with the G6PD-A⁻ variant. Consumption of fava beans is widespread in the Mediterranean area and the Middle East. The first signs of favism are malaise, severe lethargy, nausea, vomiting, abdominal pain, chills, tremor, and fever.[1] Hemoglobinuria occurs a few hours after ingestion of the beans. Persistent hemoglobinuria usually prompts the individual to seek medical attention. Jaundice can be intense. Severe favism usually affects children between the ages of 2 and 5 years. The age distribution is changing in some countries, however, due to neonatal screening and parental education. Even though favism occurs more often in males due to the X-linked nature of the disease, females are also affected depending on the proportion of enzyme deficient erythrocytes present.

Congenital Nonspherocytic Hemolytic Anemia

Congenital nonspherocytic hemolytic anemia syndrome is associated with G6PD variants (Class I) that have low in vitro activity or are markedly unstable. Hemolysis is chronic and not associated with ingestion of drugs or infections, although drugs and infections can exaggerate the hemolysis. The hemolysis is usually compensated so anemia can be mild. Reticulocytosis is in the range of 4–35%.

Leukocyte and platelet G6PD are controlled by the same gene as erythrocyte G6PD. Thus, it has been found that some patients with G6PD-deficient red cells also have leukocyte G6PD deficiency. An increase in pyogenic infections has been reported in those with <5% normal activity.[11–13] However, a group of Israeli patients with severe G6PD deficiency without an increased incidence of infections had bactericidal activity in their G6PD-deficient neutrophils within the range of healthy controls.[14] Considerable fluctuation of the enzyme activity was found to depend on the time of day it was measured. This fluctuation can produce enough NADPH to initiate the respiratory burst and prevent infection. Neutrophils also are relatively short lived, so those with unstable variants might not show functional impairment.

Neonatal Hyperbilirubinemia

Some neonates with G6PD deficiency have severe hyperbilirubinemia with the potential of kernicterus if left untreated. The prevalence of this severe jaundice accurs twice as often in G6PD-deficient male neonates than in neonates from the general population. The mechanism is unknown. Although hemolysis can be present, other factors appear to play a more important role including inability to conjugate and clear bilirubin.[15] In a recent study, G6PD deficiency was identified in at least 21% of infants who were readmitted with kernicterus.[16] Exchange transfusion and phototherapy may be required.

Neonates and preterm infants (29–32 weeks gestation) have higher G6PD activity than do adults. However, the higher activity does not affect the diagnosis of G6PD because neonates and preterm infants with G6PD deficiency have lower activity than do normal neonates.[17]

LABORATORY FINDINGS

Anemia is absent and peripheral blood findings are normal except during hemolytic attacks for most of the common G6PD variants. Patients with the congenital nonspherocytic hemolytic anemia form can exhibit chronic hemolysis. During or immediately following a hemolytic attack, polychromasia, occasional spherocytes, small hypochromic cells, erythrocyte fragments, and bite cells can be seen on the blood smear. **Bite cells,** which have a chunk of the cell removed from one side, are frequently thought to be typical of G6PD deficiency (Figure 16-2 ■). However, bite cells are more characteristic of drug-induced oxidant hemolysis in individuals with normal hemoglobin and enzyme activity.[18]

A peculiar cell referred to by a variety of descriptive terms (blister cell, irregularly contracted cell, eccentrocyte, erythrocyte hemighost, double-colored erythrocyte, and cross-bonded erythrocyte) has been described in G6PD deficiency after oxidant-related hemolysis (Figure 16-3 ■). The red cell membrane is oxidized. The hemoglobin is confined to one side of the cell and the other side is transparent. The transparent side often contains Heinz bodies and has flattened membranes in which the opposing membrane sides are juxtaposed. This cross-bonding of the membrane appears to decrease deformability and destine the cell for phagocytosis by macrophages. These cells have a decreased volume and increased MCHC.

A variety of abnormal laboratory findings related to hemolysis can be found during or after a hemolytic attack. Reticulocytosis is characteristic following a hemolytic episode.[19] Leukocytes can increase during hemolytic attacks, but platelets are usually normal. Unconjugated bilirubin and serum LD can be increased. Haptoglobin commonly decreases during the acute hemolytic phase. Absence of haptoglobin in the recovery stage indicates chronic hemolysis.

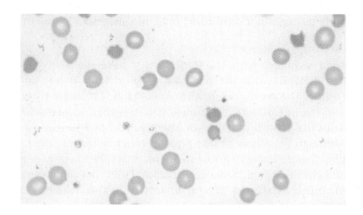

■ **FIGURE 16-2**   Heinz body hemolytic anemia. Peripheral blood from a patient with G6PD deficiency during a hemolytic episode. There are erythrocytes with a portion of the cell missing, known as bite cells. The spleen pits the Heinz body with a portion of the cell producing these misshapen erythrocytes. Some of the cells reseal and become spherocytes. (Wright-Giemsa stain; 1000× magnification)

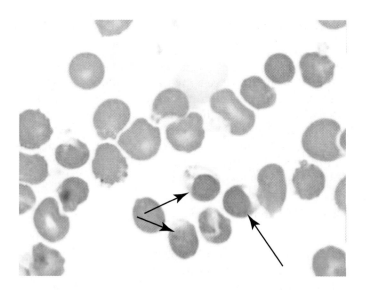

■ **FIGURE 16-3**   The arrows are pointing to "blister cells," which have been described by various names (see text). Hemoglobin is condensed to one side of the cell, leaving a transparent area (blister) on the other. These cells can be found in G6PD deficient individuals after a hemolytic attack.

Definitive diagnosis depends on the demonstration of a decrease in erythrocyte G6PD enzyme activity. In affected individuals, the enzyme activity can appear normal during and for a time after a hemolytic attack because older cells with less G6PD are preferentially destroyed during the attack and reticulocytes have normal activity. A reticulocytosis of more than 7% is generally associated with a normal enzyme screen after hemolysis.[20] For this reason, assays for G6PD should be performed 2 to 3 months after a hemolytic episode. In G6PD Mediterranean, however, even young cells have gross deficiencies of G6PD, and enzyme activity appears abnormal even with reticulocytosis. Both severe and mild types of G6PD deficiency are detected by measuring the enzyme if the patient is not undergoing hemolysis.

 CASE STUDY *(continued from page 327)*

Because of the low hemoglobin, Henry was transfused with 2 units of packed red cells. Examination of the peripheral blood smear was remarkable for occasional spherocytes and bite cells. This blood smear finding, presentation of anemia, and onset of illness coinciding with the initiation of primaquine suggested shortened RBC life span due to oxidative damage.

1. What test should be considered after finding bite cells on a blood smear?

Fluorescent Spot Test

The fluorescent spot test is a reliable and sensitive screening test for G6PD deficiency. Whole blood is added to a mixture of glucose-6-phosphate (G6P), NADP, and saponin. A drop of this mixture is placed on a piece of filter paper and examined under ultraviolet light for fluorescence. The G6PD enzyme present in erythrocytes normally metabolizes G6P, producing NADPH, which fluoresces, but NADP does not, so lack of fluorescence indicates G6PD deficiency.

Dye Reduction Test

The dye reduction screening test incubates a hemolysate of patient's blood, G6P, NADP, and the dye brilliant cresyl blue together. If the hemolysate contains G6PD, the NADP is reduced to NADPH, which in turn reduces the blue dye to its colorless form. The time it takes for this change to occur is inversely proportional to the amount of G6PD present. Normal blood is also tested as a control. The test is specific and is available in commercial kits.

Ascorbate Cyanide Test

The ascorbate cyanide test is the most sensitive screening test for detecting heterozygotes and G6PD deficiency during hemolytic attacks. The test is not specific for G6PD deficiency but also detects other defects or deficiencies in the HMP shunt. The test is also positive in PNH, pyruvate kinase deficiency, and unstable hemoglobin disorders. The test's principle is that G6PD-deficient cells fail to reduce hydrogen peroxide. A patient's blood is incubated with sodium ascorbate, sodium cyanide, and glucose. Hydrogen peroxide is generated by the interaction of ascorbate with hemoglobin. The sodium cyanide inhibits the activity of normal erythrocyte catalase, an inhibitor of the formation of hydrogen peroxide. With the inhibition of catalase, hydrogen peroxide is formed. Erythrocytes deficient in G6PD cannot reduce the peroxide, and hemoglobin is oxidized to methemoglobin, which imparts a brown tint to the solution.

Cytochemical Staining

This method detects the enzyme activity in individual cells. The G6PD in the red cells reacts with a sensitive tetrazolium salt to ultimately form formazan. The level of formazan is directly related to the G6PD activity. The activity in the cells can be scored by hand, but automated methods utilizing flow cytometry are being developed.[21]

Quantitative Rate Reduction Test

An erythrocyte hemolysate is incubated with G6P and NADP, and the rate of reduction of NADP to NADPH is measured at 340 nm in a spectrophotometer. In the case of heterozygotic females, when the quantitation of the enzyme can yield misleading results especially during or after a hemolytic episode, it is best to perform polymerase chain reaction (PCR) tests to reveal the genetic abnormality.

DNA-Based Screening Test

DNA is extracted from spots of dried blood and then submitted for PCR. Fluorescent-labeled probes are used to detect mutant G6PD alleles.

CASE STUDY *(continued from page 332)*

A spectrophotometric assay for G6PD was performed on the patient's peripheral blood. The result was borderline normal, and a preliminary diagnosis of G6PD deficiency was made. Primaquine usage was discontinued, and the patient recovered without complications. Upon follow-up, the patient was retested for G6PD deficiency and was found to be abnormal, confirming the diagnosis.

2. Why was the initial G6PD test result normal but the repeat test was abnormal?

THERAPY

Most of the patients with G6PD deficiency are asymptomatic and do not experience chronic hemolysis; thus, no therapy is indicated. However, patients should avoid exposure to the oxidant drugs and foods that can precipitate hemolytic episodes. In acute hemolytic episodes, supportive therapy including blood transfusions, treatment of infections, and removal of the precipitating agent are used. Exchange transfusion can be necessary in cases of severe neonatal jaundice. Dialysis can be indicated in patients with oliguria and severe azotemia.[9]

CASE STUDY *(continued)*

3. What was the precipitating cause of the patient's anemia?

▶ OTHER DEFECTS AND DEFICIENCIES OF THE HMP SHUNT AND GSH METABOLISM

Erythrocytes synthesize about 50% of their total glutathione every 4 days. Deficiencies in the enzymes needed for glutathione synthesis (glutathione synthetase and glutamylcysteine synthetase) have been reported to be associated with a decrease in GSH and a congenital nonspherocytic hemolytic anemia. Hemolysis increases during administration of certain drugs. Deficiencies in glutathione reductase, an enzyme that catalyzes the reduction of GSSG to GSH, are not associated with a hematologic disorder. Glutathione peroxidase catalyzes the detoxification of hydrogen peroxide by GSH. Deficiencies in this enzyme, although common, are not a cause of hemolysis. This might be explained by the fact that peroxide reduction by GSH occurs nonenzymatically at a significant rate.

▶ PYRUVATE KINASE (PK) DEFICIENCY

Pyruvate kinase deficiency is the most common enzyme deficiency in the glycolytic pathway and the second most common erythrocyte enzyme deficiency. Many pyruvate kinase enzyme mutations coincide with the disorder's variety of clinical manifestations. The more severe types are noted in infancy, whereas the milder types may not be detected until adulthood. Inheritance is autosomal recessive. Clinically significant hemolytic anemias of PK deficiency are associated with the homozygous state or double heterozygosity for two mutant enzymes. The variation in clinical phenotype associated with the genetic mutations appear to reflect not only the aberrant properties of the mutant protein but also interactions of the genotype with physiological and environmental factors including epigenetic modifications, ineffective erythropoiesis, splenic function, and coexisting polymorphisms of other enzymes.[22] Single heterozygotes are usually asymptomatic. Acquired PK deficiency is seen in some leukemias and myelodysplastic disorders.

PATHOPHYSIOLOGY

More than 180 different mutations in the PK gene (PKLR gene on chromosome 1q21) affecting the enzyme activity have been identified. Most are missense mutations, but nonsense mutations, deletions, and insertions are found also. PK catalyzes the conversion of phosphoenol pyruvate (PEP) to pyruvate, concurrent with the conversion of ADP to ATP (Figure 16-4 ■). In PK deficiency, this energy-producing reaction is prevented, resulting in a loss of two ATP molecules per molecule of glucose catabolized. The cell's inability to maintain normal ATP levels results in alterations of the erythrocyte membrane; failure of the cation pumps causing potassium loss as well as sodium and calcium gain; and dehydration (echinocytes). The decrease in echinocyte deformability enhances erythrocyte sequestration in splenic cords and phagocytosis by macrophages.

CLINICAL FINDINGS

Clinical symptoms vary depending on the degree of anemia, which is mild to severe. Individuals tolerate the anemia well because of the increase in 2,3-BPG that accompanies the distal block in glycolysis. The two to three times normal increase in 2,3-BPG enhances the release of oxygen to the tissues. Jaundice can occur with intermittant hemoglobinuria. Gallstones are a common complication.

PK deficiency can be life threatening in neonates. When anemia is present at birth, PK deficiency should be considered with and differentiated from other etiologies associated with anemia in this population (ABO/Rh incompatibility, thalassemia, G6PD deficiency, and hereditary spherocytosis).[23] Neonates with a severe phenotype usually have severe jaundice that may require exchange transfusions.[22] Splenectomy can result in stabilization of the hemoglobin and decrease the need for transfusions. Patients with milder forms of PK deficiency are commonly diagnosed in early adulthood although they could have had neonatal jaundice.[19]

LABORATORY FINDINGS

Patients with PK deficiency have a normocytic, normochromic anemia with hemoglobin levels of 6–12 g/dL. Reticulocytosis ranges from 2 to 15% and increases more after splenectomy, often above 40%. The degree of reticulocytosis before splenectomy is not proportional to the degree of anemia as it is in most other hemolytic anemias because the spleen preferentially sequesters the younger PK deficient erythrocytes. The blood smear exhibits irregularly contracted cells and occasional echinocytes before splenectomy (Figure 16-5 ■). After splenectomy, these abnormal cells present a more conspicuous finding. In contrast to G6PD deficiency, Heinz bodies and spherocytes are not found in PK defi-

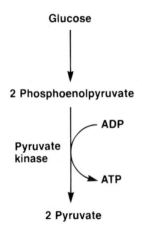

Glucose

2 Phosphoenolpyruvate

ADP

Pyruvate kinase

ATP

2 Pyruvate

■ FIGURE 16-4   Glucose is metabolized to pyruvate in the glycolytic pathway. ATP is generated as phosphoenolpyruvate and is converted to pyruvate with a net gain of 2 ATP. Two molecules of pyruvate are formed from 1 glucose molecule. In pyruvate kinase deficiency, this reaction is slowed, resulting in deficient ATP production.

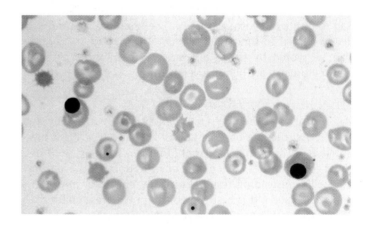

■ FIGURE 16-5   Blood smear from a patient with pyruvate kinase deficiency. Note the echinocyte, acanthocyte, target cells, and irregularly contracted cells. Howell-Jolly bodies are also present. (Wright-Giemsa stain; 1000× magnification)

ciency. Serum unconjugated indirect bilirubin and LD are increased, and haptoglobin is decreased or absent. Osmotic fragility is normal, but cells demonstrate increased hemolysis when incubated at 37°C. Autohemolysis is increased at 48 hours and is not corrected with the addition of glucose but is corrected with the addition of ATP.

In performing enzyme tests for PK, the erythrocytes are separated from leukocytes because leukocytes contain more PK than erythrocytes. Two genes located on chromosomes 15q22 and 1q21 encode for pyruvate kinase. The first locus produces PK active in muscle, leukocytes, platelets, and various other tissues. The second locus produces the PK active in erythrocytes. Thus, in erythrocyte PK deficiency (mutations of the second locus), only the erythrocytes are deficient; leukocytes are normal. The screening procedure is based on the disappearance of fluorescence as erythrocytes are incubated with phosphoenol-pyruvate (PEP), LD, ADP, and NADH.[24]

$$PEP + ADP \xrightarrow{\quad PK \quad} Pyruvate + ATP$$

$$Pyruvate + NADH + H^+ \xrightarrow{\quad LD \quad} Lactate + NAD^+$$

(fluoresces)   (no fluorescence)

Some mutant PK enzymes have normal activity at high substrate concentrations and abnormal activity at low substrate concentrations. A modification of this procedure has been developed to improve the interpretation of the endpoint.[25] In this modification, patient blood is frozen and thawed to ensure complete hemolysis of the specimen before testing.

Fluorescence in normal erythrocytes disappears in 30 minutes. In PK-deficient erythrocytes, fluorescence persists 45–60 minutes. The quantitative test for PK deficiency is performed in the same manner as the screening test except that the rate of disappearance of fluorescence is measured in a spectrophotometer at 340 nm. A rapid potentiometric method has also been developed to measure enzymatic activity by monitoring the change in pH in a reaction buffer during the conversion of the substrate to pyruvate.

THERAPY

There is no specific therapy for PK deficiency. Transfusions help maintain the hemoglobin above 8–10 g/dL. Splenectomy can improve the hemoglobin level and decrease the need for transfusions in some affected individuals; however, hemolysis continues.

✓ **Checkpoint! 4**

What are the differentiating characteristics of PK and G6PD deficiencies found on the peripheral blood smear?

▶ OTHER ENZYME DEFICIENCIES IN THE GLYCOLYTIC PATHWAY

When associated with anemia, other enzyme deficiencies in the glycolytic pathway have clinical manifestations and laboratory findings that resemble those of PK deficiency.

- **Glucose phosphate isomerase deficiency (GPI)** is the second most common disorder of the glycolytic pathway. Almost all GPI mutants are unstable, causing hemolytic anemia. Affected individuals show a partial response to splenectomy.
- **Hexokinase (HK) deficiency** is the first enzyme in the glycolytic pathway and thus is responsible for priming the glycolytic pump. There are two types of HK deficiency. One is associated with hemolytic anemia that responds to splenectomy. The other is associated not only with hemolytic anemia but also with an array of other abnormalities. A deficiency in this enzyme interferes with production of 2,3-BPG, and patients tolerate the anemia poorly.
- **Phosphoglyceratekinase (PGK) deficiency** is a sexlinked disorder that causes hemolytic anemia and mental retardation in males. Females have a milder form of the disorder.
- **Phosphofructokinase (PFK) deficiency** is indicated when subunits of the PFK enzyme are found in various tissues. Deficiency of this enzyme can appear as myopathy or hemolytic anemia or both.[26]
- **Triosephosphate isomerase (TPI) deficiency** causes severe abnormalities in erythrocytes resulting in severe hemolysis. Abnormalities are also noted in striated muscle and the central nervous system. Death in infancy is common.

▶ ABNORMAL ERYTHROCYTE NUCLEOTIDE METABOLISM

Pyrimidine 5'-nucleotidase (P5N) contributes to the degradation of nucleic acids by cleaving pyrimidine nucleotides into smaller nucleosides that can diffuse out of the cell. The buildup of pyrimidine nucleotides decreases the adenine nucleotide pool needed for normal function. P5N deficiency is an autosomal recessive disorder that leads to a severe hemolytic anemia unresponsive to splenectomy. Partially degraded mRNA and rRNA accumulate within the cell and are visualized as basophilic stippling in stained smears. Lead inhibits this enzyme, which can explain the similar coarse basophilic stippling seen in lead poisoning (∞ Chapter 9).

SUMMARY

The erythrocyte life span can be significantly shortened if the erythrocyte has intrinsic defects such as deficient metabolic machinery. Maintaining a balance of intracellular constituents is compromised when enzymes responsible for various metabolic pathways are deficient or fail to function properly. These abnormalities are almost always inherited defects. Erythrocytes with intrinsic defects are susceptible to early destruction, and when this destruction exceeds the marrow capacity to replace cells, hemolytic anemia results. These hemolytic anemias are known as *chronic* or *congenital nonspherocytic hemolytic anemias*.

Erythrocyte enzyme deficiencies can compromise the integrity of the cell membrane or hemoglobin and lead to hemolysis. The HMP shunt provides the cell reducing power, protecting it from oxidant damage. Defects in this shunt allow hemoglobin to be oxidized and denatured to Heinz bodies. The Heinz bodies damage the cell membrane. The finding of bite cells on the blood smear is evidence that Heinz bodies have been pitted from the cells. The most common deficiency in this pathway is G6PD deficiency, a sex-linked disorder. This enzyme has many different variants, some of which cause severe hemolysis and others mild hemolysis. In most cases, hemolysis is sporadic, occurring during infections or with the administration of certain drugs, and is self-limited. In these variants, the younger cells have adequate enzyme activity, but the older cells are severely deficient and selectively hemolyzed. Testing for the enzyme should be delayed until 2 months after the hemolytic episode when reticulocytes are at a steady state (normal) and the erythrocytes produced after the hemolytic episode have aged. Screening tests for the enzyme include the fluorescent dye test, cytochemical staining, dye-reduction test, and ascorbate cyanide test. Definitive testing requires quantitation of the enzyme or genetic testing for mutations.

Deficiencies of enzymes in the glycolytic pathway decrease ATP production and lead to hemolysis. There can be impaired cation pumping and increased osmotic fragility. Pyruvate kinase (PK) is the most common enzyme abnormality in this pathway. There are many PK enzyme mutants, resulting in a diverse array of clinical and laboratory findings. There can be significant reticulocytosis. The blood film is remarkable for the presence of irregularly contracted cells and echinocytes. Heinz bodies and bite cells are not found. Screening and definitive tests for the enzyme are based on fluorescence. Several other rare enzyme defects that also lead to hemolysis have been identified.

REVIEW QUESTIONS

LEVEL I

1. What are the two main metabolic pathways that erythrocytes use for glucose metabolism? (Objective 1)
   a. Krebs cycle and glycolytic
   b. hexokinase and Krebs cycle
   c. oxidative phosphorylation and glycolytic
   d. hexose-monophosphate shunt and glycolytic

2. The main protective functions of erythrocyte enzymes result from which of the following? (Objective 2)
   a. electron transport and cation pumping using ATP
   b. cation pumping using ATP and protection of hemoglobin by reduced glutathione
   c. protection of hemoglobin by reduced glutathione and electron transport
   d. cation pumping and bilirubin production

3. In G6PD deficiency, anemia ultimately results from: (Objective 2)
   a. buildup of 2,3-BPG and poor iron binding
   b. inability to maintain enough ATP to pump cations
   c. oxidative damage to hemoglobin and splenic removal of erythrocytes
   d. membrane protein defects and loss of erythrocyte flexibility

4. Which is the most common erythrocyte enzyme deficiency? (Objective 3)
   a. pyruvate kinase
   b. hexokinase
   c. glucose phosphate isomerase
   d. glucose-6-phosphate dehydrogenase

LEVEL II

1. Why should G6PD testing be delayed for an individual following a hemolytic episode? (Objective 1)
   a. The level of glucose must have time to replenish.
   b. Heinz bodies can interfere with the test method.
   c. Deficient cells have been selectively destroyed.
   d. The patient needs time to build up iron stores.

2. An 18-year-old black male was suspected of having G6PD deficiency when he experienced hemolytic anemia after administration of primaquine. An erythrocyte G6PD analysis performed on blood taken 2 days after symptoms appeared was normal. A reticulocyte count revealed 12% reticulocytes at this time. These results suggest that: (Objective 7)
   a. the patient definitely does not have G6PD deficiency but could have pyruvate kinase deficiency
   b. another G6PD test should be done in several months when the reticulocyte count returns to normal
   c. leukocytes could be contaminating the sample giving a false result
   d. the patient probably has the G6PD Mediterranean variant

3. The main consequence of enzyme defects in the glycolytic pathway is: (Objective 3)
   a. decreased ATP production
   b. Heinz body formation
   c. decreased formation of reduced glutathione
   d. decreased formation of 2,3-BPG

REVIEW QUESTIONS (continued)

LEVEL I

5. Which is true for the inheritance pattern for G6PD? (Objective 4)
   a. It is X-linked and only found in males.
   b. It is autosomal dominant and affects all offspring.
   c. It is X-linked; however, females can be affected.
   d. It is autosomal, and males are affected; females are carriers.

6. Which of the following is a quantitative test for G6PD? (Objective 6)
   a. rate reduction test
   b. fluorescent spot test
   c. dye reduction test
   d. ascorbate cyanide test

7. Following a hemolytic attack, which of the following is a common finding in G6PD deficiency? (Objective 5)
   a. reticulocytosis
   b. appearance of burr cells on the blood smear
   c. increased haptoglobin
   d. decreased unconjugated bilirubin

8. An abnormal erythrocyte resulting from splenic removal of Heinz bodies in erythrocytes is called: (Objective 7)
   a. macrocyte
   b. target cell
   c. bite cell
   d. dacryocyte

9. The type of hemolysis arising from G6PD deficiency is classified as: (Objective 2)
   a. extravascular
   b. intravascular
   c. complete
   d. rapid

10. What compound can induce anemia in G6PD deficiency? (Objective 8)
    a. aspirin
    b. vitamin C
    c. iron
    d. primaquine

LEVEL II

4. Which of the following G6PD isoenzyme variants will *not* result in hemolysis? (Objective 4)
   a. G6PD Mediterranean
   b. G6PD-B
   c. G6PD Canton
   d. G6PD-A⁻

5. The blood smear of a patient with chronic nonspherocytic hemolytic anemia reveals echinocytes, acanthocytes, target cells, and irregularly contracted cells. Which follow-up test could help define the cause of this anemia? (Objective 6)
   a. PEP fluorescent test
   b. ascorbate cyanide test
   c. fluorescent spot test
   d. quantitation of G6PD

6. Explain why bite cells are *not* characteristic of pyruvate kinase deficiency. (Objectives 3, 5, 6)
   a. The spleen removes them as they are formed.
   b. The erythrocyte forms a spherocyte as inclusions are removed.
   c. Heinz bodies are not formed in pyruvate kinase deficiency.
   d. Pyruvate kinase deficiency does not cause abnormal erythrocyte morphology.

7. Congenital nonspherocytic hemolytic anemia syndrome is associated with which G-6-PD variants? (Objective 4)
   a. Class I
   b. Class II
   c. Class III
   d. Class IV

8. Harmful peroxides in the erythrocyte are neutralized by which of the following? (Objective 2)
   a. ATP production
   b. Heinz bodies
   c. bilirubin
   d. glutathione

9. A patient is suspected of having a form of G6PD deficiency but is *not* affected by ingestion of fava beans. How can this be explained? (Objective 4)
   a. The patient has the G6PD Mediterranean type.
   b. The type of G6PD present is G6PD-B.
   c. The patient does not have G6PD deficiency.
   d. A mild form of G6PD is present.

10. Which lab test is most useful in diagnosing G6PD deficiency? (Objective 1)
    a. fluorescent spot test
    b. CBC
    c. reticulocyte count
    d. PEP fluorescent test

www.pearsonhighened.com/mckenzie
Use this address to access the interactive Companion Website created for this textbook. Find additional information, tables and figures. Evaluate your command of the chapter information using case studies and critical thinking and multiple choice questions.

REFERENCES

1. Beutler E. Disorders of red cells resulting from enzyme abnormalities. In: Lightman MA, Beutler E, Kipps TJ, Seligsohn U, Kaushansky K, Prchal JT, eds. *Williams Hematology,* 7th ed. New York: McGraw-Hill; 2006;603–31.

2. Herz F, Kaplan E, Scheye ES. Diagnosis of erythrocyte glucose-6-phosphate dehydrogenase deficiency in the Negro male despite hemolytic crisis. *Blood.* 1970;35:90.

3. Ringelhahn B. A simple laboratory procedure for the recognition of A- (Arican type) G6PD deficiency in acute haemolytic crisis. *Clin Chim Acta.* 1972;36:772.

4. Luzzatto L, Usanga EA, Reddy S. Glucose 6-phosphate dehydrogenase deficient red cells: Resistance to infection by malarial parasites. *Science.* 1969;164:839–42.

5. Cappadoro M, Giribaldi G, O'Brien E et al. Early phagocytosis of glucose-6-phosphate dehydrogenase (G6PD)-deficient erythrocytes parasitized by plasmodium falciparum may explain malaria protection in G6PD deficiency. *Blood.* 1998;92:2527–34.

6. Arese P, DeFlora A. Pathophysiology of hemolysis in glucose-6-phosphate dehydrogenase deficiency. *Sem Hematol.* 1990;27:1–40.

7. Costa E, Cabeda JM, Vieira E, Pinto R, Pereira SA, Ferraz L et al. Glucose-6-phosphate dehydrogenase averia: A de novo mutation associated with chronic nonspherocytic hemolytic anemia. *Blood.* 2000; 95:1499–501.

8. Darr S, Vulliamy TJ, Kaeda J, Mason PJ, Luzzatto L. Molecular characterization of G6PD deficiency in Oman. *Hum Hered.* 1996;46: 172–76.

9. Sarkar S et al. Acute intravascular haemolysis in glucose-6-phosphate dehydrogenase deficiency. *An Trop Paediatr.* 1993;13:391–94.

10. Nafa L et al. G6PD Aures: A new mutation (48 Ile → Thr) causing mild G6PD deficiency is associated with favism. *Hum Mol Genet.* 1993;2:81–82.

11. Vives Corrons JS, Feliu E, Pujades MA, Cardellach F, Rozman C, Carreras A et al. Severe glucose-6-phosphate dehydrogenase (G6PD) deficiency associated with chronic hemolytic anemia, granulocyte dysfunction, and increased susceptibility to infections: Description of a new molecular variant (G6PD Barcelona). *Blood.* 1982;59: 428–34.

12. Roos D, van Zwieten R, Wijnen JT, Gomez-Gallego F, deBoer M, Stevens D et al. Molecular basis and enzymatic properties of glucose-6-phosphate dehydrogenase volendam, leading to chronic nonsperocytic anemia, granulocyte dysfunction, and increased susceptibility to infections. *Blood.* 1999;94:2955–62.

13. Gray GR, Klebanoff SJ, Stamatoyannopoulous G, Austin T, Naiman C, Yoshida A et al. Neutrophil dysfunction, chronic granulomatous disease and non-sperocytic haemolytic anemia caused by complete deficiency of glucose-6-phosphate dehydrogenase. *Lancet.* 1973;2: 530–34.

14. Wolach B, Ashkenazi M, Grossmann R, Gavrieli R, Friedman Z, Bashan N et al. Diurnal fluctuation of leukocyte G6PD acitivity. A possible explanation for the normal neutrophil bactericidal activity and the low incidence of pyogenic infections in patients with severe G6PD deficiency in Israel. *Pediat Res.* 2004;55:807–13.

15. Theodorsson E, Birgens H, Hagve TA. Haemoglobinopathies and glucose-6-phosphate dehydrogenase deficiency in a Scandinavian perspective. *Scand J Clin Lab Inves.* 2007;67(1):3–10.

16. Johnson LH, Bhutani VK, Brown AK. System-based approach to management of neonatal jaundice and prevention of kernicterus. *J Pediatr.* 2002;140:396–403.

17. Mesner O, Hammerman C, Goldschmidt D, Rudensky B, Bader D, Kaplan M. Glucose-6-phosphate dehydrogenase activity in male premature and term neonates. *Arch Dis Child Fet Neonat Ed.* 2004; 89:F555–57.

18. Ward PCJ, Schwartz BS, White JG. Heinz-body anemia: "Bite Cell" variant—A light and electron microscopic study. *Amer J Hem.* 1983; l5:135–46.

19. Simmons SJ, McCann S, Glassman AB. Intracorpuscular defects II: Hereditary enzyme deficiencies. In: Harmening D., ed. *Clinical Hematology and Fundamentals of Hemostasis,* 3rd ed. Philadelphia: F.A. Davis Company; 1997:164–72.

20. Shannon K, Buchanan GR. Severe hemolytic anemia in black children with glucose-6-phosphate dehydrogenase deficiency. *Pediatr.* 1982;70(3):364–69.

21. Van Noorden, CJ, Dolbeare, F, and Aten, J. Flow cytofluorometric analysis of enzyme reactions based on quenching of fluorescence by the final reaction product: Detection of glucose-6-phosphate dehydrogenase deficiency in human erythrocytes. *Journal of Histochemistry and Cytochemistry.* 1989;37(9):1313–18.

22. Zanella A, Fermo E, Bianchi P, Chiarelli LR, Valentini G. Pyruvate kinase deficiency: The genotype-phenotype association. *Blood Rev.* 2007;21(4):217–31.

23. Pissard S, de Montalembert M, Bachir D, Max-Audit I, Goossens M, Wajcman H et al. Pyruvate kinase (PK) deficiency in newborns: The pitfalls of diagnosis. *J. Peds.* 2007;150(4):443–45.

24. Beulter E. A series of new screening procedures for pyruvate kinase, glucose-6-dehydrogenase deficiency and glutathione reductase deficiency. *Blood* 1996;28:553.

25. Tsang SS, Feng CS. A modified screening procedure to detect pyruvate kinase deficiency. *Am J Clin Pathol.* 1993;99:128–31.

26. Vora S et al. The molecular mechanism of the inherited phosphofructokinase deficiency associated with hemolysis and myopathy. *Blood.* 1980;55:629–35.

17

Hemolytic Anemia: Immune Anemias

Linda A. Smith, Ph.D.

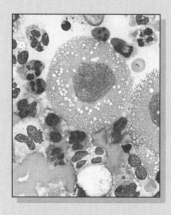

6. Interpret the results of laboratory tests for HDFN and determine whether evidence of hemolysis is present.

7. Compare and contrast the pathophysiology and clinical findings of an immediate transfusion reaction with those of a delayed reaction.

8. List the causes of the secondary types of cold agglutinin syndrome and warm autoimmune hemolytic anemia and identify key laboratory results linking the cause and the autoimmune condition.

9. Compare the typical laboratory findings in immediate versus delayed transfusion reactions.

KEY TERMS

Alloimmune hemolytic anemia
Antihuman globulin (AHG)
Autoimmune hemolytic anemia (AIHA)
Direct antiglobulin test (DAT)
Donath-Landsteiner antibody
Drug-induced hemolysis
Erythroblastosis fetalis
Hemolytic disease of the fetus and newborn (HDFN)
Hemolytic transfusion reaction
Immune hemolytic anemia (IHA)
Indirect antiglobulin test (IAT)
Kernicterus
Paroxysmal cold hemoglobinuria (PCH)

BACKGROUND BASICS

The information in this chapter builds on the concepts learned in previous chapters. Additionally, a basic understanding of immunology principles and an introduction to immunohematology will be helpful. To maximize your learning experience, you should review these concepts before starting this unit of study.

Level I

▶ Summarize the normal production, life span, and destruction of erythrocytes. (Chapter 5)

▶ List the reference interval for the hematology parameters: hemoglobin, hematocrit, erythrocyte count, and reticulocytes. (Chapters 5, 8)

▶ List the different intrinsic and extrinsic factors that can result in hemolytic anemia. (Chapter 14)

▶ Describe the basic structure of immunoglobulin and its normal physiologic role. (Chapter 7)

Level II

▶ Describe the role of erythropoietin and regulation of its production. (Chapter 5)

▶ Differentiate intravascular and extravascular destruction of erythrocytes and relate to laboratory parameters in the diagnosis of abnormal hemolysis. (Chapter 5)

▶ Choose laboratory tests to assist in diagnosing anemia in a cost-efficient and effective manner. (Chapter 8)

▶ Identify clinical signs of hemolytic anemia and changes that occur in laboratory tests that signal possible hemolytic anemia. (Chapter 14)

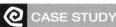
CASE STUDY

We will refer to this case study throughout the chapter.
Nancy, a 28-year-old female, makes an appointment with her physician because she is tired all the time and is short of breath with minor exertion. She indicates that the symptoms have been ongoing for about 3 weeks. She has no known history of chronic diseases. Consider the initial laboratory tests that should be done to evaluate this patient's condition based on clinical history and symptoms.

▶ OVERVIEW

This chapter compares the different types of immune mediated hemolytic anemias: autoimmune, alloimmune, and drug induced. The underlying mechanism for each of these anemias involves the reaction of an antibody with erythrocyte antigens and subsequent cell destruction either by intravascular or extravascular processes. The mechanisms of intravascular and extravascular hemolysis are compared. The tests necessary to detect erythrocyte sensitization and identify the causative antibody are described.

The pathophysiology, clinical and laboratory findings, differential diagnosis, and therapy are discussed for each of the major types of autoimmune hemolytic anemia. Hemolytic transfusion reactions and hemolytic disease of the fetus and newborn are included as examples of alloimmune hemolytic anemia. The causative antibody and clinical presentation for acute and delayed transfusion reactions are compared and the laboratory tests required to confirm hemolytic transfusion reactions are described. In the section on hemolytic disease of the newborn (HDFN), ABO-HDFN and Rh-HDFN are compared. The treatment of a fetus and the newborn with this condition as well as preventative measures is included.

▶ INTRODUCTION

When erythrocytes are destroyed prematurely by an immune mediated process (antibody and/or complement), the disorder is referred to as an **immune hemolytic anemia (IHA).** The individual, however, might or might not become

TABLE 17-1

Classification of Immune Hemolytic Anemias

Classification	Causes
Autoimmune	Warm-reactive antibodies
	Primary or idiopathic
	Secondary
	Autoimmune disorders (systemic lupus erythematosus, rheumatoid arthritis, and others)
	Chronic lymphocytic leukemia and other immunoproliferative diseases
	Viral infections
	Neoplastic disorders
	Chronic inflammatory diseases
	Cold-reactive antibodies
	Primary or idiopathic (cold hemagglutinin disease)
	Secondary
	Infectious diseases (*mycoplasma pneumoniae*, Epstein-Barr virus and other organisms)
	Lymphoproliferative disorders
	Paroxysmal cold hemoglobinuria
	Mixed-type
Drug induced	Drug adsorption
	Immune complex
	Autoantibody induction
	Membrane modification
Alloimmune	Hemolytic transfusion reaction
	Hemolytic disease of the fetus and newborn

anemic, depending on the severity of hemolysis and the ability of the bone marrow to compensate for erythrocyte loss. Initial confirmation of the underlying immune mechanism is accomplished by demonstrating attachment of antibody or complement to the patient's erythrocytes. Diagnosis of anemia (and underlying hemolysis) is determined by laboratory findings such as a decrease in hemoglobin and hematocrit an increase in reticulocytes and/or indirect bilirubin, and a decrease in serum haptoglobin. Table 14-2 (∞ Chapter 14) summarizes some common laboratory values and clinical findings characteristically seen in hemolytic anemia.

▶ CLASSIFICATION OF IMMUNE HEMOLYTIC ANEMIAS

Determining the underlying process of immune hemolysis is important because each type requires a specific treatment regimen. Initially, IHA can be classified into three broad categories based on the stimulus for antibody production[1,2] (Table 17-1 ✪): These are:

- Autoimmune hemolytic anemia
- Drug-induced hemolytic anemia
- Alloimmune hemolytic anemia

Autoimmune hemolytic anemia (AIHA) is a complex and incompletely understood process characterized by an immune reaction against self-antigens and shortened erythrocyte survival.[1,2] Individuals produce antibodies against their own erythrocyte antigens (autoantibodies). These autoantibodies are usually directed against high-incidence antigens (antigens present on the erythrocytes of most people). The autoantibodies characteristically react not only with the erythrocytes of the individual but also with the erythrocytes of other individuals carrying the antigen. The antibody in cold autoimmune hemolytic anemia is usually directed against antigens of the Ii system. The autoantibody in warm autoimmune hemolytic anemia most commonly has a complex specificity that reacts with epitopes on cells that possess Rh antigens. These complex-specific antibodies do not react with Rh null cells or some Rh deleted cells. However, some autoantibodies have a single specificity such as anti-e. In these patients, the autoantibody reacts with the patient's own cells and only with cells of individuals who possess the specific antigen. The reactions that occur with autoantibodies include erythrocyte lysis, sensitization (attachment of antibody or complement), or agglutination.

Autoimmune hemolytic anemias are further classified as warm or cold hemolytic anemia based on clinical symptoms and on the optimal temperature at which the antibody reacts (in vivo and in vitro)[1-3] (Table 17-2 ✪). Some antibodies react best at body temperature (37°C); the anemia they produce is termed *warm autoimmune hemolytic anemia* (WAIHA). About 70% of the AIHAs are of the warm type. The majority of warm autoantibodies are of the IgG class (most frequently IgG1) and cause extravascular hemolysis of the erythrocyte. A few warm-reacting autoantibodies of either the IgM or the IgA class have been identified.[4-8] Cold hemolytic anemias, on the other hand, are usually due to the presence of an IgM antibody with an optimal thermal reactivity below 30°C. Hemolysis with cold-reacting antibodies results from the binding and activation of complement by IgM. The IgM antibody attaches to erythrocytes in the cold and fixes complement. After warming, the antibody dissociates from the cell, but the complement remains, either causing direct cell lysis or initiating extravascular hemolysis. Included in the cold hemolytic anemia classification is a special condition, paroxysmal cold hemoglobinuria (PCH), which is characterized by a cold-reacting IgG class antibody.

A third major category, mixed-type autoimmune hemolytic anemia, demonstrates both warm-reacting (IgG) autoantibodies and cold-reacting (IgM) autoantibodies.

Drugs that attach to the erythrocyte membrane or alter it in some way can cause **drug-induced hemolysis.** Historically, several different mechanisms of hemolysis have been hypothesized based on whether the drug binds directly to the cell, reacts with an antibody in the circulation to form

⊕ TABLE 17-2

Characteristics of Agglutinins in Hemolytic Anemia

	Warm-Reacting Antibodies	Cold-Reacting Antibodies
Immunoglobulin (Ig) class	IgG IgM (rare) IgA (usually with IgG)	IgM IgG (PCH only)
Optimal reactivity	37°C	<30°C, usually <10°C
Mechanism of hemolysis	Attachment of membrane-bound IgG or C3b to macrophage receptors (extravascular)	Complement-mediated lysis (intravascular), or attachment of membrane-bound C3b to macrophage receptors (extravascular)
Specificity	Usually broad specificity anti-Rh	Usually autoanti-I Occasionally autoanti-i PCH-autoanti-P

PCH = paraoxysmal cold hermoglobinuria

an immune complex that binds to the cell, or alters the erythrocyte antigens to stimulate formation of autoantibodies. These mechanisms are discussed in detail later in this chapter.

Alloimmune hemolytic anemia occurs as a result of antibody development to an erythrocyte antigen that the individual lacks. When an individual is exposed to erythrocytes from another person, antigens on the transfused cells may be lacking on the erythrocytes of the recipient. Therefore, these antigens on the transfused cell can be recognized as foreign by the recipient's lymphocytes and stimulate the production of antibodies (alloantibodies). In contrast to autoantibodies, these alloantibodies react only with the antigens on the transfused cells or cells from individuals who possess the antigen. The alloantibodies do not react with the individual's erythrocytes. Examples of alloimmune hemolytic anemia are:

* Hemolytic disease of the fetus and newborn in which the mother makes antibodies that react with the antigens on the fetal erythrocytes
* Transfusion reactions in which the recipient makes antibodies to antigens on the transfused (donor) cells

The presence of alloantibodies can be demonstrated in vitro by performing an antibody screen. In this test, the patient's serum is reacted with commercial erythrocytes containing most of the clinically significant antigens. An autocontrol consisting of the patient's serum and erythrocytes can also be set up. When only alloantibodies are present, the autocontrol will show no hemolysis or agglutination while the mixture of patient's serum and the commercial cells will produce agglutination and, in rare cases, hemolysis.

✓ Checkpoint! 1

What are the three major categories of immune hemolytic anemia, and how is antibody production stimulated in each type?

⊘ CASE STUDY (continued from page 340)

Nancy's initial CBC shows a hemoglobin value of 7.0 g/dL (70 g/L) and a hematocrit of 0.21 L/L (21%). Her WBC count and platelet count are within reference interval.

1. What are some reasons that she could have a low hemoglobin value?

▶ SITES AND FACTORS THAT AFFECT HEMOLYSIS

Regardless of whether it is caused by alloantibodies or autoantibodies, hemolysis can be intravascular or extravascular, depending on the class of antibody involved and whether or not the complement cascade has been completely activated. Most immune-mediated hemolysis is extravascular. Erythrocytes sensitized with antibody or complement components attach to macrophages in the spleen or liver via macrophage receptors for the Fc portion of immunoglobulin or the C3b component of complement. These cells are then phagocytized (Figure 17-1 ■). Intravascular hemolysis occurs if the complement cascade is activated through C9 (the membrane attack complex), resulting in

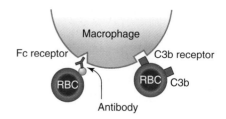

■ FIGURE 17-1   Immune mediated extravascular hemolysis. Erythrocytes sensitized with antibody or complement (C3b) attach to macrophages via specific cell receptors for these immune proteins.

TABLE 17-3

Factors Affecting the Rate of Hemolysis in Immune Hemolytic Anemias

Factor	Effect
Class of immunoglobulin coating the erythrocytes	For the IgG subclasses, the affinity of macrophage receptors and rate of hemolysis is greatest for IgG3 and IgG1
The number of Ig molecules per erythrocyte	Immunoglobulins will coat a cell with a high density of antigens (large number of antigens) more heavily than a cell with low density (fewer) antigens
Ability of the Ig to activate complement	IgM and IgG can activate complement; for IgG, the ability to activate complement, is IgG3>IgG1>gG2
Thermal amplitude of the antibody	Warm-reacting (37°C) antibodies can cause hemolysis but cold-reacting (0–4°C) antibodies usually do not
The activity level of macrophages	Suppression of F_c receptors will decrease rate of hemolysis

lysis of the cell. The rate at which hemolysis occurs in hemolytic anemia is related to several factors.[9–11] The major factors and their effects are summarized in Table 17-3 ✪. A full description of the mechanisms is found on the web (Factors Affecting Hemolysis).

✓ Checkpoint! 2

Explain how the class of immunoglobulin, amount of antibody bound, and thermal reactivity of the antibody affect hemolysis.

▶ MECHANISMS OF HEMOLYSIS

The mechanisms for hemolysis are based on whether IgM, IgG, and/or complement is/are present on the erythrocyte. Specific phagocytic cells in the spleen or liver initiate extravascular hemolysis of cells coated with IgG or complement. Complete activation of the complement cascade results in intravascular hemolysis.

IgG-MEDIATED HEMOLYSIS

IgG mediates erythrocyte destruction by first attaching to the erythrocyte membrane antigens through the Fab portion of the Ig molecule. The Fc portion of IgG is exposed to the environment. Fc receptors (FcγR-I, -II, -III) on macrophages in the red pulp of the spleen bind to the Fc portion of the attached IgG. After binding, the macrophage pits the antigen-antibody (Ag/Ab) complex, fragmenting the cell membrane. The erythrocyte membrane initially reseals itself. With repeated splenic passage, however, the erythrocyte continues to lose membrane and gradually assumes a spherocytic shape. As the cell becomes more spherocytic, it becomes rigid and less deformable and is eventually phagocytized by splenic macrophages. Alternatively, the antibody-sensitized cell can be entirely engulfed by the macrophages (phagocytosis). Natural killer (NK) cells and neutrophils also have FcγR. Neutrophils are capable of phagocytosis (FcγR-I, -III), and interaction of antibody-coated cells with NK cells usually results in antibody-dependent cell-mediated cytotoxicity (ADCC), the recognition and lysis of cells by NK cells. This occurs through binding of IgG by the FcγRIII (CD16) on NK cells. Any target cell coated with IgG can be bound to NK cells and lysed.

As the spleen becomes saturated with "sensitized" RBC (cells coated with antibody and/or complement), the liver assists in removal of the cells. Lightly opsonized cells are more efficiently removed in the spleen due to the sluggish blood flow there. The liver can also be of some importance in removing heavily sensitized cells. The splenic tissue proliferates in response to an increase in erythrocyte sequestration, accounting for splenic enlargement (splenomegaly) in chronic warm-immune hemolytic anemias. In the immune hemolytic anemias in which complement is activated, complement as well as IgG can be detected on the erythrocyte membrane. This enhances the phagocytosis of sensitized cells by increasing the likelihood of the cell binding to either the Fc and/or C3b receptors of macrophages.

COMPLEMENT-MEDIATED HEMOLYSIS

The complement system consists of more than 20 serum proteins responsible for a number of diverse biological activities including the mediation of acute inflammatory responses and destruction of cells and microorganisms. The major roles of complement in immune hemolytic anemias are sensitization and lysis of erythrocytes.[12] Sensitization occurs when only a portion of the cascade is activated and deposited on the erythrocyte membrane; lysis results when the entire system is activated.

The complement proteins are designated numerically (i.e., C1, C2, C3) or by letters or historical names. Complement proteins normally circulate in an inactive state. Under certain circumstances, the proteins become sequentially activated in a cascade-like fashion, similar to the components of the coagulation cascade. Activation of parts of the cascade is enzymatically mediated while other portions occur without enzymatic cleavage of the molecules. An activated component is identified by placing a bar over the component ($\overline{C5}$).

The complement cascade can be initiated by at least three separate mechanisms:

- Classic
- Alternate
- Lectin

The usual and most important activation pathway in IHA is the classic, although on some occasions the alternate pathway can be activated (Figure 17-2 ■). The classic complement pathway can be initiated by an antigen-antibody reaction. Antibodies of the IgM class as well as IgG1 and IgG3 (IgG2 less efficiently) subclasses can activate this pathway. The first complement component (C1q) must attach to the

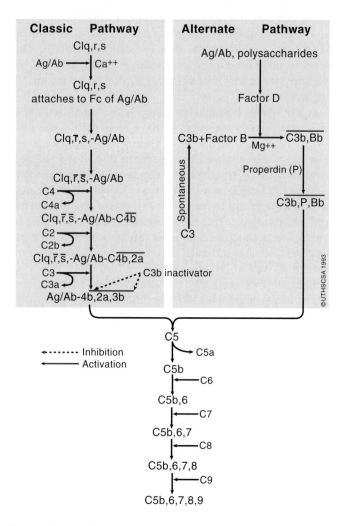

■ FIGURE 17-2   The complement cascade. The central event in complement activation is the activation of C3 by C3 convertases. This can occur by two separate but interrelated mechanisms, the classic and alternate pathways. The classic complement pathway can be initiated by an antigen-antibody reaction. The antigen-antibody complex activates the C1q, r, s complex, which in turn activates C4 by proteolytic cleavage to C4a and C4b. C2 binds to C4b and is proteolytically cleaved by C1s to form C2a and C2b. The C4b2a complex serves as C3 convertase. In the alternate pathway, C3b serves as the cofactor of the C3-cleaving enzyme complex (C3b, P, Bb), also known as C3 convertase. Thus, the C3b serves to prime its own activation. The C3b formed through the classic pathway can directly initiate the assembly of the alternate pathway C3 convertase. C3 can also be activated by spontaneous hydrolysis. The C3b complexes formed by the classic and alternate pathways activate C5 to C5a and C5b. Membrane damage is initiated by the assembly of C5b with C6, 7, 8, 9.

Fc regions of an antibody, requiring that two antibody-binding sites be in close proximity. Thus, the attachment of complement depends highly on the density or concentration of antibody molecules and their spatial arrangement on the cell surface. The IgG molecule is much less efficient than IgM in providing these side-by-side antibody Fc regions. Only one IgM molecule is required to activate the complement pathway whereas two IgG molecules are required; thus, IgM is much more likely to activate complement than IgG. Therefore, the nature of the antibody involved is an important determinant of the extent of erythrocyte destruction by complement.

Activation of the cascade is initiated when the first complement component, C1, binds to the Fc portion of an IgG or IgM antibody molecule. C1 is a tri-molecular complex that initially binds via its C1q portion and subsequently via C1r and C1s. This attachment initiates activation of the other complement components (C4, C2, C3). The complex containing C3b activates the terminal components, C5 to C9. Activation of these terminal complement components, known as the *membrane attack complex (MAC)*, is responsible for the lytic attack on the erythrocyte membrane and is common to both pathways. Membrane leakage begins at the C8-activation stage when a transmembrane pore is formed. C9 prevents the pore from resealing, resulting in osmotic lysis. The alternate pathway of complement activation can be initiated by aggregated IgG, IgA, and IgE, as well as by a number of polysaccharides and liposaccharides. In this pathway, C3 is activated directly, bypassing C1, C2, and C4 activation.

If complement activation on the erythrocyte membrane is complete (C1–C9), intravascular hemolysis will occur. However, activation of complement is not always complete (through C9) and thus does not always lead to direct cell lysis. More commonly, activation proceeds only through C3 on the erythrocyte membrane (in which case the cell is said to be *sensitized*). In this scenario, the C3 is broken down into two fragments: C3a, which is released into the plasma, and C3b, which remains attached to the cell membrane. The sensitized cell with attached C3b is totally or partially engulfed by binding to the C3b receptors (CR1, CR3) of macrophages in the liver (most complement-coated cells are removed in this organ). Because of the enzymatic action of C3b inactivator in plasma, C3b on erythrocytes can be further cleaved to form C3c and C3d before the cell encounters macrophages. C3c dissociates from the membrane, but C3d remains attached. Erythrocytes coated with C3d have a normal survival because macrophages have no receptors for this complement component. Thus, the balance between C3b deposition on the membrane and C3b inactivation determines the susceptibility of erythrocytes to phagocytosis by macrophages via the C3b receptors.

In addition to C3b inactivator, other inhibitors of complement activation exist. Some of these inactivators and their functions are listed in Web Table 17-1 ✪.

IgM-MEDIATED HEMOLYSIS

In cold immune hemolytic anemia, the IgM molecule becomes attached to the erythrocyte membrane, but these sensitized cells are not removed from circulation in the same manner as those sensitized with IgG because macrophages do not have receptors for the Fc portion of IgM. However, IgM is an efficient activator of complement, and cells can be lysed intravascularly if complement activation through C9 is complete. If activation is incomplete and only C3b coats the cells, they can be destroyed extravascularly via adherence to CR1 and CR3 receptors on macrophages. Adherence of the cell to macrophages via complement receptors and subsequent phagocytosis, however, is less efficient than immune adherence (adherence mediated via immunoglobulin) and phagocytosis via FcγR macrophage receptors. It has been estimated that more than 100,000 molecules of the complement component C3b are required on the cell surface to induce phagocytosis by macrophages via complement. C3b is also inefficient in promoting adherence to macrophages because much of the C3b is inactivated to C3d. Thus, extravascular hemolysis of cells sensitized with complement is not as severe as hemolysis of cells sensitized with IgG.

In addition to activating complement, IgM antibodies agglutinate cells. In vitro, agglutination is a useful phenomenon for detecting the presence of cold agglutinins.

Checkpoint! 3

Compare the mechanisms of IgG mediated hemolysis with those of IgM mediated hemolysis.

▶ LABORATORY IDENTIFICATION OF SENSITIZED RED CELLS

When immune hemolytic anemia is suspected, tests to detect and identify the causative antibody are indicated. In general, two distinct techniques are used:

- Agglutination in saline, which will detect antibodies of the IgM class
- **Antihuman globulin (AHG)** test, which will detect antibodies of the IgG class and/or complement

IgM antibodies can be detected by agglutination reactions between test sera and appropriate erythrocytes suspended in saline but IgG antibodies cannot. This difference in the ability of IgG and IgM to cause agglutination in saline can be explained on the basis of the difference in size of the two antibodies in relation to the zeta potential. The erythrocyte zeta potential is an electrostatic potential created by a difference in the charge density of the inner and outer layers of the ionic cloud around erythrocytes when they are suspended in saline. This force tends to keep the erythrocytes about 25 nm apart in solution. Thus, any antibody that causes agglutina-

tion of saline- or plasma-suspended cells must be large enough to span the 25 nm gap between cells. The IgM pentamer has a possible span of 35 nm; therefore, it can overcome the electrostatic forces separating the cells and cause agglutination (Figure 17-3 ■). However, the maximum span of the IgG molecule is about 14 nm, and it cannot reach antigens on two separate cells to cause agglutination. Thus, detection of IgG antibodies requires a different technique using a substance that will connect the antibody molecules on separate cells and cause agglutination. The substance used is AHG, essentially an antiserum to human IgG.

The AHG test, sometimes referred to as the *Coombs test,* is the specific laboratory procedure designed to detect erythrocytes sensitized with IgG and/or complement. AHG is a broad-spectrum antisera produced in rabbits that reacts against human immunoglobulin and complement. It contains divalent antibodies that are capable of attaching to the Fc region of immunoglobulins or to complement components on two separate cells, thus bridging the distance between cells and leading to the lattice formation known as *agglutination.*

The two applications of the AHG test are:

- Direct: detects erythrocytes coated with antibody in vivo
- Indirect: detects antibodies in the plasma or serum

DIRECT ANTIGLOBULIN TEST

The **direct antiglobulin test (DAT,** or direct Coombs test) detects erythrocytes that have been sensitized with antibody and/or complement in vivo (Web Figure 17-1 ■). This

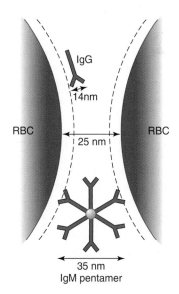

■ FIGURE 17-3   The zeta potential of erythrocytes keeps the cells about 25 nm apart when suspended in saline. IgG antibodies have a span of about 14 nm, not enough to bridge the gap between cells and cause agglutination. IgM antibodies, however, are pentamers with a span of about 35 nm, a distance sufficient to bridge the space between cells and cause agglutination.

test should always be performed in suspected cases of AIHA because it differentiates AIHA from all other types of hemolytic anemia. Specimens collected in tubes with ethylenediaminetetraacetate (EDTA) are preferred to clotted specimens for the DAT procedure because EDTA chelates Ca^{++} and Mg^{++}, preventing the in vitro binding of complement to red cells that can be mediated by naturally occurring cold reactive antibodies (e.g., anti-I). However, complement that has been bound in vivo will be detected when using an EDTA specimen. The procedure involves two steps. First, the cells are washed to remove any traces of plasma proteins not actually attached to the cell membrane. Then polyspecific AHG (anti-IgG and anticomplement) is added to the saline-washed patient cells. Agglutination of patient cells by AHG is considered positive evidence for the presence of IgG and/or complement components on the cells due to in vivo coating.

A positive test with polyspecific AHG should be followed by a DAT with monospecific AHG antiserum that reacts specifically with either immunoglobulin (IgG) or complement to determine the type of proteins bound to the erythrocyte. IgG antibodies are found with or without complement attached. Therefore, if the DAT with anti-IgG is positive, the test with anticomplement (anti-C3d or anti-C3b) can be positive or negative. If the anti-IgG test is positive, the antibody can be removed from the cell by an elution process. The resulting eluate (solution containing the antibody) is reacted with a panel of cells of known antigenic makeup to identify the specificity of the antibody.

If an autoantibody is IgM, only complement will be detected on the erythrocytes as the IgM dissociates from the cells in the warmer part of the circulation. The polyspecific and the anti-C3 monospecific DAT test will be positive; the anti-IgG will be negative. An elution procedure is not used if only complement is detected on the erythrocyte because the complement alone will not cause a reaction with screening cells and the eluate will thus give a negative reaction.

INDIRECT ANTIGLOBULIN TEST

The **indirect antiglobulin test (IAT)** is used to detect antibodies in the patient's serum. A positive IAT indicates alloimmunization (immunization to antigens from another individual) and/or the presence of free autoantibody in the patient's serum. In the IAT, free antibody is detected by incubating the patient's serum with erythrocytes of known antigenic makeup (commonly referred to as *screening cells*). An autocontrol consisting of the patient's serum and erythrocytes is also performed. After a specified incubation period, the cells are washed free of excess serum, and the AHG antiserum is added. If antibody has attached to its corresponding erythrocyte antigen during the initial incubation period, the cells will agglutinate with AHG (Web Figure 17-2 ■).

 Checkpoint! 4

Compare the purpose of the DAT and the IAT, and state the type of specimen used for each test.

NEGATIVE DAT IN AIHA

In a few cases of AIHA, antibody cannot be detected on the cells or in the serum.[13,14] This can result from an insufficient number of IgG molecules on the erythrocyte, autoantibodies of the IgA or IgM class, or the presence of autoantibodies with a low affinity for the erythrocyte.[1,15–16] The DAT will detect as few as 100–500 molecules of IgG per cell or 400–1100 molecules of complement per cell,[3] but in vivo removal of sensitized cells by macrophages can occur when cells are coated with fewer IgG molecules. Thus, the in vivo life span of the sensitized cell can be significantly shortened as evidenced by the clinical findings of a typical hemolytic anemia, but the concentration of antibodies on the cell can be insufficient to give a positive DAT. Newer, more sensitive techniques, such as enzyme linked DAT, gel tests, and flow cytometry can detect lower concentrations of antibodies than the conventional DAT technique.[17–19] IgA or IgM autoantibodies themselves are not detected using polyspecific AHG. However, if complement has been activated, it can be detected if sufficient molecules are present.

POSITIVE DAT IN NORMAL INDIVIDUALS

In contrast, some healthy blood donors and hospitalized patients can have a positive DAT but not shortened erythrocyte survival. The reason that some individuals have autoantibody coating their erythrocytes but have no evidence of hemolytic disease is not clear.[1] Factors that could be responsible for this phenomenon include the following:

1. The individual's macrophages may not be as active in removing sensitized cells as the macrophages in individuals with hemolytic disease.

2. The amount of antibody bound to cells might not be sufficient to cause decreased erythrocyte life span.

3. The subclass of antibody sensitizing the cell might not be recognized by macrophages. Macrophage Fc receptors have low affinity for the IgG2 and IgG4 subclasses. Erythrocytes coated with these immunoglobulins will give a positive direct DAT but in vivo survival of the cells will be normal.

4. The thermal amplitude of the antibody may be less than 37°C.

5. The positive DAT can be due to the presence of complement on erythrocytes. Increased amounts of C3d can be found on the erythrocytes, but because this component is not detected by macrophage receptors, erythrocytes do not have decreased survival.

6. Patients with hypergammaglobulinemia or receiving high-dose intravenous immunoglobulin (IVIG) could have a positive DAT because of nonspecific binding of immunoglobulins to the erythrocytes.

 CASE STUDY *(continued from page 342)*

When the laboratory professional examined the patient's peripheral blood smear, she noted that spherocytes were present. The reticulocyte count was elevated. She called the blood bank and found that the DAT on Nancy was positive with polyspecific AHG, anti-IgG, but negative with anticomplement.

2. What is the significance of the spherocytes?

3. Based on these results what do you suspect is going on in this patient? Explain.

► AUTOIMMUNE HEMOLYTIC ANEMIAS (AIHA)

During fetal life, a person's immune system recognizes self-antigens (those that appear on the individual's cells) and in turn does not usually mount an immune response to these antigens. The immune system normally prevents autoimmunization by ignoring self-antigenic determinants such as those that occur on an individual's erythrocytes. These antigens can, however, stimulate an immune response if injected into another individual because that person's immune system recognizes them as "foreign." The immune regulatory mechanisms that govern response to foreign or self-antigens are collectively known as *immune tolerance.*

It is generally accepted that autoimmune diseases occur because of a number of factors including genetic predisposition (familial or presence/absence of specific HLA antigens), exposure to infectious agents that can induce antibody production due to molecular mimicry, and defects in the mechanism regulating immune tolerance.[20] Suppressor T lymphocytes normally induce tolerance to self-antigens by inhibiting the antibody-producing activity of B lymphocytes to these antigens. Loss of this suppressor cell activity could result in the formation of antibodies against self. This loss of self-tolerance and resulting AIHA can occur at any age. The mechanism of antibody formation in AIHA is unknown, but because many cases of AIHA are associated with microbial infection, neoplasia, or drug administration, these agents may be involved in alteration of self-antigens and subsequent immune system response. Either warm or cold AIHA also can be categorized based on whether an underlying disease is associated with it. The two categories are:

- Primary or idiopathic: no underlying disease
- Secondary: underlying disease present

WARM AUTOIMMUNE HEMOLYTIC ANEMIA

Warm autoimmune hemolytic anemia (WAIHA) is the most common form of AIHA (70% of cases).[2] It is mediated by IgG antibodies whose maximal reactivity is at 37°C. In a majority (90%) of WAIHA cases, erythrocytes are sensitized with IgG and complement or IgG alone. Only 7% of cases are sensitized with complement alone. Most often, the antibody involved is IgG1 or IgG3. The antibody involved is rarely IgM or IgA.[4,6–8]

WAIHA can occur at any age although the incidence increases after age 40. Childhood incidence peaks in the first 4 years of life.[21,22] About 60% of the cases of warm AIHA are idiopathic.[2] In acute idiopathic WAIHA, severe anemia develops over 2 to 3 days, but the hemolysis is self-limited with duration of several weeks to several years. In other instances, the hemolysis is chronic and unabating.

The underlying disorders most frequently associated with secondary AIHA are:

- Lymphoproliferative disease, including chronic lymphocytic leukemia, and Hodgkin's disease (∞ Chapter 26). Chronic lymphocytic leukemia (CLL), found most frequently in older adults, is the disease most frequently associated with the development of secondary AIHA.[23] WAIHA often develops late in the disease when the immune dysregulation is greatest. In one study, more than 60% of the cases of WAIHA were in patients with CLL.[24] Many children with idiopathic WAIHA will eventually develop a lymphoproliferative disease.
- Neoplastic diseases
- Other autoimmune disorders, including systemic lupus erythematosus and rheumatoid arthritis, ulcerative colitis, Crohn's disease[25–29]
- Certain viral and bacterial infections[30,31]
- Vaccinations[32–34]

Presence of the underlying disorder can complicate diagnosis and treatment of hemolytic anemia. In many cases, the AIHA is resolved by treating the underlying disease.

Pathophysiology

The warm autoantibody in AIHA is reactive with antigens on the patient's erythrocytes. Most often the specificity of the antibody is directed against antigens of the Rh system, although other antigen systems can be involved. When directed against the Rh system, the antibody can be specific for a single antigen (such as autoanti-e) or, more commonly, the antibody will react with a complex Rh antigen found on all erythrocytes except Rh null cells.[1,2,35,36] The epitope against which these antibodies are directed has not been defined. Recent research suggests that the antibody can be against a component of the erythrocyte membrane such as glycophorins or protein band 4.1.[1,7,37]

Most hemolysis in WAIHA is extravascular via splenic macrophages. Although complement is not needed for cell destruction, if both antibody and complement are on the cell membrane, phagocytosis is enhanced. If erythrocyte destruction exceeds the compensatory capacity of the bone marrow to produce new cells, anemia develops. Direct complement-mediated intravascular hemolysis associated with IgM antibodies in warm AIHA is rare.

Clinical Findings

The most common presenting symptoms in idiopathic AIHA are related to anemia. Progressive weakness, dizziness, dyspnea on exertion, back or abdominal pain, and jaundice are common. In secondary AIHA, signs and symptoms of the underlying disorder can obscure the features of the hemolytic anemia. The patient can present with signs and symptoms of both the underlying disease and hemolysis or just the disease. The signs of WAIHA in a few patients can precede development of the underlying disease. While mild to moderate splenomegaly is present in more than 50% of patients with WAIHA, massive splenic enlargement suggests an underlying lymphoproliferative disorder. Hepatomegaly is found in about one-third of patients with primary WAIHA.

> ## ✓ Checkpoint! 5
>
> *What are the clinical findings and the immune stimuli for WAIHA?*

Laboratory Findings

The most common laboratory findings associated with WAIHA are listed in Table 17-4 ✪. Findings such as the positive DAT, autoantibody in the serum, and presence of spherocytes on the peripheral blood smear reflect the immune-mediated destruction of the erythrocyte.

Peripheral Blood Moderate to severe normocytic, normochromic anemia is typical. In well-compensated hemolytic disease, anemia can be mild or absent, and the only abnormal parameters can be a positive DAT and an increase in reticulocytes. Reticulocytes are invariably increased in uncomplicated hemolytic disease. The reticulocyte production index can be as high as 6 or 7. Depending on the degree of reticulocytosis, macrocytosis can be present.

The blood smear frequently shows erythrocyte abnormalities that suggest a hemolytic process. Polychromasia, nucleated red blood cells, spherocytes, schistocytes, and other poikilocytes are characteristic (Figure 17-4■). The spherocytes of AIHA are usually more heterogeneous than are the spherocytes associated with hereditary spherocytosis. This anisocytosis is readily noted upon examining the blood smear and is indicated by an increase in red cell distribution width (RDW) on automated hematology analyzers. Erythrophagocytosis by monocytes can be seen. The engulfed erythrocyte is readily detected if the cell still contains its pink-staining hemoglobin. If the hemoglobin has leaked out of the cell, however, only colorless vacuoles are seen. Leukocyte counts are normal or increased with neutrophilia in id-

✪ TABLE 17-4

Laboratory Findings Associated with WAIHA

Common findings	Positive DAT
	Normocytic, normochromic anemia
	Increased reticulocytes
	Spherocytes and other erythrocyte abnormalities
	Presence of autoantibody in the serum
	Increased serum bilirubin (total and unconjugated)
	Decreased serum haptoglobin
	Positive antibody screen with all cells including autocontrol
	Incompatible crossmatches with all donors
Other laboratory findings that can be associated with hemolysis in WAIHA	Increased osmotic fragility
	Increased urine and fecal urobilinogen
	Hemoglobinemia,* hemoglobinuria, methemoglobinemia, hemosiderinurea

*Seen only in acute hemolytic episode

iopathic WAIHA but can vary in the secondary form based on the underlying disease. Platelet counts are usually normal or slightly increased. When severe thrombocytopenia accompanies warm AIHA, the disease is called *Evan's syndrome.*

Bone Marrow Bone marrow examination is not necessary for the diagnosis of WAIHA. The bone marrow can show

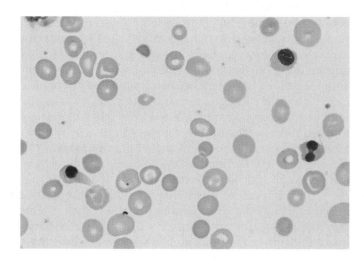

■ FIGURE 17-4 A blood smear from a patient with warm autoimmune hemolytic anemia (WAIHA). There is marked anisocytosis due to the presence of spherocytes and large polychromatophilic erythrocytes. The nucleated cells are normoblasts. (Wright stain; 1000× original magnification)

erythroid hyperplasia depending on the degree of hemolysis. Erythrophagocytosis by macrophages can be seen. Compensatory bone marrow response can be less than expected in concomitant folic acid deficiency. In chronic hemolysis, the folic acid requirement increases two to three times normal; without folic acid supplements, the stores of this vital nutrient are quickly depleted. If the patient contracts viral infections associated with bone marrow suppression, life-threatening anemia (aplastic crisis) can occur.

Other Laboratory Tests   The DAT is a useful test to distinguish the immune nature of this hemolytic anemia from non-immune-mediated hemolytic anemias. The test is usually positive with polyspecific AHG and anti-IgG monospecific AHG antiserum. Only about 30% of the cases of WAIHA have a reaction with anti-C3, either with or without the concurrent presence of IgG.[2]

Reaction of patients' serum with screening cells typically shows agglutination with all cells when AHG is added. The autocontrol (patient serum and patient erythrocytes) shows similar reactions. Other laboratory findings are nonspecific but reflect the hemolytic component of the condition (Table 17-4).

Differential Diagnosis

Warm AIHA with the presence of spherocytes can be differentiated from hereditary spherocytosis (HS) by the DAT. Antibodies are not responsible for the formation of spherocytes in hereditary spherocytosis (HS); therefore, the DAT is negative. The autohemolysis test is abnormal in both HS and in AIHA with spherocytes. In HS, autohemolysis is significantly corrected by the addition of glucose; however, glucose does not correct hemolysis in AIHA. The peripheral blood smear also gives clues to diagnosis. The spherocytes in HS appear as a rather homogeneous population, but in AIHA there is a mixture of spherocytes, microspherocytes, and normocytes.

 Checkpoint! 6

What is the DAT pattern in WAIHA? Explain why spherocytes are commonly seen in WAIHA.

Therapy

In self-limiting hemolytic disorders without life-threatening anemia, transfusion therapy is not necessary. When transfusion is indicated, finding a suitable donor is difficult because the patient's autoantibody usually reacts with all donor cells in the crossmatch. In addition, approximately 30% of patients with WAIHA have underlying alloantibodies, which can present an additional challenge to finding compatible blood because the autoantibody can mask their presence.[38,39]

If the patient has an alloantibody, blood negative for the specific antigen must be administered. If serologically compatible blood cannot be found because of the presence of the autoantibody, donor cells demonstrating the least incompat-

ibility are usually chosen. The clinical problems, however, are twofold: Donor cells are often destroyed as rapidly as the patient's own erythrocytes, and they can also stimulate the production of alloantibodies. In some cases, the use of flow cytometry can help evaluate the survival of donor cells in patients with WAIHA.[40] In other cases, such as individuals who must receive serial transfusions, finding phenotypically matched donor blood can decrease the risk of stimulating alloantibodies.[38,41–44] If the autoantibody has an identifiable single specificity (such as autoanti-e), the donor blood chosen for the compatibility test should be negative for the antigen.

Therapies for WAIHA focus on decreasing the production of autoantibodies and slowing down the destruction of erythrocytes. These include:

- **Corticosteroids.** Initial therapy for patients with AIHA is often a course of immunosuppressive drugs such as corticosteroids, which are used to produce immunosuppression by decreasing lymphocyte proliferation and suppressing macrophage sequestration of sensitized cells by affecting the Fc receptors. Few patients undergo complete remission with this therapy, but most show a decrease in erythrocyte destruction. Response usually occurs within 10–14 days, and many patients require low-dose maintenance.[44]
- **Cytotoxic drugs.** A number of alternative therapies are available for patients who do not respond to corticosteroids and/or splenectomy.[1,44] Cytotoxic drugs such as cyclophosphamide and azathioprine are used to cause general suppression of the immune system, which decreases synthesis of autoantibody.
- **High-dose intravenous immunoglobulin (IVIG).** This can block Fc receptors on macrophages and affect T and B cell function by increasing T suppressor cells or reducing B cell function. It has a variable success rate and is most often used as an adjunct therapy with corticosteroids or in selected patients with severe anemia who are refractory to drugs.[45]
- **Plasma exchange and plasmapheresis.** This can dilute or temporarily remove the autoantibody from the patient's circulation. It has been successful in reducing antibody load for a short time in some cases but is not a satisfactory long-term therapy.
- **Splenectomy.** Indicated when severe anemia is unresponsive to medical therapies including glucocorticoid therapy or other cytotoxic drugs, splenectomy provides long-term remission for some patients. Removal of the spleen decreases the destruction of IgG-coated erythrocytes that would normally adhere to Fc receptors on splenic macrophages. If, however, the antibody concentration remains high, the destruction of sensitized erythrocytes may continue in the liver. Some evidence suggests that splenectomy can be more beneficial in patients with idiopathic WAIHA than in those with the secondary type.[46]

- **Rituximab (monoclonal anti-CD20).** It has been used in the treatment of clonal B-cell malignancies including chronic lymphocytic leukemia and has been effectively used in patients with idiopathic and secondary WAIHA that are refractory to other treatments.[44,47–49]

In patients with secondary AIHA, treatment of the underlying disease is important. Often resolution of the disease leads to decreased production of the autoantibody.

COLD AUTOIMMUNE HEMOLYTIC ANEMIA (AIHA)

Cold AIHA, also termed *cold agglutinin disease* (CAD), is associated with an IgM antibody that fixes complement and is reactive below 37°C. This disorder, which comprises 16–30% of the AIHAs, is less common than anemia associated with warm antibodies and is less common in children than adults.[1,2] IgA and IgG antibodies rarely have been implicated in hemolysis in CAD.[34,50]

CAD, like warm AIHA, is either idiopathic or secondary (Table 17-5 ✪). Idiopathic CAD is usually chronic, occurring after age 50 with a peak onset after age 70.[21] The antibody involved is usually a monoclonal IgM/kappa paraprotein with autoanti-I specificity.[51] The idiopathic form has been linked to a lymphoproliferative disorder characterized by CD20+, kappa (κ)+, B cells. Trisomy and translocations have also been found in some patients.[52] The secondary type can occur after an infectious disease or be associated with lymphoproliferative disease.[21,50] The secondary type associated with infectious disease is usually an acute, self-limiting form that has an onset 1–3 weeks after infection and resolves within 2–3 weeks.[21,50] Most of these autoantibodies are polyclonal and have a specificity for antigens of the Ii system. Anti-I is usually associated with *Mycoplasma pneumoniae* infections and anti-i can be seen in infectious mononucleosis. Infectious agents including varicella (chickenpox) and rubella are associated with anti-Pr but rarely with anti-I

specificity.[34,53] HIV patients can develop anti-I.[54] The secondary chronic form of CAD, typically found in older individuals, is often associated with lymphoproliferative disorders such as lymphoma or Waldenstrom's macroglobulinemia.[50] The antibody in these cases is usually a monoclonal IgMκ protein. A more severe type of cold AIHA, paroxysmal cold hemoglobinuria (PCH), is associated with a biphasic cold-reacting IgG antibody and is discussed in the next section.

Pathophysiology

The severity of CAD is related to the thermal range of the antibody. Those cold-reacting antibodies with a wide range of thermal activity (up to 32°C) can cause problems when the peripheral circulation cools to this temperature. Complement-mediated lysis accounts for most of the erythrocyte destruction.

The cold-reacting antibody is usually directed against the I antigen, which is expressed on erythrocytes of almost all adults. The I antigen specificity of the antibody can be defined by reactivity of the patient's serum with all adult erythrocytes but minimal or no reactivity with cord cells (which lack the I antigen). In CAD associated with infectious mononucleosis and lymphoproliferative disease, however, the antibody can have anti-i specificity. These antibodies would react strongly with cord cells as the i antigen is generally expressed strongly on cord cells and erythrocytes of children younger than 2 years old and weakly or not at all with adult erythrocytes. The second most common specificity for cold autogglutinins is anti-Pr.[1] The Pr antigens are expressed on both adult and infant erythrocytes. Other specificities that have been reported include anti-M, anti-Vo, anti-Gd, anti-ZSa, and anti-Lud.[1,55]

Clinical Findings

In some instances, CAD is associated with a chronic hemolytic anemia with or without jaundice. In others, hemolysis is episodic and associated only with chilling. Erythrocyte agglutination occurs in areas of the body that cool to the thermal range of the antibody and cause sludging of the blood flow within capillaries. Vascular changes including acrocyanosis in which the hands and/or feet turn blue and cold can occur. In *Raynaud's phenomenon,* pain can be accompanied by a charascteristic pattern of color changes in the skin from white due to spasm of the vessels to blue caused by cyanosis to red, which indicates a return of blood flow to the area. These conditions primarily affect the extremities, especially the tip of the nose, fingers, toes, and ears. Hemoglobinuria accompanies the acute hemolytic attacks. Splenomegaly can be present (Table 17-6 ✪).

✪ TABLE 17-5	
Autoimmune Hemolytic Anemia Caused by Cold-Reacting Antibodies	
Cold agglutinin disease (CAD)	Primary (idiopathic)
	Secondary
	• Viral and bacterial infections
	• *Mycoplasma pneumoniae,* infectious mononucleosis
	• Lymphoproliferative diseases
Paroxysmal cold hemoglobinuria	Primary (idiopathic)
	Secondary
	• Viral infections
	• Tertiary syphilis

✓ **Checkpoint! 7**

Describe the mechanism of cell destruction in CHD.

⊘ TABLE 17-6

Criteria for Clinical Diagnosis of Cold Agglutinin Disease (CAD)	
Clinical history	Acrocyanosis
	Hemoglobinuria on exposure to cold
Laboratory findings	Serological
	• DAT: Positive with polyspecific AHG
	Negative with anti-IgG
	Positive with anti-C3
	• IAT: antibody showing characteristic reactions at <25°C
	• Cold agglutinin titer >1000 at 4°C
	False increase in MCV, MCH, and MCHC
	False decrease in erythrocyte count
	Normocytic, normochromic anemia
	Reticulocytosis
	Spherocytes, agglutinated RBCs, rouleaux, nucleated RBCs on blood smear
	Increased bilirubin (total and unconjugated)
	Decreased haptoglobin
	Hemoglobinemia, hemoglobinuria in acute hemolysis
	Hemosideccuria in chronic hemolysis

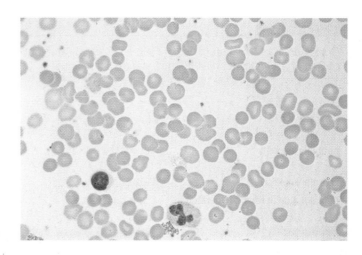

■ **FIGURE 17-5** Cold autoimmune hemolytic anemia from a patient with chronic lymphocytic leukemia. Some of the erythrocytes are in small clumps. Spherocytes are also present. (Peripheral blood; Wright stain; 1000× original magnification)

decreased C3 and/or C4 levels.[51] Patients also can have a decreased value for the CH50 assay, a functional hemolytic assay, that measures the integrity of the entire complement cascade.

> **✓ Checkpoint! 8**
>
> *Explain why the MCV, MCH, and MCHC can be falsely increased when blood from someone with CHD is tested using an automated cell counter.*

Differentiation of CAD Agglutinins from Benign Cold Agglutinins

The serum of most normal individuals exhibits the presence of cold autoantibodies when the serum and cells are incubated at 4°C. These antibodies are termed *benign cold autoagglutinins* because their thermal amplitude and concentration (titer) are not high enough to cause clinical problems. When pathologic cold agglutinins are suspected as the cause of anemia, laboratory tests should be performed to differentiate pathologic cold agglutinins from the benign ones. (Table 17-7 ⊘). The DAT with polyspecific AHG and monospecific anticomplement antiserum is positive in pathologic cold agglutinin disease but negative or only weakly positive with benign cold agglutinins. The DAT, utilizing monospecific anti-IgG, is negative both in CAD and benign cold agglutinins.

The cold agglutinin test should be performed when a diagnosis of cold AIHA is suspected. This test demonstrates the ability of the pathologic antibody to agglutinate the patient's cells at temperatures from 0°C to 20°C in saline and up to 32°C in albumin suspensions. The reaction is reversible with agglutinates dispersing at 37°C. With benign cold antibodies, agglutination occurs at 0–4°C and can occur

Laboratory Findings

The first indication of the presence of unsuspected cold agglutinins often is from blood counts performed on electronic cell counters. The erythrocyte count is inappropriately decreased for the hemoglobin content and the MCV is falsely elevated (Table 17-6). These erroneous values occur when erythrocyte agglutinates are sized and counted as individual cells. The hematocrit calculated from this erroneous erythrocyte count and the MCV is falsely low. The MCH and MCHC calculated from the erythrocyte count and hematocrit are falsely elevated. The hemoglobin assay is accurate because the cells are lysed to determine this parameter. Accurate cell counts can be obtained by warming blood and diluting reagents to 37°C. Visible autoagglutination in tubes of anticoagulated blood can be observed as the blood cools to room temperature.

When blood counts are performed at 37°C, the results indicate a mild to moderate normocytic, normochromic anemia. The blood film shows polychromasia, some spherocytes, rouleaux, or clumps of erythrocytes, and sometimes nucleated red cells (Figure 17-5 ■). Erythrophagocytosis can be seen but is more typical on smears made from buffy coats after the blood has incubated at room temperature. Leukocyte and platelet counts are usually normal. Leukocytosis can occur during acute hemolysis as the result of a bone marrow stress response. The bone marrow exhibits normoblastic hyperplasia. Patients with chronic CAD can show

TABLE 17-7

Comparison of Characteristics of Pathologic Cold Agglutinins Found in CAD with Those of Benign Cold Agglutinins Found in Normal Individuals

	Pathologic Agglutinins	Benign Agglutinins
Antibody class	IgM	IgM
Antibody specificity	Usually anti-I but in secondary CAD can be anti-i	anti-I
Antibody clonality	Monoclonal in idiopathic type and secondary type due to lymphoproliferative disease; polyclonal in secondary type due to infectious disease	Polyclonal
Thermal amplitude	0–31°C	0–4°C
Agglutination at room temperature	Significant	Not present
Titer	Usually >1:1000	<1:64
DAT	Positive with polyspecific AHG and monospecific anticomplement	Negative

up to 20°C. Agglutination is not enhanced, however, in albumin suspensions. Titers of benign cold agglutinins reach 1:64 in normal individuals; in cold agglutinin disease, the titer is usually more than 1:1000. Titers of 1:256 or more with a positive DAT using monospecific anti-C3 antisera and a negative DAT using monospecific anti-IgG antisera are highly suggestive of cold agglutinin disease.

> ### ✓ Checkpoint! 9
>
> *Compare the DAT findings and the antibody specificity in WAIHA and CHD.*

Therapy

The most effective therapy is usually achieved by keeping the individual's extremities warm. Corticosteroids are not usually effective. Chemotherapy using cyclophosphamide or chlorambucil can be instituted, especially if the CAD is associated with an underlying lymphoproliferative disease.[44,55] Plasma exchange can be used in acute hemolytic episodes because the majority of IgM is distributed in the intravascular spaces. However, it is effective for only a short time because protein regeneration half-life is ~5 days.[14,55] Splenectomy, which can be effective in WAIHA, is not effective in CAD because the C3b coated cells are destroyed primarily by Kupffer cells in the liver. In recent years, anti-CD20 (rituximab) has been used as treatment in both primary and secondary disease.[21,56,57] Patients with strongly reacting cold agglutinins can have complications if surgical procedures requiring hypothermia are undertaken.[50,55]

PAROXYSMAL COLD HEMOGLOBINURIA

Paroxysmal cold hemoglobinuria (PCH) is a rare autoimmune hemolytic disorder that can occur at any age and is characterized by massive intermittent acute hemolysis and hemoglobinuria. It is the cause of 30–40% of all AIHA in children and is most frequent in children under the age of 5 years.[1,22,58] Historically, PCH was associated with congenital or tertiary syphilis in adults. It is now most often seen in children with viral and bacterial infections although it has been reported in association with some lymphoproliferative diseases in adults.[59] The infections linked to PCH include Epstein-Barr virus, cytomegalovirus, measles, mumps, *Heamophilus influenzae,* and *Klebsiella pheumoniae.*[1,60] Parvovirus 19, which has an affinity for the P antigen, has also been linked to PCH.[61] PCH is usually a transient disorder that has its onset from 5 days to 3 weeks after onset of the infection.[58] It generally resolves spontaneously, but transfusion can be required in cases of severe anemia.

Pathophysiology

PCH was the first hemolytic anemia for which a mechanism of hemolysis was established. This hemolytic anemia is distinct from the other cold AIHA because of the nature of the antibody involved. It is caused by a biphasic complement-fixing IgG antibody, the **Donath-Landsteiner (D-L) antibody.** *Biphasic* refers to the two temperatures necessary for optimal lysis of the erythrocytes. The antibody reacts with erythrocytes in the capillaries at temperatures less than 20°C and avidly binds the early acting complement components. Upon warming to 37°C, the antibody molecule disperses from the cell, but the membrane attack complement components are activated on the cell membrane causing cell lysis. Because the antibody repeatedly attaches and detaches from erythrocytes with subsequent complement activation, it can cause significant hemolysis.[62] The PCH antibody is specific for the P-antigen (autoanti-P).

Clinical Findings

Hemoglobinuria is the most common clinical symptom. The patient can also experience jaundice, pallor, and hepatosplenomegaly. Raynaud's phenomenon can occur during acute episodes followed by jaundice.

Laboratory Findings

The degree of anemia depends on the frequency and severity of hemolytic attacks. During the attack, hemoglobin concentration drops sharply accompanied by hemoglobinemia, methemalbuminemia, and hemoglobinuria. Hemoglobin values can decrease to as low as 5 g/dl. Neutropenia, a neutrophilic shift to the left, reticulocytopenia, and spherocytes can accompany erythrocyte lysis. Serum bilirubin, BUN, and LD are elevated but serum complement and haptoglobin are decreased. Erythrophagocytosis occurs more commonly in PCH than in other types of AIHA, and the phagocytic cells usually involved are segmented neutrophils, not monocytes.[63]

Antibodies on the cells are not usually detected by the DAT because the D-L antibody elutes at warm temperatures. A weakly positive DAT with anticomplement antisera can appear and persist for several days after the hemolytic episode. The IAT can be positive if performed in the cold. Normal erythrocytes incubated with patient serum react more positively in the IAT than patient cells.

D-L antibodies are usually present in low titers (<1:32) and express a low thermal amplitude, but their presence can be verified by the D-L test, which employs a biphasic reaction (Table 17-8 ⊙). In this test the patient's blood is collected in two clot tubes; one is incubated at 4°C for 30 minutes and the other at 37°C for 30 minutes. Both tubes are then incubated at 37°C. If the D-L antibody is present, it will cause hemolysis in the tube initially incubated at 4°C and then warmed to 37°C. No hemolysis is present in the tube kept at 37°C. Hemolysis in this test can also occur in cold agglutinin disease, but the hemolysis occurs very slowly. Table 17-9 ⊙ compares PCH and CAD.

Therapy

PCH associated with acute infections terminates upon recovery from the infection. Steroids are not usually helpful. Transfusion can be required if the hemolysis is severe. In rare cases when the hemolysis persists, plasmapheresis can be used.[62] Rituximab (anti-CD20) has also been used as therapy

⊙ TABLE 17-8

Donath-Landsteiner (D-L) Test for Detecting the Presence of D-L Antibodies*

Patient's Whole Blood*	Control	Test
Incubate for 30 min at	37°C	4°C
Incubate for 30 min at	37°C	37°C
Centrifuge: observe plasma for presence of hemolysis		
Interpretation		
D-L antibodies present	No hemolysis	Hemolysis
No D-L antibodies present	No hemolysis	No hemolysis

*Two tubes of patient's whole blood are used; one tube serves as the control and the other as the test.

⊙ TABLE 17-9

Comparison of Cold Agglutinin Disease (CAD) and Paroxysmal Cold Hemoglobinuria (PCH)

	CAD	PCH
Patient	Usually adults >50 years of age	Usually children after viral infection
Clinical findings	Acrocyanosis	Chills, fever, hemoglobinuria
DAT	Positive with polyspecific AHG and monospecific C3	Positive with polyspecific AHG and monospecific C3
Donath-Landsteiner test	Negative	Positive
Antibody class	IgM	Biphasic IgG (D-L)
Antibody specificity	Anti-I	Anti-P
Thermal amplitude of antibody	Up to 31°C	Under 20°C
Hemolysis	Chronic extravascular/intravascular	Acute intravascular
Therapy	Avoid the cold	Supportive; treatment of underlying illness

in rare adult cases.[64] The chronic form of the disease is best treated by avoiding exposure to the cold.

✓ Checkpoint! 10

Compare the antibody specificity and the confirmatory test for PCH and CHD.

MIXED-TYPE AIHA

Mixed-type AIHA is characterized by the presence of a warm-reacting IgG autoantibody and a cold-reacting IgM autoantibody that has both high titer and increased thermal amplitude (reacts at >30°C). About 50% of the cases are idiopathic; most of the remainder are associated with diseases such as systemic lupus erythematosus, lymphoma, and HIV.[29,55,65] Patients frequently present with an acute, severe anemia. The IgG class antibody mediates extravascular hemolysis, and the IgM is responsible for complement fixation and intravascular hemolysis. Some patients can have a chronic course with intermittent exacerbations. Most patients respond to steroid therapy and require few or no transfusions.

In the DAT procedure, both C3 and IgG can be detected on the erythrocyte. The cold-reacting antibody often has a specificity for the Ii system antigens. The warm-reacting autoantibody is similar to those found in classic WAIHA and has a complex specificity.

Patients usually respond well to treatment with corticosteroids and do not require transfusion. Rituximab has been used in cases with underlying lymphoproliferative disease.[66,67]

DRUG-INDUCED HEMOLYTIC ANEMIAS

It is recognized that certain drugs can cause immune cytopenias that involve one or several cell lines including neutrophils, platelets, and erythrocytes. Anemia, thrombocytopenia, and agranulocytosis can occur together or separately. It has been proposed that a drug's ability to induce production of antibodies against different cell lines is related to its affinity for the cells.[68] The greater the affinity, the more likely sensitization against the drug-cell complex is to occur. Drug-induced immune hemolytic anemia is a relatively uncommon acquired condition that is precipitated by certain drugs. The drug itself does not cause erythrocyte injury, and not all individuals taking the drug develop this immune hemolytic anemia.

More than 100 drugs have been found to induce a positive DAT or an immune-mediated hemolytic anemia.[68] The classes of drugs implicated include antimicrobials, nonsteroidal anti-inflammatory drugs, antineoplastic drugs, diuretics, and antidiabetic.[69-76] Some of the specific drugs are listed in Web Table 17-2 ✪. It should be noted that second- and third-generation cephalosporins such as cefotetan and ceftriaxone constitute the majority of cases of drug-induced immune hemolytic anemia and are responsible for most fatalities.[63,72,76] Drug-induced immune hemolysis must be distinguished from both drug-induced, nonimmune hemolysis that occurs secondarily to erythrocyte metabolic defects such as G6PD deficiency and from spontaneous autoimmune disorders. This is important because drug-induced, immune hemolytic anemias are the result of an immune response to drug-induced alteration of the erythrocyte. The resolution for this immune hemolysis involves withdrawal of the offending drug and supportive treatment, not the use of immunosuppressives or other therapy.

The actual mechanisms of drug-induced hemolytic anemia are controversial. Three classic hypotheses have been proposed to explain them:[1,2,68]

- Drug absorption
- Immune complex formation
- Autoantibody induction

A fourth mechanism, membrane modification, has not been strongly correlated with immune hemolysis despite the changes noted in the erythrocyte.

Table 17-10 ✪ contains a summary of the characteristics of each mechanism. Regardless of the underlying mechanism, erythrocytes sensitized with either antibody and/or complement have a shortened life span. Each of these mechanisms will cause a positive DAT with polyspecific AHG and with either anti-IgG and/or anti-C3 AHG.

Drug Adsorption (Hapten Type)

Some drugs such as penicillin are antigenic but lack the molecular size or complexity to initiate an immune response. It is proposed that in the hapten/drug adsorption mechanism, the drug or its metabolites bind to proteins on the erythrocyte membrane, creating an immunogenic complex on the cell surface. Antibodies are produced against the drug and react with the drug complex on the erythrocyte membrane (Web Figure 17-3 ■).

Only patients receiving high doses of intravenous penicillin develop significant penicillin coating on their cells, and only a small percent of these individuals will have a positive DAT; even fewer develop hemolysis. The hemolytic anemia usually develops over a 7- to 10-day period. Hemolysis is extravascular and mediated by Fc receptors on splenic macrophages. Spherocytes can be present, and the reticulocyte count is usually elevated. Hemoglobinemia and hemoglobinuria do not occur. The DAT is usually positive. Although both IgG and IgM antibodies can be formed, only the IgG antibody causes hemolysis. Complement activation does not usually occur. Although the IAT is negative, a high

✪ TABLE 17-10

Summary of Classic Mechanisms of Drug-Induced Immune Hemolytic Anemia

Type (Prototypic Drug)	Action	Direct Antiglobulin Test	Mechanism of Cell Destruction
Drug adsorption (high-dose intravenous penicillin)	Drug bound to cell → antibody binds to drug	Polyspecific AHG positive, Anti-IgG positive, Anti-C3 may be positive	Extravascular lysis due to reaction with macrophages (Fc receptors) and phagocytosis
Immune complex (quinidine cephalosporins [2nd & 3rd generations])	Forms immune complex (drug antibody) → immune complex adsorbs to cell membrane → activates complement cascade	Polyspecific AHG positive, Anti-IgG negative, Anti-C3 positive	Intravascular complement-mediated lysis
Autoantibody induction (α-methyldopa procainamide)	Drug adheres to cell membrane → alters membrane structure → forms neoantigen → stimulates production of autoantibody	Polyspecific AHG positive, Anti-IgG positive, Anti-C3 positive or negative	Extravascular adhesion to macrophages via Fc and phagocytosis
Membrane modification (cephalosporins [first generation])	Modification of cell membrane that results in non immunologically absorbed IgG, IgA, IgM, C3	Polyspecific AHG positive, Monospecific can be positive or negative	No hemolysis

titer of the IgG penicillin antibody is present in the serum. This can be detected by incubating the patient's serum with normal erythrocytes and erythrocytes that have been coated with penicillin. If antibodies to the penicillin-protein membrane complex are present in the patient's serum, the test with the "penicillinized" erythrocytes is positive, but it is negative with cells that were not coated with penicillin.

Immune Complex Formation

In this mechanism, a drug or drug metabolite with a low affinity for the cell membrane combines with a plasma protein, forming a new antigenic complex in the plasma and stimulating either IgM or IgG antibodies. A drug/antidrug immune complex forms in the plasma, and this immune complex attaches to the erythrocyte in a nonspecific (nonimmune) manner (usually via the Fc portion of the antibody) (Web Figure 17-4■). The attached immune complex usually has the ability to activate complement. After the immune complex activates complement on the cell membrane, it can dissociate from the membrane and attach to another cell; thus, only a small amount of drug is necessary to initiate complement-mediated hemolysis. The C3b coated red cells are cleared from circulation by macrophages, or the cells may be lysed if the terminal complement components are activated. Most often the hemolytic episode is acute with signs of intravascular hemolysis (hemoglobinuria, hemoglobinemia). Spherocytes can be present on the blood smear.

The DAT with anti-C3 is positive but negative with anti-IgG because the antibody complex has dissociated from the membrane. The anti-C3 DAT can remain positive for several months after the hemolytic episode because of the persistence of inactivated complement components (C3d) on the red cell. Quinidine is the classic drug associated with this mechanism. Although a large number of drugs can cause this type of reaction, the incidence of drug-induced immune hemolysis by this mechanism has been low. However, in recent years, increased reports of fatal intravascular hemolysis by this mechanism have been reported in patients receiving intravenous third-generation cephalosporins.[72,76]

In the laboratory, the antibody is detected only if the drug and complement are present in the test system. Diagnosis is confirmed by incubating the patient's serum with normal erythrocytes in the presence of the suspected drug. If the antibody is present in the patient's serum, it combines with the drug-protein complex and the erythrocytes. Subsequently, complement is activated. Specific antiserum to complement is utilized to demonstrate the deposition of complement on the cell membrane.

Autoantibody Induction

In approximately 10–20% of patients receiving the antihypertensive drug Aldomet (α-methyldopa), a positive DAT develops after about 3–6 months. However, hemolytic anemia develops in only 1% of these patients. The mechanism by which antibody production is induced is unknown; however, evidence indicates that the drug alters normal erythrocyte antigens so they are no longer recognized as self.[77] Erythrocyte destruction is extravascular, and anemia develops gradually. If the drug is withdrawn, the antibody production gradually stops, but the DAT can remain positive for years.

The DAT is dose dependent: The larger the dose of Aldomet, the more likely the patient is to have a positive DAT. The DAT using anti-IgG is positive but because complement is rarely activated, the DAT using anti-C3 is usually negative. Patients with this form of drug-induced IHA have serum antibodies that not only react with their own cells but also with normal erythrocytes. This condition mimics warm autoimmune hemolytic anemia.

Membrane Modification

In addition to causing a positive DAT and immune hemolysis due to the drug adsorption mechanism, cephalosporins, especially the first generation drugs, are capable of modifying the erythrocyte membrane so that normal plasma proteins including immunoglobulins and complement bind to the membrane in a nonimmunologic manner. The adsorbed antibodies are not specific to any drug or drug/cell complex. The DAT is positive with polyspecific antisera and can be positive or negative with anti-IgG and anti-C3.

 Checkpoint! 11

Compare the different types of drug-induced hemolysis including the type of hemolysis, the drug usually associated with the mechanism, and the DAT profile.

Unifying Theory

A unifying theory has been proposed to explain antibody formation in drug-induced hemolytic anemias.[1,2,78] Once the drug binds to the erythrocyte membrane, antibodies that are produced can react with epitopes specifically to the drug, combined drug and erythrocyte membrane epitopes, or epitopes on the erythrocyte membrane. Patients can develop more than one type of drug-induced antibody.[79,80]

 CASE STUDY *(continued from page 347)*

Two days later, Nancy's hemoglobin dropped to 50 gm/L. The physician ordered several more tests. She had a positive IAT, and the antibody reacted with all cells including her own. Other test results indicated that this patient had systemic lupus erythematosus.

4. What type of antibody appears to be present in this patient? Explain.

5. What is the relationship of the patient's primary disease, systemic lupus erythematosus, and her anemia?

▶ ALLOIMMUNE HEMOLYTIC ANEMIA

Hemolytic anemia induced by immunization of an individual with erythrocyte antigens on the infused cells of another individual is known as *alloimmune hemolytic anemia*. The patient's erythrocytes lack the antigen(s) present on infused cells. These transfused antigens are recognized as foreign and induce the recipient to form antibodies that, in turn, react with the transfused cells. This type of immunologic destruction of erythrocytes is characteristic of transfusion reactions and hemolytic disease of the fetus and newborn (HDFN). Factors such as immunogenicity of the antigen, number of transfusions, and function of the recipient's immune system can influence the development of alloantibodies.[81]

In recent years, there has been evidence of not only the production of alloantibodies in patients undergoing solid organ and allogeneic bone marrow/stem cell transplants but also the production of autoantibodies.[82-88] Posttransplant immune-mediated hemolysis can be linked to major blood group incompatibility, passive transfer of antibody from the donor, development of autoimmunity, or passenger lymphocyte syndrome. Passenger lymphocyte syndrome is an immune hemolytic process that develops following solid organ, bone marrow, or stem cell transplant. The donor B lymphocytes that are transplanted with the organ or bone marrow produce antibodies against the recipient's blood group antigens. Although ABO incompatibility is most frequently implicated, Rh, Kell, Kidd, and/or other blood group systems can be involved. Development of autoantibodies after solid organ transplant is rare but more common after bone marrow or stem cell transplants.[82,86,87] Some evidence also suggests that blood transfusions can lead to development of autoantibodies in some patients.[83,85,88]

HEMOLYTIC TRANSFUSION REACTIONS

Transfusion of blood may cause a **hemolytic transfusion reaction** as the result of interaction of foreign (non-self) antigens on transfused erythrocytes and the patients' plasma antibodies. In contrast to AIHA, the antibodies produced in transfusion reactions cause immunologic destruction of donor cells but do not react with the erythrocytes of the person making the antibody. The two types of transfusion reactions involving antibodies to erythrocyte antigens are immediate (occurring within 24 hours) and delayed (occurring 2–14 days after transfusion) (Table 17-11 ✪). An acute or immediate hemolytic transfusion reaction results when the infused erythrocytes react with antibodies that already exist in the recipient, usually ABO system antibodies. This type of reaction usually results from clerical or other human error that results in an ABO mismatch between donor and recipient. For example, the patient is given the wrong unit of blood or is misidentified by the phlebotomist, nurse, or laboratory personnel. Most errors occur in patient care areas, not in the transfusion service area.[32] Patients given the wrong blood ex-

✪ TABLE 17-11

Comparison of Acute and Delayed Hemolytic Transfusion Reactions

	Acute	Delayed
Timing	Immediate (within 24 hours)	2–14 days
Underlying cause	Usually ABO antibodies	Other antibodies: often Kidd system (anamnestic response)
Hemolysis	Intravascular	Extravascular
Symptoms	Fever, chills, back pain, hypotension, pain at site of infusion	Uncommon (fever, hemoglobinuria)
Laboratory findings	Hemoglobinemia	Positive DAT
	Positive DAT (transient)	Antibody in eluate

hibit classic clinical signs including increased pulse rate, hypotension, chills and fever, pain, or difficulty in breathing. When an acute transfusion reaction is suspected, the transfusion must be stopped immediately because of the potential severity of the reaction. Laboratory investigation of the reaction must be performed.

The delayed hemolytic transfusion reaction is usually the result of an anamnestic response in which the donor erythrocytes contain an antigen to which the patient has been previously sensitized. In these cases, the antibody was not detectable prior to transfusion but the infused erythrocytes restimulate antibody production. The donor cells are destroyed, and the patient shows a decrease in hemoglobin. In cases of a delayed transfusion reaction, some patients show no clinical signs, and the reaction is detected only by laboratory testing. Other patients may present with dark urine or vague symptoms such as fever. Patients at highest risk for delayed reactions are those who have received multiple transfusions over their lifetime.[89]

Pathophysiology

An acute hemolytic transfusion reaction is characterized by intravascular hemolysis with hemoglobinuria as a result of complete activation of the complement cascade. This type of hemolysis of donor cells is usually mediated by IgM antibodies, although IgG antibodies are rarely involved. This type of reaction is typical of an ABO incompatibility and begins very shortly after the infusion of the donor unit has begun. As cells are lysed, the release of thromboplastic-like substances from the erythrocyte membrane can activate the intrinsic and extrinsic coagulation cascade (∞ Chapter 30). The resulting consumptive coagulopathy (disseminated intravascular coagulation) can damage the kidney by deposition of fibrin in the microvasculature (∞ Chapters 32, 33). Presence of increased tumor necrosis factor-alpha (TNF-α) and other interleukins in certain diseases can mediate some of the clinical symptoms.[90] The usual antibodies involved in an acute hemolytic transfusion reaction are anti-A or anti-B. Other antibody specificities such as anti-I, anti-P_1 have been implicated only rarely. Mortality rates from ABO acute hemolytic transfusion reactions range from 10 to 50%.

Extravascular hemolysis is typical of a delayed hemolytic transfusion reaction. This occurs when erythrocytes are coated with IgG antibodies and removed via macrophage Fc receptors in the spleen. The speed of the removal depends on the amount of antibody on the cell. Complement is not usually involved but when present can enhance phagocytosis.

Delayed transfusion reactions occur 2–14 days after a transfusion. Although the antibody cannot be detected in pretransfusion testing because the antibody concentration is lower than the test's sensitivity level, antigens on infused donor cells induce a secondary (anamnestic) antigenic stimulus. The antibody produced is usually IgG, and hemolysis is extravascular. The first indication of a delayed reaction is a sharp drop in the hemoglobin concentration several days after the transfusion. Intravascular hemolysis can also occur but is less pronounced than in acute reactions. Laboratory investigation reveals a positive DAT because of antibody-coated donor cells in the patient's circulation. Antibodies characteristically associated with a delayed transfusion reaction are in the Kidd System (anti-Jk^a, anti-Jk^b). Antibodies to antigens in the Rh system (especially anti-D, anti-E, anti-c), as well as anti-Kell, and anti-Fya have also caused delayed reactions.[81]

Clinical Findings

Symptoms of an immediate transfusion reaction begin within minutes to hours after the transfusion is begun. The reaction between antigen and antibody can trigger cytokine release, activation of the complement cascade, and the coagulation cascade. A variety of nonspecific symptoms including fever, chills, low back pain, sensations of chest compression or burning at the site of infusion, hypotension, nausea, and vomiting can occur. Unless the transfusion is immediately stopped, shock may occur. Anuria due to tubular necrosis secondary to inadequate renal blood flow and bleeding due to DIC are common complications. The severity of the reaction and extent of organ damage are directly proportional to the amount of blood infused.

Most delayed transfusion reactions cause few signs or symptoms. The most common signs are malaise and unexplained fever several days after the transfusion. Some patients notice the presence of hemoglobin in the urine.

> ✓ **Checkpoint! 12**
>
> *Compare the underlying mechanisms, pathophysiology, and clinical symptoms of an acute hemolytic transfusion reaction and a delayed one.*

Laboratory Findings

The laboratory findings vary depending on whether the transfusion reaction is acute or delayed. Intravascular hemolysis usually accompanies the acute reaction, and extravascular hemolysis usually accompanies the delayed reaction. The DAT is usually positive in both types of reaction but might not be detected until days after transfusion in the delayed type of reaction.

Acute Transfusion Reaction If an acute transfusion reaction is suspected, the transfusion should be stopped immediately and blood samples should be drawn and sent to the laboratory. Three things must be done to determine whether a transfusion reaction has occurred:[2]

- Check for clerical errors
- Perform a DAT
- Do a visual plasma hemoglobin test

The clerical check will reveal any errors in patient or specimen identification. The visual hemoglobin test involves comparing the patient's pretransfusion plasma against the posttransfusion plasma to detect signs of posttransfusion hemolysis (hemoglobinemia). If there is hemolysis, the plasma can have pink, red, or brown discoloration. The pretransfusion and posttransfusion specimens should be compared side by side to detect subtle changes between them. The DAT performed on the posttransfusion specimen will detect the presence of cell-bound immunoglobulin and/or complement. Often the DAT is only weakly or transiently positive in an acute hemolytic transfusion reaction because the antibody-coated cells are rapidly destroyed. If the DAT is positive and/or there is evidence of hemolysis and/or clerical error, an extended transfusion reaction workup is indicated.

In an extended workup, the pretransfusion specimen is retyped for ABO and Rh blood groups and retested for the presence of alloantibodies and recrossmatched with the donor units. The posttransfusion specimen will have an ABO, and Rh typing as well as an antibody screen performed. Donor units are also retyped and crossmatched with the posttransfusion specimen. Despite the fact that posttransfusion specimens drawn several hours after the reaction might not contain free hemoglobin, hemoglobinuria in the first posttransfusion urine can usually be detected if intravascular hemolysis occurred. Free red cells (hematuria) in the urine, however, are not associated with intravascular or extravascular hemolysis.

Delayed Transfusion Reaction In many cases, the clinical signs of a delayed transfusion reaction are so mild that the reaction is discovered only if the patient is crossmatched again several days later for another transfusion.[81] Hemoglobinemia and hemoglobinuria are not usually found. Other laboratory tests such as haptoglobin and bilirubin analyses can be helpful. If a reaction has occurred, the haptoglobin can be decreased and serum bilirubin increased.

In a delayed transfusion reaction, the posttransfusion specimen will show a positive DAT. A mixed field positive DAT can be seen because only donor cells, not the patient's cells, are coated by immunoglobulin or complement and agglutinated by AHG.

If the DAT is positive, an elution procedure should be performed to determine the specificity of the antibody. This procedure releases the antibody bound to the erythrocyte membrane so that the antibody can be identified. In some cases, antibody on the erythrocytes is not sufficient to provide a positive reaction when the eluate is tested against the commercial screening cells. After several days, the antibody level may be increased enough to allow identification of its specificity. Antibody produced in a delayed transfusion reaction might not be detectable in the serum until several days after the transfusion.

 Checkpoint! 13

What are the required laboratory tests for investigating a suspected transfusion reaction? Compare the characteristic laboratory findings in acute hemolytic transfusion reactions and delayed transfusion reactions.

Therapy

The most important immediate action taken when an acute transfusion reaction occurs is prompt termination of the transfusion. A major effort is made to maintain urine flow to prevent renal damage. Shock and bleeding require immediate attention. In a delayed reaction, treatment is generally not required. Future units of blood given to the patient, however, must lack the antigen to which the patient has made an antibody.

 CASE STUDY *(continued from page 355)*

The clinician wants to start Nancy on therapy and give her a transfusion.

6. How would knowing that the patient had not been transfused in the last several months help you make a decision on the underlying cause of the antibody?

7. What would you tell the clinician about giving a transfusion?

8. What kind of therapy could be used?

HEMOLYTIC DISEASE OF THE FETUS AND NEWBORN (HDFN)

Hemolytic disease of the fetus and newborn (HDFN) is an alloimmune disease associated with increased erythrocyte destruction during fetal and neonatal life and is caused by feto-maternal blood group incompatibility. The three categories of HDFN are ABO caused by anti-A, anti-B and/or antiA,B; Rh (D) caused by anti-D; and "other" caused by alloantibodies to other Rh system antigens (C,c,E,e) or antibodies to other blood group system antigens (e.g., Kell, Kidd, Duffy). More than 95% of HDFN cases are due to either anti-D or ABO system antibodies. Although HDFN caused by ABO antibodies is more common than HDFN caused by anti-D, D incompatibility causes more severe disease (Table 17-12 ✪). The antibodies most commonly associated with the remaining HDFN cases include anti-K, anti-c, anti-C, and anti-E, although any IgG antibody can be implicated.[91] HDFN caused by anti-D and anti-K are the most severe.[91]

✪ TABLE 17-12

Comparison of Hemolytic Disease of the Fetus and Newborn Caused by ABO and D			
Feature	Rh	ABO	Other
Antibody	Immune IgG	Nonimmune or immune IgG	Immune IgG
Blood group	Mother Rh negative Baby Rh positive	Mother, group O; baby, group A or B	Mother lacks antigen that is on fetal cell
Obstetric history	Only pregnancies after the first are usually affected	First pregnancy and subsequent pregnancies can be affected	Pregnancy can be first if mother previously sensitized by transfusion. If pregnancy is sensitizing event, usually second and subsequent pregnancies affected
Clinical findings	Moderate to severe anemia and bilirubinemia	Mild anemia, if present; mild to moderate bilirubinemia with a peak 24–48 hours after birth	Mild to severe anemia and bilirubinemia
Laboratory findings	DAT positive No spherocytes	DAT weakly positive or negative Spherocytes present	DAT positive
Therapy	Exchange transfusion, if severe	Phototherapy	Phototherapy and/or exchange transfusion, if severe

Pathophysiology

The pathophysiology of HDFN involves initial sensitization and antibody production, in utero effects, and postnatal effects. Four conditions must be met for HDFN to occur:

- The mother must be exposed (sensitized) to an erythrocyte antigen that she lacks.
- The fetus must possess the antigen to which the mother is sensitized.
- The mother must produce antibodies to the foreign antigens.
- The mother's antibody must be able to cross the placenta and enter the fetal circulation.

Sensitization   The mother could have been exposed to foreign (nonself) erythrocyte antigens by previous pregnancy or transfusion. Normally, the placenta does not allow free passage of erythrocytes from fetal to maternal circulation, but small numbers of erythrocytes can enter the maternal circulation during gestation. Additionally, small amounts of blood also can enter the mother's circulation during delivery. The risk of sensitization increases as the volume of the fetal bleed increases. If the fetal-maternal bleed is sufficient to stimulate the production of maternal antibodies, subsequent pregnancies could be at risk for HDFN.

Three classes of immunoglobulins can be produced during the mother's immunization—IgG, IgM, IgA—but only IgG has the ability to cross the placenta and cause HDFN. The IgG antibody is actively transported across the placenta and causes destruction of fetal erythrocytes. The fetus/newborn will have anemia and bilirubinemia of varying degrees of severity based on the strength of the immune response and degree of hemolysis.

Approximately 15% of the Group A or Group B babies born to Group O mothers will develop serologic evidence (positive DAT) of ABO-HDFN.[92] In ABO-HDFN, the mother already has the naturally occurring antibodies of the ABO system (IgG class anti-A, anti-B, and anti-A,B), which can cross the placental barrier to destroy fetal cells. In contrast to Rh-HDFN, stimulation and production of these antibodies does not require previous fetal erythrocyte sensitization; therefore, the first pregnancy can be affected.

In HDFN caused by anti-D, the mother is D negative (Rh negative) and the baby is D positive (Rh positive). The first-born is not usually affected, because the first pregnancy serves as the sensitizing event. In each subsequent pregnancy with a D positive fetus, the risk for HDFN increases as the antibody response increases.

In HDFN caused by other Rh system or other blood group system antibodies, the sensitization event is similar to that of Rh-HDFN. It has been found that anti-K can inhibit erythroid progenitor cells (that express the K antigen), contributing to the increased severity of fetal anemia.[93,94]

Prenatal Period   If destruction of fetal erythrocytes is severe enough in utero, the fetus becomes severely anemic and can develop complications as a result. Extramedullary hematopoiesis occurs in the liver and spleen, causing their enlargement. Because of hemolysis, the unconjugated (indirect) bilirubin concentration increases. In the fetus, this bilirubin traverses the placenta and is conjugated and excreted by the mother. With procedures such as amniocentesis, the amount of bilirubin in amniotic fluid can be measured to help determine the relative severity of hemolysis. Other noninvasive procedures such as Doppler ultrasound can help predict anemia based on blood flow in the fetus.[95] In recent years, noninvasive methods to obtain fetal cells or cell-free DNA from the maternal circulation have been introduced. These methods help in the prediction of Rh-HDFN and eliminate the need for invasive procedures such as amniocentesis and chorionic villus sampling. Although prenatal diagnostic procedures were initially designed to detect the D antigen, they have been expanded to detect K, Fy, and JK genotypes.[96-99]

The most serious complication of HDFN is cardiac failure and hydrops fetalis, which occurs when the fetus is unable to produce sufficient erythrocytes. **Erythroblastosis fetalis,** another term used to describe this condition, reflects the presence of large numbers of nucleated erythrocytes found in the baby's peripheral blood in very severe cases.

Postnatal Period   Erythrocyte destruction persists after birth because of maternal antibodies in the newborn's circulation. After birth, the newborn must conjugate and excrete the bilirubin on its own. In the neonate, albumin levels for bilirubin transport are limited, and liver glucuronyl transferase for bilirubin conjugation is low; therefore, considerable amounts of toxic unconjugated bilirubin can accumulate in the baby after delivery. In the unconjugated state, bilirubin is toxic because it is lipid soluble and can easily cross cell membranes. This form of bilirubin has a high affinity for basal ganglia of the CNS. Thus, the excess unconjugated bilirubin can lead to **kernicterus,** an irreversible form of brain damage. The conjugated form of bilirubin will not cause this type of problem because it is water soluble, lipid insoluble, and cannot cross cell membranes.

Clinical Findings

Anemia due to the increased cell destruction is the greatest risk to the infant with HDFN both in utero and in the first 24 hours of life. Bilirubinemia is the greatest risk thereafter. In Rh incompatibility, the cord blood hemoglobin can be low normal at birth (normal hemoglobin at birth is 14–20 g/dL), and the baby does not appear jaundiced. However, significant hemolysis occurring in the first 24 hours of life outside the womb results in anemia with pallor and jaundice. In severe cases, hepatosplenomegaly can be present. Severe anemia can be accompanied by heart failure and edema. As the level of unconjugated bilirubin rises, kernicterus can occur. In Rh-HDFN, some infants with severe kernicterus can die. The risks of hyperbilirubinemia in premature infants are even greater because of the inability of the premature liver to excrete the excess bilirubin.

ABO incompatibility is not as severe as Rh incompatibility. The clinical course is usually benign, and hemolysis is minimal. Within 24–48 hours after birth, the infant appears jaundiced but kernicterus is extremely rare. Anemia is mild and pallor is uncommon. Hepatosplenomegaly, if present, is mild. However, cases of severe ABO-HDN requiring exchange transfusion as well as phototherapy, especially in blacks and children of mixed race parents, have been reported.[92,100,101]

 Checkpoint! 14

Compare the pathophysiology and clinical findings of ABO-HDFN and Rh-HDFN.

Laboratory Findings

Laboratory tests are essential to identify the etiology of HDFN, determine prognosis, and select appropriate treatment. Classic prenatal testing on a pregnant woman includes ABO and Rh typing of the erythrocytes as well as an antibody screen (IAT) on her serum. If the IAT is positive, the antibody is identified so that an assessment of HDFN risk can be performed.

The postnatal HDFN workup consists of laboratory tests on both the mother and the infant. Classically this has included ABO and Rh typing of the mother's erythrocytes as well as an antibody screen (IAT) on her serum. The infant was typed for ABO and D antigen and had a DAT performed on the cord cells. If the DAT was positive, an elution procedure was performed, and the specificity of the antibody coating the fetal erythrocytes was identified. With the changes in the health care system and reimbursement patterns, the American Association of Blood Banks has revised its guidelines for prenatal and postnatal testing to eliminate unnecessary repeat testing or testing that does not affect treatment.[102,103] For example, testing of cord blood specimens for ABO, Rh, and DAT is not recommended unless the maternal serum has clinically significant antibodies or if there is a workup to determine RhIG candidacy for the mother.

Rh Incompatibility   The DAT is usually positive, reflecting antibody coating of the newborn's erythrocytes. About 50% of affected infants have a cord blood hemoglobin concentration of less than 14 g/dL. Because the capillary blood hemoglobin can be up to 4 g/dL higher due to placental transfer of blood at birth, the cord blood hemoglobin concentration is most useful as an indicator of anemia at birth and as a baseline to follow destruction of erythrocytes after birth. A direct relationship exists between the initial cord blood hemoglobin level and the severity of the disease. Lower cord hemoglobin levels at birth are associated with a more severe clinical course. After birth, hemoglobin levels can fall at the rate of 3 g/dL/day. Lowest hemoglobin values are present at 3–4

days. The erythrocytes are macrocytic and normochromic. Reticulocytes are markedly increased, sometimes reaching 60%. Nucleated red cells are markedly increased in the peripheral blood (10–100 × 10⁹/L), reflecting the rapid formation of cells in response to erythrocyte destruction. Normal infants also have nucleated red cells in the peripheral blood, but their values are much lower ($0.2–2.0 \times 10^9$/L).

A blood smear shows marked polychromasia, mild or absent poikilocytosis, and few, if any, spherocytes. The leukocyte count is increased to 30×10^9/L or more due to an increase in neutrophils reflecting the marrow response to stress. (The normal leukocyte count at birth is $15–20 \times 10^9$/L.) A significant neutrophilic shift to the left often occurs. The platelet count is usually normal, but thrombocytopenia can develop with an increase in disease severity.

Cord blood bilirubin is elevated but is usually less than 5.5 mg/dL. However, cord blood bilirubin does not accurately reflect the severity of hemolysis since bilirubin produced before birth readily crosses the placenta and is metabolized by the mother. The infant's serum bilirubin peaks on the third or fourth day and may reach 40–50 mg/dL if the baby is not treated. Most bilirubin is in the unconjugated form. Only unconjugated bilirubin not bound to albumin is toxic to the CNS. Full-term infants with bilirubin concentrations >10 mg/dL are at increased risk for kernicterus, and premature infants can develop it with levels as low as 8–10 mg/dL.

ABO Incompatibility   A weakly positive DAT is found in the cord blood, but it often becomes negative within 12 hours. The weak reaction is due to the small number of anti-A or anti-B antibody molecules attached to the erythrocyte. Bilirubin is not usually significantly elevated, but the bilirubin level 6 hours after birth can be used to predict development of hyperbilirubinemia in severe cases.[104] The peripheral blood smear in severe cases can show increased numbers of nucleated erythrocytes and the presence of schistocytes, spherocytes, and polychromasia.

 Checkpoint! 15

Compare the laboratory findings including the peripheral blood smear and the DAT for infants born with ABO-HDFN and those with Rh-HDFN.

Therapy

The major efforts of therapy are the prevention of hyperbilirubinemia and anemia. If the destruction of erythrocytes and degree of anemia appears to affect the viability of the fetus, an intrauterine transfusion can be given. Methods such as amniocentesis and cordocentesis and now the use of molecular methods to identify fetal DNA for detecting in utero hemolysis have allowed decisions to be made on whether an intrauterine transfusion should be given.[99] The transfused cells in an intrauterine transfusion are Group O

Rh-negative, fresh, washed, and irradiated. The cells must be compatible with the maternal serum. The antigen-negative cells lack the specific binding site for antibody and therefore have a normal life span. Transfusions often must be given on a routine basis until the fetus reaches a gestational age that will allow successful delivery.

In mild cases postnatally, the infant is treated with phototherapy, which slowly lowers the toxic bilirubin level. Although toxic levels of bilirubin are 19–20 mg/dL, exchange transfusion is usually performed before that level is reached. Exchange transfusions can also be indicated if the bilirubin is rising more than 1 mg/dL/hour or if there is significant anemia. The transfusion has several beneficial effects:

- Removes plasma containing maternal antibodies and dilutes the concentration of remaining antibodies
- Removes some of the antibody-coated erythrocytes
- Lowers the level of bilirubin
- Treats the anemia

Cells used in the exchange transfusion are usually Group O, washed and irradiated, and must be compatible with maternal serum.

Rh Immune Globulin (RhIG)

The passive injection of Rh immunoglobulin (RhIG) that contains anti-D prevents maternal immunization. About 7–8% of Rh-negative women develop antibodies to Rh positive cells after the birth of an Rh-positive ABO-compatible infant. The routine use of prophylactic RhIG in Rh-negative women during gestation (at 28 weeks) and following the birth of an Rh positive child has decreased the incidence of HDFN considerably, although other changes in prenatal care and number of pregnancies also could have contributed.[105] The majority of women (92%) who develop anti-D during pregnancy do so at 28 weeks or later. Therefore, antepartum administration of RhIG is given between weeks 28 and 30 of gestation to any woman who has not developed anti-D. The RhIG acts as an immunosuppressant, depressing the production of immune IgG. The RhIG binds to fetal cells in maternal circulation, mediating their removal in the spleen, thereby preventing the possibility of maternal sensitization to the Rh antigen.

Postnatally, a dose of RhIG given within 72 hours of birth protects against the consequences of a fetal-maternal bleed. If the Rh-positive erythrocytes of a fetus enter the mother's circulation at birth, they can stimulate the mother's immune system to make antibodies. As in the antepartum administration of RhIG, postnatal RhIG can bind fetal cells and mediate their removal in the spleen. The dose of RhIG should be determined based on the number of fetal cells in the maternal circulation. Several tests can be used for this including the Rosette and the Kleihauer-Betke tests. The Rosette test, which detects fetal Rh positive cells, can be used as a screening test for fetal maternal hemorrhage. This test detects a fetal bleed of as little as 2.5 ml of fetal blood.[102] The Klei-

hauer-Betke test, in which cells with fetal hemoglobin are detected, is the traditional method employed for quantitation of fetal-maternal bleed to determine dose of RhIg. Newer methods such as immunofluorescent flow cytometry using monoclonal antibody to fetal hemoglobin to determine the number of fetal cells present are available.[106]

SUMMARY

Immune hemolytic anemia (IHA) is mediated by antibodies and/or complement and can be classified as autoimmune, alloimmune, or drug induced, depending on the underlying process. All of these will have a positive DAT due to immunoglobulin and/or complement on the cell. The autoimmune hemolytic anemias (AIHA) are caused when the offending antibody reacts with an antigen on the patient's erythrocytes (self-antigen) and have the ability to react with erythrocytes of most other persons. AIHA are either idiopathic or secondary to an underlying disease, and are further classified as warm or cold, depending on the thermal reactivity of the causative antibody. WAIHA is most often caused by IgG antibodies that react at body temperature (37°C) and cause extravascular hemolysis. Cold hemagglutinins are IgM antibodies that generally react at less than 20°C but are efficient complement activators and can cause intravascular hemolysis. In both cases, the DAT is positive, and the antibody can be detected by the IAT procedure. PCH, another type of cold autoimmune hemolytic condition, is mediated by an IgG biphasic antibody that binds complement in the cool peripheral circulation. As the coated cells reach warmer portions of the circulation, the complement cascade is activated and intravascular hemolysis occurs.

Drug-induced immune hemolytic conditions are mediated by several mechanisms depending on the causative drug. The antibodies can be drug dependent, and the drug must be present for the antibody to react. In autoantibody formation (drug independent), the drug appears to cause a change in the erythrocyte membrane that causes the body to recognize it as foreign and produce an antibody against the cell.

Alloimmune hemolytic anemia has two presentations: transfusion reaction and hemolytic disease of the newborn. In both conditions, the antibody is stimulated by infusion of erythrocytes containing foreign (nonself) antigens. This sensitization causes the production of alloantibodies to the foreign antigens, resulting in the cell's destruction. The antibody can be detected in the serum and will cause a positive DAT.

Transfusion reactions can be acute (immediate) or delayed (2–14 days after transfusion). Acute reactions most often involve an ABO mismatch between donor and recipient and result in intravascular hemolysis as a result of complement activation. Delayed transfusion reactions are due to non-ABO antibodies such as anti-JK^a, anti-c̄, anti-K. These reactions result in extravascular lysis and are characterized by a positive DAT. The causative antibody must be identified so that future transfused erythrocytes lack the antigen corresponding to the patient's antibody.

Hemolytic disease of the fetus and newborn (HDFN) may be caused by ABO, Rh (D), or other blood group system antibodies that react with fetal erythrocytes. ABO-HDFN is generally milder than Rh-HDFN and can occur in any pregnancy because prior antigenic sensitization is not required. In Rh and other types of HDFN prior sensitization is necessary. Maternal antibodies that coat fetal cells may cause anemia or elevated bilirubin in the baby. Maternal and baby's ABO and Rh group, maternal antibody, and baby's DAT are used in evaluating HDFN.

REVIEW QUESTIONS

LEVEL I

1. The characteristic erythrocyte seen in a peripheral blood smear in WAIHA is a(n): (Objective 3)
   a. macrocyte
   b. spherocyte
   c. dacrocyte
   d. elliptocyte

2. Which of the following might be observed on a peripheral blood smear in cases of cold autoimmune hemolytic anemia? (Objective 3)
   a. helmet cells
   b. macrocytes
   c. agglutination
   d. spherocytes

3. Which of the following parameters on an automated hematology instrument could be seen in cases of cold agglutinin disease (CAD)? (Objective 3)
   a. falsely elevated MCV
   b. falsely elevated RBC count
   c. falsely decreased MCHC
   d. falsely decreased hemoglobin

4. One purpose of the DAT is to: (Objective 2)
   a. detect erythrocytes coated with immunoglobulin in vivo
   b. detect antibodies in the serum
   c. neutralize serum complement
   d. prevent agglutination by IgM antibodies

5. Intravascular hemolysis is characteristic of which of the following alloantibody situations? (Objective 5)
   a. delayed hemolytic transfusion reaction
   b. ABO-HDFN
   c. Rh-HDFN
   d. acute hemolytic transfusion reaction

6. A patient with WAIHA would most likely have serum that reacts in which of these patterns? (Objective 5)

Serum + Own Erythrocytes	Serum + Erythrocytes of Others
a. negative	negative
b. negative	positive
c. positive	positive
d. positive	negative

7. Which of the following is *not* considered a condition caused by autoantibodies? (Objective 5)
   a. PCH
   b. CAD
   c. delayed transfusion reaction
   d. drug-induced hemolytic anemia

LEVEL II

1. The drug-induced mechanism that leads to intravascular hemolysis is: (Objective 3)
   a. drug adsorption
   b. immune complex
   c. membrane modification
   d. autoantibody formation

2. A newborn shows evidence of jaundice and a workup for HDFN is started. The baby has a weakly positive DAT with anti-IgG. The mother is Group O, Rh negative. The baby is Group A, Rh negative. The blood smear shows evidence of spherocytes. What is the most likely cause? (Objective 6)
   a. Rh-HDFN
   b. ABO-HDFN
   c. combined ABO- and Rh-HDFN
   d. cold agglutinins

3. Which autoimmune syndrome is characterized by the presence of a biphasic complement-fixing IgG antibody? (Objective 4)
   a. PCH
   b. WAIHA
   c. cold agglutinin disease
   d. immune complex drug induced

4. High-dose intravenous administration of what drug is characteristically associated with the drug adsorption mechanism? (Objective 3)
   a. penicillin
   b. aldomet
   c. quinidine
   d. third-generation cephalosporins

5. Based on maternal and fetal testing, a newborn is suspected of having Rh HDFN. Which of the following peripheral blood smear morphologies might be seen? (Objective 6)
   a. microcytic, hypochromic erythrocytes, decreased reticulocytes
   b. microcytic, normochromic erythrocytes, increased nucleated red blood cells
   c. macrocytic, hypochromic erythrocytes, decreased reticulocytes
   d. macrocytic, normochromic erythrocytes, increased nucleated red blood cells

LEVEL I

8. A patient who is receiving a transfusion shows evidence of intravascular hemolysis. What antibody specificity and immunoglobulin class would most likely be involved? (Objective 6)
   a. Rh/IgG
   b. ABO/IgM
   c. Kidd system/IgG
   d. I system/IgM

9. Which of the following is *not* part of the typical peripheral blood picture in Rh-HDFN? (Objective 4)
   a. macrocytes
   b. polychromasia
   c. spherocytes
   d. increased nucleated erythrocytes

10. The antibody found in PCH is: (Objective 1)
   a. IgM
   b. IgG
   c. directed against the Rh antigens
   d. directed against the ABO antigens

LEVEL II

6. What is the *most likely* mechanism of hemolysis in WAIHA? (Objective 1)
   a. increased sensitivity to complement
   b. fixing of complement by IgM antibody
   c. biphasic reactions by IgG antibodies
   d. phagocytosis of IgG coated erythrocytes

7. A patient who received a transfusion 6 days ago is suspected of having a delayed transfusion reaction. Which of the following would *not* be a characteristic finding? (Objective 7)
   a. positive DAT
   b. positive IAT
   c. hemoglobinuria
   d. decreased hemoglobin

8. How would you interpret the following results of a Donath-Landsteiner test? (Objective 4)

   Patient incubated at 4°C and then 37°C — hemolysis

   Control incubated only at 37°C — no hemolysis
   a. positive
   b. negative
   c. invalid because of control reaction
   d. equivocal—repeat in 2 weeks

9. A 75-year-old man presents to the physician with complaints of weakness and fatigue. His leukocyte count is elevated, and his hemoglobin is 60 gm/L. The peripheral blood smear shows that a majority of the cells are small, mature lymphocytes. The diagnosis is CLL. Spherocytes are present. The physician suspects hemolytic anemia, and laboratory tests suggest a hemolytic process with an increase in reticulocytes and bilirubin. Based on this information, what is the most likely problem? (Objective 8)
   a. secondary CAD
   b. secondary PCH
   c. secondary WAIHA
   d. secondary cold agglutinins

10. The following DAT results were seen in a 35-year-old female who was being investigated for a drug-induced hemolytic anemia. She had a hemoglobin of 70 gm/L, and her serum reacted with all cells against which it was tested. What drug is the most likely cause? (Objective 3)

DAT (polyspecific)	positive
DAT anti-IgG	positive
DAT anti-C3	negative

   a. penicillin
   b. quinidine
   c. cephalosporin
   d. aldomet

REFERENCES

1. Petz LD, Garraty G. *Immune Hemolytic Anemais,* 2nd ed. Philadelphia: Churchill Livingstone; 2004.

2. Brecher ME, ed. *Technical Manual,* 15th ed. Arlington, Virginia: AABB; 2005.

3. Garratty G. Immune hemolytic anemia: A primer. *Semin Hematol.* 2005;42:119–21.

4. Sokol RJ, Booker DJ, Stamps R, Booth JR, Hook V. IgA red cell autoantibodies and autoimmune hemolysis. *Transfusion.* 1997;37:175–81.

5. Friedmann AM, King KE, Shirey RS, Resar LM, Casella JF. Fatal autoimmune hemolytic anemia in a child due to warm-reactive immunoglobulin M antibody. *J Ped Hem Onc.* 1998;20:502–5.

6. Janvier D, Sellami F, Missud F, Fenneteau O, Vilmer E, Cartron J et al. Severe autoimmune hemolytic anemia caused by a warm IgA autoantibody directed against the third loop of band 3 (RBC anion-exchange protein 1). *Transfusion.* 2002;42:1547–52.

7. Garraty G, Arndt P, Domen R, Clarke A, Sutphen-Shaw D, Clear J et al. Severe autoimmune hemolytic anemia associated with IgM warm autoantibodies directed against determinants on or associated with glycophorin A. *Vox Sang.* 1997;72:124–30.

8. Nowak-Wegrzyn A, King KE, Shirey RS, Chen AR, McDonough C, Lederman HM. Fatal warm autoimmune hemolytic anemia resulting from IgM autoagglutinins in an infant with severe combined immunodeficiency. *J Pediat Hematol Oncol.* 2001;23:250–52.

9. Wikman A, Axdorph U, Gryfelt G, Gustafsson L, Bjorkholm M, Lundahl J. Characterization of red cell autoantibodies in consecutive DAT-positive patients with relation to in vivo haemolysis. *Ann Hematol.* 2005;84:150–58.

10. Azerda daSilveira S, Kikuchi S, Fossati-Juimak L, Moll T, Salto T, Verbeek JS et al. Complement activation selectively potentiates the pathogenicity of the IgG2 and IgG3 isotypes of a high affinity anti-erythrocyte autoantibody. *J Experimental Med.* 2002;195:665–72.

11. Ruiz-Arguelles A, Llorente L. The role of complement regulatory proteins (CD55 and CD59) in the pathogenesis of autoimmune hemocytopenia. *Autoimmunity Reviews.* 2007;6:155–61.

12. Nielsen CH, Fischer EM, Leslie RGQ. The role of complement in the acquired immune response. *Immunology.* 2000;100:4–12.

13. Sachs UHJ, Roder L, Santoso S, Bein G. Does a negative direct antiglobulin test exclude warm autoimmune haemolytic anaemia? A prospective study of 504 cases. *Br J Haematol.* 2002;132:655–56.

14. Garratty G. Immune hemolytic anemia associated with negative routine serology. *Semin Hematol.* 2005;42:156–64.

15. Reardon JE, Marques MB. Laboratory evaluation and transfusion support of patients with autoimmune hemolytic anemia. *Am J Clin Pathol.* 2006;125S1:S71–7.

16. Sokol RJ, Booker DJ, Stanps R, Jalihal S, Paul B. Direct Coombs test-negative autoimmune hemolytic anemia and low-affinity IgG class antibodies. *Immunohematology.* 1997;13:115–18.

17. Wang Z, Shi J, Zhou Y, Ruan C. Detection of red blood cell-bound immunoglobulin G by flow cytometry and its application to the diagnosis of autoimmune hemolytic anemia. *Internat J Hematol.* 2001;73:188–93.

18. Chaudhary R, Das SS, Gupta R, Khetan D. Application of flow cytometry in detection of red-cell-bound igG in Coombs-negative AIHA. *Hematology.* 2006;11:295–300.

19. Lai M, Rumi C, D'Onofrio G, Voso MT, Leone G. Clinically significant autoimmune hemolytic anemia with a negative direct antiglobulin test by routine tube test and positive by column agglutination method. *Immunohematology.* 2002;18:109–13.

20. Parman P. *The Immune System,* 2nd ed. Abingdon, UK: Garland Science Publishing; 2005.

21. Ghers BC, Friedberg RC. Autoimmune hemolytic anemia. *Am J Hematol.* 2002;69:258–71.

22. Vaglio S, Arista MC, Perrone MP, Tomei G, Testi AM, Coluzzi et al. Autoimmune hemolytic anemia in childhood: serologic features in 100 cases. *Transfusion* 2007;47:50–4.

23. Mauro FR, Foa R, Cerretti R, Giannarelli D, Coluzzi S, Mandelli F et al. Autoimmune hemolytic anemia in chronic lymphocytic leukemia: Clinical, therapeutic, and prognostic features. *Blood.* 2000;95:2786–92.

24. Diehl LF, Ketchum LH. Autoimmune disease and chronic lymphocytic leukemia: Autoimmune hemolytic anemia, pure red cell aplasia, and autoimmune thrombocytopenia. *Sem. in Oncology.* 1998;25:80–97.

25. Kokori SIG, Ionnidis JPA, Voulgarelis M, Tzioufas AG, Moutsopoulos HM. Autoimmune hemolytic anemia in patients with systemic lupus erythematosus. *Am J Med.* 2000;108:198–209.

26. Plikat K, Rogler G, Scholmerich J. Coombs-positive autoimmune hemolytic anemia in Crohn's disease. *Eur J Gastroenterol Hepatol.* 2005;17:661–66.

27. Ng JP, Soliman A, Kumar B, Lam DC. Auto-immune haemolytic anaemia and Crohn's disease: A case report and review of the literature. *Eur J Gastroenterol Hepatol.* 2004;16:417–19.

28. Giannadaki E, Potamianos S, Roussomoustakaki M, Kyriakou D, Fragkiadakis N, Manousos ON. Autoimmune hemolytic anemia and positive Coombs test associated with ulcerative colitis. *Am J Gastroenterol.* 1997;92:1872–74.

29. Kao YS, Kirkley KC. A patient with mixed connective tissue disease and mixed-type autoimmune hemolytic anemia. *Transfusion.* 2005;45:1695–96.

30. Nobili V, Vento S, Comparcola D, Sartorelli MR, Luciani M, Marcellini M. Autoimmune hemolytic anemia and autoimmune hepatitis associated with Parvovirus B19 infection (letter). *Pediatr Infect Dis J.* 2004;23:184–85.

31. Sevilla J, delCarmen Escudero M, Jimenez R, Gonzalez-Vincent M, Manzanares H, Garcia-Novo D et al. Severe systemic autoimmune disease associated with Epstein-Barr virus infection. *J Pediatr Hematol Oncol.* 2004;26:831–33.

32. Downes KA, Domen RE, McCarron KF, Bringelsen KA. Acute autoimmune hemolytic anemia following DPT vaccination: Report of a fatal case and review of the literature. *Clin Pediatr.* 2001;40: 355–58.

33. Seltsam A, Shukry-Schulz S, Salama A. Vaccination-associated immune hemolytic anemia in two children. *Transfusion.* 2000;40:907–9.

34. Konig AI, Schabel A, Sugg U, Brand U, Roelcke D. Autoimmune hemolytic anemia caused by IgGλ-monotypic cold agglutinins of anti-Pr specificity after rubella infection. *Transfusion.* 2001;41:488–92.

35. Wheeler CA, Calhoun L, Blackall DP. Warm reactive autoantibodies; Clinical and serologic correlations. *Am J Clin Pathol.* 2004;122:680–85.

36. Garratty G. Specificity of autoantibodies reacting optimally at 37°C. *Immunohematology.* 1999;15:24–40.

37. DeAngelis V, DeMatteis MC, Cozzi MR, Florin F, Pradella P, Steffan A et al. Abnormalities of membrane protein composition in patients with autoimmune haemolytic anaemia. *Br J Haem.* 1996;95:273–77.

38. Buetens OW, Ness PM. Red blood cell transfusion in autoimmune hemolytic anemia. *Curr Opin Hematol.* 2003;10:429–33.

39. Branch DR, Petz LD. Detecting alloantibodies in patients with autoantibodies. *Transfusion.* 1999;39:6–10.

40. Zeiler T, Muller JT, Hasse C, Kullmer J, Kretschmer V. Flow cytometric determination of RBC survival in autoimmune hemolytic anemia. *Transfusion.* 2001;41:493–98.

41. Shirey RS, Boyd JS, Parwini AV, Tanz WS, Ness PM, King KE. Prophylactic antigen-matched donor blood for patients with warm autoantibodies: An algorithm for transfusion management. *Transfusion.* 2002;42:1435–41.

42. Petz LD. "Least incompatible" units for transfusion in autoimmune hemolytic anemia: Should we eliminate this meaningless term? A commentary for clinicians and transfusion medicine professionals. *Transfusion.* 2003;43:1503–7.

43. Petz LD. A physician's guide to transfusion in autoimmune haemolytic anaemia. *Brit J Hematol.* 2004;124:712–16.

44. Petz LD. Treatment of autoimmune hemolytic anemias. *Curr Opin Hematol.* 2001;8:411–16.

45. Vandenberghe P, Zachee P, Verstraete S, Demuynck H, Boogaerts MA, Verhoef GEG. Successful control of refractory and life-threatening autoimmune hemolytic anemia with intravenous immunoglobulins in a man with primary antiphospholipid syndrome. *Ann Hematol.* 1996;73:253–56.

46. Akpek G, McAneny D, Weintraub L. Comparative response to splenectomy in Coombs-positive autoimmune hemolytic anemia with or without associated disease. *Am J Hematol.* 1999;61:98–102.

47. Ramanathan S, Koutts J, Hertzberg MS. Two cases of refractory warm autoimmune hemolytic anemia treated with rituximab. *Am J Hematol.* 2005;78:123–26.

48. Pamuk GE, Turgut B, Demir M, Tezcan F, Vural O. The successful treatment of refractory autoimmune hemolytic anemia with rituximab in a patient with chronic lymphocytic leukemia. *Am J Hematol.* 2006;81:631–33.

49. D'Arena G, Laurenti L, Capalbo S, D'Arco AM, DeFilippi R, Marcxacci G et al. Rituximab therapy for chronic lymphocytic leukemia-associated autoimmune hemolytic anemia. *Am J Hematol.* 2006;81:598–602.

50. McNicholl FP. Clinical syndromes associated with cold agglutinins. *Transfusion Science.* 2000;22:125–33.

51. Ulvestad E, Berentsen S, Bo K, Shammas FV. Clinical immunology of chronic cold agglutinin disease. *Eur J Haematol.* 1999;63:259–66.

52. Michaux L, Dierlamm J, Wlodarska L, Criel A, Louwagie A, Ferrant A et al. Trisomy 3q11-q29 is recurrently observed in B-cell non-Hodgkin's lymphomas associated with cold agglutinin syndrome. *Ann Hematol.* 1998;76:201–4.

53. Tereda K, Tanaka H, Mori R, Kataoka N, Uchikawa M. Hemolytic anemia associated with cold agglutinin during chickenpox and a review of the literature. *J Pediatr Hematol Oncol.* 1998;20:149–51.

54. Hamblin T. Management of cold agglutination syndrome. *Transfusion Science.* 2000;22:121–24.

55. Koduri PR, Singa P, Nikolinakos P. Autoimmune hemolytic anemia in patients infected with human immunodeficiency virus-1. *Am J Hematol.* 2002;70:174–76.

56. Berentsen S, Ulvestad E, Gjertsen BT, Hjorth-Hansen H, Langholm R, Knutsen H et al. Rituximab for primary chronic cold agglutinin disease: A prospective study of 37 courses of therapy in 27 patients. *Blood.* 2004;103:2925–28.

57. Sparling TG, Andricevic M, Wass H. Remission of cold hemagglutinin disease induced by rituximab therapy. *CMAJ.* 2001;164:1405.

58. Eder AF. Review: acute Donath-Landsteiner hemolytic anemia. *Immunohematology.* 2005;21:56–62.

59. Sivakumaran M, Murphy PT, Booker DJ, Wood JK, Stamps R, Sokol RJ. Paroxysmal cold haemoglobinuria caused by non-Hodgkin's lymphoma. *Br J Haematol.* 1999;105:278–79.

60. Ziman A, Hsi R, Goldfinger D. Donath-Landsteiner antibody-associated hemolytic anemia after *Haemophilus influenzae* infection in a child. *Transfusion.* 2004;44:1127–28.

61. Chambers LA, Rauck AM. Acute transient hemolytic anemia with a appositive Donath-Landsteiner test following Parvovirus B19 infection. *J Pediatr Hematol Oncol.* 1996;18:178–81.

62. Roy-Burman A, Glader BE. Resolution of severe Donath-Landsteiner autoimmune hemolytic anemia temporally associated with institution of plasmapheresis. *Crit Care Med.* 2002;30:931–34.

63. Garratty G. Erythrophagocytosis on the peripheral blood smear and paroxysmal cold hemoglobinuria (letter). *Transfusion.* 2001;41:1073.

64. Koppel A, Lim S, Osby M, Garratty G, Goldfinger D. Rituximab as successful therapy in a patient with refractory paroxysmal cold hemoglobinuria. *Transfusion.* 2007;47:1902–04.

65. Win N, Tiwari D, Keevil VL, Needs M, Lakhani A. Mixed-type autoimmune haemolytic anaemia: Unusual cases and a case associated with splenic T-cell angioimmunoblastic non-Hodgkin's lymphoma. *Hematology.* 2007;12:159–62.

66. Morselli M, Luppi M, Potenza L, Facchini L, Tonelli S, Dini D et al. Mixed warm and cold autoimmune hemolytic anemia. Complete recovery after 2 courses of rituximab treatment. *Blood.* 2002;99:3478–79.

67. Jubinshky PT, Rashid N. Successful treatment of a patient with mixed warm and cold antibody mediated Evans syndrome and glycose intolerance. *Pediatr Blood Cancer.* 2005;45:347–50.

68. Garratty G. Review: Drug-induced immune hemolytic anemia—The last decade. *Immunohematology.* 2004;20:138–46.

69. Meyer O, Hoffman T, Asian T, Ahrens N, Kiesewetter H, Salama A. Diclofenac-induced antibodies against RBCs and platelets: Two case reports and a concise review. 2003;43:345–49.

70. Gonzalez CA, Guzman L, Nocetti G. Drug-dependent antibodies with immune hemolytic anemia in AIDS patients. *Immunohematology.* 2003;19:10–15.

71. Arndt PA, Garratty G, Hill J, Kasper M, Chandrasekaran V. Two cases of immune haemolytic anaemia, associated with anti-piperacillin, detected by the 'immune complex' method. *Vox Sang.* 2002;83:273–78.

72. Arndt PA, Garratty G. The changing spectrum of drug-induced immune hemolytic anemia. *Semin Hematol.* 2005;42:137–44.

73. Naylor CS, Steele L, Hsi R, Margolin M, Goldfinger D. Cefotetan-induced hemolysis associated with antibiotic prophylaxis for cesarean delivery. *Am J Obstet Gynecol.* 2000;182:1427–28.

74. Seltsam A, Salama A. Ceftriaxone-induced immune haemolysis: Two case reports and a concise review of the literature. *Intensive Care Med.* 2000;26:1390–94.

75. Johnson ST, Fueger JT, Gottschall JL. One center's experience: The serology and drugs associated with drug-induced immune hemolytic anemia—A new paradigm. *Transfusion.* 2007;47:697–702.

76. Arndt PA, Leger RM, Garratty G. Serology of antibodies to second- and third-generation cephalosporins associated with immune hemolytic anemia and/or positive direct antiglobulin tests. *Transfusion.* 1999;39:1239–46.

77. Garraty G, Arndt P, Prince HE, Shulman IA. The effect of methyldopa and procainamide on suppressor cell activity in relation to red cell autoantibody production. *Br J Haematol.* 1993;84:310–15.

78. Muellar-Eckhart C, Salama A. Drug-induced immunocytopenias: A unifying pathogenic concept with special emphasis on the role of drug metabolites. *Trans Med Rev.* 1990;4:69–77.

79. Habibi B. Drug-induced red blood cell autoantibodies co-developed with drug specific antibodies causing haemolytic anemias. *Brit J Haematol.* 1985;61:139–43.

80. Calhoun BW, Junsanto T, DeTolve Donoghue M, Naureckas E, Baron JM, Baron BW. Ceftizoxime-induced hemolysis secondary to combined drug adsorption and immune-complex mechanisms. *Transfusion.* 2001;41:883–97.

81. Schonewille H, van de Watering LMG, Loomans DSE, Brand A. Red blood cell alloantibodies after transfusion: Factors influencing incidence and specificity. *Transfusion.* 2006;46:250–56.

82. Sokol RJ, Stamps R, Booker DJ, Scott FM, Laidlaw ST, Vanderberghe EA et al. Posttransplant immune-mediated hemolysis. *Transfusion.* 2002;42:198–204.

83. Young PP, Uziebla A, Trulock E, Lublin DM, Goodnough LT. Autoantibody formation after alloimmunization: Are blood transfusions a risk factor for autoimmune hemolytic anemia? *Transfusion.* 2004; 44:67–72.

84. de la Rubia J, Arriaga F, Andreu R, Sanz G, Jimenez C, Vincente A et al. Development of non-ABO RBC alloantibodies in patients undergoing allogeneic HPC transplantation. Is ABO incompatibility a predisposing factor? *Transfusion.* 2001;41:106–10.

85. Chan LTG. Severe intravascular hemolysis due to autoantibodies stimulated by blood transfusion. *Immunohematology.* 1996;12:80–83.

86. Chen FE, Owen I, Savage D, Roberts I, Apperley J, Goldman JM et al. Late onset haemolysis and red cell autoimmunization after allogeneic bone marrow transplant. *Bone Marrow Transplant.* 1997;19:491–95.

87. Horn B, Viele M, Mentzer W, Mogck N, DeSantes K, Cowan M. Autoimmune hemolytic anemia inpatients with SCID after T-cell depleted BM and PBSC transplantation. *Bone Marrow Transplant.* 1999;24:1009–13.

88. Zumberg MS, Proctor JL, Lottenberg R, Kitchens CS, Klein HG. Autoantibody formation in the alloimmunized red blood cell recipient. *Arch Intern Med.* 2001;161:285–90.

89. Syed SK, Sears DA, Werch JB, Udden MM, Milam JD. Delayed hemolytic transfusion reaction in sickle cell disease. *Am J Med Sci.* 1996;312:175–81.

90. Winkelstein A, Kiss JE. Immunohematologic disorders. *JAMA.* 1997; 278:1982–92.

91. Moise KJ. Red blood cell alloimmunization in pregnancy. *Semin Hematol.* 2005;42:169–78.

92. Drabik-Clary K, Reddy VVB, Benjamin WH, Boctor FN. Case report: Severe hemolytic disease of the newborn in a Group B African-American infant delivered by a Group O mother. *Ann Clin Lab Sci.* 2006;36:205–7.

93. Vaughan JI, Manning M, Warwuck RM, Letsky EA, Murray NA et al. Inhibition of erythroid progenitor cells by anti-K antibodies in fetal alloimmune anemia. *N Engl J Med.* 1998;338:798–803.

94. Wagner T, Resch B, Reiterer F, Gassner C, Lanzer G. Pancytopenia due to suppressed hematopoiesis in a case of fatal hemolytic disease of the newborn associated with anti-K supported by molecular K1 typing. *J Pediatr Hematol Oncol.* 2004;26:13–15.

95. Oepkes D, Seaward PG, Vandenbussche F, Windrim R, Kingdom J, Beyene J et al. Doppler ultrasonography versus amniocentesis to predict fetal anemia. *N Engl J Med.* 2006;355:156–64.

96. Daniels G, Finning K, Martin P, Summers J. Fetal blood group genotyping: Present and future. *Annals of the NY Academy of Sciences.* 2006;1075:88–95.

97. Daniels G, Finning K, Martin P, Soothill P. Fetal blood group genotyping from DNA from maternal plasma: An important advance in the management and prevention of haemolytic disease of the fetus and newborn. *Vox Sang.* 2004;87:225–32.

98. Avent ND, Finning KM, Martin PG, Soothill PW. Prenatal determination of fetal blood group status. *Vox Sang.* 2000;78S2:155–62.

99. Bianchi DW, Avent ND, Costa JM, van der Schoot CE. Noninvasive prenatal diagnosis of fetal Rhesus D: Ready for prime(r) time. *Obstet Gynecol.* 2005;106:682–83.

100. McDonnell M, Hannam S, Devane SP. Hydrops fetalis due to ABO incompatibility. *Arch Dis Child Fetal Neonatal Ed.* 1998;78:220–21.

101. Ziprin JH, Payne E, Hamidi J, Roberts I, Regan F. ABO incompatibility due to immunoglobulin G anti-B antibodies presenting with severe fetal anemia. *Transfus Med.* 2005;15:57–60.

102. Judd WJ. Practice guidelines for prenatal and perinatal immunohematology, revisited. *Transfusion.* 2001;41:1145–52.

103. Dinesh D. Review or positive direct antiglobulin tests found on cord blood sampling. *J Pediatr Child Health.* 2005;41:504–7.

104. Sarici SU, Yurdakokk M, Serdar MA, Oran O, Erdem G, Tekinalp G et al. An early (sixth-hour) serum bilirubin measurement is useful in predicting the development of significant hyperbilirubinemia and severe ABO hemolytic disease in a selective high-risk population of newborns with ABO incompatibility. *Pediatrics.* 2002;109:e53.

105. Joseph KS, Kramer MS. The decline in Rh hemolytic disease: Should Rh prophylaxis get all the credit? *Am J Public Health.* 1998;88:209–15.

106. Davis BH, Olsen S, Bigelow NC, Chen JC. Detection of fetal red cells in fetomaternal hemorrhage using a fetal hemoglobin monoclonal antibody by flow cytometry. *Obstet Gynec Survey.* 1999;54:153–54.

18

Hemolytic Anemia: Nonimmune Defects

Linda A. Smith, Ph.D.

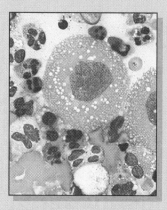

CHAPTER OUTLINE

■ OBJECTIVES—LEVEL I

At the end of this unit of study, the student should be able to:

1. Define *microangiopathic hemolytic anemia (MAHA)*; list several associated disorders and the age group most commonly affected.

2. Describe the general morphology and hematologic values associated with MAHA and criteria that distinguish disseminated intravascular coagulation (DIC), thrombotic thrombocytopenic purpura (TTP), and hemolytic uremic syndrome (HUS).

3. Recognize the characteristic erythrocyte morphology of MAHA on a stained blood film.

4. Identify several organisms that can cause erythrocyte hemolysis.

■ OBJECTIVES—LEVEL II

At the end of this unit of study, the student should be able to:

1. Summarize the general pathophysiology for MAHA.

2. Compare and contrast the clinical findings, underlying cause, treatment, and characteristic findings for erythrocytes, platelet count, and coagulation tests for each of the following types of MAHA:

   a. Hemolytic uremic syndrome (HUS)

   b. Thrombotic thrombocytopenic purpura (TTP)

   c. Disseminated intravascular coagulation (DIC)

3. Define *exercise-induced hemoglobinuria*.

4. Given a set of data and clinical history, determine whether MAHA is a probable diagnosis, or the possible etiology, and propose follow-up tests that should be performed.

5. Compare the cause of hemolysis by the following infectious agents:

   a. Plasmodium parasites (malaria)

   b. Babesia parasites

   c. Bartonella bacteria

   d. *Clostridium* bacteria

KEY TERMS

Cryosupernatant
Disseminated intravascular coagulation (DIC)
Fresh frozen plasma (FFP)
<u>H</u>emolysis, <u>e</u>levated <u>l</u>iver enzymes and <u>l</u>ow <u>p</u>latelet (HELLP) syndrome
Hemolytic uremic syndrome (HUS)
Microangiopathic hemolytic anemia (MAHA)
Plasma exchange
Thrombotic thrombocytopenic purpura (TTP)
von Willebrand factor (VWF)

BACKGROUND BASICS

The information in this chapter builds on concepts learned in previous chapters. To maximize your learning experience, you should review the following concepts:

Level I

▶ Describe the normal production, life span, and destruction of the erythrocyte. (Chapter 5)

▶ List the reference intervals for basic adult hematology parameters. (Chapters 1, 5, 6, 7, 8)

▶ Identify sources of defects that lead to hemolytic anemia. (Chapter 14)

▶ Review the immune hemolytic anemias, and describe how they differ from other hemolytic anemias. (Chapter 17)

▶ Identify the intrinsic hemolytic anemias, and describe how they differ from extrinsic hemolytic anemias. (Chapter 14)

Level II

▶ Describe the structure and function of the major proteins of the erythrocyte membrane. (Chapter 5)

▶ Identify the key tests that can be used in diagnosis of anemia, and identify clinical signs of anemia. (Chapter 8)

▶ Describe the different nonimmune mechanisms of hemolysis and how they are detected. (Chapters 5, 14, 15, 16)

▶ Identify the laboratory tests that differentiate immune from nonimmune anemia. (Chapters 14, 17)

CASE STUDY

We will refer to this case study throughout the chapter.
Mai, a 35-year-old woman, was seen by her physician. She complained of weakness, low-grade fever, periods of forgetfulness, and memory loss for the last week or so. She denied any viral illness prior to onset of symptoms. She was on oral contraceptives but was not taking any other drugs. Her initial laboratory tests showed:

Hemoglobin: 60 g/L (6g/dL)
Hematocrit: 0.18 L/L (18%)
White blood cell count: 8.9 × 10⁹/L

Consider reflex testing (further testing based on abnormal test results) that could be helpful in identifying the cause of the anemia.

▶ OVERVIEW

This chapter deals with the mechanisms of hemolysis not included in the chapters on membrane defects (∞ Chapter 15), metabolic deficiencies (∞ Chapter 16), or immune mechanisms (∞ Chapter 17). It includes microangiopathic hemolytic anemias (MAHA). Hemolytic uremic syndrome (HUS), a MAHA, is discussed in detail including disease association, pathophysiology, and clinical and laboratory findings. There is a brief overview of thrombotic thrombocytopenic purpura (TTP), which is discussed in detail in Chapter 33. Uncommon causes of hemolysis such as hypertension, mechanical heart devices, burns, exercise, and infectious agents are also discussed.

▶ INTRODUCTION

Erythrocytes that have normal hemoglobin structure, enzymes, and membranes can be prematurely destroyed by factors extrinsic to the cell. This destruction can be immune mediated via antibodies and/or complement (∞ Chapter 17). However, nonimmune factors can also cause either extravascular or intravascular hemolysis, depending on the type and extent of injury to the erythrocyte. Chapter 15 dealt with intrinsic erythrocyte membrane disorders due to abnormalities of plasma lipids and erythrocyte membrane lipids and proteins, and Chapter 16 discussed erythrocyte enzyme deficiencies. This chapter discusses the nonimmune causes that lead to premature erythrocyte destruction including different types of physical trauma to the erythrocyte and antagonists such as toxins and infectious agents (Table 18-1 ✪).

▶ HEMOLYTIC ANEMIA CAUSED BY PHYSICAL INJURY TO THE ERYTHROCYTE

Hemolytic anemia caused by traumatic physical injury to the erythrocytes in the vascular circulation is characterized by intravascular and/or extravascular hemolysis and striking abnormal shapes of the circulating peripheral blood erythrocytes, including fragments (schistocytes) and helmet cells.

MICROANGIOPATHIC HEMOLYTIC ANEMIA

Microangiopathic hemolytic anemia (MAHA) is an inclusive term referring to a hemolytic process caused by microcirculatory lesions. Damage to the endothelial lining of the small vessels results in deposits of fibrin within the vessel. As the erythrocytes are forced through the fibrin strands, the membrane can be sliced open. In some erythrocytes, the membrane seals itself, leading to abnormal erythrocyte shapes that are noted as schistocytes and keratocytes on the peripheral blood smear (∞ Chapter 8). These damaged cells are often

TABLE 18-1

Hemolytic Anemias Caused by Nonimmune Antagonists in the Erythrocyte Environment

Category	Antagonist	Mode of Hemolysis
Microangiopathic hemolytic anemia (HUS, TTP, DIC)	Thrombi in microcirculation	Physical damage to erythrocytes by microthrombi
Malignant hypertension	Unknown	Physical damage to erythrocytes
Other physical trauma		
Exercise-induced hemoglobinuria	External force	Fragmentation of erythrocytes due to excessive external force as they pass through microcapillaries
Thermal injury	Heat	Thermal damage to erythrocyte membrane proteins
Traumatic cardiac	Physical stress	Erythrocyte fragmentation
Infectious agents	*Plasmodium* sp.	Direct parasitization of erythrocyte; hypersplenism; acute intravascular hemolysis (*P. falciparum* infection)
	Babesia sp.	Invasion of the erythrocyte and cell lysis
	Bartonella sp.	Invasion of the erythrocyte and cell lysis
	Clostridium sp.	Hemolytic toxins
Animal venoms	Snake bites	Mechanical cell damage due to DIC
	Spider bites	Venom?
	Bee stings	Venom?
Chemicals and drugs	Water	Osmotic lysis
	Oxidants	Hemoglobin denaturation
	Lead	Erythrocyte membrane damage

removed in the spleen (extravascular hemolysis). Severely damaged erythrocytes can be destroyed intravascularly. Depending on the underlying pathology, leukocytes may be increased and platelets may be decreased. Evidence of intravascular coagulation and fibrinolysis may be present. The plasma concentration of markers of hemolysis (bilirubin and haptoglobin) varies depending on the type and extent of hemolysis (∞ Chapter 14).

The underlying diseases and conditions responsible for microangiopathic hemolytic anemia include hemolytic uremic syndrome (HUS), thrombotic thrombocytopenic purpura (TTP), malignant hypertension, disseminated cancer, and pregnancy (eclampsia, preeclampsia). A severe form of preeclampsia characterized by <u>h</u>emolysis, <u>e</u>levated <u>l</u>iver enzymes and <u>l</u>ow <u>p</u>latelet counts (HELLP) syndrome can also cause MAHA. HUS and TTP may present with similar initial clinical symptoms, but the underlying etiology, the age group affected, and the target organ(s) differ (Table 18-2 ✪).

✓ Checkpoint! 1

What abnormal erythrocyte characterizes microangiopathic hemolytic anemia? How is this cell formed?

✪ CASE STUDY *(continued from page 368)*

Mai's peripheral blood smear showed moderate schistocytes and polychromasia.

1. What are some conditions that result in the presence of schistocytes?

HEMOLYTIC UREMIC SYNDROME

Hemolytic uremic syndrome (HUS) is a multisystem disorder first described in the mid-1950s. It is characterized by a triad of clinical findings including hemolytic anemia with erythrocyte fragmentation, thrombocytopenia, and acute nephropathy, which can include renal failure. Most individuals, however, recover renal function.[1-3] In some cases, there can also be evidence of mild neurologic problems although only a small percentage develop severe symptoms.

HUS can be subdivided into two groups (D+ HUS and D− HUS) based on the presence or absence of a bloody diarrheal prodrome (Table 18-3 ✪). The diarrhea-associated (D+ HUS) is the most common form and represents about 90% of cases. Onset of D+ HUS tends to occur between the

✪ TABLE 18-2

Comparison of Characteristics Associated with HUS and TTP

TTP	HUS
Adults ages 20–50	Children <5 years old
Hemolytic anemia with red cell fragmentation	Hemolytic anemia with red cell fragmentation
Renal dysfunction (mild to moderate)	Acute renal failure
Thrombocytopenia	Thrombocytopenia
Severe CNS symptoms	Mild CNS symptoms
Fever	

❋ TABLE 18-3

Types of HUS and Associated Conditions That Can Precipitate HUS

Type of HUS	Associated Condition
Diarrhea related (classic)	*Eschericia coli* O157:H7
HUS (D+)	*Shigella dysenteriae serotype* I
Nondiarrhea-related HUS (D−)	Postinfectious
	S. pneumoniae
	Viral infections
	Immunosuppression related
	Chemotherapy/cytotoxic drugs
	Renal and bone marrow transplantation
	Pregnancy or oral contraceptive related
	Toxins

ages of 6 months and 10 years; however, most cases are seen in children up to the age of 5 years. It is also considered the most common cause of acute renal failure in children and can lead to chronic renal insufficiency (Table 18-2). Adult-onset D+ HUS, which is less frequently seen, occurs in those over 16 years of age, and the elderly are at highest risk for severe disease.

D+ HUS is characterized by a bloody diarrhea with more than 90% of the cases associated with gastrointestinal infections by *Escherichia coli,* which produces Shiga toxin (Stx). The other cases are associated with infection by *Shigella dysenteriae* Type 1. The incubation period from infection to onset of diarrhea is usually 3–4 days but can range from 1 to 14 days. However, only about 15% of individuals who are infected with Shiga toxin-producing *E. coli* develop HUS.[3–6]

The most common serotype of Shiga toxin-producing *E. coli* (enterohemorrhagic *E. coli*) in the United States is *E. coli* O157:H7. In other countries there are different serotypes linked to D+ HUS.[3,7] The organism is not a part of the normal flora of humans, but is found in the gastrointestinal tract of a small percentage of cattle. The majority of human infections have been traced to the ingestion of incompletely cooked beef contaminated with the organism, but the organism can also be transmitted by the fecal-oral route (inadequate hand washing).[4,8]

Other factors such as elevated neutrophil counts, increased C-reactive protein (CRP), and fever are associated with an increased risk for developing HUS.[9–12] The use of antibiotics or antimotility drugs in treating individuals with diarrhea due to *E. coli* O157:H7 has also been associated with increased risk for developing HUS.[13–15]

The second category of HUS is that of nondiarrhea-associated (D− HUS), also referred to as *atypical HUS (aHUS).* This condition has been reported in both children and adults and is

the type that is more likely to recur.[16,17] D− HUS has been attributed to various causes[17] (Table 18-3). It has been associated with connective tissue diseases such as systemic lupus erythematosus and lupus anticoagulant, as well as some types of cancer (especially stomach, colon, and breast) and diabetes.[18,19] The disease has been reported in young women with complications of pregnancy, after normal delivery, or with the use of oral contraceptives.[20] In recent years, atypical HUS also has been associated with immunosuppressive therapy used in solid organ and bone marrow transplantation.[21–24] D− HUS has been linked to invasive *Streptococcus pneumoniae* infections as well as viral infections such as Epstein-Barr virus, human immunodeficiency virus, and cytomegalovirus.[16,17,25–28]

Many drugs including antiplatelet drugs and antineoplastic agents have been reported to cause rare cases of atypical HUS.[21,29] HUS secondary to other diseases has a higher risk of recurrence and a lower survival rate than cases that are associated with colitis or have no identifiable trigger (primary).[30] In recent years, several complement regulatory gene mutations have been associated with atypical HUS; in these cases, episodes of HUS often recur. Almost 50% are mutations related to three regulatory proteins associated with the alternate complement pathway.[31–35] The three regulatory proteins, which function to control amplification of the pathway by C3bBb, are Factor H, membrane cofactor protein (MCP), and factor I. An autoantibody against Factor H has also been implicated in some cases.[36]

✓ Checkpoint! 2

What are the two types of HUS, and what organisms or diseases are most commonly associated with each type?

Pathophysiology

More than 70% of the cases of HUS have been associated with damage to the renal glomerular capillary endothelium by the Shiga toxin produced by *E. coli* O157:H7 and *S. dysenteriae* Type 1.[3,7] Once the organism enters the human gastrointestinal tract, it begins to damage the intestinal mucosa. The organism's toxin is absorbed into the circulation through damaged gastrointestinal tissue and onto the surface of neutrophils[1,37,38] (Figure 18-1). This toxin has a predisposition for endothelial cells of the microvasculature of the glomerulus and exerts a direct toxic effect.[1] The B subunits of the toxin bind to plasma membrane Gb3 receptors while the A subunit of the toxin inhibits protein synthesis at the ribosomal level, leading to cell death.[4,38] Infiltrates of inflammatory cells and production of cytokines such as IL-8 and tumor necrosis factor-α contribute to the cytotoxic damage in glomerular and renal tubular cells.[38–40] Endothelial damage leads to the release of prothrombotic-, vasoactive-, and platelet-aggregating substances that cause platelet activation with the subsequent formation of thrombi.[40,41] Although damage primarily occurs in the renal microvasculature, other

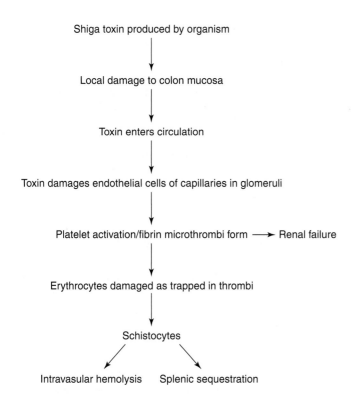

Shiga toxin produced by organism

Local damage to colon mucosa

Toxin enters circulation

Toxin damages endothelial cells of capillaries in glomeruli

Platelet activation/fibrin microthrombi form ⟶ Renal failure

Erythrocytes damaged as trapped in thrombi

Schistocytes

Intravasular hemolysis   Splenic sequestration

■ **FIGURE 18-1**   A possible mechanism for damage by Shiga-like toxin of *Escherichia coli* O157:H7.

organ systems (central nervous system, heart, liver) can be affected. The resulting thrombotic microangiopathy that traps erythrocytes and causes fragmentation is responsible for the schistocytes commonly seen in HUS.

In infections with *Streptococcus pneumoniae,* the bacterial enzyme neuraminidase is responsible for the capillary damage. Neuraminidase cleaves cell membrane glycoproteins and glycolipids, facilitating tissue invasion by the bacteria and exposing the normally hidden T-antigen (Thomsen-Friedenreich antigen) on capillary walls, platelets, and erythrocytes. Naturally occurring anti-T antibodies cause agglutination of cells and platelets leading to thrombosis in the small vessels.[26,42] Catabolic enzymes (especially leukocyte elastase) and oxidative products released from the granules of activated neutrophils have been implicated in causing additional endothelial damage.[40]

✓ **Checkpoint! 3**

Explain how infection with E. coli *O157:H7 results in intravascular hemolysis.*

Clinical Findings

D+ HUS occurs in previously healthy children with the highest incidence in the first year of life. The onset is acute with sudden pallor, abdominal pain, vomiting, foul-smelling and bloody diarrhea, and macroscopic hematuria. Other symptoms include a low-grade fever, hypertension, petechiae, bruising, and jaundice. The most important and/or serious complication of HUS is acute renal failure, which can lead to chronic renal insufficiency in some children. The duration of oliguria and anuria is variable.

Regardless of what organ is affected in addition to the kidneys, the pathology is the same (i.e., thrombosis of the microcirculation). Central nervous system symptoms, which are less severe than those associated with TTP, can result directly from microangiopathy of the central nervous system or from resulting hypertension. Lethargy and minor seizures are the most common symptoms. Hepatomegaly can be present; spelenomegaly is less common. Hyperglycemia is common in children due to pancreatic damage secondary to HUS.

Laboratory Findings

A moderate to severe normocytic, normochromic anemia is typical with hemoglobin levels as low as 3–4 g/dL (median values 7–9 g/dL) (Table 18-4 ✪). The peripheral blood smear shows fragmented and deformed cells (schistocytes, burr cells, helmet cells, spherocytes), with the degree of anemia correlated directly with the degree of morphologic change (Figure 18-2 ■). Polychromasia and an occasional nucleated erythrocyte can be seen. A leukocytosis with a shift to the left is common. Platelet counts vary from low normal to markedly decreased with a median value of 50×10^9/L. The duration of thrombocytopenia is 1–2 weeks.

Hemoglobinemia with an increase in total serum bilirubin (2–3 mg/dL) and a decrease in serum haptoglobin reflects chronic intravascular hemolysis. Serum lactate dehydrogenase is markedly elevated, and cardiac enzymes can be

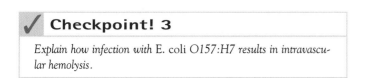

✪ TABLE 18-4	
Laboratory Findings in HUS and TTP	
Evidence of hemolysis	Decreased hemoglobin/hematocrit
	Increased reticulocytes/polychromasia
	Thrombocytopenia
	Leukocytosis with shift to the left
	Presence of schistocytes
Evidence of intravascular hemolysis	Hemoglobinemia
	Hemoglobinuria
	Decreased haptoglobin
	Increased total and unconjugated serum bilirubin
Evidence of thrombotic microangiopathy	Thrombocytopenia
	Fibrin degradation products (normal to slightly increased); D-dimer increased
	PT and APTT (normal to slightly abnormal)
	Factors I, V, VIII (normal to increased)

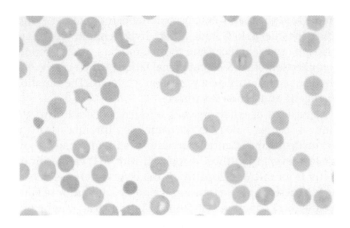

■ FIGURE 18-2   A peripheral blood smear from a patient with hemolytic uremic syndrome (HUS). The platelets are markedly decreased. Schistocytes and spherocytes are present. (Wright-Giemsa stain; 1000× magnification)

elevated due to myocardial damage.[2] Blood urea nitrogen and creatinine levels are increased, reflecting renal failure. Metabolic acidosis, hyponatremia, and hypokalemia are common.

Screening tests for coagulation abnormalities include the prothrombin time (PT) and activated partial thromboplastin time (APTT). In many cases of HUS, there is no detectable consumption of coagulation factors.[40] The PT can be normal or slightly prolonged, but the APTT is usually normal. Although fibrin split products (fragments of fibrin produced by plasmin degradation of fibrin) and D-dimer are elevated, disseminated intravascular coagulation (DIC) is rare. In DIC, when there is an uncontrolled inappropriate formation of fibrin within the blood vessels and subsequent consumption of coagulation factors, coagulation screening tests are abnormal. The direct and indirect antiglobulin tests (Coombs' tests) are usually negative reflecting a nonimmune pathology.

Urinalysis results show moderate to massive amounts of protein (1–2 g/24 hours to 10 g/24 hours), gross and microscopic hematuria, increased numbers of neutrophils (pyuria), and casts (hyaline, granular, and renal epithelial) reflecting the damage to the glomerulus. The presence of hemosiderin in the urine sediment reflects chronic intravascular hemolysis.

 Checkpoint! 4

What are the typical erythrocyte morphology and coagulation test results in children with HUS?

Therapy

Mild to moderately severe cases of D+ HUS have the best prognosis for recovery (more than 80%). With improvement in early diagnosis and supportive care, especially during oliguric or anuric phase, the mortality of the disease has been reduced to 5–15%. Supportive care includes close observation, blood transfusion, control of electrolyte and water imbalances, control of hypertension, and peritoneal dialysis in anuria. Platelet transfusions are not recommended because they can exacerbate the thrombotic process but may be required in some patients with bleeding. The beneficial use of fresh frozen plasma exchange has not been shown to be efficacious in patients with D+ HUS. In contrast, patients with atypical HUS may benefit from plasma exchange. Plasma infusions are contraindicated in patients with HUS who have a positive direct antiglobulin test or who are infected with *S. pneumoniae* due to the presence of naturally occurring anti-T in the plasma.[26,42]

A potentially promising preventative measure in individuals infected with Shiga toxin-producing *E. coli* is the use of monoclonal antibodies against Shiga toxin to provide passive immunity.[43] There is only a small window of time, 3 to 5 days, from onset of diarrhea to HUS for treatment, so detection of the toxin in stool or blood by flow cytometry must be performed.[44,45]

Thrombotic Thrombocytopenic Purpura
Thrombotic thrombocytopenic purpura (TTP) is another relatively uncommon disorder in which platelet aggregation on the microvascular endothelium results in serious complications. In most cases, it is an acute disorder that affects young adults (ages 20–50 with a peak incidence in the third decade). TTP occurs more frequently in females than males. It is characterized by several of the same clinical findings as HUS such as thrombocytopenia and microangiopathic hemolytic anemia and is often associated with mild renal dysfunction and fever. Neurological symptoms are more frequent, severe, and prominent in TTP than HUS (Table 18-2). TTP may be familial (chronic or relapsing forms) or acquired.

Various clinical events have been identified as possible precipitating factors in the acquired type (Table 18-5 ⊗). Infections are the most common precipitating factor (40%) followed by pregnancy (10–25%). Without treatment, TTP has a mortality rate in excess of 90% due to multiorgan failure. The disorder is discussed in detail in ∞ Chapter 33, but an overview comparison with HUS in this chapter highlights several key findings.

Pathophysiology   TTP is characterized by microthrombi composed of platelets and unusually large forms of **von Willebrand factor (VWF)** that occlude capillaries and arterioles in a number of organs including the kidneys, heart, brain, and pancreas. These thrombi contain platelets and sometimes immunoglobin and complement, but there is little fibrin, inflammation, or subendothelial exposure as in disseminated intravascular coagulation (DIC).[46–48]

Normally large multimers of VWF are broken into smaller forms by the circulating protease, a disintegrinlike and metalloprotease domain with thrombospondin type motifs (ADAMTS13). It is now known that a deficiency in the protease ADAMTS13 is the cause of TTP.[49–53] As a result of the

TABLE 18-5

Some Reported Clinical Conditions That Can Be Precipitating Factors in TTP

Infections

  Bacterial—enteric organisms

    Shigella sp.   *E. coli*

    Salmonella sp.   *Campylobacter* sp.

    Yersinia sp.

  Bacterial—other

    Streptococcus pneumoniae

    Legionella sp.

    Mycoplasma sp.

  Viral

    HIV   EBV

    Influenza   Herpes simplex

Pregnancy or oral-contraceptive related

Lymphomas and carcinomas

Drugs

  Antimicrobials—penicillin

  Ticlopidine

  Chemotherapeutic agents

Connective tissue diseases

  Systemic lupus erythematosus (SLE)

  Rheumatoid arthritis (RA)

  Ankylosing spondylitis

  Sjogren's syndrome

Miscellaneous

  Bee sting

  Dog bite

  Carbon monoxide poisoning

g/L (10.5 g/dL) (average 80–90 g/L). The MCV is variable, either normal, or decreased if there is marked erythrocyte fragmentation, or increased in the presence of reticulocytosis. The MCH and MCHC are normal. Nucleated erythrocytes can be found in the peripheral blood reflecting the bone marrow response to hemolysis. The most striking blood finding is the abundance of schistocytes (generally >1%).[54] Leukocytosis with counts of more than 20×10^9/L occurs in 50% of patients and is usually accompanied by a shift to the left. Thrombocytopenia is often severe ($8–44 \times 10^9$/L) due to consumption of platelets in the formation of microthrombi. Megakaryocytes are abundant in the bone marrow.

Coagulation tests are usually normal or only mildly disturbed in TTP, which helps differentiate TTP from DIC, in which there is an increase in D-dimer, as well as prolonged PT, APTT, and thrombin time increase.

Hemoglobinemia, hemoglobinuria, decreased haptoglobin levels, and increased total and unconjugated serum bilirubin are direct evidence of intravascular hemolysis.

Therapy   Studies have shown that plasma exchange with **fresh frozen plasma (FFP)** can be effective in providing the needed ADAMTS13 protease and removing autoantibody.[55–58] **Cryosupernatant**, which lacks the large VWF multimers present in FFP, yet still contains the VWF cleaving protease missing in TTP patients, can be used.[58,59] Drug treatment with monoclonal antibody (rituximab), antiplatelet or platelet-inhibiting agents, intravenous administration of steroids, or combinations of corticosteroids and plasma have been used.[56,60]

 Checkpoint! 5

How does the clinical presentation of TTP differ from that of HUS? How is it similar?

 CASE STUDY *(continued from page 369)*

As Mai was questioned further, she indicated that she noticed a large number of bruises on her extremities. Her platelet count was 31×10^9/L. She had a 2.5% reticulocyte count.

2. What is the significance of these results?

3. Why might the clinician order coagulation tests?

ADAMTS13 deficiency, these large VWF multimers remain attached to the endothelial cells and adhere to platelets, inducing platelet aggregation and formation of platelet thrombi. As erythrocytes are forced through the thrombi, fragmentation occurs. In the familial form, a mutation in the ADAMTS13 gene occurs, resulting in a deficient/dysfunctional enzyme. The acquired type is due to autoantibodies against ADAMTS13 blocking its activity. The clinical aspects of TTP are similar to those of HUS except that TTP occurs most often in young adults and involves more organ systems. Neurologic symptoms are more prominent, renal dysfunction is less severe, and the mortality rate is higher than in HUS.

Symptoms can be eliminated if treated early, although some patients recovering from TTP can have permanent manifestations of renal damage and require dialysis.

Laboratory Findings   Typical laboratory results are shown in Table 18-4. The hemoglobin is usually less than 105

Disseminated Intravascular Coagulation

Disseminated intravascular coagulation (DIC) is a complex thrombohemorrhagic condition in which the normal coagulation process is altered by an underlying condition. The more common conditions that precipitate DIC include bacterial sepsis, neoplasms, immunologic disorders or trauma[61] (Table 18-6). DIC is initiated by damage to the endothelial lining of vessels. This damage causes release of thromboplastic substances that activate the coagulation

✪ TABLE 18-6

Causes of Disseminated Intravascular Coagulation (DIC)

Bacterial sepsis	Endotoxins
	Exotoxins
Neoplasm	Solid tumors
	Myeloproliferative disorders
Serious trauma	
Immunologic disorders	Hemolytic transfusion reactions
	Transplant rejection
Miscellaneous	Venom—snake or insect
	Drugs

mechanism in vivo. As a result, platelet activation and aggregation lead to deposition of fibrin and formation of microthrombi in the microvasculature. As erythrocytes become entangled in the fibrin meshwork in the capillaries (clothesline effect), they fragment to form schistocytes. Complications that result include thrombotic occlusion of vessels, bleeding, and ultimately organ failure. Hemolysis is not usually severe, but the effects of consumptive coagulopathy (consumption of various coagulation proteins and platelets) can cause thrombocytopenia and serious bleeding complications.

The typical findings on the blood smear include the presence of schistocytes and thrombocytopenia (Figure 18-3 ■). The presence of schistocytes is not specific for DIC. However, the abnormal coagulation tests help distinguish this condition from others (TTP and HUS) that give a similar picture on a peripheral blood smear and increase diagnostic accuracy.[62,63] Abnormal coagulation tests include:

• Prolonged prothrombin time (PT), activated partial thromboplastin time (APTT), and thrombin time (TT)
• Elevated D-dimer test

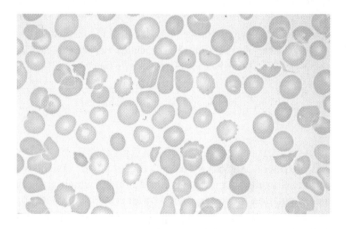

■ **FIGURE 18-3** Peripheral blood from patient with disseminated intravascular coagulation. Notice the schistocytes and thrombocytopenia. (Wright stain; 1000× magnification)

• Increase in fibrin degradation products (FDP)
• Decrease in fibrinogen

Treatment can include erythrocyte and platelet transfusions as well as infusion of fresh frozen plasma or factor concentrates to replace coagulation factors. Most important, however, are the treatment and resolution of the underlying disorder responsible for the DIC. The etiology, diagnosis, and treatment of DIC is discussed further in ∞ Chapter 32.

✓ **Checkpoint! 6**

Explain how DIC can be differentiated from TTP and HUS based on coagulation tests.

HELLP Syndrome

The **HELLP syndrome** is an obstetric complication characterized by **h**emolysis, **e**levated **l**iver enzymes, and a **l**ow **p**latelet count. The etiology and pathogenesis are not well understood but an association may exist with abnormal concentrations of vascular growth factors.[64] As with TTP and HUS, the precipitating factor is unknown, but the clinical aspects are characterized by capillary endothelial damage and intravascular platelet activation as well as microangiopathic anemia.[64,65] However, there does not seem to be an association with presence of IgM or IgG anti-cardiolipin antibodies or anti-beta2-glycoprotein-I antibodies as seen in antiphospholipid syndrome.[66] Some experts consider HELLP to be a severe form of preeclampsia and to share some of the characteristics of preeclampsia and eclampsia such as hypertension and proteinuria, but it is distinguished from them by the presence of the three aspects that gave it its name (hemolysis, elevated liver enzymes, and low platelet count). Severe cases can compromise fetal growth and survival. Approximately 10% of pregnancies with eclampsia develop HELLP syndrome with a mortality rate of about 1%.[67]

The peripheral blood findings are similar to those found in TTP, HUS, or other microangiopathic conditions. Overall, however, the hemolysis and thrombocytopenia are less severe than those associated with TTP or HUS. Liver damage is due primarily to obstruction of hepatic sinusoids and can lead to subsequent hepatic hemorrhage or necrosis.[67] There are fibrinlike deposits that resemble those in TTP/HUS. These deposits are responsible for the presence of schistocytes. Laboratory markers are used in determining the presence of HELLP. The liver enzyme most frequently measured is aspartate aminotransferase (AST), and levels >70 IU/L are common. Increased total and/or unconjugated bilirubin, increased lactic dehydrogenase (generally >600 IU/L), and decreased haptoglobin can also be seen in HELLP.[68] Coagulation tests such as the PT and APTT are usually normal until late in the course of the disease.[68,69] The platelet count is decreased (usually <100 × 10⁹/L) as a result of platelet consumption at the site of endothelial damage. Although DIC infrequently occurs as a complication of HELLP, patients can have an undetectable underlying coagulopathy.[65] Acute tubular necrosis with renal failure, hepatic rupture, and pulmonary edema can also occur as complications.[68,69]

Corticosteroid therapy may be useful in controlling cell destruction and decreasing liver enzymes if the fetus cannot be immediately delivered. Plasma exchange is rarely used as a treatment. The use of cortisone dexamethasone has eliminated the need for platelet transfusions in most patients with platelet counts $<50 \times 10^9$/L.[69-72]

 CASE STUDY *(continued from page 373)*

Mai's PT and APTT were slightly prolonged. The fibrinogen levels were slightly decreased.

4. What do these findings indicate about the underlying problem?

Malignant Hypertension

The microangiopathic hemolytic anemia associated with malignant hypertension is characterized by a low platelet count and erythrocyte fragmentation. In addition, the presence of schistocytes, platelet count, and increased LD have been used to predict renal insufficiency as well as recovery.[73] The mechanism of hemolysis is unknown. It has been suggested that it can be caused by endothelial injury, fibrinoid necrosis of arterioles, or deposition of fibrin fed by thromboplastic substances released from membranes of lysed erythrocytes.

Traumatic Cardiac Hemolytic Anemia

Hemolytic anemia is an uncommon complication following surgical insertion of prosthetic heart valves. Unlike the microangiopathic anemia seen with TTP or DIC, the platelet count is not significantly decreased. Excessive acceleration or turbulence of blood flow around the valve tears the erythrocytes apart from shear stress. The term *Waring blender syndrome* has been used to describe this disorder because of the localized turbulent blood flow. Many erythrocyte fragments are apparent on the blood smear. Some of the severely traumatized cells are removed by the spleen, but most undergo intravascular hemolysis. Newly designed prosthetic valves help decrease the shear stress and resulting erythrocyte fragmentation.[74] Rarely, hemolysis and erythrocyte fragmentation have been associated with formation of large vegetations in patients with infective endocarditis. It is theorized that the same mechanisms of turbulence and pressure as are seen in prosthetic valves cause the fragmentation in endocarditis.[75]

Thermal Injury

Hemolytic anemia occurs within the first 24–46 hours after extensive thermal burns, and the degree of hemolysis depends on the percentage of body surface area burned. He-molysis probably results from the direct effect of heat on spectrin in the erythrocyte membrane. (If erythrocytes are heated to 48°C in vitro, spectrin degradation causes a loss of elasticity and deformability.) In addition, the fatty acid and lipoprotein metabolism in both plasma and erythrocytes are altered after burn injuries, which can contribute to abnormal erythrocyte morphology.[76] Peripheral blood smears show erythrocyte budding, schistocytes, and spherocytes. After 48 hours, signs of hemolysis such as hemoglobinuria and hemoglobinemia decrease. Thermal injury to erythrocytes also has occurred during hemodialysis when the dialysate is overheated.

Exercise-Induced Hemoglobinuria

Exercise-induced hemoglobinuria (sometimes described as *march hemoglobinuria*) describes a transient hemolytic anemia occurring after strenuous exercise and often involves contact with a hard surface (e.g., running, tennis). The hemolysis is probably due to physical injury to erythrocytes as they pass through the capillaries of the feet. Plasma hemoglobin and haptoglobin results show that the primary cause of the intravascular lysis is due to footstrike.[77] However, it is not seen in every individual participating in these activities and can be seen in other physical activities such as swimming, cycling, and rowing in which footstrike is limited. In recent years, the role of exercise-induced oxidative stress and red cell age have been recognized as potential additional causes of lysis, especially in normally sedentary individuals who participate in strenuous exercise.[78] Increased osmotic fragility and decreased deformability leading to intravascular hemolysis were noted in these individuals.[79] In addition, changes in erythrocyte membrane proteins such as spectrins, especially in older cells, can increase susceptibility to extravascular hemolysis during strenuous exercise.

In contrast to the other hemolytic conditions discussed so far in this chapter, no erythrocyte fragments are seen on the peripheral blood smear, but the hallmarks of intravascular hemolysis—hemoglobinemia and hemoglobinuria—are present. The passage of reddish urine immediately after exercise and for several hours thereafter is usually the only complaint from affected individuals. Anemia is uncommon because less than 1% of the erythrocytes are hemolyzed during an attack. Individuals can present with slightly increased mean corpuscular volumes (MCV) due to increased reticulocytes.[77,80] Iron deficiency can occur if exercise and hemolysis are frequent.

Other Conditions Associated with MAHA

Several reports have linked MAHA with diabetes. It is theorized that in these cases, the cholesterol to phospholipid ratio is altered, leading to a rigidity in the erythrocyte membrane.[19] Stem cell transplant recipients can show increased evidence of transplant-associated microangiopathy (TAM) characterized by schistocytes. TAM may represent a form of graft-vs-host disease (GVHD) and result from endothelial damage induced by donor cytotoxic T cells.[22,24]

CASE STUDY *(continued from page 375)*

Mai's symptoms continued to become worse with frequent seizures, headaches, and dizziness. Her urinalysis results showed a 2+ protein and moderate blood. However, she had normal urinary volume.

5. Based on these results, what is the most likely condition associated with these clinical and laboratory results? Explain.

6. What therapy might be used?

► HEMOLYTIC ANEMIAS CAUSED BY ANTAGONISTS IN THE BLOOD

Antagonists such as drugs or venoms and infectious organisms in the environment of the erythrocyte can cause premature destruction (Table 18-1). This hemolysis is precipitated by either injury to the erythrocyte membrane or to denaturation of hemoglobin.

INFECTIOUS AGENTS

Parasites and bacteria can infect erythrocytes and directly lead to their destruction. Alternatively, toxins produced by infectious agents can cause hemolysis.

Malarial Parasites

The anemia accompanying malaria is due directly and indirectly to the intracellular malarial parasites that live part of their life cycle in the erythrocyte (Figure 18-4 ■). The anemia resulting from this infection is usually a mild, normocytic normochromic anemia but can be severe in infection with *Plasmodium falciparum* because of the high levels of parasitemia. Thrombocytopenia can also be present. Diagnosis involves finding the life cycle stage within the erythrocyte. Infection with *P. falciparum*, a cause of severe anemia in children, can be accompanied by ineffective erythropoiesis and decreased reticulocytes. The hemoglobin in these cases can reach levels as low as 5 gm/dL.[81] In addition, poor diet, malnutrition, decreased iron stores, and folate stores contribute to the severity of anemia. Exchange transfusions can be used in the severest cases to remove infected erythrocytes.[82]

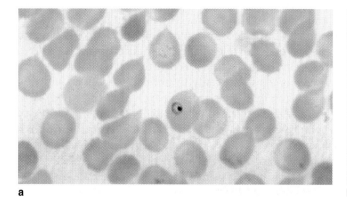

a

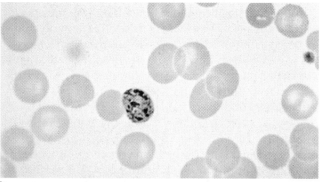

b

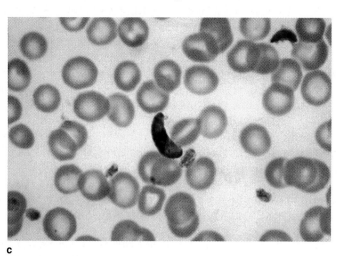

c

■ FIGURE 18-4   Peripheral blood smears from patients with malaria. a. There is a ring form of malaria in the erythrocyte. b. There is an immature schizont form of malaria in the erythrocyte. c. This is a gametocyte of *Plasmodium falciparum* in the erythrocyte. (Wright stain; 1000× magnification)

The release of the intraerythrocytic parasite from the cell results in the cell destruction. On the other hand, the spleen can remove the entire parasitized cell, or splenic macrophages can pit the parasite from the erythrocyte, damaging the cell membrane. This resulting decreased deformability can lead to removal of the cell by the spleen. Anemia can also result from an immune-mediated process. Antimalarial antibodies react with malarial antigens on the erythrocyte membrane, resulting in removal of the sensitized cell by the splenic macrophages. In some cases, the concentration of complement regulatory proteins decrease, which can facilitate complement-mediated hemolysis.[83]

Blackwater fever, an uncommon complication of infection with *P. falciparum,* is characterized by massive acute intravascular hemolysis with hemoglobinemia, hemoglobinuria, methemalbuminemia, and hyperbilirubinemia. However, the parasitemia level is often low. The mechanism that precipitates this is unclear. One possible mechanism is development of an autoantibody to the infected erythrocyte. Another is a direct reaction to the drug quinine or to repeated incomplete treatment with the drug. The drug can act as a hapten to stimulate formation of a drug-dependent antibody that has complement-fixing ability.[81] In some cases, the direct antiglobulin test (DAT) can be positive with either monospecific anticomplement or anti-IgG.[84] Use of synthetic quinine drugs has considerably decreased frequency of this complication. There is some evidence, however, that other antimalarial drugs including mefloquine can also trigger this response.[84]

Babesiosis

Babesiosis, a protozoan infection of rodents and cattle, is most commonly transmitted to humans by the bite of a hard tick. However, the organism can be acquired transplacentally and through blood transfusions. In the United States, the most common organism is *Babesia microti.* On the peripheral blood smear, the parasites appear as intracellular, pleomorphic, 1–5 μm ringlike structures resembling ring form trophozoites of *Plasmodium falciparum* (Figure 18-5 ■). Some can appear as doubles or tetrads in the form of a Maltese cross. Travel history, the absence of the characteristic banana-shaped gametocytes, and the lack of pigment help distinguish it from *P. falciparum.* Most infections are asymptomatic but some present with a flulike syndrome. Generally there is 1–10% parasitemia.[85] Extravascular hemolysis can occur in a manner similar to that seen with malaria. A mild to moderate anemia as well as thrombocytopenia can be present. Other possible laboratory findings include increased reticulocyte count, liver enzymes, and bilirubin.[86] In a rare fulminating infection, severe anemia, intravascular hemolysis, and hemoglobinuria are seen. Complications associated with intravascular hemolysis include renal failure and disseminated intravascular coagulation. Patients who are splenectomized generally have a more severe clinical presentation and higher levels of parasitemia. In severe cases of hemolysis or renal complications, exchange transfusion may be indicated.

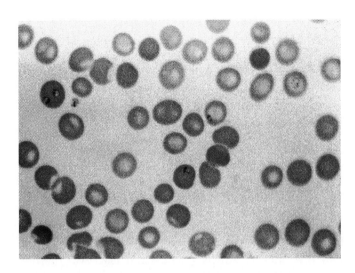

■ FIGURE 18-5 Peripheral blood smear of a patient with babesiosis. Several infected erythrocytes are in the field. One cell in the upper left contains two organisms. Infected cells are in the center and upper right. (Wright stain; 1000× magnification)

✓ **Checkpoint! 7**

Why do malaria and babesiosis result in anemia?

Bartonellosis

Organisms in the genus *Bartonella* are transmitted by blood-sucking arthropods and by direct inoculation by scratch or bite of a mammal. The organisms infect erythrocytes and endothelial cells. Infection by *Bartonella bacilliformis* is associated with Carrion's disease, which is restricted to Columbia, Peru, and Ecuador. The disease is transmitted by sandflies. One part of this biphasic disease is characterized by an often fatal syndrome consisting of myalgia, high fever, and an acute, severe hemolytic anemia (Oroya fever).[87] The disease can progress to coma and death within weeks. If the patient survives, a chronic phase will present weeks to months later. This is characterized by a granulomatous reaction with the appearance of cutaneous hemangioma-like lesions that may contain bacteria, neutrophils, macrophages, and endothelial cells. Other *Bartonella* species infect erythrocytes but are not associated with hemolytic manifestations.[87] The pleomorphic (coccobacillary) organisms are readily visualized as single, paired, or chained organisms on or within erythrocytes on Wright- or Giemsa-stained peripheral blood smears during the course of the disease. The organism releases several proteins including deformin that are responsible for inducing the pitting or invagination of the erythrocyte membrane. These structures, as well as other proteins such as hemolysins, can serve as entry portals for the bacteria and help explain the mechanism of cell destruction.[87,88]

Clostridium Perfringens

C. perfringens is a member of the normal flora of the gastrointestinal tract. Infection can present as a transient bacteremia or a life-threatening condition. It is one of the few organisms (along with *C. septicum* and *C. novyi*) that can cause a rapid, massive intravascular hemolysis. The bacteria produce potent exotoxins that affect host cell membranes. The major hemolytic toxin (α-toxin) is a phospholipase C that hydrolyzes sphingomyelin and lecithin present in the erythrocyte membrane and leads to changes in membrane integrity. Fever, thrombocytopenia, neutrophilia, hemoglobinemia, and hemoglobinuria are present.[89] Anuria or acute renal failure can develop as a result of the hemoglobinuria. Lysis of the erythrocyte or other cells can cause DIC. Bacterial neuraminidase can expose crypt antigens such as Thomsen-Friedenrich (T antigen), which can react with nonimmune autoantibody. The peripheral blood smear shows many microspherocytes and few erythrocyte fragments.

ANIMAL VENOMS

Venoms injected by bees, wasps, spiders, and scorpions can cause hemolysis in some susceptible individuals. One of the more common bites that can result in hemolysis is that of the brown recluse spider (*Loxosceles reclusa*). The characteristic symptoms of envenomation are a localized lesion that shows central thrombosis surrounded by ischemic areas. However, up to 15% of individuals, especially children, develop systemic symptoms including intravascular hemolysis that can be severe.[90,91] The mechanism of venom damage appears to involve sphingomyelinase D2, which cleaves glycophorin from the erythrocyte membrane. This decreases the structural integrity of the membrane and increases its sensitivity to complement-mediated lysis.[91,92] Although snake bites rarely cause hemolysis directly, they can cause hemolysis secondary to disseminated intravascular coagulation.[93]

Chemicals and Drugs

Various chemicals and drugs have been identified as possible causes of erythrocyte hemolysis; many of these are dose dependent. In addition to causing erythrocyte hemolysis, chemicals and drugs can also produce methemoglobinemia and cyanosis or, in some instances, aplasia of the bone marrow.

Hemoglobinemia and hemoglobinuria can occur as a result of osmotic lysis of erythrocytes when water enters the vascular system during transurethral resection or when inappropriate solutions are used during a blood transfusion.

Some drugs known to cause hemolysis in G6PD-deficient persons can also cause hemolysis in normal persons if the dose is sufficiently high. The mechanism of hemolysis is similar to that in G6PD deficiency with hemoglobin denaturation and Heinz body formation due to strong oxidants.

Lead poisoning anemia is usually classified with sideroblastic anemias because the pathophysiologic and hematologic findings are similar. Lead inhibits heme synthesis, causing an accumulation of iron within mitochondria (∞ Chapter 9). However, it is apparent that lead also damages the erythrocyte membrane. This damage is manifested by an increase in osmotic fragility and mechanical fragility.

SUMMARY

Mechanisms of nonimmune damage to the erythrocyte are varied. Of those discussed in this chapter, HUS and TTP are the more commonly encountered, presenting with a classic picture of microangiopathic hemolytic anemia with schistocytes. Classic D+ HUS is mediated by the Shiga-like toxin of *E. coli* O157:H7. The underlying cause of TTP is a deficiency in the ADAMTS13 cleaving protease. Intraerythrocytic parasitic infections with organisms such as malaria or babesiosis can cause hemolysis and anemia without the presence of schistocytes. In susceptible individuals, drugs or chemicals can also lead to hemolysis.

REVIEW QUESTIONS

LEVEL I

1. Which of the following conditions is not associated with the formation of schistocytes? (Objective 2)
   a. hemolytic uremic syndrome
   b. exercise-induced hemoglobinuria
   c. thrombotic thrombocytopenic purpura
   d. disseminated intravascular coagulation

2. One of the major criteria that distinguishes DIC from other causes of microangiopathic hemolytic anemia is: (Objective 2)
   a. the presence of schistocytes
   b. thrombocytopenia
   c. decreased hemoglobin
   d. an abnormal coagulation test

LEVEL II

1. A 43-year-old woman presents to her physician with a 3-week history of fatigue, constant headache, and low-grade fever. Selected laboratory results include:

   Hemoglobin: 7.5 g/dL (75 g/L)   Platelet count: 16×10^9/L

   Hematocrit: 0.23 L/L (23%)   Reticulocytes: 11%

   RDW: 15

   Peripheral blood smear showed schistocytes. Which of the following drugs that the patient was taking could cause these symptoms and lab values? (Objectives 2, 4)
   a. ticlopidine
   b. aspirin
   c. estrogens
   d. penicillin

REVIEW QUESTIONS (continued)

LEVEL I

3. A patient who has anemia with an increased reticulocyte count, increased bilirubin, and many schistocytes on the blood smear could have: (Objective 2)
   a. MAHA
   b. high cholesterol in the blood
   c. spur cell anemia
   d. immune hemolytic anemia

4. Which of the following organisms does *not* cause damage of the erythrocyte because of an intraerythrocytic life cycle? (Objective 4)
   a. *Plasmodium falciparum*
   b. *Babesia* sp
   c. *Bartonella* sp
   d. *Clostridium perfringens*

5. A characteristic finding on a blood smear in MAHA is the presence of: (Objective 3)
   a. target cells
   b. spur cells
   c. schistocytes
   d. echinocytes

6. All of the following are characterized as causes of MAHA *except*: (Objective 1)
   a. TTP
   b. prosthetic heart valves
   c. HUS
   d. March hemoglobinuria

7. All of the following are associated with HUS *except*: (Objective 2)
   a. thrombocytosis
   b. nucleated RBCs
   c. schistocytes
   d. reticulocytosis

8. MAHA is most frequently caused by: (Objective 1)
   a. physical trauma to the cell
   b. immune destruction
   c. antagonists in the blood
   d. plasma lipid abnormalities

9. Intravascular hemolysis in MAHA would be associated with which of the following parameters? (Objective 2)

	Bilirubin	Haptoglobin
a.	decreased	decreased
b.	decreased	increased
c.	increased	decreased
d.	increased	increased

10. MAHA due to HUS is usually seen in which age group? (Objective 1)
    a. children under 1 year old
    b. females between 20 and 50 years of age
    c. either sex under 50 years of age
    d. males older than 16 years of age

LEVEL II

2. A 34-year-old woman is brought into the ER after falling off a ladder while painting her house. Selected lab results include:

Hemoglobin: 8.0 g/dL (80 g/L)	PT: 36 seconds
Hematocrit: 0.25 L/L (25%)	APTT: >75 seconds
Platelet count: 20 × 10⁹/L	Fibrinogen: 100 mg/dL

   Peripheral blood smear shows schistocytes. Given these results, what is the most likely diagnosis? (Objectives 2, 4)
   a. HELLP syndrome
   b. TTP
   c. DIC
   d. traumatic hemolytic anemia

3. Results of tests obtained on a small child who had easy bruising, tiredness, difficulty breathing, and decreased urinary output were hemoglobin: 65 g/L; platelets: 41 × 10⁹/L; PT and PTT within normal reference intervals. His mother indicated he had an episode of bloody diarrhea about 2 weeks earlier but it had not recurred. Based on the clinical and limited laboratory findings, what is the most likely condition? (Objectives 2, 4)
   a. TTP
   b. bartonellosis
   c. *Clostridium* sp infection
   d. HUS

4. The most likely age group for developing TTP is: (Objective 2)
   a. female children under 1 year old
   b. females between 20 and 50 years of age
   c. either gender under 5 years of age
   d. males older than 16 years of age

5. Which of the following disorders is *not* characterized by the presence of schistocytes? (Objective 3)
   a. march hemoglobinuria
   b. insertion of a prosthetic valve
   c. third-degree burns
   d. malignant hypertension

6. A patient with a deficiency in the VWF protease ADAMTS13 would be at risk to develop what condition? (Objective 2)
   a. HUS
   b. spur cell anemia
   c. TTP
   d. hereditary acanthocytosis

7. The formation of schistocytes in MAHA is primarily due to: (Objective 1)
   a. pitting by splenic macrophages
   b. defective cell membranes
   c. increased membrane phospholipids
   d. shearing of erythrocytes by fibrin threads

REVIEW QUESTIONS (continued)

LEVEL I

LEVEL II

8. Plasma exchange is used as a primary treatment for which of the following? (Objective 2)
   a. HUS
   b. TTP
   c. abetalipoproteinemia
   d. DIC

9. The peripheral blood smear from a 6-months pregnant woman showed the presence of schistocytes. Platelet count was $<60 \times 10^9$/L, and her hemoglobin was 7.5 g/dL (75 g/L). She has no history of chronic disease. What laboratory test(s) might give a clue to the underlying cause? (Objective 4)
   a. haptoglobin
   b. reticulocyte count
   c. liver enzymes
   d. APTT and PT

10. Hemolytic toxins are the major cause of intravascular hemolysis in diseases or conditions caused by which of the following organisms? (Objective 5)
    a. *Plasmodium falciparum*
    b. *Babesia* sp.
    c. *Bartonella bacilliformis*
    d. *Clostridium perfringens*

www.pearsonhighered.com/mckenzie

Use this address to access the interactive Companion Website created for this textbook. Find additional information, tables and figures. Evaluate your command of the chapter information using case studies and critical thinking and multiple choice questions.

REFERENCES

1. Moake JL. Thrombotic microangiopathies. *N Engl J Med.* 2002;347: 589–600.

2. Noris M, Ramuzzi G. Hemolytic uremic syndrome. *J Am Soc Nephrol.* 2005;16:1035–50.

3. Banatvala N, Griffin PM, Greene KD, Barrett TJ, Bibb WF et al. The United States national prospective hemolytic uremic syndrome study: Microbiologic, serologic, clinical, and epidemiological findings. *J Infect Dis* 2100;183:1063–70.

4. Mead PS, Griffin PM. *Escherichia coli* O157:H7. *Lancet.* 1996;352: 1207–12.

5. Ochoa TJ, Cleary TG. Epidemiology and spectrum of disease of *Escherichia coli* O157:H7. *Curr Opin Infect Dis.* 2003;16:259–63.

6. Tarr PI, Gordon CA, Chandler WL. Shiga-toxin-producing *Escherichia coli* and haemolytic uraemic syndrome. *Lancet.* 2005; 365:1073–86.

7. Thorpe CM. Shiga toxin-producing *Escherichia coli* infection. *Clin Infect Dis.* 2004;38:1298–1303.

8. Crump JA, Sulka AC, Langer AH, Schaben C, Cruelly AS, Gage R et al. An outbreak of *Escherichia coli* O157:H7 infections among visitors to a dairy farm. *N Engl J Med.* 2002;347:555–60.

9. Anjay MA, Anoop P, Britland A. Leukocytosis as a predictor of progression to haemolytic uraemic syndrome in *Escherichia coli* O157:H7 infection. *Arch Dis Child.* 2007;92:820–23.

10. Kawamura N, Yamazaki T, Tamai H. Risk factors for the development of *Escherichia coli* O157:H7 associated with hemolytic uremic syndrome. *Pediatr Int.* 1999;41:218–22.

11. Fernandez GC, Gomez SA, Ramos MV, Bentancor LV, Fernandez-Brando RJ, Landoni VI et al. The functional state of neutrophils correlates with the severity of renal dysfunction in children with hemolytic uremic syndrome. *Pediatr Res.* 2007;61:123–28.

12. Buteau C, Proulx F, Chaibou M et al. Leukocytosis in children with *Escherichia coli* O157:H7 enteritis developing the hemolytic uremic syndrome. *Pediatr Infect Dis J.* 2000;19:642–47.

13. Wong CS, Jelacic S, Habeeb RL, Watkins SL, Tarr PI. The risk of the hemolytic-uremic syndrome after treatment of *Escherichia coli* O157:H7 infections. *N Engl J Med.* 2000;342:1930–36.

14. Beatty ME, Griffin PM, Tulu AN, Olsen SJ. Culturing practices and antibiotic use in children with diarrhea. *Pediatrics.* 2004;113: 628–29.

15. Slutsker L, Ries AA, Maloney K, Wells JG, Greene KD, Griffin PM. A nationwide-case control study of *Escherichia coli* O157:H7 infection in the United States. *J Infect Dis.* 1998;177:962–66.

16. Siegler RL, Pavla AT, Sherbotie JR. Recurrent hemolytic uremic syndrome. *Clin Pediatr.* 2002;41:705–9.

17. Siegler R, Oakes R. Hemolytic uremic syndrome: Pathogenesis, treatment, and outcome. *Curr Opin Pediatr.* 2005;17:200–4.

18. Gherman RB, Tramont J, Connito DJ. Postpartum hemolytic-uremic syndrome associated with lupus anticoagulant. *J. Reproductive Medicine.* 1999;44:471–74.

19. James SH, Meyers AM. Microangiopathic hemolytic anemia as a complication of diabetes mellitus. *So Soc for Clin Investig.* 1998;315:211–15.

20. George J. The association of pregnancy with thrombotic thrombocytopenic purpura-hemolytic uremic syndrome. *Curr Opin Hematol.* 2003;10:339–44.

21. Alexandrescu DT, Maddukuri P, Wiernik PH, Dutcher JP. Thrombotic thrombocytopenic purpura/hemolytic uremic syndrome associated with high-dose interleukin-2 for the treatment of metastatic melanoma. *J Immunotherapy.* 2005;28:144–47.

22. Matinez MT, Chucher CH, Stussi G, Heim D, Buser A, Tsakiris DA et al. Transplant-associated microangiopathy (TAM) in recipients of allogeneic hematopoietic stem cell transplants. *Bone Marrow Transplant.* 2005;36:993–1000.

23. Turner D, Schreiber R, Grant D, Hebert D, Sherman PM. Hemolytic uremic syndrome after pediatric liver transplantation. *J Pediatr Gastroenterol Nutr.* 2006;43:109–12.

24. Daly AS, Xenocostas A, Lipton JH. Transplantation-associated thrombotic microangiopathy: 22 years later. *Bone Marrow Transplant.* 2002;30:709–15.

25. Cabrera G, Fortenberry J, Warshaw BL, Chambliss CR, Butler JC, Cooperstone BG. Hemolytic uremic syndrome associated with invasive *Streptococcus pneumoniae* infection. *Pediatrics.* 1998;101:689–703.

26. Cochran JB, Panzarino VM, Maes LY, Tecklenburg FW. Pneumococcal-induced T antigen activation in hemolytic uremic syndrome and anemia. *Pediatr Nephrol.* 2004;19:317–21.

27. Huang DTN, Chi H, Lee HC, Chiu NC, Huang FY. T-antigen activation for prediction of pneumococcus-induced hemolytic uremic syndrome and hemolytic anemia. *Ped. Infect Dis J.* 2006;25:608–10.

28. Simonelli GD, Dumont-Dos Santos K, Pachlopnik JM. Hemolytic uremic syndrome linked to infectious mononucleosis. *Pediatr Nephrol.* 2003;18:1193–94.

29. Medina PJ, Sipolis JM, George JN. Drug-associated thrombotic thrombocytopenic purpura-hemolytic uremic syndrome. *Curr Opin Hematol.* 2001;8:286–93.

30. Melnyk AM, Solez K, Kjellstrand CM. Adult hemolytic-uremic syndrome: A review of 37 cases. *Arch Intern Med.* 1995;155:2077–84.

31. Zipfel PF, Misselwitz J, Licht C, Skerka C. The role of defective complement control in hemolytic uremic syndrome. *Semin Thromb Hemost.* 2006;32:146–54.

32. Zipfel PF, Skerka C. Complement dysfunction in hemolytic uremic syndrome. *Curr Opin Rheumatol.* 2006;18:548–55.

33. Cho HY, Lee BS, Moon KC, Ha IS, Cheong HI et al. Complement factor H deficiency-associted atypical hemolytic uremic syndrome in a neonate. *Pediatr Nephrol.* 2007;22:874–80.

34. Landau D, Shalev H, Levy-Finer G, Polonsky A, Segev Y, Katchko L. Familial hemolytic uremic syndrome associated with complement factor H deficiency. *J Pediatr.* 2001;138:412–17.

35. Noris M, Brioschi S, Caprioli J, Todeschini M, Bresin E et al. Familial haemolytic uraemic syndrome and an MCP mutation. *Lancet.* 2003;362:1542–47.

36. Dragon-Durey MA, Loirat C, Cloarec S, Macher MA, Blouin J et al. Anti-factor H autoantibodies associated with atypical hemolytic uremic syndrome. *J Am Soc Nephrol.* 2005;16:555–63.

37. teLoo DM, Monneus LA, vanDerDelden TJ, Vermerr MA, Preyers F et al. Binding and transfer of verocytotoxin by polymorphonuclear leukocytes in hemolytic uremic syndrome. *Blood.* 2000;95:3396–402.

38. Andreoli SP. The pathophysiology of the hemolytic uremic syndrome. *Curr Opin NephrolHypertens.* 1999:8:459–64.

39. Sassetti B, Vizcarguenaga MI, Zanaro NL, Silva MV, Kordich L, Florentini L et al. Hemolytic uremic syndrome in children: Platelet aggregation and membrane glycoproteins. *J Pediatr Hematol Oncol.* 1999;21:123–28.

40. Proulx F, Seidman EG, Karpman D. Pathogenesis of Shiga toxin-associated hemolytic uremic syndrome. *Pediatr Res.* 2001;50:163–71.

41. Chandler WL, Jelacic S, Boster DR, Ciol MA, Williams GD et al. Prothrombotic coagulation abnormalities preceding the hemolytic-uremic syndrome. *N Engl J Med.* 2002;346:23–32.

42. VonVigier RO, Seibel K, Bianchetti MG. Positive Coombs' test in Pneumococcus-associated hemolytic uremic syndrome. *Nephron.* 1999;82:183–84.

43. Ostronoff M, Ostronoff F, Calixto R, Florencio R, Domingues MC et al. Life-threatening hemolytic-uremic syndrome treated with rituximab in an allogeneic bone marrow transplant recipient. *Bone Marrow Transplant.* 2007;39:649–51.

44. Tazzari PL, Ricci F, Carnecelli D, Caprioli A, Tozzi AE et al. Flow cytometry detection of shiga toxins in the blood from children with hemolytic uremic syndrome. *Cytometry: Part B, Clinical Cytometry.* 2004;61:40–44.

45. MacConnachie AA, Todd WTA. Potential therapeutic agents for the prevention and treatment of heamolytic uraemic syndrome in Shiga toxin producing *Escherichia coli* infection. *Curr Opin Infect Dis.* 2004;17:479–82.

46. Yarranton H, Machin SJ. An update on the pathogenesis and management of acquired thrombotic thrombocytopenic purpura. *Curr Opin Neurol.* 2003;16:367–73.

47. Allford SL, Machin SJ. Current understanding of the pathophysiology of thrombotic thrombocytopenic purpura. *J Clin Pathol.* 2000;53:497–501.

48. Raife TJ, Montgomery RR. vonWillebrand factor and thrombotic thrombocytopenic purpura. *Curr Opin Hematol.* 2000;7:278–83.

49. Zheng X, Majerus EM, Sadler JE. ADAMTS13 and TTP. *Curr Opin Hematol.* 2002;9:389–94.

50. Tsai HM. Deficiency of ADAMTS13 causes thrombotic thrombocytopenic purpura. *Arterioscler Thromb Vasc Biol.* 2003;23:388–96.

51. Veyradier A, Obert B, Houllien A, Meyer D, Girma JP. Specific vonWillebrand factor—cleaving protease in thrombotic microangiopathies: A study of 111 cases. *Blood.* 2001;98:1765–72.

52. Levy GG, Nichols WC, Lian EC, Faroud T, McClintick JN et al. Mutations in a membrane of the ADAMTS gene family cause thrombotic thrombocytopenic purpura. *Nature.* 2001;413:488–94.

53. Tsai HM, Lian EC. Antibodies to vonWillebrand factor-cleaving proteins in acute thrombotic thrombocytopenic purpura. *N Engl J Med.* 1998;339:1585–94.

54. Burns ER, Lou Y, Pathak A. Morphologic diagnosis of thrombotic thrombocytopenic purpura. *Am J Hematol.* 2004;75:18–21.

55. Muncunill J. Thrombotic thrombocytopenic purpura (TTP): Is any plasma useful to treat the TTP? *ISBT Science Series.* 2007;2:233–39.

56. Ziman A, Mitri M, Klapper E, Pepkowitz SH, Goldfinger D. Combination vincristine and plasma exchange as initial therapy in patients with thrombotic thrombocytopenic purpura: One institution's experience and review of literature. *Transfusion.* 2005;45:41–49.

57. Shariatmader S, Nassiri M, Vincek V. Effect of plasma exchange on cytokines measured by multianalyte bead array in thrombotic thrombocytopenic purpura. *Am J Hematol.* 2005;79:83–88.

58. Von Baeyer H. Plasmapheresis in thrombotic microangiopathy-associated syndromes: Review of outcome data derived from clinical trials and open studies. *Therapeutic Apheresis.* 2002;6:320–28.

59. Rock G, Shumak KH, Sutton DMC, Buskard NA, Nair RC. Cryosupernatant as replacement fluid for plasma exchange in thrombotic thrombocytopenic purpura. *Br J Haematol.* 1996;94:383–86.

60. Fakhouri F, Vernant JP, Veyradier A, Wolf M, Kaplanski G et al. Efficiency of curative and prophylactic treatment with rituximab in ADAMTS13-deficient thrombotic thrombocytopenic purpura. *Blood.* 2005;106:1932–37.

61. Levi M, Ten Cate H. Current concepts: Disseminated intravascular coagulation. *N Engl J Med.* 1999;341:586–92.

62. Yu M, Nardella A, Pechet L. Screening tests of disseminated intravascular coagulation: Guidelines for rapid and specific laboratory diagnosis. *Crit Care Med.* 2000;28:1777–80.

63. Hess JR, Lawson JH. The coagulopathy of trauma versus disseminated intravascular coagulation. *J Trauma.* 2006;60:512–19.

64. Levine RJ, Maynard SE, Qian VC, Lim KH, England LJ et al. Circulatory angiogenic factors and the risk of preeclampsia. *N Engl J Med.* 2004;350:672–83.

65. Padden MO. HELLP syndrome: Recognition and perinatal management. *Am Fam Physician.* 1999;60:829–36, 839.

66. Lee RM, Brown MA, Branch W, Ward K, Silver RM. Anticardiolipin and anti-B$_2$-glycoprotein-I antibodies in preeclampsia. *Obstet Gynecol.* 2003;102:294–300.

67. Egerman RS, Sibai BM. HELLP syndrome. *Clin Obstet Gynecol.* 1999; 42:381–89.

68. Stone JH. HELLP syndrome: Hemolysis, elevated liver enzymes, and low platelets. *JAMA.* 1998;280(6):559–62.

69. OBrien JM, Barton JR. Controversies with the diagnosis and management of HELLP syndrome. *Clin Obstet Gynecol.* 2005;48:460–77.

70. Magann EF, Martin JN. Twelve steps to optimal management of HELLP syndrome. *Clin Obstet Gynecol.* 1999;42:532–50.

71. Vigil-DeGarcia P. Addition of platelet transfusions to corticosteroids does not increase the recovery of severe HELLP syndrome. *Eur J Obstet Gynecol Reprod Biol.* 2006;128:194–98.

72. Van Runnard Heimel PJ, Franx A, Schobben AF, Huisjes AJ, Derks JB et al. Corticosteroids, pregnancy, and HELLP Syndrome: A review. *Obstet Gynecol Surv.* 2005;60:57–70.

73. Van den Born BJH, Honnebier UPF, Koopmans RP, van Montfrans GA. Microangiopathic hemolysis and renal failure in malignant hypertension. *Hypertension.* 2005;45:246–51.

74. Mecozzi G, Milano ADF, DeCarlo M, Sorrentino F, Pratali S. Intravascular hemolysis in patients with new-generation prosthetic heart valves: A prospective study. *J Thorac Cardiovasc Surg.* 2002;123:550–56.

75. Gradon JD, Hirschbein M, Milligan J. Fragmentation hemolysis: An unusual indication for valve replacement in native valve infective endocarditis. *South Med J.* 1996;89:818–20.

76. Pratt VC, Tredger EE, Clandnin MT, Field CJ. Fatty acid content of plasma lipids and erythrocyte phospholipids are altered following burn injury. *Lipids.* 2001;36:675–82.

77. Telford RD, Sly GJ, Hahn AG, Cunningham RB, Bryant C, Smith JA. Footstrike is the major cause of Hemolysis during running. *J Appl Physiol.* 2003;94:38–42.

78. Senturk UK, Gunduz F, Kuru O, Kocer G, Ozkaya YG, Yesilkaya A et al. Exercise-induced oxidative stress leads hemolysis in sedentary but not trained humans. *J Appl Physiol.* 2005;99:1434–41.

79. Robinson Y, Cristancho E, Boning D. Intravascular hemolysis and mean red blood cell age in athletes. *Med Sci Sports Exerc.* 2005; 38:480–83.

80. Yusof A, Leithauser RM, Roth HJ, Finkjernagel H, Wilson MT, Beneke R. Exercise-induced hemolysis is caused by protein modification and most evident during the early phase of an ultraendurance race. *Appl Physiol.* 2007;102:582–86.

81. Casals-Pascual C, Roberts DJ. Severe malarial anaemia. *Curr Molec Med.* 2006;6:155–68.

82. Powell VI, Grima K. Exchange transfusion for malaria and babesia infection. *Transfus Med Rev.* 2002;16:239–50.

83. Waitumbi JN, Opollo MO, Muga RO, Misore AO, Stoute JA. Red cell surface changes and erythrophagocytosis in children with severe *Plasmodium falciparum* anemia. *Blood.* 2000;95:1481–86.

84. Vanden Ende J, Coppens G, Verstraeten T, VanHaegenborgh T, Depraetere K et al. Recurrence of blackwater fever: Triggering of relapses by different antimalarials. *Trop Med Int Health.* 1998;3:632–39.

85. Weinberg GA. Laboratory diagnosis of ehrlichiosis and babesiosis. *Pediatr Infect Dis J.* 2001;20:435–38.

86. Krause PJ. Babesiosis diagnosis and treatment. *Vector-Borne and Zoonootic Diseases.* 2003;3:45–51.

87. Dehio C. Molecular and cellular basis of *Bartonella* pathogenesis. *Ann Rev Microbiol.* 2004;58:365–90.

88. Hendrix LR. Contact-dependent hemolytic activity distinct from deforming activity of *Bartonella bacilliformis*. *FEMS Microbiology Letters.* 2000;182:119–24.

89. Caya JG, Truaet AL. Clostridial bacteremia in the non-infant pediatric population: A report of two cases and review of the literature. *Pediatr Infect Dis J.* 1999;18:291–98.

90. Hogan CJ, Barbero KC, Winkel K. Loxoscelism: Old obstacles, new directions. *Ann Emerg Med.* 2004;44:608–24.

91. Hostetler MA, Dribben W, Wilson DB, Grossman WJ. Sudden unexplained hemolysis occurring in an infant due to presumed Loxosceles envenomation. *J Emerg Med.* 2003;25:277–82.

92. Tambourgi DV, Morgan BP, deAndrade RM, Magnoli FC, vanDenBerg CW. Loxosceles intermedia spider envenomation induces activation of an endogenous metalloproteinase, resulting in cleavage of glycophorins from the erythrocyte surface and facilitating complement-mediated lysis. *Blood.* 2000;95:683–91.

93. Boyer LV, Seifert SA, Clark RF, McNally JT, Williams S, Nordt SP et al. Recurrent and persistent coagulopathy following pit viper envenomation. *Arch Int Med.* 1999;159:706–10.

19

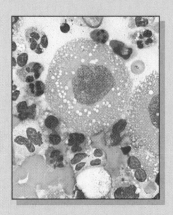

Nonmalignant Granulocyte and Monocyte Disorders

Wanda C. Reygaert, Ph.D.

CHAPTER OUTLINE

■ OBJECTIVES—LEVEL I

At the end of this unit of study, the student should be able to:

1. Recognize neutrophilia from hematologic data and name the common disorders associated with neutrophilia.

2. Explain the quantitative and qualitative neutrophil response to acute bacterial infections.

3. Identify immature granulocytes and morphologic changes (toxic granulation, Döhle bodies, intracellular organisms, and vacuoles) often seen in reactive neutrophilia.

4. Define and recognize *leukemoid reaction, leukoerythroblastosis,* and *pyknotic nuclei.*

5. Distinguish leukemoid reaction from chronic myelogenous leukemia based on laboratory data including the leukocyte alkaline phosphatase stain.

6. Identify neutropenia from hematologic data and list the common disorders associated with neutropenia.

7. Recognize the conditions associated with spurious, or false, neutropenia.

8. Identify neutrophil nuclear alterations including Pelger-Huët, hypersegmentation, and pyknotic forms.

9. Recognize as abnormal and seek assistance for identification of rare or unusual cytoplasmic abnormalities such as morulae, Alder-Reilly granules, or Chédiak-Higashi inclusions.

10. State the common conditions associated with abnormal eosinophil, basophil, and monocyte counts.

11. Define *Gaucher* and *Niemann-Pick diseases.*

■ OBJECTIVES—LEVEL II

At the end of this unit of study, the student should be able to:

1. Assess the etiology, associated conditions, and peripheral blood findings for immediate, acute, chronic, and reactive neutrophilia.

2. Contrast the hematologic and clinical features for leukemoid reaction and chronic myelogenous leukemia (CML).

3. Organize neutropenia to include etiology and associated conditions as well as blood and bone marrow findings.

■ OBJECTIVES—LEVEL II (continued)

4. Recognize, evaluate, and select appropriate corrective action for spurious or false neutropenia.

5. Appraise the nuclear abnormalities of neutrophils including Pelger-Huët, pseudo-Pelger-Huët, hypersegmentation, and pyknotic nuclei, and reconcile them with the appropriate clinical conditions of the patient.

6. Appraise the cytoplasmic abnormalities of neutrophils including toxic granulation, Döhle bodies, vacuoles, intracellular organisms, and morulae and reconcile them with the appropriate clinical conditions of the patient.

7. Recognize and summarize the clinical features of the inherited granulocyte functional disorders (Chédiak-Higashi, Alder-Reilly, May-Hegglin, and chronic granulomatous diseases) and differentiate their cellular abnormalities.

8. Evaluate alterations in the relative and/or absolute numbers of eosinophils, basophils, and monocytes and associate them with the clinical condition of the patient.

9. Evaluate the etiology, laboratory findings, and clinical features of the lysosomal storage disorders.

10. Identify and differentiate the abnormal macrophages seen in Gaucher disease, Niemann-Pick disease, and sea-blue histiocytosis.

11. Construct an efficient and cost-effective reflex testing pathway for follow-up neutrophilia, neutropenia, and qualitative granulocyte abnormalities.

12. Evaluate a case study from a patient with a nonmalignant granulocyte disorder.

KEY TERMS

Agranulocytosis
Basophilia
Döhle bodies
Egress
Eosinophilia
Hypereosinophilic syndrome (HES)
Leukemoid reaction
Leukocytosis
Leukoerythroblastic reaction
Leukopenia
Lysosomal storage disorders
Mastocytosis
Monocytopenia
Monocytosis
Morulae
Myelophthisis
Neutropenia
Neutrophilia
Pelger-Huët anomaly
Pseudoneutrophilia
Reactive neutrophilia
Shift neutrophilia
Shift to the left
Toxic granules

BACKGROUND BASICS

The information in this chapter builds on concepts learned in previous chapters. To maximize your learning experience, you should review this material before starting this unit of study.

Level I

▶ Summarize the production, kinetics, distribution, life span, and basic function of neutrophils and monocytes. (Chapter 7)

▶ Describe how leukocytes are counted and differentiated; recognize normal and immature granulocytes. (Chapter 7)

Level II

▶ Describe the role of specific neutrophil granules and enzymes in antimicrobial systems. (Chapter 7)

▶ Identify normal macrophages and discuss their role in the bone marrow and the rest of the monocyte-macrophage system. (Chapter 7)

▶ Describe leukocyte maturation and proliferation pools in the bone marrow; describe the role of cytokines in bone marrow release of leukocytes; describe the process of leukocyte egress to tissue. (Chapters 3, 7, 4)

▶ Correlate the function of the reticuloendothelial organs to leukocyte distribution and demise. (Chapter 4)

▶ OVERVIEW

This chapter discusses benign changes in granulocytes and monocytes as a response to various nonmalignant disease states and toxic challenges. These changes include both quantitative and qualitative variations that can be detected by laboratory tests. The chapter is divided into sections covering changes in quantity and morphology of neutrophils, eosinophils, basophils, and monocytes in acquired and inherited states. Emphasis is on recognition of these abnormalities by the laboratory professional and correlation to the patient's clinical condition.

▶ INTRODUCTION

It is well recognized that changes in leukocyte concentration and morphology are the body's normal responses to various disease processes and toxic challenges. Most often, one type of leukocyte is affected more than the others, providing an important clue to diagnosis. The type of cell affected depends in a large part on that cell's function (i.e., bacterial infection commonly results in an absolute neutrophilia, viral infections are characterized by an absolute lymphocytosis, and certain parasitic infections cause an eosinophilia). Thus, determination of absolute concentrations of cell types aids in differential diagnosis, especially when the total leukocyte concentration is abnormal.

Leukocytosis refers to a condition in which the total leukocyte count is more than 11.0×10^9/L in an adult. Be aware that reference ranges vary significantly among different sources and laboratories. Refer to Table B on inside cover for leukocyte and differential reference ranges compiled from numerous references.[1–4] Although leukocytosis is usually due to an increase in neutrophils, it may also be related to an increase in lymphocytes or (rarely) in monocytes or eosinophils.

Quantitative variations of different types of leukocytes are evaluated by performing a total leukocyte count and a differential count. The absolute concentration of each type of leukocyte can be calculated from these two values as follows (∞ Chapter 7):

$$\text{Absolute cells/L} = \text{Total leukocyte count/L} \\ \times \text{Percent of cell type from differential}$$

✓ Checkpoint! 1

A patient's total leukocyte count is 5.0×10^9/L. There are 60% segmented neutrophils, 35% lymphocytes, and 5% monocytes on the differential. Calculate the absolute number of each cell type. Is each of these relative and absolute cell counts normal or abnormal?

Leukopenia refers to a decrease in leukocytes below 4.5×10^9/L. This condition is usually due to a decrease in neutrophils, but lymphocytes and other cell types can also contribute.

Morphologic or qualitative variations of leukocytes are noted by examination of the stained blood smear. Some qualitative changes affect cell function while others do not. Variations in the appearance of the cell together with its concentration can provide specific clues to the pathologic process.

▶ NEUTROPHIL DISORDERS

Quantitative disorders of neutrophils are usually reflected by changes in the total leukocyte count because neutrophils are the most numerous white blood cells in the peripheral blood. Automated cell counters flag results outside the reference range. Neutrophilia is more common than neutropenia. On the other hand, automated cell counters do not detect qualitative changes in the neutrophils. Detection of these changes requires careful microscopic examination of stained blood smears. Qualitative changes may provide important diagnostic information.

QUANTITATIVE DISORDERS

Quantitative abnormalities of neutrophils occur because of a malignant or benign disorder. The malignant disorders are caused by neoplastic transformation of hematopoietic stem cells and are discussed in ∞ Chapters 21–26. Benign disorders are usually acquired and may cause an increase (**neutrophilia**) or decrease (**neutropenia**) in neutrophils, but neutrophilia is more common. Table 19-1 lists three interrelated mechanisms affecting neutrophil concentration in the peripheral blood.

Neutrophilia

The normal neutrophil concentration varies with age and race, so it is important to evaluate the count based on reference ranges for each demographic group. *Neutrophilia* refers

Factors Affecting Neutrophil Concentration in Peripheral Blood

- Bone marrow production and release of neutrophils
- Rate of neutrophil egress to tissue or survival time in blood
- Ratio of marginating to circulating neutrophils in peripheral blood

to an increase in the total circulating absolute neutrophil concentration (ANC). In adults, neutrophilia occurs when the ANC of neutrophils exceeds $7.0 \times 10^9/L$. (See Table B on inside cover for age- and race-specific reference ranges.)

Benign neutrophilia occurs most often as a result of a reaction to a physiologic or pathologic process and is called **reactive neutrophilia.** Reactive neutrophilia can be immediate, acute, or chronic and may involve any or all of the three mechanisms listed in Table 19-1.

Immediate Neutrophilia   Immediate neutrophilia can occur without pathologic stimulus and is probably a simple redistribution of the marginated granulocyte pool (MGP) to the circulating granulocyte pool (CGP). Of the neutrophils inside a blood vessel, 50% normally are freely circulating and the other 50% are loosely attached to the vessel endothelial cells (marginated) (∞ Chapter 7). Routine laboratory testing counts only freely circulating cells.

The neutrophil increase in immediate neutrophilia is immediate but transient (lasting about 20–30 minutes) and appears to be independent of bone marrow input and tissue **egress.** This type of neutrophilia is also referred to as **pseudoneutrophilia** or **shift neutrophilia** because no real change in the number of neutrophils within the vasculature occurs. The increased circulating neutrophils are typically mature, normal cells. This redistribution of neutrophils is responsible for the physiologic neutrophilia that accompanies active exercise, epinephrine administration, anesthesia, and anxiety.

Acute Neutrophilia   Acute neutrophilia occurs within 4–5 hours of a pathologic stimulus (e.g., bacterial infection, toxin). This type of neutrophilia results from an increase in the flow of neutrophils from the bone marrow storage pool to the blood. The neutrophilia is more pronounced than in pseudoneutrophilia, and the proportion of immature neutrophils may increase. More bands appear if the tissue demand for neutrophils creates an acute shortage of segmented neutrophils in the storage pool. Continued demand may result in the release of metamyelocytes and myelocytes. As bone marrow production increases and the storage pool is replenished, the leukocyte differential returns to normal.

Chronic Neutrophilia   Chronic neutrophilia follows acute neutrophilia. If the stimulus for neutrophils continues beyond a few days, the storage pool will become depleted. The mitotic pool will then increase production in an at-

tempt to meet the demand for neutrophils. In this state, the marrow shows increased numbers of early neutrophil precursors including myeloblasts, promyelocytes, and myelocytes. The blood contains increased numbers of bands, metamyelocytes, myelocytes, and (rarely) promyelocytes. An increase in the concentration of immature forms of leukocytes in the circulation is termed a **shift to the left.**

Conditions Associated with Neutrophilia

Reactive Chronic Neutrophilia   Chronic neutrophilia caused by benign or toxic conditions usually is characterized by total leukocytes less than $50 \times 10^9/L$ and a shift to the left. The immature cells are usually bands and metamyelocytes, but myelocytes and promyelocytes also may be seen. Toxic changes including toxic granulation, **Döhle bodies** (light grayish-blue cytoplasmic inclusions made up of residual endoplasmic reticulum), and cytoplasmic vacuoles are often found even if the neutrophil count is normal (Figure 19-1 ■). The leukocyte alkaline phosphatase score may be elevated (∞ Chapter 21, 34). Conditions associated with reactive chronic neutrophilia are listed in Table 19-2 ✪.

Bacterial Infection   The most common cause of neutrophilia is bacterial infection, especially with pyrogenic organisms such as staphylococci and streptococci. Depending on the virulence of the microorganism, extent of infection, and response of the host, the neutrophil count may range from $7.0 \times 10^9/L$ to $70 \times 10^9/L$. Usually, the count is in the range of $10–25 \times 10^9/L$. As the demand for neutrophils at the site of infection increases, the early response of the bone marrow is to increase output of storage neutrophils to the peripheral blood, causing a shift to the left. The inflow of neutrophils from the bone marrow to the blood continues until it exceeds the neutrophil outflow to the tissues, caus-

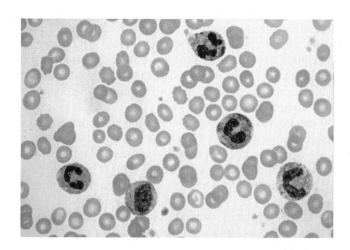

■ FIGURE 19-1   A leukemoid reaction. There is an increased leukocyte count and a shift to the left. The cells have heavy toxic granulation and Döhle bodies suggesting an infectious or toxic reactive leukocytosis. (Peripheral blood; Wright-Giemsa stain; 1000× magnification)

⊕ TABLE 19-2

Conditions Associated with Neutrophilia

Acute bacterial and fungal infections

Inflammatory processes:

    Tissue damage from burns, trauma, or surgery

    Collagen, vascular, and autoimmune disorders

    Hypersensitivity reactions

Metabolic alterations: uremia, eclampsia, and gout

Neoplasms

Acute hemorrhage or hemolysis

Rebound from bone marrow transplant or treatment with colony-stimulating growth factors

Certain chemicals, toxins, and drugs

Physiologic neutrophilia:

    Strenuous exercise, stress, pain, temperature extremes, childbirth labor, and in newborns

Chronic myeloproliferative disorders*

*In these disorders, increases in neutrophils are not reactive but due to a neoplasm of the hematopoietic stem cell.

ing an absolute neutrophilia. In very severe infections, the storage pool of neutrophils may become exhausted, the mitotic pool may be unable to keep up with the demand, and a neutropenia develops. Neutropenia in overwhelming infection is a very poor prognostic sign. Chronic bacterial infection may lead to chronic stimulation of the marrow whereby the production of neutrophils remains high and a new steady state of production develops.

Neutrophilia is neither a unique nor an absolute finding in bacterial infections. Infections with other organisms such as fungi, rickettsia, spirochetes, and parasites also may cause a neutrophilia. Certain bacterial infections are characterized by neutropenia rather than neutrophilia. In a few types of infection such as whooping cough, lymphocytosis rather than neutrophilia is typical.[5] Viral infections, although typically accompanied by a lymphocytosis, may present with neutrophilia early in their course.

ⓔ CASE STUDY *(continued from page 385)*

Laboratory results on Dennis, the trauma patient, two days after surgery are as follows:

                  WBC Differential

WBC: 14.5 × 10⁹/L   Segmented neutrophils: 5%

HGB: 12.9 g/dL (129 g/L) Band neutrophils: 50%

PLT: 180 × 10⁹/L   Lymphocytes: 40%

                  Monocytes: 5%

Urine, blood, and wound cultures were ordered.

1. What results, if any, are abnormal?

2. What is the most likely reason for these results?

Tissue Destruction/Injury, Inflammation, Metabolic Disorders Conditions other than infection that can result in a neutrophilia include tissue necrosis, inflammation, certain metabolic conditions, and drug intoxication. All of these conditions produce neutrophilia by increasing neutrophil input from the bone marrow in response to increased egress to the tissue. Examples of these conditions include rheumatoid arthritis, tissue infarctions, burns, neoplasms, trauma, uremia, and gout.

Although defenders of the body, leukocytes are also responsible for a significant part of the continuing inflammatory process. Damaged tissue releases cytokines that act as chemotactins, causing neutrophils to leave the vessels and move toward the injury site. In gout, for example, deposits of uric acid crystals in joints attract neutrophils to the area. In the process of phagocytosis and death, the leukocytes release toxic intracellular enzymes (granules) and oxygen metabolites. These toxic substances mediate the inflammatory process by injuring other body cells and propagating the formation of chemotactic factors that attract more leukocytes.

Leukemoid Reaction Extreme neutrophilic reactions to severe infections or necrotizing tissue may produce a **leukemoid reaction** (Figure 19-1). A leukemoid reaction is a benign leukocyte proliferation characterized by a total leukocyte count usually greater than 50×10^9/L with many circulating immature leukocyte precursors. In a neutrophilic-leukemoid reaction, the blood contains many bands and metamyelocytes, increased myelocytes and promyelocytes, and (rarely) blasts.

Leukemoid reactions may produce a blood picture indistinguishable from that of chronic myelocytic leukemia. (∞ Chapter 22) If the diagnosis cannot be made by routine hematologic parameters, genetic studies, molecular analysis, and leukocyte alkaline phosphatase (LAP) stain scores may be helpful (Table 19-3 ⊕). Contrary to leukemia, a leukemoid reaction is transient, disappearing when the inciting stimulus is removed. A leukemoid reaction may be seen in chronic infections (such as tuberculosis); carcinoma of the lung, stomach, breast, or liver and other inflammatory processes.[6]

✓ Checkpoint! 2

How can CML be distinguished from a leukemoid reaction?

Leukoerythroblastic Reaction **Leukoerythroblastic reaction** (Figure 19-2■) is characterized by the presence of nucleated erythrocytes and a neutrophilic shift to the left in the peripheral blood. The total neutrophil count may be increased, decreased, or normal. Often, erythrocytes in this condition exhibit poikilocytosis with teardrop shapes and anisocytosis. Leukoerythroblastosis is most often associated with chronic neoplastic myeloproliferative conditions, especially myelofibrosis, **myelophthisis** (replacement of normal

✪ TABLE 19-3

Comparison of Laboratory Results in Leukemoid Reactions and Chronic Myelocytic Leukemia (CML)

	Leukemoid Reaction	CML
Leukocyte count	Increased up to 50×10^9/L	Markedly increased (usually >50.0 $\times 10^9$/L)
Leukocyte differential	Shift to the left with bands, metamyelocytes, and myelocytes; neutrophil toxic changes	Shift to the left with immature cells including promyelocytes and blasts; increased eosinophils and basophils
Erythrocyte count	Normal	Often decreased
Platelets	Usually normal	Increased or decreased
LAP	Increased	Decreased
Philadelphia chromosome	Absent	Present
BCR/ABL mutation	Absent	Present
Clinical	Related to primary condition	Systemic (splenomegaly, enlarged nodes, bone pain)

LAP: leukocyte alkaline phosphatase

hematopoietic tissue in the bone marrow by fibrosis, leukemia, or metastatic cancer cells), and severe hemolytic anemias such as Rh hemolytic disease of the fetus and newborn (HDFN). (∞ Chapter 17).

Stimulated Bone Marrow States   When the bone marrow is stimulated to produce erythrocytes in response to hemorrhage or hemolysis, neutrophils may also become caught up in the process, resulting in neutrophilia and a slight shift to the left. Patients whose bone marrow has been stimulated by hematopoietic growth factor hormones such as granulocyte/monocyte colony-stimulating factor (GM-CSF) can demonstrate rapidly increasing total white cell counts and leukocyte precursors including blasts. Growth

cytokines are used to replenish leukocytes after bone marrow transplant, high-dose chemotherapy, bone marrow failure, or prior to autologous blood donation or stem cell apheresis[7] (∞ Chapter 27).

Corticosteroid therapy produces a neutrophilia that occurs as a result of increased bone marrow output accompanied by a decreased migration of neutrophils to the tissues (by inhibition of the ability of neutrophils to adhere to vessel walls). This inhibition of neutrophil migration to the tissues may in part explain the increased incidence of bacterial infections in patients on steroid therapy even though the blood neutrophil count is increased. Steroids also decrease the number and inhibit the function of monocytes/macrophages.[8]

Physiologic Leukocytosis   Physiologic leukocytosis and neutrophilia are present at birth and for the first few days of life (Table B inside cover). The leukocytosis can be accompanied by a slight shift to the left. Physiologic stress including exposure to extreme temperatures, emotional stimuli, exercise, and labor during delivery can cause neutrophilia generally without a shift to the left.

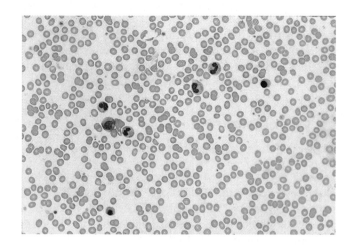

■ FIGURE 19-2   A leukoerythroblastic reaction. There are nucleated erythrocytes and a shift to the left with band neutrophils and a myelocyte. (Peripheral blood; Wright-Giemsa stain; 500× magnification)

✓ Checkpoint! 3

What is the difference between a leukemoid reaction and a leuko-erythroblastic reaction?

Neutropenia

Neutropenia occurs when the neutrophil count falls below 1.5–2.0 $\times 10^9$/L (varies with ethnic group). **Agranulocytosis,** a term that refers to a neutrophil count below 0.5 $\times 10^9$/L, is associated with high probability of infection.

Basophils and eosinophils are also commonly depleted in severe neutropenia.

True neutropenia may occur because of (1) decreased bone marrow production, (2) increased cell loss (due to immune destruction or increased neutrophil egress to the tissue), or (3) pseudoneutropenia (increased neutrophilic margination). Spurious, or false, neutropenia can result from neutrophil agglutination, disintegration and laboratory instrument problems. (See Table 19-4 ✪ for the most common causes.)

Decreased Bone Marrow Production   Neutropenia may develop as a result of decreased bone marrow production. In this case, the bone marrow shows myeloid hypoplasia, and the M:E ratio is decreased. With defective production, the bone marrow storage pool is decreased, neutrophil egress to tissues is decreased, and both the peripheral blood circulating pool and the marginal pool decrease. Immature cells may enter the blood in an attempt to alleviate the neutrophil shortage. Cells younger than bands, however, are less efficient in phagocytosis. The end result is a lack of neutrophils at inflammatory sites, resulting in a huge risk for overwhelming infections.

Stem Cell Disorders.   Decreased bone marrow production may occur with stem cell failure such as aplastic anemia, radiotherapy, or chemotherapy, or with infiltration of hematopoietic tissue by malignant cells (myelophthisis). Of new leukemia cases, 40% present with a total white count of $<10 \times 10^9$/L.[9] This occurs when normal precursor cells in the bone marrow are replaced, but the malignant cells have not yet egressed to the peripheral blood in significant numbers.

Megaloblastic Anemia.   Neutropenia is a characteristic finding in megaloblastic anemia (∞ Chapter 12) and myelodysplastic syndromes (∞ Chapter 23). In these cases, however, the marrow is usually hyperplastic. Neutropenia results not from marrow failure but from the abnormal myeloid cells being destroyed before release to the blood (ineffective granulopoiesis).

Chemicals/Drugs.   A wide variety of drugs and chemicals is associated with leukopenia and neutropenia if given in sufficient dosage (Table 19-4). Chemotherapy and radiation treatments for cancer are a common cause of neutropenia. Pancytopenia from decreased bone marrow production of granulocytes predisposes patients with malignancies to frequent and serious infections. Chemotherapy drugs act to cause apoptosis of dividing cells by a variety of mechanisms including direct DNA damage, altering folate receptors, or inhibiting enzymes needed for mitosis. Because blood cell precursors in the bone marrow are also actively dividing, their proliferation is inhibited as well. Prophylactic use of antibiotics and GM-CSF have reduced mortality in patients receiving chemotherapy, but infections due to neutropenia remain a serious complication.[7,10] Drug-induced neutropenia can also be caused by allergic (immunologic) reactions to drugs. Women, older patients, and patients with a history of allergies are more often affected.[11]

Congenital Neutropenia.   Several rare inherited disorders cause neutropenia related to decreased bone marrow production. Periodic or cyclic neutropenia is a curious form of neutropenia that begins in infancy or childhood and occurs in regular 21- to 30-day cycles. It is believed to be inherited as an autosomal dominant trait with variable expression.[12] The severely neutropenic period lasts for several days and is marked by frequent infections. Between the neutropenic attacks, the patient is asymptomatic. Severe congenital neutropenia (SCN) is a rare, often fatal autosomal recessive disorder marked by extreme neutropenia (less than 0.5×10^9/L). The total leukocyte count is often in the normal range. The basic mechanism underlying this disorder is unknown, but studies have focused on the responsiveness of neutrophil precursors to the hematopoietic growth factor G-CSF.[13] Familial neutropenia is a rare benign anomaly characterized by an absolute decrease in neutrophils but usually a normal total leukocyte count. It is transmitted as an autosomal dominant trait and is usually detected by chance. (See Table 19-5 ✪ for a more complete list of congenital neutropenic disorders.[11,14])

Increased Cell Loss   Neutropenia may occur as the result of increased neutrophil diapedesis (passage of white cells through blood vessel walls into extravascular tissue). In severe or early infection, the bone marrow may not produce cells as rapidly as they are being utilized, resulting in neutropenia. Various viral, bacterial, rickettsial, and protozoal infections induce tissue damage, increasing the demand and destruction of neutrophils. Neutropenia resulting from severe infections is often accompanied by marked toxic changes to the granulocytes. Prognosis in these cases is very poor due to the organisms prevailing over the body's immune system.

✪ TABLE 19-4

Causes of Leukopenia and/or Neutropenia

Infections, especially viral and overwhelming bacterial such as sepsis

Physical agents and chemicals (e.g., radiation and benzene)

Drugs: chemotherapy, certain drugs in the classes of sedatives, anti-inflammatory, antibacterial, antithyroid, and antihistamines*

Hematologic disorders:

    Acute leukemia

    Megaloblastic and aplastic anemia

    Splenomegaly

Alloantibodies or autoantibodies (e.g., systemic lupus erythematosus [SLE])

Hereditary or congenital disorders

*See *Wintrobe's Clinical Hematology*, 11th ed., Chapter 63, for a more complete list of drugs associated with neutropenia.

⊗ TABLE 19-5

Congenital Neutropenic Disorders

Disorder	Inheritance
Disorders of production	
Cyclic neutropenia	AD
Familial neutropenia	AD
Fanconi pancytopenia	AR
Reticular dysgenesis	AR
Severe congenital neutrophilia	AD, AR
Wiskott-Aldrich syndrome	XLR
Disorders of RNA synthesis and processing	
Cartilage-hair hypoplasia	AR
Dyskeratosis congenital	XLR, AD, AR
Shwachman-Diamond syndrome	AR
Disorders of metabolism	
Barth syndrome	XLR
Glycogen Sotrage disease, Type 1b	AR
Pearson's syndrome	Mitochondral
Disorders of vesicular transport	
Chédiak-Higashi syndrome	AR
Cohen syndrome	AR
Griscelli syndrome, Type II	AR
Hermansky-Pudlak syndrome, Type II	AR
p14 Deficiency	AR

AD: autosomal dominant, AR: autosomal recessive, XLR: X-linked recessive

Immune Neutropenia. Antibodies directed against neutrophil-specific antigens (NA) may cause a decrease in the number of neutrophils. Leukocytes are destroyed in a manner similar to erythrocytes in immune hemolytic anemia (∞ Chapter 17). In some cases, drugs precipitate an immunologic response accompanied by the sudden disappearance of cells from the circulation. The immunologic mechanism may include direct cell lysis or sensitization and subsequent sequestration in the spleen.[12] The two types of immune neutropenia are alloimmune and autoimmune.

Alloimmune neonatal neutropenia occurs when there is transplacental transfer of maternal alloantibodies directed against antigens on the infant's neutrophils (the infant's antigens are of paternal origin). Affected infants may develop infections until the neutropenia is resolved, usually in a few weeks. This immune process is similar to that found in Rh hemolytic disease of the fetus and newborn except that the firstborn child can be affected. Alloimmune neutropenia can also be the result of a transfusion reaction.

Two forms of autoimmune neutropenia (AIN) are recognized: primary and secondary. Primary AIN is not associated with other diseases. It develops as antibody-coated neu-

trophils are sequestered and destroyed by the spleen. This condition of unknown etiology occurs predominantly in young children who subsequently develop fever and recurrent infections. Spontaneous remission usually occurs after a period of 13–20 months. Secondary autoimmune neutropenia is generally found in older patients, many of whom have been diagnosed with another autoimmune disorder such as systemic lupus erythrematosus (SLE) or rheumatoid arthritis. In the secondary form of AIN, the antineutrophil antibodies are not the only cause of the neutropenia, and the actual target of the antibodies is not known.[15]

Infections associated with autoimmune neutropenia are not usually life threatening and are treated with routine antibiotic therapy. Intravenous doses of immunoglobulin may be used in severe cases. Laboratory findings are variable. The total leukocyte count may range from normal to decreased, but the neutrophil count is often quite low. GM-CSF is usually given when the neutrophil count is $<1.0 \times 10^9$/L. Immune neutropenia can be confirmed by testing for antineutrophil antibodies or neutrophil surface antigens by various methods including agglutination tests, immunofluorescense, and enzyme-linked immunosorbent assay (ELISA). The availability of these complex tests varies widely among laboratories.[16]

Hypersplenism. Hypersplenism may result in a selective splenic culling of neutrophils producing mild neutropenia. The bone marrow in this case exhibits neutrophilic hyperplasia. Thrombocytopenia and (occasionally) anemia may also accompany hypersplenism.

Pseudoneutropenia Pseudoneutropenia is similar to pseudoneutrophilia in that it is produced by alterations in the circulating and marginated pools. Pseudoneutropenia results from the transfer of an increased proportion of circulating neutrophils to the marginal neutrophil pool with no change in the total peripheral blood pool. This temporary shift is characteristic of some infections with endotoxin production and of hypersensitivity. Because of the selective margination of neutrophils, the total leukocyte count drops and a relative lymphocytosis develops.

Spurious, or False, Neutropenia It is important for the laboratory professional to recognize when neutropenia is a result of laboratory *in vitro* manipulations of blood. Table 19-6 ⊗ summarizes four *in vitro* causes of a low neutrophil count:

1. Neutrophils may (rarely) adhere to erythrocytes when the blood is drawn in EDTA, causing an erroneously low automated white count. If observed on the stained smears, blood can be recollected by fingerstick to make manual dilutions and blood smears without utilizing EDTA.

2. Neutrophils disintegrate over time faster than other leukocytes. If there is a delay in testing the blood, the neutrophil count may be erroneously decreased.

3. In some pathologic conditions, the leukocytes are more fragile than normal and may rupture with the manipulations of preparing blood for testing in the laboratory.

TABLE 19-6

Causes of False Low Neutrophil Counts in Clinical Laboratory Testing

- EDTA induced neutrophil adherence to erythrocytes
- Disintegration of neutrophils over time prior to testing
- Disruption of abnormally fragile leukocytes during preparation of the blood for testing
- Neutrophil aggregation

4. The neutrophil count may be falsely decreased if the neutrophils clump together as occurs in the presence of some paraproteins.

✓ Checkpoint! 4

How can the correct white cell count be determined when neutrophils clump in the presence of EDTA?

QUALITATIVE OR MORPHOLOGIC ABNORMALITIES OF NEUTROPHILS

Automated cell counters do not detect or flag morphologic abnormalities of neutrophils. Abnormalities are identified only by observation of cells on stained blood smears. Cytoplasmic abnormalities are more common than nuclear abnormalities. Most of these cytoplasmic changes (Döhle bodies, toxic granulation, and vacuoles) are reactive transient changes accompanying infectious states. The correct identification of alterations such as intracellular microorganisms can lead to the prompt diagnosis and treatment of life-threatening infections. Recognizing Pelger-Huët or hypersegmented neutrophils can point to the diagnosis of specific conditions that may prove elusive without the morphologic information.

Nuclear Abnormalities

Pelger-Huët   **Pelger-Huët anomaly** (Figure 19-3 ■) is a benign anomaly inherited in an autosomal dominant fashion and occurring in about 1 in 5000 individuals. The neutrophil nucleus does not segment beyond the two-lobed stage and may also appear round with no segmentation. The presence of excessive coarse clumping of chromatin in the nucleus aids in the differentiation of bilobed cells from true bands. The bilobed nucleus has a characteristic dumbbell shape with the two lobes connected by a thin strand of chromatin. Cells with this appearance are often called *"pince-nez"* cells. Rod-shaped and peanut-shaped nuclei are also found. The cell is functionally normal. The significance of recognizing this anomaly lies in differentiating the benign hereditary defect from a shift to the left occurring with infections.

Acquired, or pseudo, Pelger-Huët anomaly can be seen in myeloproliferative disorders and myelodysplastic states. The

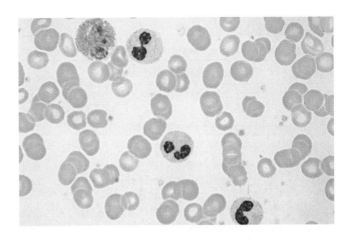

■ **FIGURE 19-3**   Pelger-Huët anomaly. Note pince-nez, or eyeglass-shaped, nuclei. These mature cells could easily be confused for bands if not for the highly clumped chromatin. (Peripheral blood; Wright-Giemsa stain; 1000× magnification)

acquired form is frequently accompanied by hypogranulation because of a lack of secondary granules, and the nuclei acquire a round rather than a dumbbell shape. The chromatin shows intense clumping, aiding in differentiation of these mononuclear cells from myelocytes.

Hypersegmentation   Larger-than-normal neutrophils with six or more nuclear segments (hypersegmented neutrophils) are a common and early indicator of megaloblastic anemia. These cells are found together with pancytopenia and macro ovalocytes that typically accompany deficiencies of folate or vitamin B_{12} (∞ Chapter 12). Rarely reported cases of hereditary hypersegmentation of neutrophils, a benign condition, are significant only by their need to be distinguished from multilobed nuclei that are associated with disease.[17]

Pyknotic Nucleus   Pyknotic, or degenerating, nuclei (Figure 19-4 ■) are found in dying neutrophils in blood or

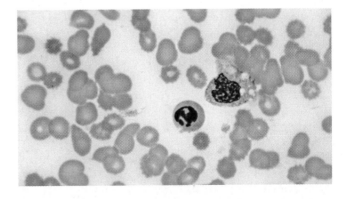

■ **FIGURE 19-4**   In the center is a dying cell with a pyknotic nucleus. Note the smooth nuclear material that is breaking up. Above this cell is a band neutrophil with vacuoles and toxic granulation. (Peripheral blood; Wright-Giemsa stain; 1000× magnification)

✪ TABLE 19-7

Cytoplasmic Inclusions Found in Neutrophils in Infectious Conditions

Inclusion	Morphologic Characteristics	Composition	Associated Conditions
Döhle body	Light gray-blue oval near cell periphery	Rough endoplasmic reticulum (RNA)	Infections, burns, cancer, toxic, or inflammatory states
Toxic granules	Large blue-black granules	Primary granules	Same as Döhle body
Cytoplasmic vacuole	Clear, unstained circular area	Open spaces from phagocytosis	Same as Döhle body
Bacteria	Small basophilic rods or cocci	Phagocytized organisms	Bacteremia or sepsis
Fungi	Round or oval basophilic inclusions slightly larger than bacteria	Phagocytized fungal organisms	Systemic fungal infections often in immunosuppressed patients
Morulae	Basophilic, granular; irregularly shaped	Clusters of *Ehrlichia* rickettsial organisms	Ehrlichiosis

body fluid preparations. The nuclear chromatin condenses and the segments disappear, becoming smooth, dark-staining spheres. If the nucleus is round, these necrotic cells may be confused with nucleated erythrocytes.[18]

✓ Checkpoint! 5

Describe the difference between hypersegmented and hyposegmented neutrophils and pyknotic nuclei. In what conditions is each seen?

Cytoplasmic Abnormalities

Cytoplasmic inclusions are often found in infectious states and, when present, give important diagnostic information to the health care provider (Table 19-7 ✪). These inclusions are Döhle bodies, toxic granules, vacuoles, and intracellular organisms.

Döhle Bodies   Döhle bodies are light gray-blue inclusions in the cytoplasm of neutrophils and eosinophils (Figure 19-5 ■). Found near the periphery of the cell, Döhle bodies are composed of aggregates of rough endoplasmic

reticulum. They may be seen in severe infections, burns and cancer, and as a result of toxic drugs. Döhle bodies should be looked for whenever toxic granulation or other reactive morphologic changes are present because they frequently occur together. Döhle bodies are similar in appearance to the cytoplasmic inclusions found in May-Hegglin anomaly.

Toxic Granules   Toxic granules are large, deep, blue-black primary granules in the cytoplasm of segmented neutrophils and sometimes in bands and metamyelocytes (Figure 19-6 ■). Primary (nonspecific) granules normally lose their basophilia as the cell matures, so even though about one-third of the granules in the mature neutrophil are primary granules, their presence is not detectable. In contrast, toxic primary granules retain their basophilia in the mature neutrophil, perhaps because of a lack of maturation. Also, primary granules may become more apparent as the secondary granules are discharged, fighting bacteria. Toxic granulation is seen in the same conditions as Döhle bodies. Toxic-like granules or inclusions can appear as artifacts with

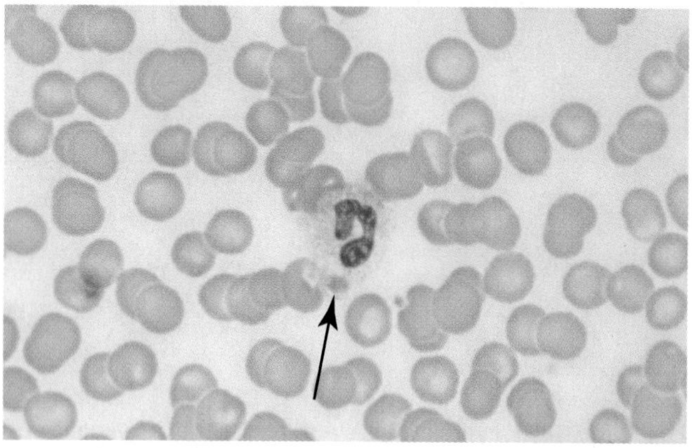

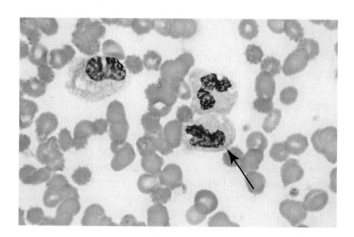

■ FIGURE 19-5   A band neutrophil with a large bluish inclusion (Döhle body). (Peripheral blood; Wright-Giemsa stain; 1000× magnification)

■ FIGURE 19-6   PMNs and a band neutrophil with vacuoles, toxic granulation. There are also Döhle bodies in the center cell, but they are difficult to see. (Peripheral blood; Wright-Giemsa stain; 1000× magnification)

increased staining time or decreased pH of the buffer used in the staining process.

Cytoplasmic Vacuoles   Cytoplasmic vacuoles appear as clear, unstained areas. Vacuoles probably represent the end stage of phagocytosis (Figure 19-6). They are usually seen in the same conditions as toxic granulation and Döhle bodies. Cytoplasmic vacuoles in neutrophils from a fresh specimen correlate highly with the presence of septicemia.

Vacuoles may also appear as an artifact in blood smears made from blood that has been collected and stored in EDTA. Vacuoles related to storage are more likely to be smaller and more uniformly dispersed than those in toxic states. This artifact can be eliminated by making smears from fresh blood without anticoagulant.

ⓔ CASE STUDY (continued from page 387)

All cultures were negative for bacteria and fungi. On further examination of the blood smear, it was noted that *no abnormal cytoplasmic features* were observed in the neutrophils. However, the nuclei of most of the bands appeared more condensed than normal, and many had two lobes in a dumbbell shape.

3. Given the leukocyte morphology and cultures, what additional condition must now be considered?

4. Explain the clinical significance of the nuclear anomaly described in this patient.

5. Why is the white cell count elevated?

Intracellular Organisms   In most infections, including septicemia, the causative agents are not demonstrable in the peripheral blood. However, microorganisms seen inside of neutrophils should always be considered a significant finding, and the physician should be notified immediately (Figure 19-7 ■).

Bacteria/Fungi.   Intracellular histoplasmosis or *Candida* are sometimes found in the blood of patients with HIV or other severe immunosuppression. Organisms found outside of cells must be interpreted with care. On stained blood smears, it is crucial to distinguish whether the microorganisms came from contaminated equipment or stain or are actually present in the patient's blood. Organisms must also be distinguished from other cytoplasmic material and precipitated stain. All bacteria and yeasts stain basophilic with Wright's stain.

Ehrlichia sp. has become a significant tick-borne pathogen in humans over the last decade. Ehrlichiosis was first described in a human in the United States in 1986. The disease is characterized by high fever, leukopenia, thrombocytopenia, and elevated liver enzymes. Most cases of ehrlichiosis occur in April through September when nymphal ticks are most active. *Ehrlichia* sp. are small, obligate intracellular, coccobacilli bacteria. They infect leukocytes, where they multiply within phagosomes. The intracellular organisms are pleomorphic, appearing as basophilic, condensed, or loose aggregates of rickettsial organisms, which tend to appear spherical. The intracellular microcolonies of *Ehrlichia*, called **morulae,** are observed in leukocytes on stained blood films (Figure 19-8 ■). The presence of morulae in leukocytes may be the first diagnostic finding of *Ehrlichia*. The leukocyte eventually ruptures and releases the organisms that then infect other leukocytes. In the United States, two known species of *Ehrlichia* infect humans. *E. chaffeensis* infects monocytes and is the causative agent of human monocytic ehrlichiosis (HME). *E. ewingii* infects granulocytes and is the causative agent of human granulocytic ehrlichiosis (HGE). The pathogenesis of ehrlichiosis may be related to direct cellular injury by the bacteria or a cascade of inflammatory or immune events.

Confirmation of infection is made through serologic determination of antibody titers using indirect fluorescent antibody (IFA) assays or by identification of DNA sequences by polymerase chain reaction (PCR). Peripheral blood cytopenia is probably the result of sequestration of infected cells in the

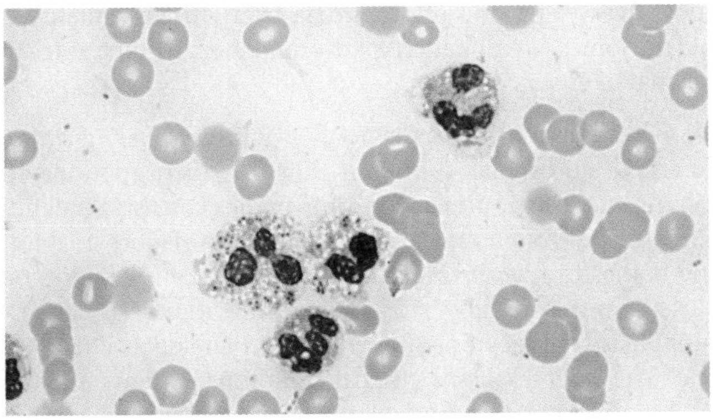

■ FIGURE 19-7   Intracellular microorganisms. Note the vacuoles and toxic granulation in the cells. (Peripheral blood; Wright-Giemsa stain; 1000× magnification)

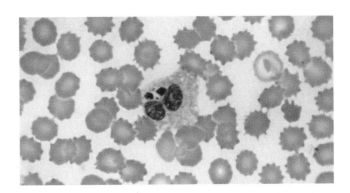

■ FIGURE 19-8   Morulae in ehrlichiosis. This segmented neutrophil from a patient with human granulocytic ehrlichiosis contains two dense, basophilic inclusions called *morulae*. (Peripheral blood; Wright-Giemsa stain; 1000× magnification)

✪ TABLE 19-8

Inherited Qualitative Neutrophil Abnormalities

Condition	Morphologic or Functional Defect	Clinical Features
Alder-Reilly anomaly	Large, dark cytoplasmic granules in all leukocytes; cells function normally	Associated with mucopolysaccharidosis such as Hurler's syndrome
Chédiak-Higashi syndrome	Giant fused granules in neutrophils and lymphs; cells engulf but do not kill microorganisms	Serious, often fatal condition with repeated pyrogenic infections
May-Hegglin anomaly	Blue, Döhle-like cytoplasmic inclusions in all granulocytes; cells function normally	Bleeding tendency from associated thrombocytopenia
Chronic granulomatous disease (CGD)	Defective respiratory burst; cells engulf but don't kill microorganisms	Recurrent infections especially in childhood
Myeloperoxidase deficiency	Low or absent myeloperoxidase enzyme; cell morphology normal	Usually benign; other bactericidal systems prevent most infections
Leukocyte adhesion deficiency (LAD)	Absence of cell-surface adhesion proteins affecting multiple cell functions; cell morphology normal	Serious condition with recurrent infections and high mortality

spleen, liver, and lymph nodes. The bone marrow is usually hypercellular.[19,20]

Inherited Functional Abnormalities

Functional neutrophil abnormalities are almost always inherited and can be accompanied by morphologic abnormalities. It is suggested that granulocyte functional abnormalities be suspected in patients with recurrent, severe infections, abscesses, delayed wound healing and in antibiotic resistant sepsis. Table 19-8 ✪ summarizes the functional defects and their clinical features.

Alder-Reilly Anomaly Alder-Reilly anomaly is an inherited condition characterized by the presence of large purplish granules in the cytoplasm of all leukocytes in disorders such as Hurler's syndrome and Hunter's syndrome. (Figure 19-9 ■). These disorders are lysosomal storage disorders (more on these later in this chapter) in which the accumulated substrates in the lysosomes are mucopolysaccharides.[21]

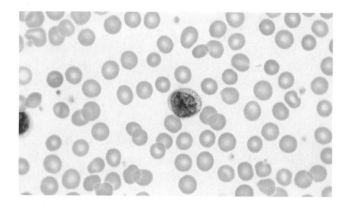

The granules can be distinguished from toxic granulation by their staining metachromatically with toluidine blue. These inclusions in lymphocytes tend to occur in clusters in the shape of dots or commas and are surrounded by vacuoles (Gasser's cells). The inclusions frequently are seen only in cells of the bone marrow, not in the peripheral blood. The blood cells function normally.

Chédiak-Higashi Syndrome Chédiak-Higashi syndrome is a rare autosomal recessive disorder in which death usually occurs in infancy or childhood because of recurrent bacterial infections (Figure 19-10 ■). Giant gray-green peroxidase-positive bodies and giant lysosomes are found in the cytoplasm of leukocytes as well as most granule-containing cells of other tissues. These bodies are formed by fusion of primary nonspecific and secondary specific neutrophilic granules. This abnormal fusion of cytoplasmic membranes prevents the granules from being delivered into the phagosomes to participate in killing of ingested bacteria. Neutropenia and thrombocytopenia are frequent complications as the disease progresses. The patients have skin hypopigmentation, silvery hair, and photophobia from an abnormality of melanosomes. Lymphadenopathy and hepatosplenomegaly are characteristic.[22]

May-Hegglin Anomaly May-Hegglin anomaly is a rare, inherited, autosomal dominant trait in which granulocytes contain inclusions similar to Döhle bodies consisting mainly of RNA from rough endoplasmic reticulum (Figure 19-11 ■). The bodies can be distinguished from true Döhle bodies because they are usually larger and more round in shape.[23] Variable thrombocytopenia with giant platelets is characteristic. The only apparent clinical symptom patients may exhibit is abnormal bleeding related to the low platelet count.

Chronic Granulomatous Disease Chronic granulomatous disease (CGD) is an inherited disorder (65% X-linked, the rest AR)[24] characterized by defects in the respi-

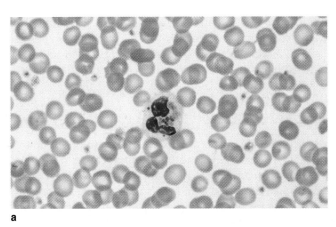
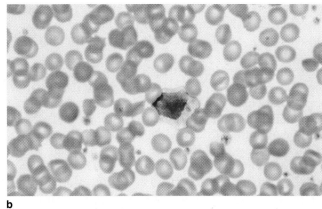

a   b

■ **FIGURE 19-10** **a.** Neutrophil from Chédiak-Higashi syndrome. **b.** Lymphocyte from the same patient as in a. Note the bluish-gray inclusion bodies. (Peripheral blood; Wright-Giemsa stain; 1000× magnification)

ratory burst oxidase system. The affected cells cannot generate antimicrobial oxygen metabolites, such as H_2O_2. The morphology of the neutrophil is normal. Affected children suffer from recurrent infections with opportunistic pathogens that result in granuloma formation. Although CGD is an inherited disorder, the onset of symptoms may not occur until early adulthood. The abnormal neutrophils can phagocytize the microorganisms but cannot kill them. Catalase-positive microorganisms are not killed because they are capable of destroying the H_2O_2 of their own metabolism. They continue to grow intracellularly where they are protected from antibiotics. Catalase-negative organisms, however, kill themselves by generating H_2O_2, which they cannot break down.[25]

The peripheral blood neutrophil count is normal but increases in the presence of infection. Immunoglobulin levels are often increased due to chronic infection.[23] Treatment involves the use of prophylactic antibiotics and early treatment of infections.

The nitroblue tetrazolium slide test (NBT) is useful in detecting the abnormal oxygen metabolism of neutrophils in CGD. Neutrophils are mixed with nitroblue tetrazolium and microorganisms. In normal individuals, the leukocytes phagocytize the microorganisms, initiating an increase in oxygen uptake. This process leads to an accumulation of oxygen metabolites that reduce the NBT to a blue-black compound, which shows up in the cell as dark crystals. Neutrophils from individuals with CGD cannot mobilize a respiratory burst, so no dark crystals are seen.[25]

The dihydrorhodamine 123 (DHR123) assay using flow cytometry is replacing the NBT test in some laboratories. In the DHR123 assay (also referred to as the *neutrophil oxidative burst assay*), granulocytes are incubated with bacteria and the dye DHR123.[26] After the neutrophils phagocytize the bacteria, they activate the NADP oxidase and produce the reactive oxygen metabolites (respiratory burst). These metabolites oxidize the DHR123 to fluorescent rhodamine 123, which is detected by flow cytometry. The mean fluorescence intensity (MFI) of control granulocytes (unstimulated) and of the bright population of stimulated granulocytes is calculated. The ratio between these two populations, called the *stimulation coefficient,* can be used to compare the respiratory burst between blood samples. In healthy adults, the reference interval for granulocytes with phagocytic activity is 80–100%.

Myeloperoxidase Deficiency Myeloperoxidase deficiency is, for the most part, a benign autosomal recessive disorder characterized by an absence of myeloperoxidase in neutrophils and monocytes. Although myeloperoxidase is involved in the bacteriocidal process in neutrophils, an increase in infections is not usually a complication of myeloperoxidase deficiency even in homozygous individuals because the cells are able to utilize an alternative system to

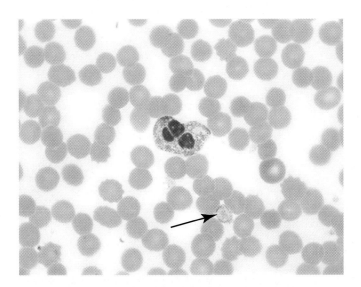

■ **FIGURE 19-11** May-Hegglin syndrome. There is a neutrophil with a Döhle-like structure in the cytoplasm and a large platelet (arrow). (Peripheral blood; Wright-Giemsa stain; 1000× magnification)

kill the microorganisms (somewhat more slowly) (∞ Chapter 7). Patients who also have diabetes mellitus may experience disseminated fungal infections (usually with *Candida albicans*).

Current hematology analyzers such as the ADVIA 2120 (Siemens) detect MPO deficiency using the intracellular myeloperoxidase enzyme of the cell in a two-stage cytochemical reaction to differentiate cells based on stain and size characteristics. Neutrophils, eosinophils, and monocytes are usually MPO positive, and basophils and lymphocytes are MPO negative. Neutrophils in the blood of MPO deficiency patients show up on the cytogram as "Large Unstained Cells," resulting in an overall decreased neutrophil count.[27] This discrepancy is flagged and can be resolved by reviewing the stained blood smear. The neutrophils are present on the stained smears and appear morphologically normal.

Leukocyte Adhesion Deficiency Leukocyte adhesion deficiency (LAD) is a rare, autosomal recessive disorder characterized by decreased or absent leukocyte cell-surface adhesion proteins (β_2-integrins), the CD11/CD18 complex (∞ Chapter 7). Neutrophils from patients with LAD have multiple defects related to adhesion to endothelial cells, chemotaxis, phagocytosis, respiratory burst activation, and degranulation. Because of defective adhesion proteins, the neutrophils cannot adhere to endothelial cells of the blood vessel walls and exit the circulation. In addition, LAD neutrophils are not able to recognize the presence of the complement C3bi fragment on microorganisms, so phagocytosis is not stimulated.

Features of LAD include recurrent soft tissue bacterial and fungal infections with persistent leukocytosis and granulocytosis due to increased stimulation of bone marrow. The frequency and severity of the infections depends on the amount of CD11/CD18 expressed by the cells. Diagnosis can be made by flow cytometric analysis of neutrophil CD11b levels using a monoclonal antibody.[25] Treatment includes prophylactic antibiotics and early, aggressive treatment of infections. Mortality rate in childhood is high, and bone marrow transplantation is recommended in severe cases.

✓ Checkpoint! 6

Explain how you can determine whether toxic granulation and vacuoles in the PMNs are due to the patient's condition or to artifact.

▶ EOSINOPHIL DISORDERS

Disorders involving exclusively eosinophils are rare. An increase in the circulating number of these cells may indicate a potentially serious condition. Because the lower limit of the reference range is very low, a decrease is difficult to determine and is probably not significant. Eosinopenia can be seen in acute infections and inflammatory reactions and with the administration of glucocorticosteroids. Glucocorticosteroids and epinephrine inhibit eosinophil release from

the bone marrow and increase margination.[28] Eosinophilia can be classified as primary (neoplastic phenotype) (∞ Chapter 22) or secondary (reactive). Primary eosinophilia can be further classified as clonal (known molecular marker) and idiopathic (unknown cause).[29]

REACTIVE (SECONDARY) EOSINOPHILIA

Eosinophilia refers to an increase in eosinophils above 0.40×10^9/L. Reactive eosinophilia appears to be induced by substances secreted from T lymphocytes. This type of eosinophilia is polyclonal and the common myeloid progenitor (CMP) cell is normal. Various conditions associated with the cellular immune response (mediated by T lymphocytes) are characterized by eosinophilia including (1) tissue-invasive parasites, (2) allergic conditions, (3) respiratory tract disorders, (4) gastrointestinal diseases, and (5) skin and connective tissue disorders and diseases.[30] Parasites are the most common cause of secondary eosinophilia worldwide. When the eosinophil concentration is high and immature forms are present, the blood picture may resemble that seen in chronic eosinophilic leukemia (∞ Chapter 22). The conditions associated with eosinophilia are listed in Table 19-9 .

 TABLE 19-9

Conditions Associated with Quantitative Changes of Eosinophils, Basophils, and Mast Cells	
Eosinopenia	Acute infections, inflammatory reactions, administration of glucocorticosteroids
Eosinophilia	
Secondary (reactive)	Parasitic infection
	Allergic conditions, especially asthma, dermatitis, and drug reactions
Primary (HES)	
Clonal	Certain clonal hematologic malignancies, Hodgkin lymphoma, CML, and eosinophilic leukemia
Idiopathic	No apparent cause
Basopenia	Inflammatory states following immunologic reactions
Basophilia	Immediate hypersensitivity reactions
	Endocrinopathies
	Infectious diseases
	Chronic myeloproliferative disorders, especially CML; chronic basophilic leukemia
Mastocytosis	Immediate hypersensitivity reactions
	Connective tissue disorders
	Infectious diseases
	Neoplastic disorders such as lymphoproliferative diseases and Hematopoietic stem cell diseases

HES = hypereosinophilic syndrome

Tissue invasion by parasites produces an eosinophilia more pronounced than parasitic infestation of the gut or blood. Eosinophils are especially effective in fighting tissue larvae of parasites. Eosinophils can readily adhere to larvae coated with IgG, IgE, and/or complement. The larva is too large for the eosinophil to phagocytose; instead, the cell molds itself around the larva. Intracellular eosinophilic granules fuse with the eosinophil membrane and expel their contents into the space between the cell and the larva. The granular substances attack the larva wall, partially digesting it.[31]

Allergic disorders (asthma, dermatitis, and drug reactions) are frequently characterized by a moderate increase in eosinophils. Large numbers can also be found in nasal discharges and sputum of allergic individuals as well as in the peripheral blood.

Pulmonary infiltrate with eosinophilia (PIE) syndrome consists of asthma, pulmonary infiltrates, central nervous system involvement, peripheral neuropathy, periarteritis nodosa, and local or systemic eosinophilia. This syndrome may be produced by parasitic or bacterial infections, allergic reactions, or collagen disorders. In some cases, no cause can be found.

PRIMARY EOSINOPHILIA

Primary eosinophilia is collectively known as **hypereosinophilic syndrome** (HES). HES is a catchall term used to describe a persistent blood eosinophilia over 1.5×10^9/L with tissue infiltration. If there is no apparent cause it is called idiopathic HES (Figure 19-12 ■). On the other hand, primary eosinophilia may be associated with a clonal molecular marker. Clonal eosinophilia, including eosinophilic leukemia, are considered myeloproliferative disorders and discussed in Chapter 22. The classification of HES is changing as genetic mutations are identified and fewer cases of HES are considered idiopathic.

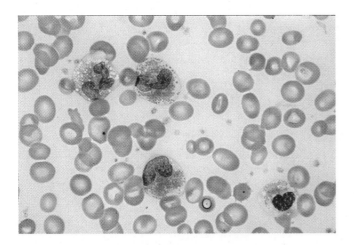

■ **FIGURE 19-12** Hypereosinophilic syndrome. Note that the cells are all mature eosinophils. (Peripheral blood; Wright-Giemsa stain; 1000× magnification)

Chronic eosinophilia may cause extensive tissue damage as the granules are released from disintegrating eosinophils. In many cases of HES, the heart is damaged by large numbers of circulating eosinophils. Charcot-Leyden crystals, which are formed from either eosinophil cytoplasm or granules, can be found in exudates and tissues where large numbers of eosinophils migrate and disintegrate. Treatment of HES with corticosteroids, hydroxyurea, and/or α-interferon is sometimes effective in reducing the eosinophil count. HES is most commonly seen in males (more than 90%) and is rarely seen in children.[29]

Idiopathic HES needs to be differentiated from reactive eosinophilias and clonal eosinophilias (such as eosinophilic leukemia). Eosinophilic leukemia usually is characterized by increased numbers of myeloblasts and eosinophilic myelocytes, whereas in idiopathic HES and reactive eosinophilia, the eosinophils are mature. In addition, an abnormal clonal chromosome karyotype or molecular mutation suggests eosinophilic leukemia or other clonal variant rather than idiopathic HES or reactive eosinophilia (∞ Chapter 22).

▶ BASOPHIL AND MAST CELL DISORDERS

Both basophils and mast cells are important in inflammatory and immediate allergic reactions because they are both able to release inflammatory mediators. Their cytoplasmic inflammatory granules can be stimulated for release by many of the same mediators. In addition, each type of cell has individual mediators. Extracellular release of inflammatory granules may be induced by physical destruction of the cell, chemical substances (toxins, venoms, proteases), endogenous mechanisms (tissue proteases, cationic proteins), and immune mechanisms. The immune mechanisms may be IgE-dependent (IgE binds to high-affinity receptors on these cells) or IgE-independent (triggered by complement fragment C5a binding to C5a receptors on these cells).

The number of basophils and mast cells increases at inflammation sites. Basophils migrate from the blood by adhering to the endothelium (mediated by several families of adhesion molecules and receptors).[32,33]

Basophilia refers to an increase in basophils above 0.20×10^9/L. Basophilia is associated with immediate hypersensitivity reactions and chronic myeloproliferative disorders (Table 19-9) (Figure 19-13 ■). An absolute basophilia is often helpful in distinguishing CML from a leukemoid reaction or other benign leukocytosis. When the basophil count exceeds 80% of the total leukocyte population and the Philadelphia chromosome and/or BCR/ABL1 gene rearrangement are not present, some hematologists prefer to call the disease *basophilic leukemia,* an extremely rare condition.

A decrease in basophils is even more difficult to establish than eosinopenia. Scanning a blood smear with 100× magnification will reveal a rare basophil in normal individuals.

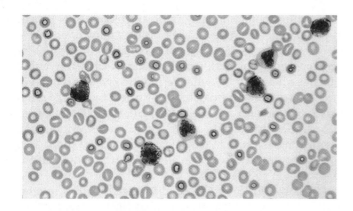

■ FIGURE 19-13   Peripheral blood from a patient with CML and 30% basophils. (Peripheral blood; Wright-Giemsa stain; 500× magnification)

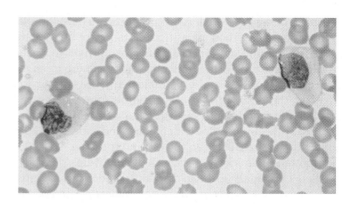

■ FIGURE 19-14   Peripheral blood from a patient with reactive monocytosis showing two reactive monocytes. (Peripheral blood; Wright-Giemsa stain; 1000× magnification)

Decreases in basophils are seen in inflammatory states and following immunologic reactions.

Mastocytosis can be found in a number of disorders in which the number of mast cells is increased up to fourfold in tissues affected by the disorder (most commonly the skin) and in conjunction with certain neoplastic disorders (Table 19-9). No clinical disorder that involves a decrease in mast cells numbers has been identified, however, long-term treatment with glucocorticoids can lower the number of mast cells.[33]

 Checkpoint! 7

Why are the basophil and eosinophil counts important when assessing the benign or neoplastic nature of a disorder?

▶ MONOCYTE/MACROPHAGE DISORDERS

Quantitative disorders are associated with monocytes whereas the qualitative disorders are associated with monocytes/macrophages. The qualitative disorders are inherited lysosomal storage disorders.

QUANTITATIVE DISORDERS

Monocytosis occurs when the absolute monocyte count exceeds 0.8×10^9/L (Figure 19-14 ■). It is seen most often in inflammatory conditions and certain malignancies (Table 19-10 ✪). Monocytosis occurring in the recovery stage of acute infections and in agranulocytosis is considered a favorable sign. Monocytes play an important role in the immune cellular response in tuberculosis.

Unexplained monocytosis has been reported to be associated with as many as 62% of all malignancies. Myelodysplastic states, acute myelocytic leukemia, and chronic myelo-

cytic leukemia are associated with monocytosis. About 25% of Hodgkin lymphomas are characterized by an increase in monocytes. In these conditions, the monocyte is probably a part of a reactive process to the neoplasm rather than a part of the clonal neoplasm itself. Neoplastic proliferation of monocytes occurs in acute monocytic leukemia and acute and chronic myelomonocytic leukemia (∞ Chapters 22, 24).

Monocytopenia refers to a concentration of monocytes below 0.2×10^9/L and is found in stem cell disorders such as aplastic anemia. A decreased number of circulating monocytes is difficult to establish because of the low normal levels of these cells.

QUALITATIVE DISORDERS

Lysosomal storage disorders are a large group of inherited disorders. All nucleated cells contain lysosomes that are part of the cell's recycling system. Lysosomes contain vari-

✪ TABLE 19-10

Conditions Associated with Quantitative Changes of Monocytes

Neoplastic	Myelodysplastic/myeloproliferative diseases
	Chronic myelomonocytic leukemia
	Juvenile myelomonocytic leukemia
	Chronic myelogenous leukemia
	Acute monocytic, myelomonocytic, and myelocytic leukemias
Reactive	Inflammatory conditions
	Collagen diseases
	Immune disorders
	Certain infections (e.g., TB, syphilis)
Monocytopenia	Stem cell disorders such as aplastic anemia

ous enzymes (including glucosidases, lipases, proteases, and nucleases) that are involved in degradative processes, and defects in any of these enzymes can lead to the accumulation of either undegraded substrates or catabolic products that are unable to be transported out of the lysosome. This accumulation can lead to cell dysfunction and pathological phenotypes. Most of these disorders are inherited in an autosomal recessive pattern.[34]

Lysosomal storage disorders can be classified by the type of storage material that accumulates (glycoproteins, glycosphingolipids, mucolipids, mucopolysaccharides, etc.). Many of these disorders cause detectable morphology in leukocytes with a few that appear in granulocytes (see Alder-Reilly anomaly earlier in this chapter) and monocytes/macrophages. The disorders that are diagnosed based on the presense of abnormal macrophages in hematologic tissue include Gaucher disease, Niemann-Pick disease, and sea-blue histiocytosis (see Histiocytoses).

Gaucher Disease

Gaucher (pronounced go-shay) disease is an inherited autosomal recessive trait that is characterized by a deficiency of glucocerebrosidase (an enzyme needed to break down the lipid glucocerebroside). In this disease, the macrophage is unable to digest the stroma of ingested cells, and the lipid glucocerebroside accumulates. The clinical findings (splenomegaly and bone pain) of the disease are related to the accumulation of this lipid in macrophages mainly in the spleen, liver, and bone marrow. The macrophages (Gaucher cells) are large (20–100 μm) with small eccentric nuclei and the cytoplasm appears wrinkled or striated (Figure 19-15 ■).[35] The spleen and liver may become greatly enlarged. Leukopenia, thrombocytopenia, and anemia may occur as the result of their sequestration by an enlarged spleen. A consistent finding useful in the diagnosis of Gaucher disease is an increase in serum acid phosphatase activity.

Cells similar to Gaucher cells may be found in the marrow of individuals with a rapid granulocyte turnover, especially in chronic myelocytic leukemia. The accumulation of lipid in these disorders does not result from a deficiency of an enzyme but from the inability of the macrophage to keep up with the flow of fat into the cell from the increased cell turnover. Gaucher disease can be confirmed by demonstrating a decreased leukocyte β-glucosidase activity whereas the enzyme level is normal or increased in myeloproliferative disorders.

Niemann-Pick Disease

Niemann-Pick disease includes a group of rare disorders that are related autosomal recessive diseases. Signs of the disease begin in infancy with poor physical development. The spleen and liver are greatly enlarged. The disease is often fatal by 3 years of age. In Niemann-Pick type A and type B disease, the defect is a deficiency of sphingomyelinase (an enzyme needed to break down lipids) resulting in excessive sphingomyelin storage. Foamy macrophages are found in lymphoid tissue and the bone marrow. (Figure 19-16■) The foam cells are large (20–100 μm) with an eccentric nucleus and globular cytoplasmic inclusions. Leukopenia and thrombocytopenia may occur from increased sequestration from the enlarged spleen, and blood lymphocytes may contain several vacuoles that are lipid-filled lysosomes.[36]

Miscellaneous Lysosomal Storage Disorders

Tay-Sachs disease, Sandhoff disease, and Wolman's disease are inherited diseases characterized by a deficiency of one or more enzymes that metabolize lipids. As a result of these enzyme deficiencies, abnormal concentrations of lipids accumulate in the lysosomes of tissue cells. These often fatal conditions affect mostly nonhematologic tissue. There are no specific findings in the peripheral blood. Lipid-laden macrophages may be present in the bone marrow.[37]

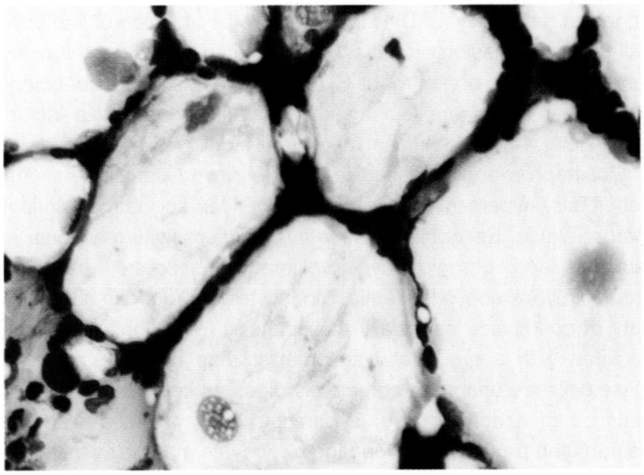

■ FIGURE 19-15 Gaucher macrophages in bone marrow. (Wright-Giemsa stain; 1000× magnification)

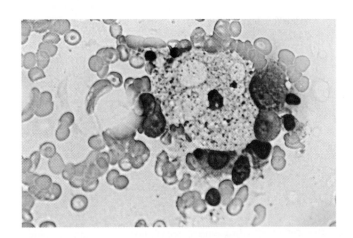

■ FIGURE 19-16 Macrophage in the bone marrow of a patient with Niemann-Pick disease. Note the foamy cytoplasm with inclusions. (Wright-Giemsa stain; 1000× magnification)

HISTIOCYTOSES

Two different types of cells are known as histiocytes: Langerhans cells/dendritic cells and monocytes/macrophages. Both types of cells are antigen processing and antigen presenting cells and share a common CD34$^+$ progenitor. The three classes of histiocytoses are class I—Langerhans cell histiocytoses (LCH); class II—non-Langerhans histiocytoses (non-LCH), which encompasses the histiocytoses of mononuclear phagocytes; and class III—malignant histiocytoses.[38]

The Langerhans cell is an immature dendritic cell that is usually found in the epidermis, oral and vaginal mucosa, and lungs. They differ from other tissue cells by characteristic racquet-shaped structural inclusions known as Birbeck granules.[39] Monocyte/macrophage histiocytes contribute to reactive (in response to an inflammatory stimulus) and malignant disorders. Reactive macrophage histiocytes can be seen in benign proliferative diseases (xanthoma disseminata, juvenile xanthogranuloma), in nonmalignant hemophagocytic diseases (fulminant hemophagocytic syndrome, histiocytosis with massive lymphadenopathy), and in several of the storage disorders (Gaucher, Niemann-Pick, and sea-blue histiocytosis).[40]

Sea-Blue Histiocytosis Syndrome   Sea-blue histiocytosis syndrome is a rare inherited disorder characterized by splenomegaly and thrombocytopenia. Sea-blue staining macrophages are found in the liver, spleen, and bone marrow (Figure 19-17 ■). The cell is large (20–60 μm in diameter) with a dense eccentric nucleus and cytoplasm that contains blue or blue-green granules. Considerable variation in clinical manifestations is present, but in most patients, the course of the disease is benign. Sea-blue histiocytes may also be seen in a variety of disorders of lipid metabolism and in association with various other disorders including Niemann-

Pick disease, some hematopoietic diseases, and in certain infections.[41]

SUMMARY

Leukocytes respond to toxic, infectious, and inflammatory processes to defend the tissues and limit and/or eliminate the disease process or toxic challenge. This may involve a change in leukocyte concentration, most often increasing one or more leukocyte types. The type of cell affected depends on the cell's function. Thus, a differential count as well as the total leukocyte count aids in diagnosis.

Neutrophilia, an increase in neutrophils, most often occurs as a result of a reaction to a physiologic or pathologic process. The most common cause is bacterial infection. Tissue injury or inflammation may also cause a neutrophilia. Web Figure 19-1 ■ summarizes the laboratory evaluation of neutrophilia.

Neutropenia, a decrease in neutrophils, is less commonly encountered. It may be caused by drugs, immune mechanisms, or decreased bone marrow production. Several inherited conditions are characterized by neutropenia and recurrent infections. Web Figure 19-2 ■ summarizes the laboratory evaluation of neutropenia.

Morphologic abnormalities of neutrophils may be found in infectious states and are important to identify on stained blood smears. These include Döhle bodies, toxic granulation, and cytoplasmic vacuoles. Other morphologic abnormalities include pince-nez cells found in Pelger-Huët anomaly and morulae found in ehrlichiosis.

A number of inherited conditions are characterized by functional and morphologic abnormalities of the leukocyte. Chronic granulomatous disease and myeloperoxidase deficiency are characterized by defects in the generation of oxidizing radicals after phagocytosing bacteria. The nitroblue tetrazolium dye test is used to detect abnormal oxygen metabolism in CGD. Peroxidase-deficient cells can be demonstrated with peroxidase stain. The neutrophil oxidative burst assay uses the dye DHR 123 to detect neutrophils that produce reactive oxidative intermediates after ingestion of bacteria. The oxygen metabolites oxidize the colorless dye into fluorescent rhodamine 123, which is detected by a flow cytometer. Leukocyte adhesion deficiency (LAD) is identified by the absence of leukocyte cell-surface adhesion proteins. Diagnosis can be made by flow cytometric analysis of neutrophil CD11/CD18 levels using monoclonal antibodies. Other rare leukocyte functional abnormalities include Alder-Reilly, Chédiak-Higashi, and May-Hegglin anomalies.

Eosinophils are increased in infections with parasites, allergic conditions, hypersensitivity reactions, cancer, and chronic inflammatory states. Basophilia is seen in hypersensitivity reactions, infections, and chronic myeloproliferative disorders, especially chronic myelogenous leukemia. Monocytosis is found in a wide variety of conditions, especially malignancies. Macrophages are associated with a group of lysosomal storage disorders in which these cells are unable to completely digest phagocytosed material because of a deficiency of a particular enzyme needed for the degradation process. Macrophage histiocytes may be seen in various reactive and malignant disorders.

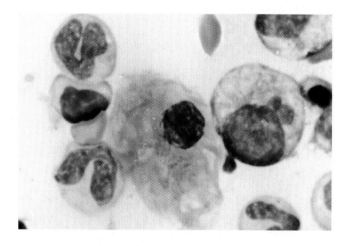

■ FIGURE 19-17   Sea-blue histiocyte from bone marrow. (Wright stain; 1000× magnification)

REVIEW QUESTIONS

LEVEL I

1. Which of the following hematologic values would you expect if the peripheral blood smear revealed toxic granulation of PMNs, Döhle bodies, and vacuoles in PMNs? (Objectives 1, 2)
   a. WBC: 4×10^9/L
   b. differential: 50% neutrophils, 15% bands, 30% lymphs, 5% monocytes
   c. 20% eosinophils
   d. Hb: 10 g/dL; platelets 20×10^9/L

2. The white count in an adult is 2.0×10^9/L. The differential has 60% segmented neutrophils. Which of the following correctly describes these results? (Objective 6)
   a. normal
   b. leukocytosis and neutrophilia
   c. leukopenia with normal number of neutrophils
   d. leukopenia and neutropenia

3. Which of the following is the most common cause of neutrophilia? (Objective 1)
   a. bacterial infection
   b. acute leukemia
   c. following chemotherapy
   d. aplastic anemia

4. Blue-gray oval inclusions composed of RNA near the periphery of neutrophils is a description of: (Objective 3)
   a. toxic granules
   b. Döhle bodies
   c. vacuoles
   d. primary granules

5. Which of the following is associated with an acute bacterial infection? (Objective 2)
   a. neutrophilia
   b. neutropenia
   c. eosinophilia
   d. leukocytopenia

6. Which of the following is a common reason for neutropenia in hospitalized patients? (Objective 6)
   a. chronic myeloproliferative disorders such as CML
   b. chemotherapy and/or radiation treatment for cancer
   c. childbirth
   d. lack of exercise

7. Which of the following causes a false neutropenia? (Objective 7)
   a. EDTA induced agglutination
   b. bone marrow aplasia
   c. splenomegaly
   d. immune neutropenia

LEVEL II

Use the following case study to answer review questions 1–5.

A patient's white count is 30.0×10^9/L. The differential is as follows:

Segmented neutrophils	54%
Band neutrophils	10%
Metamyelocytes	2%
Lymphocytes	26%
Monocytes	5%
Eosinophils	3%
6 Nucleated RBCs/ 100 WBCs	

1. Select the additional information most important to assess whether these results are normal or indicate a disease process. (Objective 1)
   a. platelet count
   b. LAP stain
   c. patient history
   d. patient age

2. Which of the following correctly describes the absolute neutrophil count (ANC) for the patient? (Objectives 1, 12)
   a. normal for both an infant and an adult
   b. neutrophilia for both an infant and an adult
   c. normal for an infant and neutrophilia for an adult
   d. normal for an adult and neutrophilia for an infant

3. Which of the following correctly describes the neutrophil concentration if the patient is an infant? (Objective 1)
   a. pseudoneutrophilia
   b. leukemoid reaction
   c. leukoerythroblastic reaction
   d. physiologic neutrophilia

4. Which of the following correctly describes the differential if the patient is an adult? (Objective 1)
   a. pseudoneutrophila
   b. leukoerythroblastic reaction
   c. agranulocytosis
   d. physiologic neutrophilia

5. A leukoerythroblastic reaction can be associated with: (Objectives 1, 2, 12)
   a. chronic granulomatous disease
   b. Chédiak-Higashi syndrome
   c. severe hemolytic anemia
   d. leukocyte adhesion deficiency

REVIEW QUESTIONS *(continued)*

LEVEL I

8. Which of the following is the most common cause of eosinophilia? (Objective 10)
   a. parasitic infection
   b. eosinophilic leukemia
   c. CML
   d. asthma and other allergies

9. What substances build up and are ingested by macrophages in the qualitative macrophage disorders such as Gaucher disease? (Objective 11)
   a. proteins
   b. carbohydrates
   c. lipids
   d. rough endoplasmic reticulum

10. Distinct, large, unidentified inclusions are found in the cytoplasm of many granulocytes. Select the best course of action. (Objective 9)
    a. Ignore them because they probably are not significant.
    b. Report them as intracellular yeast.
    c. Have a supervisor or pathologist examine the smear for rare or unusual conditions such as Chédiak-Higashi.
    d. Report them as toxic granulation.

LEVEL II

Qualitative neutrophil abnormalities can sometimes be confused with reactive or toxic conditions. For each set of conditions in questions 6–11, list all lettered features that could help evaluate the patient.
   a. presence of other toxic features (leukocytosis, toxic granulation, Döhle bodies, vacuoles)
   b. abnormal inclusions found in other cells besides neutrophils
   c. other CBC parameters abnormal (RBC, HCT, or PLT)
   d. patient symptoms
   e. patient and family history

6. Alder-Reilly versus toxic granulation. (Objectives 7, 11)

7. May-Hegglin versus toxic Döhle bodies. (Objectives 7, 11)

8. Pelger-Huët versus bands. (Objectives 5, 11)

9. Chédiak-Higashi versus intracellular yeasts or morulae. (Objectives 6, 7, 11)

10. Leukemia versus infection. (Objectives 2, 11)

11. Toxic vacuoles versus sample with prolonged storage. (Objectives 4, 6, 11)

www.pearsonhighered.com/mckenzie

Use this address to access the, interactive Companion Website created for this textbook. Find additional information, tables and figures. Evaluate your command of the chapter information using case studies and critical thinking and multiple choice questions.

REFERENCES

1. Miller DR. Normal blood values from birth through adolescence. In: Miller D, ed. *Blood Diseases of Infancy and Childhood,* 7th ed. St. Louis: Mosby; 1995:30–53.

2. McQueen, R. Pediatric and geriatric hematology. In: Rodak BF, Fritsma GA, Doig K, eds. *Hematology Clinical Principals and Applications,* 3rd ed. St. Louis: Saunders Elsevier; 2007:526–40.

3. Segel GB. Hematology of the newborn. In: Lichtman MA, Kipps TJ, Kaushansky K, Beutler E, Seligsohn U, Prchal JT, eds. *Williams Hematology,* 7th ed. New York: McGraw-Hill; 2006:81–99.

4. Perkins SL. Examination of the blood and bone marrow. In: Greer JP, Foerster J, Lukens J, Rodgers GM, Paraskevas F, Glader B, eds. *Wintrobe's Clinical Hematology,* 11th ed. Philadelphia: Lippincott Williams & Wilkins; 2004:3–25.

5. Stock W, and Hoffman R. White blood cells 1: Non-malignant disorders. *Lancet.* 2000;355(9212):1351–57.

6. Jandl JH. Granulocytes. In: Jandl JH, Minot GR, eds. *Blood Textbook of Hematology,* 2nd ed. Boston: Little, Brown; 1996:635–49.

7. Vusirikala M. Supportive care in hematologic malignancies. In: Greer JP, Foerster J, Lukens JN, Rodgers GM, Paraskevas F, Glader B, eds. *Wintrobe's Clinical Hematology,* 11th ed. Philadelphia: Lippincott Williams & Wilkins; 2004:1997–2044.

8. Sampson AP. The role of eosinophils and neutrophils in inflammation. *Clin Exp Allergy.* 2000;Suppl(30)1:22–27.

9. Whitlock JA, Gaynon PS. Acute lymphoblastic leukemia in children. In: Greer JP, Foerster J, Lukens JN, Rodgers GM, Paraskevas F, Glader B, eds. *Wintrobe's Clinical Hematology,* 11th ed. Philadelphia: Lippincott Williams & Wilkins; 2004:2143–68.

10. Hande KR. Principles and pharmacology of chemotherapy. In: Greer JP, Foerster J, Lukens JN, Rodgers GM, Paraskevas F, Glader B, eds. *Wintrobe's Clinical Hematology,* 11th ed. Philadelphia: Lippincott Williams & Wilkins; 2004:1945–69.

11. Dale DC. Neutropenia and neutrophilia. In: Lichtman MA, Kipps, TJ, Kaushansky K, Beutler E, Seligsohn U, Prchal JT, eds. *Williams Hematology,* 7th ed. New York: McGraw-Hill; 2006:907–18.

12. Watts RG. Neutropenia. In: Greer JP, Foerster J, Lukens JN, Rodgers GM, Paraskevas F, Glader B, eds. *Wintrobe's Clinical Hematology,* 11th ed. Philadelphia: Lippincott Williams & Wilkins; 2004:1777–1800.

13. Hestdal K, Welte K, Lie SO, Keller JR, Ruscetti FW, Abrahamsen TG. Severe congenital neutropenia: Abnormal growth and differentiation of myeloid progenitors to granulocyte colony-stimulating factor (G-CSF) but normal response to G-CSF plus stem cell factor. *Blood.* 1993;82:2991–97.

14. Boxer LA, Newburger PE. A molecular classification of congenital neutropenia syndromes. *Pediatr Blood Cancer.* 2007;49(5):609–14.

15. Capsoni F, Sarzi-Puttini P, Zanella A. Primary and secondary autoimmune neutropenia. *Arthritis Res Ther.* 2005;7:208–14.

16. Dale DC. Nonmalignant disorders of leukocytes. In: Dale DC, Federman DD, eds. *Hematology:VII. ACP Medicine Online.* New York: WebMD Inc.; 2004:1–16.

17. Jandl JH. Leukocyte anomalies. In: *Blood: Textbook of Hematology,* 2nd ed. Boston: Little, Brown; 1996:785–802.

18. Gall JJ. Laboratory evaluation of body fluids. In: Stiene-Martin EA, Lotspeich-Steininger CA, Koepke JA, eds. *Clinical Hematology,* 2nd ed. Philadelphia: Lippincott; 1998:400–14.

19. Bakken JS, Dumler S. Human granulocytic ehrlichiosis. *Clin Infect Dis.* 2000; 31:554–60.

20. Hamilton KS, Standaert SM, Kinney MC. Characteristic peripheral blood findings in human ehrlichiosis. *Mod Pathol.* 2004;17(5): 512–17.

21. Van Hoof F. Mucopolysaccharidosis and mucolipidoses. *J Clin Path.* 1974;27(8):64–93.

22. Dinauer MC, Coates TD. Disorders of phagocyte function and number. In: Hoffman R, Benz EJ, Shattil SJ, Furie B, Cohen HJ, Silberstein LE, McGlave P, eds. *Hematology Basic Principles and Practice,* 4th ed. Philadelphia: Churchill Livingstone; 2005:787–29.

23. Skubitz KM. Qualitative disorders of leukocytes. In: Greer JP, Foerster J, Lukens JN, Rodgers GM, Paraskevas F, Glader B, eds. *Wintrobe's Clinical Hematology,* 11th ed. Philadelphia: Lippincott Williams & Wilkins; 2004:1801–17.

24. Assari T. Chronic granulomatous disease: Fundamental stages in our understanding of CGD. *Med Immunol.* 2006;5(4):1–8.

25. Borregaard N, Boxer LA. Disorders of neutrophil function. In: Lichtman MA, Kipps, TJ, Kaushansky K, Beutler E, Seligsohn U, Prchal JT, eds. *Williams Hematology,* 7th ed. New York: McGraw-Hill; 2006: 921–50.

26. EXBIO Diagnostics. FagoFlow™ Kit. 2008. www.exbio.cz. Nov 23, 2008

27. Siemens. ADVIA 2120 White Blood Cell Technology. 2007. www.siemens.com/medical.

28. Wardlaw AJ, Kay AB. Eosinopenia and eosinophilia. In: Lichtman MA, Kipps, TJ, Kaushansky K, Beutler E, Seligsohn U, Prchal JT, eds. *Williams Hematology,* 7th ed. New York: Mc-Graw-Hill; 2006:863–78.

29. Tefferi A, Patnaik MM, Pardanani A. Eosinophilia: Secondary, clonal and idiopathic. *Br J Haematol.* 2006;133(5):468–92.

30. Ackerman SJ, Butterfield JH. Eosinophilia, eosinophil-associated diseases, chronic eosinophil leukemia, and the hypereosinophilic syndromes. In: Hoffman R, Benz EJ, Shattil SJ, Furie B, Cohen HJ, Silberstein LE, McGlave P, eds. *Hematology Basic Principles and Practice,* 4th ed. Philadelphia: Elsevier Churchill Livingstone; 2005:763–86.

31. Boggs DR, Winkelstein A. *White Cell Manual,* 4th ed. Philadelphia: F.A. Davis Co; 1983:54–57.

32. Parker, RI, Metcalfe DD. Basophils, mast cells, and systemic mastocytosis. In: Hoffman R, Benz EJ, Shattil SJ, Furie B, Cohen HJ, Silberstein LE, McGlave P, eds. *Hematology Basic Principles and Practice,* 4th ed. Philadelphia: Elsevier Churchill Livingstone; 2005:911–25.

33. Galli SJ, Metcalfe DD, Arber DA, Dvorak AM. Basophils and mast cells and their disorders. In: Lichtman MA, Kipps, TJ, Kaushansky K, Beutler E, Seligsohn U, Prchal JT, eds. *Williams Hematology,* 7th ed. New York: Mc-Graw-Hill; 2006:879–98.

34. Wraith JE. Lysosomal disorders. *Semin Neonatol.* 2002;7:75–83.

35. Jmoudiak M, Futerman AH. Gaucher disease: Pathological mechanisms and modern management. *Br J Haematol.* 2005;129:178–88.

36. Beutler E. Lipid storage diseases. In: Lichtman MA, Kipps, TJ, Kaushansky K, Beutler E, Seligsohn U, Prchal JT, eds. *Williams Hematology,* 7th ed. New York: McGraw-Hill; 2006:1009–18.

37. McGovern MM, Desnick RJ. Abnormalities of the monocyte-macrophage system: Lysosomal storage diseases. In: Greer JP, Foerster J, Lukens JN, Rodgers GM, Paraskevas F, Glader B, eds. *Wintrobe's Clinical Hematology,* 11th ed. Philadelphia: Lippincott Williams & Wilkins; 2004:1819–25.

38. Caputo R, Marzano AV, Passoni E, Berti E. Unusual variants of nono-Langerhans cell histiocytoses. *J Am Acad Dermatol.* 2007;57 (6):1031–45.

39. Lichtman MA. Inflamatory and malignant histiocytosis. In: Lichtman MA, Kipps TJ, Kaushansky K, Beutler E, Seligsohn U, Prchal JT, eds. *Williams Hematology,* 7th ed. New York: McGraw-Hill; 2006: 993–1008.

40. Cline MJ. Histiocytes and histiocytosis. *Blood.* 1994;84(9):2840–53.

41. Hirayama Y, et al. Syndrome of the sea-blue histiocyte. *Inter Med.* 1996;35(5):419–21.

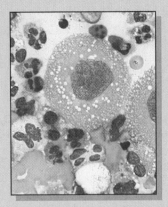

20

Nonmalignant Lymphocyte Disorders

Sue S. Beglinger, M.S.

■ OBJECTIVES—LEVEL I

At the end of this unit of study, the student should be able to:

1. Identify the infectious agent and describe the clinical symptoms and corresponding leukocyte differential in infectious mononucleosis.

2. Describe and recognize the reactive morphology of lymphocytes found in infectious mononucleosis.

3. Relate the heterophile antibody test to infectious mononucleosis.

4. Given a differential and leukocyte count, calculate an absolute lymphocyte count and differentiate it from a relative lymphocyte count.

5. Identify reactive cell morphology associated with viral infections and compare it with normal lymphocyte morphology.

6. Describe clinical symptoms of disorders in which a leukocytosis is caused by lymphocytosis.

7. State the complications associated with CMV infections.

8. Identify absolute and relative lymphocytopenia and lymphocytosis, and list conditions associated with these abnormal counts.

9. Explain the pathophysiology of HIV infections and describe how it affects lymphocytes.

10. Describe the abnormal hematological findings associated with AIDS.

■ OBJECTIVES—LEVEL II

At the end of this unit of study, the student should be able to:

1. Assess and resolve/explain conflicting results between peripheral blood morphology and serologic tests in suspected Epstein-Barr virus (EBV) infection.

2. Describe the pathophysiology of infectious mononucleosis.

3. Assess and correlate antibody titers found in infectious mononucleosis with respect to the various EBV viral antigens.

4. State the pathophysiology of toxoplasmosis infections, and explain the resulting lymphocytosis.

5. Differentiate benign lymphocytic leukemoid reactions from neoplastic lymphoproliferative disorders by laboratory results and characteristics of cell morphology.

6. Define the pathophysiology of CMV infections, and give clinical findings associated with it.

7. In *Bordetella pertussis* infections, propose the cause of lymphocytosis and recognize laboratory features associated with it.

8. Assess a patient case using the CDC AIDS case surveillance criteria and recommend appropriate laboratory testing.

9. Explain the cytopenia, identify the defect, and recognize the laboratory features in congenital qualitative disorders of lymphocytes.

10. Evaluate a case study from a patient with a lymphoproliferative disorder and conclude from the medical history and laboratory results the most likely diagnosis for the disorder.

KEY TERMS

Acquired immune deficiency syndrome (AIDS)
AIDS-related complex (ARC)
Bordetella pertussis
Cytomegalovirus (CMV)
Epstein-Barr virus (EBV)
Heterophile antibodies
Immunosuppressed
Infectious lymphocytosis
Infectious mononucleosis
Lymphocytic leukemoid reaction
Opportunistic organisms
Severe combined immunodeficiency (SCID) syndrome
Toxoplasmosis
Viral load

BACKGROUND BASICS

The information in this chapter builds on the concepts learned in previous chapters. To maximize your learning experience, you should review this material before starting this unit of study.

Level I

▶ Describe normal and reactive lymphocyte morphology; identify the distinguishing characteristics of T and B lymphocytes. (Chapter 7)

▶ Calculate absolute cell counts; summarize the relationship between the hematocrit and hemoglobin. (Chapter 8)

▶ Define *antigen* and *antibody*, and describe their roles in infectious and noninfectious diseases; summarize the immune response. (Chapter 7)

Level II

▶ Describe the process of T and B lymphocyte differentiation and the function of each subtype; summarize the structure and function of each of the immunoglobulins; describe the immune response. (Chapter 7)

▶ Describe the structure and function of the hematopoietic organs and tissue. (Chapter 4)

▶ Give the principle and application of direct antiglobulin tests in diagnosis of immune mediated anemia. (Chapter 17)

 CASE STUDY

We will refer to this case study throughout the chapter.
Heidi, a 54-day-old female, was admitted to the hospital because of recurrent respiratory distress and failure to gain weight. She was born prematurely at 35 weeks gestation by urgent Cesarean section. Her mother was immune to rubella and had negative serologic tests for syphilis. Consider why the lymphatic system should be evaluated in this child and the possible etiology of repeated respiratory problems.

▶ OVERVIEW

This chapter discusses benign conditions associated with quantitative and qualitative alterations in lymphocytes. Infectious mononucleosis and other acquired disorders characterized by lymphocytosis are described. A discussion of lymphocytopenia and immune deficiency states, both acquired and congenital, follows. Emphasis is on the laboratory features that allow the diseases to be diagnosed and differentiated from neoplastic lymphoproliferative disease.

▶ INTRODUCTION

Evidence of disease, especially infectious disease, can be observed by finding abnormal concentrations of lymphocytes and/or reactive lymphocytes on a peripheral blood smear. This finding helps direct the physician's subsequent workup of the patient and aids in the initiation of appropriate therapy. Most disorders affecting lymphocytes are acquired and are characterized by a reactive lymphocytosis. Some acquired disorders result in a lymphocytopenia that can compromise the function of the immune system. In acquired disorders affecting lymphocytes, the change in lymphocyte concentration and morphology is a reactive process. In contrast, in congenital disorders involving lymphocytes, the primary defect is within the lymphocytic system.

► LYMPHOCYTOSIS

Lymphocytosis, an increase in lymphocytes, can result from a relative or absolute increase in lymphocytes. Absolute lymphocytosis occurs in adults when the lymphocyte count exceeds 4.8×10^9/L and relative lymphocytosis is present when the lymphocyte differential exceeds 35–45% (differs with race). An absolute lymphocytosis can occur without relative lymphocytosis and a relative lymphocytosis can occur without absolute lymphocytosis. The lymphocyte concentration in children is normally higher than in adults and varies with the child's age (Table B, inside front cover). Lymphocytosis can occur without a leukocytosis.

Lymphocytosis is usually a self-limiting, reactive process that occurs in response to an infection or inflammatory condition. Both T and B lymphocytes commonly are affected but their function remains normal. Occasionally, viral infections can cause functional impairment of the lymphocytes yielding both a qualitative disorder and quantitative changes.

Once lymphocytes are stimulated by an infection or inflammatory condition, they enter various states of activation, resulting in a morphologically heterogeneous population of cells on stained blood smears (Figure 20-1 ■). These activated cells can appear large with irregular shapes and cytoplasmic basophilia, and granules and vacuoles can be seen. The nuclear chromatin usually becomes more dispersed (∞ Chapter 7). Cells with these features of activation are commonly referred to as *reactive* or *atypical lymphocytes*. Occasionally, intense proliferation of lymphoid elements in the lymph nodes and spleen occurs, causing lymphadenopathy and splenomegaly, respectively.

T lymphocytes normally compose about 60–80% of peripheral blood lymphocytes. Thus, increases in the concentration of T lymphocytes are more likely than increases in B lymphocytes to cause changes in the relative lymphocyte count. Absolute lymphocytosis is not usually accompanied by leukocytosis except in infectious mononucleosis, infectious lymphocytosis, *Bordetella pertussis* infection, cytomegalovirus infection, or lymphocytic leukemia. A relative lymphocytosis secondary to neutropenia that occurs in a variety of viral infections is more commonly found. The absolute lymphocyte count is calculated as:

Absolute lymphocyte count ($\times 10^9$/L) = % lymphocytes $\times$ WBC count ($\times 10^9$/L)

It is important to differentiate benign conditions associated with lymphocytosis from neoplastic (malignant) lymphoproliferative disorders (Table 20-1 ✪). The presence of heterogeneous reactive lymphocytes, positive serologic tests for the presence of specific antibodies against infectious organisms, and absence of anemia and thrombocytopenia favor a benign diagnosis. This section includes a discussion of the more common disorders associated with a reactive lymphocytosis.

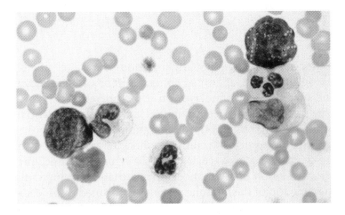

■ FIGURE 20-1   Forms of stimulated lymphocytes from a case of infectious mononucleosis. There are two immunoblasts (one o'clock and eight o'clock) and a reactive lymph (three o'clock). (Peripheral blood; Wright-Giemsa stain; 1000× magnification)

✪ TABLE 20-1

Conditions Associated with Lymphocytosis

Benign (Nonmalignant) Conditions	Neoplastic Conditions
Infectious mononucleosis	Acute lymphoblastic leukemia
Bordetella pertussis infection	Chronic lymphocytic leukemia
Toxoplasmosis	Hairy cell leukemia
Persistent polyclonal B cell lymphocytosis	Heavy chain disease
	Multiple myeloma
Viral infections	Waldenstrom's macroglobulinemia
Chicken pox	
Coxsackie virus	
Cytomegalovirus infection	
Measles	
Mumps	
Roseola infantum	
Infectious hepatitis	
Chronic infections	
Tertiary syphilis	
Congenital syphilis	
Brucellosis	
Endocrine disorders	
Thyrotoxicosis	
Addison's disease	
Panhypopituitarism	
Convalescence of acute infections	
Immune reactions	
Inflammatory diseases	

CASE STUDY *(continued from page 405)*

Admission CBC on Heidi was WBC: 7.6 × 10⁹/L; Hct: 0.55 L/L; Plt: 242 × 10⁹/L; and differential: 84% segs, 2% bands, 4% lymphocytes, 8% monocytes, and 2% eosinophils.

1. Does this patient have a leukocytosis or leukopenia?
2. Does this patient have an abnormal lymphocyte count? Explain.

INFECTIOUS MONONUCLEOSIS

Infectious mononucleosis is a self-limiting lymphoproliferative disease caused by infection with **Epstein-Barr virus (EBV)**. EBV usually affects young adults; the peak age for infection is 14–24 years. In children from lower-income groups, infection usually occurs before 4 years of age; in more affluent populations, peak infection incidence occurs during adolescence. About 80–90% of adults have had exposure and possess lifelong immunity. Not considered highly contagious, the disease is transmitted through saliva, hence, the nickname *kissing disease.*

Cellular immunity (the function of T lymphocytes) is important in limiting the growth potential of EBV-infected B lymphocytes. Immune-compromised individuals are at increased risk of serious infection. EBV-associated B cell tumors and lymphoproliferative syndromes can occur in transplant patients and patients with acquired immune deficiency syndrome (AIDS).[1] These patients have severe T lymphocyte immunodeficiency. Male children with a rare X-linked lymphoproliferative syndrome, lacking a T lymphocyte response, are unable to limit EBV infection of B lymphocytes. As a result, a fatal polyclonal B lymphocyte proliferation occurs.[2]

EBV Pathophysiology

EBV attaches to B lymphocytes by means of a specific receptor designated CD21 on the B lymphocyte membrane surface.[1] This also is the receptor for the C3d complement component. The virus infects resting B lymphocytes as well as epithelial cells of the oropharynx and cervix. The binding of the virus to the lymphocyte activates the lymphocyte, causing it to express the activation marker CD23.[3] CD23 is the receptor for a B lymphocyte growth factor. Once internalized, the virus is incorporated into the B lymphocyte genome, instructing the host cell to begin production of EBV proteins. These viral proteins are then expressed on the cell membrane. Thus, EBV-infected cells express markers of activated B lymphocytes as well as viral markers. The viral genome is maintained in the lymphocyte nucleus and passed on to the cell's progeny. This results in EBV-immortalized B lymphocytes and possible latent infection.

Acute EBV infection is controlled by a complex, multifaceted cellular immune response. In the first week of illness, a polyclonal increase in immunoglobulins occurs. During the second week, however, the number of immunoglobulin secreting B lymphocytes decreases, presumably resulting from the action of suppressor T lymphocytes. Activated cytotoxic cells that resemble activated killer cells are present early in the course of the disease. These cells are neither EBV specific nor HLA restricted (virus nonspecific). Cytotoxic T lymphocytes inhibit the activation and proliferation of EBV-infected B lymphocytes and participate in the cell-mediated immune response. The majority of the reactive lymphocytes seen in the peripheral blood are the suppressor-cytotoxic T lymphocytes.

Clinical Findings

Prodromal symptoms include lethargy, headache, fever, chills, sore throat, nausea, and anoxia. The classic triad presentation of symptoms are fever, pharyngitis, and lymphadenopathy[2] (Table 20-2 ⊙). Children younger than 10 years of age have mild disease and can be asymptomatic.[4] The cervical, axillary, and inguinal lymph nodes are commonly enlarged. Splenomegaly occurs in 50–75% of these patients, and hepatomegaly occurs in about 25%. Occasionally, jaundice can develop. Hematologic complications that can occur during or immediately after the disease include autoimmune hemolytic anemia, thrombocytopenia, agranulocytosis, and (very rarely) aplastic anemia. The disease is usually self-limiting, resolving within a few weeks.

Laboratory Findings

Hematologic findings provide important clues to diagnosis in infectious mononucleosis. Serologic tests can confirm the diagnosis.

Peripheral Blood During active viral infection, an intense proliferation of lymphocytes occurs within affected lymph nodes. The leukocyte count is usually increased (12–25 × 10⁹/L), primarily due to an absolute lymphocytosis. Lymphocytosis begins about 1 week after symptoms appear, peaks at 2–3 weeks, and remains elevated for 2–8 weeks.[5] Lymphocytes usually constitute more than 50% of the leukocyte differential. The platelet count is often mildly decreased, but concentrations of less than 100 × 10⁹/L are rare.

⊙ **TABLE 20-2**

Summary of Typical Clinical and Laboratory Findings in Infectious Mononucleosis

Clinical Findings	Laboratory Findings
Lymphadenopathy	Leukocytosis
Fever	Lymphocytosis
Lethargy	Peripheral blood smear
Sore throat	>20% reactive (atypical) lymphocytes
Splenomegaly	Immunoblasts present
	Heterophile antibodies present
	Positive antigen tests for EBV

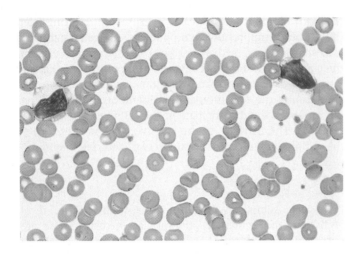

■ FIGURE 20-2 Two reactive forms of lymphocytes from a case of infectious mononucleosis. Note the cytoplasmic vacuoles and cytoplasmic basophilia and irregular shapes. (Peripheral blood; Wright-Giemsa stain; 1000× magnification)

Various forms of reactive lymphocytes (>20%) can be found in the peripheral blood (Figure 20-2 ■). Typical cells are irregular in shape and have large amounts of spreading cytoplasm with irregular bsophilia. Other reactive cells may have deep blue cytoplasm and vacuoles. Immunoblasts are usually present early in the disease. Plasmacytoid lymphocytes and an occasional plasma cell also can be found. When present, immunoblasts should be distinguished from leukemic lymphoblasts to prevent a misdiagnosis. The chromatin pattern of leukemic lymphoblasts is usually finer than the reticular chromatin of immunoblasts. In addition, immunoblasts generally have a lower N:C ratio with more abundant, sometimes vacuolated, cytoplasm. Another important criterion that helps differentiate infectious mononucleosis from leukemia is the morphologic heterogeneity of the lymphocyte population characteristic of viral infections whereas in leukemia, there is usually a homogeneous population.

Other diseases associated with a reactive lymphocytosis can be confused with the blood picture of infectious mononucleosis. These include cytomegalovirus infection, viral hepatitis, and toxoplasmosis.

Bone Marrow Bone marrow aspirations in EBV infection are not indicated, but when performed show hyperplasia of all cellular elements except neutrophils.

Serologic Tests Serologic tests (tests based on antigen/antibody reactions) are used to differentiate this disease from similar more serious diseases (i.e., diptheria, hepatitis). The blood of patients with infectious mononucleosis contains greatly increased concentrations of transient **heterophile antibodies** that agglutinate sheep or horse erythrocytes, but are not specific for EBV.[6,7] (A heterophile antibody will react with antigens that are common to multiple species.) Antibodies specific for EBV can be identified by absorbing the nonspecific heterophile antibodies from the serum with guinea pig antigen and testing the absorbed serum with horse erythrocytes. The infectious mononucleosis IgM antibodies react with horse erythrocytes. Positive agglutination between treated serum and horse erythrocytes indicates EBV infection. A negative result usually indicates infection by some other virus. The level of antibody occasionally is not yet high enough to be detected; therefore, the test should be repeated a week later if patient symptoms continue.

Rapid, specific, and sensitive slide agglutination or solid phase immunoassay tests are available to test for the presence of infectious mononucleosis heterophile antibodies. The infected individual produces antibodies specific for the viral capsid antigen (VCA) of EBV at various stages of infection which can be detected earlier than the heterophile antibodies. VCA-IgM rises first followed by VCA-IgG which, when present, signals the development of immunity.[7] Antibodies to EBV nuclear antigens (EBNA) rise during early convalescence and persist together with VCA-IgG (Table 20-3 ✪). Thus, the presence of EBNA excludes an acute infection.

A patient with all clinical manifestations and peripheral blood findings of infectious mononucleosis occasionally does not have a positive heterophile test (heterophile-negative syndrome). In 10–20% of adult cases and in 50% of children younger than 10 years of age, the test is negative in the presence of EBV infection. In other cases, the heterophile-negative syndrome is caused by a non-EBV viral infection. The likely causative agent is cytomegalovirus; however, toxoplasmosis, hepatitis, and drug intoxication also should be considered. Antibody responses might not be detected in **immunosuppressed** individuals (those in whom the immune response is suppressed either naturally, artificially, or pathologically).[7]

Other laboratory tests can be abnormal depending on the presence or absence of complications. Hepatitis of some degree is common and can be a severe complication. An increase

✪ TABLE 20-3				
Antibodies to EBV That Are Found in Infectious Mononucleosis				
Stage of Infection	Heterophile Antibodies	VCA-IgM (titer)	VCA-IgG (titer)	EBNA (titer)
Acute (0–3 months)	Present	>1:160	>1:60	Not detected
Recent (3–12 months)	Present	Not detected	>1:160	>1:10
Past (>12 months)	Present	Not detected	>1:40	>1:40

VCA = viral capsid antigen; EBNA = EBV nuclear antigen

in both direct and indirect bilirubin fractions and an increase in serum liver enzymes are common findings in the presence of hepatitis. A rare complication of infectious mononucleosis is hemolytic anemia. The anemia appears to be due to cold agglutinins directed against the erythrocyte i-antigen.

Therapy

Because the disease is normally self-limited, therapy is supportive. Bed rest is recommended if fever and myalgia are present. Strenuous exercise should be avoided for several weeks, especially if splenomegaly is present. Antibiotics are not useful except in the presence of secondary infections.

 Checkpoint! 1

A patient with lymphocytosis, showing reactive lymphocyte morphology with large, basophilic cells, fine chromatin, and a visible nucleolus has a negative infectious mononucleosis serologic test. What is a possible cause for this altered lymphocyte morphology?

TOXOPLASMOSIS

Toxoplasmosis is the result of infection with the intracellular protozoan *Toxoplasma gondii*. This obligate parasite can multiply in all body cells except erythrocytes. The infection can be congenital or acquired. Congenital infection, the most serious, results from placental transmission of organisms from the parasitized mother to the fetus. Congenital infection can cause abortion, jaundice, hepatosplenomegaly, chorioretinitis, hydrocephalus, microcephaly, cerebral calcification, and mental retardation. Acquired infection can be asymptomatic or cause symptoms resembling infectious mononucleosis. Infection in children and adults is acquired by ingestion of oocysts from cat feces or from inadequately cooked meat. Toxoplasmosis seropositivity is more common in rural children than urban children.[8] Molecular tests for *Toxoplasma gondii* DNA are available but are not yet FDA approved.

Laboratory findings assist in diagnosis. There is a leukocytosis with a relative lymphocytosis, (more rarely) an absolute lymphocytosis, and an increase in reactive lymphocytes. Most reactive cells are similar to lymphoblasts or lymphoma cells. The heterophile antibody test is negative. Biopsy of lymph nodes shows a reactive follicular hyperplasia and can play an important role in diagnosis. Diagnosis of an active infection is established by confirming a rising titer and seroconversion of antibodies to *Toxoplasma gondii*. Immunologically compromised hosts have a more severe infection. The most common hematologic complication is hemolytic anemia, which can be severe.

CYTOMEGALOVIRUS

Infection with the herpes-group virus **cytomegalovirus (CMV)** can be the result of congenital or acquired infection. Infection in neonates occurs when organisms from the infected mother cross the placenta and infect the fetus. The

newborn demonstrates jaundice, microcephaly, and hepatosplenomegaly. Only about 10% of infected infants exhibit clinical evidence of the disease. The most common hematologic findings in neonates are thrombocytopenia and hemolytic anemia.

Acquired infection is spread by close contact, blood transfusions, and sexual contact. The disease occurs in immunosuppressed individuals, in patients with malignancy, in patients after massive blood transfusions, and in previously healthy adults. It is the most common viral infection complicating tissue transplants and is a significant cause of morbidity and mortality in immunocompromised patients.[9] However, recent advances in treatment with anti-viral drugs and immunosuppressive therapy have dramatically decreased the incidence of CMV complications in organ transplantation.[10] Infected adults present with symptoms similar to those of infectious mononucleosis except pharyngitis is absent. Many cytomegalovirus infections are subclinical or cause mild flu-like symptoms.

Laboratory findings include a leukocytosis with an absolute lymphocytosis. Many of the lymphocytes are reactive, but the heterophile agglutinin test is negative. Hepatic enzymes are usually abnormal. Diagnosis is confirmed by demonstrating the virus in the urine or blood using a viral DNA (molecular) assay or by a rise in the cytomegalovirus antibody titer (except in immunocompromised patients).

CMV is thought to infect neutrophils, which serve as a means of transporting the virus to other body sites. The virus appears to suppress cell-mediated immune function and induce formation of autoantibodies that have lymphocytotoxic properties.[11] A decrease in circulating T helper lymphocytes and an increase in T suppressor/cytotoxic lymphocytes occurs.

INFECTIOUS LYMPHOCYTOSIS

Infectious lymphocytosis, previously considered an infectious, contagious disease of young children, is now referenced as the reactive immune response associated with several viruses that infect children. The most common viruses are the adenovirus and coxsackie A virus and sometimes *Bordetella pertussis*. EBV and CMV are not implicated.[12] Leukocytosis and lymphocytosis occur in the first week of illness and subsequently return to normal. The lymphocytes are small and appear normal rather than reactive.

BORDETELLA PERTUSSIS

Infection from *Bordetella pertussis* (whooping cough) causes a blood picture very similar to that of infectious lymphocytosis (Figure 20-3 ■). The leukocyte count typically rises to $15–25 \times 10^9/L$ but may reach $50 \times 10^9/L$. The rise in leukocytes is caused by an absolute lymphocytosis, although neutrophils also can be increased. Granulocytes may show toxic changes. The lymphocytes are small cells with condensed chromatin and indistinct nucleoli.

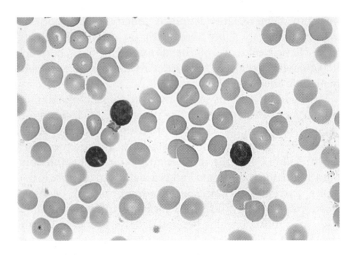

■ FIGURE 20-3 Lymphoproliferation due to *Bordetella pertussis* (whooping cough). Note the numerous small lymphocytes with condensed chromatin. This self-limiting peripheral blood picture must be distinguished from that of CLL. (Peripheral blood; Wright-Giemsa stain; 1000× magnification)

Laboratory diagnostic methods include culture, serology, and PCR.[13] Culture is the gold standard and is specific but not sensitive. The advantage of culture is that it allows antibiotic sensitivity testing and epidemiological typing. Serologic diagnosis is based on demonstrating antipertussis toxin antibodies and has high specificity. It is preferred for older children and adults who present after a prolonged coughing illness. A PCR commercial test approved by the Food and Drug Administration is not available; current tests in development have problems with variable sensitivity and specificity between laboratories. It is most useful in acutely ill infants.

Pertussis toxin stimulates lymphocytosis-promoting factor (LPF) produced by the bacteria that recruits lymphocytes into the peripheral circulation and blocks their migration back into lymphoid tissue, causing accumulation of lymphocytes in the blood. LPF interferes with lymphocyte function and appears to influence T helper cells.[13] Rapid peripheral lymphocytosis is accompanied by decreased cellularity of the lymph nodes. A recent study immunophenotyped the lymphocytes from a neonate with pertussis.[14] Results showed that the increase in lymphocytes was due to T lymphocytes with a normal CD4 to CD8 ratio. However, a dramatic loss of L-selectin expression by these T cells occurred. This could prevent the homing of T cells to lymphoid tissues and explain the buildup of lymphocytes in the peripheral blood.

Whooping cough infections rose 400% between 1990 and 2001 in the adult population, suggesting that childhood vaccinations do not yield lasting immunity. Studies show that 20–30% of adults with a cough that lingers 6–8 weeks are positive for *Bordetella pertussis*. While the infections cause a lingering cough in adults, passing it on to infants can be fatal.[15]

PERSISTENT LYMPHOCYTOSIS

Persistent lymphocytosis is a rare disorder found in young to middle-aged females who are heavy smokers. It is characterized by a persistent polyclonal B cell expansion[16] The disorder is often asymptomatic and found by chance on a routine blood analysis. Symptoms can include fever, fatigue, weight loss, recurrent chest infections, or generalized lymphadenopathy. Hematologic findings are normal except for lymphocytosis and the occasional presence of binucleated lymphocytes. There is a polyclonal increase in serum IgM but low IgG and IgA levels. Bone marrow examination reveals lymphocytic infiltrates. Patients have a benign course.

OTHER DISORDERS ASSOCIATED WITH LYMPHOCYTOSIS

Other disorders accompanied by a reactive lymphocytosis are listed in Table 20-1. The lymphocytic reactions in these disorders are characterized by an increased relative lymphocyte count with the presence of reactive or immature-appearing lymphocytes (**lymphocytic leukemoid reaction**). An absolute lymphocytosis is found occasionally. Many of the lymphocytes are large reactive cells with deep blue cytoplasm, fine chromatin, and cytoplasmic vacuoles (Figure 20-4 ■). Reactive cells are usually nonclonal T lymphocytes and large granular lymphocytes. In some viral infections, lymphocytosis is preceded by lymphocytopenia and neutropenia. As the infection subsides, plasmacytoid lymphocytes can be found (Figure 20-5 ■).

In some cases, a lymphocytic leukemoid reaction resembles chronic lymphocytic leukemia (CLL, ∞ Chapter 26). Bone marrow aspiration, however, shows minimal (if any) increase in lymphocytes in a lymphocytic leukemoid reac-

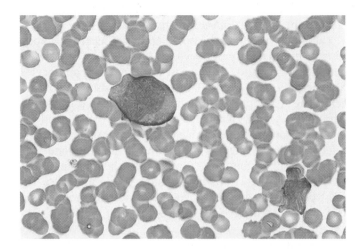

■ FIGURE 20-4 An immunoblast found in a patient with a viral infection. This cell must be distinguished from a leukemic lymphoblast. (Peripheral blood; Wright-Giemsa stain; 1000× magnification)

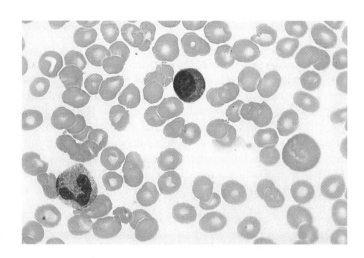

■ **FIGURE 20-5**   A plasmacytoid lymphocyte. Note the deep basophilic cytoplasm and eccentric nucleus. These cells are associated with infectious states. Note also the neutrophil with toxic granulation. (Peripheral blood; Wright-Giemsa stain; 1000× magnification)

✪ TABLE 20-4
Conditions Associated with Lymphocytopenia
• Malnutrition
• Disseminated neoplasms
• Connective tissue disease (e.g., systemic lupus erythematosus, SLE)
• Hodgkin's disease
• Chemotherapy
• Radiotherapy
• Corticosteroids
• Acute inflammatory conditions
• Chronic infection (e.g., tuberculosis, TB)
• Congenital immune deficiency diseases
• Acquired immune deficiency diseases
• Acute and chronic renal disease
• Stress

tion. In contrast to CLL, adenopathy, and splenomegaly are usually absent. In addition, patients with a lymphocytic leukemoid reaction are usually young, whereas in CLL the patients are usually older adults.

PLASMACYTOSIS

Plasma cells are not normally found in the peripheral blood. They can be present, however, with intense stimulation of the immune system as occurs in some viral and bacterial infections and in disorders associated with elevated serum gamma globulin. They are commonly found in rubeola infections. Circulating plasma cells also can be found in skin diseases, cirrhosis of the liver, collagen disorders, and sarcoidosis. Most often the presence of plasma cells is associated with the neoplastic disorders, plasma cell leukemia, and multiple myeloma.

▶ LYMPHOCYTOPENIA

Some disorders are associated with a lymphocytopenia, which occurs in adults when the absolute lymphocyte count is less than 1.0×10^9/L. In children less than 5 years old, the lower normal range varies, but it is higher than in adults (Table B, inside front cover). Generally, lymphocyte counts less than 2×10^9/L are abnormal in this population. When the lymphocyte count is decreased, there could be an impaired ability to mount an immune response, resulting in immunodeficiency.

Lymphocytopenia results from decreased production or increased destruction of lymphocytes, changes in lymphocyte circulation patterns, and other unknown causes (Table 20-4 ✪).[17] Corticosteroid therapy causes a sharp drop in circulating lymphocytes within 4 hours. The decrease is caused by sequestration of lymphocytes in the bone marrow. Values return to normal within 12–24 hours after cessation of therapy. Acute inflammatory conditions, including viral and bacterial infections, also can be associated with a transient lymphocytopenia. Carcinoma of the breast and stomach with an associated lymphocytopenia is a poor prognostic sign. Systemic lupus erythematosus is frequently associated with a lymphocytopenia presumably caused by autoantibodies produced against these cells. Chemotherapeutic alkylating drugs for malignancy, such as cyclophosphamide, cause the death of T and B lymphocytes in both interphase and mitosis. Malnutrition is the most common cause of lymphocytopenia. Starvation causes thymic involution and depletion of T lymphocytes. Both congenital and acquired immune deficiencies are associated with lymphocytopenia.

Irradiation causes a prolonged suppression of lymphocyte production. T helper lymphocytes are more sensitive to radiation than are T suppressor lymphocytes. It appears that small daily fractions of radiation are more damaging to lymphocytes than periodic large doses. With periodic radiation, the lymphocytes can renew during periods of nonradiation. Aggressive treatment of hematologic malignancies with chemotherapeutics or ionizing radiation can lead to immunodeficiency by depleting short-lived, antibody-forming B lymphocytes.

✓ **Checkpoint! 2**

Why is lymphocytopenia a concern if there is no accompanying leukopenia?

CASE STUDY *(continued from page 407)*

Heidi weighed 2 pounds 1 ounce at birth. Tests for CMV and toxoplasma infections were negative. At 4 days of age, she was transferred to a special facility for feeding and growth monitoring. She developed a diaper rash that failed to respond to many measures. No thrush was found. At 44 days, she developed pneumonia from coagulase-negative staphylococci that responded to antibiotics. Her WBC count was 12.3×10^9/L with a differential of segs 42%, bands 5%, lymphocytes 1%, monocytes 28%, eosinophils 23%, and basophils 1%.

3. What is the absolute lymphocyte count?

4. What possible causes exist for these opportunistic infections?

IMMUNE DEFICIENCY DISORDERS

Immune deficiency disorders are characterized by impaired function of one or more of the components of the immune system, T, B, or NK lymphocytes. In some disorders, the numbers of these cells also can be reduced. This results in an inability to mount a normal adaptive immune response. These disorders are characterized clinically by an increase in infections and neoplasms and can be subgrouped as acquired or congenital.

Acquired immune deficiency syndrome (AIDS) is an infectious disorder characterized by lymphocytopenia. Due to the frequency with which this disorder is encountered in the clinical hematology laboratory, it is discussed in more detail next and is followed by a discussion of the congenital immune deficiency disorders.

Acquired Immune Deficiency Syndrome

Acquired immune deficiency syndrome (AIDS) is a highly lethal immune deficiency disease first described in 1981.[18] The disease is caused by infection with a retrovirus, human immunodeficiency virus type I (HIV-1). Advances in HIV treatment with combination antiretroviral therapy delay progression to AIDS and death for people infected with HIV.[19]

AIDS is defined by the occurrence of repeated infections with multiple **opportunistic organisms** and an increase in malignancies, especially Kaposi's sarcoma, in individuals infected with HIV. Patients infected with HIV progress through three recognized stages: an asymptomatic carrier stage, an **AIDS-related complex (ARC)** stage (mild symptomatic stage), and finally, symptomatic AIDS with one of the AIDS-defining clinical conditions (discussed later).[20]

Transmission of the virus is through sexual intercourse or contact with blood and blood products. The disease occurs primarily in certain high-risk groups: those who participate in unprotected sexual intercourse with high-risk or infected individuals, homosexual and bisexual men, prostitutes, intravenous drug abusers, Haitians, and hemophiliacs. Although it is most common in men, women who have had sexual relations with someone at high risk of HIV infection also are at risk as are infants born to HIV-infected mothers. Infant infection can be perinatal or occur at birth.

Surveillance HIV Case Definition   In 1982, the Centers for Disease Control and Prevention (CDC) in the United States developed a case definition of AIDS for surveillance purposes. It is revised periodically as more is learned about the disease.[21,22] It was proposed that AIDS case definition should be as comprehensive as possible because many countries will grant social benefits or access to medical care only if HIV-infected patients have a diagnosed AIDS-defining illness[23] (Table 20-5 ⊙).

⊙ TABLE 20-5

Clinical Conditions Included in the Centers for Disease Control and Prevention Surveillance Case Definition for HIV Infection

Candidiasis of bronchi, trachea, or lungs
Candidiasis, esophageal
Cervical cancer, invasive
Coccidioidomycosis, disseminated or extrapulmonary
Cryptococcosis, extrapulmonary
Cryptosporidiosis, chronic intestinal (>1 month's duration)
Cytomegalovirus disease (other than liver, spleen, or nodes)
Cytomegalovirus retinitis (with loss of vision)
Encephalopathy, HIV related
Herpes simplex: chronic ulcer(s) (>1 month's duration) or bronchitis, pneumonitis, or esophagitis
Histoplasmosis, disseminated or extrapulmonary
Isosporiasis, chronic intestinal (>1 month's duration)
Kaposi's sarcoma
Lymphoma, Burkitt
Lymphoma, immmunoblastic (or equivalent term)
Lymphoma, primary, of brain
Mycobacterium avium complex or *M. kansasii* (disseminated or extrapulmonary)
Mycobacterium tuberculosis, any site (pulmonary or extrapulmonary)
Mycobacterium, other species or unidentified species, disseminated or extrapulmonary
Pneumocystis carinii pneumonia
Pneumonia, recurrent
Progressive multifocal leukoencephalopathy
Salmonella septicemia, recurrent
Toxoplasmosis of brain
Wasting syndrome due to HIV
Bacterial infections, multiple or recurrent*
Lymphoid interstitial pneumonia or pulmonary lymphoid hyperplasia complex*

*only among children <13 years old
(From Appendix B from *MMWR*, 41, No. RR-17, December 1992.)

However, AIDS case surveillance alone does not accurately assess the HIV epidemic. To more accurately reflect the trends in HIV infection, the CDC recommends surveillance not only for AIDS but also for HIV infection.[19] This surveillance expansion helps to identify populations with newly diagnosed HIV infection and aids in efforts to prevent HIV transmission. In 2008, the Council of State and Territorial Epidemiologists (CSTE) developed a revised case definition of HIV infection intended for public health surveillance.[24] The revised criteria apply to adults and children over 18 months of age and combine the HIV case definition, HIV classification system, and AIDS case definition into a single case definition for HIV infection. This revised case definition for HIV infection requires laboratory-confirmed evidence of HIV infection. CSTE, in cooperation with pediatricians, also described the criteria for a negative diagnosis for children <18 months old born to HIV-infected mothers. The child does *not* meet the criteria for HIV/AIDS diagnosis if antibody tests or virologic tests are negative after 4–6 months of age and the child does not have an AIDS-defining condition. The reader is directed to the primary source for details.[24]

Laboratory evidence of HIV infection includes positive serologic HIV antibody tests, positive HIV nucleic acid tests, and positive HIV cultures.[19] Almost all children born to HIV-infected mothers have anti-HIV IgG antibodies at birth due to placental transmission of maternal antibodies. However, only 15–30% are infected with HIV. Thus, anti-HIV IgG tests are not reliable until after 18 months in this population. In these cases, HIV nucleic acid detection tests performed after the infant is at least one month of age are almost always positive if the virus is present.[19]

Immune-compromised patients without one of the AIDS-defining clinical conditions but with milder symptoms, including weight loss, fever, lymphadenopathy, thrush, chronic rash, and intermittent diarrhea, are included in the ARC category.

Pathophysiology   The etiologic agent of AIDS has been identified as the retrovirus, HIV-1. This virus selectively infects helper T lymphocytes by binding to the CD4 antigen that is part of the T lymphocyte receptor (TCR), causing rapid, selective depletion of this lymphocyte subset. Cytolysis of these CD4 lymphocytes results in lymphocytopenia. Once in the cell, HIV sheds its viral coat and uses reverse transcriptase to make a DNA copy of the viral RNA. Viral DNA is then integrated into the host cell DNA where the virus replicates. Monocytes and macrophages also have the CD4 antigen and are infected but are not destroyed by the virus.

Cell-mediated immunity and humoral immunity are abnormal. Cell-mediated immunity declines as CD4 T-lymphocyte-helper function for monocytes, macrophages, and other T lymphocytes declines.[25] Humoral responses are exaggerated with polyclonal B lymphocyte proliferation and increased immunoglobulin production.[26] The B lymphocytes, however, are incapable of responding to signals that trigger resting B lymphocytes.

Laboratory Findings   Multiple hematologic abnormalities are found in AIDS, including leukopenia, lymphocytopenia, anemia, and thrombocytopenia (Table 20-6 ✪). Leukopenia is usually related to lymphocytopenia, although neutropenia also can be present.[27] Lymphocytes can include reactive forms. Mild to moderate anemia is present in the majority of HIV-infected individuals and worsens as the disease progresses.[28] Macrocytosis (MCV>110 fL) occurs in up to 70% of patients 2 weeks after receiving zidovudine.[29] Antierythrocyte antibodies can be found in up to 20% of patients with hypergammaglobulinemia. These antibodies react like polyagglutinins and cause a positive direct antiglobulin test (DAT, Coombs' test). Immune thrombocytopenia, indistinguishable from idiopathic thrombocytopenic purpura (ITP), is common (∞ Chapter 31). (ITP is characterized by immune destruction of platelets, causing a thrombocytopenia.)

Disease Monitoring   The severity of CD4 lymphocytopenia and concentration of plasma HIV-1 RNA copies correlate with the severity of disease.[20,30] The normal CD4-to-CD8 ratio in peripheral blood is about 2:1. In AIDS, this ratio reverses progressively and permanently due to destruction of the CD4 T lymphocytes. The CD4 T lymphocyte count is performed at initial diagnosis and measured periodically to monitor disease progression. AIDS (Stage 3 HIV infection) is defined by a CD4+ lymphocyte count of <200/μL or a CD4+ lymphocyte concentration <14% of total lymphocytes.[24] In addition, the **viral load** also is monitored by measuring the number of copies of HIV-1 RNA.[30]

Therapy   No cure for AIDS currently exists. Treatment with zidovudine (azodothymidine, AZT) and protease inhibitors appear to lengthen the time between HIV seropositivity and the onset of AIDS.[31] Surveillance studies between 1992 and 1997 determined that careful follow-up and new antiviral treatments decreased the incidence of opportunistic infections in over one-half of the patients on the case definition list.[32]

Health care workers with occupational exposure (e.g., needle-stick injury) to HIV should receive immediate antiretroviral therapy.[30] CDC recommends initiation of antiretroviral therapy within 2 hours of a needle-stick injury from a potential HIV source. Combination therapy should consist of two or more antiretroviral drugs and continue for 4 weeks. Laboratory evaluation for adverse effects should be considered after 2 weeks. Health care workers with questions about postexposure prophylaxis (PEP) should contact the CDC PEPline at 1(888)HIV-4911.

✪ TABLE 20-6
Common Laboratory Findings in HIV Infections

• Leukopenia	• Thrombocytopenia
• Anemia	• Decreased CD4 counts
• Macrocytosis	• Positive molecular tests for HIV-1 RNA

✓ Checkpoint! 3

Why does infection with HIV result in an increased chance for opportunistic infections?

Other Acquired Immune Deficiency Disorders

Some disorders are characterized or accompanied by functional abnormalities of lymphocytes. The lymphocyte count can be normal but in many cases is decreased. Acquired defects of either T or B lymphocytes can result in serious clinical manifestations. Some inflammatory states can transiently impede the response of T lymphocytes to antigen. These include idiopathic granulomatous disorders and malignancy. Severe infection by one microorganism sometimes impedes the ability of T lymphocytes to react to other infectious organisms. Starvation or severe protein deficiency can severely affect the functional ability of the T lymphocyte.

Congenital Immune Deficiency Disorders

Congenital disorders are usually characterized by a decrease in lymphocytes and impairment in either cell-mediated immunity (T lymphocytes), humoral immunity (B lymphocytes), or both (Table 20-7 ✪). In contrast to the reactive morphologic heterogeneity of lymphocytes associated with acquired disorders, lymphocytes in congenital disorders are usually normal in appearance. The functional impairment of the immune response is often apparent from birth or a very young age.

Severe Combined Immunodeficiency Syndrome

Severe combined immunodeficiency (SCID) syndrome includes a heterogeneous group of disorders result-ing in major qualitative immune defects involving both humoral and cellular immune functions. These disorders have diverse genetic origins with different inheritance patterns and varied severity in clinical manifestation. Most are inherited as sex-linked or autosomal-recessive traits, but sporadic forms have been reported. About 75% of individuals with SCID are males because the most common form of SCID is an X-linked disorder.

Both the T and B lymphoid lineages are functionally deficient. Subgroups of SCID are now defined on the basis of which lymphocytes are absent. If only the T cells are absent, it is termed $T^-B^+NK^+$ *SCID*; if both T and B cells are absent, $T^-B^-NK^+$ *SCID*; and in those patients (usually with the most severe lymphopenia) where all three are absent, $T^-B^-NK^-$ *SCID*. Because of the need for T cell help in generating an antibody response against protein antigens, peripheral blood B lymphocytes, even when present, are unresponsive to mitogens, and immunoglobulin production decreases. However, these B lymphocytes respond normally when incubated with normal T lymphocytes in vitro.[26] The absolute lymphocyte count is variable but often decreased to less than 1.0×10^9/L. Lymphocyte counts in SCID patients can be normal in the neonate, especially if they are able to generate B cells and NK cells, but usually eventually develop a profound lymphopenia.

Lymph node examination reveals a lack of plasma cells, B lymphocytes, and T lymphocytes. No lymphoid cells are found in the spleen, tonsils, or intestinal tract. The bone marrow also is deficient in plasma cells and lymphocyte precursors.

Frequent recurrent infections, skin rashes, diarrhea, and a failure to thrive are characteristic findings in infants with

✪ TABLE 20-7

Laboratory Findings in Selected Immunodeficiency Disorders

Disorder	Immunoglobulins	B lymphocytes	T lymphocytes	Inheritance
SCID (X-linked) $T^-B^+NK^+$ SCID	↓ IgG, IgE, IgA; N IgM	↓ or normal (number)	Mature T lymphs absent	X(q13.1−q21.1) (γ-chain of IL-7 R)
Autosomal recessive $T^-B^+NK^+$ SCID	↓ IgG, IgE, IgA; N IgM	↓ or normal (number)	Mature T lymphs absent	JAK3 (19p13.1); IL-7 α-chain (5p13); ZAP-70 (2q12)
$T^-B^-NK^+$ SCID	↓ IgG, IgM, IgA, IgE	Mature B cells and plasma cells absent	Mature T lymphs absent	ADA (20q13.11) PNP (14q13.2) RAG-1, RAG-2
$T^-B^-NK^-$ SCID Reticular dysgenesis	↓ IgG, IgM, IgA	Mature B cells and plasma cells absent	Mature T lymphs absent	Etiology unknown
Wiskott-Aldrich syndrome	↓ IgM; N/↑ IgA; ↑ IgE; N/↑ IgG	Normal	Progressive ↓	Sex-linked; X(p11.3−p11.22)
DiGeorge syndrome	Normal	Normal	↓	Gene deletion; del(22)(q11)
X-linked agammaglobulinemia	↓ IgG, IgM, IgA	↓	Normal	Sex-linked; defects at X(q21.3−q22)
Ataxia-telangiectasia	N/↑ IgM; N/↓ IgG; N/↓ IgA; ↓ IgE	Normal	Normal	Autosomal recessive; 11q22−q23

↓ = decreased; ↑ = increased; N = normal; ADA = adenosine deaminase; PNP = purine nucleoside phosphorylase; RAG = recombination activating gene.

this disorder. Death related to overwhelming sepsis usually occurs within the first 2 years of life if untreated. Bone marrow transplantation or gene therapy are the only options for successful treatment.

Sex-Linked SCID. Classic sex-linked (X-linked) SCID is the most common form of inherited severe combined immunodeficiency, accounting for ~45% of cases. This form of SCID (a T⁻B⁺NK⁺ SCID) has been mapped to the long arm of the X chromosome (Xql3.1—q21.1) and was originally associated with a loss-of-function mutation in the gene for the γ-chain of the IL-2 receptor. Because the γ-chain also is an essential subunit of the receptors for IL-4, IL-7, IL-9, and IL-15, cytokine regulation by all of these cytokines is impaired (∞ Chapter 3). IL-7/IL-7R signaling is required for T cell development and, in its absence, there is failure of T cell lymphopoiesis. Thus X-linked SCID is characterized by absent T lymphocytes and a hypoplastic thymus. B lymphocytes are normal or even increased in number but are functionally abnormal due to lack of T helper function, and immunoglobulin levels are severely depressed. Family history is important in determining the mode of inheritance of SCID, although a negative family history of the disease does not rule out an X-linked disease. Up to one-third of the cases present as a spontaneous mutation.[24,32]

Females who carry the abnormal X-linked SCID gene have normal immunity. These carriers can be detected by molecular assays for mutations in the γ-chain locus using cells other than lymphocytes. The normal mature female cell population is mosaic with one or the other X chromosome inactivated. In female SCID carriers, however, only lymphocytes carrying normal X chromosomes are found rather than the expected mixture of cells with normal and abnormal X chromosome inactivation. It has been found that random X chromosome inactivation occurs in these carriers, but the gene product of the mutant-X chromosome does not support lymphocyte maturation. Thus, lymphocytes with the mutant X chromosome fail to develop, and the only lymphocytes found in carriers have the active normal X chromosome.

 Checkpoint! 4

Would you expect female carriers of X-linked SCIDS to be more susceptible to infection than the normal population? Why or why not?

Autosomal SCID. The autosomal forms of SCID exhibit severe deficiencies of both T and B lymphocytes. The most common form, found in about 50% of autosomal-recessive SCID (15% of all SCID patients), is due to an adenosine deaminase (ADA) deficiency.[34,35] The adenosine deaminase gene is located at chromosome 20q13.11. Both point mutations and gene deletions have been associated with an ADA deficiency. Another enzyme deficiency, purine nucleoside phosphorylase (PNP), is the cause of ~2% of SCID cases. The

gene for PNP is located at chromosome 14q13.1. Both of these enzymes degrade purines. Without the enzyme, accumulation of toxic DNA metabolites (deoxyadenosine triphosphate/dATP and deoxyguanosine triphosphate/dGTP) occurs, inhibiting normal T and B cell development. In both cases, the result is a T⁻B⁻NK⁺ type of SCID. Other defects include a deficiency of MHC class II gene expression, interleukin-2 (IL-2) deficiency, mutations in the *RAG-1* and *RAG-2* genes (which catalyze VDJ recombination), and defective assembly of the T lymphocyte receptor/CD3 complex.[26] (∞ Chapter 7)

 CASE STUDY *(continued from page 412)*

All of Heidi's immunoglobulin levels were decreased. T and B lymphocyte counts were severely decreased. The peripheral blood smear showed anisocytosis, poikilocytosis (schistocytes), polychromatophilia, and 2 nucleated RBCs/100 WBCs. Her thymus was not detectable on chest films.

5. Is this child more likely to have a congenital or acquired immune deficiency?

6. If she has a congenital immune deficiency, is it more likely she has X-linked or autosomal SCIDS?

7. Are the lymphocytes more likely to be morphologically heterogeneous or homogeneous? Why?

8. What confirmatory test is indicated?

Wiskott-Aldrich Syndrome Wiskott-Aldrich syndrome (WAS) is a sex-linked recessive disease characterized by the triad of eczema, thrombocytopenia, and immunodeficiency resulting in recurrent infections. About two-thirds of affected children have a family history of the disease; one-third reflects a spontaneous mutation. Most children die before 10 years of age due to infection or bleeding. Those who survive longer can develop neoplasms of the histiocytic, lymphocytic, or myelocytic systems.

Laboratory findings play an important role in the diagnosis of WAS (Table 20-8 ✪). There is progressive decrease in thymic-dependent immunity and depletion of paracortical areas in the lymph nodes leading to abnormal lymphocyte function. The absolute numbers of helper and suppressor T lymphocytes and their ratio is normal to variable. Typically, CD8 T lymphocytes are decreased, but numbers vary over time for individuals. Circulating B lymphocyte concentrations are normal, but antibody production is abnormal.[36] Serum IgM levels are decreased, but IgE and IgA levels are increased. IgG concentrations are usually normal.

One of the most consistent findings is low or absent levels of circulating antibodies to the blood group antigens.[36] This is due to the inability of these children to produce antibodies to polysaccharide antigens. This T-lymphocyte-independent phenomenon suggests that there is an intrinsic B lymphocyte abnormality.

⊛ **TABLE 20-8**

Laboratory Features in Wiskott-Aldrich Syndrome

- Platelets: decreased concentration; small size
- Lymphocytes: decreased or normal concentration; T lymphocytes variable; B lymphocytes usually normal
- Immunoglobulin: IgM decreased, IgE and IgA increased, IgG normal/increased
- Antibodies to blood group antigens absent
- PCR detects WAS gene mutation

A low platelet count with abnormal bleeding in the neonatal period is one of the first clinical signs of WAS. Patients have a severe thrombocytopenia ($<70,000/mm^2$) with small sized platelets.[35] Bleeding times are abnormal, but the prothrombin time and activated partial thromboplastin time are normal, indicating the coagulation factor proteins are adequate (∞ Chapters 29 and 30). Megakaryocytes in the bone marrow are normal or increased in number. Genetic mutations involve the WAS gene on the short arm of the X chromosome between Xp11.3 and Xp11.22. Females are carriers; affected males cannot pass the deficiency to their male children. PCR techniques detect 98% of affected males and are the primary diagnostic tests when WAS is suspected.[35] Molecular analysis using restriction fragment length polymorphisms reveals that female carriers have selective inactivation of the WAS X chromosome rather than random inactivation of paternal or maternal X chromosomes. This nonrandom inactivation pattern is found in the carrier's T and B lymphocytes, granulocytes, monocytes, and megakaryocytes, indicating all hematopoietic cells in WAS express the defect.

Therapy includes treatment for bleeding and infection. Splenectomy usually results in correction of the platelet count and significantly reduces the risk of bleeding complications. Bone marrow transplantation has been used with some success.

 Checkpoint! 5

What laboratory findings suggest WAS in a child, and how is the diagnosis confirmed?

DiGeorge Syndrome   DiGeorge syndrome is a congenital immunodeficiency marked by the absence or hypoplasia of the thymus, hypoparathyroidism, heart defects, and dysmorphic facies. Hypocalcemia is typical, and the presenting symptom can be seizure due to hypocalcemia. There is usually a decrease in peripheral blood T lymphocytes as well as a decrease in the cellularity of the thymic-dependent regions of peripheral lymphoid tissue. The low lymphocyte count is related to a decreased number of CD4 lymphocytes. T lymphocyte function varies. Those children with a hypoplastic thymus may be able to produce enough lymphocytes with

normal function to maintain immunocompetence. B lymphocytes are normal in number and function, and immunoglobulin levels are normal. Infants exhibit increased susceptibility to viral, fungal, and bacterial infections that are frequently overwhelming. Death occurs in the first year unless thymic grafts are performed.

Cytogenetic studies on these children reveal a deletion within chromosome 22q11.[37] This defect also is found in a parent of a child with DiGeorge syndrome in 25% of the cases.

Sex-Linked Agammaglobulinemia   Sex-linked (X-linked) agammaglobulinemia (Bruton's disease) is inherited as a sex-linked disease characterized by frequent respiratory and skin infections with extracellular, catalase-negative, pyogenic bacteria. Molecular analysis has revealed that the genetic defect is on the long arm of the X chromosome (q21.3—q22).[26] More than 90% of patients have a loss-of-function mutation of a tyrosine kinase gene named *Bruton tyrosine kinase* (*BTK*). The genetic mutation results in a block in B lymphocyte maturation at the pre-B-lymphocyte stage. The variable and constant regions of the IgM immunoglobin chain fail to connect. Peripheral blood lymphocyte counts are normal as are T lymphocytes; there is, however, a decrease in B lymphocytes and an absence of plasma cells in lymph nodes. The serum concentrations of IgG, IgM, and IgA are decreased or absent. Cell-mediated immune function is normal. Monthly injections of gamma globulin are effective in preventing severe infections.

Female carriers of this disease have normal immunity. All of their B lymphocytes carry the paternal, normal X chromosome. This suggests the normal X chromosome confers a growth advantage to the normal cells.

Ataxia-Telangiectasia   Ataxia-telangiectasia (AT) is inherited as an autosomal-recessive disease that results from mutations in the ataxia-telangiectasis mutated gene (ATM) at chromosome 11(q22—q23). The ATM protein is involved in the repair of DNA double-stranded breaks. The disease is characterized by progressive neurologic disease, immune dysfunction, and predisposition to malignancy. Affected individuals are ataxic and develop telangiectasias in childhood or adolescence. Telangiectasia is a vascular lesion formed by a dilation of a group of blood vessels that appears as a red line or radiating limbs (spider). Chronic respiratory infection and lymphoid malignancy are the most common causes of death.

These patients have a defect in cell-mediated immunity with hypoplasia or dysplasia of the thymus gland and depletion of thymic-dependent areas in the lymph nodes. B lymphocyte function also is abnormal. Lymphocytopenia with a reversed CD4:CD8 ratio exists along with deficiencies in IgA, IgG and IgE. IgM levels are increased. Cytogenetic analysis reveals excessive chromosome breakage and rearrangements in cultured cells and clonal abnormalities of chromosome 7 or 14.[38]

SUMMARY

Lymphocytes mount an immune response in inflammatory or infectious states. In these states, the lymphocyte morphology often includes various reactive forms, immunoblasts, and possibly plasmacytoid cells. Quantitative changes in the total lymphocyte concentration occur, which can be either increased or decreased. Although the lymphocyte induces an immune response to eliminate foreign antigens, the cell itself also can serve as the site of infection for some viruses that use lymphocyte membrane receptors to attach to and invade the cell.

Infectious mononucleosis is a common self-limiting lymphoproliferative disorder caused by infection with EBV. Laboratory diagnosis of this disorder includes serologic testing for heterophile antibodies and identification of reactive lymphocytes on Romanowsky-stained blood smears.

AIDS is a disease caused by infection of the CD4 lymphocyte with the retrovirus HIV-1. The virus suppresses the immune response by replicating within and destroying CD4 lymphocytes. CD4 lymphocyte levels and viral loads monitor the disease's progression. Antiviral treatments in combination with protease inhibitors slow the progression of the disease process. This disease has no cure.

Congenital qualitative disorders of lymphocytes include a wide variety of immunodeficiency disorders. Either the T or B lymphocyte or both can be affected. These are usually very serious defects with most affected individuals succumbing to the disease in childhood. Diagnosis involves genetic tests. Bone marrow transplant is the only treatment in many cases.

REVIEW QUESTIONS

LEVEL I

1. The infectious agent in infectious mononucleosis is: (Objective 1)
   a. CMV
   b. HIV
   c. EBV
   d. *Toxoplasmosis gondii*

2. Large reactive (atypical) lymphocytes with dispersed chromatin and irregular cytoplasmic membranes are associated with: (Objective 2)
   a. infectious lymphocytosis
   b. infectious mononucleosis
   c. cytomegalovirus infection
   d. hepatitis

3. Which of the following best describes the lymphocytes seen in viral infection? (Objective 5)
   a. large cells with high N:C ratio, immature nucleus, and vacuoles
   b. small cells with high N:C ratio and vacuolated cytoplasm
   c. large cells with deep basophilic cytoplasm and decreased N:C ratio
   d. large cells with immature nuclei and high N:C ratio

4. The CD4:CD8 ratio of T lymphocytes in a patient with AIDS is: (Objectives 9, 10)
   a. 2:1
   b. increased
   c. decreased
   d. equal

5. The type of antibodies found in infectious mononucleosis that are used to confirm a diagnosis are: (Objective 3)
   a. heterophile antibodies
   b. cold agglutinins
   c. PIG antibodies
   d. HIV antibodies

LEVEL II

Use this case study for questions 1–3.

A 39-year-old male was seen at the clinic with complaints of nagging cough, weight loss, diarrhea, and low-grade temperature. Results of physical examination showed lymphadenopathy, congested lungs, and increased heart rate. Slight splenomegaly and hepatomegaly were noted. A CBC and flow cytometry studies were ordered. Histologic examination of sputum with Gomori's methenamine silver nitrate stain revealed *Pneumocystis carinii*.

Laboratory Data:

Erythrocyte count	3.86×10^{12}/L		
Hb	13.6 g/dL (136 g/L)		
Hct	0.41 L/L		
Platelet count	104×10^9/L		
Leukocyte count	2.8×10^9/L		
Differential			
Segmented neutrophils	68%	Monocytes:	10%
Lymphocytes	21%	Eosinophils:	1%
Positive for HIV-1 antibodies			

1. What clinical condition does this patient have? (Objectives 8, 10)
   a. congenital immune deficiency
   b. infectious mononucleosis
   c. ARC
   d. AIDS

2. Which lymphocytes are periodically counted to monitor the disease? (Objective 8)
   a. infected B lymphocytes
   b. CD4 T lymphocytes
   c. CD8 T lymphocytes
   d. natural killer lymphocytes

REVIEW QUESTIONS (continued)

LEVEL I

6. The HIV-1 virus infects what type of lymphocyte? (Objective 9)
   a. B lymphocyte
   b. suppressor T lymphocyte
   c. CD4+ T lymphocyte
   d. CD8+ T lymphocyte

7. A 2-year-old child has a total leukocyte count of 10×10^9/L and 60% lymphocytes. Which of the following best describes the child's blood count? (Objectives 4, 8)
   a. absolute lymphocytosis
   b. relative lymphocytosis
   c. normal lymphocyte count for the age given
   d. absolute lymphocytopenia

Use this case study for questions 8–10.

A 19-year-old female college student went to student health complaining of lethargy and a sore throat over the last two weeks. Physical exam shows pharyngitis, lymphadenopathy, and splenomegaly with a total leukocyte count of 11×10^9/L and 70% lymphocytes (50% of lymphs are reactive).

8. She probably has: (Objective 1)
   a. HIV
   b. hepatitis
   c. X-linked SCIDS
   d. infectious mononucleosis

9. Her absolute lymphocyte count is: (Objective 4)
   a. 10×10^9/L
   b. 11×10^9/L
   c. 5.5×10^9/L
   d. 7.7×10^9/L

10. The best description of this patient's leukocyte count is a(n): (Objectives 4, 8)
    a. relative lymphocytopenia
    b. relative neutrophilia
    c. absolute lymphocytosis
    d. absolute neutrophilia

LEVEL II

3. Which laboratory test is used to follow this patient's disease? (Objective 8)
   a. HIV-1 viral load
   b. throat swab
   c. serologic test for heterophile antibody
   d. PCR for genetic mutations

4. A clue to differentiating the lymphocytes of infectious mononucleosis from those found in neoplastic lymphocytic disorders is that in neoplastic disorders, the lymphocytes are: (Objective 5)
   a. morphologically similar
   b. heterogeneous morphologically
   c. not increased
   d. reactive

5. A 17-year-old male has a sore throat and lymphadenopathy. He is lethargic and has a temperature of 99.5°F. Laboratory tests reveal a leukocyte count of 13×10^9/L with 65% lymphocytes, most of which are reactive. The heterophile antibody test is positive, the VCA-IgM titer is 1:640, VCA-IgG titer is 1:120, and EBNA is not detectable. What is the most likely explanation for these results? (Objectives 3, 10)
   a. acute EBV infection
   b. EBV infection within the last 3–12 months
   c. EBV infection more than a year ago
   d. no EBV infection present now or in the past

6. In female carriers of sex-linked, severe combined immunodeficiency gene, the lymphocytes carry: (Objective 9)
   a. a normal X chromosome in the T lymphocytes
   b. the mutant X chromosome in T and B lymphocytes
   c. the mutant X chromosome in T lymphocytes
   d. the mutant X chromosome in 50% of T lymphocytes

7. *Bordetella pertussis* infection is characterized by: (Objective 7)
   a. positive heterophile antibody test and lymphocytosis
   b. lymphocytopenia and reactive lymphocytes
   c. lymphocytosis with normal appearing lymphocytes
   d. lymphocytosis with reactive lymphocytes

8. Occasionally, a patient who has been exposed to EBV shows clinical symptoms and reactive lymphocytes but has a negative serologic test. This could be due to: (Objective 1)
   a. infection with a parasite
   b. infection with *Bordetella pertussis*
   c. infection with syphilis
   d. early infection with no detectable antibody

9. Documentation and surveillance for AIDS in patients includes those who are positive for: (Objective 8)
   a. HIV viral DNA
   b. EBV viral RNA
   c. heterophile antibodies
   d. any bacterial infection

REVIEW QUESTIONS *(continued)*

LEVEL I

LEVEL II

10. Which of the following nonmalignant conditions is associated with a lymphocytosis? (Objectives 5, 7, 9)
    a. whooping cough
    b. AIDS
    c. X-linked immunodeficiency syndrome
    d. SCIDS

www.pearsonhighered.com/mckenzie

Use this address to access the interactive Companion Website created for this textbook. Find additional information, tables and figures. Evaluate your command of the chapter information using case studies and critical thinking and multiple choice questions.

REFERENCES

1. Straus SE, Cohen JI, Tosato G, Meier J. Epstein-Barr virus infections: Biology, pathogenesis, and management. *Ann Intern Med.* 1993; 118:45–58.

2. Foerster J. Infectious mononucleosis. In: Lee GR, Foerster J, Lukens JN, Paraskevas F, Greer JP, Rodgers GM, eds. *Wintrobe's Clinical Hematology, vol. 2,* 10th ed. Baltimore, Md: Williams & Wilkins; 1999:1926–55.

3. Bailey RE. Diagnosis and treatment of infectious mononucleosis. *Am Fam Physician.* 1994;49:879–85.

4. Nathwani D, Wood MJ. Herpes virus infections in childhood: 2. *Br J Hosp Med.* 1993;50:301–8.

5. Peterson L, Hrisinko MA. Benign lymphocytosis and reactive neutrophilia. *Clin Lab Med.* 1993;13:863–77.

6. Paul JR et al. The presence of heterophile antibodies in infectious mononucleosis. *Am J Med Sci.* 1932;83:90–104.

7. Ebell M. Epstein-Barr virus infectious mononucleosis. *Am Fam Physician.* 2004;70:1279–87.

8. Taylor M, Lennon B, Holland C, Caffrey M. Community study of toxoplasma antibodies in urban and rural school children age 4 to 8 years. *Arch Dis Child.* 1997;77:406–9.

9. Dropului L. The impact of cytomegalovirus infections on solid organ transplantation. *Adv Stud Med.* 2006;6:303–4, 319–28.

10. Steininger C. Clinical relevance of cytomegalovirus infection in patients with disorders of the immune system. *Clin Micro Infec.* 2007; 13(10):953–63.

11. Mustafa MM. Cytomegalovirus infection and disease in the immunocompromised host. *Pediatr Infect Dis J.* 1994;13:249–57.

12. Arnez M, Cizman M, Jazbec J, Kotnik A. Acute infectious lymphocytosis caused by coxsackievirus B2. *Pediatr Infect Dis J.* 1996;15: 1127–28.

13. Crowcroft N, Pebody R. Recent developments in pertussis. *Lancet.* 2006;367:926–36.

14. Hudnall SD, Molina CP. Marked increase in L-selectin-negative T cells in neonatal pertussis. *Amer J Clin Path.* 2000;114:35–40.

15. Dworkin MS. Adults are whooping, but are internists listening? *Ann Intern Med.* 2005;142:832–35.

16. Bain B, Mantutes E, Catovsky D. Teaching cases from the Royal Marsden and St. Mary's Hospitals. Case 14: persistent lymphocytosis in a middle aged smoker. *Leuk Lymphoma.* 1998;28:623–25.

17. Schoentag RA, Cangiarella J. The nuances of lymphocytopenia. *Clin Lab Med.* 1993;13:923–36.

18. Gottlieb MS et al. *Pneumocystis carinii* pneumonia and mucosal candidiasis in previously healthy homosexual men: Evidence of a new acquired cellular immunodeficiency. *N Engl J Med.* 1981;305: 1425–31.

19. Centers for Disease Control and Prevention. Guidelines for national human immunodeficiency virus case surveillance, including monitoring for human immunodeficiency virus infections and acquired immunodeficiency syndrome. *MMWR.* 1999;48(RR-13):1–27,29–31.

20. Centers for Disease Control and Prevention. Prevention and treatment of tuberculosis among patients infected with human immunodeficiency virus: Principles of therapy and revised recommendations. *MMWR.* 1998;47(RR-20):1–51.

21. Gold JWM. HIV-1 Infection. *Med Clin North Am.* 1992;76:1–18.

22. Centers for Disease Control and Prevention. 1993 revised classification system for HIV infection and expanded surveillance case definition for AIDS among adolescents and adults. *MMWR.* 1992;41(RR-17):1–19.

23. Albrecht H. Redefining AIDS: Towards a modification of the current AIDS case definition. *Clin Infec Diseases.* 1997;24(1):64–74.

24. Center for Disease Control and Prevention. Revised Surveillance Case Definitions for HIV Infection Among Adults, Adolescents, and Children aged <18 months for HIV infection and AIDS among children aged 18 months to <13 years . . . United States, 2008. *MMWR.* 2008;57(RR-10):1–10.

25. Said JW. Pathogenesis of HIV infection. In: Nash G, Said JW, eds. *Pathology of AIDS and HIV Infection.* Philadelphia: WB Saunders Co.; 1992; 26:15–18.

26. Insel RA. Disorders of lymphocyte function. In: Hoffman R, Benz EJ, Shattil SJ, Furie B, Cohen HJ, Silberstein LE, eds. *Hematology: Basic Principles and Practice.* Philadelphia: Churchill Livingstone; 1995:819–38.

27. Brynes RK, Gill PS. Clinical characteristics, immunologic abnormalities, and hematopathology of HIV infection. In: Joshi VV, ed. *Pathology of AIDS and Other Manifestations of HIV Infection.* New York: Igaku-Shoin; 1990:21–42.

28. Doukas MA. Human immunodeficiency virus associated anemia. *Med Clin North Am.* 1992;76:699–709.

29. Aboulafia DM, Mitsuyasu RT. Hematologic abnormalities in AIDS. *Hematol Oncol Clin North Am.* 1991;5:195–214.

30. Centers for Disease Control and Prevention. Updated U.S. Public Health Service guidelines for the management of occupational exposures to HIV and recommendations for postexposure prophylaxis. *MMWR.* 2005;54(RR-09):1–17.

31. Hammer SM, Eron JJ, Reiss P, et al. Antiretroviral treatment of adult HIV infection. *JAMA* 2008;300(5):555–570.

32. Centers for Disease Control and Prevention. Surveillance for AIDS-defining opportunistic illnesses, 1992–1997. *MMWR.* 1999;47 (SS-2):1–22.

33. Puck JM. Prenatal diagnosis and genetic analysis of X-linked immunodeficiency disorders. *Pediatr Res.* 1993;33(Suppl 1):29–33.

34. Hershfield M. Adenosine deaminase deficiency. *GeneReviews.* 2006; www.ncbi.nlm.nih.gov/bookshelf/br.fcgi?book=gene&part=ada. Accessed March 15, 2009.

35. Rosen FS, Bhan AK. Weekly clinicopathological exercises, case 18-1998: A 54-day-old premature girl with respiratory distress and persistent pulmonary infiltrates. *New Eng J Med.* 1998;338:1752–58.

36. Filipovich AH, Johnson J, Zhang K. WAS-related disorders. *GeneReviews.* 2004; www.ncbi.nlm.nih.gov/bookshelf/br.fcgi?book=gene&part=was. Accessed March 15, 2009.

37. Wilson DI, Burn J, Scanbler P, Goodship J. DiGeorge syndrome: Part of CATCH 22. *J Med Genet.* 1993;30:852–56.

38. Forte WC, Menezes MC, Dionigi PC, Bastos CL. Different clinical and laboratory evolutions in ataxia-telangiectasia syndrome: Report of four cases. *Allergol Immunopathol.* 2005;33(4):199–203.

Introduction to Hematopoietic Neoplasms

Shirlyn B. McKenzie, Ph.D.

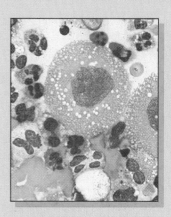

■ OBJECTIVES—LEVEL I

At the end of this unit of study, the student should be able to:

1. Define and differentiate the terms *neoplasm* and *malignant* and identify hematopoietic disorders that can be included in each category.

2. Compare and contrast the general characteristics of the myelodysplastic syndromes (MDS), myeloproliferative disorders (MPD), and acute and chronic leukemias.

3. Name and describe the classification systems used for MDS, MPD, and the leukemias.

4. List the various methods used to categorize the leukemias.

5. Compare and contrast the laboratory findings of the acute and chronic leukemias and myeloid and lymphoid leukemias.

6. Differentiate proto-oncogenes and oncogenes and summarize their relationship to neoplastic processes.

7. Correlate patient age to the overall incidence of the hematopoietic neoplasms.

8. Explain the usefulness of immunological techniques, chromosome analysis, molecular analysis, and cytochemistry in the diagnosis and prognosis of hematopoietic neoplasms.

9. Predict the prognosis and survival rates of the hematopoietic neoplasms.

■ OBJECTIVES—LEVEL II

At the end of this unit of study, the student should be able to:

1. Explain how proto-oncogenes are activated and the role that oncogenes and tumor suppressor genes and their protein products play in the etiology of hematopoietic neoplasms.

2. Describe the effects of radiation on the incidence of leukemia.

3. Differentiate between the acute and chronic leukemias based on their clinical and hematologic findings.

4. Reconcile the use of chemotherapy for treatment of leukemia.

5. Compare and contrast treatment options for the hematopoietic neoplasms including possible complications.

■ OBJECTIVES—LEVEL II *(continued)*

6. Name the leukemogenic factors of leukemia and propose how each contributes to the development of leukemia.

7. Compare and contrast laboratory features of MDS, MPD, and acute leukemia (AL), and justify a patient diagnosis based on these features.

8. Define the principles of, explain the applications of, and select appropriate cytochemical stains for bone marrow evaluation.

9. Select laboratory procedures appropriate for confirming cell lineage and diagnosis in hematopoietic neoplasms.

10. Explain the role of epigenetics in cancer.

11. Define *cancer stem cell* and explain its similarities to the hematopoietic stem cell (HSC).

KEY TERMS

Acute lymphocytic leukemia (ALL)
Acute myeloid leukemia (AML)
Aleukemic leukemia
Auer rods
Benign
Cancer-initiating cell
Cancer stem cells
Chronic lymphocytic leukemia (CLL)
Chronic myelogenous leukemia (CML)
Consolidation therapy
Cytogenetic remission
Epigenetics
French-American-British (FAB)
Hematologic remission
Induction therapy
Leukocyte alkaline phosphatase (LAP)
Leukemia
Leukemic hiatus
Leukemic stem cell
Lymphoma
Maintenance chemotherapy
Malignant
Minimum residual disease (MRD)
Molecular remission
MPO
Myelodysplastic syndromes (MDS)
Myeloproliferative disorders (MPD)
Neoplasm
Nonspecific esterases
PAS
Specific esterases
Tartrate resistant acid phosphatase (TRAP)

BACKGROUND BASICS

The information in this chapter serves as a general introduction to the hematopoietic neoplasms (Chapters 22, 23, 24, 25, 26). To maximize your learning experience you should review these concepts before starting this unit of study.

Level I

▶ Summarize the origin and differentiation of the hematopoietic cells. (Chapters 3, 4)
▶ Describe the morphologic characteristics of the hematopoietic cells. (Chapters 5, 7)
▶ Define *oncogenes* and *proto-oncogenes*. (Chapter 2)

Level II

▶ Describe the actions of growth factors and oncogenes. (Chapter 2, 3)
▶ Summarize the cell cycle and identify factors that affect it. (Chapter 2)
▶ Describe the normal structure and function of the bone marrow, spleen, and lymph nodes. (Chapter 4)

⊘ CASE STUDY

We will refer to this case study throughout the chapter.

Agnes, a 72-year-old female, was seen by her physician for a persistent cough and fatigue. She had always been in good health and played golf regularly. Upon examination, she was noted to be pale and had slight splenomegaly. A CBC revealed the WBC was 83.9×10^9/L. Consider possible explanations for this test result and select reflex tests that should be performed.

► OVERVIEW

This chapter provides a general introduction to the neoplastic hematopoietic disorders discussed in detail in Chapters 22–26. It discusses oncogenesis including how oncogenes are activated and their association with hematopoietic disease. This is followed by a description of how neoplasms are classified and characterized according to cell lineage and the degree of cell differentiation, morphology, cytochemistry, immunophenotype, and genetic abnormalities. The etiology and pathophysiology of the leukemias are examined with general clinical and laboratory findings. Finally, prognosis and treatment modalities are considered for the disorders.

► INTRODUCTION

Neoplasm (tumor) literally means "new growth." Neoplasms arise as a consequence of dysregulated proliferation of a single transformed cell. Genetic mutations in the transformed cell reduce or eliminate the cell's dependence on external growth factors to regulate proliferation.

Neoplasms are either malignant or benign. **Benign** neoplasms are formed from highly organized, differentiated cells and do not spread or invade surrounding tissue. *Malignancy* means "deadly" or "having the potential for producing death." A **malignant** neoplasm is a clone of abnormal, anaplastic, proliferating cells, which often have the potential to metastasize. Only malignant tumors are correctly referred to as cancer. Although cancer is actually a malignancy of epithelial tissue, common use of the term includes all malignant neoplasms. A benign neoplasm can be premalignant and progress with further genetic mutations to a malignant neoplasm.

Neoplasms of hematopoietic cells in the bone marrow are phenotypically grouped as lymphoid or myeloid. Both groups include benign (premalignant) and malignant neoplasms. The premalignant myeloid neoplasms include the **myeloproliferative disorders (MPD)** and **myelodysplastic syndromes (MDS).** (Figure 21-1■) The premalig-

nant lymphoid disorders include the chronic lymphoproliferative disorders and plasma cell disorders. The lymphoid and myeloid malignant bone marrow neoplasms are collectively known as **leukemia.** Malignant cells may or may not circulate in the peripheral blood. The term *leukemia* is used when abnormal cells are seen in both the bone marrow and peripheral circulation. If the abnormal cells are found only in the bone marrow, the term **aleukemic leukemia** is used.

Abnormal proliferation of lymphoid cells sometimes occurs within the lymphatic tissue or lymph nodes. These solid tumors are referred to as **lymphoma.** If the lymphoma affects the bone marrow and the lymphoma cells are found in the peripheral circulation, the leukemic phase of *lymphoma* is present.

Failure of normal hematopoiesis is the most serious consequence of malignant neoplasms. As the neoplastic cell population increases, the concentration of normal cells decreases, resulting in the inevitable cytopenias of normal blood cells (Figure 21-2■). If the neoplasm is not treated, the patient usually succumbs to infections secondary to granulocytopenia or bleeding secondary to thrombocytopenia.

The next section briefly discusses these major groups of hematopoietic neoplasms. More detailed information is available in Chapters 22–26.

LEUKEMIAS

The two broad groups of leukemia are myeloid and lymphoid, which are based on the origin of the leukemic stem cell clone. If myelocytic cells or other cells derived from the common myeloid progenitor cell (CMP) predominate, the disease is called *myelogenous leukemia.* If lymphoid cells predominate, the disease is termed *lymphocytic leukemia.* These two groups are further classified based on the aggressiveness of the illness and degree of differentiation of the leukemic

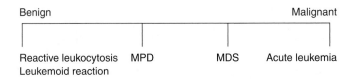

Benign   Malignant

Reactive leukocytosis   MPD   MDS   Acute leukemia
Leukemoid reaction

■ **FIGURE 21-1** The spectrum of granulocytic proliferation disorders ranges from benign to malignant processes. Benign granulocyte proliferation is usually a reactive process. Myeloproliferative disorders, myelodysplastic syndromes, and acute myeloid leukemia (AML) are neoplastic clonal stem cell defects characterized by autonomous proliferation of hematopoietic cells. (Adapted from McKenzie, S. Chronic myelocytic leukemia. *Tech Sample.* H-4 Chicago, ASCP; 1990.)

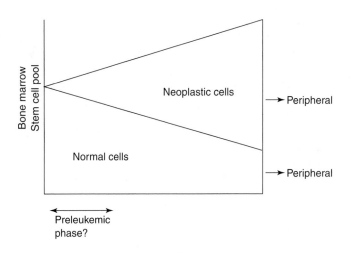

■ **FIGURE 21-2** Clonal expansion of neoplastic cells in the bone marrow in leukemia over a period of time.

⊙ TABLE 21-1

Comparison of Acute and Chronic Leukemias

	Acute	Chronic
Age	All ages	Adults
Clinical onset	Sudden	Insidious
Course of disease (untreated)	Weeks to months	Months to years
Predominant cell	Blasts, some mature forms	Mature forms
Anemia	Mild–severe	Mild
Thrombocytopenia	Mild–severe	Mild
WBC	Variable	Increased

cells: (1) acute, an aggressive disease (**acute myeloid [myelogenous** or **myelocytic] leukemia, AML; acute lymphoid [lymphoblastic** or **lymphocytic] leukemia, ALL**); and (2) chronic, a less aggressive form (**chronic myelogenous leukemia, CML; chronic lymphocytic leukemia, CLL**) (Table 21-1 ⊙).

In acute leukemia, there is an apparent gap in the normal maturation pyramid of cells with many blasts and some mature forms but an apparent decrease in intermediate maturational stages. This is referred to as the **leukemic hiatus.** The mature cells seen in the bone marrow and peripheral blood arise from proliferation of the residual normal hematopoietic stem cells (HSC) in the bone marrow. The apparent excess of blasts reflect primarily proliferation of the abnormal malignant clone, which fails to undergo maturation. Eventually, the immature neoplastic cells fill the bone marrow and spill over into the peripheral blood, producing leukocytosis. In the laboratory, the diagnosis of acute leukemia is suggested when examination of the peripheral blood smear reveals the presence of many undifferentiated or minimally differentiated cells (Figure 21-3 ■). Chronic leukemias are characterized by leukocytosis and although blasts may be present in the peripheral blood, there is a predominance of more mature cells (Figure 21-4 ■).

Subtypes of acute leukemia (ALL, AML) can be identified based on morphologic, cytochemical, immunologic, and genetic criteria of the malignant cells. Acute leukemias involving the granulocytic, monocytic, erythrocytic, or megakaryocytic cell lines are classified as subtypes of acute myeloid leukemia (also known as *acute nonlymphocytic leukemia, ANLL*) because these cell types develop from the common myeloid progenitor cell, CMP. The ALL group can be subtyped based on immunophenotype of the neoplastic lymphoid cell, as T or B cell neoplasms.

In the past, chronic leukemias were commonly classified as a distinct group of hematopoietic disorders. More recently, they have been grouped with other chronic neoplastic stem cell disorders, MPD, MDS, and chronic lymphoproliferative disorders. The bone marrow in chronic leukemias typically exhibits an accumulation of differentiated lymphocytic (CLL) or myelocytic (CML) elements (<20% blasts). The differential count of the bone marrow and of peripheral blood is similar with all stages of maturation present but with a predominance of the more mature forms. These chronic leukemias will be discussed in ∞ Chapters 22 and ∞ 23 with MPD and MDS and in ∞ Chapter 26 with lymphoproliferative disorders.

✓ **Checkpoint! 1**

A patient has 50% monoblasts in the bone marrow. Which of the four major types of leukemia—AML, CML, ALL, or CLL—does he have?

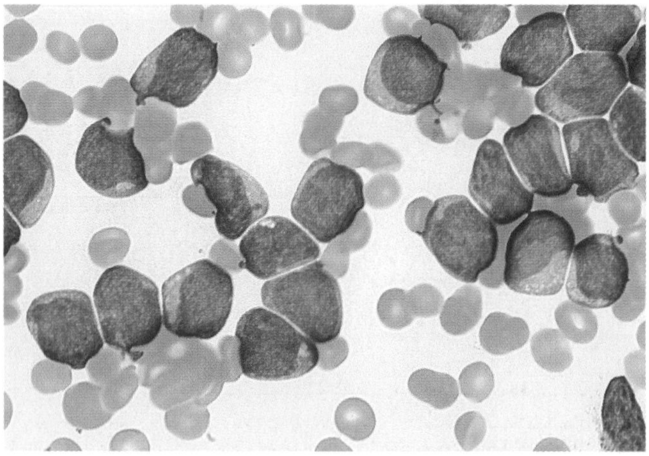

■ **FIGURE 21-3** Acute myelocytic leukemia. Note the large number of myeloblasts with no mature granulocytes present. (Wright stain, 1000×, PB).

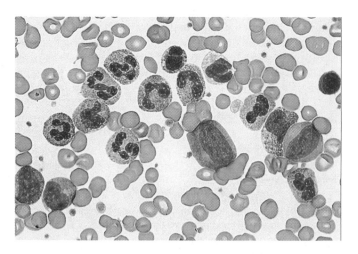

■ **FIGURE 21-4** Chronic myelogenous leukemia. Note the large number of granulocytic cells in various stages of granulocytic maturation including blasts, metamyelocyte, bands and segmented neutrophils. (Wright stain, 1000×, PB).

MYELOPROLIFERATIVE DISORDERS

The MPDs are characterized by a hypercellularity of the bone marrow and erythrocytosis, granulocytosis, and/or thrombocytosis in the peripheral blood due to unregulated cell proliferation. One cell line is usually more prominent than the others, a feature used to subgroup these clonal stem cell disorders. Acquired abnormalities of tyrosine kinases or other proteins involved in cell cycle signaling are commonly found in these disorders. The MPDs are found most often in adults. These disorders will be discussed in ∞ Chapter 22.

MYELODYSPLASTIC SYNDROMES

The MDS are characterized by a hypercellular, dysplastic bone marrow and peripheral blood cytopenias with variable dysplasia of the various lineages. The peripheral blood cytopenias are the result of ineffective hematopoiesis and increased apoptosis. The transformed neoplastic cell is thought to be the pluripotential HSC. The MDS are subgrouped based on percentage of blasts, presence or absence of ringed sideroblasts, and number of cytopenias and dysplastic cell lines. These disorders are found most commonly in the elderly. The MDS will be discussed in ∞ Chapter 23.

MYELODYSPLASTIC SYNDROMES/ MYELOPROLIFERATIVE DISORDERS

This group of disorders is characterized by the proliferative features of MPD and dysplastic features of MDS. They are subgrouped by lineage of the involved neoplastic cell. These disorders will be discussed in ∞ Chapter 23.

▶ ETIOLOGY/PATHOPHYSIOLOGY

Hematopoietic neoplasms are believed to occur as the result of a somatic mutation of a single hematopoietic stem or progenitor cell. Evidence for the clonal evolution of neoplastic cells comes from cytogenetic studies. More than 50% of individuals with leukemia show an acquired abnormal karyotype in hematopoietic cells whereas other somatic cells are normal. Using these specific cytogenetic markers, normal and malignant cells can be demonstrated to populate the marrow simultaneously. In untreated leukemias and during relapse, the leukemic cells dominate whereas during remission, only normal cells can usually be detected. The MPD, MDS, and lymphomas are also associated with nonrandom genetic abnormalities.

The cell in which a genetic mutation(s) occurs can be a committed lymphoid or myeloid progenitor cell (CMP, CLP) or a more primitive precursor cell that has the potential of differentiating into either lymphoid or myeloid cells, the hematopoietic stem cell (HSC), or the multipotential progenitor cell (MPP).[1] The cell from which the cancer originally

arises is sometimes called the *cell of origin* or the **cancer-initiating cell** (Figure 21-5 ■). A hallmark of hematologic malignancies is the capacity for unlimited self-renewal of the cancer initiating cell, which is also a characteristic of normal HSC (∞ Chapter 3). *Normal* MPP, CMP, and CLP do not have the self-renewal capacity. Because malignant cells share the capacity for self-renewal with the HSC, it would seem logical that the HSC was the source of the transforming (mutation) event. However, if more restricted progenitor cells acquired or reactivated the self-renewal program(s), they could be the cancer-initiating cells.[2] Many of the signaling pathways that play a role in cancer cell proliferation have been shown to regulate normal stem cell development.[1,2]

Studies in the field of cancer cell biology over the past several years have resulted in the hypothesis that **cancer stem cells** exist.[1,2] Most cancers are not truly clonal but

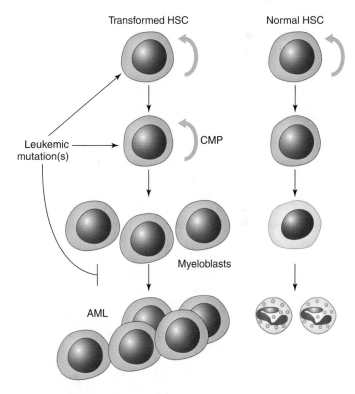

Clonal evolution of a neoplasm

■ FIGURE 21-5   Clonal evolution of a neoplasm from a single transformed (mutated) cell (the "cell of origin"). The genetic mutation(s) that transform a normal hematopoietic precursor cell to a malignant cell can occur at either the hematopoietic stem cell (HSC) or committed progenitor cell (CMP, common myeloid progenitor) stage, producing the leukemic "cell of origin." If the cell of origin is the CMP, the mutations must include the reacquisition of the capacity for self-renewal (broad curved arrow). If the mutation(s) also results in a block to terminal differentiation (⊥), the resulting malignancy will be acute myeloid leukemia (AML). Residual "normal" HSC and CMP in the marrow will still be capable of producing mature granulocytes.

consist of heterogeneous cell populations. Only a small subset of cells within a tumor is capable of extensive proliferation in vitro (in colony-forming assays) and in vivo (in transplantation models). These cancer stem cells are believed to be rare cells with infinite proliferative potential that drive the formation and growth of tumors. In leukemias, identification of the leukemic stem cell (LSC) for each type of leukemia has become a major focus of research.

The mutation(s) resulting in malignant transformation can often be identified as a chromosome alteration (abnormal karyotype) when cells in mitosis are studied. When chromosome studies are normal, aberrations in DNA at the molecular level occasionally can be found. The mutation leads to a survival and/or proliferation advantage over normal cells and to the neoplastic expansion of the affected stem cell and its progeny. In acute leukemia, this unregulated proliferation is accompanied by an arrest in maturation at the blast cell stage.

✓ Checkpoint! 2

A 62-year-old male presents with an elevated leukocyte count, mild anemia, and a slightly decreased platelet count. His physician suspects leukemia. Explain why the erythrocytes and platelets are affected.

ONCOGENES

Until recently, the actual pathogenic mechanisms of neoplasms remained obscure. Enormous progress in our understanding of the pathogenesis of these disorders has been made in the last several decades.

In 1976, J. Michael Bishop and Harold Varmus of the University of California, San Francisco, discovered that normal cells contain genes that can cause cancer/tumors if they become altered or activated.[3] These altered cell genes that cause tumors are referred to as *oncogenes* (*onco* means "tumor"), and the normal unaltered cellular counterparts of oncogenes are known as *proto-oncogenes* (∞ Chapter 2). Proto-oncogenes can become activated to oncogenes as a consequence of gene mutation, gene rearrangement (translocations, inversions, deletions), and gene amplification. This alters gene expression or activity/structure of its protein product. In the normal cellular state, proto-oncogenes direct cellular growth, proliferation, differentiation, or apoptosis by encoding proteins that are involved at every level of growth regulation. When altered, these genes are capable of inducing and maintaining cell transformation.

The protein products encoded by proto-oncogenes include:

• Growth factors
• Growth factor receptors
• Proteins involved in signal transduction
• Transcription factors (nuclear)

When a proto-oncogene is activated to an ocogene, either a qualitative or quantitative change occurs in the gene's protein product. Protein changes include increased protein activity, unregulated protein control and increased protein production. These changes allow cells to proliferate without the normal controls.

Another type of gene recognized as playing a role in neoplastic transformation of cells is the anti-oncogene, or tumor-suppressor gene (TSG). The TSG products function by suppressing cellular proliferation and, hence, neoplastic transformation. For example, they can trigger apoptosis if DNA cannot be repaired, or they can block the progression of the cell cycle if DNA is damaged. In terms of oncogenic potential, these genes are considered recessive because one copy is usually sufficient to provide a reasonable amount of normal functioning protein to keep cell growth in check. Mutations to both copies, however, eliminate the block and facilitate tumor growth. Recently, a number of tumor-suppressor genes have been shown to be associated with malignancy when only a single mutated allele was present, indicating that for these TSG, haploinsufficiency (loss of one copy of the gene) can be tumorigenic.

ROLES OF ONCOGENES AND TUMOR-SUPPRESSOR GENES IN NEOPLASIA

Neoplasia is a multistep process that involves a series of progressive changes. Both oncogenes and TSG play a role in this process. Activation of an oncogene or loss of a TSG is only one step in tumor development. Alterations of multiple oncogenes and TSGs acting together probably are necessary for a malignant neoplasm to develop. This concept of multiple genetic mutations helps explain the high incidence of leukemia in nonhematopoietic disorders associated with hereditary genetic mutations such as Down syndrome. In these conditions, the genetic mutation associated with the nonhematopoietic disorder can be one of the first of multiple steps leading to malignancy. Thus, these individuals are at a higher risk of developing a neoplasm. Some benign neoplasms progress to more malignant disorders as additional genetic mutations occur over the course of the disease. For instance, myelodysplasia and chronic leukemia often evolve to acute leukemia as progressive genetic abnormalities occur.

The role of oncogenes and TSGs in the pathogenesis of neoplasms continues to be investigated. Oncogenes (∞ Chapter 2) have been identified at the breakpoints of chromosomal aberrations that are commonly present in specific types of leukemias and lymphomas. Chromosome breaks and translocations appear to activate these genes and result in the aberrant expression of the protein product (Table 21-2 ✪). Also, breaks and translocations *within* a gene sequence can produce a hybrid (fusion) gene and a new protein product. For example, the balanced translocation between chromosmes in chronic myelogenous leukemia (CML)

✪ TABLE 21-2

Common Genetic Abnormalities in Hematopoietic Neoplasms (for a more complete listing see Tables 38-6, 38-7, 38-8)

Malignancy	Genetic Abnormality	Involved Genes	Product/Activity
Myeloid neoplasm			
CML	t(9;22)	BCR/ABL	Fusion protein/tyrosine kinase
PV	9p (V617F mutation)	JAK2	Increased tyrosine kinase activity
AML-M2	t(8;21)	ETO/AML1	Fusion protein/transcription deregulation
AML-M3	t(15;17)	PML/RAR-α	Fusion protein/transcription deregulation
CMMoL	t(5;12)	PDGFRB/TEL	Fusion protein/activation of signal transduction pathways
B cell neoplasm			
ALL	t(9;22)	ABL/BCR	Fusion protein/increased tyrosine kinase activity
Pre-B ALL	t(1;19)	E2A/PBX1	Fusion protein/transcription dysregulation
CLL	t(14;19)	IGH/BCL3	Deregulated expression
Lymphomas			
Burkitt lymphoma	t(8;14)	MYC/IGH	Transcription deregulation
Mantle cell lymphoma	t(11;14)	BCL1/IGH	Transcription deregulation
T cell lymphoma	t(8;14)	MYC/TCR	Transcription deregulation
Mixed lineage leukemia	11q23	MLL	Fusion protein/transcription deregulation

CML = chronic myelogenous leukemia; AML = acute myeloid leukemia; PV = polycythemia vera; CMMoL = chronic myelomonocytic leukemia; ALL = acute lymphoblastic leukemia; CLL = chronic lymphocytic leukemia

9 and 22 results in the formation of a *BCR-ABL* fusion gene that results in synthesis of an abnormal tyrosine kinase (TK) protein.[4] This protein is constitutively activated and involved in cell cycle signaling and increased resistance to apoptosis. Consequently, the cell is in a continual state of proliferation. As the molecular basis of malignant disorders is disclosed, as in CML, therapy is becoming more targeted. Imatinib (Gleevec), the first-line drug therapy for CML, competitively binds to and prevents cell signal transduction by the mutant BCR-ABL kinase. It is not a cure, but it inhibits the TK activity of the aberrant protein.

ACTIVATION OF ONCOGENES

From studies on laboratory animals, several factors have been proposed as playing roles in the activation of oncogenes: (1) genetic susceptibility, (2) somatic mutation, (3) viral infection, and (4) immunologic dysfunction (Table 21-3 ✪).

Genetic Susceptibility

Strong evidence suggests that hereditary factors and abnormal genetic material have important leukemogenic effects. A number of individuals who have congenital abnormalities associated with karyotypic abnormalities have a markedly increased risk of developing acute leukemia. Each of these genetic events has the potential to activate proto-oncogenes or eliminate the function of a TSG. The best known of the genetic abnormalities associated with leukemia is Down syndrome.[5,6]

Various other congenital disorders also are associated with an increased risk for leukemia; these include Fanconi anemia, Kleinfelter syndrome, Bloom syndrome, Wiskott-Aldrich syndrome, and Blackfan-Diamond syndrome.

✪ TABLE 21-3

Factors Proposed to Play a Role in Leukemogenesis

Factor	Example
Genetic susceptibility	Down syndrome
	Fanconi anemia
	Kleinfelter syndrome
	Bloom syndrome
	Wiskott-Aldrich syndrome
	Blackfan-Diamond syndrome
	Xeroderma pigmentosum
	Li-Fraumeini syndrome
Somatic mutation	Radiation
	Chemicals
	Drugs
Viral infection	Retroviruses—HTLV-I, II, V, HIV-1
Immunologic disorders	Wiskott-Aldrich syndrome
	Bruton's type X-linked agammaglobulinemia
	Ataxia telangiectasia
	Immunosuppressive therapy

Further evidence supporting the association of genetic factors with the occurrence of leukemia comes from family studies in which increased incidence has been reported in family groups.[7,8]

Somatic Mutation

A somatic cell mutation is an acquired change in the genetic material of cells other than those involved in reproduction. Mutations in the chromosome near proto-oncogenes likely play a role in the development of neoplasms. More than 50% of patients with leukemia can be demonstrated to have acquired abnormal karyotypes. As data accumulated from cytogenetic studies, specific, consistent mutations have been found in certain subgroups of hematopoietic neoplasms.[9]

Radiation, some chemicals, and drugs can cause chromosome mutations. Ionizing radiation has long been recognized as capable of inducing leukemia, which is evident from observations of human exposure to radiation from nuclear reactions, therapeutic radiation, and occupational exposure to radiation. An increase in leukemia has been observed after treatment with alkylating agents and other chemotherapeutic drugs used in treatment of many kinds of malignancy. The only specific chemical implicated in causing leukemia other than those used as medications is benzene.

Viral Infection

Retroviruses have been shown to cause leukemia in laboratory animals, and a few malignancies can be traced to a viral infection of cells in humans.[10] Retroviruses contain a reverse transcriptase that allows them to produce a DNA copy of the viral RNA core. The DNA can then be copied to produce more viral cores or can be incorporated into the host cell's nuclear DNA. The strongest support for the existence of a leukemogenic virus in humans comes from the isolation of several human retroviruses known as *human T cell leukemia/lymphoma virus* (HTLV-I, II, V) and *human immunodeficiency virus* (HIV-1) from cell lines of patients with mature T cell malignancies.[11] Exactly how viruses induce leukemia is unclear, but it is suspected that the incorporation of the viral genome into host DNA can lead to activation of proto-oncogenes.

Immunologic Dysfunction

An increased incidence of lymphocytic leukemia has been observed in both congenital and acquired immunologic disorders. These disorders include the hereditary immunologic diseases Wiskott-Aldrich syndrome, Bruton's type X-linked agammaglobulinemia, and ataxia telangiectasia. An association between long-term treatment of patients with immunosuppressive drugs (e.g., renal transplant) and leukemia also has been observed. Possibly, a breakdown in the cell-mediated immunologic self-surveillance system and/or deficient production of antibodies against foreign antigens leads to the emergence and survival of neoplastic cells.

Miscellaneous Factors

Certain hematologic diseases appear to pose a leukemogenic risk. The development of leukemia sometimes appears to be related to the treatment used for the primary disease, but in other patients no such relationship can be found. The highest incidence of acute leukemia is found in individuals with other neoplastic disorders, such as MPD and MDS,[12] prompting some hematologists to use the word *preleukemia* for these disorders. Additional genetic mutations (or epigenetic alterations, see below) occur as the preleukemic disease progresses to the frank malignancy, leukemia. Other hematopoietic diseases with an increased incidence of leukemia include paroxysmal nocturnal hemoglobinuria (PNH), aplastic anemia, and multiple myeloma. It is interesting to note that all of these hematologic disorders are considered stem cell disorders in which the primary hematologic defect lies in the myeloid or lymphoid progenitor cells or in the pluripotential stem cells.

No single factor is responsible for the activation of oncogenes that result in hematopoietic neoplasms, but the malignancy is produced by a variety of etiologic factors including genetic factors and environmental exposures.[13,14] The cause probably varies from patient to patient, and some individuals could be more susceptible than others to oncogene activation.

EPIGENETICS AND MALIGNANCY— SILENCING OF TUMOR SUPPRESSORS

Research in the past two decades has revealed that genetic changes (mutations either at the molecular level or chromosomal alterations) and epigenetic changes both contribute to the development of a malignancy.[15] **Epigenetics** is defined as the heritable (i.e., stable from one cell generation to the next during mitosis) changes in gene expression not due to changes in DNA sequence (∞ Chapter 2). Epigenetic alterations involve chemical modifications of the DNA polynucleotide chains (e.g., CpG methylation) or the nuclear histone proteins (acetylation, methylation, phosphorylation). These chemical changes alter the configuration of the chromatin, affecting its packaging and accessibility for transcription within the nucleus.[16] The best understood epigenetic modifications are DNA methylation and histone deacetylation, both of which result in gene silencing. Although gene silencing plays an important role in normal cellular differentiation, silencing can become dysregulated in various disease processes including cancer. Epigenetic events resulting in altered gene expression, particularly silencing genes involved in regulating cell growth and differentiation, can result in a cellular growth advantage, progressive uncontrolled growth, and the development of a cancer. Many cancers are associated with epigenetic silencing of TSG (i.e., p16, Rb, p53), which play a major role in tumorigenesis.[15,17,18]

✓ Checkpoint! 3

Does a 3-year-old child with Down syndrome have an increased risk of developing leukemia? Why or why not?

▶ EPIDEMIOLOGY

The Leukemia and Lymphoma Society predicted that in the year 2008, about 44,270 new cases of leukemia would be reported in the United States.[19] Most cases occur in older adults with more than half occurring after age 67.

Approximately 50% of all leukemias are diagnosed as acute. Although some difference in the incidence of the acute leukemias exists between countries and regions of countries, the differences are not great. However, all leukemias are more prevalent in Jews of Russian, Polish, and Czech ancestry than in non-Jews. Acute leukemia also is more common in whites than in blacks.

Of particular interest is the incidence and morphologic variation of leukemia among age groups (Table 21-4 ✪). Although acute leukemia occurs at all ages, peak incidence occurs in the first decade, particularly from the ages of 2 to 5 followed by a decreasing incidence in the second and third decade. Thereafter, the incidence begins to increase, rising steeply after age 50. The cellular type of leukemia occurring at these peak periods differs significantly. Most childhood acute leukemias are of the lymphoid type, whereas those occurring in adults are typically myeloid in origin. Chronic leukemias are rare in children. Most chronic myelogenous leukemias occur in young to middle-aged adults, and chronic lymphocytic leukemia is found primarily in older adults. MPD and MDS occur most often in middle-aged to older adults.

▶ CLINICAL FINDINGS

Failure of normal hematopoiesis is the most serious consequence of hematopoietic neoplasms. The most frequent symptoms are related to erythropenia, thrombocytopenia, or neutropenia. The major clinical problems are anemia, infection, and bleeding episodes occurring as frank hemorrhages, petechiae, or ecchymoses. Bone pain due to marrow expansion and weight loss are also common complaints. Physical examination can show hepatosplenomegaly and, occasionally, lymphadenopathy. Organomegaly is more common in chronic leukemias than in the acute forms.

Although the disease originates in the bone marrow, neoplastic cells can infiltrate any tissue of the body, especially the spleen, liver, lymph nodes, central nervous system, and skin. The lesions produced vary from rashes to tumors. Skin infiltration is most commonly found in AML, particularly those with a monocytic component. Central nervous system (CNS) involvement is common in ALL of childhood. Chloromas, which are green tumor masses of immature leukocytes, are associated with AML and CML. They are usually found in bone but can be found throughout the body. The green color, which fades to a dirty yellow after exposure to air, is responsible for the descriptive name given to this unique clinical finding. Presumably, the green color results from the myeloperoxidase content of the malignant cells.

▶ HEMATOLOGIC FINDINGS

Cell counts and morphology are variable in the hematopoietic neoplasms (Table 21-5 ✪). A normocytic (occasionally macrocytic) normochromic anemia is usually present at diagnosis. If not present initially, it invariably develops during progression of the disease.

Thrombocytopenia is usually present at diagnosis in acute leukemia. Thrombocytosis is a common initial finding in MPD. The platelet count in MDS is variable. In both MPD and MDS, however, the platelet count decreases with progression of the disease. Platelet morphology and function also can be abnormal. Large hypogranular forms are common, and circulating micromegakaryocytes occasionally are present.

The leukocyte count can be normal, increased, or decreased. More than 50% of patients with AML do not have a significant leukocytosis at diagnosis. However, if left untreated, leukocytosis eventually develops. On the other hand, in the chronic myeloproliferative and lymphoproliferative neoplasms, leukocytosis at diagnosis is a prominent finding. Normal or decreased leukocyte counts are typical in MDS. Regardless of the leukocyte count, an increase in immature precursors is found in most cases. Blasts are especially prominent in the acute leukemias. Unique pink-staining granular inclusions called **Auer rods** can be found in the blast cells and promyelocytes of some acute myeloid leukemias. These Auer rods are believed to be formed from fused primary granules. When AML is suspected, the finding of Auer rods can help establish the diagnosis because these inclusions are not found in ALL.

✪ TABLE 21-4	
Age Groups Typically Found in Acute and Chronic Leukemias	
ALL	Children 2–5 years old
CLL	Adults >50 years old
AML	Adults
CML	Adults

✪ TABLE 21-5

Characteristic Hematologic Findings in Acute Leukemia (AL), Myelodysplastic Syndrome (MDS), and Myeloproliferative Disorders (MPD)

Neoplasm	Leukocytes	Platelets	Bone Marrow	Other
AL	Normal or increased Blasts present	Decreased	Hypercellular, >20% blasts	Auer rods in AML
MDS	Normal or decreased Blasts may be present	Variable	Hypercellular, <20% blasts	Dysplastic
MPD	Increased Shift to left but predominance of mature forms	Usually increased	Hypercellular, <20% blasts, (occasionally hypocellular)	
MDS/MPD	Increased blasts and other immature forms	Usually decreased	Hypercellular, <20% blasts	Dysplastic

The bone marrow is hypercellular, although occasionally normocellularity or hypocellularity is found. Reticulin is increased, often worsening with progression of the disease. Blasts are usually increased. The cutoff of <20% blasts is used to differentiate MPD and MDS from AL.

Maturation abnormalities are commonly present in all three cell lines. Megaloblastoid erythropoiesis can be prominent but is unresponsive to vitamin B_{12} or folic acid treatment.

Because of the intense increase in cell turnover, other laboratory tests reflecting cell destruction could be abnormal. An increase in uric acid, which is a normal product of nucleic acid metabolism, is a consistent finding in all types of leukemia. The rate of excretion can increase to 50 times normal. Serum lactic dehydrogenase (LD) levels appear to correlate closely with the concentration of leukemic cells. Isoenzyme studies reveal that the LD is derived from immature leukocyte precursors. Muramidase (lysozyme) is a lysosomal enzyme present in monocytes and granulocytes. The serum and urine muramidase concentration in leukemia is highly variable and is related to the cellular type. The highest concentrations are found in neoplasms with a monocytic component.

 Checkpoint! 4

Why is the finding of Auer rods an important factor in the diagnosis of leukemia?

▶ HEMATOPOIETIC NEOPLASM CLASSIFICATION

Two classification systems of hematopoietic neoplasms are currently recognized: the French-American-British (FAB) and the World Health Organization (WHO). The newer WHO classification system is widely accepted and is replacing the older FAB classification. The FAB system is discussed for historical information, but the WHO classification is used in this text.

Classifications of hematopoietic neoplasms are considered to be important for three reasons:

1. They allow clinicians and researchers a way to compare various therapeutic regimens.

2. They allow a system for identification and comparison of clinical features and laboratory findings.

3. They permit meaningful associations of cytogenetic abnormalities with disease.

FAB CLASSIFICATION

The French-American-British system classifies neoplastic disorders into three main groups: myeloproliferative disorders (MPD), myelodysplastic syndromes (MDS), and acute leukemia (AL).

In 1976, in an effort to improve and standardize the classification of AL, a group of **French, American, and British** physicians proposed a classification and nomenclature system based on cell lineage as determined by the morphologic characteristics of blast cells on Romanowsky-stained smears and the results of cytochemical stains.[20] In the FAB classification, a blast count >30% is diagnostic of AL. In 1984, the FAB group proposed a classification for the MDS using the blast count (<30%) and degree of dysplasia in subgrouping the MDS. The MDS are characterized by peripheral blood cytopenias (except chronic myelomonocytic leukemia). Dameshek recognized the MPDs in 1951. Myeloproliferative disorders are characterized by neoplastic increases in erythrocytes, leukocytes, and/or platelets.

In the FAB system, both MPD and MDS have a blast count <30% and can have a chronic or acute course and the potential to evolve into acute leukemia (Figure 21-1). Of the three groups of neoplastic bone marrow disorders, acute leukemias represent the frankly malignant hematopoietic neoplasms with a proliferation of blast cells.

Malignant lymphoproliferative disorders can occur in the hematopoietic system (bone marrow and peripheral blood) or in the lymphatic system (lymph nodes and spleen). When the malignant proliferation involves the bone marrow and peripheral blood, the disease is referred to as *acute* or *chronic lymphocytic leukemia*. When the malignant proliferation is in the lymphoid tissue, the disease is referred to as a *lymphoma* (∞ Chapter 26). Lymphomas can eventually spread to the bone marrow, and the malignant cells can then be found in the peripheral blood. The acute lymphoblastic leukemias are discussed in ∞ Chapter 25. Classification and description of the other malignant lymphoproliferative diseases are discussed in ∞ Chapter 26.

Each of the three primary FAB groups of neoplastic disorders can be further divided into subgroups based on blast count and degree of differentiation as well as degree of dysplasia and cell lineage(s) involved. These subgroups are listed in Table 21-6 ✪.

✪ TABLE 21-6

FAB Classification of Hematologic Neoplasms

Acute Nonlymphocytic Leukemias

M0	Acute myeloblastic leukemia without differentiation
M1	Acute myeloblastic leukemia with minimal differentiation
M2	Acute myeloblastic leukemia with maturation
M3	Promyelocytic leukemia, hypergranular
M3m	Promyelocytic leukemia, microgranular variant
M4	Acute myelomonocytic leukemia
M4eo	Acute myelomonocytic leukemia with abnormal eosinophils
M5a	Acute monoblastic leukemia without differentiation
M5b	Acute monoblastic leukemia with differentiation
M6	Acute erythroleukemia
M7	Megakaryocytic leukemia

Acute Lymphoblastic Leukemias

L1	Lymphoblastic leukemia with homogeneity
L2	Lymphoblastic leukemia with heterogeneity
L3	Burkitt type lymphoblastic leukemia

Myelodysplastic Syndromes

Refractory anemia (RA)

Refractory anemia with ringed sideroblasts (RARS)

Refractory anemia with excess blasts (RAEB)

Refractory anemia with excess blasts in transformation (RAEB-T)

Chronic myelomonocytic leukemia (CMML)

Myeloproliferative Disorders

Chronic myelogenous (or myelocytic, myeloid, granulocytic) leukemia (CML or CGL)

Polycythemia vera (PV)

Essential thrombocythemia (ET)

Agnogenic myeloid metaplasia (AMM), also known as *myelofibrosis with myeloid metaplasia* (MMM).

THE WHO CLASSIFICATION

Genetic features, prior therapy, and a history of myelodysplasia recently have been recognized to have a significant impact on the clinical behavior of the hematopoietic neoplasms. The Society for Hematopathology and the European Association of Hematopathologists developed the WHO to better define the hematopoietic neoplasms. This classification uses features similar to those in the FAB classification including morphology, cytochemistry, and immunophenotype of the neoplastic cells to determine cell lineage and degree of maturation. However, it also uses genetic and clinical features such as prior therapy and history of MDS to define distinct subgroups[21] (Table 21-7 ✪).

The classification according to lineage of the neoplastic cells includes four groups: myeloid, lymphoid, mast cell, and histiocytic. Mast cells are derived from hematopoietic progenitor cells and possess myeloid cell characteristics. Thus, mast cell disease can be considered a myeloid disorder. The four major groups of myeloid disease are defined by morphology, genetic abnormalities, immunophenotyping, and clinical features:

- Myeloproliferative disorders (MPD)
- Myelodysplastic/myeloproliferative disorders (MDS/MPD)
- Myelodysplastic syndromes (MDS)
- Acute myeloid leukemia (AML)

Although this classification is similar to the FAB classification of myeloid disorders, the criteria for subgroups within these four major groups differ. WHO also adds the MDS/MPD category that includes diseases that have features of both MDS and MPD such as chronic myelomonocytic leukemia. Each major group with subgroups is discussed in ∞ Chapters 22–26.

A significant change in the WHO classification relates to the bone marrow blast count used to define and differentiate AML from the other myeloid neoplasms. This classification uses the standard of >20% blasts to define AML versus the FAB standard of >30% blasts. This is based on the observation that patients with 20–30% blasts have a prognosis similar to those with >30% blasts. The percentage of blasts is determined as the number of blasts in all nucleated marrow cells (except for acute erythroleukemia).[22] If AML exists concurrently with another nonmyeloid hematologic neoplasm, the cells from the nonmyeloid neoplasm are not included when performing the differential.[22]

The WHO classification also defines the criteria for blasts differently than previous classifications. When counting blasts for a diagnosis of AML, the following are included in addition to myeloblasts:[22]

- Monoblasts and promonocytes in acute monoblastic/ monocytic and acute and chronic myelomonocytic leukemia
- Megakaryoblasts in acute megakaryoblastic leukemia
- Abnormal promyelocytes in acute promyelocytic leukemia
- Erythroblasts only in pure erythroleukemia

⭐ **TABLE 21-7**

2001 WHO Classification of Hematologic Neoplasms*

Myeloproliferative Diseases

Chronic myelogenous leukemia (CML), Philadelphia chromosome, (9;22)(q34;q11), BCR/ABL1 positive

Chronic neutrophilic leukemia (CNL)†

Chronic eosinophilic leukemia (CEL)/hypereosinophilic syndrome (HES)†

Chronic idiopathic myelofibrosis (CIMF)

Polycythemia vera (PV)

Essential thrombocythemia (ET)

Myeloproliferative disease, unclassifiable (MDP-U)†

Myelodysplastic/Myeloproliferative Diseases†

Chronic myelomonocytic leukemia (CMML)

Atypical myelogenous leukemia (aCML)

Juvenile myelomonocytic leukemia (JMML)

Myelodysplastic Syndromes

Refractory anemia (RA)

Refractory anemia with ringed sideroblasts (RARS)

Refractory cytopenia with multilineage dysplasia (RCMD)†

Refractory cytopenia with multilineage dysplasia with ringed sideroblasts (RCMD-RS)†

Refractory anemia with excess blasts-1

Refractory anemia with excess blasts-2

MDS associated with isolated del (5q)†

Myelodysplastic syndrome, unclassifiable (MDS-u)†

Acute Myeloid Leukemia‡

Acute myeloid leukemias with recurrent genetic abnormalities†

Acute myeloid leukemia with multilineage dysplasia†

Acute myeloid leukemia and myelodysplastic syndromes, therapy related†

Acute myeloid leukemia not otherwise categorized§

Acute leukemia of ambiguous lineage

Acute Lymphoid Leukemias (precursor B- and T-cell neoplasms)

Precursor B cell acute lymphoblastic leukemia† (classified by cytogenetic subgroups)

Precursor T cell acute lymphoblastic leukemia†

B Cell Neoplasms (mature cell neoplasms)‡

T Cell Neoplasms (mature cell neoplasms)‡

Hodgkin lymphoma‡

*The 2008 WHO classification is on the Website.
†Not included in FAB classification.
‡Subgroups not listed.
§Includes subgroups of AML in FAB classification.

In the lymphoid neoplasms, the proposed WHO classification adopts the *revised European-American lymphoid neoplasm* (REAL) classification, which uses morphology, immunophenotype, genetic, and clinical features. There are three groups of lymphoid neoplasms: B cell, T/NK cell, and Hodgkin's disease. The T and B cell neoplasms are grouped into precursor (lymphoblastic) and mature neoplasms. The ALLs are in the precursor group and include B cell and T cell ALL and Burkitt cell leukemia (L3 in FAB). The mature neoplasms include B cell chronic lymphocytic leukemia (CLL) and hairy cell leukemia. The REAL classification for lymphoid neoplasms is in general use (∞ Chapter 26).

ℯ **CASE STUDY** *(continued from page 422)*

The CBC results on Agnes were:

WBC	83.9×10^9/L	
RBC	3.15×10^{12}/L	
Hb	9.5 g/dL (95 g/L)	
Hct	0.29 L/L	
Platelets	130×10^9/L	
Differential	segs	12%
	lymphs	88%

1. Given the patient's laboratory results, would this most likely be considered an acute or chronic leukemia? Explain.

2. What group of leukemia (cell lineage) is suggested by the patient's blood cell differential results?

3. What would you expect the blast count in the bone marrow to be?

▶ **LABORATORY PROCEDURES FOR DIAGNOSING AND CLASSIFYING NEOPLASMS**

As mentioned, the hematopoietic neoplasms are initially classified into myeloid (nonlymphocytic) and lymphoid groups, depending on the predominant cell types present. In the acute leukemias, identification of the cell lineage (myeloid or lymphoid) of leukemic blasts is often difficult by morphology alone unless Auer rods are present. However, the distinction of cell lineage is important for selecting the appropriate therapy. Distinction of MDS and MPD is not as difficult as in acute leukemias because in MDS and MPD, the maturation of the neoplastic cell is not blocked and the cell matures into recognizable blood cells.

Differentiation of leukemic blasts allows classification of acute leukemia into cell lineage (lymphoid or myeloid) and various subtypes (Table 21-8 ✪). Differentiation can be determined by morphology, immunologic marker analysis (im-

TABLE 21-8

Comparison of Acute Lymphoblastic Leukemia (ALL) and Acute Nonlymphocytic Leukemia (ANLL)

	ALL	ANLL
Age	Common in children	Common in adults
Hematologic presentation	Anemia, neutropenia, thrombocytopenia, lymphoblasts, prolymphocytes	Anemia, neutropenia, thrombocytopenia, myeloblasts, promyelocytes
Prominent cell morphology	Small to medium lymphoblasts, fine chromatin with scanty to abundant cytoplasm, indistinct nucleoli	Medium to large myeloblasts with distinct nucleoli, fine nuclear chromatin and abundant basophilic cytoplasm, Auer rods can be present
Cytochemistry	PAS positive, peroxidase negative, Sudan black B negative, TdT positive	PAS negative, peroxidase positive, Sudan black B positive, TdT negative or positive

munophenotype), cytochemical stains, and/or chromosome analysis. Immunophenotyping and cytochemistry are not usually necessary in classification of MDS and MPD, but genetic studies are helpful in subgrouping.

CYTOCHEMICAL ANALYSIS

Cytochemistry in hematology refers to in vitro staining of cells that allows microscopic examination of the cells' chemical composition. Cell morphology is not significantly altered in the staining process. Most cellular cytochemical markers represent organelle-associated enzymes and other proteins. The cells are incubated with substrates that react with specific cellular constituents. If the specific constituent is present in the cell, its reaction with the substrate is confirmed by the formation of a colored product. The stained cells are examined and evaluated on smears with a light microscope, although electron microscopy occasionally is necessary to identify very weak reactions at the subcellular level. The results of these cellular reactions in normal and disease states are well established. Cytochemistry is particularly helpful in differentiating the lymphoid or myeloid lineage of the blasts in acute leukemias when morphologic identification on Romanowsky-stained smears is difficult (Table 21-9 ✪). Cytochemistry is also helpful in subgrouping the AML.

It is important to remember that the blast cells seen in leukemias are neoplastic cells and can therefore differ from normal blasts in both morphology and metabolic activity. Leukemic cells often display nuclear/cytoplasmic asynchrony similar to that of megaloblastic cells. As a result, although the nucleus appears very immature, the cytoplasm of leukemic blasts can contain constituents normally present only in more mature cells or can lack one or more constituents expressed by their normal counterparts. In addition, there can be abnormal accumulation and distribution of cellular metabolites.

The cytochemical staining reactions are either enzymatic or nonenzymatic. The enzymatic group includes stains for myeloperoxidase, esterases, alkaline and acid phosphatases. The nonenzymatic stains include Sudan black B for lipids,

TABLE 21-9

Cytochemical Stains Useful in Differentiating Acute Myeloid Leukemia (AML) from Acute Lymphoblastic Leukemia (ALL)

Stains	Myeloblasts	Lymphoblasts	Cell constituent stained
MPO/SBB	Positive	Negative	MPO: myeloperoxidase SBB: lipids
Chloroacetate esterase (specific)	Positive	Negative	Esterases
PAS	Negative or diffusely positive	Negative or chunky positive	Glycogen
TdT	10–20% positive	Over 90% positive	DNA polymerase

Note: When all cytochemical stains are negative, the differential diagnosis is usually between ALL and AML with minimal differentiation. TdT is not helpful in differentiating the two because it can be positive in 90% of cases of AML with minimal differentiation. Thus, distinction of AML with minimal differentiation from ALL is not possible by cytochemical stains. Flow cytometric analysis is required in this situation. AML with minimal differentiation expresses myeloid antigens (CD13, CD15, and CD33), while ALL expresses lymphoid markers (CD19, CD20, and CD22 or CD3, CD2, CD5, CD7, etc.).

periodic acid-Schiff (PAS) for glycogen, and toluidine blue O for mucopolysaccharides.

Myeloperoxidase (MPO) and Sudan black B (SBB)

The **MPO** and SBB stains are generally performed first to differentiate the myeloid and lymphoid blasts. The myeloblasts are positive, but lymphoblasts are negative. Additional staining can be necessary to assist in subgrouping the AML and ALL.

Esterases

The esterase stains are generally used to differentiate monoblasts and myeloblasts. Myeloblasts are positive for **specific esterases** (chloroacetate esterase), and monoblasts are positive for **nonspecific esterases** (alpha-naphthyl acetate esterase, ANAE).

Periodic Acid Schiff (PAS)

The **PAS** stain is helpful in diagnosing ALL and acute erythroid and megakaryoblastic leukemias. Normal erythroblasts do not stain with PAS. However, PAS activity is strongly positive in erythroid leukemia. Leukemic lymphoblasts can demonstrate blocklike or coarse granular activity. This typical positivity of lymphoblasts in ALL can sometimes be seen in AML (monocytic, erythroleukemia, and megakaryoblastic). The PAS stain reaction is not useful in differentiating other acute leukemias (∞ Chapter 34).

Leukocyte Alkaline Phosphatase (LAP)

Leukocyte alkaline phosphatase (LAP) is an enzyme present within the specific (secondary) granules of maturing granulocytes (from the myelocyte stage onward). The enzyme is not present in eosinophils and basophils. Activated neutrophils contain an increased amount of LAP. Therefore, the LAP score is useful in distinguishing leukemoid reactions/reactive neutrophilia (high LAP) from chronic myelogenous leukemia (low LAP).[23,24]

Acid Phosphatase

A constituent of lysosomes and present in most human cells, acid phosphatase activity is present in most normal leukocytes, but the acid phosphatase activity in T cell ALL is characteristic, exhibiting focal polarized acid phosphatase activity. Hairy cells in hairy cell leukemia are positive, but the activity is not inhibited by **tartrate resistant acid phosphatase (TRAP)**, differentiating them from other leukocytes whose activity is inhibited by tartrate.[25,26]

Terminal Deoxynucleotidyl Transferase (TdT)

TdT, a DNA polymerase found in cell nuclei, is a primitive cell marker and is of value in distinguishing ALL from malignant lymphoma.[27,28] It is also helpful in identifying leukemic cells in body fluid specimens. TdT is present in 90–95% of ALL (T cell ALL and precursor B cell ALL, but not in mature B cell ALL). TdT staining might not be beneficial in evaluating acute leukemias because up to 20% of AMLs can show TdT positivity, and more than 90% of minimally differentiated AML can be TdT positive.

Toluidine Blue

Toluidine blue is specifically positive for basophils and mast cells and is useful in diagnosing mast cell disease and rare cases of AML with basophilic differentiation.[29,30,31] The granules in basophils and mast cells have a strong affinity for toluidine blue. A negative reaction should not rule out neoplasm of these cells because the acid mucopolysaccharides can be scarce or negative in neoplastic disorders.

Reticulin Stain and Masson's Trichrome Stain

These stains are used to evaluate both the presence and extent of fibrosis. However, the presence of fibrosis can be suspected on hematoxylin and eosin (H&E) stained sections. The Gomori methenamine silver–staining method is more suitable for detecting reticulin. Masson's trichrome stain is useful to evaluate the degree of collagenous fibrosis. Increased staining can be seen in myelofibrosis and indicates severe and dense fibrosis.

IMMUNOLOGIC ANALYSIS

Immunologic analysis is based on identifying specific membrane antigens (surface markers) that are characteristically found on a particular cell lineage. Immunologic techniques with monoclonal antibodies are widely used to identify cell membrane antigens on a variety of cells (∞ Chapter 37). The development of a large number of monoclonal antibodies that react with surface antigens on normal and neoplastic cells and technical advances in flow cytometry, have greatly enhanced the ability to define leukemic cell lineage, the stage of cell development, and clonality. By utilizing a panel of monoclonal antibodies, a more complete picture of the cells' lineage can be determined.

The routine use of immunologic markers to characterize AML subtypes and myeloid antigenic development has lagged behind the use of these markers in ALL. There are two possible explanations for this lag.[32] The first is that AML unlike ALL has two specific cytochemical markers—peroxidase and nonspecific esterase—that help to identify the myeloid origin of the cells. The second is that to subtype AML, markers for myeloblasts, erythroblasts, monoblasts, and megakaryoblasts need to be identified. An increasing repertoire of antibodies to myeloid antigens has been developed. These antibodies have helped not only in subtyping the myeloid leukemias but also in identifying the lineage of those leukemias that lack specific morphologic and cytochemical characteristics. A more thorough discussion of monoclonal antibodies and their use in the identification of neoplastic hematopoietic disorders can be found in ∞ Chapter 37.

GENETIC ANALYSIS

Cytogenetics

Advances in cytogenetics have allowed cytogeneticists to identify characteristic nonrandom abnormal karyotypes in the majority of the acute leukemias and in some MPD and MDS.[33] Some specific chromosome changes are consistently associated with a particular neoplastic subgroup and thus are helpful in diagnosis. For example, the t(15;17)(q22;q11) is diagnostic of acute promyelocytic leukemia, and the Philadelphia chromosome characterized by t(9;22) (q34;q11.2) confirms a clinical diagnosis of chronic myelogenous leukemia (CML). In the lymphoid leukemias, nonrandom chromosome changes are often associated with either the B or T lymphocyte lineage and provide important prognostic as well as diagnostic information. Chromosomal rearrangements and their accompanying molecular abnormalities can identify distinct clinical groups with a predictable clinical course and response to specific therapy. In addition to helping physicians evaluate their patients, cytogenetic studies provide new insights into the pathogenesis of neoplastic diseases.

When cytogenetic abnormalities are present before therapy, their presence or absence can be used to identify remission, relapse, and minimal residual disease after therapy. If the cytogenetic abnormality identified before therapy is identified after therapy, it is evidence that the neoplastic cells are still present in the bone marrow. In some cases, additional chromosome aberrations can be identified during the course of the disease or after a period of remission. This is usually a signal of disease progression. Thus, patients can have multiple cytogenetic analyses (∞ Chapter 24).

Molecular Analysis

Molecular genetic analysis, the process of using DNA technology to identify genetic defects at the molecular level, is being used increasingly as a diagnostic tool in studying neoplasms. In some cases, the chromosome karyotype is normal, but a genetic mutation can be identified. About 5% of patients with CML do not show the typical Philadelphia chromosome on karyotyping, but the *BCR-ABL* mutation can be identified by molecular techniques. When present, this helps establish or confirm the diagnosis.

Molecular analysis also is helpful in providing clues to the pathogenesis of hematopoietic neoplasms. For example, the specific t(15;17) (q22;q11) mutation found in acute promyelocytic leukemia produces an abnormal form of the nuclear hormone receptor, retinoic acid receptor-alpha (RAR-α). The receptor in its normal form is important in the transcription of certain target genes. The abnormal receptor is involved in the maturation blockade seen in these cells. When patients who have this mutation are treated with retinoic acid derivatives, the cells are induced to differentiate into mature granulocytes.

One of the limitations of molecular genetic analysis is that the specific genetic aberration must be identified first so that probes can be made to detect the gene abnormality. Currently, this technology is helpful in diagnosis of M3-AML, CML, PV, and T and B ALL. Another limitation of molecular techniques is that only a single gene mutation usually can be identified using a given probe, so other gene mutations are not detected. Thus, it is important for the clinical laboratory scientist to understand the advantages and limitations of each diagnostic procedure and recommend the appropriate combination as well as sequence of testing. ∞ Chapter 39 discusses molecular genetic techniques and their application in diagnosis of hematopoietic diseases.

Quantitative molecular methods are used to monitor treatment of CML. Baseline levels of mRNA transcripts of BCR/ABL are obtained before treatment is started and then at intervals (3–6 months) to determine whether patients are responding to treatment.[34,35]

 Checkpoint! 5

A patient has 35% blasts in the bone marrow. They do not show any specific morphologic characteristics that will allow them to be classified according to cell lineage. What are the next steps that the clinical laboratory scientist should take with this specimen?

▶ PROGNOSIS AND TREATMENT OF NEOPLASTIC DISORDERS

PROGNOSIS

Before the 1960s, a patient diagnosed with acute leukemia could expect to die within a few months. With new treatment modalities, remission rates for both ALL and AML have improved dramatically. Remission was defined originally as a period of time in which there were no clinical or hematologic signs of the disease. More recently with the various diagnostic and monitoring modalities available, several levels of remission can be defined. For treatment purposes, complete remission (response) is defined as the total absence of disease according to the test utilized (e.g., hematologic versus cytogenetic versus molecular). **Hematologic remission** refers to the absence of neoplastic cells in the peripheral blood and bone marrow and the return to normal levels of hematologic parameters. **Cytogenetic remission** refers to the absence of recognized cytogenetic abnormalities associated with a given neoplastic disease.

Molecular remission refers to the absence of detectable molecular abnormalities using PCR or related molecular technologies.

Sensitive molecular testing such as PCR can detect the presence of less than 1 in 10^6 tumor cells (∞ Chapter 39) whereas the sensitivity of detection of malignant cells using cytogenetics is much lower. Thus, a complete molecular response is highly desirable and the most promising evidence that the neoplasm has been eliminated. A combination of negative "traditional" tests (peripheral blood and bone marrow blast count and cytogenetics) and positive molecular tests (PCR/FISH) is sometimes referred to as a state of **minimum residual disease (MRD).** The designation "partial response" is used when the relevant laboratory values have a significant decrease without achieving a total absence of disease. A "major response" can include either a complete or partial response.

Therapeutic success rates differ by disease and the patient's condition at time of diagnosis. Often a complete hematologic or cytogenetic remission is achieved initially only to be followed by a return of the disease (relapse) after a period of time. It has been recognized recently that most currently used treatment regimens are targeting the actively proliferating cancer cells and might not, in fact, be effective against the leukemic stem cells (LSC). Thus, the relapse seen in some patients following a complete remission is likely due to the reemergence of the disease from a quiescent LSC, which was not eliminated by the treatment regimen utilized.

Survival in acute leukemias varies with age and group—ALL or AML. Approximately 80% of children treated for ALL can be expected to enter a prolonged remission with an indefinite period of survival. The prognosis for ALL in adults is not so good as for children. Two years is the median survival for adults after remission has been achieved. Only 10–25% of patients typically achieve a 5-year survival. The remission rate for AML is about 55–65%. Approximately 50% of these patients remain in remission for more than 3 years. Patients who receive bone marrow or stem cell transplants, especially younger ones, have a better prognosis. Patients who had a previous myelodysplastic syndrome or chronic myeloproliferative disorder respond poorly to standard chemotherapy.

Survival in the chronic neoplasms is longer. The International Randomized Study of Interferon and STI571 (IRIS) reported that for CML patients receiving imatinib as initial therapy, overall survival at 60 months was 89%.[36] After onset of blast crisis, survival is generally only 1–2 months.[37] Survival in CLL depends on the severity of the disease at diagnosis and ranges from 30 to more than 120 months. Patients with other MDS and MPD diseases usually survive for a year or more and even longer for some subtypes without treatment. Prognosis for the lymphomas depends on the cell type and can range from 6 months to 10 years or longer.

CASE STUDY (continued from page 432)

4. Would you expect Agnes to survive more than 3 years or succumb fairly quickly after treatment?

TREATMENT

Chemotherapeutic drug and radiotherapy protocols have been developed by cancer and leukemia groups (CALG) and are used by cooperative oncology groups (COG) to access statistically valid data in a highly efficient fashion.

Chemotherapy

Chemotherapy remains the treatment of choice for many leukemias. The goal of this therapy type is to eradicate all malignant cells within the bone marrow, allowing repopulation by residual normal hematopoietic precursors. The problem with this type of therapy is that the drugs used in treatment are not specific for leukemic cells. Thus, treatment also kills many normal cells. Complications of traditional therapy include bleeding due to decreased platelet counts, infections due to suppression of granulocyte counts, and anemia due to erythrocyte suppression in the marrow. Supplemental support with recombinant growth factors can be used to mitigate the cytopenias.

Most drugs used to treat leukemia are included in three groups: antimetabolites, alkylating agents, and antibiotics. The antimetabolites are purine or pyrimidine antagonists, which inhibit the synthesis of DNA. These drugs kill cells in cycle, affecting any rapidly dividing cell. In addition to leukemic cells, the antimetabolites also kill cells lining the gut, germinal epithelium of the hair follicles, and normal hematopoietic cells. This leads to complications of gastrointestinal disturbances, loss of hair, and life-threatening cytopenias. The alkylating agents (chemical compounds containing alkyl groups) are not specific for cells in cycle but kill both resting and proliferating cells. The drug attaches to DNA molecules, interfering with DNA synthesis. These drugs as a class are mutagenic and carcinogenic; they fragment and clump chromosomes, inactivate DNA viruses, and inhibit mitosis but not protein function. The side effects of these compounds include myelosuppression, stomatitis, nausea, and vomiting. Antibiotics bind to both DNA and RNA molecules, interfering with cell replication. Toxic effects of this therapy are similar to those of alkylating agents.

Since the 1970s, various drug combinations have been found to be more effective than single drug administration. The drugs commonly used and their modes of action are included in Table 21-10 ✪.

Therapy for most leukemias is divided into several phases. The **induction therapy** phase is designed to induce the disease into complete remission (i.e., eradicating the leukemic blast population). Once a complete remission has been achieved, it is often followed by a continuation of

✪ TABLE 21-10

Chemotherapeutic Agents Usually Used in Acute Leukemia (AL) Treatment

Drug	Class	Action
Doxorubicin	Anthracycline antibiotic	Inhibits DNA and RNA synthesis
Daunorubicin	Anthracycline antibiotic	Inhibits DNA and RNA synthesis
Idarubicin	Anthracycline antibiotic	Inhibits DNA and RNA synthesis
5-azacytidine	Pyrimidine antimetabolite	Inhibits DNA and RNA synthesis
6-thioguanine	Purine antimetabolite	Inhibits purine synthesis
Methotrexate	Folic acid antimetabolite	Inhibits pyrimidine synthesis
6-mercaptopurine	Purine antimetabolite	Inhibits pyrimidine synthesis
Cytosine arabinoside	Pyrimidine antimetabolite	Inhibits DNA synthesis
Prednisone	Synthetic glucocorticoid	Lyses lymphoblasts
Vincristine	Plant alkaloid	Inhibits RNA synthesis and assembly of mitotic spindles
Asparaginase	*E. coli* enzyme	Depletes endogenous asparagines
Cyclophosphamide	Synthetic alkylating agent	Cross-links DNA strands

✪ TABLE 21-11

Treatment and Prognosis of Myeloproliferative Disorders (MPD) and Myelodysplastic Syndromes (MDS)

Neoplasm	Treatment	Prognosis
Myeloproliferative disorders		
CML	Imatinib; stem cell transplant	>5 years
PV	Phlebotomy, chemotherapy, or no treatment	8–15 years
ET	Chemotherapy, or no treatment	>10 years
CIMF	Chemotherapy, bone marrow transplant	2–10 years
Myelodysplastic syndromes	Not curable except with stem cell transplant, chemotherapy; demethylating agents	5–50 months, depending on classification of MDS

CML = chronic myelogenous leukemia; PV = polycythemia vera; ET = essential thrombocythemia; CIMF = chronic idiopathic myelofibrosis

treatment, referred to as **maintenance chemotherapy,** or **consolidation therapy.** The purpose of maintenance therapy is to eradicate any remaining leukemic cells.

The treatment regimen for AML and ALL is similar, although the combination of antileukemic agents differs. However, the purpose of chemotherapy is the same: to eradicate the leukemic blasts. CNS involvement is a common feature of ALL but not AML. Therefore, CNS prophylactic treatment (cranial irradiation and/or intrathecal chemotherapy) is part of the therapy regimen for ALL.

Permanent remission in CLL is rare. Treatment is conservative and usually reserved for patients with more aggressive forms of the disease. Treatment for the MPD and the MDS is also primarily supportive and designed to improve the quality of the patient's life (Table 21-11 ✪). Drugs designed to reverse epigenetic alterations in MDS recently have been introduced (see below).

Molecular-Targeted Therapy

As the genetic mysteries of hematologic neoplasms are being resolved, novel therapies that target the genetic mutation are being developed to silence the gene's expression or that of the mutated protein or to reactivate silenced genes. The therapies appear to be tolerated better than the traditional chemotherapy regimens. Two targeted therapies are in current use as first-line therapy: imatinib for CML and all trans retinoic acid (ATRA) for acute promyelocytic leukemia.[36] Although hematopoietic stem cell transplantation had been recommended as first-line therapy for CML because it was the only treatment that had the potential for cure, recent studies reveal that survival is superior in patients receiving drug treatment (interferon and/or imatinib).[38] These therapies are discussed in ∞ Chapters 22 and 24.

Epigenetic Therapies

With the recognition of the contribution of epigenetic alterations to the neoplastic process, a number of drugs have been developed and are in various stages of clinical trials. Both demethylating agents (e.g., azacitidine) and histone deacetylase inhibitors (HDAC-I) (e.g., valproic acid, phenylbutyrate) are being evaluated with promising early results.[15,39,40]

Bone Marrow Transplant

Bone marrow transplants have provided hope as a possible cure for hematopoietic disorders; the highest rate of success in transplant patients has occurred with those younger than 40 years of age in a first remission with a closely matched donor. In this procedure, drugs and irradiation are used to induce remission and eradicate any evidence of leukemic cells. Bone marrow from a suitable donor is then transplanted into the patient to supply a source of normal stem cells.

Autologous transplants have been used when a compatible donor cannot be found. This procedure involves removing some of the patient's marrow while the patient is in complete remission. The marrow specimen is then treated in vitro with monoclonal antibodies or 4-hydroperoxycyclophosphamide to remove any residual leukemic cells (purged) and cryopreserved. Chemotherapy and/or radiotherapy is administered to the patient to remove all traces of leukemia, and the treated marrow is given back to the patient.

Autologous bone marrow transplantation has been applied to patients in remission and to those in early relapse. Overall survival appears to be better in those transplanted during the first complete remission. Bone marrow transplantation appears to be successful in many cases; the number of patients who are undergoing this type of therapy is increasing.

Stem Cell Transplants

Peripheral blood as well as bone marrow stem cells can be used to reestablish hematopoiesis in the marrow after intensive chemotherapy or radiotherapy in a process called *stem cell transplantation*. In this procedure, apheresis is used to collect stem cells from the peripheral circulation, usually after they have been mobilized (induced to exit the marrow) by cytokines such as G-CSF. These stem cells can come from either the patient (autologous) or from a suitable donor (allogeneic). People who receive allogeneic stem cells are given drugs to prevent rejection. Production of new blood cells becomes established usually in 10–21 days following infusion of the stem cells. Stem cell transplantation is still a fairly new and complex treatment for leukemia. A more thorough discussion of hematopoietic stem cell transplantation can be found in ∞ Chapter 27.

 CASE STUDY *(continued from page 436)*

5. Is Agnes a suitable candidate for a bone marrow transplant? Why or why not?

Hematopoietic Growth Factors

Recombinant hematopoietic growth factors are used in the supportive care of AL patients. Erythropoietin was introduced in 1989 and has been used in the treatment of chemotherapy-related anemia.[41] Granulocyte colony-stimulating factor (G-CSF) and granulocyte-macrophage colony-stimulating factor (GM-CSF) have been available since 1991 to aid in decreasing the incidence of severe neutropenia and infection in patients receiving myelosuppressive chemotherapy.[41] Interleukin-11, introduced for use in 1997,[42] promotes the maturation of megakaryocytes by stimulating stem cells and megakaryocyte progenitor cells. Research in the area of identifying additional hematopoietic growth-stimulating

factors continues in the hope of accelerating hematopoietic recovery in chemotherapy patients.

Complications of Treatment

Treatment for leukemia actually can aggravate the patient's clinical situation. Although uric acid levels are commonly elevated in leukemia from an increase in cell turnover, the concentration of this constituent can increase manyfold during effective therapy because of the release of nucleic acids by lysed cells. Uric acid is a normal end product of nucleic acid degradation and is excreted mainly by the kidney. In excessive amounts, the uric acid precipitates in renal tubules, leading to renal failure (uric acid nephropathy). Lysed cells also can release procoagulants into the vascular system, precipitating disseminated intravascular coagulation. In this case, the resulting decrease in platelets and coagulation factors can lead to hemorrhage. This complication is especially prevalent in acute promyelocytic leukemia. The granules of the promyelocytes contain potent activators of the coagulation factors (∞ Chapter 33).

Chemotherapeutics destroy normal as well as leukemic cells. The cytopenias that develop during aggressive chemotherapy can lead to death from infection, bleeding, or complications of anemia. To prevent these life-threatening episodes, the patient may need supportive treatment including transfusions with blood components and/or cytokines as well as antimicrobial therapy.

 CASE STUDY *(continued)*

6. What types of treatment are available for our patient Agnes?

SUMMARY

A neoplasm is an unregulated production of cells that can be either malignant or benign. The WHO classification of neoplastic disorders of the bone marrow hematopoietic cells groups the disorders according to lineage of the neoplastic cells: myeloid, lymphoid, mast cell, histiocytic. The four major groups of myeloid disease are defined by morphology, genetic abnormalities, immunophenotype and clinical features. They include: myeloproliferative disorders, myeloproliferative/myelodysplastic disorders, myelodysplastic syndromes and acute myeloid leukemia.

The myeloproliferative disorders are characterized by an overproduction of erythrocytes, leukocytes, and/or platelets. Myelodysplastic syndromes show peripheral blood cytopenias and dysplasia of cell maturation. Both MPD and MDS can follow a chronic or acute course, and both have the potential to evolve into an acute leukemia. The abnormal proliferation of cells sometimes occurs within the lymphatic tissue or lymph nodes. These solid tumors are referred to as *lymphoma.*

Leukemia is a progressive malignant disease of hematopoietic stem cells characterized by an inability of these cells to mature into functional peripheral blood cells. Leukemias can be classified as acute or chronic based on the aggressiveness of the disease and degree of differentiation of the cells. Acute leukemias are characterized by accumulation of immature cells and have a rapidly progressive course. Chronic leukemias are characterized by an accumulation of more differentiated cells and have a slowly progressive course. The chronic leukemias are classified with other chronic neoplastic stem cell disorders: MPD, MDS, and chronic lymphproliferative disorders.

The role of oncogenes in the pathogenesis of hematopoietic disorders remains under intense investigation. Oncogenes are altered cellular proto-oncogenes known to contribute to tumorigenesis. Many proto-oncogene protein products are involved in regulating cell growth and include hematopoietic growth factors as well as their cellular receptors, signaling proteins, and transcription factors. Proto-oncogenes can be mutated to oncogenes by mutagens, viruses, or chromosome breaks and translocations. Oncogenes can cause production of abnormal growth factors, abnormal amounts of growth factors, abnormal growth factor receptors, or other abnormalities in the regulatory mechanisms of cell proliferation and differentiation. Epigenetic alterations also play an important role in silencing tumor-suppressor genes in neoplastic cells.

Differentiation and classification of acute leukemias depend on accurate identification of the blast cell population. Because the lineage of blast cells is sometimes difficult to differentiate using only morphologic characteristics, immunologic phenotyping using monoclonal antibodies and cytochemical analysis are employed routinely to help identify blast phenotypes and stage of cell differentia-tion. Chromosome and molecular analyses are helpful because specific mutations often are associated with specific types of leukemias.

Hematologic findings of hematopoietic neoplasms include anemia, thrombocytopenia (in acute leukemia and MDS), and often leukocytosis. A leukocytic shift to the left is consistently found with a combination of blasts and mature cells in acute leukemia. In the chronic leukemias and other chronic neoplastic stem cell disorders, cells appear more on a continuum from immature to mature. Morphologic abnormalities of neoplastic cells are not unusual. Auer rods can be found in blasts of AML.

Historically, hematopoietic neoplasms have been treated using a combination of cytotoxic drugs (chemotherapy). The goal is to induce remission by eradicating the leukemic cells. Hematopoietic stem cell transplants are being used increasingly to restore the marrow after intense chemotherapy or radiotherapy. New approaches include drugs to reverse epigenetic modifications characteristic of neoplastic cells and other drugs targeted at the exact molecular abnormality associated with the neoplastic cell. Treatment with hematopoietic growth factors is used in some cases to stimulate leukemic cells to proliferate, making these cells more susceptible to cytotoxic drugs. This therapy also has been used to decrease the neutropenic, anemic, and thrombocytopenic period after chemotherapy or radiotherapy.

The WHO classification of neoplastic hematologic diseases was updated in 2008, but it was too late for inclusion in the printed version of this text. For the updates, refer to the book's Website.

REVIEW QUESTIONS

LEVEL I

1. A gap in the normal maturation pyramid of cells with many blasts and some mature forms is known as: (Objectives 2, 5)
   a. leukemic hiatus
   b. chronic leukemia
   c. mixed cell lineage
   d. lineage restricted

2. Auer rods are inclusions found in: (Objective 5)
   a. myeloblasts
   b. lymphoblasts
   c. erythrocytes
   d. prolymphocytes

3. Chromosome changes in hematologic neoplasms are: (Objective 8)
   a. present in AL but not MPD or MDS
   b. nonrandom
   c. associated with a poor outcome
   d. not usually present

4. Genes that can cause tumors if activated are: (Objective 6)
   a. cancer genes
   b. proto-oncogenes
   c. preleukemia genes
   d. tumor-suppressor genes

LEVEL II

1. This stain is helpful in distinguishing myeloblasts from lymphoblasts: (Objective 8)
   a. myeloperoxidase
   b. TRAP
   c. LAP
   d. esterase

2. Oncogenes can cause leukemia by: (Objective 1)
   a. suppressing proliferation of normal cells
   b. activating retroviruses
   c. encoding for an aberrant growth protein
   d. encoding proteins that cause DNA damage

3. The PAS stain is helpful in diagnosis of: (Objectives 3, 8)
   a. CLL
   b. CML
   c. MDS
   d. ALL

4. Which of the following factors has **not** been proposed as playing a role in the causation of leukemia? (Objective 6)
   a. benzene
   b. therapeutic radiation for Hodgkin's disease
   c. living at high altitudes
   d. chromosome translocations

REVIEW QUESTIONS (continued)

LEVEL I

5. A common characteristic of acute lymphoblastic leukemia is: (Objective 2)
   a. found primarily in the elderly
   b. bone and joint pain
   c. many blast cells with Auer rods
   d. leukocytopenia

6. The FAB classification is used to divide acute leukemias into groups according to: (Objective 3)
   a. immunology
   b. clinical presentation
   c. cytogenetics
   d. morphology

7. A leukemia that shows a profusion of granulocytes at all stages of development from blasts to segmented neutrophils is: (Objectives 2, 5)
   a. AML
   b. CML
   c. ALL
   d. CLL

8. Acute lymphoblastic leukemia occurs with greatest frequency in which age group? (Objective 7)
   a. 2–5 years
   b. 10–15 years
   c. 20–30 years
   d. over 50 years

9. Chronic leukemias primarily affect: (Objectives 2, 7)
   a. all ages, progress rapidly, and have immature cells in peripheral circulation
   b. children, progress rapidly, and have mature cells in peripheral circulation
   c. young adults, progress slowly, and have immature cells in peripheral circulation
   d. adults, progress slowly, and have mature cells in circulation

10. A 19-year-old patient's bone marrow is classified by the WHO system as a precursor B-cell leukemia. Which of the following best describes this leukemia? (Objectives 2, 3, 5)
    a. CLL
    b. ALL
    c. AML
    d. CML

11. Immunologic phenotyping of the blast cells is important to: (Objective 8)
    a. help determine cell lineage
    b. identify the etiology of the leukemia
    c. determine whether cytogenetic analysis is necessary
    d. replace the need to do multiple cytochemical stains

LEVEL II

5. A 3-year-old child with Down syndrome presents with pallor, fatigue, lymphadenopathy, and hepatosplenomegaly. The initial CBC results were: (Objectives 3, 7)

		WBC differential	
WBC	18.7×10^9/L		10 segs
RBC	2.34×10^{12}/L		27 lymphs
Hb	5.8 g/dL (58 g/L)		63 blasts
Hct	0.174 L/L		
PLT	130×10^9/L		

These findings are suggestive of:
   a. acute lymphoblastic leukemia
   b. chronic lymphocytic leukemia
   c. acute myeloid leukemia
   d. chronic myelogenous leukemia

6. A patient with a hypercellular, dysplastic bone marrow, and anemia and neutropenia in peripheral blood most likely has which of the following neoplasms? (Objective 7)
   a. MPD
   b. MDS
   c. AML
   d. ALL

7. A 52-year-old female was admitted to the hospital for minor elective surgery. Her preop CBC was:

WBC	49.4×10^9/L
RBC	4.50×10^{12}/L
Hb	12.7 g/dL (127 g/L)
Hct	0.38 L/L
PLT	213×10^9/L
WBC differential	3% segs
	97% lymphs

What is the best explanation for this patient's leukocytosis and lymphocytosis? (Objectives 3, 7)
   a. ALL
   b. AML
   c. CLL
   d. CML

Use the following information to answer questions 8–10:

A 43-year-old male had been working with the Peace Corps in Mexico for the past 10 years. His primary responsibilities were taking X-rays and doing laboratory work at the various clinics. He had been complaining of weakness and fatigue for about a month and had several severe nosebleeds. His CBC upon admission to the hospital was:

		WBC differential	
WBC	25.6×10^9/L		75% blasts
RBC	3.11×10^{12}/L		with Auer rods
Hb	8.9 g/dL (89 g/L)		20% lymphs
Hct	0.267 L/L		3% monos
PLT	13×10^9/L		2% segs

LEVEL I

12. The minimum percentage of blast cells required for a diagnosis of acute leukemia using the WHO classification is: (Objective 3)
    a. 50%
    b. 40%
    c. 30%
    d. 20%

LEVEL II

8. Which leukemia is this patient most likely to have acquired? (Objectives 3, 7)
   a. ALL
   b. AML
   c. CLL
   d. CML

9. What would be the most likely causative agent of the leukemia? (Objective 2)
   a. virus
   b. age
   c. hepatitis
   d. ionizing radiation

10. What treatment would result in the *best* prognosis for this patient if there were no complicating factors? (Objective 5)
    a. hematopoietic growth factors
    b. stem cell transplantation
    c. radiation therapy
    d. chemotherapy

11. You are doing several cytochemical stains on a bone marrow from a patient who was recently diagnosed with acute leukemia. You are looking at the MPO, and the blasts are negative. However, the reagent is getting close to the expiration date, and you are not sure if the stain worked properly. What cells found in the bone marrow normally express myeloperoxidase and could be used to assess the stain's integrity? (Objectives 8, 9)
    a. neutrophils
    b. red cell precursors
    c. megakaryocytes
    d. lymphocytes

12. Use this information to answer questions 12 and 13.

    A pathologist is looking at the bone marrow aspirate of a 26-year-old male. The marrow is packed with undifferentiated blasts. After careful searching, she could not find any Auer rods. She thinks that the patient most probably has acute lymphoblastic leukemia but cannot rule out AML by using morphology. She is thinking of ordering a TdT stain on the slides. Is that going to be useful? (Objectives 8, 9)
    a. Yes, TdT is always positive in acute lymphoid leukemia but never in myeloid leukemia.
    b. Yes, TdT is always positive in acute myeloid leukemia but never in lymphoid leukemia.
    c. No, TdT is positive in the majority of acute lymphoid leukemias but approximately 20% of acute myeloid leukemias can be positive.
    d. No, Tdt is positive in the majority of acute myeloid leukemias, but approximately 20% of acute lymphoid leukemias can be positive.

REVIEW QUESTIONS *(continued)*

LEVEL I

LEVEL II

13. Which stain would you suggest the pathologist order in question 12? (Objectives 8, 9)
    a. PAS
    b. myeloperoxidase
    c. nonspecific esterase
    d. trichrome

14. Heritable changes in gene expression not due to changes in DNA are is known as: (Objective 10)
    a. mutations
    b. molecular genetics
    c. epigenetics
    d. cytogenetics

www.pearsonhighered.com/mckenzie

Use this address to access the interactive Companion Website created for this textbook. Find additional information, tables and figures. Evaluate your command of the chapter information using case studies and critical thinking and multiple choice questions.

REFERENCES

1. Reya T, Morrison SJ, Clarke MF, Weissman IL. Stem cells, cancer, and cancer stem cells. *Nature.* 2001;414:105–11.

2. Passegue E, Jamieson CHM, Ailles LE, Weissman IL. Normal and leukemic hematopoiesis: Are leukemias a stem cell disorder or a reacquisition of stem cell characteristics? *Proc Natl Acad Sci USA.* 2003;100:11842–49.

3. Stehelin D, Varmus HE, Bishop JM, Vogt PK. DNA related to the transforming gene(s) of avian sarcoma viruses is present in normal avian DNA. *Nature.* 1976;260:(5547)170–73.

4. Deininger MW, Goldman JM, Melo JV. The molecular biology of chronic myeloid leukemia. *Blood.* 2000;96:3343–56.

5. Toll T, Estella J, Illa J, Alcorta I, Mateo M. Acute leukemia in Down syndrome children. *Cytogenet Cell Genet.* 1997;7(Suppl 1):25–26.

6. Ross JA, Spector LG, Robison LL, Olshan AF. Down syndrome and leukemia: State of the art series epidemiology of leukemia in children with Down syndrome. *Pediatr Blood Cancer.* 2005;44(1):8–12.

7. Gao Q et al. Susceptibility gene for familial acute myeloid leukemia associated with loss of 5q and/or 7q is not localized on the commonly deleted portion of 5q. *Genes Chromosomes Cancer.* 2000;28:164–72.

8. Fearon ER. Human cancer syndromes: Clues to the origin and nature of cancer. *Science.* 1997;278:1043–50.

9. Jaffe ES, Harris NL, Stein H, Vardiman JW. *Pathology & Genetics. Tumours of Haematopoietic and Lymphoid Tissues.* World Health Organization Classification of Tumours. Washington, DC: IARC Press; 2001.

10. Wyke J. Principles of viral leukemogenesis. *Semin Hematol.* 1986;23:189–200.

11. Manzari V et al. HTLV-V: A new human retrovirus in a Tac-negative T cell lymphoma/leukemia. *Science.* 1987;238(4833):1581–83.

12. Kumar T, Mandla SG, Greer WL. Familial myelodysplastic syndrome with early age of onset. *Am J Hematol.* 2000;64:53–58.

13. Occhipinti E, Correa H, Yu I, Craver R. Comparison of two classifications for pediatric myelodysplastic and myeloproliferative disorders. *Pediatr Blood Cancer.* 2005;44:240–44.

14. Paltiel O, Friedlander Y, Deutsch L, Yanetz R, Calderon-Margalit R, Tiram E et al. The interval between cancer diagnosis among mothers and off-spring in a population-based cohort. *Familial Cancer.* 2007;6(1):121–29.

15. Jones PA, Baylin SB. The epigenomics of cancer. *Cell.* 2007;128:683–92.

16. Devaskar SU, Raychaundhuri S. Epigenetics—A science of heritable biologic adaptation. *Pediatric Research.* 2007;61:1R–4R.

17. Robertson KD, Wolffe AP. DNA methylation in health and disease. *Nat Reviews.* 2000;1:11–19.

18. Marks PA, Miller T, Richon VM. Histone deacetylases. *Curr Opin Pharm.* 2003;3:344–51.

19. Leukemia and Lymphoma Society. *Leukemia facts and statistics.* http://www.leukemia-lymphoma.org/hm_11s (accessed Nov 29, 2008).

20. Bennet JM et al. Proposals for the classification of the acute leukaemias. French-American-British (FAB) Co-operative Group. *Br J Haematol.* 1976;33:451–58.

21. Harris NL et al. World Health Organization classification of neoplastic diseases of the hematopoietic and lymphoid tissues: Report of the Clinical Advisory Committee meeting, Airlie House, Virginia, November 1997. *J Clin Oncol.* 1999;17:3835–49.

22. Vardiman JW, Harris NL, Brunning RD. The World Health Organization (WHO) classification of the myeloid neoplasms. *Blood.* 2002;100(7):2292–2302.

23. National Committee for Clinical Laboratory Standards. *Proposed Standard: Histochemical Method for Leukocyte Alkaline Phosphatase.* Villanova, PA: *NCCLS;* 1984;4 (14).

24. Sigma Diagnostics. *Alkaline Phosphatase, Leukocyte: Histochemical Semiquantitative Demonstration in Leukocytes*. St. Louis: Sigma Diagnostics; 1990.

25. Yam LT, Li CY, Lam KW. Tartrate-resistant acid phosphatase isoenzyme in the reticulum cells of leukemic reticuloendotheliosis. *N Engl J Med*. 1971;284:357–60.

26. Yam LT, Janckila AJ, Li CY, Lam KW. Cytochemistry of tartrate-resistant acid phosphatase: Fifteen years' experience. *Leukemia*. 1987; 1:285–88.

27. Bollum FJ. Terminal deoxynucleotidyl transferase as a hematopoietic cell marker. *Blood*. 1979;54:1203–15.

28. Kung PC, Long JC, McCaffrey RP, Ratliff RL, Harrison TA, Baltimore D. Terminal deoxynucleotidyl transferase in the diagnosis of leukemia and malignant lymphoma. *Am J Med*. 1978;64:788–94.

29. Yam LT, Li CY, Crosby WH. Cytochemical identification of monocytes and granulocytes. *Am J Clin Pathol*. 1971;55:283–90.

30. Li CY, Yam LT. Cytochemical characterization of leukemic cells with numerous cytoplasmic granules. *Mayo Clin Proc*. 1987;62:978–85.

31. Wick MR, Li CY, Pierre RV. Acute non-lymphocytic leukemia with basophilic differentiation. *Blood*. 1982;60:38–45.

32. Keren DF. *Flow Cytometry*. Chicago: ASCP; 1989.

33. First MIC Cooperative Study Group. Morphologic, immunologic, and cytogenetic (MIC) working classification of acute lymphoblastic leukemias. *Cancer Genet Cytogenet*. 1986;23:189–97.

34. Hughes T. ABL kinase inhibitor therapy for CML: Baseline assessments and response monitoring. *Hematology*. 2006;211–18.

35. Hughes T, Deininger M, Hochhaus A, Branford S, Radich J, Kaeda J et al. Monitoring CML patients responding to treatment with tyrosine kinase inhibitors: Review and recommendations for harmonizing current methodology for detecting BCR-ABL transcripts and kinase domomain mutations and for expressing results. *Blood*. 2006; 108:28–37.

36. Drucker BJ, Guilhot F, O'Brien SG, Gathmann I, Kantarjian H, Gattermann N et al. Five year follow-up of patients receiving imatinib for chronic myeloid leukemia. *N Engl J Med*. 2006;355:2408–17.

37. Collins RH Jr et al. Donor leukocyte infusions in 140 patients with relapsed malignancy after allogeneic bone marrow transplantation. *J Clin Oncol*. 1997;15:433–44.

38. Hehlmann R, Berger U, Pfirrmann M, Heimpel H, Hochhaus A, Hasford J. Drug treatment is superior to allografting as first-line therapy in chronic myeloid leukemia. *Blood*. 2007;109(11):4686–92.

39. Garcia-Manero G, Issa J-P. Histone Deacetylase inhibitors: A review of their clinical status as antineoplastic agents. *Cancer Invest*. 2005; 23:635–42.

40. Garcia-Manero G. Modifying the Epigenome as a therapeutic strategy in myelodysplasia. *Hematology Am Soc Hematol Educ Pro*. 2007; 405–11.

41. Parsons SK. Oncology practice patterns in the use of hematopoietic growth factors. *Curr Opin Pediatr*. 2000;12:10–17.

42. Kaushansky K. Use of thrombopoietic growth factors in acute leukemia. *Leukemia*. 2000;14:505–8.

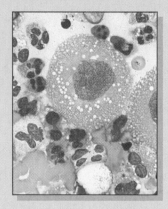

22

Myeloproliferative Disorders

Sue S. Beglinger, M.S.
Shirlyn B. McKenzie, Ph.D.

■ OBJECTIVES—LEVEL I

At the end of this unit of study, the student should be able to:

1. Interpret the leukocyte alkaline phosphatase (LAP) activity found in patients with chronic myelogenous leukemia (CML).

2. Identify the major lineages involved with the various myeloproliferative disorders (MPD): chronic myelogenous leukemia, CML; polycythemia vera, PV; essential thrombocythemia, ET; and chronic idiopathic myelofibrosis, CIMF.

3. Recognize abnormal complete blood count (CBC) results that suggest an MPD.

4. Explain the diagnostic chromosome abnormality associated with CML and its significance in acute lymphoblastic leukemia (ALL).

5. Identify the peak incidence of CML according to age and sex distribution.

6. Describe and recognize the peripheral blood findings in CML patients.

7. List and recognize laboratory findings typically associated with CIMF.

8. Define criteria that indicate a transformation of an MPD into a blast crisis.

9. Compare the lab findings in primary PV to secondary polycythemia.

10. Describe and recognize the characteristic peripheral blood picture found in essential thrombocythemia (ET).

■ OBJECTIVES—LEVEL II

At the end of this unit of study, the student should be able to:

1. Differentiate the subgroups of myeloproliferative disorders (MPD) from other reactive and neoplastic diseases based on laboratory findings in the peripheral blood, bone marrow, and other diagnostic laboratory tests.

2. Contrast laboratory findings in MPD and myelodysplastic syndromes (MDS) as well as acute leukemia (AL).

3. Describe molecular gene mutations in MPD and hypothesize how these changes in the pluripotential stem cell lead to MPD and blast crisis (Ph-chromosome; *BCR/ABL1* rearrangement; *p53, p16* mutations, *FIP1L1/PDGFRA*, and *JAK2* (V617F) mutations and expression of growth factor receptors).

4. Differentiate chronic myelogenous leukemia (CML) from a benign leukemoid reaction using laboratory tests.

5. Assess the role of platelet-derived growth factor (PDGF) in the fibrosis found with CIMF.

6. Assess laboratory results including the evaluation of peripheral blood and bone marrow smears using the diagnostic criteria associated with CIMF.

7. Compare clinical and laboratory findings, and interpret laboratory findings in relative polycythemia and absolute polycythemia.

8. Infer the significance of finding one form of the glucose-6-phosphate dehydrogenase (G6PD) isomer in myeloproliferative disorders.

9. Use laboratory results and clinical findings to differentiate essential thrombocythemia from nonmalignant conditions that result in thrombocytosis.

10. Use the criteria suggested for diagnosing variants of CML, chronic eosinophilic leukemia, CEL; chronic basophilic leukemia, CBL; and chronic neutrophilic leukemia, CNL to evaluate laboratory results of patients.

11. Differentiate unclassifiable myeloproliferative disease from other subgroups of MPD based on laboratory features.

12. Describe systemic mastocytosis by giving the criteria for diagnosis.

13. Using peripheral blood and bone marrow findings and patient medical history, determine the classification of MPD.

KEY TERMS

Chronic basophilic leukemia (CBL)
Chronic eosinophilic leukemia (CEL)
Chronic idiopathic myelofibrosis (CIMF)
Chronic myelogenous leukemia (CML)
Chronic neutrophilic leukemia (CNL)
Essential thrombocythemia (ET)
Hypereosinophilic syndrome (HES)
Janus kinase 2 (*JAK2*) gene
Leukemic hiatus
Mastocytosis
Myelophthisic anemia
Panmyelosis
Plethora
Polycythemia vera (PV)
Spent phase

BACKGROUND BASICS

The information in this chapter builds on concepts learned in previous chapters. To maximize your learning experience, you should review these concepts before starting this unit of study.

Level I

▶ Outline the cell cycle; describe stem cell differentiation and maturation for the various myeloid lineages. (Chapters 2, 3)

▶ Describe and recognize morphology for the various stages of myeloid maturation. (Chapter 7)

▶ Calculate red cell indices. (Chapter 8)

▶ Use appropriate morphologic terms to describe size and chromia of red cells in anemic states. (Chapter 8)

▶ Outline and explain the classification of hematopoietic neoplasms. (Chapter 21)

Level II

▶ Describe the influence of growth factors on hematopoietic cell proliferation. (Chapter 2)

▶ Explain the evaluation of red cell mass based on changes in fluid volume. (Chapter 8)

▶ Explain the hemoglobin–oxygen dissociation curve. (Chapter 6)

▶ Describe how cell marker panels can be used to differentiate hematopoietic neoplasms. (Chapter 21)

▶ Discuss the value of cytogenetic studies in suspected hematologic malignancies. (Chapter 21)

▶ Explain how the utilization of molecular tests can assist in diagnosis of hematopoietic neoplasms. (Chapter 21)

CASE STUDY

We will refer to this case throughout the chapter.

Roger, a 52-year-old man with hyperuricemia, was seen at the clinic for a follow-up evaluation for splenomegaly. His palpable spleen, noted 18 months earlier, had been gradually enlarging. He originally denied fatigue, fever, and discomfort. He was examined, and a CBC was ordered. The results revealed leukocytosis, thrombocytosis, and anemia. Consider reflex laboratory testing that can assist in diagnosing this patient.

▶ OVERVIEW

This chapter is a study of the group of neoplastic but not frankly malignant disorders called *myeloproliferative disorders* (MPD). The MPD must be distinguished from other neoplastic and benign hematologic disorders for the physician to select appropriate therapy for the patient. The chapter begins with the classification, pathophysiology, and general characteristics of the MPD, which provide the groundwork for a more detailed explanation and description of each subgroup. More specific pathophysiology, clinical findings, laboratory findings, and therapy are included for each subgroup. These are followed by an explanation of how to differentiate the MPD from diseases with similar laboratory findings. Systemic mastocytosis (SM) considered to be a type of MPD but included in a separate WHO group is also briefly discussed.

▶ INTRODUCTION

As discussed (∞ Chapter 3), hematopoiesis is a highly regulated process whereby a normal steady-state production of hematopoietic cells in the bone marrow and destruction of senescent cells in the tissues maintain a constant peripheral blood cell concentration. Acquired mutations in hematopoietic stem cells that allow them to escape the regulatory controls for proliferation and/or differentiation in the bone marrow result in hematopoietic neoplasms.

In the French-American-British (FAB) classification, neoplastic disorders of hematopoietic cells typically are grouped into three main categories: MPD, myelodysplastic states or syndromes (MDS), and acute leukemias (AL) including both myeloid and lymphoid. This classification uses the blast count, lineage commitment, and level of differentiation of the neoplastic cells to classify the diseases. The classification uses cell morphology, cytochemistry, and immunophenotyping. Recently, the World Health Organization (WHO) proposed a newer classification for hematopoietic neoplasms that integrates cytogenetics and clinical features with cytochemistry and immunophenotyping. The WHO myeloid classification includes the same three categories as the FAB—acute myelogenous leukemia (AML), MPD, and MDS—and adds a fourth category, *the myelodysplastic/myeloproliferative disorders* (MDS/MPD), which has both myeloproliferative and myelodysplastic features, and a fifth category, mast cell disease (mastocytosis). In the WHO classification, the percentage of blasts, degree of cell maturation, and dysplasia are critical initial assessments used to classify the hematopoietic neoplasms. A blast count ≥20% is necessary for a diagnosis of AML. The other groups have <20% blasts. Each group has subcategories based on clinical history, genetic and other laboratory findings.

Although not clearly malignant, MPD and MDS, are characterized by an autonomous, neoplastic clonal proliferation of hematopoietic precursors. MPD generally can be distinguished from MDS because in MPD, both the bone marrow and peripheral blood show increases in erythrocytes, leukocytes, and/or platelets. MDS, on the other hand, are most commonly characterized by a hyperproliferative bone marrow, dysplastic maturation, and increased apoptosis that yields peripheral blood cytopenias. Both MPD and MDS have a chronic and acute course with the potential of evolving into AL. Some hematologists believe that MDS are actually acute leukemias diagnosed at an early stage. The WHO proposed MDS/MPD category includes neoplasms that are proliferative like MPD but have dysplastic features like MDS. The MDS/MPD will be discussed in Chapter 23 with MDS.

▶ CLASSIFICATION OF MYELOPROLIFERATIVE DISORDERS (MPD)

The term *myeloproliferative syndrome*, coined by William Dameshek in 1951, describes a group of disorders that result from an unchecked, autonomous clonal proliferation of cellular elements in the bone marrow.[1] Myeloproliferative disorders are generally characterized by panhypercellularity (**panmyelosis**) of the bone marrow accompanied by erythrocytosis, granulocytosis, and/or thrombocytosis in the peripheral blood. Although trilineage cell involvement (erythrocytic, granulocytic, thrombocytic) is characteristic of MPD, one cell line is usually more prominently affected than the others. Hematologic classification is based on the most affected cell line (Table 22-1 ✪). In the WHO classification, the spectrum of myeloproliferative disorders includes:

- Chronic myelogenous leukemia (CML) Ph positive, t(9;22)(q34;q11)
- Chronic neutrophilic leukemia (CNL)
- Chronic eosinophilic leukemia (CEL)/hypereosinophilic syndrome (HES)
- Chronic idiopathic myelofibrosis (CIMF) also known as *myelofibrosis with myeloid metaplasia* (MMM)
- Polycythemia vera (PV)
- Essential thrombocythemia (ET)
- Myeloproliferative disease, unclassifiable (MPD-u).

✪ TABLE 22-1

Classification of Myeloproliferative Disorders (MPD) by Predominance of Cell Types

Involved Cell Line	Myeloproliferative Disorder
Erythroid	Polycythemia vera (PV)
Myeloid	Chronic myelogenous leukemia (CML) and chronic neutrophilic leukemia (CNL)
Megakaryocytic	Essential thrombocythemia (ET)
Fibroblast*	Chronic idiopathic myelofibrosis (CIMF) with extramedullary hematopoiesis
Eosinophil	Chronic eosinophilic leukemia (CEL)
Basophil	Chronic basophilic leukemia (CBL)
Mast cell	Mast cell disease (mastocytosis)
Variable	Myeloproliferative disease, unclassifiable (MPD-u)

*The fibroblast in CIMF is not a part of the neoplastic process but is increased due to a reactive process.

The most important change from the FAB to the WHO classification of the MPD is that only cases with the Philadelphia (Ph) chromosome are included as CML in the WHO classification. The Ph chromosome negative cases with myelodysplastic and myeloproliferative features are included in the WHO MDS/MPD group and called *atypical CML (aCML)*. Another rare neoplasm, chronic basophilic leukemia, is also considered an MPD and will be discussed in this chapter.

The classification of these disorders is not always clear because of overlapping clinical and laboratory features between subgroups at different times during the course of the disease (Table 22-2 ✪).

▶ PATHOPHYSIOLOGY

The primary defect in MPD appears to be in the pluripotential hematopoietic stem cell (HSC) (Figure 22-1 ■). Studies indicate that in myeloproliferative diseases, increased numbers of stem cells and progenitor cells are found in the precursor cell compartment.[2] A clone of abnormal hematopoietic stem cells and their progeny preferentially expands until normal hematopoietic cell growth is inhibited and the majority of functioning bone marrow is derived from the abnormal clone. Excessive proliferation of hematopoietic cells occurs through various mechanisms that require multiple genetic mutations[3,4] (∞ Chapter 3). Commitment, differentiation, and maturation of the abnormal clone are generally preserved, leading to increased numbers of mature cells in the peripheral blood, usually with one lineage (erythroid, myeloid, or megakaryocytic) predominating.

The finding of uniform biochemical, cytogenetic, or molecular genetic abnormalities in hematopoietic cells from the bone marrow or peripheral blood of patients with MPD suggests a clonal origin for these disorders. The most useful biochemical marker for demonstrating monoclonality of MPD is the glucose-6-phosphate dehydrogenase (G6PD) enzyme. G6PD isoenzymes (A and B) are coded for by a gene on the X chromosome. The inactivation of one X chromosome in a cell containing two or more X chromosomes is random. Hence, each cell has only one active G6PD gene. Females heterozygous for isoenzyme A and isoenzyme B produce both enzymes. Approximately half of the cells contain isoenzyme A; the remaining cells contain isoenzyme B. The blood cells of G6PD heterozygous females with MPD, however, contain either one or the other isoenzyme in their granulocytes, erythrocytes, and platelets, reflecting their origin from a common HSC (i.e., "clonal" hematopoiesis).

✪ TABLE 22-2

Differential Features of Myeloproliferative Disorders

Parameter	CML	CIMF	PV	ET	CEL	CNL
Peripheral blood:						
Hematocrit	N or ↑	↓	↑↑↑	N or ↓	N	N or ↑
Leukocyte	↑↑↑	↑ or ↑↑	N or ↑	N or ↑	↑	↑
Platelets	↑ or ↓	N,↑,↓	↑	↑↑↑	N	N or ↑
Immature granulocytes	↑↑↑	↑↑	Absent or ↑	Rare	N or ↑	Slight ↑ (<10%)
LAP	↓	N,↑,↓	N or ↑	N or ↑	−	↑
Philadelphia chromosome	Present	Absent	Absent	Absent	Absent	Absent
Spleen size	N or ↑	↑↑↑	↑	N or ↑	N	↑
Bone marrow fibrosis	Absent or ↑	↑↑↑	Absent or ↑	Absent or ↑	Absent or ↑	Absent

N = normal; ↓ = decreased; ↑, ↑↑, ↑↑↑ = slight, moderate, marked increase; CML = chronic myelogenous leukemia; CIMF = chronic idiopathic myelofibrosis; PV = polycythemia vera; ET = essential thrombocythemia; CEL = chronic eosinophilic leukemia; CNL = chronic neutrophilic leukemia

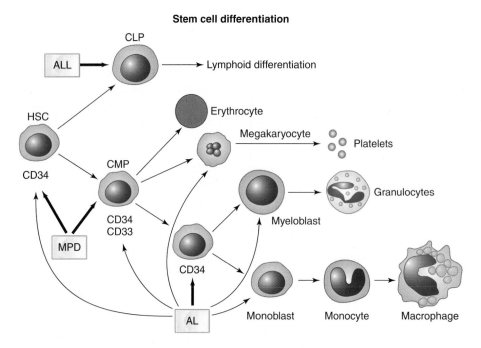

Stem cell differentiation

■ FIGURE 22-1   This schematic of hematopoietic cell development shows that a mutation in the pluripotential hematopoietic stem cell, HSC (CD34$^+$), results in clonal proliferation of the progeny of that cell, all containing the mutation. Thus, all cell lines will be
affected. This is thought to be the original neoplastic cell in CML and other MPDs. The
common lymphoid progenitor cell is thought to be the original neoplastic cell in ALL. In
AML, the cell of origin can be the common myeloid progenitor cells (CMP), the committed myeloid progenitor cells or occasionally the HSC. (ALL = acute lymphocytic
leukemia; MPD = myeloproliferative disorder; AL = acute leukemia)

In addition, many individuals with a MPD have identical
karyotypic abnormalities in all hematopoietic lineages, also
suggesting that these cells were derived from a single mutant
stem cell. These abnormalities are not present in other somatic cells, indicating that the mutations are acquired rather
than inherited. The most consistent chromosome abnormality, the Ph chromosome, is found in all hematopoietic blood
cells in patients with CML. Recently, the **Janus kinase 2
(JAK2) gene,** which codes for a tyrosine kinase involved in
cell signaling was found to be mutated in almost all cases of
PV and some cases of ET and CIMF. These mutations are discussed in more detail later in the chapter. The application of
molecular biology in the study of hematopoietic neoplasms
has been useful in identifying the specific genetic abnormality at the DNA, mRNA, and protein levels. These studies
have supported the clonality hypothesis of MPD.

▶ GENERAL FEATURES

Myeloproliferative disorders usually occur in the middle-
aged and older adults (peak frequency in the fifth to seventh
decades of life). They are rare in children. The onset of the
disease is gradual, evolving over months or even years. The

MPD frequently overlap in clinical, laboratory, and morphologic findings among the specific entities.

Clinical findings can include hemorrhage, thrombosis,
infection, pallor, and weakness. Anemia or polycythemia,
leukoerythroblastosis, leukocytosis, and thrombocytosis
with bizarre platelets are common laboratory findings that
can occur in almost any of the subtypes of MPD. Anemia,
when present, is caused by ineffective erythropoiesis, marrow fibrosis, and/or a shortened cell survival due to
splenomegaly.

Decreased bone marrow iron, not reflective of true iron
deficiency, is a consistent finding in MPD.[5] For this reason,
serum ferritin and serum iron are more reliable estimates of
iron deficiency in the presence of MPD than is the evaluation of bone marrow iron.

Thrombocytosis can be a common occurrence in MPD.
When thrombocytosis is classified as the primary disorder, it
is believed to result from an autonomous, unregulated proliferation of megakaryocytes. The level of interleukin-6
(IL-6) and thrombopoietin (TPO), cytokines that promote
megakaryopoiesis, is normal in MPD, whereas the level is
usually increased in secondary or reactive thrombocytosis.[6]
Platelet membrane proteins—glycoprotein IIb/IIIa, von
Willebrand factor (VWF), fibrinogen, fibronectin, and vitronectin—are significantly decreased in many patients with

MPD.[7,8] Genetic changes altering growth factor receptors, including the thrombopoietin receptor (MPL), and mutations in the Janus kinase (JAK) signaling pathways result in increased megakaryopoiesis and enhanced activation and aggregation of platelets.[9]

The bone marrow is usually hypercellular at onset of the MPD but often becomes fibrotic during the course of the disease. Fibroblasts are a part of the bone marrow stroma, which provides a suitable microenvironment for developing hematopoietic cells (∞ Chapter 3). Fibroblasts produce reticular fibers that form a three-dimensional supporting network for vascular sinuses and hematopoietic elements. *Fibrosis* refers to an increase in fibroblasts and reticular fibers. Fibrosis in MPD is thought to be a reactive process that is secondary to the increased production of cytokines from the abnormal hematopoietic cells (primarily megakaryocytes). As evidence of their benign proliferation, fibroblasts exhibit normal karyotypes and G6PD mosaicism in female heterozygotes. Although often considered the hallmark of CIMF, fibrosis can be seen in the other MPD entities as well.

Reactive fibrosis can result from the intramedullary release of cytokines from platelets, megakaryocytes, and malignant cells that are mitogenic for fibroblasts. Human platelet-derived growth factor (PDGF) stimulates growth and cell division of fibroblasts as well as other cells. The platelet concentration of PDGF in patients with MPD is significantly decreased. Although this could be due to either decreased synthesis or excessive release, assays of circulating PDGF in MPD suggest that the mechanism is excessive release. The serum PDGF level is significantly higher in patients with CIMF and ET than in other MPD or in normal controls. Not surprisingly, CIMF and ET are the two MPD with the most significant degree of fibrosis.[4] Increased fibroblasts lead to an increase in collagen, laminin, and fibronectin in the medullary cavity.

When marrow fibrosis supervenes over the course of the disease, the major sites of hematopoiesis become the extramedullary tissues, particularly the liver and spleen. Hepatosplenomegaly is a common clinical finding. Extramedullary hematopoiesis can also occur in benign diseases such as chronic hemolytic anemias, but the hematopoiesis in these disorders is confined to the erythrocyte lineage. In contrast, all cell lineages are present in the extramedullary masses that accompany the MPD. It has been hypothesized that marrow fibrosis causes distortion of marrow sinusoids, which permit hematopoietic stem cells to escape into the sinusoids and gain entry to the peripheral blood.[10] These stem cells then lodge in extramedullary sites, such as the spleen, to proliferate and differentiate.

MPD carry a significant risk of terminating in acute leukemia. This transition is commonly seen in CML. The question has been raised as to whether acute leukemia is a natural transition of MPD or is the result of leukemogenic chemotherapy and radiotherapy for the original myeloproliferative disorder.

✓ Checkpoint! 1

In essential thrombocythemia, all hematopoietic lines have increased cell proliferation. Which lineage has the greatest increase?

▶ CHRONIC MYELOGENOUS LEUKEMIA (CML)

Chronic myelogenous leukemia (CML), also known as *chronic granulocytic leukemia (CGL)* and *chronic myeloid leukemia,* is the best defined MPD. It is characterized by a neoplastic growth of primarily myeloid cells in the bone marrow with an extreme elevation of these cells in the peripheral blood. Extramedullary granulocytic proliferation in the spleen and liver is progressive. Erythrocytic and megakaryocytic lineages can also expand.

The natural history of the disease has three phases: chronic followed by one or both of two aggressive transformed stages—accelerated transition and blast crisis. The initial chronic phase responds well to therapy. Normal health can usually be restored and maintained for months or years. CML eventually transforms into an accelerated phase and blastic leukemia, either AML or acute lymphoblastic leukemia (ALL). After progression to blast crisis, the prognosis is poor with a survival of less than 6 months. With the newer treatment protocol using Gleevec, survival time has been increased to more than 5 years.

ETIOLOGY AND PATHOPHYSIOLOGY

The Ph chromosome, an acquired chromosome abnormality, is present in all neoplastic hematopoietic cells in CML except T lymphocytes and sometimes B lymphocytes (Figure 22-2 ■) (∞ Chapters 21, 38). This was the first chromosome abnormality found consistently associated with a malignant disease. It is not found in somatic cells or fibroblasts.

In some cases, the Ph chromosome was detected months before the diagnosis of CML. Once the chromosome abnormality is present, it rarely disappears, even in patients in remission. Because all hematopoietic cells are involved in the neoplastic process, the original neoplastic cell (cell of origin) is most likely a pluripotential HSC common to all lineages (Figure 22-1).

Molecular biology has dramatically increased our understanding of the role of the Ph chromosome in this disease. The Ph chromosome results from a balanced reciprocal translocation between the longarms of chromosomes 9 and 22, t(9;22)(q34;q11.2) (Figure 22-3 ■). On chromosome 9, the break point is spread across 90 kb within the first exon of *ABL*, translocating the 3' end of exon 1 and exons 2–11 (in which the tyrosine kinase domains reside) to chromosome 22. The break point in chromosome 22 occurs within the *BCR* gene, a large 70-kb gene with 20 exons. The break point usually involves a 5.8-kb area known as the *major break point*

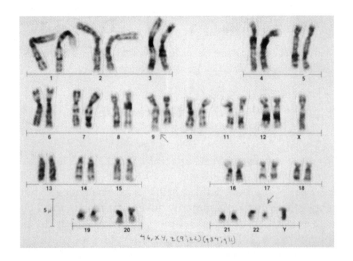

■ **FIGURE 22-2** Karyotype from a patient with CML showing the Philadelphia chromosome translocation, t(9:22)(q34;q11.2). The Philadelphia chromosome is chromosome 22.

cluster region (M-BCR) between either exons b2 and b3 or b3 and b4. Two different fusion genes can be formed, both joining the translocated portion of the *ABL* gene with either exon b2 of *BCR* or exon b3 of *BCR*. The resulting Ph chromosome has a 5' end of *BCR* from chromosome 22 and a 3' end

of *ABL* sequences from chromosome 9 (Figure 22-4 ■). This hybrid gene is then transcribed into an 8.5-kb mRNA, in contrast to the normal *ABL*, which is transcribed to a 6- or 7-kb mRNA.[11–13]

Translation of the 8.5-kb mRNA creates a new, abnormal protein, with a molecular mass of 210 kD (p210) with enhanced tyrosine kinase activity, increasing autophosphorylation within the cell (∞ Chapter 2). (Tyrosine kinase proteins regulate metabolic pathways and some serve as receptors for growth factors [RTK—receptor tyrosine kinase]). The normal ABL protein codes for a 145-kD protein. The oncogenic role of p210 is found in association with increased granulocyte colony–stimulating factor (G-CSF) and PDGF. Studies also suggest that this activation of tyrosine kinase activity suppresses apoptosis in hematopoietic cells.[13] Over a period of several years, the t(9;22) cell line replaces the normal marrow cells, and CML is expressed. The reciprocal fusion gene, *ABL/BCR1* is transcribed in approximately two-thirds of CML patients, although its significance is not clear. Characteristics of the *ABL* and *BCR* proto-oncogenes, as well as the *ABL/BCR1* fusion oncogene, are described in Table 22-3 ☉.

Detection of the *BCR* gene rearrangement has several clinical uses in the diagnosis and prognosis of CML (Table 22-4 ☉).[14] About 5–10% of patients with the CML phenotype lack the Ph chromosome. In these cases, the translocation is not detected at the karyotypic level by cytogenetic studies, but molecular analyses by reverse transcriptase polymerase chain reaction (RT-PCR) or fluorescent in situ hybridization (FISH) show that the molecular *BCR/ABL1* rearrangement has occurred (∞ Chapter 21). The malignant

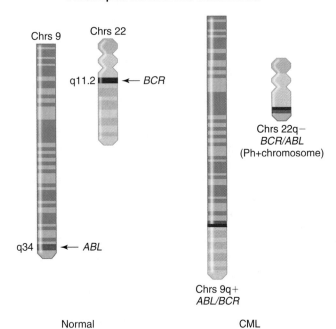

■ **FIGURE 22-3** The Philadelphia translocation in CML. Arrows indicate the chromosome breakpoints at 9q34 (*ABL* gene) and 22q11.2 (*BCR* gene) in the genes directly involved in the translocation. The translocation results in a lengthened 9q+ chromosome and a shortened 22q− chromosome (Philadelphia chromosome).

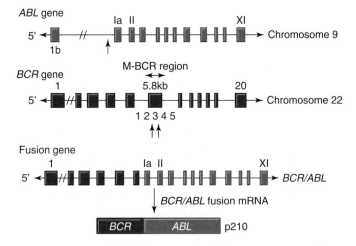

■ **FIGURE 22-4** Exon maps of the normal *BCR* and *ABL1* genes, and the *BCR/ABL1* fusion gene formed by the Philadelphia-chromosome translocation found in CML resulting in a protein of 210 kilodaltons. Upward arrows show breakpoints in the major *BCR* (M-BCR) region of the *BCR* gene and in exon 1 of the *ABL1* gene that results in the *BCR/ABL1* fusion gene.

⊘ TABLE 22-3

Characteristics of the Proto-Oncogenes and Oncogenes Involved in the *BCR/ABL* Gene Rearrangements in CML

Gene	Size	No. Exons	Break Point	Transcript(s)	Protein	Location	Activity
ABL	>230 kb	11	5′ of exon II (100–200 kb)	6 kb; 7 kb	p145	Nucleus	Tyrosine kinase (normal)
BCR	>100 kb	20	bcr (5.8 kb)	4.5 kb; 6.7 kb	p160	Unknown	Unknown
BCR/ABL1 fusion	Varies	Varies	Fusion hybrid	8.5 kb	p210	Plasma membrane	Tyrosine kinase (increased)

cells in these cases also express the 8.5-kb chimeric mRNA and the p210 protein (Table 22-5 ⊘).

Cases of phenotypic CML that are Ph chromosome and *BCR/ABL1*-negative are aCML or possibly cases of CMML (if absolute monocytosis and leukocytosis are present); both of these disorders are now considered myelodysplastic/myeloproliferative disorders.[15] Other chronic myeloproliferative diseases, similar to CML, include chronic eosinophilic leukemia, chronic basophilic leukemia, and chronic neutrophilic leukemia. All have high proliferative rates, but are Ph-chromosome negative.[16,17]

Disease Progression and Additional Chromosome/Molecular Mutations

Progression of CML is marked by an accelerated or acute phase (blast crisis). In more than 75% of patients, this progression is preceded or accompanied by the development of additional chromosomal abnormalities (Table 22-6 ⊘).[18] Thus, repeated chromosome analysis in patients with CML can be helpful in predicting impending blast crisis.

At the molecular level, mutations in the *p53* gene (∞ Chapter 2), a tumor suppressor antioncogene, are found in at least 30% of patients in blast crisis, especially in those with myeloid or megakaryocytic blast crisis.[19] Mutations/alterations of this gene in the chronic state of CML are rare.

RAS proteins, found on the inner surface of the cell membrane where they associate with cell surface receptors, also are altered in CML. *RAS* genes encode for proteins that bind guanosine diphosphate (GDP) in their neutral (unactivated) state. When the cell surface receptor is activated by a cytokine, the RAS protein is activated by expelling the GDP and binding GTP in its place. By binding G-proteins, RAS proteins transfer cell activation signals from the cytokine/receptor complex into the nucleus in a process that is carefully regulated. Oncogenic forms of RAS have a reduced ability to be deactivated, thus sending unregulated proliferation signals to the cell nucleus. Both normal and oncogenic RAS proteins must have a farnesyl group added in a post-translational modification of the protein to be fully active. One of the new treatment approaches for those malignancies with elevated RAS activity is a "farnesyl transferase inhibitor" drug, which reduces or blocks activation of RAS and decreases the proliferative stimulus.

⊘ TABLE 22-4

Clinical Uses of Molecular Analysis for the *BCR* Gene Rearrangement

- Diagnosis of CML when the Ph chromosome is absent
- Differentiation of CML in blast crisis from de novo ALL when the Ph chromosome is present
- Confirmation of a diagnosis of CML when the patient presents in the blast crisis phase of CML
- Differentiation of CML from other myeloproliferative diseases and myelodysplastic syndromes when overlapping clinical and/or morphological features are present
- Monitoring of CML patients on therapy for minimal residual disease

Adapted from: Mattson J, Crisan D, Wilner F, Decker D, Burdakin J. Clinical problem solving using bcl-2 and BCR gene rearrangement analysis. *Lab Med.* 1994;25:648–53.

⊘ TABLE 22-5

Genetic Rearrangements and Related Proteins Found in Philadelphia Chromosome Positive CML, ALL, and Philadelphia Chromosome Negative MPD, or ALL

Clinical Condition	Involvement of Ph/BCR	PTK
Normal	Ph−, BCR−	145 kD
CML	Ph+, BCR+	210 kD
	Ph−, BCR+	210 kD
Other MPD	Ph−, BCR−	145 kD
ALL	Ph+, BCR+	210 kD (CML blast crisis)
	Ph+, BCR−	190 kD (? de novo ALL)
	Ph−, BCR−	145 kD (? de novo ALL)

PTK = protein tyrosine kinase; CML = chronic myelogenous leukemia; ALL = acute lymphoblastic leukemia; Ph+ = Philadelphia chromosome positive; Ph− = Philadelphia chromosome negative; BCR+ = rearrangement within the M-BCR region; BCR− = no rearrangement within the M-BCR region

⊕ TABLE 22-6

Additional Mutations in Blast Crisis of CML
Frequent
Duplication of Ph chromosome
Trisomy 8
Isochromosome 17
Loss of Y chromosome
Rare
Translocation (15;17)
Translocation (3;21)(q26;q22)
Translocation (3;3)/inversion (3)
Very Rare
Deletion of chromosome 5(−5) or the long arm (5q−)
Deletion of chromosome 7(−7) or the long arm (7q−)

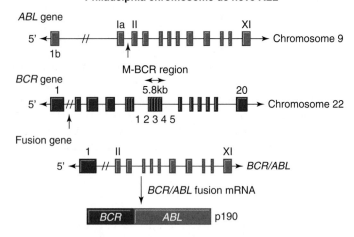

Philadelphia chromosome de novo ALL

■ **FIGURE 22-5** Exon maps of the normal *BCR* and *ABL* genes and the *BCR/ABL* gene rearrangement in the Philadelphia translocation of de novo acute leukemias resulting in a protein of 190 kilodaltons. Upward arrows show breakpoints in intron 1 of the BCR gene, upstream of the common major breakpoint region (M-BCR), and in exon II of *ABL* that result in the *BCR/ABL* gene rearrangement.

Philadelphia (Ph) Chromosome in Acute Leukemias

About 2–5% of childhood ALL, 25% of adult ALL, and some cases of AML have the Ph chromosome. Ph-positive AML cases can actually be CML in blast crisis that were not diagnosed in the chronic (CML) stage. In about 50% of the Ph-positive ALLs, the molecular defect is identical to that found in CML and the BCR/ABL protein, p210, is present. These cases probably represent the blast crisis phase of CML. In the remaining 50% of Ph-positive ALL, the break points on chromosome 22 fall 5′ to the *BCR* but are still within the first intron of the *BCR* gene. These leukemias express a distinct translation product of the mRNA hybrid termed the *p190kD protein* (Figure 22-5 ■).[13,20] These Ph-positive ALLs can actually be de novo acute leukemia cases (Table 22-5). Like p210, the p190 protein also shows an increased tyrosine kinase activity, but its role in the development of the ALL phenotype is unclear.

 Checkpoint! 2

A patient has the CML phenotype, but the genetic karyotype does not show the Ph chromosome. If this is truly a CML, what should molecular analysis show?

CLINICAL FINDINGS

CML is the most common MPD, accounting for 15–20% of all leukemia cases. It can occur at any age, but the incidence increases dramatically among those 55 years of age and older. It is most prevalent in the seventh, eighth, and ninth decades of life. It is almost equally distributed between sexes and can occur in young adults more so than other MPD. Although rare, CML can occur in childhood. More economically advanced countries report higher incidences of CML.

The question arises, however, as to whether the higher incidences reflect the ability to detect and diagnose the disease because of increased availability of advanced medicine and diagnostic tools in these countries.

The disease has an insidious onset with the most common symptoms being increased weakness, loss of stamina, unexplained fever, night sweats, weight loss, and feelings of fullness in the abdomen (hepatosplenomegaly). Gastrointestinal tract bleeding or retinal hemorrhages are occasionally the first signs of the disease. Physical examination reveals pallor, tenderness over the lower sternum, splenomegaly, and occasionally hepatomegaly. Lymphadenopathy is not typical; when present, it suggests an onset of the acute phase of the disease. Petechiae and ecchymoses reflect the presence of quantitative and/or qualitative platelet abnormalities. Some individuals are asymptomatic, and CML is found incidentally during examination for other medical problems or in a routine physical.

Any organ eventually can be infiltrated with myeloid elements, but extramedullary masses in areas other than the spleen and liver are uncommon findings in the chronic phase. On fresh incision, extramedullary masses appear green, presumably due to the presence of the myeloid enzyme myeloperoxidase. These greenish tumors have been called *chloromas*. The green color fades to a dirty yellow on exposure of the tissue to air.

Without intervention, symptoms worsen over the next 3–5 years, and increased debilitation heralds the onset of the blast phase. When the onset of blast crisis has been reached, response to therapy is poor and survival is less than 6 months.

LABORATORY FINDINGS

Peripheral Blood

The most striking abnormality in the peripheral blood is the extreme leukocytosis. The white count is usually more than 100×10^9/L with a median of about 170×10^9/L. Patients diagnosed earlier may have a leukocyte count of $25-75 \times 10^9$/L. Thrombocytosis, which can exceed 1000×10^9/L and variation in platelet shape are found in more than half of the patients. If thrombocytosis is a new observation, blast crisis is probably imminent. During blast crisis, thrombocytopenia is often a common finding. Platelet function also is frequently abnormal. Megakaryocyte fragments and micromegakaryocytes can be found (Figure 22-6 ■).

At the time of diagnosis, a moderate normocytic, normochromic anemia is typical with a hemoglobin concentration in the range of 9–l3 g/dL. The severity of anemia is proportional to the increase in leukocytes. Erythrocyte morphology is generally normal, but nucleated erythrocytes can be found. Reticulocytes are normal or slightly increased.

Blood smears exhibit a shift to the left with all stages of granulocyte maturation present (Figure 22-7 ■). The predominant cells are the segmented neutrophils and myelocytes. Promyelocytes and blasts do not usually exceed 20% of the leukocytes. Eosinophils and basophils are often increased in both relative and absolute terms. Increasing blast concentrations or progressive basophilia herald blast crisis. Monocytes are moderately increased. Signs of myeloid dysplasia including pseudo–Pelger-Huët anomaly (hyposegmentation of PMN nucleus) and decreased leukocyte alkaline phosphatase (LAP) are frequent (∞ Chapters 21, 34). Low or absent LAP is characteristic but not specific for CML. Monocytosis, myeloid dysplasia, and micromegakaryocytes are overlapping features found in both CML and chronic myelomonocytic leukemia (CMML). The presence of the Ph chromosome helps differentiate the two disorders.

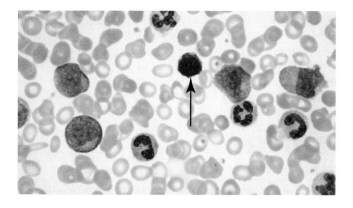

■ FIGURE 22-6   Arrow points to the micromegakaryocyte in the peripheral blood of a patient with chronic myelocytic leukemia. (Peripheral blood; Wright-Giemsa stain; 1000× magnification)

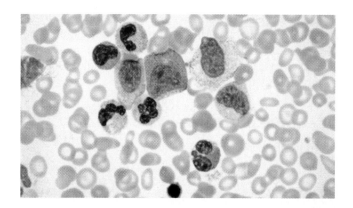

■ FIGURE 22-7   Chronic myelocytic leukemia (CML) with leukocytosis and a shift to the left. (Peripheral blood; Wright-Giemsa stain; 1000× magnification)

Bone Marrow

The bone marrow is 90–100% cellular with a striking increase in the myeloid:erythroid ratio (10:1 to 50:l). The active red marrow can extend into the long bones. Thinning of the cortex and erosion of the trabeculae can be present. The hematopoietic marrow cells are primarily immature granulocytes with <20% blasts by WHO classification, an important characteristic that distinguishes CML from AL.[21] The marrow differential count of leukocyte precursors often is within the normal range. The typical **leukemic hiatus** (gap) between the number of immature cells (blasts) and mature cells (segmented neutrophils) characteristic of AL is not present in CML. Auer rods can be found in the myeloblasts during blast crises, but this is an unusual finding. Erythropoiesis is normoblastic, but normoblasts can be decreased. Megakaryocytes are usually increased with frequent immature and atypical forms. In contrast to the large megakaryocytes found in other subgroups of MPD, CML typically reveals small megakaryocytes.

Gaucher-like cells (histiocytes) have been observed in the bone marrow (∞ Chapter 18). However, these cells, with the typical wrinkled tissue paper appearance of the cytoplasm, are not due to the lack of the β-glucocerebrosidase enzyme as in Gaucher's disease but to the overload of cerebrosides caused by increased cell turnover. The histiocytes in CML have normal to increased amounts of the β-glucocerebrosidase, but the cell cannot process the cerebrosides fast enough to prevent them from accumulating in the cell.

The marrow can become fibrotic late in the course of the disease. If a physician does not see the patient until the fibrosis is prominent, a diagnosis of CIMF may be considered. At this point, only chromosome analysis can establish the correct diagnosis.

Other nonspecific findings related to the increased proliferation of cells can be present. Total serum cobalamin and the unsaturated cobalamin binding capacity are increased. Serum transcobalamin I is often elevated. These findings are probably related to the increased number of granulocytes that are thought to synthesize the cobalamin-binding proteins. Uric acid and lactic dehydrogenase (LD) are elevated, secondary to increased cell turnover. Muramidase is normal or only slightly increased.

✓ Checkpoint! 3

Describe the peripheral blood differential of a CML patient.

@ CASE STUDY (continued from page 446)

Physical examination revealed a slightly enlarged liver and palpable spleen. Roger had hyperuricemia. Blood counts showed:

Hb 11.6 g/dL Hct 0.35 L/L RBC 3.6 × 10^{12}/L
WBC 26.2 × 10^9/L Platelets 853 × 10^9/L

The blood cell differential showed marked anisocytosis, poikilocytosis with many teardrops, and numerous NRBC. Immature myeloid cells were found along with basophilia and large platelets.

1. What are Roger's MCV and MCHC?

2. How would you classify his anemia morphologically?

3. Based on Roger's history and current laboratory data, what other tests should be performed?

TERMINAL PHASE

Historically, about 3–5 years after the diagnosis of CML, the typical course of the disease is transition to the accelerated stage (Figure 22-8 ■). This transitional, accelerated stage can occur at any time after the initial diagnosis and often precedes blastic transformation. Transition is heralded by one or more of the changes listed in Table 22-7 ✪. Marked granulocytic dysplasia or dysplastic megakaryocytes in clusters/sheets with increased fibrosis in the marrow suggests the accelerated phase. Additional chromosomal abnormalities also

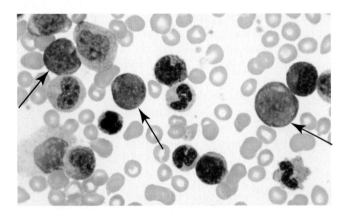

■ FIGURE 22-8 Peripheral blood film from a patient with CML in accelerated phase. There is an increase in blasts. Arrows point to blasts (Wright-Giemsa stain; 1000× magnification)

✪ TABLE 22-7

Accelerated Phase of CML

Characterized by the Presence of One or More of the Following

- 10–19% myeloblasts in peripheral blood or bone marrow
- ≥20% basophils in peripheral blood
- Platelet count < 100 × 10^9/L unrelated to therapy
- Persistent thrombocytosis >1000 × 10^9/L unresponsive to therapy
- Increasing WBC count and spleen size unresponsive to therapy
- Additional clonal genetic aberrations not present in the chronic phase
- Megakaryocytic proliferation in sheets and clusters associated with marked reticulin or collagen fibrosis and/or severe granulocytic dysplasia*

*Not yet evaluated as a criteria in large clinical studies
Adapted from: Vardiman JW, Harris NL, Brunning RD. The World Health Organization (WHO) classification of the myeloid neoplasms. *Blood.* 2002;100[7]: 2292–2302

can be found. Clinical features reflect an increase in debilitation including pyrexia, night sweats, weight loss, increased weakness, malaise, bone pain, and lymphadenopathy. About 30% of those patients in the accelerated phase die before developing a blastic crisis.

Although blast crisis typically develops after a short accelerated phase, about one-third of cases abruptly develop a blastic transformation. After onset of blast crisis, survival is about 1–2 months. The clinical features in blast crisis are similar to those of acute leukemia.

The hematologic criteria for identifying a blast crisis is made by finding moderate to marked diffuse bone marrow fibrosis and 20% or more blasts[21,22] in the peripheral blood or bone marrow of a patient previously diagnosed as having CML (Table 22-8 ✪ and Figure 22-9 ■). Any type of blast involvement is possible including myeloid, lymphoid, erythroid, or megakaryocytic cells. Because blast morphology alone is often not sufficient to identify the type of blast involved, cytochemical, enzymatic, ultrastructural, and immunophenotyping studies are helpful (∞ Chapter 21). About 65–75% of blast crises are myeloblastic, and 25–35% of blast crises are lymphoblastic. The lymphoblasts in blast crisis immunologically type common acute lymphocytic leukemia antigen positive (CALLA+) (∞ Chapters 7, 21, 37) and demonstrate an elevated terminal deoxynucleotidyl transferase (TdT), findings indicating that these cells belong to

✪ TABLE 22-8

Blast Crisis Phase of CML

Characterized by the Presence of One or More of the Following

- ≥20% blasts in the bone marrow or nucleated cells in the peripheral blood
- Extramedullary blast proliferation
- Presence of large clusters of blasts in the bone marrow biopsy specimen

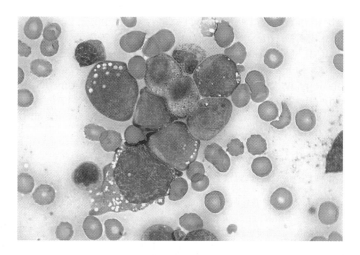

■ **FIGURE 22-9**   Peripheral blood from a patient with CML in blast crisis. Note the cluster of blasts with vacuoles. (Wright stain; 1000× magnification)

the B lymphocyte lineage (∞ Chapter 37). Erythroblastic and megakaryoblastic crises are uncommon.

THERAPY

Therapy for CML seeks to reduce the leukocyte mass, restore bone marrow function, reduce splenomegaly, and abolish symptoms. Leukapheresis is sometimes used initially to reduce the leukocyte mass when excessive numbers of cells result in a significant increase in blood viscosity. Supportive measures during therapy regimens include transfusion to treat severe anemia and antibiotics to treat infections.

Before the discovery of molecularly targeted therapy for malignant diseases, interferon-α plus cytarabine were considered standard therapy for patients with CML who were not candidates for an allogeneic HSC transplant. Interferon-α, a glycoprotein produced by a variety of cells in response to viral infection, immune stimulation, or chemical inducers, has a myelosuppressive effect directly inhibiting myeloid progenitor cells.[13,23] It induces a remission in 55–75% of CML patients and, in some cases, eliminates the Ph chromosome clone. A cytogenetic response is more favorable in patients who are treated early in the chronic phase of the disease.[13,29]

Now imatinib mesylate (Gleevec), formerly known as STI571, is considered the first treatment option except in pregnant patients. It is a molecular-targeted therapy. Imatinib competitively binds to the ATP binding site of the tyrosine kinases of ABL (BCR/ABL and TEL/ABL), C-KIT, stem cell factor receptor and platelet derived growth factor receptor (PDGFR) thus inhibiting kinase activity and preventing cell signal transduction. Gleevec is well tolerated with mild to moderate side effects, primarily involving the gastrointestinal track and skin. However, it is teratogenic in laboratory animals. Results of a 5-year study using imatinib indicate that 96% of patients have a complete hematologic response by 12 months and 98% at 60 months.[24] The rates of major cytogenetic response (<35% Ph+ metaphases) and complete cytogenetic response (0 Ph+ metaphases) were 92% and 87%, respectively.[24] Imatinib also has been shown to be effective in delaying progression of disease in patients in blast crisis.[25] Current research is assessing the benefits of combining treatment options (i.e., imatinib and interferon alpha).

Patients initially responsive to imatinib therapy can develop resistance (secondary resistance or loss of response), but other patients might not respond even in the early phase of the disease (primary resistance). Patients in the advanced stages of CML might not respond to imatinib.

Primary resistance is defined as a:

• Complete hematologic response (CHR) is not achieved by 3 months
• Cytogenetic response is not achieved by 6 months (>95% Ph+ metaphases persist)
• Major cytogenetic response is not achieved by 12 months (>35% Ph+ metaphases persist)

Loss of response is defined as:

• Loss of a complete hematologic response
• Loss of a major cytogenetic response
• Increasing levels of *BCR/ABL* as assessed by real-time PCR

Loss of response is related to development of additional mutations in the kinase domain of *BCR/ABL*.[26] A first therapeutic option in loss-of-response patients is increasing the dose of imatinib. Other options include switching to another tyrosine kinase inhibitor (TKI) such as desatinib or nilotinib.

Baseline assessment for CML patients before imatinib therapy should include bone marrow morphology, cytogenetics, and RT-PCR to determine baseline level of *BCR/ABL* transcripts. Measuring BCR/ABL mRNA levels in plasma has been found to correspond with patient tumor burden and is suggested as a monitoring standard for patients.[27] The RT-PCR assay of blood should be performed at least every 3 months after therapy begins, or a single assay at 6 months can be performed if the patient is responding.[28] Bone marrow cytogenetics should be performed every 6 months until a major cytogenetic response (MCyR) is achieved. A complete cytogenetic response and *BCR/ABL*-negative results (complete molecular response) in treated patients predict a favorable outcome. Incomplete response and *BCR/ABL*-positive results indicate the presence of minimal residual disease and the potential for disease relapse.

Mutation screening is suggested for those who do not have an adequate initial response or loss of response to imatinib because the position of the mutation within the kinase domain can be clinically relevant. Some mutations have inferior survival (P-loop mutations) compared to mutations at other sites.[27] A particular ABL mutant, T315I, in which threonine is mutated to isoleucine at the gatekeeper position of the kinase domain is not responsive to any of the TKIs currently used in CML therapy.[29]

Allogenic HSC transplantation can be an option for patients who meet the bone marrow transplant criteria.[13] Limitations are based on patient age (<60 years) and availability of a compatible donor.[13] High-dose chemoradiotherapy is followed by transplantation of HSC from syngeneic or allogenic donors. Stem cell transplantation is most successful when administered during the first chronic phase of CML. Of patients receiving HLA-matched sibling stem cells, 80% have cure rates that exceed 5 years of leukemic-free survival.[24]

DIFFERENTIAL DIAGNOSIS

Many infectious, inflammatory, or malignant disorders and severe hemorrhage or hemolysis can cause a leukemoid reaction (∞ Chapter 19) with subtle distinctions from the picture of CML (Table 22-9 ✪). At times, the clinical findings permit an accurate diagnosis, but in some cases, differential diagnosis requires further investigation. In a leukemoid reaction, leukocytosis is generally accompanied by a predominance of segmented neutrophils and bands on the blood smear. Myelocytes and metamyelocytes can be present, but if so, they are few in number compared to CML. Although blasts and promyelocytes are easily found in CML, these cells are rarely present in a leukemoid reaction. Toxic granulation, cytoplasmic vacuoles, and Döhle bodies in granulocytes often accompany benign toxic leukocytosis due to infection. These findings are not common at the time of diagnosis in CML. Monocytes, eosinophils, and basophils are generally not elevated in a leukemoid reaction, but typically are in CML.

Other diagnostic tests are helpful in differentiating a leukemoid reaction from CML. In a leukemoid reaction, the LAP score is typically elevated and the Ph chromosome is absent. Splenomegaly is uncommon in a leukemoid reaction. A bone marrow examination rarely is necessary to make a differential diagnosis. The marrow can be hypercellular, but in contrast to CML the maturation of granulocytic cells is orderly.

CML occasionally resembles CIMF. Distinguishing features of CIMF include markedly abnormal erythrocyte morphology with nucleated erythrocytes and immature leukocytes (leukoerythroblastic reaction), an increased LAP score, frank bone marrow fibrosis, and the absence of the Ph chromosome.

✓ Checkpoint! 4

What clinical, peripheral blood, and genetic features differentiate CML from an infectious process?

▶ ## CHRONIC NEUTROPHILIC LEUKEMIA (CNL)

Chronic neutrophilic leukemia (CNL) is an MPD characterized by a sustained increase in neutrophils in the peripheral blood with a slight shift to the left. Monocytosis and basophilia are absent. The bone marrow is hypercellular due to increased neutrophilic granulocyte proliferation. Dysplasia is not present. The BCR/ABL mutation is also absent. All causes of a reactive neutrophilia and other MPD must be ruled out for a diagnosis of CNL, so it is a diagnosis of exclusion. The diagnostic criteria for CNL are defined in Table 22-10 ✪.[30]

ETIOLOGY AND PATHOPHYSIOLOGY

The cause of CNL has not been identified. About 20% of cases are associated with an underlying neoplasm, particularly multiple myeloma. However, clonality of the neutrophils when neutrophilia is associated with multiple myeloma has not been demonstrated. Thus, neutrophil proliferation can be related to abnormal cytokine production in

---

✪ TABLE 22-9

Comparison of Peripheral Blood Features of CML and Leukemoid Reactions

Laboratory Parameter	CML	Leukemoid Reaction
Leukocytes	Blasts and promyelocytes in peripheral blood; toxic changes usually absent; eosinophilia and basophilia; neutrophils with single-lobed nuclei and hypogranular forms may be present	Toxic granulation; Döhle bodies and vacuoles present; blasts and promyelocytes rare; no absolute basophilia or eosinophilia
Platelets	Often increased with abnormal morphological forms present; occasional micromegakaryocytes	Usually normal
Erythrocytes	Anemia usually present; variable anisocytosis; poikilocytosis; NRBC present	Anemia may be present, but NRBC not typical
LAP	Low	Increased
Chromosome karyotype	Ph chromosome or *BCR/ABL* translocation present	Normal

❂ TABLE 22-10

Diagnostic Criteria for CNL

- Peripheral blood leukocytosis ≥25 × 10^9/L
  Bands and segmented neutrophils >80% white blood count (WBC)
  Immature granulocytes <10% WBC
  Myeloblasts <1% WBC
- Hypercellular BM with increased percent of neutrophilic granulocytes;
  <5% myeloblasts, normal neutrophil maturation pattern
- Hepatosplenomegaly
- No cause identified for physiologic neutrophilia
  Absence of infection/inflammation
  No underlying tumor or if present, demonstration of clonality of myeloid
  cells by cytogenetics/molecular diagnostics
- Absence of Ph chromosome or BCR/ABL mutation
- No evidence of other MPD
- No evidence of a MDS or MDS/MPD disorder; monocytes <1 × 10^9/L

From: Imbert M et al. Chronic neutrophic leukemia. In: Jaffe ES, Harris NL, Stein H, Vardiman JW. *World Health Organization Classification of Tumours: Tumours of the Haematopoietic and Lymphoid Tissues.* Lyon, France: IARC Press; 2001:27.

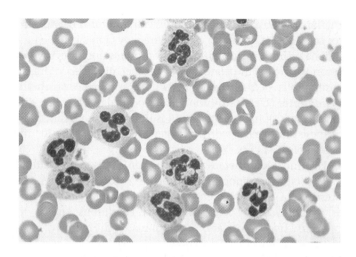

■ **FIGURE 22-10**   Peripheral blood from a patient with CNL. Note the increased numbers of mature neutrophils. (Wright stain; 1000× magnification)

this setting. CNL's cell of origin is probably a bone marrow stem cell with limited myeloid lineage potential colony forming unit granulocyte monocyte (CFU-GM) or colony forming unit-granulocyte (CFU-G).

CLINICAL FINDINGS.

CNL is a rare MPD with less than 150 reported cases. The median age at diagnosis is 67 years. The male:female ratio is about 1:1. Most patients are asymptomatic at the time of diagnosis, but fatigue, weight loss, easy bruising, bone pain, and night sweats can occur. Hepatosplenomegaly is usually present.

LABORATORY FINDINGS

The most notable feature is neutrophilia (>25 × 10^9/L) (Figure 22-10 ■). Mature segmented forms and bands predominate, and more immature cells account for <10% of the WBC. Neutrophils can appear toxic but not dysplastic. Both red blood count (RBC) and platelet morphology are normal. Platelets are usually present in normal concentration, but thrombocytopenia can develop as the disease progresses and the spleen enlarges. Bone marrow is hypercellular with an M:E ratio that can reach 20:1 or higher. Granulocytic hyperplasia is present, but dysplasia, Auer rods in blasts, and increased number of blasts are absent. Excessive erythroid and megakaroyocytic proliferation can be present. The LAP score is usually increased.

GENETICS

Cytogenetics are normal in most patients but up to 25% have mutations including 20q–, 21+, 11q–, and +8, +9.[31] The Ph chromosome and BCR/ABL fusion gene are absent. If

plasma cell proliferation is present, clonality of the neutrophils should be established by cytogenetic or molecular studies for a diagnosis of CNL.

THERAPY

Hydroxyurea is a first-line therapy for CNL. Response lasts for about 12 months. Second-line therapy is interferon-α. Allogeneic stem cell transplantation is a potentially curative treatment for those patients who are eligible.

Median survival is 2 years. CNL also has a an accelerated phase. The accelerated phase is marked by progressive neutrophilia unresponsive to treatment, anemia, thrombocytopenia, and splenomegaly.[31] Blasts and other immature cells can be present in the peripheral blood.

DIFFERENTIAL DIAGNOSIS

CNL must be differentiated from CML and physiologic causes of neutrophilia such as infection or inflammation. Differential diagnosis from other myeloid neoplasms requires an absence of circulating blasts, absolute monocytosis, eosinophilia, and basophilia.

▶ HYPEREOSINOPHILIC SYNDROME (HES)

Eosinophils are derived from the CFU-GEMM (CMP) through the action of eosinophilic cytokines, GM-CSF, IL-3, and IL-5. IL-5 is relatively lineage specific for eosinophils (∞ Chapters 3, 7). The cells are released into the peripheral blood and rapidly migrate to tissues where they have a short survival.

The accumulation of eosinophils can result from a progenitor cell disorder (primary) often defined by clonal genetic mutations or from increased production of eosinophil cytokines secondary to or associated with another diagnosis. Primary eosinophilia is collectively known as **hypereosinophilic syndrome (HES).** Eosinophilia associated with other diseases is polyclonal, and the CMP is normal. The classification of these disorders is evolving as genetic mutations are identified (Table 22-11 ✪).

HES includes a heterogeneous group of disorders defined by a sustained eosinophil count of 1.5×10^9/L or higher, the presence of eosinophil-associated organ/tissue damage such as cardiomyopathy, and absence of conditions known to cause reactive (secondary) eosinophilia. Until recently, most of these disorders had no known pathogenesis and were referred to as "idiopathic" HES (I-HES). As new molecular mutations and immunologic markers as well as clinical subtypes are being defined, these disorders are being reclassified (Figure 22-11 ■). Two major subtypes include the myeloproliferative (M-HES) and lymphocytic (L-HES) variants. These account for about 50% of HES.[32] Some of the remaining cases have clinical features that allow them to be classified into subgroups, but in most, the underlying cause is unknown, so they are considered I-HES. **Chronic eosinophilic**

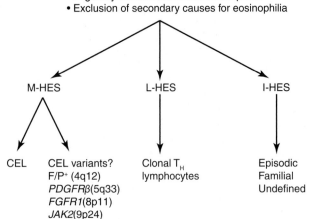

■ **FIGURE 22-11** Hypereosinophilic syndrome classification. The two major variants are myeloid and lymphoid. The myeloid includes chronic eosinophilic leukemia (CEL) and other variants that have clonal genetic mutations. It is not clear whether these other variants should be classified as CEL. The lymphoid variant is characterized by an abnormal clonal T cell proliferation that produces IL-5, which is a growth factor for eosinophils. The idiopathic HES is a group of disorders in which the pathogenesis is not known and the genetic basis for the disease has not been identified. (M-HES = myeloid-hypereosinophilic syndrome; L-HES = lymphocytic hypereosinophilic syndrome; I-HES = idiopathic hypereosinophilic syndrome; CEL = chronic eosinophilic leukemia; T_H = T-helper; F/P+ = FIP1L1/PDGFRA mutation)

leukemia (CEL) is classified under M-HES whose nomenclature is controversial.

Diseases typically associated with secondary eosinophilia must be ruled out before considering a diagnosis of HES. Associated diseases are included in Table 22-11. Testing for these disorders are listed in Table 22-12 ✪. It is especially important to do serology to rule out infection with *Strongyloides* sp. because patients with this infection given corticosteroids (common treatment for HES) can experience dissemination of the disease, which can be fatal.[33]

MYELOPROLIFERATIVE VARIANT (M-HES)

The molecular basis of some MPD-type eosinophilias have been determined, forming the basis for a semimolecular classification of these disorders.[31,35] Most of the clonal molecular abnormalities result in constitutive activation of tyrosine kinases, and the resulting phenotype is an eosinophil-associated MPD. Because the WHO classification specifies that if patients who would have been classified as having I-HES have clonal genetic abnormalities, the diagnosis is CEL, these M-HES variants could fit the criteria for CEL. However, the diagnostic terminology has not been agreed upon.

✪ TABLE 22-11

Classification of Eosinophilia

Hypereosinophilic syndrome (HES, primary)
- Myeloproliferative variant of HES (M-HES)
  - Chronic eosinophilic leukemia (CEL), not defined molecularly
  - Platelet derived growth factor receptor-*α* (*PDGFRA*) or platelet derived growth factor receptor-*β* (*PDGFRB*) mutations
  - *FGFR1*(8p11)
  - JAK2(9p24) mutation
  - Eosinophilia associated with other primary neoplasms, including AML, ALL, CML, MDS, MPD
- Lymphocytic variant of HES (L-HES)
- Idiopathic HES (I-HES)
  - Episodic
  - Familial
  - Undefined

Eosinophilia secondary to or associated with another primary diagnosis
- Parasitic infection
- Asthma
- Allergies
- Skin diseases
- Loeffler's syndrome
- Malignancy
- Immune diseases
- Vasculitis
- Drug hypersensitivity
- Nonhematologic malignancies
- Connective tissue and cutaneous disorders
- Lymphoma

✪ TABLE 22-12

Suggested Information and Testing to Exclude Diseases Associated with Secondary Eosinophilia

Clinical
- Patient history
- Physical examination

Laboratory tests
- Complete blood count and differential
- Bone marrow aspiration and biopsy
- Routine chemistries
- Serum IgE
- Vitamin B$_{12}$
- HIV serology
- Serology testing and stool analysis for parasites

Other tests
- Pulmonary function tests
- Chest and abdominal CT scan

From: Klion AD. Recent advances in the diagnosis and treatment of hypereosinophilic syndromes. Hematology 2005. *Amer Soc Hematol Program Book.* 2005;209–14.

FIP1L1/PDGFRA (F/P) Fusion Gene

This variant was discovered when some HES patients who were unresponsive to corticosteroid therapy were found to respond to imatinib therapy. This led to the identification of a fusion between the FIP1-like1 gene and the platelet-derived growth factor receptor α gene (*FIP1L1/PDGFRA* [*F/P*]), which gives rise to an abnormal tyrosine kinase protein that is constitutively activated. Although some of these mutations can be identified by cytogenetics, most require molecular analysis because the mutation is a small interstitial deletion in chromosome 4, del(4)(q12q12). This can be demonstrated by reverse transcriptase-polymerase chain reaction (RT-PCR) or FISH techniques (∞ Chapter 38).

Most of the cases involving this mutation are found in males.[32] There is evidence of eosinophil-related tissue damage and tissue fibrosis. Splenomegaly is present. Increased serum tryptase, anemia, eosinophilia, thrombocytopenia, and bone marrow hypercellularity are typical. These findings also are present in a significant number of patients who have systemic mastocytosis with increased atypical (spindle-shaped) mast cells in the bone marrow and a codon 816KIT mutation. However in M-HES with atypical mast cells, the codon 816KIT mutation is not present, the *F/P* fusion gene is present, and the bone marrow has no mast cell aggregates.[36] It has not yet been established whether this syndrome should be considered a variant of CEL or systemic mastocytosis.[36,37] The *F/P* mutation is sensitive to imatinib therapy. Other molecular mutations identified in M-HES are listed in Table 22-13 ✪.

✪ TABLE 22-13

Genetic Abnormalities Found in M-HES*

- *FIP1L1/PDGFRA* at 4q12 (F/P⁺)[†]
- *PDGFRB* at 5q31-33[†]
- *FGFR1* at 8p11 (8p11 Myeloproliferative syndrome)
- Janus Kinase 2 (*JAK2*) at 9p24

*In 2008, the WHO placed genetic abnormalities of PDGFRA, PDGFRB or FGFR1 in a new category of "Myeloid and lymphoid neoplasms with eosinophilia" regardless of morphologic classification. See Website for an update on the WHO classification of MPD.
[†]Imatinib therapy is effective.

Chronic Eosinophilic Leukemia

CEL is a Ph-chromosome-negative variant of CML that is difficult to distinguish from other subgroups of HES. CEL is defined as a clonal eosinophilia with an HES phenotype. The diagnostic criteria are listed in Table 22-14 ✪. Note that since these criteria were established, the genetic clonal aberrations noted previously in this section have been identified. Thus, whether the categories with clonal mutations described in M-HES (e.g., F/P⁺) should actually be considered CEL if the other criteria are met is controversial.[34]

When clonality cannot be established, CEL can be diagnosed based on clinical and hematologic features including splenomegaly, hepatomegaly, increased blast cells in the peripheral blood and/or bone marrow, increased bone marrow cellularity, dysplastic blood cells, increased vitamin B$_{12}$ and tryptase, and no increase in IL-5.

Etiology and Pathophysiology   The cell of origin for this leukemia may be the hematopoietic stem cell (HSC), multipotential progenitor cell (MPP), or a committed

✪ TABLE 22-14

Diagnostic Criteria for Chronic Eosinophilic Leukemia and Hypereosinophilic Syndrome

- Required: Persistent eosinophilia ($\geq 1.5 \times 10^9$/L in blood; increased eosinophils in bone marrow), and <20% blasts in blood or bone marrow
- Exclude all secondary causes of eosinophilia
- Exclude neoplastic disorders with secondary eosinophilia
- Exclude neoplastic disorders when eosinophils are a part of the neoplastic clone (e.g., AML)
- Exclude presence of an aberrant phenotypic T-cell population
- With all of the preceding conditions and evidence of clonality or >2% blasts in the peripheral blood and >5% blasts in the bone marrow, diagnosis is CEL
- With no identified causes of eosinophilia, no abnormal T-cell population, and no evidence of eosinophil clonality, diagnosis is HES

From: Bain BJ. Relationship between idiopathic hypereosinophilic syndrome, eosinophic leukemia, and systemic mastocytosis. *Amer J Hematol.* 2004;77:82–85.

eosinophilic progenitor cell (CFU-Eo). In some cases, cytogenetic abnormalities can be identified.

Clinical Findings CEL is most often diagnosed in middle-aged men (male: female ratio is 9:1). Presenting symptoms include fever and significant weight loss. Clinical features include central nervous system (CNS) irregularities, hepatosplenomegaly, congestive heart failure, pulmonary fibrosis, and occasionally lymphadenopathy. Release of excessive eosinophilic granules in the blood cause fibrosis of the endothelial cells resulting in peripheral vasculitis, gangrene of digits, and organ damage, particularly of the heart and lungs.[39,40]

Laboratory Findings CEL is characterized by a peripheral blood eosinophilia of 1.5×10^9/L or more. There are cytogenetic abnormalities and/or >2% blasts in the peripheral blood or 5–19% blasts in the bone marrow. The leukocyte count is usually $>30 \times 10^9$/L with 30–70% eosinophils. Anemia and thrombocytopenia can be present. The LAP score is normal, but the serum cobalamin, uric acid, and muramidase are frequently elevated. The bone marrow shows a left shift with many eosinophilic myelocytes. Marrow fibrosis is a common finding.

Genetics Cytogenetic abnormalities can include del(4q12), +8, t(10;11)(p14;q21), t(7;12)(q11;p11), monosomy 7, and 20q−. The case should be classified as CML if the Ph chromosome or molecular evidence of the *BCR/ABL* translocation is found.

Therapy When therapy is ineffective, the prognosis is poor. Most patients do not live beyond 1 year of diagnosis. The major cause of death is congestive heart failure due to tissue injury.

Differential Diagnosis Ruling out conditions associated with eosinophilia is important. CEL should also be differentiated from clonal eosinophilia found in other hematologic disorders (Table 22-15 ✪).

LYMPHOCYTIC-HES (L-HES)

About one-third of patients with HES are estimated to have an underlying T cell disorder.[41] Eosinophilia in this condition is associated with the expansion of a population of nonmalignant helper T cells with an aberrant phenotype (CD34+) with a type 2 cytokine profile (TH2).[42] The L-HES is also referred to as *T cell-related eosinophilia*. The activated T cells produce IL-3, IL-5, and IL-13, resulting in eosinophilia. Because the increase in eosinophils is due to increased secretion of IL-5 by aberrant lymphocytes, this variant could be considered secondary. It is currently referred to as *lymphocytic-HES*.

The T cells are often clonal and can have chromosomal abnormalities. The eosinophils are polyclonal. Demonstration of T cell clonality by T cell receptor rearrangement (α/β or δ/γ receptor genes) supports the diagnosis.[41] Evidence of TH2 activation includes elevated serum IgE and **t**hymus and **a**ctivation-**r**egulated **c**hemokine (TARC). Patients have cutaneous manifestations. Therapy is aimed at blocking production of eosinophiliopoietic cytokines by the aberrant T cells and controlling the T cell's proliferation. Glucocorticoids can reduce the production of type 2 cytokines, but their effect on controlling aberrant T cell proliferation is not clear. Progression to a T cell lymphoma is common.

IDIOPATHIC HES (I-HES)

Idiopathic HES is a diagnosis of exclusion. I-HES is characterized by persistant eosinophilia and usually with organ-associated involvement, no evidence of clonality or T cell abnormality. Pathogenesis is unknown. As more molecular mutations are found and more diagnostic techniques become available, this diagnosis has been made less frequently. Subgroups can be identified based on clinical features.

Episodic

This disorder is characterized by monthly episodes of eosinophilia preceded by cyclic increases in eosinophilic cytokines. The primary patient complaint is swelling and weight gain. Also referred to as Gleich's syndrome.

Familial

Multiple family members may have a history of persistant eosinophilia. It appears to be inherited in an autosomal dominant manner: Marked eosinophilia is present from birth. When clinical disease is present, it is similar to F/P^- HES.

Undefined

A number of disorders with eosinophilia could have organ involvement and not meet the criteria for a L-HES or M-HES.

EOSINOPHILIA SECONDARY TO OR ASSOCIATED WITH ANOTHER PRIMARY DIAGNOSIS

This group of disorders includes conditions in which eosinophilia is thought to be secondary to another primary diagnosis such as parasitic infection in which the body's nat-

✪ TABLE 22-15

Hematologic Disorders That Can Be Associated with Clonal Eosinophilia

- Acute myelogenous leukemia (AML)
- Chronic myelogenous leukemia (CML)
- Myelodysplastic syndrome (MDS)
- Myeloproliferative disorders (MPD)
- Atypical MPD
  - Systemic mastocytosis (SM)
  - Chronic myelomonocytic leukemia (CMML)
  - Myeloproliferative disease, unclassified (MPD-u)

ural response is to produce eosinophils to help eliminate the parasites. Other conditions have clinical findings and test results that overlap with HES such as a persistent eosinophilia, but they might not meet all criteria for HES (eosinophil damage may affect only one organ or type of tissue (e.g., eosinophil-associated gastrointestinal disease, EGID).

TREATMENT

First-line therapy for most patients with HES is the use of corticosteroids except in F/P^+ HES.[43] In F/P^+ patients, the treatment is imatinib. Patients refractory to corticosteroid therapy can receive cytotoxic therapy, most commonly hydroxyurea. Immunomodulatory therapy (i.e., IFN-α, cyclosporine) is also utilized in patients with corticosteroid-refractory HES. These agents affect type 2 cytokine production (IL-4 and IL-5) and T cell proliferation.[34] An anti-IL5 monoclonal antibody results in a prolonged decreased eosinophil count after a single dose. As additional molecular mutations are identified, new therapies (such as imatinib) aimed at the specific defect likely will become available.

▶ CHRONIC BASOPHILIC LEUKEMIA (CBL)

Chronic basophilic leukemia (CBL) is the rarest entity of the MPD and is not included in the WHO classification of MPD. More recently, CBL has been identified as a distinct pathologic entity.[44] It is considered an atypical myeloproliferative disease (aMPD).[31] The disease needs to be distinguished from the basophilia in CML that commonly precedes the blast crisis and from the basophilia found in other myeloproliferative disorders and mast cell leukemia.

ETIOLOGY AND PATHOPHYSIOLOGY

The etiology and pathophysiology of CBL are not known. The cell of origin appears to be a bipotential progenitor cell capable of differentiation into either basophil or eosinophil lineages or differentiation into basophil or mast cell lineages.[44]

CLINICAL FINDINGS

CBL occurs in middle-aged individuals with a slight predominance in males. Its onset can be insidious or abrupt, and clinical features are similar to those found in CML. Many patients have symptoms related to hyperhistaminemia such as wheezing, urticaria, diarrhea, pruritis, and peripheral edema. These symptoms are related to the massive increase in histamine-containing granules derived from basophils.[31] Massive release of basophil granules can occur following effective therapy resulting in shock or severe disseminated intravascu-

lar coagulation (DIC). The disease is aggressive with the potential to transform into acute leukemia.

LABORATORY FINDINGS

The leukocyte count can be normal but is most often increased. The most striking finding on the blood smear is an extreme increase in basophils, usually between 40% and 80% of the WBC with some immature forms present. The basophils are abnormal, resembling tissue mast cells. Fine uniform granules cover most of the nucleus and cytoplasm. Eosinophils are usually increased as well. Abnormal neutrophils, monocytes, and eosinophils also can be found. The LAP score is normal or low. Serum and urine histamine levels are from 10 to 15 times normal. The bone marrow is hypercellular with trilineage hyperplasia. There is a slight shift-to-the-left in granulocyte maturation, and myeloblasts can be increased. Often there is dysmegakaryopoiesis with small mononucleated and binucleated forms.[44]

GENETICS

No clonal genetic mutations have been associated with the disorder. The Ph chromosome and the *BCR/ABL* fusion gene are absent.[44]

THERAPY

Patients do not respond well to conventional therapy modalities. Allogenic bone marrow transplant can result in long-term survival. Table 22-16 summarizes the similarities and differences of CML, CNL, CEL, and CBL.

✓ Checkpoint! 5

What one feature separates other forms of MPD from CML?

▶ CHRONIC IDIOPATHIC MYELOFIBROSIS (WITH MYELOID METAPLASIA)

Chronic idiopathic myelofibrosis (CIMF), also known as *myelofibrosis with myeloid metaplasia (MMM)*, is a clonal hematopoietic stem cell disorder with splenomegaly, leukoerythroblastosis, extramedullary hematopoiesis (myeloid metaplasia), and progressive bone marrow fibrosis.[45] The fibroblast, collagen-producing cell, is an important component of normal bone marrow, where the fibroblasts provide a support structure for hematopoietic cells. Fibroblast proliferation in CIMF is reactive and secondary to the underlying disorder. Fibrotic tissue eventually disrupts the normal architecture and replaces hematopoietic tissue marrow. The proliferation of hematopoietic cells is neoplastic. Myeloid metaplasia usually occurs in both the spleen and the liver. These

TABLE 22-16

Comparison of CML Features with CML Variants

Disorder	Predominant Age in Years/Sex	Leukocyte Count (× 10^9/L)	Leukocyte Differential	LAP Score	Ph Chromosome
Chronic myelogenous leukemia	Middle age; 60–80 peak, rarely in adolescence, equal sex distribution	100–500	Left shift; less than 20% blasts	Decreased	Present
Chronic eosinophilic leukemia	Middle age/male predominance	>30	30–70% eosinophils with immature forms; left shift in neutrophils	Normal	Absent
Chronic basophilic leukemia	Middle age/slight male predominance	Normal or increased	40–80% basophils with immature forms present	Normal or slight decrease	Absent
Chronic neutrophilic leukemia	Over 50/equal between sexes	Marked increase	Mature cells	Increased	Absent

organs can become massive in size due to islands of proliferating erythroid, myeloid, and megakaryocytic elements. The extramedullary hematopoiesis is similar to that occurring during embryonic hematopoiesis.

CIMF has been known by many synonyms. Most of the different names were attempts to describe the typical blood, bone marrow, and spleen abnormalities. Some of the terms that have been used include *agnogenic myeloid metaplasia*, *myelofibrosis with myeloid metaplasia*, *primary myelofibrosis*, *aleukemic myelosis*, *myelosclerosis*, *splenomegalic myelophthisis*, and *leukoerythroblastic anemia*.

PATHOPHYSIOLOGY

About 50% of CIMF patients can be found to have a somatic mutation, either a point mutation in the Janus kinase 2 *(JAK2)* tyrosine kinase gene or a mutation of the thrombopoietin membrane receptor *(MPL)* gene. These mutations constitutively activate cell signaling and DNA replication.[46] G6PD isoenzyme and cytogenetic studies demonstrate clonality of the neoplastic cells. Chromosome aberrations, when present, are restricted to cells derived from the mutated HSC. Some of these cells are highly sensitive to or independent from regulation by their respective stimulatory factors. The disorder has been reported to terminate in ALL as well as AML in some patients.

In most cases, only megakaryocytes and granulocytes are involved, but all three lineages, including erythrocytes, can be involved in the disease process. CIMF is often preceded by a hypercellular phase of variable duration. The disease evolves from this prefibrotic stage with minimal reticulin fibrosis to a fibrotic stage with marked reticulin or collagen fibrosis. Thus, at the time of diagnosis, the bone marrow can exhibit varying degrees of fibrosis. The fibrosis is not considered part of the primary abnormal clonal proliferation but is a secondary reactive event occurring in response to the progeny of the clonal hematopoietic cells. Fibroblasts do not contain the chromosome abnormalities found in the hematopoietic cells, and they exhibit heterozygosity rather than homozygosity for the G6PD isoenzymes in females.

Our understanding of this disease has increased considerably with a better understanding of normal bone marrow structure and the changes that occur in myelofibrotic marrow associated with megakaryocyte growth factors that mediate fibrogenesis.[47] The bone marrow extracellular matrix or microenvironment (stroma) supports hematopoietic cell proliferation. Myelofibrotic stroma is characterized by an increase in total collagen, fibroblasts, vitronectin (a cytoadhesion molecule), fibronectin (a cytoadhesion molecule normally limited to megakaryocytes and walls of blood vessels), and laminin (a glycoprotein that supports adhesion and growth of cells).

CIMF is associated with a profound hyperplasia of morphologically abnormal megakaryocytes (dysplastic and necrotic). Evidence indicates that the megakaryocytes play an important role in the pathogenic development of the abnormal CIMF marrow. In areas of megakaryocyte necrosis, fibroblast proliferation and collagen deposition often are prominent. This stromal reaction is a cytokine-mediated process.[44]

PDGF, epidermal growth factor (EGF), and transforming growth factor beta (TGF-β) are contained in the α-granules of megakaryocytes and platelets, and all stimulate the growth and proliferation of fibroblasts. Reduced platelet concentrations of PDGF and increased levels of serum PDGF are characteristic of CIMF. This condition is thought to represent the abnormal release or leakage of the growth factor from the platelet. PDGF does not stimulate synthesis of collagen, laminin, or fibronectin, but TGF-β stimulates increased expression of genes for fibronectin and collagen while decreasing synthesis of collagenase-like enzymes. Thus, the net effect is the accumulation of bone marrow stromal elements.[45,47]

In 2005, a gain in function mutation in the *JAK2* tyrosine kinase gene, *JAK2*(V617F), was identified in many patients with CIMF. The normal JAK 2 protein is a cytoplasmic protein kinase closely associated with cytokine receptors and thus is distributed almost exclusively near the cell membrane. When a receptor binds cytokines, the JAK2 protein is transphosphorylated and activated. In turn, JAK2 phosphorylates **s**ignal **t**ransducers and **a**ctivators of **t**ranscription (STAT5) proteins. The JAK-receptor complex also activates other signaling pathways. Several inhibitory control mechanisms constrain the normal JAK2/STAT5 activation pathway. The JAK2 protein has 2 homologous domains: JH1, which has functional (kinase) activity, and JH2, which lacks kinase activity. JH2 normally interacts with the JH1 domain to inhibit kinase activity and to modulate or regulate receptor signaling.

In the mutated *JAK2*(V617F) gene, a point mutation replaces valine with phenylalanine at codon 617 in the JH2 domain.[46,47,48] This mutation results in a conformational change in the tyrosine kinase protein, which allows it to phosphorylate STAT5 molecules independent of cytokine interaction with the receptor (i.e., autonomous signaling). This gain-of-function mutation gives the cells a proliferation advantage. The mutation also results in increased responsiveness to erythropoietin (EPO) and IL-3. *JAK2*(V617F) is found in ~50% of patients with CIMF, ~50% of patients with essential thrombocythemia (ET), and most patients with polycythemia vera.[46,48]

Research also has identified a mutation in the *MPL*. This mutation, *MPL*-W515L, leads to a myeloproliferative disorder similar to CIMF with thrombocytosis, extramedullary hematopoiesis, and increased reticulin fibrosis in mice that are negative for the *JAK2*(V617F) mutation.[49]

 ## Checkpoint! 6

What growth factors are primarily responsible for stimulating fibrogenesis in the bone marrow?

CLINICAL FINDINGS

CIMF generally affects individuals over 50 years of age. It rarely occurs in childhood. It appears to occur equally between sexes. The onset is gradual and the disease is chronic. Early in the disease process, the patient might have no symptoms, making the time of onset difficult to determine. If symptoms are present, they are usually related to anemia or pressure from an enlarged spleen. Bleeding occasionally is a presenting symptom. Patients complain of weakness, weight loss, loss of appetite, night sweats, pain in the extremities, and discomfort in the upper left quadrant. The major physical findings are splenomegaly, hepatomegaly, pallor, and petechiae. Myeloid metaplasia is found in the spleen and frequently in the liver and can be found in the kidney, adrenal glands, peritoneal and extraperitoneal surfaces, skin, lymph nodes, and spinal cord. Osteosclerosis is a frequent finding and, when found in association with splenomegaly, suggests a diagnosis of myelofibrosis.

An atypical acute form of the disease has been described with a rapid and progressive course of a few months to one year. Anemia develops rapidly, and the leukocyte count is decreased. The bone marrow in these cases exhibits a proliferation of reticular and collagen fibers.

Patients with systemic lupus erythematosus (SLE) can present with myelofibrosis morphologically indistinguishable from the myelofibrosis of CIMF. These patients also have various peripheral blood cytopenias similar to those found in CIMF, but splenomegaly is not found. The myelofibrosis in SLE has been referred to as *autoimmune myelofibrosis*. It has been suggested that all patients with myelofibrosis and an absence of splenomegaly should have an antinuclear antibody (ANA) test to rule out SLE.[50]

LABORATORY FINDINGS

Peripheral Blood

The typical peripheral blood findings for CIMF reflect both qualitative and quantitative cellular abnormalities. Although peripheral blood findings are variable, a moderate leukoerythroblastic anemia with striking anisocytosis and poikilocytosis is characteristic (Figure 22-12■). The anemia is usually normocytic, normochromic, but hypochromia can be found after a history of hemorrhage or hemolysis. Folic acid deficiency can develop as a result of increased utilization by the neoplastic clone and is associated with a macrocytic anemia. Anemia uncomplicated by iron deficiency or folic acid deficiency correlates directly with the extent of bone marrow fibrosis and the effectiveness of extramedullary hematopoiesis. The anemia becomes more severe with the progression of the disease and is aggravated in some patients by the combination of splenomegaly, which causes sequestration of erythrocytes, and expanded plasma volume, (dilutional anemia).

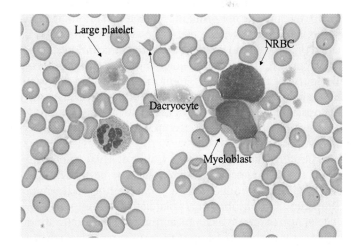

■ FIGURE 22-12 Peripheral blood from a patient with CIMF. Leukoerythroblastic picture with nucleated erythroblast at about 1 o'clock and a myeloblast below it. The arrow points to a large platelet at about 11 o'clock. Other abnormal platelets are present. Note the poikilocytosis with dacryocytes. (Wright stain; 1000× magnification)

The presence of abnormal erythrocyte morphology is an important feature of CIMF. The most typical poikilocyte is the dacryocyte, although elliptocytes and ovalocytes are also present (Figure 22-12). A few nucleated erythrocytes are usually found and sometimes can be numerous. Basophilic stippling is a common finding. Reticulocytosis is typical, ranging from 2% to 15%. The majority of patients have an absolute reticulocyte count $> 60 \times 10^9$/L.

The leukocyte count is usually elevated but can be normal or less often decreased. The count generally ranges from 15 to 30×10^9/L. A leukocyte count above $60-70 \times 10^9$/L prior to splenectomy is rare. The leukocyte concentration is rather constant and does not decrease with the progression of the disease as is typical of erythrocytes and platelets. An orderly progression of immature granulocytes is characteristically found. Blasts generally compose less than 5% of circulating leukocytes. Other common findings include basophilia, eosinophilia, and pseudo–Pelger-Huët anomaly. The LAP is elevated or normal but occasionally is decreased. Low LAP scores correlate with leukopenia. When elevated, the LAP score helps to differentiate this disease from CML. The Ph chromosome is not present.

Platelets can be decreased, normal, or increased. Higher counts are associated with early disease stages; thrombocytopenia is usually found in the later stages. Thrombocytopenia is often attributed to excessive splenic pooling. The platelets can appear dysplastic: typically giant, bizarre, and frequently hypogranular. Circulating megakaryocyte fragments, mononuclear micromegakaryocytes, and naked megakaryocyte nuclei can be found. The micromegakaryocytes can present a problem in identification because they frequently resemble lymphocytes. However, an important differentiating feature is the presence of demarcation membranes with bull's-eye granules in the cytoplasm, characteristic of megakaryocytes. Qualitative platelet abnormalities including abnormal aggregation, adhesiveness, and defective platelet factor-3 (PF3) released on exposure to collagen are consistent findings.

Of patients, 15% have major hemolytic episodes during the course of their disease.[51] Hemosiderinuria and decreased haptoglobin are found in about 10% of patients, suggesting intravascular hemolysis. The cause of hemolysis can be hypersplenism, PNH-like defective erythrocytes, and antierythrocyte antibodies.

A bleeding diathesis ranging from petechiae and ecchymoses to life-threatening hemorrhage can be found in patients. It likely results from a combination of thrombocytopenia and/or abnormal platelet function. Defective platelet aggregation is a common finding. Hemostatic abnormalities suggestive of chronic DIC can be present, including decreased platelet count, decreased concentration of factors V and VIII, and increased fibrin degradation products.[51]

Other laboratory tests are frequently abnormal in this disease. Serum uric acid and LD are elevated in most patients. Serum cobalamin can be slightly increased but is usually normal.

✓ Checkpoint! 7

What erythrocyte morphologic feature is a hallmark for myelofibrosis?

Bone Marrow

The bone marrow is difficult to penetrate and frequently yields a dry tap. If aspiration is successful, smears may show no abnormalities; biopsy specimens are needed to reveal the extent of fibrosis. In most CIMF cases, the marrow is hypercellular with varying degrees of diffuse fibrosis and focal aggregates of megakaryocytes (Figure 22-13 ■).

Three bone marrow histologic patterns have been described: (1) panhyperplasia with absence of myelofibrosis but a slight increase in connective tissue reticulin, (2) myeloid atrophy with fibrosis, prominent collagen, and reticulin fibers, and cellularity less than 30%, and (3) myelofibrosis and myelosclerosis with bony trabeculae occupying 30% of the biopsy and extensive fibrosis.

CASE STUDY *(continued from page 454)*

(continued from page 454)

During the office visit, Roger stated that he had symptoms of fatigue, weakness, dyspnea, bone pain, and abdominal discomfort. A bone marrow biopsy was ordered. The aspiration was unsuccessful, but the marrow biopsy showed moderate to marked hyperplasia, clusters of platelets, abnormal megakaryocyte morphology, and fibrotic marrow spaces.

4. What diagnoses are suggested?

5. Give a reason for the unsuccessful, dry-tap bone marrow aspiration.

6. What characteristic peripheral blood morphologies correlate with the bone marrow picture and physical exam?

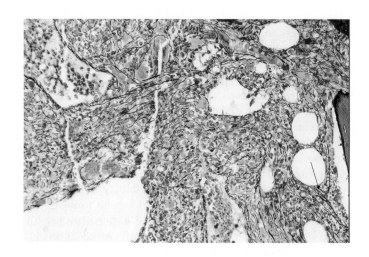

■ **FIGURE 22-13** Bone marrow stained with reticulum stain shows increased collagen (black staining fibers) in a patient with CIMF. (BM bipsy; reticulum stain; 100× magnification)

Genetics

Cytogenetic analysis is important to differentiate myelofibrosis from other myeloproliferative disorders, in particular CML, which also can have some degree of fibrosis. The Ph chromosome is not present in CIMF. Although no specific cytogenetic abnormality is diagnostic for CIMF, *JAK2* (V617F) is found in about 50% of patients, and a trisomy or deletion of Group C chromosomes is also associated with myelofibrosis. Complete or partial loss of chromosomes 5, 7, and 20 is associated with CIMF patients treated with chemotherapy.

PROGNOSIS AND THERAPY

The average survival time after diagnosis is 4–5 years. The main causes of death are infection, hemorrhage, thrombosis, and cardiac failure. About 10–15% of patients terminate with an acute myelogenous leukemia and some with acute lymphoid leukemia.

In the past, corticosteroids and androgens were used to stimulate erythropoiesis, but most patients required periodic transfusions. Cytokine therapy (interferon-α with erythropoietin and/or GM-CSF) is now used with variable success.[51] When anemia cannot be controlled, splenectomy can be considered. Irradiation has been suggested to decrease spleen size in an attempt to relieve symptoms or to decrease excessive erythrocyte destruction. Alkylating agents have been used but have the potential to cause severe pancytopenia. Allogeneic stem cell transplantation is the only curative therapy for CIMF, but due to the advanced age of many patients, the mortality rate is high. Thalidomide derivatives, protease inhibitors, and antibodies to growth factors show some promise for patients resistant to conventional treatment.[48,52] Drugs to control hyperuricemia have been used to prevent or decrease problems with gout and nephropathy.

DIFFERENTIAL DIAGNOSIS

Differentiation of CIMF from other conditions associated with fibrosis is essential to ensure appropriate therapy regimens (Table 22-17 ✪). Splenomegaly, anemia, and a leukoerythroblastic blood picture are significant findings in both myelofibrosis and CML. In myelofibrosis, the leukocyte count is generally lower—less than 50×10^9/L, in CML, the count is expected to be higher. In myelofibrosis, the shift to the left is less pronounced and poikilocytosis is striking. The bone marrow in myelofibrosis is fibrous with large numbers of megakaryocytes. In CML, the bone marrow can also exhibit some fibrosis, but the most abnormal finding is the myeloid hyperplasia. The serum cobalamin level is not as elevated in myelofibrosis as it is in CML. The LAP score in myelofibrosis is variable, but when elevated, it is strong evidence against CML. The most reliable test to differentiate CML and CIMF is cytogenetic analysis for the Ph chromosome.

✪ **TABLE 22-17**

Conditions Associated with Marrow Fibrosis

- Chronic idiopathic myelofibrosis (CIMF)
- Chronic myelogenous leukemia (CML)
- Polycythemia vera (PV)
- Essential thrombocythemia (ET)
- Megakaryocytic leukemia
- Metastatic carcinoma
- Miliary tuberculosis
- Fungus infection
- Hairy cell leukemia
- Lymphoma
- Hodgkin's disease
- Granulomas
- Marrow damage by radiation or chemicals

Differentiation of myelofibrosis from polycythemia vera (PV, see below), especially in the later stages, is more difficult. The later stages of PV can be accompanied by increased marrow fibrosis, or actual transformation to myelofibrosis can occur.

When thrombocytosis is the principal initial hematologic finding, myelofibrosis can be confused with ET. A bone marrow biopsy aids in the differentiation, revealing a frank fibrosis in myelofibrosis.

Myelophthisic anemia, or leukoerythroblastosis is found with a fibrotic bone marrow and extramedullary hematopoiesis. *Myelophthisic anemia* refers to the reduction of cells formed in normal bone marrow resulting from a neoplastic disease process. Various disease processes including bone marrow tumors and metastatic disease from solid tumors are associated with myelophthisic anemia. Although myelophthisic anemia can have a morphologic peripheral blood picture very similar to myelofibrosis, the leukocyte count in myelophthisic anemia is usually normal or decreased. Bone marrow examination from more than one site may be necessary to rule out a secondary reaction due to tumor or other cells replacing the marrow.

 CASE STUDY *(continued from page 464)*

Over the next several months, Roger experienced increasing splenomegaly and abdominal discomfort. Cytogenetic studies revealed a trisomy 8.

7. What is the most likely explanation for the increased splenomegaly?

8. What are possible outcomes of this disorder?

► POLYCYTHEMIA VERA

The term *polycythemia* literally means an increase in the cellular elements of the blood; however, it is most commonly used to describe an increase in erythrocytes exclusive of leukocytes and platelets. **Polycythemia vera (PV)** is a myeloproliferative disorder characterized by an unregulated proliferation of the erythroid elements in the bone marrow and an increase in erythrocyte concentration in the peripheral blood. In addition to erythroid cells, other progeny of the HSC can also be simultaneously or sequentially involved in the autonomous proliferation, resulting in a pancytosis (increase in all hematopoietic cells in the blood). Polycythemia vera has several synonyms, including *polycythemia rubra vera*, *primary polycythemia*, *erythremia*, and *Osler's disease*.

CLASSIFICATION

Polycythemia is a general term used to describe erythrocytosis resulting in an increase in both hemoglobin concentration and red cell mass (RCM) or hematocrit. Hemoglobin, hematocrit, and erythrocyte count are parameters measured in relative terms (e.g., the ratio of hemoglobin or erythrocytes to plasma volume), not in absolute concentrations. When evaluating a patient for polycythemia, it is important to determine whether these parameters are elevated because of an absolute increase in total erythrocyte mass (absolute erythrocytosis) or from a decrease in plasma volume (relative erythrocytosis) (Figure 22-14 ■). Although an absolute erythrocytosis suggests a diagnosis of PV, polycythemia that is secondary to tissue hypoxia, cardiac or pulmonary disease, and abnormal hemoglobins should also be considered.

In an attempt to clarify the pathogenesis of the disorder, polycythemia is classified into three different groups: polycythemia vera, secondary polycythemia, and relative polycythemia (Table 22-18 ✪). PV and secondary polycythemia

✪ TABLE 22-18	
Classification of Polycythemia	
Classification	**Associated Conditions**
Polycythemia vera (primary)	Normal or decreased erythropoietin levels; autonomous cell proliferation
Secondary polycythemia (erythropoietin-driven)	High altitude
	Chronic obstructive pulmonary disease
	Obesity (Pickwickian syndrome)
	Inappropriate erythropoietin production
	Tumors (e.g., hepatoma, uterine fibroma, renal carcinoma)
	Renal ischemia
	Familial erythrocytosis
	Hemoglobins with high oxygen affinity
	Congenital decrease in erythrocyte 2,3-BPG
Relative polycythemia	Gaisböck's syndrome (stress polycythemia, spurious polycythemia, pseudopolycythemia)
	Dehydration

both result from an absolute increase in the total body RCM. Secondary polycythemia can be distinguished from PV by a distinct, although not always apparent, physiologic stimulus for erythrocytosis—hence, the name *secondary polycythemia*—and is associated with elevated plasma EPO levels. PV results from a primary, unregulated or dysregulated increase in erythrocyte production with no identifiable inciting cause. Relative polycythemia is characterized by a normal or even decreased RCM and occurs as a result of a decreased plasma volume. It is generally a mild polycythemia due to dehydration, hemoconcentration, or a condition known as *Gaisböck's syndrome*.

PATHOPHYSIOLOGY

The panhyperplasia often associated with PV suggests a clonal stem cell defect. The clonal nature of the disease is confirmed by G6PD isoenzyme and cytogenetic studies. Evidence of clonality persists in cells even during complete remission.

Although all lineages in the peripheral blood can be increased in PV, an increase in erythropoiesis is the outstanding feature. Possible mechanisms for this increase are suggested in Table 22-19 ✪.[16,53] In vitro studies using cell culture systems show that PV bone marrow cells from some patients form erythroid colonies without the addition of erythropoietin (endogenous erythroid colonies/EEC), suggesting that increased proliferation is due to an unregulated neoplastic proliferation of stem cells. Other patients' bone marrow cells show increased sensitivity to EPO, insulin like growth factor I, and IL-3, forming in vitro colonies at significantly reduced

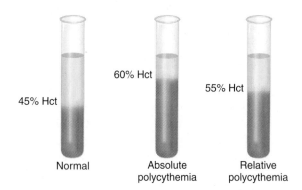

45% Hct

60% Hct

55% Hct

Normal   Absolute polycythemia   Relative polycythemia

■ FIGURE 22-14   The hematocrit can be increased due to an absolute increase in erythrocyte mass, a condition known as *absolute polycythemia* (center) or a decrease in plasma volume, a condition known as *relative polycythemia* (right).

TABLE 22-19

Possible Mechanisms for Increased Erythropoiesis in Polycythemia Vera

- Erythropoietin-independent proliferation of neoplastic progenitor cells
- Hypersensitivity of erythroid progenitor cells to erythropoietin
- Hypersensitivity of erythroid progenitor cells to growth factors other than erythropoietin
- Inhibition of apoptosis in progenitor cells

cytokine concentrations. This increased sensitivity to cytokine stimulation gives PV progenitor cells a growth advantage.[54–58] The erythroid maturation is morphologically normal and the erythrocytes function normally and have a normal lifespan.

Several mutations have been identified in patients with PV. The *JAK2*(V617F) mutation, which codes for a mutated protein kinase activator of cell signal transduction, is found in almost all patients with PV. The mutated protein binds to the cytoplasmic domain of the EPO receptor and promotes receptor activation independent of EPO binding and signaling. PV patients also have an increased level of Bcl-x_L, an antiapoptotic protein member of the Bcl-2 family, which inhibits apoptosis of progenitor cells (∞ Chapter 2).[55] This defect in programmed cell death creates an accumulation of altered, hypersensitive stem and progenitor cells. Similar thrombopoietin receptor hyper-responsiveness and resistance to apoptosis are found in the megakaryocytic lineage, resulting in the common finding of thrombocytosis associated with PV.[9,16,55–57]

CLINICAL FINDINGS

The annual incidence of PV varies geographically from 2 cases per million in Japan to 13 per million in Australia and Europe. The annual incidence in the United States averages 8–10 per million population. It occurs most often between the ages of 40 and 60 years with a peak incidence in the sixth decade of life. The disease is rare in children. It occurs more frequently in males than females and is more common in whites than blacks, particularly in those of Jewish descent.[53] PV has been reported to occur in several members of the same family, suggesting a possible genetic predisposition for the disease.

The onset of the disease is usually gradual with a history of mild symptoms for several years. In some cases, PV is found in asymptomatic individuals. When symptoms are present, they are typically related to the increased erythrocyte mass and the associated cardiovascular disease due to hyperviscosity of the blood. Headache, weakness, pruritus, weight loss, and fatigue are the most common symptoms. Pruritus is attributed to hyperhistaminemia that can be spontaneous or induced by hot showers or baths. Itching is generalized with absence of a rash.

About one-third of the patients experience thrombotic or hemorrhagic episodes. Myocardial infarctions, retinal vein thrombosis, thrombophlebitis, and cerebral ischemia can occur at any stage of the disease and occasionally is the first indication of the disease.

When the hematocrit exceeds 60%, the blood viscosity increases steeply, decreasing blood flow and increasing peripheral vascular resistance. These interactions produce hypertension in about 50% of the patients with PV. **Plethora** (a florid complexion due to an excessive amount of blood), especially on the face but also on the hands, feet, and ears, is a common finding on physical examination.

After a period of 2–10 years, the patient may develop bone marrow failure accompanied by an increase in splenomegaly. At this time, anemia and bleeding may be the primary clinical findings, secondary to a decreased platelet count and decreasing hematocrit. This is known as the **spent phase** and is often a transition to AML. Postpolycythemic myelofibrosis and myeloid metaplasia develop in about 30% of PV cases. Splenomegaly is characteristic at this stage. Acute leukemia develops as an abrupt transition in 5–10% of patients. Leukemia appears to develop at a higher rate in patients treated with myelosuppressive drugs than in those treated with phlebotomy alone.

LABORATORY FINDINGS

Peripheral Blood

The most striking peripheral blood finding in PV is an absolute erythrocytosis in the range of $6–10 \times 10^{12}$/L, with a hemoglobin concentration >18.5 g/dL in males and >16.5 g/dL in females. The hematocrit in females is usually >0.48 L/L (48%) and in males >0.52 L/L (52%). The total RCM is increased >25% of mean normal; the plasma volume can be normal, elevated, or decreased. Early in the disease, the erythrocytes are normocytic, normochromic; however, after repeated therapeutic phlebotomy, iron-deficient erythropoiesis can result in microcytic hypochromic cells. Patients with PV occasionally present with iron deficiency secondary to occult blood loss as a result of abnormal platelet function. This can create a confusing peripheral blood picture because the concentration of erythrocytes is normal to increased with significant microcytosis, simulating a thalassemia (∞ Chapter 11). Nucleated erythrocytes can be found. On the blood smear, the erythrocytes typically appear crowded even at the feathered edge. The reticulocyte count is normal or slightly elevated. The erythrocyte sedimentation rate (ESR) does not exceed 2–3 mm/hour.

Leukocytosis in the range of $12–20 \times 10^9$/L occurs in about two-thirds of the cases because of an increase in granulocyte production. Early in the disease there can be a relative granulocytosis and a relative lymphopenia with a normal total leukocyte count. A shift to the left can be found with the presence of myelocytes and metamyelocytes, but finding promyelocytes, blasts, or excessive numbers of immature myeloid cells is unusual. Relative and absolute basophilia is common. The LAP score is usually higher than 100.

Megakaryocytic hyperplasia in the bone marrow accompanied by an increase in platelet production is a consistent finding in PV. In some patients, the megakaryocytes proliferate without expressing the receptor for thrombopoietin (those patients with a mutation in the *MPL* gene) and have decreased apoptosis as do the erythroid progenitor cells.[16,55,57] The platelet count is $>400 \times 10^9/L$ in 20% of PV patients and occasionally exceeds $1,000 \times 10^9/L$. Giant platelets can be found on the blood smear. Qualitative platelet abnormalities are reflected by abnormal aggregation to one or more aggregating agents—epinephrine, collagen, adenosine diphosphate (ADP), or thrombin (∞ Chapter 31). Lack of aggregation with epinephrine is the most common abnormality. The prothrombin time (PT) and activated partial thromboplastin time (APTT) are usually normal (∞ Chapter 39). Abnormal multimeric forms of VWF are found in about half of PV patients and can lead to a diagnosis of acquired von Willebrand's disease (VWD)[56] (∞ Chapter 31).

Advanced disease is accompanied by striking morphologic changes in erythrocytes (Figure 22-15 ■). The peripheral blood picture can resemble that seen in myelofibrosis with a leukoerythroblastic anemia, poikilocytosis with dacryocytes, and thrombocytopenia. In cases that advance to acute leukemia, the blood picture exhibits anemia with marked erythrocyte abnormalities, thrombocytopenia, and blast cells.

Bone Marrow

Most patients with PV have a moderate to marked increase in bone marrow cellularity. The hypercellularity is greater than is seen in secondary polycythemia, and hematopoietic marrow can extend into the long bones. Granulopoiesis as well as erythropoiesis is often increased; consequently, the myeloid:erythroid ratio is usually normal. The relative number of myeloblasts is not increased. One of the most significant findings is an increase in megakaryocytes. Eosinophils are also often increased. Sometimes bone marrow biopsies reveal a slight to marked increase in fibrotic material or reticulin, generally directly proportional to the degree of cellularity (e.g., more cellular marrows demonstrating more reticulin). Iron stores are usually absent, presumably due to a diversion of iron from storage sites to the large numbers of developing erythroblasts.

In the postpolycythemic stage, the bone marrow reveals reticulin and collagen fibrosis. Cellularity varies but is often hypocellular with prominent clusters of megakaryocytes. Erythropoiesis and granulopoiesis decrease. A shift to the left can be present, but blasts are usually <10% and dysplasia is unusual.

Other Laboratory Findings

EPO levels are normal or low in PV, and arterial oxygen saturation levels are normal. In secondary polycythemia resulting from tissue hypoxia, EPO levels are elevated, and arterial oxygen saturation levels are decreased. When secondary polycythemia occurs due to an inappropriate increase in EPO, oxygen saturation levels are usually normal.

Other laboratory tests also can be abnormal. Serum uric acid is >7 mg/dL in two-thirds of the patients and can cause symptoms of gout. The increase probably reflects an increase in the turnover of nucleic acids from blood cells. Serum cobalamin-binding capacity in most of the untreated PV patients is increased, primarily due to the increase in transcobalamin III derived from granulocytes. Serum cobalamin also is increased but not in proportion to the unsaturated binding capacity.

Genetics

The nonspecific molecular mutation, *JAK2*(V617F), is found in >90% of patients with PV and in about 50% of CIMF and ET patients.[16,48,59,60] Due to the frequency of this mutation in PV, peripheral blood screening for *JAK2*(V617F) in the initial evaluation of patients suspected of having PV has been recommended.

Cytogenetic abnormalities including chromosomal aneuploidy and deletions can be found. The most consistent abnormality is an extra Group C chromosome, especially a trisomy 8 or 9, an abnormally long chromosome 1 due to additional chromosomal material on the long arms with a partial deletion of chromosome 13 and 20. The frequency of multiple karyotypic abnormalities increases after years of treatment to more than 80% in patients who develop acute leukemia. Thus, progression from a normal to an abnormal karyotype is an adverse prognostic indicator.[58]

PROGNOSIS AND THERAPY

There is no known cure for PV but treatment usually prolongs survival. Two types of therapy, phlebotomy and myelosuppressive therapy generally have been used. Thera-

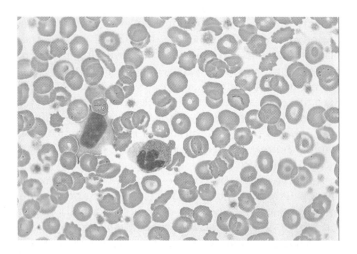

■ FIGURE 22-15   Peripheral blood from a patient with polycythemia vera showing thrombocytosis and large platelets. There is a reactive lymphocyte and segmented neutrophil in the center. (Wright-Giemsa stain; 600× original magnification)

peutic phlebotomy is performed to keep the hematocrit below 0.45 L/L (45%) and to reduce iron supplies. It is expected that lack of iron will slow the production of erythrocytes. Myelosuppressive therapy with chemotherapy and/or radiotherapy is utilized to reduce the amount of proliferating hematopoietic cells. Hydroxyurea inhibits ribonucleotide reductase and carries less risk of secondary leukemia than busulphan, an alkylating agent.

Without treatment, 50% of the patients survive about 18 months. With only phlebotomy as the palliative treatment, survival extends to about 14 years. Thrombosis is the most frequent complication, and often patients are given antiplatelet therapy.[56] Patients receiving myelosuppressive therapy with or without phlebotomy have a mean survival of 9 years with chlorambucil therapy and 12 years with ^{32}P therapy. However, these patients show a progressive incidence of malignant complications. Research is ongoing to find a molecularly targeted therapy specific for the abnormal JAK2 kinase similar to the use of imatinib in CML.

DIFFERENTIAL DIAGNOSIS

It is essential that PV be differentiated from the more benign causes of secondary erythrocytosis and relative polycythemia so that effective therapy can be initiated.

Secondary Polycythemia

Secondary polycythemia can be classified into the following groups:

1. Polycythemia due to an increase in EPO as a normal physiologic response to tissue hypoxia

2. Polycythemia due to an inappropriate, nonphysiologic increase in erythropoietin

3. Familial polycythemia associated with high oxygen-affinity hemoglobin variants

4. Neonatal polycythemia associated with intrauterine hypoxia or late cord clamping

Tissue Hypoxia A decreased arterial oxygen saturation and subsequent tissue hypoxia are the most common cause of secondary polycythemia. The polycythemia disappears when the underlying cause is identified and effectively treated. Residents of high-altitude areas demonstrate a significant increase in hemoglobin and hematocrit that is progressively elevated at higher altitudes. The decrease in barometric pressure at high altitudes decreases the inspired oxygen tension. As a result, less oxygen enters the erythrocytes in the alveoli, and the arterial blood oxygen saturation decreases (∞ Chapters 5, 6). The reduced pO_2 in the lungs is partially compensated for by a chronic hyperventilation. Compensation at the cellular level involves an increase in 2,3-BPG, facilitating the transfer of oxygen to the tissues. Tissue hypoxia secondary to a decrease in arterial blood oxygen saturation can also occur in severe obstructive lung disease and in obesity. The hematocrit is generally not higher than 0.57 L/L in these cases.

Inappropriate Increase in Erythropoietin A nonphysiologic increase in EPO (inappropriate) has been described in association with certain tumors that appear to secrete EPO or an EPO-like substance. About 50% of these patients have renal tumors. Other tumors that have been associated with erythrocytosis include those of the liver, cerebellum, uterus, adrenals, ovaries, lung, and thymus. In almost all cases, EPO levels return to normal and the erythrocytosis disappears after resection of the tumor. Renal cysts are also associated with polycythemia, possibly because of localized pressure and hypoxia to the juxtaglomerular apparatus, resulting in increased EPO secretion. In some patients with hypertension, renal artery disease, and renal transplants, renal ischemia can occur, resulting in erythrocytosis secondary to increased EPO production.

Familial Polycythemia Inherited hemoglobin variants with increased oxygen affinity cause tissue hypoxia and are associated with a secondary erythrocytosis. Because of the increased oxygen affinity, less oxygen is released to the tissues, stimulating erythropoietin production. Inherited deficiency of 2,3-BPG also results in decreased oxygen release to tissues. These inherited conditions are usually found in young children and in other family members as well.

Neonatal Polycythemia Hematocrits >0.48 L/L are common in neonates. The etiology is attributed to placental transfusion that occurs as a result of late cord clamping (7–10 seconds after delivery) and/or increased erythropoiesis stimulated by intrauterine hypoxia.[61]

 Checkpoint! 8

Renal tumors can produce an inappropriate amount of EPO, resulting in what type of polycythemia?

Relative Polycythemia

Relative polycythemia is a mild polycythemia due to dehydration, hemoconcentration, or a condition known as *Gaisböck's syndrome*. Gaisböck's syndrome is known by several synonyms, including *spurious polycythemia, pseudopolycythemia,* and *stress erythrocytosis*. These patients have a relative polycythemia and hypertension with nephropathy or relative polycythemia associated with emotional stress[56] RCM is essentially normal. High hematocrit and hemoglobin concentrations appear to result from a combination of high-normal erythrocyte concentrations with a low-normal plasma volume. The most common symptoms are light-headedness, headaches, and dizziness. Plethora is common but splenomegaly is rare. These patients have a high incidence of thromboembolic complications and cardiovascular disease. Although the hemoglobin, hematocrit, and erythrocyte counts are increased, leukocytes and platelets are normal.

Bone marrow cellularity is normal with no increase in megakaryocytes or reticulin. Bone marrow iron stores are absent in 50% of the patients, but serum iron studies are normal. Chromosome karyotypes are almost always normal.

Laboratory Differentiation of Polycythemia

The WHO-defined diagnostic criteria for PV includes initial determination of total RCM or hemoglobin to establish the presence of an absolute polycythemia (Table 22-20 ●).[62] However, it has been shown that in some cases with hemoglobin levels below the value used for a diagnosis of PV and thrombocytosis, the RCM was higher than that required, thus revealing an occult erythrocytosis.[63] Without the RCM, these cases would have been diagnosed as essential thrombocythemia. This suggests that RCM is an important test to perform when PV is suspected. Determination of serum EPO levels is important because it helps to distinguish between primary and secondary polycythemia. If EPO levels are low, screening for the *JAK2*(V617F) mutation and bone marrow histology should be done.[51,58] An elevated EPO indicates secondary polycythemia.

A diagnostic algorithm for PV using initial peripheral blood screening for the *JAK2*(V617F) mutation and serum EPO has been suggested. Depending on the results of these tests, bone marrow biopsy might not be indicated.[64] However, the diagnostic utility of this algorithm must be determined in large studies.

Checkpoint! 9

Which of these conditions—iron deficiency, smoking, emphysema, pregnancy, dehydration—are associated with an absolute increase in RCM?

Erythropoietin Measurement   EPO is critical in differentiating PV from secondary polycythemias. With the *JAK2*(V617F) mutation, erythropoiesis occurs without the need for EPO stimulation. Serum EPO levels are usually very low or not detectable in PV. Secondary causes of polycythemia are related to elevated EPO levels either because of hypoxia or an inappropriate release of EPO from the kidneys (tumors and renal carcinomas).

Genetic Studies   Studies should include molecular analysis for the *JAK2*(V617F) along with karyotype screening for trisomies of chromosome 8 and 9 as well as deletions of 13 or 20. In addition, molecular markers can show a decreased expression of thrombopoietin receptor, MPL, and an overexpression of polycythemia rubra vera-1(*PRV-1*) in mRNA of granulocytes.[65]

Bone Marrow Changes   A bone marrow assessment can be helpful in patients in whom EPO is not low and *JAK2*(V617F) is not detected, but an elevated RCM and clinical symptoms suggest PV. Histologic changes for PV include hypercellularity with increased erythroid precursors, megakaryocytes with megakarocyte clusters, and reticulin fibrosis.[51]

It is always imperative in any classification scheme to recognize the possibility of two coexisting disease states. For instance, a patient can have both PV and a secondary polycythemia as occurs in chronic obstructive pulmonary disease. Differentiating features of polycythemia vera from secondary and relative polycythemia are found in Table 22-21 ●).

► ESSENTIAL THROMBOCYTHEMIA (ET)

Essential thrombocythemia (ET) is a myeloproliferative disorder affecting primarily the megakaryocytic lineage. Sustained proliferation of megakaryocytes in the marrow and extreme thrombocytosis in the peripheral blood with thrombocytopathy (a qualitative disorder of platelets) occurs. In the past, considerable controversy has existed concerning the inclusion of ET as a specific entity in the myeloproliferative disorders because thrombocytosis is often a component of CML, CIMF, and PV. However, ET is now firmly estab-

---

✪ TABLE 22-20

Diagnostic Criteria for Polycythemia Vera as Defined by WHO

Diagnosis of PV requires 2 of category A criteria and one other A criterion or 2 B criteria[62]

Category A: Two Diagnostic Criteria Required

1. Increased RBC mass >25% mean normal or Hb >18.5 g/dL in men or >16.5 g/dL in women or >99th percentile of method-specific reference range for sex, age, altitude
2. Causes of secondary polycythemia ruled out:
   a. Familial erythrocytosis
   b. No increase of EPO due to:
      i. Hypoxia
      ii. High oxygen–affinity Hb
      iii. Truncated EPO receptor
      iv. Inappropriate EPO production by tumor
3. Splenomegaly
4. Clonal genetic abnormality other than BCR/ABL in bone marrow
5. Endogenous erythroid colony (EEC) formation in vitro

Category B: Two Diagnostic Criteria Required

1. Platelet count >400 × 10⁹/L
2. Leukocyte count >12 × 10⁹/L in absence of obvious infection or fever
3. Low EPO levels
4. Bone marrow biopsy shows panmyelosis with prominent erythroid and megakaryocytic proliferation

From: Pierce RV, Vardemann JW, Imbert M, Brunning RD, Thiele J, Flandrin G, Polycythemia vera. In: Jaffe ES, Harris NL, Stein H, Vardiman JW. *World Health Organization Classification of Tumours: Tumours of the Haematopoietic and Lymphoid Tissues.* Lyon, France: IARC Press; 2001:32.

TABLE 22-21

Differential Features of Polycythemia

Feature	PV	Secondary	Relative
Spleen size	↑	N	N
RCM	≥36 mL/Kg (males) ≥32 mL/Kg (females)	↑	N
Leukocyte count	↑	N	N
Platelet count	↑	N	N
Serum cobalamin	↑	N	N
Arterial O₂ saturation	N	↓	N
Bone marrow	Panhyperplasia; reticulin deposits	Erythroid hyperplasia	N
LAP	N to ↑	N	N
Iron stores	↓	N	N
EPO	N, ↓	N, ↑	N
Chromosome studies	Abnormal; >90% JAK2(V617F)+	N	N

N = normal; ↑ = increased; ↓ = decreased; LAP = leukocyte alkaline phosphatase; EPO = erythropoietin.

lished as a hematologic malignancy with distinct clinical manifestations and complications.[66]

Synonyms for ET include *primary thrombocythemia, hemorrhagic thrombocythemia, primary thrombocytosis,* and *idiopathic thrombocytosis.*

PATHOPHYSIOLOGY

ET is a neoplastic disorder of the HSC usually resulting in clonal hematopoiesis affecting all three lineages, but in some cases, only the megakaryocytes are involved.[66] Normal megakaryocyte colony formation from CFU-Meg depends on the addition of cytokines in in vitro cultures. Although spontaneous megakaryocyte colony formation in serum-containing cultures has been reported, data on spontaneous colony formation in serum-free conditions are conflicting.[66] Early studies suggested that TPO and/or its receptor (MPL) were not directly associated with the underlying pathology in ET. Expression of MPL and its mRNA are generally decreased in ET, yet proliferation of progenitor cells ensues.[65] Serum levels of thrombopoietin are normal or slightly elevated in most patients.[16,67] The clonal population of cells appears hypersensitive to some cytokines, including IL-3 and IL-6, but the clones are not hypersensitive to GM-CSF. However, sensitivity to the inhibitory effects of TGF-β is decreased, thus minimizing inhibition of thrombopoiesis.

Thus, a combination of increased sensitivity to some cytokines that promote platelet production coupled with a decreased sensitivity to negative regulators could account for the increased megakaryocyte proliferation characteristic of ET.

The recently discovered *JAK2*(V617F) mutation has been shown to be present in about 50% of patients with ET.[68] Because the cytokine receptors for EPO, MPL, and CSF-G have been associated with disease transformation mediated by *JAK2*(V617F), mutations in these receptors may activate JAK2 in those cases that are *JAK2*(V517F)-negative. Recent studies have revealed a mutation in *MPL* (MPLW515L) in some patients with *JAK2*(V617F)-negative ET and CIMF. This mutation results in cytokine-independent growth and constitutive downstream signaling pathways.[68]

CLINICAL FINDINGS

A rare disorder, ET's incidence peaks primarily from 50 to 60 years of age and secondarily from 20 to 30 years of age. The older group of patients has no gender predilection, but the younger age peak predominantly involves women. The overall incidence is ~1.5–2.4/100,000 people annually.[66]

The presenting symptoms of patients with ET are variable. With the inclusion of platelet counts as a part of a routine CBC by most instrumentation now, extreme thrombocytosis is being detected more frequently than previously recognized. Many of these patients are asymptomatic, and their diagnosis is made incidentally.[69] Symptomatic patients most commonly present with thrombosis (primarily involving the microvasculature) or minor bleeding. Neurologic complications are common (e.g., headache, paresthesias of the extremities) and are associated with platelet-mediated ischemia and thrombosis. Circulatory insufficiency involving the microvasculature of the toes and fingers is frequent and is associated with pain and occasionally gangrene. Hemorrhagic episodes can occur, primarily involving the gastrointestinal tract, skin, urinary tract, and oral mucosal membranes. These problems appear to be more frequent in patients over 59 years of age with thrombosis occurring more frequently than bleeding at the lower values of thrombocytosis.[9,17,67,70,71]

About half the patients have a palpable spleen, but splenomegaly is usually slight. Occasionally, splenic atrophy resulting from repeated splenic thrombosis and silent infarctions is seen. When this occurs, it is associated with typical morphologic alterations on the peripheral blood smear as discussed in the next section.

LABORATORY FINDINGS

Peripheral Blood

The most striking finding in the peripheral blood is extreme and consistent thrombocytosis (Figure 22-16 ■). Platelet counts are more than 600 × 10⁹/L and usually range from

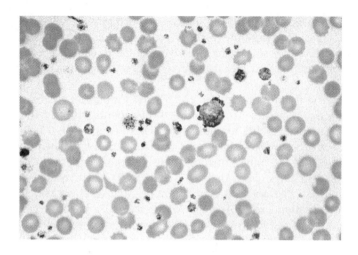

■ FIGURE 22-16   Essential thrombocythemia. Platelets are markedly increased, and a giant form is present. (Peripheral blood; 1000× magnification; Wright-Giemsa stain)

$1000–5000 \times 10^9$/L. The peripheral blood smear can show giant bizarre platelets, and platelets can appear in aggregates. Megakaryocytes and megakaryocyte fragments also can be found. However, in many cases, platelet morphology appears normal. Abnormalities in platelet aggregation and adhesion suggest defects in platelet function (see Tests of Hemostasis).

Anemia, if present, is generally proportional to the severity of bleeding and is usually normocytic; however, longstanding or recurrent hemorrhagic episodes can lead to iron deficiency and a microcytic, hypochromic anemia. In about one-third of the patients, slight erythrocytosis is present, which can cause confusion with polycythemia vera. Aggregated platelets can lead to an erroneous increase in the erythrocyte count on automated cell counters. Therefore, hemoglobin determinations are better to assess the patient's anemic status. Histograms can reveal a high tail on the leukocyte histogram because of platelet clumps. The reticulocyte count can be increased if bleeding is present and mild polychromatophilia is noted. Peripheral blood abnormalities secondary to autosplenectomy may occur if the spleen has been infarcted. These abnormalities include Howell-Jolly bodies, nucleated erythrocytes, and poikilocytosis.

A leukocytosis from 22 to 40×10^9/L is almost always present. Occasional metamyelocytes and myelocytes can be found with ET. Mild eosinophilia and basophilia also are observed. The LAP score can be normal or increased; it rarely is low. Nucleated erythrocytes are found in 25% of patients.

Bone Marrow

The bone marrow exhibits marked hyperplasia with a striking increase in megakaryocytes often with clustering of megakaryocytes along the sinusoidal borders. The background of stained slides shows many platelets. The megakaryocytes are large with abundant mature cytoplasm and frequently increased nuclear lobulation. Mitotic forms are increased. Erythroid and myeloid hyperplasia also are evident. Stains for iron reveal normal or decreased stores but normal serum ferritin levels. In ~25% of cases, reticulin is increased, but significant fibrosis is generally not seen.[66]

Tests of Hemostasis

Laboratory tests alone are unreliable in predicting bleeding or thrombotic complications in ET. The PT and APTT are usually normal, but evidence of low-grade DIC can be present. Platelet aggregation studies are frequently abnormal with the most common findings including defective platelet aggregation with epinephrine, ADP, and collagen. A loss of platelet α-adrenergic receptors associated with reduced epinephrine-induced aggregation is characteristic of an MPD and is useful in differentiating ET from secondary thrombocytosis. Spontaneous in vitro platelet aggregation or hyperaggregability is a common finding. In vivo platelet aggregation is suggested by finding increased plasma levels of β-thromboglobulin and platelet factor 4 (released from platelet α-granules). Other platelet abnormalities that have been described in association with ET are included in Table 22-22 ✪.[72] A form of acquired VWD has been described in association with excessively high platelet counts and ET. The increase in number of circulating platelets is associated with adsorption of larger VWF multimers and their removal from the circulation. The laboratory features are characteristic of Type II VWD with a decrease or absence of large VWF multimers and reduced levels of ristocetin cofactor activity (∞ Chapter 32).

Genetics

A low incidence of clonal chromosomal cytogenetic abnormalities (about 5%) are found in ET. No diagnostic abnormality has been reported, but trisomies of Group C chromosomes can be seen. However, in 25–50% of cases, molecular screenings yield a *JAK2*(V617F) or *MPL* (W515L or W515K) mutation.[16]

✪ TABLE 22-22
Platelet Abnormalities Found in Essential Thrombocythemia
• Decreased MPL receptors for thrombopoietin (TPO)
• Shortened platelet survival
• Increased beta-thromboglobulin (β-TG)
• Increased urinary thromboxane B_2 (TxB_2)
• Acquired Von Willebrand disease
• Defective epinephrine, collagen, ADP-induced platelet aggregation
• Decreased ATP secretion
• Acquired storage pool deficiency due to abnormal in vivo platelet activation

Other Laboratory Findings

Other laboratory tests can be abnormal. Serum cobalamin and the unsaturated cobalamin binding capacity are increased. An increase in cell turnover can cause serum uric acid, LD, and acid phosphatase to be elevated. Serum potassium can be elevated as a result of in vitro release of potassium from platelets (pseudohyperkalemia). The spurious nature of this hyperkalemia can be verified by performing a simultaneous potassium assay on plasma, which should be normal. Arterial blood gases can reveal a pseudohypoxia if the sample is not tested promptly due to the in vitro consumption of oxygen by the increased numbers of platelets.

PROGNOSIS AND THERAPY

About 64–80% of the patients with ET survive 10 years. The prognosis appears to be better in younger patients. One large study found no significant difference in survival probability compared to the control population. The most common causes of death are thrombosis and bleeding. Occasionally, the disease transforms to AML, PV, or CIMF (usually <10% of patients for each type of transformation).[73]

Controversy exists as to which patients with ET require therapy. It is generally agreed that patients with a history of thrombosis or cardiovascular risk factors require therapy to reduce the platelet count. Plateletpheresis is utilized to quickly reduce the platelet count below 1000×10^9/L for control of vascular accidents. Anticoagulants and drugs to inhibit platelet function are used to control thrombosis.[70]

The benefit of specific therapy in asymptomatic patients has not been established. Therapeutic trials with β-interferon show improvement of both hematologic parameters and clinical symptoms on nearly all patients.[70] Withdrawal of interferon, however, leads to recurrence of thrombocytosis. Chronic megakaryocyte suppression can be achieved by radiation or chemotherapy. However, the leukemogenic potential of these therapeutic agents is of concern.

DIFFERENTIAL DIAGNOSIS

Although the other MPDs have certain diagnostic markers, ET is largely a diagnosis of exclusion. Essential thrombocytosis must be differentiated from a secondary, reactive thrombocytosis (Table 22-23 ✪). Secondary thrombocytosis is associated with many acute and chronic infections, inflammatory diseases, carcinomas, and Hodgkin's disease. The platelet count in ET exceeds 1000×10^9/L and is persistent over a period of months or years. Secondary or reactive thrombocytosis rarely reaches 1000×10^9/L and is transitory. In addition, in secondary thrombocytosis, platelet function is normal, leukocytes and erythrocytes are normal, and splenomegaly is absent.

Differentiating ET from PV can be difficult. However, marked erythrocytosis with clinical findings suggestive of hypervolemia is more typical of PV.

✪ TABLE 22-23

Conditions Associated with Thrombocytosis

- Essential thrombocythemia (ET)
- Polycythemia vera (PV)
- Chronic myelogenous leukemia (CML)
- Chronic idiopathic myelofibrosis (CIMF)
- Chronic inflammatory disorders
- Acute hemorrhage
- Hemolytic anemia
- Hodgkin's disease
- Metastatic carcinoma
- Lymphoma
- Postsplenectomy
- Postoperative
- Iron deficiency

The Polycythemia Vera Study Group (PVSG) proposed a set of diagnostic criteria for ET, which were adopted as diagnostic criteria in the WHO classification (Table 22-24 ✪). The first criterion, a platelet count of more than 600×10^9/L, excludes many cases of secondary thrombocytosis. The second criterion of increased megakaryocytes in the bone marrow is necessary to confirm the diagnosis of ET and rule out other causes of clonal thrombocythemia.[31] The third, a hemoglobin of less than 18.5 g/dL in males and less than 16.5 g/dL in females, and the fourth, presence of iron in the bone marrow or failure of response to iron therapy, exclude cases of PV. The fifth criterion, absence of the Ph chromosome, was designed to rule out CML, and the sixth, absence of collagen fibrosis, rules out CIMF. The seventh, absence of dysplasia and related genetic mutations, rules out MDS. The eighth criterion excludes conditions associated with reactive thrombocytosis.

✓ Checkpoint! 10

Is a patient who has a platelet count of 846×10^9/L, splenomegaly, and abnormal platelet function tests of hyperaggregation likely to have reactive or essential thrombocytosis? Explain.

► CHRONIC MYELOPROLIFERATIVE DISEASE, UNCLASSIFIABLE (CMPD-U)

Chronic myeloproliferative disease, unclassified (CMPD-U) is the diagnosis for cases that have the characteristic clinical, laboratory, and morphologic features of an MPD but do not meet the specific criteria for one of the other MPD categories or have features that overlap two or more categories. The Ph

✪ TABLE 22-24

WHO Diagnostic Criteria for Essential Thrombocythemia (ET)

Diagnostic Criteria for ET	Helps Differentiate ET From:
Sustained platelet count >600 × 10⁹/L	Secondary thrombocytosis
Bone marrow biopsy shows megakaryocytic hyperplasia (enlarged, mature megakaryocytes)	
Hemoglobin ≤18.5 g/dL in males, <16.5 g/dL in females or normal RCM	PV
Stainable iron in the marrow, normal serum ferritin, or normal MCV or failure of iron therapy to increase the RCM or raise the hemoglobin to the PV level after one month of iron therapy	PV
Absence of the Ph chromosome or BCR/ABL fusion gene	CML
Absent collagen fibrosis of marrow and minimal or absent reticulin fibrosis	CIMF
No evidence of myelodysplastic syndrome (absent del[5q]; t[3;3][q21;q26]; inv[3][q21q26]; absence of granulocytic dysplasia and micromegakaryocytes	MDS
No known cause for reactive thrombocytosis	Reactive thrombocytosis

RCM = red cell mass

Adapted from: Murphy S, Peterson P, Iland H, Lazlo J. Experience of the Polycythemia Vera Study Group with essential thrombocythemia: A final report on diagnostic criteria, survival, and leukemic transition by treatment. *Semin Hematol.* 1997;34:29–39, and Imbert M, Vardiman JW, Pierre RV et al. Essential thrombocythemia. In Jaffe ES, Harris NL, Stein H, Vardiman JW, eds. *World Health Organization Classification of Tumours: Tumours of the Haematopoietic and Lymphoid Tissues.* Lyon, Frace: International Agency for Research on Cancer (IARC) Press; 2001:17–44.

chromosome and BCR/ABL are absent. The cell of origin is most likely the pluripotent HSC.

Most cases of CMPD-U are either very early stages of PV, CIMF, or ET or are at a late stage of advanced MPD in which extensive myelofibrosis, osteosclerosis, or transformation to an aggressive stage obscures the true disorder. Follow-up at intervals can permit an accurate diagnosis. A specific diagnosis should be made as soon as possible because of the therapeutic implications for each of the neoplastic disorders.

The incidence of CPMD-U is unknown but can be as high as 20% of MPDs. Clinical features are similar to those found in other MPD including splenomegaly and hepatomegaly.

LABORATORY FINDINGS

WBC and platelets can be increased. Hemoglobin is variable. The bone marrow is hypercellular with megakaryocytic hy-perplasia and variable granulocytic and erythroid proliferation. In advanced stages, the BM is fibrotic or osteomyelosclerotic. If there are 10–19% blasts in the peripheral blood, the disease is diagnosed as an accelerated stage.

GENETICS

No specific cytogenetic or molecular abnormalities are identified with this disorder.

▶ MAST CELL DISEASE (MASTOCYTOSIS)

Mast cell disorders are heterogeneous. They are characterized by the abnormal proliferation of mast cells in one or more organ systems. Mast cells share a common progenitor cell with myelomonocytic cells. Based on current knowledge about mast cells, it has been suggested that mast cell disorders be classified as myeloproliferative disorders, but classification schemes for them have not been universally accepted. The WHO classification is included in Table 22-25 ✪.

The two major groups of mast cell disorders are cutaneous and systemic. Cutaneous disease is based on the presence of histological skin lesions and typical clinical signs but no systemic involvement. It is typically found in children.

Systemic disease is characterized by multifocal histological lesions in the bone marrow and other organs. There may be anemia and an increase or decrease in leukocytes and platelets. Eosinophilia can be marked.

Genetic studies reveal that systemic mastocytosis (SM) is a clonal disorder. It is characterized by a somatic mutation of the *KIT* (CD117) protooncogene. *KIT* codes for the tyrosine kinase receptor for SCF, which is a major regulator of mast cell development, and hematopoietic stem cells. When mutated, the receptor is constitutively activated giving the cell a proliferative advantage.[74]

✪ TABLE 22-25

WHO Classification of Mast Cell Disorders (Mastocytosis)

- Cutaneous mastocytosis
- Indolent systemic mastocytosis
- Systemic mastocytosis associated with other clonal, nonmast cell hematologic disorders
- Aggressive systemic mastocytosis
- Mast cell leukemia
- Mast cell sarcoma
- Extracutaneous mastocytoma

Adapted from: Valent P, Harry HP, Escribano L, Longley BJ, Li CY, Schwartz LB et al. Diagnostic criteria and classification of mastocytosis: A consensus proposal. *Leuk* Res. 2001;25(7):603–25.

One subgroup of systemic mast cell disease is mast cell leukemia, (MCL) an aggressive disease with a short survival. The criteria for a diagnosis of MCL include criteria for systemic mastocytosis fulfilled; circulating mast cells in the peripheral blood (≥10%) and >20% of the nucleated cells in bone marrow are mast cells; and multiorgan failure (Table 22-26 ✪). The aleukemic mast cell leukemia variant has <10% mast cells in the peripheral blood. The bone marrow mast cells can be immature and blastlike. Mast cells with bilobed or polylobed nuclei can be found. Signs of myeloproliferation and dysplasia, can be present but the criteria for another hematologic disorder are not. The mast cells are tryptase positive and express KIT. Serum tryptase levels are elevated. Pancytopenia characterizes later stages of the disease when the bone marrow fails.

Most patients are adults with symptoms related to proteins or mediators released from mast cells and include hypotension, flushing, and diarrhea. Weight loss, bone pain, and organomegaly occur later in the disease. There is no standard therapy or long-term cure. Antimediator drugs such as aspirin and antihistamines are used to relieve symptoms. Experience with chemotherapy and bone marrow transplant is lacking.[74]

SUMMARY

The myeloproliferative disorders (MPD) are characterized as a group of clonal stem cell disorders differentiated by neoplastic production of one or more of the hematopoietic lineages in bone marrow and peripheral blood. The WHO classification of MPD includes the subgroups chronic myelogenous leukemia (CML), chronic neutrophilic leukemia (CNL), chronic eosinophilic leukemia (CEL), chronic idiopathic myelofibrosis (CIMF) with myeloid metaplasia, polycythemia vera (PV), and essential thrombocythemia (ET).

Although all hematopoietic cell lineages can be involved in the unregulated proliferation in MPD, one lineage is usually involved more than the others. The myeloid cells are primarily affected in CML, CEL, and CNL; the erythrocytes are affected in PV; and the platelets/megakaryocytes are affected in ET. The most characteristic finding of CIMF is a nonmalignant proliferation of fibroblasts in the bone marrow. Splenomegaly, bone marrow fibrosis, and megakaryocytic hyperplasia are findings common to all subgroups. The underlying pathophysiology appears to be chromosomal rearrangements that occur in the regions of proto-oncogenes leading to qualitative or quantitative alterations in gene expression and abnormal control of cell growth. *JAK2*(V617F) and *MPL* (W515) mutations that lead to constitutive phosphorylation, signal transduction, DNA transcription, and decreased apoptosis have been identified.

Abnormal karyotypes in hematopoietic cells can be found in any of the subgroups. The most well-characterized abnormality is the Philadelphia (Ph) chromosome found in up to 95% of individuals with CML. The Ph chromosome is the result of a translocation of genetic material between chromosomes 9 and 22 [t(9;22) (q34;q11.2)]. Molecular testing of CML patients who are Ph chromosome negative by cytogenetics, reveals a *BCR/ABL1* fusion gene encoding for an abnormal tyrosine kinase protein, p210, comparable to that produced by the Ph chromosome. This protein plays a role in the pathogenesis of CML. Trisomies within the Group C chromosomes, trisomy 8 or trisomy 9, are common findings in progressive MPD.

The survival of MPD patients varies according to the subgroup and complications of thrombosis. Patients with PV and ET appear to survive longer than patients with CML or CIMF. Any of the subgroups can evolve into acute leukemia with or without specific therapy. Currently no cure exists for any of the MPDs, although stem cell transplantation, molecular-targeted therapy, and antiplatelet drugs give favorable outlooks for improving prognosis.

✪ TABLE 22-26
Criteria for Diagnosis of Systemic Mastocytosis (SM) and Mast Cell Leukemia (MCL).
SM requires the major criteria and 1 minor criteria or 3 minor criteria. MCL requires criteria for SM plus those listed for MCL in this table.
Major criteria:
• Bone marrow or other organs that show multifocal, dense infiltrates of tryptase positive mast cells
Minor criteria:
• Biopsy of bone marrow or other organs shows spindle-shaped or atypical morphology in >25% of mast cells or >25% of all mast cells in the bone marrow are immature or atypical
• Presence of KIT point mutation (codon 816) in mast cells from bone marrow or other organ
• Mast cells in peripheral blood, bone marrow, or other tissue coexpress CD117 with CD2 +/or CD25
• In absence of associated clonal myeloid disorder, total serum tryptase is >20 ng/mL
Mast cell leukemia criteria
• Criteria for SM fulfilled
• Diffuse infiltration by atypical immature mast cells shown in bone marrow biopsy
• Bone marrow aspirate with ≥20% mast cells
• Peripheral blood with ≥10% mast cells

REVIEW QUESTIONS

LEVEL I

1. The most prominent cell line in CML is the: (Objective 2)
   a. erythroid
   b. myeloid
   c. megakaryocyte
   d. fibroblast

2. The most prominent cell line found in polycythemia vera (PV) is the: (Objective 2)
   a. erythroid
   b. myeloid
   c. megakaryocyte
   d. fibroblast

3. The Philadelphia chromosome is a gene fusion resulting from a translocation of: (Objective 4)
   a. chomosomes 8 and 14
   b. chomosomes 9 and 22
   c. chomosomes 12 and 17
   d. chomosomes 15 and 17

4. The peak age for CML is: (Objective 5)
   a. less than 5 years
   b. 15–30 years
   c. 40–59 years
   d. over 60 years

5. The Philadelphia chromosome can be found in patients with: (Objective 4)
   a. CML
   b. ALL
   c. ET
   d. polycythemia vera

6. Which of the following represent a characteristic peripheral blood finding in patients with CIMF? (Objective 7)
   a. elliptocytes
   b. dacrocytes
   c. target cells
   d. schistocytes

7. Polycythemia vera (PV) can be distinguished from secondary polycythemia by measuring: (Objective 9)
   a. hematocrit
   b. plasma volume
   c. hemoglobin concentration
   d. erythropoietin

8. A 50-year-old man was admitted to the emergency room for chest pain and a blood count was ordered. The results showed erythrocyte count 6.5×10^{12}/L; hematocrit 0.60 L/L; leukocyte count 15×10^9/L; platelet count 500×10^9/L. These results indicate: (Objective 3)
   a. the need for further investigation of a possible diagnosis of MPD
   b. normal findings for an adult male
   c. that the patient has experienced a thrombotic episode
   d. a malfunction of the cell counting instrument

LEVEL II

Use this case study to answer questions 1–5.

A 45-year-old Caucasian female was admitted to the hospital from the emergency room. She had experienced pain in the upper quadrant and bloating for the past several weeks. She had multiple bruises on her legs and arms. She also stated that her gums bled easily when she brushed her teeth. She had been unusually tired and lost about 10 pounds in the last 2 months. Results of physical examination showed a massive spleen. The following laboratory results were noted on blood count admission.

Hb	7.4 g/dL (74 g/L)
Erythrocyte count	2.9×10^{12}/L
Hct	.22 L/L
RDW	18.0
Leukocyte count	520×10^9/L
Platelet count	960×10^9/L
Differential	31% segmented neutrophils
	26% bands
	8% metamyelocytes
	11% myelocytes
	4% promyelocytes
	2% blasts
	4% lymphocytes
	3% monocytes
	5% eosinophils
	6% basophils
	4 nucleated erythrocytes/100 leukocytes
	Occasional micromegakaryocytes

There was moderate anisocytosis and poikilocytosis.

A bone marrow aspiration was performed. The marrow was 90% cellular with a myeloid:erythroid ratio of 10:1. The majority of the cells were neutrophilic precursors. There was an increase in eosinophils and basophils. Myeloblasts accounted for 10% of the nucleated cells. Megakaryocytes were increased.

1. What findings suggest that this patient has a defect in the pluripotential stem cell rather than a benign proliferation of hematopoietic cells? (Objective 4)
   a. the presence of a leukoerythroblastic blood picture
   b. the involvement of several cell lineages in the proliferative process including neutrophilic cells and platelets
   c. the shift to the left in the neutrophilic cell line
   d. an increase in the RDW

2. Molecular analysis by (RT-PCR) revealed the presence of a BCR/ABL fusion product. Based on this information, what myeloproliferative disorder is present? (Objectives 1, 3)
   a. CML
   b. PV
   c. ET
   d. CIMF

REVIEW QUESTIONS (continued)

LEVEL I

9. A patient previously diagnosed with CML now has a platelet count of 540×10^9/L and a leukocyte count of 350×10^9/L with a peripheral blood differential showing 15% segmented neutrophils, 23% bands, 2% metamyelocytes, 35% blasts, 6% lymphocytes, 4% monocytes, 6% eosinophils, and 8% basophils. These results are most consistent with: (Objective 6)
   a. chronic CML
   b. ET
   c. CML in blast crisis
   d. CIMF

10. A patient presenting in the ER with a platelet count of more than 1000×10^9/L and a leukocyte count of 25×10^9/L with a normochromic, normocytic anemia should be evaluated for: (Objective 10)
    a. Philadelphia chromosome
    b. essential thrombocythemia
    c. CIMF
    d. primary polycythemia

LEVEL II

3. What cytochemical stain is used to help differentiate a leukemoid reaction from CML? (Objectives 1, 4)
   a. myeloperoxidase
   b. new methylene blue
   c. leukocyte alkaline phosphatase
   d. Perl's Prussian blue

4. Which of the following terms most accurately describes the peripheral blood picture of this patient? (Objectives 10, 13)
   a. leukemoid reaction
   b. leukoerythroblastic
   c. leukopenia
   d. myelodysplastic

5. What is the best description of the bone marrow? (Objective 1)
   a. decreased M:E ratio and increased cellularity
   b. increased M:E ratio and decreased cellularity
   c. increased M:E ratio and increased cellularity
   d. decreased M:E ratio and decreased cellularity

6. Extensive bone marrow fibrosis, leukoerythroblastic peripheral blood, and the presence of anisocytosis with dacryocytes are most characteristic of which MPD? (Objective 6)
   a. CML
   b. PV
   c. ET
   d. CIMF

7. A 68-year-old man was seen in the clinic for lethargy, dyspnea, and light-headedness. Results of his blood counts were erythrocyte count 5.0×10^{12}/L; hematocrit 0.55 L/L; leukocyte count 60×10^9/L; platelet count 70×10^9/L. His differential showed a shift to the left in myeloid elements with 40% eosinophils. The bone marrow revealed 10% blasts. Philadelphia chromosome was negative. He most likely has: (Objective 10)
   a. polycythemia vera
   b. CML in blast crisis
   c. essential thrombocythemia
   d. chronic eosinophilic leukemia

8. A molecular test should be performed on the patient in question 7 for which mutation? (Objective 3)
   a. JAK2(V617F)
   b. BCR/ABL
   c. FIP1L1/PDGFRA
   d. *MPL*(W515)

9. Which of the following does *not* cause secondary polycythemia? (Objective 7)
   a. chronic obstructive pulmonary disease
   b. smoking
   c. emphysema
   d. dehydration

REVIEW QUESTIONS (continued)

LEVEL I

LEVEL II

10. Evidence of clonal proliferation in myeloproliferative disorders can be identified by: (Objective 8)
    a. G6PD isomers
    b. myeloperoxidase stain
    c. Perl's Prussian blue
    d. trisomy 8

www.pearsonhighered.com/mckenzie

Use this address to access the interactive Companion Website created for this textbook. Find additional information, tables and figures. Evaluate your command of the chapter information using case studies and critical thinking and multiple choice questions.

REFERENCES

1. Dameshek W. Some speculations on the myeloproliferative syndromes. *Blood.* 1951;6:372–75.

2. Douer D, Fabian I, Cline MJ. Circulating pluripotent haemopoietic cells in patients with myeloproliferative disorders. *Br J Haematol.* 1983;54:373–81.

3. Gilbert HS, Praloran V, Stanley ER. Increased circulating CSF-1 (M-CSF) in myeloproliferative disease: Association with myeloid metaplasia and peripheral bone marrow extension. *Blood.* 1989;74:1231–34.

4. Gersuk GM, Carmel R, Pattengale PK. Platelet derived growth factor concentrations in platelet poor plasma and urine from patients with myeloproliferative disorders. *Blood.* 1989;74:2330–34.

5. Cervantes F, Salgado C, Rozman C. Assessment of iron stores in hospitalized patients. *Am J Clin Pathol.* 1991;1:105–6.

6. Tefferi A, Ho TC, Ahmann GJ, Katzmann JA, Greipp PR. Plasma interleukin-6 and C-reactive protein levels in reactive versus clonal thrombocytosis. *Am J Med.* 1998;97:374–78.

7. Landolfi R, De Cristofaro R, Castagnola M, De Candia E, D'Onofrio G, Leone G. Increased platelet-fibrinogen affinity in patients with myeloproliferative disorders. *Blood.* 1988;71:978–82.

8. Mazzucato M, De Marco L, De Angelis V, De Roia D, Bizzaro N, Casonato A. Platelet membrane abnormalities in myeloproliferative disorders: Decrease in glycoproteins Ib and IIb/IIIa complex is associated with deficient receptor function. *Br J Haematol.* 1989;73:369–74.

9. Kaushansky K. Hematopoietic growth factors, signaling and the chronic myeloproliferative disorders. *Cytokine Growth Factor Rev.* 2006;17:423–30.

10. Dickstein JI, Vardiman JW. Issues in the pathology and diagnosis of the chronic myeloproliferative disorders and the myelodysplastic syndromes. *Am J Clin Pathol.* 1993;99:513–25.

11. Epner DE, Roeffler HP. Molecular genetic advances in chronic myelogenous leukemia. *Ann Intern Med.* 1990;113:3–6.

12. Guo JQ, Wang JY, and Arlinghaus RB. Detection of BCR-ABL proteins in blood cells of benign phase chronic myelogenous leukemia patients. *Cancer Res.* 1991;51:3048–51.

13. Cortes JE, Talpaz M, Kantarjian H. Chronic myelogenous leukemia: A review. *Am J Med.* 1996;100:555–70.

14. Mattson JC, Crisan D, Wilner F, Decker D, Burdakin J. Clinical problem solving using BCL-2 and BCR gene rearrangement analysis. *Lab Med.* 1994;25:648–53.

15. Hasle H, Niemeyer CM, Chessells JM, Baumann I, Bennett JM, Kerndrup G, Head DR. A pediatric approach to the WHO classification of myelodysplastic myeloproliferative diseases. *Leukemia.* 2003;17(2):277–82.

16. Bennett M, Stroncek DF. Recent advances in the bcr-abl negative chronic myeloproliferative diseases. *J Trans Med.* 2006;4:41. www.translational-medicine.com/content/4/1/41. PubMed accessed February 4, 2007.

17. Tefferi A, Barbui T. BCR/ABL negative, classic myeloproliferative disorders: Diagnosis and treatment. *Mayo Clin Proc.* 2005;80:1220–32.

18. Ahuja H, Bar-Eli M, Arlin Z, Advani S, Allen SL, Goldman J et al. The spectrum of molecular alterations in the evaluation of chronic myelocytic leukemia. *J Clin Invest.* 1991;87:2042–47.

19. Imamura J, Miyoshi I, Koeffler HP. p53 in hematologic malignancies. *Blood.* 1994;84:2412–21.

20. Li S, Ilaria RL Jr, Million RP, Daley GQ, Van Etten RA. The P190, P210, and P230 forms of the BCR/ABL oncogene induce a similar chronic myeloid leukemia-like syndrome in mice but have different lymphoid leukemogenic activity. *J Exp Med.* 1999;189:1399–1412.

21. Vardiman JW, Harris NL, Brunning RD. The World Health Organization (WHO) classification of the myeloid neoplasms. *Blood.* 2002;100:2292–302.

22. Xu Y, Wahner AE, Nguyen PL. Progression of chronic myeloid leukemia to blast crisis during treatment with imatinib mesylate. *Arch Pathol Lab Med.* 2004;128:980–85.

23. Cornelissen JJ, Ploemacher RE, Wognum BW, Borsboom A, Kluin-Nelemans HC, Hagemeijer A, Lowenberg B. An in vitro model for cytogenetic conversion in CML: Interferon-alpha preferentially inhibits the outgrowth of malignant stem cells preserved in long-term culture. *J Clin Invest.* 1998;102:976–83.

24. Druker BJ, Guilhot F, O'Brien SG, Gathmann I, Kantarjian H, Gattermann N et al. Five-year follow-up of patients receiving imatinib for chronic myeloid leukemia. *N Engl J Med.* 2006;355:2408–17.

25. Nadal E, Olavarria E. Imatinib mesylate (Gleevec/Glivec) a molecular-targeted therapy for chronic myeloid leukaemia and other malignancies. *Int J Clin Pract.* 2004;58:511–16.

26. Gorre ME, Mohammed M, Ellwood K et al. Clinical resistance to STI-571 cancer therapy caused by BCR-ABL gene mutation or amplification. *Science.* 2001;293(5531):876–80.

27. Ma W, Tseng R, Gorre M, Jilani I, Keating M, Kantarjian H et al. Plasma RNA as an alternative to cells for monitoring molecular response in patients with chronic myeloid leukemia. *Haematologica.* 2007;92:170–75.

28. Hughes T et al. Monitoring CML patients responding to treatement with tyrosine kinase inhibitors: Review and recommendations for harmonizing current methodology for detecting BCR-ABL transcripts and kinase domain mutations and for expressing results. *Blood.* 2006;108(1):28–37.

29. Zhou T, Parillon L, Li F et al. T315I ABL mutant-threonine mutated to isoleucine at gatekeeper position of kinase domain. *Chem Biol Drug Des.* 2007;70(3):171–81.

30. Imbert M et al. Chronic neutrophilic leukemia. In: Jaffe ES, Harris NL, Stein H, Vardiman JW, eds. *World Health Organization Classification of Tumours: Tumours of the Haematopoietic and Lymphoid Tissues.* Lyon, France: IARC Press; 2001:27.

31. Tefferi A, Elliott MA, Pardanani A. Atypical myeloproliferative disorders: Diagnosis and management. *Mayo Clin Proc.* 2006;81(4):553–63.

32. Roufosse F, Goldman M, Cogan E. Hypereosinophilic syndrome: Lymphoproliferative and myeloproliferative variants. *Sem Resp Crit Care Med.* 2006;27:158–70.

33. Weller P. The pivotal role of IL-5 in HES: Eosinophils, Th2-mediated immune responses, and clinical implications for HES. Hypereosinophilic syndromes. *ASH seminar,* 2007.

34. Klion AD. Recent advances in the diagnosis and treatment of hypereosinophilic syndromes. *Hematology Am Soc Hematol Educ Program* 2005;209–14.

35. Gotlib J. Molecular classification and pathogenesis of eosinophilic disorders: 2005 update. *Acta Haematologica.* 2005;114(1):7–25.

36. Klion AD, Noel P, Akin C, Law MA, Gilliland G, Cools J et. al. Elevated serum tryptase levels identify a subset of patients with a myeloproliferative variant of idiopathic hypereosinophilic syndrome associated with tissue fibrosis, poor prognosis, and imatinib responsiveness. *Blood.* 2003;101(12):1660–66.

37. Bain BJ. Relationship between idiopathic hypereosinophilic syndrome, eosinophilic leukemia, and systemic mastocytosis. *Amer J Hematol.* 2004;77:82–85.

38. Bain BJ et al. Chronic eosinophilic leukemia and hypereosinophilic syndrome. In: Jaffe ES, Harris NL, Stein H, Vardiman JW, eds. *World Health Organization Classification of Tumours: Tumours of the Haematopoietic and Lymphoid Tissues.* Lyon, France: IARC Press; 2001:27.

39. Gotlib J, Cross NC, Gilliland DG. Eosinophilic disorders: Molecular pathogenesis, new classification, and modern therapy. *Best Pract Res Clin Haematol.* 2006;19:535–69.

40. Gotlib V, Darji J, Bloomfield K, Chadburn A, Patel A, Braunschweid I. Eosinophilic variant of chronic myeloid leukemia with vascular complications. *Leuk Lymphoma.* 2003;44:1609–13.

41. Roche-Lestienne C, Lepers S, Soenen-Cornu V et al. Molecular characterization of the idiopathic hyposinophilic syndrome (HES) in 35 French patients with normal conventional cytogenetics. *Leukemia.* 2005;19:792–98.

42. Roufosse F, Cogan E, Goldman M. The hypereosinophilic syndrome revisited. *Annu Rev Med.* 2003;54:169–84.

43. Klion AD, Bochner BS, Gleich GJ, Nutman TB, Rothenberg ME, Simon H et al. Approaches to the treatment of hypereosinophilic syndromes: A workshop summary report. *J Allergy Clin Immunol.* 2006;117(6):1292–302.

44. Pardanani AD, Morice WG, Hoyer JD, Tefferi A. Chronic basophilic leukemia: A distinct clinicopathologic entity. *Europ J Haematol.* 2003;71(1):18–22.

45. Tefferi A. Medical progress: Myelofibrosis with myeloid metaplasia. *N Engl J Med.* 2000;342:1255–65.

46. Tefferi A, Gilliland DG. The JAK2(V617F) tyrosine kinase mutation in myeloproliferative disorders: Status report and immediate implications for disease classification and diagnosis. *Mayo Cl Proc.* 2005;80:947–58.

47. Arana-Yi C, Quintas-Cardama A, Giles F, Thomas D, Carrasco-Yalan A, Cortes J et al. Advances in the therapy of chronic idiopathic myelofibrosis. *Oncologist.* 2006;11:929–43.

48. Zhao R, Xing S, Li A, Fu X, Li Q, Krantz SB, Zhao JZ. Identification of an acquired JAK2 mutation in polycythemia vera. *J Bio Chem.* 2005;280:22788–92.

49. Pikman Y, Lee BH, Mercher T, McDowell E, Ebert BL, Gozo M et al. *MPLW515L* is a novel somatic activating mutation in myelofibrosis with myeloid metaplasia. *Plos Medicine.* 2006;3:1140–51. www.plosmedicine.org. PubMed accessed January 26, 2007.

50. Paquette RL, Meshkinpour A, Rosen PJ. Autoimmune myelofibrosis. *Medicine.* 1994;73:145–52.

51. Hoffman R, Ravandi-Kashani F. Idiopathic myelofibrosis. In: Hoffman R, Benz EJ, Shattil SJ, Furie B, Cohen H, Silberstein LE, McGlave P, eds. *Hematology: Basic Principles and Practice,* 4th ed. Philadelphia: Churchill Livingstone; 2005:1255–76.

52. Cervantes F. Modern management of myelofibrosis. *Br J Haematol.* 2005;128:583–92.

53. Tefferi A, Spivak JL, Polycythemia vera: Scientific advances and current practice. *Semin Hematol.* 2005;42:206–20.

54. Remy I, Wilson IA, Michnick SW. Erythropoietin receptor activation by a ligand-induced conformation change. *Science.* 1999;283:990–93.

55. Silva M, Richard C, Benito A et al. Expression of Bcl-x in erythroid precursors from patients with polycythemia vera. *N Engl J Med.* 1998;338:564–71.

56. Tefferi A. Polycythemia vera: A comprehensive review and clinical recommendations. *Mayo Clin Proc.* 2003;78:174–94.

57. Moliterno AR, Hankins WD, Spivak JL. Impaired expression of the thrombopoietin receptor by platelets from patients with polycythemia vera. *N Engl J Med.* 1998;338:572–80.

58. Cao M, Olsen RJ, Zu Y. Polycythemia vera. *Arch Pathol Lab Med.* 2006;130:1126–32.

59. Khwaja A. The role of Janus kinases in haemopoiesis and haematological malignancy. *Br J Haematol.* 2006;134:366–84.

60. Tefferi A et al. Proposals and rationale for revision of the World Health Organization diagnostic criteria for polycythemia vera, essential thrombocythemia, and primary myelofibrosis: Recommendations from an ad hoc international panel. *Blood.* 2007;110(4):1092–97.

61. Danish EH. Neonatal polycythemia. *Prog Hematol.* 1986;14:55–98.

62. Pierre RV, Vardemann JW, Imbert M, Brunning RD, Thiele J, Flandrin G. Polycythemia vera. In: Jaffe ES, Harris NL, Stein H, Vardiman JW, eds. *World Health Organization Classification of Tumours: Tumours of the Haematopoietic and Lymphoid Tissues.* Lyon, France: IARC Press; 2001:32.

63. Cassinat B, Laguillier C, Gardin C, de Beco V, Burcheri S, Fenaux P, Chomienne C et al. Classification of myeloproliferative disorders in the JAK2 era: Is there a role for red cell mass? *Leukemia.* 2008;22:452–53.

64. Tefferi A. Classification, diagnosis and management of myeloproliferative disorders in the JAK2V617F era. *Hematology:* Amer Soc Hematol Educ Program. 2006;240–45.

65. Horikawa Y, Matsumura I, Hashimoto K, Shiraga M, Kosugi S, Tadokoro S et al. Markedly reduced expression of platelet c-Mpl receptor in essential thrombocythemia. *Blood.* 1997;90:4031–38.

66. Fruchtman SM, Hoffman R. Essential Thrombocythemia. In: Hoffman R, Benz EJ, Shattil SJ, Furie B, Cohen H, Silberstein LE, McGlave P, eds. *Hematology: Basic Principles and Practice,* 4th ed. Philadelphia: Churchill Livingstone; 2005:1277–96.

67. Wang JC, Chen C, Novetsky AD, Lichter SM, Ahmed F, Friedberg NM. Blood thrombopoietin levels in clonal thrombocytosis and reactive thrombocytosis. *Am J Med.* 1998;104:451–55.

68. Levine RL, Wenig G. Role of JAK-STAT signaling in the pathogenesis of meyloproliferative disorder. *Hematology.* 2006;233–39.

69. Cortelazzo S, Viero P, Finazzi G et al. Incidence and risk factors for thrombotic complications in a historical cohort of 100 patients with essential thrombocythemia. *J Clin Oncol.* 1990;8:556–62.

70. Michiels JJ, Berneman Z, Schroyens W, Koudstall PJ, Lindemans J, Neumann HA et al. Platelet-mediated erythromelalgic, cerebral, ocular and coronary microvascular ischemic and thrombotic manifestations in patients with essential thrombocythemia and polycythemia vera: A distinct aspirin-responsive and coumadin-resistant arterial thrombophilia. *Platelets.* 2006;17:528–44.

71. Briere JB. Essential thrombocythemia. *Orphanet J Rare Dis.* 2007;2:3. www.ojrd.com/content/2/1/3. PubMed accessed February 17, 2007.

72. Imbert M, Vardiman JW, Pierre RV, Brunning RD, Theile J, Flandrin G. Essential thrombocythaemia. In: Jaffe ES, Harris NL, Stein H, Vardiman JW. *World Health Organization Classification of Tumours: Tumours of the Haematopoietic and Lymphoid tissues.* Lyon, France: IARC Press; 2001:27.

73. Rozman C, Giralt M, Felia E et al. Life expectancy of patients with chronic nonleukemic myeloproliferative disorders. *Cancer.* 1991;67:2658–63.

74. Valent P, Horny HP, Escribano L, Longley BJ, Li CY, Schwartz LB et al. Diagnostic criteria and classification of mastocytosis: A consensus proposal. *Leuk Res.* 2001;25(7):603–25.

23

Myelodysplastic Syndromes

Louann W. Lawrence, DrP.H.

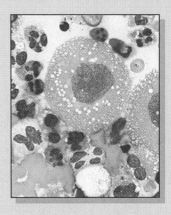

■ OBJECTIVES—LEVEL I

At the end of this unit of study, the student should be able to:

1. Define *myelodysplastic syndromes* (MDS) and list general characteristics of these diseases.
2. List the six subgroups of MDS recognized by the World Health Organization (WHO) Classification System and identify key morphological and clinical criteria that distinguish each group.
3. Describe laboratory findings and recognize changes in morphology that are characteristic of this group of disorders.
4. Define the WHO category of myelodysplastic/myeloproliferative diseases, and list its general/characteristics.
5. List the four subgroups of myelodysplastic syndromes/myeloproliferative diseases (MDS/MPD), and identify key morphological and clinical criteria as well as laboratory findings that distinguish each group.

■ OBJECTIVES—LEVEL II

At the end of this unit of study, the student should be able to:

1. Describe the pathophysiology of MDS.
2. Distinguish among Type I, Type II, and Type III blasts and promyelocytes.
3. Summarize the treatment and prognosis of MDS.
4. Explain the relationship between MDS and acute leukemia.
5. Assess the results of cytogenetic and molecular tests and correlate them with a diagnosis of MDS.
6. List and briefly describe the MDS variants not listed in the six WHO subgroups.
7. Differentiate MDS from myeloproliferative disorders, acute leukemia, and other hematologic abnormalities using peripheral blood, bone marrow, and cytogenetic characteristics.
8. Differentiate MDS/MPD from MDS, MPD, acute leukemia, and other hematologic abnormalities using peripheral blood, bone marrow, and cytogenetic characteristics.
9. Select laboratory tests that are helpful in diagnosing and differentiating MDS and MDS/MPD.
10. Evaluate a patient's laboratory and clinical findings, and propose a diagnostic MDS or MDS/MPD subgroup.

KEY TERMS

Atypical chronic myeloid leukemia (aCML)
Chronic myelomonocytic leukemia (CMML)
Dysplasia
Dyspoiesis
Endomitosis
Juvenile myelomonocytic leukemia (JMML)
Micromegakaryocyte
Myelodysplastic syndromes (MDS)
Myelodysplastic/myeloproliferative diseases
   (MDS/MPD)
Refractory anemia (RA)
Refractory anemia with excess blasts (RAEB)
Refractory anemia with ringed sideroblasts (RARS)
Refractory cytopenia with multilineage dysplasia
   (RCMD)
Refractory cytopenia with multilineage dysplasia
   and ringed sideroblasts (RCMD-RS)
Ringed sideroblasts

BACKGROUND BASICS

The information in this chapter builds on the concepts learned in previous chapters. To maximize your learning experience, you should review these concepts before starting this unit of study.

Level I

▶ Create a schematic depicting derivation of different types of blood cells from the pluripotent hematopoietic stem cell. (Chapter 3)

▶ Describe and recognize the cell morphology described by these terms: ringed sideroblasts (Chapter 9), Pelger-Huët anomaly (Chapter 19), and megaloblastoid erythropoiesis. (Chapter 12)

▶ Explain what *ineffective hematopoiesis means*. (Chapters 8, 22)

▶ Summarize the history and basis of the classification system to classify malignant leukocyte disorders. (Chapter 21)

▶ Review normal leukocyte development, differentiation, and concentrations in the peripheral blood. (Chapter 7)

Level II

▶ Describe the use of cytochemical and immunological features that distinguish the different types of blasts. (Chapters 21, 37)

▶ Explain how oncogenes and hematopoietic growth factors affect cellular maturation and proliferation. (Chapters 3, 21)

▶ Explain the role of epigenetics in cellular development (Chapter 2)

▶ Explain the use of cytogenetics and flow cytometry in the diagnosis of malignant disorders. (Chapters 37, 38)

 CASE STUDY

We will refer to this case study throughout the chapter.
Hancock, a 65-year-old white male, was seen in triage with complaints of fatigue, malaise, anorexia, and hemoptysis of recent onset. A CBC was ordered and revealed anemia and a shift to the left in granulocytes. Hematopoietic cells showed dysplastic features. Consider diagnostic probabilities and reflex testing that could provide differential diagnostic information.

▶ OVERVIEW

This chapter describes the neoplastic hematopoietic disorders known as the *myelodysplastic syndromes* (MDS). It begins with the classification of the disorders into morphologic subgroups according to the classification of both the French-American-British (FAB) and more recently, the WHO. This is followed by a description of the pathogenesis, incidence, and general clinical and laboratory features including peripheral blood and bone marrow findings. Each subgroup is then described with specific features that allow it to be classified. Variants are also described. Genetic findings common to the MDS are discussed. The chapter concludes with prognosis and therapy.

▶ INTRODUCTION

The **myelodysplastic syndromes (MDS)** are considered primary, neoplastic, pluripotential stem cell disorders. They are characterized by one or more peripheral blood cytopenias with prominent maturation abnormalities (**dyspoiesis** or **dysplasia**) in the bone marrow. The peripheral blood cytopenias are the result of ineffective hematopoiesis and increased apoptosis as evidenced by an accompanying bone marrow hyperplasia. These relatively common entities evolve progressively, leading to the aggravation of the cytopenias and, in some cases, transformation into a condition indistinguishable from acute leukemia. MDS occurs most commonly in the elderly, although it is being diagnosed with increased frequency in children.

Before the 1980s, much confusion and disagreement existed in the literature concerning the criteria for defining, subgrouping, and naming the MDSs. Because of the predisposition of MDS to terminate in leukemia, the term *preleukemia* commonly has been used to describe these disorders. However, the evolution of MDS to acute leukemia is not obligatory, and in fact, many patients die of intercurrent disease or complications of the cytopenia before evolving to leukemia.[1] Whether or not these patients would have developed leukemia had they survived the cytopenic complications is, of course, unknown. In addition, the diagnosis of preleukemia can be made only in retrospect (i.e., after the patient develops leukemia). Thus, the term *myelodysplasia* is more appropriate until the patient actually develops overt leukemia. In the past, MDS has also been described under the terms *refractory anemia with excess blasts, chronic erythremic myelosis, hematopoietic dysplasia, refractory anemia with or without sideroblasts, subacute or chronic myelomonocytic leukemia,* and *smoldering leukemia.* Most hematologists currently consider the terms *dysmyelopoietic syndrome* and *myelodysplastic syndrome* to be more acceptable than *preleukemia* or other synonyms in describing these hematologic disorders. In this book, the term *myelodysplastic syndrome* is used.

▶ PATHOGENESIS

The spectrum of clinical and hematological features in MDS is a result of the gradual expansion of abnormal hematopoietic cells and an accompanying increase in premature destruction (apoptosis) of these abnormal cells, resulting in ineffective hematopoiesis. Cytogenetic, G6PD isoenzyme studies and molecular diagnostic tests support the theory that the abnormal cells in MDS are clones derived from an abnormal pluripotent stem cell.[2–10] Chromosome abnormalities are present in more than 50% of patients at diagnosis. These abnormalities detected by standard karyotyping are present in granulocytic, monocytic, erythrocytic, and/or megakaryocytic lineages.[9–11] Recent studies have suggested that lymphocytes could be part of the leukemic clone, but other evidence has been contradictory.[2,12] Normal clones are found to coexist in the marrow with the abnormal clones. As the disease progresses, additional alterations can affect the abnormal cells, providing them a growth advantage and allowing the abnormal clone to predominate.[2] In MDS cases that progress to acute leukemia, additional abnormalities in cell culture and karyotypes can be demonstrated. Therefore, it appears that after the abnormal clone is established, additional genetic events can be required for the transformation into acute myeloid leukemia (AML).[9]

THE ROLE OF ONCOGENES

Control of cellular differentiation, maturation, and proliferation occurs through the interaction of hematopoietic growth factors with specific cellular receptors (∞ Chapter 3). This interaction causes a complex series of protein and tyrosine kinase phosphorylations, eventually resulting in DNA synthesis. Cellular proto-oncogenes control the entire process. When these genes are mutated to oncogenes, they can disrupt the process, causing disordered control and neoplasia.[13]

The abnormal MDS clone is characterized by altered gene functions resulting from either single gene mutations, chromosomal abnormalities, or gene silencing (epigenetic changes). Many of these chromosomal alterations involve gene deletions suggesting that tumor suppressor genes or DNA repair genes are altered. Changes involving tumor suppressor or DNA repair genes usually require two events: mutation of the target gene and loss of the second allele through deletion or recombination.[10]

"Unbalanced" genetic abnormalities (which result in a larger or smaller amount of DNA in the cell, such as trisomies or whole or partial chromosomal deletions) that are characteristically seen in the MDS are thought to be responsible for the ineffective hematopoiesis and cytopenias.[14] These chromosomal abnormalities are in contrast to the balanced abnormalities (which maintain the normal quantity of DNA, e.g., reciprocal translocations) seen primarily in AML.

The most frequent chromosome abnormalities in MDS involve chromosomes 5, 7, and 8, all of which carry proto-oncogenes. Chromosome 5 carries the *FOS, RAS,* and *FMS* proto-oncogenes; chromosome 7 carries the *ERB-B* proto-oncogene; and chromosome 8 carries the *MYC* proto-oncogene. The RAS gene family has been studied most often in MDS. Of patients with MDS, 10–40% have *RAS* mutations. The most common mutation is a single base change at codon 12 of the *N-RAS* (neuroblastoma-ras) family. The *N-RAS* mutation is associated with a higher risk of AML transformation and a worse prognosis. New drugs aimed to target this specific mutation are being studied.[2] The *RAS, MYC,* and *FOS* proto-oncogenes have been implicated in growth factor-mediated signaling pathways. If these proto-oncogenes are activated, the abnormal clone in MDS can become immortalized by losing the normal control mechanisms that regulate growth. Other gene mutations described in MDS involve the *P53* tumor suppressor gene (seen in 5–10% of cases) and *FLT3* oncogene receptor kinase (seen in 5% of cases).[2]

MATURATION AND PROLIFERATION ABNORMALITIES

Impaired cellular maturation and function due to intrinsic defects in cells of the neoplastic clone are fundamental pathophysiologic abnormalities in MDS as well as in AML. Erythrocyte precursors in MDS patients have been shown to have decreased sensitivity to erythropoietin. Neutrophils can have decreased myeloperoxidase activity leading to increased risk of infection even when cells are quantitatively normal. Platelets can also have functional defects.[11] Progression of MDS to acute leukemia is characterized by a gradual or sudden increase in the blast population with a block in maturation. This progression often is accompanied by the finding of additional chromosome karyotype abnormalities or epigenetic changes.[15]

Recent in vitro studies suggest that excessive premature intramedullary cell death of hematologic precursors via apoptosis contributes to ineffective hematopoiesis and peripheral blood cytopenias seen in early MDS. The various gene alterations of the MDS clone result in an intrinsic increase in susceptibility of the clone to apoptosis.[2] Increased levels of tumor necrosis factor alpha (TNF-α) and other cytokines such as IL-1, IL-6, and IL-8 in the serum and bone marrow of MDS patients have been linked to increased apoptosis of the MDS clone and normal hematopoietic cells.[2,16] Progression to leukemia is associated with a reduction in apoptosis, thereby allowing the expansion of the neoplastic clone.[17]

SECONDARY MDS

Originally, all MDS cases were classified as idiopathic (primary myelodysplasia). Evidence now indicates that a portion of MDS cases, especially those occurring in patients under 50 years of age, are probably secondary to chemotherapy, radiation therapy (therapy-related myelodysplasia, t-MDS), or exposure to toxic substances, such as benzene.[18-20] In children, MDS can be associated with predisposing conditions such as constitutional chromosome disorders (e.g., Down syndrome) and immunodeficiency disorders.[21] Complex karyotypes (presence of three or more different cytogenetic abnormalities) are present in 90% of therapy-related MDS as compared to 10–20% of primary MDS.[2]

▶ INCIDENCE

MDS occurs primarily in individuals of more than 50 years of age and has a slight male predominance (approximately 60%).[11] The risk increases sharply with age. Due to the lack of definition and classification of MDS before 1982, the actual incidence of these disorders has not been accurately assessed by large-scale epidemiological studies. Morbidity and mortality statistics are also lacking, partly because MDS was not included as a separate code in the International Classification of Diseases (ICD) until recently. The difficulty in making correct diagnoses in the early stages of the disease also contributes to unreliable incidence figures. One source estimated the overall incidence as 6–10 cases per 100,000 per year with increasing incidence beyond age 60.[2] The incidence in persons of more than 70 years has been estimated as 15–50 cases per 100,000 per year.[9] MDS is more common than AML in patients between 50 and 70 years of age, and the incidence appears to be rising. This rise could be due to an increase in the awareness of MDS on the part of physicians and clinical laboratory professionals, an increased ap-

plication of diagnostic procedures in elderly individuals, and in the number of elderly in the population.[9]

Myelodysplasia is rare in children. Problems in diagnosis can contribute to an underestimation of incidence. The approximate incidence has been reported as 1.0–1.8 cases per million per year.[12,22] The median age of children at presentation of MDS is about six years, and the male/female ratio is about 1.6:1.

▶ CLINICAL FINDINGS

The most frequent presenting symptoms, fatigue and weakness, are related to an anemia that is nonresponsive to treatment. Less commonly, hemorrhagic symptoms and infection precede diagnosis. These symptoms are related to thrombocytopenia and neutropenia. Many individuals can be asymptomatic, and their disease is discovered on routine laboratory screening.[4] Infection is a common and life-threatening complication in patients with diagnosed MDS. Neutropenia ($<1 \times 10^9$/L) and the more aggressive subgroups are associated risk factors for infectious complications.[23] Infection is the most common cause of death. Splenomegaly and/or hepatomegaly are uncommon.

▶ LABORATORY FINDINGS

The MDS present with a range of abnormal morphologic features that can be demonstrated on stained peripheral blood and bone marrow smears. Criteria for classification of MDS into subtypes is presented in a later section of this chapter. Included here are the general hematologic features used to initially define the presence of an MDS (Table 23-1 ✪).

PERIPHERAL BLOOD

The peripheral blood characteristics of MDS are cytopenias and dysplasia. Findings include anemia, neutropenia, and thrombocytopenia. Anemia is the most consistent finding, which occurs as an isolated cytopenia in 35% of the cases.

✪ TABLE 23-1			
Hematologic Abnormalities in Myelodysplastic Syndromes			
Findings	Erythroid Series	Myeloid Series	Thrombocyte Series
Peripheral blood	Anemia; macrocytes; oval macrocytes; dimorphism; basophilic stippling; nucleated RBC; Howell-Jolly bodies; sideroblasts; anisocytosis; poikilocytosis; reticulocytopenia	Neutropenia; hypogranulation; abnormal granulation; shift to the left; nuclear abnormalities including pseudo–Pelger-Huët and ring nuclei, monocytosis	Thrombocytopenia, or thrombocytosis; giant forms; hypogranulation; micromegakaryocytes; functional abnormalities
Bone marrow	Megaloblastoid erythropoiesis; nuclear fragmentation and budding; karyorrhexis; multiple nuclei; defective hemoglobinization; vacuolization; ringed sideroblasts	Abnormal granules in promyelocytes; increase in Type I and Type II blasts; absence of secondary granules; nuclear abnormalities; decreased myeloperoxidase; Auer rods in blasts	Micromegakaryocytes; megakaryocytes with multiple, separated nuclei; large mononuclear megakaryocytes; hypogranulation or large abnormal granules in megakaryocytes

Bicytopenia occurs in 30% of the cases and pancytopenia in 19%.[24] Less commonly, an isolated neutropenia or thrombocytopenia is found. Dysplastic features of one or more cell lines are typical. Because of the critical importance of recognizing dysplasia in the diagnosis of MDS, smears should be made from samples that have been anticoagulated two hours or less.[25] Morphologic changes due to prolonged exposure to anticoagulant can easily be confused with dysplastic changes in cells. Functional abnormalities of hematologic cells are also common.[26] Studies show that the higher the degree and number of cytopenias, the worse is the prognosis.[27]

Erythrocytes

The degree of anemia is variable, but the hemoglobin is generally <10 g/dL. The erythrocytes are usually macrocytic (Figure 23-1■) and less often normocytic. Oval macrocytes similar to those in megaloblastic anemia are frequently present, but patients have normal vitamin B_{12} and folate levels. A dimorphic anemia with both oval macrocytes or normocytes and microcytic hypochromic cells is also a common initial finding in the refractory anemia with ringed sideroblasts (RARS) subgroup. Reticulocytes show an absolute decrease in number but can appear normal if only the uncorrected or relative number (percent) is reported. In addition to anemia, qualitative abnormalities indicative of dyserythropoiesis are present. These include anisocytosis, poikilocytosis, basophilic stippling, Howell-Jolly bodies, and nucleated erythrocytes. Often hemoglobin F is increased (5–6%) and distributed in a heterogeneous pattern. Acquired hemoglobin H has also been found in MDS.[12] Other erythrocyte changes include altered A, B, and I antigens, enzyme changes, and an acquired erythrocyte membrane change similar but not identical to that found in paroxysmal nocturnal hemoglobinuria (PNH)[4,12](∞ Chapter 15).

Leukocytes

Neutropenia is the second most common cytopenia observed in MDS. Neutropenia can be accompanied by a shift to the left with the finding of metamyelocytes and myelocytes on the peripheral blood smear. Blasts and promyelocytes can also be present.

Morphologic abnormalities in granulocytes indicative of dysgranulopoiesis are considered a hallmark finding in MDS. Dysgranulopoiesis is characterized by agranular or hypogranular neutrophils, persistent basophilia of the cytoplasm, abnormal appearing granules, hyposegmentation (pseudo–Pelger-Huët) (Figure 23-2■) or hypersegmentation of the nucleus and donut- or ring-shaped nuclei. Care should be taken to distinguish neutrophils with the pseudo–Pelger-Huët anomaly and hypogranulation from lymphocytes and to distinguish neutrophilic-band forms with hypogranulation from monocytes. Neutrophils also can demonstrate enzyme defects, such as decreased myeloperoxidase (MPO) and decreased leukocyte alkaline phosphatase (LAP). In some cases, neutrophils exhibit severe functional impairment, including defective bactericidal, phagocytic, or chemotactic properties. Absolute monocytosis is a common finding even in leukopenic conditions.

Platelets

Qualitative and quantitative platelet abnormalities are often present. The platelet count can be normal, increased, or decreased. Approximately 25% of patients have mild to moderate thrombocytopenia when diagnosed.[12] Giant platelets, hypogranular platelets, and platelets with large fused granules can be seen in the peripheral blood (Figures 23-3■ and 23-4■). Functional platelet abnormalities include abnormal adhesion and aggregation. As a result, platelet function tests can be abnormal.

Micromegakaryocytes

Sometimes circulating **micromegakaryocytes** (small abnormal megakaryocytes), also called *dwarf megakaryocytes*,

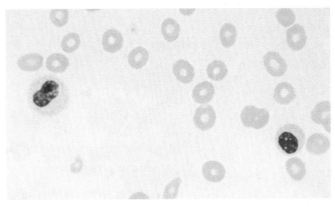

■ FIGURE 23-2   Peripheral blood film from a patient with MDS showing neutrophils with the pseudo–Pelger-Huët nucleus. One cell's nucleus is peanut shaped and the other is single lobed. The nuclear chromatin is condensed, and the cells contain granules, making identification possible. In many cases, these types of neutrophils are agranular, making differentiation of them from lymphocytes difficult. (Peripheral blood; Wright-Giemsa stain; 1000× magnification)

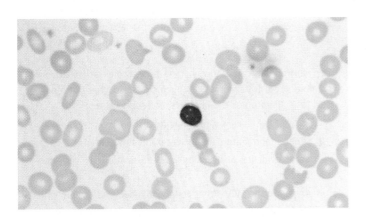

■ FIGURE 23-1   A peripheral blood film of a patient with MDS. Note macrocytic cells, and anisocytosis. (Peripheral blood; Wright-Giemsa stain; 1000× magnification)

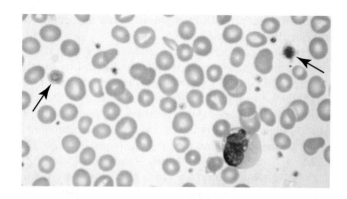

■ FIGURE 23-3   A peripheral blood film from a patient with MDS showing large platelets. (Wright-Giemsa stain; 1000× magnification)

can be found in the MDS and myeloproliferative syndromes. Micromegakaryocytes can be difficult to identify and are frequently overlooked unless cytoplasmic tags or blebs are present (Figure 23-5 ■). Micromegakaryocytes are believed to represent abnormal megakaryocytes that have reduced ability to undergo **endomitosis**. (Megakaryocytes undergo a unique maturation process whereby the DNA content duplicates without cell division, resulting in a polyploid nucleus [endomitosis]) (∞ Chapter 29). Most micromegakaryocytes have a single-lobed nucleus and are the size of a lymphocyte. Morphologically, they can be confused with lymphocytes but can be distinguished by cytoplasmic tags of one or more platelets attached to a nucleus. Some can have pale blue, foamy, or vacuolated cytoplasm that resembles a nongranular platelet. The nuclear structure is variable, but many cells have very densely clumped chromatin and stain dark blue-black with Wright-Giemsa stain. Others can have a finer, looser chromatin. These cells are also found in the bone marrow.

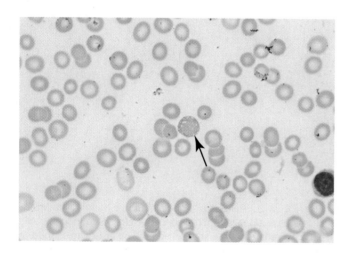

■ FIGURE 23-4   Peripheral blood from a patient with MDS showing large agranular platelet. (Wright-Giemsa stain; 1000× magnification)

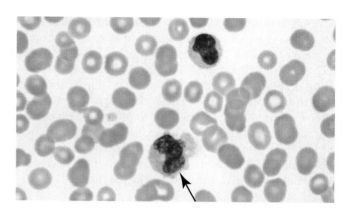

■ FIGURE 23-5   Micromegakaryocyte in peripheral blood film from a patient with MDS. Note the dense chromatin structure and the irregular rim of cytoplasm with cytoplasmic tags. An agranular platelet in the field matches the appearance of the micromegakaryocyte cytoplasm. (Wright-Giemsa stain; 1000× magnification)

✓ Checkpoint! 1

How does the typical peripheral blood picture in MDS differ from that in aplastic anemia? (∞ Chapter 13)

ⒸCASE STUDY (continued from page 482)

The results of the CBC on Hancock were:

RBC	1.60×10^{12}/L	Differential
Hb	5.8 g/dL (58 g/L)	44% segmented
Hct	0.17 L/L	neutrophils
WBC	10.5×10^9/L	7% band
Platelets	39×10^9/L	neutrophils
Reticulocyte count	0.8%	6% lymphocytes
		28% eosinophils
		1% metamyelocytes
		1% myelocytes
		9% promyelocytes
		4% blasts

The neutrophilic cells show marked hyposegmentation and hypogranulation. RBC morphology includes anisocytosis and poikilocytosis, teardrop cells, ovalocytes, and schistocytes.

1. In what cell lines is cytopenia present?
2. What abnormalities are present in the differential?
3. What evidence of dyspoiesis is seen in the leukocyte morphology?
4. Calculate the MCV. What peripheral blood findings are helpful to rule out megaloblastic anemia?
5. What features of the differential resemble CML? What helps to distinguish this case from CML?

BONE MARROW

Bone marrow examination is necessary to identify the dyshematopoietic element, to determine cellularity, and to establish a diagnosis. In most cases, the bone marrow is hypercellular with erythroid hyperplasia, although normocellular and hypocellular marrows can occur. The hypercellular bone marrow with a peripheral blood picture of cytopenia is the result of premature cell loss in the marrow (increased apoptosis and ineffective hematopoiesis).[12] The cellularity of the marrow should be interpreted in relation to the patient's age because MDS is commonly found in the elderly. The number of myeloblasts can range from normal to 19% (promonocytes, erythroblasts, promyelocytes, and megakaryoblasts are not included in the blast count). Generally, all cell lines exhibit evidence of dyshematopoiesis.

Bone marrow trephine biopsy can be helpful in establishing the diagnosis of MDS in difficult cases.[28] (Trephine biopsy is the removal of a disc of bone using a cylindrical saw.) Abnormal localization of immature myeloid precursors (ALIP) clustering centrally can be seen in biopsy before an increase in myeloblasts is detected in bone marrow smears.[29] ALIP has been shown to indicate increased risk for transformation to leukemia and is associated with poor survival. In patients with less than 5% blasts, ALIP can indicate evolution to a more aggressive disease. However, these claims have not been validated in large studies.[4] A biopsy also gives a better assessment of cellularity and an indication of the amount of reticulin fibers present. On the other hand, ringed sideroblasts, nuclear fragmentation and budding, Auer rods, irregular cytoplasmic basophilia, and abnormal staining of primary granules in promyelocytes are more easily identified in bone marrow aspirate smears. Thus, both aspirate smears and biopsy preparations are necessary for accurate diagnosis.

Dyserythropoiesis

The most common bone marrow finding in MDS is nuclear-cytoplasmic asynchrony similar to that seen in megaloblastic anemia (∞ Chapter 12). However, the chromatin is usually hypercondensed. This nuclear chromatin pattern is often described as megaloblastoid (Figure 23-6 ■). The abnormal erythrocytic maturation is not responsive to vitamin B_{12} or folic acid therapy. Giant, multinucleated erythroid precursors can be found (Figure 23-7 ■). Other nuclear abnormalities include fragmentation, abnormal shape, budding, karryohexis, and irregular staining properties. The cytoplasm of erythroid precursors can show defective hemoglobinization, vacuoles, and basophilic stippling. The presence of ringed sideroblasts, reflecting the abnormal erythrocyte metabolism, is a common finding. **Ringed sideroblasts** are defined as erythroblasts in which mitochondrial iron deposits encircle at least one-third or more of the nucleus.

Dysgranulopoiesis

Granulopoiesis is usually normal to increased unless the overall marrow is hypocellular. Abnormal granulocyte matu-

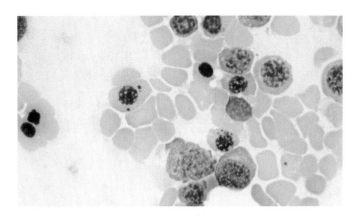

■ FIGURE 23-6   Megaloblastoid erythroblasts in the bone marrow of a patient with MDS. Note the condensed chromatin and Howell-Jolly bodies. (Wright-Giemsa stain; 1000× magnification)

ration (dysgranulopoiesis), however, is almost always present (Figure 23-8 ■). One of the major findings of dysgranulopoiesis in the bone marrow is abnormal staining of the primary granules in promyelocytes and myelocytes. Sometimes the granules are larger than normal and at other times are absent. Secondary granules can be absent in myelocytes and other more mature neutrophils, giving rise to the hypogranular peripheral blood neutrophils. Irregular cytoplasmic basophilia with a dense rim of peripheral basophilia is also characteristic. Nuclear abnormalities similar to those found in the peripheral blood granulocytes can be present in bone marrow granulocytes.

Dysmegakaryopoiesis

Megakaryocytes can be decreased, normal, or increased. The presence of micromegakaryocytes, large mononuclear megakaryocytes, and megakaryocytes with other abnormal

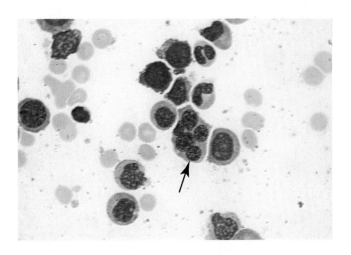

■ FIGURE 23-7   Multinucleated polychromatophilic erythroblast in the bone marrow of a patient with MDS. It is also megaloblastoid. (Wright-Giemsa stain; 1000× magnification)

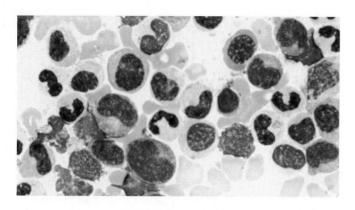

■ FIGURE 23-8   Bone marrow from a patient with MDS. Note the metamyelocytes and bands with a lack of secondary granules. The bands have light bluish-pink cytoplasm, and the metamyelocytes have a darker bluish cytoplasm. (Wright-Giemsa stain; 1000× magnification)

nuclear configurations (Figure 23-9 ■) reflect abnormalities in maturation. The lack of granules or presence of giant abnormal granules is also characteristic.

OTHER LABORATORY FINDINGS

Serum iron is normal or increased, and the TIBC is normal or decreased, distinguishing MDS from IDA (iron-deficiency anemia). Cobalamin (vitamin B_{12}) and folic acid levels are normal to increased, a feature that helps to differentiate MDS with megaloblastoid features from megaloblastic anemias with the typical megaloblastic features.

Immunologic analysis has revealed that MDS is associated with a significant decrease in the total number of T lymphocytes and a decrease in both CD4 and CD8 lymphocyte sub-

sets.[30] The responses of T lymphocytes to mitogens, Phyto-hemaglutinin A, and Concanavalin A can be significantly decreased. Although B lymphocytes are quantitatively normal, serum immunologlubulins are often increased, and circulating immune complexes are frequently present. In addition, granulocytic oxidative metabolism as measured by the nitroblue tetrazolium reduction test can be abnormal and chemotaxis impaired.

 Checkpoint! 2

Why is serum vitamin B_{12}, serum folate level, or bone marrow iron stain important in the diagnosis of MDS?

 CASE STUDY *(continued from page 486)*

A bone marrow was performed on Hancock. The marrow showed a cellularity of about 75%. There was myeloid hyperplasia with 9% blasts, 26% promyelocytes, 18% myelocytes, 6% metamyelocytes, 4% bands, and 37% eosinophils. The M:E ratio was 12:1. The myelocytes were hypogranular, and some had two nuclei. The erythroid precursors showed megaloblastoid changes. Megakaryocytes were adequate in number but showed abnormal forms with nuclear separation and single nucleated forms.

6. Which of the hematopoietic cell lines exhibit dyshematopoiesis in the bone marrow?

7. How would you classify the bone marrow cellularity?

8. What does the M:E ratio indicate?

9. Identify at least two features of the bone marrow that are compatible with a diagnosis of MDS.

10. What chemistry tests would be helpful to rule out megaloblastic anemia?

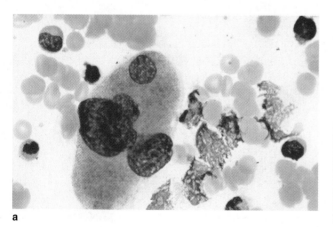

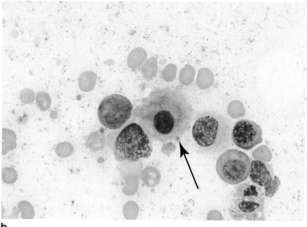

a   b

■ FIGURE 23-9   **a.** Abnormal megakaryocyte from a patient with MDS. **b.** Micromegakaryocyte in the bone marrow of a patient with MDS. Note the megaloblastoid features of the surrounding cells. (Both: Bone marrow; Wright-Giemsa stain; 1000× magnification)

► BLAST CELL CLASSIFICATION

The blast count appears to be the most important prognostic indicator of survival and progression to acute leukemia in MDS. The maximum number of blasts compatible with a diagnosis of MDS is 19% (<30% in the FAB classification; see below). The minimum criterion for a diagnosis of acute leukemia is at least 20% blasts (>30% in the FAB classification). In MDS, correctly identifying blasts and type and degree of dysplasia is important because these characteristics are the basis of classifying subtypes and differentiating them from AML. Experts recommend performing a 200-cell differential on peripheral blood and identifying at least 500 cells in the bone marrow.[25]

MORPHOLOGIC IDENTIFICATION OF BLASTS

The dysgranulopoiesis that affects primary azurophilic granules in neoplastic blasts changes the standard criteria for identification and classification of blast cells and promyelocytes. The standard criteria for a blast cell include a cell with a central nucleus with fine nuclear chromatin, prominent nucleoli, a high nuclear:cytoplasmic ratio, and deeply basophilic and agranular cytoplasm. It is now recognized that in MDS and acute leukemia, there are some blast-like cells that contain primary azurophilic granules. These early azurophilic granules do not indicate differentiation but abnormal neoplastic cells.[31] Consequently, two types of blasts that could be found in the bone marrow and peripheral blood in MDS and AML were recognized: Type I and Type II. More recently, it has been suggested to recognize a third type of blast cell (Type III) in MDS to improve predictions of progression to acute leukemia and survival.[31] Typical agranular blasts are included in the Type I category. Type II and Type III blasts have typical blast features except that they contain primary azurophilic granules. The following morphologic criteria have been established for identifying Type I blasts, Type II blasts, Type III blasts, and promyelocytes in MDS and acute leukemia.[31]

Type I Blasts
The Type I blast cells (Figure 23-10a ■) include typical myeloblasts and unclassifiable cells. The nuclear chromatin is finely dispersed with prominent nucleoli. The nuclear cytoplasmic ratio is variable but is higher in the smaller blasts than the larger ones. The cytoplasm contains no granules.

Type II Blasts
Type II blast cells (Figure 23-10b ■) resemble Type I blasts except that the cytoplasm contains primary granules (fewer than 20) and the nucleus is in a more central position. The nuclear cytoplasmic ratio tends to be lower than that of Type I blasts.

Type III Blasts
These cells are similar to Type II blasts except that they contain more than 20 granules in the cytoplasm (Figure 23-10c ■).

Promyelocytes
The nucleus is eccentrically placed, and the chromatin pattern is more condensed. The Golgi apparatus is obvious as a clear area adjacent to the nucleus. The nuclear cytoplasmic ratio is lower due to the increase in cytoplasm. Many primary granules are present. In some MDS cases the promyelocyte appears hypogranular or even agranular. In these cases, the abnormal cell can be identified as a promyelocyte by the other nuclear and cytoplasmic criteria. If the azurophilic granules are clumped and heterogeneous in size, the promyelocyte is classified as abnormal.

Using these criteria for distinguishing blasts and promyelocytes, the minimum criteria for a diagnosis of acute leukemia is 20% blasts including any combination of Type I, Type II, and Type III blasts (exclusive of promyelocytes) in the bone marrow. The maximum proportion of blasts compatible with a diagnosis of MDS is 19% including any combination of Type I, Type II, and Type III blasts. Often the blast count in the blood is higher than that in the marrow. It has been suggested that when the blast count exceeds 19% in the blood but the bone marrow concentration is less than 19%, the case should be regarded as acute leukemia. With the exception of subgroup RAEB-2 (refractory anemia with excess blasts, subgroup 2), the blasts in MDS usually do not have Auer rods present.

✓ Checkpoint! 3

Why is it important to correctly identify the number of blasts when evaluating the peripheral blood or bone marrow smear of a patient suspected of having MDS?

CYTOCHEMICAL AND IMMUNOLOGICAL IDENTIFICATION OF BLASTS

Although the blast cells in MDS are derived primarily from myeloid or monocytic precursors, a panel of cytochemical and immunocytochemical reactions should be performed and interpreted to enhance the accuracy of diagnosis[32] (∞ Chapters 21, 34, 37). Cytochemical stains help to identify the origin of atypical and bizarre dyspoietic cells that are often seen in MDS.[4] Peroxidase and Sudan black B identify blasts with a myeloid origin; however, in MDS, the blasts can have lower peroxidase activity than normal blasts. Combined esterase stains can be performed on both peripheral blood and bone marrow for a more accurate assessment of monocytic cells. Iron stain can reveal abnormal iron metabolism in erythroblasts with the presence of increased iron stores and ringed sideroblasts. The presence of blocks of PAS-positive material in erythrocyte precursors indicates abnormal carbohydrate metabolism. Abnormal small megakaryoblasts can be difficult to

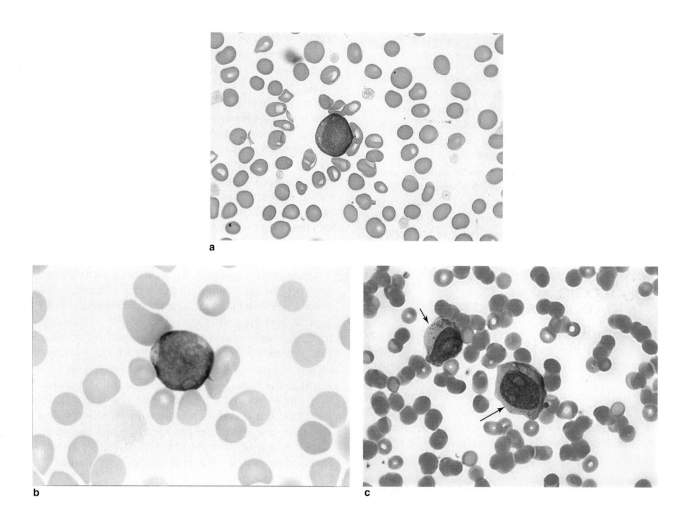

■ FIGURE 23-10   **a.** Type I myeloblast. **b.** Type II myeloblast with <20 granules in the cytoplasm. **c.** Type III myeloblasts with >20 granules. (Both: Peripheral blood; Wright-Giemsa stain; 1000× magnification)

distinguish from lymphoblasts or Type I myeloblasts. They can be readily identified, however, by immunochemistry with antibodies against platelet-specific glycoproteins IIb/IIIa (CD41), GPIIIa (CD61) or by antibody against factor VIII in histiologic sections. Diaminobenzidine can be utilized to identify platelet peroxidase in electron micrographs.[32]

Immunophenotyping is being used increasingly to aid in diagnosis and prognosis of MDS patients.[33] Immunophenotyping is most useful when marrow morphology and cytogenetics are inconclusive and to distinguish MDS cases with a hypoplastic bone marrow from other bone marrow failure disorders, such as aplastic anemia.[34] It has been suggested that increased expression of markers found on immature myeloid cells such as CD13, CD33, CD34, and HLA-DR and decreased expression of NAT-9 (found on mature myeloid cells) can be associated with a worse prognosis and with progression to AML.[34–36] MDS patients with a low percentage of bone marrow cells expressing CD11b had a higher risk of evolution to AML and shorter survival compared to patients with more than 53% of marrow cells expressing CD11b.[36]

CD7-positivity also has been associated with short survival in MDS patients.[37] Standardization of methods so that comparable results are obtained by different laboratories must be achieved before surface marker studies can be more fully utilized as diagnostic tools in MDS.[36,37]

Immunological phenotyping using monoclonal antibodies can be useful in identifying the lineage of blasts in those cases of acute leukemia derived from therapy-related MDS. Many of these cases show trilineage dysplasia and are difficult to define by morphology and cytogenetics.[38] The specific cellular markers found on different cell lineages in acute leukemia are described in ∞ Chapters 24, 25, 37.

► CLASSIFICATION

In 1982, the French-American-British (FAB) group proposed a classification scheme for the myelodysplastic syndromes.[39] This classification defined five subgroups based on morphological characteristics, such as the blast count and degree of dyspoiesis in the peripheral blood and bone marrow. The five subgroups included:

- Refractory anemia (RA)
- Refractory anemia with ringed sideroblasts (RARS)
- Refractory anemia with excess blasts (RAEB)
- Chronic myelomonocytic leukemia (CMML)
- Refractory anemia with excess blasts in transformation (RAEB-t)

Specific criteria for each FAB subgroup are shown in Table 23-2 ✪.

Although the FAB classification system has been the benchmark for diagnosing the MDS for the past two decades, it does not incorporate the newer diagnostic technologies such as cytogenetics and immunophenotyping.[2,3] In 2001, the World Health Organization (WHO) published a new classification system developed by a group of American and European pathologists, hematologists, and oncologists. This new system incorporates morphology, immunophenotype, and genetics with clinical and prognostic features into a classification of all neoplastic diseases of the hematopoietic and lymphoid tissues (∞ Chapter 21). This resulted in significant changes in the classification of the MDS.[3]

The WHO Classification System criteria for each subgroup of MDS are shown in Table 23-3 ✪. Chronic myelomonocytic leukemia (CMML) was removed from the MDS group of diseases and placed in a newly created category, **myelodysplastic/myeloproliferative diseases (MDS/MPD)** because it has features of both MDS and MPD. RAEB-t was eliminated due to lowering the blast count necessary for a diagnosis of AML from 30% to 20%. It was believed that patients with 20–29% blasts have a prognosis similar to that of patients with ≥30% blasts. Three new categories were added to the WHO classification of MDS: refractory cytopenia with multilineage dysplasia (RCMD), 5q–syndrome, and MDS unclassified (MDS-U). RCMD was created for cases of MDS with less than 5% blasts that have significant dysplasia involving granulocytic and/or megakaryocytic lineages as well as erythrocytic. Recent studies have shown that these cases are more likely to result in death due to bone marrow failure or to progress to acute leukemia than other cases that do not have these distinct features. This category also helps to distinguish these cases from RA and RARS, which typically involve dysplasia in only the erythroid lineage.

Recent studies to evaluate the clinical usefulness of the WHO classification conclude that it clearly identifies more homogenous subgroups and enables clinicians to select the best treatments and better predict prognosis and clinical responses.[2,4,5] Although at this time both classification systems can be found in clinical practice, most clinicians are adopting the WHO classification system, and it will be followed in this chapter.

▶ DESCRIPTION OF SUBGROUPS OF MDS

The WHO Classification System identifies six MDS subgroups:

- Refractory anemia (RA)
- Refractory anemia with ringed sideroblasts (RARS)
- Refractory cytopenia with multilineage dysplasia (RCMD)
- Refractory anemia with excess blasts (RAEB)
- MDS associated with isolated del(5q–)
- Myelodysplastic syndrome, unclassified (MDS-U)

REFRACTORY ANEMIA

Refractory anemia (RA) occurs with anemia as the primary clinical finding. The anemia is refractory (nonresponsive) to all conventional forms of therapy. Erythrocytes usually appear macrocytic but occasionally are microcytic or normocytic. The peripheral blood shows reticulocytopenia and signs of dyserythropoiesis, but leukocytes and platelets are usually quantitatively and qualitatively normal. Blast cells are usually absent in the peripheral blood, but, if present, they constitute less than 1% of the nucleated cells.

✪ TABLE 23-2

Differentiating Characteristics of FAB Subtypes of Myelodysplastic Syndromes					
Characteristic	RA	RARS	CMML	RAEB	RAEB-t
Blasts in PB (%)	<1	<1	<5	<5	≥5
Blasts in BM (%)	<5	<5	≤20	5–20	21–30 and/or Auer rods
Ringed sideroblasts (%)	<15	≥15	Variable	Variable	Variable
Monos in PB	—	—	>1 × 10^9/L	—	—
Monos in BM	—	—	≥20%	—	—

RA = refractory anemia; RARS = refractory anemia with ringed sideroblasts; CMML = chronic myelomonocytic leukemia; RAEB = refractory anemia with excess blasts; RAEB-t = refractory anemia with excess blasts in transformation; PB = peripheral blood; BM = bone marrow; monos = monocytes or immature cells of monocytic origin

(Adapted, with permission, from Greer JP, et al. *Wintrobe's Clinical Hematology*, 11th ed., Philadelphia: Lippincott, Williams and Wilkins, 2004; p. 2208.)

⊘ TABLE 23-3

World Health Organization Classification Criteria for Myelodysplastic Syndromes

Classification	Peripheral Blood	Bone Marrow
Refractory anemia (RA)	Anemia Rare or no blasts (<1%)	Erythroid dysplasia only <5% blasts <15% ringed sideroblasts
Refractory anemia with ringed sideroblasts (RARS)	Anemia Rare or no blasts (<1%)	>15% ringed sideroblasts Erythroid dysplasia only <5% blasts
Refractory cytopenia with multilineage dysplasia (RCMD)	Cytopenias (bicytopenia or pancytopenia) Rare or no blasts No Auer rods <1 × 10^9/L monocytes	Dysplasia in >10% of the cells of two or more myeloid lineages <5% blasts in marrow No Auer rods <15% ringed sideroblasts
Refractory cytopenia with multilineage dysplasia and ringed sideroblasts (RCMD-RS)	Cytopenias (bicytopenia or pancytopenia) Rare or no blasts No Auer rods <1 × 10^9/L monocytes	Dysplasia in >10% of the cells of two or more myeloid lineages <5% blasts in marrow >15% ringed sideroblasts No Auer rods
Refractory anemia with excess blasts 1	Cytopenias <5% blasts No Auer rods <1 × 10^9/L monocytes	Unilineage or multilineage dysplasia 5–9% blasts No Auer rods
Refractory anemia with excess blasts 2	Cytopenias 5–19% blasts Auer rods present <1 × 10^9/L monocytes	Unilineage or multilineage dysplasia 10–19% blasts Auer rods present
5q–syndrome	Anemia Usually normal or increased platelet count <5% blasts	Normal to increased mega karyocytes with hypolobulated nuclei <5% blasts Isolated del(5q–) cytogenetic abnormality No Auer rods
Myelodysplastic syndrome, unclassified	Cytopenias Rare or no blasts No Auer rods	Unilineage dysplasia: one myeloid cell line <5% blasts No Auer rods

(Adapted, with permission, from Greer JP, et al. *Wintrobe's Clinical Hematology*, 11th ed., Philadelphia: Lippincott, Williams and Wilkins, 2004; p. 2208.)

The bone marrow is hypercellular with erythroid hyperplasia and signs of dyserythropoiesis. Megaloblastoid erythropoiesis is present but unresponsive to folic acid or cobalamin. Ringed sideroblasts are absent or present in low numbers (<15% of erythroblasts). Maturation of neutrophils and megakaryocytes is generally normal. Blast cells compose less than 5% of marrow cells.

Cytogenetic abnormalities are useful in diagnosis and can be observed in up to 25% of cases. However, no specific abnormality is associated with this subgroup. Approximately 6% of cases progress to acute leukemia.[25]

REFRACTORY ANEMIA WITH RINGED SIDEROBLASTS

Refractory anemia with ringed sideroblasts (RARS), or acquired idiopathic sideroblastic anemia (AISA), is similar to RA except that ringed sideroblasts account for more than

15% of the erythroid precursor cells in the bone marrow. The anemia is usually macrocytic but is less often normocytic. Sometimes evidence of a dual population of normochromic and hypochromic cells exists. The peripheral blood shows reticulocytopenia and often leukopenia. The occurrence of leukopenia in one study was 33% with neutropenia occuring in 7%.[24] The platelet count occasionally is increased. A few cases exhibit granulocyte and platelet morphologic abnormalities.

The bone marrow is hypercellular with megaloblastoid dyserythropoiesis. If dysgranulopoiesis and dysmegakaryopoiesis are present, it is mild. Fewer than 5% blast cells are in the marrow. Chromosomal abnormalities are seen in less than 10% of cases. Approximately 1–2 % of cases evolve into AML. Secondary causes of ringed sideroblasts, such as exposure to toxic substances, certain drugs, and alcoholism should be ruled out.[25]

REFRACTORY CYTOPENIA WITH MULTILINEAGE DYSPLASIA

Refractory cytopenia with multilineage dysplasia (RCMD) is a new category established in the WHO classification system for patients with dysplastic features in at least 10% of the cells in two or more cell lines, less than 5% blasts in the bone marrow, and less than 1% blasts in the peripheral blood. Studies have shown that these individuals have a worse prognosis than those with dysplasia in only one cell line and thus a new subgroup was needed.[3] They usually display cytopenias in two or more cell lines and have less than 1×10^9/L monocytes present in the peripheral blood. Ringed sideroblasts must compose less than 15% of the nucleated red blood cells in the marrow. If more than 15% ringed sideroblasts are present, the case is categorized as **refractory cytopenia with multilineage dysplasia and ringed sideroblasts (RCMD-RS)**.[25] Chromosomal abnormalities can be present in up to 50% of cases in this category, some being complex. The frequency of evolution to AML is approximately 11%.[25]

REFRACTORY ANEMIA WITH EXCESS BLASTS

In **refractory anemia with excess blasts (RAEB)**, cytopenia occurs in at least two lineages and conspicuous qualitative abnormalities in all three lineages. The anemia is normocytic or slightly macrocytic with reticulocytopenia. Evidence of dysgranulopoiesis is prominent. The peripheral blood has 0–19% blasts. Monocytosis without leukocytosis can be present, but the absolute monocyte count does not exceed 1×10^9/L, and serum and urinary lysozyme levels are normal. Platelet abnormalities include giant forms, abnormal granularity, and functional aberrations. Sometimes, circulating micromegakaryocytes can be found.

The bone marrow is hypercellular but less often is normocellular with varying degrees of granulocytic and erythrocytic hyperplasia. All three lineages show signs of dyshematopoiesis. The proportion of blasts varies from 5% to 19%. Abnormal promyelocytes can be present. These abnormal cells have blastlike nuclei with nucleoli and no chromatin condensation, and the cytoplasm contains large bizarre granules. Ringed sideroblasts may be increased, but the elevated blast count differentiates RAEB from RARS. In some cases, differentiating RAEB from acute leukemia is difficult. Serial examinations are sometimes necessary to make an accurate diagnosis.

A difference in survival for patients having 5–9% blasts and those having 10–19% blasts has been shown. Those with more than 9% blasts have a worse outcome. The separation of these two groups into RAEB-1 (5–9% blasts in bone marrow, <5% blasts in the peripheral blood) and RAEB-2 (10–19% blasts in the bone marrow, 5–19% blasts in the peripheral blood) provides a more accurate prognostic classification.[25,31] Cases with 5–19% blasts in the peripheral blood and <10% blasts in the bone marrow are also placed in RAEB-2.[25]

Between 30–50% of cases show cytogenetic abnormalities, some complex. Immunophenotyping reveals that blasts express one or more myeloid antigens (CD13, CD33, CD117). Approximately 25% of RAEB-1 and 33% of RAEB-2 progress to AML.[25]

THE 5q-SYNDROME

MDS patients with an isolated deletion of the long arm of chromosome 5 (del 5q or 5q–) and no other chromosomal abnormalities appear to have a unique disease course characterized by a favorable prognosis and low risk of transformation into AML. Women have a marked predominance of cases (70%), and the mean age at presentation is 66 years. The main features are macrocytic anemia, moderate leukopenia, normal to increased platelet count, hypolobulated megakaryocytes, and less than 5% blasts in the peripheral blood and bone marrow.[25] The bone marrow is usually hypercellular or normocellular with normal to increased megakaryocytes, some with hyperlobulated nuclei.[25] A number of genes coding for hematopoietic growth factors and their receptors are localized on the long arm of chromosome 5. It has been suggested that loss of these genes and/or tumor suppressor genes may be involved in the pathogenesis of this disease.[11,40]

MDS, UNCLASSIFIABLE (MDS-U)

When the MDS does not fit any of the defined WHO subgroups, it is placed in this category. Blasts in the blood and bone marrow are not increased, and there are no specific morphological findings. Usually neutropenia or thrombocytopenia is seen. Dysplastic cells can be found in either the neutrophilic or megakaryocytic lineages and can be severe. The bone marrow is usually hypercellular but can be normocellular or rarely hypocellular. No specific cytogenetic findings are present. Cases demonstrating unilineage dysplasia in the granulocytic or megakaryocytic lineages are rare but would be placed in this category.[25]

 CASE STUDY *(continued from page 488)*

Review Hancock's peripheral blood and bone marrow features previously identified.

11. What is the most likely MDS subgroup? Based on what criteria?

▶ VARIANTS OF MDS

A number of patients have blood and/or marrow findings that cause problems in diagnosis and/or classification. Some of these findings occur often enough to consider them as variants of MDS.

HYPOPLASTIC MDS

Although most cases of MDS are associated with hypercellular or normocellular bone marrows, about 10% have hypocellular marrows. In these cases, trephine biopsy is necessary to exclude a diagnosis of aplastic anemia or hypoplastic acute myeloid leukemia (AML). This distinction is important because the diagnosis has an influence on treatment and prognosis.

Hypocellular MDS should be considered when the bone marrow cellularity is less than 30% or less than 20% in patients over 60 years of age.[41] The criteria for MDS must be met in hypoplastic cases as well as the hypercellular or normocellular cases. Dysplasia can be difficult to identify, and dyserythropoiesis has been described in aplastic anemia. Dysmegakaryopoiesis and dysgranulopoiesis, however, are most characteristic of MDS and can be helpful findings. In addition, ALIP, indicating an abnormal bone marrow architecture, is typical of MDS. If present, chromosomal abnormalities help distinguish MDS from aplastic anemia. The distinction of MDS from AML can be made based on the blast count. A count over 19% indicates AML. Although the pathophysiology of hypoplastic MDS is unknown, secretion of inhibitory cytokines by autoreactive or clonal-involved T-cells is believed to suppress normal hematopoiesis.[20]

MDS WITH FIBROSIS

Mild to moderate fibrosis has been described in up to 50% of patients with MDS; marked fibrosis can be seen in 10–15% of cases.[42] The incidence of fibrosis appears to be even higher in

therapy-related MDS. If fibrosis is present, other diagnoses including chronic idiopathic myelofibrosis (CIMF) (∞ Chapter 22), chronic myelogenous leukemia (∞ Chapter 22), and acute megakaryoblastic leukemia (∞ Chapter 24) should be considered and excluded. MDS patients with fibrosis typically have pancytopenia, hypocellular bone marrow with fibrosis, trilineage dysplasia, small megakaryocytes with hypolobulated nuclei, and the absence of hepatomegaly and prominent splenomegaly.[11,43] The increased fibrosis is thought to be produced by liberation of cytokines such as transforming growth factor-β (TGF-β) and platelet-derived growth factor (PDGF) from dysplastic megakaryocytes.[12]

THERAPY-RELATED MYELODYSPLASIA

Myelodysplasia secondary to alkylating chemotherapy and/or radiotherapy for other malignant or nonmalignant diseases is frequently referred to as *therapy-related* or *treatment-related MDS* (*t-MDS*). It should be kept in mind, however, that MDS can develop as a second primary disorder unrelated to therapy, especially if MDS develops a very short or a very long time after therapy.

A study of 65 patients with t-MDS or acute leukemia suggests that panmyelosis related to therapy develops in three stages: (1) pancytopenia with myelodysplastic changes and less than 5% blasts, (2) frank MDS, which resembles RAEB, and (3) overt AML.[38] Not all stages are found in all patients; some present with overt AML, but others expire from infection, hemorrhage, or other disease before developing MDS or AML. Development of MDS or acute leukemia appears to be related to the duration, amount, and repetition of the therapy as well as the patient's age.

The highest incidence of t-MDS occurs 3–8 years after treatment, and long-term use of DNA alkylating agents appears to present the highest risk.[4,20] Currently, there is no way to predict which patients will develop MDS after treatment; therefore, posttherapy monitoring is not recommended.[4]

t-MDS tends to have a younger age of onset, an increased frequency and severity of thrombocytopenia, and a higher percentage of patients presenting with RAEB than does primary MDS.[9] In most cases, the qualitative changes are marked with trilineage involvement, typical of RAEB. The number of blasts, however, is usually less than 5%, typical of RA. Despite the low percentage of blasts, the clinical course of the disease reflects profound marrow failure, and the outcome is very unfavorable (a median survival of 4–6 months).[38] About 25% of patients have blast counts of 5–19%, which with the marked qualitative changes in all cell lines, qualify for the RAEB classification. The bone marrow is most often hypercellular or normocellular. The finding of increased megakaryocytes is associated with increased fibrosis. Complex karyotypes are present in the majority of t-MDS cases. Similar to primary MDS, about 30% of t-MDS evolve to acute leukemia.[38]

CHILDHOOD MDS

Few cases of MDS in children have been reported. This may be due to the lack of a widely accepted classification system and clear diagnostic criteria. Both the FAB and WHO classification systems are based on review of adult cases. A new classification system that allows for the special problems of diagnosis in children and based on WHO criteria has been recently proposed.[22] Dysplasia in children with MDS is less pronounced, and the more aggressive subtype (RAEB) predominates; progression to acute leukemia is faster than in adults.[21] Age of 2 years or less and a hemoglobin F level of 10% or higher are associated with a poor prognosis.[11] Cytogenetic abnormalities are seen in approximately 70% of cases, and monosomy 7 is the most common cytogenetic change. Unlike adults, abnormalities of chromosome 7 do not seem to be associated with a poor prognosis in children. One-third of children with MDS suffer from genetic predisposition syndromes, such as trisomy 21 or trisomy 8.[44] Thus, childhood MDS is believed to have a different etiology and pathogenesis than the adult form and genetic predisposition is a factor.[44]

► CYTOGENETICS AND MOLECULAR TESTING

Abnormal karyotypes can be demonstrated in up to 50% of individuals with MDS (Table 23-4 ✪). These are acquired clonal aberrations as are those seen in patients with AML.[35] However, the types of chromosomal abnormalities seen in MDS are usually unbalanced (deletions or extra chromosomes) in contrast to the inversions or translocations seen in AML. None of the chromosomal abnormalities seen in MDS are unique to the disease.[20] The more frequent cytogenetic

✪ TABLE 23-4

Most Frequent Cytogenetic Abnormalities in MDS Patients

Numerical	Translocations	Deletions
+8 (19%)	inv 3 (7%)	del 5q (27%)
−7 (15%)	t(1;7) (2%)	del 11q (7%)
+21 (7%)	t(1;3) (1%)	del 12q (5%)
−5 (7%)	t(3;3) (1%)	del 20q (5%)
	t(6;9) (<1%)	del 7q (4%)
	t(5;12) (<1%)	del 13q (2%)

+ = additional chromosome; − = loss of chromosome; inv = inversion; t = translocation; del = deletion; % = frequency of chromosomal aberration

Reprinted, with permission, from Hofmann WK, Koeffler HP. Myelodysplastic syndrome. *Ann Rev Med*. 2005;56:5.

abnormalities involve structural or numeric abnormalities of chromosomes 5 and 7 and trisomy 8.

The most well described and common chromosome defect in MDS is the deletion of the long arm of chromosome 5, known as the 5q–syndrome, discussed previously. Another common abnormality is deletion of the long arm of chromosome 7 (7q–) or deletion of the whole chromosome (–7). The long arm contains the proto-oncogene *ERB-B*, which codes for the epidermal growth factor (EGF) receptor. This abnormality is most common in pediatric MDS.[45] Trisomy 8 (+8) is found in about 10–15% of the MDS abnormal karyotypes. Chromosome 8 contains the *MYC* proto-ongogene that codes for a nuclear transcription factor.

Adult MDS patients with chromosome aberrations have a worse prognosis than do patients with a normal karyotype and show increased incidence of progression to acute leukemia and complications of marrow failure. The emergence of new abnormal clones is associated with transformation to a more aggressive subgroup of AML.

The t-MDS have more frequent and complex abnormalities than those found in primary MDS. Chromosome changes are almost always present in t-MDS and are usually multiple at diagnosis. The majority of the karyotypic abnormalities include abnormalities of chromosomes 5 and/or 7 either singly or in combination with other abnormalities.[46] In contrast to primary MDS, the karyotypic aberrations can be extremely variable with no two cells exhibiting the same abnormality.

Examination of the bone marrow for cytogenetic abnormalities is a critical part of the diagnosis and evaluation of the MDS. New techniques such as fluorescence in situ hybridization (FISH) have improved the identification of chromosome abnormalities using specific DNA probes. Certain abnormal karyotypes have been associated with characteristic morphological dysplastic changes. The 5q–syndrome frequently demonstrates hyperlobulated megakaryocytes. Deletion of chromosome 17p has been associated with pseudo–Pelger-Huët cells and small vacuolated neutrophils. Cytogenetic-morphological correlations can become more and more useful to help distinguish subgroups of MDS in the future.[25]

Molecular diagnostic techniques are also becoming important tools for identifying genetic abnormalities that can aid in more reliable classification and treatment of these diseases. Gene profiles are being studied using microarray analysis. Thousands of genes can be analyzed simultaneously to eventually identify gene profiles that can help identify the subgroups of MDS and lead to more effective treatment. For example, researchers in one study were able to differentiate between AML blasts and MDS blasts by their gene profiles. Deltalike gene (*DLK*), *TEC* gene, and inositol 1,2,5-triphosphate receptor type 1 gene were among the genes highly specific for MDS.[2] Presently, the only specific gene mutation known to be common in MDS patients is a point mutation in the oncogene *RUNX/AML1*. It is found in up to 50% of patients depending on the karyotype, prior radiation exposure, and subtype of MDS.[4] Gene patterns associated with alterations of specific cellular pathways or signal cascades are also being studied in an effort to develop drugs to intervene with these alterations.[2] In the future, the MDS as well as acute leukemias will be classified according to specific molecular genetic abnormalities along with the corresponding clinical symptoms.

▶ PROGNOSIS

The median survival for all types of MDS is less than 2 years; however, some patients can survive many years with continuous transfusion therapy. The mortality rate varies from 58% to 72%. Leukemic transformation ranges in incidence from 10% to 40%.[47] The likelihood of transformation to AML increases with the presence of severe cytopenias, more overt dysplastic features of cells, and complex chromosome abnormalities.[12]

The International Prognostic Scoring System (IPSS)[48,49] (Table 23–5) was developed in 1997 to assist physicians in predicting prognosis and selection of optimal therapy for this heterogenous group of disorders.[50] This system was developed using data from seven large studies that had previously generated prognostic systems and is accepted worldwide. The major variables having an impact on disease outcome and risk of evolution to acute leukemia were:

- Cytogenetic abnormalities
- Percentage of blasts in the bone marrow
- Number of cytopenias.

With these three variables, patients can be divided into four risk groups with distinct risks of death and leukemic transformation. Low scores indicate prolonged survival. The IPSS complements the WHO classification system, and both can be useful when counseling patients. One criticism of the IPSS is that it does not include secondary MDS cases, such as t-MDS.[4] Even though it has some disadvantages, the IPSS has been extensively validated in independent patient populations and has become a benchmark for clinical trials and clinical decision making.[51]

⊘ CASE STUDY (continued from page 494)

The patient's karyotope showed multiple complex abnormalities.

12. Using the IPSS, what is the prognosis for this patient?

▶ THERAPY

In patients with pancytopenia, morbidity is associated with infection, bleeding, and anemia. The most common causes of death are hemorrhage and infection. Supportive care includes transfusions with leukocyte-depleted erythrocytes and platelets and prophylactic or curative antibiotic therapy. Hematopoietic cytokines and growth factors are sometimes effective supportive treatment for MDS. Studies with GM-CSF, G-CSF, and IL-3 show that the growth factors improve the neutrophil count in most cases.[52] Erythropoietin is effective in some patients, leading to decreased requirement for red cell transfusions. A combination of erythropoietin and either G-CSF or GM-CSF appears to have a synergistic effect in MDS patients, resulting in an increased response rate when given in combination.[11,20] Stimulation of megakaryopoiesis is least successful.[53] Use of cytokines that stimulate

⊘ TABLE 23-5

International Prognostic Scoring System (IPSS) for the Myelodysplastic Syndromes

Score Value	Cytopenias	BM Blasts (%)	Karyotype	Total Score	Risk Group	Median Survival (Years)
0	0–1	<5	Normal, −Y only,	0	Low	5.7
			del (5q) only	0.5–1.0	Int. 1	3.5
			del (20q) only	1.5–2.0	Int. 2	1.2
0.5	2–3	5–10	Other abns.	>2.5	High	0.4
1.0	—	—	Complex			
			>2 abns.			
			chr 7 abns.			
1.5	—	11–20	—			
2.0	—	21–30	—			

Cytopenias = hemoglobin <10 g/dL, platelets <100 × 10⁹/L, or neutrophils <1.8 × 10⁹/L in the peripheral blood; BM = bone marrow; abns. = abnormalities; Int. = intermediate; chr. = chromosome

(Adapted, with permission, from: Greenberg PL, Sanz GF, Sanz MA: Prognostic scoring system for risk assessment in myelodysplastic syndromes. *Forum: Trends in Experimental and Clinical Medicine.* 1999;9(1):17.)

platelet production (IL-11) has had variable results. More studies are needed using combinations of growth factors.

Patients with poor prognosis can be treated more aggressively with AML-type chemotherapeutic regimens. Only about one-third of patients in this risk category can endure high-intensity therapy because of their increased age. Almost all patients who respond to this type of therapy and achieve remission relapse in a short period of time. Only about 5% are alive at 3 years, but there are a few long-term responders.[4]

Bone marrow transplant is the only curative treatment available and is the treatment of choice for those 55–60 years of age or younger. Allogeneic stem-cell transplantation has been the most successful procedure for medically appropriate patients with HLA-matched donors.[11] The overall long-term disease-free survival is 60% in low risk patients, 40% for those in the intermediate risk category, and 20% for high-risk individuals.[20]

A better understanding of the pathophysiology of MDS has led to the development of unique drugs that target both the MDS cell and its interactions with the abnormal marrow microenvironment. Hypomethylating agents (to reactivate silenced genes), immunomodulatory drugs, and farnesyltransferase inhibitors (which inhibit RAS activation and function) have produced promising results in terms of response and survival in MDS patients.[54] A more thorough review of these new agents can be found on the website.

► MYELODYSPLASTIC/ MYELOPROLIFERATIVE DISEASES (MDS/MPD)

The category of MDS/MPD diseases is new in the WHO classification and is not found in the FAB classification system. It includes clonal hematopoietic neoplasms that, at the time of initial presentation, have some clinical, laboratory, or morphologic findings of both a MDS and a MPD.[25] Typically, patients with MDS/MPD have a hypercellular bone marrow associated with proliferation in one or more of the myeloid lineages. Frequently, the proliferation is effective and results in increased numbers of circulating cells. However, these cells commonly are morphologically and functionally dysplastic. While one or more lineages can show hyperproliferation, one or more other lineages can exhibit ineffective proliferation and resulting cytopenia(s). The percentage of blasts in the bone marrow and peripheral blood is always <20%. Splenomegaly and hepatomegaly are commonly found, but the clinical presentation is highly variable. The disorders included in MDS/MPD are listed in Table 23-6 ☉.

The major clinical and laboratory findings in MDS/MPD disorders are due to abnormalities in the regulation of myeloid proliferation, maturation, and cell survival. Clinical symptoms can be due to cytopenia(s) when present, dysplastic cells that do not function properly, and leukemic infiltration of various organs. At present, there are no identified genetic defects specific for any of the entities included in this category. However, recurring chromosomal and molecular abnormalities have been described (see table below). The incidence varies widely depending on the specific disease as do the prognosis and tendency for clonal evolution and disease progression (see following sections on subgroups).

CHRONIC MYELOMONOCYTIC LEUKEMIA (CMML)

Chronic myelomonocytic leukemia (CMML) is a clonal hematopoietic neoplasm associated with a persistent monocytosis ($> 1 \times 10^9$/L in the peripheral blood) (Figure 23-11 ■). The blood or bone marrow has <20% blasts. Determination of the percentage of blasts includes myeloblasts,

☉ TABLE 23-6

The Myelodysplastic/Myeloproliferative Diseases (MDS/MPD)

Classification	Peripheral Blood	Bone Marrow	Genetics	Immunophenotype
Chronic myelomonocytic leukemia (CMML-1)	Monocytosis >1 × 10⁹/L; <5% blasts	<10% blasts; dysplasia of ≥1 myeloid lineages	Absence of Ph chromosome, BCR/ABL1	CD33, CD13 +; CD14, CD68, CD64 +; lysozyme +
CMML-2	5–19% blasts	10–19% blasts	(same as CMML-1)	(same as CMML-1)
Atypical chronic myeloid leukemia (aCML)	Leukocytosis (<10% monocytes); <5% blasts; promyelocytes, myelocytes, metamyelocytes 10–20%	Hypercellular; <20% blasts; dysgranulopoiesis; occasionally dyserythropoiesis	Absence of Ph chromosome, BCR/ABL1 neg	CD33, CD13 +; MPO +
Juvenile myelomonocytic leukemia (JMML)	Monocytosis >1 × 10⁹/L; <20% blasts	Hypercellular; <20% blasts; dysgranulopoiesis; occasionally dyserythropoiesis	Absence of Ph chromosome, BCR/ABL1 neg	CD33, CD13 +; CD14, CD68, CD64 +; lysozyme +
Myelodysplastic/ myeloproliferative disease, unclassifiable (MDS/MPD-u)	Anemia, leukocytosis and/or thrombocytosis; <20% blasts	Hypercellular; proliferation is any or all myeloid lineages	Absence of Ph chromosome, BCR/ABL1 neg	Nondiagnostic

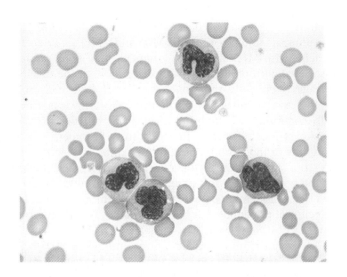

■ FIGURE 23-11 Increased monocytes in the peripheral blood from a patient with CMML. (Wright stain; 1000× magnification)

monoblasts, and promonocytes. Usually dysplasia involving one or more myeloid lineages is present. Most patients with CMML are older than 50 years (median age at diagnosis ~70 years) with an annual incidence of ~3/100,000. Median survival time is 20–40 months, and progression to acute leukemia is seen in 15–30% of cases. The cell of origin is believed to be the HSC.

In approximately 50% of patients, the WBC count is normal or slightly decreased with monocytosis and neutropenia (more myelodysplastic in presentation). In the remaining patients, the WBC count is increased at the time of diagnosis (more myeloproliferative in presentation). Splenomegaly and hepatomegaly are more common in patients with an elevated WBC count. The liver, spleen, skin, and lymph nodes are common sites of extramedullary leukemic infiltration.

Peripheral blood monocytosis is always present and can range from 2 to 80 × 10⁹/L. The monocytes are generally morphologically normal mature cells. They occasionally exhibit abnormal granulation, unusual nuclear lobulation, or dispersed chromatin. If blasts and promonocytes account for ≥20% of the WBC, the diagnosis is AML rather than CMML. If the WBC count is increased, accompanying neutrophilia with <10% neutrophil precursors (promyelocytes, myelocytes) are often present. Mild basophilia and occasionally mild eosinophilia are sometimes present. Dysgranulopoiesis (hypolobulated, abnormal granulation) is present in most cases but usually is less prominent in patients with leukocytosis. Mild normocytic (occasionally macrocytic) anemia is usually present. Although platelet counts vary, moderate thrombocytopenia is usually present with occasional atypical, giant forms.

The bone marrow is usually hypercellular (> 75% of patients) but occasionally is normocellular or hypocellular. Cytochemistry (both specific and nonspecific esterase stains) could be necessary to identify both the myelocytic and mono-

cytic cells (∞ Chapter 21). Dysgranulopoiesis similar to that found in the peripheral blood and dyserythropoiesis (megaloblastoid changes, ringed sideroblasts) are found in more than 50% of the patients. Micromegakaryocytes are common. Variable fibrosis is seen in the marrow of ~30% of patients.

The WHO classification recommends that CMML be further divided into two subcategories depending on the number of blasts in the peripheral blood and bone marrow. CMML-1 is defined as <5% blasts in the blood and <10% in the marrow. CMML-2 is defined as 5–19% blasts in the blood or 10–19% in the marrow. An additional subset, CMML with eosinophilia, has been described; in addition to the criteria for CMML, it includes a peripheral blood eosinophil count of >1.5 × 10⁹/L.

Clonal cytogenetic abnormalities are found in 20–40% of patients, but none is specific. The most frequently reported abnormalities include +8, −7/del(7q), structural abnormalities of 12p, and isochromosome 17q [i(17q)]. Point mutations of the *RAS* protooncogenes are found in ~40% of patients. The Philadelphia chromosome and *BCR/ABL* fusion gene are absent.

ATYPICAL CHRONIC MYELOID LEUKEMIA (ACML)

Atypical chronic myeloid leukemia (aCML) is a variant of MDS/MPD characterized by primary involvement of the neutrophil series with leukocytosis involving immature and mature neutrophils that are dysplastic. Multilineage dysplasia is common. The peripheral blood and bone marrow are always involved. While splenic and hepatic involvement are also common, skin infiltration is not. Most patients with aCML are older with the median age at diagnosis in the 7th to 8th decade and an annual incidence of ~3/100,000. Median survival time is <20 months, and progression to acute leukemia is seen in 25–40% of cases. The cell of origin is believed to be the common myeloid progenitor cell (CMP).

The peripheral blood WBC is variable, generally ranging from 35–96 × 10⁹/L, although counts in excess of 300 × 10⁹/L have been reported. Blasts are usually <5%, and always <20% of the peripheral blood white cells. Immature neutrophils (promyelocytes, myelocytes, and metamyelocytes) are usually 10–20% of the white cell differential. A mild monocytosis and basophilia occasionally are present. Dysgranulopoiesis can be pronounced, including acquired Pelger-Huët and other nuclear abnormalities as well as abnormal cytoplasmic granularity. Moderate anemia is frequent and can show dyserythropoietic changes including macro-ovalocytosis. The platelet count is variable but is often thrombocytopenic.

The bone marrow is usually hypercellular due to the granulocytic proliferation. Blasts account for <20% of the marrow cells. Dysgranulopoiesis is a constant finding while dyserythropoiesis is variable. The M:E ratio usually is >10:1. Megakaryocytes can be increased, decreased, or normal in number and occasionally are dysplastic. Increased fibrosis is seen occasionally. Immunophenotype and cytochemistry results are typical for the neutrophil lineage although leukocyte alkaline phosphatase (LAP) scores can be elevated, normal, or low.

Up to 80% of patients with aCML have been reported to have cytogenetic abnormalities, but none is specific. Reported cytogenetic abnormalities include +8, +13, del(20q), i(17q), and del(12p). The Philadelphia chromosome and *BCR/ABL* fusion gene are absent.

JUVENILE MYELOMONOCYTIC LEUKEMIA (JMML)

Juvenile myelomonocytic leukemia (JMML) is a clonal hematopoietic neoplasm of childhood characterized by proliferation of the granulocytic and monocytic lineages. Erythroid and megakaryocytic abnormalities are also frequently present. Myelomonocytic proliferation is evident in the blood and bone marrow. The liver, spleen, skin, lymph node, and respiratory tract can have leukemia infiltration. The annual incidence of JMML is 0.13/100,000 children (age 0–14 years of age). JMML accounts for <2–3% of all leukemia in children. The age at diagnosis is variable (from 1 month to early adolescence), but 75% of cases are diagnosed in children <3 years of age. A significant association of JMML with neurofibromatosis type 1 (NF-1) exists with ~10% of cases of JMML occurring in children with this diagnosis. The cell of origin is believed to be the HSC. The overall prognosis is poor with median survival times of 5 months to >4 years; the prognosis varies inversely with patient age at diagnosis. Most children die from organ failure due to leukemic infiltration; only 10–20% progress to acute leukemia.

JMML is characterized by a peripheral blood monocytosis ($>1 \times 10^9$/L) with <20% blasts (including promonocytes). Leukocytosis ($25-100 \times 10^9$/L), anemia, and often thrombocytopenia usually occur. Both immature neutrophils and monocytes can be present. Eosinophilia and basophilia rarely are observed.

The bone marrow is usually hypercellular with granulocytic and monocytic proliferation. Rare patients have a significant increase in erythroid precursors. Monocytes can account for 5–30% of the marrow cells. Blasts (myeloblasts, monoblasts, and promonocytes) account for <20% of the marrow cells (Auer rods are never seen). Evidence of dyspoiesis includes pseudo–Pelger-Huët, hypogranularity of the neutrophils, and megaloblastoid erythroblasts but rarely megakaryocytic dysplasia.

Cytochemistry and immunophenotype results are as expected for the mixed granulocytic and monocytic cell population. Cytogenetic abnormalities occur in 30–40% of patients, but none are specific for JMML. The Ph chromosome and *BCR/ABL* fusion gene are absent. Point mutations of *RAS* are reported in the neoplastic cells of 20% of patients.

MYELODYSPLASTIC/MYELOPROLIFERATIVE DISEASE, UNCLASSIFIABLE (MDS/MPD-u)

This subcategory, MDS/MPD-u is used for cases that have clinical, laboratory, and morphologic features that support a diagnosis of both MPD and MDS but do not meet the criteria of the other entities included in the MDS/MPD category. Typically, the patient has the clinical, laboratory, and morphologic features of one of the categories of MDS (RA, RARS, RCMD, RAEB) with <20% blasts in the blood and bone marrow and prominent myeloproliferative features associated with either thrombocytosis or leukocytosis. The bone marrow and peripheral blood are always involved; extramedullary tissues (liver, spleen) are sometimes also involved. Blasts account for <20% of the nucleated cells of the marrow and peripheral blood.

The disorders categorized as MDS/MPD-u are characterized by the proliferation of one or more of the myeloid lineages that are ineffective and/or dysplastic. Proliferation of the other myeloid lineages is generally effective with or without dysplasia. Anemia (with or without macrocytosis) usually occurs, occasionally with a dimorphic population of RBC. The bone marrow is hypercellular and can show proliferation in any or all of the myeloid lineages. Dysplastic features are present in at least one lineage.

No cytogenetic or molecular genetic findings are specific for this group. The presence of the Ph chromosome and *BCR/ABL* fusion gene must always be excluded.

SUMMARY

The myelodysplastic syndromes are pluripotential hematopoietic stem cell disorders characterized by one or more peripheral blood cytopenias and prominent cellular maturation abnormalities. The bone marrow is usually normocellular or hypercellular, indicating a high degree of ineffective hematopoiesis. Proto-oncogene mutations are commonly found in patients with MDS indicating that oncogenes most likely play a role in the pathogenesis of MDS.

Although anemia is the most common cytopenia, neutropenia and thrombocytopenia also occur. Erythrocytes are macrocytic or less frequently normocytic. Erythropoiesis in the bone marrow is abnormal with megaloblastoid features commonly present. Neutrophils can show hypolobulation of the nucleus and hypogranulation. Megakaryocytes also show megaloblastoid features and hypolobulation of the nucleus. Platelets can be large and agranular.

The WHO group has classified the MDS into six subgroups depending on the blast count, degree of dyspoiesis and cytopenias, and presence of abnormal cytogenetic findings. These include RA, RARS, RCMD, RAEB, 5q–syndrome and MDS-unclassified. Subgroups with higher blast counts and involvement of multiple lineages in dyspoiesis and complex cytogenetic abnormalities are more aggressive disorders. MDS frequently terminate in acute leukemia. Treatment is primarily supportive unless the patient is a candidate for a bone marrow transplant.

The myelodysplastic/myeloproliferative category (MDS/MPD) includes disorders that have features of both a myeloproliferative and a myelodysplastic disorder simultaneously. This category includes CMML, JMML, aCML, and MDS/MPD-unclassifiable. An important diagnostic consideration is absence of the Ph chromosome or *BCR/ABL1* fusion gene in these patients.

REVIEW QUESTIONS

LEVEL I

1. In addition to the number of blasts, what other criterion is essential for a diagnosis of RARS? (Objective 2)
   a. ≥15% ringed sideroblasts
   b. ≥30% ringed sideroblasts
   c. dyshematopoiesis in all three cell lineages
   d. pancytopenia

2. A patient with suspected MDS exhibits anemia, neutropenia, anisocytosis, poikilocytosis, oval macrocytes, Howell-Jolly bodies, hypogranular neutrophils, and a few pseudo–Pelger-Huët cells. The differential shows a few immature granulocytes but no blasts. Which MDS subgroup would be most likely? (Objective 2)
   a. RA
   b. RARS
   c. RCMD
   d. RAEB

3. The WHO classification system incorporates: (Objective 2)
   a. the presence of cellular dysplasia
   b. cytogenetics
   c. morphology
   d. all of the above

4. The type of anemia usually seen in MDS is: (Objective 1)
   a. macrocytic, normochromic
   b. normocytic, normochromic
   c. microcytic, hypochromic
   d. normocytic, hypochromic

5. The most common cytopenia(s) seen in MDS is(are): (Objective 3)
   a. leukopenia
   b. thrombocytopenia
   c. anemia
   d. a combination of two of the above

6. The typical bone marrow cellularity in MDS is: (Objective 3)
   a. hypocellular
   b. normocellular
   c. hypercellular
   d. fibrotic

7. Atypical CML is classified as: (Objective 5)
   a. MDS
   b. AML
   c. MPD
   d. MDS/MPD

LEVEL II

1. According to the WHO classification system, what is the minimum percentage of bone marrow blasts needed for a diagnosis of acute leukemia? (Objective 4)
   a. 19%
   b. 30%
   c. 5%
   d. 20%

2. The t-MDS differ from primary MDS in that t-MDS: (Objective 6)
   a. are usually the less aggressive subgroup
   b. have more peripheral blood blasts
   c. have fewer and less complex abnormal karyotypes
   d. usually have a younger age of onset

3. Progression of MDS to acute leukemia is characterized by: (Objective 4)
   a. an increase in blast population
   b. decreased bone marrow cellularity
   c. a decreased M:E ratio
   d. splenomegaly

4. A cell resembling a blast that contains 18 primary granules and a centrally located nucleus would be classified as a: (Objective 2)
   a. Type I blast
   b. Type II blast
   c. Type III blast
   d. promyelocyte

5. The contrast between a hypercellular bone marrow and a cytopenic peripheral blood film seen in MDS is attributed to: (Objective 1)
   a. premature destruction of abnormal cells in the bone marrow (ineffective hematopoiesis)
   b. production of blood cells outside the bone marrow (extramedullary hematopoiesis)
   c. immune destruction of cells in the peripheral blood
   d. splenic sequestration

6. Which of the following would be most helpful to differentiate RA from 5q–syndrome? (Objective 10)
   a. percentage of bone marrow blasts
   b. elevated leukocyte count
   c. presence of nucleated RBCs
   d. karyotype

REVIEW QUESTIONS (continued)

LEVEL I

8. The most common dyserythropoietic finding in the bone marrow in MDS is: (Objective 3)
   a. megaloblastoid development
   b. impaired hemoglobinization
   c. pseudo–Pelger-Huët cells
   d. agranular cytoplasm

9. Which abnormality demonstrates myelocytic dysplasia? (Objective 3)
   a. dimorphism
   b. pseudo–Pelger-Huët cells
   c. sideroblasts
   d. all of the above

10. This group of neoplasms is characterized by a hypercellular bone marrow, effective proliferation of one or more myeloid lineages but morphologically and functionally dysplastic cells. (Objective 4)
    a. MDS
    b. MPD
    c. MDS/MPD
    d. AML

LEVEL II

7. The most effective treatment for MDS is currently considered to be: (Objective 3)
   a. chemotherapy
   b. immunotherapy
   c. hematopoietic growth factors
   d. bone marrow transplant

Use the following case history to answer questions 8–10.

A patient presents with the following laboratory data:

RBC	2.30×10^{12}/L
Hgb	7.8 g/dL (78 g/L)
Hct	0.24 L/L
MCV	104 fL
RDW	20
WBC	8.5×10^9/L
PLT	140×10^9/L

The differential was normal except for 2% metamyelocytes. Oval macrocytes, a few abnormal NRBC, and a few siderocytes were seen. The bone marrow contained 3% blasts and exhibited hypercellularity with megaloblastoid development in erythroid cells.

8. What is the most probable MDS subgroup? (Objective 10)
   a. RA
   b. RARS
   c. RCMD
   d. RAEB

9. What other hematologic disorder does this peripheral blood picture resemble? (Objective 7)
   a. aplastic anemia
   b. megaloblastic anemia
   c. iron-deficiency anemia
   d. anemia of chronic disease

10. What laboratory test(s) would be helpful to distinguish MDS from megaloblastic anemia? (Objective 7)
    a. serum lysozyme
    b. serum ferritin
    c. serum folate and vitamin B_{12}
    d. combined esterase stain

www.pearsonhighered.com/mckenzie
Use this address to access the interactive Companion Website created for this textbook. Find additional information, tables and figures. Evaluate your command of the chapter information using case studies and critical thinking and multiple choice questions.

REFERENCES

1. Coiffier B, Bryon PA, Fiere D et al. Dysmyelopoietic syndromes: A search for prognostic factors in 193 patients. *Cancer.* 1983;52:83–90.

2. Bennett JM, Komrokji RS. The myelodysplastic syndromes: Diagnosis, molecular biology and risk assessment. *Hematology.* 2005;10 (Suppl 1): 258–69.

3. Harris NL, Jaffe ES, Diebold J et al. The World Health Organization classification of neoplastic diseases of the haematopoietic and lymphoid tissues: Report of the Clinical Advisory Committee Meeting, Airlie House, Virginia, November 1997. *Histopathology.* 2000;36:69–87.

4. Steensma DP, Bennett JM. The myelodysplastic syndromes: Diagnosis and treatment. *Mayo Clin Proc.* 2006;81(1):104–30.

5. Germing U, Gattermann N, Strupp C et al. Validation of the WHO proposals for a new classification of primary myelodysplastic syndromes: A retrospective analysis of 1600 patients. *Leuk Res.* 2000;24: 983–92.

6. Musilova J, Michalova K. Chromosome study of 85 patients with myelodysplastic syndrome. *Cancer Genet Cytogenet.* 1988;33:39–50.

7. Prchal JT, Throckmorton DW, Carroll AJ III, Fuson EW, Garns RA, Prchal JF et al. A common progenitor for human myeloid and lymphoid cells. *Nature.* 1978;274:590–91.

8. Weimar IS, Bourhis JH, DeGast GC, Gerritsen WR. Clonality in myelodysplastic syndromes. *Leuk Lymph.* 1994;13:215–21.

9. Aul C, Bowen DT, Yoshida Y. Pathogenesis, etiology, and epidemiology of myelodysplastic syndromes. *Haematologica.* 1998;83:71–86.

10. Hofmann WK, Lubbert M, Hoelzer D, Koeffler P. Myelodysplastic syndromes. *The Hematology Journal.* 2004;5:1–8.

11. Heaney ML, Golde DW. Myelodysplasia. *New Engl J Med.* 1999;340 (21):1649–60.

12. Lichtman MA, Liesveld JL. Myelodysplastic syndromes. In: Lichtman MA, Beutler E, Kipps TJ et al, eds. *Williams Hematology,* 7th ed. New York: McGraw-Hill, 2006;1157–81.

13. Besa EC. Myelodysplastic syndromes (refractory anemia): A perspective of the biologic, clinical, and therapeutic issues. *Med Clin North Am.* 1992;76:599–617.

14. Willman CL. Molecular genetic features of myelodysplastic syndromes. *Leukemia.* 1998;12 (Suppl 1):S2–S6.

15. Dormer P, Hershko C, Wilmanns W. Mechanisms and prognostic value of cell kinetics in the myelodysplastic syndromes. *Br J Haemat.* 1987;67:147–52.

16. Yoshida Y, Mufti GJ. Apoptosis and its significance in MDS: Controversies revisited. *Leukemia Research.* 1999;23:777–85.

17. Mufti GH, Parker JE. Ineffective haemopoiesis and apoptosis in myelodysplastic syndromes. *British J of Haematology.* 1998;101:220–30.

18. Degnan T, Weiselberg L, Schulman P, Budman DR. Dysmyelopoietic syndrome. *Am J Med.* 1984;76:122–28.

19. Ciccone G, Mirabelli D, Levis A et al. Myeloid leukemias and myelodysplastic syndromes: Chemical exposure, histologic subtype, and cytogenetics in a case-control study. *Cancer Genet Cytogenet.* 1993;68:135–39.

20. Hofmann WK, Koeffler HP. Myelodysplastic syndrome. *Annu Rev Med.* 2005;56:1–16.

21. Gadner H, Haas OA. Experience in pediatric myelodysplastic syndromes. *Hematol/Oncol Clin North Am.* 1992;6:655–72.

22. Hasle H, Niemeyer CM, Chessells JM et al. A pediatric approach to the WHO classification of myelodysplastic and myeloproliferative diseases. *Leukemia.* 2003;17:277–82.

23. Pomeroy C, Oken MM, Rydell RE, Felice GA. Infection in the myelodysplastic syndromes. *Am J Med.* 1991;90:338–44.

24. Juneja SK, Imbert M, Jouault H, Scoazec JY, Sigaux F, Sultan C. Haematological features of primary myelodysplastic syndromes (PMDS) at initial presentation: A study of 118 cases. *J Clin Pathol.* 1983;36:1129–35.

25. Jaffe ES, Harris NL, Stein H, Vardiman JW, eds. Pathology and genetics of tumours of haematopoietic and lymphoid tissues. In: Kleihues P, Sobin LH, eds. *World Health Organization Classification of Tumours.* Lyon, France: IARC Press; 2001, 63–73.

26. Noel P, Solberg LA. Myelodysplastic syndromes: Pathogenesis, diagnosis, and treatment. *Crit Rev Oncol/Hematol.* 1992;12(3):193–215.

27. Sanz GF, Sanz MA. Prognostic factors in myelodysplastic syndromes. *Leuk Res.* 1992;16:77–86.

28. Rios A, Canizo MC, Sanz MA et al. Bone marrow biopsy in myelodysplastic syndromes: Morphological characteristics and contribution to the study of prognostic factors. *Br J Haemat.* 1990;75: 26–33.

29. Yoshida Y, Stephenson J, Mufti GJ. Myelodysplastic syndromes: From morphology to molecular biology. Part K. Classification, natural history and cell biology of myelodysplasia. *Int J Hematol.* 1993; 57:87–97.

30. Colombat PH, Renoux M, Lamagnere J, Renous G. Immunologic indices in myelodysplastic syndromes. *Cancer.* 1988;61:1075–81.

31. Goasguen JE et al. Prognostic implication and characterization of the blast cell population in the myelodysplastic syndrome. *Leuk Res.* 1991;15:1159–65.

32. Third MIC Cooperative Study Group Recommendations for a morphologic, immunologic, and cytogenetic (MIC) working classification of the primary and therapy-related myelodysplastic disorders. *Cancer Genet Cytogenet.* 1988;32:1–10.

33. Pagnucco G, Giambanco C, Gervasi F. The role of flow cytometric immunophenotyping in myelodysplastic syndromes. *Ann NY Acad Sci.* 2006;1089:383–94.

34. Stetler-Stevenson M, Arthur DC, Jabbour N et al. Diagnostic utility of flow cytometric immunophenotyping in myelodysplastic syndrome. *Blood.* 2001;98(4):979–87.

35. Kristensen JS. Immunophenotyping in acute leukemia, myelodysplastic syndromes, and hairy cell leukemia. *Dan Med Bulle.* 1994;41: 52–65.

36. Elghetany MT. Surface marker abnormalities in myelodysplastic syndromes. *Haematologica.* 1998;83:1104–15.

37. Ogata K, Yoshida Y. Clinical implications of blast immunophenotypes in myelodysplastic syndromes. *Leuk Lymph.* 2005;46(9): 1269–74.

38. Michels SD, McKenna RW, Arthur DC, Brunning RD. Therapy related acute myeloid leukemia and myelodysplastic syndromes: A clinical and morphologic study of 65 cases. *Blood.* 1985;65:1364–72.

39. Bennett JM, Catovsky D, Daniel MT et al. Proposals for the classification of the myelodysplastic syndromes. *Bri. J Haematol.* 1982;51: 189–99.

40. Boultwood J, Lewis S, Wainscoat JS. The 5q–syndrome. *J of American Society of Hematology.* 1994;84(10):3253–60.

41. Dickstein JI, Vardiman JW. Issues in the pathology and diagnosis of the chronic myeloproliferative disorders and the myelodysplastic syndromes. *Am J Clin Pathol.* 1993;99:513–25.

42. List AF, Sandberg AA, Doll DC. Myelodysplastic syndromes. In Greer JP, Foerster J, Lukens JN et al, eds. *Wintrobe's Clinical Hematology*, 11th ed. Philadelphia: Lippincott Williams and Wilkins; 2004, 2207–34.

43. Kampmeier P, Anastasi J, Vardiman JW. Issues in the pathology of the myelodysplastic syndromes. *Hematol/Oncol Clin North Am.* 1992; 6:501–22.

44. Haas OA, Gadner H. Pathogenesis, biology, and management of myelodysplastic syndromes in children. *Seminars in Hematology.* 1996;33(3):225–35.

45. Noel P, Tefferi A, Pierre RV, Jenkins RB, Dewald GW. Karyotypic analysis in primary myelodysplastic syndromes. *Blood Rev.* 1993;7: 10–18.

46. Iurlo A, Mecucci C, Van Orshoven A et al. Cytogenetic and clinical investigations in 76 cases with therapy-related leukemia and myelodysplastic syndrome. *Cancer Genet Cytogenet.* 1989;43:227–41.

47. Ganser A, Hoelzer D. Clinical course of myelodysplastic syndromes. *Hematol/Oncol Clin North Am.* 1992;6:607–18.

48. Greenberg P, Cox C, LeBeau MM et al. International scoring system for evaluating prognosis in myelodysplastic syndromes. *Blood.* 1997;89(6):2079–88.

49. Greenberg PL, Sanz GF, Sanz MA. Prognostic scoring systems for risk assessment in myeloproliferative syndromes. *Forum.* 1999;9(1): 17–31.

50. List AF, Vardiman J, Issa, JPJ, DeWitte TM. Myelodysplastic syndromes. *Hematology Am Soc Hematol Educ Program.* 2004;297–317.

51. Malcovati L, Della Porta MG, Pascutto C et al. Prognostic factors and life expectancy in myelodysplastic syndromes classified according to WHO criteria: A basis for clinical decision making. *J Clin Oncol.* 2005;23:7594–7603.

52. Ganser A, Hoelzer D. Treatment of myelodysplastic syndromes with hematopoietic growth factors. *Hematol/Oncol Clin North Am.* 1992;6: 633–53.

53. Arcenas AG, Vadhan-Rah S. Hematopoietic growth factor therapy of myelodysplastic syndromes. *Leuk Lymph.* 1993;11(Suppl 2):65–69.

54. Meletis J, Viniou N, Terpos E. Novel agents for the management of myelodysplastic syndromes. *Med Sci Monit.* 2006;12(9):RA194–206.

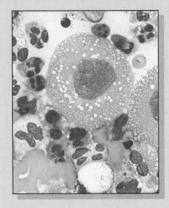

CHAPTER OUTLINE

24
Acute Myeloid Leukemias

Susan J. Leclair, Ph.D.
J. Lynne Williams, Ph.D.

■ OBJECTIVES—LEVEL I

By the end of this unit of study, the student should be able to:

1. Define *acute leukemia,* and explain the difference between acute myeloid leukemia (AML) acute lymphoblastic leukemia (ALL) and myelodysplastic syndrome (MDS).

2. List and define the common variants of AML as defined by the WHO classification.

3. Describe and recognize the typical peripheral blood picture (erythrocytes, leukocytes, and thrombocytes) seen in AML.

4. Describe the M:E ratio in bone marrow in acute leukemia (AL).

5. Give the typical results of cytochemical stains in AML.

6. Identify Auer rods and describe their significance.

■ OBJECTIVES—LEVEL II

At the end of this unit of study, the student should be able to:

1. Compare and contrast the various presentations of AML.

2. Predict the most likely leukemia type based on patient history, physical assessment, and laboratory findings.

3. Correlate cellular presentation of AML with prognosis and common complications.

4. Correlate Wright-stain morphology of the AML subgroups with cytochemical stains, flow cytometry, and genetic testing.

5. Evaluate peripheral blood results in relation to oncological therapy (i.e., complete or partial remission, relapse, engraftment).

6. Evaluate patient data from the medical history and laboratory results to determine whether a disorder can be classifed, and, if not, specify the additional testing to be performed.

7. Compare the WHO and FAB classifications of AML.

KEY TERMS

Acute leukemias (AL)
Auer rods
Biphenotypic leukemia
FAB classification
Faggot cells
CD33, CD13, CD34
CD10, CD19, CD20, CD22
CD2, CD3, CD5, CD7
Mixed lineage leukemia
Pseudo–Pelger-Huët cell
WHO classification

BACKGROUND BASICS

The information in this chapter builds on concepts learned in previous chapters. To maximize your learning experience, you should review and have an understanding of these concepts before starting this unit of study.

Level I

▶ Describe the origin and differentiation of hematopoietic cells. (Chapter 3)
▶ Summarize the leukocyte's maturation, differentiation, and function. (Chapter 7)
▶ Outline the classification and general laboratory findings of the acute leukemias (Chapter 21).
▶ List and describe the criteria used to differentiate acute leukemias (Chapter 21).

Level II

▶ Summarize the role of oncogenes and growth factors in cell proliferation, differentiation, and maturation. (Chapters 3 and 21)
▶ Describe the role of molecular analysis in diagnosis and treatment of acute leukemia. (Chapter 21)
▶ Describe the use of immunophenotyping in acute leukemia. (Chapter 21)
▶ Describe the role of cytogenetics in diagnosis and treatment of acute leukemia. (Chapter 21)

CASE STUDY

We will refer to this case study throughout the chapter.
Guillermo, a 34-year-old Latin-American male, had been in excellent health until two weeks prior to admission when he had a mild sore throat. He was seen at a neighborhood clinic and was prescribed penicillin. He was able to return to work and felt better until four days prior to admission when he developed a fever and experienced easy bruising. He noticed other bleeding symptoms including gingival bleeding and petechiae. He reported to the emergency room. A CBC revealed a WBC count of 26.2×10^9/L and 6% blasts. He was admitted for further evaluation. Consider what additional laboratory testing could assist in the diagnosis of this patient.

▶ OVERVIEW

This chapter describes the acute myeloid (also referred to as *myelocytic* or *myelogenous*) leukemias (AML), also known as acute nonlymphocytic leukemias (ANLL). It begins with an account of the general laboratory findings in AML followed by a specific description of each subgroup in the WHO (World Health Organization) classification (with some reference to the older French-American-British [FAB] classification). Clinical and laboratory findings are described with an emphasis on defining characteristics. The chapter concludes with a look at the current types of therapy used to treat AML.

▶ INTRODUCTION

All **acute leukemias (AL)** are stem cell disorders characterized by malignant neoplastic proliferation and accumulation of immature and nonfunctional hematopoietic cells in the bone marrow. The neoplastic cells show increased proliferation and/or decreased programmed cell death (apoptosis). The net effect is expansion of the leukemic clone and a decrease in normal cells.[1]

Because leukemia is a clonal expansion of a single transformed cell, all ALs begin long before any clinical signs and symptoms appears. A tumor burden of 10^{12} cells is believed to be sufficient for recognizable signs and symptoms. Lethal levels of tumor burden occur at neoplastic cell numbers of 10^{13-14} or higher. As the tumor burden expands, the normal functional marrow cells decrease. The classic triad of anemia, infection, and bleeding seen in acute leukemia occur as a result of "normal" hematopoietic cell cytopenias. Death often occurs from either infection or hemorrhage in weeks to months unless therapeutic intervention occurs.[2]

The two major categories of acute leukemias are classified according to the cellular presentation of the primary stem cell defect: AML and ALL. If the defect primarily affects the maturation and differentiation of the common myeloid progenitor (CMP) cell, the leukemia is classified as AML or ANLL. If the defect primarily affects the common lymphoid progenitor (CLP) cell, the leukemia is classified as ALL.

The most reliable parameters for defining and classifying neoplastic cells in AML into subtypes are immunologic probes to define cell markers (cell surface or internal antigens) and cytogenetic and molecular studies to identify genetic abnormalities (∞ Chapters 37, 38, and 39). In the late 1970s, the first internationally accepted classification for the acute leukemias, the FAB classification, was based on a combination of neoplastic cell morphology and cytochemical cellular reactions.[3] This classification remained essentially unchanged until 1999 when the WHO and the International Society of Hematology proposed a new classification.[4] Many health care practitioners have dropped the use of the old FAB system in favor of the **WHO classification,** but because some individuals continue to use the older system, the FAB nomenclature is reviewed here.

► BASIC BIOLOGY OF AML

AML is a disease characterized by two fundamental features: the ability to proliferate continuously and aberrant or arrested development.[5] Excessive overproliferation can be the result of mutations affecting growth factors, growth factor receptors, signaling pathway components, and transcription factors that regulate genes involved in cell survival and proliferation. The majority of the genetic mutations that have been identified in AML involve transcription factors and other signaling pathway molecules. More than half of the cases of AML display cytogenetic abnormalities. Most are balanced, reciprocal chromosomal translocations with many of the translocation break points located at the loci for genes encoding transcription factors. The most common consequence of the translocation is the generation of a fusion gene that encodes for a novel fusion protein. The fusion proteins that are formed usually alter the normal function of one or both of the rearranged genes and modify the normal programs of cell proliferation, differentiation, and survival. In addition, other types of genetic abnormalities (e.g., epigenetic alterations) likely interact with the cytogenetic mutations (called the *multistep origin* of malignancy) resulting in the full leukemic transformation.[5,6]

► LABORATORY FINDINGS

PERIPHERAL BLOOD

The peripheral blood picture is quite variable in AML. Although it is traditional to describe leukemias as having elevated leukocyte counts, 50% of the cases can have decreased counts or counts within the reference range at the time of diagnosis. The leukocyte count ranges from less than 1×10^9/L to more than 100×10^9/L. Regardless of the leukocyte concentration, the presence of blasts on the blood smear suggests the AL diagnosis. The current WHO definition of AL requires ≥20% blasts in the peripheral blood or bone marrow in contrast to the older FAB requirement of more than 30%. Experienced clinical laboratory professionals are often able to determine the lineage of the leukemic cells by bright-field microscopy on Romanowsky-stained preparations. The remaining cases must be identified through cytochemical, immunologic, and/or genetic methods. Typically, the myeloblast seen in AML is approximately 20 μ in diameter with variably prominent nucleoli in a nucleus composed primarily of dispersed chromatin (euchromatin or transcriptionally active DNA). A Golgi apparatus is present but is not easily visualized. Although blasts normally do not have granules visible by bright-field microscopy, neoplastic blasts do not always develop normally and can have a

few granules in the RNA-rich cytoplasm. The FAB group defined neoplastic blasts as Type I, Type II, and Type III; Type I has typical blast features without granules, Type II has <20 granules, and Type III has numerous granules (∞ Chapter 23). Although the common presentation includes a variety of immature granulocyte forms, occasionally only myeloblasts are found on the peripheral blood smear. Abnormalities in cell granules, nuclear structure, and function are frequent.

Erythrocytes are typically decreased, and a hemoglobin value less than 10g/dL is common. Erythrocytes can be slightly macrocytic because of the inability to successfully compete with neoplastic cells for folate or vitamin B_{12} and/or early release of marrow reticulocytes. The RDW often is elevated. Erythrocyte inclusions such as Howell-Jolly bodies, Pappenheimer bodies, and basophilic stippling reflective of erythrocyte maturation defects can be present. Nucleated erythrocytes can be present in proportion to the anemia or marrow damage.

Platelets are typically decreased. Hypogranular platelets and occasional enlarged forms (giant platelets) can be present. As the disease progresses, more immature platelet forms such as megakaryocytic fragments can be seen. The platelet count might not correlate with the potential complication of bleeding because qualitative platelet defects also can be present.

If the physician suspects AL but no blast cells are detected on the peripheral blood smear or if the leukocyte count is low ($<2 \times 10^9$/L), a buffy-coat smear should be prepared. This often reveals the presence of blast cells when they are present in very low concentrations. Finding blasts with azurophilic granules is helpful in identifying the myeloid nature of the leukemia. The presence of granules or **Auer rods** (fused or coalesced primary granules) in blasts excludes a diagnosis of ALL. Auer rods are primarily found in myeloblasts; on rare occasions, they are found in monoblasts or more differentiated monocytic or myelocytic cells.

Other abnormal findings on the blood smear often include monocytosis and neutropenia. Monocytosis frequently precedes overt leukemia. Neutrophils can demonstrate signs of myelodysplasia including **pseudo–Pelger-Huët cells,** hypogranulation, and small nuclei with hypercondensed chromatin. Signs of myelodysplasia are especially common in promyelocytic leukemia.[7] Eosinophils and basophils can be mildly to markedly increased. When present, basophilia can help to differentiate leukemia from a leukemoid reaction. Absolute basophilia is not present in a leukemoid reaction.

BONE MARROW

Bone marrow testing should include both aspirate and biopsy specimens. The quality of marrow specimen is critical for all subsequent analyses. Typically, the bone marrow presentation is hypercellular with decreased fat content (relative to age-related normals), a predominance of blasts, and sometimes an increase in fibrosis. According to the WHO criteria for AL, blasts must compose ≥20% of the nonerythroid nucleated cells to distinguish AL from myelodysplastic syndromes. Frequently, the blast count is close to 100%. Auer rods are present in bone marrow blasts in about half the cases of AML.

Cells can be clumped together, occasionally forming sheets of infiltrate that disturb the usual marrow architecture. In addition to light microscopy morphologic evaluation, bone marrow samples should be tested for immunologic markers and genetic mutations.

 Checkpoint! 1

What results would you expect to find on the CBC and differential in a suspected case of AL?

OTHER LABORATORY FINDINGS

Other laboratory findings can reflect the increased proliferation and turnover of cells. Hyperuricemia and increased lactate dehydrogenase (LD) are common findings resulting from the increased cell turnover. Hypercalcemia, when present, is thought to be caused by increased bone resorption associated with leukemic proliferation in the bone marrow. Increased serum and urine muramidase are typical findings in leukemias with a monocytic component.

CASE STUDY *(continued from page 505)*

Admission laboratory data on Guillermo are as follows:

RBC	3.2×10^{12}/L
Hb	9.7 g/dL
Hct	30.5 L/L
PLT	31×10^9/L
WBC	26.2×10^9/L
Differential	
Blasts	6%
Promyelocytes	79%
Myelocytes	5%
Lymphocytes	11%

Erythrocyte morphology: Erythrocytes are normochromic and normocytic with rare schistocytes seen.

1. What clues do you have that this patient could have an acute leukemia?

2. Based on the presenting data, what additional testing might be of value?

▶ **CLASSIFICATION**

As mentioned (∞ Chapter 21), investigations have shown that the mutant neoplastic "stem" cell can occur at multiple points in the differentiation scheme of the myeloid lineages[8]

(Figure 24-1 ■). The original classification of leukemias was based solely on bright-field microscopy and the patient's signs and symptoms at the time of diagnosis. With the inability to categorize all leukemias by bright-field microscopy, the **FAB classification** developed in 1976 combined morphology and cytochemistry to help identify the neoplastic blast lineage. This classification (Table 24-1 ✪) required ≥30% blasts to establish a diagnosis of AML. The FAB classification

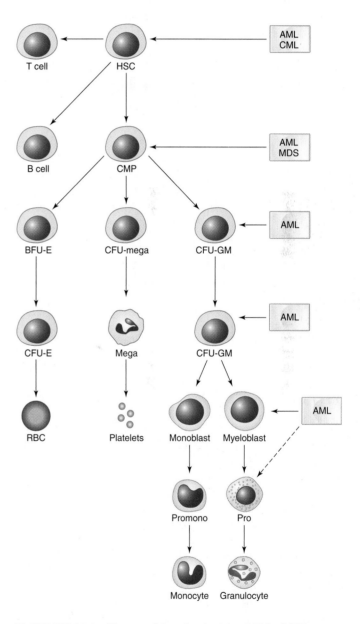

■ FIGURE 24-1   The possible cells of origin of AML. (HSC = hematopoietic stem cell; CMP = Common myeloid progenitor cell; CFU = colony forming unit; mega = megakaryocyte; GM = granulocyte, monocyte; BFU-E = burst-forming unit, erythroid; CFU-E = colony-forming unit, erythroid; AML = acute myelocytic leukemia; CML = chronic myelocytic leukemia.) (Adapted from: Griffin JD, Lowenberg B. Clonogenic cells in acute myeloblastic leukemia. *Blood.* 1986;68[6]:1305.)

⚙ TABLE 24-1

FAB Cytochemical Classification of Acute Leukemia

	Morphology	Myeloperoxidase (MPO)	Sudan Black B (SBB)	Chloroacetate esterase (specific esterase)	α-naphthyl Butyrate esterase (nonspecific esterase)	PAS	Platelet Peroxidase
M0	Acute myelobastic leukemia: minimally differentiated	> 30% blasts; no granules	-	-	-	-	-	-
M1	Acute myelobastic leukemia with no maturation	> 30% blasts; few granules; +/− Auer rods	+	+	+/−	-	-	-
M2	Acute myelobastic leukemia with maturation	> 30% blasts; granules common; + Auer rods	+	+	+/−	-	-	-
M3	Acute promyelocytic leukemia	> 30% blasts; prominent granules; ++Auer rods	++	++	+	-	-	-
M4	Acute myelomonocytic leukemia	> 30% blasts; >20% monocytes; +Auer rods	+	+	+	+	-	-
M4 eo	Acute myelomonocytic leukemia with eosinophilia	> 30% blasts; >20% monocytes; >5% abnormal eosinophils; +Auer rods	+	+	+	+	-	-
M5 a/b	Acute monoblastic leukemia with or without maturation	> 30% blasts; >80% monocytes with/without differentiation	+/−	+/−	-	++	-	-
M6	Acute erythroleukemia	> 30% myeloblasts; >50% megaloblasts; +Auer rods	+ (myeloblasts)	+ (myeloblasts)	+ (myeloblasts)	-	+ (erythroblasts)	-
M7	Acute megakaryocytic leukemia	> 30% megakaryoblasts; cytoplasmic budding	-	-	+/−	-	-	+

++ = strongly present; − = usually not present; +/− = can be present

groups the acute leukemias into AML with eight subgroups, M0–M7 (M4 and M5 have subgroups), and ALL with 3 subgroups, L1–L3.

The newer WHO classification is the result of a worldwide consensus on classification of the hematopoietic neoplasms and expands the parameters used to classify the neoplastic disorders.[10,11,12,13] The parameters include not only microscopic morphology and cytochemistry but also immunologic probes of cell markers, cytogenetics, molecular genetic abnormalities, and clinical findings. In this classification, ≥20% blasts establishes the diagnosis of AL. The WHO four major AML subgroups, each with variants or subtypes, are:

- *AML with recurrent genetic abnormalities.* AML with specific genetic abnormalities, distinctive clinical findings, and characteristic hematologic morphology are defined as subgroups
- *AML with multilineage dysplasia.* The two variants are those with prior history of myelodysplastic syndrome (MDS) and without prior MDS.
- *AML and MDS therapy-related.* These AMLs are distinctly different from de novo (primary) AML in terms of response to therapy and prognosis.
- *AML not otherwise categorized.* Includes any AML not included in the preceding subgroups.

The subgroups of the WHO AML classification are included in Table 24-2 .

 Checkpoint! 2

What is the major difference between the FAB and WHO classification systems in differentiating acute leukemia from the other neoplastic hematologic disorders?

IDENTIFICATION OF CELL LINEAGE

Because blast cells are immature cells, they are often difficult to identify by morphology alone using light microscopy. Cytochemistry, molecular testing, and immunophenotyping give additional information that can help define cell lineage (∞ Chapters 37, 38, 39). When both cytochemistry and immunophenotyping are used, most cases of AL can be classified as being of lymphoid or myeloid origin. Rarely, a population of malignant blasts is cytochemically negative by conventional and ultrastructural methods and nonreactive with both lymphoid and myeloid monoclonal antibodies. Such leukemias are classified as undifferentiated.[14]

The "acute leukemias of ambiguous lineage" are characterized by a blast population with both myeloid and lymphoid markers on the same cell (**biphenotypic leukemia**) or with two separate populations of malignant blasts (i.e., one myeloid and the other lymphoid—(a **mixed lineage leukemia**). The WHO classification defines mixed lineage leukemia. Some believe that the presence of both myeloid

✪ TABLE 24-2

2001 WHO Classification of Acute Myeloid Leukemias (AML)*

Group	Subgroups
AML with recurrent genetic abnormalities	AML with t(8;21)(q22;q22), *AML1(CBFα)/ETO*
	Acute promyelocytic leukemia, AML with t(15;17)(q22;q12), (*PML/RARα*), and variants (FAB M3)
	AML with abnormal bone marrow eosinophils: inv(16)(p13q22) or t(16;16)(p13;q22), (*CBFβ/MYH11*)
	AML with 11q23(*MLL*) abnormalities
AML with multilineage dysplasia	Following myelodysplastic syndrome or myelodysplastic syndrome/myeloproliferative disorder
	Without prior myelodysplastic syndrome
AML and MDS—therapy-related	Alkylating agent related
	Topoisomerase type II inhibitor-related (some can be lymphoid)
	Other types
AML not otherwise categorized	AML minimally differentiated (FAB M0)
	AML without maturation (FAB M1)
	AML with maturation (FAB M2)
	Acute myelomonocytic leukemia (FAB M4)
	Acute monoblastic and monocytic leukemia (FAB M5)
	Acute erythroid leukemia (FAB M6)
	Acute megakaryoblastic leukemia (FAB M7)
	Acute basophilic leukemia
	Acute panmyelosis with myelofibrosis
	Myeloid sarcoma

*The 2008 WHO Classification has some revisions and is on the book's Website.

and lymphoid markers on the same cell is an example of lineage infidelity of malignant cells.[15]

Cytochemistry

The common cytochemical stains originally used in the FAB classification include the myeloperoxidase, Sudan black B, naphthol AS-D chloroacetate esterase (specific esterase), and alpha-naphthyl esterases (nonspecific esterase) (∞ Chapter 34). These stains are still the foundation of cytochemical analysis. Granulocytic cells stain positive with myeloperoxidase and with Sudan black B; lymphoblasts are negative. Thus, these stains help differentiate the acute myeloid leukemias from the acute lymphoblastic leukemias. The esterase stains help differentiate precursor granulocytic cells from precursor monocytic cells. Granulocytic cells stain positive with naphthol AS-D chloroacetate esterase, and cells of monocytic lineage stain positive with nonspecific esterase (Table 24-1). Many institutions have begun using immunophenotyping and cytogenetics as first line tests to define cell lineage. However, cytochemistry can be helpful in cases undefined by these methods and in the identification of some subgroups.[16]

Immunofluorescence or cytochemistry can be used to demonstrate terminal deoxynucleotidyl transferase (TdT) in individual cells. Although originally thought to be a lymphoid specific marker, TdT is found on more immature hematopoietic cells including those of myeloid lineage.[17] Therefore, TdT should not be the sole determinant of lymphoid lineage.

 CASE STUDY *(continued from page 507)*

3. Based on the peripheral blood examination, what cytochemical stain results would you expect to find on Guillermo's neoplastic cells?

Immunophenotyping

Immunophenotyping has become a necessary component of AL classification, particularly when the morphological appearance and cytochemical reactions do not clearly define cell lineage or when the presence of more than one neoplastic cell population is suspected.[18] A specific sequence of testing with monoclonal antibodies is followed.[9,19] The use of extensive panels is costly and time consuming. In most cases, lineage can be determined using a limited, representative panel of monoclonal antibodies. Common cell markers used in identification include CD2, CD3, CD5, CD7, CD10, CD13, CD14, CD15, CD19, CD22, CD33, MPO (myeloperoxidase), HLA-DR, CD34, CD56, CD45, and CD117.[9]

The first panel of monoclonal antibodies should be those that differentiate AML from ALL and T cell ALL (T-ALL) from B cell ALL (B-ALL). More than 90% of AML can be discriminated from ALL using a panel of antibodies such as that listed in Table 24-3. Individual facilities have their own preferred panels of antibodies. Immunophenotyping using monoclonal antibodies for differentiating AML from ALL should include typing for the myeloid antigens, the B lymphoid restricted cell antigens (**CD10, CD19, CD20,** and **CD22**), and the T lymphoid cell antigens (**CD2, CD3, CD5,** and **CD7**). Human leukocyte antigen (HLA)-DR is present on both myeloid and B lymphoid cells. Several aberrant antigens are sometimes found on neoplastic cells (e.g., the CD7 [T-lymphoid] antigen can be found on neoplastic myeloid cells in AML). The **CD34** marker is also present on the least differentiated myeloid cells and early lymphoid cells. These blasts are considered myeloid in nature if immunophenotyping reveals at least one lineage-specific myeloid antigen.[14]

The monoclonal antibodies that react with most cases of AML include CD13, CD15, CD33, and CD117.[20] In addition, the monoclonal antibody that identifies myeloperoxidase is helpful, especially when cytochemistry for myeloperoxidase is negative. Myeloperoxidase occasionally is identified in blasts at the ultrastructural level (i.e., electron microscopy) when negative by light microscopy cytochemistry.

The CMP cell is capable of differentiation into granulocytes, erythrocytes, monocytes, and megakaryocytes. Thus, if the neoplastic clone has "early" myeloid antigens, a second panel of monoclonal antibodies should include antibodies to subtype the AML into granulocytic, monocytic, erythrocytic, and megakaryocytic lineages (Tables 24-4 and 24-5).

✪ TABLE 24-3

Differentiation of ALL from AML Using Immunophenotyping with Selected Monoclonal Antibodies

Leukemia Type	Cell Marker				
	HLA-DR	CD13, CD33	CD19, CD20, CD22	CD10	CD2, CD3, CD5, CD7
AML	+	+	−	−	−
B lymphocyte	+	−	+	+	−
T lymphocyte	−	−	−	+/−	+

TABLE 24-4

The Pattern of Reactivity with Monoclonal Antibodies Most Commonly Observed in the Category AML not Otherwise Categorized (TdT is usually used to identify early lymphoid precursors but can also be found in 10–20% of AML.)

AML Subgroup	Cell Markers with Monoclonal Antibodies								
	HLA-DR	CD34	CD13	CD33	CD11b	CD14	CD71 Glycophorin A	CD41, CD42, CD61	Other Markers That May Be Present
AML minimally differentiated	+	+	+	Usually +	Usually −	Usually −	−	−	−
AML without maturation	+	Usually +	Usually +	+	+ or −	Usually −	−	−	−
AML with maturation	+	Usually −	+	+	+ or −	Usually −	−	−	CD19
Acute myelomonocytic leukemia	−	−	+	+	+	+	−	−	CD11c
Acute monoblastic leukemia/acute monocytic leukemia	+	Usually −	+ or −	+	+	+	−	−	CD11c
Acute erythroid leukemia	+ or −	−	+ or −	+ or −	−	−	+	−	−
Acute megakary-oblastic leukemia	Usually +	+	−	+ or −	−	−	−	+	−

 CASE STUDY *(continued from page 510)*

4. If the cells from Guillermo's bone marrow were immunophenotyped, would you expect CD 13, CD33, CD34, CD19, CD10, CD7, or CD2 to be positive?

CYTOGENETIC ANALYSES

Two-thirds of patients with AML have detectable cytogenetic abnormalities.[21] Of these, approximately 60% are found to have specific, consistent aberrations. Additional abnormalities can develop in subclones as the disease progresses. A clone is present if two or more cells show the identical structural chromosomal change or additional chromosomes or if three cells show the same missing chromosome.[22] The WHO category of AML with recurrent genetic abnormalities has characteristic cytogenetic abnormalities. Therapy-related AML (secondary to alkylating agent therapy) and AML with a history of a previous myelodysplastic disorder also have characteristic cytogenetic abnormalities (and are classified as separate groups of AML in the WHO classification). The nonrandom chromosome abnormalities most commonly associated with these WHO subgroups are discussed in subsequent sections. If the expected abnormal karyotype is not found, molecular analysis is sometimes helpful because the genetic alteration may be detected only at the molecular level (see the following discussion of acute promyelocytic leukemia).

✔ **Checkpoint! 3**

Explain why molecular analysis is not performed on all suspected cases of acute leukemia.

ASSESSMENT OF BONE MARROW

When a diagnosis of AML or MDS is suspected, the first step is to estimate the bone marrow cellularity followed by an assessment of the percentage of erythroblasts. Further evaluation of the bone marrow depends on the number of erythroblasts present (>50% or <50% of all nucleated marrow cells). If erythroblasts compose more than 50% of all nucleated bone marrow cells, the percentage of nonerythroid blast cells (i.e., myeloblasts, monoblasts) is determined by

★ TABLE 24-5

Morphologic, Immunophenotypic, and Cytochemical Results Used to Classify AML (WHO)

	Morphology	Immunophenotype	Cytochemistry
1. AML with recurrent genetic abnormalities			
AML with t(8;21)(q22;q22), *AML1(CBFα)/ETO*	Maturation in the neutrophil lineage Auer rods, pseudo–Pelger Huët nuclei	CD13, CD33, CD34, MPO, CD56 + Occasional CD19 + Occasional TdT +	Myeloperoxidase + Sudan black B +
Acute promyelocytic leukemia, AML with t(15;17)(q22;q12), (*PML/RARα*), and variants (old FAB M3)	Hypergranular variant Promyelocytes dominate Abnormal hypergranulation Multiple Auer rods in one cell Microgranular variant Butterfly shaped nuclei No visible granularity	CD33, CD13 + (CD2 and CD9 +/–) CD15, CD34, HLADR–	Myeloperoxidase + + Sudan black B + + Nonspecific esterase = weakly +
AML with abnormal bone marrow eosinophils: inv(16)(p13q22) or t(16;16)(p13;q22), (*CBFβ/MYH11*)	Maturation in both the neutrophil and monocytic lineage; abnormal eosinophils (AMML Eo) Eosinophils≥5% Abnormal eosinophilic granules present in promyelocyte or myelocyte stage	CD13, CD33, MPO + CD14, CD4, CD11b, CD 11c, CD64, CD36, and lysosyme +	Myeloperoxidase + Sudan black B +
AML with 11q23(*MLL*) abnormalities	Monoblasts and promonocytes predominate. Pseudopods frequent	CD 13, CD 33 variable CD14, CD4, CD11b, CD11c, CD64, CD36, and lysosyme + for monocytic cells	Myeloperoxidase +/– Sudan black B +/– Nonspecific esterase +
2. AML with multilineage dysplasia			
Following myelodysplastic syndrome or myelodysplastic syndrome/myeloproliferative disorder Without prior MDS	Dysplasia required in ≥50% of two cell lines Hypogranular neutrophils, pseudo–Pelger-Huët nuclei Dyserythropoiesis with megaloblastoid changes, ringed sideroblasts, nuclear fragments or vacuoles Dysmegakaryopoiesis with micromegakaryocytes, hypolobulated nuclei, and other dysplastic signs	CD34, CD13, CD33 + CD56 and CD7 +/– Multi-drug resistance glycoprotein receptor (MDR-1) +/–	Myeloperoxidase + Sudan black B + Increased iron in ring formation + Periodic Acid Schiff (PAS +)
3. AML and MDS, therapy related			
Alkylating agent related	Pancytopenia or isolated cytopenia Ringed sideroblasts Obvious multiple dysplasias	CD 34+ CD13 and CD33 + CD56 and CD7 +/–	Myeloperoxidase + Sudan black B + Increased iron in ring formation + PAS +
Topoisomerase type II inhibitor-related (some can be lymphoid)	Dominant monocytic component Neutrophil maturation possible		Myeloperoxidase +/– Specific esterase + Nonspecific esterease +

4. AML not otherwise categorized

AML minimally differentiated (FAB M0)	Minimal evidence of myeloid differentiation No maturation seen Agranular cytoplasm	CD13, CD33, CD117 + CD34, CD38, HLA-DR +	Myeloperoxidase−(<3% of blasts) Sudan black B−(<3% of blasts) Specific esterase −
AML without maturation (FAB M1)	Evidence of myeloid differentiation, no maturation seen, Auer rods or some granulation	C13, CD33, CD117, CD34, lysosyme +	Myeloperoxidase + (>3% of blasts) Sudan black B + (>3% of blasts) Specific esterase +
AML with maturation (FAB M2)	All stages of neutrophil maturation Pseudo–Pelger–Huët Hypogranulation Eosinophilic precursors possible	CD13, CD33, CD 15 + CD 117, CD34, HLA-DR +/− CD 11b, CD11c, CD14 − ; CD 3, CD 20, CD79a −	Myeloperoxidsae + Sudan black B + Specific esterase +
Acute myelomonocytic leukemia AMML (FAB M4)	Neutrophil and monocytic precursors present Vacuolization	CD13, CD33 CD14, CD4, CD11b, CD11c, CD64, CD36 lysosyme +	Myeloperoxidase + Nonspecific esterase +/− Specific esterase +
Acute monoblastic and monocytic leukemia (FAB M5)	Monoblast/monocyte dominance Hemophagocytosis present Nuclear lobulation	CD13, CD33, CD117 + CD14, CD4, CD11b, CD11c, CD64, CD68, CD36, lysosyme +	Myeloperoxidase − Nonspecific esterase + Specific esterase −
Acute erythroid leukemia (FAB M6)	>50% erythroid precursors and >20% myeloblasts in the nonerythroid cell population Megaloblastoid morphology Auer rods +/−	CD13, CD33, CD117 + Glycophorim A +	Myeloperoxidase + Sudan black B + Nonspecific esterase +/− PAS + (erythroblasts)
Acute megakaryoblastic leukemia (FAB M7)	Cytopenia with or without thrombocytopenia Basophilic agranular blasts with pseudopods Micromegakaryocytes	CD41 and/or CD61 + CD13, CD 33, and CD 42 +/−	Myeloperoxidase − Sudan black B − Nonspecific esterase +/− Specific esterase − PAS + Platelet peroxidase +
Acute basophilic leukemia	Basophilic precursors Vacuolization	C13, CD33, CD 34, and class II HLA-DR +	Metachromatic positivity with toluidine blue
Acute panmyelosis with myelofibrosis	Pancytopenia Dysplastic changes in neutrophils and platelets	CD13, CD33, CD117 + Lysosyme, CD41, CD61 and glycophorin A +/−	Myeloperoxidase +
Myeloid sarcoma	Biopsy of specific lesion	CD13, CD33, CD117 +	Myeloperoxidsae + Specific esterase +

Specific esterase = Napthol AS-D chloroacetate esterase; nonspecific esterase = Alpha-naphthyl esterase

performing a differential count on the nonerythroid cells. This differential count is used in determining the percentage of myeloblasts in the AML category of erythroleukemia. If fewer than 50% erythroblasts are in the bone marrow, it is not necessary to exclude the erythroid cells from the differential count in determining the percentage of myeloblasts or monoblasts for a diagnosis of AL or MDS (Figure 24-2■). The diagnosis of the myeloblastic/monoblastic AL is made when ≥20% of all nucleated bone marrow cells are leukocytic blasts. The WHO classification does not include the RAEB-t subgroup of MDS, which is in the FAB classification (20–29% blasts) but reclassifies it as AL (∞ Chapter 23). Additional assessment of the subtypes of AML evaluates only the myeloid cells, not lymphocytes, plasma cells, mast cells, macrophages, or nucleated erythrocytes.

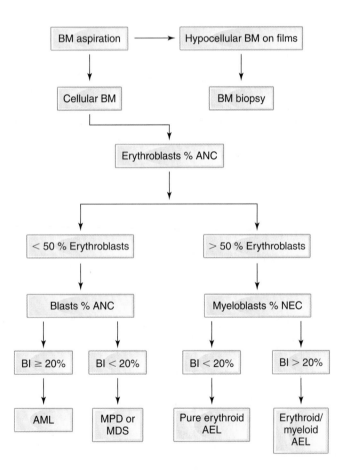

■ FIGURE 24-2   Suggested steps in the analysis of a bone marrow aspirate to reach a diagnosis. (ANC = all nucleated cells; NEC = nonerythroid cells; AML = acute myelocytic leukemia; MDS = myelodysplastic syndrome; MPD = myeloproliferative disorders; AEL = acute erythrocytic leukemia; M1–M5 = FAB subtypes of AML; Bl = leukocytic blasts.) (Adapted from: Bennett JM, et al. Proposed revised criteria for the classification of acute myeloid leukemia. *Ann Intern Med.* 1985;103:620.)

WHO CLASSIFICATION OF AML

AML with Recurrent Cytogenetic Abnormalities

This classification consists of presentations with recurrent chromosome abnormalities, usually balanced (reciprocal) translocations (see below). In most cases, the chromosomal rearrangements create a fusion gene, encoding a novel fusion (chimeric) protein. Molecular techniques (RT-PCR) have a higher sensitivity than cytogenetics for diagnosing and following the progression of the disease. The AMLs in this category generally have a high rate of complete remission and a more favorable prognosis.

AML with t(8;21)(q22;q22);(*AML1/ETO*)   This subcategory generally presents morphologically as AML with maturation. Myeloblasts are usually large with abundant basophilic cytoplasm containing numerous azurophilic granules and Auer rods. Promyelocytes, myelocytes, and mature neutrophils with variable dysplasia are usually present in the bone marrow. Eosinophilia can be present. Cytochemical and immunophenotypic results are typical for myeloblasts (Table 24-5). The leukemic "cell of origin" is believed to be the hematopoietic stem cell (HSC). This cytogenetic category accounts for 5–12% of cases of AML.[13]

Core binding factor (CBF), a transcription factor critical for hematopoietic development, is composed of two subunits: CBFα (also known as *AML1* or *RUNX1*) and CBFβ. The t(8;21) translocation results in a chimeric protein containing the N-terminal portion of AML1 (chromosome 21) and most of the ETO protein from chromosome 8 (a nuclear protein involved in the regulation of transcription). The fusion protein blocks the normal function of AML-1 and induces abnormal gene activation and gene repression. This presumably contributes to the leukemic phenotype of increased proliferation with blocked differentiation.[5]

AML with abnormal bone marrow eosinophils inv(16)(p13;q22) or t(16;16)(p13;q22) (*CBFβ/MYH11*)   This subcategory generally presents morphologically as AML with monocytic and granulocytic maturation and the presence of abnormal eosinophils in the bone marrow. The combination of acute myelomonocytic leukemia (AMML) with abnormal eosinophils is morphologically *AMML Eo.* The most striking abnormality of the eosinophils is the presence of immature (basophilic) granules, predominantly evident at the promyelocyte and myelocyte stages. The immunophenotypic and cytochemical results reflect the presence of both neutrophilic and monocytic lineages (Table 24-5). The leukemic cell of origin is believed to be an HSC. This type accounts for 10–12% of all cases of AML.[13]

The inv(16)(p13;q22) and t(16;16)(p13;q22) both result in the fusion of the *CBFβ* gene (16q22) to the smooth muscle myosin heavy chain gene SMMHC (*MYH11*) at 16p13. Because of difficulties in correctly identifying these mutations with traditional cytogenetics, fluorescent in situ hybridization (FISH) or RT-PCR may be necessary to document the mutation. The CBFβ/SMMHC fusion protein binds to AML1/CBFα and represses its function as a transcription factor.[5]

AML with 11q23(*MLL*) abnormalities.

These leukemias are usually associated with monocytic features (monoblasts and promonocytes). They can occur at any age but are more common in children. Identical cytogenetic abnormalities can also be found in therapy-related AML (see below). Patients can have extramedullary monocytic sarcomas (malignant tumors that originate in connective tissue) and tissue infiltration (gingiva, skin) and may present with disseminated intravascular coagulation. Monoblasts and promonocytes can have scattered azurophilic granules and vacuoles and give cytochemical and phenotypic results typical for the monocytic lineage (Table 24-5). The leukemic cell of origin is believed to be the HSC. AML with 11q23 (MLL) abnormalities is found in 5–6% of cases of AML.[13]

The *MLL* gene (11q23) is involved in a number of leukemia-associated translocations with different partner chromosomes. The MLL protein is a DNA-binding protein that interacts with other nuclear proteins and permits the association of transcription factors which help regulate transcription. The most common translocations involving 11q23 seen in childhood AML are t(9;11)(p21;q23), t(11;19)(q23;p13.1), and t(11;19)(q23;p13.3). Other translocations involving ~20 different partner chromosomes have also been observed. In addition, some *MLL* gene rearrangements can be identified only by molecular studies, not by conventional cytogenetics.[5]

AML with t(15;17)(q22;q12)(*PML/RARα*) and Variants

One of the most well-studied leukemias is acute promyelocytic leukemia (APL) with t(15;17)(q22;q12), an AML in which abnormal promyelocytes predominate. Both hypergranular ("typical" APL) and hypogranular or microgranular presentations are seen. APL can occur at any age, but most patients are adults in middle life. APL constitutes 5–8% of AML[13]

The presenting signs for both hypergranular and hypogranular APL often include acute disseminated intravascular coagulation (DIC).[23] (See ∞ Chapter 32 for a review of the pathophysiology of DIC.) The most common clinical finding at initial diagnosis is bleeding. It is believed that the release of procoagulant material from promyelocytic granules initiates DIC, a serious complicating factor of the disease.[24] Therapy for the leukemia can potentiate or aggrevate this complication because lysed promyelocytes release large amounts of this material. In addition, a significant release of tissue factor–containing particles from dying cells can occur during cytotoxic therapy. Evidence of secondary fibrinolysis as a component of the DIC syndrome is also present. Heparin therapy can be administered with initiation of chemotherapy to prevent or modulate the DIC. Other abnormalities of coagulation can be present.

Hypergranular APL   Most patients with the hypergranular subtype are leukopenic or exhibit only slightly increased leukocyte counts. Most cells in the bone marrow are abnormal promyelocytes with heavy azurophilic granulation. The granules can be so densely packed that they obscure the nucleus (Figure 24-3a■). Some cells filled with fine dustlike granules also can be present. Cells with multiple Auer rods, sometimes occurring in bundles (**faggot cells**), are characteristic with cytoplasm that is frequently clear and pale blue, but cells can contain only a few azurophilic granules or lakes

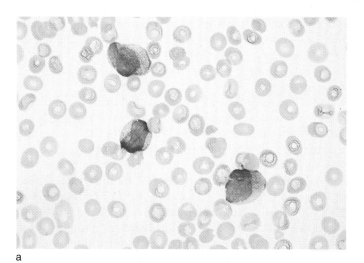

a

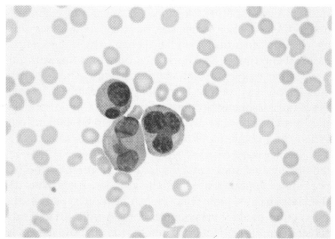

b

■ FIGURE 24-3   **a.** Peripheral blood film from a patient with acute promyelocytic leukemia (APL), hypergranular variant. These promyelocytes have an irregularly shaped nucleus and numerous azurophilic granules. **b.** Peripheral blood film from a patient with APL, microgranular variant. Note the bilobed nuclei and absent or fine granules in these abnormal promyelocytes. (Wright-Giemsa stain; 1000× magnification)

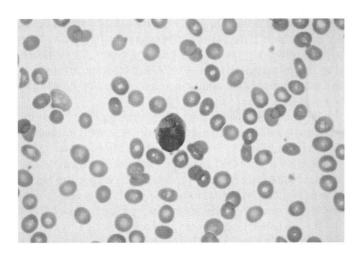

■ FIGURE 24-4   A faggot cell from promyelocytic leukemia. Notice the bundle of Auer rods. (Wright-Giemsa stain; 1000× magnification)

of clear pink material[25] (Figure 24-4 ■). In some cases, the typical hypergranularity of promyelocytes is less evident in the peripheral blood than in the bone marrow.[26] The nucleus varies in shape but is often folded or indented or sometimes bilobed. Often a large number of promyelocytes appear to be disrupted on the blood smear with free azurophilic granules and Auer rods intermingled with intact cells. Anemia and thrombocytopenia are typical findings.

Microgranular APL Variant   In contrast to typical APL, the leukocyte count in microgranular APL is usually markedly increased.[27] The predominant cell in the peripheral blood is a promyelocyte with a bilobular, reniform, or multilobed nucleus (resembling that of a monocyte) and cytoplasm with an apparent paucity of granules on Romanowswky-stained smears (Figure 24-3b ■). The apparent absence of granules is due to their submicroscopic size, but they are readily visible by electron microscopy and cytochemistry (myeloperoxidase, MPO positive). The nuclear chromatin is fine with nucleoli often visible. A small abnormal promyelocyte with a bilobed nucleus, deeply basophilic cytoplasm, and sometimes cytoplasmic projections is present as a minor population in most cases but occasionally is the predominant cell. When cytoplasmic projections are present, the cells can resemble megakaryoblasts. Faggot cells are scarce or absent, but single Auer rods can be found. In contrast to the hypogranular appearance of peripheral blood promyelocytes, the bone marrow promyelocytes can be more typical of the cells found in the hypergranular form of APL. Cytochemical and immunophenotypic results for APL are given in Table 24-5.

A form of APL in which some promyelocytes contain metachromatic granules (when stained with toluidine blue) has been described.[27] Distinctive features include folded nuclei, hypergranular cytoplasm, and coarse metachromatic granules.

Diagnostic Gene Rearrangement   The t(15;17) rearrangement is consistently associated with APL. The break point involves the retinoic acid receptor alpha (*RARα*) gene on chromosome 17 and the *PML* gene on chromosome 15 and is limited to the neoplastic cells. Some APL patients have a cytogenetically normal karyotype, but molecular analysis has shown submicroscopic insertion of *RARα* into *PML,* leading to the expression of the PML/RARα transcript. No major differences exist between t(15;17) positive patients and PML/RARα positive patients without t(15;17).[13] These findings suggest that the t(15;17) translocation/fusion protein is involved in the pathogenesis of the disease. However, other variant translocations have been reported in PML, all involving the *RARα* gene translocated with different target genes, including *PLZF* on chromosome 11(t[11;17][9q23;q21]), *NuMA* on chromosome 15 (t[11;17][q13;q21]), *NPM* on chromosome 5 (t[5;17][q23;q12]), and *STAT5b* on chromosome 17 (t[17;17]).[13]

The typical t(15;17) gene rearrangement results in a fusion *PML/RARα* gene and a reciprocal *RARα/PML* gene. The PML/RARα mRNA has been identified in all APL patients while the RARα/PML mRNA is found in about two-thirds of APL patients.[28] Molecular analysis of the *PML/RARα* gene is important in monitoring therapy and relapse because the gene disappears with successful treatment but returns as an early marker of relapse. Also, some patients have molecular evidence of the fusion protein product (fusion gene) in the absence of a detectable cytogenetic abnormality.

The RARα protein is a nuclear hormone receptor that binds to specific DNA sequences (RA responsive elements) and controls transcription of specific target genes under the control of the retinoid hormones. RARα forms a complex with a second protein, retinoid-X receptor (RXRα). In the absence of RA, the RARα/RXRα complex represses transcription by recruiting corepressor proteins and inducing histone deacetylation.[29] Physiologic concentrations of RA normally induce a conformational change in the RARs, causing release of the corepressor molecules and recruitment of coactivator molecules, resulting in gene transcription and granulocytic differentiation.[30]

PML is a growth suppressor nuclear protein normally found in complex macromolecular structures containing numerous other nuclear proteins. The PML/RARα fusion protein binds to the RA responsive elements of the target genes. Like the native protein, the fusion protein recruits corepressor molecules and in the absence of RA inhibits transcription of RA-responsive genes. Although the fusion protein can bind RA, physiologic concentrations of RA are not sufficient to induce the release of the corepressor proteins from PML/RARα, and repression of gene transcription is maintained.[30] Thus, the cells do not differentiate into granulocytes.

Pharmacological concentrations of RA (all-transretinoic acid—ATRA) have proven to be an effective treatment for inducing complete hematologic remission in APL (but the remission is generally short lived). ATRA induces the neoplastic promyelocytes to differentiate to mature granulocytes, thus overcoming the maturation arrest.[31] It is thought that a high concentration of RA, as is given in induction therapy for APL, overcomes the interference with receptor activation (it promotes release of the corepressor molecules and assembly of the coactivator molecules on the target genes, allowing gene transcription and cellular differentiation). Cells previously unable to mature and initiate apoptosis are then able to do so, causing a transitory situation known as *hyperleukocytosis.*

Unfortunately, the stem cells bearing the t(15;17) translocation are unaffected by ATRA and continue to proliferate, resulting in relapse of the disease. The current approach to therapy is to induce hematologic remission with ATRA and then administer traditional chemotherapy (to try to eradicate the leukemic stem cells). When the promyelocytes are first induced to differentiate and are no longer present in large numbers, the subsequent chemotherapy does not result in the massive death of promyelocytes (and the release of procoagulants), thus avoiding or minimizing the life-threatening effects of DIC. Instead, the chemotherapy destroys the dividing stem cells that bear the t(15;17) translocation and induces a durable remission.

About 25% of patients given RA therapy become acutely ill associated with the death and lysis of the large number of cells. The mortality rate in these individuals can be high. The illness is similar to capillary leak syndrome with fever, respiratory disease, renal impairment, and hemorrhage.[32]

 Checkpoint! 4

Why is it important to do molecular studies on patients with acute promyelocytic leukemia?

AML with Multilineage Dysplasia (With or Without Prior Myelodysplastic Syndrome)

AML with multilineage dysplasia is an acute leukemia (≥20% blasts) with dysplasia in two or more myeloid cell lines. It occurs de novo (anew) or following a myelodysplastic/myeloproliferative disorder (MDS/MPD). Diagnosis requires dysplasia in ≥50% of the cells of at least two lineages.[13] Examples of dysplasia include hypogranular PMNs, psuedo–Pelger-Huët anomaly, megaloblastic erythrocytes, erythrocytes with multinuclearity or nuclear fragmentation, ringed sideroblasts, micromegakaryocytes, and/or megakaryocytes with monolobed nuclei or multiple separated nuclei. No significant difference in the disease progression and prognosis between AMLs arising from myelodysplasia or from de novo AMLs with multilineage dysplasia has been identified.[11]

Immunophenotypic and cytochemical results for this category of AML are included in Table 24-5. The cytogenetic abnormalities are variable and are similar to those seen in MDS including: −7/del(7q); −5/del(5q); +8, +9, +11, del(11q), del(12p), −18, +19, del(20q) and +21.[13] The cell of origin is believed to be the HSC. This type of AML (with multilineage dysplasia) generally has a poor prognosis.[13]

AML and Myelodysplastic Syndrome, Therapy-Related

These disorders arise as a result of cytotoxic chemotherapy and/or radiation therapy. Two major subtypes are described, those following alkylating agent/radiation treatment and those following topoisomerase II inhibitor treatment.[13]

AML can develop 5–6 years following alkylating agent therapy (range 1–10 years). The disease often presents initially with a myelodysplastic syndrome, eventually evolving to AML. Cytogenetic abnormalities are similar to those seen in AML with multilineage dysplasia and de novo MDS (unbalanced translocations or deletions involving chromosomes 5 and 7). Other chromosomes involved include 1, 4, 12, 14, and 18.

AML develops an average of ~3 years following therapy with a topoisomerase II inhibitor (range 1–15 years). In this instance, AML usually presents without a preceding MDS phase. Cytogenetic abnormalities are most commonly associated with a balanced translocation involving 11q23 (the *MLL* gene).

The cell of origin is thought to be the HSC. Therapy-related AML is generally refractory to treatment and is associated with shortened survival.[33]

Acute Myeloid Leukemias not Otherwise Categorized

This AML category includes cases of AML that do not fulfill criteria for any of the other described groups.[13] The subcategories in this group are primarily differentiated on morphology and cytochemical features. The defining criteria for all is ≥20% blasts (the blast percentage includes promyelocytes in APL and promonocytes in AML with monocytic differentiation). For pure erythroid leukemias, the blast percentage is based on the percentage of abnormal erythroblasts. Immunophenotypic and cytochemical results for this category of AML are included in Table 24-5.

AML—Minimally Differentiated This rather rare leukemia is characterized by lack of evidence of myeloid differentiation by morphology (absence of granules) or cytochemistry (<3% of the blasts are positive for SBB or MPO).[13] This subtype accounts for less than 5% of all AMLs and is generally associated with a poor prognosis. The blasts, however, demonstrate myeloid differentiation by immunologic markers for the myeloid lineage (CD13 and CD33) and/or ultrastructural cytochemistry studies.[34] Most cases are also CD34, CD38, and HLA-DR +. No unique chromosomal abnormalities are associated with this subtype, but trisomy 13, 8, and 4 as well as monosomy 7 have been reported. Cells that fulfill these criteria but also have evidence for ultrastructural platelet peroxidase and/or show the glycoprotein IIb/IIIa (CD41) immunophenotype should be classified as acute megakaryoblastic leukemia.[35] Because the blasts in the minimally differentiated AML group have no morphologic differentiating features, immunophenotyping should also be used to exclude the lymphoid lineage. The cell of origin is thought to be a hematopoietic precursor cell at the earliest stage of myeloid differentiation.[13]

AML Without Maturation   Characterized by a high percentage of bone marrow blasts without significant evidence of maturation to more mature neutrophils, the variant AML without maturation may occur at any age but most commonly in adulthood. It accounts for ~10% of the cases of AML.[13] Leukocytosis is present in about 50% of patients at the time of initial diagnosis. The defining feature is its lack of cellular maturation (<10% of all granulocytic cells show evidence of maturation beyond the myeloblast stage) (Figure 24-5 ■).

The predominant cell in the peripheral blood is usually a poorly differentiated myeloblast with fine lacy chromatin and nucleoli. Myeloblasts are usually ≥90% of nonerythroid cells in the bone marrow with >3% of blasts positive for MPO and/or SBB. The blasts may have azurophilic granules, Auer rods, and vacuoles. If no evidence of granules or Auer rods is present, the blasts can resemble lymphoblasts and must be differentiated by immunophenotype. Patients frequently present with anemia, thrombocytopenia, and neutropenia. Cytochemical staining reactions for Auer rods are similar to reactions for myeloblasts (Table 24-6 ✪). About 50% of patients demonstrate clonal chromosome aberrations in the leukemic cells, which are of variable origin. If the karyotype is abnormal, the prognosis is significantly worse for this subtype of AML. The cell of origin is thought to be a hematopoietic precursor cell at the earliest stage of myeloid differentiation.[13]

✓ Checkpoint! 5

What hematologic features help differentiate AML minimally differentiated from AML without maturation?

✪ TABLE 24-6

Cytochemical Reactions for Auer Rods

SBB	+
MPO	+
Napthol AS-D chloroacetate esterase	±
PAS	±
Romanowsky	+ or − (occasionally seen only with MPO or SBB)

AML With Maturation.   AML with maturation is characterized by ≥20% blasts with evidence of maturation to more mature neutrophils (>10% of cells at differentiated stages of maturation: promyelocytes, myelocytes, metamyelocytes). Monocytes and their precursors constitute <20% of the marrow cells. This type of AML occurs in all age groups (20% of patients are <25 years of age, and 45% are >60 years of age) and accounts for about 30% of AML cases.[13] Patients often present with anemia, thrombocytopenia, and neutropenia.

Blasts with and without azurophilic granulation can be present, and blasts frequently contain Auer rods. Variable dysplasia can be seen, including myeloid hypogranulation, granulocytic hypo- and hyper-segmentation, and occasionally binucleated myeloid cells (Figure 24-6 ■). The bone marrow is hypercellular, and myeloblasts make up from 20 to 89% of the non-erythroid nucleated cells. Eosinophils and sometimes basophils can be increased. The cell of origin is thought to be a hematopoietic precursor cell at the earliest stage of myeloid differentiation.[13]

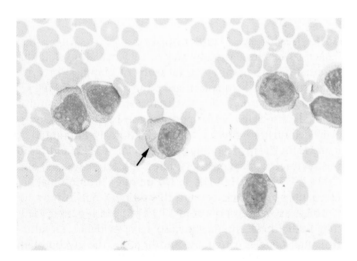

■ FIGURE 24-5   Peripheral blood film from a patient with AML without maturation. The large mononuclear cells are myeloblasts. The cell in the center (arrow) is a myeloblast with an Auer rod. Note the high nuclear-to-cytoplasmic ratio, the fine lacy chromatin, and the prominent nucleoli. (Wright-Giemsa stain; 1000× magnification)

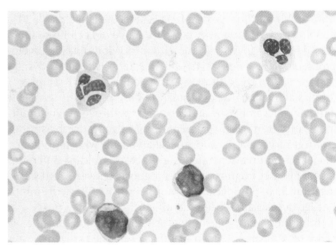

■ FIGURE 24-6   Peripheral blood film from a patient with AML-with maturation. Myeloblasts are at the bottom and hypogranulated segmented neutrophils are at the top. (Wright-Giemsa stain; 1000× magnification)

Checkpoint! 6

A patient with AML has a peripheral blood differential that includes 91% myeloblasts, 4% promyelocytes, 3% granulocytes, and 2% monocytes. Which category of AML is the most likely diagnosis? Explain.

Acute Myelomonocytic Leukemia (AMML) Characterized by proliferation of both myelocytic and monocytic precursors, the bone marrow in *AMML* is hypercellular with ≥20% blasts; neutrophils and their precursors as well as monocytes and their precursors compose ≥20% of marrow cells. AMML is one of the most common AML variants, accounting for 15–25% of AML cases. Some patients have a history of chronic myelomonocytic leukemia. Infiltrations of leukemic cells in extramedullary sites are more frequent than in the pure granulocytic variants. Serum and urinary levels of muramidase (lysozyme) are usually elevated because of the monocytic proliferation.

The peripheral blood leukocyte count in AMML is usually increased. Monocytic cells (monoblasts, promonocytes, monocytes) are increased to ≥5 × 10⁹/L (Figure 24-7 ■). Anemia and thrombocytopenia are present in almost all cases. The myeloblasts appear similar to blasts in AML with differentiation. Monoblasts are usually large with abundant bluish-gray cytoplasm and can show pseudopods. Scattered fine azurophilic granules and vacuoles can be present. The nucleus is round or convoluted with delicate chromatin and one or more prominent nucleoli. The monoblasts and myeloblasts demonstrate the expected cytochemical and immunophenotypic results for their respective lineages (Table 24-5). The bone marrow can reveal erythrophagocytosis by monocytes. The cell of origin is thought to be a hematopoietic precursor cell with the potential to differentiate into neutrophil and monocytic lineages (CFU-GM).¹³

Additional laboratory testing is required when (1) the bone marrow findings are as previously described but the peripheral blood monocyte count is <5 × 10⁹/L and (2) the peripheral blood monocyte count is ≥5 × 10⁹/L but the bone marrow has <20% monocytic cells. In these cases, ancillary laboratory tests such as lysozyme levels or cytochemical methods can be utilized to confirm the presence of a significant monocytic component and establish a diagnosis of AMML (Table 24-7 ✪).

Acute Monoblastic Leukemia and Acute Monocytic Leukemia These subtypes are myeloid leukemias in which ≥ 80% of the leukemic cells are monocytic (including monoblasts, promonocytes, and monocytes). The neutrophilic component, if present, is <20% of the cells. The majority of the monocytic cells (usually >80%) found in acute monoblastic leukemia are monoblasts (Figure 24-8a ■ and b ■). The majority of the monocytic cells in acute monocytic leukemia are promonocytes (Figure 24-9a ■ and b ■). Acute monoblastic leukemia accounts for 5–8% of AML cases, and acute monocytic leukemia accounts for 3–6% of the cases.¹³ This disease is usually seen in children or young adults.

The most common clinical findings are weakness, bleeding, and a diffuse erythematous skin rash. One notable aspect of this disease is the degree of extramedullary leukemic proliferation (gingival and cutaneous infiltration, central nervous system involvement). As with AMML, serum and

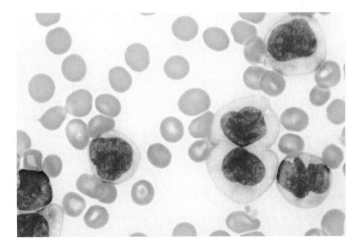

■ FIGURE 24-7 Peripheral blood film from a case of acute myelomonocytic leukemia (AMML). Monoblasts and promonocytes are present. (Wright-Giemsa stain; 1000× magnification)

✪ TABLE 24-7

Nonimmunophenotypic Criteria for Diagnosis of AMML	
I. Bone marrow	Blasts ≥20% of nonerythroid cells
	Monocytic cells ≥20% of nonerythroid cells
	Granulocytic cells ≥20% of nonerythroid cells
and Peripheral blood	≥5 × 10⁹/L monocytic cells
or if Peripheral blood	<5 × 10⁹/L monocytic cells
Requires ancillary tests	Serum or urinary lysozyme 3 × normal;
	or naphthol AS-D chloroacetate esterase *and* alpha-naphthyl acetate esterase (+) in blasts;
	or naphthol AS-D acetate esterase with and without NaFl reveal >20% monocytic cells in bone marrow
II. Peripheral blood	≥5 × 10⁹/L monocytic cells
and Bone marrow	Blasts ≥20% of nonerythroid cells
	Monocytic cells <20% of nonerythroid cells
Requires ancillary tests	Serum or urinary lysozyme 3 × normal;
	or naphthol AS-D chloroacetate esterase *and* alpha-naphthyl acetate esterase (+) in blasts;
	or naphthol AS-D acetate esterase with and without NaFl reveal >20% monocytic cells in bone marrow

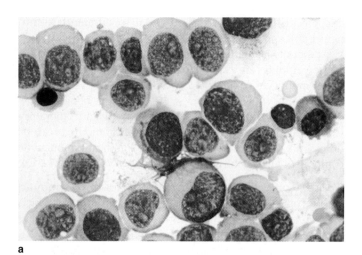
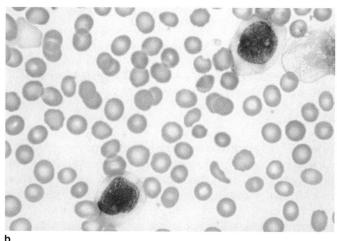

a

b

■ FIGURE 24-8   a. A smear from a bone marrow aspirate of a patient with acute monoblastic leukemia. The cells are predominately monoblasts and promonocytes. b. Monoblasts in peripheral blood from a case of acute monoblastic leukemia. (Wright-Giemsa stain; 1000×
magnification)

urine muramidase are moderately elevated. Monocytic cells account for 80% or more of cells in the bone marrow. Monocytes in the peripheral blood are increased, and monoblasts are often present. The monoblasts are large (up to 40 μ) with abundant, variably basophilic cytoplasm. Pseudopods with translucent cytoplasm are common and fine azurophilic granules can be present. The nucleus is round or oval with delicate chromatin and one or more prominent nucleoli, but Auer rods are usually not found. Dyshematopoiesis is not conspicuous. Promonocytes have a more irregular and convoluted nucleus, and nucleoli can be present. The cytoplasm is less basophilic than that of the monoblast with a ground glass appearance. Fine azurophilic granules are often present.

Abnormalities of the long arm of chromosome 11 with translocations or deletions are often found in monocytic leukemias. The t(8;16) abnormality is also found and is associated with hemophagocytosis. The expression of *c-FOS* proto-oncogene on chromosome 14 appears to be enhanced in acute leukemias with monocytic lineage involvement.[36] This gene has been linked to normal monocyte-macrophage differentiation. The cell of origin for this AML subtype is believed to be a hematopoietic precursor cell committed to monocytic differentiation (CFU-M).[13]

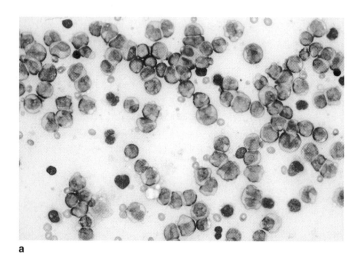
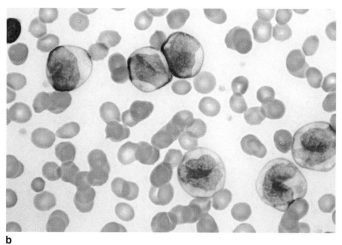

a

b

■ FIGURE 24-9   a. A smear from a bone marrow aspirate of a patient with acute monocytic leukemia. There is a predominance of
promonocytes and monoblasts. (Wright-Giemsa stain; 400× magnification) b. Monocytic cells in peripheral blood, including
promonocytes and monoblasts, from acute monocytic leukemia. (Wright-Giemsa stain; 1000× magnification)

Acute Erythroid Leukemia (AEL) Acute erythroid leukemias have a predominant erythroid population. The two subtypes described are differentiated by the presence or absence of a sigificant myeloid component. The erythroid/myeloid variant of erythroid leukemia is defined by ≥50% erythroid precursors in the bone marrow (percent of all nucleated cells) with ≥ 20% myeloblasts in the nonerythroid cell population. Pure erythroid leukemias show neoplastic proliferation exclusively in the erythroid lineage (>80% of total marrow cells).[37] Erythroid/myeloid leukemia is predominantly a disease of adults and acounts for 5–6% of cases of AML. Pure erythroid leukemia is extremely rare and can occur at any age.[13]

The most dominant changes in the peripheral blood are anemia with striking poikilocytosis and anisocytosis with a large number of nucleated red blood cells (RBC). Nucleated erythrocytes are dysplastic with megaloblastoid nuclei and/or bi- or multinucleated cells in the more immature stages. The cytoplasm frequently contains vacuoles. Myeloblasts can be seen in the peripheral blood in the mixed lineage form of AEL (Figure 24-10 ■).

The bone marrow erythroblasts are distinctly abnormal with bizarre morphological features. Giant multilobular or multinucleated forms are common (Figures 24-11 ■ and 24-12 ■). Other features include nuclear budding and fragmentation, cytoplasmic vacuoles, Howell-Jolly bodies, ringed sideroblasts, and megaloblastoid changes. Erythrophagocytosis of the abnormal erythroblasts is a common finding. Auer rods can be found in the myeloblasts in the mixed lineage variant. Dysmegakaryopoiesis is common with mononuclear forms or micromegakaryoblasts present. Neutrophils can exhibit hypogranularity and pseudo–Pelger-Huët anomaly. The

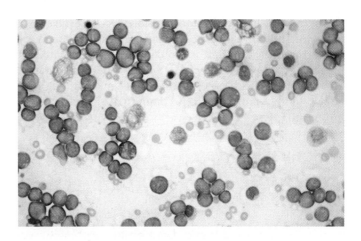

■ FIGURE 24-11   Smear of a bone marrow aspirate from a patient with erythroid/myeloid AEL. Most cells are myeloblasts. (Wright-Giemsa stain 400× magnification)

leukocyte alkaline phosphatase score is normal or increased. Leukocytes and platelets are usually decreased.

Normoblasts are typically PAS negative; however, in erythroleukemia, erythroblasts can demonstrate coarse positivity in either a diffuse or granular pattern. PAS-positive erythroblasts are occasionally also found in MDS, other subgroups of AML, iron-deficiency anemia, thalassemia, severe hemolytic anemia, and sometimes in megaloblastic anemia. The myeloblastic component shows reactions similar to those found in other subtypes of AML in both morphology and chromosomal aberrations. Erythroblasts usually react positively with antibodies to glycophorin A or hemoglobin A.

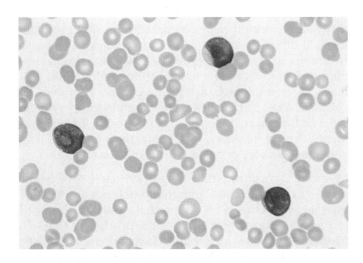

■ FIGURE 24-10   Myeloblasts in the peripheral blood from a patient with the erythroid-myeloid variant of acute erythroid leukemia (AEL). The blast morphology is typical of AML-without differentiation. (Wright-Giemsa stain; 1000× magnification)

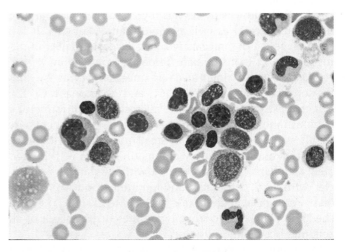

■ FIGURE 24-12   Erythroblasts with megaloblastoid features in the bone marrow from a case of AEL. (Wright-Giemsa stain; 1000× magnification)

The mixed lineage variant occasionally can evolve to a predominantly myeloblastic leukemia. The cell of origin for the mixed lineage variant is thought to be a multipotential progenitor cell with wide myeloid differentiation potential. The cell of origin for pure erythroid leukemia is thought to be a primitive progenitor cell committed to the erythroid lineage (BFU-E or CFU-E).[13]

 Checkpoint! 7

What differentiating hematologic feature of acute erythroid leukemia causes it to be classified into two subgroups?

Acute Megakaryoblastic Leukemia The megakaryoblastic subgroup of AML is an acute leukemia in which ≥50% of the leukemic blasts are of the megakaryocytic lineage. It occurs in both adults and children and constitutes ~3–5% of all AML cases.[13] It can occur de novo or as an acute leukemic transformation of chronic myeloid leukemia (CML) and myelodysplastic syndromes.[38]

Patients usually present with cytopenias; although most have thrombocytopenia, some can have thrombocytosis. Dysplastic features in the neutrophils and platelets can be present. There is no significant organomegaly. The bone marrow megakaryoblasts are usually medium to large (12–18 μ) with basophilic, often agranular, cytoplasm. The cells frequently show distinct pseudopod formation. Small blasts resembling lymphoblasts can also be present. On careful examination of the peripheral blood smear, circulating micromegakaryocytes and undifferentiated blasts can be found. However, the finding of cytoplasmic blebs suggests that these cells are megakaryocytic. Megakaryocytic fragments also can be present.

Bone marrow aspiration often results in a dry tap due to extensive marrow fibrosis associated with an expanded megakaryocyte lineage. In these cases, marrow biopsy may be required and usually reveals increased fibroblasts and/or increased reticulin as well as more than 20% blasts. It has been suggested that megakaryocytes secrete a number of mitogenic factors that stimulate fibroblast proliferation.

Blasts can be identified as megakaryocytic by immunophenotyping (CD41, CD61, and occasionally CD42), cytochemistry, and electron microscopy (ultrastructural demonstration of platelet peroxidase [PPO]). The blasts are highly variable, ranging from small round cells with scant cytoplasm and dense heavy chromatin to cells with moderately abundant cytoplasm with or without granules and nuclei with lacy chromatin and prominent nucleoli. Some blasts can have cytoplasmic blebs. Megakaryocytes with shedding platelets occasionally are present. Dysplasia of all cell lines is a common finding.

No unique chromosomal abnormality is associated with acute megakaryoblastic leukemia in adults. Abnormalities of chromosome 2l have been described, but similar abnormalities are also found in other types of acute myeloid leukemias. Children with acute megakaryoblastic leukemia often have a t(1;21)(p13;q13) translocation and a particularly poor prognosis. Individuals with Down syndrome have an increased predisposition to develop acute leukemia, particularly AML. Most often, the subtype of AML is acute megakaryoblastic. The disorder usually manifests in the neonatal period, frequently with significant leukocytosis and >30% blasts in the peripheral blood. In addition to trisomy 21 (Down syndrome), these patients often have additional clonal abnormalities including trisomy 8 or a chromosome 21 translocation.[39]

The cell of origin is believed to be a hematopoietic precursor cell committed to the megakaryocytic lineage (CFU-Mk) or a bipotential precursor able to differentiate into both erythroid and megakaryocytic lineages (CFU-EMk).

Acute Basophilic Leukemia The primary differentiation of this acute leukemia is along the basophil lineage. Some cases develop as a blast transformation phase of chronic myelocytic leukemia (CML). This is a very rare form of AML with few reported cases (<1% of all AML cases). The most characteristic feature by cytochemistry is metachromatic positivity with toluidine blue.[13] The blasts can show diffuse staining with acid phosphatase and occasionally PAS positivity. They are usually negative for typical cytochemical stains for myeloid cells but express myeloid markers (e.g., CD13, CD33). No consistent chromosomal abnormality has been identified with this subtype of AML. The cell of origin is believed to be a myeloid precursor committed to the basophil lineage.

Acute Panmyelosis with Myelofibrosis This disorder is associated with an acute panmyeloid proliferation and fibrosis of the bone marrow. A rare form of AML, it occurs primarily in adults. It can occur de novo or following alkylating-agent chemotherapy and/or radiation. The major differential diagnosis is with acute megakaryoblastic leukemia (with fibrosis) or other types of AML with associated marrow fibrosis and/or with chronic idiopathic myelofibrosis. This diagnosis is indicated when the proliferative process involves all major myeloid lineages (granulocytes, erythroid cells, and megakaryocytes [i.e., panmyelosis]). Immunohistochemistry is necessary to identify the multilineage involvement. The cell of origin is believed to be the CMP.

Myeloid Sarcoma This designation refers to a disease process in which a tumor mass of myeloblasts or immature myeloid cells occurs in an extramedullary site or in bone. It can occur concurrently with acute or chronic myeloid leukemias or other myeloproliferative or myelodysplastic disorders. The immunophenotype and cytochemistry reflect the specific myeloid cell(s) involved in the malignant process (i.e., myeloblasts, promyelocytes, occasionally monocytes). The cell of origin is believed to be the CMP.

CASE STUDY *(continued from page 511)*

A bone marrow aspirate and biopsy were performed on Guillermo to aid in diagnosis. The bone marrow biopsy revealed a hypercellular marrow. The bone marrow aspirate revealed an M:E ratio of 7.8:1. The predominant cell was an abnormal immature cell with an indented or lobulated nuclear configuration. Heavy cytoplasmic granulation was present, and multiple Auer rods were in several cells. The cells were strongly positive with myeloperoxidase.

5. Based on the morphology and cytochemical staining of these cells, what is the most likely AML classification?

6. What is the major complication associated with this leukemia?

7. What chromosome abnormality is associated with this leukemia?

▶ THERAPY

Traditional chemotherapy for AML is designed to reduce tumor load as rapidly as possible (∞ Chapter 21). Newer treatment modalities include molecularly targeted therapies (e.g., ATRA), epigenetic-targeted therapies (demethylating agents, histone deacetylase inhibitors), and autologous or allogeneic bone marrow transplants and infusions of donor lymphocyte cells together with total body irradiation to increase leukemic cell destruction. Current research is focusing on novel therapies including the use of monoclonal antibodies and gene therapy and the destruction of the cellular matrix that supports the neoplastic tissue.

Evaluation of peripheral blood counts is essential to support patients during chemotherapy. Development of at-risk stages such as pancytopenia, severe granulocytopenia, and/or thrombocytopenia must be monitored so that early intervention can occur (growth factors to stimulate hematopoietic cell recovery and/or transfusions).

Bone marrow transplantation (∞ Chapter 27), whether allogeneic or autologous, remains the only therapeutic choice that currently provides the potential for a prolonged (10+ years) disease-free survival for most patients with AML.

 CASE STUDY *(continued)*

8. If this patient were treated with all transretinoic acid, what would you expect to find two weeks later when the blood count was repeated?

✓ **Checkpoint! 9**

Predict the peripheral blood picture of a patient on antifolate chemotherapy.

SUMMARY

The acute leukemias (AL) compose a heterogeneous group of neoplastic stem cell disorders characterized by unregulated proliferation and blocked maturation. The two major groups of AL are AML and ALL. These two major groups are further classified into subtypes based on morphologic criteria, cytochemical stains, immunologic analysis, and cytogenetic and molecular abnormalities. The WHO classification system, which separates those AML types with recurrent chromosomal abnormalities, those with multilineage dysplasia, and those following cytotoxic therapy from the classic FAB categories has replaced the FAB classification system. It also recognizes new subcategories of acute basophilic leukemia, acute panmyelosis with myelofibrosis, and myeloid sarcoma.

Peroxidase and/or Sudan black B cytochemical staining help differentiate AML (peroxidase positive) from ALL (peroxidase negative). Subgrouping the AMLs further requires additional cytochemical stains, immunophenotyping, and cytogenetic analysis. The most common cytogenetic abnormality is the t(15;17) found in acute promyelocytic leukemia. This abnormality has been shown at the molecular level to involve the retinoic acid receptor (*RAR*) gene and the *PML* gene.

AL's onset is usually abrupt; without treatment, it progresses rapidly. Symptoms are related to anemia, thrombocytopenia, and/or neutropenia. Splenomegaly, hepatomegaly, and lymphadenopathy are common findings. Hematologic findings include a macrocytic or normocytic, normochromic anemia, thrombocytopenia, and a decreased, normal, or increased leukocyte count. Blasts are almost always found in the peripheral blood. A bone marrow examination is always indicated if leukemia is suspected. The bone marrow reveals ≥20% blasts. An update of the WHO classification for AML is on the Website, Chapter 24.

REVIEW QUESTIONS

LEVEL I

1. A differential report notes the presence of more than 20% blasts. This number supports the diagnosis of: (Objective 1)
   a. CML
   b. AML
   c. CLL
   d. MDS

2. The presence of blasts with no evidence of myeloid differentiation by morphology and <3% positive for SBB or MPO is commonly seen in: (Objective 2)
   a. AML—minimally differentiated
   b. AML—without maturation
   c. Acute basophilic leukemia
   d. Myeloid sarcoma

3. Which M:E ratio is most characteristic of acute leukemia ? (Objective 4)
   a. 1:1
   b. 10:1
   c. 1:5
   d. 4:1

4. A large cell with an immature nucleus containing multiple prominent nucleoli and few azurophilic granules is a: (Objective 3)
   a. type 1 myeloblast
   b. type 2 myeloblast
   c. promyelocyte
   d. promyelocyte with hypogranulation

5. The leukemia that belongs to the WHO classification of AML with recurrent genetic abnormalities is: (Objective 2)
   a. APL
   b. megakaryoblastic leukemia
   c. erythroleukemia
   d. AML minimally differentiated

6. PAS stain differs from the traditional stains used in cytochemistry in that PAS: (Objective 5)
   a. requires a fresh, nonanticoagulated specimen
   b. is reported as positive or negative in different cell lines
   c. produces characteristic patterns of positivity in different cell lines
   d. is better used in conjunction with monoclonal antibody testing

7. Auer rods have been determined to be: (Objective 6)
   a. diagnostic for AML
   b. composed of histamine
   c. positive for proteolytic esterases
   d. present in high numbers in adolescent AML

LEVEL II

1. In attempting to subtype a case of acute leukemia, the clinical laboratory scientist noted that the blasts were negative with myeloperoxidase, Sudan black B, naphthol AS-D chloroacetate esterase, and alpha-naphthyl butyrate esterase but positive when stained with alpha-naphthyl esterase and PAS. Peroxidase was positive at the ultrastructural level. These blasts should show positivity with the following monoclonal antibodies: (Objectives 2, 4)
   a. CD41, CD42, CD61
   b. CD24
   c. CD7
   d. glycophorin A

2. The WHO classification of AML is based on: (Objectives 2, 7)
   a. genetic abnormalities
   b. morphology and cytochemistry of blasts
   c. immunophenotyping of blasts
   d. A, B, and C

3. Which of the following leukemias is associated with faggot cells? (Objective 2)
   a. APL
   b. AML with multilineage dysplasia
   c. AML t(8;21)
   d. AML therapy related

4. These leukemic blasts demonstrate CD71 positivity and have coarse positivity with PAS: (Objective 4)
   a. erythroblasts
   b. myeloblasts
   c. megakaryoblasts
   d. monoblasts

5. A bone marrow from a 20-year-old male revealed 40% agranular blasts.Cytochemical stains were negative for myeloperoxidase, SBB, specific and nonspecific esterases. What immunophenotype panel should be used to help identify the blast cell lineage? (Objective 6)
   a. CD13, CD33, CD34, CD10, CD19, CD2, CD3, CD5
   b. CD11a, CD14, CD10, CD2, CD3, CD71, CD61
   c. CD13, CD33, CD34, CD11b, CD71, CD41
   d. CD41, CD61, CD13, CD15, CD38, CD117

REVIEW QUESTIONS (continued)

LEVEL I

8. A bone marrow contains many blast cells that stain positively for alpha-naphthyl acetate esterase. This reaction indicates that these cells are more likely of what lineage? (Objective 5)
   a. erythroblastic
   b. lymphoblastic
   c. monoblastic
   d. myeloblastic

9. When Auer rods are found in blasts of a case of acute leukemia, the leukemia is most probably: (Objective 6)
   a. undifferentiated
   b. B lymphocytic
   c. T lymphocytic
   d. myelocytic

10. Circulating micromegakaryocytes typically can be found in which of the following acute leukemias? (Objectives 2, 3)
   a. AML with t(8;21)
   b. APL
   c. AML therapy related
   d. acute megakaryoblastic

LEVEL II

6. A patient has a leukocyte count of 75×10^9/L. A large number of blast cells are present in the peripheral blood smear. Cytochemical stains reveal the following:
   - Periodic acid Schiff   negative
   - Sudan black B   positive
   - Naphthol AS-D chloroacetate esterase   positive
   - Alpha-naphthyl acetate esterase   negative

   Based on the staining reaction, these cells would be considered: (Objective 4)
   a. myeloblasts
   b. stem cells
   c. monoblasts
   d. promyelocytes

7. A patient with leukemia is receiving chemotherapy that includes a drug that is an antagonist to folic acid metabolism. Which of the following types of erythrocytes will be produced? (Objective 5)
   a. spherocytes
   b. microcytes
   c. macrocytes
   d. codocytes

8. In neutrophils, the myeloperoxidase activity is located in the: (Objective 4)
   a. primary granules
   b. secondary granules
   c. mitochondria
   d. nucleoli

9. The presence of CD34, CD13, and CD14 is typically associated with a positive: (Objective 4)
   a. periodic acid Schiff stain
   b. TdT
   c. CD71
   d. myeloperoxidase

10. All transretinoic acid therapy is used in leukemia patients with this genetic abnormality: (Objectives 3, 5)
   a. t(9;22)
   b. t(8;21)
   c. t(15;17)
   d. trisomy 8

www.pearsonhighered.com/mckenzie
Use this address to access the interactive Companion Website created for this textbook. Find additional information, tables and figures. Evaluate your command of the chapter information using case studies and critical thinking and multiple choice questions.

REFERENCES

1. Lowenberg B, Touw IP. Hematopoietic growth factors and their receptors in acute leukemia. *Blood.* 1993;81:281–92.

2. Lechner K, Geissler K, Jager U, Greinix H, Kalhs P. Treatment of acute leukemia. *Ann Oncol.* 1999;10(Suppl 6):45–51.

3. Bennett JM, Catovsky D, Daniel MT, Flandrin G, Galton DA, Gralnick HR, Sultan C. Proposals for the classification of the acute leukaemias. French-American-British (FAB) co-operative group. *Br J Haematol.* 1976;33(4):451–58.

4. Harris NL, Jaffe ES, Diebold J, Flandrin G, Muller-Hermelink HK, Vardiman J, Lister TA, Bloomfield CD. The World Health Organization Classification of neoplastic diseases of the hematopoietic and lymphoid tissues. *Ann Eur Soc Med Onc.* 1999;10(12):1419–32.

5. Scandura JM, Boccuni P, Cammenga J, Nimer SD. Transcription factor fusions in acute leukemia: Variations on a theme. *Oncogene.* 2002;21:3422–44.

6. Look TL. Oncogenic transcription factors in the human acute leukemias. *Science.* 1997;278:1059–64.

7. Orazi A. Histopathology in the diagnosis and classification of acute myeloid leukemia, myelodysplastic syndromes, and myelodysplastic/myeloproliferative diseases. *Pathobiology.* 2007;74(2):97–114.

8. Hope KJ, Jin L, Dick, JE. Acute myeloid leukemia originates from a hierarchy of leukemic stem cell classes that differ in self-renewal capacity. *Nat Immunol.* 2004;5:738–43.

9. Pereira FG, Metze K, Costa FP, Lima CS, Lorand-Metze I. Phenotypic quantitative features of patients with acute myeloid leukemia. *Neoplasma.* 2006;53(2):155–60.

10. First MIC Cooperative Study Group. Morphologic, immunologic, and cytogenetic (MIC) working classification of acute lymphoblastic leukemias. Report of the workshop held in Leuven, Belgium, April 22–23, 1985. *Cancer Genet Cytogenet.* 1986;23:189–97.

11. Second MIC Cooperative Study Group. Morphologic, immunologic, and cytogenetic (MIC) working classification of the acute myeloid leukaemias. *Br J Haematol.* 1988;68:487–94.

12. Harris NL et al. World Health Organization classification of neoplastic diseases of the hematopoietic and lymphoid tissues: Report of the Clinical Advisory Committee meeting, Airlie House, Virginia, November 1997. *J Clin Oncol.* 1999;17:3835–49.

13. Jaffe ES, Harris NL, Stein H, Vardiman JW. *Pathology & Genetics. Tumours of Haematopoietic and Lymphoid Tissues. World Health Organization Classification of Tumours.* Lyon, France: IARC Press; 2001.

14. Bacher U, Kern W, Schnittger S, Hiddemann W, Schoch C, Haferlach T. Further correlations of morphology according to FAB and WHO classification to cytogenetics in de novo acute myeloid leukemia: A study on 2,235 patients. *Ann Hematol.* 2005 Nov;84 (12):785–91.

15. Owaidah TM, Al Beihany A, Iqbal MA, Elkum N, Roberts GT. Cytogenetics, molecular and ultrastructural characteristics of biphenotypic acute leukemia identified by the EGIL scoring system. *Leukemia.* 2006;20(4):620–26.

16. Kheiri SA, MacKerrell T, Bonagura VR, Fuchs A, Billett HH. Flow cytometry with or without cytochemistry for the diagnosis of acute leukemias? *Cytometry.* 1998;15;34(2):82–86.

17. Krober SM, Horny HP, Steinke B, Kaiserling E. Adult hypocellular acute leukaemia with lymphoid differentiation. *Leuk Lymphoma.* 2003;44(10):1797–801.

18. Haferlach T, Bacher U, Kern W, Schnittger S, Haferlach C. Diagnostic pathways in acute leukemias: A proposal for a multimodal approach. *Ann Hematol.* 2007;86(5):311–27.

19. Kaleem Z, Crawford E, Pathan MH, Jasper L, Covinsky MA, Johnson LR, White G. Flow cytometric analysis of acute leukemias. Diagnostic utility and critical analysis of data. *Arch Pathol Lab Med.* 2003; 127(1):42–48.

20. Powari M, Varma N, Varma S, Marwaha RK, Sandhu H, Ganguly NK. Flow cytometric characterization of phenotype, DNA indices and p53 gene expression in 55 cases of acute leukemia. *Anal Quant Cytol Histol.* 2002;24(3):159–65.

21. Bacher U, Kern W, Schnittger S, Hiddemann W, Haferlach T, Schoch C. Population-based age-specific incidences of cytogenetic subgroups of acute myeloid leukemia. *Haematologica.* 2005;90(11): 1502–10.

22. Duesberg P, Rasnick D. Aneuploidy, the somatic mutation that makes cancer a species of its own. *Cell Motil Cytoskeleton.* 2000;47 (2):81–107.

23. Deschler B, Lubbert M. Acute myeloid leukemia: Epidemiology and etiology. *Cancer.* 2006;107(9):2099–107.

24. Meijers JC, Oudijk EJ, Mosnier LO, Bos R, Bouma BN, Nieuwenhuis HK, Fijnheer R. Reduced activity of TAFI (thrombin-activatable fibrinolysis inhibitor) in acute promyelocytic leukaemia. *Br J Haematol.* 2000;108:518–23.

25. Lemez P. A case of acute promyelocytic leukaemia with "faggot cells" exhibiting strong alpha-naphthylbutyrate esterase activity. *Br J Haematol.* 1988;68:138–39.

26. Castoldi GL, Liso V, Specchia G, Tomasi P. Acute promyelocytic leukemia: Morphological aspects. *Leukemia.* 1994;8:1441–46.

27. Bennett JM et al. A variant form of hypergranular promyelocytic leukaemia (M3). *Br J Haematol.* 1980;44:169–70.

28. Iqbal S, Grimwade D, Chase A, Goldstone A, Burnett A, Goldman JM, Swirsky D. Identification of PML/RARalpha rearrangements in suspected acute promyelocytic leukemia using fluorescence in situ hybridization of bone marrow smears: A comparison with cytogenetics and RT-PCR in MRC ATRA trial patients. MRC Adult Leukaemia Working Party. *Leukemia.* 2000;14:950–53.

29. Grignani F, DeMattels S, Nervi C et al. Fusion proteins of the retinoic acid receptor-a recruit histone deacetylase in promyelocytic leukemia. *Nature.* 1998;391:815–18.

30. Gianni M, Ponzanelli I, Mologni L, Reichert U, Rambaldi A, Terao M, Garattini E. Retinoid-dependent growth inhibition, differentiation and apoptosis in acute promyelocytic leukemia cells: Expression and activation of caspases. *Cell Death Differ.* 2000;7:447–60.

31. Sun SY, Wan H, Yue P, Hong WK, Lotan R. Evidence that retinoic acid receptor beta induction by retinoids is important for tumor cell growth inhibition. *J Biol Chem.* 2000;275(22):17149–53.

32. Tallman MS, Andersen JW, Schiffer CA, Appelbaum FR, Feusner JH, Ogden A, Shepherd L, Rowe JM, Francois C, Larson RS, Wiernik PH. Clinical description of 44 patients with acute promyelocytic leukemia who developed the retinoic acid syndrome. *Blood.* 2000; 95:90–95.

33. Larson RA. Is secondary leukemia an independent poor prognostic factor in acute myeloid leukemia? *Best Pract Clin Haematol.* 2007; 20(1):29–37.

34. Lewis RE, Cruse JM, Webb RN, Sanders CM, Beason K. Contrasting antigenic maturation patterns in M0-M2 versus M3 acute myeloid leukemias. *Exp Mol Pathol.* 2007; [Epub prior to print].

35. Dunphy CH, Orton SO, Mantell J. Relative contributions of enzyme cytochemistry and flow cytometric immunophenotyping to the evaluation of acute myeloid leukemias with a monocytic component and of flow cytometric immunophenotyping to the evaluation of absolute monocytoses. *Am J Clin Pathol.* 2004;122(6): 865–74.

36. Mavilio F, Testa U, Sposi NM, Petrini M, Pelosi E, Bordignon C, Amadori S, Mandelli F, Peschle C. Selective expression of fos proto-oncogene in human acute myelomonocytic and monocytic leukemias: A molecular marker of terminal differentiation. *Blood.* 1987;69:160–64.

37. Huang Q. Pure erythroid leukemia. *Arch Pathol Lab Med.* 2004;128 (2):241–42.

38. Kinugawa N, Okimoto Y, Hata J. Simultaneous detection of platelet-associated antigen and platelet peroxidase on buffy coat cells from bone marrow in two patients with pediatric acute megakaryocytic leukemia. *J Pediatr Hematol Oncol.* 1999;21:451–52.

39. Bennett JM. World Health Organization classification of the acute leukemias and myelodysplastic syndrome. *Int J Hematol.* 2000;72: 131–33.

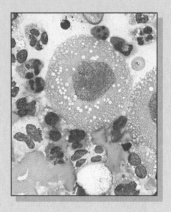

25

Acute Lymphoblastic Leukemias

Susan J. Leclair, Ph.D.
J. Lynne Williams, Ph.D.

■ OBJECTIVES—LEVEL I

At the end of this unit of study the student should be able to:

1. Define *acute lymphoblastic leukemia* (ALL) and differentiate it from acute myeloid leukemia (AML).

2. List and define the common variants seen in ALL as defined by the FAB and WHO classifications.

3. Describe and recognize the typical peripheral blood picture (erythrocytes, leukocytes, blasts and thrombocytes) seen in ALL.

4. Give the typical results of cytochemical stains in ALL.

5. Summarize the clinical signs and symptoms and the most frequent age groups associated with ALL.

6. Define the rare acute leukemias that are not included in AML and ALL groups.

■ OBJECTIVES—LEVEL II

At the end of this unit of study the student should be able to:

1. Compare and contrast the various presentations of ALL.

2. Predict the most likely WHO or immunophenotype subgroup based on patient history, physical assessment, and laboratory findings.

3. Correlate cellular presentation with prognosis and common complications in ALL.

4. Correlate Wright stain blast morphology in the ALL subgroups with cytochemical stains, flow cytometry, and genetic testing results.

5. Evaluate peripheral blood results in relation to oncological therapy (i.e., complete or partial remission, relapse).

6. Identify AL from a peripheral blood smear and recommend laboratory tests that may be useful in differentiation of AML and ALL and in classification of subtypes.

KEY TERMS

Acute undifferentiated leukemia (AUL)
B cell ALL
Bilineage acute leukemia
Biphenotypic acute leukemia
Burkitt cell
Consolidation therapy
Induction therapy
Maintenance chemotherapy
Natural killer (NK) cell acute leukemia
T cell ALL

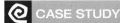 CASE STUDY

We will refer to this case study throughout this chapter.

Dan, a 4-year-old white male, is seen by his physician for symptoms of easy fatigue and bruising. His mother states that until one month ago he was a "typical kid." Since then she has noticed increased lassitude, a regression to more baby-like behavior, and loss of appetite. For the past two days, his temperature has been 100°F. Upon physical examination, the child presented as a pale, quiet child of appropriate size for his age. Most systems were unremarkable with the exception of several small firm lymph nodes felt in the cervical and auxiliary regions. His CBC revealed a WBC count of 40.2 × 10⁹/L with 90% blasts. Consider the laboratory testing that may help in the diagnosis of Dan's illness.

BACKGROUND BASICS

The information in this chapter will build upon concepts learned in previous chapters. To maximize your learning experience you should review and have an understanding of these concepts before starting this unit of study.

Level I

▶ Summarize the origin and differentiation of hematopoietic cells. (Chapter 3)
▶ Describe the maturation, differentiation, and function of the lymphocyte. (Chapter 7)
▶ Outline the classification and general laboratory findings of the acute leukemias. (Chapter 21)
▶ Summarize the typical laboratory findings that define acute myeloid leukemia. (Chapter 24)

Level II

▶ Summarize the role of oncogenes and growth factors in cell proliferation, differentiation, and maturation. (Chapters 3, 21)
▶ Diagram the maturation pathway for T and B lymphocytes. (Chapter 7)
▶ Describe the role of molecular analysis in diagnosis and treatment of acute leukemia. (Chapter 39)
▶ Describe the use of immunophenotyping in acute leukemia. (Chapters 21, 37)
▶ Describe the role of cytogenetics in diagnosis and treatment of acute leukemia. (Chapters 21, 37)

▶ OVERVIEW

This chapter is a study of the acute lymphoblastic leukemias (ALL). A summary of clinical signs and symptoms as well as hematologic findings associated with ALL are discussed. A description of the classification systems including the morphologic FAB system and the World Health Organization (WHO) system follows. Lastly, the rare acute leukemias that are not grouped into either AML or ALL are briefly reviewed.

▶ INTRODUCTION

Lymphocyte malignancies include a wide spectrum of syndromes, from disorders that primarily involve the bone marrow and peripheral blood (leukemias) to those that initially present as tumorous masses (lymphomas) primarily involving the lymphoid organs (lymph nodes, tonsils, spleen, thymus, and lymphoid tissue of the gastrointestinal tract). The neoplastic transformation (cell of origin) may involve the common lymphoid progenitor cell (CLP), or more differentiated progenitors of the T, B or NK (natural killer) cell lineage.

Generally, T cell and NK cell malignancies tend to have more aggressive clinical behavior than B cell malignancies. T cell malignancies often involve extranodal and extramedullary sites including the skin, central nervous system, or the mediastinum. Neoplastic B cells can secrete monoclonal proteins (immunoglobulins; i.e. IgM, IgA, IgG) inappropriately, which may increase the viscosity of the blood and impair blood flow through the microcirculation (the hyperviscosity syndrome). The monoclonal immunoglobulins can interact with cell surfaces and impair granulocyte or platelet function, or induce the formation of erythrocyte rouleaux in vivo and in vitro. They can also interact with the coagulation proteins, resulting in impaired hemostasis. Production of autoantibodies spontaneously or by the B-cell neoplasia may lead to autoimmune hemolytic anemia, autoimmune thrombocytopenia, or autoimmune neutropenia.

This chapter discusses a group of lymphoid malignancies known as acute lymphoblastic leukemia. Other lymphoproliferative diseases are discussed in ∞ Chapter 26. There are two major categories of acute leukemias, classified according to the cellular origin of the primary defects: acute myeloid leukemia (AML) and acute lymphoblastic leukemia (ALL) (∞ Chapters 21 and 24). If the defect affects primarily the common lymphoid progenitor cell (CLP) or its progeny, it is classified as ALL. If the defect affects primarily the common myeloid progenitor cell (CMP) or its progeny, it is classified as AML. ALL falls within the WHO classification category of "Precursor B- and T-cell neoplasms" (see below).

▶ BASIC BIOLOGY OF ALL

Similar to AML (∞ Chapter 24), the ALLs are hematologic disorders characterized by malignant neoplastic proliferation and accumulation of immature and dysfunctional hematopoietic cells in the bone marrow. The basic abnormality appears to be multiple somatically acquired genetic mutations within a lymphoid precursor cell at one of several possible stages of development, giving rise to a clone of malignant lymphocytes. These lymphoid cells proliferate in an unregulated manner (i.e. they have altered responses to growth and antigrowth signals) and have a block in differentiation at various stages in their maturation sequence. They do not develop into mature cells, have an enhanced ability of self-renewal, and have increased resistance to apoptosis. Thus the leukemic clone expands.[1] The trigger for the original leukemic genetic mutations is unknown but may be a combination of leukemogenic factors (∞ Chapter 21). As in AML, impairment of normal hematopoiesis is the primary cause of concern.

The types of genetic alterations include chromosomal rearrangements and abnormalities of leukemic cell ploidy, both of which result in abnormal karyotypes detected by cytogenetic analysis, as well as point mutations affecting a variety of oncogenes or tumor suppressor genes, detectable by molecular techniques (RT-PCR, FISH).[2]

Initially diagnosis of ALL required the presence of ≥30% lymphoblasts and the parameters for classifying the neoplastic cells in ALL were defined by the morphologically-based FAB classification.[3] The World Health Organization's classification utilizes cellular cytochemical reactions, immunophenotyping, and genetic abnormalities as well as cell morphology to discriminate among the various lymphoproliferative disorders. WHO recommends that a diagnosis of ALL should not be made if the blast count is less than 20%.[4]

▶ CLINICAL FINDINGS

Acute lymphoblastic leukemia (ALL) is primarily a disease of young children, with a peak incidence between the ages of 2 and 5 years, and gradually decreasing rates during later childhood and adolescence. The incidence rises again in the sixth decade, reaching a second, smaller peak in the elderly. In the younger population, the onset of signs and symptoms can be insidious or abrupt, and often nonspecific in nature. Without treatment survival is short, but with current treatment regimens, most children enter a period of prolonged remission and many appear to be "cured."[5] For an adult with ALL, the onset of signs and symptoms is generally more rapid, with more significant complaints of fatigue, infections, and bruising. Adult onset ALL does not respond to treatment as well as childhood ALL, and morbidity and mortality statistics are significantly worse.[6]

The clinical presentation generally reflects the degree of marrow failure and the extent of extramedullary disease. Symptoms are related to anemia, thrombocytopenia, and neutropenia, due to replacement of normal marrow elements by leukemic lymphoblasts. Common complaints include fatigue, pallor, fever, weight loss, irritability, and anorexia. Fever is often related to a concomitant infection. Petechiae and ecchymoses are present in over half the patients; actual hemorrhage is less common. Bone pain is noted in about 80% of patients, especially tenderness of the long bones, and is associated with expansion of the marrow cavity by leukemic cells. Often this complaint is dismissed as "growing pains." When severe, the child may refuse to walk or stand. Occasionally children have symptoms related to CNS involvement, including headaches and vomiting. Splenomegaly, hepatomegaly, and lymphadenopathy are common findings, associated with leukemic infiltrations.

 Checkpoint! 1

Compare the typical age groups in which AML and ALL are found.

▶ LABORATORY FINDINGS

Evaluation of the peripheral blood and bone marrow is critical to making a diagnosis of ALL.

PERIPHERAL BLOOD

The leukocyte count may be increased, decreased, or normal (from 0.1 to >50 × 10^9/L). The median leukocyte count at presentation is 10–12 × 10^9/L.[1] About 50% of the patients have leukocytosis due to an abundance of circulating leukemic lymphoblasts. Even though the total leukocyte count is usually elevated, neutropenia is often marked, and is

✪ TABLE 25-1	
Initial Laboratory Findings Characteristic of ALL	
Peripheral Blood	Leukocyte count usually increased but may be normal or decreased
	Neutropenia
	Lymphoblasts
	Normocytic, normochromic anemia
	Thrombocytopenia
Bone Marrow	Hypercellular
	≥20% lymphoblasts (WHO)

associated with increased risk of infection. The platelet count is usually decreased (median 48–52 × 10^9/L).[1] Normocytic, normochromic anemia is almost always present and can be severe. Anisocytosis, poikilocytosis, and nucleated erythrocytes, however, are not usually present.[7] (Table 25-1 ✪).

Morphologic evaluation of peripheral blood smears usually reveals the presence of blasts. The most common presentation in children is one in which there is homogeneity in the morphology of the lymphoblasts. The blasts are typically small, up to twice the size of a small lymphocyte, with scant to moderate amounts of light basophilic or blue-grey cytoplasm. The nucleus is round or slightly indented, with finely granular to slightly clumped chromatin, and inconspicuous or absent nucleoli (Figure 25-1 ■). The chromatin pattern can vary from case to case, but is homogeneous within cases. In adults, the more common presentation is one in which the lymphoblast morphology is heterogeneous. Larger lymphoblasts with moderate amounts of basophilic cytoplasm, irregularly shaped nuclei and prominent nucleoli can be intermixed with smaller blasts, producing a heterogeneous population of leukemic

cells (Figure 25-2 ■). The cytoplasm can contain amphophilic granules that stain fuchsia, which may make it difficult to distinguish these lymphoblasts from the myeloblasts seen in AML. Cytochemical staining should help clarify the cellular origin of the leukemic blasts (see below). There is significant variability in cell size, nuclear chromatin condensation, and cytoplasmic basophilia. This marked heterogeneity of morphology is seen both within a given case and between cases. The FAB classification distinguished between those diseases with a homogeneous blast population (L1) and those with a heterogeneous blast population (L2). The WHO classification does not. The distribution of ALL into L1 and L2 subtypes has little relevance in predicting outcome and thus, the FAB classification is being replaced by the WHO classification.

ℯ CASE STUDY *(continued from page 529)*

The physician ordered a CBC on Dan. The results are as follows:

WBC	40.2 × 10^9/L
RBC	3.45 × 10^{12}/L
Hb	9.7 g/dL
Hct	0.32 L/L
MCV	92.7 fL
MCH	28.1 pg
MCHC	30.3
RDW	17.3
PLT	63 × 10^9/L

The differential showed 90% lymphoblasts, 8% neutrophils, 1% monocytes, and 1% eosinophils. Rare nucleated erythrocytes are seen on scan. The platelets appear decreased in number.

1. Based upon this data, what would be the initial interpretation of John's presentation?

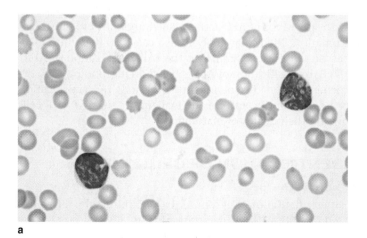

a

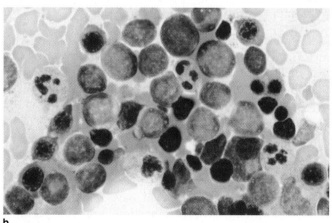

b

■ FIGURE 25-1 **a.** Lymphoblasts in peripheral blood from acute lymphoblastic leukemia, homogeneous morphology. Notice the nuclear cleavage. **b.** Lymphoblasts in the bone marrow in a case of ALL, homogenous morphology. (Both Wright-Giemsa stain; 1000× magnification)

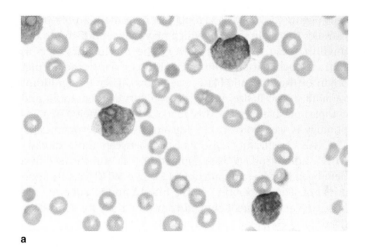

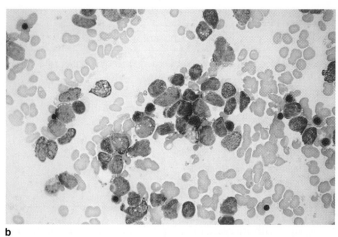

a

b

■ FIGURE 25-2   **a.** Lymphoblasts in peripheral blood from acute lymphoblastic leukemia, heterogeneous morphology. **b.** Lymphoblasts in the bone marrow of a patient with heterogeneous lymphoblasts. (a. Wright-Giemsa stain; 1000× magnification; b. Wright-Giemsa stain; 500× magnification)

BONE MARROW

The hypercellular bone marrow reveals replacement of normal hematopoietic cells by neoplastic lymphoid cells. Although the WHO criteria requires ≥20% lymphoblasts, most patients present with >65% blasts. The morphology of the blasts can be variable as described for peripheral blood blasts. The more homogenous presentation is frequently seen in pediatric patients, while the heterogeneous population of blasts is more frequently seen in adult patients. Auer rods (∞ Chapter 24) are not present in lymphoblasts. Intra-cytoplasmic inclusions have been described in the lymphoblasts of patients with ALL, and cytochemistry suggests they are probably lysosomal in origin.[8]

OTHER LABORATORY FINDINGS

As with AML, other laboratory findings are consistent with increased cellular metabolism, and in general the extent of abnormality of the various laboratory parameters is proportional to tumor burden. Hyperuricemia and an increased lactate dehydrogenase are common findings resulting from the increase in cell turnover. Hypercalcemia, when present, is thought to be caused by increased bone resorption associated with leukemic proliferation in the bone marrow. Impairment of renal function is often seen, due to leukemic infiltration of the kidneys, as well as a uric-acid induced nephropathy. These patients will have serum chemistries consistent with impaired renal function (elevated creatinine, urea nitrogen, uric acid, and phosphorus).

Because the central nervous system (CNS) is a frequent site for extramedullary spread of ALL, cerebrospinal fluid (CSF) is usually analyzed for the presence of circulating lymphoblasts. Although CNS involvement is relatively uncommon at diagnosis, most patients will eventually develop overt CNS disease unless adequate preventive therapy is administered.

▶ CLASSIFICATION

The first step in classifying acute leukemia (AL) is to differentiate ALL from AML. This can usually be done by evaluating cell morphology and interpreting cytochemical results. Further classification into subgroups relies on analysis of the leukemic cells. Immunophenotyping of ALL helps to differentiate the lineage of the neoplastic cells into T, B, or NK cells. It can also determine the cells' maturation stage. Cytogenetics and molecular analysis can provide evidence of clonality, reveal distinct genetic abnormalities associated with subgroups of ALL and provide important prognostic information. Molecular analysis also can help determine neoplastic cell lineage. Similar to the FAB classification of AML, the FAB classification of ALL is based on morphology and cytochemistry of the malignant cell. The WHO classification relies on identification of the malignant cells as T or B cells and on their degree of maturation.

IDENTIFICATION OF CELL LINEAGE

Cytochemistry
Differentiation of ALL from AML (AML minimally differentiated or AML without maturation) is usually not possible by Romanowsky stained smears alone. Cytochemistry helps identify the lymphoid nature of these abnormal cells (see Table 21-9, p. 433). In lymphoblasts, the myeloperoxidase, Sudan black B and nonspecific esterase stains are negative. The PAS reaction usually demonstrates a coarse granular or block-like positivity. Some myeloid leukemias can also

demonstrate PAS reactivity, but in AML the granular pattern (if present) is superimposed on a diffusely positive background, whereas in lymphoblasts there is no background positivity. Lymphoblasts often demonstrate acid phosphatase positivity, especially those with a T cell immunophenotype. However, neither PAS nor acid phosphatase reacts exclusively with leukemic lymphoid cells.

Immunophenotyping

As described above, leukemic lymphoblasts lack specific morphologic and cytochemical features. Thus immunophenotyping is essential to not only differentiate ALL from AML minimally differentiated, but also to identify the immunologic subtype (T, B, or NK cell) of the neoplastic lymphoblast. This information has important prognostic implications.[1] Immunophenotyping is also useful in recognizing leukemias of mixed cell lineages, and in identifying minimal residual disease.

In normal lymphoid cells, the appearance of specific cellular markers or antigens is developmentally regulated (∞ Chapter 7). Some antigenic determinants appear at a very early developmental stage and disappear with maturity, whereas others appear on more mature cells. Malignant lymphoblasts share many of the features of their normal lymphoid counterparts.[9] Studies of surface markers and intracellular markers reveal that lymphoblasts in ALL can be subclassified according to recognized stages of normal maturation. However, immunophenotyping has also demonstrated that while some leukemic cells have phenotypes of normal cells, others can show asynchronous gene expression, resulting in an inappropriate combination of antigens[10] (Figure 25-3 ■). Occasionally, B lineage lymphoblasts will express low levels of the myeloid-associated antigens CD13 and CD33.

Terminal Deoxynucleotidyl Transferase (TdT)

In addition to identification of lymphocytes by immunophenotyping, certain intracellular enzymes are helpful in identifying cellular subtypes. The most important of these is terminal deoxynucleotidyl transferase (TdT), a DNA polymerase found in cell nuclei. Its presence can be determined by direct enzyme assay, by indirect immunofluorescence, or with monoclonal antibodies. This enzyme is not present in normal mature lymphocytes but can be found in 65% of the total thymic population of lymphocytes, with the TdT cells localized in the cortex.[11] It can also be found in very early B cells and occasionally very early myeloblasts (myeloblasts minimally differentiated, or without differentiation). About 1–3% of normal bone marrow cells are TdT positive. Its value in ALL is to identify early precursor lymphoblasts from more mature cells.

Cytogenetic Analysis

Karyotyping of the ALLs is important for providing prognostic information. Specific abnormalities are associated with certain subgroups. Chromosomal translocations are found in 75% of ALL cases, and in many instances the breakpoints involve transcription factor genes such as *MYC*, *TAL1*, *HOX11*, *HOX11L2*, *E2A*, *MLL*, *TEL*, and *AML1*.[2] Abnormalities appear to be more common in B-cell ALL than in T-cell ALL. In addition to translocations, hyperdiploidy (>46 chromosomes) and hypodiploidy (<46 chromosomes) have been described. Generally, hyperdiploidy is a better prognostic finding than hypodiploidy. Patients who have hyperdiploid chromosome counts >50 have a better prognosis with long-term remission. Patients with hyperdiploid chromosome counts <50 have a worse prognosis.[2]

Molecular Analysis

Point mutations of major cell cycle regulator proteins are seen in ALL, such as p53; various cyclin-dependent kinase inhibitors (CDKi), including p16, p15, p14; and activating mutations of proto-oncogenes involved in signaling pathways that govern cell proliferation, such as RAS (∞ Chapter 2).[2] These are often detectable by standard molecular techniques such as quantitative real-time PCR (RT-PCR) or fluorescent in-situ hybridization (FISH).

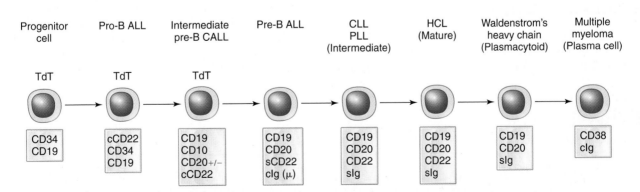

■ FIGURE 25-3   B lymphocyte maturation pathway with leukemic and other lymphoproliferative counterparts. (ALL = acute lymphoblastic leukemia; CLL = chronic lymphocytic leukemia; PLL = prolymphocytic leukemia; HCL = hairy cell leukemia; Clg = cytoplasmic immunoglobulin; Slg = surface immunoglobulin)

Another application of molecular analysis in acute lymphoid malignancies is to detect DNA rearrangements of the immunoglobulin (Ig) heavy and/or light chain genes, or the proteins which constitute the T-cell receptor (TCR), the α, β, δ, and γ chain (∞ Chapter 7). Rearrangement of Ig heavy chain genes occurs before cellular protein expression, and is an early genetic marker of B-lymphocyte ontogeny.[12] Likewise, rearrangement of the TCR polypeptide genes is an early marker of T-lymphocyte ontogeny. Molecular analysis to establish rearrangements of Ig or TCR genes can be used to establish clonality of the T or B cell populations, as well as to determine lineage derivation.[13] However, Ig gene rearrangement is seen in some instances of T-cell ALL, and TCR gene rearrangement occurs in some cases of B-cell precursor ALL. Thus molecular phenotyping to determine B- or T-cell lineage is not 100% reliable.[14]

 CASE STUDY *(continued from page 531)*

2. What is the correct choice of tests that should be used in the initial follow up in this case?

 Checkpoint! 2

Contrast the malignant neoplastic cells in ALL with those found in AML.

FAB CLASSIFICATION

The FAB classification divides ALL into three types (Table 25-2 ☼). L1 is characterized by a population of small, homogenous blasts with scant cytoplasm and inconspicuous nucleoli. It is seen primarily in children. L2 is characterized by a heterogenous population of cells with more abundant cytoplasm, less condensed nuclei, and more conspicuous nucleoli. L2 is more frequently seen in adults. L3, also known as Burkitt's type leukemia, is characterized by large basophilic lymphoblasts with abundant cytoplasm and vacuoles.

WHO CLASSIFICATION

The WHO classification defines two subgroups of ALL: 1) Precursor B- and T-cell neoplasms (leukemia/lymphoma) (which includes the FAB categories of L1 and L2) and 2) Burkitt type ALL (FAB category L3). The WHO classification considers acute lymphoblastic leukemias and lymphoblastic lymphomas to be a single disease with different clinical presentations. Thus, precursor T-cell and precursor B-cell neoplasms with bone marrow and peripheral blood involvement are acute lymphoblastic leukemias, while precursor T-cell and precursor B-cell neoplasms presenting as solid tumors are lymphoblastic lymphomas (∞ Chapter 26). The morphology and heterogeneity of bone marrow lymphoblasts help to define these categories (Table 25-3 ☼).

The cell features evaluated include:

* cell size
* nuclear chromatin
* nuclear shape
* nucleoli
* amount of cytoplasm
* cytoplasmic basophilia
* cytoplasmic vacuolation

Precursor B-Cell Leukemia

Precursor B-cell leukemia (B-cell ALL) is a neoplasm of lymphoblasts committed to the B-cell lineage, involving the bone marrow and peripheral blood. Occasionally, the disease may present with primary involvement of the lymph nodes or extranodal sites, in which case it is called B lymphoblastic lymphoma (B-LBL). Although arbitrary and with exceptions, if a patient has a mass lesion and 25% or fewer lymphoblasts in the bone marrow, the term *lymphoma* is preferred.

B-ALL accounts for 80–85% of the cases of ALL in children, and ~70% of the cases of ALL in adults. In general children diagnosed with precursor B-cell ALL have a good prognosis (long term event-free survival of >80%). Adult event-free survival is lower, between 30 and 50 percent, depending on the disease subtype, and patient age at diagnosis (there is an inverse relationship between age and prognosis). Although the morphologic appearance of the blasts is usually homogeneous, a heterogeneous morphology can be seen in some cases, particularly in adult patients.

Molecular testing may be helpful in establishing the B-cell lineage for B-ALL. B cell lineage is detected by rearrangement of immunoglobulin genes (Ig).[12,13] The assembly of the D-J light chain segments is the first genetic event that identifies a B cell progenitor (∞ Chapter 7). Clonal gene rearrangement helps to differentiate neoplastic B cells from normal B

☼ TABLE 25-2				
FAB Classification of ALL				
	Morphology		**TdT**	**CALLA (CD 10)**
ALL – L1	Small lymphoblasts scanty cytoplasm; Moderately clumped chromatin; Inconspicuous nucleoli		+	+
ALL – L2	Small and medium size lymphoblasts; Mixed chromatin patterns; Inconspicuous nucleoli		+	+
ALL – L3 Burkitt-type	Large lymphoblasts; Large nucleus with nucleoli; Cytoplasmic vacuolization; Intense cytoplasmic basophilia		−	+/−

⊘ TABLE 25-3

WHO Criteria for the Subtypes of ALL

Morphologic Feature	ALL	Burkitt Type ALL
Cell size	Small or large, heterogeneous	Large
Nuclear chromatin	Ranges from fine or clumped to variable-among cells within a single case	Fine and homogeneous
Nuclear shape	Occasional clefting or indentation common	Regular, oval to round
Nucleoli	Range from not visible or small and inconspicuous to large and prominent	Prominent, one or more
Cytoplasm Amount	Variable from scant to abundant	Moderately abundant
Basophilia	Variable	Very deep
Vacuolation	Variable	Often prominent

(WHO Criteria for the Subtypes of ALL Harris NL, Jaffe ES, Diebold J, Flandrin G, Muller-Hermelink HK, Vardiman J, Lister TA, Bloomfield CD. World Health Organization classification of neoplastic diseases of the hematopoietic and lymphoid tissues: report of the Clinical Advisory Committee meeting-Airlie House, Virginia, November 1997. *J Clin Oncol.* 1999 Dec;17(12):3835–49.)

cells. Ig gene rearrangement is seen in some instances of T-cell ALL, and thus additional markers of B lineage commitment are required for diagnosis.

Immunophenotyping of precursor B-cell ALL reveals that the lymphoblasts may have variable degrees of differentiation, which has clinical and prognostic implications (Table 25-4 ⊘, see Figure 25-3).[1,10] The precursor B-lymphoblasts are TdT+, HLA-DR+, and almost always CD19+ and CD79a+. The earliest B-cell differentiation stage, the "pro-B," is identified by this immunophenotype. In the next differentiation stage, the "intermediate pre-B" stage or common ALL, the blasts also express CD10 (the common ALL antigen, or CALLA).[15] B-ALL cases expressing the CD10/CALLA antigen appear to have the best prognosis of the immunologic subtypes.[16] In the most mature precursor B differentiation stage, ("pre-B" stage), the blasts may be CD10 negative, but express CD 20, surface CD22 (sCD22) and cytoplasmic mu chains (cytμ). Surface immunoglobulin is usually absent. Malignancies of later stages of B lymphocyte differentiation are included in the classification of chronic neoplastic lymphoproliferative disorders (∞ Chapter 26).

The CD19, CD22, CD10, and TdT phenotype is the same as the phenotype of most normal immature B cells in the bone marrow. Therefore, the distinction of normal and neoplastic B cells may be difficult unless the neoplastic cell also has an abnormal phenotypic marker.[17] This distinction is important for the detection of minimal residual disease after treatment. In some cases, the neoplastic cells lose antigens that usually show synchronous expression, or express two antigens that are usually not found on the same differentiation stage. Up to 50% of cases of B ALL co-express a myeloid-associated antigen, CD13 or CD33. This abnormal finding makes it easier to differentiate the neoplastic cells from normal cells and thus detect MRD.

Cytogenetic abnormalities associated with B-ALL include translocations, hypodiploidy, and hyperdiploidy.[1,2] However, there appears to be no recurrent abnormality in terms of the specific genes or chromosomes involved. The most common translocation in childhood B-ALL, present in ~25% of the cases, is t(12;21)(p13;q22), producing the *TEL-AML1* fusion gene.[2] Both the *TEL* and *AML1* genes are translocated in other types of leukemia, including t(5;12), t(8;21), and t(3;21)

⊘ TABLE 25-4

Cellular Markers Useful in Diagnosis and Classification of B-ALL

Subgroup	HLA-DR	TdT	CD34	CD19	CD22	CD10	CD20	CD2, 3, 4, 5, 7	cIg(μ)	sIg	Rearrangement of Ig genes	Rearrangement of TCR genes
Pro-B (early precursor)	+	+	+	+	+(c)	−	−	−	−	−	+/−	−
Intermediate Pre-B (common ALL)	+	+	+/−	+	+(c)	+	+/−	−	−	−	+	−
Pre-B ALL	+	+	−	+	+(s)	+/−	+	−	+	−	+	−

(c) cytoplasmic; (s) surface; − = absent; +/− = can be present; + = present

found in various subtypes of AML. *TEL-AML-1* expression in B-ALL is associated with an excellent prognosis, with event-free survival approaching 90%. Hyperdiploid B-ALL is also a common cytogenetic abnormality, found in ~30% of patients at diagnosis. In addition, ~20% of hyperdiploid B-ALL also have mutations in the receptor tyrosine kinase *FLT-3*, resulting in constitutive activation of the receptor. Hyperdiploid B-ALL is also associated with an extremely good prognosis, with event-free survival rates near 90%.

Other cytogenetic abnormalities include: t(4;11)(q21;q23) (*AF4/MLL*)(9%), t(1;19)(q23;p13.3) (*PBX/E2A*)(5%), t(9;22) (q34;q11.2) (*BCR/ABL*)(4%) and hypodiploidy (5%). All are considered poor prognostic factors in B-ALL. The t(9;22) (*BCR/ABL*) translocation is more common in adults than children (10–15%) with B-ALL, and is generally associated with a poor prognosis.[18] In most childhood cases, the *BCR/ABL* translocation results in a p190 kD fusion protein, while in adults, about half of the translocations produce the p210 kD protein that is present in CML. (∞ Chapter 22 for a detailed discussion of the Philadelphia chromosome.) The remainder produce the p190 protein.

Precursor B-ALL generally has a good prognosis. In the pediatric population, the complete remission rate approaches 95%, and in adults, it is 60–85%.[3] Long term, event-free survival is lower for both patient groups (~80% and 30–50%, respectively). Positive predictive factors in children include age 4–10, hyperdiploid chromosomes or t(12;21), and a low or normal WBC count at diagnosis. Adverse factors include very young age (<1 year), high WBC counts at diagnosis, and the other cytogenetic abnormalities listed above.

Precursor T-Cell Leukemia

Precursor T-cell leukemia (T-ALL) is a neoplasm of lymphoblasts committed to the T-cell lineage, involving the bone marrow and peripheral blood. Occasionally, the disease will present with primary involvement of the lymph nodes or extranodal sites, in which case it is called T lymphoblastic lymphoma (T-LBL). T-ALL accounts for about 15% of the cases of childhood ALL. It is more common in adolescents than younger children, and more common in males than females. It accounts for ~25% of the cases of adult ALL.

T cell lineage can be detected by rearrangement of the T-cell receptor (TCR) genes using molecular methods. There are four TCR genes capable of rearranging, coding for the α, β, γ, and δ chains of the TCR. A neoplastic T-cell may exhibit rearrangement of one or more of these genes. Detection of a monoclonal TCR gene rearrangement suggests a neoplasm of the T cell lineage, but a small number of B-cell ALL will also demonstrate TCR gene rearrangement.

Precursor T-ALL usually presents with a high WBC count, and often a mediastinal mass (leukemic infiltration of the thymus) or other tissue masses. The lymphoblasts are similar to those seen in B-ALL, although there is more likely to be variability in size, and cytoplasmic vacuoles may be present. The cytochemistry is also similar to that seen in B-ALL, but acid phosphatase can show focal intense positivity in T-ALL.

The lymphoblasts in T-ALL are TdT+, and usually CD7+ and CD3+. They can have variable expression of CD1, CD2, CD4, Cd5, CD8, and CD10.[10] Lymphoblasts frequently co-express CD4 and CD8, indicative of the cortical stage of thymocyte differentiation ("double-positive cells").[19] At the medullary stage of differentiation, the cells are either CD4+ or CD8+. CD79a, generally considered to be a B-lineage marker, has been observed in some cases. One or more of the myeloid-associated markers CD13 and CD33 can be seen. As in B-ALL, T-ALL also can be stratified into differentiation stages, with cytoplasmic CD3, CD2, and CD7 appearing in the earliest stage, followed by CD5, CD1a, and subsequently, the appearance of membrane CD3 (Table 25-5).

✓ **Checkpoint! 3**

Why is it necessary to immunophenotype the lymphoblasts in ALL if they have been identified as lymphoblasts morphologically?

⊗ TABLE 25-5

Cellular Markers Useful in Diagnosis and Classification of T-ALL

Subgroup	HLA-DR	TdT	CD34	CD2	CDIa	CD3	CD7	CD8	CD4	CD10	CD19 CD20 CD22	Rearrangement of Ig genes	Rearrangement of TCR genes
Pro T	+/−	+/−	+/−	−	−	+(c)	+	−	−	+/−	−	−	+/−
Pre T	+/−	+/−	+/−	+	−	+(c)	+	−	−	+/−	−	−	+/−
Cortical T	+/−	+/−	−	+	+	+(c)	+	+	+	+/−	−	−	+/−
Medullary T	+/−	+/−	−	+	−	+(c)	+	+* or −	+* or −	+/−	−	−	+/−

*Either CD4 or CD8 positive; (c) = cytoplasmic; − = absent; + = present; +/− may be present; Ig = immunoglobulin; TCR = T cell receptor

Cytogenetic studies reveal translocations in T-ALL as well as B-ALL. About one-third of the cases of T-ALL have translocations involving the alpha and delta T-cell receptor loci (14q11.2), the beta locus (7q35) or the gamma locus (7p14–15). The translocations involve a variety of partner genes including the transcription factors *MYC* (8q24.1), *TAL1* (1p32), *RBTN1* (11p15), *RBTN2* (11p13), *HOX11* (10q24) and *HOX11L2* (5q35).[4,9] The result is usually a dysregulation of the partner gene, resulting in growth enhancement. In addition, molecular mutations of the *NOTCH1* gene are found in >50% of cases of T-ALL.[9] NOTCH1 encodes a transmembrane receptor that is involved in the regulation of normal T-cell development.

Historically, T-ALL was considered a high risk disease with a poorer prognosis than B-ALL. However, with current therapeutic protocols, survival is comparable for the two types of ALL.

 Checkpoint! 4

A patient has 50% blasts in his bone marrow. Cytochemical stains are negative with peroxidase and Sudan black B. Immunophenotyping is CD19 positive, but CD20, CD2, CD10, and CD7 negative. What additional testing may be helpful to distinguish the immunologic subgroup of this leukemia?

Acute Lymphoblastic Leukemia—Burkitt Type

This rare form of ALL occurs in both adults and children, and is considered to be the leukemic phase of Burkitt lymphoma. The lymphoblasts are homogeneous or monomorphic in appearance. The cells are large with abundant, intensely basophilic cytoplasm, with prominent cytoplasmic vacuolization (Figure 25-4 ■). The cytoplasmic vacuoles correspond to lipid vacuoles. The nucleus is oval to round with stippled chromatin and relatively clear parachromatin. They contain multiple basophilic nucleoli. Classically, this tumor

has a high proliferation rate, and many mitotic figures may be seen in the bone marrow smear. A "starry sky" pattern has been described, consisting of fields of basophilic leukemic blasts interrupted by benign macrophages that have ingested apoptotic tumor cells.

Burkitt cells show clonal rearrangement of the immunoglobulin heavy and light chain genes, as appropriate for B cells at this stage of differentiation. In addition, all cases have a translocation of the *MYC* gene (8q24) to the heavy chain region on chromosome 14 [t(8;14)] or to light chain loci on chromosome 2p12 [t(2;8)] or chromosome 22q11 [*t*(8;22)].[20,2] As a result of the translocation, the *MYC* gene is under the control of the Ig promoters on chromosomes 14, 2, or 22, and is constitutively expressed. Overexpression of *MYC* drives cells through the cell cycle, and also activates genes involved in apoptosis.[2] A summary of the cytogenetic findings associated with subgroups of ALL can be found in Table 25-6 .

Treatment for Burkitt leukemia is substantially different from treatment for precursor B-ALL or T-ALL. Treatment consists of very intense chemotherapy of relatively short duration. Most patients have a good prognosis, with 80–90% survival.

 Checkpoint! 5

Contrast the morphology of blasts found in the two subtypes of ALL.

CASE STUDY *(continued from page 534)*

3. If the flow cytometry pattern showed a positive CD10, what would be the classification of this acute leukemia?

4. In this situation, would the therapeutic outcome be considered as favorable or bleak? Why?

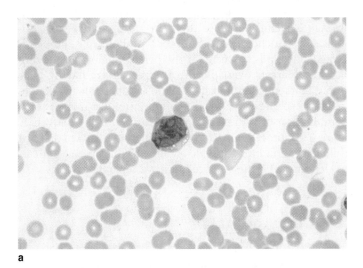

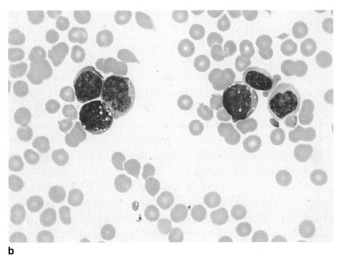

a   b

■ FIGURE 25-4   a. Lymphoblast in peripheral blood from Burkitt type acute lymphoblastic leukemia. Notice the vacuoles. b. Lymphoblasts in the bone marrow from the patient in Figure 25-4a. (Wright-Giemsa stain; 1000× magnification)

TABLE 25-6

The WHO Classification of Acute Lymphoblastic Leukemias (ALL) Using Chromosomal and Molecular Aberrations

	Cytogenetic Abnormality	Genetic Alteration
Precursor B-cell ALL	t(9;22)(q34:q11)	*BCR/ABL*
	t(11;v)(11q23;var)	*MLL* rearranged
	t(1;19)(q23:p13)	*E2A/PBX1*
	t(12;21)(p12:q22)	*TEL/AML1*
	T(17;19)	*E2A/HLF*
Precursor T-cell ALL	t(1;14)	*MYC/TCRα/δ*
	t(11;14)(p15;q11)	*LMO1/TCRα/δ*
	t(11;14)(p13;q11)	*LMO2/TCRα/δ*

v = various

✓ Checkpoint! 6

A 3-year-old patient has 45% lymphoblasts in the bone marrow. The blasts are slightly larger than lymphocytes and appear to be a homogeneous population. The nuclear membrane is regular and nucleoli are not prominent. There is a small amount of moderately basophilic cytoplasm. What is the most likely WHO group of this leukemia? If the cells tested positive for CD19, CD10, and CD34, what is the most likely immunologic subgroup? Why should cytogenetics be done on this patient?

ACUTE LEUKEMIAS OF AMBIGUOUS LINEAGE

This WHO group of leukemias include malignant neoplasms in which the morphology, cytochemistry, and immunophenotype lack sufficient information to classify them within a given lineage, or neoplasms in which the blasts have morphologic and/or immunophenotypic characteristics of more than one lineage.

Acute Undifferentiated Leukemia

The **acute undifferentiated leukemia (AUL)** category includes acute leukemias in which the morphology, cytochemistry, and immunophenotype of the proliferating blasts lack sufficient information to classify them as myeloid or lymphoid origin. In this case, the leukemia is classified as "acute undifferentiated leukemia."[4] Electron microscopic studies can sometimes detect ultrastructural evidence of primary granules and/or peroxidase, a finding which would indicate acute non-lymphocytic leukemia. Determination of the myeloid or lymphoblastic origin of the cell is important for treatment decisions. Absence of primary granules and/or peroxidase with electron microscopy together with the other negative or ambiguous findings indicates a diagnosis of AUL. AUL is predominantly found in adults, and only about 1/3 of patients respond to the chemotherapy regimens of AML and ALL.

Acute Leukemias with Lineage Heterogeneity

This category includes those leukemias in which the blasts have morphologic and/or immunophenotypic characteristics of both myeloid and lymphoid cells (or of both T and B lymphocytes). If two distinct populations of blasts are identifiable, each expressing markers of a distinct lineage (i.e., one population myeloid and one population lymphoid, or one population T-lymphoid and one population B-lymphoid) the disease is considered a "**bilineage acute leukemia.**" If the blasts coexpress myeloid and T or B lineage specific markers, or concurrent T and B lineage markers, the disease is considered a "**biphenotypic acute leukemia.**"[4] A more recently recognized leukemia with lineage heterogeneity is the "myeloid/**natural killer (NK) cell** acute leukemia," which has markers of both NK cells (CD56+), and myeloid lineage cells (CD13 +/− CD33 +/− MPO).[21]

The biphenotypic designation is reserved for those cases in which there is ambiguity of lineage assignment. It should not be used in situations in which an ALL aberrantly expresses one or two myeloid antigenic markers, or an AML aberrantly expresses one or two lymphoid antigenic markers. These are considered "myeloid antigen positive ALL" and "lymphoid antigen positive AML" respectively. Because many markers are only lineage-associated and not lineage-specific, co-expression of only one or two cross-lineage antigens is insufficient for a diagnosis of biphenotypic leukemia.[4,22]

Lack of lineage specificity (lineage infidelity) could be the result of genetic misprogramming, or the leukemic clone could represent a bipotential cell that has retained both lymphoid and myeloid markers during development.[4] Although mixed-lineage leukemias are uncommon, it is important to identify them in order to determine their actual occurrence, to identify appropriate therapy, and to correlate karyotypic abnormalities.[23] A high percentage of the acute leukemias of ambiguous lineage have associated cytogenetic abnormalities. The cell of origin is thought to be the MPP.

Immunological phenotyping is necessary to define mixed lineage leukemias because there are no definitive morphological or cytochemical features for lymphoid cells. Biphenotypic leukemia is suspected if the percentage of cells having myeloid markers overlaps with the percentage having lymphoid markers. More specific diagnosis is possible if a double labeling technique utilizing two immunologic markers or a combination of cytochemistry and immunologic markers is used. This procedure distinguishes between mixed lineage (bilineage) and biphenotypic acute leukemias because it can be determined if the same cell has two separate markers.

✓ Checkpoint! 7

A patient with acute leukemia has two morphologically different types of blasts. One population is positive for CD7 and CD2. The other is positive for CD33 and CD13. What is the most appropriate classification of this leukemia?

► THERAPY

A significant number of acute leukemias express inappropriate combinations of antigens making diagnosis challenging. Treatment protocols and prognosis are proving to be more effective and accurate when the leukemic cell lineage is immunologically classified correctly. In addition, therapy response and detection of residual leukemic cells (minimal residual disease/MRD) is possible using immunophenotyping and genetic testing.

Before the 1960s, a patient diagnosed with acute leukemia could expect to die within a few months. With new treatment modalities, remission rates for ALL (T- and/or B-ALL) have improved dramatically. Approximately 80% of children treated for ALL can be expected to enter a prolonged remission with an indefinite period of survival. The prognosis of ALL in adults is not as good as in children. Only 10–25% have achieved a 5-year survival. Poor prognostic factors are listed in Table 25-7 ✪.

Chemotherapy for ALL is divided into several phases. The **induction therapy** phase is designed to reduce the disease into complete remission (i.e., eradicating the leukemic blast population). This is followed by the CNS prophylactic phase. CNS leukemia is the most common form of relapse in young children who have not undergone specific treatment to the brain and spinal column early in remission. The two potential modes of treatment in the CNS prophylactic phase are cranium irradiation and/or intrathecal chemotherapy. Cranial irradiation is seldom a component of most current treat-

ment protocols, due to the risk of neurocognitive deficits, endocrinopathy, and the risk of inducing a second cancer. The third phase is **maintenance chemotherapy**, also called cytoreductive therapy or remission **consolidation therapy.** The need for this type of therapy is controversial. Some studies have shown a slight increase in survival with its use, whereas others reveal no improvement. Before the institution of CNS prophylactic treatment, there was a high incidence of relapse. The maintenance therapy was designed to prevent this relapse and prolong remission. The purpose of maintenance therapy is to eradicate any remaining leukemic cells. Drug treatment usually continues for 2–3 years. The relapse rate after cessation of all therapy is about 25% in the pediatric patient population.

✪ TABLE 25-7

Poor Prognostic Indicators in Acute Lymphoblastic Leukemia (ALL)

Clinical findings
   Infants (<1 year old)
   Patients past puberty
   CNS or mediastinal involvement
Laboratory findings
   High blast counts
   Presence of Philadelphia chromosome

✪ TABLE 25-8

Summary of Laboratory Features Helpful in Classification of ALL

Characteristic	Pro-B	Common ALL (Intermediate Pre-B)	Pre-B	Precursor T
Gene rearrangement				
Immunoglobulin (Ig)	+/−	+	+	−
T cell receptor (TCR)	−	−	−	+
Immunologic features				
Cytoplasmic μ	−	+	+	−
Surface Ig	−	−	+/−	−
Immunophenotype				
CD34	+	+/−	−	+
CD19	+	+	+	−
CD22	+(c)	+(c)	+(s)	−
CD10	−	+	+/−	−
CD20	−	+/−	+	−
CD2, CD3, CD5, CD7	−	−	−	+
Cytochemistry				
TdT	+	+	+	+
PAS	−	−	−	+

+ = positive; − = negative; (c) = cytoplasmic; (s) = surface

Allogeneic stem cell transplantation (HSCT) remains controversial. There is an incremental improvement in long term event-free survival in adults treated with HSCT in first remission (40–60%) versus treatment with chemotherapy alone (30–40%).[1] Currently, most clinicians consider HSCT to be of benefit to some high-risk adult patients. Patients who relapse while on therapy, or after only a short remission, are often considered candidates for HSCT. The use of umbilical cord blood as a source of HSC is being considered more frequently, especially in the pediatric patient population, as it does not require the same degree of histocompatibiity as do transplants using peripheral blood or marrow stem cells.

Relapse is defined as the reappearance of leukemic cells anywhere in the body, although the bone marrow is the most common site. Leukemic relapse occasionally occurs at extramedullary sites. Most relapses occur during treatment, or within the first two years after completion. Rarely, relapses have been observed up to ten years post remission induction. Relapse indicates a poor outcome for most patients, especially if it occurs while on therapy, or after only a brief initial remission.

SUMMARY

The acute leukemias (AL) are a heterogeneous group of neoplastic hematopoietic cell disorders characterized by unregulated proliferation, blocked maturation, and/or blocked apoptosis. The two major groups of AL are acute myeloid leukemia (AML) and acute lymphoblastic leukemia (ALL). These two major groups are further classified into subtypes using the World Health Organization (WHO) Classification based on patient presentation, morphological criteria, cytochemical stains, immunologic analysis, and cytogenetic and molecular abnormalities (Table 25-8 ⊗). This classification describes two subtypes for ALL, precursor B and precursor T leukemia. Immunophenotyping in ALL helps subtype the blasts into B- or T-ALL. The B cell lineage ALL includes Burkitt type leukemia.The peroxidase and/or Sudan black B may help differentiate AML (peroxidase positive) from ALL (peroxidase negative).

Acute leukemia with lineage heterogeneity is used to describe ALs in which blasts have characteristics of both myeloid and lymphoid cells or T and B lymphoid cells. *Biphenotypic leukemia* is used to describe ALs with blasts that possess markers of multiple lineages on the same leukemic cells while bilineage is used to describe leukemia with two different populations of blasts.

Regardless of subtype, the onset of AL is usually abrupt and, without treatment, progresses. Symptoms are related to anemia, thrombocytopenia, and/or neutropenia. Splenomegaly, hepatomegaly, and lymphadenopathy are common findings.

Hematologic findings of AL include a normocytic, normochromic anemia, thrombocytopenia, and a decreased, normal, or increased leukocyte count. Blasts are almost always found in the peripheral blood. A bone marrow examination is always indicated if leukemia is suspected. Using the WHO criteria, the bone marrow and/or peripheral blood must have more than 20% blasts.

REVIEW QUESTIONS

LEVEL I

1. Which of the following descriptions is more closely associated with the lymphoblasts seen in ALL of childhood? (Objective 3)
   a. heterogeneous with a deeply basophilic cytoplasm
   b. homogeneous and small with moderate basophilia in the cytoplasm
   c. heterogeneous with granules
   d. homogeneous with granules

2. Acute lymphoblastic leukemia is most often seen in patients: (Objective 5)
   a. over the age of 60
   b. age 35–60 years
   c. age 10–35 years
   d. below 5 years

3. The WHO classification of ALL is primarily based on: (Objective 2)
   a. cytogenetic and morphology abnormalities
   b. morphology and cytochemistry of blasts
   c. immunophenotyping of blasts and genetic analysis
   d. molecular genetic abnormalities and cytochemistry of blasts

LEVEL II

1. Cells that are positive for the 8;14 translocation are characteristic of which of the following? (Objective 4)
   a. T cell ALL
   b. reactive lymphocytosis
   c. B cell ALL
   d. Burkitt type ALL

2. Monoclonal rearrangement of the TCR genes is associated with blasts that have the following immunophenotype: (Objective 2)
   a. CD10+, CD22+, CD2−
   b. CD2−, CD3−, CD10+
   c. CD19+, CD22+, CD3−
   d. CD2+, CD3+, CD7+

3. In a case of ALL, the lymphoblasts showed strong localized positivity with acid phosphatase and were positive for CD7 and CD2, negative for CD19, CD24, and CD20. These blasts are most likely: (Objective 4)
   a. T lymphoblasts
   b. B lymphoblasts
   c. lymphoid stem cells
   d. biphenotypic blasts

LEVEL I

4. An acute leukemia has morphologically undifferentiated blasts that are negative with cytochemical stains and lineage-marker associated immunophenotyping. This should be classified as: (Objective 6)
   a. acute undifferentiated leukemia
   b. mixed lineage acute leukemia
   c. myeloid/NK cell acute leukemia
   d. bilineal acute leukemia

5. Acute leukemia blasts that have myeloid and lymphoid markers on the same cells most likely define what subgroup of leukemia? (Objective 6)
   a. bilineage
   b. myeloid/NK
   c. biphenotypic
   d. undifferentiated

6. The following are included in the WHO classification of ALL: (Objective 2)
   a. T and B cell lymphoma
   b. ALL and Burkitt type ALL
   c. L1, L2, and L3
   d. bilineal and biphenotypic ALL

7. This finding in ALL can help differentiate it from AML: (Objective 1)
   a. presence of Auer rods
   b. positivity for myeloperoxidase
   c. >20% blasts
   d. positivity for CD19 and CD22

8. Blasts that are positive for block like PAS positivity are most likely: (Objectives 1, 4)
   a. myeloblasts
   b. monoblasts
   c. megakaryoblasts
   d. lymphoblasts

9. Which of the following laboratory results are most commonly found in ALL? (Objective 3)
   a. Eosinophilia and basophilia
   b. Neutropenia and thrombocytopenia
   c. Neutrophilia and thrombocytopenia
   d. Lymphocytosis and thrombocytosis

10. Which of the following signs is common in the presentation of childhood ALL? (Objective 5)
    a. gum infiltration
    b. bone and joint pain
    c. large, painful nodes
    d. eosinophilia

LEVEL II

4. While performing a differential count on a 2-year-old child, the clinical laboratory scientist identifies 78% blasts and notes the following other data: (Objectives 4, 6)

Hb	9.5 gm/dL
WBC	50.3×10^9/L
PLT	43×10^9/L

   Which of the following tests most likely is positive?
   a. Sudan black B
   b. CD19
   c. myeloperoxidase
   d. CD5

5. An adult patient with splenomegaly has an increase in mononuclear cells in the peripheral blood. The bone marrow was filled with a heterogeneous collection of blasts with no granulation. The cells in the marrow were negative for myeloperoxidase and Sudan black B. Flow cytometry shows a positive CD20 and CD10 and negative surface immunoglobulin. Which of the following conditions is most likely? (Objective 4)
   a. pro-B ALL
   b. common ALL (CALLA)
   c. pre-T cell ALL
   d. cortical T cell ALL

6. BCR/ABL can be seen in: (Objective 2)
   a. AUL
   b. Burkitt type ALL
   c. precursor B cell ALL
   d. precursor T cell ALL

7. The CD10 antigen found in ALL is also known as the: (Objective 4)
   a. BALL antigen
   b. TALL antigen
   c. Burkitt cell antigen
   d. CALLA antigen

8. What condition is suggested by the following laboratory findings? (Objectives 2, 4)

WBC	50.4×10^9/L
Diff	75% blasts
	20% segmented cells
	2% lymphs
	3% monos
Peroxidase	Negative
Alpha-naphthyl esterase	Negative
CD 19, CD22, CD34	Positive

   a. acute lymphoblastic leukemia
   b. acute myeloid leukemia
   c. chronic myelogenous leukemia
   d. chronic lymphocytic leukemia

REVIEW QUESTIONS *(continued)*

LEVEL I

LEVEL II

9. A 4-year-old male is admitted with the following findings:

WBC	60×10^9/L
Segs	15%
Bands	5%
Blasts	80%

The blasts are positive for TdT, CD2, cytoplasmic CD3, and CD7. What type of cell is involved? (Objectives 2, 4)

a. null cells

b. T cells

c. B cells

d. NK cells

10. A patient with ALL underwent chemotherapy. Results from hematologic, cytogenetic, and molecular analyses indicated that he entered complete remission. Four years later on his routine followup, the peripheral blood results were in the normal range and cytogenetic analysis revealed no abnormalilties, but molecular analysis showed BCR/ABL transcripts that were found in the blasts at diagnosis 4 years ago. This patient can be said to: (Objective 5)

a. be in complete remission

b. be in molecular and cytogenetic remission

c. have minimal residual disease

d. have partial cytogenetic remission

www.pearsonhighered.com/mckenzie

Use this address to access the interactive Companion Website created for this textbook. Find additional information, tables and figures. Evaluate your command of the chapter information using case studies and critical thinking and multiple choice questions.

REFERENCES

1. Pui C-H. Acute lymphoblastic leukemia. In: Lichtman MA, Beutler E, Kipps TJ, Seligsohn U, Kaushansky K, Prchal JT, eds. *Williams Hematology,* 7th ed. New York: McGraw-Hill; 2006:1321–42.

2. Ferrando AA, Look AT. Pathobiology of acute lymphoblastic leukemia. In: Hoffman R, Benz EJ, Shattil SJ, Furie B, Cohen HJ, Silberstein LE, McGlave P, eds. *Hematology: Basic Principles and Procedures,* 4th ed. Philadelphia: Churchill Livingstone; 2005:1135–54.

3. Bennet JM et al. Proposals for the classification of the acute leukaemias. French-American-British (FAB) Co-operative Group. *Br J Haematol.* 1976;33:451–58.

4. Jaffe ES, Harris NL, Stein H, Vardiman JW. *Pathology & Genetics. Tumours of Haematopoietic and Lymphoid Tissues.* World Health Organization Classification of Tumours. Lyon, France: IARC Press; 2001.

5. Howard SC, Pedrosa M, Lins M et al. Establishment of a pediatric oncology program and outcomes of childhood acute lymphoblastic leukemia in a resource-poor area. *JAMA.* 2004;291(20):2471–75.

6. Bleyer A. Adolescent and young adult (AYA) Oncology: The first A. *Pediatr Hematol Oncol.* 2007;57(4):242–55.

7. Majumder D, Banerjee D, Chandra S et al. Red cell morphology in leukemia, hypoplastic anemia and myelodysplastic syndrome. *Pathophysiology.* 2006;13(4):217–25.

8. Pitman SD, Huang Q. Granular acute lymphoblastic leukemia: A case report and literature review. *Am J Hematol.* 2007;82(9):834–37.

9. Kersey J, Newbit M, Hallgren H et al. Evidence for origin of certain childhood acute lymphoblastic leukemias and lymphomas in thymus-derived lymphocytes. *Cancer.* 1975;36:1348–52.

10. Hurwitz CA, Loken MR, Graham ML et al. Asynchronous antigen expression in B-lineage acute lymphoblastic leukemia. *Blood.* 1988; 72:299–307.

11. Kaleem Z, Crawford E, Pathan MH et al. Flow cytometric analysis of acute leukemias. Diagnostic utility and critical analysis of data. *Arch Pathol Lab Med.* 2003; 127(1):42–48.

12. Korsmeyer SJ, Hieter PA, Ravetch JV et al. Developmental hierarchy of immunoglobulin gene rearrangements in human leukemic pre-B cells. *Proc Natl Acad Sci USA.* 1981;78:7096–7100.

13. Korsmeyer SJ, Arnold A, Bakshi A et al. Immunoglobulin gene rearrangement and cell surface antigen expression in acute lymphocytic leukemias of T-cell and B-cell origins. *J Clin Invest.* 1983;71: 301–13.

14. Tawa A, Hozumi N, Minden M et al. Rearrangement of the T-cell receptor B-chain gene in non-T-cell, non-B-cell acute lymphoblastic leukemia of childhood. *N Engl J Med.* 1985;313:1033–37.

15. Basso G, Case C, Dell'Orto MC. Diagnosis and genetic subtypes of leukemia combining gene expression and flow cytometry. *Blood Cells Mol Dis.* 2007;39(2):164–68.

16. Schultz KR, Pullen DJ, Sather HN et al. Risk- and response-based classification of childhood B-precursor acute lymphoblastic leukemia: A combined analysis of prognostic markers from the Pediatric Oncology Group (POG) and Children's Cancer Group (CCG). *Blood.* 2007;109(3):926–35.

17. Dworzak MN, Fritsch G, Fleischer C et al. Comparative phenotype mapping of normal vs. malignant pediatric B-lymphopoiesis unveils leukemia-associated aberrations. *Exp Hematol.* 1998;26(4): 305–13.

18. Arico M, Valsecchi MG, Camitta B et al. Outcome of treatment in children with Philadelphia chromosome-positive acute lymphoblastic leukemia. *N Engl J Med.* 2000;342(14):998–1006.

19. Lewis RE, Cruse JM, Sanders CM et al. The immunophenotype of pre-TALL/LBL revisited. *Exp Mol Pathol.* 2006;81(2):162–65.

20. Truffinet V, Pinaud E, Cogné N et al. The 3' IgH locus control region is sufficient to deregulate a c-myc transgene and promote mature B cell malignancies with a predominant Burkittlike phenotype. *J Immunol.* 2007;179(9):6033–42.

21. Scott AA, Head DR, Kopecky KJ et al. HLA-DR⁻, CD33⁺, CD56⁺, CD16⁻ myeloid/natural killer cell acute leukemia: A previously unrecognized form of acute leukemia potentially misdiagnosed as French-American-British acute myeloid leukemia-M3. *Blood.* 1994; 84:244–55.

22. Owaidah TM, Al Beihany A, Iqbal MA et al. Cytogenetics, molecular and ultrastructural characteristics of biphenotypic acute leukemia identified by the EGIL scoring system. *Leukemia.* 2006;20(4): 620–26.

23. Garcia Vela JA, Monteserin MC, Delgado I et al. Aberrant immunophenotypes detected by flow cytometry in acute lymphoblastic leukemia. *Leuk Lymphoma.* 2000;36(3-4):275–84.

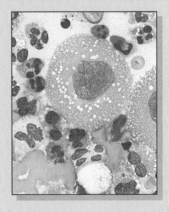

26

Lymphoid Malignancies: Chronic Lymphoid Leukemias, Lymphomas, and Plasma Cell Neoplasms

Fiona Craig, M.D.

CHAPTER OUTLINE

■ OBJECTIVES—LEVEL I

At the end of this unit of study, the student should be able to:

1. Describe the clinical presentation of patients with lymphoid malignancies.
2. Describe how the diagnosis of lymphoid malignancy is made.
3. Differentiate among chronic lymphocytic leukemia (CLL), lymphoma, and multiple myeloma based on peripheral blood findings and ancillary studies.
4. Describe the histology of a normal lymph node.
5. Summarize the causes of lymphadenopathy.
6. Describe the morphologic differences between Hodgkin and non-Hodgkin lymphoma.
7. List and describe the chronic leukemic lymphoproliferative disorders.
8. Recognize and differentiate abnormal and normal lymphocytes on a stained peripheral blood smear and associate their presence with a clinical diagnosis.
9. Describe and apply a multidisciplinary approach to the classification and staging of lymphoid and plasma cell neoplasms.
10. Compare the laboratory and clinical findings of multiple myeloma and Waldenström macroglobulinemia.
11. Define *monoclonal gammopathy*.

■ OBJECTIVES—LEVEL II

At the end of this unit of study, the student should be able to:

1. Describe the use of immunophenotyping and genotyping in detecting clonality and list the results characteristic of the more common lymphoid malignancies.
2. Contrast the features of low-grade and high-grade lymphoma.

3. Compare and contrast the laboratory features characteristic of the following non-Hodgkin lymphomas:
   a. Small lymphocytic lymphoma
   b. Follicular lymphoma
   c. Mantle cell lymphoma
   d. MALT lymphoma
   e. Waldenström macroglobulinemia
   f. Diffuse large B cell lymphoma
   g. Burkitt lymphoma
   h. Lymphoblastic lymphoma
   i. Peripheral T cell lymphoma
   j. Anaplastic large cell lymphoma

4. Compare and contrast the laboratory features characteristic of Hodgkin lymphoma (HL) subtypes.

5. Compare and contrast the clinical and laboratory features characteristic of the following chronic leukemic lymphoproliferative disorders:
   a. Chronic lymphocytic leukemia (CLL)
   b. Prolymphocytic leukemia (PLL)
   c. Hairy cell leukemia (HCL)
   d. Circulating lymphoma
   e. Large granular lymphocyte leukemia (LGLL)
   f. Sézary syndrome

6. Compare and contrast the laboratory features characteristic of the following plasma cell disorders:
   a. Plasmacytoma
   b. Multiple myeloma
   c. Monoclonal gammopathy of undetermined significance

7. Recognize and identify the peripheral blood abnormalities associated with CLL, PLL, HCL, LGLL, Sézary syndrome, multiple myeloma, and non-Hodgkin lymphoma.

8. Describe the etiology and pathogenesis of lymphoid neoplasms.

9. Differentiate reactive from malignant proliferations of lymphoid cells using clinical and laboratory data.

KEY TERMS

Anaplastic large cell lymphoma (ALCL)
BCL-2 gene
Bence-Jones proteinuria
Butt cell
Clonality
Dutcher body
Hairy cell
Lacunar cell
Lymphoepithelial lesion
Lymphoma
Plasma cell neoplasm
Popcorn cell (L&H cell)

Prolymphocyte
Reed-Sternberg (R-S) cell
Richter's transformation
Rouleaux
Sézary cell
Small lymphocytic lymphoma (SLL)
Smudge cell
Stage
Starry-sky appearance
Tingible body macrophages
Tartrate resistant acid phosphatase (TRAP)

BACKGROUND BASICS

The information in this chapter builds on concepts learned in previous chapters. To maximize your learning experience, you should review these concepts before starting this unit of study:

Level I

▶ Describe the structure and function of lymph nodes. (Chapter 4)

▶ Outline the classification and summarize the general characteristics of acute leukemia. (Chapter 21)

Level II

▶ Explain the pathogenesis of neoplasia. (Chapters 2 and 21)

▶ Identify the etiology of acute leukemia. (Chapter 21)

 CASE STUDY

We will address this case study throughout the chapter.
Julia, a 56-year-old female, presented with a 4-month history of generalized painless lymphadenopathy and fatigue. A CBC revealed leukocytosis due to lymphocytosis. Consider laboratory features that can help differentiate a reactive lymphocytosis from a neoplastic lymphocytosis.

▶ OVERVIEW

This chapter discusses the classification of lymphoid malignancies, the formation of a diagnosis and the unique features of selected subtypes. The etiology and pathogenesis of the disorders are discussed first followed by the classification and diagnosis this broad group of diseases. The remainder of the chapter describes characteristics of the more common types of chronic leukemic lymphoid malignancy, malignant lymphoma, and plasma cell neoplasms.

▶ INTRODUCTION

Lymphoid malignancies represent a heterogeneous group of disorders composed of cells that resemble one or more stages of normal lymphocyte development. This broad group can be divided into four categories based on the maturity of the neoplastic cells and the distribution of disease:

• Acute lymphoblastic leukemia
• Chronic leukemic lymphoid malignancies
• Malignant lymphoma
• Plasma cell neoplasms

Leukemia is a malignant neoplasm that primarily involves the bone marrow and peripheral blood. Acute lymphoblastic leukemia is a proliferation of blasts belonging to the lymphoid lineage (∞ Chapters 21, 25). The chronic leukemic lymphoid malignancies are composed of mature lymphocytes and usually have an insidious onset and more indolent course than the acute leukemias.

The **lymphomas** are malignant neoplasms that present as tumorous masses that primarily involve the lymphoid organs including lymph nodes, tonsils, spleen, thymus, and lymphoid tissue of the gastrointestinal tract. Although most lymphomas are composed of mature lymphoid cells, blastic malignancies (lymphoblastic lymphoma) do occur. The distinction between leukemia and lymphoma is not always clear cut. Leukemia primarily involves the bone marrow and peripheral blood, but tissue involvement can occur. Lymphoma primarily involves tissue, but bone marrow and peripheral blood involvement can occur. Lymphoblastic lymphoma and acute lymphoblastic leukemia probably represent different clinical manifestations of a single disease entity. Therefore, the World Health Organization (WHO) classification groups them.[1]

The **plasma cell neoplasms** are considered a group of diseases composed of immunoglobulin-secreting cells. The boundary between this group and the malignant lymphomas is not sharp. Lymphoma can contain a subset of cells demonstrating plasma cell differentiation, as occurs in lymphoplasmacytic lymphoma. Despite these difficulties in classification, the lymphoid malignancies can usually be divided into groups that provide information about prognosis and help direct treatment.

▶ ETIOLOGY AND PATHOGENESIS

The genesis of lymphoid malignancy is thought to be a multistep process involving acquired genetic, inherited genetic, and environmental factors.

ACQUIRED GENETIC FACTORS

As described for the leukemias, acquired alterations of proto-oncogenes and tumor suppressor genes have been associated with the development of lymphoid malignancy. Additional targets for genetic damage are the genes involved in programmed cell death (apoptosis) (e.g., *BCL-2*, ∞ Chapter 2). The ***BCL-2* gene** on chromosome 18 is involved in the pathogenesis of follicular lymphoma. Translocation of the *BCL-2* gene to the region of the immunoglobulin heavy chain gene, t(14;18), causes overexpression of the *BCL-2* gene. The resulting increase in BCL-2 protein leads to an inhibition of apoptosis. Decreased cell death results in an accumulation of lymphocytes within the lymph node. Therefore, low-grade follicular lymphoma appears to arise from cell persistence rather than uncontrolled cell proliferation.

INHERITED GENETIC FACTORS

Some inherited immunodeficiency syndromes such as Wiskott Aldrich and ataxia telangiectasia are associated with a higher incidence of malignant lymphoma.

ENVIRONMENTAL FACTORS

The Epstein-Barr virus (EBV) is associated with the development of several forms of lymphoid malignancy including African Burkitt lymphoma, B cell malignant lymphoma in HIV-infected individuals, and Hodgkin lymphoma (HL). Latent infection with EBV is only one of multiple steps involved in the genesis of these types of lymphoma. EBV infection is acquired orally and is often manifest clinically as infectious mononucleosis. The virus infects B lymphocytes where it remains latent under the immune system's control. The EBV-infected cells can proliferate if the host becomes immunocompromised and/or the B lymphocytes acquire additional genetic abnormalities such as the *C-MYC* translocation.

Another infectious agent associated with the development of non-Hodgkin lymphoma is *Helicobacter pylori*. Patients with *Helicobacter pylori*-induced inflammation of the stomach have a high incidence of gastric lymphoma of <u>m</u>ucosa <u>a</u>ssociated <u>l</u>ymphoid <u>t</u>issue (MALT) lymphoma type. Chronic *Helicobacter* infection leads to antigen-driven T lymphocyte stimulation and subsequent B lymphocyte activation. The B lymphocytes initially are polyclonal and depend entirely on T lymphocyte stimulation. With time, the B cell population can proliferate autonomously. If the B lymphocyte proliferation still depends on T lymphocyte stimulation, the lymphoma can regress following removal of the antigenic stimulus with antimicrobial therapy. Lymphoma that is proliferating independent of antigenic stimulation probably requires more drastic therapy including excision and/or chemotherapy.

> ✓ **Checkpoint! 1**
>
> *How does the BCL-2 gene rearrangement differ from most other oncogenes?*

▶ DIAGNOSIS OF LYMPHOID MALIGNANCY

Knowledge of the distribution of lymphoid malignancy at presentation and of the morphologic appearance and growth pattern of the neoplastic cells is essential for correctly diagnosing it. The phenotype and genotype of the malignant cells often assist in diagnosis and classification, determination of prognosis, and detection of residual disease following treatment.

MORPHOLOGIC APPEARANCE

The diagnosis of a lymphoid malignancy is established by examination of a specimen of peripheral blood, bone marrow, and/or other tissue in the laboratory. For most cases of leukemia, this examination involves a CBC and bone marrow sample (aspirate and biopsy). A diagnosis of lymphoma is usually rendered from biopsy or a fine-needle aspirate of a mass. In general, normal or reactive proliferations of lymphocytes contain a mixture of cells varying in size, shape, and staining characteristics. The cells present in lymphoid malignancies are usually more homogeneous than normal or reactive lymphocytes because of the expansion of a single cell type. Less frequently, malignant lymphoid cells can be recognized because of an abnormal or bizarre appearance.

ANCILLARY STUDIES

Sometimes morphology alone is not sufficient to diagnose or subclassify lymphoid malignancies. Several additional studies are available to assist in the diagnosis: immunophenotyping, molecular diagnostics, and cytogenetics. These studies can detect abnormal lymphocytes and/or **clonality** (the presence of identical cells derived from a single progenitor). The cells of malignant lymphoma are thought to derive from a single precursor cell (i.e., the cell of origin). The progeny from this cell belong to a clone that shares morphologic, immunophenotypic, and genotypic features. In most circumstances, clonality is synonymous with malignancy. Clonality can be detected by the identification of only one of the immunoglobulin light chains (kappa or lambda) on B cells or the presence of a population of cells with an abnormal phenotype such as CD5 negative T lymphocytes (∞ Chapter 37). Clonal rearrangement of immunoglobulin or T cell receptor genes or the presence of an abnormal translocation can also be used to identify malignant lymphocytes. The presence of characteristic translocations can assist in the diagnosis of a subtype of lymphoid malignancy as in the *BCL-2* gene rearrangement in follicular lymphoma (∞ Chapters 2, 21).

CLASSIFICATION

The World Health Organization (WHO) scheme currently classifies lymphoid malignancies into distinct disease entities that have similar morphologic, phenotypic, and genotypic features (Table 26-1).[1] Most disease entities have an expected clinical course and response to treatment. This predicted clinical behavior is referred to as the lymphoma grade. Low-grade lymphoma (e.g., small lymphocytic lymphoma) usually has a long indolent course; patients often die of disorders other than their lymphoma. High-grade lymphoma (e.g., Burkitt lymphoma) is clinically aggressive and kill the patient rapidly if not treated. Ironically, current therapeutic regimens are more effective against high-grade than low-grade lymphoid malignancies. Therefore, many patients with high-grade lymphoma who are treated are cured of their disease. Often patients with low-grade lymphoma are treated for symptomatic relief rather than the intent to cure. In general, histologic sections from lower grade lymphoma more often demonstrate a nodular growth pattern, smaller cells, lower mitotic activity, and an absence of apoptosis. Higher grade lymphoma usually has a diffuse growth

TABLE 26-1

WHO Classification of Lymphoid Neoplasms

B cell neoplasms	Precursor B cell neoplasms
	Precursor B lymphoblastic leukemia/lymphoma
	Mature B cell neoplasms
	Chronic lymphocytic leukemia/small lymphocytic lymphoma
	B cell prolymphocytic leukemia
	Waldenström macroglobulinemia
	Splenic marginal zone lymphoma
	Hairy cell leukemia
	Plasma cell myeloma
	Monoclonal gammopathy of undetermined significance
	Extranodal marginal zone B cell lymphoma of mucosa associated lymphoid tissue (MALT) lymphoma
	Nodal marginal zone B cell lymphoma
	Follicular lymphoma
	Mantle cell lymphoma
	Diffuse large B cell lymphoma
	Mediastinal large B cell lymphoma
	Intravascular large B cell lymphoma
	Primary effusion lymphoma
	Burkitt lymphoma leukemia
T cell and Natural Killer (NK) cell neoplasms	Precursor T cell neoplasm
	Precursor T lymphoblastic leukemia/lymphoma
	Mature T cell neoplasms
	Leukemic/Disseminated
	T cell prolymphocytic leukemia
	T cell large granular lymphocytic leukemia
	Aggressive NK cell leukemia
	Adult T cell lymphoma/leukemia,
	Cutaneous
	Mycosis fungoides/Sézary syndrome
	Anaplastic large cell lymphoma, primary cutaneous type
	Other extranodal
	Extranodal NK/T cell lymphoma, nasal type
	Enteropathy-type T cell lymphoma
	Hepatosplenic T cell lymphoma
	Subcutaneous panniculitis-like T cell lymphoma
	Nodal
	Angioimmunoblastic T cell lymphoma
	Anaplastic large cell lymphoma, primary systemic type
	Peripheral T cell lymphoma, not otherwise characterized
Hodgkin lymphoma (disease)	Nodular lymphocyte predominant Hodgkin lymphoma
	Classical Hodgkin lymphoma
	Nodular sclerosis classical Hodgkin lymphoma
	Mixed cellularity classical Hodgkin lymphoma
	Lymphocyte-rich classical Hodgkin lymphoma
	Lymphocyte depleted Hodgkin lymphoma

pattern, is often composed of larger cells, and displays more numerous mitoses and apoptotic bodies.

In addition to the prognostic information provided by identifying the disease entities defined in the WHO classification, some diseases can be divided into further prognostic groups. The entity follicular lymphoma, for instance, is divided into three grades defined by the number of large cells (centroblasts). Many prognostic markers including expression of the proteins CD38 and ZAP-70, presence of cytogenetic abnormalities, and degree of mutation of the immunoglobulin heavy chain variable region are used for chronic lymphocytic leukemia. Diffuse large B cell lymphoma is divided into germinal and nongerminal center types.

STAGING

The prognosis of a patient with a lymphoid malignancy is not only related to the lymphoma grade but also to the extent and distribution of disease (**stage**). Patients with widespread lymphoma usually have a worse prognosis. Determining the stage of disease usually involves radiologic studies, peripheral blood examination, and bone marrow aspiration and biopsy. The Ann Arbor scheme is often used to stage malignant lymphoma (Table 26-2 ✪). Bone marrow involvement indicates disseminated disease, stage IV.

The remainder of this chapter describes examples of lymphoid malignancies that illustrate the characteristics of the chronic leukemic lymphoid malignancies, malignant lymphoma, and plasma cell neoplasms.

> ✓ **Checkpoint! 2**
>
> *How does staging differ from grading in characterizing the lymphoid malignancies?*

► CHRONIC LEUKEMIC LYMPHOID MALIGNANCIES

The chronic leukemic lymphoid malignancies compose a heterogeneous group of disorders displaying a variety of morphologic appearances and immunophenotypes.[2] They

TABLE 26-2

Ann Arbor Staging System for Malignant Lymphoma

I	Single lymph node region or single extralymphatic site (I_E)
II	Two or more lymph node regions on same side of diaphragm or with involvement of limited contiguous extralymphatic site (II_E)
III	Lymph node regions on both sides of diaphragm, which can include spleen (III_S) and/or limited contiguous extralymphatic site (III_E)
IV	Multiple or disseminated foci of involvement of one or more extralymphatic organs or tissues with or without lymphatic involvement

are grouped together because they are primarily located in the blood and bone marrow and the malignant cells are mature lymphocytes. Although these malignancies are usually more indolent than the acute leukemias, the prognosis varies with the subtype. The features of the following more common subtypes of chronic leukemic lymphoid malignancies—B cell chronic lymphocytic leukemia, prolymphocytic leukemia, hairy cell leukemia, large granular lymphocyte leukemia (LGLL), Sézary's syndrome, and circulating lymphoma—(Table 26-3 ✪) are discussed further.

B CELL CHRONIC LYMPHOCYTIC LEUKEMIA

Chronic lymphocytic leukemia (CLL) is a disease of adults with a median age of 70 years at diagnosis. The incidence of CLL in men is twice that in women. The disease can be detected in an asymptomatic patient because of lymphocytosis found on a CBC performed for another reason. When present, symptoms are often related to anemia, thrombocytopenia, and neutropenia. These cytopenias can arise from a variety of causes including replacement of the bone marrow hematopoietic cells by neoplastic lymphocytes, hypersplenism, poor nutritional status, and immune mediated cell destruction (∞ Chapter 17). Lymphadenopathy is frequently present at diagnosis or can develop during the course of the disease. Indeed, CLL and small lymphocytic lymphoma (see below) are thought to represent different clinical presentations of a single disease entity.

A diagnosis of CLL requires a sustained absolute lymphocytosis $>5 \times 10^9$/L with characteristic morphologic and phenotypic findings. The lymphocytes are small and mature appearing with scant cytoplasm. The nuclei are usually round, and the chromatin is regularly clumped (block-type chromatin). Nucleoli are inconspicuous (Figure 26-1a ■). A few large **prolymphocytes** are usually present but represent less than 10% of all lymphocytes (Figure 26-1b ■). Prolymphocytes have abundant pale-staining cytoplasm and a large central prominent nucleolus. The neoplastic cells in CLL appear to be more fragile than normal lymphocytes and often burst open during smear preparation to produce **smudge cells.** However, smudge cells also can be found in reactive lymphocytosis and in other neoplasms; therefore, their presence should not be used to diagnose CLL. In fact, smudge cells can make diagnosing CLL more difficult by preventing visualization of the lymphocytes. The number of smudge cells can be reduced by mixing a drop of albumin with a drop of blood prior to making the smear.

The differential diagnosis of CLL includes reactive lymphocytosis and the other chronic leukemia lymphoproliferative disorders (Table 26-3). Although a provisional diagnosis usually can be made following smear examination, immunophenotyping is often used to establish a definitive diagnosis. B cell CLL is characterized by aberrant expression of the T lymphocyte antigen CD5. Expression of CD23 and lack

✪ TABLE 26-3	
Key Features of Subgroups of Chronic Leukemic Lymphoid Malignancies	
B cell chronic lymphocytic leukemia (CLL)	Lymphocytosis
	Smudge cells
	Prolymphocytes <10%
	CD19+, CD5+, CD20+ weak intensity, CD23+, FMC-7−
	Surface Ig weak intensity
B cell prolymphocytic leukemia (PLL)	Splenomegaly
	Marked lymphocytosis
	Prolymphocytes >55%
	CD19+, CD20+, CD22+, CD5−/+, FMC-7+
	Surface Ig strong intensity
T cell PLL	Splenomegaly
	Skin lesions
	Marked lymphocytosis
	Varied morphologic appearance
	CD3+, CD2+, CD5+, CD4+, CD8−/+
	inv(14)q11q32
Hairy cell leukemia	Pancytopenia
	Circulating hairy cells
	TRAP+
	CD19+, CD5−, CD20+ strong intensity, CD22+, CD103+, CD11c+, CD25+
	Surface Ig strong intensity
	Bone marrow dry tap
	Bone marrow "fried egg" appearance
T cell large granular lymphocyte (LGL) leukemia	Lymphocytosis
	Anemia
	Neutropenia
	Thrombocytopenia
	Rheumatoid factor often present
	CD2+, CD3+, CD4−, CD5+, CD7+, CD8+, CD16+, CD56−/+, CD57+/−
	T cell receptor (TCR) clonally rearranged
	Indolent course
Sézary's syndrome	Erythroderma (red skin)
	Cutaneous T cell lymphoma
	Circulating malignant cells
	CD2+, CD3+, CD4+, CD5+, CD7−, CD8−

of FMC-7 positivity distinguishes CLL from leukemic mantle cell lymphoma (MCL). FMC-7 is a monoclonal antibody that binds to an epitope of CD20 formed when this surface antigen is present at high density. The CLL cells usually have weak surface expression of monoclonal immunoglobulin.

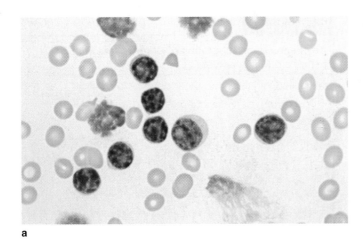
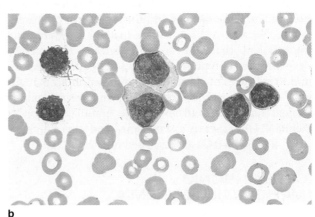

a   b

■ FIGURE 26-1   a. Chronic lymphocytic leukemia. Small round lymphocytes with clumped chromatin, a larger prolymphocyte with a prominent nucleolus, and numerous smudge cells. b. Prolymphocytic leukemia. Numerous large lymphoid cells with prominent nucleoli (prolymphocytes). (Peripheral blood, Wright stain, 1000× magnification)

CLL had been considered a low-grade disease with a uniformly indolent course that could not be cured and was only treated for relief of symptoms. More recently it has been recognized that CLL is actually a rather heterogeneous disorder that includes a subset of patients that requires earlier treatment and has a shorter overall survival. Several prognostic markers have been associated with this difference in clinical behavior and are often evaluated at diagnosis in an attempt to predict outcome. These prognostic markers include the proteins CD38 and ZAP-70 and the mutational status of the immunoglobulin (Ig) heavy chain gene variable region (V_H).[3] During normal B cell development, rearranged immunoglobulin variable gene segments undergo somatic hypermutation. CLL cases can be divided into two groups, those with "mutated" V_H genes and those with "unmutated" V_H genes. CLL with a more aggressive behavior is associated with higher levels of expression of CD38 and ZAP-70 as determined by flow cytometry and an "unmutated" Ig V_H gene.

Cytogenetic abnormalities were initially difficult to detect in CLL because the leukemic cells were not easy to induce to proliferate in culture. However, with improved cytogenetic methods such as fluorescence in situ hybridization (FISH), approximately half of all CLL patients are found to have clonal chromosomal abnormalities. The most common chromosomal abnormality, del 13q14-23.1, is associated with a relatively good prognosis. The following chromosomal abnormalities, listed in order of decreasing frequency, are associated with a worse prognosis:

• Trisomy 12
• Del 11q22.3-23.1
• Del 6q21-23
• Deletions at 17p13.1 (*p53* aberrations)
• 14q abnormalities and complex chromosomal abnormalities

Translocations are rarely observed in CLL. Patients with abnormal karyotypes survive for a significantly shorter period than do patients with normal karyotypes.

Less than 10% of patients with CLL develop transformation of their disease into one with a worse prognosis. **Richter's transformation** is the transition to an agressive large B cell lymphoma, which occurs in ~3% of patients with CLL. Prolymphocytoid transformation of CLL is associated with an increased number of prolymphocytes (usually prolymphocytes account for <10% of the leukemic cell population).

PROLYMPHOCYTIC LEUKEMIA

Prolymphocytic leukemia (PLL) is an aggressive leukemic disorder that often does not respond to treatment. Its incidence is ~10% that of CLL. It can have either a mature B or T cell phenotype.

B Cell PLL

Approximately 70% of cases of PLL are of a B cell lineage. B cell PLL is a disease of adult patients with a 4:1 male:female predominance. Although most cases arise de novo, PLL can develop from CLL (see above). However, preceding CLL may be asymptomatic and go unrecognized. Unlike CLL, patients with PLL usually have marked splenomegaly but minimal lymphadenopathy.

The CBC in patients with PLL reveals marked absolute lymphocytosis, often >300 × 10⁹/L, anemia, and thrombocytopenia. The neoplastic cells have a characteristic appearance: large cells with moderate amounts of pale basophilic cytoplasm, moderately condensed chromatin, and a single prominent nucleolus (Figure 26-1b). Prolymphocytes represent less than 10% of the lymphocytes seen in CLL and more than 55% of the lymphocytes present in PLL. Cases with 11–55%

prolymphocytes are classified as CLL/PL and have an unpredictable course. The phenotype of prolymphocytes often differs from the cells of CLL in demonstrating stronger intensity expression of surface immunoglobulin and CD20, strong intensity CD22, positivity with FMC-7, and variable expression of CD5 and are often negative for CD23. The karyotype abnormalities in B cell PLL include 14q+, trisomy 12, 6q– and rearrangements affecting chromosomes 1 and 12. Inactivating mutations in the *p53* gene are seen in 75% of cases of PLL.

T Cell PLL

T cell PLL is a rare disorder of adults that, like B cell PLL, usually presents with marked lymphocytosis and splenomegaly. However, patients with T cell PLL have more frequent lymphadenopathy, hepatomegaly, and skin lesions (infiltrations) than do patients with B cell PLL. In addition, the morphologic appearance of T cell PLL is more variable than that of B cell PLL. The cells of T cell PLL usually have a prominent nucleolus but are medium in size and can have convoluted nuclear outlines. T cell PLL has a mature phenotype with expression of CD3, CD2, CD5, and CD7. Most cases are CD4 positive. Like T cell acute lymphocylic leukemia (ALL), some cases of PLL express both CD4 and CD8, but PLL is negative for TdT. The majority of cases of T cell PLL have cytogenetic abnormalities, most frequently inv(14)q11q32, del(11q), i(8q), and trisomy 8q. T cell PLL is an aggressive disorder with a median survival time of only 7.5 months, although some response has been seen with anti-CD52 monoclonal antibody therapy (CAMPATH).

HAIRY CELL LEUKEMIA

Hairy cell leukemia (HCL) is an uncommon B cell malignancy presenting in middle age. Males have a higher incidence (male : female = 7 : 1). At presentation, patients usually have massive splenomegaly but lack lymphadenopathy. Extensive bone marrow involvement often exists; therefore, patients with HCL usually present with pancytopenia. The white blood cell (WBC) count is low due to both neutropenia and monocytopenia; patients thus have an increased susceptibility to infection, especially with mycobacterial organisms. Although neoplastic cells are usually present on a peripheral smear, they are usually too few to elevate the WBC. The neoplastic cells (**hairy cells**) have a characteristic abnormal appearance with abundant pale-staining cytoplasm, circumferential cytoplasmic projections ("hairs"), usually oval or reniform nuclei, and relatively fine chromatin (Figure 26-2a ■). Flow cytometric immunophenotyping is used to establish a diagnosis of HCL. HCL cells are mature B lymphocytes that are positive for CD19, CD20 (strong intensity), CD22, CD25, CD103, and CD11c. Although there is usually strong intensity monoclonal surface immunoglobulin, demonstrating it can be difficult because of nonspecific binding of the antibodies used to detect surface antigens. In addition, the cells of HCL show acid phosphatase staining after tartrate (**tartrate resistant acid phosphatase [TRAP]**) incubation.

Bone marrow involvement is often diffuse, and the neoplastic cells are usually surrounded by fibrosis, preventing their aspiration from the bone marrow (resulting in a "dry tap"). Bone marrow biopsy sections reveal a monotonous infiltrate of abnormal lymphocytes with small nuclei and abundant pale-staining cytoplasm ("fried egg" appearance) (Figure 26-2b ■). Immunohistochemical stains for the B cell antigen CD20 can be used to highlight the infiltrate. Splenectomy specimens reveal marked expansion of the red pulp because of an infiltrate of abnormal cells with the fried egg appearance described in the bone marrow. Lakes of erythrocytes are often formed between the tumor cells (pseudosinuses).

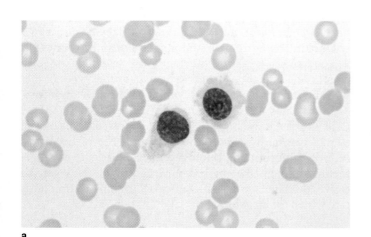

a

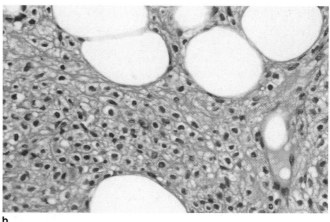

b

■ FIGURE 26-2   a. Hairy cell leukemia. Two abnormal lymphocytes with abundant pale-staining cytoplasm with hairlike projections and relatively finely distributed chromatin. b. Hairy cell leukemia. Replacement of hematopoietic precursors by abnormal small lymphocytes with abundant clear cytoplasm ("fried-egg" appearance). (a. Peripheral blood, Wright stain, 1000× magnification; b. Bone marrow, H&E stain, 100× magnification)

Hairy cell leukemia is an indolent disease. Long-lasting complete remissions are often obtained with the chemotherapy agents 2-chlorodeoxyadenosine (2-CDA/cladribine) and deoxycoformycin (pentostatin).

LARGE GRANULAR LYMPHOCYTE LEUKEMIA (LGLL)

Only 5% of chronic leukemic lymphoproliferative disorders express T cell antigens. These cases were previously referred to as *T cell CLL;* the vast majority of them are now classified as *large granular lymphocyte* (LGL) *leukemia* (LGLL). LGLL is characterized by a modest lymphocytosis composed of cells with abundant pale-staining cytoplasm, azurophilic cytoplasmic granules, and nuclei with mature clumped chromatin (Figure 26-3■). LGLs are normal components of the peripheral blood (10–15% of mononuclear cells) and are usually NK-like T cells (CD3+) or NK cells (CD3–). Therefore, distinction of LGLL from reactive lymphocytosis requires demonstration of an abnormal phenotype or evidence of clonality using molecular diagnostic or cytogenetic studies.

Two categories of LGLL that differ in their phenotype and clinical course are recognized: T lymphocyte and NK cell types.

Approximately 80% of patients with LGLL fall into the T-LGL leukemia category. The neoplastic cells of T-LGL leukemia are T lymphocytes with the following phenotype: CD2+, CD3+, CD4−, CD5+, CD7+, CD8+, CD16+, CD56−/+, CD57+/− (usually CD56−/CD57+). The cells can demonstrate an abnormal phenotype with loss of pan T cell antigens. Molecular diagnostic studies can be used to confirm the diagnosis by demonstration of clonal T cell receptor rearrangement. In addition to lymphocytosis, patients with T-LGL leukemia often have anemia, neutropenia, and thrombocytopenia. Anemia can be related to bone marrow infiltra-

tion or aplasia of erythroid precursors (pure red cell aplasia). Neutropenia and thrombocytopenia can be the result of immune destruction, splenic sequestration, or marrow infiltration. Although splenomegaly is common, lymphadenopathy and hepatomegaly are uncommon. Approximately 25% of patients with T-LGL leukemia have symptomatic rheumatoid arthritis, and many more are positive for rheumatoid factor. Therefore, many patients with T-cell LGL leukemia have the triad defining Felty's syndrome (rheumatoid arthritis, splenomegaly, and neutropenia). The median age at presentation for patients with T-LGL leukemia is 55 years. Patients with T-LGL leukemia usually have an indolent course with more than 80% actuarial overall survival after 10 years. Death is often due to concurrent infection.

LGLL with a NK phenotype has a morphologic appearance similar to T-LGL leukemia but is usually associated with a more acute presentation and aggressive course with death within 2 months of diagnosis. The median age at presentation is 39 years. Patients often present with fever, hepatomegaly, splenomegaly, involvement of the GI tract, and a bleeding disorder. Although anemia is common, neutropenia is rare. The neoplastic cells of NK-LGL leukemia have an NK phenotype: CD2+, CD3−, CD4−, CD8−, CD7+, CD16+, CD56+/−, CD57−/+ (usually CD56+/CD57−). Conventional molecular diagnostic studies cannot be used to determine clonality because NK cells do not rearrange the T cell receptor gene.

SÉZARY'S SYNDROME

Cutaneous T cell lymphoma (CTCL) composes a group of malignant T-cell lymphomas that are primary to the skin. Mycosis fungoides (MF) is the most common variant of CTCL. A few patients with MF/CTCL present with Sézary's syndrome (erythroderma and circulating **Sézary cells**). Sézary cells are malignant T lymphocytes that have a very irregular, convoluted (cerebriform) nuclear outline and finely distributed chromatin (Figure 26-4■). Abnormal cells can be counted in a blood smear leukocyte differential to determine a Sézary count. The differential diagnosis includes other types of mature and immature malignant lymphoproliferative disorders.

Sézary cells are mature memory helper T cells (CD3+, CD4+) but are usually CD7 negative. Molecular diagnostic studies can be used to confirm the presence of neoplastic cells by demonstrating clonal T cell receptor gene rearrangement. Although the marked nuclear convolutions can be easily identified on electron microscopy, this technique is rarely used for diagnosis.

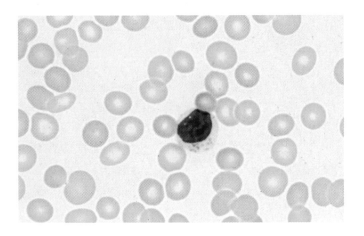

■ FIGURE 26-3   Large granular lymphocyte leukemia. Lymphocyte with abundant clear-staining cytoplasm and azurophilic cytoplasmic granules. (Peripheral blood, H&E stain, 1000× magnification)

CIRCULATING LYMPHOMA CELLS

Patients with non-Hodgkin lymphoma can develop peripheral blood involvement. Circulating lymphoma cells must be distinguished from normal lymphocytes and the cells of chronic leukemic lymphoproliferative disorders. Although

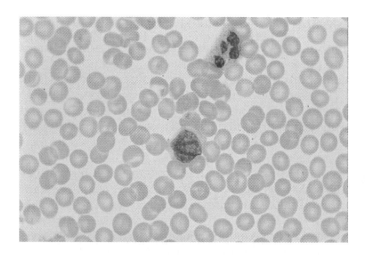

■ **FIGURE 26-4**   Sézary syndrome. Abnormal large lymphocyte with relatively finely distributed chromatin and numerous nuclear folds (Sézary cell). (Peripheral blood, H&E stain, 1000× magnification)

the most frequent type of lymphoma to circulate is low-grade follicular lymphoma, others also can have a leukemic phase (mantle cell lymphoma, diffuse large B-cell lymphoma, Burkitt lymphoma). The circulating neoplastic cells of follicular lymphoma often have very irregular nuclear outlines and a deep indentation (cleft) of the nuclear membrane ("buttock" or **"butt" cells**) (see Follicular Lymphoma). Flow cytometric immunophenotyping can assist in the differential diagnosis by demonstrating monoclonal surface immunoglobulin and a phenotype characteristic of the particular subtype of lymphoma.

> ✓ **Checkpoint! 3**
>
> *Chronic leukemic lymphoid malignancies compose a heterogeneous group. What characteristics allow these malignancies to be grouped together?*

 CASE STUDY *(continued from page 546)*

A CBC revealed a WBC of 20×10^9/L with 60% lymphocytes. Examination of the peripheral blood revealed mature lymphocytes with scant cytoplasm, clumped chromatin, and irregular nuclear outlines.

1. What is the differential diagnosis?
2. What studies could be performed to establish the diagnosis?

▶ **MALIGNANT LYMPHOMA**

The two basic types of lymphoma are Hodgkin and non-Hodgkin lymphoma, which differ in clinical presentation, morphologic appearance, phenotype, and treatment (Table 26-4 ✪ and Table 26-5 ✪).

B CELL NON-HODGKIN LYMPHOMA

Within the United States, non-Hodgkin lymphoma of a B cell phenotype has the highest incidence of all lymphoid malignancies. Non-Hodgkin lymphoma of a T cell or NK cell phenotype has a lower incidence. B cell non-Hodgkin lymphoma is a heterogeneous group of neoplasms composed of cells that resemble those found in the normal compartments of the lymph node. The following subtypes of B cell non-Hodgkin lymphoma have been selected for further discussion either because they are more common or illustrate important concepts: small lymphocytic lymphoma, follicular lymphoma, mantle cell lymphoma, MALT lymphoma, Waldenström macroglobulinemia, diffuse large B cell lymphoma, Burkitt lymphoma, and lymphoblastic lymphoma. A more complete description of lymphoma subtypes is available in the cited reference.[4]

 TABLE 26-4

Differences Between Hodgkin and Non-Hodgkin Lymphomas		
Parameter	**Hodgkin Lymphoma**	**Non-Hodgkin Lymphoma**
Stage	Usually localized	Usually widespread
Distribution	Usually central nodes	Usually involves peripheral nodes
Mode of spread	Contiguous	Noncontiguous
Extranodal disease	Uncommon	Common
Peripheral blood	Never involved	Can be involved
Cell type	Abnormal bizarre cells	Resembles normal lymphoid cells
Treatment regimen	Often ABVD	Often CHOP

ABVD = doxorubicin (adriamycin), bleomycin, vinblastine, dacarbazine; CHOP = cyclophosphamide, doxorubicin, vincristine, and prednisolone

✪ TABLE 26-5

Key Features of Malignant Lymphomas

Follicular lymphoma	Nodular growth pattern
	Lack of tingible body macrophages
	CD19+, CD20+, CD5−, CD10+
	Surface Ig strong intensity
	t(14;18)
	BCL-2 protein overexpression
	BCL-2 gene rearrangement
Mantle cell lymphoma (MCL)	Lack of large cells
	CD19+, CD20+, CD5+, CD23−, FMC-7+
	Surface Ig+ strong intensity
	Cyclin-D1 overexpression
	t(11;14)
	BCL-1 rearrangement
MALT lymphoma	Accompanied by infectious or autoimmune disease
	Often localized
	Extranodal
	Lymphoepithelial lesions
	Benign follicles
	Heterogeneous neoplastic infiltrate
	Phenotype and genotype not specific
Waldenström macroglobulinemia	Lymphoid malignancy with plasmacytic differentiation
	IgM
	Hyperviscosity syndrome
Burkitt lymphoma	Can be associated with EBV
	Starry sky growth pattern
	CD19+, CD20+, CD5−, CD10+
	Strong surface Ig
	t(8;14)
	C-MYC gene rearrangement
Anaplastic large cell lymphoma (ALCL)	Bizarre, anaplastic cells can resemble HD
	T cell or null phenotype
	LCA+/−, CD30+, CD15−, EMA+/−, EBV−, Alk-1+/−
	t(2;5)
Classic Hodgkin lymphoma (HL)	Reed-Sternberg cells
	LCA−, CD15+, CD30+, Alk-1−
	Often EBV positive
Lymphocyte predominant (LP) Hodgkin lymphoma	Growth pattern frequently nodular
	L&H cells
	LCA+, CD20+, CD15−, CD30−, EBV−

Ig = immunoglobulin; MALT = mucosa associated lymphoid tissue; LCA = leukocyte common antigen; EMA = epithelial membrane antigen; EBV = Epstein-Barr virus; L&H = lymphocytic and/or histiocytic; Alk-1 = anaplastic large cell kinase

SMALL LYMPHOCYTIC LYMPHOMA

Small lymphocytic lymphoma (SLL) is the tissue equivalent of CLL. The two disorders appear to belong to one disease entity with different clinical manifestations. Patients with CLL present with peripheral blood lymphocytosis but often develop lymph node involvement. Patients with SLL present with lymphadenopathy but often develop peripheral blood and bone marrow disease.

A lymph node biopsy performed in either CLL or SLL reveals an essentially diffuse infiltrate of small mature lymphocytes. The small lymphocytes have dense, regularly clumped chromatin and lack nucleoli (Figure 26-5 ■). At low power, a vague nodularity is often present due to aggregates of paler large cells (proliferation centers) (Figure 26-5). Proliferation centers contain larger cells with abundant pale-staining cytoplasm and prominent eosinophilic nucleoli (including prolymphocytes). The immunophenotype, cytogenetic findings, and survival are identical to those of CLL (see previous CLL discussion).

FOLLICULAR LYMPHOMA

Follicular lymphoma is a neoplasm composed of cells originating within the germinal center. It is the most common type of non-Hodgkin lymphoma within the United States. The median age at presentation is 50–60 years. There is no sex predilection. Patients usually present with generalized painless lymphadenopathy, some have peripheral blood involvement (Figure 26-6a ■), and most have advanced stage disease with bone marrow involvement (Figure 26-6b ■). Involvement of other extranodal sites is unusual.

Lymph node biopsy of follicular lymphoma reveals an infiltrate of lymphoid cells forming poorly circumscribed nod-

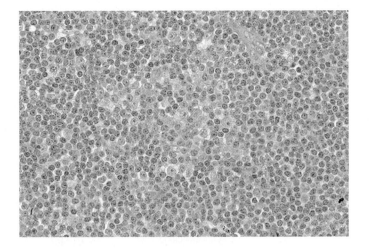

■ FIGURE 26-5 Small lymphocytic lymphoma. The periphery of the image displays many small lymphocytes with round nuclei and clumped chromatin. The center of the image contains a vague nodule containing paler staining larger cells (proliferation center). (Lymph node biopsy, H&E stain, 50× magnification)

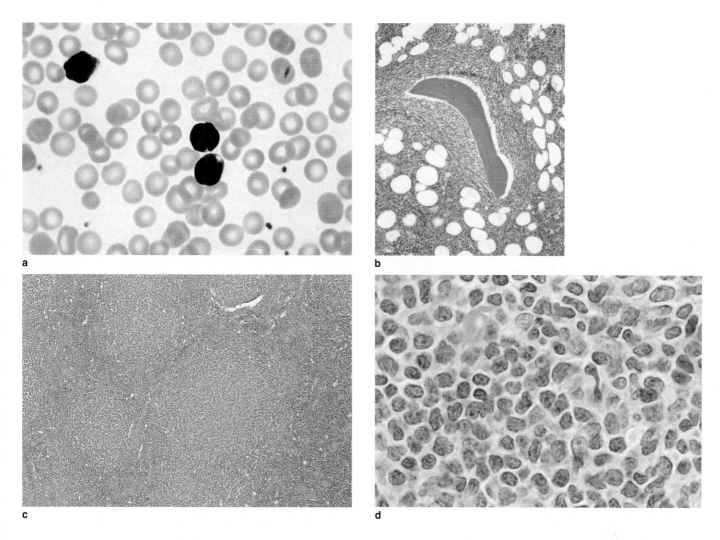

■ FIGURE 26-6   Follicular lymphoma, grade 1. **a.** Circulating lymphoma cells with irregular nuclear outlines (Peripheral blood, Wright stain, magnification 1000×). **b.** Bone marrow involvement by low grade follicular lymphoma displaying a characteristic paratrabecular growth pattern (Bone marrow biopsy, H&E stain, magnification 20×). **c.** Loss of the normal lymph node architecture. The abnormal infiltrate forms numerous poorly defined nodules (follicles) (Lymph node biopsy, H&E stain, magnification 20×). **d.** Neoplastic follicle composed of a relatively homogeneous population of small lymphoid cells containing angulated, twisted nuclei. (Lymph node biopsy, H&E stain, magnification 200×)

ules that resemble follicular germinal centers (Figure 26-6c ■). In addition, the lymphoma cells grow in a diffuse pattern in some areas. Neoplastic follicles differ from reactive follicles in lacking apoptosis of lymphocytes. This is manifest on histologic sections as a lack of macrophages engulfing fragments of dead cells (**tingible body macrophages,** which are usually found in areas of extensive apoptosis (reactive germinal centers and high-grade lymphoma). The neoplastic infiltrate always contains a mixed population of small cleaved (centrocytes) and large cells (centroblasts) but is often more homogeneous than a normal germinal center (Figure 26-6d ■). The proportion of large cells varies and is used to separate follicular lymphoma into three grades (1, 2, or 3) (Table 26-6 ✪). The presence of more large cells is often associated with a more aggressive clinical course.

Most diagnoses of follicular lymphoma are made using conventional histologic evaluation. Immunophenotyping can be used to confirm the presence of lymphoma (monoclonal lymphocytes) and confirm the subtype of lymphoma (CD10 positive). Most cases of follicular lymphoma arise because of a chromosome translocation t(14;18) involving the *BCL-2* gene that leads to overexpression of BCL-2 protein in lymphocytes. BCL-2 protein inhibits individual cell death (apoptosis), allowing follicle center cells to accumulate and produce lymphadenopathy.

Most patients with follicular lymphoma have an indolent disease with a median survival of 7–9 years. Patients with grade 3 follicular lymphoma are sometimes cured. However, the lower-grade follicular lymphomas (grades 1 and 2) are incurable with current therapies and are therefore treated for

TABLE 26-6

Grading of Follicular Lymphoma

Grade	Definition
1	0–5 centroblasts per defined high power field
2	6–15 centroblasts per defined high power field
3	>15 centroblasts per defined high power field

relief of symptoms. Low-grade follicular lymphoma can progress to a diffuse large cell lymphoma with a median survival of less than 1 year.

CASE STUDY *(continued from page 553)*

A cervical lymph node biopsy reveals effacement of the normal architecture by a lymphoid infiltrate with a nodular growth pattern. The nodules contain a relatively homogeneous population of small lymphocytes and a few admixed large cells. The infiltrating lymphoid cells have irregular nuclear outlines. Tingible body macrophages are lacking, and very few mitotic figures are present.

3. What is the cause of the lymphadenopathy?

4. Is this process low grade or high grade?

MANTLE CELL LYMPHOMA (MCL)

MCL is a neoplasm thought to be derived from the cells of the mantle zone of the lymphoid follicle. The median age at presentation is approximately 60 years, and male predominance exists. Most patients present with disseminated disease involving multiple lymph node groups, bone marrow, peripheral blood, spleen, liver, and gastrointestinal tract. Gastrointestinal tract involvement can present as multiple polyps involving the small bowel (lymphomatous polyposis) (Figure 26-7a■).

On histologic sections, MCL can demonstrate either a diffuse or vaguely nodular growth pattern (Figure 26-7b■). The neoplastic infiltrate occasionally surrounds a reactive germinal center (mantle zone pattern). The neoplastic cells are usually small to intermediate in size with round to slightly irregular nuclear outlines; in contrast to small lymphocytic lymphoma and follicular lymphoma, MCL usually lacks a large cell component (Figure 26-7c■). However, it has a rare morphologic variant referred to as *blastic MCL* composed of either large cells resembling diffuse large B cell lymphoma or cells with finely distributed chromatin resembling lymphoblastic lymphoma.

Diagnosing MCL often requires the use of ancillary studies. The following immunophenotype is characteristic of MCL: CD19+, CD5+, CD23−, FMC-7+, and sIg+ (strong intensity). Immunohistochemistry reveals nuclear staining for cyclin-D1 protein in approximately 90% of cases of MCL

(Figure 26-7d■). Cyclin D-1 is involved in regulating progression of cells from the G1 to S phase of the cell cycle (∞ Chapter 2). Overexpression of cyclin-D1 in MCL is usually the result of a chromosome translocation, t(11;14), that involves the *BCL-1* gene. The *BCL-1* translocation is thought to lead to neoplastic transformation through loss of cell cycle control. This translocation can be demonstrated by fluorescence in situ hybridization (FISH) studies in the vast majority of cases of MCL. Although molecular diagnostic studies are available, only approximately 60% of MCL cases are routinely identified because of the wide range of break points involved in the t(11;14) translocation.

MCL is a relatively aggressive lymphoma with a poor response to current therapies. The overall median survival is approximately 3–4 years. The blastic variant has a median survival of only 18 months. Therefore, distinction of MCL from the other small lymphoid B cell neoplasms (follicular lymphoma, SLL, and MALT lymphoma [see below]) is important.

MUCOSA ASSOCIATED LYMPHOID TISSUE (MALT) LYMPHOMA

MALT lymphoma is a B cell neoplasm derived from mucosa associated lymphoid tissue. Patients with MALT lymphoma usually present with localized extranodal disease (e.g., involving the stomach, salivary gland, lacrimal gland, thyroid, and lung). A preceding chronic inflammatory disorder such as chronic gastritis due to *Helicobacter pylori* infection or autoimmune disease (Sjögren's syndrome or Hashimoto's thyroiditis often occurs).

A biopsy of MALT lymphoma reveals an infiltrate of small to intermediate size lymphocytes intimately associated with epithelial cells (e.g., gastric mucosa, salivary gland ducts). Epithelial structures infiltrated by neoplastic lymphocytes are referred to as **lymphoepithelial lesions** (Figure 26-8a■). MALT lymphoma is composed of small lymphocytes with round or slightly cleaved nuclei that often have abundant pale-staining cytoplasm and are referred to as *monocytoid B cells* because of their resemblance to monocytes (Figure 26-8b■). MALT lymphoma can demonstrate differentiation to plasma cells. In addition to the neoplastic cells, the infiltrate often contains benign germinal centers. Infiltration of benign germinal centers by neoplastic cells is referred to as *follicular colonization*. The differential diagnosis includes other lymphomas composed of small lymphocytes, including SLL, MCL, and follicular lymphoma. Ancillary studies can assist in obtaining the correct diagnosis. Monoclonality of immunoglobulin light chains can be demonstrated by either flow cytometry immunophenotyping (surface immunoglobulin on lymphocytes) or paraffin section immunohistochemistry (cytoplasmic immunoglobulin in cells demonstrating plasma cell differentiation). In contrast to follicular lymphoma and small lymphocytic lymphoma, MALT lymphoma is usually negative for CD10 and CD5.

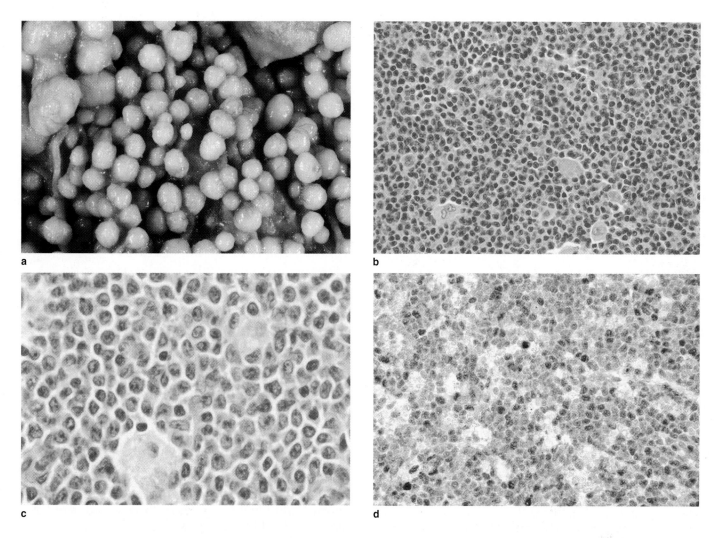

■ FIGURE 26-7   Mantle cell lymphoma. **a.** Gross photograph of the large intestine in a patient with lymphomatous polyposis of gastrointestinal tract. **b.** Abnormal lymphoid infiltrate in a lymph node displaying a vaguely nodular growth pattern. **c.** Uniform infiltrate of small lymphoid cells with slightly irregular nuclear outlines. **d.** Cyclin D-1 overexpression. (b. Lymph node biopsy, H&E stain, 20× magnification; c. lymph node biopsy, H&E stain, 100× magnification; d. lymph node biopsy, immunohistochemistry stain, 100× magnification)

MALT lymphoma is an indolent disease previously considered to be a reactive condition mimicking lymphoma (pseudolymphoma) but is now considered malignant because like other non-Hodgkin lymphomas, it is composed of monoclonal lymphocytes and has the potential to transform to higher grade, large B cell lymphoma. However, patients with *Helicobacter pylori*-associated gastric MALT lymphoma are often cured with antimicrobial therapy. MALT lymphoma that is unresponsive to antimicrobial therapy or that occurs at other sites is often treated with local excision or radiation therapy.

WALDENSTRÖM MACROGLOBULINEMIA

Waldenström macroglobulinemia is a lymphoid malignancy that produces immunoglobulin IgM. High plasma levels of the large pentamer IgM result in hyperviscosity that can lead

to poor circulation in small blood vessels, visual impairment, headache, dizziness, and deafness. Although several different subtypes of lymphoid malignancy can produce this clinical disorder, including MALT lymphoma, Waldenström macroglobulinemia is often associated with the lymphoplasmacytic subtype of lymphoma. The differential diagnosis includes other types of lymphoid malignancy and neoplasms composed entirely of plasma cells (plasma cell neoplasms).

Patients with lymphoplasmacytic lymphoma usually have peripheral blood and bone marrow involvement and often have lymphadenopathy, hepatomegaly, and splenomegaly at presentation. Unlike the plasma cell neoplasm multiple myeloma, patients with lymphoplasmacytic lymphoma lack lytic bone lesions. Histologic sections demonstrate a diffuse infiltrate composed of lymphocytes, plasma cells, and lymphoid cells that demonstrate some evidence of differentiation toward plasma cells (plasmacytoid lymphocytes).

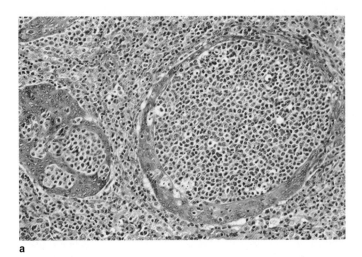 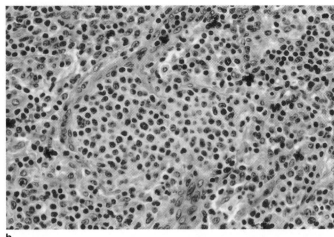

a

b

■ FIGURE 26-8   MALT lymphoma. **a.** Parotid salivary gland involved by low-grade lymphoma of MALT type. Two lymphoepithelial lesions are present demonstrating infiltration of ducts by neoplastic lymphocytes. **b.** Heterogeneous lymphoid infiltrate of MALT lymphoma. Many of the infiltrating cells have abundant clear-staining cytoplasm (i.e., monocytoid B cells). (a. Parotid gland biopsy, H&E stain, 50× magnification; b. Parotid gland biopsy, H&E stain, 100× magnification)

Immunohistochemistry can be performed to demonstrate the presence of cytoplasmic monoclonal immunoglobulin light chain (kappa or lambda) and IgM heavy chain.

The median survival for patients with Waldenström macroglobulinemia is 4 years. Plasmapheresis can alleviate many symptoms related to increased plasma viscosity.

DIFFUSE LARGE B CELL LYMPHOMA

Diffuse large B cell lymphoma (DLBCL) is a heterogeneous group of tumors composed of large B-lymphoid cells (Figure 26-9 ■). Some DLBCL develop as a result of transformation from a lower grade lymphoma (e.g., follicular lymphoma or small lymphocytic lymphoma) while others arise de novo. The possibility of blastic mantle cell lymphoma should be excluded using staining for cyclin-D1. The immunophenotype of DLBCL is quite variable and has been associated with the clinical course. Diffuse large B cell lymphoma with a phenotype similar to follicular lymphoma (germinal center-like phenotype) often has a better prognosis than diffuse large B cell lymphoma with a nongerminal centerlike phenotype. With multiagent chemotherapy and anti-CD20 monoclonal antibody therapy (Rituxan), some patients can be cured of their lymphoma.

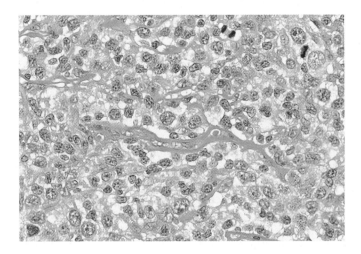

■ FIGURE 26-9   Diffuse large B cell lymphoma. Abnormal infiltrate composed of large lymphoid cells with pale-staining, vesicular chromatin, irregular nuclear outlines, and basophilic nucleoli. Several mitotic figures are present. (Lymph node biopsy, H&E stain, 200× magnification)

ⓔ CASE STUDY *(continued from page 556)*

The previous biopsy had established a diagnosis of low-grade non-Hodgkin lymphoma, follicular type. Julia received multiagent chemotherapy for symptomatic relief. Two years following the diagnosis, she returned with rapidly expanding lymph nodes in her neck. Repeat biopsy revealed effacement of the lymph node architecture by a diffuse infiltrate of large B cells.

5. What is the diagnosis?

6. What is the relationship of this disease to the previous diagnosis?

BURKITT LYMPHOMA

Burkitt lymphoma is a high-grade non-Hodgkin lymphoma having a high incidence in Africa (endemic subtype). It represents approximately one-third of all pediatric lymphomas occurring outside Africa (sporadic Burkitt lymphoma). Many adult cases occur in immunocompromised individuals such as those infected with the HIV virus. Burkitt lymphoma often involves extranodal sites. Endemic Burkitt lymphoma has a predilection for involvement of the facial bones and jaw; sporadic Burkitt lymphoma often presents with disease involving the intestine, ovaries, or kidney. EBV is thought to play a role in the pathogenesis of Burkitt lymphoma. DNA of EBV is present in most cases of endemic Burkitt lymphoma and approximately one-third of the HIV-associated tumors. EBV is found less frequently in the sporadic form.

A biopsy of Burkitt lymphoma usually reveals a diffuse infiltrate of neoplastic cells demonstrating a *"starry sky" appearance* (Figure 26-10■). The "sky" represents the blue nuclei of the neoplastic lymphocytes; the "stars" are formed by scattered pale-staining tingible body macrophages. The infiltrating lymphoid cells are intermediate in size with nuclei approximately the same size as the nuclei of the tingible body macrophages. Multiple small nucleoli are usually present, and mitotic figures and apoptotic bodies are frequent. The latter two features are characteristic of high-grade lymphoma.

The differential diagnosis for Burkitt lymphoma includes lymphoblastic lymphoma and DLBCL. The presence of surface immunoglobulin and absence of TdT allow distinction of Burkitt lymphoma from acute lymphoblastic leukemia (ALL) (∞ Chapter 25). Distinguishing Burkitt lymphoma from DLBCL is often more difficult because the two can share the same immunophenotype: CD19+, sIg+, CD10+, CD5−. Most cases of Burkitt lymphoma have the t(8;14) or less frequently t(2;8) or t(8;22) chromosome translocations leading to rearrangement of the *C-MYC* gene. *C-MYC* gene rearrangement occurs in only 5% of DLBCL.

Burkitt lymphoma is a highly aggressive tumor but is curable with aggressive combination chemotherapy. The therapeutic regimen used for Burkitt lymphoma usually differs from that used for DLBCL.

LYMPHOBLASTIC LYMPHOMA

Lymphoblastic lymphoma is the tissue equivalent of ALL. Children are more often affected than adults. Approximately 80% of lymphoblastic lymphomas are of a T cell lineage, and the remaining cases have an immature B cell phenotype. T cell lymphoblastic lymphoma often affects adolescent males who present with a rapidly enlarging mediastinal mass due to involvement of the thymus. Neoplastic blasts can also be seen in the peripheral blood, bone marrow, pleural fluid, and cerebrospinal fluid. A tissue biopsy of lymphoblastic lymphoma usually reveals intermediate to small cells with scant cytoplasm, finely distributed chromatin, and small nucleoli (Figure 26-11■).

Immunophenotyping is required to distinguish lymphoblastic lymphoma from other types of non-Hodgkin lymphoma, to distinguish lymphoblastic lymphoma from tissue infiltration by AML (extramedullary myeloid sarcoma), and to identify a T or B cell phenotype. TdT is present in the majority of cases of lymphoblastic lymphoma and can be used to help distinguish it from Burkitt lymphoma.

PERIPHERAL T CELL OR NATURAL KILLER (T/NK) CELL LYMPHOMA

Non-Hodgkin lymphoma with a mature T cell or NK (T/NK) cell phenotype represents only 15% of lymphomas in the United States. Several subtypes of peripheral T/NK cell

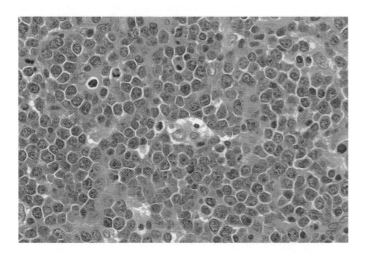

■ FIGURE 26-10 Burkitt lymphoma. Intermediate size lymphocytes with multiple nucleoli and scant cytoplasm. Numerous mitotic figures are present. The presence of apoptotic bodies indicates individual cell necrosis. There is a "starry-sky" appearance due to pale-staining tingible body macrophages scattered in an infiltrate that appears basophilic due to staining of the tumor cell nuclei. (Lymph node biopsy, H&E stain, 100× magnification).

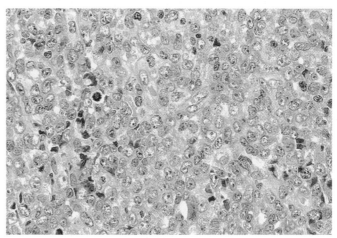

■ FIGURE 26-11 Lymphoblastic lymphoma. Intermediate size lymphocytes with irregular nuclear outlines and finely distributed, speckled, chromatin. A mitotic figure is present. (Lymph node biopsy, H&E stain, 500× magnification)

lymphoma are defined using a combination of parameters including the clinical presentation, distribution of disease (nodal or extranodal), association with Epstein-Barr virus, and immunophenotype (CD4+ or CD8+, and presence of NK-associated or cytotoxic markers). However, a large category of peripheral T-cell lymphoma cannot be put into one of the other subtypes (peripheral T cell lymphoma, unspecified). In general, peripheral T/NK cell lymphoma is an aggressive disease with frequent relapses. However, some patients are cured by combination chemotherapy.

Although the morphologic appearance of peripheral T/NK cell lymphoma is quite variable, a number of morphologic features suggest this diagnosis. Peripheral T/NK cell lymphoma usually has a diffuse growth pattern and is rich in blood vessels. The tumor cells vary in size and can display abundant clear or pale-staining cytoplasm and irregular nuclear outlines. The infiltrate is often heterogeneous with histiocytes, plasma cells, and eosinophils in addition to the neoplastic cells. However, immunophenotyping is essential for distinction from B cell non-Hodgkin lymphoma and, in some cases, Hodgkin lymphoma. Peripheral T/NK cell lymphoma demonstrates expression of pan-T cell antigens with frequent abnormal lack of staining for one or more of the expected antigens (e.g., CD5– and/or CD7–). The presence of an abnormal immunophenotype or clonal rearrangement of the T cell receptor can assist in the distinction of T cell lymphoma from a reactive process.

Anaplastic large cell lymphoma (ALCL) is one of the best characterized subtypes of T/NK cell lymphoma. Most ALCL cases are composed of large bizarre anaplastic cells that can resemble Reed-Sternberg cells and Hodgkin variant cells (Figure 26-12 ■). Like Hodgkin lymphoma and some large cell non-Hodgkin lymphomas, ALCL is usually positive for the CD30 antigen (initially referred to as the *Ki-1*

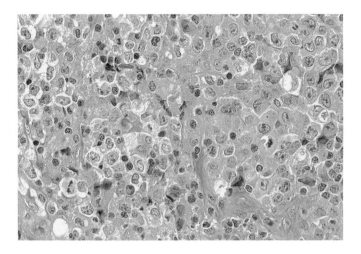

■ FIGURE 26-12 Anaplastic large cell lymphoma. Abnormal infiltrate of large cells with abundant eosinophilic cytoplasm. (Lymph node biopsy, H&E stain, 100× magnification)

antigen). However, in contrast to classical Hodgkin lymphoma, ALCL usually lacks CD15 expression and evidence of Epstein-Barr virus infection and is often positive for leukocyte common antigen (LCA) and epithelial membrane antigen (EMA). Although ALCL is derived from T-cells, frequent loss of T-cell antigen expression can result in a null phenotype (lack of expression of either T or B cell antigens).

Most, but not all, ALCL cases involving lymph nodes contain the translocation t(2;5) that joins the nucleophosmin (NPM) and anaplastic large cell kinase (ALK) genes. This leads to abnormal expression of ALK protein that can be detected by immunohistochemistry. The presence of ALK protein expression can assist in the distinction of ALCL from HL and most other subtypes of NHL. However, absence of staining for ALK-1 protein does not exclude a diagnosis of ALCL. Most cases of cutaneous ALCL are ALK negative.

Primary cutaneous ALCL can be treated successfully by local excision or radiation therapy. Approximately 70% of patients with systemic ALCL go into remission with systemic multiagent chemotherapy, but the rate of relapse is high.

HODGKIN LYMPHOMA (HL)

HL differs from non-Hodgkin lymphoma in its clinical presentation and histologic appearance (Table 26-4). Separation of these two broad categories of lymphoma is important because they are treated with different combinations of chemotherapeutic agents.

HL is composed of large tumor cells that do not resemble a normal cell counterpart and are accompanied by many reactive cells. HL has several histologic subtypes that differ in phenotype, appearance of the large neoplastic cells, and nature of the reactive component. The main histologic types are lymphocyte predominant (LP) HL and classical HL. Classical HL is further classified into nodular sclerosis (NS), mixed cellularity (MC), lymphocyte rich (LR), and lymphocyte depletion (LD) subtypes (Table 26-7 ✪).

LP HL is composed of numerous reactive small lymphocytes and rare tumor cells that often grow in loose nodular aggregates. The tumor cells in LP HL (L&H cells) characteristically have a large multilobated nucleus with delicate nuclear membranes, finely granular chromatin, and small indistinct nucleoli (**popcorn cells; L&H cells**) (Figure 26-13 ■). Unlike the neoplastic cells of classical HL, those of LP HL have a B cell phenotype: LCA+, CD 45+, CD20+, CD30–/+, CD15– (Table 26-5). Therefore, the phenotype of LP HL overlaps that of B cell non-Hodgkin lymphoma. The reactive small lymphocytes that surround the neoplastic cells of LP HL often include an unusual subset of CD57 positive T cells.

The tumor cells in classical HL have large prominent eosinophilic nucleoli and coarse nuclear membranes. One variant of tumor cell is found in all cases of classic Hodgkin lymphoma: the **Reed-Sternberg (R-S) cell,** which has two

⊙ TABLE 26-7

Classification of Classic Hodgkin Lymphoma

Subtype	Sclerosis	Lymphocytes	Tumor Cells	Variants	Cell Type
LP	–	++++	+	L&H	B-cell
NS	Present	++	++	Lacunar	?
MC	–	++	++	–	?
LR	–	++++	+	–	?
LD	–/+	+	++++	–	?

NS = nodular sclerosis classical HL; MC = mixed cellularity classical HL; LD = lymphocyte depletion classical HL; LR = lymphocyte rich classical HL; LP = lymphocyte predominance HL; L&H = malignant cells characteristic of LP HL; ? = uncertain cell of origin; + = few; ++++ = many

or more nuclear lobes containing inclusion-like nucleoli and an area of perinucleolar clearing imparting an owl's eye appearance (Figure 26-14a ■). The reactive cells accompanying the neoplastic cells of classical HL include a heterogeneous mixture of small lymphocytes, histiocytes, eosinophils, and plasma cells. The tumor cells of classical HL are negative for LCA and ALK but positive for the CD30 antigen. They can also be positive for CD15 and/or EBV.

Classical HL is further divided into histologic subtypes based on the presence of sclerosis (fibrosis), type of tumor cell variants, and proportion of reactive lymphocytes. The NS subtype of Hodgkin lymphoma is characterized by C-shaped bands of birefringent fibrous tissue (Figure 26-14b ■), nodular aggregates of cells, and tumor cell variants with cytoplasmic clearing and delicate, multilobated nuclei (**lacunar cells**) (Figure 26-14c ■). The LR form of classical HL has a background of reactive cells that includes many small lymphocytes, but in contrast to LP HL, the neoplastic

cells have the phenotype of classical HL. LD HL is a rare subtype that has many tumor cells and only rare reactive lymphocytes. A diagnosis of MC HL is made after excluding the other classic subtypes: NS, LR, and LD. However, the histologic subtypes of classical HL do not have independent prognostic significance. The stage of HL is one of the most important prognostic markers. The 5-year survival for patients with stage I or IIA Hodgkin lymphoma currently is approximately 90% and for stage IV 60–70%.

✓ **Checkpoint! 4**

Name and describe the cell that is characteristic of Hodgkin lymphoma.

▶ **PLASMA CELL DISORDERS**

Plasma cell neoplasms are diverse disorders that rarely involve lymph nodes and usually secrete monoclonal immunoglobulin into the serum and/or urine. They can be divided into disease entities based on the distribution and extent of disease (solitary versus multiple lesions and bone versus extramedullary) and the characteristics of the immunosecretory protein produced (class of heavy chain and the presence of amyloid production, immunoglobulin heavy, or light chain) (Table 26-8 ⊙). Primary amyloidosis is a neoplasm of plasma cells producing an abnormal immunoglobulin that becomes deposited in a beta pleated sheet configuration in tissues (amyloid). The heavy chain diseases are characterized by the production of immunoglobulin heavy chain fragments only and vary in their clinical presentation, morphologic features, and class of heavy chain produced. The more common plasma cell neoplasms, multiple myeloma and plasmacytoma, are discussed in more detail along with the precursor lesion monoclonal gammopathy of undetermined significance. Their key features are outlined in Table 26-9 ⊙.

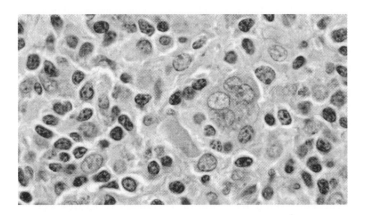

■ FIGURE 26-13 Hodgkin lymphoma, lymphocyte predominant subtype. Large L&H ("popcorn") cell with multilobated nucleus, delicate nuclear membranes, and small basophilic nucleoli. The background contains many small lymphocytes and histiocytes with pale-staining, eosinophilic cytoplasm. (Lymph node biopsy, H&E stain, 200× magnification)

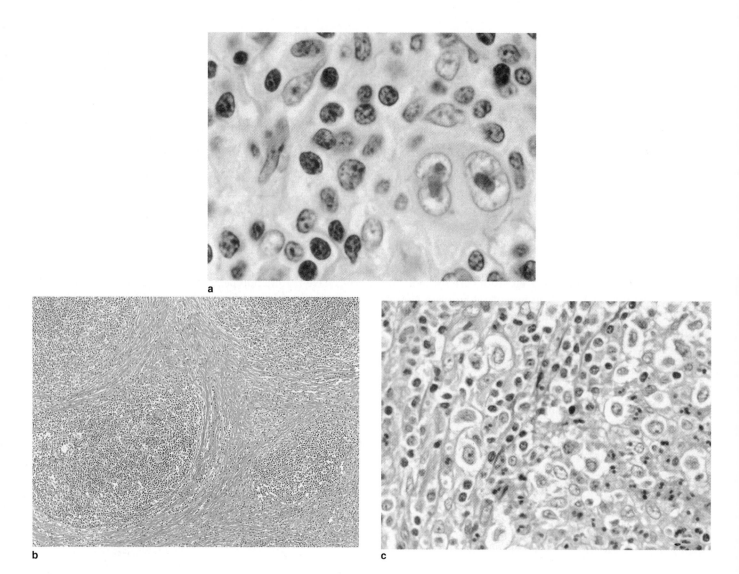

■ FIGURE 26-14 Hodgkin lymphoma, classic type, nodular sclerosis subtype. **a.** Reed-Sternberg cell with two nuclear lobes and prominent, eosinophilic nucleoli giving an owl's eye appearance. The background contains many small lymphocytes and a few pale eosinophilic histiocytes. **b.** Bands of fibrous tissue isolate nodules containing an abnormal cellular infiltrate (nodular sclerosing pattern). **c.** Lacunar cells with abundant clear-staining cytoplasm, delicate nuclear membranes, and small basophilic nucleoli. (a. Lymph node biopsy, H&E stain, 200× magnification; b. Lymph node biopsy, H&E stain, 20× magnification; c. Lymph node biopsy, H&E stain, 100× magnification)

✪ TABLE 26-8
Plasma Cell Disorders
• Plasma cell myeloma (multiple myeloma)
• Plasmacytoma
• Primary amyloidosis
• Heavy chain disease
• Monoclonal gammopathy of undetermined significance (MGUS)

MULTIPLE MYELOMA

Multiple myeloma is a plasma cell neoplasm that forms multiple tumors throughout the skeletal system (lytic bone lesions) (Figure 26-15a■). The median age at diagnosis is 65 years, and there is a male predominance. Patients often present with bone pain and/or pathologic fractures due to tumor infiltration.

Examination of the bone marrow from a lytic lesion or the posterior iliac crest reveals an abnormal infiltrate of plasma cells replacing the normal hematopoietic cells. In multiple myeloma, plasma cells usually represent more than 30% of all bone marrow cells (Figure 26-15b■). Although neoplastic plasma cells can appear normal, abnormal forms

⊘ TABLE 26-9

Key Features of Plasma Cell Disorders

Neoplasm	Features
Multiple (plasma cell) myeloma	Lytic bone lesions
	"M" spike on serum/urine electrophoresis
	Rouleaux on blood smear
	>30% plasma cells in bone marrow
Plasmacytoma	Localized mass
	Monoclonal plasma cells
Monoclonal gammopathy of undetermined significance	Monoclonal serum protein
	Monoclonal protein <3 gm/dL
	Lytic bone lesions absent
	Bone marrow plasma cells <10%

with more finely distributed chromatin, nucleoli, or intranuclear inclusions that contain immunoglobulin (**Dutcher bodies**) are often present. Neoplastic plasma cells rarely circulate in the blood, but the peripheral smear is often abnormal due to stacking of the erythrocytes (**rouleaux** formation) (Figure 26-15c ■). In addition, the stained blood smear often has a blue background due to increased serum protein.

Serum protein electrophoresis (SPEP) reveals increased protein with a narrow range of electrophoretic mobility (M spike) (Figure 26-16 ■). The M spike can be further characterized by immunofixation electrophoresis (IFE) to confirm the presence of a monoclonal protein and determine the immunoglobulin class (Figure 26-16c). The monoclonal protein usually contains one immunoglobulin light chain (kappa or lambda) and one heavy chain with the following incidence: IgG > IgA > IgM > IgD > IgE. Normal immunoglobulin production is usually decreased leading to functional hypogammaglobulinemia. Plasma cell neoplasms can produce an excess of immunoglobulin light chains, light chains only, heavy chains

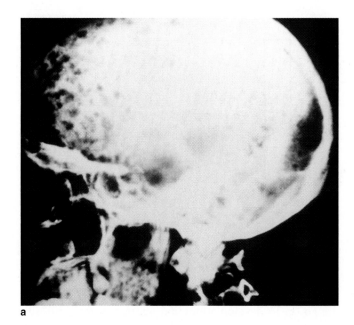

a

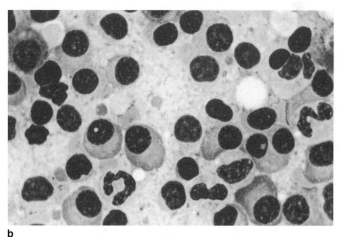

b

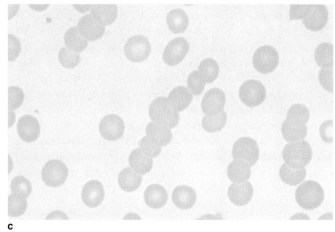

c

■ FIGURE 26-15   Multiple myeloma. **a** Skull X-ray demonstrating multiple lytic bone lesions giving a "moth-eaten" appearance. **b.** Replacement of hematopoietic precursors by an infiltrate of plasma cells. Plasma cells appear normal but represent >30% of the cells present. **c.** Stacking of the erythrocytes due to the presence of increased immunoglobulin (Rouleaux). (b. Bone marrow aspirate, Wright stain, 1000× magnification; c. Peripheral blood, Wright stain, 1000× magnification)

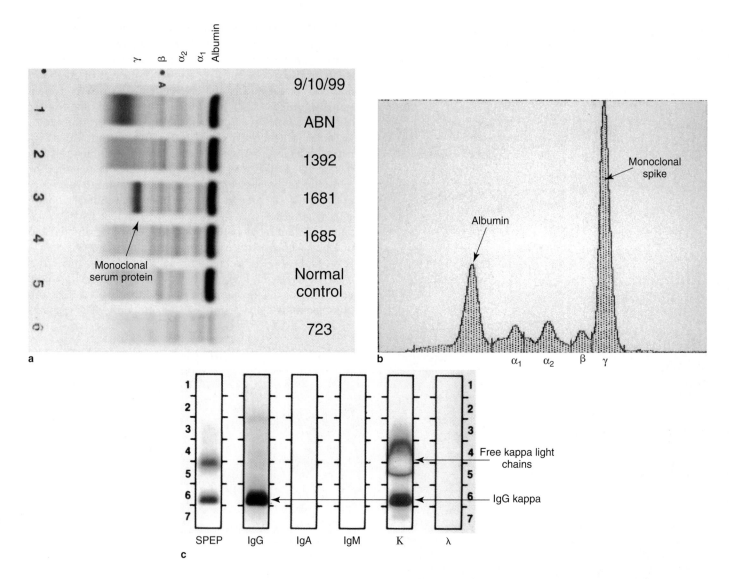

■ FIGURE 26-16   Monoclonal gammopathy. **a.** Serum protein electrophoresis. Sample 1681 displays a band in the early gamma region. **b.** Densitometry scan reveals a "spike" in the gamma region. A similar spike was found in the urine. **c.** Immunofixation electrophoresis performed on a urine sample reveals two monoclonal bands composed of IgG kappa and free kappa light chains (Bence-Jones proteins).

only, or no immunoglobulin (non-secretory). Patients with light chain only disease can have a normal SPEP because the protein passes into the urine. Free light chains in the urine are referred to as **Bence-Jones proteins.**

The prognosis of multiple myeloma is poor with a median survival of only 6 months without therapy. The median survival can be increased to 3 years with chemotherapy, and an increased survival has been reported with autologous bone marrow and peripheral blood stem cell transplants. Infection is a major cause of death.

PLASMACYTOMA

A *plasmacytoma* is a localized, tumorous collection of monoclonal plasma cells. The prognosis of a plasmacytoma is related to its location. Many patients with plasmacytoma of

bone go on to develop additional plasmacytomas and ultimately meet the criteria for multiple myeloma. In contrast, plasmacytoma of the upper respiratory tract has a good prognosis with only rare recurrence after excision and a low incidence of dissemination.

MONOCLONAL GAMMOPATHY OF UNDETERMINED SIGNIFICANCE (MGUS)

Identification of a monoclonal spike is not diagnostic of multiple myeloma. The term *monoclonal protein of undetermined significance (MGUS)* is used to describe a low level of serum monoclonal protein without evidence of an overt neoplasm. Therefore, MGUS is a diagnosis that requires exclusion of other plasma cell and lymphoid malignancies. The prevalence of a monoclonal serum spike increases with age and is present in 3% of asymptomatic patients over 70 years of age. There is no treatment for MGUS. Although most patients have stable disease and die of other causes, an overt plasma cell dyscrasia such as multiple myeloma develops in approximately 25% of patients.

 Checkpoint! 5

What clinical finding differentiates multiple myeloma from other plasma cell neoplasms?

SUMMARY

The lymphoid malignancies compose a diverse group of neoplasms that vary in clinical presentation, morphologic appearance, immunophenotype, and genotype. The malignant cells resemble one or more of the stages of normal lymphocyte development. The lymphoid malignancies can be classified as acute lymphoblastic leukemia, chronic leukemic lymphoid malignancies, and lymphoma. The leukemic entities are characterized by peripheral blood and bone marrow involvement; lymphomas have tumorous masses involving the lymph nodes and other lymphoid tissue. The diagnosis often requires a combination of conventional morphology and ancillary studies. Ancillary studies include immunophenotyping, molecular diagnostics, and cytogenetics.

Although the classification of lymphoid malignancies is complicated, it is important to separate distinct disease entities that have a predictable outcome and response to specific therapy.

REVIEW QUESTIONS

LEVEL I

1. Which of the following is the most likely distribution of disease in a patient with leukemia? (Objective 3)
   a. a lytic bone lesion
   b. a tumorous mass involving lymph nodes
   c. a tumorous mass involving the tonsil
   d. widespread involvement of the bone marrow

2. A 60-year-old male being evaluated for insurance purposes was found to have lymphocytosis. Peripheral smear revealed a uniform population of small mature lymphocytes. Which of the following is the most likely diagnosis? (Objectives 3, 7)
   a. acute lymphoblastic leukemia
   b. chronic lymphocytic leukemia
   c. infectious mononucleosis
   d. malignant lymphoma

3. Which of the following indicate(s) the presence of a lymphoid malignancy? (Objective 2)
   a. clonal immunoglobulin gene rearrangement
   b. population of lymphocytes expressing only one immunoglobulin light chain
   c. population of lymphocytes expressing an abnormal phenotype
   d. all of the above

4. A patient with non-Hodgkin lymphoma is found to have bone marrow involvement. What stage is the lymphoma? (Objective 9)
   a. I
   b. I$_E$
   c. III
   d. IV

LEVEL II

1. Which of the following is involved in the pathogenesis of low-grade follicular lymphoma? (Objective 8)
   a. genes involved in apoptosis
   b. inherited immunodeficiency
   c. proto-oncogenes
   d. tumor suppressor genes

2. Which type of lymphoma can be cured by antimicrobial therapy? (Objective 8)
   a. Burkitt lymphoma
   b. Hodgkin lymphoma
   c. MALT lymphoma
   d. HIV-associated non-Hodgkin lymphoma

3. A lymph node biopsy is performed in a patient with lymphadenopathy. Which of the following findings would support the diagnosis of a reactive proliferation rather than malignant lymphoma? (Objective 9)
   a. a mixed population of cells varying in size, shape, and color
   b. clonality
   c. presence of large, bizarre cells
   d. mitotic activity

4. A CBC performed on a 65-year-old female reveals lymphocytosis. A bone marrow reveals replacement of the hematopoietic precursors by an infiltrate of mature lymphocytes. Which of the following is the most likely course of the disease? (Objective 5)
   a. cure following therapy
   b. rapid progression
   c. slow progression
   d. spontaneous remission

REVIEW QUESTIONS (continued)

LEVEL I

5. A lymph node biopsy reveals a nodular infiltrate of small, mature lymphoid cells with an absence of mitoses and apoptosis. Which of the following is the correct classification of this lymphoma? (Objective 9)
   a. high grade
   b. high stage
   c. low grade
   d. low stage

6. Which of the following lymphoid malignancies is most likely to have circulating neoplastic cells? (Objectives 3, 6)
   a. chronic lymphocytic leukemia
   b. high-grade lymphoma
   c. low-grade lymphoma
   d. Hodgkin lymphoma

7. The WHO classification of lymphoid malignancies recommends which of the following studies? (Objective 9)
   a. genotype
   b. morphology
   c. phenotype
   d. all of the above

8. A bone marrow sample obtained for staging purposes revealed involvement by non-Hodgkin lymphoma. This finding indicates that the disease is: (Objective 9)
   a. high grade
   b. high stage
   c. low grade
   d. low stage

9. A peripheral smear performed on a 35-year-old male with lymphocytosis reveals numerous smudge cells. Which of the following does this finding indicate? (Objectives 3, 8)
   a. chronic lymphocytic leukemia
   b. infectious mononucleosis
   c. acute lymphoblastic leukemia
   d. none because the finding is not diagnostic

10. Peripheral smear examination of a patient with chronic lymphocytic leukemia reveals 8% prolymphocytes. This finding is consistent with which of the following diagnoses? (Objective 8)
    a. chronic lymphocytic leukemia
    b. prolymphocytic leukemia
    c. prolymphocytoid transformation
    d. Richter's transformation

LEVEL II

5. Which of the following phenotypes is characteristic of chronic lymphocytic leukemia? (Objective 1)
   a. CD19+, CD5+, CD23+
   b. CD19+, CD5−, CD23+
   c. CD19+, CD5+, CD23−
   d. CD19+, CD5−, CD23−

6. A CBC performed on an 80-year-old female reveals an absolute lymphocyte count of 8×10^9/L. Examination of the peripheral blood smear reveals a uniform population of small lymphocytes. Which of the following procedures would be most likely to establish a diagnosis? (Objectives 1, 5)
   a. cytogenetics
   b. flow cytometry immunophenotyping
   c. immunoglobulin gene rearrangement
   d. lymph node biopsy

7. A patient presents with a lymphocyte count of 350×10^9/L. Peripheral blood examination reveals large cells with moderate amounts of pale basophilic cytoplasm, moderately condensed chromatin, and prominent nucleoli. Which of the following is the most likely clinical finding? (Objective 5)
   a. massive splenomegaly
   b. lymphadenopathy
   c. lytic bone lesions
   d. lymphomatous polyposis

8. A CBC performed on a 60-year-old male with a history of rheumatoid arthritis revealed neutropenia and an absolute lymphocytosis. Examination of the peripheral smear revealed many lymphocytes with abundant pale-staining cytoplasm and cytoplasmic granules. Which of the following is the most likely phenotype? (Objectives 1, 5)
   a. CD3+, CD2+, CD57+
   b. CD19+, CD5+, CD57−
   c. CD2+, CD3−, CD56+
   d. CD19+, CD10+, CD34+

9. A patient previously diagnosed with small lymphocytic lymphoma (SLL) is found to have peripheral blood lymphocytosis. The lymphocytes are small and have round nuclei with clumped chromatin. Which of the following is the most appropriate interpretation? (Objective 3)
   a. This represents the same disease process (SLL).
   b. The patient has a new lymphoid malignancy: chronic lymphocytic leukemia.
   c. The lymphoma has transformed.
   d. The patient has developed a therapy-related malignancy.

REVIEW QUESTIONS *(continued)*

LEVEL I

LEVEL II

10. A lymph node biopsy revealed an infiltrate of small lymphoid cells with a vaguely nodular growth pattern. Flow cytometry revealed a monoclonal population of B cells expressing CD5. Immunohistochemistry revealed nuclear staining for cyclin-D1 protein. Which of the following is the most likely diagnosis? (Objective 3)
    a. mantle cell lymphoma
    b. small lymphocytic lymphoma
    c. chronic lymphocytic leukemia
    d. follicular lymphoma

www.pearsonhighered.com/mckenzie

Use this address to access the interactive Companion Website created for this textbook. Find additional information, tables and figures. Evaluate your command of the chapter information using case studies and critical thinking and multiple choice questions.

REFERENCES

1. Jaffe ES, Harris NL, Stein H, Vardiman JW. *Pathology & Genetics. Tumours of Haematopoietic and Lymphoid Tissues. World Health Organization Classification of Tumours.* Lyon, France IARC Press; 2001.

2. Kipps TJ. Chronic lymphocytic leukemia and related diseases. In: Lichtman MA, Beutler E, Kipps TJ, Seligsohn U, Kaushansky K, Prchal JT, eds. *Williams Hematology,* 7th ed. New York: McGraw-Hill; 2006:1343–83.

3. Chiorazzi N, Rai KR, Ferrarini M. Chronic lymphocytic leukemia. *New Engl J Med.* 2005;352:804–15.

4. Harris NL, Jaffe ES, Stein HS et al. A revised European-American classification of lymphoid neoplasms: A proposal from the International Lymphoma Study Group. *Blood.* 1994;84:1361–92.

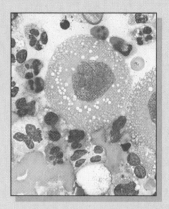

27

Hematopoietic Stem Cell Transplantation

Aamir Ehsan, M.D.

■ OBJECTIVES—LEVEL I

At the end of this unit of study, the student should be able to:

1. Describe the sources of hematopoietic stem cells and characteristics of each source.
2. Identify the diseases that can be treated with different sources of hematopoietic stem cells.
3. List characteristics of stem cells.
4. Describe the significance of ABO and HLA antigens for stem cell transplant.
5. Identify the infections that are serious complications during the peritransplant period.
6. Describe the significance and effects of graft-versus-host disease (GVHD) and compare them to those of the graft-versus-leukemia (GVL) process.

■ OBJECTIVES—LEVEL II

At the end of this unit of study, the student should be able to:

1. Summarize the collection and processing of hematopoietic stem cells and assess the success of these procedures.
2. Explain the role of the clinical laboratory professional in stem cell transplantation.
3. Select and outline methods to enumerate hematopoietic stem cells.
4. Explain the complications of stem cell transplant, and assess the patient's risk of developing them.
5. Formulate the sequence of events for a patient who will receive a stem cell transplant.
6. Select laboratory tests used to determine engraftment and assess engraftment given results of these tests.

KEY TERMS

Allogeneic
Apheresis
Autologous
Chimerism
Clonogenic
Conditioning regimen
Cryopreserved
Engraftment
Graft-versus-host disease (GVHD)
Graft-versus-leukemia (GVL)
In situ hybridization
Polymorphic
Purging
Syngeneic transplantation
Variable number tandem repeats (VNTR)

BACKGROUND BASICS

This chapter builds on concepts learned in previous chapters. To maximize your learning experience, you should review the following material before starting this unit of study.

Level I

▶ Describe the origin and differentiation of hematopoietic cells. (Chapters 2, 3)
▶ Outline the classification and explain the etiology and pathophysiology of neoplastic hematologic disorders. (Chapter 21)
▶ Explain the role of chemotherapy and radiotherapy in treatment of neoplastic hematologic disorders. (Chapters 21, 22, 23, 24, 25, 26)

Level II

▶ Describe the role of cytokines and bone marrow microenvironment in maturation and differentiation of hematopoietic stem cells; explain the role of oncogenes in cancer development. (Chapters 2, 3)
▶ Explain the use of molecular genetic technology and cytogenetics in diagnosis and prognosis of neoplastic hematopoietic disorders. (Chapters 38, 39)
▶ Correlate subgroups of neoplastic hematologic disorders with laboratory findings and prognosis. (Chapter 21)

CASE STUDY

We will refer to this case study throughout the chapter.

Brandon, a 35-year-old male (weight 80 kg), was recently diagnosed with AML with maturation and received induction chemotherapy. Day 21 bone marrow reveals no evidence of residual leukemia. Two weeks later, circulating blasts were seen in the peripheral blood. Brandon is being evaluated for a stem cell transplant. Consider the laboratory's role in evaluating the transplant, collecting and processing the stem cells, and determining engraftment.

▶ OVERVIEW

The use of stem cells in the therapy of neoplastic hematopoietic disorders has become commonplace. The laboratory's role in this therapy is critical and requires that the clinical laboratory professional know not only the associated laboratory tests but also why the tests are necessary and how they relate to the overall process of stem cell transplantation. This chapter reviews the sources of hematopoietic stem cells (HSCs); the use of allogeneic, autologous, and umbilical cord stem cells in treating a variety of malignant and nonmalignant disorders; the mobilization, collection, and enumeration of mononuclear cells (MNCs) and CD34 positive cells; the procedures used to assess transplant success (**engraftment**); and the role of the clinical laboratory professional during this process.

▶ INTRODUCTION

Hematopoietic stem cell transplantation (HSCT) is a recognized therapeutic modality for leukemias, lymphomas, solid organ tumors, and a variety of metabolic and immunologic disorders (Table 27-1 ✪). The concept of stem cell transplantation (SCT) came from experiments done five decades ago when it was observed that mice given intravenous marrow infusions could overcome lethal doses of radiation.[1,2] Later, in the 1960s, the first successful bone marrow transplant was performed on a leukemia patient using marrow donated by the leukemic patient's brother.

After the early successful **allogeneic** bone marrow SCTs (transplantation of stem cells between genetically dissimilar but human-leukocyte-antigen-matched [HLA-matched] individuals) using fresh anticoagulated bone marrow from HLA-matched siblings or family members, clinical practice has expanded to include the use of **autologous** bone marrow stem cells (transplantation or infusion of a person's own stem cells), autologous and allogeneic peripheral blood stem cells (PBSCs), and umbilical cord stem cells. HLA genes control the body's ability to mount an immune response. These genes code for histocompatible antigens found on the surface of essentially all nucleated cells (∞ Chapter 7).

▶ ORIGIN AND DIFFERENTIATION OF HEMATOPOIETIC STEM CELLS

HSCs are rare cells that can be found in the bone marrow and occasionally in the peripheral blood of healthy individuals. Self-renewal and multilineage differentiation are the two distinct biologic properties that make HSCs remarkable. Pluripotent stem cells differentiate into myeloid and lymphoid stem cells (Figure 3-2). Myeloid stem cells produce three types of committed/progenitor cells that differentiate into erythroid, granulocyte-macrophage, and megakaryocytic cell pathways. The lymphoid stem cells differentiate into T cells, B cells, and

⊗ TABLE 27-1

Diseases That Can Be Treated with Stem Cell Transplantation

Hematologic		Nonhematologic
Neoplastic	Non-neoplastic	
Acute lymphoblastic leukemia	Aplastic anemia	Solid organ malignancies (breast, ovarian, neuroblastoma, Wilms' tumor, germ cell)
Acute myeloid leukemia	Paroxysmal nocturnal hemoglobinuria	
Chronic myelogenous leukemia	Thalassemia	Inborn error of metabolism (e.g., Hurler's syndrome)
Idiopathic myelofibrosis	Sickle cell disease	Severe combined immunodeficiency disease
Chronic lymphocytic leukemia	Fanconi's anemia	Wiskott-Aldrich syndrome
Myelodysplastic syndrome	Congenital pure red cell aplasia	Congenital leukocyte dysfunction syndromes
Non-Hodgkin lymphoma		Malignant osteopetrosis
Hodgkin lymphoma		
Multiple myeloma		

possibly natural killer cells. The committed progenitor cells have been called *colony-forming units (CFUs)* because they give rise to colonies of differentiated progeny in vitro (∞ Chapter 2). From these CFUs arise morphologically recognizable precursors of differentiated cells (pronormoblast, myeloblast, monoblast, megakaryoblast) that further differentiate into mature cells. In summary, pluripotent stem cells have the capacity to self-renew and differentiate. With additional divisions, their progeny, the committed progenitor cells, become progressively restricted to proliferation and differentiation into a single cell line. The committed cell lacks the property of self-renewal.

▶ **SOURCES OF HEMATOPOIETIC STEM CELLS AND TYPES OF STEM CELL TRANSPLANTS**

HSCs for clinical use[3] can be harvested from the bone marrow, peripheral blood, and umbilical cord blood (UCB). Fetal bone marrow and liver are also rich in stem cells, but use is limited due to ethical issues. Unlike other tissues and organs destined for transplant, HSCs are not routinely taken from cadavers. One reason for this is that in most situations, the stem cell donor receives hematopoietic cytokines for a few days before the stem cells are harvested to maximize stem cell yield.

ALLOGENEIC STEM CELL TRANSPLANTATION

Allogeneic stem cell transplantation is the infusion of HSCs from another individual (donor) into the patient (recipient). In the past, the usual source of stem cells has been the bone marrow, but now allogeneic transplants using PBSCs are more common. Allogeneic transplants are often indicated when the disease process involves the patient's own stem cells, making them potentially unsuitable for transplant (Table 27-2 ⊗). Allogeneic transplant is usually performed for therapy of acute leukemias, chronic myelogenous leukemia (CML), aplastic anemia, hemoglobinopathies, immune deficiencies, and metabolic genetic disorders.[4,5]

⊗ TABLE 27-2

Type of Transplant, Sources of Stem Cells, and Diseases in Which These Stem Cells Are Used

Type of Transplant	Source of Stem Cells	Diseases
Allogeneic	Bone marrow	Acute leukemias, CML, non-neoplastic hematologic conditions (see Table 27-1), immunologic and inherited
	Peripheral blood	diseases
	Cord blood	
Autologous	Peripheral blood	HL, NHL, solid organ tumors, MM
	Bone marrow	
Syngeneic	Peripheral blood	Any disorder treated by allogeneic/autologous transplant except a genetic disease
	Bone marrow	

CML = chronic myelogenous leukemia; HL = Hodgkin lymphoma; NHL = non-Hodgkin lymphoma; MM = multiple myeloma

Three important factors must be considered in order to achieve successful allogeneic SCT. Adequate numbers of HSCs should be present in the graft so that when infused into the recipient's circulation, engraftment in the marrow microenvironment will occur. The recipient's immune system should tolerate donor stem cells so that graft rejection does not occur, and the donor's immune cells should tolerate host tissue to avoid severe **graft-versus-host disease (GVHD)**. GVHD occurs when immunocompetent donor T lymphocytes recognize nonself HLA antigens on the host cells and initiate cell injury.

Highly incompatible tissues are almost certain to be rejected. Compatibility is based on the immune system's recognition of certain cell markers as "self." The most critical of these cell markers appear to be the HLAs, also known as the *major histocompatibility complex* (*MHC*). The HLA system is highly **polymorphic** (occurring in several forms).

Genes present on the short arm of chromosome 6 encode HLA antigens. Class I HLA antigens are encoded by three loci: HLA-A, HLA-B, and HLA-C. Class II HLA antigens are encoded by another three loci: HLA-DR, HLA-DP, and HLA-DQ. Serological and molecular testing methods are available to HLA-type individuals.[6,7] Although the candidate donors and recipients are tested for HLA-A, -B, -C, -DR, and -DQ antigens, an HLA match requires only that the donor and recipient have compatible HLA-A, HLA-B, and usually HLA-DR antigens. An optimum clinical result occurs when the donor and recipient are matched at the HLA-A, HLA-B, and HLA-DR loci. Even with a complete match, graft rejection and GVHD can occur, indicating the possibility current testing methods may not recognize antigens that are incompatible or not encoded by MHC. On the other hand, successful transplant can occur even with some degree of HLA mismatch.[8,9]

Approximately 30% of patients requiring allogeneic transplant have a matched sibling donor and another 2 to 5% have a partially matched related donor.[10] If family members do not match or are not available, the search for an unrelated HLA-matched donor is made through the National Marrow Donor Program (NMDP).[11] This type of transplant is called a *matched unrelated donor (MUD)* transplant. The NMDP was established in 1987 and currently has more than 3 million registered donors. Even with such a large donor pool in the NMDP, the MUD transplant has certain limitations. First, because of HLA polymorphisms, locating HLA-matched donors is difficult. Second, the length of time to find a compatible allograft is about 4–6 months. Third, the cost of a donor search/procurement is high. Fourth, the racial distribution in the NMDP is unbalanced, limiting its usefulness for patients of minority origins, particularly those of African, Mexican, and Asian heritage. However, considerable efforts are being made to recruit minority donors. Finally, the chance of graft failure, GVHD, and opportunistic infections with MUD transplant increases.

The initial donor selection for an allogeneic transplant is based on HLA compatibility with the recipient. The ABO blood group antigens of the donor and recipient do not need to be matched to accomplish successful transplantation because these antigens are not expressed on HSCs. Stem cell donors are tested for the same infectious diseases as are required by the Food and Drug Administration (FDA) for volunteer blood donors. Most transplant centers absolutely exclude donors only if they are found to have serologic evidence of HIV infection. Before receiving the allogeneic HSC infusion, the recipient is treated with conditioning chemotherapy and/or total body irradiation.[12] Depending on the underlying disease, this regimen can serve two purposes. First, it provides an antitumor effect, and second, it is immunosuppressive to enable the recipient to better tolerate the donor cells. The goal of giving high-dose chemotherapy/radiotherapy is to destroy all malignant cells but the therapy is also toxic to normal bone marrow cells. The patient's marrow is then rescued with normal cells by infusing the donor stem cells. As in solid organ transplantation, recipients must also be given additional immunosuppressive therapy such as cyclosporine or tacrolimus to minimize graft rejection and GVHD.

Syngeneic transplantation is the use of bone marrow or PBSCs from an identical twin. This type of transplant is rare but could be used for any disorder treated by allogeneic or autologous transplant except genetic diseases that affect both twins. This uncommon situation should have no risk of rejection or GVHD, and no special immunosuppressive drugs need be given.

 CASE STUDY *(continued from page 569)*

Brandon had a bone marrow examination, and 6% blasts were present. He has four siblings.

1. Is Brandon a candidate for a stem cell transplant?
2. If yes, what form of transplant is required for him?
3. What testing should be done on Brandon to proceed with the transplant?

AUTOLOGOUS STEM CELL TRANSPLANTATION

Autologous stem cell transplantation infuses the patient's own bone marrow or PBSCs. These stem cells are collected prior to intensive or myeloablative chemotherapy and/or radiotherapy, which are aimed at eliminating the malignant cells. After therapy, the collected stem cells are infused into the patient to re-establish hematopoiesis. Autologous transplantation is usually indicated when the patient's stem cells are not affected by the disease and the underlying disease is potentially responsive to high-dose chemotherapy and/or radiotherapy. This type of transplant is commonly utilized for Hodgkin lymphoma; non-Hodgkin lymphoma; multiple myeloma; solid organ tumors including breast, ovarian, and testicular cancers; and pediatric neoplasms such as neuroblastoma and Wilms' tumor (Table 27-2).

Autologous PBSC transplant also can be performed if the disease involves the patient's own marrow. However, in this case, a number of other factors should be evaluated: age, underlying disease, degree of marrow involvement, response to previous chemotherapy, and donor availability. The use of autologous stem cells for transplant in a subset of acute leukemias, myeloproliferative disorders, and myelodysplastic syndrome (MDS) has been attempted but without great success.[13–15]

Autologous stem cell transplantation has both advantages and disadvantages. One important advantage is that it is not necessary to identify HLA-matched donors. Immunosuppression is not used, so graft rejection and GVHD are not an issue. Peritransplant mortality is low, and older patients tolerate the procedure relatively well. Some disadvantages of autologous transplant include the possibility of neoplastic cells in the stem cell product that could cause disease recurrence; difficulty in obtaining adequate stem cells if the patient has received extensive prior therapy; and the **graft-versus-leukemia (GVL)** effect sometimes seen with allogeneic transplant is not possible. (GVL effect is a favorable effect seen when immunocompetent donor T cells present in the allograft destroy the recipient's leukemic cells. The significance of GVL is described later in the chapter.)

 Checkpoint! 1

A physician is evaluating a 28-year-old patient with a history of acute lymphoblastic leukemia for PBSC transplantation. The laboratory professional found circulating leukemic blasts in the peripheral blood. Is this patient a candidate for an autologous PBSC transplant?

UMBILICAL CORD STEM CELL TRANSPLANTATION

Umbilical cord blood contains sufficient numbers of HSCs to provide short-term and long-term engraftment in related and unrelated recipients.[16–18] The first cord blood transplantation was performed in a 5-year-old boy with Fanconi's anemia in 1988.[19] Clinical data indicate that cord blood from siblings and unrelated donors can be used to reconstitute hematopoiesis in patients with malignant and nonmalignant disorders.[16–18,20] As a result of the early successes with cord blood transplantation from sibling donors, pilot programs for banking unrelated donor cord blood were initiated in various countries around the world. Cord blood contains sufficient numbers of HSCs for engraftment in most recipients weighing less than 40 kg. However, cord blood transplants have been attempted with some success in patients weighing more than 40 kg. See Table 27-3 ✪ for the advantages and disadvantages of using cord blood over marrow.

 Checkpoint! 2

What would be the best form of transplant for a patient with CML who needs a stem cell transplant, and what antigen type needs to be matched?

✪ **TABLE 27-3**

Advantages and Disadvantages of Using Cord Blood Stem Cells versus Marrow Stem Cell Donors

Advantages	Disadvantages
• Cord blood is abundantly available. • Cord blood stem cells can be collected without risk to the mother or infant. • Cord blood can be frozen and readily available on demand. • Ethnic balance of a given population of donors can be maintained. • The risk of latent viral contamination (CMV, EBV) is low. • Cord blood does not contain mature T cells and therefore is likely to be less immunogenic and will reduce the incidence of GVHD.	• Total number of stem cells is generally inadequate for most adult transplant patients. • GVL effect can be reduced. • Only one unit is available for each transplant procedure.

GVL = graft versus leukemia; CMV = cytomegalovirus; EBV = Epstein Barr virus

▶ COLLECTION AND PROCESSING OF HEMATOPOIETIC STEM CELLS

Collecting and processing HSC requires a team of clinical laboratory professionals as well as physicians.

BONE MARROW

Collection of bone marrow stem cells (allogeneic or autologous) is a surgical procedure performed in the operating room using general or local anesthesia. The marrow is taken from the posterior iliac crest with harvest needles and syringes. Approximately 1 liter of marrow is harvested to provide an adequate number of mononuclear cells (MNCs). When the marrow is harvested, it contains a mixture of red blood cells, white blood cells, MNCs, platelets, plasma, and fat particles. If a marrow recipient is ABO compatible with the donor, the marrow can be infused immediately after filtering the fat and small bone particles. Otherwise the marrow can be further processed to remove a mononuclear cell layer that can be frozen and stored. Stem cell collection by this method is rarely used now and is being replaced by peripheral stem cell collection (see below).

PERIPHERAL BLOOD

Because stem cells are rare in the peripheral blood (less than 0.01%), various regimens have been tried to mobilize stem cells in the marrow to enter the peripheral blood and increase the number of circulating MNCs. Transplanting more stem cells means more rapid hematopoietic recovery.[21] For autologous PBSC collection, patients can receive cytotoxic chemotherapy (e.g., Cytoxan); hematopoietic cytokines (e.g., granulocyte colony-stimulating factor [G-CSF]; granulocyte-macrophage colony-stimulating factor [GM-CSF]); or a combination of chemotherapy and cytokines to mobilize stem cells.

After cytotoxic and cytokine therapy, the stem cells in the marrow rebound and are mobilized to the peripheral blood where they can be collected by **apheresis,** an automated procedure that uses a blood cell separator. Whole blood is withdrawn from the donor and anticoagulated. The components are separated using centrifugation or filtration, and the desired component is collected (in this case, mononuclear cells that contain the hematopoietic stem cells). The remaining components are combined and infused back into the donor.

The optimum timing for collection of PBSCs after cytotoxic and growth factor therapy is sometimes unpredictable, and the time of harvest varies depending on the mobilization protocol. Some centers determine timing of PBSC collection based on a preapheresis peripheral blood CD34 count.[22]

For allogeneic PBSC collection, hematopoietic cytokines (G-CSF or GM-CSF) are given to normal, healthy donors to mobilize stem cells, and then the MNCs are collected by apheresis.

CASE STUDY *(continued from page 571)*

An HLA-matched sibling has agreed to be a donor for Brandon.

4. Should the source of stem cells be peripheral blood or bone marrow? Why?

UMBILICAL CORD BLOOD

If UCB is collected as a source of stem cells, the mother must sign an informed consent, and a complete medical history of the parents is obtained. Cord blood is usually collected from a delivered placenta or sometimes from an undelivered placenta (after the baby is delivered and the cord is being clamped). A large-bore needle is inserted into the umbilical vein to collect blood in a sterile collection bag containing anticoagulant. Several methods are used to separate MNCs from the whole cord blood: Ficoll-Hypaque, modified Ficoll-Hypaque gradient method, and addition of hydroxyethyl starch (HES).[23,24] The cord blood is not usually processed if certain conditions are present (Table 27-4).

PURGING

Purging is a technique to remove undesirable cells present in the product. Purging is performed on the stem cell product that has been collected by apheresis. Depending on the source of stem cells and clinical conditions in which these

⊗ TABLE 27-4

Conditions in Which Stem Cells Are Not Usually Collected and/or Processed from the Cord Blood

- Inadequate volume collected from an individual placenta (less than 40 mL)
- Preterm delivery (less than 36 weeks)
- Fever higher than 100°F (38°C) in mother
- Premature rupture of membranes
- Meconium staining of the fluid
- Family history of inherited diseases
- Congenital anomalies in the infant

cells are used, various purging techniques (mechanical, immunological, and pharmacological) are available.[25]

When a patient with a history of solid tumor is undergoing an autologous transplant, the bone marrow and PBSCs to a lesser extent can be contaminated with occult tumor cells. Therefore, removal of tumor cells, if present, is theoretically highly desirable.

GVHD is an immunologic response that results from the presence of donor origin CD8-positive T suppressor cells that can interact with the host's CD4-positive T helper cells. In an allogeneic transplantation, GVHD is a potential complication. Purging the donor T lymphocytes from the allograft can prevent GVHD or reduce its severity. However, some of these T cells seem to be necessary for marrow engraftment and for achievement of the GVL effect. A favorable response, GVL is usually seen because the T cells present in the graft can have an active role in destroying the residual leukemic cells of the recipient. In support of this possibility, patients receiving T cell-depleted grafts are known to be at higher risk for disease relapse than patients receiving unmanipulated grafts for the same disease.

CRYOPRESERVATION AND STORAGE OF HSCS

HSCs from bone marrow, PBSCs, or cord blood can be effectively **cryopreserved** (stored at very low temperatures) to maintain cell viability for months or years. When the stem cells are frozen or thawed, cell injury or loss of stem cell viability results from intracellular crystal formation and cellular dehydration.

To achieve the optimum cryopreservation without compromising the cell viability, a cryoprotectant agent is used.[25] The most common cryoprotectants are either 10% DMSO (dimethylsulfoxide) or 5% DMSO with 6% HES. The DMSO diffuses rapidly into the cells and increases intracellular solute concentration, thus decreasing intracellular ice crystal formation and preventing cell lysis.

After optimizing the concentration of the stem cells in the presence of cryoprotectant, tissue culture media and autologous plasma are frozen in many small plastic bags. The freezing rate seems to be an important factor for viable cell recovery. The freezing is usually performed in the chamber of a programmable device into which liquid nitrogen is pumped to maintain the desired rate. When the freezing program has been completed, the bags are removed from the chamber and placed in a liquid nitrogen refrigerator in either liquid or vapor phase at −196°C.

INFUSION OF HSCS

The patient to be infused is premedicated with antihistamine and antiemetic (sometimes diuretics and/or steroids). The frozen bags are immediately thawed in a 37°C water bath just before the infusion. The infusion is carried out as quickly as possible to dilute the cell suspension with the patient's blood volume because DMSO in liquid phase can be toxic to stem cells. The most common adverse reactions associated with cryopreserved stem cells are chills, nausea, vomiting, fever, allergic reactions, transient cough, and shortness of breath. Adverse events from infusion can be related to DMSO-induced histamine release; therefore, some centers thaw and dilute or wash the cell suspension to remove the DMSO, but cell loss and clumping can be a problem.

► QUANTITATION OF HEMATOPOIETIC STEM CELLS

The number of stem cells or CD34+ cells that can be obtained varies greatly from donor to donor. For PBSCs, one or more apheresis procedures are needed to acquire the appropriate dose for engraftment and hematopoietic recovery. Because the engraftment outcome depends on the number of stem cells present in the product, the HSCs (from bone marrow, PBSCs, or cord blood) are quantitated by one of the three methods described next.

DETERMINATION OF MONONUCLEAR CELL COUNT

Stem cells are mononuclear cells as are other cells (such as immature myeloid cells, lymphocytes, and monocytes); thus, counting MNCs provides a very indirect estimate of the number of stem cells present in the sample (Figure 27-1 ■). The volume of cells necessary to achieve a satisfactory dose for successful engraftment can be determined from the MNC count. The dose is usually specified as the number of MNCs per kilogram of the recipient's body weight. Laboratories use automated cell counters or hemacytometers to count the MNCs.

CD34 ENUMERATION BY FLOW CYTOMETRY

Enumerating stem cells that express CD34 antigen and using immunophenotyping has become a routine practice. When bound to fluorescent dyes, anti-CD34 antibodies offer a

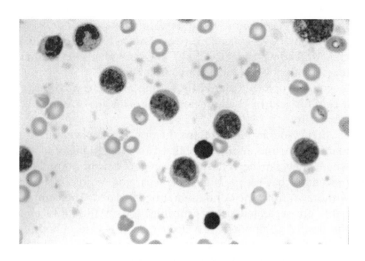

■ FIGURE 27-1   Wright's stain slide prepared for the manual differential count from the stem cell product showing myeloid precursors and mononuclear cells. (Peripheral blood; Wright's stain, 1000× magnification)

rapid method of enumerating stem cells using a flow cytometer. Flow cytometric enumeration of CD34+ cells has been shown to be the most useful indicator of the hematopoietic reconstitutive capacity of SCT.

The major difficulty with the analysis of CD34+ cells is the low number of cells present in the specimen. The method's sensitivity is 1 in 10,000. Procedures to measure CD34+ cells vary widely. Optimally, 100 CD34+ cells and 75,000 CD45+ (leukocytes) events should be acquired to optimize the accuracy of analysis.[26,27] The CD34 count is calculated in conjunction with the total leukocyte counts.[27,28] These results should be reported as soon as possible because the clinical decision to collect more stem cells depends on CD34 yield. CD34 counts can be performed on peripheral blood and stem cell product. Some centers determine the timing of PBSC collection based on a peripheral blood CD34 count.[22] If the CD34+ cells are lower than required, the decision can be made to perform more (or postpone) apheresis or "prime" the patient in a different manner.

CELL CULTURE FOR COLONY FORMING UNITS (CFU)

Flow cytometry analysis identifies cells only by their antigenic markers and thus cannot identify cells that are clonogenic; only culture techniques can demonstrate clonogenecity. An in vitro clonogenic assay is a culture system containing stem cells and various growth factors. The culture is incubated for 14–15 days on a semisolid medium (agar or methylcellulose). The colonies generated from committed myeloid and erythroid hematopoietic progenitors can be differentiated and counted (Figure 27-2 ■).

The advantage of the clonogenic assay is that this system tests the capacity of progenitor cells to divide and can pre-

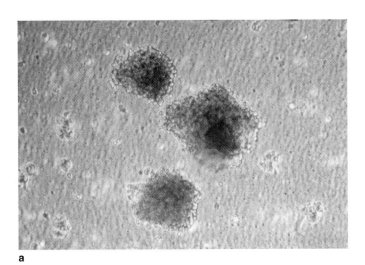

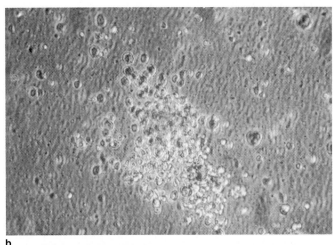

a   b

■ FIGURE 27-2   Cell culture colonies: **a.** erythroid colonies and **b.** myeloid colonies (on semisolid medium).

dict the engraftment potential of the stem cell product.[29,30] The 2-week incubation period needed in this method is a distinct disadvantage when data are needed for immediate clinical decisions. The results of clonogenic assay systems from different institutions vary greatly due to variance in reagent lots and the level of staff expertise. Commercial kits are now available to aid in the standardization of clonogenic assays.

 Checkpoint! 3

You receive a peripheral blood specimen in the hematology laboratory with a request for a mononuclear cell count and analysis of CD34+ cells. Without any further information, why should you consider this a STAT request?

▶ COLLECTION TARGET FOR STEM CELLS

The recipient's body weight determines the adequate dose of stem cells, the exact number of which is needed to ensure engraftment is not known, but cell doses of $2.5–5.0 \times 10^6$ CD34+ cells per kilogram recipient weight are desirable; earlier engraftment are observed with even higher doses.[31,32] For a transplant using umbilical cord blood, more than 3.0×10^7 of total nucleated cells per kilogram recipient weight is desirable.

ⓔ CASE STUDY *(continued from page 573)*

PBSCs were collected by apheresis from the sibling. Enumeration of CD34 count indicates that the total CD34+ cells collected are 6×10^6/kg.

5. Is this an adequate dose for SCT?

▶ HEMATOPOIETIC ENGRAFTMENT

The **conditioning regimen** given to patients for SCT causes severe myelosuppression in recipients and can affect T and B cell immunity (usually in an allogeneic setting). After the conditioning regimen, the HSCs are usually given to restore the marrow function. A period of pancytopenia typically follows during which the patient is prone to develop infections and bleeding complications. To reduce the pancytopenia period, growth factors such as G-CSF or GM-CSF can be given.[32,33]

EVIDENCE OF SHORT-TERM ENGRAFTMENT

After transplant, the time for engraftment depends on the number of CD34+ cells in the graft. The period of pancytopenia can last from a few days to 2–4 weeks. Myeloid recovery is followed by platelet and red cell recovery. Short-term evidence of hematopoietic engraftment exists when the absolute neutrophil count is more than $500/\mu L$ and platelet count is more than $20,000/\mu L$ with no need for platelet transfusion. The pancytopenia period after PBSC transplant, when compared to bone marrow transplant, is somewhat shorter. After cord blood transplants, neutrophil recovery can take 5–6 weeks, and the platelets usually engraft late (median time 80 days).[20]

EVIDENCE OF LONG-TERM ENGRAFTMENT

When testing reveals that all hematopoietic cells in a SCT recipient are derived from an allogeneic donor, the condition is referred to as full **chimerism** (the presence of donor hematopoietic cells in a recipient). When a recipient's hematopoietic cells persist together with donor cells after SCT, the condition is referred to as *partial chimerism*.

To evaluate the long-term engraftment of HSCs, various laboratory methods have evolved.[34] Detection of red cell antigens was among the first tests used to evaluate donor cell engraftment. For example, if the recipient's blood group is O and the donor's blood group is A, then after hematopoietic engraftment with complete chimerism, the recipient can type as group A. However, because of the long life span of red cells and multiple blood transfusions during transplantation, the red cell antigens are no longer used for chimerism studies.

The most widely used tests for evaluating long-term engraftment currently are in situ hybridization (ISH) with sex chromosomes and the typing of **variable number tandem repeat (VNTR)** polymorphism by DNA amplification (∞ Chapter 39). **In situ hybridization** is a technique for detecting specific DNA or RNA sequences in tissue sections or cell preparations using a labeled complementary nucleic acid sequence probe. The ISH is applicable only when the donor and recipient are of the opposite sex. Variable number tandem repeats are DNA sequences that are tandemly repeated in a genome and can vary among different individuals. DNA amplification for chimerism is applicable in allogeneic transplant settings when testing a person's VNTRs can distinguish donor and recipient cells.

In summary, the clinical applications of chimerism tests in marrow transplantation are to document donor cell engraftment, evaluate the persistence of donor cells, and assess the recurrence of disease.

 Checkpoint! 4

A physician wants to evaluate the engraftment on a male patient who received SCT from his brother four months ago. What laboratory tests should be performed to make this assessment?

 CASE STUDY *(continued from page 575)*

Stem cells were collected and frozen for Brandon.

6. Does Brandon need to undergo any form of therapy before the transplant?

▶ ROLE OF THE CLINICAL LABORATORY PROFESSIONAL IN STEM CELL TRANSPLANTATION

When the decision to undertake an SCT has been made, collecting and processing stem cells involves a dedicated clinical laboratory staff that works as a team (Figure 27-3 ■). The SCT process involves the clinical laboratory professionals working in the department of hematology, apheresis, blood bank, microbiology, flow cytometry, molecular/HLA, cytogenetics, and bone marrow transplant laboratories (Figure 27-4 ■).

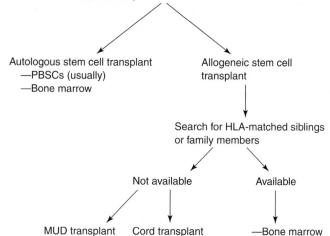

Factors to be considered for the SCT

1. Age of the patient
2. Underlying disease
3. Involvement of patient's own bone marrow or stem cells
4. Degree of marrow involvement
5. Response to previous chemotherapy
6. Donor availability

Autologous stem cell transplant
—PBSCs (usually)
—Bone marrow

Allogeneic stem cell transplant

Search for HLA-matched siblings or family members

Not available   Available

MUD transplant   Cord transplant if patient is a child or adult weighing <40kg   —Bone marrow —PBSCs

PBSCs: Peripheral blood stem cells
MUD: Matched unrelated donor

■ **FIGURE 27-3**   Decision-making process in stem cell transplantation. The evaluation of the patient for SCT is usually done at the time of primary diagnosis. For allogeneic SCT, a donor is selected based on HLA compatibility. If family members do not match or are not available, the search for an unrelated HLA-matched donor is made through the NMDP. If the patient is a child or small adult (less than 40 kg), the cord blood registry/banks is also an option. In general, if the disease involves the patient's own stem cells, allogeneic transplant is a valid option. Autologous transplant is planned when the disease has not affected the patient's own stem cells. On the other hand, autologous PBSC transplant may be performed even if the disease involves the patient's marrow, but a number of other factors should be evaluated, as shown in this algorithm.

Let's consider a patient for whom the clinical decision for autologous SCT has been made. This patient will receive cytotoxic chemotherapy, or G-CSF, or both. For PBSC collection, the patient will undergo apheresis. (In an allogeneic transplant setting, both the donor and recipient cells are typed for HLA antigens in the molecular/HLA laboratory before collecting stem cells.) The apheresis staff will spend 4–6 hours with the patient to get a good yield of MNCs. After collecting the product, the sample will be sent to the hematology and flow cytometry labs where WBC/MNCs and CD34 counts will be performed on a sample collected by apheresis.

The bone marrow transplant laboratory staff will process and cryopreserve the stem cells for future use. The cells' via-

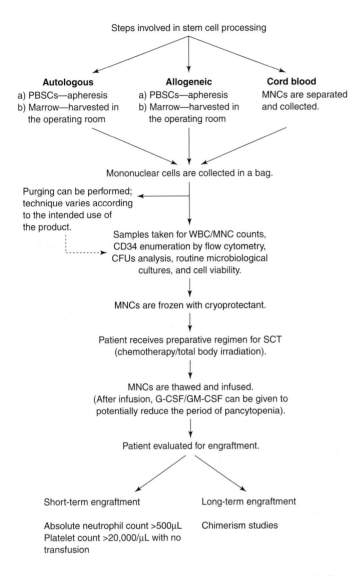

Steps involved in stem cell processing

Autologous
a) PBSCs—apheresis
b) Marrow—harvested in
the operating room

Allogeneic
a) PBSCs—apheresis
b) Marrow—harvested in
the operating room

Cord blood
MNCs are separated
and collected.

Mononuclear cells are collected in a bag.

Purging can be performed;
technique varies according
to the intended use of
the product.

Samples taken for WBC/MNC counts,
CD34 enumeration by flow cytometry,
CFUs analysis, routine microbiological
cultures, and cell viability.

MNCs are frozen with cryoprotectant.

Patient receives preparative regimen for SCT
(chemotherapy/total body irradiation).

MNCs are thawed and infused.
(After infusion, G-CSF/GM-CSF can be given to
potentially reduce the period of pancytopenia).

Patient evaluated for engraftment.

Short-term engraftment

Long-term engraftment

Absolute neutrophil count >500μL
Platelet count >20,000/μL with no
transfusion

Chimerism studies

■ FIGURE 27-4   Steps involved from the time the patient is diagnosed with the disease to the final infusion of stem cell product. For autologous transplant, the stem cells are usually collected from peripheral blood or sometimes harvested from the bone marrow. If the stem cells are collected from the peripheral blood, the patient can receive cytotoxic chemotherapy or growth factors, or both to mobilize stem cells into the blood; the stem cells are then collected by apheresis. For an allogeneic transplant, an HLA-matched family member donor or an HLA-matched donor from the NMDP is considered. The stem cells are collected from the iliac crests in a surgical procedure. In an allogeneic setting, stem cells can also be collected by apheresis from peripheral blood after mobilizing the donor with growth factors. Whatever the method of collection, after collecting the required number of stem cells from peripheral blood, bone marrow, or cord blood, samples are taken for appropriate tests and stem cells are cryopreserved for later infusion. Before the transplant, the patient receives a high dose of chemotherapy and/or radiotherapy to destroy the tumor cells. This therapy can be toxic to normal organs including bone marrow. The marrow is rescued by transplanting frozen stem cells that have been reserved for a particular patient.

bility will be checked, samples for bacterial cultures taken, and the cell culture can set up for enumeration of CFUs. On the day of transplant, the clinical laboratory staff (usually of the bone marrow lab) will thaw the units for the infusion.

After the transplant, hematology will evaluate short-term engraftment with a complete blood count. For evaluation of long-term engraftment, the sample will be sent to the cytogenetic and molecular/HLA laboratories to perform chimerism studies. Throughout the course of the transplant, the blood bank personnel will provide special blood components required during the transplantation process.

▶ GRAFT-VERSUS-HOST DISEASE AND GRAFT-VERSUS-LEUKEMIA EFFECT

The exact mechanism for GVHD is not yet clearly known. However, the suggested pathogenesis of GVHD is that immunocompetent donor T lymphocytes recognize HLA antigens on the host (recipient) cells and initiate secondary inflammatory injury mediated by inflammatory cytokines (interleukin-1, tumor necrosis factor [TNF]). This leads to tissue injury.[35,36]

Three factors necessary to set the stage for GVHD are the presence of immunocompetent donor T lymphocytes, HLA alloantigens, and an immunosuppressed host. GVHD is more frequent and severe in recipients of partially HLA-matched sibling allografts or in grafts from unrelated donors.[8] However, GVHD also occurs after HLA-identical sibling donor allografts, indicating the role of other HLA minor antigens or factors that are not usually tested at the time of transplant.

Overall, the risk of acute GVHD for the degree of HLA mismatch is less in recipients of cord SCT than in recipients of marrow transplant perhaps because of the immature nature of cord blood cells. GVHD can be prevented or its severity reduced by decreasing the number of donor T lymphocytes from the graft and/or administration of medications such as cyclosporine A, methotrexate, steroids, cyclophosphamide, antithymocyte globulin, and tacrolimus.[37,38]

Recipients of T cell-depleted marrow less frequently experience GVHD but have a higher incidence of relapse and higher graft failure than patients with unmanipulated marrow for the same disease. T lymphocytes are known to be essential for marrow engraftment and for achieving desirable GVL effect, which is seen when immunocompetent donor T cells present in the allograft destroy the recipient's leukemic cells.[39] For example, in allograft recipients with CML who relapse after allogeneic SCT, donor lymphocyte infusion (DLI) of small numbers of lymphocytes collected by apheresis from the original graft donor[40] can induce a potent GVL effect and reestablish complete remission in most patients.

The critical issue of how many T lymphocytes need to be removed from the allograft to avoid GVHD yet allow marrow engraftment and GVL effect is controversial. Any number should be interpreted with caution because the T cell concentration required to achieve long-term engraftment, control of GVHD, and beneficial GVL effect also depends on the disease and the degree of HLA disparity.

► COMPLICATIONS ASSOCIATED WITH STEM CELL TRANSPLANTATION

SCT complications can be categorized as early and late. Complications that usually occur during the first 100 days after transplantation are considered early and those that occur from a few months (>3 months) to several years post-transplantation are late.

EARLY COMPLICATIONS

Early complications include graft rejection, graft-versus-host disease, peritransplant infections, and recurrence of malignant disease.

Graft Rejection

Primary graft failure is the failure to establish hematologic engraftment and can be defined as failure to attain an absolute neutrophil count above 500 μL by 28 days post-transplant. *Secondary graft failure* is the loss of an established graft and is defined as the redevelopment of pancytopenia at any time after primary engraftment. These complications can be seen in the allogeneic transplant setting and rarely in the autologous setting. Causes of graft failure are listed in Table 27-5 ✪.

Graft-versus-Host Disease

GVHD can be either acute or chronic. Acute GVHD generally occurs in the first three months after allogeneic SCT and usually involves the recipient's skin (maculopapular dermatitis), liver (elevation of bilirubin, abnormal liver function tests), and gastrointestinal tract (nausea, vomiting, diarrhea). Chronic GVHD is defined as symptoms appearing 80–100 days post-transplantation.

Peritransplant Infections

In the peritransplant period, when the patient has been immunosuppressed and has a low neutrophil count, the risk of opportunistic infection is very high. Infections can be bacterial, protozoal, fungal, and/or viral. These infections during

✪ TABLE 27-5

Causes of Graft Failure

- Inadequate number of stem cells
- HLA disparity between donor and recipient
- Significant T cell depletion of the allograft
- Decreased degree of immunosuppression

the first 3 months post-transplant can be serious but rarely life threatening. Reactivated cytomegalovirus (CMV), a group of the herpes virus family, and herpes simplex are the most common. In the United States, CMV prevalence in the population ranges from 50 to 85%. SCT patients are particularly vulnerable to CMV infection, which can be primary, but superinfection with a second strain or a reactivation of latent disease also can occur. The complications include pneumonitis, gastroenteritis, and retinitis. Fatal CMV pneumonia occurs in 10–15% of patients.

The relative risk for CMV infection among SCT patients depends on the serostatus of both the donor and the recipient.[41] A seronegative recipient of seropositive transplant is at significant risk of primary transfusion-transmitted CMV infection. Seropositive recipients of seropositive transplants can develop reactivation or superinfection of CMV.

A donor for a CMV negative patient should be an HLA-compatible person who is seronegative for CMV. SCT patients who are at significant risk for acquiring transfusion-transmitted CMV also should receive cellular components that carry a reduced risk of CMV. It has been shown that CMV resides in leukocytes, and studies have indicated that leukocyte-reduced cellular blood components can prevent CMV infection.[42–44] However, equivalent efficacy of leukocyte-reduced and CMV-seronegative cellular components in preventing transfusion associated (TA)-CMV has not yet been completely resolved. Most transplant physicians believe that if a CMV-seronegative recipient receives stem cells from a CMV-seronegative donor, all subsequent blood components received should be CMV-seronegative. If the CMV-negative blood component is not available, transfusing a leukocyte-reduced filtered component can effectively prevent the transmission of CMV disease.

Recurrence of Malignant Disease

Patients who undergo autologous transplantation are more at risk of dying from disease recurrence than from transplant-related complications. After autologous transplant, recurrence of the original disease can occur because of incomplete eradication of malignant cells or the presence of residual neoplastic cells in the autograft that have not been adequately eliminated by purging techniques. Patients who receive an allogeneic transplant rather than an autologous transplant for hematologic malignancies have a lower relapse rate; however, the risk of leukemic relapse varies from 5 to 70%. This variability depends on the diagnosis and stage of the disease, the degree of immunosupression, the match or mismatch of the allograft, and the presence or absence of GVHD.

Other Complications

Symptoms and clinical signs of toxicity related to chemotherapy and radiotherapy can occur after SCT including mucositis, myocarditis, pericarditis, pneumonitis, hemorrhagic cystitis, and adverse drug reactions. A serious liver disorder that complicates up to 50% of marrow transplants is called *veno-occlusive disease;* it is characterized by right upper quadrant pain, weight gain, and jaundice and is diagnosed clinically. Other features include ascites, hepatomegaly, hyperbilirubinemia, encephalopathy, and renal failure or multiorgan failure.

LATE COMPLICATIONS

Late complications can be secondary to pretransplantation chemotherapy/radiotherapy, continued effects of acute complications, and/or immunosuppressive states leading to delayed infections. These complications include hypothyroidism, hypogonadism, cataracts, growth retardation in pediatric patients, neuropathies, and sometimes development of post-transplant lymphoproliferative disorders and second malignancies (myelodysplastic syndrome and leukemia).

 Checkpoint! 5

A CMV-seronegative patient requires SCT. Two HLA-matched donors are available. Is it important to know the stem cell donor's CMV status? If the stem cell donor is CMV-seronegative and the patient requires red cell transfusion during the peritransplant period, what blood components (in terms of CMV status) would you select for this patient?

 CASE STUDY *(continued from page 576)*

Brandon received stem cells from his HLA-matched sibling that successfully engrafted. Three months later, he developed diarrhea, skin rash, and jaundice.

   7. What could be the possible cause for this?

GENE THERAPY

In addition to the HSCT, gene therapy is a technology that offers the possibility for a complete cure for genetic disease.[45]

The discussion of this technology is beyond the scope of this book. Suffice it to say that its goal is to introduce a functional copy of the patient's defective gene into a sufficient number of the appropriate cell types (such as stem cells) and to have sufficient expression of that gene so that its product functions to correct the deficiency. Attempts have been made to use genetically engineered viruses to carry the DNA of interest into host cells. Viral genes required for propagation are replaced with a working copy of the human gene. This form of therapy has been used (with variable success) to treat conditions such as adenosine deamianse deficiency, chronic granulmatous disease, and X-linked combined severe immune deficiency. Before gene therapy using stem cells finds more widespread clinical utility, several important issues such as the isolation of the appropriate cell population for transduction and association of other side effects (such as leukemia-like condition) with gene therapy must be overcome.

SUMMARY

HSCT is a recognized therapeutic modality for leukemias, lymphomas, solid organ tumors, and a variety of metabolic/immunologic disorders. Sources of HSCs can be bone marrow, peripheral blood, and umbilical cord blood. For an autologous transplant, the patient's own stem cells are collected, frozen, and used later for hematopoietic reconstitution. For an allogeneic transplant, the donor is selected based on the best HLA match from either family members or an unrelated donor. In the future, embryonic stem cells could become a source of hematopoietic stem cells.

Determining the number of stem cells can be performed by counting the MNCs, CD34+ cells, and CFUs. Before transplant, the patient undergoes conditioning chemotherapy/radiotherapy, and then the stem cells are infused. Routine blood counts and chimerism studies (in allogeneic SCT only) can be performed to assess the engraftment. Complications of SCT include graft rejection, GVHD, opportunistic infections, and recurrence of malignant disease.

REVIEW QUESTIONS

LEVEL I

1. Which of the following properties is (are) attributable to stem cells? (Objective 3)
   a. self-renewal
   b. multilineage differentiation
   c. mononuclear morphology
   d. all the above

LEVEL II

1. What does the term *chimerism* mean? (Objective 6)
   a. recovery of recipient's red cells
   b. absence of malignant cells
   c. presence of donor hematopoietic stem cells in a recipient
   d. recovery of patient's white cells and platelets only

REVIEW QUESTIONS (continued)

LEVEL I

2. What is (are) the source(s) of hematopoietic stem cells? (Objective 1)
   a. bone marrow
   b. peripheral blood
   c. umbilical cord blood
   d. all of the above

3. What form of transplant can be used for inherited genetic diseases? (Objective 2)
   a. autologous stem cell transplant
   b. allogeneic stem cell transplant
   c. syngeneic stem cell transplant
   d. stored autologous cord blood

4. What is a syngeneic transplant? (Objective 1)
   a. infusion of stem cells from any donor into the recipient
   b. infusion of patient's own stem cells
   c. infusion of stem cells from an identical twin
   d. infusion of stem cells from different species

5. What cells are usually CD34-positive? (Objective 3)
   a. maturing myeloid cells
   b. stem cells
   c. B lymphocytes
   d. T lymphocytes

6. Which of the following is correct regarding allogeneic stem cell transplant and ABO antigens? (Objective 4)
   a. ABO antigens do not need to be matched.
   b. ABO antigens are strongly expressed on stem cells.
   c. The O group patient should not receive stem cells from A or B blood group donors.
   d. ABO antigens should always be matched.

7. What is the single most important factor considered in donor selection for an allogeneic transplant? (Objective 4)
   a. HLA compatibility with the recipient
   b. ABO compatibility with the recipient
   c. CMV status of the donor
   d. HLA and ABO compatibility with the recipient

8. Which of the following infections can be serious in the peri-transplant period? (Objective 5)
   a. bacterial
   b. fungal
   c. cytomegalovirus
   d. all of the above

9. Severe GVHD usually is seen in which group of patients? (Objective 6)
   a. syngeneic SCT
   b. autologous SCT
   c. unmatched allogeneic SCT
   d. umbilical cord stem transplant

LEVEL II

2. What is the most appropriate form of transplant in an adult patient with CML weighing 80 kg? (Objective 4)
   a. autologous SCT
   b. umbilical cord SCT
   c. allogeneic SCT
   d. none of the above; transplant is not indicated in patients with CML

3. A risk for GVHD is carried by a patient who has: (Objective 4)
   a. received allogeneic SCT
   b. received autologous SCT
   c. received both allogeneic and autologous SCT
   d. received autologous SCT for only solid organ tumors

4. What are the three factors necessary to set the stage for GVHD? (Objective 4)
   a. immunocompetent donor T lymphocytes, ABO antigens, and immunosuppressed host
   b. immunosuppressed donor T lymphocytes, HLA alloantigens, and immunosuppressed host
   c. immunocompetent donor B lymphocytes, HLA alloantigens, and immunosuppressed host
   d. immunocompetent donor T lymphocytes, HLA alloantigens, and immunosuppressed host

5. What procedure usually is used to quantify HSCs? (Objective 3)
   a. lymphocyte count
   b. CD4 count by flow cytometry
   c. monocyte count by automated cell counter
   d. CD34 count by flow cytometry

6. Which of the following infections can be serious in patients after SCT? (Objective 4)
   a. pseudomonas
   b. cytomegalovirus
   c. fungal
   d. all of the above

7. This test is appropriate to determine long-term engraftment of HSCs only when donor and recipient are of the opposite sex. (Objective 6)
   a. detection of RBC antigens
   b. ISH with sex chromosomes
   c. typing of VNTR polymorphism by DNA amplification
   d. platelet and neutrophil counts

8. GVL effect is seen after SCT in patients who: (Objective 4)
   a. have received autologous transplant
   b. have received allogeneic transplant
   c. have received either autologous or allogeneic transplant
   d. have received umbilical cord transplant

REVIEW QUESTIONS (continued)

LEVEL I

10. What organ(s)/tissue(s) is (are) usually involved in GVHD? (Objective 6)
    a. skin only
    b. skin, liver, and/or the gastrointestinal tract
    c. liver only
    d. gastrointestinal tract only

LEVEL II

9. For autologous peripheral SCT, the patient usually undergoes therapy in which sequence? (Objective 5)
    a. myeloablative therapy, apheresis, and then G-CSF
    b. G-CSF followed by myeloablative therapy and then apheresis
    c. cytotoxic chemotherapy followed by G-CSF and then apheresis to collect CD34+ cells
    d. myeloablative therapy and then apheresis to collect CD34+ cells

10. What is the sequence in which successful engraftment occurs after SCT? (Objective 6)
    a. Neutrophils are increased first followed by an increase in platelets.
    b. Platelets are increased first followed by an increase in neutrophils.
    c. Red cells are increased first followed by an increase in platelets.
    d. Red cells and platelets are increased followed by an increase in neutrophils.

www.pearsonhighered.com/mckenzie

Use this address to access the interactive Companion Website created for this textbook. Find additional information, tables and figures. Evaluate your command of the chapter information using case studies and critical thinking and multiple choice questions.

REFERENCES

1. Jacobson LO, Marks EK, Robson MJ, Gaston E, Zirkle RE. Effect of spleen protection on mortality following x-irradiation. *J Lab Clin Med.* 1949;34:1538–43.

2. Lorenz E, Uphoff D, Reid TR, Shelton E. Modification of irradiation injury in mice and guinea pigs by bone marrow injections. *J Natl Cancer Inst.* 1951;12:197–201.

3. Wilson A, Trumpp A. Bone marrow hematopoietic stem cell niches. *Nat Rev Immunol.* 2006;6(2):93–106

4. Speck B, Bortin MM, Champlin R, Goldman JM, Herzig RM, McGlave PB et al. Allogeneic bone-marrow transplantation for chronic myelogenous leukaemia. *Lancet.* 1984;1:665–68.

5. Copeland EA. Hematopoietic stem cell transplantation. *N Engl J Med.* 2006;354(17):1813–26

6. Begovich AB, Erlich HA. HLA typing for bone marrow transplantation: New polymerase chain reaction-based methods. *JAMA.* 1995; 273:586–91.

7. Beatty PG. The immunogenetics of bone marrow transplantation. *Transfus Med Rev.* 1994;8:45–58.

8. Beatty PG, Clift RA, Mickelson EM, Nispero SBB, Flournoy N, Martin PJ et al. Marrow transplantation from related donors other than HLA-identical siblings. *N Engl J Med.* 1985;313:765–71.

9. Vogelsang GB, Hess AD, Santos GW. Acute graft-versus-host disease: Clinical characteristics in the cyclosporine era. *Medicine.* 1988;67: 163–74.

10. Kernan NA, Bartsch G, Ash RC, Beatty PG, Champlin R, Filipovich A et al. Analysis of 462 transplantations from unrelated donors facilitated by the National Marrow Donor Program. *N Engl J Med.* 1993;328:593–602.

11. National Marrow Donor Program Survey. www.marrow.org. Accessed Dec. 19, 2008.

12. Copelan EA, Penza SL. Preparative regimens for stem cell transplantation. In: Hoffman R, Benz EJ Jr, Shattil SJ, Furie B, Cohen HJ, Silberstein LE, McGlave P, eds. *Hematology: Basic Principles and Practice,* 3rd ed. Philadelphia: Churchill Livingstone; 2000:1628–42.

13. Stein AS, Forman SJ. Autologous hematopoietic stem cell transplantation for acute myeloid leukemia. In: Thomas ED, Blume KG, Forman SJ, eds. *Hematopoietic Stem Cell Transplantation,* 2nd ed. Boston: Blackwell Science; 1999:963–77.

14. Armitage JO. Bone marrow transplantation. *N Engl J Med.* 1994;330: 827–38.

15. Blaise D, Gaspard MH, Stoppa AM, Michel G, Gastaut JA, Lepeu G, Tubiana N, Blanc AP, Rossi JF, Novakovitch G et al. Allogeneic or autologous bone marrow transplantation for acute lymphoblastic leukemia in first complete remission. *Bone Marrow Transplant.* 1990;5(1):7–12.

16. Ballen KK. New trends in umbilical cord blood transplantation. *Blood.* 2005;105(10):3786–92.

17. Wagner JE, Rosenthal J, Sweetman R, Shu XO, Davies SM, Ramsay NK et al. Successful transplantation of HLA-matched and HLA-mismatched umbilical cord blood from unrelated donors: Analysis of engraftment and acute graft-versus-host disease. *Blood.* 1996;88: 795–802.

18. Gluckman E, Rocha V, Boyer-Chammard A, Locatelli F, Arcese W, Pasquini R et al. Outcome of cord-blood transplantation from related and unrelated donors. Eurocord Transplant Group and the European Blood and Marrow Transplantation Group. *N Engl J Med.* 1997;337:373–81.

19. Gluckman E, Broxmeyer HE, Auerbach AD, Friedman HS, Douglas GW, Devergie A et al. Hematopoietic reconstitution in a patient with Fanconi's anemia by means of umbilical-cord blood from an HLA-identical sibling. *N Engl J Med.* 1989;321:1174–78.

20. Rubinstein P, Carrier C, Scaradavou A, Kurtzberg J, Adamson J, Migliaccio AR et al. Outcomes among 562 recipients of placental-blood transplants from unrelated donors. *N Engl J Med.* 1998;339:1565–77.

21. Papayannopoulou T. Current mechanistic scenarios in hematopoietic stem/progenitor cell mobilization. *Blood.* 2004;103(5):1580–85.

22. Schots R, Van Riet I, Damiaens S, Flament J, Lacor P, Staelens Y et al. The absolute number of circulating CD34+ cells predicts the number of hematopoietic stem cells that can be collected by apheresis. *Bone Marrow Transplant.* 1996;17:509–15.

23. Rubinstein P, Dobrila L, Rosenfield RE, Adamson JW, Migliaccio G, Migliaccio AR et al. Processing and cryopreservation of placental/umbilical cord blood for unrelated bone marrow reconstitution. *Proc Natl Acad Sci USA.* 1995;92:10,119–22.

24. Harris DT, Schumacher MJ, Rychlik S, Booth A, Acevedo A, Rubinstein P et al. Collection, separation, and cryopreservation of umbilical cord blood for use in transplantation. *Bone Marrow Transplant.* 1994;13:135–43.

25. Wissel ME, Lasky LC. Progenitor processing and cryopreservation. In: Brecher ME, Lasky LC, Sacher RA, Issitt LA, eds. *Hematopoietic Progenitor Cells: Processing, Standards, and Practice.* Bethesda, MD: AABB; 1995:109–24.

26. Sims LC, Brecher ME, Gertis K, Jenkins A, Nickischer D, Schmitz JL et al. Enumeration of CD34-positive stem cells: Evaluation and comparison of three methods. *J Hematother.* 1997;6:213–26.

27. Sutherland DR, Anderson L, Keeney M, Nayar R, Chin-Yee I. The ISHAGE guidelines for CD34+ cell determination by flow cytometry. International Society of Hematotherapy and Graft Engineering. *J Hematother.* 1996;5:213–26.

28. Keeney M, Chin-Yee I, Weir K, Popma J, Nayar R, Sutherland DR. Single platform flow cytometric absolute CD34+ cell counts based on the ISHAGE guidelines. International Society of Hematotherapy and Graft Engineering. *Cytometry.* 1998;34:61–70.

29. Lasky LC, Johnson NL. Quality assurance in marrow processing. In: Areman EM, Deeg HJ, Sacher RA, eds. *Bone Marrow and Stem Cell Processing: A Manual of Current Techniques.* Philadelphia: FA Davis; 1992:386–443.

30. Douay L, Gorin NC, Mary JY, Lemarie E, Lopez M, Najman A et al. Recovery of CFU-GM from cryopreserved marrow and in vivo evaluation after autologous bone marrow transplantation are predictive of engraftment. *Exp Hematol.* 1986;14:358–65.

31. Bensinger W, Appelbaum F, Rowley S, Storb R, Sanders J, Lilleby K et al. Factors that influence collection and engraftment of autologous peripheral-blood stem cells. *J Clin Oncol.* 1995;13:2547–55.

32. Haas R, Mohle R, Fruhauf S, Goldschmidt H, Witt B, Flentje M et al. Patient characteristics associated with successful mobilizing and autografting of peripheral blood progenitor cells in malignant lymphoma. *Blood.* 1994;83:3787–94.

33. Siena S, Schiavo R, Pedrazzoli P, Carlo-Stella C. Therapeutic relevance of CD34 cell dose in blood cell transplantation for cancer therapy. *J Clin Oncol* 2000;18(6):1360–77.

34. Bryant E, Martin PJ. Documentation of engraftment and characterization of chimerism following hematopoietic cell transplantation. In: Thomas ED, Blume KG, Forman SJ, eds. *Hematopoietic Stem Cell Transplantation,* 2nd ed. Boston: Blackwell Science; 1999:197–206.

35. Jadus MR, Wepsic HT. The role of cytokines in graft-versus-host reactions and disease. *Bone Marrow Transplant.* 1992;10:1–14.

36. Krenger W, Ferrara JL. Dysregulation of cytokines during graft-versus-host disease. *J Hematother.* 1996;5:3–14.

37. Cao TM, Shizuru JA, Wong RM, Sheehan K, Laport GG, Stockerl-Goldstein KE, Johnston LJ, Stuart MJ, Grumet FC, Negrin RS, Lowsky R. *Blood.* 2005;105(6):2300–6.

38. Chao NJ, Schmidt GM, Niland JC, Amylon MD, Dagis AC, Long GD et al. Cyclosporine, methotrexate, and prednisone compared with cyclosporine and prednisone for prophylaxis of acute graft-versus-host disease. *N Engl J Med.* 1993;329:1225–30.

39. Porter D, Antin J. Graft-versus-leukemia effect of allogeneic bone marrow transplantation and donor mononuclear cell infusions. In: Winter J, ed. *Blood Stem Cell Transplantation.* Norwell, MA: Kluwer Academic; 1996:57–85.

40. Mackinnon S, Papadopoulos EB, Carabasi MH, Reich L, Collins NH, Boulad F et al. Adoptive immunotherapy evaluating escalating doses of donor leukocytes for relapse of chronic myeloid leukemia after bone marrow transplantation: Separation of graft-versus-leukemia responses from graft-versus-host disease. *Blood.* 1995;86:1261–68.

41. Bowden RA, Slichter SJ, Sayers MH, Mori M, Cays MJ, Meyers JD. Use of leukocyte-depleted platelets and cytomegalovirus-seronegative red blood cells for prevention of primary cytomegalovirus infection after marrow transplant. *Blood.* 1991;78:246–50.

42. Leukocyte reduction for the prevention of transfusion-transmitted cytomegalovirus. Association Bulletin #97-2. Bethesda, MD. 1997: AABB.

43. Bowden RA, Slichter SJ, Sayers M et al. A comparison of filtered leukocyte-reduced and cytomegalovirus (CMV) seronegative blood products for the prevention of transfusion-associated CMV infection after marrow transplant. *Blood.* 1995;86:3598–603.

44. Preiksaitis JK. The cytomegalovirus-"safe" blood product: Is leukoreduction equivalent to anibody screening? *Transfus Med Rev.* 2000;14:112–36.

45. Chinen J, Puck JM. Perspectives of gene therapy for primary immunodeficiencies. *Curr Opin Allergy Clin Immunol.* 2004;4(6):523–27.

28

Morphologic Analysis of Body Fluids in the Hematology Laboratory

C. Nanette Clare, M.D.

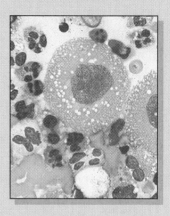

■ OBJECTIVES—LEVEL I

At the end of this unit of study, the student should be able to:

1. List the types of body fluids studied in the clinical laboratory, and describe the body cavities in which they are found.

2. List and describe the normal tissue cells seen in each body fluid type.

3. Describe various artifact types that can be seen in body fluid preparations including those in cytocentrifuged specimens.

4. Define *transudate, exudate,* and *chylous fluid,* and differentiate among these fluid types given laboratory data.

5. Describe the appearance of bacterial and fungal organisms in Wright-stained preparations, and suggest methods to confirm them.

6. List the morphologic features of malignant cells on Wright-stained preparations.

7. List the types of crystals that can be found in joint fluids, and associate them with pathologic conditions.

■ OBJECTIVES—LEVEL II

At the end of this unit of study, the student should be able to:

1. Identify the procedure used to obtain each type of body fluid.

2. Describe the production of cerebrospinal fluid (CSF).

3. Compare and contrast how each of the following fluids is formed: transudate, exudate, and chylous fluid.

4. Evaluate the significance of microorganisms present in Wright-stained body fluid preparations.

5. Compare and contrast the morphologic distinction between benign tissue cells and malignant cells in cytocentrifuged, Wright-stained preparations of body fluids, and identify these cells when seen.

6. Recognize erythrophagocytosis, and explain its significance in CSF.

7. Define *birefringence,* and explain its use in examining body fluids.

8. Identify and differentiate the various types of crystals that can be found in joint fluids, and associate them with particular disorders.

9. Use peripheral blood and CSF cell counts to differentiate true hemorrhage from a traumatic tap.

KEY TERMS

Arachnoid mater
Ascites
Ascitic fluid
Birefringence
Cardiac tamponade
Central nervous system (CNS)
Cerebrospinal fluid (CSF)
Chylous
Dura mater
Effusion
Exudate
Meninges
Pericardial cavity
Pericardium
Peritoneal cavity
Peritoneum
Pia mater
Pleura
Pleural cavity
Pseudochylous
Synovium
Transudate

BACKGROUND BASICS

Although the study of body fluids is not generally included in textbooks of hematology, most clinical hematology laboratories have the responsibility of performing total cell counts and differential cell counts on body fluid samples. Much of this chapter can be read independently of the other chapters. However, the chapter builds on the general knowledge of hematologic morphology and hematologic neoplasms. You should review the following concepts before beginning this chapter.

Level I

▶ Recognize the common types of normal cells found in the peripheral blood. (Chapters 1, 5, 7)
▶ List the major types of neoplastic hematopoietic disorders. (Chapter 21)
▶ Describe the major types of lymphoma. (Chapter 26)

Level II

▶ Recognize reactive hematopoietic cells found in the peripheral blood. (Chapters 7, 19, 20)
▶ Describe and recognize the hematopoietic precursors found in the normal bone marrow. (Chapters 5, 7, 35)
▶ Describe and identify the cells associated with the various types of acute leukemia. (Chapters 24, 25)
▶ Compare and contrast the various types of lymphoproliferative disorders. (Chapter 26)

 CASE STUDY

We will address this case study throughout the chapter.
Carolyn, a 51-year-old woman who is otherwise in her usual state of good health, has flulike symptoms. After two weeks, her cough and fever persist. Antibiotics are started, and two days later she has severe right-side chest pain and worsening shortness of breath. Radiologic studies show a large effusion in the right pleural cavity. A thoracentesis is performed, and 1 liter of thick, yellow fluid is aspirated. As you read and study this chapter, think about the type of fluid this could be and the laboratory studies that should be done on the fluid to assist in diagnosis.

▶ OVERVIEW

The hematology laboratory usually receives body fluids for cell counts and morphologic evaluation. The types of cells found and their concentration are helpful information for the clinician in arriving at a diagnosis. The cells that can be found in these fluids include white blood cells (WBCs) and red blood cells (RBCs) as well as tissue and tumor cells. The cytocentrifuge is used to prepare slide preparations for morphologic review, and Wright's stain is used to stain the cells on the slide. Identifying and differentiating the various types of cells seen in body fluids requires experience. However, all laboratory professionals who perform body fluid analysis should be able to differentiate most malignant cells from benign cells. This chapter describes the sites where body fluids are found, the methods in which the fluids are obtained, and an explanation of why fluids accumulate at these sites. The focus of the chapter is the description of the types of cells and inclusions that can be found in each fluid. The artifacts that can be found and the way to differentiate them from significant inclusions are also described and depicted. This chapter is presented in atlas format, because this is the most helpful way to discuss the morphology of body fluid cells. This chapter does not discuss other studies, such as those performed in the chemistry and microbiology laboratories.

▶ INTRODUCTION

The hematology laboratory plays an increasingly important role in the morphologic evaluation of body fluids. This is primarily due to the use of the cytocentrifuge, which markedly improves morphology over the previously used direct smear technique. The cytocentrifuge is an instrument used to prepare slides from body fluid specimens other than peripheral blood. The sample is centrifuged directly onto a glass slide and yields a concentrate of cells with excellent morphology.

The Wright-stained, cytocentrifuge-prepared slide is made in the hematology laboratory for the purpose of performing a differential WBC count. However, this slide also is valuable in making many important diagnoses, both benign and malignant. Most malignant cells, including hematopoietic malignancies, carcinomas, and sarcomas, can be recognized microscopically. The hematopoietic malignancies are generally easier to diagnose from the Wright-stained slide than from the routine cytology preparation, which is prepared by alcohol fixation of cells and Papanicolaou stain. Another advantage of the slides made in the hematology laboratory is that these slides are prepared within an hour of specimen receipt, whereas cytology preparations take longer. Additionally, important nonmalignant findings, such as intracellular bacteria and fungi, that can be diagnosed on Wright's stain are frequently not seen on cytology slides. Hematologic slides, however, should not replace cytology preparations, which have better retention of nuclear detail and are superior to hematologic slides when attempting to determine the specific type of carcinoma or sarcoma present. Both techniques are necessary and aid in arriving at the most accurate diagnosis.

▶ TYPES OF BODY FLUIDS

The body fluids discussed in this chapter are most commonly sampled. They are derived from the pleural, pericardial, and peritoneal cavities and from the central nervous system (CNS) and joint spaces (Table 28-1 ✪). The pleural, pericardial, and peritoneal cavities are actually potential spaces and do not contain any appreciable amount of fluid in the normal setting. The CNS, however, normally contains a specific amount of fluid to protect the brain and spinal cord. The joint spaces also have a consistent amount of fluid present for the continual lubrication of the bone surfaces and delivery of nutrients.

The **pleural cavities** (left and right) consist of the space between the lung and the inside portion of the chest wall. A thin membrane, called the **pleura,** lines these cavities. The pleura is composed of a continuous single layer of mesothelial cells (derived from embryonic mesoderm) and submesothelial connective tissue (Figure 28-1 ■). The pleural lining that covers the lung is the visceral pleura, and the lining that covers the inside of the chest wall is the parietal pleura. The pleural lining's purpose is to provide a moist surface to minimize friction between the lung and chest wall as respiration occurs. In disease states, the mesothelial cells multiply, the lining thickens, and fluid collects in the cavity. The contents of the fluid depend on the pathologic process causing the fluid accumulation.

The heart is enclosed in a saclike structure called the *pericardial sac,* which also is lined by mesothelial cells. The **pericardial cavity** is the anatomic region between the outermost aspect of the heart and the innermost aspect of the pericardial sac. The **pericardium** is a thin membrane that provides a continuous covering of the pericardial cavity composed of a single layer of mesothelial cells and submesothelial connective tissue. The lining covering the outside of the heart is the visceral pericardium, and the lining covering the inside of the pericardial sac is the parietal pericardium (Figure 28-1).

During certain pathologic events, fluid can accumulate in the pericardial sac. If the fluid accumulates rapidly (a minimum of 250 mL) or if a relatively large amount (1000 mL) accumulates over a longer time, there may be a serious restriction to the normal heart beat and venous return to the heart, creating a life-threatening event. This pathologic compression of the heart due to an accumulation of fluid is called **cardiac tamponade.** In this event, fluid must be removed quickly either by pericardial aspiration or surgery to save the patient's life.

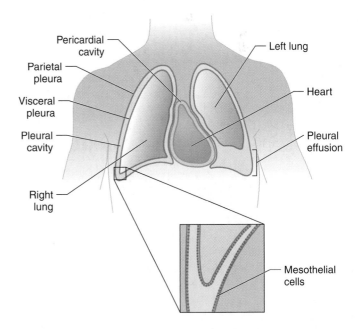

■ **FIGURE 28-1**   Diagram of right lung illustrating the pleural cavity and inset showing mesothelial cells of the parietal and visceral pleura. Illustration of heart shows the pericardial cavity. Diagram of the lung shows the abnormal accumulation of fluid (effusion) in the pleural cavity compressing the lower left lung.

✪ TABLE 28-1		
List of Site of Origin of Body Fluids with Terminology of Procedure to Obtain Fluid and Type of Fluid		
Anatomic Site	**Procedure**	**Fluid Obtained**
Pleural cavity	Thoracentesis	Pleural fluid
Pericardial cavity	Pericardial aspiration	Pericardial fluid
Peritoneal cavity	Paracentesis	Peritoneal fluid (ascitic fluid)
Joint space	Joint aspiration (arthrocentesis)	Synovial fluid
Spinal cord	Spinal tap, lumbar puncture	Cerebrospinal fluid

The **peritoneal cavity** consists of the space between the inside of the abdominal wall and the outside of the stomach, small and large intestine, liver, and superior aspect of the urinary bladder and uterus. The kidneys are positioned posterior to the peritoneal lining (the **peritoneum**) and are referred to as *retroperitoneal*. Other retroperitoneal organs include the pancreas, duodenum, some lymph nodes, and the abdominal aorta. The peritoneal lining, consisting of one layer of mesothelial cells and submesothelial connective tissue, is identical to the pleural lining. The lining covering the inside of the abdominal wall is the parietal peritoneum, and the lining covering the organ surfaces is the visceral peritoneum (Figure 28-2 ■). In disease states, the cell layers will thicken and fluid can accumulate; this is referred to as **ascitic fluid** or **ascites.**

The **central nervous system (CNS)** consisting of the brain and spinal cord is normally lined by special membranes referred to as *meningeal membranes,* or *meninges,* that protect it. The **meninges** consist of a relatively thick **dura mater,** the outermost membrane; a thinner **arachnoid mater,** the middle membrane; and an innermost **pia mater** that lies directly on the surface of the brain and spinal cord.

The **cerebrospinal fluid (CSF)** occupies the subarachnoid space between the arachnoid mater and pia mater and protects the brain and spinal cord (Figure 28-3 ■). The choroid plexus cells and ependymal lining cells found in the ventricles produce the CSF. This CSF fluid circulates through the ventricular system in the cerebrum, cerebellum, and brain stem and completely covers the surface of the brain and spinal cord. The CSF is a product of ultrafiltration and active secretion and is made at a rate of approximately 21 mL/hour.[1] The CSF is reabsorbed by the arachnoid cells. The total volume of CSF in adults is 90–150 mL. Neonates have a CSF volume of 10–60 mL. In certain disease states, the CSF's content changes.

 ## Checkpoint! 1

To obtain a sample of CSF for analysis, the needle must be inserted into what area of the central nervous system?

Some bony joints of the body are lined by special membranes called the **synovium** that normally consist of a single layer of synovial cells (Figure 28-4 ■). The joint space contains synovial fluid that acts as a lubricant and a transport medium for nutrients to get to the joint's bone surfaces. The synovial fluid is produced in part by the synovial cells and is an ultrafiltrate of plasma. Synovial fluid also contains a mucopolysaccharide called *hyaluronic acid,* which sometimes makes the fluid so thick that it hampers laboratory studies.

► COMMON CELL TYPES SEEN IN BODY FLUIDS

Segmented neutrophils (segs) are frequently seen in the pleural, pericardial, and peritoneal fluids in varying numbers. The neutrophils have the same appearance as in peripheral blood smears. Sometimes, however, cytocentrifuge artifactual changes can be seen with nuclear segments being thrown to the periphery of the cytoplasm, creating a hypersegmented appearance (Figure 28-5 ■). Degeneration of neutrophils is seen more frequently in body fluid samples than in peripheral blood smears. The dying cells show cytoplasmic vacuolization and separation of nuclear segments with dense-staining chromatin (Figure 28-6 ■). These cells can be mistaken for nucleated RBC and even yeast organisms. Neutrophilic precursors, such as promyelocytes, myelocytes, and metamyelocytes, are not commonly seen but if present can represent a chronic inflammatory process or true marrow disorder, such as myeloproliferative disorders, myelodysplastic states, and leukemia. Myeloblasts are usually seen only in the latter three.

Lymphocytes are frequently present in all types of fluids in variable numbers. The lymphocytes vary in morphology from small to large and transformed (reactive). In cytocentrifuge preparations, the lymphocyte nucleoli can be artifactually more prominent than in peripheral blood smears, the nuclear shape can be irregular, and the cytoplasm can have artifactual projections[2] (Figures 28-7 ■ and 28-8 ■). If the lymphocytes are neoplastic (leukemias, lymphomas), the morphology depends on the type of neoplasm, and the cells are homogeneous in appearance. Flow cytometry or

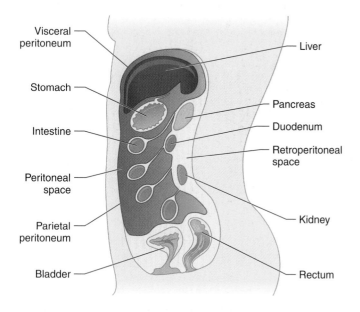

■ FIGURE 28-2   Abdominal cavity illustrating the peritoneal space between the inside of the abdominal wall and the outside of the liver, stomach, intestines, and dome of the bladder.

Visceral peritoneum
Liver
Stomach
Pancreas
Intestine
Duodenum
Retroperitoneal space
Peritoneal space
Parietal peritoneum
Kidney
Bladder
Rectum

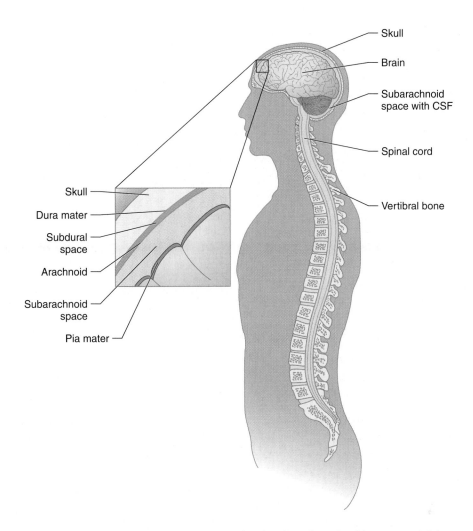

■ FIGURE 28-3   Central nervous system showing the subarachnoid space containing cerebral spinal fluid (CSF) covering the brain and spinal cord. Inset illustrates the meninges: dura mater, arachnoid mater, and pia mater.

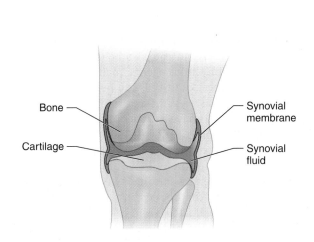

■ FIGURE 28-4   Knee joint illustrating synovial membrane lining and synovial fluid.

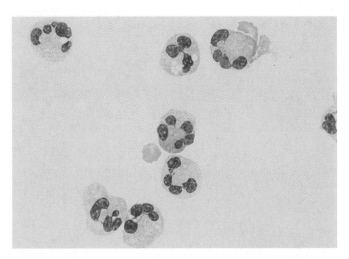

■ FIGURE 28-5   Artifactual change in neutrophils showing nuclear lobes thrown to the periphery of the cytoplasm. (Slides in this chapter are all cytocentrifuge prepared body fluids, Wright-stained. Magnification 1000× unless otherwise noted.)

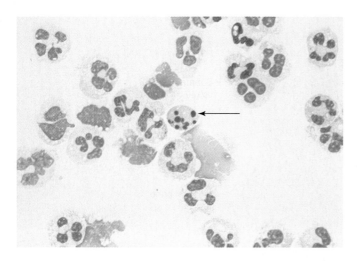

■ FIGURE 28-6   In the center is a degenerating neutrophil with separation of nuclear lobes and dense staining of the chromatin.

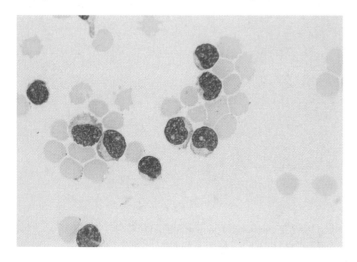

■ FIGURE 28-7   Artifactual change in lymphocytes with overly prominent nucleoli.

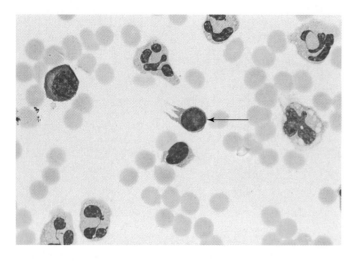

■ FIGURE 28-8   Artifactual change in lymphocytes with cytoplasmic projections.

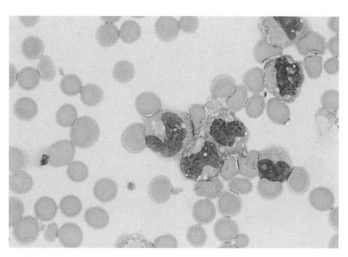

■ FIGURE 28-9   Monocytes in pleural fluid.

immunoperoxidase techniques can be helpful in distinguishing benign versus malignant lymphocytes.

Monocytes in body fluids can appear similar to that seen in peripheral blood smears or can be larger with abundant, vacuolated cytoplasm (histiocyte), or they can have actual phagocytosed material (macrophage, phagocyte) (Figures 28-9 ■, 28-10 ■, and 28-11 ■). The distinction among the three morphologic types (monocytes, histiocytes, and macrophages) is not clinically important; however, in some cases, the phagocytosed cells or organisms can be diagnostically important. When large vacuoles fuse, a "signet ring" appearance with the nucleus flattened against the cell membrane occurs (Figure 28-12 ■). Only a few monocytes are present in CSF, and histiocytes/macrophages usually are seen in the CSF only in pathologic states. Plasma cells are not seen in normal fluids and usually are present only in chronic inflammatory disorders (Figure 28-13 ■).

Eosinophils, basophils, and mast cells can be present in small numbers in pleural, pericardial, peritoneal, or joint fluids. Increased numbers of these cell types are seen in various disorders and may correlate with peripheral eosinophilia or basophilia.[3] Eosinophils are frequently seen in nonspecific or idiopathic effusions but can also be present in effusions caused by various infectious agents, malignancies, and connective tissue disorders. Mast cells can be distinguished from basophils because mast cells have a round (not segmented) nucleus, and mast cells have a higher number of cytoplasmic granules than basophils. The granules in mast cells are smaller than those seen in basophils (Figures 28-14 ■ and 28-15 ■). An increase in the number of basophils can correlate with myeloproliferative disorders involving body fluids.

Benign tissue cells can be seen in any of the body fluids and must be differentiated from malignant cells (Table 28-2 ✪). Benign mesothelial cells can be seen in the pleural, pericardial, and peritoneal fluids. These are large cells that have a moderate to abundant amount of cytoplasm. The cytoplasm can be light or dark blue and occasionally contain

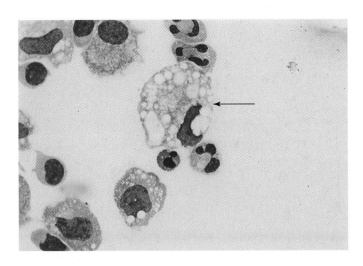

■ FIGURE 28-10 Histiocyte in pleural fluid.

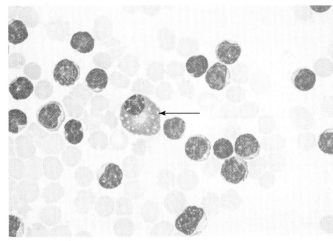

■ FIGURE 28-13 Plasma cell in pleural fluid.

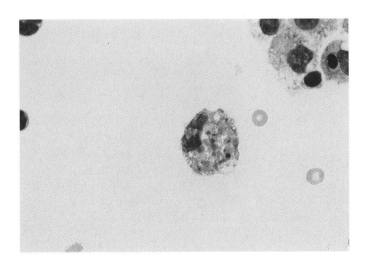

■ FIGURE 28-11 Macrophage in pleural fluid.

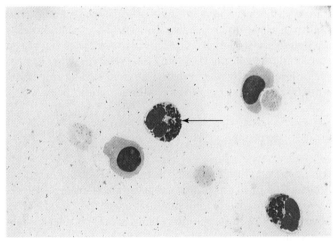

■ FIGURE 28-14 Basophil in pleural fluid.

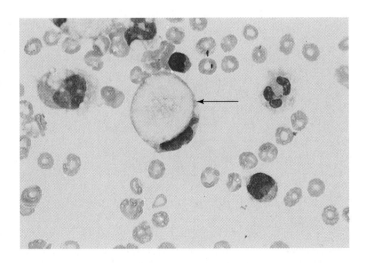

■ FIGURE 28-12 Macrophage in pleural fluid with single large vacuole giving a "signet ring" appearance.

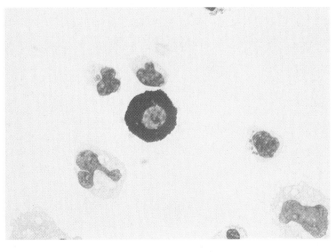

■ FIGURE 28-15 Mast cell in pleural fluid.

☼ TABLE 28-2

Normal Existing Tissue Cells Found in the Various Body Fluids

Fluid Type	Normal Tissue Cells
Cerebrospinal	Ependymal, choroid plexus cells, arachnoid
Pleural, pericardial, peritoneal	Mesothelial
Joint	Synovial

granules or phagocytosed debris. The nucleus is eccentric with a homogeneous chromatin pattern. Nucleoli can be seen, and if present, are blue with a smooth membrane (Figure 28-16 ■). The tissue cells present in joint fluids are synovial and have a similar appearance to mesothelial cells with a somewhat denser cytoplasm (Figure 28-17 ■). The tissue cells (choroid plexus and ependymal) that can be seen in CSF tend to cluster and can have cytoplasmic granules and slightly irregular nuclei (Figure 28-18 ■). The arachnoid cells are frequently seen as a syncytium with a mass of cytoplasm containing several nuclei (Figure 28-19 ■). These benign tissue cells are usually seen only in CSF from infants and adults who have had recent neurosurgery or a shunt in place.

▶ MORPHOLOGIC FINDINGS DUE TO ARTIFACT

Some artifactual findings such as peripheral displacement of the nucleus in neutrophils, cytoplasmic extensions of lymphocytes, and overly prominent nucleoli of lymphocytes have already been mentioned (Table 28-3 ☼). Other artifactual changes can resemble actual pathologic findings, and interpretation must be made cautiously. Starch particles can be an in vitro contaminant in any type of body fluid. This

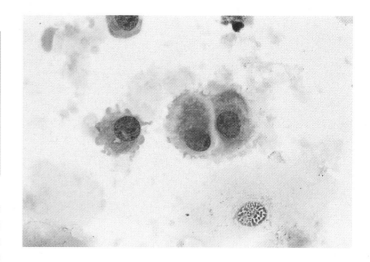

■ FIGURE 28-17   Synovial cells in joint fluid.

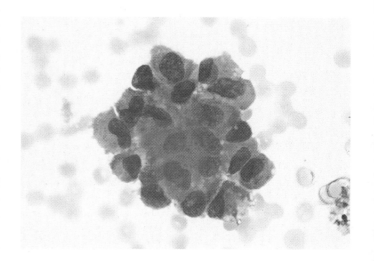

■ FIGURE 28-18   Choroid plexus cells in CSF.

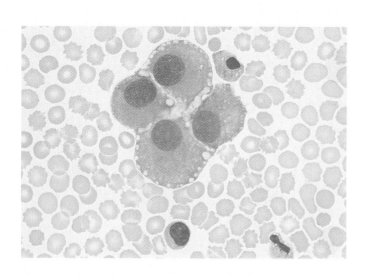

■ FIGURE 28-16   Benign mesothelial cells in pleural fluid.

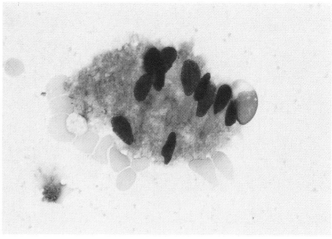

■ FIGURE 28-19   Arachnoid cell syncytium in CSF.

⊘ TABLE 28-3

Artifacts That Can Be Seen with Wright-Stained Cytocentrifuge Prepared Slides and the Potential Mistaken Interpretation

Artifact	Mistaken Interpretation
Peripheral localization of nuclear lobes in neutrophils	Hypersegmented neutrophils
Degenerating neutrophil	Yeast organisms, nucleated RBC
Overprominence of nucleoli in lymphocytes	Blast cells
Cytoplasmic projections of lymphocytes	Hairy cell leukemia
Single large vacuole in histiocyte	Signet ring cell carcinoma
Starch particles	Yeast organisms, crystals
Stain precipitate	Bacterial organisms
Degenerating tissue cells	Malignant cells

starch is on sterilized surgical gloves used by the physician obtaining fluid from the patient. Starch particles can look like yeast organisms, even budding yeasts if two particles are closely associated. Starch particles usually have a refractile center that is not a feature of yeast and are birefringent (discussed later), showing up as bright Maltese crosslike figures with polarized light (Figure 28-20 ■). Stain precipitate can look like bacterial organisms. If the precipitate appears to be intracellular, changing the fine focus usually shows the precipitate to be in a different plane of focus from the cell. True intracellular bacteria are in the same plane of focus as the cell. Stain precipitate is darker than bacteria and variable in size and can be seen extracellularly, sometimes in distant areas of the slide (Figure 28-21 ■). In difficult cases, an extra slide should be prepared for a gram stain. Early cellular degeneration is exaggerated by the cytocentrifuge and shows irregular nuclear margins and separating chromatin. This can be mistaken for malignant cells (Figure 28-22 ■).

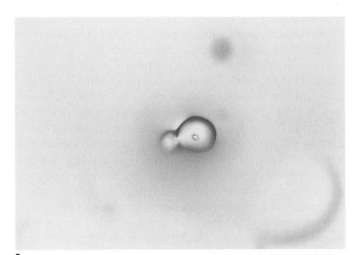

a

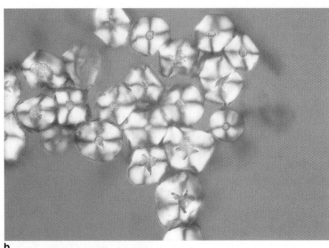

b

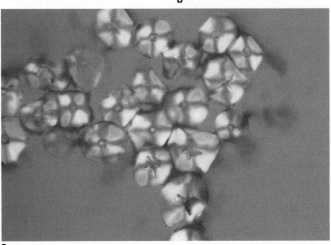

c

■ **FIGURE 28-20**   **a.** Starch particle with plain light resembling yeast. **b.** Starch particles as seen with polarized light appearing as a Maltese cross shape. **c.** Starch particles with polarized light and quartz compensator.

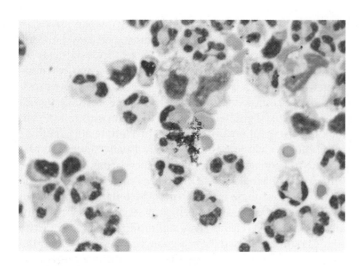

■ FIGURE 28-21   Stain precipitate on top of the cell with precipitate in focus and cells slightly out of focus.

▶ PLEURAL, PERICARDIAL, AND PERITONEAL FLUIDS

Fluids obtained from the pleural, pericardial, and peritoneal cavities have similar findings in various pathologic states and are discussed together. The pleural, pericardial, and peritoneal spaces normally contain a minimal amount of fluid (less than 2.5 mL in the pleural cavity), only enough to keep the lining membranes moist. The fluid is produced by the parietal lining and absorbed by the visceral lining. Fluid is produced by plasma filtration through capillary endothelial cells and depends on four factors: capillary hydrostatic pressure, plasma oncotic pressure, lymphatic resorption, and capillary permeability.[2] Any pathologic state affecting one or several of these four factors can result in abnormal fluid col-

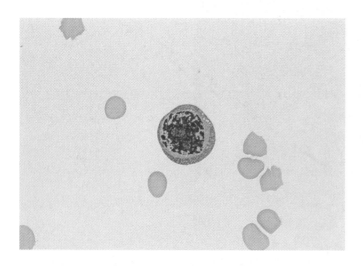

■ FIGURE 28-22   Early cell degeneration.

lection, or **effusion,** in the pleural, pericardial, and peritoneal spaces. In the pleural spaces, accumulation of at least 300 mL is necessary to be detected on chest x-ray, and in the peritoneal cavity accumulation of at least 500 mL is necessary to be detected by abdominal x-ray.[2]

An effusion can accumulate due to a systemic disease state (**transudate**) or a primary pathologic state of the area (**exudate**).[4] Transudates are frequently a result of increased capillary hydrostatic pressure as seen with congestive heart failure or of decreased plasma oncotic pressure as seen with hypoproteinemia due to nephrotic syndrome or liver failure. A transudate most often has a specific gravity of 1.015 or less, a total protein of 3.0 g/dL or lower, a ratio of effusion total protein to serum total protein of less than 0.5, a ratio of effusion lactate dehydrogenase (LD) to serum LD of less than 0.6, and usually a total leukocyte count <1000/μL.[1,2]

An exudate is formed by increased capillary permeability and/or decreased lymphatic resorption. An exudative effusion can be caused by many different pathologic processes, such as bacterial infections, viral infections, neoplasms, and collagen vascular diseases. An exudate has a specific gravity >1.015, a total protein >3.0 g/dL, a ratio of total fluid protein to serum protein >0.5, a ratio of fluid LD to serum LD >0.6, and usually a total leukocyte count >1000/μL.[1,2]

A **chylous** effusion has a characteristic milky, opaque appearance that remains in the supernatant after centrifugation. Chylous effusions result from leakage of lymphatic vessels. In the pleural cavity (chylothorax), this is due to leakage of the major thoracic duct. In the peritoneal cavity, chylous effusions result from blockage of the lymphatic vessels. In both the pleural and peritoneal cavities, chylous effusion most often results from malignancy such as lymphoma or carcinoma or from trauma. This type of fluid is rich in chylomicrons and has elevated triglycerides (>110 mg/dL), and its predominant cells are lymphocytes.[2,5] A **pseudochylous** effusion is also milky and results from a chronic, long-standing effusion due to such conditions as tuberculosis and rheumatoid pleuritis.[2] Pseudochylous effusions do not contain chylomicrons and usually have triglycerides <50 mg/dL. There is a mixed reactive cell population with many inflammatory and necrotic cells.

ⓔ CASE STUDY *(continued from page 584)*

Radiologic studies show a large effusion in the right pleural cavity. A thoracentesis is performed, and 1 liter of thick, yellow fluid is aspirated. Laboratory studies show a total protein of 4.5 g/dL (serum = 6 g/dL), lactate dehydrogenase 40 U/L (serum = 50 U/L), and total leukocyte count of 20,000/μL with 90% segmented neutrophils, 10% histiocytes, and many degenerating cells.

1. Is this a transudate or exudate?
2. Is this a chylous fluid?

NONSPECIFIC REACTIVE CHANGES

The term *nonspecific reactive changes* refers to effusions that have an inflammatory cell response that is not diagnostic for any specific disorder. In various pathologic states, certain types of WBCs can be present in increased numbers. Bacterial infections have a predominance of segmented neutrophils while viral, fungal, and mycobacterial infections can have a predominance of lymphocytes or show a mixed inflammatory response. As in peripheral blood, neutrophils can have toxic granulation, Döhle bodies, and cytoplasmic vacuoles.

Lymphocytes are frequently reactive and transformed, simulating lymphoma cells. The most helpful feature in distinguishing reactive lymphocytes from lymphoma cells is that the former consist of a heterogeneous population of cells with varying nuclear shape, amount of cytoplasm, and degree of cytoplasmic basophilia (Figures 28-23 ■ and 28-24 ■). Lymphoma cells are homogeneous with the same nuclear and cytoplasmic features. The morphology of the lymphoma cells depends on the particular type of lymphoma.

In rare cases, spontaneous formation of lupus erythematosus (LE) cells is apparent. An LE cell is a macrophage, either neutrophil or monocyte, that has phagocytosed a nucleus showing a homogeneous, smooth chromatin pattern (Figure 28-25 ■). The finding of these cells is suspicious but not diagnostic for systemic lupus erythematosus (SLE). Other autoimmune type disorders can also show the LE cell phenomenon. Nevertheless, the identification of these cells can be extremely helpful in arriving at a difficult diagnosis. The LE cell should not be mistaken for simple phagocytosis of cells by macrophages, which is frequently seen. The chromatin of the usual phagocytosed cell is not smooth or homogeneous.

Mesothelial cells can show nonspecific reactive changes, which include multinuclearity, presence of nucleoli, mitotic activity, and sometimes an increase in cell size (Figures 28-26 ■ and 28-27 ■). There also occasionally is an increased

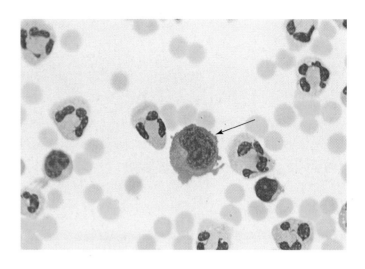

■ FIGURE 28-24   Reactive lymphocyte in pleural fluid.

nuclear-cytoplasmic ratio and nuclear folding simulating carcinoma. Reactive mesothelial cells also can tend to cluster and appear cohesive; however, nuclear molding is not seen (Figure 28-28 ■). In cases when distinguishing reactive mesothelial cells from malignant cells is very difficult, cytology preparations usually are definitive because alcohol fixation and Papanicolaou stain yield better nuclear detail.

✓ Checkpoint! 2

A 32-year-old woman has right-side chest pain and shortness of breath that has worsened over a two-week period. Chest radiologic studies reveal a right pleural effusion, and a thoracentesis is performed. The pleural fluid specimen on a cytocentrifuged, Wright-stained slide reveals cells similar to that seen in Figure 28-7. What is the best interpretation of this finding? If there is a strong concern that this can represent a low-grade lymphoma, what would be the best way to determine whether these are benign on malignant lymphocytes?

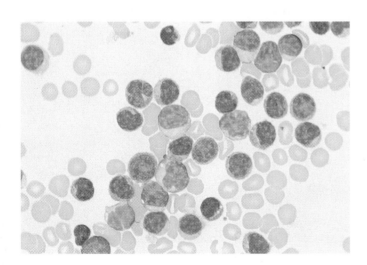

■ FIGURE 28-23   Reactive lymphocytes in pleural fluid.

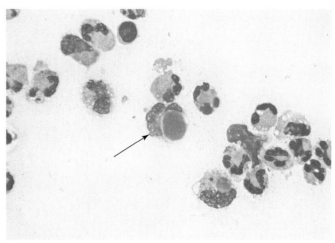

■ FIGURE 28-25   Spontaneous LE cell formation in pleural fluid.

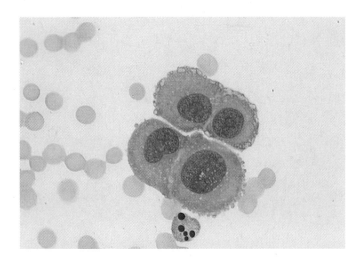

■ FIGURE 28-26 Reactive mesothelial cells in pleural fluid.

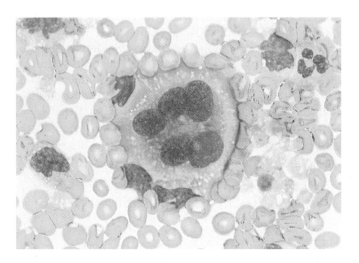

■ FIGURE 28-27 Multinucleated reactive mesothelial cells in pleural fluid.

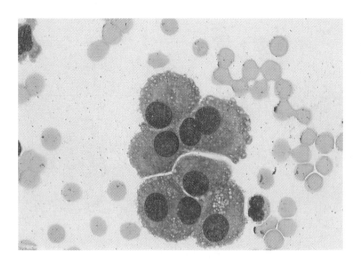

■ FIGURE 28-28 Reactive mesothelial cells in pleural fluid.

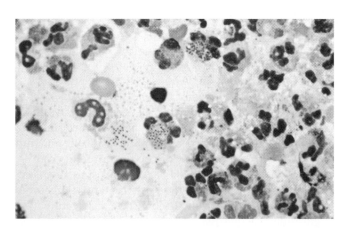

■ FIGURE 28-29 Intracellular and extracellular bacterial cocci, joint fluid.

MICROORGANISMS

Most types of pathogenic bacterial and fungal organisms stain with Wright's stain and are detectable on a routine cytocentrifuge preparation. Bacteria stain blue regardless of the gram stain features. Demonstrating the organisms intracellularly is important because this indicates true pathogenicity rather than in vitro contamination (Figures 28-29■ and 28-30■). Once bacteria have been recognized with Wright's stain, preparing a second cytocentrifuge slide for a gram stain is helpful to confirm the presence of bacteria and to be able to give additional information to the physician while cultures are pending.

Most pathogenic yeasts are found in CSF rather than in pleural, pericardial, or peritoneal fluids. These organisms can be found intracellularly. The different types of pathogenic yeast show some distinguishing features on Wright's stain. This morphologic variance can be used as a clue for an ini-

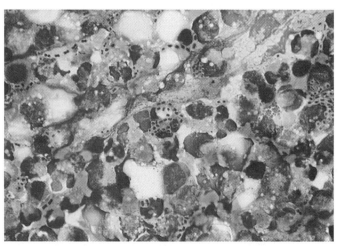

■ FIGURE 28-30 Intracellular and extracellular bacteria, bacilli, peritoneal fluid.

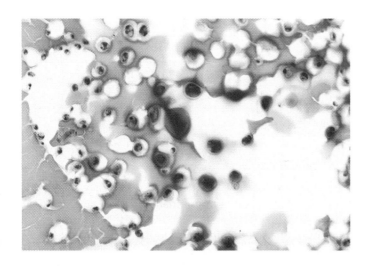

■ FIGURE 28-31   *Cryptococcus neoformans,* CSF.

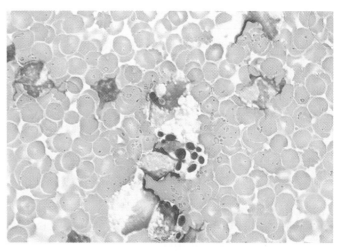

■ FIGURE 28-33   *Candida albicans,* CSF.

tial impression of the specific type of yeast, but cultures must be obtained for definitive identification. The most frequently seen fungal organisms in fluids are *Cryptococcus, Histoplasma, Candida albicans,* and *Candida tropicalis* (Figures 28-31 ■, 28-32 ■, 28-33 ■, and 28-34 ■). Refer to Table 28-4 ✪ for a comparison of morphology.

> **CASE STUDY** *(continued from page 592)*

A cytocentrifuged, Wright-stained slide is prepared and a photomicrograph is taken (Figure 28-35 ■).

3. What would be an appropriate next step to determine whether the material seen is debris or true organisms?

Some of the large tissue cells showed features of degeneration and features suspicious for malignancy.

4. How should this be interpreted?

MALIGNANT CELLS IN FLUIDS

The pleural, pericardial, and peritoneal fluids can contain malignant cells, and their identification is critical for making an accurate diagnosis.[6,7,8] In some patients, a diagnosis of malignancy can already have been established by other tissue sampling (biopsy or excision), and finding the malignant cells in fluid establishes a condition of tumor metastasis. For other patients, finding malignant cells in fluid can be the initial diagnosis of a malignancy, and if a sample is not sent to cytology, the recognition of malignancy on the hematology laboratory preparation is critical in establishing an early diagnosis. Malignant cells in fluids can usually be distinguished as hematopoietic in origin (leukemia, lymphoma) versus nonhematopoietic (carcinoma, sarcoma), and in some cases further specification of cell type is also possible. It is important to look at the entire cellular area of the slide with a low power objective (10×) to detect suspicious

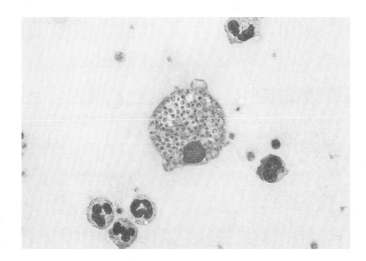

■ FIGURE 28-32   *Histoplasma capsulatum,* multiple organisms in histiocyte; buffy coat, peripheral blood.

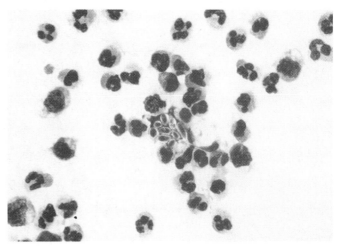

■ FIGURE 28-34   *Candida tropicalis,* peritoneal fluid.

⊙ TABLE 28-4

Comparison of Morphology of Pathologic Yeast as Seen with Wright Stain

Histoplasma	Cryptococcus	Candida Albicans	Candida Tropicalis
Usually small, often intracellular, distinct nonstaining cell wall, partially staining interior	Wide variation in size, usually extracellular, capsule not visible on air-dried preparations, either solidly stained with "wrinkled" appearance or partial internal staining	Can be extracellular and intracellular, moderate in size, stain solid, rarely can see pseudohyphae formation	Can be extracellular and intracellular, moderate in size, dark blue with red internal staining

clusters of cells. In any one sample, there may be only a few malignant cells that are difficult to find.

General features that can be seen in almost any type of malignant cell include an irregular nuclear membrane, unevenly distributed chromatin, and nucleoli that also have an irregular membrane (Table 28-5 ⊙).[7] The nuclear-cytoplasmic ratio varies, with small cell carcinoma cells having minimal cytoplasm and adenocarcinoma cells having as much or more cytoplasm as a benign mesothelial cell. The nuclear membrane irregularity can be jagged or show multiple folds. When nucleoli are present, they are frequently prominent and irregular in shape (Figure 28-36 ■). Mitotic activity by itself is not a reliable sign of malignancy because their reactive mesothelial cells can undergo mitosis, nor are cytoplasmic vacuoles a reliable finding for malignancy because their presence can be seen as a part of early degeneration in many cells. None of the features described can be used alone to diagnose malignancy. All of the features must be looked for and evaluated together. For example, one type of malignancy can show smooth nuclear membranes but with unevenly distributed chromatin and irregular nucleoli (Table 28-6 ⊙).

The most common nonhematopoietic malignancies seen in body fluids are small cell carcinoma and adenocarcinoma. Small cell carcinoma cells have the same general morphologic findings of malignant cells but can be distinguished from other types of carcinoma cells because of the characteristic high nuclear-cytoplasmic ratio, blastlike chromatin, absence of nucleoli or nonprominent nucleoli, and frequent nuclear molding (Figure 28-37 ■), which is the process of the nucleus of one cell molding around the shape of an adjacent cell. Nuclear molding occurs with cohesive growth of cells requiring the presence of tight junctions between the cytoplasmic membranes of the cells. Therefore, nuclear molding can be seen in any type of carcinoma but is most often seen with small cell carcinoma. Some cells also can have a paranuclear "blue body," which is an inclusion that has not yet been characterized and can represent early cell degeneration or phagocytosed material. Depending on the cell's orientation, the blue body can appear to be intranuclear and has been described in small cell carcinoma and rarely in sarcoma.[9] The blue body is seen only with air-dried, Wright-stained preparations (Figure 28-38 ■). If the malignant cells are noncohesive, small cell carcinoma could be mistaken for a hematopoietic malignancy, and the finding of a blue body would be a good clue for the diagnosis of small cell carcinoma.

Adenocarcinoma differs from small cell carcinoma in that the overall size of an adenocarcinoma cell is larger than a small cell carcinoma cell with a moderate to abundant amount of cytoplasm (Figure 28-39 ■). The nuclear chromatin is partially clumped and heterogeneous and has prominent nucleoli. The presence of cytoplasmic vacuoles is not specific and can represent early cell degeneration.

Other types of carcinoma and sarcoma can be found in body fluids (Figures 28-40 ■, 28-41 ■, 28-42 ■, and 28-43 ■).

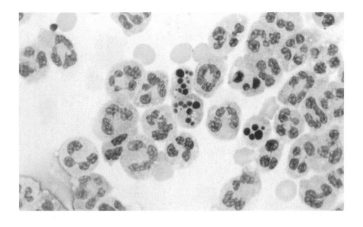

■ FIGURE 28-35   Pleural fluid. (Case Study questions 3 and 4.)

⊙ TABLE 28-5

Comparison of Morphologic Features of Reactive Mesothelial Cells versus Malignant Cells

Cell Features	Reactive Mesothelial Cells	Malignant Cells
Nuclear membrane	Smooth	Irregular, jagged
Chromatin	Evenly distributed	Unevenly distributed
Nucleoli	Absent or present with smooth membrane	Prominent, frequently multiple, irregular membrane
Nuclear molding	None	Present in nonhematopoietic malignancies

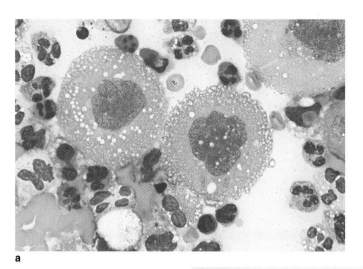

a

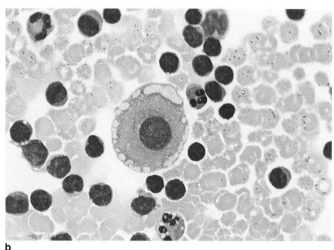

b

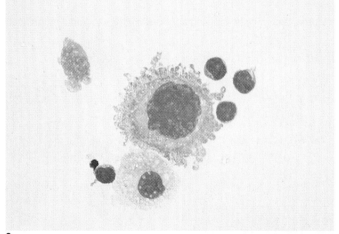

c

■ FIGURE 28-36 **a.** Malignant cells (adenocarcinoma), pleural fluid. **b.** Benign mesothelial cell to contrast with features of malignant cell. **c.** Single malignant cell (adenocarcinoma), pleural fluid.

✪ TABLE 28-6

General Morphologic Findings of Benign Mesothelial Cells and Malignant Cells

Any given cell can show variable features so that all must be evaluated before deciding whether a body fluid sample is benign or malignant. No single feature can be used to diagnose malignancy.

	Mesothelial Cell	Adenocarcinoma	Small Cell Carcinoma	Large Cell Lymphoma	Leukemic Blasts
Cell size	Large, 15–30 μ	Large to giant	Moderate to large	Moderate to large	Small to moderate
Chromatin	Loose, homogeneous	Partially clumped, heterogeneous	Slightly course, homogeneous	Partially clumped, heterogeneous	Smooth, lace-like, homogeneous
Nucleoli	None to small and regular	Prominent, multiple, irregular	None to small, not prominent	Small to prominent, irregular	Variable
Nuclear membrane	Smooth	Irregular, jagged	Irregular, jagged, folded	Irregular, jagged, folded	Smooth or irregular, folded
N:C ratio	Low, 1:3–5	Low, 1:3 or less	High, 1:1.25	High to moderate 1:1.25–1:2	High to moderate 1:1.25–1:1.75
Intercell relationship	Individual or clumped, no nuclear molding	Usually clumped, ± nuclear molding	Clumped with nuclear molding, occasionally individual	Individual, no clumping, no nuclear molding	Individual, no clumping, no nuclear molding

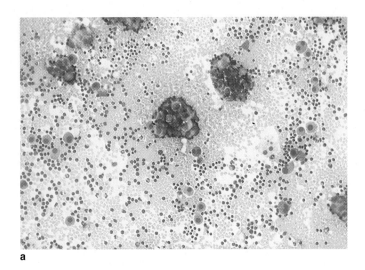

a

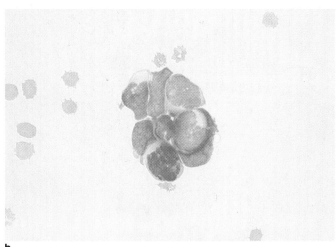

b

■ FIGURE 28-37   **a.** Small cell carcinoma, pleural fluid showing tight cell clusters (original magnification, 25×). **b.** Small cell carcinoma.

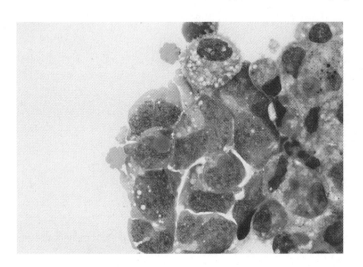

■ FIGURE 28-38   Small cell carcinoma, paranuclear "blue body" in malignant cell.

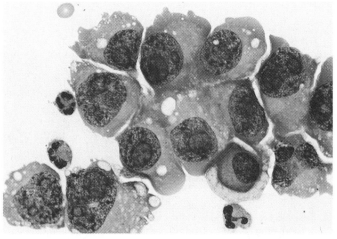

■ FIGURE 28-40   Pancreatic carcinoma in peritoneal fluid.

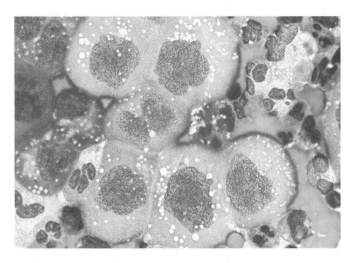

■ FIGURE 28-39   Adenocarcinoma in pleural fluid.

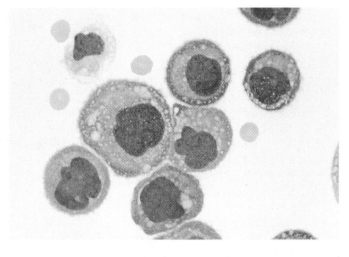

■ FIGURE 28-41   Gastric adenocarcinoma in pleural fluid.

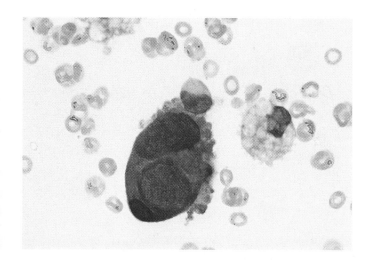

■ FIGURE 28-42   Liposarcoma in pleural fluid.

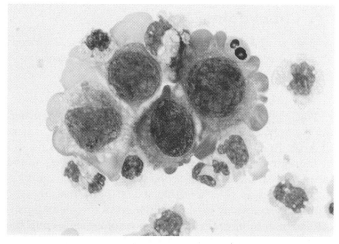

■ FIGURE 28-44   Squamous cell carcinoma in pleural fluid.

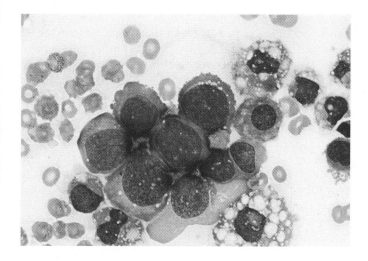

■ FIGURE 28-43   Germ cell tumor (spermatocytic seminoma) in pleural fluid.

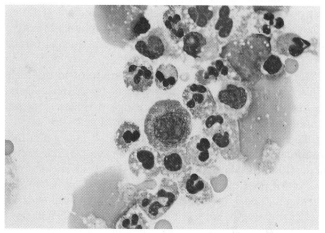

■ FIGURE 28-45   Malignant melanoma in pleural fluid with melanin pigment in malignant cells.

The features seen with Wright's stain are not as specific as from a cytology preparation; the latter is necessary to specifically identify the type of malignancy. For example, squamous cell carcinoma can look like adenocarcinoma with Wright's stain; however, in most cases, the two are readily distinguishable on cytology preparations (Figure 28-44 ■). Certain types of malignant cells can contain clues for the cellular origin. Melanoma cells can have melanin pigment that is demonstrable with Wright's stain, and hepatocellular carcinoma can have bile pigment (Figures 28-45 ■ and 28-46 ■). The presence of these pigments can be suspected with Wright's stain but must be confirmed with more specific staining techniques.

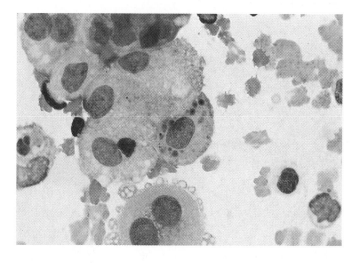

■ FIGURE 28-46   Bile pigment in macrophage in peritoneal fluid due to cholangiocarcinoma.

✔ Checkpoint! 3

When examining a cytocentrifuged, Wright-stained slide of a body fluid specimen, what are the best features to use in determining whether tissue cells are benign or malignant?

Practically any type of hematopoietic malignancy, including lymphocytic and nonlymphocytic leukemias, lymphomas, Hodgkin disease, and plasma cell[10] neoplasms, can be found in body fluids. Generally, the abnormal cells found in the body fluids in these disorders have the same morphologic features as peripheral blood and bone marrow. The acute leukemias only occasionally involve the pleural, pericardial, or peritoneal cavities and more often are seen in the CSF. Blasts appear larger on cytocentrifuge preparations than on peripheral blood smears, and the nuclear membrane can be surprisingly irregular. Auer rods can be seen, and, if necessary, unstained slides can be prepared for cytochemistry stains and terminal deoxynucleotidyl transferase (TdT) to differentiate the blasts (∞ Chapter 21). Lymphoblasts have a very high nuclear-cytoplasmic ratio, and the nucleus can be folded or convoluted.

The morphology of non-Hodgkin lymphoma in the body fluids depends on the particular type of lymphoma. Again, the nuclear membrane can be surprisingly irregular. Large cell lymphoma has cells that are moderate to large in size with irregular nuclei, partially clumped chromatin, and sometimes prominent nucleoli (Figure 28-47 ■). The cytoplasm is low to moderate in amount and basophilic. The cells are discohesive, but if the fluid is very cellular, the cells can be thrown together and have the appearance of carcinoma cell clusters; nuclear molding is not seen. Burkitt lymphoma (small noncleaved cell) has intermediate size cells with more than one nucleoli and an immature blastlike chromatin (Figure 28-48 ■). Prominent cytoplasmic vacuoles frequently are ap-

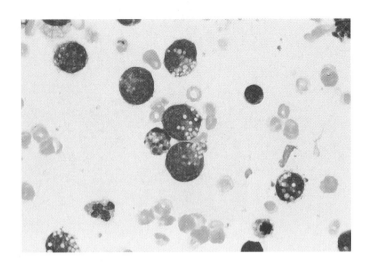

■ FIGURE 28-48   Burkitt lymphoma (small noncleaved cell) in pleural fluid.

parent. Small cell lymphoma is the most difficult to diagnose and can look like a benign lymphocytic infiltrate. In these cases, flow cytometry is valuable in demonstrating a clonal population of cells (∞ Chapter 37). T cell lymphoma can show markedly irregular, convoluted nuclei; however, marker studies are necessary to confirm T or B cell origin of the neoplastic cells (Figures 28-49 ■, and 28-50 ■). Cell origin can be accomplished by flow cytometry or immunoperoxidase techniques on cytocentrifuge-prepared slides.

Primary effusion (body cavity) lymphoma is a high-grade type found only in a body cavity without an associated solid tumor mass. This unique malignancy has been reported in patients who are immunocompromised, usually HIV positive, and is associated with HHV-8 (human Herpes virus 8, also known as *Kaposi sarcoma* associated Herpes virus, KSHV).[11,12,13] The morphology of the cells in the effusion is similar to the

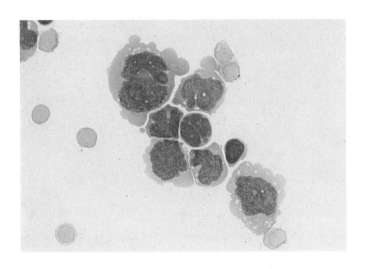

■ FIGURE 28-47   Large cell lymphoma in pleural fluid.

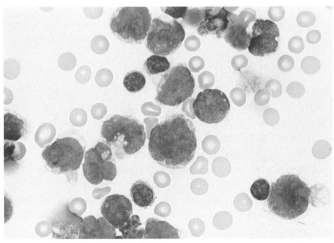

■ FIGURE 28-49   Lymphoblastic lymphoma, T cell type, in pleural fluid.

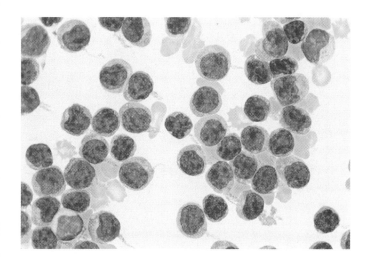

■ FIGURE 28-50   Small lymphocytic lymphoma.

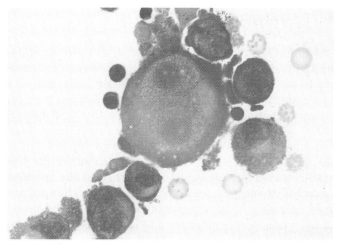

■ FIGURE 28-52   Hodgkin disease with Reed-Sternberg cell, pleural fluid.

morphology of cells found in anaplastic large cell lymphoma, immunoblastic lymphoma, or small noncleaved cell lymphoma. These malignant cells are usually B cell derived but lack surface-associated antigens for T or B cell lineage.

Hodgkin lymphoma can occasionally be seen to involve pleural fluid (Figures 28-51■ and 28-52■). The malignant Hodgkin cell is large with a moderate to abundant amount of cytoplasm, large nuclei, and prominent nucleoli. If the nucleus is bilobated or if the cell has two nuclei, it can be a Reed-Sternberg cell. The other cells present consist of varying numbers of small lymphocytes, eosinophils, histiocytes, and plasma cells. If other tissue biopsy has already established a patient's Hodgkin disease diagnosis, the malignant cells (either Hodgkin, Reed-Sternberg, or multinucleated variants) must still be identified in the effusion sample to diagnose the fluid's involvement.

CASE STUDY (continued from page 595)

After 3 weeks, Carolyn improved significantly, but the chest pain and effusion did not resolve. A repeat thoracentesis was performed. Laboratory studies show protein 4.7 g/dL (serum = 6 g/dL), lactate dehydrogenase 50 U/L (serum = 60 U/L), and total nucleated cell count 3,000/μL. A cytocentrifuged, Wright-stained slide is examined, and the differential count shows 30% segmented neutrophils, 20% lymphocytes, 10% histiocytes, and 40% tissue cells. A photomicrograph of the tissue cells is seen in Figure 28-53■.

5. Is this an exudate or transudate?

6. What is the most appropriate interpretation of these findings?

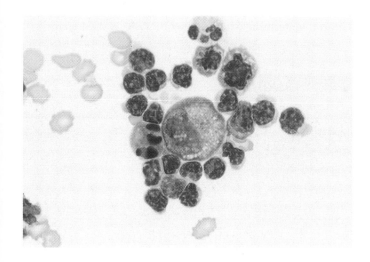

■ FIGURE 28-51   Hodgkin disease, pleural fluid.

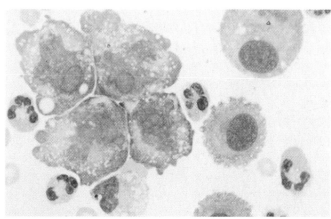

■ FIGURE 28-53   Pleural fluid. (Case Study question 6.)

► CEREBROSPINAL FLUID

CSF differs from the pleural, pericardial, and peritoneal fluids in that it exists in the normal state. However, CSF is normally acellular so that the presence of any cells even at a low count suggests a pathologic state. A common problem when evaluating CSF is to distinguish a true CNS hemorrhage versus a spinal tap procedure that causes hemorrhage (traumatic tap). Both of these present as grossly bloody fluids. If the total erythrocyte count (RBC count) in the first tube collected is significantly higher than in the last tube collected, it suggests a traumatic tap. Xanthochromia is a pink to orange fluid supernatant produced by the breakdown products of hemoglobin and is usually thought to indicate true CNS hemorrhage. Xanthochromia occurs, however, if a grossly bloody fluid from a traumatic tap sits for some time before it is centrifuged. A definitive sign of CNS hemorrhage is phagocytosis of erythrocytes by histiocytes (erythrophagocytosis) (Figure 28-54 ■). It takes approximately 18 hours for histiocytes to mobilize and phagocytose erythrocytes after a hemorrhage. If the hemorrhage is older, hematoidin crystals can be seen intracellularly or extracellarly (Figure 28-55 ■). Hematoidin is a product of hemoglobin catabolism.

✓ Checkpoint! 4

A 47-year-old man is found comatose at home by his wife. During examination in the emergency room, a spinal tap is performed and grossly bloody spinal fluid is obtained. The total RBC count in the first tube is the same as that in the third tube. A cytocentrifuged, Wright-stained slide shows findings similar to that seen in Figure 28-54. What is the most appropriate interpretation?

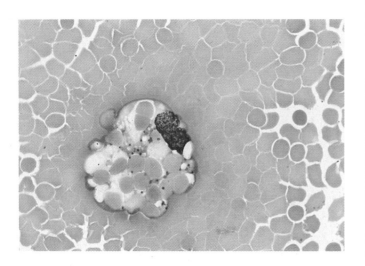

■ FIGURE 28-54   Erythrophagocytosis.

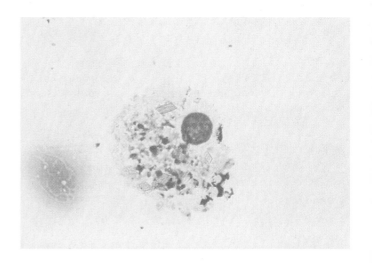

■ FIGURE 28-55   Hematoidin crystals in macrophage in CSF.

NONSPECIFIC REACTIVE CHANGES

The normal leukocyte counts of CSF have been difficult to determine (Table 28-7 ✪).[1,2] The reference ranges listed for pediatric ages are somewhat controversial because they have a high upper limit. Most important for interpretation is to consider the types of white blood cells present and to correlate them with clinical findings.

The total WBC count cannot be interpreted without the total RBC count. When a specimen is obtained as a traumatic tap, the WBC and RBC reflect the same WBC/RBC ratio as the patient's peripheral blood. A general rule is to expect 1 to 2 WBC for every 1000 RBC in the CSF. For example, if the total WBC in a CSF specimen is $10/\mu L$ and the RBC is $10,000/\mu L$, there is no significant increase of WBC (pleocytosis). If, however, the total RBC is $100/\mu L$ with a WBC of $10/\mu L$, a significant increase of WBC indicates a pathologic state.[14] When a patient has an elevated or decreased peripheral blood WBC or RBC, it is best to use the following calculation to determine whether the CSF WBC is significant:[1,2]

✪ TABLE 28-7

Reference Range for Leukocytes in CSF per μL	
Age	**Reference Range**
Adults	0–5
5–puberty	0–10
1–4	0–20
<1	0–30

Based on data from: Smith GP, Kieldsberg CR. Cerebrospinal, synovial, and serous body fluids. In: Henry SB, ed. *Clinical Diagnosis and Management by Laboratory Methods,* 20th ed. Philadelphia: W.B. Saunders; 2001; and Kieldsberg C, Knight J. *Body Fluids,* 3rd ed. Chicago: ASCP Press; 1993.

Corrected CSF WBC =

$$\text{Total WBC of fluid} - \frac{\text{WBC of blood} \times \text{RBC of fluid}}{\text{RBC of blood}}$$

For example, a 21-year-old man has fever, headache, and a stiff neck. A spinal tap is performed. Laboratory studies reveal the following:

	Total RBC	Total WBC
CSF	$50,000/\mu L$	$250/\mu L$
Peripheral blood	$3.5 \times 10^{12}/L$	$3.5 \times 10^{9}/L$

The physician asks if the CSF WBC count represents peripheral blood contamination or a true increase indicating meningitis. Because the patient has peripheral leukopenia and anemia, the formula should be used to answer this question.

$$\text{Corrected CSF WBC} = 250/\mu L - \frac{(3.5 \times 10^{9}/L) \times (50,000/\mu L)}{3.5 \times 10^{12}/L}$$

$$\text{Corrected CSF WBC} = 250/\mu L - 50/\mu L$$

$$\text{Corrected CSF WBC} = 200/\mu L$$

Hence, there is a significant increase in the CSF WBC.

In general, the type of predominant WBC present has the same diagnostic indication as is seen in the peripheral blood. For example, a predominance of neutrophils most often indicates a bacterial meningitis, a predominance of lymphocytes correlates with viral or fungal meningitis, and an increase of eosinophils can indicate a parasitic infection or allergic and drug reactions. More detailed correlations of possible diagnosis and type of cell increase is available in other sources.[1,2,15]

As with the pleural, pericardial, and peritoneal fluids, reactive lymphocytes must be distinguished from lymphoma cells (Figure 28-56■). Hematopoietic precursors, including megakaryocytes, are present if the spinal tap needle penetrated the vertebral bone, drawing back a portion of bone marrow. This is most often seen in infants but can occur in adults with osteoarthritis.[16]

Mesothelial cells are not present in CSF, but other tissue cells such as arachnoid and choroid plexus can be seen. These are most often present in CSF from infants and adults who have had some type of manipulation such as surgery or shunt placement. It is very unusual to see these cells from a simple spinal tap procedure in an adult.

MICROORGANISMS

The same types of microorganisms described in pleural, pericardial, and peritoneal fluids can be present in CSF samples. As mentioned earlier, distinguishing intracellular bacteria from stain precipitate is critical. A Gram stain is most helpful in this situation. The most common yeast organism seen in CSF is cryptococcus (Figure 28-31). When cryptococcus is suspected from the cytocentrifuge-prepared slide, the microbiology laboratory should perform an India ink preparation to confirm the presence of the characteristic large capsule of cryptococcus. If very few organisms are present, however, the India ink preparation can be negative because unconcentrated CSF is used for the India ink. Cultures must be obtained to confirm the type of organism present.

MALIGNANT CELLS

Much of the description of malignant cells in pleural, pericardial, and peritoneal fluids also holds true for spinal fluid examination.[17] Carcinoma cells tend to be less cohesive in spinal fluid than in other fluids and can simulate hematopoietic malignancies. Because mesothelial cells do not exist in the CSF, the presence of any large tissue cells should be considered suspicious for malignancy (Figures 28-57■, 28-58■, and 28-59■). Malignant cells, however,

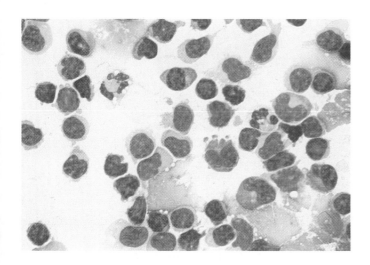

■ FIGURE 28-56   Reactive lymphocytes, CSF.

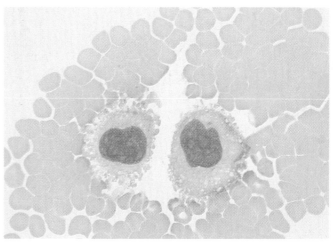

■ FIGURE 28-57   Adenocarcinoma, CSF.

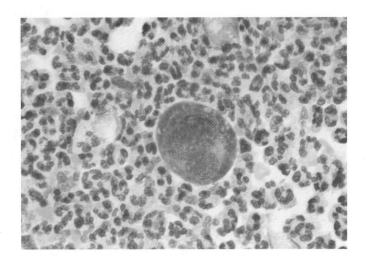

■ FIGURE 28-58   Large cell undifferentiated carcinoma with intense chemical acute meningitis, CSF.

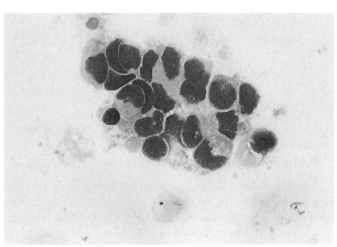

■ FIGURE 28-60   Medulloblastoma, CSF.

must be differentiated from the benign choroid plexus cells, ependymal cells, and arachnoid cells by evaluating the cells for standard features of malignancy as described earlier. Cytology preparations are usually definitive. Benign tissue cells usually are seen only in CSF from infants and from adults who have recent neurosurgery or a shunt or reservoir in place.

Cells from primary CNS neoplasms rarely are be found in the CSF. Medulloblastoma is a malignant tumor usually occurring in the cerebellum of pediatric patients and has a morphologic appearance similar to that of small cell carcinoma (Figure 28-60■). Patient history from the physician would be necessary to distinguish the tumor's origin.

Acute lymphocytic leukemia more often involves the CNS than acute nonlymphocytic leukemia (Figures 28-61■, 28-62■, and 28-63■). When erythrocytes are present, care

must be taken not to overinterpret the presence of blasts that simply represent peripheral blood contamination. If no erythrocytes are present, even a low number of blasts (1% to 2%) can indicate CNS involvement.[18] Special studies such as cytochemistry stains, TdT, and surface markers by immunoperoxidase stains or flow cytometry can be helpful[19] (∞ Chapters 14, ∞ 37).

Any type of lymphoma can involve the CNS, but the high-grade lymphomas such as lymphoblastic, immunoblastic, and Burkitt lymphoma (small noncleaved cell) are more often seen. Primary CNS lymphoma is seen more often in patients who are HIV-positive. The lymphomas in these patients are high grade and frequently correspond to Burkitt lymphoma (small noncleaved cell) or B immunoblastic (Figure 28-64■).

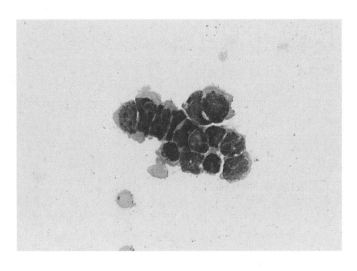

■ FIGURE 28-59   Small cell carcinoma, CSF.

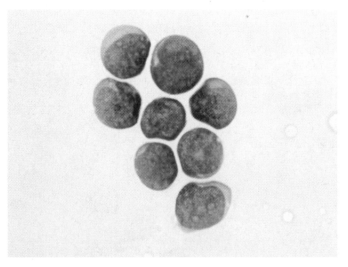

■ FIGURE 28-61   Acute lymphocytic leukemia, CSF.

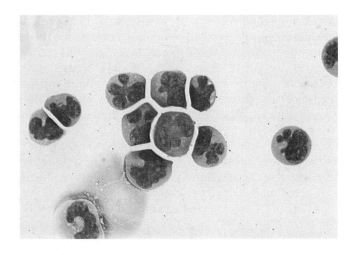

■ FIGURE 28-62   Acute myelomonocytic leukemia, CSF.

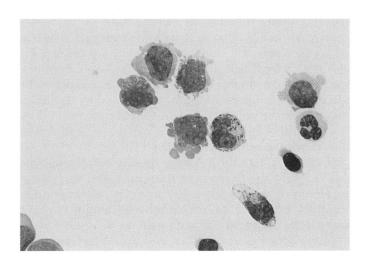

■ FIGURE 28-63   Blast crisis of chronic myelocytic leukemia with myeloblasts in CSF.

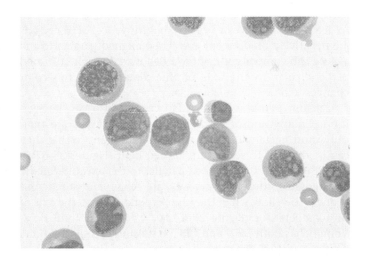

■ FIGURE 28-64   High-grade lymphoma, small noncleaved cell type, CSF.

CASE STUDY *(continued from page 601)*

After an extensive work up, Carolyn is found to have a primary adenocarcinoma of the right upper lung lobe. A surgical resection is performed. Six months later, the patient has severe headaches. A spinal tap is performed, and a photomicrograph of the cells is as seen in Figure 28-65■.

7. What is the most appropriate interpretion of these cells?

▶ JOINT FLUID

Synovial fluids tend to be thick and viscous due to the presence of hyaluronic acid, a mucopolysaccharide substance secreted by the lining synovial cells. If the fluid is too thick to proceed with cell counts, the use of hyaluronidase can be very helpful to loosen the fluid. Joint fluid is most often aspirated to distinguish crystal-inducing diseases (gout, pseudogout) from septic processes. Other disease states can induce an inflammatory response; however, diagnosing these by joint-fluid examination alone is usually not possible. Certain diagnoses can be suspected when comparing the total WBC count with percent of segmented neutrophils present; however, there is great overlap, and morphologic examination by cytocentrifuge preparations can be extremely helpful (Table 28-8 ✪).[20,21]

Joint fluids that have a total WBC of 50,000 to 200,000/μL suggest an infectious or crystal-induced etiology. If the differential count shows 90% or more segmented neutrophils, an infectious agent is most likely and cultures must be obtained. Microorganisms can be seen in joint fluid if present in sufficient numbers and have the same

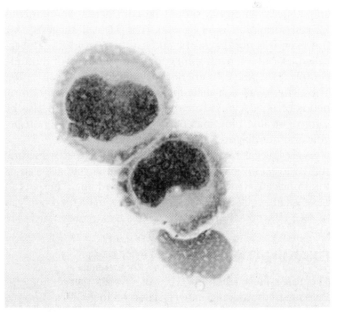

■ FIGURE 28-65   Cerebral spinal fluid. (Case Study question 7)

✪ TABLE 28-8

General Grouping of Diagnosis by Total WBC and Percent Neutrophils in Synovial Fluid Analysis

There is some overlap of diagnostic groups, and other studies are necessary to reach an accurate diagnosis.

Total WBC	% Neutrophils	Diagnostic Groups
0–5,000/μL	<30% neutrophils	Osteoarthritis, traumatic arthritis, neuropathic arthropathy, pigmented villonodular synovitis
2,000–200,000/μL	>50% neutrophils	Rheumatoid arthritis, Lupus erythematosus, Reiter's syndrome, rheumatic fever, ankylosing spondylitis
50,000–200,000/μL	>90% neutrophils	Infectious—bacterial, mycobacterial, fungal
500–200,000/μL	<90% neutrophils	Crystal induced—gout, pseudogout, apatite arthropathy
50–10,000/μL	<50% neutrophils, RBC present	Hemorrhagic—trauma, hemophilia, anticoagulant, pigmented villonodular synovitis, neuropathic arthropathy, hemangioma

morphology as previously described. Bacterial organisms are more common, and pathogenic yeasts are only rarely seen.

When the total WBC is in the range of 2,000 to 200,000/μL with more than 50% neutrophils in the differential count, entities such as rheumatoid arthritis (RA), SLE, and Reiter's syndrome should be considered. Spontaneous LE cell formation rarely occurs. The LE cell suggests SLE; however, it is not diagnostic and can be seen in RA. The so-called RA cell is a neutrophil containing granules of immune complexes. These cells are not specific for a diagnosis of RA. The Reiter's cell is a macrophage with vacuoles containing debris of phagocytosed neutrophils. The debris can also be unrecognizable blue material. These cells are also nonspecific and not diagnostic for Reiter's disease.

Synovial cells can become proliferative in a reactive setting similar to mesothelial cells. Reactive synovial cells also can be multinucleated and occur in clusters, and their nuclei can have small, regular nucleoli. Theoretically, malignant cells can be seen in synovial fluid; however, this is extremely rare.[22]

EXAMINATION FOR CRYSTALS

The three most common types of crystals present in joint fluid are monosodium urate crystals seen in gout, calcium pyrophosphate crystals seen in pseudogout, and cholesterol crystals present in different types of chronic arthritides such as

RA.[23] Examination for crystals on a cytocentrifuge-prepared slide is superior to a standard wet preparation because the cytocentrifuge concentrates the specimen. Samples that are negative with wet preparation can actually show crystals on the concentrated cytocentrifuge slide. Using cytocentrifuge prepared slides also decreases the biologic hazard when handling wet preparations. If sufficient numbers of crystals are present, they can be seen with plain light microscopy on a Wright-stained cytocentrifuge slide. However, polarized light must be used to confirm birefringence[24] (described later). If fewer crystals are present, polarization is necessary to see them initially. Every joint fluid sent to the hematology laboratory for cell counts should have a crystal examination.[25] Some Wright's stain techniques result in the dissolution of the monosodium urate crystals. Therefore, preparing two cytocentrifuge slides, one for Wright's stain and one left unstained, is best. Both slides should be examined for crystals on multiple specimens to determine whether a particular stain technique dissolves the monosodium urate crystals (Table 28-9 ✪).

Birefringence refers to a particular material's ability to refract light rays. It is determined by using a polarizing microscope. A fixed light filter (analyzer) is placed above the specimen and a rotating filter (polarizer) is placed below the specimen. Both filters allow light to pass in only one direction. When the polarizer is rotated 90 degrees to the analyzer, no light can pass, yielding a "dark field." If the specimen contains birefringent material, it changes the direction (refract) of the light rays, allowing them to pass through the analyzer, and the birefringent material is seen as a bright particle or crystal.[24] A quartz compensator is used to further identify a crystal by determining the velocity of the light rays passing through the crystal's grain (axis).

Monosodium urate (MSU) crystals should be reported as intracellular and/or extracellular. MSU crystals are typically long, thin, and needlelike with pointed ends (Figure 28-66a ■). They can be seen singly or in bundles. MSU crystals are strongly birefringent and are brilliant with polarized light (Figure 28-66b ■). A quartz compensator must be used to determine positive or negative birefringence. MSU crystals are negatively birefringent and when aligned parallel to the axis of the compensator, show a yellow color; when turned perpendicular to the axis of the compensator, the color changes to blue (Figure 28-66c ■).[1,2,24]

Calcium pyrophosphate (CPP) crystals also can be seen intracellularly and/or extracellularly. CPP crystals are typically short, rectangular, and weakly birefringent so that they can be difficult to see with polarized light (Figures 28-67a ■ and 28-67b ■). When aligned parallel to the axis of a quartz compensator, the CPP crystals are blue, and the color changes to yellow when they are perpendicular to the axis of the compensator (Figure 28-67c ■).[1,2,24] A joint fluid occasionally has both MSU and CPP crystals; the presence of one does not exclude the other.

Cholesterol crystals have a characteristic notched-plate shape and are birefringent (Figure 28-68 ■). These crystals

⊘ TABLE 28-9

Morphologic Comparisons of Commonly Seen Birefringent Crystals and Particles

Crystal	Birefringence	Color Parallel to Quartz Compensator	Morphology
Monosodium urate	Strong	Yellow	Long, thin, needlelike, intra- and extracellular
Calcium pyrophosphate	weak	Blue	Short, rectangular, intra- and extracellular
Cholesterol	Strong	Variable	Large platelike, notched, extracellular
Steroids	Strong	Variable	Amorphous, intra- and extracellular
Talc particles	Strong	Yellow and blue	Maltese cross shape, extracellular

are present in chronically inflamed joints as are seen in rheumatoid arthritis.

Starch particles are distinguished from pathogenic crystals by a characteristic Maltese cross shape with polarized light (Figure 28-20). If a joint has been injected with steroids, the steroid particles can be seen intracellularly and extracellulary. Steroid particles do not have a crystal shape and are amorphous but birefringent.

✓ Checkpoint! 5

A 57-year-old man has an acutely swollen, painful, reddened joint in his left great toe. Joint fluid is aspirated, and a photomicrograph is taken (Figure 28-69 ■). This picture is taken with polarized light using a quartz compensator. What is the most appropriate interpretation of this finding?

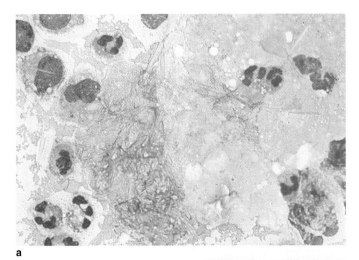

a

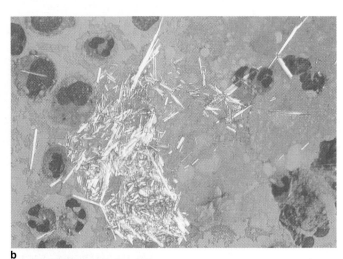

b

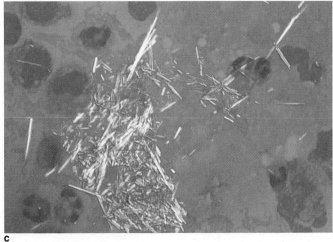

c

■ FIGURE 28-66   MSU crystal with **a.** plain light, **b.** polarized light, and **c.** quartz compensator with crystal showing yellow parallel to quartz line and crystal with blue perpendicular to quartz line.

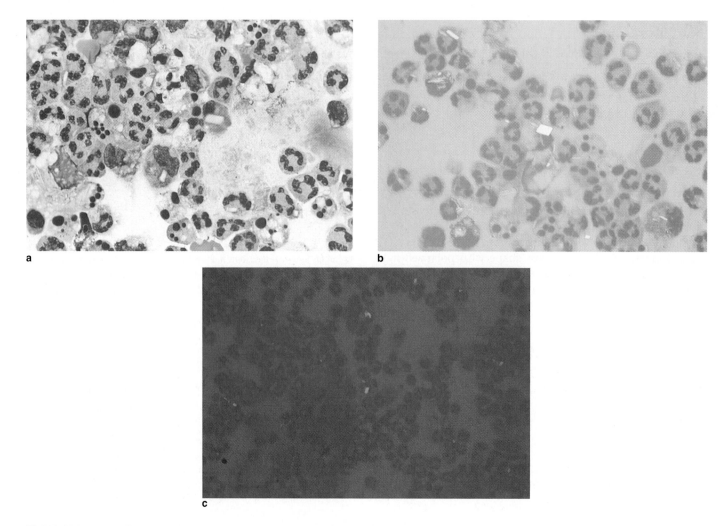

■ FIGURE 28-67 CPP crystal with **a.** plain light, **b.** polarized light, **c.** quartz compensator with yellow crystal perpendicular to quartz line and blue crystal parallel to quartz line.

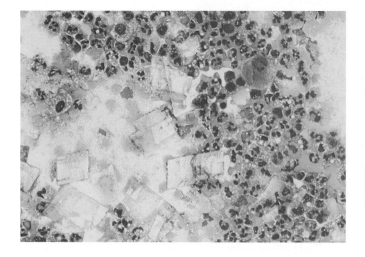

■ FIGURE 28-68 Cholesterol crystals in joint fluid.

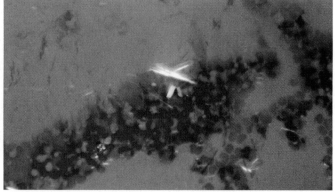

■ FIGURE 28-69 Synovial fluid. (Figure for Checkpoint 5.)

SUMMARY

The fluids discussed in this chapter are those most commonly sampled: pleural, pericardial, peritoneal, synovial, and CSF. In pathologic conditions, the amount of fluid can increase (effusion). An effusion can be a transudate or an exudate. Chylous effusions are milky and result from leakage of lymphatic vessels. Common cell types seen in these fluids include white blood cells, tissue cells, and malignant cells. Examination of cellular morphology in body fluids, a critically important procedure for hematology laboratories,

is performed for not only a differential leukocyte count but also a possible demonstration of diagnostic findings such as microorganisms and malignant cells. The cytocentrifuge-prepared Wright-stained slide yields excellent morphology of cells and can significantly aid in making a timely diagnosis of patients with effusions of unknown etiology. The hematology laboratory must take an active role in correlating morphologic findings such as cultures, special stains, and cytology with additional studies that can be necessary.

REVIEW QUESTIONS

LEVEL I

1. The types of body fluids other than peripheral blood that are frequently sent to the hematology laboratory include which of the following? (Objective 1)
   a. cerebrospinal fluid
   b. pleural fluid
   c. pericardial fluid
   d. all of the above

2. The pleura, pericardium, and peritoneum are composed of what type of cell? (Objective 2)
   a. white blood cell
   b. epithelial cell
   c. mesothelial cell
   d. squamous cell

3. Anatomically, where is the visceral pleura located? (Objective 1)
   a. innermost aspect of the abdominal wall
   b. outermost portion of the heart
   c. innermost aspect of the chest wall
   d. outermost portion of the lung

4. Which of the following cell type(s) seen in cerebrospinal fluid can be considered normal, not a sign of pathologic disease? (Objective 2)
   a. arachnoid cells
   b. choroid plexus cells
   c. ependymal cells
   d. all of the above

5. The finding of possible bacterial organisms on a cytocentrifuged, Wright-stained slide would be easiest to confirm by which of the following? (Objective 5)
   a. gram stain
   b. silver stain
   c. culture
   d. electrophoresis

6. Which of the following can be seen as artifact on a cytocentrifuged, Wright-stained slide? (Objective 3)
   a. hypersegmentation of neutrophils
   b. stain precipitate
   c. cytoplasmic projections of lymphocytes
   d. all of the above

LEVEL II

1. A specimen labeled "ascites" is sent to the laboratory. What type of procedure was used to obtain this fluid? (Objective 1)
   a. thoracentesis
   b. lumbar puncture
   c. pericardial aspiration
   d. paracentesis

2. Which of the following cell types is responsible for the production of cerebrospinal fluid? (Objective 2)
   a. choroid plexus
   b. arachnoid
   c. neutrophils
   d. mesothelial

3. A 25-year-old woman develops a left-sided pleural effusion while recovering from bacterial pneumonia. A thoracentesis is performed, and the following laboratory results are reported:

	Serum	Fluid
Protein	6.5 g/dL	5 g/dL
LD	75 U/L	60 U/L

   These results would be best interpreted as which of the following? (Objective 3)
   a. chylous
   b. exudate
   c. pseudochylous
   d. transudate

4. A 56-year-old woman has a 3-week history of abdominal pain. A peritoneal effusion is found. After paracentesis, a sample is sent to the laboratory. Examination of the cytocentrifuged, Wright-stained slide shows clusters of large cells that have abundant cytoplasm, smooth nuclear membranes, evenly distributed chromatin, and no nucleoli. An occasional multinucleated cell is found with the same features. These cells most likely represent: (Objective 5)
   a. reactive mesothelial cells
   b. adenocarcinoma cells
   c. small cell carcinoma
   d. ependymal cells

REVIEW QUESTIONS (continued)

LEVEL I

7. Which of the following best characterizes a chylous fluid? (Objective 4)
   a. transparent, yellow, low nucleated cell count
   b. opaque, bloody, many neutrophils
   c. cloudy, yellowish-green, many histiocytes
   d. opaque, white, many lymphocytes and chylomicrons

8. A 45-year-old man has pleural effusions on the right and left side. A right-sided thoracentesis is performed and a sample is sent to the laboratory. The fluid-serum protein ratio is 0.3, the fluid-serum LD ratio is 0.4, and the total nucleated cell count is low. Which of the following best describes this fluid? (Objective 4)
   a. chylous
   b. exudate
   c. pseudochylous
   d. transudate

9. Malignant tissue cells have which of the following morphologic feature characteristic(s)? (Objective 6)
   a. irregular nuclear membrane
   b. evenly distributed chromatin
   c. prominent, irregular nucleoli
   d. a and c only

10. The finding of which of the following in joint fluid is most helpful to establish a diagnosis of gout? (Objective 7)
    a. monosodium urate
    b. cholesterol
    c. starch particles
    d. neutrophils

LEVEL II

5. A 60-year-old man who has smoked cigarettes since the age of 16 years has left-sided chest pain. A thoracentesis sample is sent to the laboratory. The cytocentrifuged, Wright-stained slide is examined, and clusters of large cells have irregular, jagged nuclear membranes, prominent and irregular nucleoli, and unevenly distributed chromatin. These cells most likely represent: (Objective 5)
   a. reactive mesothelial cells
   b. adenocarcinoma cells
   c. large cell lymphoma
   d. reactive histiocytes

6. Referring to the case in question 5, the protein, LD, and other studies would most likely reveal that this is a(n): (Objective 3)
   a. exudate
   b. chylous fluid
   c. transudate
   d. pseudochylous fluid

7. A 65-year-old woman has a painful, swollen elbow. A joint aspiration is performed, and a sample is sent to the laboratory. A cytocentrifuged slide is examined with polarized light and a quartz compensator. Birefringent crystals are seen intracellular and extracellular; they are needlelike in appearance and are yellow when oriented parallel to the quartz compensator. These crystals would be best identified as which of the following? (Objective 8)
   a. calcium pyrophosphate
   b. cholesterol
   c. monosodium urate
   d. steroids

8. Referring to the case in question 7, which of the following is the most likely diagnosis? (Objective 8)
   a. gout arthritis
   b. pseudogout arthritis
   c. rheumatoid arthritis
   d. systemic lupus erythematosus

9. A 55-year-old man is brought to the emergency room in a comatose state. He was found at home by his son and appears to have fallen from a ladder. A spinal tap is performed and reveals the following:

Color	Red
Appearance	Bloody
RBC	100×10^9/L
WBC	0.10×10^9/L
Differential WBC	80% segmented neutrophils
	15% lymphocytes
	5% monocytes

REVIEW QUESTIONS (continued)

LEVEL I

LEVEL II

Which of the following would be the most specific finding in this patient for a true CNS hemorrhage versus traumatic spinal tap? (Objective 6)

a. crenated red blood cells

b. xanthochromia of the supernatant

c. erythrophagocytosis by histiocytes

d. WBC of 0.1×10^9/L

10. Referring to the patient in question 9, what is the significance of the WBC count of 0.1×10^9/L? (Objective 9)

a. This is diagnostic for bacterial meningitis.

b. This is diagnostic for early viral meningitis.

c. This is expected for the amount of hemorrhage.

d. This is diagnostic for fungal meningitis.

www.pearsonhighered.com/mckenzie

Use this address to access the interactive Companion Website created for this textbook. Find additional information, tables and figures. Evaluate your command of the chapter information using case studies and critical thinking and multiple choice questions.

REFERENCES

1. Smith GP, Kieldsberg CR. Cerebrospinal, synovial, and serous body fluids. In: Henry SB, ed. *Clinical Diagnosis and Management by Laboratory Methods,* 20th ed. Philadelphia: W. B. Saunders; 2001.

2. Kieldsberg C, Knight J. *Body Fluids,* 3rd ed. Chicago: ASCP Press; 1993.

3. Lau MS, Pien FD. Eosinophilic pleural effusions. *Hawaii Med J.* 1990; 49:206–7.

4. Light RW. Pleural effusion. *N Engl J Med.* 2002;346:1971–76.

5. Horn KD, Penchansky L. Chylous pleural effusions simulating leukemic infiltrate associated with thoracoabdominal disease and surgery in infants. *Am J Clin Path.* 1999;111:99–104.

6. Ultmann J. Malignant effusions. *CA-Cancer.* 1991;41:166–79.

7. Clare N, Rone R. Detection of malignancy in body fluids. *Lab Med.* 1986;17:147–50.

8. Kendall B, Dunn C, Solanki P. A comparison of the effectiveness of malignancy detection in body fluid examination by the cytopathology and hematology laboratories. *Arch Pathol Lab Med.* 1997;121: 976–79.

9. Wittchow R, Laszewski M, Walker W, Dick F. Paranuclear blue inclusions in metastatic undifferentiated small cell carcinoma in the bone marrow. *Mod Pathol.* 1992;5:555–58.

10. Mitchell MA, Horneffer MD, Standiford TJ. Multiple myeloma complicated by restrictive cardiomyopathy and cardiac tamponade. *Chest.* 1993;103:946–47.

11. Nador RG, Cesarman E, Chadburn A et al. Primary effusion lymphoma: A distinct clinicopathologic entity associated with the Kaposi's sarcoma-associated herpes virus. *Blood.* 1996;88:645–56.

12. Knowles D, Chadburn A. Lymphadenopathy and the lymphoid neoplasms associated with the acquired immune deficiency syndrome. In: Knowles D, ed. *Neoplastic Hematopathology,* 2nd ed. Philadelphia: Lippincott Williams and Wilkins, 2001.

13. Jaffe ES, Harris NL, Stein H, Vardiman JW, eds. *Pathology and Genetics of Tumours of Haematopoietic and Lymphoid Tissues.* Lyon: IARC Press, 2001.

14. Bonadio WA, Smith DS, Goddard S, Burroughs J, Khaja G. Distinguishing cerebrospinal fluid abnormalities in children with bacterial meningitis and traumatic lumbar puncture. *J Infect Dis.* 1990; 162:251–54.

15. Greenlee JE. Approach to diagnosis of meningitis: Cerebrospinal fluid evaluation. *Infect Dis Clin North Am.* 1990;4:583–98.

16. Craver RD, Carson TH. Hematopoietic elements in cerebrospinal fluid in children. *Am J Clin Pathol.* 1991;95:532–35.

17. Bigner SH. Cerebrospinal fluid (CSF) cytology: Current status and diagnostic applications. *J Neuropathol Exp Neurol.* 1992;51:235–45.

18. Odom L, Wilson H, Jamieson B et al. Significance of blasts in low cell count cerebrospinal fluid specimens from children with acute lymphoblastic leukemia. *Cancer.* 1990;66:1748–54.

19. Homans AC, Barker BE, Forman EN, Cornell CJ Jr, Dickerman JD, Truman JT. Immunophenotypic characteristics of cerebrospinal fluid cells in children with acute lymphoblastic leukemia at diagnosis. *Blood.* 1990;76:1807–11.

20. Shmerling RH, Delbanco TL, Tosteson A, Trentham D. Synovial fluid tests: What should be ordered? *JAMA.* 1990;264:1009–14.

21. Freemont AJ, Denton J, Chuck A, Holt PJ, Davies M. Diagnostic value of synovial fluid microscopy: A reassessment and rationalisation. *Ann Rheum Dis.* 1991;50:101–7.

22. Li CY, Yam LT. Blast transformation in chronic myeloid leukemia with synovial involvement. *Acta Cytol.* 1991;35:543–45.

23. O'Connell JX. Pathology of the synovium. *Am J Clin Pathol.* 2000; 114:773–84.

24. Judkins S, Cornbleet PJ. Synovial fluid crystal analysis. *Lab Med.* 1997;28:774–79.

25. Rabinovitch A, Cornbleet J. Body fluid microscopy in US laboratories: Data from two College of American Pathologists surveys, with practice recommendations. *Arch Pathol Lab Med.* 1994;118:13–17.

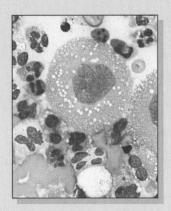

SECTION SEVEN
HEMOSTASIS

29

Primary Hemostasis

Barbara A. O'Malley, M.D.

■ OBJECTIVES—LEVEL I

At the end of this unit of study, the student should be able to:

1. Define *hemostasis, blood coagulation,* and *thrombosis.*

2. Explain the general interaction of the systems involved in maintaining hemostasis.

3. Distinguish the events that occur in primary hemostasis from those that occur in secondary hemostasis.

4. Differentiate the primary hemostatic plug from the secondary hemostatic plug.

5. Name the three types of blood vessels and explain the general roles of the vasculature and normal endothelial cells in aiding and preventing activation of the hemostatic system.

6. Describe the normal morphology and number of platelets on a peripheral blood smear and state the normal concentration in the blood.

7. Name and describe the cell that is the precursor of platelets in the bone marrow.

8. Identify and define the steps in the normal sequence of events of platelet activation following injury to the endothelium.

9. Describe the role of the primary hemostatic plug in the cessation of bleeding.

■ OBJECTIVES—LEVEL II

At the end of this unit of study, the student should be able to:

1. Identify key histologic features of each type of blood vessel and explain the metabolic functions of endothelial cells in hemostasis.

2. Describe the development of megakaryocytes and platelets in the bone marrow to include the action of humoral factors, the stem cell and progenitor cell compartment, the recognizable features of the morphologic stages, and the mechanism of release from the marrow to peripheral blood.

3. Define *endomitosis* and *polyploidy.*

4. Identify three key substances that are stored in the platelet dense bodies and five key substances stored in the platelet alpha granules and explain the role of each in hemostasis.

5. Outline steps the platelets undergo in forming the primary hemostatic plug, including the biochemical mediators necessary for platelet adhesion, platelet aggregation, and platelet secretion.

6. Correlate various platelet ultrastructural features with their functions.

7. Identify platelet agonists and predict their effect on platelet function.

8. Describe the biochemical roles of the secreted contents of the platelet granules in hemostasis.

KEY TERMS

Agonist
Alpha granule (αG)
Arachidonic acid (AA)
Clot retraction
Demarcation membrane system (DMS)
Dense bodies (DB)
Dense tubular system (DTS)
Endomitosis
Glycocalyx
Glycoprotein Ib (GPIb)
Glycoprotein IIb/IIIa (GPIIb/IIIa)
Hemostasis
Open canalicular system (OCS)
Platelet activation
Platelet adhesion
Platelet aggregation
Platelet procoagulant activity
Platelet secretion (Platelet release reaction)
Polyploid
Primary hemostatic plug
Secondary hemostatic plug
Thrombogenic/nonthrombogenic
Thrombopoietin (TPO)
Thrombosis

BACKGROUND BASICS

The information in this chapter builds on the concepts learned in previous chapters. To maximize your learning experience, you should review these concepts before starting this unit of study.

Level I

▶ Describe the bone marrow production of blood cells. (Chapters 3, 4)

Level II

▶ Summarize the hierarchy of stem and progenitor cells in the bone marrow and the growth factors that direct the proliferation and maturation of blood cells. (Chapter 3)

▶ Describe the general biology of integrins and other adhesion molecules. (Chapter 7)

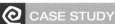
CASE STUDY

We will refer to this case study throughout the chapter.
Michael, a 20-year-old male with acute lymphocytic leukemia (ALL) is receiving chemotherapy. Two weeks after his second treatment, he notices small reddish-purple spots on his lower legs and ankles. A CBC reveals Hb 9 g/dL; WBC 2×10^9/L; platelets 19×10^9/L. Consider what could be responsible for the pancytopenia and the potential consequences of this condition.

▶ OVERVIEW

This chapter is the first of a section describing the processes involved when blood clots in response to vascular injury. The actions of the blood vessels and platelets in hemostasis are collectively called *primary hemostasis*; the actions of the protein coagulation factors are called *secondary hemostasis*. This chapter discusses primary hemostasis and first describes the physical structure and functions of the blood vessels in hemostasis. It discusses platelets in hemostasis next under the major subtopics of production, structure, and functions.

▶ INTRODUCTION

Blood normally flows through the circulatory system, a closed system of vessels. The blood vessels and their constituents are critical in controlling the physiologic functions of the circulatory system. A traumatic injury such as a cut to the finger severs vessels, resulting in bleeding. To minimize blood loss, the normally inert circulating platelets and dissolved plasma proteins mobilize to form a "clot," an insoluble mass or structural barrier (thrombus), which occludes the injured vessel and prevents further loss of blood. The formation of the clot is limited to the area of injury so that normal circulation is maintained in vessels elsewhere in the body. In other words, the hemostatic system is activated when and where it is needed. The same elements provide a continuous surveillance system that prevents leakage of plasma and cells into the tissues in normal circumstances.

Hemostasis is the property of the circulation that maintains blood as a fluid within the blood vessels and the system's ability to prevent excessive blood loss upon injury. Hemostasis is from the Greek words *heme,* meaning blood, and *stasis,* meaning to halt. The barrier mass formed to limit blood loss is known as the *hemostatic plug, blood clot,* or *thrombus.* Hemostasis requires the interaction of three compartments: the blood vessels, the platelets, and a group of soluble plasma proteins, the coagulation factors. Blood coagulation ("clotting") is the mechanism that transforms the fluid plasma into a gel by converting the soluble protein fibrinogen to the insoluble form, fibrin.

Hemostasis occurs in stages called *primary hemostasis, secondary hemostasis,* and *fibrinolysis.* During primary hemostasis, the platelets interact with the injured vessels and with each other. This interaction results in a clump of platelets known as the **primary hemostatic plug,** which temporarily arrests bleeding, but it is fragile and easily dislodged from the vessel wall.

Subsequently, insoluble strands of fibrin become deposited on and within the primary platelet plug to reinforce and stabilize it and to allow the wound to heal without further blood loss. Generation of fibrin constitutes the stage of secondary hemostasis. Fibrin is formed by a series of complex biochemical reactions involving soluble plasma proteins (coagulation factors) as they interact with the injured blood vessels and the platelet plug (∞ Chapter 30). The plug, or thrombus, is then called the **secondary hemostatic plug** (Figure 29-1 ■). The blood has changed from a liquid to a semisolid gel at the site of injury.

After the wound has healed, additional components of the hemostatic system break down and remove the clot in the fibrinolytic stage. Physiologic and biochemical inhibitors control all phases and components of the hemostatic system.

Injury also can occur to intact, unsevered blood vessels. In this case, blood clot formation can occur on an interior surface of the damaged vessel wall and result in the abnormal condition **thrombosis.**

In summary, hemostasis occurs because of the interaction of the blood vessels, platelets, and certain plasma proteins (Table 29-1 ✪). Proteins of hemostasis include those that form fibrin, those that are involved with fibrinolysis, and those that inhibit all stages of the process. Defects in one hemostatic compartment can be overcome by effective utilization of the other two; defects in two of the three compartments generally results in pathologic hemostasis and bleeding. This chapter focuses on primary hemostasis. It describes the structure and functions of the blood vessels (vascular system, or vasculature) and the platelets as they form the primary hemostatic plug. Chapter 30 describes secondary hemostasis (fibrin formation) and fibrinolysis. Chapters 31 and 32 discuss the disorders of hemostasis that result in bleeding symptoms and Chapter 33 discusses disorders that result in thrombosis.

ℓ CASE STUDY *(continued from page 613)*

1. Does Michael have a defect in primary or secondary hemostasis?

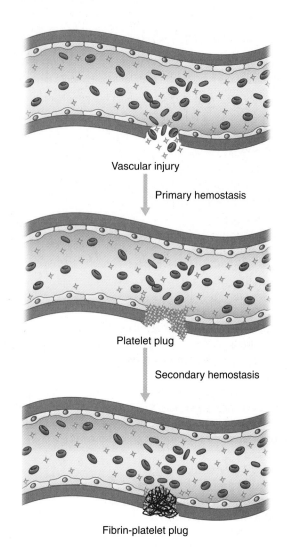

■ **FIGURE 29-1**   Stages of hemostasis after vascular injury. Bleeding occurs after an injury to a blood vessel. The hemostatic system is activated to prevent excessive blood loss. Hemostasis occurs in two stages: (1) primary hemostasis when the platelets aggregate at the site of the injury and form the platelet plug (primary hemostatic plug) and (2) secondary hemostasis when fibrin develops to strengthen the platelet plug forming the fibrin-platelet plug (secondary hemostatic plug).

Vascular injury

Primary hemostasis

Platelet plug

Secondary hemostasis

Fibrin-platelet plug

✪ TABLE 29-1
Components of Hemostasis
• Vasculature
• Platelets
• Proteins
Fibrin-forming proteins
Fibrinolytic proteins
Inhibitors

ROLE OF THE VASCULAR SYSTEM

The vascular system forms an extensive distribution system for blood, carrying nutrients to all the body's cells and tissues and transporting waste products for disposal. To perform this function, the system must provide an uninterrupted flow of blood (i.e., a nonleaking circuit) and maintain blood in a fluid state. The vascular system consists of three types of blood vessels: arteries, veins, and capillaries (Table 29-2 ✪). The arteries carry blood from the heart to the capillaries. The veins return blood from the capillaries to the heart. The vessels in which hemostasis occurs are primarily the smallest veins (*venules*) and, to a lesser degree, the smallest arteries (*arterioles*). Venules and arterioles are 20–200 μm in diameter.

STRUCTURE OF BLOOD VESSELS

The structure of all blood vessels is similar (Figure 29-2 ■) consisting of a central cavity, the lumen, through which the blood flows. The lumen is lined with a continuous, single layer of flattened endothelial cells that separate the blood from the underlying tissues and provide a protective environment for the blood's cellular elements. Overlapping portions of their cytoplasm interconnect the individual endothelial cells.

The luminal surface of the endothelial cells (on the inside of the vessel) has a thin coating of complex protein and carbohydrate substances (mucopolysaccharides) called the **glycocalyx**. The abluminal surface (on the tissue side) is attached to a basement membrane that consists of a unique form of collagen, type IV, embedded in a matrix of adhesive proteins.

Three layers of tissue in the vessel wall vary in thickness and composition depending on the size and type of vessel. Histologically on cross-section, the layers of the walls of veins and arteries appear distinct (Figure 29-2a). The innermost layer, tunica intima, consists of the endothelial cell monolayer, the basement membrane, and subendothelial connective tissue that holds them together; arteries also have an organized internal elastic membrane.

The middle layer, tunica media, is thicker in arteries than in veins. In arteries, smooth muscle cells predominate and are surrounded by loose connective tissue primarily consisting of elastin fibers, collagen fibers, reticular fibers, and proteoglycans. The tunica media of veins contains only a few smooth muscle cells, fewer elastin fibers, and a similar matrix of connective tissue. In response to a variety of physiologic stimuli, the smooth muscle cells of the tunica media contract and expand, which constricts or dilates the lumen.

The tunica adventitia, the outer coat, is thicker in veins than in arteries. A few fibroblasts are embedded in collagen and other connective tissues in this layer. The fibroblasts

✪ TABLE 29-2

Structure and Functions of Blood Vessels of the Microcirculation

Blood Vessel	Structural Characteristics	Functions
Arterioles	20–200 μm in diameter	Serve as site of hemostatic activity following injury
	Basement membrane	Regulate blood pressure by change in diameter
	Primary component is smooth muscle	Perform endothelial cell hemostatic functions
	Fibroblasts	
	Thicker wall of collagen and extracellular matrix	
Venules	20–200 μm diameter	Serve as major site of hemostatic activity following traumatic injury
	Basement membrane	Exchange nutrients, oxygen, and waste products
	Few smooth muscle cells	Regulate vascular permeability
	Few fibroblasts	Perform endothelial cell hemostatic functions
	Primary component, thin layer of collagen and extracellular matrix	
	No elastic fibers	
Capillaries	5–10 μm diameter	Have no hemostatic function except those of endothelial cells
	Single endothelial cell lumen	Exchange nutrients, oxygen, and waste products
	Basement membrane	
	No smooth muscle cells	
	No collagen fibers	
	No elastic fibers	

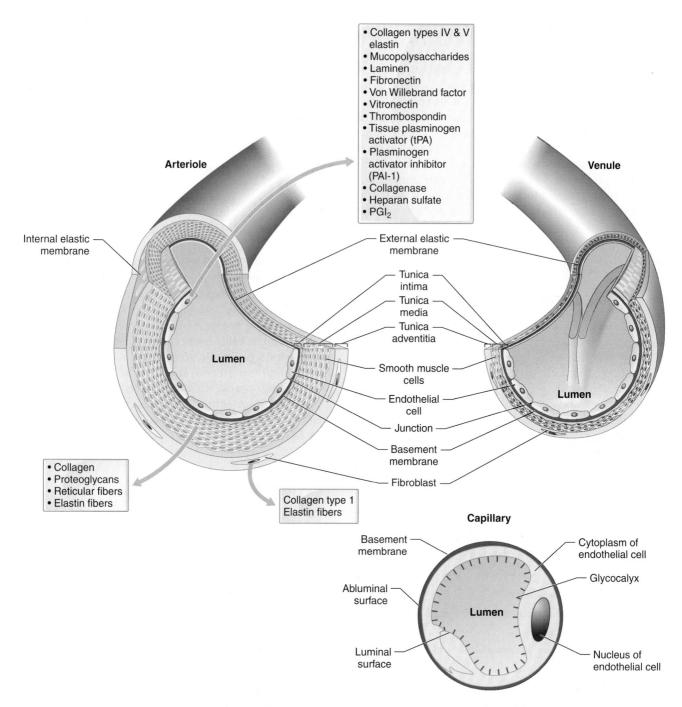

- Collagen types IV & V elastin
- Mucopolysaccharides
- Laminen
- Fibronectin
- Von Willebrand factor
- Vitronectin
- Thrombospondin
- Tissue plasminogen activator (tPA)
- Plasminogen activator inhibitor (PAI-1)
- Collagenase
- Heparan sulfate
- PGI_2

Arteriole

Venule

Internal elastic membrane

External elastic membrane

Tunica intima

Tunica media

Tunica adventitia

Smooth muscle cells

Endothelial cell

Junction

Basement membrane

Fibroblast

Lumen

Lumen

- Collagen
- Proteoglycans
- Reticular fibers
- Elastin fibers

Collagen type 1
Elastin fibers

Capillary

Basement membrane

Abluminal surface

Lumen

Luminal surface

Cytoplasm of endothelial cell

Glycocalyx

Nucleus of endothelial cell

■ **FIGURE 29-2** Structure and function of the blood vessel wall, comparing and contrasting arterioles, venules, and capillaries. **a.** Arterioles and venules. Endothelial cells, smooth muscle cells, and fibroblasts synthesize and secrete the components of the subendothelial matrix of connective tissue and the basement membrane proteins. The wall of arterioles is primarily composed of smooth muscle cells and contains elastin in contrast to the venule, which has only sparse smooth muscle cells. The media of arterioles is the most prominent layer; the adventitia layer is the largest in venules. **b.** A capillary consists primarily of endothelial cells and basement membrane with very little connective tissue.

synthesize and secrete the fibers and other components of the matrix. Mast cells are present in some layers of veins (∞ Chapter 7).

The third type of blood vessel, the capillary (Figure 29-2b), connects the arterioles and venules. Capillaries collectively compose by far, the largest surface area of all types of blood vessels, although they are individually the smallest. They are approximately $5-10 \, \mu m$ in diameter, just large enough for single blood cells to traverse. Single endothelial cells form the lumen of a capillary with their cytoplasm wrapped around in a circular form. The endothelial cells communicate with surrounding pericytes through gap junctions.[1] The tissue beneath a capillary's basement membrane is sparse and contains no smooth muscle cells.

FUNCTIONS OF BLOOD VESSELS

After an injury, the damaged vessels initiate hemostasis. The first response of vessels to injury is constriction or narrowing of the lumen of the arterioles to minimize the flow of blood into the wound area and the escape of blood from the wound site. Vasoconstriction also brings the hemostatic components of the blood (the platelets and the plasma proteins) closer to the vessel wall, facilitating their interactions. Vasoconstriction occurs immediately and lasts a short time.

The mechanism of vasoconstriction is complex. It is caused in part by neurogenic factors and in part by several regulatory substances that interact with receptors on the surface of cells of the blood vessel wall. The regulating substances include serotonin and thromboxane A_2 (both products of platelet activation) and endothelin-1 (which is produced by damaged endothelial cells). These substances can aid in prolonging vasoconstriction.[2]

In contrast, healthy intact endothelial cells synthesize and secrete a prostaglandin, PGI_2, also called *prostacyclin*. PGI_2 counteracts constriction by causing vasodilation of the arterioles.[3] Vasodilation increases blood flow into the injured area to bring fresh supplies of plasma-blood clotting substances and causes redness of the skin at the wound site.

Also after injury, endothelial cells of the venules contract, producing gaps between them and allowing plasma leakage into the tissues causing swelling or edema (increased vascular permeability). The increased blood flow into the area (vasodilation) and the increased vascular permeability are components of the *inflammatory response*, a normal physiologic response to injury.

✓ Checkpoint! 1

Think about the last time that you injured your finger with a paper cut. Did your finger bleed immediately? If not, what might have prevented immediate bleeding?

FUNCTIONS OF ENDOTHELIAL CELLS

Endothelial cells lining the lumina of blood vessels are the principal elements regulating many vascular functions. Some functions modulated by the endothelial cells are hemostatic; others are nonhemostatic in nature (Table 29-3 ⊙). The endothelial lining of normal, healthy blood vessels is **nonthrombogenic** and antithrombotic, preventing inappropriate clotting. Damaged endothelial cells become **thrombogenic**, promoting the formation of a thrombus or blood clot (Figure 29-3 ■).

Hemostatic functions that inhibit clot formation include the provision of a nonreactive environment for the components of the hemostatic system. Components of the hemostatic system (platelets and coagulation proteins) are inert in the presence of normal endothelium. Both physiologic and biochemical interactions provide the nonreactive environment.[4] Physiologically, the surface of the endothelial cells is negatively charged and repels circulating proteins and platelets, which also are negatively charged. Biochemically, a wide variety of substances is synthesized and secreted by the endothelial cells, which contribute to the nonreactive environment. These include substances that:

- inhibit platelet function (PGI_2, nitric oxide [NO], and ADPase)
- inhibit coagulation (heparan sulfate/glycosaminoglycans [cofactor for antithrombin], thrombomodulin [protein C activation], tissue factor pathway inhibitor [TFPI])
- activate fibrinolysis (tissue plasminogen activator [tPA] and urinary-type plasminogen activator [uPA])

(See ∞ Chapter 30 for a discussion of the functions of these components.)

Damaged endothelium becomes thrombogenic, producing substances that activate platelets and coagulation proteins and inhibit fibrinolysis. Damaged endothelial cells:

- produce and secrete von Willebrand factor (VWF) (∞ Chapters 30 and 32), which aids platelets in the initial stage of primary hemostasis
- produce tissue factor that is released during injury and initiates the formation of fibrin for secondary hemostasis (∞ Chapter 30)
- expose collagen in the subendothelium and secrete platelet activating factor (PAF), which activate platelets
- release plasminogen activator inhibitor (PAI-1), which inhibits fibrinolysis

Nonhemostatic functions of the endothelial cells are described on the Chapter 29 Website.

When endothelial injury occurs and bleeding starts, platelets and coagulation proteins in the plasma physically contact exposed subendothelial tissues. Interactions then occur between the vessel wall, platelets, and hemostatic proteins in the plasma to form a blood clot to stop the bleeding.

The amount of blood lost from a vessel depends on its size and type as well as on the efficiency of the hemostatic

✪ TABLE 29-3

Functions of Endothelial Cells

Component/Characteristic	Function
Hemostatic functions	
Nonthrombogenic	
Negatively charged surface	Repels platelets and hemostatic proteins
Heparan sulfate	Inhibits fibrin formation (cofactor for antithrombin)
Thrombomodulin	Inhibits fibrin formation (cofactor in activation of protein C)
PGI_2 (Prostacyclin)	Vasodilates; inhibits platelet aggregation
Tissue plasminogen activator (tPA)	Activates fibrinolytic system
Nitric oxide	Vasodilates
Thrombogenic	
Endothelin	Vasoconstricts
von Willebrand factor production and processing	Carries factor VIII (F-VIII) in plasma; causes platelet adhesion
Tissue factor	Initiates fibrin formation
Plasminogen activator inhibitor (PAI-1)	Inhibits activation of fibrinolytic system
Nonhemostatic functions	
Selective blood/tissue barrier	Keeps cells and macromolecules in vessels; allows nutrient and gas exchange
Processing of blood-borne antigens	Contributes to cellular immunity
Synthesis and secretion of connective tissue:	
Basement membrane collagen	Provides backup protection for endothelial cells
Collagen of the matrix	Is responsible for platelet adhesion
Elastin	Vasodilates and vasoconstricts
Fibronectin	Binds cells to one another
Laminin	Contributes to platelet adhesion after injury
Vitronectin	Binds cells to one another; ? platelet adhesion
Thrombospondin	Binds cells to one another; ? platelet adhesion

? = possibly

mechanism. Hemostasis is most effective in arterioles and venules. Capillaries lack the tissue layers beyond the basement membrane and do not effectively contribute to hemostasis. When larger vessels are severed, hemostatic plug formation takes longer and might not be sufficient to stop bleeding. The pressure within arteries is much higher, and the blood flow can be so rapid that clotting cannot occur effectively (e.g., within the upper aorta).

✓ Checkpoint! 2

What actions of the endothelial cells prevent clotting from occurring within the blood vessels?

▶ PLATELETS IN HEMOSTASIS

The second major component of the hemostatic system is the blood platelet. Bizzozero first established the platelet's role in hemostasis in 1882.[5] He noted that they were clumped together as part of thrombi in the mesenteric vessels of rabbits and guinea pigs.

Platelets appear on a Romanowsky-stained peripheral blood smear as small, anuclear cells with prominent reddish purple granules (Figure 29-4). They circulate as discoid-shaped structures, approximately $2-3~\mu m$ in diameter and have a lifespan of 9–12 days. The normal concentration of platelets in the blood is $150-440 \times 10^9/L$. The spleen and liver remove nonviable or aged platelets. (∞ Chapter 35 describes methods of counting platelets.)

The following sections of this chapter discuss the production of platelets in the bone marrow, their structure, and the various functions in hemostasis.

PLATELET PRODUCTION

Platelets are produced in the bone marrow from the same progenitor cell as the erythroid and myeloid series (CMP/CFU-GEMM) (∞ Chapter 3). The bipotential CFU-E/Mk ultimately gives rise to precursor cells committed to

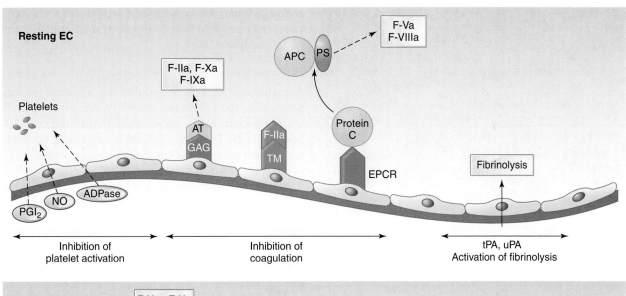

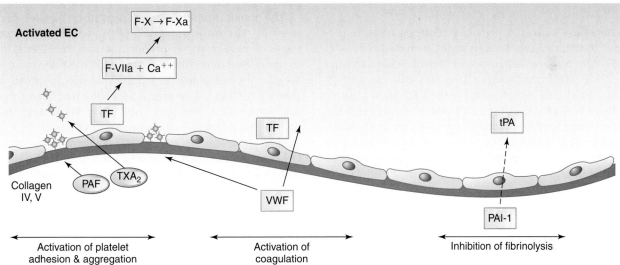

■ **FIGURE 29-3** Antithrombotic characteristics of resting endothelium versus the prothrombotic effects of damaged or activated endothelium. Resting endothelium provides an environment that inhibits activation of hemostasis. This includes secretion of substances that (1) inhibit platelet activation (PGI_2, NO, ADPase), (2) inhibit coagulation (heparan sulfate/GAG as a cofactor for AT, TM for activation of Protein C, which inactivates activated F-Va and F-VIIIa, and TFPI), and (3) activate fibrinolysis (tPA, uPA). When endothelium is damaged, it secretes substances that (1) activate platelets (TXA_2, PAF) and bind them to the vessel wall (VWF), (2) activate coagulation (TF, which initiates formation of fibrin), and (3) inhibit fibrinolysis (PAI-1). EC = endothelial cells; PGI_2 = prostacyclin; NO = nitric oxide; GAG = glycosaminoglycans; AT = antithrombin; TM = thrombomodulin; APC = activated protein C; EPCR = endothelial protein C receptor; PS = protein S; tPA = tissue type plasminogen activator; uPA = urinary type plasminogen activator; PAF = platelet activating factor; TXA_2 = thromboxane; TF = tissue factor; VWF = von Willebrand factor; PAI-1 = plasminogen activator inhibitor-1; → = stimulation; ⋯→ = inhibition

megakaryocytic development (Figure 29-5 ■). The morphologically identifiable platelet precursor cell is a megakaryocyte. Platelets are fragments of the cytoplasm of mature megakaryocytes. The cells of the megakaryocytic lineage include actively proliferating progenitor cells and postmitotic megakaryocytes undergoing maturational development.

Megakaryocyte Progenitor Cell Compartment

Megakaryocyte progenitor cells are responsible for expanding the megakaryocyte numbers and proliferating in response to a number of hematopoietic cytokines. The CFU-GEMM differentiates into a committed megakaryocyte progenitor cell (∞ Chapter 3). Using cell culture techniques to grow human adult bone marrow precursor cells,

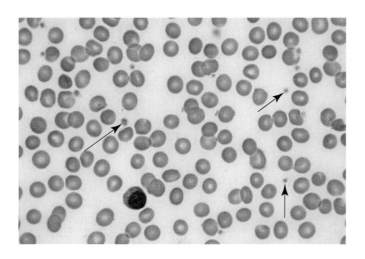

■ **FIGURE 29-4**   Peripheral blood smear. The arrows point to platelets. (Wright-Giemsa stain; 1000× magnification)

researchers have defined a hierarchy of megakaryocyte progenitor cells that develop through stages identified as *BFU-Mk* and *CFU-Mk*. Surface antigens and growth characteristics differentiate the two stages. The BFU-Mk is CD34+, HLA-DR−, c-kit+ (SCF receptor), while the CFU-Mk is positive for all three antigens. In culture, BFU-Mk produce multifocal colonies (bursts) of 100–500 megakaryocytes while the CFU-Mk produce single colonies of 4–32 megakaryocytes. A progenitor cell that is more primitive than the BFU-Mk has been grown in cultures of fetal bone marrow called the *high prolif-*

erative potential cell-megakaryocyte (HPPC-Mk).[6] Morphologically, early progenitor cells appear as small indistinguishable lymphoid-like cells.[7]

Regulation of Platelet Production

A regulatory process maintains an adequate number of platelets in the peripheral blood. Production of platelets by the bone marrow can increase or decrease according to the body's needs. The major stimulus regulating production is the platelet mass in the circulating blood plus the megakaryocyte mass in the bone marrow.[8]

Similar to their action on other myeloid cell lines,[8,9] cytokines and growth factors such as interleukin-3 (IL-3), GM-CSF, and stem cell factor influence the progenitor stages of megakaryocytes to proliferate. Interleukins-6 and -11 also affect megakaryocyte development, particularly the maturation phases, but only when they work in synergy and with other cytokines.[10]

The major humoral factor regulating platelet development is **thrombopoietin (TPO)**, which influences all stages of megakaryocyte production from the HPPC-Mk level to the release of mature platelets from the bone marrow.[11,12] Megakaryocytes grown in culture undergo apoptosis in the absence of TPO.[13] The presence of TPO had been suspected since the 1950s, but not until 1994 did several research groups first isolate it.[9] The gene for TPO was cloned shortly after its discovery. By 1997, TPO was made by recombinant DNA techniques, and its effects have been studied in vitro and in clinical trials to treat patients with certain platelet

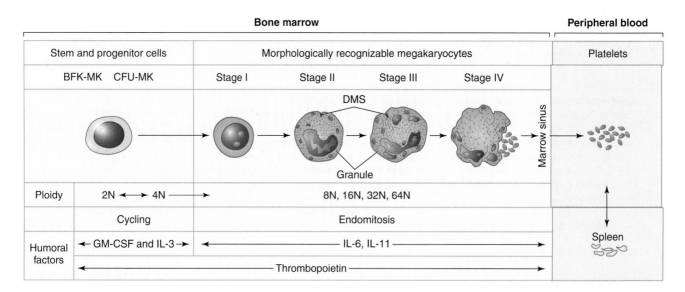

■ **FIGURE 29-5**   Production of platelets. Progenitor cells become committed to the megakaryocyte lineage. Committed progenitor stages are BFU-Mk and CFU-Mk. Megakaryoblasts undergo a series of endomitoses until nuclear maturation is complete at 8N to 64N ploidy levels. Cytoplasmic maturation occurs at ploidy levels of 8N or higher. Morphologic features of each stage of cytoplasmic maturation are described in the text. Growth factors SCF, GM-CSF, and IL-3 influence proliferation of the stem and progenitor cells. Thrombopoietin influences all stages of megakaryocyte production. IL-6 and IL-11 also support megakaryocyte production, primarily maturation. Platelets are first released between the endothelial cells of the marrow sinuses as proplatelets. Proplatelets break into mature platelets and are released into the peripheral blood.

disorders.[14] TPO is produced in the liver, the kidneys, and the spleen, and possibly in the bone marrow in patients who have low platelet counts.[8,11] Thrombopoietin is structurally related to the erythrocyte growth factor, erythropoietin.[8]

TPO maintains a constant number of platelets in the peripheral blood via a unique mechanism. Cellular production of TPO is relatively consistent from day to day. TPO binds to its receptor, Mpl (CD110), on circulating platelets and bone marrow megakaryocytes and progenitors.[8] TPO bound to circulating platelets is internalized and degraded and is not available to stimulate proliferation of bone marrow progenitor cells. Therefore, the higher the peripheral platelet count, the more TPO is bound and less TPO remains free in the plasma. This reduces both the stimulation of megakaryocyte progenitor cells in the bone marrow and platelet production. When the platelet count decreases, more TPO is free to bind to megakaryocyte progenitor cells in the bone marrow, increasing platelet production.[11] TPO appears to work both independently and in synergy with the other growth factors mentioned. The effects of TPO in patients with low platelet numbers are to increase the number of megakaryocytes in the bone marrow, the size and DNA content (ploidy level) of megakaryocytes, and the rate of maturation of the megakaryocytes.[12] The number of circulating platelets can increase from 3 to 10 times the baseline level by administration of TPO.[11] (To access more information on the Mpl receptor online, see <www.ncbi.nlm.nih.gov/prow/guide/11586825_g.htm>.)

✓ Checkpoint! 3

What would be the effect on the platelet count if a patient had a mutation in the gene for thrombopoietin that resulted in the gene's inability to code for functional mRNA?

CASE STUDY *(continued from page 614)*

2. If Michael were given TPO, how would you expect his bone marrow and peripheral blood picture to change?

Stages of Megakaryocyte Development

When TPO and other growth factors stimulate progenitor cell receptors, megakaryocyte differentiation results. The blast cell undergoes a maturation sequence that differs from that of other marrow lineages in that nuclear maturation takes place first and is largely complete before cytoplasmic maturation begins. Following an initial series of proliferative (mitotic) cell divisions, the precursor cells begin a unique nuclear maturation process consisting of a series of endomitoses. With each **endomitosis**, the cell's DNA content doubles, but cell division and nuclear division do not take place.[10] The resulting cells become **polyploid**, meaning that the DNA content, or ploidy level within a single nuclear envelope (normally 2N), can range from 4N to 64N or higher.

Endomitosis begins in megakaryoblasts and is completed by the end of stage II megakaryocytes. The 8N stage is generally the first recognizable stage on a bone marrow smear because by this stage, the megakaryocytes are becoming significantly larger than other cells in the bone marrow. The 16N stage is the most common ploidy class in adult humans.

Cytoplasmic maturation can be initiated at nuclear ploidy levels of 8N or more, but the stage at which maturation occurs varies from cell to cell. In general, nuclear maturation ceases when cytoplasmic maturation begins. The reason for variability in cytoplasmic maturation at different ploidy levels is not known. Clinical conditions associated with the presence of large platelets on the peripheral blood smear are noted to have more megakaryocytes with lower ploidy (shifted left). These large platelets are sometimes called *stress platelets* analogous to stress reticulocytes seen in anemias. Increased ploidy of an individual megakaryocyte's nucleus generally results in more cytoplasm and, thus, more platelets from that megakaryocyte.

Four arbitrary stages of megakaryocyte development are described according to their morphologic appearance on Romanowsky-stained bone marrow smears. Differentiating characteristics include nuclear morphology, cytoplasmic appearance, and relative size of the cell as determined by the ploidy class. The four stages are described in Table 29-4 ⊗. Figure 29-6■ shows an early megakaryocyte and a mature megakaryocyte. The nucleus transforms from a single (round) lobe with fine chromatin and visible nucleoli to lobulated with coarse chromatin and no visible nucleoli. In general, as the megakaryocyte matures, the cytoplasm increases in volume and changes from basophilic, nongranular, and scant in the blast stage (Stage I) to completely granular and acidophilic in the mature stage. The cytoplasm in the early stages (Stage I and II) may have a few granules appearing in the region of the Golgi apparatus whereas the cytoplasm of the mature cell (Stage IV) appears completely filled with azurophilic granules.

In addition to granules, the cytoplasm of a maturing megakaryocyte develops an internal membrane system of channels called the **demarcation membrane system (DMS).** The demarcation membrane is not visible in the light microscope and is first seen in electron micrographs at the promegakaryocyte stage. It is derived by invagination of the megakaryocyte's outer membrane and eventually develops into a highly branched, interconnected system of channels that maintain open communication with the extracellular space. As the DMS forms, small areas of the megakaryocyte cytoplasm are compartmentalized (Figure 29-7a■). These areas eventually become the platelets, and the DMS becomes the outer membrane of the platelets.[9] The separated cytoplasmic areas can be seen on the edges of the cell pictured in Figure 29-6b.

In the practical day-to-day evaluation of bone marrow specimens, distinguishing the maturation stages of megakaryocytes is not necessary. It is, however, important to recognize a cell as being of the megakaryocyte lineage.

✪ TABLE 29-4

Developmental Stages of Megakaryocytes

	Name	Characteristics
Stage I	Megakaryoblast	6–24 μm diameter
		Scant basophilic cytoplasm
		No visible granules
		Round nucleus
		Visible nucleoli
Stage II	Promegakaryocyte (basophilic megakaryocyte)	14–30 μm diameter
		Increased cytoplasm, primarily basophilic
		Few visible azurophilic cytoplasmic granules
		Indented or bilobed nucleus
		Beginning of demarcation membranes (visible with electron microscopy)
Stage III	Granular megakaryocyte	25–50 μm diameter
		Numerous cytoplasmic granules
		Abundant acidophilic cytoplasm
		Large, multilobed nucleus
		No visible nucleoli
Stage IV	Mature megakarocyte	40–60 μm diameter
		Abundant acidophilic, very granular cytoplasm
		Demarcation zones present
		Multilobulated nucleus
		No visible nucleoli

✓ Checkpoint! 4

If a patient has a mutation in the gene for TPO that resulted in the inability to code for mRNA, how would you expect the number of megakaryocytes on bone marrow smears to be affected?

Release of Platelets

The primary site of megakaryocyte development and platelet production (megakaryocytopoiesis) is in the bone marrow. Mature megakaryocytes are typically situated less than 1 μm from the abluminal surface of the marrow sinus endothelial cells and shed platelets directly into the sinuses. Platelets appear to be released from megakaryocytes in groups called *proplatelets,* which are long slender protrusions of megakaryocyte cytoplasm called *pseudopods* or *filopodia* (Figure 29-7b ■). Each megakaryocyte extrudes multiple cytoplasmic extensions between endothelial cells into the marrow sinuses as proplatelets, which then break up into individual platelets. The megakaryocyte nucleus remains in the marrow and is engulfed by the marrow macrophages. Localized apoptosis (caspase activation) is thought to play a role in the final stages of platelet formation and release.[15,16] Whole intact megakaryocytes occasionally are released from the marrow, circulate in the peripheral blood, and become trapped in capillary beds in the spleen and lungs. These cells also can release platelets to the peripheral blood.[17] One mature megakaryocyte produces between 1000–3000 platelets.

Development of a megakaryoblast to the platelet-producing stage requires approximately 7 days. Two-thirds of the platelets that are released into the peripheral blood circulate in the bloodstream; the remaining third is sequestered in the spleen and is in equilibrium with those platelets in the circulation. The average life span of platelets in peripheral blood is ~9.5 days.

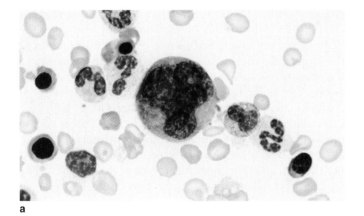

a

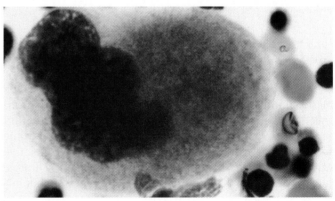

b

■ FIGURE 29-6 **a.** Early megakaryocyte. **b.** Mature megakaryocyte. (Bone marrow; Wright-Giemsa stain; 1000× magnification)

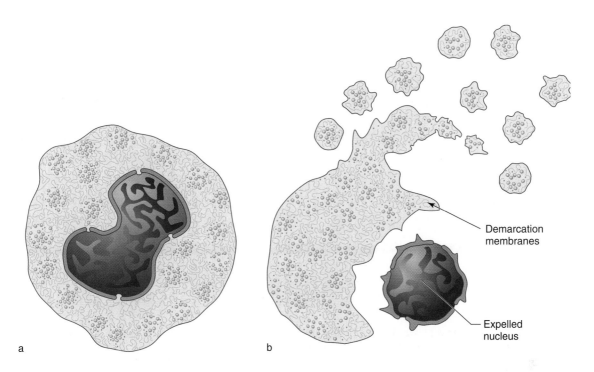

■ **FIGURE 29-7** **a.** Mature megakaryocyte showing future platelets. **b.** Platelet release from mature megakaryocyte. Outward extrusion of cytoplasm, eventually breaking up into individual platelets delineated by demarcation membrane system (arrow). Expelled nucleus is phagocytized by marrow macrophages.

Demarcation
membranes

Expelled
nucleus

a

b

PLATELET STRUCTURE

Circulating inert platelets are disc shaped anucleate cell fragments with smooth surfaces. Unlike the exterior surfaces of erythrocytes and leukocytes, the surface membranes of platelets have several openings resembling holes in a sponge. The openings are membranous channels that extend deep into the interior of the cells.

Circulating platelets repel one another and the surfaces of the endothelial cells that line the interior lumen of blood vessels. After an injury, many changes affecting the platelet morphology and biochemistry occur, causing the platelets to become "activated" after which they interact with the vessel wall and other platelets to form the primary hemostatic plug. To understand the activation process, the ultrastructure of normal platelets must be considered.

The platelet ultrastructure is divided into four arbitrary regions or zones: peripheral zone, structural zone, organelle zone, and membrane systems[12] (Figure 29-8 ■ and Table 29-5 ✪). The components of each region have specific functions in activated platelets and are discussed in the following sections.

Peripheral Zone

The peripheral zone of the platelet consists of a phospholipid membrane covered on the exterior by a fluffy surface coat and on the interior by a thin submembranous region

between the cytoplasmic membrane and the next layer. Microfilaments are present in the submembranous region, the nature of which is described below.

The surface coat, or glycocalyx, is thicker on platelets than on most other cells (~14–20 nm). It consists of glycolipids, membrane glycoproteins, proteins, mucopolysaccharides, and adsorbed plasma proteins, including coagulation factor V (F-V), VWF, and fibrinogen (∞ Chapters 30 and 31). The glycocalyx is responsible for the platelet surface's negative charge and is found on the surface membrane of the interior channels. Some surface proteins are receptors for substances that cause **platelet activation**.

The cytoplasmic membrane has a typical trilaminar structure of a bilayer of phospholipid and embedded integral proteins. It functions to maintain cytoplasmic integrity and to mediate interactions between platelets and the vasculature and plasma proteins. The membrane is the former demarcation membrane of the parent megakaryocyte. The surface membrane of platelets invaginates to give rise to a system of channels, the *surface-connected open canalicular system (OCS)*.

An asymmetrical arrangement of the phospholipids is an important factor in the function of platelets. Phosphatidylcholine (PC) and sphingomyelin (SM), which are neutral in charge, are concentrated on the outer half while negatively charged phospholipids (phosphatidylserine [PS], phosphatidylinositol [PI], and phosphatidylethanolamine [PE]) predominate on the inner half of the bilayer.[2] The phospholipid

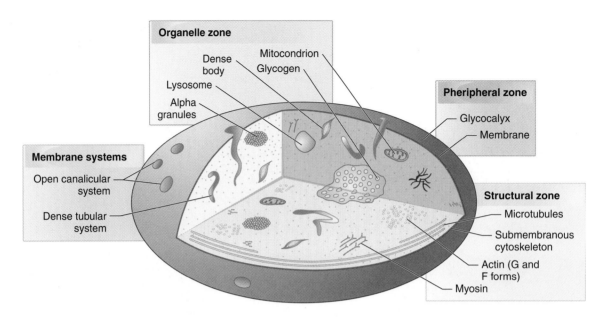

■ FIGURE 29-8   Diagram of platelet ultrastructure. (Modified, with permission, from Thompson AR, Harker LA. *Manual of Hemostasis and Thrombosis*, 3rd ed. Philadelphia: F.A. Davis; 1982.)

asymmetry is maintained in resting platelets by an ATP-dependent amino phospholipid translocase that actively pumps PE and PS from the outer to the inner leaflet.[18] The negatively charged phospholipids accelerate several steps in the plasma protein coagulation sequence. The placement of these phospholipids on the platelet membrane's inner leaflet separates them from the plasma coagulation proteins and prevents inappropriate coagulation. However, during platelet activation, these phospholipids become exposed on the platelet surface, facilitating their interactions with plasma procoagulant proteins.

The cytoplasmic membrane contains integral proteins that are receptors for stimuli involved in platelet function. Approximately 30 proteins have been identified as glycoproteins, and a nomenclature system has been developed using GP for glycoprotein and a Roman numeral from I to IX according to electrophoretic migration by decreasing molecular weight. Glycoproteins Ib, IIb, IIIa, and IX play a major role in platelet function and pathophysiology (∞ Chapter 31).

Glycoprotein Ib (GPIb) is the major platelet receptor for VWF (Figure 29-9a ■). It is noncovalently associated with GPIX and GPV in the membrane (in a ratio of 2:2:1). The function of GPV is not known, and no clinical bleeding problems are associated with its absence. GPV is not required for either membrane expression of the GPIb/IX complex or for interaction between GPIb/IX and VWF. The function of GPIX is also unknown, but it is required for efficient surface expression of GPIb. Rare bleeding disorders are associated with abnormalities of GPIb and with GPIX. The complex (also known as CD42) is referred to in this text as *GPIb/IX*.

Glycoprotein Ib consists of two chains, α and β. The GPIbα chain is larger and contains the binding sites for VWF, thrombin, and ristocetin (used in the platelet aggregation test described in ∞ Chapter 40). The binding sites are located on the major extracellular portion of GPIb called *glycocalicin*. The glycocalicin portion of the chain extends from the platelet surface and can be cleaved by proteolytic enzymes. Plasma levels of glycocalicin correlate with platelet production and can be used to differentiate thrombocytopenia due to decreased platelet production (low plasma glycocalicin) from that resulting from increased platelet destruction (elevated glycocalicin).[19,20] The remainder of GPIbα is associated with the GPIbβ chain and spans the phospholipid bilayer. On the cytoplasmic side, both the α and the β portions are associated with actin-binding protein. Each platelet contains approximately 25,000 GPIb/IX complexes.[17] GPIb/IX functions in the platelet adhesion process (as explained later).

Glycoproteins IIb and IIIa associate in the membrane, forming a complex (**GPIIb/IIIa**), which is the major plasma membrane receptor for fibrinogen (Figure 29-9b ■). The GPIIb/IIIa complex also binds other subendothelial adhesive proteins such as VWF, thrombospondin, vitronectin, and fibronectin. Each platelet has approximately 80,000–100,000 copies of this receptor on its external membrane, and another 30,000 copies are present within platelets on the internal membranes of the α-granules, dense bodies, and OCS.[21] These internal receptors join the plasma membrane when platelets are activated and undergo secretion.[18]

Glycoprotein IIb, the larger of the two subunits, is a two-chain protein. The α chain is embedded in the phospholipid bilayer, and the β chain protrudes from the platelet surface. Part of the β chain carries the HPA-3 (formerly Bak^a) platelet

TABLE 29-5

Platelet Ultrastructure and Functions

Zone and Component	Function/Role
Peripheral zone	Adhesion and aggregation
Glycocalyx	
Proteins, glycoproteins, mucopolysaccharides	
Phospholipid bilayer	
Phospholipids	Asymmetric arrangement; source of arachidonic acid
Integral proteins	
Glycoproteins Ib/IX, IIb/IIIa	Adhesion and aggregation
Enzymes	Activation
Structural zone	Structure and support
Microtubules (tubulin)	
Cytoskeletal network	
Microfilaments (Actin)	
Intermediate filaments (filamin/ actin-binding protein, talin, vimetin)	
Organelle zone	Secretion and storage
Granules	
Dense bodies	Nonprotein mediators (ADP, ATP, serotonin)
Alpha granules	Protein mediators
Lysosomes	Enzymes
Peroxisomes	Lipid metabolism
Mitochondria	Oxidative energy metabolism
Glycogen	
Membrane systems	Secretion and storage
Open canalicular system	Secretion of granule contents
Dense tubular system	Storage of calcium

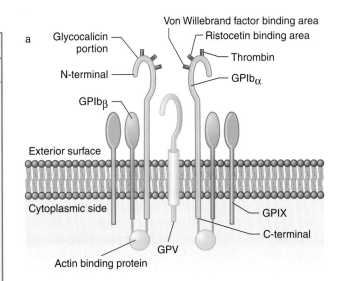

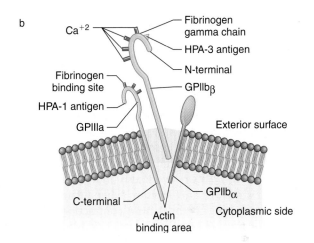

FIGURE 29-9 Structure of platelet membrane glycoproteins. **a.** Glycoprotein Ib is composed of an alpha and a beta chain. Both span the phospholipid bilayer. The alpha chain is larger and contains the binding sites for thrombin, ristocetin, and VWF. Actin-binding protein is attached to the cytoplasmic side. Glycoprotein IX and glycoprotein V associate with glycoprotein Ib in the platelet membrane. **b.** Glycoproteins IIb and IIIa associate in a complex after platelet activation. Binding sites for fibrinogen as well as platelet-specific antigens are present. Cytoplasmic portions of each component have binding areas for actin.

✓ **Checkpoint! 5**

If a patient inherited a mutation of the gene for glycoprotein IIIa that resulted in its absence, what two platelet antigens would be decreased or absent?

Structural Zone

alloantigen. Glycoprotein IIIa is a single chain polypeptide and is associated with the GPIIb portion that lies within the phospholipid bilayer. The small surface portion of GPIIIa contains the HPA-1 (formerly Pl^{A1}) alloantigen. The cytoplasmic tails of the two proteins are associated with actin in the platelet cytoskeleton. The GPIIb/IIIa complex is a latent receptor "hidden" in resting platelets and has low affinity for fibrinogen binding. When agonists activate platelets, the GPIIb/IIIa complex is converted to a high-affinity ligand-binding conformation. The high-affinity configuration is required for platelet aggregation (described later). GPIIb/IIIa is an $\alpha_{IIb}\beta_3$ integrin (CD41/CD61). The GPIIb/IIIa receptors appear to be responsible for the uptake of fibrinogen from plasma into megakaryocytes and platelets.

The structural zone consists of *microtubules* and a submembranous and cytoplasmic network of *microfilaments* and *intermediate filaments.* The structural zone's functions are to support the plasma membrane, stabilize the resting discoid shape of the platelet, and provide a means of shape change when the platelet is activated.

Microtubules (MT) are composed of the protein tubulin. Each is a bundle of 8 to 24 hollow tubules (25 nm diameter) located beneath the submembranous region of microfilaments and completely surrounds the circumference of the resting platelet.

The submembranous protein network consists of actin microfilaments, actin-binding protein, and several other structural proteins (intermediate filaments) that form a cytoskeleton supporting the plasma membrane (Web Figure 29-1 ■). Actin, the most abundant protein in platelets, accounts for 15–20% of the total protein content. It has two forms, monomeric G (globular) actin and F (filamentous) actin. The F form consists of several polymerized G molecules. Approximately 30–40% of the actin in a resting platelet is in the F form with the remainder in the G form. Actin-binding protein is attached to the cytoplasmic side of the GPIb/IX complex and anchors actin to the membrane.[19] Upon platelet activation, the submembranous microfilaments and intermediate filaments reorganize, polymerize, and form the characteristic filapodia (pseudopods) seen in activated platelets.

Actin also is part of a network of structural support proteins dispersed throughout the cytoplasm. In the cytoplasm, actin is associated with myosin and several other contractile proteins similar to those of smooth muscle. Unlike smooth muscle, in which the ratio of actin: myosin is about 7:1, the platelet ratio is ~100:1. This network also undergoes significant changes in structure and location when platelets become activated, resulting in the central contraction of MT and relocation of organelles during platelet activation and shape change.

Organelle Zone

The organelle zone is beneath the MT layer and consists of mitochondria, glycogen particles (which support the platelet's metabolic activities), and four types of granules dispersed within the cytoplasm. The granules are *dense bodies, alpha granules, lysosomal granules,* and *peroxisomes;* they serve as storage sites for proteins and other substances essential for platelet function. Generally, mature platelets have very little ribosomes or rough endoplasmic reticulum.

Platelets contain 3–8 electron-dense organelles, 20–30 nm in diameter. These **dense bodies (DB)** are so named because they appear denser in electron microscope preparations than the other types of granules due to their high Ca^{2+} content. These bodies contain mediators of platelet function and hemostasis that are not proteins: ADP, ATP, and other nucleotides as well as phosphate compounds, calcium ions, and serotonin (Table 29-6 ✪). The ADP in the dense bodies is known as the *nonmetabolic,* or *storage, pool* of ADP to distinguish it from metabolic ADP found in the cytoplasm. The ratio of ADP:ATP in the DB is higher than that found in the cytoplasm (3:2 vs 1:8 in the cytoplasm). The metabolic pool

✪ TABLE 29-6

Composition and Functions of Platelet Dense Body Contents

Component	Role
ADP (nonmetabolic)	Agonist for platelets
ATP (nonmetabolic)	Agonist for cells other than platelets; activates Ca^{2+} influx channel in outer membrane
Other nucleotides	Unknown
Inorganic phosphates	Unknown
Calcium	Platelet activation
Serotonin	Vasoconstriction; platelet agonist

provides energy for normal platelet metabolism, whereas the storage pool is important in the platelet aggregation reactions. Serotonin is taken up from the plasma and stored in the DB.

Alpha granules (αG) are the most numerous of the four types of granules, numbering ~50–80 per platelet. They contain two major groups of proteins (Table 29-7 ✪): One group consists of proteins similar to hemostatic proteins found in the plasma. Some, such as VWF, are synthesized in the megakaryocyte as the platelets develop.[22] Others, such as fibrinogen, immunoglobulins, and albumin, are absorbed from the plasma by megakaryocytes and packaged in the αG during thrombopoiesis.[10] The second group includes proteins with a variety of functions. Some are found exclusively in platelets (e.g., platelet factor 4 and β-thromboglobulin). Some proteins are growth factors that affect the growth and gene expression of smooth muscle cells in the blood vessel wall (e.g., platelet derived growth factor). Plasminogen activator inhibitor is present in platelet αG in addition to being synthesized by endothelial cells. Platelet αG also contain a number of adhesive proteins including fibronectin, VWF, vitronectin, and thrombospondin.

Lysosomal granules contain several hydrolytic enzymes and are similar to the lysosomes found in other cells. The peroxisomes are thought to be involved in lipid metabolism.[18]

Platelets contain all of the necessary enzymes for the glycolytic and tricarboxylic acid cycles and for glycogen synthesis and degradation. About 50% of the platelet's energy (ATP) is derived from the glycolytic pathway, and about 50% is derived from the tricarboxylic acid cycle.

Membrane Systems

The fourth structural zone of the platelet is composed of two systems of membranes. One, the **surface-connected open canalicular system** (SCCS or OCS) is an elaborate, interconnected series of conduits leading from the platelet surface to its interior. This OCS is derived from the demarcation membrane system of the parent megakaryocyte and serves several functions in platelets. It provides for both the entry of external substances into the interior of platelets and a

TABLE 29-7

Composition and Functions of Platelet Alpha Granule Proteins

Protein	Role
Group I—hemostatic proteins	
Fibrinogen	Platelet aggregation
	Conversion to fibrin
F-V, F-XI	Fibrin formation
Protein S, tissue factor pathway inhibitor, α_1 protease inhibitor, C1 esterase inhibitor	Inhibition of coagulation
von Willebrand factor	Platelet adhesion
	Carries F-VIII in plasma
Plasminogen	Conversion to plasmin (fibrinolysis)
PAI-1, α_2-PI	Fibrinolytic inhibitors
Group II—nonhemostatic proteins	
Platelet-specific	
β-thromboglobulin	Chemoattractant for neutrophils, fibroblasts
	Neutralizes heparin
Platelet factor 4	Neutralizes heparin
	Weak neutrophil and fibroblast chemoattractant
Platelet-derived growth factor (PDGF)	Promotes regrowth of smooth muscle cells (wound repair)
Transforming growth factor— beta (TGF$_\beta$), epidermal growth factor (EGF), insulin-like growth factor (IGF)	Mitogenic factors
Vascular endothelial growth factor (VEGF)	Angiogenic factor
Not platelet specific	
Albumin	Unknown
Thrombospondin, fibronectin, vitronectin	Adhesive glycoproteins

route for the release of granule contents to the outside. The OCS also represents an extensive internal store of membranes. Activated platelets undergoing shape change, filopodia formation and spreading require a dramatic increase in surface membrane compared to resting platelets, which OCS membranes provide. Because the OCS membranes contain many of the same glycoproteins as the surface membrane, it also serves as a source for additional plasma membrane glycoproteins during platelet activation.[18]

A second type of membrane is the **dense tubular system (DTS)**, which originates from the residual endoplasmic reticulum of the megakaryocyte. The channels of the DTS do not connect with the surface of the platelet. The DTS is a storage site for ionized calcium within platelets analogous to the sarcoplasmic reticulum of muscle cells and releases Ca^{2+} when platelets are activated.[23] The concentration of calcium ions within the platelet cytoplasm is important in regulating platelet metabolism and activation. The DTS is also a major site of prostaglandin and thromboxane synthesis.[24]

PLATELET FUNCTION

Platelet Roles in Hemostasis

Platelets are involved in several aspects of hemostasis (Table 29-8). One role appears to be performing passive surveillance of the blood vessel endothelial lining for gaps and breaks. Although the exact nature of this role is somewhat controversial, it has been shown that platelets maintain the vessels' continuity or integrity by filling in the small gaps caused by the separation of endothelial cells. Platelets attach to the underlying exposed collagen fibers of the subendothelium and prevent blood from escaping. A decrease in the number of platelets in the peripheral blood results in blood leaking through these gaps into the tissues.

When injury occurs and an actual break in the continuity of the lining of the vessels occurs, the platelets react by forming the primary hemostatic plug. By sticking first to exposed collagen and other components of the subendothelium and then to each other, the platelets form a mass that mechanically fills openings in the vessels and limits the loss of blood from the injury site.

Following platelet plug formation, membrane phospholipids of the aggregated platelets provide a reaction surface for the proteins that make fibrin. Fibrin stabilizes the initial platelet plug, and the entire mass of fibrin and platelets constitutes the secondary hemostatic plug.

As a fourth role, platelet-derived growth factors stimulate smooth muscle cells and fibroblasts to divide and replace the cells that were damaged, thus promoting healing of the injured tissues.

The steps and mechanisms that result in primary and secondary hemostatic plug formation are described next.

Formation of the Primary Hemostatic Plug

Platelets circulating in blood vessels do not interact with other platelets or other cell types. Circulating platelets are disc-shaped and inert in the environment of normal endothelium (Figure 29-10a ▪). Injury to the blood vessels

TABLE 29-8

Platelet Roles in Hemostasis

- Perform surveillance of blood vessel continuity
- Platelet-platelet interactions (primary hemostatic plug)
- Platelet-coagulation protein interactions (secondary hemostatic plug)
- Aid in healing injured tissue

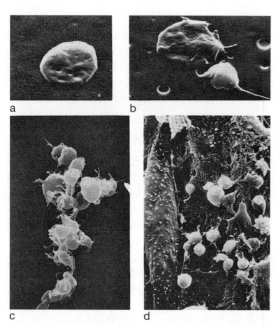

■ FIGURE 29-10 Stages of platelet activation. **a.** "Resting," disc-shaped platelet. **b.** Partially activated platelet (upper left) and fully activated platelet (spiny sphere—lower right). **c.** Aggregate of activated platelets. **d.** Platelets (P) adherent to exposed subendothelium (SE). EC = intact endothelial cells (Figure courtesy of Dr. Marion Barnhart, Wayne State University School of Medicine).

causes a change in the normal environment, and in response, activate the platelets. The primary hemostatic plug is the result of the transformation of the platelets from an inactive to an active state. The formation of a platelet plug requires several platelet activation events, including adhesion, contraction or shape change, secretion, and aggregation (Figure 29-11 ■).

Platelet Adhesion The major function of platelets is to seal openings in the vascular network. The initial stimulus for platelet activation and deposition is exposure of subendothelial components of the vessel walls that are normally hidden from circulating platelets. The subendothelium contains a large number of adhesive proteins, and the platelet has receptors for many of them. The first step in primary hemostatic plug formation, **platelet adhesion**, is the attachment of platelets to collagen and other components of the subendothelium. Platelets contain two collagen receptors: GPIaIIa and GPVI, which mediate direct collagen binding at

■ FIGURE 29-11 Diagram of platelets forming the primary hemostatic plug. Tissue injury causes platelets to adhere to subendothelial collagen. Shape change, secretion of granule contents, and aggregation follow. Additional platelets become activated by the secreted substances and clump together, eventually forming a mechanical barrier that halts the flow of blood from the wound.

Tissue injury

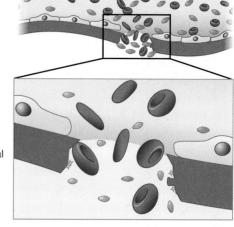

Platelet adhesion (subendothelial collagen)

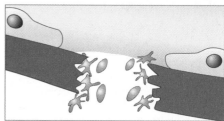

Shape change

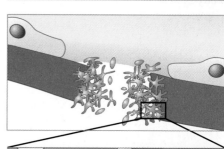

Platelet aggregation

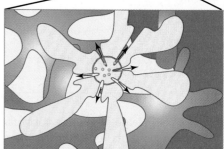

Secretion

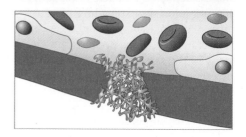

Primary hemostatic plug

low shear rates. Platelet adhesion to collagen at high shear rates, however, requires the presence of VWF and the platelet VWF receptor, GPIb/IX.

VWF, which is synthesized by endothelial cells and megakaryocytes, is both stored in intracellular granules (Weibel Palade bodies in endothelial cells and αG in platelets) and secreted into the plasma. It is deposited in the subendothelium, where it is bound to collagen (Web Figure 29-2 ■ and ∞ Chapter 31). VWF is a multimeric protein made up of a series of identical subunits, each containing binding sites for both GPIb/IX on the platelet surface and collagen in the subendothelium. Circulating VWF will not bind to GPIb/IX. However, high shear rates cause conformational changes in immobilized VWF and/or GPIb, and platelets readily adhere to VWF immobilized on collagen via their GPIb/IX receptors.[25,26] VWF thus becomes a "bridge" connecting the platelet to the collagen fibers (Web Figure 29-2).

While the tissues have numerous other adhesion molecules and the platelet surface has many other receptors, their contributions to platelet adhesion in vivo remain uncertain. Platelets preferentially bind to collagen via VWF under conditions of high shear rates. The GPIb/IX receptor is functionally available in the resting platelet, and binding does not require platelet activation or Ca^{2+}. Once its ligand becomes available, adhesion occurs; it is a passive, non energy-requiring process and is potentially reversible in its early stages. Many platelets adhere in a similar manner until a monolayer of platelets covers the exposed surface of the subendothelium (Figure 29-10d ■).

Much of what is known about this phase of platelet function has been learned from studying patients with two diseases in which platelets fail to adhere properly: Bernard-Soulier disease and von Willebrand disease (VWD). Patients with Bernard-Soulier disease have mutations in one of the genes of the GPIb/IX complex that cause either decreased amounts of the receptor complex on the platelet surface or abnormal function of the complex (∞ Chapter 31). Patients with VWD have mutations in the gene encoding VWF (∞ Chapter 32).

✓ Checkpoint! 6

If a patient with Bernard-Soulier disease or VWD cut a finger, would you expect bleeding to stop as fast as the bleeding stops when you cut your own finger? Why or why not?

Platelet Activation Adhesion of platelets to subendothelial components via VWF triggers a series of morphologic and functional changes known as *platelet activation.* Activation is a complex process that includes changes in metabolic biochemistry, platelet morphology (shape), surface receptors, and membrane phospholipid orientation. Key outcomes of activation are the generation of active GPIIb/IIIa receptors for fibrinogen binding, the secretion of the contents of the platelet granules into the surrounding tissue, and the formation of platelet aggregates. Only activated platelets are able to proceed with the subsequent steps in the formation of the primary hemostatic plug. Once activated, the platelet response becomes self-perpetuating and irreversible. Through strict control mechanisms, platelet activation remains localized to the injured area. The cellular changes associated with activation are described first, followed by the changes in platelet biochemistry. Activation of platelets is summarized schematically in Figure 29-12 ■ and in Web additional files.

Platelet Agonists A number of substances have been shown to stimulate platelets and to activate them. An agent

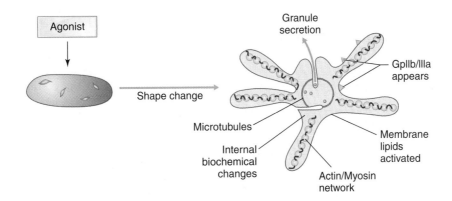

■ FIGURE 29-12 Platelet shape change after stimulation by an agonist. Pseudopods develop on the platelet surface and contain a network of actin and myosin; the microtubule circumferential ring contracts; the membrane phospholipids are activated; glycoprotein IIb/IIIa receptors appear; internal biochemical changes occur; and granule secretion follows.

that induces platelet activation is called an **agonist**. Each agonist binds to the platelet surface at its specific platelet receptor. A signal is transmitted (transduced) internally by the receptor, and a series of reactions in the interior of the platelet leads to subsequent platelet responses. The signal transduction mechanisms in the platelet are similar to those of other cells.

Some agonists (Table 29-9 ✪) are generated by the platelets themselves and some by other cells or molecules at the site of injury. Some agonists are normally present within cells and are released when the cells are injured or activated; others are synthesized de novo with activation. Agonists are often grouped as "strong" or "weak." Strong agonists (e.g., collagen, thrombin) can activate the full range of platelet functions themselves (shape change, secretion, aggregation). Weak agonists initiate platelet activation but require platelet synthesis and release of endogenous TXA_2 (i.e., activation of the platelet cyclooxygenase pathway) to drive full activation through secretion and aggregation. Thrombin is probably the most potent activator of platelets in vivo.[17]

Platelet Shape Change   Activation of platelets by a number of agonists is accompanied by a change in the platelet's shape from flattened disc-shaped cells to spiny spheres with long projections from the surface called *pseudopods* or *filopodia* (Figure 29-10b). Shape change involves reorganization of proteins in the structural zone including the MT, submembranous cytoskeletal proteins, and actin and myosin cytoplasmic filaments. The MTs contract centrally within the activated platelet, concentrating the platelet organelles in the center of the cell (causing the change to a spherical rather than flattened cell). This brings the platelet granules into closer proximity to the OCS, facilitating secretion. The protrusive force for developing filopodia is due to actin polymerization and is an energy-requiring process. After platelets adhere to the subendothelium, they undergo variable degrees of "spreading," resulting in the development of broad lamellipodia rather than spikelike filopodia.[27] As a result of the shape change, each platelet has

a larger membrane surface area for biochemical reactions and a larger area for contact with the injured tissue and other platelets.

The cytoskeletal rearrangements, resulting in shape change and spreading, alter membrane glycoproteins. GPIb/IX receptors are moved from the platelet surface to the OCS and internalized while active GPIIb/IIIa receptors increase in density on the platelet surface as they are mobilized from αG and OCS membranes.[28] The result is to convert the activated platelet from an "adhesive" state to an "aggregation" state.

Shape change leads to succeeding responses if the stimulus from the agonists is strong enough. In the absence of a sufficiently strong stimulus, the platelet returns to its original discoid shape.

Platelet Secretion (Release)   Following the centralization of organelles by the contractile process responsible for shape change, platelets begin to discharge granule contents into the surrounding area, a process known as **platelet secretion** or **platelet release reaction**. Secretion is an energy-dependent process requiring ATP. The open canalicular system fuses with membranes of granules that have been centralized deep within the platelets interior during platelet shape change, and the contents are then extruded through the OCS to the exterior of the platelet. Alternatively, secretion can occur by direct fusion with the plasma membrane.[18]

Secretion provides a positive feedback mechanism in platelet activation. Some of the substances released from the platelet granules (e.g., serotonin, ADP) function as agonists that stimulate membrane receptors on additional platelets. The binding of secreted ligands to platelet receptors repeats itself, resulting in the recruitment of additional layers of platelets and ultimately the formation of a platelet plug. These positive feedback mechanisms ensure an adequate hemostatic response.

Roles of the Granule Contents   The DB release their contents into the surrounding tissue (Table 29-6). The DB release of ADP is considered to be of primary importance because ADP functions as an agonist, producing a positive feedback mechanism in the continued stimulation and recruitment of additional platelets. The receptors for ADP are designated $P2Y_1$, $P2Y_{12}$, and P2X1 receptors.[18] Stimulation by ADP results in the typical response of increased cytoplasmic calcium, more platelet release, and the appearance of active fibrinogen receptors (GPIIb/IIIa).

DB release calcium extracellularly with the ADP. This calcium is nonmetabolic and is not involved in the internal stimulation processes. The extruded calcium is believed to provide a high concentration outside the platelets necessary for fibrinogen attachment and for other enzymatic reactions that take place on the platelet exterior surface. Other components and their functions are listed in Table 29-6.

The αG contain a wide variety of proteins (see Table 29-7 for a partial list of αG components). Some are specific for the

---

✪ TABLE 29-9

Platelet Agonists

Platelet-derived agonists
- ADP
- Serotonin
- Platelet-activating factor (PAF)
- Thromboxane A_2 (TXA_2)

Other (nonplatelet-derived) agonists
- Collagen*
- Thrombin*
- Epinephrine

*strong agonists (full activation of platelet does not require cyclooxygenase activity)

platelet, and others are similar to hemostatic proteins found in the plasma. The platelet-specific proteins include platelet factor 4 (PF4) and β-thromboglobulin (βTG). Both have heparin-neutralizing activity, although βTG does not bind heparin as avidly as PF4. Heparin is an anticoagulant used to treat patients who are hypercoagulable (have increased tendency to form clots) or who are at increased risk of thrombosis (∞ Chapter 33). PF4 performs many other actions including chemotactic activity for neutrophils, monocytes, and fibroblasts. βTG, which is actually a family of proteins, also is a chemoattractant for fibroblasts and can promote wound healing.

Thrombospondin constitutes about 20% of the protein released from the platelet αG. It is also synthesized by other cells including endothelial cells and is found in the extracellular connective tissue. It may function to stabilize the aggregated platelets.[21]

Platelets contain a number of growth factors, including PDGF, TGF$_\beta$, EGF, and IGF. All function as mitogens and are thought to contribute to healing injured tissue.[18]

F-V, VWF, and fibrinogen are proteins in the αG that are similar to hemostatic proteins of the plasma. F-V can function as a receptor on the platelet surface for hemostatic proteins (F-Xa and prothrombin, ∞ Chapter 30) and is a cofactor in the process of fibrin formation. Platelets contain ~20% of the F-V in whole blood,[29] which, like fibrinogen, appears to be taken up from plasma.[30] The functions of VWF and fibrinogen have been discussed previously. Plasminogen activator inhibitor (PAI-1) and α_2-antiplasmin, when released from activated platelets, appear to protect newly formed clots from lysis. When released from the platelet granules, these hemostatic proteins can serve as an additional source of these components for secondary hemostasis.

Platelet Aggregation During platelet adhesion, VWF binding to GPIb/IX triggers intracellular signaling that results in activation of GPIIb/IIIa in the platelet membrane, which then binds soluble fibrinogen. The active GPIIb/IIIa complex appears soon after platelet activation with any agonist. Resting platelets do not express functional GPIIb/IIIa complex and are unable to bind fibrinogen. This prevents unactivated platelets from aggregating as they circulate in the plasma. With the development of the high-affinity, ligand-binding form of GPIIb/IIIa, the platelet is functionally able to undergo platelet aggregation.[18]

Platelet aggregation is the attachment of platelets to one another (Figure 29-10c). Newly arriving platelets flowing into the area become activated by contact with agonists such as ADP and TXA$_2$ (released by the initial adherent and activated platelets), products from the damaged tissue and endothelial cells, and thrombin (a procoagulant enzyme generated by tissue factor/F-VIIa) (∞ Chapter 30). With activation, the new platelets undergo shape change and exposure of their active GPIIb/IIIa sites. The fibrinogen bound to activated platelets serves as a bridge, cross-linking GPIIb/IIIa molecules on two adjacent platelets.

Fibrinogen is able to link two platelets because of its molecular structure (∞ Chapter 30). Briefly, it is a dimeric molecule composed of two each of three polypeptide chains: Aα_2,Bβ_2,γ_2. One fibrinogen molecule attaches to the GPIIb/IIIa receptors on two adjacent platelets via binding sites at the carboxy terminal end of each of the γ chains[31] (Figure 29-13 ■). The α chains also contain sequences for platelet binding. Approximately 40,000–50,000 molecules of fibrinogen are bound to each activated platelet. Fibrinogen binding is reversible for a time, but after about 10 to 30 minutes, it becomes irreversible. Ca^{2+} is needed for platelet aggregation to occur whereas platelet adhesion does not require Ca^{2+}.

Fibrinogen and Ca^{2+} are supplied by both the plasma and internal platelet storage sites (αG, DB, DTS), which provide high concentrations of both constituents in the injured area.

The importance of GPIIb/IIIa receptors in platelet aggregation was demonstrated by studying patients with Glanzmann thrombasthenia (∞ Chapter 31). Persons with this rare disease lack functional GPIIb/IIIa receptors, and their platelets do not aggregate in response to various agonists in platelet aggregation tests (∞ Chapter 40). Patients who have decreased levels of fibrinogen also have abnormal platelet aggregation (∞ Chapter 31). Other adhesive proteins such as VWF, thrombospondin, and fibronectin also bind to the GPIIb/IIIa receptor, but their roles in platelet aggregation in vivo are unclear.

Within in vitro test systems, aggregation occurs in two phases, primary and secondary aggregation (∞ Chapter 40).

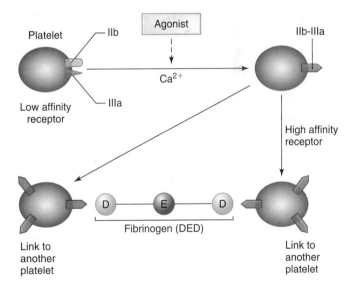

■ FIGURE 29-13 Platelet aggregation. Agonist stimulation in the presence of Ca^{+2} causes high-affinity fibrinogen receptors, activated glycoprotein IIb/IIIa, to appear on the platelet surface. Fibrinogen binds horizontally to two platelets by peptide sequences at the terminal end of its gamma and alpha chains in the D domains, one gamma chain to GPIIb/IIIa receptors on each platelet. Fibrinogen thus becomes a bridge between the two platelets.

During primary aggregation, platelets adhere loosely to one another. If the stimulus by agonists is weak, primary aggregation is reversible. Secondary aggregation follows and results in irreversible platelet aggregation. It begins as the platelets start to release their own ADP and other granule contents and to synthesize and release TXA_2 (to be described). The released substances act as additional agonists, which supplement the platelet stimulation. If platelets are unable to release ADP and/or to synthesize TXA_2, secondary aggregation does not occur, and the platelets disaggregate. Generally, the in vivo result in such situations increases the time to stop bleeding from a wound.

 Checkpoint! 7

Your finger is still bleeding at this point, but the platelets are aggregating to form the primary hemostatic plug. Let's review the key events:

  a. *To what do platelets first adhere?*
  b. *What bridge and what platelet membrane receptor are needed for platelet adhesion?*
  c. *What bridge and what platelet membrane receptor are needed for platelets to attach to one another?*
  d. *What is the attachment of platelets to one another called?*

Biochemistry of Platelet Activation   Platelets become activated after agonists bind to receptors on the platelet surface, initiating signaling events within the platelets. These signaling events eventually lead to the reorganization of the platelet cytoskeleton, granule secretion, and aggregation.

G Proteins   Actions of most of the familiar agonists (collagen, ADP, thrombin, epinephrine, TXA_2, and arachidonic acid) and their receptors are linked with guanine nucleotide-binding (G) proteins on the inner leaflet of the phospholipid membrane. G proteins are molecular switches, which are inactive when GDP is bound, but active after GTP is bound. When the platelet adheres to collagen, G proteins are activated and, in turn, activate enzymes in the platelet membrane and cytoplasm. Some activated enzymes cleave specific membrane phospholipids. The resulting lipid products are "second messengers" that transmit the signal to interior parts of the cells.

Phospholipase C and the Phosphoinositide Pathway
One second messenger pathway important in platelet activation involves activation of the enzyme phospholipase C (PLC) (Figure 29-14 ■). Activated G proteins activate PLC, which cleaves phosphatidyl inositol bis-phosphate (PIP_2) into IP_3 and DAG. PIP_2 is the doubly phosphorylated product of the membrane lipid phosphatidyl inositol (PI) produced by PI kinase. The cleavage products released from PIP_2 by PLC function to mobilize calcium ions from storage sites in the DTS (IP_3) and to activate a kinase enzyme, protein kinase C/PKC (DAG). Activated PKC in turn phosphorylates proteins, contributing to granule secretion and fibrinogen receptor exposure.[18]

Role of Ca^{2+}   Platelet activation is accompanied by an increase in the cytosolic free Ca^{2+} concentration. Ca^{2+} serve as intracellular second messengers and affect enzyme activity and protein-protein interactions. Resting platelets have very low levels of ionic calcium in the cytoplasm (Figure 29-15 ■). Many cellular enzyme systems that are inactive at the Ca^{2+} concentration in resting platelets become activated by the increase in Ca^{2+} that occurs with platelet activation. These enzymes include phospholipase A2 (PLA_2), phospholipase C (PLC), PI kinase, and myosin light chain kinase (MLCK), important in the assembly of the contractile mechanism responsible for platelet shape change. The increase in calcium ions is due to both the release from internal stores (by IP_3) and the influx from outside the cell. A direct relationship exists between the amount of cytoplasmic-free calcium and the extent of platelet stimulation.

Arachidonate Pathway   Phospholipase A_2 is activated by the increase in cytoplasmic calcium and hydrolyzes arachidonic acid from the second carbon of the glycerol backbone of membrane phospholipids. **Arachidonic acid**

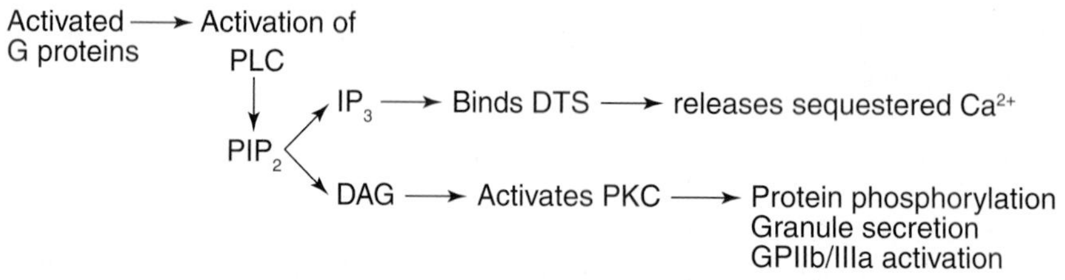

Activated → Activation of
G proteins   PLC
                 ↓
               PIP_2 → IP_3 → Binds DTS → releases sequestered Ca^{2+}
                      ↘ DAG → Activates PKC → Protein phosphorylation
                                               Granule secretion
                                               GPIIb/IIIa activation

■ **FIGURE 29-14**   Phospholipase C/phosphoinositide pathway. Activated G proteins activate PLC. Activated PLC cleaves PIP_2, releasing IP_3 and DAG. IP_3 in turn triggers release of Ca^{2+} from the DTS. DAG activates PKC, inducing granule secretion and activation of GP IIb/IIIa, the fibrinogen receptor. PLC = phospholipase C; PIP_2 = phosphatidyl bis-phosphate; IP_3 = inositol triphosphate; DAG = diaceyl glycerol; DTS = dense tubularsystem; PKC = protein kinase C

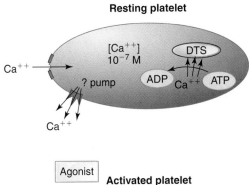

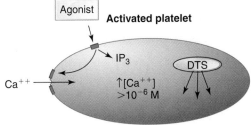

■ **FIGURE 29-15** Ca^{2+} regulation in platelets. Resting platelets maintain low levels of cytoplasmic Ca^{2+} via active uptake by the DTS and active extrusion, probably via a Ca^{2+} pump. These mechanisms counter a passive diffusion of Ca^{2+} into the platelet along a concentration gradient. With activation, platelets increase intracellular cytoplasmic Ca^{2+} due to release from the DTS (by IP_3) and increase Ca^{2+} influx (probably mediated via ATP). DTS = dense tabular system

(**AA**) is an unsaturated fatty acid and once released from the membrane phospholipids serves as a precursor of a variety of regulatory substances including prostaglandins and leukotrienes. In the platelet, thromboxane $A_2(TXA_2)$ is synthesized from AA by the enzymes cyclo-oxygenase and thromboxane synthase. In endothelial cells, prostacyclin (PGI_2) is synthesized from AA by cyclo-oxygenase and prostacyclin synthase (Figure 29-16 ■).

TXA$_2$ is a potent platelet agonist and can stimulate platelet activation and secretion. Platelet activation by "weak" agonists does not produce platelet secretion if TXA_2 synthesis is blocked, which seriously impairs subsequent steps in platelet function. Aspirin (acetyl-salicylic acid) irreversibly inhibits cyclooxygenase and prevents affected platelets from synthesizing TXA_2 (∞ Chapter 31). Because aspirin's inhibition of cyclooxygenase is irreversible, the effect lasts for the lifetime of the platelets exposed. TXA_2 also is released from activated platelets and enhances vasoconstriction and functions as a platelet agonist, perpetuating the activation process. TXA_2 is a labile compound quickly converted into an inert form, TXB_2, shortly after its synthesis.

Cyclic AMP (cAMP) Pathway   cAMP is an important negative regulator of platelet activation (Figure 29-17 ■). It inhibits shape change, platelet secretion, and integrin activation (conversion of GPIIb/IIIa to an active form). The

platelet membrane enzyme adenyl cyclase is activated when PGI_2 from endothelial cells contacts platelet membrane receptors. Activated adenyl cyclase produces cAMP within the platelet cytoplasm, resulting in the activation of protein kinase enzymes that, in turn, inhibit platelet aggregation. This is one way to limit and localize the formation of the primary hemostatic plug.[18] ADP functions as a platelet agonist by inhibiting adenyl cyclase, thus lowering cAMP levels and permitting platelet activation. The platelet inhibitory drug, dipyridamole, inhibits phosphodiesterase, the enzyme responsible for the degradation of cAMP to AMP, thus stabilizing platelet cAMP levels and inhibiting platelet activation.

Platelet activation and biochemical reactions leading to aggregation are summarized in Figures 29-16 and 29-18 ■.

Primary Hemostatic Plug   The platelets eventually form a barrier (the primary hemostatic plug) that seals the injury and prevents further blood loss. When the primary hemostatic plug is formed, the bleeding stops. The time for bleeding to cease depends on the depth of the injury and the size of the blood vessel involved. Superficial wounds in which only capillaries and small vessels are affected usually stop bleeding within 10 minutes.

✓ **Checkpoint! 8**

Your finger has now stopped bleeding. Outline the steps of primary hemostasis that have occurred.

@ **CASE STUDY** *(continued from page 621)*

3. The physician explained to Michael that the reddish purple spots on his legs and ankles were tiny pinpoint hemorrhages into the skin. Explain the relationship of these hemorrhages to the platelet count.

Platelets and Secondary Hemostasis
The final aspect of platelet activation involves the changes in the platelet membrane that allow platelets to function in secondary hemostasis. Activated platelets accelerate thrombin formation, a function known as **platelet procoagulant activity**. Fibrin-forming proteins (coagulation factors) bind to the surface of activated platelets by binding either to specific receptors on platelets or nonspecifically to negatively charged phospholipids.[18] The resulting platelet-coagulation factor interactions result in formation of the secondary hemostatic plug.

The primary platelet plug is relatively unstable and is easily dislodged. During secondary hemostasis, fibrin forms amid and around the aggregated platelets. Platelets enhance the fibrin-forming processes by mechanisms explained in ∞ Chapter 30. The proteins that interact enzymatically to

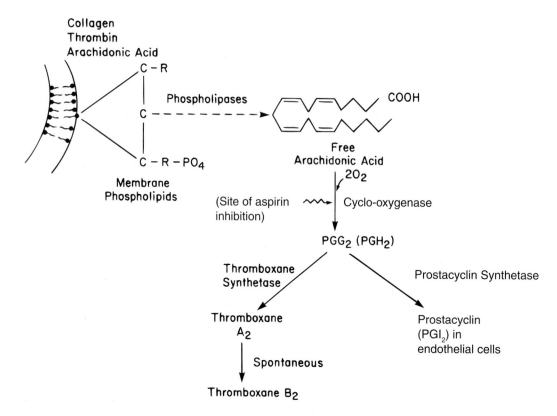

■ FIGURE 29-16   Biochemical pathways of TXA_2 formation in the platelet. Stimulation of platelet membranes (both intracellular granule and cytoplasmic membranes) by agonists (e.g., collagen, thrombin, arachidonic acid) results in liberation of arachidonic acid from membrane phospholipids. Cyclo-oxygenase incorporates two molecules of oxygen-forming prostaglandin PGG_2 (PGH_2 in the reduced form). Thromboxane synthetase converts PGG_2 to TXA_2 and TXA_2 is spontaneously converted to inactive thromboxane B_2. Alternatively, PGG_2 can be converted to (PGI_2) in endothelial cells, a powerful platelet inhibitor. TXA_2 = thromboxane A_2; PGI_2 = prostacyclin

form fibrin must be assembled on a lipid surface where the reactions take place. The membrane phospholipids of activated platelets are the primary source of this lipid surface.

Fibrin-forming proteins do not bind to resting platelet surfaces in the circulation. In resting platelets, the negatively charged phospholipids are almost exclusively found in the inner half of the membrane bilayer. During the activation of platelets, the membrane phospholipids flip-flop, and the negatively charged phospholipids move to the outer leaflet, perhaps via a Ca^{2+}-activated "scramblase" enzyme that reverses the asymmetric distribution of phospholipids.[18] This phospholipid rearrangement provides the phospholipid surface allowing coagulation factors to bind, become activated, and initiate fibrin formation. Platelets can assemble both the Xase and prothrombinase complexes (∞ Chapter 30). *Platelet factor 3* activity is an older name for this platelet procoagulant activity. The fibrin-platelet plug is the secondary hemostatic plug.

The entire platelet-fibrin mass then contracts to a firmer, more cohesive clot. This contraction is called **clot retraction**. An adequate number of functional platelets are needed for clot retraction to occur, a process that can be observed in a test tube of blood when no anticoagulant is added. After blood is placed into the test tube, the formation of fibrin results in a network or mesh of fibrin strands that extends throughout, trapping essentially all of the blood cells with some serum. The mass of fibrin and trapped cells

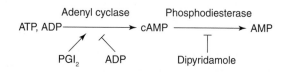

■ FIGURE 29-17   Role of cAMP in platelets. cAMP is a negative regulator of platelet function, inhibiting various steps of platelet activation. Adenyl cyclase converts ATP or ADP to cAMP. Subsequently, phosphodiesterase breaks cAMP down into inactive AMP. PGI_2, a platelet-activation antagonist, activates adenyl cyclase, while ADP, a potent platelet agonist, inhibits adenyl cyclase. Dipyridamole, a platelet inhibitory drug, functions by inhibiting phosphodiesterase, thereby stabilizing cAMP and preventing platelet activation. cAMP = cyclic AMP;
→ = stimulation; —| = inhibition.

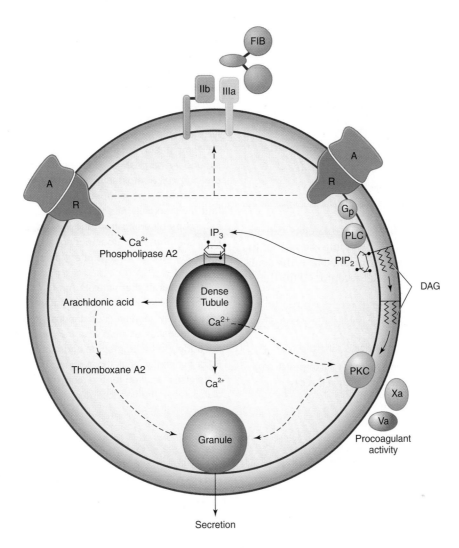

■ **FIGURE 29-18** Schematic diagram showing platelet biochemical changes after activation. An agonist (A) binds to a receptor (R) on the platelet. The GPIIb/IIIa complex appears soon after platelet activation with an agonist. Gp on the inner part of the phospholipid membrane (linked with R) becomes activated which in turn activates PLC. PLC cleaves PIP_2 to form IP_3 and DAG. Subsequently, Ca^{2+} is mobilized into the cytoplasm from the DTS. Many enzymes are activated by the increase in Ca^{2+} including phospholipase A2. Arachidonic acid released from the membrane phospholipids is converted to thromboxane which stimulates platelet secretion. DAG activates PKC which contributes to granule secretion. Coagulation factors (e.g., Xa, Va) bind to the platelet surface leading to fibrin formation. Key: IIb, IIIa = GPIIb/IIIa receptor; FIB = fibrinogen; DAG = diacylglycerol; Gp = guanine nucleotide binding protein; IP_3 = inositol-3-phosphate; PLC = phospholipase C; PKC = protein kinase C; PIP_2 = phosphatidylinositol phosphate.

contracts over a period of 2–24 hours, extruding much of the serum from the fibrin mass.

Clot retraction is believed to occur by the association of adjacent platelet pseudopods with each other and the fibrin strands. Actin and other contractile proteins within the pseudopods cause the platelets to retract. A comparable phenomenon is believed to occur in vivo, consolidating the thrombus into a cohesive mass of platelets and fibrin that seals the wounded vessel and prevents further blood loss. Contraction can also decrease thrombolysis efficiency and enhance wound healing.[32] The stabilized platelet-fibrin mass remains in place until fibroblast repair of the wound results in permanent healing, and fibrinolysis dissolves the mass.

Physiologic Controls of Platelet Activation

Several inhibitory mechanisms balance platelet activation and prevent excessive platelet deposition (Table 29-10 ✪). The platelet contacts with agonists are minimized due to the endothelial cell (EC) barrier. The flowing blood produces a dilutional effect, removing platelet agonists, loosely associated platelets, and coagulation proteins from the developing platelet aggregate. ECs produce NO and PGI_2, two potent inhibitors of platelet activation. ECs also have an ADPase enzyme that cleaves ATP and ADP to AMP, limiting the agonist effects of ADP. Physiologic controls that limit thrombin activity (∞ Chapter 30) also limit platelet aggregation because thrombin is a potent platelet activator. Many agonists have

⊗ TABLE 29-10

Physiologic Controls of Platelet Activation
• Minimal platelet contact with agonists (endothelial cell barrier)
• Dilutional effect of flowing blood
• Limited platelet responsiveness to agonists (endothelial cell production of NO; $PGI_2 \rightarrow \uparrow$cAMP; ADPase; antithrombin)
• Limited duration of agonist receptor activity (short half-life of agonists)
• Maintenance of tight controls on cytosolic $[Ca^{2+}]$
• Inability of "resting" GPIIbIIIa to bind fibrinogen

short half-lives, limiting their effects, and platelets can become desensitized to stimulation by some agonists. Intraplatelet calcium levels are tightly controlled as is the availability of the active form of the platelet receptor GPIIb/IIIa.

 CASE STUDY *(continued from page 633)*

4. What is the most likely cause of Michael's pancytopenia?

5. Why would the administration of growth factors such as erythropoietin (EPO) and TPO be considered in this case?

SUMMARY

After an injury, blood clots as the result of a series of complex biochemical reactions called *hemostasis*. Its purpose is to temporarily reconstruct continuity of injured vessels to minimize loss of blood. The components of hemostasis are found in the plasma and in the tissues that compose the blood vessel walls. All of the components are inert until the injury activates them.

Hemostasis occurs in phases called *primary hemostasis*, *secondary hemostasis*, and *fibrinolysis*. This chapter discussed the primary hemostasis phase during which the blood vessels and the platelets cooperatively form an aggregate of platelets that mechanically fills the openings in the injured blood vessels and stops bleeding from the wound site. The injured blood vessels contribute by constricting and secreting a variety of biochemical mediators that affect all of the subsequent hemostasis steps.

The roles of the platelets are to adhere to the injured areas of the blood vessel walls and to aggregate by attaching to one another and by secreting substances stored in their granules. The secreted substances help to attract and activate new platelets that are added to the aggregate and that help the growth of new tissue to permanently heal the wound. The surface of the aggregated platelets is required for the reactions of secondary hemostasis; it is discussed in the next chapter.

REVIEW QUESTIONS

LEVEL I

1. The definition of hemostasis is the: (Objective 1)
   a. process of maintaining the body temperature
   b. termination of bleeding following a traumatic injury
   c. process of forming a hematoma
   d. regulation of kidney function

2. Which of the following is the primary element that prevents blood from clotting inside blood vessels? (Objective 5)
   a. fibrinogen
   b. arteriole
   c. endothelial cells
   d. platelets

3. What bone marrow cell is the precursor of platelets? (Objective 7)
   a. neutrophil
   b. erythrocyte
   c. endothelial
   d. megakaryocyte

4. What is the action of the blood vessels in hemostasis immediately after an injury? (Objective 5)
   a. thrombosis
   b. aggregation
   c. vasoconstriction
   d. vasodilation

LEVEL II

1. What are the cells called that line the central cavity of all blood vessels and related tissues? (Objective 1)
   a. epithelial cells
   b. endothelial cells
   c. capillaries
   d. smooth muscle cells

2. What is the normal life span of platelets in the peripheral blood? (Objective 11)
   a. 8 hours
   b. 1 day
   c. 10 days
   d. 100 days

3. Platelet dense bodies are storage organelles for which of the following that are released after activation? (Objective 4)
   a. calcium, ADP, and serotonin
   b. fibrinogen, glycoprotein Ib, and VWF
   c. ADP, thromboxane A_2, and F-V
   d. lysosomal granules, ATP, and factor-VIII

4. Which of the following is the platelet receptor needed for platelet adhesion? (Objective 5)
   a. glycoprotein IIb/IIIa
   b. actin
   c. VWF
   d. glycoprotein Ib/IX

REVIEW QUESTIONS (continued)

LEVEL I

5. Which of the following has happened when a cut finger initially stops bleeding? (Objectives 8, 9)
   a. vasoconstriction of vessels proximal to the cut
   b. vasodilation of vessels distal to the cut
   c. formation of the primary hemostatic plug by aggregated platelets
   d. completion of fibrin formation and formation of the secondary hemostatic plug

6. What is a reasonable reference range for platelets in the peripheral blood? (Objective 6)
   a. $1.5-4.0 \times 10^9$/L
   b. $150-400 \times 10^9$/L
   c. $4.0-11.0 \times 10^{12}$/L
   d. $4.0-11.0 \times 10^9$/L

7. What is the first step in platelet function after an injury? (Objective 8)
   a. fibrin formation
   b. release of ADP
   c. platelet aggregation
   d. platelet adhesion to collagen

8. What is the process called when platelets bind to one another? (Objective 8)
   a. platelet secretion
   b. fibrin formation
   c. platelet adhesion
   d. platelet aggregation

9. Which of the following best describes the normal morphology of platelets on a peripheral blood smear? (Objective 6)
   a. They are larger than erythrocytes.
   b. They are filled with azurophilic granules.
   c. They are light blue in color without granules.
   d. They have large nuclei.

10. Each of the following is involved in hemostasis *except:* (Objective 2)
   a. vasoconstriction by the blood vessels
   b. adhesion and aggregation by the platelets
   c. fibrin formation by proteins in the plasma and platelets
   d. regulation of blood pressure

LEVEL II

5. The platelet glycoprotein IIb/IIIa complex is: (Objective 5)
   a. a membrane receptor for fibrinogen
   b. secreted from the DB
   c. secreted by endothelial cells
   d. also called *actin*

6. The formation of thromboxane A2 in the activated platelet: (Objective 8)
   a. is needed for platelets to adhere to collagen
   b. is caused by the alpha granule proteins
   c. requires the enzyme cyclooxygenase
   d. occurs via a pathway involving VWF

7. What effect does thrombopoietin have on the megakaryocyte? (Objective 2)
   a. decreases the number of platelets formed
   b. speeds maturation in the bone marrow
   c. induces the cell's release to the peripheral blood
   d. decreases the rate of endomitosis and ploidy

8. The function of microtubules in the resting platelet is to: (Objective 6)
   a. keep a high level of calcium in the cytoplasm
   b. store and sequester calcium
   c. provide a negative charge on the platelet surface
   d. maintain the disc shape

9. The contents of the platelet granules are released from the platelet: (Objective 5)
   a. through the open membrane system after fusion with the granules
   b. through the microtubules after fusion with the granules
   c. by disintegration of the platelet plasma membrane
   d. by the mitochondria

10. Which of the following is true about the relationship between ADP and platelets? (Objective 7)
   a. ADP is necessary for platelet adhesion.
   b. ADP released from the DB is required for adequate platelet aggregation.
   c. ADP is synthesized in the platelet from arachidonic acid.
   d. ADP is released from the alpha granules of the platelets.

www.pearsonhighered.com/mckenzie
Use this address to access the interactive Companion Website created for this textbook. Find additional information, tables and figures. Evaluate your command of the chapter information using case studies and critical thinking and multiple choice questions.

REFERENCES

1. Karsan A, Harlan JM. The blood vessel wall. In: Hoffman R, Benz EJ Jr, Shattil, SJ, Furie B, Cohen HJ, Silberstein LE, McGlave, P, eds. *Hematology Basic Principles and Practice,* 4th ed. Philadelphia: Churchill Livingstone/Elsevier; 2005: 1915–16.

2. Jandl JH. *Textbook of Hematology,* 2nd ed. Boston: Little, Brown; 1996.

3. Hajjar KA, Esmon NL, Marcus AJ, Muller WA. Vascular function in hemostasis. In: Beutler E, Lichtman MA, Coller BS, Kipps TJ, Seligsohn U, eds. *William's Hematology,* 6th ed. New York: McGraw-Hill; 2001: 1451–69.

4. Rodgers GM. Endothelium and the regulation of hemostasis. In: Lee GR, Foerster J, Lukens J, Paraskevas F, Greer JP, Rodgers GM, eds. *Wintrobe's Clinical Hematology,* 10th ed. Baltimore: Williams & Wilkins; 1999: 765–73.

5. Bizzozero J. Ueber einen neuen Formbestandtheil des Blutes und dessen Rolle bei der Thrombose und der Blutgerinnung. *Virchows Arch Pathol Anat.* 1882;90:261–332.

6. Bruno E, Hoffman R. Human megakaryocyte progenitor cells. *Semin Hematol.* 1998;35:182–91.

7. Gerwirtz AM. Human megakaryocytopoiesis. *Semin Hematol.* 1986; 23:27–42.

8. Wendling F. Thrombopoietin: Its role from early hematopoiesis to platelet production. *Haematologica.* 1999;84:158–66.

9. Italiano JE, Hartwig JH. Megakaryocyte and platelet structure. In: Hoffman R, Benz EJ Jr, Shattil SJ, Furie B, Cohen HJ, Silberstein LE, McGlave P, eds. *Hematology: Basic Principles and Practice,* 4th ed. Philadelphia: Churchill Livingstone/Elsevier; 2005: 1872–80.

10. Cramer EM. Megakaryocyte structure and function. *Curr Opin Hematol.* 1999;6:354–61.

11. Long MW. Thrombopoietin stimulation of hematopoietic stem/progenitor cells. *Curr Opin Hematol.* 1999;6:159–63.

12. Stenberg PE, Hill RJ. Platelets and megakaryocytes. In: Lee GR, Foerster J, Lukens J, Paraskevas F, Greer JP, Rodgers GM, eds. *Wintrobe's Clinical Hematology,* 10th ed. Baltimore: Williams & Wilkins; 1999: 615–60.

13. Osada M, Komeno Y, Todokoro K et al. Immature megakaryocytes undergo apoptosis in the absence of thrombopoietin. *Exp Hematol.* 1999;27:131–38.

14. Kaushansky K. Megakaryopoiesis and thrombopoiesis. In: Lichtman MA, Beutler E, Kipps TJ, Seligsohn U, Kaushansky K, Prchal JT, eds. *Williams Hematology,* 7th ed. New York: McGraw-Hill; 2006: 1571–85.

15. Li J, Kuter DJ. The end is just the beginning: Megakaryocyte apoptosis and platelet release. *Int J Hematol.* 2001;74:365–74.

16. De Botton S, Sabri S, Daugas E et al. Platelet formation is the consequence of caspase activation within megakaryocytes. *Blood.* 2002; 100:1310–17.

17. Plow EF, Abrams CS. Molecular basis for platelet function. In: Hoffman R, Benz EJ Jr, Shattil SJ, Furie B, Cohen HJ, Silberstein LE, McGlave P, eds. *Hematology: Basic Principles and Practice,* 4th ed. Philadelphia: Churchill-Livingston/Elsevier; 2005: 1881–97.

18. Parise LV, Smyth SS, Shet AS, Coller BS. Platelet morphology, biochemistry and function. In: Lichtman MA, Beutler E, Kipps TJ, Seligsohn U, Kaushansky K, Prchal JT, eds. *Williams Hematology,* 7th ed. New York: McGraw-Hill; 2006: 1587–663.

19. Steinberg MH, Kelton JG, Coller BS. Plasma glycocalicin. An aid in the classification of thrombocytopenic disorders. *N Engl J Med.* 1987;317:1037–42.

20. Beer JH, Buchi L, Steiner B. Glycocalicin: A new assay—The normal plasma levels and its potential usefulness in selected diseases. *Blood.* 1994;83:691–702.

21. Parise LV, Boudignon-Proudhon C, Keely PJ, Naik UP. Platelets in hemostasis and thrombosis. In: Lee GR, Foerster J, Lukens J, Paraskevas F, Green JP, Rodgers GM, eds. *Wintrobe's Clinical Hematology,* 10th ed. Baltimore: Williams & Wilkins; 1999: 661–83.

22. Parise LV, Smyth SS, Coller BS. Platelet morphology, biochemistry, and function. In: Beutler E, Lichtman MA, Coller BS, Kipps TJ, Seligsohn U, eds. *Williams Hematology,* 6th ed. New York: McGraw-Hill; 2001: 1357–1408.

23. Menashi S, Davis C, Crawford N. Calcium uptake associated with an intracellular membrane fraction prepared from human blood platelets by high-voltage, free-flow electrophoresis. *FEBS Lett.* 1982; 140:298–302.

24. Gerrard JM, White JG, Rao GHR, Townsend D. Localization of platelet prostaglandin production in the platelet dense tubular system. *Am J Pathol.* 1976;83:283–98.

25. Roth GJ. Developing relationships: arterial platelet adhesion, glycoprotein Ib, and leucine-rich glycoproteins. *Blood.* 1991;77:5–19.

26. Andrews RK, Shen Y, Gardiner EE et al. The glycoprotein Ib-IX-V complex in platelet adhesion and signaling. *Thromb Haemost.* 1999; 82:357–64.

27. Hartwig JH, Barkalow K, Azim A, Italiano J. The elegant platelet: Signals controlling actin assembly. *Thromb Haemost.* 1999;82:392–98.

28. George JN, Pickett EB, Saucerman S et al. Platelet surface glycoproteins. Studies on resting and activated platelets and platelet membrane microparticles in normal subjects, and observations in patients during adult respiratory distress syndrome and cardiac surgery. *J Clin Invest.* 1986;78:340–48.

29. Tracy PB, Eide LL, Bowie EJ, Mann KG. Radioimmunoassay of factor V in human plasma and platelets. *Blood.* 1982;60:59–63.

30. Camire RM, Pollak ES, Kaushansky K, Tracy PM. Secretable human platelet-derived factor V originates from the plasma pool. *Blood.* 1998;92:3035–41.

31. Hawiger J. Adhesive ends of fibrinogen and its antiadhesive peptides: The end of a saga? *Semin Hematol.* 1995;32:99–109.

32. Kunitada S, Fitzgerald GA, Fitzgerald DJ. Inhibition of clot lysis and decreased binding of tissue-type plasminogen activator as a consequence of clot retraction. *Blood.* 1992;79:1420–27.

30

Secondary Hemostasis and Fibrinolysis

J. Lynne Williams, Ph.D.

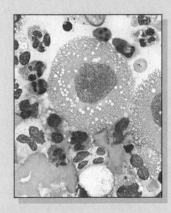

■ OBJECTIVES—LEVEL I

At the end of this unit of study, the student should be able to:

1. Define *hemostasis.* Identify the three physiologic compartments involved in the hemostatic mechanism.
2. Differentiate primary and secondary hemostasis.
3. List the coagulation factors using Roman numerals and determine how each is evaluated in lab testing.
4. Classify the coagulation factors into groups and discuss their characteristics.
5. Evaluate the importance of vitamin K in hemostasis.
6. Describe the mechanism of action of the coagulation proteins.
7. Diagram the sequence of reactions in the coagulation cascade according to the historic concepts of intrinsic, extrinsic, and common pathways.
8. Identify the factors involved in contact activation.
9. Diagram the physiologic pathway of blood coagulation.
10. Define *fibrinolysis,* identify the major components of the fibrinolytic system, and explain why fibrinolysis is a necessary component of hemostasis.
11. List the fragments resulting from fibrinolytic degradation; compare and contrast the fragments resulting from the degradation of fibrinogen and fibrin.
12. List the major biochemical inhibitors that regulate secondary hemostasis.

■ OBJECTIVES—LEVEL II

At the end of this unit of study, the student should be able to:

1. Explain the interactions of the three physiologic compartments involved in hemostasis.
2. Describe the domain structure of the coagulation factors, determine how this structure affects the action of the serine proteases, and explain the significance of the noncatalytic regions.
3. Summarize the formation of complexes on a phospholipid surface and explain the significance of these complexes to hemostasis.
4. Integrate the role of contact factors with other systems (complement activation, fibrinolysis, inflammation).
5. Describe the multiple roles of thrombin in hemostasis.

■ OBJECTIVES—LEVEL II *(continued)*

6. Explain the physiologic functions of ADAMTS-13, LRP, EPCR, UPAR.

7. Compare and contrast physiologic and systemic fibrinolysis.

8. Describe the physiologic controls of hemostasis including blood flow, feedback inhibition, liver clearance, and inhibitors (antithrombin, tissue factor pathway inhibitor, protein C, protein S, and TAFI).

9. Evaluate a case study from a patient with a defect in hemostasis and, using the medical history and laboratory results, determine the diagnosis.

KEY TERMS

ADAMTS-13
Coagulation factor
Common pathway
Contact group
Endothelial cell protein C receptor (EPCR)
Extrinsic pathway
Extrinsic Xase complex
Fibrin degradation (split) products (FDP or FSP)
Fibrinogen group
Fibrinolysis
γ–Carboxylation
Intrinsic pathway
Intrinsic Xase complex
LRP receptor (LDL receptorlike protein)
PIVKA
Plasminogen activator inhibitor (PAI)
Plasminogen activator (PA)
Prothrombinase complex
Prothrombin group
Serine protease
Serpin
Thrombin activatable fibrinolysis inhibitor (TAFI)
Thrombomodulin (TM)
Tissue factor pathway
Tissue factor pathway inhibitor (TFPI)
Tissue-type plasminogen activator (tPA)
Transglutaminase
Urokinase-type plasminogen activator (uPA)
(Urokinase)
UPAR (uPA receptor)
Vitamin K dependent
Zymogen

BACKGROUND BASICS

The information in this chapter builds on the concepts learned in previous chapters. To maximize your learning experience, you should review these concepts before starting this unit of study.

Level I

▶ Define and summarize the events in *primary hemostasis*. (Chapter 29)

Level II

▶ Describe the structure of the platelet phospholipid membrane. (Chapter 29)

▶ Review protein structure, protein domains, and properties of enzymes. (Chapter 2 and previous chemistry and biology courses)

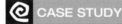 CASE STUDY

We will address this case throughout the chapter.

Shawn, a 10-year-old boy, was seen by his physician for recurrent nosebleeds and anemia. History revealed that the epistaxis began when he was about 18 months old. The nosebleeds occurred one or two times a month and began spontaneously. His mother reported that he seemed to bruise easily. No lesion was found in the nose. No history of drugs was noted. The family history indicated that the boy's grandparents were cousins. The patient had a brother who died of intracranial hemorrhage at 10 years of age. Parents and all other relatives showed no bleeding problems.

► OVERVIEW

Hemostasis requires the interaction of platelets, blood vessels, and coagulation proteins. The previous chapter described primary hemostasis (platelets and blood vessels). This chapter introduces the plasma protein systems contributing to secondary hemostasis. It begins with an overview of hemostasis and discusses the distinctions between primary and secondary hemostasis. The coagulation proteins are presented in related groups for initial discussion of general properties, mechanisms of action, and protein structure. The chapter describes the functional interactions of these procoagulant proteins from the classical perspective of intrinsic, extrinsic, and common pathways. The fibrinolytic system (components, activators, and inhibitors) is presented, and the products of fibrinolytic degradation are defined. The various components contributing to the control of hemostasis are discussed including physiologic processes (blood flow, liver clearance), positive and negative feedback mechanisms, and natural inhibitors. The chapter concludes with an updated perspective of the hemostatic system referred to as the *physiologic pathway*.

► INTRODUCTION

Hemostasis is a carefully balanced process by which the body maintains blood in a fluid state within the vasculature and prevents loss of blood from the vascular system upon injury. Although often thought of as "clot" formation, hemostasis also includes fibrin (clot) dissolution and vessel repair. Hemostasis involves a series of complex and highly regulated events linking platelets, vascular endothelial cells, and coagulation proteins (**coagulation factors**). The interaction of these three components at the cellular and molecular levels determines whether the equilibrium between bleeding (hemorrhage) and clotting (thrombosis) is maintained (Figure 30-1 ■).

As discussed (∞ Chapter 29), hemostasis consists of two stages: primary and secondary. Primary hemostasis (∞ Chapter 29), the formation of the unstable platelet plug, is the first response to vascular injury. Secondary hemostasis, the rapid reinforcement of the unstable platelet plug with chemically stable fibrin, follows and includes a series of interdependent, enzyme-mediated reactions. The endpoint of these reactions is the generation of thrombin that transforms the soluble protein fibrinogen to insoluble fibrin to stabilize the platelet plug.

The process of fibrin formation is well balanced and controlled, limiting fibrin formation to the area of vessel injury. This localization prevents widespread or systemic coagulation activation. The procoagulant reactions are amplified to the appropriate degree, while natural inhibitors limit the proteolytic activity of the activated clotting factors. Negative feedback also controls fibrin formation: large amounts of thrombin, the last enzyme formed, destroy coagulation cofactors in

The Coagulation System

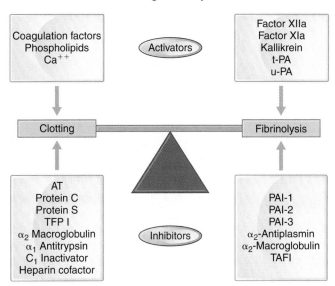

■ FIGURE 30-1 The coagulation system is kept in balance by activators and inhibitors of clotting and fibrinolysis. Clotting occurs when blood vessels are damaged and activators of coagulation factors are exposed or released. Clotting is controlled because fibrinolysis is initiated in response to clotting activation. Inhibitors of both clotting and fibrinolysis serve to bring the system back into balance. An imbalance in the activation or inhibition of either clotting or fibrinolysis causes thrombosis or bleeding.

the rate-limiting steps of its own production. The platelet-fibrin plug seals the injured vessel preventing blood loss, the vessel begins to repair itself, and the fibrin is ultimately digested by plasmin, an enzyme of the fibrinolytic system.

Hemostasis is complex, involving many interrelating components and control mechanisms. No part of the system acts alone. However, each part is discussed individually and then the concepts are integrated into a cohesive theory of hemostasis.

► COAGULATION MECHANISM

The reactions involved in coagulation were originally described as occurring in a cascade[1] or waterfall-like[2] fashion in which circulating, inactive coagulation factor precursors, called **zymogens,** are sequentially activated to their active enzyme forms. Each zymogen serves first as the substrate for the preceding enzyme in the cascade and, when activated, serves as an enzyme for the subsequent zymogen. A simplified diagram of the cascade is shown in Figure 30-2 ■. In vitro, initiation of the cascade occurs via two pathways: The **intrinsic pathway** requires enzymes and protein cofactors that are present in plasma; the **extrinsic pathway** requires enzymes and protein cofactors present in plasma as well as

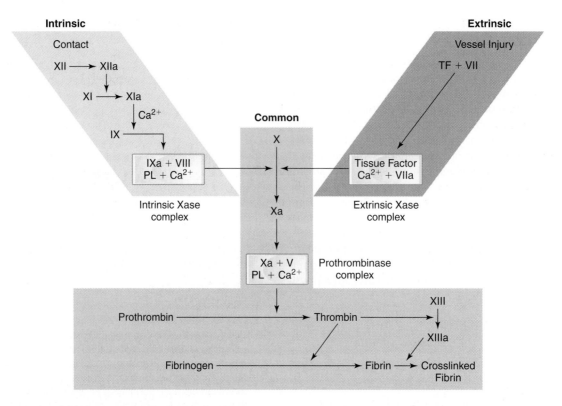

■ FIGURE 30-2   A simplified version of the coagulation cascade showing the cascade or waterfall-like sequence of reactions. Boxes indicate complex formation. PL = platelet phospholipid; TF = tissue factor

an activator—tissue factor—not found in blood under normal conditions. Both converge in a third path called the **common pathway** to generate the fibrin clot. The traditional analysis of the coagulation process assigns each of the coagulation factors to the intrinsic, extrinsic, or common pathway as indicated in Table 30-1 ✪.

The concept of intrinsic, extrinsic, and common pathways evolved from observations of reactions occurring in vitro (in test tubes) and has contributed to our knowledge of how coagulation occurs in vivo. For clinical laboratory professionals, understanding hemostasis from an in vitro diagnostic perspective is important. The concept of the three pathways, combined with available tests for in vitro evaluation of the intrinsic system (activated partial thromboplastin

time [APTT]) and the extrinsic system (prothrombin time [PT]) are invaluable in diagnosing clinical hemorrhagic disorders. Although the model of intrinsic, extrinsic, and common pathways still serves as the basis of our understanding of this complicated system, the system in vivo functions quite differently and is not so compartmentalized. Physiologic hemostasis is basically a single pathway, now called the **tissue factor pathway**.[3]

 Checkpoint! 1

What is the major distinction between the so-called extrinsic and intrinsic pathways?

✪ TABLE 30-1

Coagulation Factors in Intrinsic, Extrinsic, and Common Pathways

Intrinsic Pathway	Extrinsic Pathway	Common Pathway
Prekallikrien (PK)	VII	X
HK	Tissue factor (TF; III)	V
XII		II
XI		I
IX		
VIII		

CASE STUDY *(continued from page 640)*

Screening tests for evaluating hemostasis were done on Shawn. The child was found to have a platelet count of 242×10^9/L. Bleeding time was 8 minutes. The PT was 29.5 seconds with a control of 12.0 seconds. The APTT was 51.0 seconds with a control of 55.4 seconds. Liver function tests were normal.

1. What do the results of the screening tests (platelet count, bleeding time, PT, and APTT) indicate?

2. What component of the hemostatic mechanism is most likely affected?

▶ PROCOAGULANT FACTORS

The coagulation factors are the procoagulant proteins involved in hemostasis. The International Committee on Nomenclature of Blood Coagulation Factors[4] has assigned Roman numerals I through XIII to some of the factors. Each Roman numeral was assigned according to the order of discovery of the respective factor, not its place in the reaction sequence. Each factor had one or more common names or synonyms in addition to the Roman numeral designation, although the common names are rarely used today (Table 30-2 ✪). The letter *a* following the Roman numeral indicates the activated form of the factor (i.e., it is no longer a zymogen but has enzymatic activity). There are, however, several exceptions to this terminology. In its activated form, factor II (prothrombin) is preferentially known as *thrombin* rather than F-IIa. When fibrinogen (F-I) is cleaved by thrombin, it is preferentially called *fibrin*. Tissue factor (TF) was assigned F-III, and calcium was assigned F-IV, but these Roman numeral designations are seldom used. F-VI is no longer included in the coagulation sequence because it was originally assigned to a procoagulant activity subsequently found to be activated F-V. High molecular weight kininogen (HK) and prekallikrein (PK) were never assigned Roman numerals.

Most coagulation factors were discovered when physicians saw patients with a life-long history of bleeding problems. Studies of the affected patient's blood revealed that certain proteins were functionally deficient. These proteins have been isolated and characterized as to their composition (including full amino acid sequences), biochemical functions, and the chromosomal location of their genes, providing useful information for understanding hereditary problems (Table 30-2).

CASE STUDY *(continued from above)*

3. What evidence exists to indicate that Shawn has a hereditary bleeding disorder?

4. Are the nosebleeds significant in considering the diagnosis?

PROPERTIES OF THE BLOOD COAGULATION FACTORS

Similarities among the structural and functional properties of the coagulation factors permit division into three groups: the **prothrombin group**, the **fibrinogen group**, and the **contact group** (Table 30-3 ✪).

Prothrombin Group

The prothrombin group of proteins includes prothrombin (F-II) and factors VII, IX, and X. These factors have a molecular mass ranging from 50,000 to 100,000 Daltons (Da.). The factors in the prothrombin group are produced in the liver, and all contain the γ-carboxyglutamic acid-rich region called the *GLA-domain* that is critical for the calcium-binding properties of these proteins. The prothrombin group is also referred to as **vitamin K dependent** because its members require vitamin K (see later section) to be functional. Other vitamin K-dependent proteins include protein C, protein S, and protein Z (see section on biochemical inhibitors).

Fibrinogen Group

The fibrinogen group includes fibrinogen (F-I) and F-V F-VIII, and F-XIII. Thrombin acts on all during coagulation. They have the highest molecular weights of all the factors, ranging from 300,000 to 350,000 Da. These factors are not found in serum because they are consumed during clotting.

Contact Group

The contact group includes F-XI and F-XII, PK, and high molecular weight kininogen (HK). The proteins have molecular weights ranging from 80,000 to 173,000 Da. The contact group is involved in the initial activation of the intrinsic pathway and requires contact with a negatively charged surface for activation. With the exception of F-XI, the contact factors do not appear to play an essential role in hemostasis in vivo.[5] However, this group of factors is integrally related to other physiologic systems. In addition to the coagulation system, the activated forms of the contact group can activate the fibrinolytic, kinin, and complement systems and play an important role in the inflammatory response. These factors are found in serum because they are not consumed during clotting.

MECHANISM OF ACTION OF THE COAGULATION FACTORS

The coagulation proteins can be grouped functionally as cofactors, substrates, or enzymes. The enzymes can be further grouped as either serine proteases or a transglutaminase.

Cofactors

F-V and F-VIII function as *cofactors* for activated coagulation proteases F-Xa and F-IXa, respectively. F-Va and F-VIIIa have no enzymatic activity of their own. HK functions as a cofactor for the contact activation phase of coagulation (F-XIIa and F-XIa), protein S is a cofactor for activated protein C (see

Summary of the Properties of Coagulation Factors

Factor	Common Name(s)	Description	T$_{1/2}$ (hours)	Role	Plasma Concentration	Chromosome
I	Fibrinogen	6-chain glycoprotein MW 340,000	72–120	Substrate; fibrin precursor	2000–4000 μg/mL 10 nM	4
II	Prothrombin	Single-chain glycoprotein MW 72,000	60–70	Serine protease Thrombin precursor	100–150 μg/mL 1.4 nM	11
III	Tissue factor	Single-chain, transmembrane lipoprotein MW 45,000	NA	Cofactor in extrinsic Xase complex not found in circulation	NA	1
IV	Calcium	Element	NA	Cofactor in some coagulation reactions	8.8–10.5 mg/dL	—
V	Proaccelerin	Single-chain glycoprotein MW 330,000	12–36	Cofactor in prothrombinase complex	5–10 μg/mL 30 nM	1
VII	Proconvertin, stable factor	Single-chain glycoprotein MW 50,000	3–6	Serine protease; constituent of extrinsic Xase complex	0.5 μg/mL 30 nM	13
VIII	Antihemophilic factor	Heterodimer glycoprotein MW 80,000 (light chain) 90–200,000 (heavy chain)	8–12	Complex with VWF in the circulation; cofactor in intrinsic Xase complex	0.15 μg/mL	X
VWF	von Willebrand factor	Multimeric glycoprotein MW 250,000 (subunit)	12	Platelet adhesion; stabilization of circulating F-VIII	8–10 μg/mL	12
IX	Plasma thromboplastin component	Single-chain glycoprotein MW 57,000	18–24	Serine protease; constituent of intrinsic Xase complex	4 μg/mL 70 nM	X
X	Stuart factor	Two-chain glycoprotein MW 56,000	30–40	Serine protease; constituent of prothrombinase complex	4–6 μg/mL 100 nM	13
XI	Plasma thromboplastin antecedent	Two-chain glycoprotein MW 160,000	52	Serine protease; contact factor	4–6 μg/mL 30 nM	4
XII	Hageman factor	Single-chain glycoprotein MW 80,000	60	Serine protease; contact factor	23–39 μg/mL 375 nM	5
XIII	Fibrin-stabilizing factor	Multimeric glycoprotein MW 320,000	240	Transglutaminase; stabilizes fibrin	14–28 μg/mL 65 nM	6 (A-chain) 1 (B-chain)
HK	Fitzgerald factor, Williams factor, Flaujeac factor	Monomeric α-globulin MW 120,000	156	Cofactor; complexed with PK and F-XI; contact factor	70–90 μg/mL 670 nM	3
PK	Fletcher factor	Monomeric γ-globulin MW 100,000	35	Serine protease complexed with HK; contact factor	35–45 μg/mL 410 nM	4

T$_{1/2}$ = biologic half-life; MW = molecular weight in da.; HMWK = high molecular weight kininogen; PK = prekallikrein

Coagulation Factor Groups Based on Physical Characteristics

	Contact Group	Prothrombin Group	Fibrinogen Group
Characteristics	Requires contact with a surface for activation	Requires vitamin K for synthesis; needs Ca^{++} to bind to a phospholipid surface; is adsorbed from plasma by BaSO$_4$	Has large molecules; is absent from serum (consumable)
Factors/Proteins included	XII, XI, PK, HK	II, VII, IX, X, protein C, protein S, protein Z	I, V, VIII, XIII

later section), and TF is a cofactor for F-VIIa. Each protease has some activity in the absence of its cofactor, but interaction with cofactor significantly enhances proteolytic function. The full activity of F-VIIa, F-IXa, and F-Xa is expressed only when they are a part of a procoagulant complex named for their physiologic substrate. Thus, the F-VIIa/TF complex is termed *extrinsic tenase* (named for the extrinsic factor complex's enzymatic action on F-X), the F-IXa/F-VIIIa complex is termed the *intrinsic tenase* (named for the intrinsic factor complex's enzymatic action on F-X), and the F-Xa/F-Va complex is termed the *prothrombinase* complex (named for the complex's enzymatic action on prothrombin).

Substrate

Fibrinogen is classified as a *substrate* because it is acted upon by the enzyme thrombin. It is the only coagulation protein that, as a substrate, does not become an activated enzyme.

Enzymes

The coagulation proteins that have enzymatic activity are secreted as zymogens, which are proenzymes or inactive precursors that must be modified to become active. Activation can involve either (1) a conformational change of the molecule or (2) proteolytic cleavage of one or more specific zymogen peptide bond(s). The coagulation zymogens are rapidly activated in a cascade-like sequence. Initially, a small number of zymogens are activated, and each sequentially activates the next zymogen in the cascade, resulting in the amplification of the initial stimulus.

Members of the family of **serine proteases,** including thrombin, factors VIIa, IXa, Xa, XIa, and XIIa, have a functional serine in their active sites and a common catalytic mechanism. They selectively hydrolyze arginine- or lysine-containing peptide bonds in their substrates. Each serine protease involved in the coagulation cascade is highly specific for its substrate(s).

F-XIIIa is the only coagulation protein with **transglutaminase** activity. It catalyzes the formation of isopeptide bonds between glutamine and lysine residues on fibrin, forming stable covalent cross-links.

VITAMIN K-DEPENDENT COAGULATION PROTEINS

Seven of the blood coagulation proteins, including prothrombin, factors VII, IX, and X, and proteins C, S, and Z, require vitamin K to become functional. Vitamin K is a fat-soluble vitamin found in green leafy vegetables, fish, and liver. Some gram-negative intestinal bacteria also synthesize it. Vitamin K is necessary for the **γ-carboxylation** of glutamic acid residues in the GLA domains of these proteins. The addition of an extra carboxyl group (COOH) to the γ-carbon of the glutamic acid residues (a reaction known as γ-carboxylation) is a post-translational modification of the protein carried out by a

specific γ-glutamyl carboxylase in the endoplasmic reticulum (ER) of the liver. The γ-carboxylation is essential for binding the factor to negatively charged phospholipid surfaces (e.g., exposed phospholipids on activated platelets) via Ca^{2+} bridges.[6] The carboxylase requires the reduced form of vitamin K (hydroquinone form) for its action. The carboxylation reaction converts reduced vitamin K to the epoxide form, which is converted back to the reduced form by the enzyme vitamin K epoxide reductase. Conversion back to the reduced form allows recycling of the vitamin K. Vitamin K antagonist drugs such as warfin/coumadin inhibit the activity of the vitamin K epoxide reductase and prevent recycling of vitamin K back to the reduced form. Warfarin/coumadin overdose can be reversed by vitamin K administration (Figure 30-3 ■).

In the absence of vitamin K, the liver synthesizes the proteins, which can be found in the plasma. However, they are nonfunctional because they lack the γ-COOH groups necessary for Ca^{2+}/phospholipid binding. The vitamin K-dependent factors lacking the COOH modification have previously been referred to as **PIVKA** (**p**rotein **i**nduced by **v**itamin **k** **a**bsence or antagonists) or des-γ-carboxy form. The International Committee on Thrombosis and Haemostasis recommends using the term *acarboxy* form. Warfarin/coumadin, which inhibits the γ-carboxylation process, results in the production of inactive proteins by the liver. The nonfunctional and functional forms of the factors are identical with respect to amino acid composition and antigenic determinants.

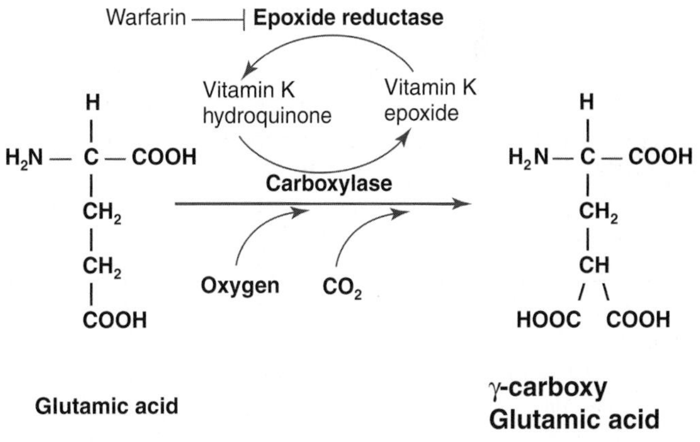

■ **FIGURE 30-3** The vitamin K-dependent γ-carboxylation of glutamic acid. The coagulation factors in the prothrombin group must undergo this postribosomal carboxylation of glutamic acid residues in order to become functional. A specific carboxylase converts glutamyl residues to γ-carboxy glutamyl residues in a reaction requiring oxygen, carbon dioxide, and reduced vitamin K (hydroquinone). In the process, reduced vitamin K is converted to an epoxide and must be recycled to its reduced form by the enzyme epoxide reductase. This latter reaction is blocked by vitamin K antagonist drugs such as warfarin or coumadin.

STRUCTURE OF THE BLOOD COAGULATION PROTEINS

The blood coagulation proteins are made up of multiple functional units called *domains,* which can be classified as catalytic or noncatalytic depending on their function.[7] Catalytic domains contain the active site of the enzyme and are involved in activating other proteins. Noncatalytic domains contain regulatory elements. Structural similarities occur among proteins involved in the hemostatic mechanism, many of which are believed to be derived from common ancestral genes (Web Figure 30-1 ■).

The *catalytic domain* of the serine proteases involved in blood clotting is highly homologous to trypsin. The main function of this domain is the conversion of an inactive proenzyme to an active enzyme by cleavage of a peptide bond in its target substrate, a process known as *zymogen activation by limited proteolysis.*

The noncatalytic domains give each coagulation factor its own unique identity, making each highly specific in its activity and activation. They are regulatory elements serving to bind calcium and promoting interaction with phospholipids, cofactors, receptors, and substrates. Some of the more common types of noncatalytic domains include the signal peptide, propeptide, γ-carboxyglutamic acid-rich (GLA) domain, epidermal growth factor domain, apple domain, finger domain, and kringle domain.

The *signal peptide* is a short domain that permits translocation of the protein to the endoplasmic reticulum. Vitamin K-dependent proteins have a *propeptide* between the signal peptide and the GLA domain, which contains the recognition site that directs γ-carboxylation of the vitamin K-dependent proteins after synthesis. The GLA domain contains 9–12 γ-carboxyglutamic acid residues and is essential for Ca^{2+} binding. When bound, Ca^{2+} mediates the association of a coagulation factor with a phospholipid surface.

The *epidermal growth factor (EGF) domain, finger domain,* and *apple domains* are thought to be involved in binding to cofactors, activators, or substrates. The *kringle domain* is a lysine-binding site responsible for the affinity of certain proteins (plasminogen, plasmin, tissue plasminogen activator) for fibrin. There are other domains whose functions are as yet unknown (Web Figure 30-2 ■).

► COAGULATION CASCADE

The coagulation cascade is composed of four interacting sets of reactions: complex formation on phospholipid membranes, intrinsic pathway activation, extrinsic pathway activation, and the common pathway.

COMPLEX FORMATION ON PHOSPHOLIPID MEMBRANES

The coagulation cascade occurs on cell surface membranes. Clotting factors bind to the phospholipid membrane surface, forming a complex including enzyme, substrate, and cofactor.[8] Subendothelial tissue, exposed when blood vessel injury occurs, and the activated platelet surface provide the critical phospholipids for coagulation in vivo. The phospholipid surface serves to decrease the Km of the reaction between enzyme and substrate and to localize the reaction to the site of injury.[9]

Three procoagulant complexes, the **extrinsic Xase** (also called *extrinsic tenase*), **intrinsic Xase** (also called *intrinsic tenase*), and **prothrombinase complexes** assemble on the phospholipid membrane (Figure 30-4 ■). Extrinsic Xase is formed when TF, an integral membrane lipoprotein, is exposed to blood when vessel injury occurs. TF binds F-VII or F-VIIa in the presence of Ca^{2+}, giving rise to the F-VIIa/TF complex that activates F-X. The intrinsic Xase is formed on membrane surfaces when F-IXa and F-VIIIa bind to phospholipid in the presence of Ca^{2+}. This complex also activates F-X to Xa. In a similar way, F-Xa and F-Va bind to negatively charged membranes in the presence of Ca^{2+} to form the prothrombinase complex. This complex converts prothrombin, also bound to the membrane, to thrombin. The rate of prothrombin activation by the prothrombinase complex is about 300,000 times faster than activation by F-Xa alone.[10]

THE INTRINSIC PATHWAY

Contact Factors/the Surface Mediated Pathway

The four contact factors include F-XII, F-XI, PK, and HK. The contact factors are activated when exposed to and adsorbed on negatively charged surfaces such as glass, kaolin, celite, and ellagic acid. Activation of these factors does not require Ca^{2+}; thus, in vitro activation (or "pre-activation") can occur in citrated patient samples stored in glass tubes for prolonged periods before testing. Patients deficient in F-XII, PK, and HK have no apparent clinical bleeding disorder despite a markedly prolonged APTT; thus, it is unlikely that these factors play an important role in coagulation in vivo. They do, however, contribute significantly to fibrinolysis, inflammation, complement activation, angiogenesis, and kinin formation. About 50% of patients with F-XI deficiency have clinically evident bleeding abnormalities, suggesting that F-XI

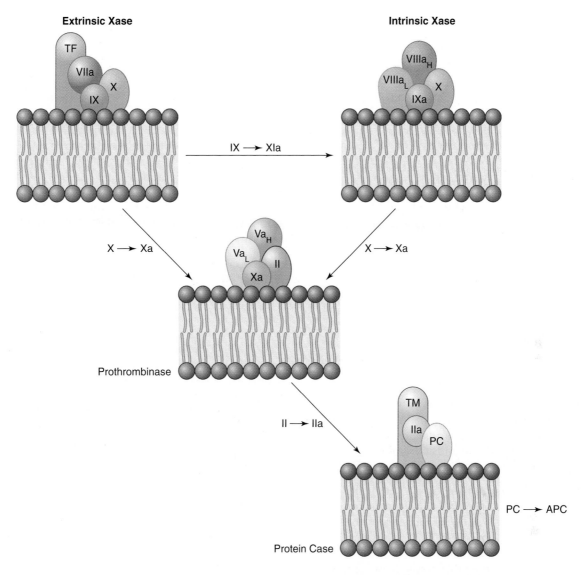

■ **FIGURE 30-4** Schematic illustration of the coagulation complexes forming on a phospholipid surface. The vitamin K-dependent proteases (F-VIIa, F-IXa, and F-Xa and thrombin) are shown associated with their cofactors (TF, F-VIIIa, F-Va, and thrombomodulin [TM], respectively) and substrates (F-IX and F-X, prothrombin, and protein C [PC], respectively) on the membrane surface. APC = activated protein C

could be an important accessory to blood coagulation, but it is probably not essential.

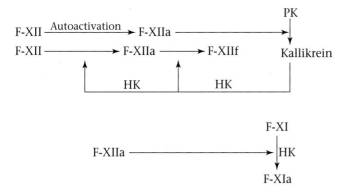

Factor XII The liver produces F-XII (Hageman factor). Zymogen single-chain F-XII is converted into the two-chain active serine protease F-XIIa by proteolysis by kallikrein, plasmin (PLN), or by "autoactivation." Autoactivation of F-XII occurs by contact with negatively charged surfaces. Binding to the negatively charged surface induces a conformational change that makes the protein more susceptible to autocatalysis. Many nonphysiologic substances (glass, kaolin, ellagic acid)[11] have been associated with in vitro F-XII autoactivation. The nature of the physiologic surfaces responsible for autoactivation is still in question but is most likely negatively charged cellular membranes or subendothelial structures (collagen, basement membrane).

Bound F-XIIa proteolytically cleaves PK to kallikrein, which with HK as a cofactor can then reciprocally proteolytically activate surface-bound F-XII to F-XIIa (Web Figure 30-3 ■). The generation of F-XIIa and kallikrein by reciprocal activation amplifies the reactions. F-XIIa can be further cleaved by kallikrein yielding smaller F-XII fragments (F-XIIf) that have little or no procoagulant activity.[12]

In addition to activating PK to kallikrein, F-XIIa has other enzymatic functions in hemostasis. As the first enzyme in the intrinsic pathway, it converts F-XI to its active form, F-XIa, in a reaction that requires HK as a cofactor. Second, F-XIIa activates the fibrinolytic and complement systems. F-XIIa, F-XIa, and kallikrein activate plasminogen directly, although much less efficiently than tissue plasminogen activator (tPA) or urokinase (uPA) (see later section) (Figure 30-5 ■). F-XIIa also activates the first component of the complement cascade (C-1).

Prekallikrein   PK predominantly circulates in plasma bound to HK (75% bound, 25% free).[12] F-XIIa activates PK to the serine protease kallikrein. In addition to reciprocal activation of F-XII and initiation of "intrinsic" coagulation, kallikrein can activate the kinin, fibrinolytic, and complement systems. Kallikrein cleaves bradykinin from HK. It directly activates plasminogen to PLN and converts prourokinase (scuPA) to uPA, which in turn can activate plasminogen. PLN subsequently can activate the first and third components of the complement cascade (Figure 30-5). Kallikrein also serves as a chemoattractant and activator for neutrophils and monocytes, facilitating the inflammatory response.

High Molecular Weight Kininogen (HK)   HK serves as a nonenzymatic cofactor in activation of the contact factors and is the source of kinins. HK accelerates the rate of surface-dependent activation of F-XII and the rate of PK activation by F-XIIa. HK binds to platelets, endothelial cells, and granulocytes, assembling the other components of the con-

tact activation pathway. Two forms of kininogen are found in plasma, HK and low molecular weight kininogen (LK). The liver produces both forms by alternative splicing of a single gene. In addition, HK is found in endothelial cells, platelets, and granulocytes. HK, the preferred substrate for kallikrein, is a single-chain glycoprotein that can be cleaved by kallikrein into a two-chain disulphide-bonded molecule with the release of a small nonapeptide, bradykinin, a potent bioactive peptide. Bradykinin has many functions including increasing vessel permeability, dilating small vessels, contracting smooth muscle, and causing pain. Bradykinin stimulates vasodilation, increasing blood flow, and stimulates endothelial cell profibrinolytic, antithrombotic and antiplatelet properties by stimulating endothelial cell prostacyclin (PGI_2), nitric oxide (NO) and tPA synthesis and secretion (∞ Chapter 29).

Factor XI   F-XI is activated to a serine protease by F-XIIa and cofactor HK (Web Figure 30-4 ■).

$$\text{F-XI} \xrightarrow{\text{XIIa, HK}} \text{XIa}$$

Like PK, F-XI circulates in the plasma primarily as a complex with HK. In addition to activation by F-XIIa, F-XI can be activated by both thrombin and F-XIa itself in a positive feedback reaction. Thrombin is likely the physiologically relevant activator of F-XI with minimal need for activation by F-XIIa in vivo. Both F-XI and thrombin bind to the surface of activated platelets where in vivo activation most likely occurs.[13] The substrate for F-XIa is F-IX. Although patients with deficiencies of other contact factors (F-XII, PK, and HK) do not have bleeding problems, about 50% of patients with a F-XI deficiency experience abnormal bleeding after surgery or injury. Plasma levels of F-XI are not the only determinant of whether bleeding occurs because patients who have bleeding problems and those who do not have similar plasma concentrations of F-XI.

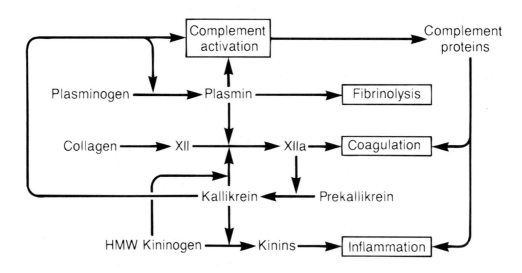

■ FIGURE 30-5   Role of contact factors in physiologic systems.

Other Factors in the Intrinsic Pathway

Factor IX   F-IX is a single-chain vitamin K-dependent zymogen containing 12 Gla residues. F-IX is activated by F-XIa in the presence of Ca^{2+} and does not require any other cofactor (Web Figure 30-5 ■). Activation is associated with cleavage of two bonds in F-IX, releasing a 35 amino acid activation peptide and a two-chain molecule, F-IXa.

$$\textbf{XIa}$$
$$\downarrow$$
$$\textbf{IX} \xrightarrow[\textbf{Ca}^{2+}]{} \textbf{IXa}$$

When activated, F-IXa forms a complex (intrinsic Xase) with cofactor F-VIIIa and Ca^{2+} on the surface of activated platelets to activate F-X (Figure 30-6 ■).

$$\textbf{IXa} + \textbf{VIIIa}$$
$$\textbf{activated platelet surface}$$
$$\textbf{Ca}^{2+}$$
$$\downarrow$$
$$\textbf{X} \longrightarrow \textbf{Xa}$$

The extrinsic pathway complex F-VIIa/TF also activates F-IX (see later section). This extrinsic pathway for F-IX activation bypasses the contact activation system.

F-IXa (but not F-IX) binds to phospholipid surfaces on activated platelets in the presence of calcium; it does not bind to resting platelets. It is one of two coagulation proteins (F-VIII and F-IX) whose genes are encoded on the X chromosome. The severe bleeding that results from a deficiency of F-IX (Hemophilia B) indicates that it plays a critical role in blood coagulation.

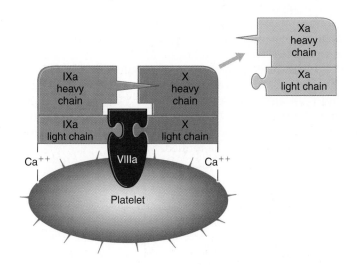

■ **FIGURE 30-6**   The complex formed by the sequential activation of the intrinsic pathway (F-IXa, F-VIIIa, Ca^{2+}) activates F-X. The cofactor, F-VIIIa, binds to the platelet phospholipids and serves to orient F-IXa and F-X to enhance activation of F-X. F-IXa and F-X are bound to the platelet surface via Ca^{2+} bridges. Spikes on platelet indicate activated platelet.

Factor VIII   F-VIII is synthesized primarily in the liver and circulates in plasma in association with von Willebrand factor (VWF) (Figure 32-1). Each protein in this complex is under separate genetic control and has distinct biologic functions and immunologic properties (∞ Chapter 32). Binding to VWF stabilizes F-VIII and protects it from inhibition or degradation. F-VIII circulates in the plasma in an inactive form until it is activated by thrombin (or F-Xa), yielding F-VIIIa, which serves as a cofactor for the F-IXa activation of F-X.

F-VIII is synthesized as a large precursor protein consisting of the linear array of A1:A2:B:A3:C1:C2 domains (Figure 32-3). A signal peptide is cleaved on translocation into the lumen of the ER. F-VIII is further processed on secretion from the cell with the cleavage of part of the B domain and the release of a heterodimer composed of heavy-chain (A1:A2 and part of B domain) and light-chain (A3:C1:C2 domains) polypeptides. In the plasma, F-VIII associates with VWF, which stabilizes F-VIII and prolongs its circulating half-life from ~2 hours to ~12 hours.[14] In addition to increasing F-VIII survival, VWF also is involved in regulating F-VIII activity. VWF prevents F-VIII from binding to phospholipids and activated platelets and protects against inactivation by activated protein C. It does not, however, prevent thrombin activation of F-VIII but rather facilitates thrombin proteolytic activation.[15] Thrombin cleaves both the heavy and the light chains of F-VIII, creating a three polypeptide molecule (F-VIIIa) with subunits derived from the A1, A2, and A3:C1:C2 domains). The A1 and A3:C1:C2 subunits remain linked as a stable dimer while the A2 subunit, associated primarily by weak electrostatic interactions, readily dissociates. As a result, F-VIII is labile, and its activity is rapidly lost at room temperature. Thrombin activation of F-VIIIa by proteolytic cleavage dissociates F-VIIIa from VWF, permitting F-VIIIa interaction with the platelet surface. F-VIIIa has no enzymatic activity but as part of the intrinsic Xase complex functions as a cofactor for F-IXa activation of F-X. However, large amounts of F-Xa and thrombin destroy the procoagulant function of F-VIIIa. Like F-IX, the gene for F-VIII is located on the X chromosome, and the factor is critical for normal blood coagulation. A deficiency of F-VIII results in Hemophilia A.

von Willebrand Factor (VWF)   VWF is a large multimeric glycoprotein synthesized by endothelial cells and megakaryocytes (Figure 32-1). VWF is synthesized as a proprotein with a signal peptide, a propeptide (pp), and the mature VWF protein. VWF undergoes extensive intracellular modifications during trafficking through the ER and Golgi including removal of the signal peptide, formation of dimers and subsequently higher multimers, glycosylation, and protein folding.[16] In the Golgi, the propeptide is cleaved from pro-VWF, releasing the VWFpp and the mature VWF monomer.[17] The VWF monomer consists of areas of internal homology or domains, resulting in a structure with A-, B-, C-, and D-domains (Figure 32-2). The propeptide, also called VWF antigen II, is required for the VWF multimerization process as well as the regulated intracellular storage of VWF. Although synthesized as a monomer of 250,000 Da. VWF circulates in the plasma as a family of molecules (multimers) of a wide range of sizes (0.5– > 20 million Da.) with the largest forms being most effective in promoting platelet adhesion. However, all multimers can bind F-VIII in a 1:1 molar ratio.

Mature VWF multimers are stored within α-granules (αG) of platelets and in Weibel-Palade bodies of endothelial cells. They are released from these intracellular stores following injury or stimulation by thrombin, histamine, or the vasopressin analog 1-desamino-8-D-arginine vasopressin (DDAVP). Platelet and endothelial cell VWF generally consists of larger multimers, called *ultralarge VWF multimers* (*ULVWF*), than are found in plasma. Degradation of ULVWF to the normal plasma forms is accomplished by the VWF-cleaving protease, ADAMTS-13 (a member of the ***a d**isintegrinlike **a**nd **m**etalloprotease with **t**hrombo**s**pondin repeats proteins).[18] The ULVWF are released from the Weible-Palade bodies and remain tethered to the endothelial cell surface, forming long stringlike structures. When tethered, ULVWF is exposed to the shear forces of the flowing blood, and the protein unfolds and exposes the cleavage site for ADAMTS-13.[19] If the ULVWF is released directly into plasma, platelets can spontaneously aggregate, resulting in thrombosis (∞ Chapter 33).

VWF contributes to both primary and secondary hemostasis. It mediates adhesion of platelets to the vessel wall in areas of high flow rate and high shear force by the simultaneous binding of VWF to GPIb/IX on platelet surfaces and to collagen and elastin in the subendothelium (∞ Chapter 29). High molecular weight multimers of VWF contain the highest number of platelet and other cell surface-binding sites. VWF also can bind to the GPIIb/IIIa receptor on platelets (the normal physiologic receptor for fibrinogen) and thus can promote platelet aggregation. These molecules serve as *intercellular bridges* between platelets, between platelets and subendothelium, and between platelets and endothelial cells. In secondary hemostasis, VWF carries F-VIII in the plasma, binding to and stabilizing F-VIII via a noncovalent interaction between the two molecules. The two proteins circulate as a VWF/F-VIII complex.

 Checkpoint! 4

Which components of the intrinsic pathway are believed to be essential for in vivo hemostasis?

THE EXTRINSIC PATHWAY

F-X can also be activated by the extrinsic pathway involving F-VII and its cofactor, TF, or tissue thromboplastin. When vessel injury occurs, nonvascular cells (fibroblasts, smooth muscle cells) with TF on their surface are exposed to the blood. TF binds F-VII and F-VIIa in the presence of calcium,

forming the F-VIIa/TF complex. Once formed, this complex initiates the extrinsic pathway of blood coagulation. The F-VIIa/TF complex (extrinsic Xase) converts F-X to F-Xa, similarly to the intrinsic Xase complex. The F-VIIa/TF complex also can activate F-IX of the intrinsic pathway, bypassing the need for contact activation of this pathway. F-Xa can feed back to activate more F-VII to F-VIIa.

$$
\begin{array}{cc}
\textbf{VIIa/TF} & \textbf{VIIa/TF} \\
\downarrow \textbf{Ca}^{2+} & \downarrow \textbf{Ca}^{2+} \\
\textbf{X} \longrightarrow \textbf{Xa} & \textbf{IX} \longrightarrow \textbf{IXa}
\end{array}
$$

Tissue Factor

TF is the cellular receptor and cofactor for F-VII and F-VIIa. It is a transmembrane lipoprotein originally named *F-III* or *tissue thromboplastin*. TF is expressed constitutively on the plasma membrane of most nonvascular cells. It is not normally expressed by cells that are in contact with flowing blood, but monocytes and endothelial cells can be stimulated to produce TF by endotoxin, complement component 5a, immune complexes, interleukin-1, and tumor necrosis factor.[20] TF and the platelet phospholipid surface have similar functions in coagulation; both attract calcium ions to facilitate the formation of procoagulant enzyme complexes at the injury site.

Factor VII

F-VII is one of the vitamin K-dependent proteins produced by the liver and has 12 Gla residues. F-VII circulates in two forms: the inactive zymogen, F-VII, and low levels of the active enzyme, F-VIIa (~1% of the total plasma F-VII).[21] Free F-VIIa is a weak enzyme in the absence of TF. However, these trace levels of circulating F-VIIa are sufficient to initiate the coagulation cascade when injury exposes TF. F-VII is a single-chain molecule activated to two-chain F-VIIa by proteolytic cleavage of a single peptide bond, with the two cleavage peptides remaining tethered by a disulfide bond. No cleavage peptide is released.

As with intrinsic activation of coagulation, there is positive feedback in activating the extrinsic pathway. When TF and F-VII are bound in a complex, F-VIIa can autocatalyze more F-VII to F-VIIa. Additionally, F-Xa associated with a phospholipid surface can feed back to activate F-VII, increasing the amount of F-VIIa formed.[22]

 Checkpoint! 5

Historically, the major importance for initiating coagulation was assigned to either the intrinsic or extrinsic pathway. What are some observations that suggest that the classic concepts were not accurate?

THE COMMON PATHWAY

The intrinsic and extrinsic pathways converge on the common pathway as both pathways activate F-X.

Factor X Activation

F-X can be activated by the F-VIIa/TF/Ca^{2+} complex (extrinsic Xase) or the F-IXa/F-VIIIa/Ca^{2+}/phospholipid complex (intrinsic Xase).

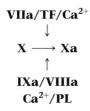

Thrombin Generation

F-Xa then forms a complex with cofactor F-Va, phospholipid, and Ca^{2+}. This prothrombinase complex acts to optimally activate prothrombin to thrombin.

$$\begin{array}{c} \mathbf{Xa/Va/Ca^{2+}/PL} \\ \downarrow \\ \mathbf{Prothrombin \longrightarrow Thrombin} \end{array}$$

Factor X   F-X is another vitamin K-dependent protein produced by the liver; it contains 11 Gla residues. It circulates as a two-chain disulfide-linked zymogen. A 52-amino acid activation peptide is released from the F-X heavy chain to generate F-Xa.

Factor V   F-V is a large glycoprotein produced by the liver. It is also called *labile factor* because, like F-VIIIa, its activity deteriorates quickly at room temperature. About 25% of F-V in the blood is found in the αG of platelets from which it is secreted during platelet activation.[23] F-V circulates in the plasma as a single-chain molecule with a domain organization similar to F-VIII (A1:A2:B:A3:C1:C2). Activation of F-V to F-Va, with full cofactor activity, requires cleavage of several bonds. Both thrombin and F-Xa can activate F-V, although thrombin is the primary activator in vivo. Cleavage produces a two-chain heterodimer consisting of a heavy chain (A1:A2 domains) noncovalently linked through Ca^{2+} to a light chain (A3:C1:C2 domains). The B domain is released as a result of activation. F-Va binds to specific sites on the activated platelet surface, serving as the attachment site for F-Xa (Figure 30-7 ■). Most of the F-V that participates in the prothrombinase complex on the platelet membranes probably is supplied as the result of secretion from activated platelet αG.

Prothrombin   Prothrombin is a vitamin K-dependent protein produced by the liver; it contains 10 Gla residues. Zymogen F-II circulates as a single-chain molecule and is cleaved by the prothrombinase complex in two places. Cleavage releases the C-terminal half of the molecule that contains the catalytic domain (prethrombin) from the remainder of the molecule (the activation peptide, prothrombin fragment 1.2). Assays for fragment 1.2 reflect the level of in vivo prothrombin activation. Prethrombin (single-chain)

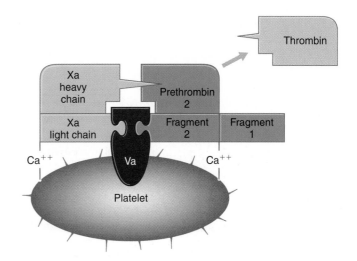

■ **FIGURE 30-7**   The prothrombinase complex (F-Xa, F-Va, Ca^{2+}, PL) activates prothrombin to thrombin. F-Va binds to the platelet phospholipid surface and orients F-Xa and prothrombin to enhance the formation of thrombin. F-Xa and prothrombin are bound to the platelet surface via Ca^{2+} bridges. This complex is very similar to the complex formed by the intrinsic pathway (F-IXa, F-VIIIa, Ca^{2+}, PL). Spikes on platelet indicate activated platelet.

is cleaved to thrombin, which is composed of an α- and a β-chain linked by a disulfide bond. It does not contain the GLA domain of prothrombin and thus does not bind to negatively charged phospholipids (Figure 30-8 ■). As a result, thrombin does not remain tethered to the phospholipid surface on which it was formed but can dissociate and move to other areas or surfaces (e.g., thrombomodulin on nearby intact endothelial cells).

Roles of Thrombin

Thrombin generation is critical for normal hemostasis and it has a number of diverse roles (Figure 30-9 ■). This protein functions as a procoagulant by cleaving fibrinopeptides A and B from fibrinogen to create fibrin monomer; it also generates other procoagulant activities, activating factors Va, VIIIa, and XIIIa to greatly amplify its own formation; it stimulates endothelial cells to release VWF and plasminogen activator inhibitor (PAI-1) and to express TF[24]; it also activates platelets, stimulating platelet aggregation. Thrombin can suppress fibrinolysis by activating the **thrombin activatable fibrinolysis inhibitor (TAFI)**. Conversely, thrombin also has antithrombotic functions that dampen its own formation. Thrombin binds to thrombomodulin and activates protein C, and it stimulates endothelial cells to release tissue plasminogen activator and endothelium-derived relaxing factor (EDRF, also known as nitric oxide). In addition to its role in hemostasis, thrombin has mitogen and cytokine-like activities and plays a role in inflammation, wound healing, and atherosclerosis.

Prothrombin Conversion to Thrombin

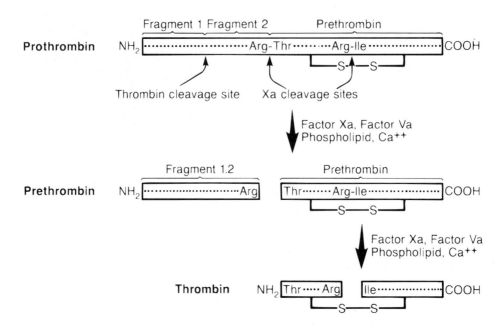

FIGURE 30-8 The prothrombin molecule is a single-chain glycoprotein that can be divided into the "pro" portion (fragments 1 and 2 or fragment 1.2) and the thrombin portion (prethrombin). Factor Xa proteolytically cleaves the molecule between the "pro" and thrombin portions releasing fragment 1.2 and prethrombin. Prethrombin is further cleaved into two disulfide bonded chains forming the potent enzyme thrombin.

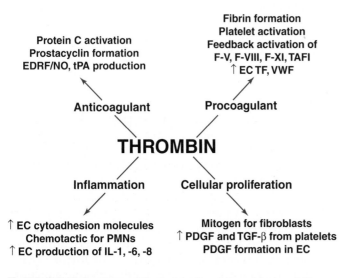

FIGURE 30-9 The multifactorial roles of thrombin. In addition to its multiple roles as a procoagulant protease, thrombin also has anticoagulant functions as well as important activities in promoting inflammation and cellular proliferation. (EDRF= endothelium-derived relaxing factor; NO = nitric oxide; tPA= tissue plasminogen activator; TAFI = thrombin activable fibrinolysis inhibitor; EC = endothelial cell; TF = tissue factor; VWF = von Willebrand factor; PMNs = polymorphonuclear neutrophils; PDGF = platelet-derived growth factor)

CASE STUDY *(continued from page 643)*

5. What coagulation factors are included in the extrinsic pathway?

6. What factors are included in the intrinsic pathway?

7. What factors are included in the common pathway?

8. An abnormal PT and a normal APTT would indicate a problem with which factor?

Formation of Fibrin

The insoluble fibrin clot is formed from soluble fibrinogen in three distinct steps:

1. *proteolytic cleavage* of arginine-glycine bonds by thrombin, releasing fibrinopeptides A and B from the α and β chains, forming fibrin monomer

2. spontaneous *polymerization* of fibrin monomers to form fibrin polymers

3. *stabilization* of the fibrin polymers by F-XIIIa-catalyzed cross-linking.

Fibrinogen The fibrinogen molecule is a large (350,000 Da.), trinodular glycoprotein found in plasma and platelet αG. Megakaryocytes and platelets do not synthesize the protein but absorb it from plasma. Fibrinogen is the most abundant coagulation protein with a plasma concentration of 2–4 mg/mL (representing about 2% of the total plasma protein concentration). Fibrinogen is encoded by three separate genes located on chromosome 4, and the production of the three chains is coordinately regulated. Fibrinogen is also one of several hepatic proteins whose production is increased as part of the acute phase response mediated by IL-6.

Fibrinogen is a dimeric protein composed of three pairs of nonidentical polypeptide chains referred to as Aα, Bβ, and γ-chains (a molecule of fibrinogen would be described as $A\alpha_2B\beta_2\gamma_2$)[25] (Figure 30-10■). This nomenclature refers to the fact that small polypeptides (fibrinopeptides A and B) are released from Aα and Bβ chains by thrombin, producing a single molecule of fibrin, $\alpha_2\beta_2\gamma_2$. Twenty-nine disulfide bonds join the three pairs of chains. Electron microscopy has demonstrated the folding of the molecule into a trinodular structure.[26] The central nodule, the E domain, is referred to as the *N-terminal disulfide knot* (*N-DSK*) because the amino terminal ends of all six polypeptide chains join to form this region. The E domain contains the fibrinopeptides A and B. The two outer nodules, the D domains, are made up of the carboxy-terminal ends of the β and γ chains and a short sequence of the α chain. The Aα chain has a long polar appendage at the carboxy-terminal end that folds back toward the N-DSK, which is the site of initial PLN hydrolysis (see below). The D and E domains are separated from each other by 111–112 amino acids forming a triple-stranded α-helical structure called the *coiled-coil domain* (supercoiled region).

Release of FPs A and B. Thrombin binds to the central E domain of fibrinogen and cleaves specific arginine-glycine bonds, releasing four peptides from the fibrinogen molecule. It releases a short peptide containing 16 amino acids from each Aα chain (fibrinopeptide A [FPA]) as well as a 14 amino acid peptide from each Bβ chain (fibrinopeptide B [FPB]). The resulting molecule is called a *fibrin monomer.* Release of FPA alone is sufficient for the fibrin assembly process.

Assembly of Fibrin Polymers. The cleavage of FPA and FPB exposes binding sites in the central E domain that interact with complementary sites on the γ-chain of the D domain of other fibrin monomers, creating a D-E contact. The polymerization sites on the D domain are always available and interact with complementary sites on the E domain

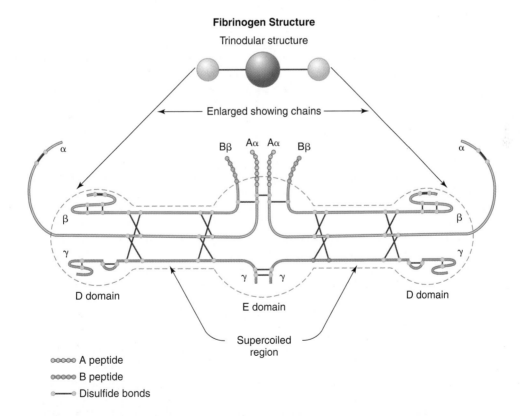

■ FIGURE 30-10   Fibrinogen is a trinodular structure composed of three pairs (Aα, Bβ, γ) of disulfide bonded polypeptide chains. The central nodule is known as the *E domain.* Thrombin cleaves small peptides, A and B, from the α and β chains in this region to form fibrin. The central nodule is joined by supercoiled α-helices to the terminal nodules also known as the *D domains.*

after thrombin cleavage. The polymerization continues by the addition of a third monomer forming a D-D contact as well as another D-E contact. The use of x-ray crystallography to study fibrinogen has provided insights into the mechanism by which fibrin self-assembles. The crystal structures show a mechanism for electrostatic steering to guide the alignment of fibrin polymers during polymerization.[27] The noncovalent interaction of the nodules leads to the initial formation of two-stranded polymers termed *protofibrils*. The polymer strands aggregate in an overlapping pattern called *half-staggered array* in which the second strand is offset from the first by half of the length of a single fibrin molecule. The protofibrils then aggregate into thick fibers through lateral associations held together by weak noncovalent and electrostatic interactions. During fibrin monomer polymerization, other plasma proteins including components of the fibrinolytic system (plasminogen, plasminogen activators, and fibrinolytic inhibitors) can also bind to the fibrin surface. Thrombus extension in vivo can be blunted by unactivated fibrinogen molecules or fibrin degradation products (FDPs) which can bind to and cap the ends of a protofibril.

Fibrin Stabilization.   Spontaneously polymerized fibrin strands are unstable, but the α and γ chains of adjacent fibrin strands are subsequently covalently cross-linked by F-XIIIa. The cross-linking strengthens the clot and provides resistance to chemical (5 M urea) and enzymatic (plasmin) digestion compared to the uncross-linked polymer (Figure 30-11 ■).

Factor XIII   The final reaction in fibrin formation is the stabilization of the fibrin polymer catalyzed by F-XIIIa. F-XIII circulates as a heterotetramer (A_2B_2), which is the product of two separate genes coding for the A and B chains. F-XIII is found evenly distributed between plasma and platelets. Platelet F-XIII exists as an A_2 dimer lacking the B subunit. The plasma F-XIII A chain is primarily synthesized by bone marrow cells, megakaryocytes, monocytes, and macrophages and is stored in the soluble (nongranular) fraction of the platelet. The A chain contains the active site of the enzyme, the fibrin binding and substrate recognition domains. The B chains are secreted by hepatocytes and complex rapidly with the A chains in the plasma, stabilizing them and prolonging their plasma survival. The B chains also promote plasma F-XIII association with fibrinogen.

When fibrin is polymerized, plasma F-XIII is bound as the A_2B_2 complex. Fibrin binding provides a mechanism to localize F-XIII to sites of thrombin generation and fibrin polymerization, allowing for efficient activation of the zymogen F-XIII. Thrombin cleavage of the A chains, dissociating the B chains and releasing an activation peptide, activates F-XIII to F-XIIIa. The expression of F-XIIIa activity requires its interaction with calcium ions, which induce a conformational change, exposing its active center and promoting catalysis.

F-XIIIa is thus a calcium-dependent transglutaminase that catalyzes the formation of covalent isopeptide bonds within

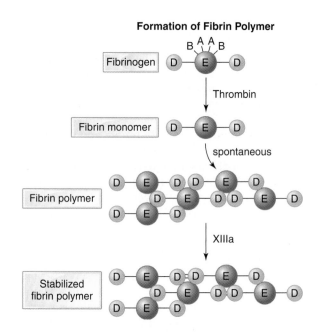

Formation of Fibrin Polymer

■ **FIGURE 30-11**   Thrombin cleaves the A and B fibrinopeptides from the E domain of fibrinogen to form fibrin monomer. The cleavage apparently changes the negative charge of the E domain to a positive charge. This permits the spontaneous growth of fibrin polymers as the positively charged E domain assembles with the negatively charged D domains of other fibrin monomers. The polymer is initially joined by hydrogen bonds. F-XIIIa in the presence of Ca^{2+} is responsible for catalyzing the formation of covalent bonds between glutamine and lysine residues of adjacent monomers (D domains), thus stabilizing the lattice formation.

the fibrin polymer. These bonds are formed between the terminal domains of γ chains of two adjacent fibrin monomers within a protofibril, forming longitudinal end-to-end cross-links. More slowly, cross-links form between polar appendages of α chains of neighboring monomers. The covalently cross-linked fibrin network produces a fibrin clot with increased mechanical strength and increased resistance to proteolytic digestion by plasmin. The presence of these unique bonds is responsible for the liberation of specific fibrin degradation products (D-dimers, see below) when plasmin digests the clot. In contrast to the hydrogen-bonded polymers, the F-XIIIa–stabilized fibrin polymer is not soluble in 5M urea or monochloroacetic acid (∞ Chapter 40). In addition to forming covalent cross-links between molecules of fibrin, F-XIIIa also cross-links fibrinolytic inhibitors to the fibrin clot, including α_2-antiplasmin, plasminogen activator inhibitor-2 (PAI-2), and TAFI.[28] The localization of these fibrinolytic inhibitors to the fibrin clot results in the inhibition of plasmin formation and augmentation of fibrin stabilization. F-XIIIa also cross-links fibrin to extracellular matrix molecules, helping to anchor the fibrin clot to the vessel wall and promoting wound healing.

Checkpoint! 6

What are the three steps in the formation of an insoluble fibrin clot?

▶ THE FIBRINOLYTIC SYSTEM

The fibrinolytic system is activated in response to the activation of the coagulation cascade. This system functions to remove fibrin from the vascular system in a controlled manner once it has fulfilled its function and to prevent excessive fibrin accumulation. This system, which digests the fibrin clot through proteolysis, must be regulated so that proteolytic activity is limited to the area of fibrin formation and does not occur prior to healing of the vascular lesion.

INTRODUCTION

Fibrin formation occurs both intravascularly and extravascularly as a consequence of coagulation, inflammation, and tissue repair. When no longer needed, fibrin must be removed so that normal vessel and tissue structure and function can be restored. The process of removing fibrin is called **fibrinolysis.** The fibrinolytic system is responsible for dissolving thrombi and maintaining a patent vascular system. The key components in this system are (1) the inactive proenzyme, plasminogen, (2) plasminogen activators (PA), (3) the active enzyme PLN, (4) fibrin, (5) fibrin/fibrinogen degradation (split) products, and (6) inhibitors of plasminogen activators and PLN (Table 30-4 ⊙).

Like the coagulation system, the fibrinolytic system normally acts locally at sites of fibrin accumulation without causing systemic effects. If the fibrinolytic system's activity increases (e.g., deficiencies of inhibitors α_2-antiplasmin or PAI-1), stability of the hemostatic plug can be compromised or premature dissolution can occur resulting in an increased bleeding tendency. Conversely, decreased activity of the system (e.g., deficiency of plasminogen, plasminogen activators, or elevated inhibitors) can result in delayed or inadequate fibrin dissolution and thromboembolic tendencies.

Fibrin formation essentially initiates fibrinolysis. Fibrin acts to assemble the various fibrinolytic components to optimize and localize their interactions. When clotting begins, the zymogen plasminogen binds to fibrin throughout the developing thrombus. tPA also binds to fibrin, which increases its enzymatic activity so it can efficiently convert plasminogen (PLG) to PLN. The formation of a ternary complex between the activator (tPA), the zymogen (PLG), and the substrate (fibrin) results in the targeted, specific degradation of fibrin (not fibrinogen or other plasma proteins). PLN then digests fibrin to soluble degradation products, producing several well-characterized fibrin fragments. The system is inhibited by the action of PAIs and by the PLN inhibitor, α_2-antiplasmin (α_2-AP).

When associated with the fibrin surface, plasmin is protected from rapid inhibition by α_2-AP so that efficient degradation of a fibrin clot can occur (Figure 30-12 ■). If free PLN leaks into the circulation, these PLN molecules are rapidly inactivated by α_2-AP. Thus, the activity of this potentially dangerous proteolytic enzyme is localized to the fibrin clot. The relative proportions and locations of profibrinolytic (PLG and PA) molecules and the antifibrinolytic molecules influence the timing and degree of clot dissolution.

 Checkpoint! 7

Why is the process of fibrinolysis a vital part of the hemostatic mechanism? Why must it be closely regulated and controlled?

PLASMINOGEN AND PLASMIN

PLG is a single-chain glycoprotein synthesized by the liver. It has five kringle domains that are critical in regulating fibrinolysis. The kringles contain lysine-binding sites that are responsible for the binding affinity of PLG and PLN for fibrin, cell surface receptors, and other proteins including α_2-antiplasmin. PLG preferentially binds to C-terminal lysines as opposed to intramolecular lysines. **Plasminogen activators (PA)** convert PLG into its active two-chain form, the serine protease PLN, by hydrolysis of a single peptide bond. PLN exhibits much broader substrate specificity than the procoagulant serine proteases and has the potential to degrade and destroy most proteins. In addition to fibrin, PLN can degrade essentially all proteins susceptible to trypsin including fibrinogen, F-V and F-VIII, complement, and several hormones. However, PLN formation and inactivation is highly regulated in vivo, and the enzyme is active only temporarily and locally (in the vicinity of the fibrin clot). PLG binds to fibrin, and activation occurs much more efficiently at the fibrin surface, targeting the proteolytic action of the enzyme PLN to its substrate.

The active enzyme PLN has a positive feedback effect on fibrinolysis. Intact plasma PLG has an amino terminal glutamic acid residue (Glu-PLG). PLN can cleave the Glu-PLG, producing a smaller PLG molecule with a lysine N-terminal amino acid (Lys-PLG). Lys-PLG has a higher affinity for binding to fibrin and greater reactivity with PAs, thus accelerating and improving the efficiency of PLN formation.[29]

ACTIVATORS OF FIBRINOLYSIS

The two major PA that occur in the circulating blood are tissue-type PLG activator (tPA) and urokinase-type PLG activator (uPA), also called *urokinase* (UK). The contact phase of coagulation produces serine proteases (F-XIIa and kallikrein), which also can promote PLG activation.

Contact Phase PA

PAs are generated during the contact phase of the intrinsic pathway, although the physiologic importance of these

⊗ TABLE 30-4

Summary of Properties of the Components of the Fibrinolytic System

Component	Description	Role	t1/2	Concentration	Chromosome
I. Fibrinolytic component					
Plasminogen (PLG)	Single-chain glycoprotein MW 92,000	Zymogen; precursor of plasmin	2.2 days	200 μg/mL 2000 nM	6
Plasmin (PLN)	Dimeric glycoprotein MW 92,000	Serine protease; cleaves fibrin	0.1 sec	—	—
II. Activators of plasminogen					
Tissue plasminogen activator (tPA)	Glycoprotein MW 70,000	Serine protease; complexed with inhibitor PAI-1; activates plasminogen	4 min	0.005 μg/mL 0.07 nM	8
Urokinase type plasminogen activator (uPA)	Single-chain glycoprotein (scuPA) MW 54,000	Serine protease; low enzymatic activity until cleaved to tcuPA by PLN; activates plasminogen	7 min	0.004 μg/mL 0.07 nM	10
III. Inhibitors					
Plasminogen activator Inhibitor-1 (PAI-1)	Single-chain glycoprotein MW 52,000	Proteinase inhibitor (SERPIN): inhibits tPA and uPA	8 min	0.001–0.04 μg/mL 0.1–0.4 nM	7
Plasminogen activator inhibitor-2 (PAI-2)	Glycoprotein—Two forms: MW 60,000 (secreted); 47,000 (intracellular)	Proteinase inhibitor (SERPIN): inhibits tPA, uPA	—	Trace (normal plasma) 0.250 μg/mL in late pregnancy	18
α_2-antiplasmin (AP)	Single-chain glycoprotein MW 70,000	Complexes with PLN; also inhibits kallikrein, thrombin, tPA	3 days	70 μg/mL 1000 nM	17
Thrombin activated fibrinolysis inhibitor (TAFI)	Single-chain protein MW 60,000	Carboxypeptidase B: inhibits plasminogen activation by cleaving lysine AA from fibrin	10 min	5 μg/mL 75 nM	13
IV. Cell surface receptors					
UPAR	Glycoprotein receptor MW 60,000	Binds uPA—localizes on surface of EC, monocytes, and macrophages	—	—	19
Annexin 2	Heterotetramer MW 36,000	Binds tPA, PLG; found on EC, monocytes, and macrophages, SMC	—	—	15
Low-density-lipoprotein Receptor-like protein (LRP)	MW 600,000	Clearance receptor for uPA/PAI-1 & PAI-2, tPA/PAI-1, PLN/α_2PI	—	—	12

MW = molecular weight in Da.; SERPIN = serine protease inhibitor; UPAR = urinary plasminogen activator (uPA) receptor; EC = endothelial cells; SMC = smooth muscle cells

activators is uncertain. F-XIIa, F-XIa, and kallikrein all have the ability to directly activate PLG to PLN, although somewhat slowly. They normally account for no more than 15% of total PLN-generating activity in plasma.[30] Kallikrein can affect fibrinolysis by converting scuPA to its more active two-chain form, uPA, and by liberating bradykinin from HK. Bradykinin can then stimulate release of tPA from endothelial cells, further enhancing fibrinolysis. In vivo, the importance of intrinsic activators is likely mediated via kallikrein conversion of scuPA to uPA, which has increased ability to activate plasminogen.

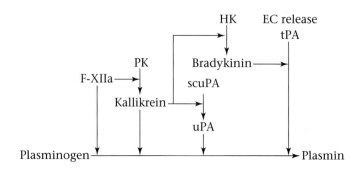

The Fibrinolytic System

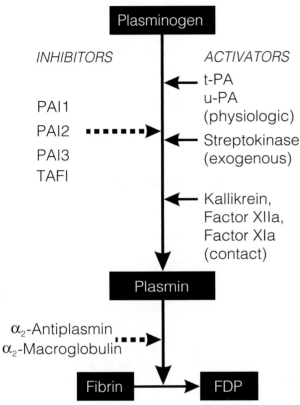

■ FIGURE 30-12   The fibrinolytic system can be activated by the physiologic activators, tissue plasminogen activator (tPA) derived from endothelial cells, and urokinase-type plasminogen activator (uPA) or the contact activators, kallikrein, F-XIIa, and F-XIa. Exogenous activator, streptokinase, can also activate the system. Plasmin (PLN), the product of activation, controls coagulation by digesting fibrin to fibrin degradation products (FDP) and by degrading factors V, VIII, and XII. The inhibitors of plasminogen activation, plasminogen activator inhibitor-1 (PAI-1), plasminogen activator inhibitor-2 (PAI-2), plasminogen activator inhibitor-3 (PAI-3), thrombin activatable fibrinolysis inhibitor (TAFI), and the inhibitors of plasmin (α_2-antiplasmin and α_2-macroglobulin) serve to control the fibrinolytic system. The fibrinolytic system, like the clotting system, is intricately regulated by these activators and inhibitors.

Physiologic PLG Activators

The two important physiologic plasma PAs are **tissue-type plasminogen activator (tPA)** and **urokinase-type plasminogen activator (uPA)**. Both are serine proteases that have a high degree of specificity for converting PLG to PLN by cleavage of a single bond (Arg561-Val). Each has different structural, functional, and immunologic properties.

Vascular endothelial cells of small vessels mainly produce tPA, which seems to be the predominant PA activity in the circulatory system. In vivo, single-chain tPA (sctPA) is released from the endothelial cells by stimuli such as thrombin, bradykinin, histamine, exercise, venous stasis, shear

stress, and DDAVP administration.[31] tPA has two kringle domains containing lysine-binding sites (LBS). LBS are involved in fibrin binding, fibrin-specific plasminogen activation, rapid clearance in vivo, and binding to endothelial receptors.[32] tPA is unique among the serine proteases because it does not circulate as a zymogen but is fully active toward its substrate plasminogen in its single-chain form. However, PLG activation by tPA in plasma (in the absence of fibrin) is relatively inefficient. The activation of PLG by tPA is markedly increased when both proteins are bound to fibrin via their respective LBS. Single-chain tPA can be converted to a two-chain molecule by cleavage of a single peptide bond by kallikrein, PLN, or F-Xa. However, the single-chain form is nearly as effective as the two-chain form in the presence of fibrin.[33]

In addition to binding to and functioning on a fibrin surface, tPA also associates with the membrane of endothelial cells. The endothelial cell receptor for tPA is annexin II, which functions as a coreceptor for both tPA and PLG. Binding and activation of tPA and PLG help maintain a fibrinolytic potential on undamaged vascular surfaces.

uPA is produced primarily by renal tubular epithelium and vascular endothelium and is found in urine and plasma. However, it functions mainly in the tissues where it plays an important role in digesting the extracellular matrix, enabling cells to migrate.[34] This process is important in wound healing, embryogenesis, inflammation, and cancer metastasis. uPA is secreted as a single-chain molecule (scuPA) but has little proteolytic activity until it is converted to a two-chain form by PLN, F-XIIa, or kallikrein.[35] uPA differs from tPA because it lacks high-affinity binding for fibrin, although it can activate both fibrin-bound and circulating PLG. The localized generation of small amounts of fibrin-bound PLG converts scuPA to uPA, bringing about the reciprocal activation of PLG and scuPA.

A specific receptor for uPA, **urokinase plasminogen activator receptor (uPAR)**, plays an important role in localizing uPA-catalyzed PLG activation. The receptor binds scuPA and uPA to the endothelial cell surface and facilitates activation of scuPA to uPA and of PLG. Binding uPA to uPAR increases the activation of plasminogen sixfold by colocalization of uPA and PLG and contributes to a fibrinolytic potential on undamaged endothelium.

Lipoprotein(a) (Lp[a]), an LDL-like particle similar in structure to PLG, has been shown to inhibit the activation of PLG by tPA and uPA[36] Lp(a), which also possesses LBS, competes with PLG and tPA for fibrin binding, interfering with PLG activation. Thus, elevated levels of Lp(a) are antifibrinolytic and are considered a thrombotic risk factor (∞ Chapter 33).

Exogenous Activators

In addition to these physiologically important endogenous PLG activators, several bacterial species also produce efficient PLG activators. Streptokinase (SK), derived from β-hemolytic streptococci, is not a serine protease but acts by forming a 1:1 complex with PLG. When bound to SK, PLG undergoes a conformational change, exposing an altered active site in PLG, which can then autocatalytically convert to PLN. SK is used as a therapeutic agent to dissolve clots. However, SK has no preferential action toward PLG bound to fibrin and thus acts equally well on plasminogen molecules in the circulation, resulting in extensive systemic plasmin activation and a generalized proteolytic state. Plasminogen activators are also produced by *Staphyloccus aureus* (staphylokinase [SAK]) and by *Yersinia pestis*. Like SK, SAK is not an enzyme but forms a 1:1 complex with PLG. However, SAK does not activate PLG in the absence of fibrin. Trace amounts of PLN can convert the SAK:PLG complex to SAK:PLN that is a highly fibrin-specific PA.

FIBRIN DEGRADATION

PLN is responsible for the asymmetric, progressive degradation of fibrin (or fibrinogen), forming distinct protein fragments referred to as **fibrin degradation (split) products** (**FDP** or **FSP**). The liver rapidly clears these fragments from the circulation. Their detection in the plasma is of diagnostic value for some hemostatic disorders.

The sites of PLN proteolytic action are similar in fibrinogen and cross-linked fibrin. PLN digestion of fibrinogen has been widely studied and has been used as the model to explain the digestion of fibrin. The products formed include fragments X, Y, D, and E (Figure 30-13 ■). Fragment X is formed when plasmin cleaves a few small peptides from the exposed polar appendages in the C-terminal region of the α chains of fibrinogen and liberation of β1-42 from the N-terminal portion of the β chain occurs. Next, cleavage in one coiled region midway between one D terminal domain and the E central domain produces a uninodular fragment D and a binodular fragment E-D (fragment Y). PLN then cleaves fragment Y in the coiled region between the remaining E and D domains, producing free fragment E and another fragment D. Each fibrinogen molecule ultimately is degraded into two D fragments, one E fragment, and a few small peptides.

PLN degradation of fibrin monomer and noncross-linked fibrin polymer is essentially identical to that of fibrinogen. PLN degradation of cross-linked fibrin, however, is slower and produces unique degradation products because of the intermolecular bonds induced by F-XIIIa. The smallest unique degradation product, the D-D fragment, consists of two fragment D segments of two adjacent cross-linked fibrin monomers. To completely separate adjacent D and E domains on neighboring molecules, six cleavages must occur (2α, 2β, and 2γ chains cleaved). Digestion severing all connections is not always complete. Therefore, some of the cross-linked D-D degradation products are found within molecules of various molecular weights. They can consist of X, Y, D, and E fragment complexes from two or more cross-linked fibrin monomers (e.g., DD/E, YD/DY, YY/DXD) (Figure 30-14 ■). A test for breakdown products, the D-dimer

Plasmin Degration of Fibrinogen

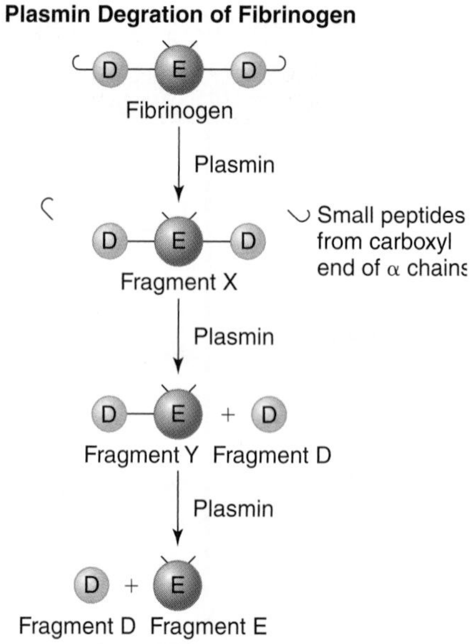

■ FIGURE 30-13   The degradation of fibrinogen by plasmin occurs in well-defined sequential steps. First, small peptides are cleaved from the carboxyl ends of α-chains producing fragment X. The E domain retains the A and B peptides. The fragment X is still capable of reacting with thrombin to form fibrin. Next, one of the D domains is cleaved from the fragment X, producing fragment Y (DE) and a fragment D. Further cleavage of the fragment Y produces D and E fragments.

test, is a specific marker for PLN degradation of fibrin (∞ Chapter 40).

The fibrin fragments, if present in sufficient concentration, can exert an anticoagulant effect on the clotting system. Fragment X can still react with and bind thrombin but very slowly. Fragment X can compete with fibrinogen for thrombin so that less fibrin is formed. Fragments Y, D and E inhibit the polymerization of fibrin monomers. The fragments can also interfere with primary hemostasis by inhibiting platelet aggregation.

If free in plasma, PLN can cause proteolytic degradation of numerous plasma proteins including fibrinogen; factors V, VIII, and XII; and components of the kinin and complement systems. The rapid formation of complexes between free PLN and its inhibitor, α₂-antiplasmin (P-AP), controls this potentially dangerous proteolytic process. If inactivation of PLN is not sufficiently controlled, a systemic fibrinolytic state results, characterized by PLG activation, depletion of α₂-antiplasmin, and fibrinogen breakdown. Physiologic fibrinolysis, which occurs when PLN is attached to fibrin, is highly fibrin specific and not associated with a systemic fibrinolytic/proteolytic state.

✓ Checkpoint! 8

Why are the PLN degradation products of fibrinogen and fibrin different?

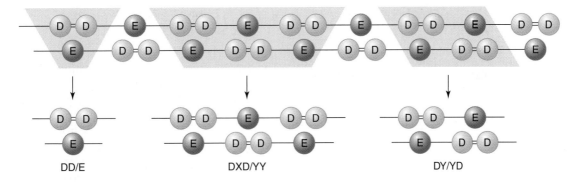

■ **FIGURE 30-14** Fibrin digestion by plasmin occurs at cleavage sites identical to those of fibrinogen. However, because of the covalent bonds of the F-XIIIa-stabilized polymer, digestion is slower. Derivatives also are different as some sites are not accessible in the lattice formation. This schematic drawing depicts some of the derivatives of plasmin digestion of fibrin. (Adapted, with permission, from: Beutler E et al., eds. *Williams Hematology.* New York: McGraw Hill; 1995).

INHIBITORS OF FIBRINOLYSIS

The fibrinolytic proteins are held in check by fibrinolytic inhibitors, which modulate the fibrinolytic system to prevent systemic proteolysis (Table 30-4). They act at the PLG activation step or directly on plasmin.

Plasminogen Activator Inhibitors (PAI)

Several inhibitors control the activation of PLG. Most belong to a family of serine-protease inhibitors called **serpins** that inhibit target molecules by formation of a 1:1 stoichiometric complex. The primary regulators are the **plasminogen activator inhibitors (PAIs)**. Five proteins with PAI activity have been identified: PAI-1, PAI-2, PAI-3, protease nexin-1, and neuroserpin. Of these, only PAI-1 appears to play a significant role in regulating PA activity in blood and most tissues.[29] The interaction of PAI-1 with tPA is >1000 times higher than the interaction of tPA with the other PAIs.

PAI-1, which appears to be the primary physiological inhibitor of tPA and uPA, is produced by endothelial cells, monocytes, macrophages, megakaryocytes, hepatocytes, smooth muscle cells, and adipocytes. PAI-1 reacts with tPA, sctPA, and uPA but not scuPA. In plasma, about 70% of the tPA circulates in complex with PAI-1. Release of PAI-1 from activated platelets into the developing hemostatic plug ensures that the initial fibrin matrix is not prematurely lysed by tPA activation of PLG. PAI-1 is an acute phase reactant protein. Thrombin, IL-1, TGF-β, TNFα, and endotoxin all induce dramatic increases in plasma PAI-1 levels. Elevated PAI-1 results in a decrease in tPA activation of PLG and a shift in the hemostatic balance toward hypercoagulability (∞ Chapter 33). Deficiency of PAI-1 results in a serious bleeding disorder due to unregulated and excessive fibrinolysis.

PAI-2, the second plasminogen activator inhibitor, is found in greatest amounts in placentas and in macrophages. Plasma levels are very low except in pregnancy when it is drastically elevated. PAI-2 inhibits both tPA and uPA but is less effective toward sctPA.

PAI-3 is probably the activated protein C (APC) inhibitor. These two molecules are immunologically and functionally identical.

PA/PAI complexes are removed from the circulation by binding to the low-density lipoprotein receptor-like protein (LRP) receptors on hepatocytes and macrophages. LRPs mediate clearance of free tPA, tPA/PAI-1, uPA/PAI-1, tPA- or uPA-PAI-2, and $\alpha_2$macroglobulin/protease complexes.[29]

Thrombin Activatable Fibrinolysis Inhibitor (TAFI)

TAFI is a recently discovered plasma protein that inhibits fibrinolysis when activated. TAFI is a procarboxypeptidase B, activated to TAFIa by the thrombin/thrombomodulin complex.[37] Activation requires formation of a ternary complex involving TAFI-thrombin-thrombomodulin. PLG binding to fibrin occurs primarily at carboxy-terminal lysine residues. New C-terminal lysines are generated during initial plasmin degradation of fibrin. TAFIa suppresses fibrinolysis by removing C-terminal lysine and arginine residues from fibrin, thereby eliminating the fibrin-binding sites for plasminogen[38] (Figure 30-15 ■). TAFIa protects the fibrin clot from degradation by inhibiting binding and activation of PLG. Because of TAFIa's short half-life, this effect is temporary, delaying activation of fibrinolysis until the fibrin clot can be established and stabilized. Thus, thrombin generation initially results in the suppression of fibrinolysis by activating TAFI. TAFIa, in turn, plays a major role in the balance between fibrin deposition and removal. Thrombomodulin also has a role in down-regulating coagulation by activating protein C (see later section).

α_2-Antiplasmin

The liver produces and secretes α_2-antiplasmin (AP), which is also found in platelet αG. It is the principal physiologic

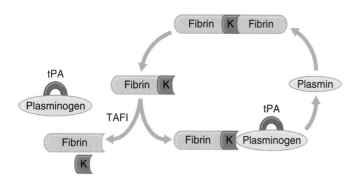

■ **FIGURE 30-15** Down regulation of plasmin formation by TAFI. Fibrinolysis is initiated when plasminogen is converted to plasmin by tPA. Both plasmin and tPA preferentially bind to carboxy-terminal lysine (K) residues of fibrin. The formation of plasmin is enhanced by a positive feedback loop. New C-terminal lysine residues generated after limited plasmin cleavage provide new binding sites for continued tPA and plasminogen binding. TAFIa cleaves off the C-terminal lysine residues from partially degraded fibrin and thereby eliminates/decreases the fibrin cofactor function in the tPA/plasminogen/fibrin complex, inhibiting the formation of plasmin and the degradation of the fibrin clot. (TAFI = thrombin activatable fibrinolysis inhibitor; tPA= tissue plasminogen activator)

inhibitor of PLN, binding via LBS on PLN and rapidly inhibiting the enzyme. In the circulation, AP reacts quickly with free PLN, but PLN bound to fibrin is protected from inactivation because fibrin occupies the same binding sites on PLN as would AP. Circulating AP thus makes an important contribution to limiting systemic fibrinolysis. AP can also bind PLG, interfering with the absorption of PLG to fibrin. Some AP molecules are cross-linked to fibrin by F-XIIIa during clotting, thus increasing the initial resistance of fibrin to the action of PLN. This allows repair processes to start before clot lysis is initiated.

α_2-Macroglobulin

α_2-Macroglobulin is an inhibitor with wide specificity that reacts with many different proteases. It is a backup inhibitor for several proteases including PLN and the other hemostatic serine proteases. If the fibrinolytic system has been extensively activated and a large amount of PLN has been generated, inhibitory capacity of AP's would be exhausted. α_2-Macroglobulin then operates as a second line of defense to inactivate remaining PLN. Antithrombin, α_1-antitrypsin, and C1 inhibitor all have some antiplasmin activity in vitro but are probably of minimal significance in vivo.

> **CASE STUDY** *(continued from page 652)*
>
> 9. Does any evidence exist to indicate a problem with Shawn's fibrinolytic system?

PHYSIOLOGIC CONTROL OF HEMOSTASIS

The dynamic process of fibrin formation is normally limited to the site of vascular injury. However, the disruptive force of blood flow presents an extraordinary problem for regulating hemostasis. Activated factors and/or platelets must be kept at the site of injury and must be controlled so they are inactive when distant from the site of vessel damage. Cellular localization and plasma protease inhibitors are essential in confining the coagulation reactions to sites of injury so that blood remains fluid in uninvolved vessels. Other physiologic mechanisms involved in controlling hemostasis include the control of blood flow, liver clearance of activated proteins, and negative and positive feedback of activated clotting factors.

BLOOD FLOW

Vasoconstriction and activation of clotting factors are necessary for clot formation to begin. Vessel constriction initially enhances clot formation by slowing blood flow through the injured vessel. As blood pools, creating an area of stasis, platelets and coagulation factors are brought in proximity to the vessel wall, promoting the initiation of primary and secondary hemostasis. Neither stasis alone nor the activation of circulating coagulation factors in flowing blood results in clot formation. Vasoconstriction of the injured vessel is an important initial step for adequate fibrin formation. Return to normal blood flow through an area of injury then limits coagulation by diluting the concentration of activated factors. Activated factors carried away from the fibrin clot are bound by inhibitory proteins with loss of their coagulant potential.

LIVER CLEARANCE

The liver is the site of production of many clotting factors, making it a vital organ for normal hemostasis. The liver removes activated coagulation factors complexed with their inhibitors from the circulation as well as PLN-antiplasmin complexes and fibrin degradation products. A major receptor for removal of these complexes is the LRP receptor found on hepatocytes and liver macrophages. Liver disease can result in hemorrhage due to decreased production of coagulation factors. It can also contribute to systemic fibrinolysis or thrombosis associated with the failure to remove activated proteases.

POSITIVE FEEDBACK AMPLIFICATION

The hemostatic system has several positive feedback mechanisms. Some of the most important are (1) thrombin, which, as a major activator of platelets, promotes the release of platelet F-Va and the exposure of negatively charged phospholipid surfaces used for assembly of coagulation protein complexes, (2) thrombin activates F-Va and F-VIIIa, (3) F-Xa feeds back to activate F-VII, and (4) F-Xa has limited ability to activate F-VIII in a reaction that can be important before significant quantities of thrombin are produced (Figure 30-16■).

NEGATIVE FEEDBACK INHIBITION

Some of the activated factors have the potential to destroy other factors in the coagulation cascade. This process of feedback inhibition limits further production of the enzymes and dampens the coagulation cascade. Thrombin has the ability to activate F-Va and F-VIIIa but at higher concentrations can inactivate them via activated protein C (APC). F-Xa first activates F-VIIa and then, through the action of tissue factor pathway inhibitor, is itself inactivated in a reaction that requires F-VIIa/TF. Fibrin, the end product of the cascade, also indirectly controls clotting. Fibrin has a strong affinity for thrombin. Once adsorbed onto the fibrin meshwork, thrombin is very slowly released, limiting the amount of thrombin available to cleave more fibrinogen to fibrin. In addition, FDPs produced by PLN digestion function as inhibitors of fibrin formation by interfering with the conversion of fibrinogen to fibrin and the polymerization of fibrin monomers.

BIOCHEMICAL INHIBITORS

Naturally occurring inhibitors are soluble plasma proteins that regulate the enzymatic reactions of serine proteases.

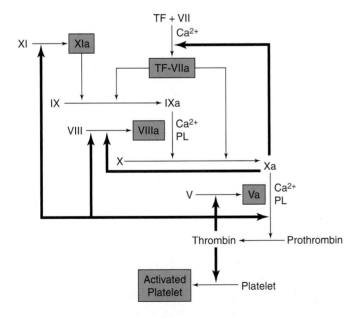

■ FIGURE 30-16 Positive feedbacks in coagulation. Positive feedbacks are indicated by heavy arrows. Shaded boxes indicate targets. (Adapted, with permission, from: Beutler E et al., *William's Hematology.* New York: McGraw-Hill; 1995)

They prevent the initiation or amplification of the coagulation cascade (Table 30-5 ✪) (Figure 30-17■). The natural inhibitors include:

1. antithrombin (AT)
2. heparin cofactor II (HCII)
3. protein C (PC) and protein S (PS)
4. tissue factor pathway inhibitor (TFPI)
5. protein Z-dependent protease inhibitor (ZPI) and protein Z (PZ)
6. α_2-Macroglobulin (α_2-M)
7. α_1-antitrypsin (α_1-protease inhibitor [α_1PI])
8. C1-inhibitor
9. Thrombin activatable fibrinolysis inhibitor (TAFI see under fibrinolysis)
10. α_2-antiplasmin (α_2AP; see under fibrinolysis)

Antithrombin, α_1-antitrypsin, heparin cofactor II, C1-inhibitor, ZPI and AP are all members of the serpin family of **ser**ine **p**rotease **in**hibitors (Serpins), which inhibit their target enzymes by forming a covalent complex between the active site serine of the enzyme and the reactive center of the serpin. Conformational changes are induced in both molecules, trapping the enzyme with the serpin and resulting in loss of activity of both proteins.

Antithrombin

AT, formerly called *AT III,* is a serpin protease inhibitor and is clinically the most important inhibitor of procoagulant serine proteases. AT can neutralize all serine proteases including thrombin; factors XIIa, XIa, IXa, and Xa; kallikrein; and plasmin. AT molecules circulating in the blood have limited inhibitory activity. AT forms a 1:1 complex with each target protease, but the reaction is slow in the absence of heparin. Inhibition of the target proteases is accelerated three to four orders of magnitude by the cofactor heparin. Originally, two antithrombin activities, the progressive antithrombin (in the absence of heparin) and heparin cofactor (in the presence of heparin) activities, were described and were thought to be due to two separate plasma proteins. Subsequently, however, both activities were shown to be associated with a single protein, AT.[39] Procoagulant proteases associated with surface-activating complexes (prothrombinase, tenase) are protected against AT/heparin inactivation.

AT is produced by hepatocytes, endothelial cells, and possibly megakaryocytes. In vivo, heparin is located in the granules of mast cells and basophils although under normal circumstances, it is not released from these cells into the circulation and cannot be detected in plasma. While only small amounts of naturally occurring heparin are found in the plasma, vascular endothelium is rich in heparin-like molecules called *heparan sulfate proteoglycans (HSPGs).* These endothelial cell-associated proteins have heparan side chains with the correct carbohydrate sequences needed for AT recognition. Both thrombin and AT can bind to HSPGs and

✪ TABLE 30-5

Summary of Naturally Occurring Inhibitors

Component	Description	Role	Concentration in Plasma	t1/2	Chromosome
Protein C (PC)	Two-chain glycoprotein MW 62,000	Serine protease: inactivates F-Va and F-VIIIa	4–6 μg/mL 70 nM	6 hr	2
Protein S (PS)	Single-chain glycoprotein MW 75,000	Cofactor for APC inhibition of F-Va and F-VIIIa	20–25 μg/mL 300 nM	42 hr	3
Thrombomodulin (TM)	Transmembrane protein MW 450,000	Cofactor/modulator: EC receptor for thrombin; cofactor for thrombin activation of PC; stimulates EC to release tPA and EDRF	0.02 μg/mL	–	20
Antithrombin (AT)	Single-chain glycoprotein MW 58,000	SERPIN: inhibits thrombin, factors Xa, IXa XIa, XIIa, kallikrein, plasmin, tPA	150–400 μg/mL 2500 nM	61–72 hr	1
Heparin cofactor II (HCII)	Glycoprotein MW 66,000	SERPIN: inhibits thrombin	40–70 μg/mL 1000 nM	60	22
C1 esterase inhibitor	Single-chain glycoprotein MW 105,000	SERPIN: inhibits kallikrein, plasmin, C1, factors XIIa, XIa	180 μg/mL 1700 nM	70	–
Protein C inhibitor (PAI-3)	Single-chain protein MW 57,000	Proteinase inhibitor (SERPIN): inhibits APC	5.3 μg/mL 100 nM	23 days	–
α_1-antitrypsin (α_1-proteinase inhibitor, α_1PI)	Protein MW 55,000	SERPIN: inhibits F-XIa, thrombin, kallikrein, plasmin, tPA	2500 μg/mL 45,000 nM	144 hr	–
Tissue factor pathway Inhibitor (TFPI)	MW 40,000	Proteinase inhibitor: inhibits F-VIIa and F-Xa	0.05–0.15 μg/mL 2.5 nM	1–2 min	–
α_2-Macroglobulin	Dimeric protein MW 725,000	Proteinase inhibitor: inhibits kallikrein, PLN, thrombin, tPA	2500 μg/mL 3400 nM	–	12
Protein Z dependent Protease Inhibitor (ZPI)	Single-chain glycoprotein MW 72,000	SERPIN: inhibits F-Xa with cofactor Protein Z; inhibits F-XI	1.0–1.6 μg/mL 20 nM	–	–
Protein Z	Vitamin K-dependent glycoprotein MW 62,000	Cofactor for ZPI inhibition of F-Xa	2–3 μg/mL 50 nM	60	13

SERPIN = serine protease inhibitor; tPA = tissue plasminogen activator; MW = molecular weight in Da.; APC = activated protein C; EC = endothelial cells; PAI = plasminogen activator inhibitor; EDRF = endothelium derived relaxing factor; PLN = plasmin.

are brought close together. Upon binding, AT undergoes a conformational change, making its reactive site more accessible to the active site serine of thrombin (or other protease targets). The thrombin/AT (TAT) complex then dissociates from the proteoglycan, and the heparan sites are free to bind other thrombin/AT molecules. Dermatan sulfate, another glycosaminoglycan located in the vessel wall and the tissues, has little catalytic effect on AT but is a potent catalyst for heparin cofactor II. Vessel wall HSPGs bind and localize plasma AT, which contributes to the anticoagulant and antithrom-

botic properties of the endothelium by inhibiting free thrombin and other activated proteases.

As an anticoagulant, heparin molecules are structurally and functionally heterogeneous, ranging in size from 5000 to 30,000 Da. In commercial preparations of heparin, only about one-third of the molecules have catalytic activity. Among naturally occurring heparin-like proteoglycans, less than 10% are active. Heparin inhibits platelet function by inhibiting VWF binding and reducing platelet adhesion to subendothelium and thus can produce hemorrhagic side ef-

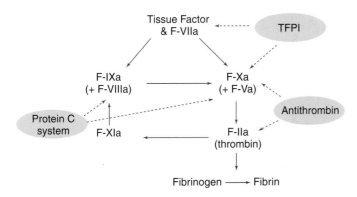

■ **FIGURE 30-17** Major naturally occurring inhibitors of coagulation. Solid lines indicate proteolytic pathways. Dashed lines show direction of inhibition. Shaded ovals indicate inhibitors. TFPI = tissue factor pathway inhibitor

fects if not monitored during therapeutic administration. Also, heparin can produce a mild thrombocytopenia (heparin-associated thrombocytopenia [HAT] ∞ Chapter 31), resulting from direct interactions between heparin and platelets. The low-molecular-weight (LMW) heparins (alternative therapeutic antithrombotic agents) can inactivate F-Xa but are less effective in inactivating thrombin. As the size of the heparin molecules decreases, the ratio of inactivation of F-Xa versus thrombin increases. LMW heparins are also less likely to induce thrombocytopenia and HAT. Heparin has no action as an anticoagulant in the absence of AT. When AT levels are significantly reduced, patients can become unresponsive to antithrombotic therapy with heparin.

Heparin Cofactor II

HCII is a second plasma protease inhibitor whose activity is accelerated by heparin. Unlike AT, HCII is not a broad-spectrum inhibitor. It inhibits thrombin but has little activity against other coagulation proteases (F-Xa, F-IXa, F-VIIa). Because HCII's affinity for heparin is less than that of AT, a higher concentration of heparin is needed to accelerate its thrombin inhibition. Therefore, HCII probably contributes a minimal anticoagulant effect in heparinized patients. It has been suggested that HCII might function as a second-line inhibitor of thrombin. It likely is to be involved in thrombin inhibition in extravascular locations because its activity (unlike that of AT) is accelerated significantly by extravascular dermatan sulfate. HCII can also play a role in protection from thrombosis during pregnancy.[40]

Protein C and Protein S

The protein C (PC) pathway is a major inhibitory mechanism involved in controlling blood coagulation. Unlike the other inhibitory mechanisms directed at the proteases of the coagulation cascade, activated protein C (APC) inhibits two of the nonproteolytic regulatory cofactors of coagulation: Va and VIIIa.

PC and its cofactor, protein S (PS), are vitamin K-dependent proteins synthesized in the liver. PC circulates as a two-chain disulfide-linked zymogen containing 9 Gla residues. PS is a single-chain glycoprotein with 11 Gla residues. Unlike the other vitamin K-dependent factors, PS does not contain a serine protease domain and thus lacks protease activity. The protein C pathway is illustrated in Figure 30-18 ■.

Thrombin is generated at the site of injury. Excess thrombin binds to thrombomodulin on adjacent EC surfaces. **Thrombomodulin (TM)** is an integral membrane protein named for its ability to change the activity of thrombin from procoagulant to anticoagulant so that thrombin loses its ability to clot fibrinogen, activate F-V, or activate platelets but instead rapidly activates PC in the presence of Ca²⁺.[41,42] TM binding appears to cause a conformational change in the thrombin molecule that accounts for its altered activity. APC is released from the T:TM complex and in association with its cofactor PS, proteolytically inactivates F-Va and F-VIIIa. The precursor F-V and F-VIII molecules are resistant to the action of APC. The inactivation of these cofactors prevents effective, sustained thrombin generation. Thus, via activation of PC, thrombin creates a self-dampening effect that limits the growth of the fibrin clot.

To function effectively, APC must interact with PS, forming a 1:1 stoichiometric complex in the presence of Ca²⁺ and a phospholipid surface. PS circulates in the blood in two forms: (1) free PS (40% of the total circulating protein) and (2) protein that is noncovalently associated with the complement regulatory protein, C4b-binding protein (C4b-BP). The free form of PS is the only effective cofactor for APC. When bound to a cell surface, the complex of PC–PS is capable of inactivating F-Va and F-VIIIa. APC cleaves Arg 306 and Arg 506 in F-Va, dissociating the A2 fragment, and the analogous Arg 336 and Arg 562 in F-VIIIa. Inactivation of F-VIIIa is stimulated significantly by F-V. APC also produces a profibrinolytic effect, presumably due to the decreased generation of thrombin resulting in the lack of activation of TAFI.

An **endothelial protein C receptor (EPCR)** is found on the endothelial cells of larger vessels.[43] When EPCR binds PC, it augments PC activation by increasing the affinity of the T:TM complex for PC.[44] When activated by the T:TM in the microcirculation, APC rapidly dissociates from the endothelial cells but dissociates more slowly from the endothelium of larger vessels because of binding to EPCR. When bound to EPCR, APC is not capable of inactivating F-Va (and probably F-VIIIa). When APC dissociates from EPCR, APC can bind PS and then inactivate F-Va. APC bound to EPCR induces a profound anti-inflammatory effect, mediated at least in part via activation of protease-activated receptor-1 (PAR-1) on the EC membrane.[45]

APC is neutralized by PC inhibitor (PCI, or PAI-3), α₁-antitrypsin, and α₂-M. PCI is a serpin that produces a procoagulant effect due to its blocking the anticoagulant effect of the PC system. Deficiency of either PC or PS results in a tendency for thromboembolic disease. Patients have been

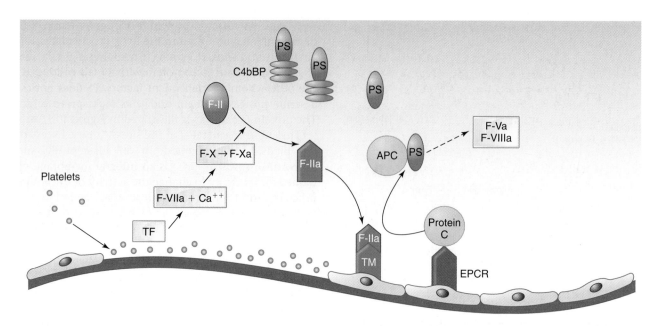

■ FIGURE 30-18 Protein C pathway. Thrombin forms on the vessel wall at the site of injury. Thrombomodulin on the endothelial cell forms a complex with thrombin. This complex activates protein C, which then in association with free protein S inactivates F-Va and F-VIIIa. TF = tissue factor; PC = protein C; PS = protein S; F-II = prothrombin; F-IIA = thrombin; TM = thrombomodulin; APC = activated protein C; C4b-BP = complement binding protein; EPCR = endothelial cell protein C receptor

described with normal amounts of PC and PS in their plasma yet activation of PC fails to inactivate F-Va. This abnormality (F-V Leiden), referred to as *APC resistance,* is due to a mutation in one of the cleavage sites of F-Va (∞ Chapter 33).[46]

Tissue Factor Pathway Inhibitor

TFPI, also called *extrinsic pathway inhibitor, lipoprotein-associated coagulation inhibitor,* and *antithromboplastin,* inhibits the F-VIIa-TF complex, suppressing the activity of the extrinsic pathway.

The endothelium is the major source of TFPI synthesis in vivo. A significant portion of TFPI is bound to heparan sulfate on the surface of endothelial cells with most of the remainder in blood bound to low density lipoproteins (LDL).[47] Heparin administration releases the EC-bound TFPI and raises the plasma level severalfold.[48] The range of TFPI concentrations is broad among normal individuals. Plasma concentrations of TFPI activity vary with LDL levels because the interaction of TFPI with lipoproteins reduces the measurable anticoagulant activity.[49]

TFPI is unique among the protease inhibitors because it is a potent inhibitor of both F-Xa and F-VIIa. First, TFPI binds to and inhibits the active site of F-Xa. Subsequently, this binary complex reacts with F-VIIa in complex with TF, forming a quarternary compound (VIIa-TF-Xa-TFPI) on a membrane surface, inactivating both proteases.[50] TFPI can neutralize F-Xa when bound in a prothrombinase complex, but its activity against F-VIIa requires F-VIIa to be complexed with TF[51] (Figure 30-19 ■).

The molecular basis for TFPI's capacity to neutralize two proteases simultaneously is due to the fact that TFPI has three inhibitor domains: the first domain binds to and inhibits the F-VIIa/TF complex and the second inhibits F-Xa. The target of the third inhibitory domain is unknown.[52]

Because TFPI inhibition of F-VIIa/TF requires F-Xa, the extrinsic pathway is not shut off until a significant amount of

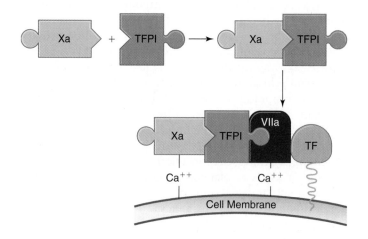

■ FIGURE 30-19 The inhibition of F-VIIa/TF by tissue factor pathway inhibitor (TFPI) occurs as the result of a multistep process. First, TFPI binds to F-Xa and neutralizes it, resulting in a conformational change of TFPI that promotes binding of the F-Xa/TFPI complex with the F-VIIa/TF complex in a calcium-dependent reaction.

F-Xa is generated. Once F-Xa is produced, TFPI prevents continued activation of F-X by the F-VIIa/TF complex, and further activation of F-X must occur through the intrinsic pathway by the F-IXa-F-VIIIa complex. While initial activation of F-Xa occurs via the extrinsic pathway, sustained activation requires activation of F-IXa via the intrinsic pathway.[53] This explains the bleeding associated with factor deficiencies of the intrinsic pathway. Even in the event of tissue damage and tissue factor generation, deficiencies of factors VIII and IX will not permit sufficient activation of F-Xa to maintain normal hemostasis.

α_2-Macroglobulin

α_2-M is capable of inhibiting several serine proteases including thrombin, F-Xa, plasmin, and kallikrein. The inhibition rate is relatively slow when compared to other inhibitors, and protease activity is not completely neutralized. It serves as a secondary or backup inhibitor for many coagulant and fibrinolytic enzymes.

The glycoprotein α_2-M is widely distributed in the body. Its concentration changes with age with the highest levels in infants and children. It also can be elevated in pregnancy, in women using oral contraceptives, and in a number of other disorders. Following initial binding to the target enzyme, α_2-M undergoes a conformational change essentially trapping the enzyme within the inhibitor, preventing binding to its substrate. However, the catalytic site of the protease is left intact. This suggests that α_2-M may function primarily as a clearance mechanism for serine proteases rather than as an inhibitor of enzymatic activity because the α_2-M/protease complexes are rapidly cleared from plasma via binding to LRP receptors in the liver.

α_1-Antitrypsin

The glycoprotein α_1-antitrypsin (α_1 protease inhibitor [α_1PI]) has the capacity to inhibit a number of proteases and is the major inhibitor of F-XIa. Its activity is thought to be more important at the tissue level, particularly in its role as an inhibitor of neutrophil elastase. α_1PI deficiency results in emphysema due to unopposed elastase activity damaging lung alveoli.[54]

C1-Inhibitor

C1-inhibitor was first recognized as an inhibitor of the esterase activity of C1 from the complement cascade. As well, it inhibits the contact system proteases F-XIIa, F-IXa, kallikrein, and PLN. C1-inhibitor is the major plasma protease inhibitor of F-XIIa, accounting for more than 90% of the plasma inhibitory activity.

Protein Z and ZPI

PZ is a vitamin K-dependent protein that markedly enhances the inhibitory function of protein ZPI against F-Xa. ZPI is a plasma serpin that inhibits F-Xa in a PZ-dependent manner.[55] It also inhibits F-XIa in the absence of PZ. The physiologic importance of ZPI and PZ in the regulation of coagulation is still unclear.

 Checkpoint! 9

Why are naturally occurring inhibitors important in the hemostatic mechanism?

 CASE STUDY *(continued from page 660)*

10. Why were liver function tests done on Shawn?
11. What is the significance of normal results in a patient with hemostatic disease?

▶ THE PHYSIOLOGIC PATHWAY OF COAGULATION

Although it has been traditional to divide the coagulation mechanism into intrinsic and extrinsic pathways, it is now accepted that the two pathways do not operate independently of each other. Current thought is that TF is the key initiator of coagulation in vivo because it can activate both F-X and F-IX (Figure 30-20 ■).

TF is not normally expressed on cells in contact with blood but is found on the surface of a variety of cell types outside the vasculature. Upon injury, cells expressing TF are exposed to the blood. Membrane-bound TF binds F-VII or F-VIIa with high affinity, anchoring the complex to the site of injury. F-VIIa/TF then activates F-X to F-Xa, and the common pathway continues. The extrinsic activation of F-X seems to make the activation of F-X by the intrinsic Xase complex (F-IXa, F-VIIIa, PL, and Ca^{2+}) unnecessary, but clinical observations have demonstrated the absolute necessity of these factors for normal hemostasis. Patients with F-VIII and F-IX deficiencies have major bleeding problems (∞ Chapter 32) as do patients with severe deficiencies of factors II, V, VII, and X. The observation that F-VIIa/TF also activates F-IX to IXa demonstrates that extrinsic pathway activation could result in activation of F-X through both "intrinsic" and "extrinsic" mechanisms (Figure 30-20). The roles of TFPI and the positive feedback effects of thrombin also contribute to explaining physiologic coagulation.

When coagulation is triggered, a series of events occurs, described as the *initiation, propagation,* and *termination* phases of coagulation. Coagulation is initiated when TF-bearing cells are exposed to blood at a site of vascular injury. TF binds and activates F-VII, and the TF-VIIa complex binds and activates F-X and F-IX on the surface of the TF-bearing cells. The result is the generation of a small amount of thrombin, which may or may not be sufficient to induce fibrin formation. However, it is sufficient to set in motion the events that will result in a subsequent burst of thrombin generation.

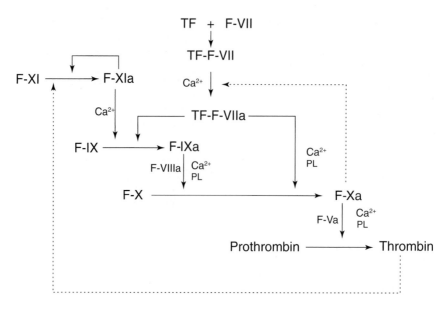

■ **FIGURE 30-20** Tissue factor initiation of the physiologic pathway by activation of F-IX and F-X. Dotted lines indicate positive feedback activation of TF-F-VII by Xa and activation of F-XI by thrombin. TF = tissue factor

The small amounts of thrombin formed during the initiation phase initiate a series of events, associated with the multiple roles of thrombin in hemostasis that culminate in the acceleration or propagation of the coagulation mechanism. These events include the activation of (1) platelets, (2) F-V, F-VIII, and F-XIII, and (3) F-XI. The F-Xa that is produced on the TF-bearing cell is almost immediately inhibited by TFPI, which quickly inhibits the F-VIIa/TF complex. Formation of thrombin through the extrinsic pathway is transient and subsequent propagation of the coagulation cascade occurs on the surface of activated platelets (activated by either the initial injury or thrombin generated during the initiation phase). Further activation of F-X and the coagulation cascade occurs through the "intrinsic" pathway by the F-IXa-F-VIIIa complex generated by F-VIIa/TF activation of F-IXa and thrombin activation of F-XIa. The result is massive prothrombin activation and with the surge in thrombin generation, activation of protein C and TAFI (via thrombin binding to thrombomodulin).

Once the platelet/fibrin clot has formed, the coagulation process must be terminated to prevent clot extension into noninjured areas of the vasculature. The termination phase is the phase in which the coagulation reactions subside. Activated by the burst of thrombin generation in the propagation phase, the PC/PS/TM system inactivates F-Va and F-VIIIa, preventing the generation of additional thrombin. The intact endothelium adjacent to the area of injury also has AT and TFPI bound to heparin sulfate molecules on the surface, which inactivates any proteases that venture beyond the injury area. Circulating protease inhibitors directly inhibit proteases that escape into the fluid phase.

Thus, patients with hereditary deficiencies of F-XII, PK, and HK have a markedly prolonged partial thromboplastin time (PTT), suggesting an abnormality in the intrinsic pathway, but they do not have abnormal bleeding in vivo because in vivo hemostasis requires only F-VIIa/TF activation of F-IX and F-X and thrombin activation of F-XI. The severe bleeding seen in patients with deficiencies of F-VIII or F-IX is due to their inability to generate the "burst" of thrombin generation associated with the propagation phase of coagulation. Linked to a level of thrombin generation insufficient to generate an adequate fibrin clot is the failure to activate TAFI and its suppression of fibrinolysis.

ⓒ CASE STUDY *(continued from page 665)*

A specific assay for F-VII activity was done on Shawn and both of his parents. His F-VII activity was found to be 3% of that in normal plasma. Prothrombin and F-X activities were normal. The F-VII activity of Shawn's father and mother was 50% and 47%, respectively. (The reference range of F-II activity is 70–120%.)

12. Do these findings explain the patient's bleeding history?

SUMMARY

The hemostatic system functions to keep blood fluid within the vasculature and to prevent excessive blood loss upon vascular injury. Platelets, vascular endothelial cells, and numerous coagulation proteins interact to maintain a balance between bleeding and clotting in vivo. Primary hemostasis occurs through activation of platelets and results in the formation of an unstable platelet plug. The formation of fibrin (coagulation) subsequently reinforces this resulting in stabilization of the platelet plug, or secondary hemostasis.

The process of fibrin formation is carefully controlled, limited to areas of damage within the vascular network. Localization of the response to the site of injury prevents widespread coagulation activation. Activation of the coagulation system occurs on phospholipid membrane surfaces (activated platelets) or on exposed subendothelial tissue at sites of vessel injury. Coagulation involves a series of sequential activations of inactive proenzymes to active enzyme products. Classically, activation of the coagulation system has been described as being initiated via one of two possible pathways, the intrinsic and the extrinsic. Currently, however, it is believed that this distinction, while useful in discussing the system, is probably not physiologically relevant. In vivo, activation of coagulation is believed to be initiated by F-VIIa/TF activation of F-X and IX.

Each sequential activation step in the coagulation cascade, involving the generation of an active clotting enzyme, is modified and/or controlled by cofactors that accelerate the activation and inhibitory mechanisms that slow activation. The net result of these two opposing forces is a well-balanced physiologic process designed to control activation of the system to an appropriate degree. The final activation step results in the formation of the enzyme thrombin, which is responsible for converting the soluble plasma protein, fibrinogen, into an insoluble state, fibrin.

Once the fibrin clot has been formed and hemostasis achieved, repair of the damaged vascular tissue is initiated. The final step in the process requires the dissolution of the fibrin clot once it is no longer needed by the plasma fibrinolytic system. Like clotting, fibrinolysis involves the activation of an inactive proenzyme precursor (plasminogen) to the active enzyme plasmin. This process is also regulated by both activators (plasminogen activators) and inhibitors (plasminogen activator inhibitors and α_2-antiplasmin).

REVIEW QUESTIONS

LEVEL I

1. Which of the following is (are) involved in hemostasis? (Objective 1)
   a. only blood clotting
   b. clot formation, clot dissolution, vessel repair
   c. only blood clotting and bleeding
   d. only keeping blood in the fluid state

2. Which describes the events involved in secondary hemostasis? (Objective 2)
   a. lead to the formation of a chemically stable fibrin clot
   b. usually occur independently of primary hemostasis
   c. are uncontrolled
   d. occur in a random fashion

3. Which factor is known as the antihemophilic factor? (Objective 3)
   a. F-IX
   b. F-XI
   c. F-VIII
   d. F-XII

4. The prothrombin group includes which of the following coagulation proteins? (Objective 4)
   a. factors I, V, VIII, XIII
   b. PK, HK, F-XI, F-XII
   c. factors II, VII, IX, X
   d. factors I, II, V, X

5. Which of the following function as cofactors in hemostasis? (Objective 6)
   a. fibrinogen, prothrombin
   b. F-Va, F-VIIIa
   c. factors IXa, XIa, XIIa
   d. platelet phospholipid, Ca^{2+}

LEVEL II

1. Hemostasis depends on the balance of which of the following? (Objective 1)
   a. the interaction of blood vessels, platelets, and coagulation proteins
   b. the interaction between platelets and coagulation proteins
   c. the interaction between blood vessels and coagulation proteins
   d. the rate of complex formation

2. Which statement most accurately describes the domains of coagulation proteins? (Objective 2)
   a. The catalytic region distinguishes each of them from trypsin.
   b. The catalytic region gives each protein its own identity.
   c. The noncatalytic regions are identical in all coagulation proteins.
   d. The domains impart specificity and recognition to control hemostasis.

3. Which of the following is true concerning the formation of protein complexes that occur during coagulation? (Objective 3)
   a. slows the rate of reaction
   b. does not require the presence of Ca^{2+} ions
   c. is not necessary for normal coagulation
   d. localizes the reaction to the site of injury

LEVEL I

6. What activates the extrinsic pathway? (Objective 7)
   a. exposure to negatively charged surfaces
   b. contact with tissue factor
   c. the intrinsic pathway
   d. F-XIIa

7. Which factors are involved in the initial activation of the coagulation system and require contact with a negatively charged surface for their activation? (Objectives 7, 8)
   a. factors II, V, VII, X
   b. factors XII, XI, PK, HK
   c. factors II, VII, IX, X
   d. factors I, V, VIII, XIII

8. Which of the following is *not* involved in the fibrinolytic system? (Objective 10)
   a. plasminogen activator inhibitors
   b. plasmin
   c. thrombin
   d. F-XII, kallikrein

9. Which of the following is (are) end products in the breakdown of fibrin? (Objective 11)
   a. fragment X
   b. fragments Y and D
   c. fragments D and E
   d. fibrin monomer

10. Which of the following pairs the correct protein with its inhibitor? (Objective 12)
    a. thrombin–antithrombin
    b. tissue factor–TFPI
    c. heparin–heparin cofactor II
    d. fibrin–TAFI

LEVEL II

4. Which of the following describes the contact factors (PK, HK, F-XI, F-XII)? (Objective 4)
   a. have a significant role in initiating hemostasis in vivo
   b. all cause a serious bleeding problem when defective or deficient
   c. contribute to fibrinolysis, inflammation, and complement activation
   d. can be assayed by the prothrombin time

5. What is the role of ADAMTS-13 in hemostasis? (Objective 6)
   a. activate protein C to activated protein C
   b. cleave ULVWF to multimers normally found in the circulation
   c. serve as a receptor for uPA on hepatocytes
   d. inhibit activated hemostatic proteases

6. What is the hepatic cell receptor which binds and clears tPA/PAI-1, plasmin/AP, and uPA/PAI-1 complexes from the circulation? (Objective 6)
   a. UPAR
   b. LRP
   c. annexin-2
   d. thrombomodulin

7. What is the procoagulant function of thrombin? (Objective 5)
   a. activate of F-XII
   b. inactivate protein C
   c. suppress platelet activation
   d. activate F-V and F-VIII

8. What is needed for fibrinolysis to occur at a physiologically significant rate? (Objective 7)
   a. tPA must bind to fibrin
   b. circulating plasminogen must be activated to plasmin
   c. PAI-1 must be inhibited by α_2-antiplasmin
   d. plasminogen must be bound to fibrinogen

9. Which is true of TFPI? (Objective 8)
   a. is found in platelets
   b. is unique because two different proteases are inhibited at the same time
   c. does not require Ca^{2+}
   d. inhibits the entire coagulation cascade by inhibiting the extrinsic pathway

10. The following results were reported on a 10-year-old male with a history of bleeding problems: prothrombin time—29.5 seconds (control 12.5 seconds); partial thromboplastin time—51.0 seconds (control 55.4 seconds). What do these results indicate? (Objective 9)
    a. a F-VII defect or deficiency exists
    b. a defect in the intrinsic system exists
    c. the child has hemophilia A
    d. platelet testing should be done

www.pearsonhighered.com/mckenzie

Use this address to access the interactive Companion Website created for this textbook. Find additional information, tables and figures. Evaluate your command of the chapter information using case studies and critical thinking and multiple choice questions.

REFERENCES

1. MacFarlane RG. An enzyme cascade in the blood clotting mechanism and its function as a biochemical amplifier. *Nature.* 1991; 202:498–99.

2. Davie EW, Ratnoff OD. Waterfall sequence for intrinsic blood clotting. *Science.* 1964;145:1310–12.

3. Morrissey JH, Mutch NJ. Tissue factor structure and function. In: Colman RW, Marder VJ, Clowes AW, George JN, Goldhaber SZ, eds. *Hemostasis and Thrombosis. Basic Principles and Clinical Practice,* 5th ed. Philadelphia: Lippincott Williams & Wilkins; 2006: 91–106.

4. Wright IS. The nomenclature of blood clotting factors. *Thromb Diath Haemorrh.* 1962;27:381.

5. Rapaport, SI. Blood coagulation and its alterations in hemorrhagic and thrombotic disorders. *West. J. Med.* 1993;158:153–61.

6. Mann KG. Prothrombin. *Methods Enzymology.* 1976;45:123–56.

7. Furie B, Furie BC. The molecular basis of blood coagulation. *Cell.* 1998;53:505–18.

8. Scully MF. The biochemistry of blood clotting: The digestion of a liquid to form a solid. *Essays Biochem.* 1992;27:17–36.

9. Hemker HC, Kessels H. Feedback mechanisms in coagulation. *Haemost.* 1991;21:189–96.

10. Nesheim ME, Taswell JB, Mann KG. The contribution of bovine factor V and factor Va to the activity of prothrombinase. *J Biol Chem.* 1979;245:10,952–62.

11. Ratnoff OD. The biology and pathology of the initiation of coagulation. In: Broom EB, Moore CV, eds. *Progress in Hematology.* New York: Grune & Stratton; 1966:204:204–45.

12. Colman RW. Contact activation (kallikrein-kinin) pathway: Multiple physiologic and pathophysiologic activities. In: Colman RW, Marder VJ, Clowes AW, George JN, Goldhaber SZ, eds. *Hemostasis and Thrombosis. Basic Principles and Clinical Practice,* 5th ed. Philadelphia: Lippincott Williams & Wilkins; 2006: 107–30.

13. Walsh PN, Gailani D. Factor XI. In: Colman RW, Marder VJ, Clowes AW, George JN, Goldhaber SZ, eds. *Hemostasis and Thrombosis. Basic Principles and Clinical Practice,* 5th ed. Philadelphia: Lippincott Williams & Wilkins; 2006: 221–33.

14. Brinkhous KM, Sandberg H, Garris JB et al. Purified human factor VIII procoagulant protein: Comparative hemostatic response after infusions into hemophilic and von Willebrand disease dogs. *Proc Natl Acad Sci USA.* 1985;92:9752–56.

15. Kaufman RJ, Antonarakis SE, Fay PJ. Factor VIII and hemophilia. In: Colman RW, Marder VJ, Clowes AW, George JN, Goldhaber SZ, eds. *Hemostasis and Thrombosis. Basic Principles and Clinical Practice,* 5th ed. Philadelphia: Lippincott Williams & Wilkins; 2006: 151–75.

16. Haberichter SL, Montgomery RR. Structure and function of von Willebrand factor. In: Colman, RW, Marder VJ, Clowes AW, George JN, Goldhaber SZ, eds. *Hemostasis and Thrombosis. Basic Principles and Clinical Practice,* 5th ed. Philadelphia: Lippincott Williams & Wilkins; 2006: 707–22.

17. Wise RJ, Barr PJ, Wong PA et al. Expression of a human proprotein processing enzyme: Correct cleavage of the von Willebrand factor precursor at a paired basic amino acid site. *Proc Natl Acad Sci USA.* 1990;87:9378–82.

18. Fijikawa K, Suzuki H, McMullen B et al. Purification of human von Willebrand factor-cleaving protease. *Blood.* 2001;98:1662–66.

19. Dong JF, Moake JL, Nolasco L et al. ADAMTS-13 rapidly cleaves newly secreted ultra-large von Willebrand factor multimers on the endothelial surface under flowing conditions. *Blood.* 2002;100: 4033–39.

20. Vercellotti GM. Effects of viral activation of the vessel wall on inflammation and thrombosis. *Blood Coagul Fibrinolysis.* 1998–99; Suppl 2: S3–S6.

21. Morrissey JH, Macik BG, Neuenschwander PF, Comp PC. Quantitation of activated factor VII levels in plasma using tissue factor mutant selectively deficient in promoting factor VII activation. *Blood.* 1993;81:734–44.

22. Radcliffe R, Nemerson Y. Activation and control of factor VII by activated factor X and thrombin: Isolation and characterization of a single chain form of factor VII. *J Biol Chem.* 1975;250:388–95.

23. Tracy PB, Eide LL, Bowie EJ, Mann KG. Radioimmunoassay of factor V in human plasma and platelets. *Blood.* 1982;60:59–63.

24. Brox JH, Osterus B, Bjorklid E et al. Production and availability of thromboplastin activity in endothelial cells: The effects of thrombin, endotoxin, and platelets. *Brit J Haematol.* 1984;57:239–46.

25. Doolittle RF. The structure and evolution of vertebrate fibrinogen. *Ann NY Acad Sci.* 1983;408:13–27.

26. Fowler WE, Erickson HP. Trinodular structure of fibrinogen: Confirmation by both shadowing and negative stain electron microscopy. *J Mol Biol.* 1979;134:241–49.

27. Yee VC, Pratt KP, Cote HC, Trong IL, Chung DW, Stenkamp RE, Teller DC. Crystal structure of a 30kDa C-terminal fragment from the gamma chain of human fibrinogen. *Structure.* 1997;5:125–38.

28. Greenberg CS, Sane DC, Lai T-S. Factor XIII and fibrin stabilization. In: Colman RW, Marder VJ, Clowes AW, George JN, Goldhaber SZ, eds. *Hemostasis and Thrombosis. Basic Principles and Clinical Practice,* 5th ed. Philadelphia: Lippincott Williams & Wilkins; 2006: 317–34.

29. Booth NA, Bachmann F. Plasminogen-plasmin system. In: Colman RW, Marder VJ, Clowes AW, George JN, Goldhaber SZ, eds. *Hemostasis and Thrombosis. Basic Principles and Clinical Practice,* 5th ed. Philadelphia: Lippincott Williams & Wilkins; 2006: 335–64.

30. Hajjar KA, Francis CW. Fibrinolysis and thrombolysis. In: Lichtman MA, Beutler A, Kipps TJ et al., eds. *Williams Hematology,* 7th ed. New York: McGraw-Hill; 2006: 2089–115.

31. Francis CW, Marder VJ. Mechanisms of fibrinolysis. In: Beutler E et al., eds. *William's Hematology,* 5th ed. New York: McGraw-Hill Inc; 1995: 1256.

32. Colman RW et al. *Hemostasis and Thrombosis,* 4th ed. Philadelphia: Lippincott Wlliams & Wilkins; 2001: 284–85.

33. Rijken DC, Hoylaerts M, Collen D. Fibrinolytic properties of one-chain and two-chain human extrinsic (tissue-type) plasminogen activator. *J Biol Chem.* 1982;257:2920–25.

34. Sepanova V, Bobik A, Bibilashvily R et al. Urokinase plasminogen activator induces smooth muscle cell migration: Key role of growth factor-like domain. *FEBS Lett.* 1997;414:471.

35. Lijnen HR, Zamarron C, Blaber M et al. Activation of plasminogen by pro-urokinase. I. Mechanism. *J Biol Chem.* 1986;261:1,253–58.

36. Scanu AM, Lawn RM, Berg M. Lipoprotein (a) and atherosclerosis. *Ann Intern Med.* 1991;115:209–18.

37. Bajzar L, Morser J, Nesheim M. TAFI, or plasma procarboxypeptidase B, couples the coagulation and fibrinolytic cascades through the thrombin-thrombomodulin complex. *J Biol Chem.* 1996;271: 16,603–8.

38. Wang W, Boffa MB, Bajzar L, Walker JB, Nesheim ME. A study of the mechanism of inhibition of fibrinolysis by activated thrombin-activatable fibrinolyis inhibitor. *J Biol Chem.* 1998;273:27,176–81.

39. Abildgaard U. Highly purified antithrombin III with heparin cofactor activity prepared by disc electrophoresis. *Scand JClin Lab Invest.* 1968;125:89–91.

40. Andrew M, Mitchell L, Berry L et al. An anticoagulant dermatan sulfate proteoglycan circulates in the pregnant woman and her fetus. *J Clin Invest.* 1992;89:321–26.

41. Esmon CT, Esmon NL, Harris K. Complex formation between thrombin and thrombomodulin inhibits both thrombin-catalyzed fibrin formation and factor V activation. *J Biol Chem.* 1982;257: 7,944–47.

42. Esmon NL, Carroll RC, Esmon CT. Thrombomodulin blocks the ability of thrombin to activate platelets. *J Biol Chem.* 1983;258: 12,238–42.

43. Fukudome K, Esmon CT. Identification, cloning, and regulation of a novel endothelial cell protein C/activated protein C receptor. *J Biol Chem.* 1994;269:26,486–91.

44. Stearns-Kurosawa DJ, Kurosawa S, Mollica JS, Ferrell GL, Esmon CT. The endothelial cell protein C receptor augments protein C activation by the thrombin–thrombomodulin complex. *Proc Natl Acad Sci USA.* 1996;93:10,212–16.

45. Hajjar KA, Esmon NL, Marcus AJ, Muller W. Vascular function in hemostasis. In: Lichtman MA, Beutler A, Kipps TJ et al., eds. *Williams Hematology,* 7th ed. New York: McGraw-Hill; 2006:1715–37.

46. Dahlbeck B, Hildebrand B. Inherited resistance to activated protein C is corrected by anticoagulant cofactor activity found to be a property of factor V. *Proc Natl Acad Sci USA.* 1994:91:1396–1400.

47. Hansen JB, Huseby NE, Sandset PM et al. Tissue factor pathway inhibitor and lipoproteins. Evidence for association with and regulation by LDL in human plasma. *Arterioscler Thromb Vasc Biol.* 1995;15:879–85.

48. Sandset P, Abildgaard U, Larsen M. Heparin induces release of extrinsic coagulation pathway inhibitor (EPI). *Thromb Res.* 1988;50: 803–13.

49. Caplice NM, Panetta C, Peterson TE et al. Lipoprotein (a) binds and inactivates tissue factor pathway inhibitor: A novel link between lipoproteins and thrombosis. *Blood.* 2001;98:2980–87.

50. Sandset PM, Abilgaard U. Extrinsic pathway inhibitor: The key to feedback control of blood coagulation initiated by tissue thromboplastin. *Haemost.* 1991; 21:219–39.

51. Griffin JH. Control of coagulation reactions. In: Lichtman MA, Beutler A, Kipps TJ et al., eds. *Williams Hematology,* 7th ed. New York: McGraw-Hill; 2006: 1695–714.

52. Broze GJ, Girard TJ, Novotny WF. The lipoprotein-associated coagulation inhibitor. *Prog Hemost Thromb.* 1991;10:243–68.

53. Hoffman M, Monroe DM, Oliver JA, Roberts HR. Factors IXa and Xa play distinct roles in tissue factor-dependent initiation of coagulation. *Blood.* 1995;86:1794–1801.

54. Scott CF, Schapira M, James HL et al. Inactivation of factor XIa by plasma protease inhibitors: Predominant role of alpha 1-protease inhibitor and protective effect of high molecular weight kininogen. *J. Clin Invest.* 1982;69:844–52.

55. Broze GJ. Protein Z and protein Z-dependent protease inhibitor. In: Colman, RW, Marder VJ, Clowes AW, George JN, Goldhaber SZ, eds. *Hemostasis and Thrombosis. Basic Principles and Clinical Practice,* 5th ed. Philadelphia: Lippincott Williams & Wilkins; 2006: 215–20.

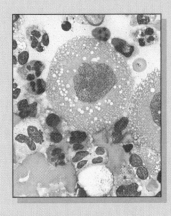

31

Disorders of Primary Hemostasis

Barbara A. O'Malley, M.D.

■ OBJECTIVES—LEVEL I

At the end of this unit of study, the student should be able to:

1. Define and differentiate among *thrombocytopenia, thrombocytosis,* and *thrombocythemia* and state an expected range of platelet count in each.
2. Define and differentiate among *petechiae, purpura, ecchymosis, hematoma,* and *easy bruisability.*
3. Identify laboratory tests that can be ordered to screen for abnormalities of the hemostatic system.
4. Explain the expected clinical consequences when a patient has an abnormality of platelets or blood vessels.
5. Correlate quantitative variations in the platelet count with disease manifestations.
6. Recognize hematologic disorders that are characterized by the presence of thrombocytopenia or thrombocytosis.
7. Describe the etiology, pathophysiology, and laboratory findings of the thrombocytopenias.
8. Differentiate primary (malignant) from secondary (reactive) thrombocytosis.
9. Explain the effect of aspirin and its duration on platelet function.
10. Identify the cause and describe the clinical and laboratory features of hereditary disorders of platelet function.

■ OBJECTIVES—LEVEL II

At the end of this unit of study, the student should be able to:

1. Categorize each specific disorder of hemostasis by body system affected (e.g., vasculature, platelets).
2. Predict the type of bleeding symptoms in patients with disorders of primary hemostasis.
3. Describe the expected symptomatology, etiology, pathophysiology, and laboratory test results in patients with disorders of the vasculature.
4. Organize thrombocytopenic and thrombocytosis conditions by etiology and pathophysiology and explain laboratory findings in each condition.
5. Differentiate acute from chronic immune thrombocytopenic purpura by significant clinical and laboratory data.
6. Explain the pathophysiology of thrombocytopenia and thrombocytosis in hematologic disorders.
7. Organize the hereditary and acquired qualitative platelet defects by etiology and pathophysiology, and predict the clinical and laboratory features.

8. Explain the biochemical mechanism of the effect of aspirin on platelet function and recommend a time frame for patients to refrain from taking aspirin and related anti-inflammatory drugs prior to platelet function testing.

9. Summarize the effect of aspirin, alcohol, and antibiotics on platelet function.

KEY TERMS

Bernard-Soulier syndrome (BSS)
Congenital amegakaryocytic thrombocytopenia (CAMT)
Congenital thrombocytopenia with radioulnar synostosis (CTRUS)
δ-storage pool disease
Disseminated intravascular coagulation (DIC)
Ecchymoses
Epistaxis
Fanconi anemia (FA)
Glanzmann's thrombasthenia (GT)
Gray platelet syndrome (α storage pool disease)
Hematoma
Hemolylic uremic syndrome (HUS)
Heparin-associated thrombocytopenia (HAT)
Heparin-induced thrombocytopenia (HIT)
Immune thrombocytopenic purpura (ITP)
Ischemia
May-Heggelin anomaly (MHA)
Necrosis
Neonatal alloimmune thrombocytopenia (NAIT)
Nonthrombocytopenic purpura
Petechiae
Primary thrombocytosis
Purpura
Quebec platelet disorder
Scott syndrome
Secondary (reactive) thrombocytosis
Thrombocytopenia with absent radii (TAR)
Thrombotic thrombocytopenic purpura (TTP)
Vasculitis
Wiskott-Aldrich syndrome (WAS)
X-linked thrombocytopenia (XLT)

BACKGROUND BASICS

The information in this chapter builds on the concepts learned in previous chapters. To maximize your learning experience, you should review these concepts before starting this unit of study.

Level I

▶ Hemostasis: Describe how a blood clot forms after an injury, especially the role of platelets in cessation of bleeding. (Chapter 29)

▶ Immunology: Define and describe antigen/antibody reactions, classes of immunoglobulins, and the process of immune complex formation. (Chapter 7)

▶ Immune hemolytic anemia: Summarize the pathophysiology of the immune hemolytic anemias. (Chapter 17)

▶ Laboratory methods: Correlate the automated platelet count with the platelet count estimate on a peripheral blood smear. (Chapters 34 and 41)

▶ Laboratory methods: Identify artifacts that can cause spuriously increased or decreased automated platelet counts. (Chapters 34 and 41)

Level II

▶ Hemostasis: Correlate the functions of the blood vessels, platelets, and coagulation factors in forming a blood clot. (Chapters 29 and 30)

▶ Neoplastic leukocyte disorders: Summarize the consequences of malignant diseases of the bone marrow, particularly as they relate to the production of platelets. (Chapters 21–26)

▶ Cytokines: Describe how cytokines and growth factors regulate the production of blood cells. (Chapter 3)

▶ Flow cytometry: Recognize and correctly utilize the CD nomenclature of cellular antigens. (Chapter 37)

CASE STUDY

We will address this case study throughout the chapter.
Mohammed, a 15-year-old male from Saudi Arabia, was admitted to the emergency room after an automobile accident with several superficial cuts and bruises to the head and arms. He was bleeding profusely, having more severe bleeding than would be expected from the nature of his wounds. Consider possible causes of this abnormal bleeding and the laboratory tests that might be used to differentiate and diagnose the cause.

▶ OVERVIEW

This chapter is the first of two that describe abnormalities of the hemostatic system that result primarily in bleeding. It begins with a discussion of general clinical and laboratory aspects of hemostatic disorders. Following the general topics, defects in primary hemostasis, including the vascular system and platelets, are discussed. The pathophysiologic basis and clinical manifestations for each defect are presented, but the major emphasis is on laboratory involvement in the diagnosis and/or treatment of the conditions. It is important to correctly identify the cause of the hemostatic defect so that appropriate treatment or preventive measures can be implemented.

▶ INTRODUCTION

As discussed in ∞ Chapters 29 and 30, hemostasis minimizes blood loss from disruptive injuries to blood vessels and prevents blood loss from intact vessels. The hemostatic response includes vasoconstriction of blood vessels, primary hemostatic plug formation by platelet activation, fibrin formation by activation of soluble plasma proteins, and function of inhibitors that prevent inappropriate or excessive activation of hemostasis and regulate the system to allow activation only when and where it is needed. Adequate hemostasis depends on a large number of intricately balanced mechanisms. Abnormalities of one or more components in the process of clot formation (i.e., the blood vessels, platelets, or clotting factors) can lead to excessive bleeding. Failure to regulate excessive clot formation leads to thrombosis.

▶ DIAGNOSIS OF BLEEDING DISORDERS

CLINICAL MANIFESTATIONS OF BLEEDING DISORDERS

A patient with a clinically significant bleeding disorder presents to the physician with hemorrhagic symptoms. Bleeding symptoms can range from easy bruisability to life-threatening hemorrhage. The severity of the bleed is generally proportional to the severity and type of hemostatic defect.

The type of bleeding can indicate which component of the hemostatic system is defective. A defect in a component of primary hemostasis (vasculature, platelets) usually results in bleeding from the skin or mucous membranes, such as epistaxis (nose bleeds), gingival mucosa (gums), or menorrhagia (abnormal menstrual bleeding). Bleeding symptoms in patients with coagulation factor abnormalities, on the other hand, are usually internal, involving deeper tissues and joints.

Bleeding from subcutaneous blood vessels (capillaries) into intact skin can be visualized as petechiae, ecchmyoses, or hematomas (Figure 31-1 ■). **Petechiae** are small red to purple spots in the skin less than 3 mm in diameter resulting from blood leakage through the endothelial lining of capillaries. Petechiae usually occur on the extremities because of the high venous pressure. When arising spontaneously, without trauma, they are painless. Several petechiae in one area can merge into a larger bruised area. Petechial lesions are characteristic of abnormalities of platelets and blood vessels and usually are not seen in coagulation factor disorders.

Ecchymoses are bruises that are larger than 1 cm in diameter and are caused by blood escaping through the endothelium into subcutaneous tissue, commonly from a vessel larger than a capillary. They are red or purple when first formed and become yellowish green as they heal and hemoglobin degrades into bilirubin and biliverdin. Ecchymoses can appear spontaneously or with trauma and can be painful and tender. They can occur when there are abnormalities of blood vessels, platelets, or coagulation factors.

Intermediate lesions (>3 mm but <1 cm) are called *intermediate purpura*. The word **purpura,** meaning purple, is used ambiguously but generally refers to all bruises from petechiae to ecchymoses. Purpura is also used as part of the name of diseases in which these typical symptoms occur such as immune thrombocytopenic purpura (ITP). A bruise is called a **hematoma** when blood leaks from an opening in a vessel and collects beneath intact skin. It is blue or purple and slightly raised. Hematomas can occur in any organ or tissue.

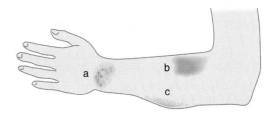

■ FIGURE 31-1   Schematic drawing of bleeding manifestations in intact skin. **a.** Petechiae. **b.** Ecchymosis. **c.** Hematoma.

When ecchymoses and petechiae are found in higher than normal numbers and with less than usual trauma, the condition is termed *easy bruisability.* Another term used often in describing clinical manifestations of bleeding disorders is *excess bleeding,* which occurs from superficial cuts and scratches when platelets fail to form an effective primary hemostatic plug. Excess bleeding means that the bleeding is more prolonged and/or is more profuse than normal for the patient or as compared with a normal person. Blood can escape from visceral organs into any body cavity or from mucous membranes into any body orifice. Frank bleeding is characteristic of both platelet and coagulation abnormalities.

PHYSICIAN EVALUATION OF A PATIENT WITH ABNORMAL BLEEDING

Excessive bleeding can be caused by a local disruption of the vasculature, such as a bleeding ulcer, or by generalized failure of the hemostatic mechanism. In some cases both are present, compounding the effect of the vascular disruption. It is the physician's responsibility to determine the cause of the bleeding and to institute proper treatment. This requires obtaining an accurate medical history, performing a thorough physical examination, and ordering and interpreting the results of appropriate laboratory tests.

The patient's history should include:

- age of onset of hemorrhagic symptoms
- type of symptoms
- family history
- presence of other diseases
- complete drug history (including over-the-counter drugs and herbal supplements)
- exposure to toxins

The answers should enable the physician to decide whether a bleeding disorder exists, determine the probability of an inherited versus an acquired condition, and help define the affected portion of the hemostatic system. The age at which symptoms first appeared provides a clue to the disorder's etiology. Bleeding occurring at birth or shortly thereafter often indicates an inherited disorder, although onset later in life does not rule this out. Bleeding from the umbilical cord and/or from the circumcision site suggests a coagulation factor defect.

The persistence and severity of symptoms—whether occurring throughout life, a single event, or intermittently—is also informative. Bleeding in excess of that expected from a tonsillectomy, tooth extraction, trauma, injury, surgery, or childbirth can provide clues.

Family history is helpful in determining whether other family members have had similar symptoms. A pedigree analysis can help to establish the pattern of inheritance (X-linked, autosomal, dominant, or recessive). Patients with inherited abnormalities do not always have a positive family history, however, because spontaneous mutations occur in several hemostatic disorders.

The presence of an associated disease, such as a malignancy, aplastic anemia, leukemia, liver disease, uremia, or infection, must be considered. These conditions can be associated with secondary or acquired platelet disorders and/or coagulation defects.

A history of drug exposure is important to consider because many drugs are known to affect the hemostatic mechanism, and various drugs affect different portions of the system. Aspirin, chemotherapeutic drugs, coumadin, and other anticoagulants are examples, but there are many others. The reader is referred to the Website (∞ Chapter 40) and to other texts that provide extensive lists of specific drugs that have been implicated in acquired hemostatic defects.[1,2]

Finally, past or present exposure to toxic chemicals such as benzene, insect sprays, and hair dyes should be investigated.

On physical examination, the type and sites of bleeding are noted, as well as whether the bleeding is from single or multiple sites, and whether it is spontaneous or the result of trauma. Using the information from the history and physical examination, the physician orders appropriate laboratory tests to confirm and classify the presence of abnormal hemostasis.

LABORATORY EVALUATION OF ABNORMAL BLEEDING

Although laboratory testing plays an important role in evaluating a patient with a suspected hemostatic abnormality, it should never be a substitute for good clinical assessment of the patient. No single laboratory test can fully evaluate defective hemostasis, so initially a battery or group of screening tests is usually ordered. Based on their results, the physician can determine whether a detectable abnormality of hemostasis does exist and order the confirmatory tests necessary to define the disorder. Minimum screening tests include:

- platelet count
- prothrombin time (PT)
- activated partial thromboplastin time (APTT)

The results of one or more of these tests is abnormal in most patients with hemostatic disorders, and they are usually within the reference ranges if the patient does not have a defect in the hemostatic system. However, screening tests are not helpful in predicting *bleeding risk* for the patient. In patients with disorders of primary hemostasis, the PT and APTT are usually normal, and the platelet count may or may not be abnormal.

When the results of these screening tests are normal in a patient with a history of clinically significant bleeding, a vascular disorder or functional platelet defect is likely. Confirmatory tests of platelet function can then be ordered. These include the closure time (measured by platelet function analyzer, PFA-100®), platelet aggregation tests, flow cytometry for platelet antigens, and the template bleeding time, which measures the time it takes for an incision to stop bleeding (if available on the laboratory test menu) (∞ Chapter 40). The PFA-100 is an alternative or supplement to the bleeding time test. It provides automated assessment of platelet dysfunction. It aspirates a blood sample through a capillary at high shear flow to simulate the hemodynamic conditions of platelet adhesion and aggregation at a vascular lesion. The instrument uses cartridges with membranes that are coated with collagen and ADP or collagen and epinephrine. When the blood encounters the coated membranes, platelet adhesion, activation, and aggregation are triggered, leading to the occlusion of an aperature and cessation of blood flow. In the absence of abnormal results of platelet function testing, the physician can investigate the possibility of a vascular disorder.

Abnormality of the PT and/or APTT denotes a coagulation factor disorder (∞ Chapter 32). Numerous confirmatory tests are available to specify the diagnosis (∞ Chapter 40).

In some patients with mild hemostatic disease, the screening tests may not be sensitive enough to detect an abnormality. Other patients may have conditions that do not affect the screening tests. In such cases, a knowledgeable physician in the field of bleeding disorders can direct the clinical investigation using the information obtained from the clinical history and physical examination.

Laboratory testing for the hemostatic system consists of a number of tests, each of which evaluates a specific part of the hemostatic system. It is important for a clinical laboratory professional to correlate and understand the significance of the results of all hemostasis tests and to correlate the results with the patient's history, if available. In this way, potentially erroneous results can be identified, and/or additional testing procedures can be recommended.

 Checkpoint! 1

Assume that you are the clinical laboratory professional collecting a blood specimen from a patient with a suspected bleeding disorder. You noticed petechiae and several bruises on the patient's arm. What screening tests would the physician likely have ordered? What results of these tests would you expect (normal or abnormal) in this patient?

▶ DISORDERS OF THE VASCULAR SYSTEM

Because the blood vessels are actively involved in hemostasis in a variety of ways (∞ Chapter 29), a structural abnormality or damage either to the endothelial lining of blood vessels or the subendothelial structures can result from, or lead to, a variety of clinical manifestations and disease conditions. These disorders can be either inherited or acquired secondary to another condition. The hereditary vascular diseases are caused by abnormal synthesis of subendothelial connective tissue components[3–8] (Table 31-1 ✪). Either abnormal subendothelium or altered endothelial cells cause acquired vascular disorders (Table 31-2 ✪).

Symptoms seen in vascular disorders are, for the most part, superficial bleeding, such as easy bruising, petechiae, or lesions that mimic them but are actually not caused by bleeding. In the majority of patients with a primary vascular disorder, hemostatic testing is entirely normal. Thus, the diagnosis of blood vessel disorders is most often made by exclusion (i.e., by finding no positive evidence for a disorder of platelets, coagulation factors, or fibrinolysis in a patient who has a history or physical examination suggesting a bleeding problem). The platelet count and screening tests for coagulation factors are usually normal in blood vessel disorders. The

✪ TABLE 31-1

Characteristics of Inherited Disorders of the Vascular System

Disorder	Gene	Effect	Chromosome	Laboratory Findings
Hereditary hemorrhagic telangiectasia (HHT)	Endoglin (HHT-1) Activin A receptor (HHT-2)	↑ VEGF → enhanced microcirculatory growth	9q (HHT-1) 12q (HHT-2)	Normal
Ehlers-Danlos syndromes	Multiple collagen genes (9 subtypes)	Fragility of blood vessels; joint hypermobility	Multiple	BT increased
Marfan syndrome	Fibrillin-1	Decreased strength and elasticity of blood vessels	15	BT increased
Osteogenesis imperfecta	Type I procollagen (COLA1 & 2)	Patchy, defective bone matrix	2	Not significant
Pseudoxanthoma elasticum	ABCC6	Degeneration of elastin; calcification of vessels	Unknown	Not significant

BT = Bleeding time

⊗ TABLE 31-2

**Classification of Acquired Disorders
of the Vascular System**

Purpura due to decreased connective tissue
- Senile purpura
- Cushing syndrome and corticosteroid therapy
- Scurvy

Purpura associated with paraprotein disorders
- Paraproteins
- Amyloidosis

Purpura due to vasculitis
- Henoch-Schönlein purpura
- Infections
- Drugs

Miscellaneous causes of purpura
- Mechanical purpura
- Artificially induced purpura
- Easy bruising syndrome
- Purpura fulminans

template bleeding time and other platelet function testing are also usually normal but can be prolonged in some vascular disease states.

When platelets are normal in number and function, purpura are considered to be caused by damage to the blood vessels, a condition called **nonthrombocytopenic purpura.**

HEREDITARY DISORDERS OF THE VASCULAR SYSTEM

Table 31-1 summarizes the hereditary disorders of the vascular system. They are very rare, and although bleeding is a common symptom, hemostasis tests are not informative in making the diagnosis. Some vascular disorders are associated with abnormal vessel wall integrity, but others manifest as vascular proliferative lesions. *Hemangiomas* are arteriovenous malformations caused by either upregulation of growth-promoting factors and/or inhibition of apoptosis. Most hemangiomas appear in infancy and spontaneously involute over the next several years. In contrast, the telangestasia lesions seen in hereditary hemorrhagic telangectasia slowly progress over decades. A more complete description of these disorders is available on this chapter's Companion Website.

ACQUIRED DISORDERS OF THE VASCULAR SYSTEM

Acquired disorders of the vascular system are seen quite often and are characterized by bruising and petechiae. Defects of either the vessel wall or the endothelial cells can be caused by (1) conditions that decrease the supportive connective tissue in blood vessel walls, (2) presence of abnormal proteins in the vascular tissues, (3) infections or allergic conditions, and (4) mechanical stress. Acquired disorders of the vasculature are shown in Table 31-2.

Purpura Due to Decreased Connective Tissue
The diseases in this category are due to a decreased amount of supportive connective tissue in the blood vessel walls.

Senile Purpura   Senile purpura are ecchymoses that appear with unrecognized or minor trauma in older individuals. With age, the extracellular matrix components of the skin degenerate, especially in body areas that have been exposed to sunlight. This decreases the supportive collagen fibrils and allows small blood vessels, particularly capillaries, to burst and form bruises with minor pressure. The bruises do not heal easily and can last for months.

Cushing Syndrome and Corticosteroid Therapy
Excess endogenous glucocorticosteroids (Cushing syndrome) or exogenous (therapeutic) glucocorticoids result in excessive breakdown of collagen, thin fragile skin, vessel wall fragility, and bruising.[9] Small blood vessels can be mechanically broken and bleed into the skin.

Scurvy   Scurvy is a disease caused by a deficiency of vitamin C, which is needed for collagen synthesis. In its absence, collagen production is abnormal, resulting in vascular fragility and bleeding. Bleeding gums and bleeding around hair follicles on arms and legs are characteristic; ecchymoses and intramuscular hemorrhages are also seen. Treatment is oral vitamin C.

Purpura Associated with Paraprotein Disorders
The diseases in this category are due to the presence of abnormal proteins in the vascular system.

Paraproteins   Paraproteins are monoclonal immunoglobulins produced by monoclonal neoplastic plasma cells. They occur in a variety of malignant conditions such as multiple myeloma, Waldenstrom's macroglobulinemia, and lymphoproliferative disorders (∞ Chapter 26). Hemostatic symptoms include purpura, bleeding, and thrombosis. The mechanisms leading to these symptoms are varied and complex including qualitative platelet defects, acquired inhibitors and deficiencies of coagulation factors, binding of calcium by paraprotein leading to interference with coagulation, and deposition of light chain protein in the vascular wall. Thrombocytopenia can be present because of the underlying disease and contributes to the bleeding. Bleeding symptoms include epistaxis, petechiae, purpura, and hemorrhages into other organs, particularly the retina.[9] Puncture wounds, such as a finger stick, bleed profusely.

Amyloidosis   Amyloidosis occurs as a primary disorder, as well as secondary to paraproteinemias, such as multiple myeloma. It is a condition in which deposits of amyloid (modified or misfolded proteins) form in the skin, perivascular tissue, and vessel walls. It leads to fragility of the vessels and to bruising. Bleeding into visceral organs can also occur, and thrombosis is common.

Purpura Due to Vasculitis

Vasculitis is inflammation of the small blood vessels. It occurs when immune complexes attach either to the endothelial cells or the underlying subendothelial structures and activate complement.[5] The activation fragments of complement initiate several processes: (1) Neutrophils migrate to the area by chemotaxis and phagocytize the immune complexes. Enzymes, free oxygen radicals, and other substances are then released from the neutrophils and damage the vascular tissue. (2) Complement components C3a and C5a cause increased vascular permeability, resulting in vasodilation and edema. (3) The lytic complement cascade can be completed, resulting in damage to the vascular cell membranes.

Antigen–antibody complexes also cause aggregation of platelets and activation of factor XII (F-XII) (∞ Chapter 30), both of which contribute to thrombosis. Thrombi can occlude blood vessels (**ischemia**) and could result in the destruction of the tissue supplied by the occluded vessels (**necrosis**). Activated F-XII results in the activation of kallikrein and the release of kinins from high molecular weight kininogens, which contribute to the vasodilation and edema associated with inflammation. The damaged vessels can rupture and produce localized purpura. The purpura caused by vasculitis are called *palpable purpura* because small nodules form at the site of the inflammation.[10]

The cause of the vasculitis in most patients is never found. Some conditions that are associated with vasculitis are:

- Henoch-Schönlein purpura
- infections
- drugs

Details of these conditions can be found on this text's Companion Website.

Miscellaneous Causes of Purpura

Other causes of purpura may or may not be related to abnormalities of the hemostatic system.

Mechanical Purpura   Increased pressure within the lumen of capillaries after intense exercise, coughing spasms, or epileptic seizures can cause petechial hemorrhages in the skin.

Artificially Induced Purpura   Artificially induced bruises can be self-inflicted (factitious purpura) or result from abuse by others. The cause is difficult to distinguish from a true physiologic (pathologic) process. Artifically induced purpura and bleeding occasionally are the result of unnecessary, secretive overuse of anticoagulant drugs such as

heparin and coumadin. Health professionals with psychological problems who are aware of the consequences of anticoagulant drugs and have the means to obtain them have been guilty of abusing these drugs. Petechial purpura can be induced by placing negative pressure on the skin for a prolonged period as, for instance, sucking the air from a glass held to the mouth. Petechiometers used for the capillary fragility test were based on this principle.

Easy Bruising Syndrome   A benign condition called *easy bruising syndrome* (or *purpura simplex*) commonly occurs in young women. Spontaneous small ecchymoses appear on the skin of the thighs or upper arms and have been called *devil's pinches*. The cause of this condition is not fully understood at the molecular level but is thought to be due to hormonal effects on the blood vessel and/or its surrounding tissue.[11]

Purpura Fulminans   Purpura fulminans is a devastating type of purpura seen in newborns and others associated with abnormalities of certain clotting factors or their inhibitors and in some patients who are on therapy for thrombotic conditions (∞ Chapter 33). In purpura fulminans, thrombi form in the small vessels supplying the skin and subcutaneous tissues. The vessels become occluded, the skin becomes necrotic, and the condition can rapidly lead to death.

Psychogenic Purpura   Psychogenic purpura refers to severe recurrent erythema and ecchymoses, often accompanied by pain and swelling. This was once theorized to be an allergic reaction to blood cells or DNA but no longer. It is generally believed to be a form of factitious purpura associated with a psychiatric illness. Most patients have normal coagulation studies and no evidence of underlying medical illness.[5]

⊘ CASE STUDY *(continued from page 673)*

Petechiae were noted on Mohammed's extremities. Blood work was ordered.

1. What laboratory tests, hematology and hemostasis, that would be most informative in interpreting the cause of the patient's bleeding would likely be ordered immediately?

2. Does the patient most likely have a disorder of primary or of secondary hemostasis? Why?

▶ PLATELET DISORDERS

Platelets function in hemostasis to maintain the integrity of the blood vessels and to form the primary hemostatic plug in response to injury so that blood loss is minimized (∞ Chapter 29). Bleeding from a cut finger stops when the primary hemostatic plug has sealed the openings in the injured vessels. Formation of the primary hemostatic plug requires an adequate number of normally functioning platelets. If

⊘ **TABLE 31-3**

Types of Bleeding in Disorders of Primary Hemostasis

- Petechiae
- Ecchymoses
- Epistaxis
- Excessive bleeding from superficial wounds
- Bleeding into the retina
- Gastrointestinal bleeding
- Bleeding in the urinary tract
- Hypermenorrhea
- Gingival bleeding (gums)
- Increased bleeding after tooth extraction
- Intracranial bleeding

platelet numbers are decreased or if platelet function is abnormal, an injury can bleed excessively.

Platelet disorders are classified as quantitative (numerical) or qualitative (functional). *Quantitative disorders* are those in which the platelet count is either below (thrombocytopenia) or above (thrombocytosis) the reference range. *Qualitative disorders* involve an abnormality of some aspect of platelet function.

Characteristic manifestations of the hemostatic defect seen in patients with platelet disorders are petechiae and excess bleeding from superficial areas of the body such as the skin and mucous membranes. **Epistaxis** (nose bleeds), excessive bleeding from cuts in the skin, and easy bruisability

are commonly experienced. Other possible sites of bleeding are listed in Table 31-3 ⊘. The bleeding symptoms reflect the decreased ability of the platelets to form the primary hemostatic plug.

Manifestations of increased platelet counts generally reflect the underlying problem that caused the thrombocytosis; occasionally there is increased likelihood of thrombosis (or rarely, hemorrhage).

QUANTITATIVE PLATELET DISORDERS

Quantitative abnormalities of platelets include thrombocytopenia or thrombocytosis. A reference range of $150–450 \times 10^9/L$ (Table C, front cover) is similar to that established by most laboratories. Platelets are usually counted by automated instruments, although some laboratories use manual counting methods as a backup. Methods of counting platelets and of correlating the automated platelet count with the number of platelets found on a peripheral blood smear are described in ∞ Chapter 34.

The blood smear can also include the presence of morphologically abnormal forms of platelets, such as platelets larger (macrothrombocytes) or smaller (microthrombocytes) than normal, those with decreased or absent granules (hypogranular or agranular), or a combination of variables. Platelet variants should be recognized and reported by the clinical laboratory professional. Platelets are reported as macrothrombocytes if they are larger than normal and as giant forms (megathrombocytes) if they are larger than erythrocytes. Some laboratories use the term *giant platelet* to describe all abnormally large platelets (Figure 31-2 ■).

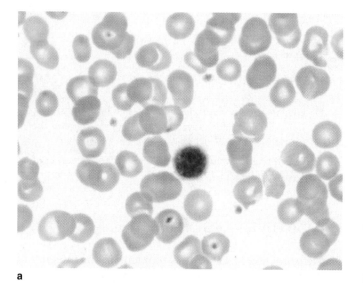

a

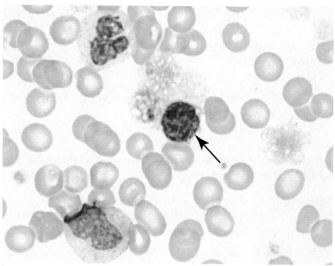

b

■ FIGURE 31-2   **a.** Large granular platelet. **b.** Increased numbers of platelets, some of which have normal morphology, some of which are hypogranular or agranular, and one giant agranular platelet. (*Note:* The central nucleated cell [arrow] is a micromegakaryocyte.) (Peripheral blood, Wright-Giemsa stain, 1000× magnification)

TABLE 31-4

Significant Laboratory Tests in Defects of Primary Hemostasis

	Screening Tests			
	Platelet Count	Prothrombin Time	APTT	Template BT
Vascular disorders	Normal	Normal	Normal	Normal or abnormal
Thrombocytopenia	Decreased	Normal	Normal	Abnormal
Platelet dysfunction	Usually normal	Normal	Normal	Normal or abnormal

✓ Checkpoint! 2

If you observed an average of 14 platelets per high power field on a peripheral blood smear prepared from the needle tip and your laboratory allowed correlation between the direct instrument count and the blood smear estimate of 20%, what range would you expect the instrument count to be? Is this platelet estimate within an acceptable reference range?

Thrombocytopenia

The lower limit of the reference range for platelets is approximately 150×10^9/L, but clinical symptoms are usually not seen unless the count falls below 50×10^9/L. When it is below 50×10^9/L, the severity of clinical manifestations can, to some degree, parallel the platelet count. At levels less than 30×10^9/L, possible symptoms include petechiae, menorrhagia, or spontaneous bruising with little or no trauma. The possibility of severe and spontaneous bleeding is quite high when the platelet count is below 10×10^9/L.[11] Fatal bleeding into the central nervous system as well as spontaneous bleeding from mucous membranes (e.g., the gastrointestinal tract, the genitourinary tract, and the nose) can occur. The extent of symptoms at all platelet levels varies from patient to patient and can be affected by medications, the blood vessel status, platelet activity, and concurrent disease.

When the patient has thrombocytopenia without other complicating factors, the bleeding time is generally prolonged proportionally at platelet counts between 10 and 100×10^9/L. The linear relationship is altered, however, if patients have abnormalities of platelet function in addition to the thrombocytopenia. The bleeding time is no longer available in most hospital laboratories. Laboratory tests for coagulation factors (PT and APTT) and for fibrinolysis are unaffected by thrombocytopenia. Table 31-4 ✪ compares typical laboratory screening test results in thrombocytopenia, disorders of abnormal platelet function, and vascular disorders.

Thrombocytopenia, the most common cause of excess or abnormal bleeding, is not a disease per se but a symptom of an underlying condition as is anemia. The finding of a decreased platelet count with or without abnormalities of other hematologic parameters alerts the physician to search for a cause so that the condition can be appropriately treated. A decreased platelet count can be the primary feature or a secondary manifestation of several conditions. This text classifies thrombocytopenia into five major categories based on pathophysiology (Table 31-5 ✪).

Increased Destruction The most common cause of thrombocytopenia is increased destruction of platelets, resulting in a decreased platelet life span after they have been released into the peripheral blood. If the bone marrow is normal, it attempts to compensate for the decreased platelet numbers in the peripheral blood by increasing production. Consequently, bone marrow megakaryocytes are normal to increased in number. However, the platelets may be eliminated from the circulation faster than the bone marrow can produce them, resulting in thrombocytopenia (Figure 31-3 ■).

TABLE 31-5

Classification of Quantitative Platelet Abnormalities

Thrombocytopenia
- Increased destruction
    - Immune
    - Nonimmune
- Decreased production
    - Megakaryocyte hypoplasia
    - Replacement of normal marrow
    - Ineffective thrombopoiesis
    - Inherited disorders
- Increased splenic sequestration
- Dilutional thrombocytopenia
- Conditions with multiple mechanisms of thrombocytopenia

Thrombocytosis
- Primary thrombocytosis
- Secondary thrombocytosis
- Transient thrombocytosis

Artifacts in the quantitative measurement of platelets

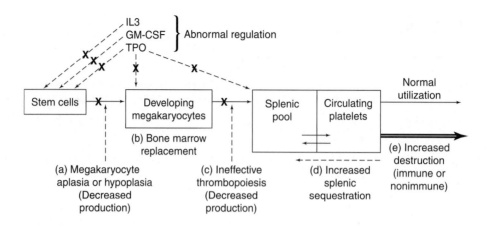

■ FIGURE 31-3   Schematic drawing showing various causes of thrombocytopenia.
IL3 = Interleukin 3; GM-CSF = granulocyte macrophage colony-stimulating factor;
TPO = thrombopoietin; X = abnormal or absent

Causes of increased destruction include both immune mediated destruction and those processes that are nonimmune in nature (Table 31-6 ✪).

Immune Mediated Destruction.   Immune platelet destruction is caused by antibodies and is analogous to the destruction of erythrocytes in immune hemolytic anemias (∞ Chapter 17). Platelets become sensitized with antibody, and the mononuclear phagocyte system, primarily in the spleen, destroys them. Monocytes and macrophages possess Fc receptors (FcγR) by which they recognize platelets coated

with antibody (Figure 31-4 ■). In addition, liver macrophages can remove platelets when coated with large amounts of antibody. The length of time that antibody-coated platelets survive in the peripheral blood can range from a few minutes to 2 or 3 days as measured by ^{51}Cr assays.

Antibodies attach to platelets either by their Fab regions, binding to specific epitopes on GP IIb/IIIa or Ib/IX, or by nonspecific attachment of immune complexes to platelet Fc receptors (Figure 31-4). The antibodies can be IgG, IgA, or rarely IgM,[12] and complement may become activated. The level to which the platelet count becomes decreased depends on the concentration and activity of the antibody, the function of the macrophages Fc and complement receptors, and the ability of the bone marrow to increase platelet production to compensate for the increased loss.[13]

Unlike the immune hemolytic anemias, routine laboratory tests designed to quantitate the amount of immunoglobulin on platelets of thrombocytopenic patients are not available. Several laboratory procedures have been developed to measure the immunoglobulin on the surface (**p**latelet **a**ssociated **i**mmun**o**g**l**obulin [PAIg]), as well as the total platelet immunoglobulin. Circulating platelets contain two distinct pools of IgG: surface associated and intracellular, within α-granules (αG). Normally, the platelet surface has fewer than 200 Ig molecules, while the αG contain approximately 20,000 Ig molecules. The internal immunoglobulin is absorbed from the plasma in proportion to the plasma concentration and, therefore, does not necessarily correlate with an immune process that is destroying the platelets.[1] Although the amount of platelet immunoglobulin is increased in many patients with immune thrombocytopenia, platelet immunoglobulins are also increased in several conditions not associated with the immune destruction of platelets.[2]

If performed, bone marrow aspiration evaluates the megakaryocytes and rules out other causes of thrombocytopenia.[1] The granulocyte and erythrocyte precursors show

✪ TABLE 31-6
Classification of Thrombocytopenia Caused by Increased Destruction
Immune mechanisms of destruction
• Immune thrombocytopenic purpura
Acute
Chronic
Transplacental
• Alloimmune thrombocytopenia
Neonatal (NAIT)
Post-transfusion purpura
• Drugs
Quinidine/quinine
Heparin
• Other diseases
Nonimmune mechanisms of destruction
• Disseminated intravascular coagulation
• Thrombotic thrombocytopenic purpura
• Hemolytic uremic syndrome
• Mechanical destruction by artificial heart valves

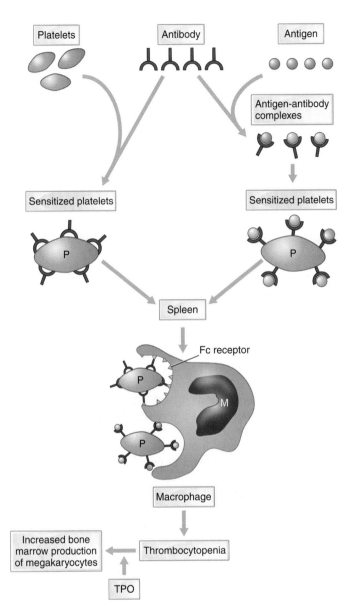

■ **FIGURE 31-4** Mechanisms of thrombocytopenia caused by immune destruction of platelets. In immune thrombocytopenic purpura, antibody-sensitized platelets are recognized by Fc receptors of the splenic mononuclear phagocyte system and eliminated from the circulation. The bone marrow is stimulated by thrombopoietin and produces increased numbers of megakaryocytes. Thrombocytopenia develops if immune destruction exceeds the compensatory capacity of the marrow. The antibody can also injure megakaryocytes.

normal development with no abnormal cells present. Megakaryocytes are increased, often markedly, reflecting stimulation by thrombopoietin (TPO) to increase platelet production. In cases of severe thrombocytopenia, the marrow can increase production up to five times normal. The ploidy of megakaryocytes also can be increased, resulting in a larger cytoplasmic mass and an increased number of platelets produced per megakaryocyte (∞ Chapter 29). How-

ever, a majority of the megakaryocytes often are young forms showing scant cytoplasm and lack of lobulation of the nucleus. Vacuoles in the cytoplasm have been described, which likely reflect the rapid turnover of megakaryocytes rather than abnormal morphology.

The mean platelet volume (MPV), as measured electronically, is increased in immune thrombocytopenia and can be a helpful clue for diagnosis. The peripheral blood smear has increased numbers of platelets that are $>2.5 \mu m$ in diameter.[1] An inverse relationship generally exists between the platelet count and the number of large platelets when the count is less than $50 \times 10^9/L$. TPO levels are generally normal in immune thrombocytopenias.

Autoimmune Thrombocytopenia   The most common form of thrombocytopenia is **immune thrombocytopenic purpura (ITP),** formerly called idiopathic thrombocytopenic purpura. ITP is an autoimmune disorder in which autoreactive antibodies bind to platelets, shortening the platelet life span. The clinical presentation can vary from an asymptomatic thrombocytopenia to severe mucosal bleeding. Because of the difficulty in identifying platelet-specific antibodies, the diagnosis of ITP is made by exclusion (i.e., ruling out all other causes of thrombocytopenia). It is based on the patient's history and physical examination, complete blood counts, and examination of the blood smear. Except for thrombocytopenia, the findings on a peripheral blood smear are within normal limits for the age of the patient unless an underlying condition exists. Other tests are usually not indicated.

The clinical features of ITP in children and adults are different. Children usually have an acute form of ITP, while adults have a chronic form of the disease (Table 31-7 ❖). Acute ITP occurs most often in children 2–4 years of age, shows no gender preference, and often follows a viral infection by 1–3 weeks. Nonspecific upper respiratory infections, chickenpox, rubella, cytomegalovirus, and viral hepatitis are some diseases that have been associated with ITP in children.

The platelet count is often less than $20 \times 10^9/L$. There can be an increase in the number of lymphocytes or mild eosinophilia in some cases, most likely related to the preceding infection. The marrow typically shows normal to increased numbers of megakaryocytes,[14] but it is recommended that a bone marrow examination not be done on children with acute ITP unless the thrombocytopenia has persisted for at least 6 months and unless therapy was not helpful.

Symptoms of acute ITP include the abrupt onset of easy bruising, petechiae on the extremities, and bleeding from mucous membranes. Spontaneous bleeding into the central nervous system occurs in fewer than 1% of children whose platelet count is less than $20 \times 10^9/L$ but is the most dreaded consequence of ITP.[15] The spleen is not enlarged, and the patient is afebrile.

Most patients (93%) with acute ITP experience a spontaneous remission within 2–6 weeks of the onset of the illness,[1,14] and the disease does not recur in these patients.

⊘ TABLE 31-7

Comparative Features of Acute and Chronic ITP

Feature	Acute ITP	Chronic ITP
Peak age incidence	Children 2–4 years	Adults 20–40 years
Platelet count, initial	$<20 \times 10^9$/L	$30–80 \times 10^9$/L
Onset of bleeding	Abrupt	Insidious
Type of bleeding	Petechiae and superficial	Petechiae and superficial
Antecedent infection	Common 1–3 weeks prior	Unusual
Gender predilection	None	Females 3:1
Eosinophilia	Common	Rare
Lymphocytosis	Common	Rare
Hemorrhagic bullae in mouth	Present in severe cases	Usually absent
Duration	2–6 weeks	Months or years (lifetime)
Spontaneous remissions	Occur in 93% of cases	Rare; course of disease fluctuates
Therapy	Corticosteroids, anti-D, IVIg	Corticosteroids, splenectomy

IVIg = intravenous immunoglobulin

Some patients fail to achieve a remission by 6 months and are then said to have the chronic form of the disease.

Treatment for patients with acute ITP includes prevention of trauma to reduce the risk of bleeding and simple observation to see that the symptoms subside and the platelet count increases. Because of the high spontaneous remission rate, most patients usually require no specific treatment. The goal of treating patients, if needed, is to raise the platelet count to a level that supports adequate hemostasis as rapidly as possible while preventing life-threatening bleeding. The type of therapy recommended depends on whether the patient is actively bleeding or is *at risk* of bleeding. In general, replacement therapy with platelet transfusions should be used only in life-threatening situations. Some physicians give steroids in an attempt to reduce the risk of bleeding into the central nervous system, but steroids have undesirable side effects.[1] The platelet count increases at a faster rate if a pooled preparation of immunoglobulins (IVIg) or anti-D prepared from donors with high titers of anti-D antibodies (WinRho®) is given. Anti-D binds to D-positive erythrocytes, and splenic mononuclear phagocytes then destroy the sensitized red cells instead of the sensitized platelets.[16] This therapy is limited, therefore, to Rh positive individuals.

✓ Checkpoint! 3

How many platelets per 1000× field would you expect to observe on the peripheral smear of a patient with acute ITP?

Chronic ITP is defined as persistent thrombocytopenia lasting more than 6 to 12 months.[14] The chronic form of ITP differs from acute ITP in several aspects including typical patient age, female predominance, insidious onset, and initial platelet count (Table 31-7). Chronic ITP rarely has a spontaneous resolution.

The diagnosis is made based on the patient's history, physical examination, peripheral blood counts, and blood smear examination. From 30% to 40% of adult patients with ITP are asymptomatic and are diagnosed only by the incidental finding of a low platelet count.[17] Bleeding symptoms are rare unless the thrombocytopenia is severe. As in acute ITP, the erythrocyte and leukocyte morphology are usually normal with thrombocytopenia being the only significant finding.[14] Bone marrow examination is not recommended unless it is necessary to rule out other diseases with similar presentation, such as acute leukemia, aplastic anemia, or myelodysplastic syndrome. No other testing is recommended unless the patient is at risk for HIV infection.[18]

Antiplatelet autoantibodies can be identified in 58–80% of patients with chronic ITP. Most are directed toward epitopes on either GPIIb/IIIa or GPIb/IX; however, the exact antigenic stimulation is unknown.[13] Although the numbers of megakaryocytes in the bone marrow are normal or increased, platelet production is generally decreased to low normal (rather than a compensatory increase as might be expected) probably due to the effect of antiplatelet antibodies on the marrow megakaryocytes.[17] Most patients have normal platelet function, but some patients have impaired platelet function, likely due to antibody binding to the GPIIb/IIIa or GPIb/IX receptors (producing in essence an "acquired" Glanzmann thrombasthenia or Bernard Soulier syndrome).

The goal of ITP treatment is to reach a safe platelet count, not a normal platelet count.[17] Patients with chronic ITP are treated only if their platelet counts are less than 30×10^9/L or if symptoms necessitate it. Corticosteroids are recommended and result in a durable complete response in two-thirds of patients. Splenectomy is advised for patients who are unresponsive and symptomatic after treatment with corticosteroids because the spleen is a major site of antibody production as well as the destruction of the platelets.[18] Splenectomy is successful in a majority of patients, although relapse occurs in 10% to 12% within 1–5 years. The decision to splenectomize the patient usually rests on the patient's previous responses to different treatment modalities. The major risk of splenectomy is overwhelming bacterial sepsis; thus, immunization against encapsulated bacteria at least two weeks prior to surgery is recommended.[13]

Some patients are refractory to both corticosteroid therapy and splenectomy. IVIg improves the platelet count temporarily, but anti-D is not recommended for patients with chronic ITP.[14] For patients who are refractory to this therapy, the most aggressive treatments include chemotherapeutic agents such as vincristine or vinblastine or immunosuppressive therapies such as cyclosporin. Rituximab, an anti-CD20 monoclonal antibody, is a targeted immunotherapy directed specifically toward B lymphocytes. It has been reported to induce complete or partial response in 50% of patients.

The clinical course of ITP in some patients consists of alternate periods of remission within 6 months of the onset followed by relapse after at least 3 months. This is referred to as an *intermittent* form of the disease.

Transplacental (or neonatal) ITP is an immune form of thrombocytopenia that occurs in newborn infants of mothers with ITP. It is estimated to affect 1–2 of every 10,000 pregnancies.[19] Approximately 15% to 65% of newborns of mothers with ITP have thrombocytopenia at birth. Between 6% and 70% of them will have severe thrombocytopenia with platelet counts of less than 50×10^9/L. The maternal platelet count does not correlate with that of the fetus, so there is no way to predict which neonates will be at risk. The major hazard is intracranial bleeding during delivery. Thrombocytopenia lasts an average of 3–4 weeks postdelivery until the maternal antibody is cleared from the newborn's system.[19]

Alloimmune Thrombocytopenias Immune platelet destruction can be caused by alloantibodies stimulated by foreign antigens during pregnancy or after blood transfusions. **Neonatal alloimmune thrombocytopenia (NAIT)** is similar to hemolytic disease of the newborn except that the antibodies are directed toward platelet antigens rather than erythrocyte antigens. Platelet destruction in the newborn is due to maternal alloantibodies formed against a platelet-specific antigen the baby inherited from the father and that the mother lacks.[13]

The most frequently encountered platelet antigen causing NAIT is HPA-1a (PLA1). Approximately 97% of Caucasian people have the HPA-1a antigen, but 3% are homozygous for the alternate allele HPA-1b (PLA2) and will be immunized if exposed to HPA-1a.[13] When maternal IgG antiplatelet antibodies cross the placenta, immune destruction of the infant's platelets occurs. Figure 31-5a ■ shows a proposed

mechanism of attaching alloimmune or autoimmune antibodies to the platelet surface.

Symptoms appear at or shortly after birth and are self-limited. There is, however, a high mortality rate due to bleeding into the central nervous system. This may be a result of birth trauma that is complicated by the natural low levels of certain coagulation proteins in the fetus and newborn (∞ Chapter 32). Thus, it is important to recognize NAIT and treat it with IVIg or transfusion with HPA-1a negative platelets as soon as possible.[12]

Rarely patients develop severe alloimmune thrombocytopenia 7–10 days after blood transfusion (post-transfusion purpura). Symptoms such as bleeding from mucous membranes and purpura begin abruptly and last 2–6 weeks. The alloantibody is usually directed against the HPA-1a antigen, but other platelet-specific antigens have been implicated as well. The mechanism of alloantibody destruction of autologous platelets negative for the antigen is controversial, and more than one mechanism may be operative.[13]

Drug-Induced Thrombocytopenia Drug-induced thrombocytopenia is relatively common, and a number of drugs have been implicated as a cause of thrombocytopenia in a small percentage of patients who take them.[1,2] A list of the drugs that have been identified as causing thrombocytopenia is accessible at http://w3.ouhsc.edu/platelets. There is little experimental evidence to establish that some drugs are the actual cause of the decreased platelet count because the thrombocytopenia occurs weeks to months after the drug was first taken. Some drugs can cause a generalized hematopoietic suppression; others cause selective suppression of platelet production. Other drugs cause thrombocytopenia by increasing platelet destruction with circulating immunoglobulins apparently being the cause of the platelet destruction.

More than 200 drugs have been reported to cause thrombocytopenia. Some most commonly reported to cause immunologic thrombocytopenia are quinidine, quinine, gold salts, sulfonamides and derivatives, and heparin. The experimental and clinical association for these drugs is more substantial. In some cases, the offending agent is a metabolite of the drug formed in vivo rather than the original form of the drug.

Symptoms of excess bleeding appear suddenly and can be severe. The platelet count can be very low, often less than 10×10^9/L. Bleeding manifestations include petechiae, purpura, and, occasionally, intracranial hemorrhage. On first exposure, symptoms appear 6–7 days after taking the drug. After the patient has been sensitized, symptoms can occur immediately after taking a dose. Usually the only necessary treatment is withdrawal of the offending drug. When the drug is removed, the drug-dependent antibody cannot bind to the platelets, and the platelet count rises and symptoms subside.[20] The exception is the thrombocytopenia induced by α-methyldopa and gold, a condition in which the antibodies bind to platelets even in the absence of the drug.

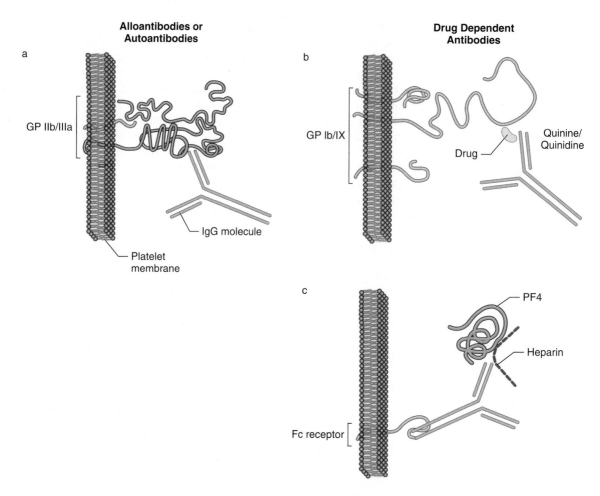

■ FIGURE 31-5   Variations in antibody binding to platelets. **a.** Platelet autoantibodies or alloantibodies bind to epitopes on GPIIb/IIIa, GPIb/X, most frequently, or to other glycoproteins resulting in ITP. **b.** Quinine/quinidine-dependent antibodies bind to a complex of drug and glycoprotein, usually either GP-Ib/IX or IIb/IIIa. **c.** Heparin binds platelet factor 4 and the heparin/PF4 complex attaches to IgG antiheparin antibodies via the Fab combining site. The Fc portion of the antibody binds to platelet IgG Fc$_\gamma$IIa receptors.

Three pathways have been proposed to explain drug-induced immune-mediated platelet destruction. The first mechanism, the *hapten theory,* proposes that the drug binds covalently with platelets to form a drug-platelet antigenic complex, and the drug acts as a hapten. A drug-dependent antibody is formed that recognizes and binds to this complex. However, few studies support the hapten model of antibody formation except for perhaps the thrombocytopenia seen with large doses of penicillin. The second model was the *innocent bystander mechanism* in which the drug binds to a plasma protein and elicits an antibody response. Antibody binding to the drug-protein complex forms an immune complex that nonspecifically binds to circulating platelet Fc receptors (Figure 31-5c ■). Again, with the exception of some heparin-induced thrombocytopenias, most drugs do not appear to work via this mechanism.

The most common mechanism is the formation of drug-dependent antibodies against epitopes created by the association of the drug with proteins on the platelet surface. The association can be a specific ligand-receptor interaction, often with GPIIb/IIIa molecules, or a nonspecific noncovalent interaction. Some drugs can create neoepitopes for antibody formation by interacting with the platelet surface glycoproteins. Antibodies to quinidine and quinine bind to either drug/GPIb/IX or drug/GPIIb/IIIa complexes on the platelet surface by their Fab portions (Figure 31-5b ■).

The mechanism of platelet destruction is similar to that described previously: antibodies bind to the platelet, and the mononuclear phagocyte system removes the platelet. Drug-induced thrombocytopenias occasionally are caused by inhibition of megakaryocyte proliferation and platelet production as well as destruction of platelets in the circulation.

Heparin can cause thrombocytopenia via two mechanisms, one immune mediated (**heparin-induced thrombocytopenia [HIT]**) and the other nonimmune mediated (**heparin-associated thrombocytopenia [HAT]**). Heparin is used for the prevention or treatment of thrombosis (∞ Chapter 33). In some patients, heparin causes a direct platelet activation effect, a nonimmune mediated thrombocytopenia, resulting in HAT. *HIT* refers to the situation characterized by immune-mediated destruction of platelets due to heparin-dependent, platelet-activating IgG antibodies that recognize complexes of platelet factor 4 (PF-4) bound to heparin. PF-4 is released from platelet αG during platelet activation, binds to heparin in the circulation, and antibodies are produced to the heparin/PF-4 complex. The antibody/heparin/PF-4 complex then attaches to the platelet surface via the platelet FcγIIa receptors, resulting in increased platelet clearance and thrombocytopenia. Occasionally the antibody-heparin-PF4 complexes can induce platelet activation (Figure 31-5c). The most serious complication of HIT is the activation of the clotting system and thrombosis (∞ Chapter 33). Thrombocytopenia develops in approximately 3% of patients who receive heparin, and thrombosis occurs in one-third of those.[21] For this reason, patients receiving heparin therapy should be monitored with daily platelet counts. For a complete discussion of the role of HIT in inducing thrombosis, ∞ Chapter 33.

Miscellaneous Immune Thrombocytopenias   Immune thrombocytopenia occurs as a secondary feature in many diseases. Although a variety of mechanisms can contribute to thrombocytopenia in these disease states, there appears to be an immune element in collagen diseases, other autoimmune disorders including systemic lupus erythematosus and rheumatoid arthritis, lymphoproliferative disorders such as Hodgkin disease and chronic lymphocytic leukemia, and solid tumors.

Patients with infections can develop an immune-mediated thrombocytopenia. Many infectious agents have been implicated, including the Epstein-Barr virus in infectious mononucleosis, cytomegalovirus, rubella, mumps, HIV, hepatitis, and nonspecific viral infections. Thrombocytopenia occurs in more than one-third of patients with bacterial septicemia, although the platelet count is usually not less than 50×10^9/L and resolves when the infection is treated. Typical features of an immune process accompany the reduced platelet count in infections: shortened platelet survival, increased megakaryocytes in the bone marrow, and large platelets on the peripheral blood smear.[21]

✓ Checkpoint! 4

A 6-year-old boy was brought to his pediatrician because the mother noticed small pinkish spots on his legs. Examination discovered several bruises on his arms and legs. Laboratory tests were ordered. His platelet count was 20×10^9/L, and the PT and APTT were within normal limits. The CBC was normal except for the low platelet count. The boy had no previous history of bleeding. The mother said she had noted the spots after he was given the hepatitis vaccine. What is the most probable type of thrombocytopenia? Should other coagulation tests be performed at this time?

Nonimmune Destruction.   Increased destruction of platelets may occur by processes other than immune-related mechanisms. Platelets can be activated and consumed by aggregation within the circulation. **Disseminated intravascular coagulation (DIC)** is a disorder in which fibrin formation within the blood vessels is associated with platelet activation and consumption (∞ Chapter 32). **Thrombotic thrombocytopenic purpura (TTP)** and **hemolytic uremic syndrome (HUS)** are conditions in which platelets are activated without generalized activation of the coagulation cascade. These are discussed in ∞ Chapter 33 with other hypercoagulable disorders and briefly in ∞ Chapter 20 with other causes of hemolytic anemias (erythrocyte destruction is also a classic feature of these disorders).

Mechanical destruction of platelets occurs in patients with artificial heart valves or vascular grafts. Platelets are destroyed by adhering to the artificial prosthesis or by mechanical rupture as the valves open and close against them.

Decreased Production   A second category of disorders causing thrombocytopenia is characterized by failure of the bone marrow to deliver adequate numbers of platelets to the peripheral blood. The bone marrow function in these disorders is abnormal, and thombocytopenia develops secondarily. Examination of bone marrow smears and sections aids in the identification of the primary condition. The decreased platelet count occurs because of one of the following: (1) megakaryocyte hypoplasia exists in the bone marrow, (2) there is ineffective thrombopoiesis, or (3) the patient has a hereditary condition that affects the ability of the bone marrow to support megakaryocyte growth (Table 31-8 ✪).

Megakaryocyte Hypoplasia Syndromes.   Hypoplasia of megakaryocytes (Figure 31-3) can result from either decreased proliferation of megakaryocytes in the bone marrow or replacement of the bone marrow by neoplastic disease, fibrosis, or granulomatous inflammation. All three myeloid cell lineages can be affected or only the megakaryocytes.

Decreased Megakaryocyte Proliferation   The most frequent cause of marrow hypoplasia is drug or radiation therapy for malignant disease. Chemotherapeutic agents and radiotherapy produce generalized marrow suppression affecting all three lineages. The marrow usually regenerates shortly after the therapy is stopped, but the megakaryocytes are often the last lineage to recover.

Aplastic Anemia   Megakaryocytes are decreased in aplastic anemia, a bone marrow disease characterized by pancytopenia and bone marrow hypoplasia. Acquired and constitutional aplastic anemias are discussed in ∞ Chapter 13. In acquired aplastic anemia, a decreased platelet count may appear before hypoplasia of other cell lineages and may be the last lineage to return to normal after recovery. Platelet size (mean platelet volume [MPV]) is normal in aplastic conditions in contrast to the increased MPV seen in immune-mediated thrombocytopenia. Platelets can, however,

⊗ TABLE 31-8

Causes of Decreased Platelet Production

Hypoplasia of megakaryocytes
- Decreased megakaryocyte proliferation
    - Chemotherapy and radiation therapy for malignant disease
    - Aplastic anemias
        - Acquired
        - Congenital/Hereditary
            - Fanconi anemia
            - Congenital amegakaryocytic thrombocytopenia (CAMT)
            - Congenital thrombocytopenia with radioulnar synostosis (CTRUS)
        - Isolated megakaryocyte hypoplasia
        - Thrombocytopenia with absent radii (TAR)
- Replacement of normal marrow
    - Leukemias and lymphomas
    - Myelodysplastic syndromes
    - Other neoplastic diseases at times
    - Fibrosis or granulomatous inflammation

Ineffective thrombopoiesis
- Megaloblastic anemia

Hereditary thrombocytopenia
- Wiscott-Aldrich syndrome/X-linked thrombocytopenia
- Bernard-Soulier syndrome
- May-Hegglin anomaly

---

demonstrate an increased variation in size as indicated by the platelet distribution width (PDW) on electronic instruments. TPO levels are increased in patients with aplastic anemia in contrast to normal levels in immune-mediated platelet destruction.

Several hereditary disorders result in a congenital aplastic anemia. **Fanconi anemia (FA)** (∞ Chapter 13) is a congenital disorder characterized by chromosomal instability, defective DNA repair mechanisms, and progressive bone marrow hypoplasia, eventually resulting in aplastic anemia in ~90% of affected patients. At least eight different genes have been associated with the development of FA.[22]

Congenital amegakaryocytic thrombocytopenia (CAMT) presents with isolated hypomegakaryocytic thrombocytopenia during the first years of life but eventually converts into bone marrow failure and aplastic anemia, usually between the ages of 3–20.[23] The molecular basis for most patients has been identified as a mutation within the gene for the thrombopoietin receptor, TPO-R (c-mpl). The evolution from an isolated thrombocytopenia to complete marrow hypoplasia underscores the importance of TPO and its receptor in the maintenance of hematopoietic stem cells.

Congenital thrombocytopenia with radioulnar synostosis (CTRUS) is also a congenital disorder presenting as an isolated amegakaryocytic thrombocytopenia that evolves into aplastic anemia.[23] Most patients have a mutation within the *HOXA11* gene, resulting in a truncated HOXA11 protein, an important regulatory protein for development of both hemopoietic and bone tissue. The abnormal bone morphology usually presents as a union of the ulna and radius by osseous tissue.

Thrombocytopenia with absent radii (TAR) is an inherited condition characterized by isolated hypoplasia of the megakaryocyte lineage, thrombocytopenia, and bilateral radial aplasia. Other skeletal malformations occasionally may be seen. The thrombocytopenia is usually severe only during the first years of life with a gradual improvement in platelet count to within normal values in adulthood. No mutations within the genes for TPO or TPO-R have been identified, and the defect is assumed to be an abnormality in the TPO/TPO-R signaling pathway.[23]

Replacement of Normal Marrow. Abnormal cells, malignant or nonmalignant, can replace normal marrow causing decreased numbers of megakaryocytes (as well as the precursor cells for the other marrow lineages). Some myelodysplastic syndromes have decreased platelets as part of their pathology (∞ Chapter 23). The bone marrow may have normal or increased numbers of megakaryocytes, many of which are micromegakaryocytes and dysplastic forms. Peripheral blood platelets also can have abnormal morphology and abnormal function as indicated in the platelet aggregation tests. Marrow replacement by solid tumors or by fibrous tissue, as in chronic idiopathic myelofibrosis, sometimes results in thrombocytopenia, although thrombocytosis is more common. Abnormal platelet morphology, such as large and/or hypogranular forms, can be present.

Ineffective Thrombopoiesis. Megaloblastic anemias caused by a deficiency of vitamin B_{12} or folic acid are characterized by ineffective thrombopoiesis as well as ineffective erythropoiesis and granulopoiesis (Figure 31-3) (∞ Chapter 12). Pancytopenia is often seen in these diseases. The bone marrow contains normal or increased numbers of megakaryocytes, but the number of platelets entering the peripheral blood is decreased.

Hereditary Thrombocytopenia. Wiskott-Aldrich syndrome, Bernard-Soulier syndrome, and May-Hegglin anomaly are inherited disorders in which platelet production is decreased. These disorders also demonstrate other abnormalities.

The **Wiskott-Aldrich Syndrome (WAS)**, an X-linked disorder, is characterized by very small platelets, thrombocytopenia, and severe immune dysregulation (eczema and infections) due to a progressive decline in T lymphocyte number and function.[23] The *WAS* gene codes for a protein expressed exclusively in hematopoietic cells that is involved in cell signaling and regulation of the cytoskeleton. **X-linked thrombocytopenia (XLT)** results from mutations within the *WAS* gene, which manifest as an isolated thrombocytopenia without the immune dysfunction seen in WAS. WAS platelets show decreased aggregation to ADP, epinephrine and collagen, and reduced numbers of dense granules.

Bernard-Soulier syndrome (BSS) is characterized by both thrombocytopenia and dysfunctional platelets and is discussed later in this chapter. **May-Hegglin anomaly (MHA)** is characterized by a moderate macrothrombocytopenia and Döhle-like inclusions in leukocytes and is one of a group of disorders associated with abnormalities of the *MYH9* gene (nonmuscle myosin gene). MHA is discussed in ∞ Chapter 19.

 Checkpoint! 5

What is the pathophysiology of thrombocytopenia in megaloblastic anemia?

Increased Splenic Sequestration The spleen normally stores ~one-third of the platelets produced and released by the bone marrow in a pool that is in equilibrium with circulating platelets. In some conditions in which the spleen is enlarged (congestive splenomegaly and reactive splenomegaly or hypersplenism), the proportion of platelets sequestered also is increased and can reach 90% of the total platelet mass.[19] Because the bone marrow production remains constant, the number of circulating platelets decreases. The platelet count is usually above 20×10^9/L, and symptoms of excess bleeding usually are not seen.

Most causes of thrombocytopenia resulting from splenomegaly are complicated by other factors that also contribute to it. It is rare for splenomegaly to occur as an isolated event. Examples of diseases in which splenomegaly is found include hepatic cirrhosis with portal hypertension, hemolytic anemia, Gaucher's disease and other storage diseases, Felty's syndrome, leukemias, and lymphomas. Bone marrow infiltration with the malignant cells can complicate the decreased platelet count in lymphomas.

Some myeloproliferative disorders are characterized by splenomegaly but increased platelet counts. In these conditions, the number of platelets sequestered increases, but the spleen also can be involved in producing platelets (extramedullary hematopoiesis).

Hypersplenism is a condition in which the spleen is enlarged and is hyperactive with an increase in the number of macrophages. Platelets are removed by increased pooling and by increased phagocytosis. Platelet size in hypersplenism is normal. The enlarged spleen can simultaneously sequester erythrocytes and neutrophils.

Dilutional Thrombocytopenia Patients who experience massive hemorrhage requiring replacement of 10 or more units of blood within 24 hours can develop thrombocytopenia if stored banked blood alone is used for transfusion. Because of the relatively short half-life of platelets, minimal viable platelets are in banked blood. Bleeding occurs in 20% to 60% of patients who receive 20 units or more

of transfused blood. Certain coagulation factors are also deficient in stored blood, possibly contributing to the bleeding diathesis. Recommendations for patients receiving massive transfusions are to monitor the platelet count, PT, and APTT and to administer platelet concentrates to maintain the platelet count at 75×10^9/L.[24]

Conditions with Multiple Mechanisms of Thrombocytopenia Thrombocytopenia in some conditions is the result of more than one mechanism (Table 31-9 ✪). In alcoholic patients without cirrhosis, the major effect of ethanol is on the platelets. When cirrhosis is present, coagulation factors can also be affected. Alcohol reduces platelet numbers and causes defects of aggregation, release, and procoagulant activity. Platelet production is suppressed by a direct toxic effect of alcohol on the bone marrow, which can be compounded by ineffective production associated with a deficiency of folate. Also, decreased TPO production by the liver contributes to a reduced thrombopoiesis. Patients with cirrhosis have enlarged spleens due to passive congestion, also contributing to thrombocytopenia.

In lymphoproliferative disease, when the tumor affects the bone marrow, production of platelets is impaired. Additionally, the production of autoantibodies can enhance platelet destruction. If splenomegaly is present, increased sequestration by the spleen can contribute to the thrombocytopenia.

During cardiopulmonary bypass surgery, the patient's blood circulates through a pump outside the body to be oxygenated. Hemostasis is altered in a variety of ways. The platelet count is decreased to approximately one-half of the presurgical level because of the dilution by IV fluids and donor blood if transfusions were necessary. Platelet counts

✪ **TABLE 31-9**

Conditions with Multiple Mechanisms
of Thrombocytopenia

Alcoholism
- Suppress platelet production
- Ineffective platelet production
- Increased destruction
- Splenomegaly

Lymphoproliferative disease
- Impaired production
- Immune destruction
- Splenomegaly

Cardiopulmonary bypass surgery
- Mechanical destruction
- Increased utilization
- Dilutional thrombocytopenia
- Inadequate neutralization of heparin

usually remain above 100×10^9/L during the procedure but can take several days to correct to the patient's normal concentration. Platelets can be activated or mechanically damaged by the artificial surfaces encountered during the procedure.[25] Additional effects of extracorporeal circulation are discussed in later sections.

⊘ CASE STUDY *(continued from page 677)*

Mohammed's laboratory results were:

Hematology	Hemostasis
WBC 10.5×10^9/L	Prothrombin time 11.2 sec
RBC 2.3×10^{12}/L	APTT 25.6 sec
Hb 6.6 g/dL (66 g/L)	
Hct 0.193 L/L	
Platelet count 133×10^9/L	

3. Explain how these laboratory tests confirm that the patient's bleeding is related to a defect in primary hemostasis rather than secondary hemostasis.

4. Is the bleeding more likely related to problems with the vascular system or with platelets? Why?

5. Is this profuse bleeding with the presence of petechiae consistent with the platelet count? Why?

6. What additional testing would be helpful to identify the cause of the patient's excess bleeding?

Thrombocytosis

Thrombocytosis is the general term for a platelet count that is elevated above the established reference range. On the peripheral smear, more than 20 platelets are seen per $100 \times$ oil immersion field, and they can appear in large clumps on capillary or first drop smears. They can be more concentrated on the featheredge of a smear.

Sustained increases in platelet numbers are the result of increased production by the bone marrow because the platelet's life span is not increased. Bone marrow megakaryocytes are increased on histologic sections and can be found in clusters. On buffy coat smears from the marrow, significant numbers of megakaryocytes can be present on the featheredge and throughout the body of the smear. Table 31-10 ⊘ shows primary and secondary conditions associated with thrombocytosis.

Primary Thrombocytosis   In **primary thrombocytosis,** megakaryocyte proliferation and maturation bypass the normal regulatory mechanisms. Uncontrolled or autonomous production of megakaryocytes in the bone marrow results in a marked increase in the number of circulating platelets. The platelet count is usually more than 1000×10^9/L. In the bone marrow, megakaryocyte hyperplasia as well as giant megakaryocytes with increased ploidy are seen.

⊘ TABLE 31-10

Causes of Thrombocytosis

Primary thrombocytosis
- Essential thrombocythemia
- Chronic myelogenous leukemia
- Polycythemia vera
- Chronic idiopathic myelofibrosis
- Refractory anemia with ringed sideroblasts
- 5q– syndrome

Secondary (reactive) thrombocytosis
- Acute hemorrhage
- Surgery
- Post splenectomy
- Recovery from thrombocytopenia
    Alcohol-induced thrombocytopenia
    Chemotherapeutic drugs
    Therapy of cobalamin deficiency
- Malignant diseases
- Chronic inflammatory diseases
- Iron-deficiency anemia
- Hemolytic anemia

Transient thrombocytosis
- Vigorous exercise
- Epinephrine
- Childbirth

Thrombocytosis occurs in both the chronic myeloproliferative disorders and myelodysplasia (∞ Chapters 22 and 23). In essential thrombocythemia (∞ Chapter 22), the megakaryocyte lineage predominates. Thirty-five percent of patients with refractory anemia with ringed sideroblasts and some patients with the 5q– syndrome have thrombocytosis, but the platelet count is usually less than 1000×10^9/L (∞ Chapter 23).[26]

Patients with myeloproliferative disorders can have either hemorrhagic or thrombotic episodes; the cause of these episodes is not always known. Although thrombotic complications are slightly more frequent than bleeding symptoms in general, patients with chronic myelogenous leukemia only rarely develop thrombosis. Hemorrhagic symptoms are present in approximately one-fourth of patients despite the increased numbers of platelets. Epistaxis and bleeding from the gastrointestinal tract and from other mucous membranes can be quite profuse.

The bleeding time is only rarely prolonged, even in patients with bleeding symptoms, but most patients have abnormal in vitro platelet aggregation. Abnormal platelet aggregation has been demonstrated most frequently with epinephrine but can also be abnormal with ADP and collagen.[26] Screening tests for clotting factors are normal.

Secondary (Reactive) Thrombocytosis

Secondary, thrombocytosis is also called **reactive thrombocytosis** because another disease or condition causes the increased platelet count by normal regulatory mechanisms. The platelet count returns to the reference range by treating the primary condition. The clinical picture is generally related to the underlying condition rather than the thrombocytosis.

Differentiating primary from secondary thrombocytosis can be difficult. Although platelet counts are usually lower than 1000×10^9/L in reactive thrombocytosis, they can be as high as in primary thrombocytosis. The bleeding time and platelet aggregation tests are normal, and hemorrhagic and thrombotic complications are infrequent.[27] IL-6 is increased in most patients with secondary thrombocytosis but not in primary thrombocytosis, however routine testing procedures are not available for this cytokine.

Several conditions associated with reactive thrombocytosis are shown in Table 31-10. The etiology of the increased platelet count varies. After acute hemorrhage or surgery, the platelet count can rise to 600×10^9/L or more but returns to the reference range within a short time. After splenectomy, the platelet count rises, sometimes to more than 1000×10^9/L and can remain elevated for several months. The rise in platelet count exceeds that expected for the loss of the splenic reservoir function, indicating that the spleen plays a role in regulating platelet production. Rebound thrombocytosis can follow recovery from thrombocytopenia in alcoholics and patients on chemotherapeutic drugs, or after therapy for vitamin B_{12} deficiency. Platelet counts in patients with iron deficiency anemia vary from thrombocytopenic to $>1000 \times 10^9$/L. In adults with iron deficiency anemia due to chronic blood loss, thrombocytosis is commonly reported (50–75% of patients), and the platelet count returns to normal after iron replacement. Thrombocytosis is thought to occur in hemolytic anemias due to the stimulation of the bone marrow by hematopoietic growth factors to produce erythrocytes resulting in stimulation of other lineages as well.

Transient Thrombocytosis

Platelet counts rise transiently in the conditions listed in Table 31-10.

 Checkpoint! 6

Explain why primary thrombocytosis is often associated with abnormal platelet function while secondary thrombocytosis is not.

Artifacts in the Quantitative Measurement of Platelets

The laboratory must be aware of artifacts responsible for erroneously (spuriously) low or high platelet counts in automated electronic platelet counting.[28] Recognition of these artifacts can prevent misdiagnosis and inappropriate or unnecessary diagnostic procedures and therapy. In many cases, these errors can be reduced by examining a blood smear. Pseudothrombocytopenia is an in vitro artifact of automated cell counting seen when blood is collected in EDTA. Aggregates of platelets, or platelet satellitism (platelets bound to neutrophils), are common findings on the peripheral smear. (∞ Chapters 34 and 41 describe these artifacts in more detail and offer suggestions for resolving the descrepancies.)

 CASE STUDY *(continued from page 688)*

Mohammed's hematology report included a finding that at least 65% of the platelets were large and giant forms with intense granulation.

7. Is there a possibility that the patient's platelet count is spuriously increased or decreased? Why?

QUALITATIVE (FUNCTIONAL) PLATELET DISORDERS

The functions of platelets in primary hemostasis were discussed in ∞ Chapter 29. The platelet's roles in hemostasis include platelet adhesion, contraction, release of ADP, generation of thromboxane A_2, aggregation, and procoagulant activity. Inherited or acquired abnormalities in any phase of platelet function can lead to defective formation of a primary hemostatic plug and abnormal bleeding.

Clinical symptoms vary from asymptomatic to mild, easy bruisability to severe, life-threatening hemorrhaging depending on the nature of the defect. The type of bleeding is similar to that seen in thrombocytopenic disorders. Common manifestations include petechiae, easy and spontaneous bruising, bleeding from mucous membranes such as the nose or gastrointestinal tract, abnormal vaginal bleeding, and prolonged bleeding from trauma.

Laboratory screening test results are similar to those found in thrombocytopenia except that the platelet count is usually normal. A mildly decreased platelet count, however, is characteristic of some conditions. The bleeding time is often prolonged, and in patients who are also thombocytopenic, is increased more than expected for the degree of thrombocytopenia. Screening tests for coagulation factors (PT, APTT) and tests for fibrinolysis are normal. Special laboratory tests for platelet function reflect the nature of the platelet defect.

Platelet functional disorders are classified as hereditary or acquired. The inheritance pattern in the hereditary types is usually autosomal recessive.

Hereditary Disorders of Platelet Function

Hereditary platelet defects are rarely encountered clinically. However, much of the present knowledge of platelet

⊙ TABLE 31-11

Inherited Disorders of Platelet Function

Disorders of adhesion (defects in platelet-vessel wall interaction)
- von Willebrand disease (deficiency/defect in plasma VWF)
- Bernard-Soulier syndrome (deficiency/defect in GPIb/IX)

Disorders of aggregation (defects in platelet–platelet interaction)
- Congenital afibrinogenemia (deficiency of plasma fibrinogen)
- Glanzmann thrombasthenia (deficiency/defect in GP IIb/IIIa)

Disorders of platelet secretion and abnormalities of granules
- Storage pool deficiency (δSPD; αSPD)
- Quebec platelet disorder

Disorders of platelet secretion and signal transduction
- Receptor defects (defects in platelet-agonist interaction) (Receptor defects: TXA_2, ADP, collagen, epinephrine, serotonin)
- Defects in G-protein activation
- Defects in phosphatidylinositol metabolism (phospholipase C deficiency)
- Defects in protein phosphorylation (PKC deficiency)
- Abnormalities in arachidonic acid pathways and TXA_2 synthesis (deficiency of phospholipase A2, cyclooxygenase, thromboxane synthase)

Disorders of platelet coagulant-protein interaction (Scott syndrome)

function has been derived from the study of patients with such anomalies. Defects in each phase of platelet function have been described (Table 31-11 ⊙). A convenient classification scheme is based on the steps in platelet function. Abnormalities in function can be related to affected portions of the platelet ultrastructure (Figure 31-6 ■).

Disorders of Platelet Adhesion   Adhesion to collagen requires the presence of both an adequate amount of functional von Willebrand factor (VWF) and the presence of functional GPIb/IX on the platelet membrane (∞ Chapter 29). VWF is a bridge binding the platelet via GPIb/IX to collagen. Disorders of platelet adhesion include deficiencies of either VWF (von Willebrand Disease) or GP Ib/IX (Bernard-Soulier syndrome). Because adhesion to collagen is the major mechanism initiating platelet function, aggregation and formation of the primary hemostatic plug are also defective.

Bernard-Soulier Syndrome.   **Bernard-Soulier syndrome (BSS)** is a rare autosomal-recessive disorder first described by Bernard and Soulier in 1948.[29] The incidence is less than 1 in 1,000,000.[30] BSS is characterized by a moderate to severe thrombocytopenia and abnormal platelet function. Homozygous patients have a lifelong bleeding tendency that can begin in infancy. Bleeding symptoms are similar to those

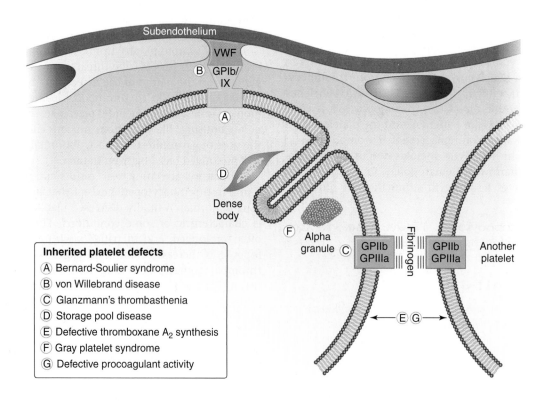

Inherited platelet defects
- (A) Bernard-Soulier syndrome
- (B) von Willebrand disease
- (C) Glanzmann's thrombasthenia
- (D) Storage pool disease
- (E) Defective thromboxane A_2 synthesis
- (F) Gray platelet syndrome
- (G) Defective procoagulant activity

■ FIGURE 31-6   Ultrastructural components associated with inherited disorders of platelet function.

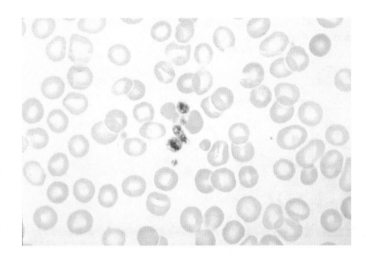

■ **FIGURE 31-7**   Platelet morphology in Bernard-Soulier syndrome. (Peripheral blood, Wright-Giemsa stain, 1000× magnification)

described for thrombocytopenia. Heterozygous persons usually have no significant bleeding symptoms.[30]

BSS is sometimes called the *giant platelet syndrome* because of the appearance of the platelets on a peripheral blood smear. More than 60% and up to 80% of platelets are increased in size with a diameter between 2.5 and 8.0 μm, occasionally up to 20 μm (Figure 31-7 ■). The cause and signifi-

cance of the large size is unknown. Platelets also have an increase in the number of dense granules proportional to their increase in size.[30]

The defect in BSS is a quantitative decrease or abnormal function of the GPIb/IX complex. It results from a mutation in one of the genes that code for the proteins in the complex: GPIbα, GPIbβ, or GPIX. Lack of functional GPIb/IX prevents interaction of the platelets with VWF and the subsequent platelet adhesion to collagen (Figure 31-6a). More than 600 genetic mutations associated with BSS have been identified (see www.bernardsoulier.org).

Laboratory tests are required to diagnose this disease and differentiate it from other platelet functional disorders and other causes of thrombocytopenia (Table 31-12 ✪). Examination of the peripheral blood smear typically reveals thrombocytopenia and the abnormal platelet morphology. The platelet count can be normal or slightly decreased and is variable over time in the same patient. The bleeding time is prolonged more than expected for the degree of thrombocytopenia, indicating a coexistent disorder of platelet function. Platelet aggregation studies are normal with ADP, collagen, and epinephrine. However, agglutination with ristocetin, which requires VWF and GPIb/IX, is abnormal[30] (Figure 31-8a ■) (∞ Chapter 40).

Similar platelet aggregation results are obtained in patients with VWD. To differentiate them, a modification of

✪ TABLE 31-12

Laboratory Test Results in Selected Platelet Disorders

Disorder	Defective Platelet Component	Platelet Count	Bleeding Time Test	Platelet Aggregation	Closure Time (PFA*)	Other
Bernard-Soulier syndrome	Glycoprotein Ib/IX	Normal or decreased	Increased	Abnormal with ristocetin Normal with ADP, collagen, epinephrine	Increased	Giant platelets
Glanzman thrombasthenia	Glycoprotein IIb/IIIa	Normal	Increased	Abnormal with ADP, collagen, epinephrine Normal with ristocetin	Increased	
δ-storage pool disease	Dense granule deficiency	Normal	Increased	Abnormal secondary aggregation with ADP, epinephrine; abnormal with collagen Normal primary aggregation	Variable	
Gray platelet syndrome	Alpha granule deficiency	Variably decreased	Variable	Normal	Variable	Agranular platelet
Defective thromboxane A_2 synthesis	Deficiency of cyclooxygenase, or TXA_2 synthase	Normal	Increased	Abnormal secondary aggregation with ADP, abnormal with collagen Normal primary aggregation	Increased	

*PFA = Platelet Function Analyzer

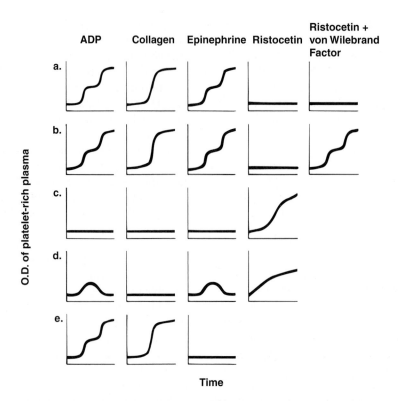

■ FIGURE 31-8   Platelet aggregation patterns in disorders of platelet function. **a.** Bernard-Soulier syndrome. **b.** von Willebrand disease. **c.** Glanzmann's thrombasthenia. **d.** δ-storage pool disease, aspirin ingestion, uremia, thromboxane A$_2$ deficiency. **e.** Myeloproliferative disease.

the ristocetin agglutination test is used. The addition of VWF (e.g., normal plasma) to the patient's platelet suspension does not correct the abnormal ristocetin agglutination in BSS patients but corrects the agglutination defect in VWD (Figure 31-8b■). Also, flow cytometry can characterize the platelet surface GPIb/IX proteins (CD42b/CD42a).

BSS has no specific treatment. Supportive measures such as erythrocyte and platelet transfusions are used as needed.

von Willebrand Disease.   VWD is characterized by a decrease in production of VWF or production of a dysfunctional protein (Figure 31-6b). Because it is a plasma protein disorder rather than a platelet functional disorder, VWD is discussed in ∞ Chapter 32.

Disorders of Platelet Aggregation   Platelet aggregation requires the presence of fibrinogen and the GPIIb/IIIa receptor on the platelet membrane. In the absence of either of these components, platelets do not interact with one another to produce primary or secondary aggregation. The congenital disorder in which the GPIIb/IIIa complex is defective is **Glanzmann's thrombasthenia (GT).** The absence of fibrinogen is discussed in ∞ Chapter 32.

GT is a rare autosomal recessive disease first described in 1918.[31] Clinical manifestations are apparent only in homozygotes.[32] Platelets of patients with GT are deficient in

the GPIIb/IIIa complex (Figure 31-6c), the site of attachment of fibrinogen to the platelet surface. Fibrinogen "bridges" two platelets in the presence of calcium, initiating platelet aggregation (∞ Chapter 29).

Glycoproteins IIb and IIIa are encoded by separate genes closely linked on the long arm of chromosome 17. A deficiency of the whole complex in the platelet membrane occurs when either gene is defective because both proteins are required to form a functional complex. More than 100 different molecular defects of the two genes have been identified (see www.sinaicentral.mssm.edu/intranet/research/glanzmann). Three subtypes of GT[33] have been described: GT Type I is characterized by undetectable or trace amounts (<5%) of GP-IIb/IIIa; GT Type II patients have GPIIb/IIIa of up to 15% of normal; GT Type III is a qualitative defect of GPIIb/IIIa with laboratory diagnostic features of GT except that GPIIb/IIIa levels are 50–100% of normal. Obligate carriers (heterozygotes) of a quantitative defect have 50% to 60% of the complex but are phenotypically normal.[34]

Aggregation in GT does not occur because the platelets lack the site for attachment of fibrinogen. Aspects of platelet function that do not depend on aggregation, such as adhesion and secretion, are usually normal. At low agonist concentrations, however, decreased secretion and TXA$_2$ synthesis can occur. Additional abnormalities of platelets occur in patients with GT, including deficiencies of antigens such as HPA-1a and HPA-1b that are normally present on the GPIIb/IIIa complex. Some patients have a deficiency of fibrinogen in the αGs, presumably due to decreased GPIIb/IIIa-mediated endocytosis of fibrinogen from the plasma.

Bleeding symptoms can begin in infancy and involve superficial areas of the body characteristic of platelet abnormalities. Although they are usually described as moderate in severity, deaths have occurred.

Laboratory tests are necessary to differentiate this disorder from other platelet defects (Table 31-12). The platelet count and morphology are normal, but the bleeding time is markedly prolonged, and clot retraction is abnormal, indicating platelet dysfunction. Platelet aggregation tests show no response to agonists such as ADP, epinephrine, or collagen because the platelets lack the site of attachment of fibrinogen; thus, aggregation cannot occur. Normal agglutination, however, occurs with ristocetin (Figure 31-8c■). Deficiencies of GPIIb or IIIa are identified by flow cytometry of platelets utilizing anti-CD41 or anti-CD61 antibodies and/or observing a quantitative decrease of the proteins using polyacrylamide gel electrophoresis to separate platelet glycoproteins.

No specific treatment is available for thrombasthenic patients. Supportive platelet transfusions are used when needed, and bone marrow transplantation has been performed in rare cases.

Disorders of Platelet Secretion, Granule Abnormalities, and Signal Transduction

Disorders of platelet secretion and signal transduction include a heterogeneous group of disorders that have in common impaired secretion of granule contents and abnormal aggregation during platelet activation. In aggregation studies, the second wave of aggregation has been found to be reduced or absent. The abnormal platelet functions occur either because the granules or their contents are decreased (storage pool deficiency) or because of an abnormality in the activation mechanisms regulating secretion and aggregation. Symptoms vary from moderate to mild bleeding tendencies depending on the abnormality. Manifestations can be easy bruising, hemorrhage, and excess bleeding after surgery or childbirth.[35] The platelet count is normal, and the bleeding time is variable.

Deficiencies of Granules (Storage Pool Diseases/SPD).

An autosomal dominant trait characterized by an isolated decrease in dense granules (DG) is called δ-**storage pool disease.** The platelets in this disorder show a decrease or absence of platelet DG on electron microscopy (Figure 31-6d), but the morphologic appearance of the platelets on stained peripheral blood smears is normal. The bleeding time is usually prolonged (Table 31-12), and platelet aggregation tests are abnormal with ADP, epinephrine (normal primary wave of aggregation, absent or blunted secondary wave) and low levels of collagen (markedly reduced response) (Figure 31-8d■). The platelet aggregation abnormali-

ties are due to the lack of ADP release from the DG so that secondary aggregation does not occur with ADP or epinephrine. The platelet aggregation curve induced by collagen is normally produced by release of endogenous DG products ("secondary aggregation" only) and is therefore absent. The ratio of total platelet ATP:ADP is increased (>2.5).[34] Platelet agglutination studies using ristocetin demonstrate normal results.

Deficiencies of DG also occur as one of the features of several rare autosomal recessive disorders including Chediak-Higashi syndrome, Hermansky-Pudlak syndrome, Wiscott-Aldrich syndrome, and TAR syndrome.

Gray Platelet Syndrome (GPS).

Selective deficiency of platelet α-granules is called the **gray platelet syndrome,** or α-**storage pool disease.** Because αG are so numerous, their absence causes the platelets to appear agranular on a peripheral blood smear. By electron microscopy, αG are absent or markedly decreased. Recent studies indicate that megakaryocyte synthesis of αG contents is normal, and the defect may be in targeting endogenously synthesized proteins to the developing αG.[35] In contrast to δ-storage pool disease, platelet aggregation studies are generally normal, and clinical manifestations are usually mild. Patients can have a mild thrombocytopenia, and the bleeding time can be prolonged (Table 31-12).

Quebec Platelet Disorder.

Quebec platelet disorder is a rare autosomal dominant disorder associated with abnormal proteolysis of αG proteins due to increased levels of platelet urinary-type plasminogen activator.[35] In contrast to GPS, the structure of the αG is preserved, and platelets are morphologically normal by light microscopy. Platelet counts often are moderately decreased, and patients experience a variable bleeding history.

Abnormalities of the Platelet Secretory Mechanism.

These disorders are typically associated with a mild to moderate bleeding history. Patients usually have a prolonged bleeding time, absence of second wave of platelet aggregation with ADP or epinephrine, and decreased aggregation with collagen. They must be differentiated from acquired abnormalities of platelet secretion induced by drugs such as aspirin (see below). Although rare, these disorders as a group are far more common than thrombasthenia (GT), BSS, or SPD.[36]

Defective Thromboxane A_2 (TXA$_2$) Synthesis.

Liberation of arachidonic acid from membrane phospholipids and its conversion to TXA$_2$ is an important positive feedback loop enhancing the platelet activation process (∞ Chapter 29). A defect in the pathway of TXA$_2$ synthesis produces a platelet aggregation pattern similar to that seen in δ-storage pool disease (Figure 31-6d, Table 31-12). Defects can occur in the liberation of arachidonic acid from phospholipids (phospholipase A$_2$ deficiency) and in TXA$_2$ synthesis (cyclooxygenase deficiency or thromboxane synthase deficiency).[37] Platelet secretion and secondary aggregation do not occur.

Signal Transduction Defects.   Various heterogeneous disorders are grouped together as signal transduction defects. The defect can involve platelet-agonist interaction (i.e., defect of the platelet receptor for a specific agonist). In these disorders, patients typically have impaired platelet responses to a single agonist in platelet aggregation assays. Documented receptor defects include receptors for $TXA_2(TP\alpha)$, ADP ($P2Y_{12}$), collagen (GPIa/IIa or GP-VI), epinephrine, and serotonin.[35,36] Other potential defects in platelet secretion and signal transduction are listed in Table 31-11.

Disorders of Platelet Procoagulant Activity

Defective procoagulant activity of platelets has been described as an additional finding in several of the previously mentioned disorders and as a single entity in some patients. **Scott syndrome** is a rare autosomal recessive disorder characterized by abnormal Ca^{2+}-induced phospholipid scrambling. The activated platelets secrete and aggregate normally but fail to transport phosphatidyl serine from the inner to the membrane's outer phospholipid leaflet. As a result, the platelet surface is unable to bind coagulation factors, and thrombin formation is defective.[38,39]

✓ Checkpoint! 7

Compare the results of platelet aggregation studies in platelet adhesion, aggregation, and secretion disorders.

Acquired Disorders of Platelet Function

Platelet dysfunction is induced in a variety of conditions and with the ingestion of certain drugs. Clinical manifestations and the results of laboratory tests vary with the cause and the resulting effect on the platelet mechanism.

Chronic Renal Failure

A bleeding tendency in uremia recognized for many years was first associated with a platelet functional abnormality in 1956. The platelet defect's pathogenesis and severity is related to the accumulation of waste products in the blood, although which of the metabolites produces harmful effects is unclear. The bleeding time is prolonged and seems to correlate with the severity of the renal failure. The platelet aggregation test with collagen and secondary aggregation with ADP and epinephrine is decreased, indicating an abnormal secretory response (Figure 31-8d). Platelet procoagulant activity also is defective.

Bleeding symptoms in uremic patients can be severe. Ecchymoses, gastrointestinal bleeding, and hemorrhages into serous cavities can be seen. The bleeding time shortens, and clinical symptoms decrease with dialysis treatment.

Hematologic Disorders

The bleeding and thrombotic problems in myeloproliferative disorders were described earlier in this chapter. An abnormal response to epinephrine in the platelet aggregation test is a fairly consistent abnormality as well. The response to ADP and collagen appears to be variable (Figure 31-8e).

Defective platelet aggregation has been noted in patients with acute leukemia and myelodysplasia. Bleeding problems in these conditions, however, are usually the result of thrombocytopenia.

In addition to impaired vascular function in patients with dysproteinemias such as multiple myeloma and macroglobulinemia described earlier, abnormal platelet function is observed (∞ Chapter 26). Severe bleeding symptoms can result. Thrombocytopenia and hyperviscosity are the major causes of the bleeding tendency, but platelet function is abnormal because the paraprotein coats the platelet surface and interferes with the membrane reactions of platelet activation. The bleeding symptoms and the abnormal platelet function are proportional to the amount of abnormal protein in the plasma. Abnormal tests include bleeding time, platelet aggregation, and platelet procoagulant activity. The results of the abnormal tests, however, do not correlate with the severity of clinical bleeding.

Drugs

Many drugs have been shown to contribute to platelet dysfunction. The effect of drugs on platelets of persons with normal hemostatic function is usually clinically unnoticeable. However, those with significant abnormalities of the hemostatic system are at greater risk for developing severe bleeding symptoms.

Drugs can variably alter the bleeding time and platelet aggregation studies, but the effects on these laboratory tests do not necessarily correlate with clinical symptoms. The mechanisms of inhibiting platelet function also are variable and are not completely understood. The effects of three drugs—aspirin, alcohol, and certain antibiotic agents—are discussed next.

Aspirin.

Aspirin affects platelet function by irreversibly acetylating, and thus inactivating, the cyclooxygenase enzyme, thereby preventing the formation and release of TXA_2. As a result, platelet secretion is decreased. A single dose of 650 mg of aspirin can inhibit 95% of the function of cyclooxygenase in circulating platelets. The platelets affected by aspirin continue to circulate but are nonfunctional. Laboratory tests of platelet function, therefore, can be altered in patients taking aspirin. Platelet function tests return to normal as new platelets are produced and released from the marrow. Tests typically become normal 7 days after the last dose.

The bleeding time in normal persons can be increased by 1–2 minutes after taking a single dose of aspirin and can be affected for as long as 7 days. In healthy persons, though, it rarely becomes prolonged beyond the reference range. In persons with a functional abnormality of platelets (either hereditary or acquired) or VWD, aspirin ingestion can lead to serious bleeding complications. It is recommended that patients should not ingest aspirin or any of the numerous aspirin-containing products for 7 days before having platelet function tests.

Abnormalities in platelet aggregation tests reflect the lack of TXA_2 synthesis and are similar to results from patients with hereditary deficiencies of enzymes in this pathway. A first wave of aggregation is seen with ADP and epinephrine, but no secondary wave is present. Aggregation does not occur with collagen, and agglutination is normal with ristocetin (Figure 31-8d). For further discussion of the effects of drugs on platelet function testing, ∞ Chapter 40.

✓ Checkpoint! 8

Why are the bleeding time test and closure time abnormal for up to 7 days following ingestion of aspirin?

Alcohol. Ingestion of large amounts of alcohol over a long period of time can lead to platelet dysfunction in some individuals. Several mechanisms have been proposed: inhibition of prostaglandin synthesis and alteration of the storage pool of nucleotides or membrane stabilization. The platelet aggregation test can show decreased primary aggregation with ADP.

Antibiotics. Antibiotics, particularly penicillins and cephalosporins (which affect bacterial cell wall synthesis), alter platelet function. Patients taking these drugs show no aggregation with ADP either in the primary or secondary wave. Bleeding time can also be prolonged. The drug is believed to coat the platelet membrane, blocking ADP and epinephrine receptors, and resulting in platelet inability to respond to agonist. Serious bleeding complications can occur.

Cardiopulmonary Bypass Surgery In addition to thrombocytopenia, as discussed previously, platelet function is altered during cardiopulmonary bypass surgery. The platelets are believed to become activated temporarily by the abnormal surfaces to which they are exposed.

Significant bleeding develops in approximately 3% to 5% of patients after bypass surgery. In approximately one-half of these cases, the bleeding is due to inadequate surgical technique and can require additional surgery to correct. The remaining one-half can be due to a variety of defects of hemostasis, the most common of which is acquired abnormal platelet function.

Flow cytometry has been used to study platelet activation during cardiopulmonary bypass surgery in pediatric patients. Results using monoclonal antibodies to CD62P and GPIb/IX are correlated with the extent of platelet activation and with the risk of bleeding. CD62P is contained within the αG and is expressed on the platelet surface only after platelets have undergone the release reaction. After platelets have been activated, GPIb decreases in density on the platelet surface.[40]

 CASE STUDY *(continued from page 689)*

When asked if he had had bleeding problems in the past, Mohammed recounted having petechiae, lots of bruises off and on since childhood, frequent nosebleeds, and bleeding for a long time after cuts. A bleeding time, platelet function analyzer closure time, and platelet aggregation studies were ordered. The results are bleeding time, greater than 20 minutes and closure time increased. Platelet aggregation studies showed normal aggregation with ADP, collagen, epinephrine and thrombin. Agglutination with ristocetin was abnormal and was not corrected when VWF was added.

8. Is Mohammed's problem more likely acquired or inherited? Why?
9. What is the significance of these platelet function tests?
10. What is Mohammed's most likely condition?
11. What additional testing would be considered?

SUMMARY

This chapter described disorders of primary hemostasis. Patients affected by these conditions usually have an imbalance in the hemostatic system and experience bleeding of some type. Although bleeding can occur in any organ, most patients experience excess bleeding from superficial cuts, easy skin bruising, and the presence of petechiae. Occasional disorders result in excess clotting, that is, thrombosis rather than excess bleeding.

Vascular disorders are diverse in origin and can be inherited or acquired. Diagnosis of vascular disorders is usually done by excluding other causes of bleeding and observing symptoms consistent with the underlying disorders. Laboratory tests of hemostasis with the exception of the bleeding time are usually normal.

Platelet disorders are broadly categorized as quantitative disorders in which the platelet count is too low or too high or as functional abnormalities in which an aspect of platelet function is altered. Thrombocytopenia is caused by conditions that affect the bone marrow production of megakaryocytes, conditions that cause increased destruction of platelets after they are released into the peripheral blood, conditions in which the spleen is increased in size or by dilution during transfusion of multiple units of banked blood within a short period of time. Thrombocytosis is seen in myeloproliferative disorders and a number of other diseases. Functional platelet abnormalities are caused by mutations in genes that produce platelet membrane or granule constituents or can be acquired by ingestion of certain drugs such as aspirin. Laboratory tests that are helpful in establishing the cause of a platelet disorder include platelet counts, template bleeding time, closure time (PFA-100®), and platelet aggregation studies.

REVIEW QUESTIONS

LEVEL I

1. Which of the following platelet counts indicates thrombocytopenia? (Objective 1)
   a. 200×10^9/L
   b. 2000×10^9/L
   c. 200×10^{12}/L
   d. 20.0×10^9/L

2. What laboratory test(s) is (are) most often ordered to screen for abnormalities of the hemostatic system? (Objective 3)
   a. platelet count
   b. prothrombin time
   c. activated partial thromboplastin time
   d. all of the above

3. An average of 20 platelets per field was counted on a blood smear from an EDTA specimen with a 1000× magnification. What is the platelet count estimate? (Background Basics 4)
   a. 300×10^9/L
   b. 150×10^9/L
   c. 400×10^9/L
   d. 200×10^9/L

4. What are purple lesions that are larger than 1 cm in diameter that are *not* raised called? (Objective 2)
   a. petechiae
   b. ecchymoses
   c. hematoma
   d. thrombocytosis

5. In which hematologic disorder would you expect to observe a decreased platelet count? (Objective 6)
   a. acute leukemia
   b. chronic myelocytic leukemia
   c. hemolytic anemia
   d. iron-deficiency anemia

6. How long should a patient be off aspirin or aspirin-containing products before having platelet function testing? (Objective 9)
   a. 2 hours
   b. 2 days
   c. 7 days
   d. 30 days

7. Which of the following can result in a falsely decreased platelet count on an automated hematology counter? (Background Basic)
   a. large number of schistocytes
   b. iron-deficiency anemia
   c. aplastic anemia
   d. platelet satellitism

LEVEL II

Use the following history for questions 1–5.

The mother of a 4-year-old boy noticed several bruises on his arms, legs, and torso. Upon closer examination, she saw several pinpoint, brownish purple spots on his ankles. Just before leaving home for the doctor's office, the child had a moderately severe nosebleed. There had been no previous episodes of this type.

The child's physical examination was unremarkable except for the bruises. The child had not recently taken any medication but was recovering from the chicken pox.

Laboratory results showed:

RBC	4.25×10^{12}/L
Hb	10.8 g/dL (108 g/L)
Hct	.34 L/L
MCV	80 fL
MCH	25.4 pg
MCHC	301 g/L
WBC	5.2×10^9/L
Platelet count	4.0×10^9/L

A bone marrow examination was scheduled but was later cancelled.

1. What disorder is most probably indicated by the boy's history? (Objectives 4, 5)
   a. acute leukemia
   b. Bernard-Soulier syndrome
   c. idiopathic thrombocytopenic purpura
   d. Marfan syndrome

2. If a bone marrow examination had been performed, what morphology would it likely have shown? (Objective 4)
   a. normal to increased numbers of megakaryocytes
   b. large numbers of blast cells
   c. decreased numbers of erythrocyte precursors
   d. absence of all myeloid precursors and replacement by fat

3. What is the mechanism of platelet destruction in immune thrombocytopenia? (Objective 4)
   a. lysis by complement in the peripheral blood
   b. increased sequestration of platelets by the spleen
   c. removal of antibody-coated platelets by splenic macrophages
   d. activation and increased utilization by forming aggregates in the blood stream

REVIEW QUESTIONS *(continued)*

LEVEL I

8. What level of platelet count is associated with a risk of life-threatening bleed into the central nervous system? (Objective 5)
   a. 200×10^9/L
   b. 500×10^9/L
   c. 100×10^9/L
   d. 5×10^9/L

9. Thrombocytosis is: (Objective 8)
   a. a platelet count within the reference range for age
   b. abnormal platelet function
   c. the presence of a blood clot in a leg vein
   d. a platelet count above the reference range

10. Platelet satellitism and platelet agglutination seen on a peripheral blood smear occur only: (Background Basic 5)
   a. in blood collected in sodium citrate anticoagulant
   b. in blood collected in EDTA anticoagulant
   c. after the blood has sat on the countertop for 24 hours
   d. on a smear made from a capillary puncture

LEVEL II

4. The small purple spots seen on this boy's ankles are most probably: (Objective 2)
   a. petechiae
   b. ecchymoses
   c. allergic purpura
   d. hematoma

5. What is the boy's expected prognosis? (Objective 2)
   a. imminent death from overwhelming infection
   b. complete spontaneous recovery within 6 months
   c. similar problems for the rest of his life
   d. recovery after a long period of steroid therapy

6. Which of the following is characteristic in a patient with Bernard-Soulier syndrome? (Objective 7)
   a. abnormal glycoprotein IIb/IIIa
   b. increased prothrombin time
   c. increased platelet count
   d. abnormal platelet aggregation with ristocetin

7. Which of the following is found in Glanzmann's thrombasthenia? (Objective 7)
   a. mutation in the gene for VWF
   b. acquired abnormality of fibrinogen
   c. genetic abnormality of glycoprotein IIb or IIIa
   d. acquired vascular disorder

8. Hereditary telangiestasia is characterized by which of the following? (Objective 3)
   a. abnormal platelet adhesion to collagen
   b. thrombocytosis
   c. deficiency of platelet dense bodies
   d. skin lesions that are arterioles connected directly to venules

9. Platelet aggregation studies were performed and showed a primary wave of aggregation with ADP that returned to the baseline with no secondary wave. Which of the following conditions are consistent with these results? (Objectives 7, 8)
   a. senile purpura
   b. chronic idiopathic thrombocytopenic purpura
   c. aspirin effect
   d. Bernard-Soulier syndrome

10. Reactive thrombocytosis is associated with: (Objectives 4, 6)
   a. post-surgery
   b. MPD
   c. aspirin ingestion
   d. heparin therapy

www.pearsonhighered.com/mckenzie
Use this address to access the interactive Companion Website created for this textbook. Find additional information, tables and figures. Evaluate your command of the chapter information using case studies and critical thinking and multiple choice questions.

REFERENCES

1. Levine SP. Thrombocytopenia: Pathophysiology and classification. In: Lee GR, Foerster J, Lukens J, Paraskevas F, Greer JP, Rodgers GM, eds. *Wintrobe's Clinical Hematology,* 10th ed. Williams & Wilkins; 1999:1579–1611.

2. Lopez JA, Thiagarajan P. Acquired disorders of platelet function. In: Hoffman R, Benz EJ Jr, Shattil SJ, Furie B, Cohen HJ, Silberstein LE, McGlave P, eds. *Hematology: Basic Principles and Practice,* 4th ed. Philadelphia: Elsevier; 2005:2347–67.

3. Hanes FM. Multiple hereditary telangiectasias causing hemorrhage (hereditary hemorrhagic telangiectasia). *Bull John Hopkins Hosp.* 1999;20:63–73.

4. Shovlin CL. Molecular defects in rare bleeding disorders: Hereditary haemorrhagic telangiectasia. *Thromb Haemost.* 1997;78:145–50.

5. Zumberg M, Kitchens CS. Primary vascular disorders. In: Colman RW, Marder VJ, Clowes AW, George JN, Goldhaber SZ, eds. *Hemostasis and Thrombosis Basic Principles and Clinical Practice,* 5th ed. Philadelphia: Lippincott, Williams & Wilkins; 2006:1011–23.

6. Byers PH. Ehlers-Danlos syndrome type IV: A genetic disorder in many guises. *Invest Dermatol.* 1995;105:311–13.

7. Manusov EG and Martucci E. The Marfan syndrome: An underdiagnosed killer. *Arch Fam Med.* 1994;3:822–26.

8. Cole WG. The molecular pathology of osteogenesis imperfecta. *Clin Orthop.* 1997;343:235–48.

9. Bick RL. *Disorders of Thrombosis and Hemostasis: Clinical and Laboratory Practice.* Chicago: ASCP Press; 1992.

10. Lightfoot RW. Palpable purpura: Identifying the cause. *Hosp Pract.* 1992;27(12):39–47.

11. Hermes B, Haas N, Henz BM. Immunopathologic events of adverse cutaneous reactions to coumarin and heparin. *Acta Derm Venereol.* 1997;77:35–38.

12. Levine SP. Thrombocytopenia caused by immunologic platelet destruction. In: Lee GR, Foerster J, Lukens J, Paraskevas F, Greer JP, Rodgers GM, eds. *Wintrobe's Clinical Hematology,* 10th ed. Baltimore: Williams & Wilkins; 1999:1579–1613.

13. Bussel JB, Cines D. Immune thrombocytopenic purpura, neonatal alloimmune thrombocytopenia, and post transfusion purpura. In: Hoffman R, Benz EJ Jr, Shattil SJ, Furie B, Cohen HJ, Silberstein, LE, McGlave P, eds. *Hematology: Basic Principles and Practice,* 4th ed. Philadelphia: Elsevier; 2005:2269–85.

14. George JN, Woolf SH, Raskob GE et al. Idiopathic thrombocytopenic purpura: A practice guideline developed by explicit methods for the American Society of Hematology. *Blood.* 1996;88:3–40.

15. Davis, GL. Quantitative and qualitative disorders of platelets. In: Steine-Martin EA, Lotspeich-Steininger CA, Koepke JA, eds. *Clinical Hematology: Principles, Procedures, Correlations,* 2nd ed. Philadelphia: Lippincott; 1998:717–34.

16. Ware RE, Zimmerman SA. Anti-D: Mechanisms of action. *Semin Hemat.* 1998;35:14–22.

17. George JN, Kojouri K. Immune Thrombocytopenic Purpura. In: Colman RW, Marder VJ, Clowes AW, George JN, Goldhaber SZ, eds. *Hemostasis and Thrombosis Basic Principles and Clinical Practice,* 5th ed. Philadelphia. Lippincott, Williams & Wilkins; 2006:1085–93.

18. George JN, Raskob GE. Idiopathic thrombocytopenic purpura: A concise summary of pathophysiology and diagnosis in children and adults. *Semin Hemat.* 1998;35:5–8.

19. McCrae KR, Samuels P, Schreiber AD. Pregnancy associated thrombocytopenia: Pathogenesis and management. *Blood.* 1992;80:2697–2714.

20. Kelton JG. The serological investigation of patients with autoimmune thrombocytopenia. *Thromb Haemost.* 1995;74:228–33.

21. Warkentin TE. Heparin-induced thrombocytopenia: A ten-year retrospective. *Annu Rev Med.* 1999;50:129–47.

22. Segel GB, Lichtman MA. Aplastic anemia. In: Lichtman MA, Beutler E, Kipps TJ et al., eds. *Williams Hematology,* 7th ed. New York: McGraw-Hill; 2006:419–36.

23. Nurden P, George JN, Nurden AT. Inherited thrombocytopenias. In: Colman RW, Marder VJ, Clowes AW, George JN, Goldhaber SZ, eds. *Hemostasis and Thrombosis Basic Principles and Clinical Practice,* 5th ed. Philadelphia: Lippincott Williams & Wilkins; 2006:975–86.

24. Levine SP. Miscellaneous causes of thrombocytopenia. In: Lee GR, Foerster J, Lukens J, Paraskevas F, Greer JP, Rodgers GM, eds. *Wintrobe's Clinical Hematology,* 10th ed. Baltimore: Williams & Wilkins; 1999:1623–32.

25. Woodman RC, Harker LA. Bleeding complications associated with cardiopulmonary bypass. *Blood.* 1990;76:1680–97.

26. Fruchtman SM, Hoffman R. Primary thrombocythemia. In: Hoffman R, Benz EJ Jr, Shattil SJ, Furie B, Cohen HJ, Silberstein LE, McGlave P eds.. *Hematology: Basic Principles and Practice,* 4th ed. Philadelphia: Elsevier; 2005:1277–96.

27. Levine SP. Thrombocytosis. In: Lee GR, Foerster J, Lukens J, Paraskevas F, Greer JP, Rodgers GM, eds. *Wintrobe's Clinical Hematology,* 10th ed. Baltimore: Williams & Wilkins; 1999:1648–60.

28. Evans VJ. Platelet morphology and the blood smear. *J Med Tech.* 1984;1:689–95.

29. Bernard J, Soulier JP. Sur une nouvelle varieté de dystrophie thrombocytaire hémorragipare congénitale. *Sem Hôp Paris.* 1948;24:2317.

30. Lopez JA, Andrew RK, Afshar-Karghan V, Berndt MC. Bernard-Soulier syndrome. *Blood.* 1998;91:4397–418.

31. Glanzmann E. Hereditare hamorrhagische thrombasthenie: Ein Beitrag zur Pathologie der Blutplattchen. *J Kinderkranken.* 1918;88:113.

32. Fausett B, Silver RM. Congenital disorders of platelet dysfunction. *Clin Obstet Gynecol.* 1999;42:390–405.

33. Nurder AT, George JN. Inherited abnormalities of the platelet membrane: Glanzmann thrombasthenia, Bernard-Soulier syndrome, and other disorders. In: Colman RW, Marder VJ, Clowes AW, George JN, Goldhaber SZ, eds. *Hemostasis and Thrombosis Basic Principles and Clinical Practice,* 5th ed. Philadelphia: Lippincott Williams & Wilkins; 2006:987–1010.

34. Coller BS. Hereditary qualitative platelet defects. In: Beutler E, Lichtman MA, Coller BS, Kipps TJ, eds. *William's Hematology,* 5th ed. New York: McGraw-Hill; 1995:1364–85.

35. Rao AK. Hereditary disorders of platelet secretion and signal transduction. In: Colman RW, Marder VJ, Clowes AW, George JN, Goldhaber SZ, eds. *Hemostasis and Thrombosis Basic Principles and Clinical Practice,* 5th ed. Philadelphia: Lippincott Williams & Wilkins; 2006:961–74.

36. Rao AK, Jalagadugula G, Sun L. Inherited defects in platelet signaling mechanisms. *Semin Throm Hemost.* 2004;30:525–35.

37. Bennett JS. Hereditary disorders of platelet function. In: Hoffman R, Benz EJ Jr, Shattil SJ, Furie HJ, Cohen HJ, Silberstein, LE, McGlave P, eds. *Hematology: Basic Principles and Practice,* 4th ed. Philadelphia: Elsevier; 2005:2327–45.

38. Weiss HJ. Scott syndrome: A disorder of platelet coagulant activity. *Semin Hemat.* 1994;31:312–19.

39. Nurden, AT. Inherited abnormalities of platelets. *Thromb Haemost.* 1999;82:468–80.

40. Rinder HM. Platelet function testing by flow cytometry. *Clin Lab Sci.* 1998;11:365–72.

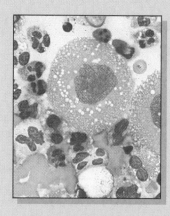

32

Disorders of Secondary Hemostasis

Shannon Carpenter, MD, MS
Beverly Kirby, EdD

■ OBJECTIVES—LEVEL I

At the end of this unit of study, the student should be able to:

1. Define *deficiency* as it relates to the proteins of secondary hemostasis.

2. Describe the expected results of laboratory screening tests that detect abnormalities of the proteins of secondary hemostasis.

3. Describe the expected laboratory results, pathophysiology, and clinical symptoms in patients with classic (type I) von Willebrand disease.

4. Identify hemostatic proteins that are deficient in hemophilias A and B.

5. Characterize deficiencies of factors VIII and IX by inheritance pattern, clinical symptoms, and laboratory findings.

6. Differentiate classic (type 1) von Willebrand disease and deficiencies of factors VIII and IX based on results of laboratory tests and clinical symptoms.

7. Identify clinical conditions associated with acquired disorders of the hemostatic proteins and describe the expected results in laboratory screening tests for hemostasis.

8. Characterize disseminated intravascular coagulation (DIC) by etiology, pathophysiology, and the results of laboratory testing.

9. Explain physiologic variations in the reference ranges of laboratory hemostatic screening tests in newborns.

10. Describe the expected general clinical consequences in a patient with an abnormality of the proteins of secondary hemostasis.

■ OBJECTIVES—LEVEL II

At the end of this unit of study, the student should be able to:

1. Explain the clinical symptoms characteristic of deficiencies of the fibrin-forming proteins, and contrast them with the symptoms associated with disorders of primary hemostasis.

2. Compare and contrast the results of laboratory tests for hemostasis in disorders of primary and secondary hemostasis.

3. Describe genetic mutations and diagram the inheritance pattern that results in deficiencies of the hemostatic proteins.

4. Differentiate von Willebrand disease subtypes, deficiencies of factors VIII and IX, and the inherited deficiencies of the remaining proteins of fibrin formation by inheritance pattern, pathophysiology, clinical symptoms, and laboratory findings.

■ OBJECTIVES—LEVEL II *(continued)*

5. Select and interpret the results of laboratory tests, and identify clinical symptoms that differentiate von Willebrand disease subtypes, deficiencies of factors VIII and IX, Bernard-Soulier disease, and Glanzmann's thrombasthenia.

6. Describe the pathophysiology of the conditions that result in acquired abnormalities of the hemostatic system, and select confirmatory laboratory procedures.

7. Select and describe the laboratory screening methods for distinguishing between deficiencies and inhibitors of hemostatic proteins.

8. Describe the significance and clinical implications of the development of circulating anticoagulants, and select laboratory procedures that confirm and differentiate between specific and nonspecific factor inhibitors.

9. Choose laboratory methods that differentiate between excessive primary and secondary fibrinolysis, and support your selection.

KEY TERMS

Acquired inhibitor (circulating anticoagulant)
Afibrinogenemia
Consumption coagulopathy
Cross-reacting material/positive (CRM+)
Cross-reacting material/negative (CRM−)
Disseminated intravascular coagulation (DIC)
Dysfibrinogenemia
Hemophilia A
Hemophilia B
Hemorrhagic disease of the newborn (HDN)
Hypofibrinogenemia
Lupus anticoagulant (LA)
Platelet-type-pseudo-VWD
Primary fibrinogenolysis
Ristocetin-induced platelet agglutination (RIPA)
VWF multimers
von Willebrand disease (VWD)
von Willebrand factor:ristocetin cofactor activity (VWF:RCo)
von Willebrand factor antigen (VWF:Ag)

BACKGROUND BASICS

The information in this chapter builds on the concepts learned in previous chapters. To maximize your learning experience, you should review these concepts before starting this unit of study.

Level I

▶ Secondary hemostasis: Describe the formation of fibrin and the process of fibrinolysis. (Chapter 30)
▶ Laboratory testing in coagulation: Review coagulation screening tests. (Chapter 40)

Level II

▶ Molecular genetics: Summarize the principles and the use of molecular diagnostic tests. (Chapter 39)

 CASE STUDY

We will address this case throughout the chapter.

Scott, a 2-year-old male, developed a severe bleed into a knee joint and was seen in the emergency room of his local hospital. Consider which of the three physiologic compartments involved in hemostasis could be responsible for his bleeding and how this diagnosis could be established.

▶ OVERVIEW

This chapter discusses disorders of clotting factors that result in excess bleeding. Deficiencies of most of the fibrin-forming proteins are included in this category as are some proteins associated with the fibrinolytic system. The pathophysiologic basis and clinical manifestations for each defect are presented. A major emphasis is on the laboratory involvement in the diagnosis and treatment of the defects. Because the levels of coagulation proteins are different in neonates when compared with adults and testing presents a unique challenge, a section on newborn hemostasis also is included.

▶ INTRODUCTION

The process of secondary hemostasis (∞ Chapter 30) results in the formation of fibrin, which stabilizes the primary hemostatic plug. Production of an effective fibrin clot requires the interaction of several plasma proteins (procoagulant proteins) that become activated by the injured tissue in a cascade sequence. In addition, other proteins are required to inhibit or inactivate the procoagulant proteins so that clot formation is limited to the injured area. Fibrin subsequently is broken down, or lysed, as the wound heals.

If one or more of these proteins are defective, either quantitatively or qualitatively, the balance between clot formation and clot lysis is upset. Fibrin formation is impaired if the fibrin-forming proteins are faulty. If proteins of the fibrinolytic system malfunction, either too much fibrin is formed or lysis of fibrin is inadequate or excessive. The results of such imbalances in the system are symptoms of either excessive bleeding or inappropriate and excessive clotting. This chapter discusses disorders of the plasma proteins that result in excess bleeding. Plasma protein disorders resulting in excessive clotting (thrombosis) are discussed in ∞ Chapter 33.

▶ DISORDERS OF THE PROTEINS OF FIBRIN FORMATION

Disorders of the proteins of fibrin formation arise either by inheritance of a defective gene that directs the synthesis of a hemostatic protein or by acquisition of a deficiency secondary to another condition during the individual's lifetime. In the hereditary disorders, the genetic defect causes either the failure of synthesis of one of the proteins or the production of a malfunctioning molecule (Web Figure 32-1 ■). In both situations, the rate of fibrin formation is slowed and ineffective, and the patient can experience abnormal bleeding.

Early investigators of coagulation disorders assumed that if a patient bled excessively, a coagulation protein was absent or decreased in quantity and called the defect a deficiency. The word *deficiency* currently is applied to either hereditary or acquired disorders and is understood to relate either to the absence of a coagulation protein (quantitative disorder) or to a protein that is present in the plasma but that is functionally defective (qualitative disorder). The defect affects fibrin formation both in vivo and in vitro in laboratory screening tests such as the prothrombin time (PT) and the activated partial thromboplastin time (APTT) (∞ Chapter 40).

Laboratory screening tests are based on the length of time that it takes a clot to form in plasma. They depend, therefore, on the presence of an adequate amount of the clot forming proteins (quantity) and how well the proteins function (quality). They do not differentiate qualitative from quantitative defects. A functionally defective coagulation factor prolongs the clotting screening test but can still be recognized by immunologically based procedures in the laboratory, which utilize antibodies to detect the presence of the protein. Individuals who have these functionally defective factors that can be detected immunologically are said to be positive for **cross-reacting material (CRM+)** (i.e., the protein is present although it is nonfunctional). Patients in whom the clotting factor is quantitatively decreased and thus have abnormal results in both functional and immunological assays are negative for **cross-reacting material (CRM−)** (Web Figure 32-1).

Clinical bleeding symptoms in patients with coagulation factor deficiencies differ from those seen in platelet defects (Table 32-1 ✪). These patients bleed from the rupture of small arterioles rather than from capillaries, and the sites of bleeds are into deep muscular tissues and joints rather than the superficial areas seen in platelet disorders. Hematomas

✪ TABLE 32-1

Bleeding Characteristics in Disorders of Secondary Hemostasis

Symptoms typical of secondary hemostatic disorders
- Delayed bleeding
- Deep muscular bleeding
- Spontaneous joint bleeding

Symptoms common to primary and secondary hemostatic disorders
- Ecchymoses
- Gastrointestinal bleeding
- Hematuria
- Hypermenorrhea
- Gingival (gums) bleeding
- Increased bleeding after tooth extraction
- Intracranial bleeding
- Epistaxis

are common and can be massive. Patients also experience delayed bleeding from cuts. Patients with coagulation factor defects usually have normal platelets; therefore, a typical primary hemostatic plug is formed after a superficial cut. This initially arrests the blood flow, and the bleeding stops. Delayed bleeding occurs because, in the absence of stabilization with fibrin formation, the plug dislodges and the wound begins to bleed again later. The subsequent bleed usually continues for a longer time with the loss of a larger amount of blood. Patients with disorders of secondary hemostasis do not bleed faster but for a prolonged period of time.

Patients with coagulation factor deficiencies can experience ecchymoses, excess bleeding from traumatic injuries, and bleeding from the body sites listed in Table 32-1. Some of these symptoms are also seen in patients with platelet disorders. Retroperitoneal bleeding and hematuria also are common, but petechiae are not usually seen in disorders of secondary hemostasis.

The physician's evaluation and laboratory investigation of a bleeding patient proceeds as described in ∞ Chapter 31. The battery of screening tests in a factor deficiency usually show a normal platelet count, but the PT, the APTT, or both are usually prolonged (Table 32-2 ✪). In the case of von Willebrand disease (VWD), at times the only abnormal laboratory test is the bleeding time or PFA-100®, or the patient can have no abnormal lab results and only a strong family or personal history of bleeding (see discussion of VWD testing, ∞ Chapter 40). The thrombin clotting time can be the only abnormal test in disorders of fibrinogen. Abnormalities of factor (F) XIII require specific testing. When the history and results of the screening tests indicate, additional testing is ordered to more specifically define the problem. Coagulation factor assays, fibrinogen levels, a D-dimer test, and/or antithrombin levels can be useful confirmatory procedures (∞ Chapter 40).

This chapter discusses the hereditary disorders of each of the coagulation factors on the basis of inheritance pattern. The most common types of VWD demonstrate an autosomal dominant pattern of inheritance; hemophilias A and B show

✪ TABLE 32-2

Coagulation Screening Test Results in Congenital Deficiencies

Platelet Count	PT	APTT	PFA-100	TT	Suspected Congenital Deficiency
N	N	N	N	N	Factor XIII, mild deficiencies of any factor, α_2-antiplasmin, Plasminogen Activator Inhibitor-1
N	A	N	N	N	Factor VII
N	N	A	N	N	Factors XII, XI, IX, VIII, prekallikrein, high molecular weight kininogen
N	A	A	N	N	Factors X, V, II (prothrombin)
N	A	A	N	A	Fibrinogen
N	N	A or N	A or N	N	von Willebrand disease

N = normal; A = abnormal; PT = prothrombin time; APTT = activated partial thromboplastin time; TT = thrombin time

X-linked recessive inheritance. Deficiencies of the remaining clotting factors exhibit an autosomal recessive inheritance pattern. Acquired disorders of the clotting factors follow and are classified as consumption disorders, liver disease, vitamin K deficiencies, and acquired pathologic inhibitors.

The amino acid sequences of most of the hemostatic proteins and their inhibitors have been determined as has the nucleotide sequences of most of their genes. Research laboratories are involved in characterizing the molecular sites and types of mutations that lead to coagulation factor deficiencies. Specific molecular defects in many genes and their corresponding proteins have been established, and various mutations have been characterized. Point mutations, alterations of splice junctions, deletions, insertions, inversions, and mutations resulting in premature stop codons are a few of the known molecular defects. Researchers are gathering information in an attempt to correlate sites and types of mutations with the clinical symptoms seen in patients.

HEREDITARY DISORDERS OF SECONDARY HEMOSTASIS

Secondary hemostasis disorders can be inherited as autosomal dominant, X-linked recessive, and autosomal recessive disorders. Inherited coagulation factor disorders usually involve a single coagulation protein, and if bleeding occurs, it is generally from one site at a time.

Autosomal Dominant Inheritance

An autosomal dominant inheritance of a defective protein causes two coagulation disorders: von Willebrand disease (types 1, 2A, 2B, and 2M) and dysfibrinogenemia. Dysfibrinogenemia will be discussed with the other disorders of fibrinogen in the autosomal recessive category. von Willebrand disease is considered here.

von Willebrand Disease **von Willebrand disease (VWD)** is a quantitative or qualitative deficiency of von Willebrand factor (VWF) arising from mutations in the VWF gene. Inherited defects in VWF can result in defective protein processing or disruption of specific ligand-binding sites.

Based on the nature of the mutation and inheritance patterns, VWD is subdivided into three types with type 2 containing 4 subtypes. The results of laboratory tests in VWD can sometimes be confused with a deficiency of F-VIII. The similarities and differences between VWD and F-VIII deficiency will be addressed later.

Chapter 29 described the role of VWF in primary hemostasis. VWF serves as a bridge between GPIb/IX receptors on activated platelets and subendothelial collagen exposed when the vessel is injured (primary hemostatic plug formation).[1] VWF also plays a role in secondary hemostasis, complexing with and stabilizing circulating coagulation F-VIII in the plasma (∞ Chapter 30). The function of VWF in both primary hemostasis and fibrin formation is altered in most patients with clinically symptomatic VWD.

The autosomal dominant pattern of inheritance is important in the clinical expression of type 1 VWD. Clinical symptoms occur when one gene is defective and the production of VWF is reduced by about one-half. Circulating levels of F-VIII generally are reduced in proportion to the reduction in VWF. The platelet-associated function of VWF is independent of the presence or absence of F-VIII. While the inheritance pattern of most patients with VWD is autosomal dominant, more severely affected patients (with types 2N and 3) demonstrate an autosomal recessive or compound heterozygous pattern. Symptomatic patients with these inheritance patterns have mutations in both the VWF genes (i.e., are homozygotes or double heterozygotes).

Nature of von Willebrand Factor. Figure 32-1 ■ depicts the synthesis of the F-VIII/VWF complex. The structure of the mature VWF molecule is a chain of identical subunits called *multimers*. Normally, the number of subunits in individual molecules varies so that the molecular weights range from 0.5 to more than 20 million Daltons (Da). Although VWF in plasma consists of a wide range of sizes, most VWF molecules bind only one F-VIII molecule; thus, the molar ratio of VWF:F-VIII is ~1:1 (∞ Chapter 30). A detailed description of the synthesis of VWF, which occurs in endothelial cells and megakaryocytes, can be found on this text's Companion Website.

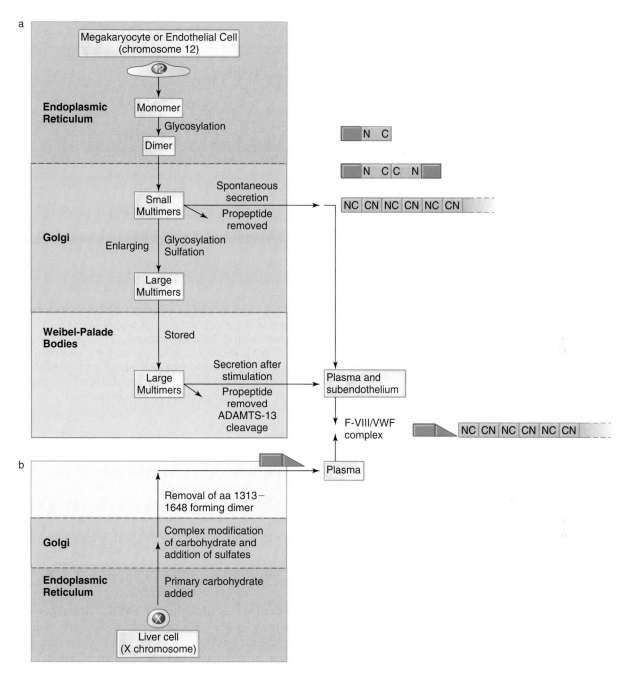

A schematic diagram of the structure of a VWF subunit is shown in Figure 32-2 ■. It consists of four types of domains, A through D, which are repeated and numbered in the arrangement shown. Sites of interaction with F-VIII, GPIb/IX, GPIIb/IIIa, collagen, and heparin have been identified.[1,2]

Clinical Findings.   Dr. von Willebrand first described the disease that carries his name after studying an extended family in the Åland Islands of Finland in 1926.[3] The first patient studied died during her fourth menstrual period, and four sisters also had died from bleeding. At the time, available laboratory tests included the platelet count, coagulation

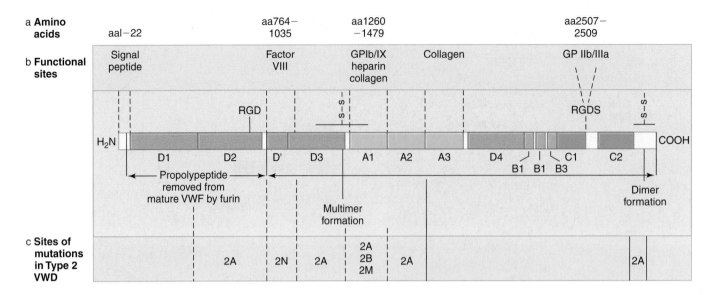

a Amino acids   aal−22   aa764−1035   aa1260−1479   aa2507−2509

b Functional sites

c Sites of mutations in Type 2 VWD

■ FIGURE 32-2   A diagrammatic depiction of the domain structure of a VWF monomer precursor protein. The precursor protein consists of 2813 amino acids. **a.** The amino acids (aa) involved in the functions at **b.** aa 1–22 is the signal peptide; domains D1 and D2 (aa 23–741) are the propeptide removed during processing; domain D' (aa 764–1035) plus part of domain D3 are the binding site for F-VIII; domain A1 (aa 1260–1479) contains binding sites for GP Ib, heparin and collagen; domain A3 contains the major binding site for collagen; domain C1 contains the binding site for GP IIb/IIIa; disulfide bridges at D3 and the C terminal end are the sites of attachment when forming multimers and dimers, respectively. The mature protein with the propeptide removed contains 2050 amino acids. **c.** Sites of mutations of the subtypes of type 2 VWD. R = arginine; G = glycine; D = aspartic acid; S = serine

time, and clot retraction, all of which were normal. With further studies, von Willebrand concluded that the disease was related to platelet dysfunction.

VWD is the most common inherited bleeding disorder. It is estimated that about 125 in 1 million persons have VWD with clinical (bleeding) symptoms and another 1% of the population is asymptomatic and thus not aware of having the disease.[4]

Bleeding symptoms, if present, are usually mild. Those patients who are homozygous or doubly heterozygous for VWD can exhibit severe symptoms and have the potential for life-threatening bleeding. The typical type of bleeding is hemorrhage in mucosal and cutaneous tissues. Approximately 60% of patients report epistaxis, and 50% report menorrhagia and bleeding after dental extraction. Thirty-five percent of patients report gingival bleeding and easy bruising.[5,6] These clinical features resemble those seen in platelet disorders. Excessive bleeding at childbirth is comparatively rare because in pregnancy the activity of the entire F-VIII/VWF complex increases, but postpartum bleeding can occur in 21–59% of patients.[7] In type 3 VWD (homozygous), the symptoms can include hemarthroses and spontaneous deep bleeding resembling coagulation factor deficiencies due to the concomitant decrease in F-VIII levels. An individual's ABO blood type affects VWF antigen levels (discussed later), which may affect the severity of bleeding symptoms although the impact is still somewhat controversial.[8,9]

One hallmark of the disease is its variability. The severity of bleeding symptoms differs in individuals within the same kindred, among kindreds, and, from time to time, within the same individual. Symptoms might not begin until the second decade of life in mild forms of the disease. In the severe forms, symptoms begin early in life and often decrease with age. Laboratory test results vary, often requiring repeated testing of the same individual (∞ Chapter 40).[3] The severity of clinical symptoms does not necessarily correlate with the level of VWF activity. However, some VWD subtypes demonstrate unique symptoms related to the nature of the mutations.

Laboratory Evaluation of VWD. The common laboratory tests for fibrin formation do not directly evaluate VWF. The laboratory diagnosis of VWD is based on the results of a battery of tests after identification of a patient with a lifelong clinical history of the typical bleeding symptoms and/or a history of similar symptoms in other family members. Screening tests include the platelet count, APTT, PT, the template bleeding time, and/or the PFA-100®. The recently developed platelet function analyzer (PFA-100), a device that uses a membrane coated with collagen and a platelet agonist to which platelets adhere, has replaced the bleeding time in many institutions. Typical results of these tests in VWD are shown in Table 32-3 ✪ and are compared with the results in the hemophilias (discussed in the next section).

The template bleeding time, a crude measure of platelet function, is abnormal not because the platelets are abnormal but because in the absence of VWF, the platelets are unable to adhere to collagen and initiate the formation of the pri-

⊕ TABLE 32-3

Laboratory Evaluation of von Willebrand Disease (VWD) and the X-Linked Recessive Disorders

	VWD, Type 1	Factor VIII Deficiency	Factor IX Deficiency
Platelet tests			
Platelet count	N	N	N
Template bleeding time	N/Increased	N	N
Platelet function analyzer	N/Increased	N	N
Platelet aggregation test			
ADP	N	N	N
Collagen	N	N	N
Epinephrine	N	N	N
Ristocetin	Decreased/Absent*	N	N
Coagulation factor tests			
Prothrombin time	N	N	N
Activated partial thromboplastin time	N or increased	Increased	Increased
Thrombin time	N	N	N
Factor VIII assay	N/Decreased	Decreased	N
Factor IX assay	N	N	Decreased
VWF:Ag assay	Decreased	N	N
Fibrinolysis tests	N	N	N

*Except for type 2B VWD in which aggregation with ristocetin is increased. Decreased or absent when VWF:A ≤30%.
N = normal

mary hemostatic plug (∞ Chapter 29 and Figure 31-6b). The platelet function analyzer has been shown to be abnormal with collagen/ADP and collagen/epinephrine cartridges for similar reasons.[9,10] The APTT is used as an indirect screening test for VWF because of the correlation of VWF and F-VIII levels. An abnormal APTT occurs only when the level of F-VIII is near or below the sensitivity of the APTT reagent (for most commercial reagents ≤30% of normal). Therefore, bleeding time (BT), PFA, and APTT results may produce discordant normal/abnormal results (∞ Chapter 40). The PT, which does not depend on either F-VIII or VWF, is normal.

If the screening test results and the patient's clinical history suggest VWD, specific tests are required to establish the diagnosis and to determine the type or subtype of VWD. The specific tests quantitate VWF and F-VIII activity and determine various functional and structural aspects of the VWF protein (∞ Chapter 40).

Because VWF cannot be measured by clotting assays, immunologic tests are used to quantitate the amount of VWF protein in the plasma as **von Willebrand factor antigen (VWF:Ag).** Various immunologic methodologies (e.g., ELISA) are available and use commercially prepared monoclonal antibodies to VWF. F-VIII activity is determined by a standard factor assay method (∞ Chapter 40). F-VIII levels usually correlate with the amount of VWF antigen. The patient's ABO blood type should also be determined because blood type significantly affects the normal level of VWF protein (Table 40-6). Type B plasma has up to twice the VWF antigen as type O plasma. Some laboratories have developed different reference ranges for each blood type. Also, because VWF is an acute phase reactant, levels of protein are increased during inflammatory states, stress, or pregnancy.

The ability of VWF to function in platelet adhesion is determined by the **von Willebrand factor:ristocetin cofactor activity (VWF:RCo).** The VWF:RCo assay is performed on a platelet aggregometer and measures the ability of the patient's VWF to support agglutination of platelets by ristocetin (∞ Chapter 40).

The diagnosis of VWD is established by finding a decreased plasma level of VWF activity, VWF antigen, F-VIII levels (which usually correlate with the quantity of VWF), and/or a prolonged bleeding time or prolonged closure time. Classic (type 1) VWD results from a partial quantitative deficiency and typically leads to abnormal results in all of these tests. In some cases, however, one or more of the tests is normal, making diagnosis more difficult. The functional VWF:RCo activity might not correspond to the VWF antigen levels, depending on whether the patient has a quantitative or a qualitative defect as described later. Patients with qualitative defects usually have decreased concentrations of VWF antigen but more markedly abnormal functional tests than would be expected by the amount of VWF present.

When the diagnosis of VWD is established by decreased VWF:Ag and/or abnormal function of VWF, the final step in the laboratory diagnosis of VWD is to establish the subtype. The structure of **VWF multimers** is studied by electrophoresis using 1% agarose gels in the presence of sodium dodecyl sulfate (SDS). The multimers are separated by size and visualized as bands. These tests can be performed on platelet- or plasma-derived VWF. Other tests of VWF functional activity include ELISA tests designed to measure the ability of the patient's VWF to bind to either F-VIII or to collagen, described as VWF:CB (collagen binding) and VWF:VIIIB (F-VIII binding) assays.[11,12] The **ristocetin-induced platelet agglutination test (RIPA)** detects the ability of the patient's VWF to bind patient's platelet GPIb/IX. In patients with rare qualitative mutations, one or more of these abilities is decreased. Theoretically, DNA analysis to establish the specific gene mutation would be desirable but is difficult because the VWF gene is very complex and most molecular defects have not yet been identified. Databases for VWD mutations have been established.[9] An online database is accessible at www.shef.ac.uk/vwf/index.html. In the future, with improvements in methodology, DNA analysis could become the test of choice for differentiating the qualitative types of VWD because the sites of mutations are more predictable than in the quantitative types of VWD.[6]

Classification.   A classification system for VWD proposed in 1994 simplifies previous schemes and is based on the phenotype of the VWF protein determined using the laboratory tests described previously.[13] This classification was updated in 2006 to include our improved understanding of the metabolism of VWF.[14] This scheme has three major categories, types 1, 2, and 3, which depend on whether the patient has a quantitative or a qualitative defect and, in the case of quantitative defects, the extent of the quantitative deficiency. Types 1 and 3 VWD are both quantitative deficiencies of VWF. Type 1, the most common type (the "classic" type), is a mild form of VWD in which patients have a partial quantitative deficiency of VWF. Type 3 patients have an absolute absence of VWF (a severe form of the disease). Type 2 patients have qualitatively abnormal VWF of various kinds; the type is further subdivided into four variants, Types 2A, 2B, 2M, and 2N.[15] The structure of a VWF protein with sites of mutations is depicted in Figure 32-2. Some characteristics of the VWF types are shown in Table 32-4 ✪. These subtypes are discussed in more detail on the text's Companion Website and on the ∞ Chapter 40 Website. Table 32-5 ✪ summarizes laboratory test results in all types and subtypes of VWD. Discriminating qualitatively normal and abnormal VWF by routine laboratory testing is difficult. A common approach used by many laboratories is to compare values obtained in functional assays (VWF:RCo, VWF:CB, VWF:FVIIIB) with VWF:Ag. A ratio <0.6[11] or <0.7[12] the VWF:Ag value is considered to be abnormal (i.e., a dysfunctional protein).

✓ Checkpoint! 1

a. *Why do patients with type 1 VWD have 25–50% of VWF in their plasma?*

b. *Why do they have a corresponding decrease in F-VIII in their plasma?*

Two additional forms of VWD are **platelet-type-pseudo-VWD** and acquired von Willebrand syndrome. While clinical bleeding symptoms and laboratory test results are similar to those in VWD, they are not caused by mutations in the VWF gene.

Pseudo-VWD is a platelet disorder that results in increased affinity of the platelet GPIb/IX receptor for VWF.

✪ TABLE 32-4

Description of von Willebrand Disease (VWD) Subtypes

Type	Description	% of VWD	Mutation Sites; Functional Abnormalities
1	Partial quantitative deficiency with normal structure and function of the multimers	70–80	Multiple
2	Qualitative disorder with functionally abnormal VWF		
2A	Decreased platelet adhesion because of absence of largest multimers	10–15	A2, A1, D2,D3 domains—either defective synthesis of largest multimers or increased proteolysis
2B	Increased affinity for platelet GPIb and absence of largest multimers	<5	A1 domain—spontaneous binding to platelets and removal from circulation
2M	Decreased platelet adhesion via GPIb/IX not due to absence of largest multimers	Rare	A1 domain—inactivation of specific binding sites for ligands on platelets or in connective tissue
2N	Decreased affinity for F-VIII (autosomal recessive)	Rare	D′, part of D3 domains—platelet-dependent functions preserved, loss of function as carrier of F-VIII
3	Absence of VWF in platelets and plasma	0.5–5 per million	Varied; 64% characterized

⊕ TABLE 32-5

Differentiation of Subtypes of von Willebrand Disease (VWD)[7]

Type	1	3	2A	2B	2M	2N
Mode of inheritance	Autosomal dominant	Homozygous or double heterozygous	Autosomal dominant	Autosomal dominant	Autosomal dominant	Autosomal recessive
Screening tests						
Platelet count	Normal	Normal	Normal	Decreased	Normal	Normal
Bleeding time	Normal or increased	Increased	Increased	Increased	Increased	Normal
Closure time	Normal or increased	Increased	Increased	Increased	Increased	Normal
Diagnostic tests						
VWF:Ag assay	Decreased	Absent	Normal or decreased	Normal or decreased	Normal or decreased	Normal
Factor VIII assay	Normal or decreased	Severely decreased	Normal or decreased	Normal or decreased	Normal or decreased	Decreased
VWF:RCo	Decreased	Absent	Decreased relative to VWF:Ag	Normal to decreased	Decreased relative to VWF:Ag	Normal
Tests to determine subtype						
RIPA	Normal or decreased	Absent	Decreased relative to VWF:Ag	Increased	Decreased relative to VWF:Ag	Normal
Multimer analysis	Normal	Absent	Absence of large and intermediate	Absence of large	Normal	Normal

VWF:Ag = von Willebrand factor:antigen; VWF:RCo = von Willebrand factor:ristocetin cofactor activity; RIPA = ristocetin-induced platelet aggregation

Pseudo-VWD is clinically similar to VWD type 2B, but its defect is in the platelet receptor for VWF, usually resulting in spontaneous binding of the larger multimers of plasma VWF to platelet GPIb. This results in a decrease of large VWF multimers and F-VIII in the plasma. In addition, GPIIb/IIIa receptors are exposed and platelets aggregate, resulting in thrombocytopenia.

Acquired VW syndrome (AVWS) is called a *syndrome* rather than a *disease* because it is not caused by VWF mutations. AVWS is very rare and has been reported in fewer than 100 patients. It is associated primarily with lymphoproliferative diseases such as multiple myeloma, lymphoma, and chronic lymphocytic leukemia. The pathogenic mechanism of AVWS varies from patient to patient, although most are associated with loss of VWF due to neutralizing anti-VWF antibodies, proteolytic or mechanical degradation of the protein, or adsorption to cell surfaces. AVWS is diagnosed with the same laboratory tests used for inherited VWD: F-VIII coagulant activity, VWF:Ag, and VWF:RCo.[16] Elevated levels of the VWF propeptide (VWFpp or VWF antigen II) can sometimes help distinguish between acquired and congenital disease (normal or elevated in AVWS, decreased in VWD), although this result is not completely specific for acquired VWS because some forms of congenital disease also result from increased clearance of VWF.[17]

Prenatal Diagnosis.   Prenatal diagnosis of VWD is available but is usually reserved for patients with severe types of the disease. Type 2 is easily identified prenatally by PCR techniques, but diagnosis of type 3 is more difficult.[4]

VWD Therapy.   Patients with mild VWD who are not experiencing clinical bleeding do not require therapy. For VWD patients who are actively bleeding, several preparations are available to raise the level of VWF in their plasma. The classic treatment for VWD was to inject cryoprecipitate preparations that contain all molecular forms of VWF including the large multimer forms, as well as F-VIII and fibrinogen. A drawback to using cryoprecipitate is that it cannot be treated to inactivate blood-borne viruses and, therefore, carries a risk of transmission of blood-borne disease.

The current preferred method of treatment is a modified antidiuretic hormone, desamino-D-vasopressin (DDAVP), which was found to induce endothelial cell release of VWF from the Weibel-Palade bodies. It temporarily increases the levels of VWF and F-VIII and is used in treating patients who are bleeding. Transmission of blood-borne disease is not a risk with DDAVP. About 20–25% of VWD patients, including all type 3 patients and about 10–15% of type 1 patients, do not respond to DDAVP. The response to DDAVP can be variable in type 2 subtype patients. It should be used with caution to treat patients with type 2B VWD because it can cause a dangerous reduction in the platelet count. Patients with type 2A do not respond consistently.

The preferred form of therapy for those who do not respond to DDAVP is concentrated "intermediate purity" preparations of F-VIII that contain intermediate-size VWF molecules. High purity or monoclonal F-VIII preparations do not contain sufficient VWF to be useful in treating VWD. F-VIII concentrates are virus inactivated by a variety of methods. A potential complication of using products containing both F-VIII and VWF is the elevation of plasma F-VIII levels, sometimes to as high as 400 IU/mL. Excessively high levels of F-VIII can be associated with venous thrombosis (∞ Chapter 33). A highly purified VWF concentrate that contains little F-VIII has been used successfully in treating European patients with VWD but is not yet available in the United States.[18]

Checkpoint! 2

If a patient with VWD has an equal decrease in F-VIII activity, VWF:RCo, and VWF:Ag assay, does this more likely indicate that there is a true decrease in the amount of VWF, or does it indicate that the patient has a type of VWD that is characterized by a functional abnormality of VWF? Support your answer.

What type of VWD is most likely in a patient with these laboratory results?

 CASE STUDY *(continued from page 700)*

Scott's mother was questioned about how the bleeding had begun in the joint and about other bleeding history. She answered that Scott had taken a slight tumble, but that it had not seemed to her enough to cause such severe bleeding. She also mentioned that when Scott had minor cuts, they seemed to stop bleeding quickly but often would bleed again in a day or two.

1. What term is used to describe the type of bleeding from minor cuts that Scott's mother is describing?
2. Does this history seem to be typical of a platelet disorder or of a coagulation factor disorder? Why?

X-Linked Recessive Disorders

The hemophilias are hereditary bleeding disorders resulting from congenital deficiencies of proteins involved in blood coagulation. The clinically most common deficiencies are associated with mutations in the genes for factors VIII and IX on the X chromosome. These proteins participate as a cofactor (F-VIII) and serine protease (F-IX) in the intrinsic pathway of fibrin formation (∞ Chapter 30). Deficiency of F-VIII is known as **hemophilia A;** deficiency of F-IX is called **hemophilia B** (also known as *Christmas disease*). Both deficiencies demonstrate X-linked recessive inheritance patterns.

X-linked recessive disorders are usually inherited by sons from their carrier (heterozygous) mothers who have an abnormal allele on one X chromosome and a normal allele on the other. Each son has a 50% chance of inheriting the affected gene. Males have only one X chromosome (hemizygous); thus, if they inherit an abnormal allele on that chromosome, they are affected with hemophilia. In the case of F-VIII or F-IX deficiency, males are able to synthesize little or none of the clotting factor, depending on the particular mutation inherited.

Hemophilia A is a deficiency of the F-VIII portion of the F-VIII/VWF complex as opposed to VWD in which the VWF portion of the complex is abnormal (discussed previously). Patients with hemophilia A have normal circulating levels and functionally normal VWF. Thus, their platelets adhere properly to collagen, and the formation of an effective primary hemostatic plug is not disrupted. Patients with hemophilia B have an intact F-VIII/VWF complex and likewise have normal primary hemostatic plug formation. The abnormal bleeding in both diseases is caused by delayed and inadequate fibrin formation with a secondary increase in fibrinolysis. These patients generate a normal tissue-factor driven *initiation* phase of coagulation but fail to generate the massive amounts of thrombin during the *propagation* phase of coagulation (∞ Chapter 30). As a result, in addition to inadequate thrombin and fibrin production, thrombin activation of TAFI fails to occur, resulting in excessive fibrinolysis compounding the bleeding associated with inadequate fibrin formation.

The clinical presentations in both deficiencies are identical. They can be distinguished only by laboratory testing. The common clinical and laboratory aspects of the hemophilias are discussed later after a discussion of the genetic mutations specific for F-VIII and F-IX.

Hemophilia has been known for several thousand years. It has contributed to world history by its presence in the royal families of Europe, particularly Great Britain, Russia, and Spain, through Queen Victoria, who was a carrier for hemophilia A. Originally, all patients with X-linked bleeding disorders were believed to have the same disease. This idea was challenged when, in 1947, Pavlovsky observed that prolonged recalcification times (the test available then) on two patients with hemophilia were corrected when the test was performed on mixtures of the two plasmas.[19] In 1952, three groups of investigators reported patients who were missing a new clotting factor that became known as F-IX.

Hemophilia A accounts for 80–85% of all cases of hemophilia with a prevalence of approximately 1 in 5,000–10,000 male births. Most of the remaining 15–20% of hemophilia patients are deficient in F-IX (affecting ~1 in 30,000 males). Hemophilia A is second to VWD in the overall frequency of inherited bleeding disorders. Approximately 30% of the affected individuals have no positive family history of the disease, indicating that de novo genetic mutations occur often.

Factor VIII Nomenclature   In 1985, the International Committee on Thrombosis and Hemostasis published rec-

TABLE 32-6

Nomenclature of the F-VIII/von Willebrand Factor Complex

von Willebrand factor—deficient in von Willebrand disease (VWD)

VWF	von Willebrand factor protein
VWF:Ag	Antigenic properties of von Willebrand factor
	Measured by monoclonal antibodies with immunologic procedures
VWF:RCo	Functional activity of the VWF molecule as measured by ristocetin cofactor activity

Factor VIII—deficient in hemophilia A

F-VIII	F-VIII protein
F-VIII:C	Functional activity of F-VIII as a procoagulant in fibrin formation (as measured by APTT)
F-VIII:Ag	Antigenic properties of F-VIII

Checkpoint! 3

What abbreviation is acceptable for:

   a. the antigenic properties of VWF?
   b. the functional activity of F-VIII?
   c. the complex of F-VIII and VWF?

ommendations that defined nomenclature for the F-VIII/VWF complex.[20] Prior to these recommendations, the literature referring to F-VIII and VWF was quite confusing. By the mid-1980s, the genes for both F-VIII and VWF had been identified and cloned. The 1985 committee recommendations recognized that two distinct proteins were associated as the F-VIII/VWF complex, each having unique immunologic and functional properties. The currently accepted definitions and abbreviations for the F-VIII/VWF complex components are shown in Table 32-6.[20] The original name for F-VIII, *antihemophilic factor,* is still an acceptable synonym.

F-VIII Mutations The molecular structure and key sites of functional activities of F-VIII are shown in Figure 32-3 ■.[21] Genetic defects in the F-VIII gene cause hemophilia A. Using restriction enzyme techniques, the polymerase-chain reaction, and other methods, the molecular defects have been determined in more than 4500 patients. The Hemophilia A Mutation Database (www.europium.csc.mrc.ac.uk/WebPages/Main/main.htm) lists >1200 different mutations.[22] Genetic defects include point mutations (more than 50% of the identified defects), gross deletions, and regulatory defects spread throughout the gene.[23,24] Mutations result in either quantitative or qualitative defects of the F-VIII protein. The majority of mutations result in a CRM− or CRM reduced phenotype (~95%). The clinical severity of the disease depends on the site of mutation within the gene and the molecular functions of the protein that are disrupted. One unique type of mutation involving intron 22, called the *F-VIII inversion mutation,* occurs in almost 50% of patients with a severe phenotype. The same mutation occurs in all members of a family, resulting in a similar clinical expression of disease in affected members of the family.

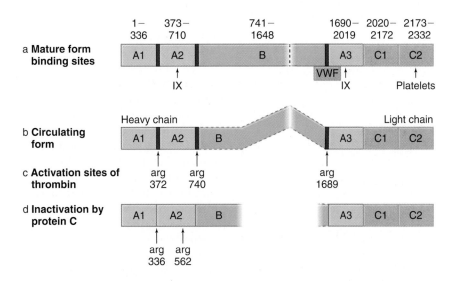

■ FIGURE 32-3 Schematic diagram depicting F-VIII. **a.** The mature protein with domains A1, A2, B, A3, C1, and C2. **b.** The circulating form of F-VIII with variable portions of the B domain removed; attaches to VWF at the acidic region preceeding domain A3. **c.** Sites of activation by thrombin at Arg residues 372, 740, and 1689. The heavy chain is cleaved, forming a 3-chain structure, and F-VIII is released from VWF. **d.** Sites of proteolytic inactivation of F-VIII by activated protein C (APC) at Arg 336 and Arg 562. Arg = arginine

Factor IX Mutations   F-IX deficiency, or hemophilia B, is also known as *Christmas disease* (*Christmas* was the surname of the first reported affected family). Heterogeneous mutations in the F-IX gene or its regulatory components result in hemophilia B. A database of mutations, available at www.kcl.ac.uk/ip/petergreen/haemBdatabase.html, includes more than 1050 unique mutations in 2891 patients.[25,26] Point mutations (mis-sense and nonsense), deletions of various portions of the gene, and insertions are the main types of molecular events. The clinical severity depends on the type of mutation and the region of the gene affected. Some F-IX deficient patients are CRM−, approximately one-third are CRM+, and some have reduced levels of antigen (CRM^R). CRM+ hemophilia B patients have a mutation in the structural gene resulting in production of an abnormal molecule. These patients have normal levels of F-IX antigen and variably reduced levels of F-IX activity. Patients who are CRM− can have large deletions of the gene and are at risk for developing inhibitors and anaphylactic reactions to replacement therapy.

Clinical Aspects of the Hemophilias   Clinical manifestations of hemophilia vary with the amount of factor present and are classified as severe, moderate, or mild disease (Table 32-7 ⊘). Generally individuals with >30% activity do not have hemophilia symptoms. The variation in clinical symptoms is largely the result of the type and site of the mutation (e.g., F-VIII deficient patients who have mutations at the thrombin-cleavage sites of F-VIII are unable to activate it, and patients with the inversion mutation have no F-VIII activity and severe bleeding symptoms).

Clinical symptoms in severe disease can begin at circumcision. Hemarthrosis is the most common feature of severe hemophilia. Bleeding into a joint can be triggered by even minor trauma and is accompanied by intense pain. The joint fills with blood, some of which is not reabsorbed, causing chronic inflammation, pain, and eventually destruction of the joint. Joint bleeds, particularly into the knee and ankle, generally occur when the child starts to walk. Subcutaneous hematomas can begin with slight trauma and spread to involve a large mass of tissue, causing purple discoloration of the skin. Epistaxis is rare in hemophilia. Other manifestations include hematuria, deep muscle bleeding, excess bleeding from dental extractions, bleeding with intramuscular injections, and delayed bleeding after minor cuts. The most common cause of death (after exclusion of viral infections transmitted by the replacement product) is intracranial hemorrhage, which can occur spontaneously or after trauma.

Hemarthrosis and severe spontaneous crippling bleeding into muscles are usually found in patients with severe disease. These symptoms are not commonly seen in those with moderate or mildly severe disease. More characteristic of moderate hemophilia is excessive bleeding after traumatic injury. Mild deficiencies of F-VIII or F-IX can be asymptomatic and unsuspected until a surgical procedure or major traumatic injury results in severe bleeding. Although the site of bleeding varies from individual to individual, the clinical severity of deficiencies of both factors remains similar within families.

Laboratory Evaluation of the Hemophilias   Laboratory tests are required to screen for abnormalities of coagulation factors and then to confirm and quantitate the specific factor that is deficient (∞ Chapter 40). Screening tests (APTT) are expressed as time, usually in seconds. Confirmatory assays are expressed in units of activity with normal plasma considered to have 1 unit (U) activity per mL , or 100 U per dL. The reference range for both F-VIII and F-IX is ~50–150% of normal (0.5-1.5 U/mL).

See Table 32-2 for the results of screening tests in a variety of hemostatic disorders. The APTT is prolonged in both F-VIII and F-IX deficiencies; it is lengthened inversely to the level of factor present in the patient's plasma when the level is below the sensitivity of the testing methodology. Levels of ≤20 U/dL of F-IX and ≤30 U/dL of F-VIII consistently prolong the APTT (∞ Chapter 40 and its associated website).

Definitive diagnosis is made on the basis of the results of specific factor assays. These precautions should be used in interpreting results: (1) F-VIII levels are lower in persons with blood group O than other blood groups (corresponding to the level of VWF) so the blood type must be considered when diagnosing F-VIII deficiency. (2) F-VIII level varies as an acute phase reactant and increases with exercise, inflammation, and so on. Estrogen-containing contraceptives also increase F-VIII levels. (3) Screening test systems might not be sensitive enough to detect mild deficiencies at levels between 20 and 50 U/dL. In these cases, the physician can order a factor assay on the basis of the patient's history. (4) The newborn range for F-IX is lower than that in adults

⊘ TABLE 32-7

Clinical Findings in Deficiencies of Factors VIII and IX

Factor VIII or IX Level, Units/dL	Severity	Symptoms
<1	Severe	Frequent spontaneous hemarthrosis with crippling
		Frequent severe, spontaneous hemorrhage (intracranial, intramuscular)
1–5	Moderate	Bleeding at circumcision
		Infrequent spontaneous joint and tissue bleeds
		Excessive bleeding after surgery or trauma
		Serious bleeding from minor injuries
6–30	Mild	Rare spontaneous bleeds
		Excessive bleeding after surgery or trauma
		Might not be discovered until bleeding episode occurs

(20–50% of normal), so one must refer to age-appropriate ranges when making the diagnosis of hemophilia B.

The results of additional laboratory tests shown in Table 32-3 are compared with the results in type 1 VWD. All platelet testing results are normal in the hemophilias. The thrombin time and PT are normal because neither assay depends on F-VIII or F-IX. One abnormal molecular variant, F-IXBm, does cause prolongation of the PT when bovine brain thromboplastin is used instead of rabbit thromboplastin.[27] Tests for fibrinolysis also are normal.

Hemophilia A must be distinguished from deficiencies of F-IX or F-XI and from VWD types 2N and 3. Hemophilia A is distinguished from hemophilia B by factor assays and from F-XI deficiency by both factor assays and inheritance pattern. Mixing studies in which the patient's plasma is mixed with normal plasma (1:1 ratio) with subsequent APTT testing should also be performed to eliminate the possibility of an inhibitor rather than the genetic disorder prior to performing the factor assay. In the event of an inhibitor, the APTT remains prolonged whereas with a factor deficiency, mixing corrects the defect. Type 2N VWD is caused by abnormalities of the D' domain of VWF that prevent F-VIII from binding.[3] Both hemophilia and type 2N VWD demonstrate low F-VIII levels and normal structure and functional tests for VWF:Ag, ristocetin cofactor activity, and VWF multimeric structure. Specialized testing is required to distinguish hemophilia A from VWD type 2N, and patients with type 2N VWD would not respond well clinically to F-VIII replacement therapy. Patients with type 2N VWD exhibit autosomal recessive inheritance. Type 3 VWD could be differentiated on the basis of an autosomal inheritance pattern and by a decrease of VWF:Ag in both platelets and plasma.

✓ Checkpoint! 4

Referring to Table 32-3, explain why the platelet function tests are abnormal in VWD but not in F-VIII or F-IX deficiencies.

Carrier Detection and Prenatal Diagnosis
Daughters of hemophilic males are obligate carriers of the disease and generally do not require further testing. Daughters of obligate carriers may inherit either one of their mother's X chromosomes and thus can be either carriers or normal. Hemophiliac males can inherit the disorder from carrier mothers or represent a spontaneous mutation. Female carriers of X-linked disorders are usually asymptomatic because they have one functional allele. Inactivation of one of the X chromosomes occurs randomly in each somatic cell of a female. Theoretically, in a carrier of an X-linked disorder, random inactivation results in approximately 50% of the cells having a functional X chromosome active, while the remaining 50% would have the X chromosome bearing the mutant allele. A female carrier of F-VIII or F-IX deficiency is expected to have approximately 50% of the normal plasma level of the factor in question. Detection of the carrier state cannot, however, be based merely on finding half of the normal activity in a factor assay because the normal reference range is 50–150%. Approximately 6% to 20% of women studied could be erroneously classified for two reasons. First, inactivation of the X chromosomes is not always randomly distributed. A carrier can have functional F-VIII- or F-IX-bearing X chromosomes in more than 50% of her hepatocytes, in which case her activity level would fall within the reference range. Conversely, if more than 50% of the hepatocytes have the normal X chromosomes inactivated, she could show clinical signs of mild hemophilia. Second, the F-VIII protein is an acute phase reactant and is physiologically increased in pregnancy, exercise, fever, and several other conditions, which can result in a transient rise of F-VIII to within the reference range. Both F-VIII and F-IX coagulant activity can rise with the use of oral contraceptives.

Detection of carriers is sometimes possible by analysis for both VWF antigen and F-VIII activity levels. VWF:Ag levels in carriers should be ~2 times the F-VIII:C.[28] The preferred method of detection of carriers is genetic testing when a proband is available to establish the genetic mutation. In families with a severe phenotype, DNA testing using the Southern blot technique is available for screening for the inversion mutation in intron 22, the most commonly encountered mutation in severe deficiencies. Potential carriers of F-IX deficiency can be detected by direct gene sequencing.[29,30]

Prenatal diagnosis by genotypic analysis has certain advantages over phenotypic analysis. Results are not affected by X chromosome inactivation, ABO blood type, or VWF levels, and testing can be done earlier in gestation. Various methods are available for prenatal diagnosis; the method of choice varies with the type of mutation anticipated. A chorionic villus biopsy can be done at 11 weeks of gestation and tested with DNA studies such as restriction enzymes (restriction fragment length polymorphism [RFLP]) or PCR methods. Because of the enormous variety of different molecular defects and the considerable size of the F-VIII gene, direct DNA diagnosis (PCR) is not available for all families. Direct DNA analysis is also limited by the fact that as many as one-third of hemophilia cases arise from new mutations. If the precise genetic defect is not known, it is difficult to do direct molecular analysis, but indirect DNA analysis (RFLP) can still be informative.

Direct sampling of fetal blood from the umbilical vein is possible at many institutions, and a factor assay can be performed on the blood sample. Some mutations require the simultaneous analysis of both antigen and activity levels for identification. Ultrasound analysis for determining the gender of the fetus is also available. Patients often elect to undergo prenatal diagnosis (even when pregnancy termination is not being considered) so that physicians can take precautions at birth to prevent bleeding if the fetus is at risk for hemophilia.[31] Intracranial hemorrhage during vaginal delivery is a potentially life-threatening complication.

Therapy for Hemophilia The goal of treatment for bleeding in hemophilia is replacement of the clotting factor to a level sufficient to achieve hemostasis. Typically, hemostasis for minor bleeding can be achieved at plasma factor levels of 25–30% of normal, whereas severe bleeding requires at least 50% of normal activity. Patients with severe trauma or surgery require plasma levels of 75–100% of normal. For patients who are actively bleeding, several preparations are available to raise the level of F-VIII or F-IX in the patient's plasma (Table 32-8 ✪).

F-VIII deficiencies were originally treated with cryoprecipitate preparations or F-VIII concentrate. F-VIII concentrates are prepared from plasma by a lyophilization process that results in a slight reduction of the activity of F-VIII, and loss of the largest VWF multimers. In the past, major problems were encountered with the use of plasma-derived concentrates of F-VIII, because the plasma from up to 20,000 donors is pooled to prepare one lot of product. Most patients who received this therapy before 1984 were exposed to hepatitis B, hepatitis C, and the HIV viruses. Since 1984, heat or solvent-detergent treatments have been used to inactivate the viruses, and concentrates are now considered safe. However, for a time, 90% of patients with severe F-VIII deficiency had HIV antibodies and antibodies to hepatitis B surface antigen (indicating exposure to both viruses). Since 1987, no new cases of HIV have been attributed to the administration of clotting factor concentrates in North America, and transmission of hepatitis has been documented only rarely.

To prevent virus transmission, F-VIII products can be prepared using monoclonal antibodies or recombinant technologies. Recombinant F-VIII (rF-VIII), however, also has hazards. Human albumin was added to the "first generation" rF-VIII preparations to stabilize the protein, and this has been associated with transmission of the B19 parvovirus (although there have been no significant clinical sequelae from these transmissions). Full-length F-VIII products stabilized by sucrose, not human albumin, are also available. Another form of F-VIII replacement therapy is a rF-VIII in which the B domain is deleted. This type of rF-VIII does not require albumin additive for stabilization. Concentrates can be used by hemophiliacs at home as prophylactic therapy to prevent extensive bleeding; they have markedly reduced the crippling hemarthropathy and improved the quality of life for patients with severe disease.

An alternative form of therapy in patients capable of producing some F-VIII (mildly affected hemophilia A) is the hormone, DDAVP, which stimulates storage cells to release F-VIII and VWF into the plasma.

F-IX deficiency can be treated with whole plasma or with concentrates that also contain factors II, VII, and X (prothrombin complex concentrates [PCC]). Another complication of therapy with intermediate purity products (PCC) in addition to viral infections is thrombosis because these concentrates contain variable amounts of activated factors VII, X, and prothrombin. Purified F-IX concentrate called Mononine is prepared from plasma using monoclonal antibodies. Purified F-IX concentrates are heat treated to inactivate the hepatitis and HIV viruses as described for F-VIII. Recombinant F-IX (Benefix®) is also available and is now the preferred form of therapy, avoiding complications of both viral transmission and hypercoagulability.

To achieve cure for both F-VIII and F-IX deficiencies, gene therapy is being researched. Because of the larger size of the F-VIII molecule (~200 kDa) compared to the F-IX protein (44 kDa), it has been more difficult to successfully express F-VIII using gene transfer protocols. The first clinical trials in F-IX deficiency were promising, but limited benefits and complications resulted in the trials' termination prematurely.[32] Progress in the development of gene therapy for the hemophilias has been slow. The increases in clotting factor activity are transient, and problems have been associated with the viral vectors used in the early studies. However, most researchers in the field believe that the likelihood of eventual success is high.[33]

Some hemophilia patients form neutralizing antibodies, also called *inhibitors,* to their deficient factor after factor-replacement therapies. In vivo antibody formation causes destruction of the infused factor, neutralizes the coagulant effects of therapy, and complicates treatment of the patient. An inhibitor to F-VIII or F-IX is clinically suspected when a bleeding episode fails to respond to an adequate dose of factor concentrate. Inhibitors develop primarily in severely affected patients. Approximately 5–20% of F-VIII-deficient patients and 1–3% of hemophilia B patients have inhibitors. There is no way to accurately predict which patients will form inhibitors. The prevalence of antibody formation is higher in patients with severe disease than those with moderate or mild disease. F-VIII inhibitors occur twice as commonly in African Americans than in Caucasians. Scandinavians are at higher risk than other populations to develop F-IX inhibitors. Severe gene lesions, resulting in CRM− or

✪ TABLE 32-8
Therapy for Hemophilia
Modes of therapy for F-VIII deficiency
• Recombinant F-VIII (rF-VIII)
• F-VIII concentrates
• Cryoprecipitate
• Desamino-D-vasopressin (DDAVP) (for some)
• Gene therapy (in research phase)
Modes of therapy for F-IX deficiency
• Recombinant F-IX (Benefix)
• Prothrombin complex concentrates (e.g., Konyne, Proplex)
• F-IX concentrates (e.g., Mononine)
• Gene therapy (in research phase)

reduced phenotypes are associated with a higher risk of developing inhibitors compared to CRM+ phenotypes. Patients with large F-VIII gene deletions (affecting >1 domain of the F-VIII molecule) have a threefold higher risk of developing an inhibitor compared with single domain deletions.[33]

 CASE STUDY *(continued from page 708)*

Scott's mother was questioned regarding the family history. She stated that her father and his brother had had similar bleeding symptoms. Her father died from a brain hemorrhage, and his brother died from complications associated with HIV. These brothers had sisters, none of whom had bleeding problems.

3. What type of inheritance is most probably present in this family?

4. Is this history typical of that of a patient with von Willebrand disease? Why?

5. What could have caused the patient's great uncle to have acquired HIV infection?

Autosomal Recessive Disorders

Autosomal recessive traits are expressed only in those individuals homozygous for the defective gene who inherit an abnormal allele from each parent. Each parent is likely to be heterozygous for the trait. Individuals who are homozygous generally have bleeding symptoms; those who are heterozygous usually have normal hemostasis.

Hereditary deficiencies of the remainder of the coagulation factors are rare in most of the world's populations. In areas of the world where consanguinity (mating between relatives) is more common, the prevalence of autosomal recessively inherited factor deficiencies is higher and can approach that of hemophilia B.[34]

The genetic mutations for all the proteins to be discussed are diverse between families but unique and constant within each family group. The mutation type and site within the molecule determines the severity of bleeding symptoms. Some mutations result in CRM+, and others result in CRM− phenotypes.

The clinical expression of the autosomally inherited deficiencies varies. Deficiencies of some factors result in severe bleeding symptoms while others are not associated with any bleeding abnormalities. Bleeding phenotype even among individuals with the same disorder can vary significantly. Deficiencies of some fibrinolytic inhibitors can also result in bleeding symptoms. The conditions are discussed under the appropriate categories.

Coagulation Factor Disorders with Bleeding Symptoms The diagnosis of the bleeding disorder is suspected from the results of the PT and APTT and confirmed with subsequent specific factor assays (Table 32-2). The degree of abnormality suggested by both PT and APTT can be small in cases of mild deficiency. Tests for platelet number and function are normal as are tests for fibrin split products and the thrombin time with some exceptions. Before a hereditary disease is considered, though, all possible causes for acquired coagulation factor deficiencies must be ruled out.

The autosomal recessive bleeding disorders are discussed in numerical order beginning with fibrinogen (factor I) deficiencies. Rare hereditary deficiencies of hemostatic proteins other than those involved in fibrin formation are presented briefly. Additional information including clinical bleeding characteristics and therapy can be found on this text's Companion Website. Table 32-9 ✪ shows the results of laboratory tests in these disorders.

Fibrinogen (Factor I) Deficiency. Two forms of fibrinogen deficiency are inherited as autosomal recessive traits. First reported in 1999, **afibrinogenemia** is a homozygous form of the disease in which no chemically, antigenically, or functionally detectable fibrinogen is found. **Hypofibrinogenemia** is a heterozygous form in which plasma levels of fibrinogen are ~50% of normal (reference range: 200–400 mg/dL). Consanguinity is found in about half of the families with afibrinogenemia. The prevalence of afibrinogenemia is estimated to be 1 in 1,000,000. More than 30 novel mutations have been identified in patients with afibrinogenemia.[35] A database of mutations is available at www.geht.org/databaseang/fibrinogen/l.

Clinically, afibrinogenemia is the more severe disease with patients having a severe bleeding disorder. At birth, umbilical cord and mucosal bleeding are frequent symptoms and can lead to death, but in general, patients have a milder course than do severe hemophiliacs and can go long periods without bleeding episodes. Joint or uterine bleeding is seen in 50% of patients.[34] Fatal bleeds from intracranial hemorrhages in infants have been reported. Patients with hypofibrinogenemia have a milder bleeding course. They are often asymptomatic, but bleeding can follow invasive procedures. Both disorders are associated with recurrent pregnancy loss as well as antepartum and postpartum hemorrhage.[36]

In afibrinogenemia, all laboratory tests based on production of a fibrin clot (PT, APTT, and thrombin time) are abnormal, and all are corrected in mixing studies with normal plasma. The bleeding time is prolonged in about half of the patients because fibrinogen is required for primary platelet aggregation. Platelet aggregation tests are also abnormal (Table 32-9). The diagnosis is confirmed using antigenic and functional assays for fibrinogen, which usually reveal <1mg/dL of the protein. The platelet count is also decreased in ~20% of patients. The erythrocyte sedimentation rate approaches zero because of the lack of fibrinogen in the plasma.

The presence of heparin, fibrin degradation products, or circulating anticoagulants in the plasma, which also prolong the hemostasis screening tests, must be considered in the differential diagnosis of afibrinogenemia. Mixing studies, the

⊘ TABLE 32-9

Laboratory Screening Tests in Autosomal Recessive Coagulation Factor Disorders

Factor	Platelet Tests		Coagulation Factor Tests				Tests for	
	Count	CT	PT	APTT	TT	FibA	FDP	Other
Afibrinogenemia	±N	±A	A	A	A	Absent	N	Abnormal platelet aggregation with ADP and epinephrine
Hypofibrinogenemia	N	N	N	N	A	N	N	
Dysfibrinogenemia	N	N	N	N	A	Variable	N	
Factor II	N	N	A	A	N	N	N	
Factor V	N	±N	A	A	N	N	N	
Factor VII	N	N	A	N	N	N	N	
Factor X	N	N	A	A	N	N	N	Abnormal Russell's viper venom test
Factor XI	N	N	N	A	N	N	N	
Factor XII	N	N	N	A	N	N	N	No bleeding tendency
Prekallikrein	N	N	N	A	N	N	N	No bleeding tendency; APTT corrected with 10-minute incubation with kaolin reagents
HK	N	N	N	A	N	N	N	No bleeding tendency
Factor XIII	N	N	N	N	N	N	N	

CT = closure time; PT = prothrombin time; APTT = activated partial thromboplastin time; TT = thrombin time; FibA = fibrinogen assay; FDP = fibrin degradation products; N = normal; A = abnormal; HK = high molecular weight kininogen

patient's history, and tests for FDPs are helpful in distinguishing inherited afibrinogenemia from acquired conditions in which fibrinogen can be decreased (∞ Chapters 30 and 40).

Replacement therapy with cryoprecipitate or fresh frozen plasma is used when patients are actively bleeding or to prevent excessive hemorrhage during surgical procedures.

A third form of fibrinogen abnormality is **dysfibrinogenemia,** in which the patient has normal levels (mg/dL) of fibrinogen but has abnormal fibrinogen molecules in the plasma. Dysfibrinogenemia is a relatively rare disorder that most commonly occurs in a heterozygous state. More than 300 novel mutations have been associated with dysfibrinogenemia.[35] Mutations have been identified in all three genes encoding the fibrinogen peptide chains (α, β, or γ chains).[36,37] Similar to abnormal hemoglobins, the fibrinogen abnormalities are often named for the city in which they were discovered. Some individuals have both reduced antigen levels and variant fibrinogen molecules and constitute a subcategory called *hypodysfibrinogenemias.*[35]

Dysfibrinogenemia is inherited as an autosomal dominant trait. Clinically, ~50% of individuals with dysfibrinogenemia have no bleeding symptoms or other clinical manifestations and are discovered incidentally when laboratory tests are ordered for unrelated reasons and unexpected abnormal results are found. Approximately 25% of individuals have bleeding complications, and 25% have thrombosis (∞ Chapter 33). It is suspected that the number of identified patients with dysfibrinogenemia is a small percentage of the actual number present in the population. In those patients who do exhibit

hemorrhagic symptoms, the bleeding is mild and generally occurs only after trauma. Dysfibrinogenemia has also been associated with hereditary renal amyloidosis.[35,38] Clinical manifestations depend on the type and the location of the mutation in the protein.

The functions or properties of fibrinogen are also affected by the type and site of mutation. In general, these mutations impair either the conversion of fibrinogen to fibrin monomer (proteolysis step), the conversion of fibrin monomers to polymers (spontaneous polymerization step), or the cross-linking of the fibrin polymers. Some mutations affect either thrombin binding or fibrinopeptide cleavage and are associated with abnormal release of either fibrinopeptides A or B. Other mutations affect the polymerization sites within the N-terminus of the α or β chain or the C-terminal region of the γ or β chains (∞ Chapter 30).

Laboratory tests for hemostasis in patients with dysfibrinogenemia are usually normal with the exception of the thrombin time, clot-based quantitative fibrinogen assays, and reptilase time, which are prolonged in most patients. However, determinations of fibrinogen antigenically or by a biochemical technique of precipitation and quantitation of fibrinogen are normal. Bleeding times and other platelet tests also are normal.

 Checkpoint! 5

Explain why the thrombin time is abnormal in patients with afibrinogenemia and dysfibrinogenemia.

Prothrombin (Factor II) Deficiency. Deficiencies of prothrombin occur at an estimated prevalence of 1 in 2,000,000, making it likely the rarest inherited bleeding disorder. Prothrombin deficiency is genetically heterogeneous with both quantitative (type I) and qualitative (type 2) deficiencies identified (www.archive.uwcm.ac.uk/uwcm/mg/hgmd0.html). Combined defects have also been reported. Heterozygotes have prothrombin levels of ~50% of normal; complete absence of prothrombin appears to be incompatible with life.[39] Both the PT and APTT are typically prolonged while the thrombin time and bleeding time are normal (Tables 32-2 and 32-9). The degree to which the PT and APTT are prolonged varies from patient to patient, and results can occasionally be within the reference range. The diagnosis is established using a specific factor assay for functional prothrombin and immunologic tests for antigen levels.

Factor V Deficiency. The first reported case of F-V deficiency was presented by Owren in 1947.[40] The prevalence of F-V deficiency is 1:1,000,000, and both quantitative (type 1) and qualitative (type 2) disorders have been described (www.hgmd.org; in Search enter "119896" for keyword). The specific genetic defect in most patients has not been identified.[39] Like prothrombin and F-X, F-V functions in the common pathway, so the PT and APTT are both prolonged, but thrombin time (TT) is normal (Table 32-2). Abnormal bleeding times are reported in about one-third of patients and may be related to a deficiency of F-V in platelet alpha granules.[34] Other screening tests are normal (Table 32-9). Definitive diagnosis requires an F-V assay (functional and immunologic).

Factor VII Deficiency. F-VII deficiency is the only plasma coagulation factor deficiency in which the PT alone is prolonged (Tables 32-2 and 32-9). The incidence is estimated as 1 in 300,000 to 1 in 500,000. To date, more than 150 cases have been reported, and both quantitative (type 1) and qualitative (type 2) disorders have been described (http://193.60.222.13/). A quantitative F-VII determination by standard factor assay methods (functional and immunologic) provides a definitive diagnosis. Homozygous patients usually have less than 10 U/dL of the factor; heterozygous individuals (who are generally asymptomatic) have 40–60 U/dL. It is important to use age- and gestational-related reference ranges because F-VII is naturally low at birth.[36]

 Checkpoint! 6

Explain why the prothrombin time but not the APTT is prolonged in F-VII deficiency.

Factor X Deficiency. The incidence of F-X deficiency is 1 in 1,000,000 in the general population.[36] F-X deficiency is genetically heterogeneous, and both quantitative (type 1) and qualitative (type 2) disorders have been described (www.hgmd.org; in Search enter "119890" for keyword).[41,42] Both the PT and APTT screening tests are usually prolonged

(Tables 32-2 and 32-9). However, in three mutations, the PT is prolonged, but the APTT is normal; the opposite is true in another variant.[43] The Russell's viper venom (RVV) test, which directly activates F-X, is prolonged, although it too can be normal in some variants. A F-X assay (functional and immunologic) is the definitive test although it is important to exclude vitamin K deficiency before confirming the diagnosis.

Factor XI Deficiency. F-XI deficiency is the fourth most common inherited bleeding disorder[34] with an estimated frequency in the general population of 1 in 100,000.[44] F-XI deficiency has a high frequency in the Ashkenazi Jewish population; approximately 0.2% of these individuals are homozygous, and 11% are heterozygous for this disorder.[45]

Laboratory screening tests reveal a prolonged APTT and normal PT, although the APTT can be normal in heterozygous patients with mild deficiency. Other tests are normal (Table 32-9). Deficiencies of factors XII, XI, VIII, and IX, prekallikrein (PK), and high molecular weight kininogen (HK) are considered when the APTT is the sole abnormal screening test. The clinical and family histories are useful in determining which factor assay to perform. The specific assay for F-XI is the definitive test for this deficiency. Homozygous individuals have from less than 1 U/dL up to 10 U/dL F-XI activity. Most patients have equivalent decreases in antigenic and functional activity, indicative of a type I (quantitative) disorder. A few F-XI mutations are associated with production of a dysfunctional protein.[46] More than 80 mutations in the F-XI gene have been associated with F-XI deficiency, although three different point mutations account for >90% of the affected patients (www.med.unc.edu/isth/mutations-databases/Factor_XI.htm).

Laboratory testing for F-XI activity requires precautions in collecting and handling the specimen. If the blood sample is collected in glass tubes, F-XI can become activated (glass pre-activation of contact proteins, ∞ Chapter 30) and can lead to false normal results and missed diagnosis of mild deficiencies. It is recommended that blood be drawn in plastic to minimize glass-contact activation. Multiple freezing and thawing of the specimen and/or a delay in running the assay (prolonged plasma storage) have been reported to cause pre-activation of F-XI and can cause normalization of an abnormal APTT. However, a single quick freeze and quick thaw appear to have minimal effect on F-XI levels (∞ Chapter 40, and associated web pages). The type of activator used by different manufacturers can also affect a test system's ability to detect a deficiency. Patients with mild F-XI deficiencies may react variably with different activators. Abnormal results may be obtained with one reagent and normal results with another.

Factor XIII Deficiency. F-XIII deficiency is very rare with an estimated prevalence of 1 in 2,000,000. F-XIII deficiency is a highly heterogeneous disorder, and a wide variety of genetic mutations affecting either the A or B chain of

F-XIII have been reported. Patients generally lack both plasma and platelet F-XIII.[47] Platelet F-XIII contains only the A_2 form of F-XIII (∞ Chapter 30), which carries the active enzymatic site. However, inherited deficiencies of the B chain also result in low plasma F-XIII levels because the B chains are required for the stabilization and survival of F-XIII (A_2B_2) in plasma. Low plasma levels of F-XIII (<5% of normal) are sufficient to control bleeding. The hallmark of F-XIII deficiency is bleeding from the umbilical cord site, after circumcision, or spontaneous intracranial bleeding after delivery. Miscarriage is very common because stabilization of fibrin at the maternal-fetal interface is required to maintain pregnancy.[47]

Because F-XIII functions after formation of fibrin, a deficiency does not affect the usual screening tests (PT, APTT, TT). However, in vitro clot formation is abnormal. One can observe excess red cells at the bottom of a whole blood clot tube after clot retraction. Laboratory diagnosis still relies on a screening test for F-XIII based on dissolution of the fibrin clot in 1% monochloroacetic acid or 5M urea. This clot solubility test is positive (i.e., the clot dissolves) when the F-XIII concentration is 0.5 U/dL or less. The clot is insoluble at levels as low as 1–2 U/dL (∞ Chapter 40). Because this screening test is not sensitive to mild deficiencies that can result in clinical sequelae, efforts have been made to develop more sensitive tests.[48] Specific assays are available, some that measure enzymatic activity and others that use immunologic techniques. One recently developed ELISA assay was used to establish the first reference range for F-XIII at 14–28 mg/L.[48]

Combined Factor V and Factor VIII Deficiency. In this rare disorder (< 100 families identified), both F-V and F-VIII levels are reduced (5% to 30% of normal levels).[49] The antigen and clotting activity are usually concordant. This disorder is also called *familial multiple clotting factor deficiency type 1*. Bleeding is mild to moderate and similar to that observed in other coagulation disorders. Combined F-V/VIII deficiency is due to a mutation of either of two genes.[39] The first gene produces a protein of the endoplasmic reticulum-Golgi intermediate compartment (ERGIC 53), also called *LMAN1* (*L-mannose 1*), and mutations of this protein are found in ~70% of patients with this disorder. The second is the multiple coagulation factor deficiency 2 (*MCFD2*) gene, which accounts for the remaining 30% of patients. The LMAN1-MCFD2 proteins form a complex, which functions to facilitate transport of F-V and F-VIII from the ER to the Golgi apparatus. The decrease in F-V and F-VIII results from defective intracellular transport and secretion in a pathway unique to these two coagulation factors.[39] The PT and APTT are prolonged in this disorder with the prolongation of APTT out of proportion to that of the PT.

Combined Deficiencies of Vitamin K-Dependent Clotting Factors. Vitamin K clotting factor deficiency (VKCFD) is caused by mutations of either the carboxylase enzyme responsible for the γ-carboxylation reaction (γ-glutamyl carboxylase, VKCFD1) or one of the enzymes of the pathway for vitamin K metabolism (e.g., vitamin K epoxide reductase, VKCFD2).[39] VKCFD is characterized by deficient activity of all vitamin K-dependent clotting factors. γ-carboxylation is required for the production of functional forms of these clotting factors and enables them to interact with phospholipids in the formation of the prothrombinase and Xase complexes (∞ Chapter 30). In this disorder, the proteins are produced but are nonfunctional due to their lack of γ-carboxylation. Affected individuals resemble patients on coumadin therapy with drastically prolonged PT and APTT tests and normal TT.

✓ Checkpoint! 7

Explain why the laboratory screening tests are normal in patients with F-XIII deficiency.

Factor Deficiencies without Clinical Bleeding The combination of a normal PT, a prolonged APTT, and a negative history of bleeding suggests deficiencies of either F-XII, PK, or HK. No bleeding symptoms are associated with deficiencies of these proteins even after severe trauma or during surgery. When an abnormal APTT is found in presurgical or screening testing, it must be resolved.[45] Although deficiencies of F-XII, PK, or HK display abnormal in vitro plasma coagulation, none is associated with in vivo bleeding. However, these deficiencies must be distinguished from those of F-VIII, F-IX, and F-XI, which are accompanied by defective hemostasis. The abnormal APTT is corrected by 1:1 mixing studies with normal plasma. All other hemostatic screening tests are normal (Table 32-9). The three deficiencies are differentiated by specific factor assays performed by the traditional modification of the APTT or by chromogenic substrate assays (∞ Chapter 40).

The specific factor assay can be preceded by a laboratory screening procedure (a modified APTT) to presumptively identify whether PK is the deficient factor and to choose assay procedures to perform. If the patient's plasma is incubated with a kaolin- or celite-containing APTT reagent for 10 minutes (rather than the usual 2 or 3 minutes), the prolonged APTT is corrected to normal in a PK deficiency.[45] The APTT remains prolonged in F-XII or HK deficiencies.

A deficiency of HK (also called *Fitzgerald, Williams,* or *Flaujac factor*) is one of a group of disorders involving not only HK but also variable deficiencies of low molecular weight kininogens (LK). LK does not affect the hemostatic system, so an isolated LK deficiency would not affect laboratory coagulation tests. Concurrent absence of the LK aids in classifying the disorders, however. "Williams" trait was characterized by a deficiency of both HK and LK; "Fitzgerald" and "Flaujac" traits were deficient in only HK.[50]

Because there is no clinical bleeding, therapy is usually not needed for these conditions. However, F-XII deficiency can be associated with defective fibrinolysis (due to decreased plasminogen activator activity) and an increased risk of thromboembolism (∞ Chapter 33).

Disorders of Fibrinolytic Protein Inhibitors with Bleeding Symptoms   Congenital deficiencies of these disorders are rare.[51] Deficiencies of α_2-antiplasmin (AP) and plasminogen activator inhibitor-1 (PAI-1) result in impaired regulation of fibrinolysis with excess plasmin activity. This disturbs the balance between coagulation and fibrinolysis, resulting in a bleeding disorder. Initial hemostasis is typically normal, but delayed bleeding can occur because of premature lysis of hemostatic plugs. Futher information is available on this text's Companion Website.

CASE STUDY *(continued from page 713)*

Screening hemostasis tests were performed on Scott's blood in the hemostasis laboratory. The results follow (see reference ranges in table E on cover):

Platelet count	250×10^9/L
Prothrombin time	12 sec
Activated partial thromboplastin time	95 sec

6. Name the coagulation factor deficiencies that are possible with these laboratory results.

7. What is the most likely factor deficiency? Why?

ACQUIRED DISORDERS OF HEMOSTASIS ASSOCIATED WITH BLEEDING

Acquired deficiencies of hemostatic proteins that result in bleeding symptoms can occur in individuals who were previously normal. Acquired deficiencies are far more common than the hereditary disorders of coagulation factors. Acquired coagulation disorders are also more complicated than the inherited conditions because multiple factors usually are defective, and bleeding is often simultaneous from more than one site. In addition to acquired deficiencies of the fibrin-forming proteins, there are also deficiencies of naturally occurring inhibitors.

Acquired disorders occur in response to another disease process and are produced by a variety of mechanisms. The conditions in which these disturbances occur are classified into the following categories: disseminated intravascular coagulation, primary fibrinogenolysis, liver disease, vitamin K deficiency, and acquired pathologic inhibitors.

Disseminated Intravascular Coagulation
Disseminated intravascular coagulation (DIC) is a condition in which the normal balance of hemostasis is altered, allowing the uncontrolled and inappropriate formation and lysis of fibrin within the blood vessels. Activation of coagulation occurs systemically rather than locally at sites of vascular injury. Fibrin is deposited diffusely within the capil-laries as well as in arterioles and venules. As fibrin is formed, several clotting proteins and naturally occurring inhibitors and platelets are consumed faster than they are synthesized (**consumption coagulopathy**). The result is an acquired deficiency of multiple hemostatic components. Fibrinolysis follows fibrin formation as a natural sequence of the hemostatic process, the same processes that occur in normal hemostasis except that they are happening at the wrong time and in the wrong place. As a result of consumption of coagulation factors and platelets and the formation of fibrin degradation products (FDP), the patient often bleeds at the same time that disseminated clotting is occurring.

Incidence   DIC occurs in approximately 1 in 1000 hospitalized patients. About 20% of the cases are asymptomatic and suspected only on the basis of laboratory data. It can occur at any age, although it is more often seen in the very young and the elderly.

Etiology   DIC is a syndrome, not a disease. It is a group of symptoms that is always triggered by a primary condition that does not necessarily involve coagulation. A number of diverse disease states can trigger the DIC syndrome; they often involve the introduction of tissue factor (TF) into the blood stream, resulting in the initiation of fibrin formation. TF can enter the blood from mechanical injury to tissues or from injury to the endothelial cells.

Conditions most often associated with triggering DIC are summarized in Table 32-10 ✪, the most common of which are infections, particularly those associated with septicemia. The trigger mechanism of infections is likely cytokines (IL-1, IL-6, and/or tumor necrosis factor TNF) released into the tissues by the inflammatory response, which activate endothelial cells. Resting endothelium does not express TF, but endothelial cells or monocytes activated by inflammatory cytokines or injured by endotoxin express TF activity. The full DIC response is seen in 30–50% of patients with Gram-negative or Gram-positive septicemia.[52]

Complications of pregnancy likely cause DIC because amniotic fluid acts as a thromboplastin to activate fibrin formation pathways. With massive tissue or blood cell injury, it is thought that TF-like substances, such as fat and phospholipids, enter the circulation and activate coagulation. In one study, most patients with head trauma had laboratory evidence of DIC caused by procoagulants entering the circulation from the injured brain tissue.[53] The trigger mechanism of malignant cells is a variation of tissue injury. Some malignant cells express a TF-like substance, and others have been shown to produce a cysteine protease capable of directly activating F-X.[52,54] Figure 32-4 ■ summarizes the potential activation sites in the hemostatic system.

Pathophysiology   After the initiating event has occurred, thrombin is formed within the circulation. Unlike the physiologic formation of the hemostatic plug in which thrombin generation remains limited and localized at the site of vessel injury, DIC results in generalized or systemic activation of

TABLE 32-10

Clinical Conditions Associated with the Development of Disseminated Intravascular Coagulation (DIC)

Infections	Bacterial (endotoxins)
	Viral
	Fungal
	Rickettsial
	Protozoal
Complications of pregnancy	Abruptio placentae
	Amniotic fluid embolism
	Retained placenta
	Toxemia
	Intrauterine fetal death
	Septic abortion
Neoplasms (malignant)	Solid tumors
	Leukemia, particularly Acute Promyelocytic
Massive tissue injury	Burns
	Trauma
	Head injury
	Extensive surgery
	Extracorporeal circulation
Vascular injury	Shock
	Hypotension
	Hypoxia
	Acidosis
Miscellaneous	Snake bite
	Heat stroke
	Any disease

coagulation. The circulating thrombin acts on its substrates as they circulate in the same manner as it does after an injury-induced localized formation of fibrin (∞ Chapter 30). This unregulated generation of thrombin results in consumption of fibrinogen; factors V, VIII, and XIII (the natural substrates of thrombin); and depletion of prothrombin (the precursor zymogen). Thrombin is a potent agonist of platelets inducing platelet activation and aggregation. Thrombin also binds to receptors on endothelial cells, inducing endothelial release of tissue plasminogen activator (tPA), which in the presence of the newly formed fibrin activates plasminogen to plasmin and triggers an aggressive secondary fibrinolysis. As plasmin is generated, plasminogen becomes depleted. DIC results from a failure of the mechanisms that limit blood clotting and thrombin generation (the normal inhibitory pathways to prevent the systemic effects of thrombin).

The coagulation inhibitors antithrombin (AT), heparin cofactor II (HC II), and thrombomodulin (TM), normally effective in regulating the localized generation of thrombin, are overwhelmed in DIC. Deficiencies of AT, protein C (PC),

and protein S (PS) are induced because they are utilized in removing their activated substrates from the circulation. Also, IL-1 and TNF (elevated in sepsis) decrease TM expression on endothelium, resulting in decreased activation of the PC/PS inhibitory mechanism (∞ Chapter 30).

Plasma levels of fibrinopeptides A and B (FPA and FPB) and D-dimer are elevated because of the actions of thrombin on fibrinogen and of plasmin on fibrin. FDPs interfere with fibrin formation and platelet function, contributing to the bleeding tendency.

All of these events can result in bleeding as the clotting mechanism is activated and procoagulant components become depleted. The pathogenesis of DIC is summarized in Figure 32-5 ■.

Clinical Aspects of DIC   The symptoms seen in patients with DIC result from the presence and activation of thrombin, plasmin, platelets, endothelium, and proteolytic inhibitors within the bloodstream and vary from patient to patient because of the complex interactions between these components. Because clotting factors and platelets are consumed, bleeding symptoms are favored in some patients. In other patients, thrombosis is the dominant process. In addition, the intensity and duration can result in either an acute or chronic clinical course. Patients with acute disease tend to manifest hemorrhagic symptoms whereas in those with chronic disease thrombosis is more likely to predominate.[54] The more commonly recognized acute form begins with sudden onset of severe bleeding and is seen in 80–90% of patients with DIC. In the chronic form (10–20% of patients), the stimulus that triggers clotting is weaker, and the natural homeostatic mechanisms are sufficient to replace depleted hemostatic components.

Hemorrhages and thrombosis occur predominantly in the microvasculature and are responsible for the clinical manifestations. In patients with acute DIC whose disease course is hemorrhagic, bleeding begins abruptly and generally occurs from three or more sites simultaneously.[45] Sites of bleeding tend to correspond to the tissues involved in the triggering event. Possible bleeding manifestations include hematuria; gastrointestinal and respiratory tract bleeding; intracranial bleeding; epistaxis; oozing from needle puncture sites, surgical drains, or sutures; and spontaneous bruising and petechiae. Bleeding can be profuse, leading to death.

At the same time, small strands of fibrin (microclots) form inside blood vessels and obstruct the microvasculature. Because blood vessels are occluded, tissue anoxia and microinfarcts in various organs can occur. Manifestations can include renal failure, coma, liver failure, respiratory failure, skin necrosis, gangrene, and venous thromboembolism.

Shock is a common feature and can be either a cause or an effect of DIC. The association of shock with DIC is complex and not well understood. Shock is likely induced because cytokine generation and products of the kinin and complement systems cause increased vascular permeability and hypotension. The mortality rate of DIC is 50–60%.

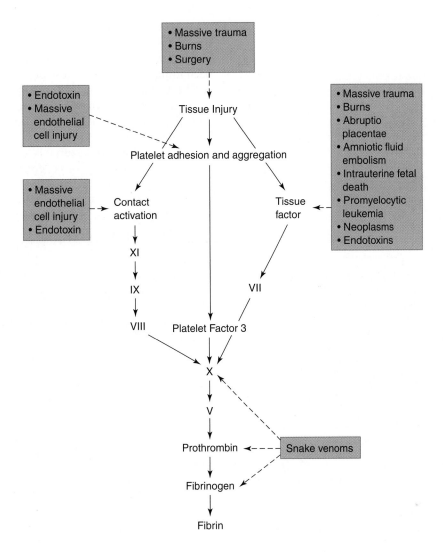

■ FIGURE 32-4   Conditions that initiate DIC activate the hemostatic pathways in a variety of ways. Normal hemostasis is shown by solid arrows. Processes that trigger DIC are shown in the boxes, and broken arrows indicate proposed sites of activation. (Adapted with permission from: Grosset AMB, Rodgers GM. Acquired coagulation disorders. In: Lee GR, Foerster J, Lukens J, Paraskevas F, Greer JP, Rodgers GM, eds. *Wintrobe's Clinical Hematology*, 10th ed. Baltimore: Williams & Wilkins; 1999: 1733–80.)

Laboratory Evaluation of DIC   The physician makes the diagnosis of DIC primarily based on the patient's clinical symptoms. No single laboratory test will establish a diagnosis of DIC, nor are any combination of tests specific for DIC. Laboratory tests are ordered to confirm a suspected clinical diagnosis. Screening tests that are usually ordered by the physician include a platelet count, blood smear, PT, APTT, fibrinogen level, and D-dimer test. Some laboratories include a test for AT. These tests demonstrate the generation of both thrombin and plasmin and can reflect the severity of the consumption of hemostatic components. Table 32-11 ✪ shows the typical laboratory results in patients with DIC.

The platelet count, the most useful parameter, can fall to levels of 40–75 × 10^9/L. It is decreased in 97% of patients.

Identifying a decrease in the platelet count can be difficult in patients whose usual platelet count is in the upper reference range, and serial platelet counts clearly demonstrating decreasing values are more useful than a single determination.

The PT and APTT can be prolonged because of the decrease in factors II, V, and VIII and fibrinogen, although their alterations are not as consistent as the platelet count. One or more of these tests are prolonged in 60–75% of patients with DIC.[45] Early in the disease process, these tests occasionally may be shorter than normal, perhaps due to the presence of factors that are already activated, and which would require less time for clot formation in vitro.[45]

In severe disease, the fibrinogen level can drop to 10–50 mg/dL but is decreased in only 23–71% of patients.[52] Fibrinogen

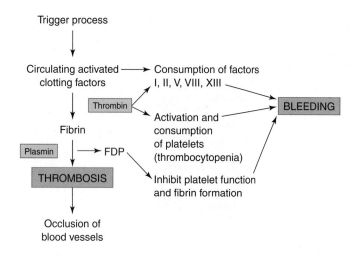

FIGURE 32-5   Pathogenesis of DIC. Activation of hemostasis by triggering processes leads to clotting and bleeding simultaneously. Intravascular fibrin formation results in occlusion of vessels. During clotting, several coagulation factors and platelets are consumed, leading to bleeding. (Adapted from: Grosset AMB, Rodgers GM. Acquired coagulation disorders. In: Lee GR, Foerster J, Lukens J, Paraskevas F, Greer JP, Rodgers GM, eds. *Wintrobe's Clinical Hematology,* 10th ed. Baltimore: Williams & Wilkins; 1999: 1733–80.)

is an acute phase reactant, and the protein increases in inflammatory conditions. Because many patients with DIC have underlying disease, their fibrinogen levels could have been initially elevated because of the acute phase response.

The D-dimer test to demonstrate the presence of fibrin-derived FDPs, and therefore generation of both thrombin and plasmin, is elevated in 93% of patients and provides good evidence supporting the diagnosis of DIC.[45] D-dimers, which are present only after F-XIII stabilization of fibrin, confirm that activation of coagulation has taken place, but they are not specific for DIC. The D-dimer test can be positive in several other clinical conditions such as after surgery and in patients with renal disease or pulmonary emboli. Most laboratories use the D-dimer test, which has replaced a similar latex test for fibrin degradation products that fails to distinguish between plasmin degradation products of fibrinogen and fibrin (∞ Chapter 40).

Some clinicians have recommended a test to demonstrate a decrease in AT. AT decreases in concentration early in the disease process as it combines with and inactivates thrombin and other serine proteases. It is decreased in 89% of patients. Examination of the blood smear reveals the presence of schistocytes in 50% of patients. Schistocytes are produced as

TABLE 32-11

Typical Laboratory Findings in Acquired Disorders of Hemostasis Associated with Bleeding

Test	DIC	Primary Fibrinogenolysis	Severe Liver Disease	Vitamin K Deficiency	Specific Factor Inhibitor	Lupus Anticoagulant*
Screening tests						
Platelet count	Dec	N	Dec	N	N	N
PT	Inc	Inc	Inc	Inc	N (inc with inhibitor against F-VII)	N (occasionally inc)
APTT	Inc	Inc	Inc	Inc	Inc (except if inhibitor against F-VII)	Inc
TT	Inc	Inc	Inc	N	N	N
Definitive tests						
Fibrinogen	Dec	Dec	Dec	N	N	N
D-dimer	Inc	N	N	N	N	N
Latex FSP test	Inc	Inc	N/inc	N	N	N
Plasminogen	Dec	Dec	N/dec	N	N	N
Fibrinopeptide A	Inc	N	N	N	N	N
Natural inhibitors						
Antithrombin	Dec	N	Dec	N	N	N
Protein C	Varies	N	Dec	Dec	N	N
Protein S	Varies	N	Dec	Dec	N	Varies
Miscellaneous						
Blood smear	Schistocytes	N	Macrocytes, target cells, acanthocytes	N	N	N

*Not a hemostatic disorder associated with bleeding but necessary to consider in the differential diagnosis.
Inc = increased; Dec = decreased; N = normal; PT = prothrombin time; APTT = activated partial thromboplastin time; TT = thrombin time; FSP = fibrin split products.

blood cells are forced through the fibrin webs that clog the microvessels. However, fragmented red blood cells rarely constitute >10% of the red cells on the peripheral smear.

Other laboratory tests that could be abnormal in DIC but generally are not necessary for a diagnosis in most cases are the TT and serial specific factor assays for F-V, F-VIII, or prothrombin (to demonstrate decreased factor levels/increased consumption). The TT is increased because of the presence of FDPs and the decreased fibrinogen level and is abnormal in 58% of patients. Additional tests of thrombin generation include tests for fibrin monomers, FP-A and -B, thrombin-AT complexes (TAT), and prothrombin fragment 1.2 (∞ Chapter 40). They are all potentially useful parameters but at present are mainly research tools.

Therapy for DIC The first step in the treatment for DIC is to eliminate the underlying cause, if possible. After that it is controversial. The acute form is often self-limited and disappears when the fibrin is completely lysed. Replacement therapy using platelets, red cells, cryoprecipitate, or fresh frozen plasma are used when indicated (patients with clear laboratory evidence of DIC and bleeding).[55] Low molecular weight heparins have been found helpful in those patients with strong clinical and laboratory evidence of DIC and predominant thromboembolic manifestations or in patients in whom replacement therapy fails to alleviate excessive bleeding and increase the level of clotting factors. Newer approaches to therapy are to replace the depleted physiologic inhibitors (AT, PC, and TFPI) with concentrates. Clinical trials are being conducted on some of these products. Under most circumstances, patients with DIC should not be treated with fibrinolytic inhibitors.

The chronic form of DIC is usually seen secondary to disseminated malignancy in which case elimination of the precipitating event can be difficult. Heparin therapy sometimes is helpful if thrombosis is life threatening because it will stop intravascular fibrin formation. It must be administered with caution, however, because fatal bleeding has occurred with its use.

✓ Checkpoint! 8

a. *Why is thrombocytopenia usually present in a patient with DIC?*

b. *Which hemostasis laboratory screening tests (PT and APTT), if any, will the following affect:*
Decreased F-V
Decreased F-VIII
Decreased fibrinogen
Decreased antithrombin

c. *Which laboratory test results would distinguish DIC from hemophilia A?*

Primary Fibrinogenolysis

This syndrome is sometimes referred to as *primary fibrinolysis,* but this is technically inaccurate because the proteolytic action of plasmin is on fibrinogen, not fibrin. **Primary fibrinogenolysis** is a condition clinically similar to DIC, but it requires differentiation so that proper treatment can be instituted. In primary fibrinogenolysis, plasminogen becomes inappropriately activated to plasmin without concomitant thrombin generation. Plasmin then circulates and, if it overwhelms the antiplasmin inhibitors, degrades fibrinogen; factors V, VIII, and XIII; and other coagulation factors (and other proteins). An acquired deficiency of the proteins eventually develops and leads to bleeding symptoms that resemble DIC.

Similar pathologies can cause the two conditions, but liver disease is one of the most common triggers of primary fibrinogenolysis. Differentiating the two conditions with laboratory tests is sometimes difficult. Patients with primary fibrinogenolysis can have an abnormal PT, APTT, TT, fibrinogen assay, and increased fibrin(ogen) degradation products but normal D-dimer and fibrin monomer tests because stabilized fibrin is not formed. The level of fibrinopeptide A is normal in primary fibrinogenolysis but is elevated in DIC.[56] Table 32-11 compares laboratory test results in these two conditions with other acquired hemostatic disorders.

Therapy for primary fibrinogenolysis is epsilon aminocaproic acid (EACA), a specific inhibitor of plasmin. EACA is dangerous if administered to patients with DIC; therefore, the diagnosis of DIC needs to be excluded before the drug is given.[56]

Liver Disease

Liver disease affects all hemostatic functions. Most hemostatic proteins (those involved in fibrin formation, fibrinolysis, as well as hemostatic inhibitors) are synthesized in the liver (∞ Chapter 30; Web Table 32-1 ⊙). The liver macrophages play a major role in the removal of activated factors, products of activation such as the fibrinopeptides, fibrin degradation products, and plasminogen activators. A diseased liver diminishes these functions.[56]

Laboratory test results on a patient with liver disease can resemble those obtained from a patient with DIC. Differentiating the two conditions may be a difficult task for the physician. Table 32-11 compares the results of laboratory testing. The decreased production of proteins involved in fibrin formation can prolong all screening coagulation tests including the PT, APTT, and TT. The fibrinogen concentration is usually normal but can stabilize in the low reference range. An abnormal fibrinogen molecule that has an increased content of sialic acid and can cause defective clot formation may be synthesized.

The platelet count can be decreased for several reasons including hypersplenism (backing up of the portal blood supply when it is unable to enter the liver), alcohol toxicity of the bone marrow, decreased thrombopoietin production, and consumption of the platelets if DIC is also present.

FDPs are increased because the liver cells are unable to remove them from the circulation. Incomplete removal of plasminogen activators can result in systemic formation of plasmin and subsequent proteolysis of fibrinogen, contributing to the increase of FDPs. Excess fibrin or fibrinogen degradation products can impair blood coagulation and result in platelet dysfunction. The D-dimer test is usually normal and can be one way to differentiate DIC from liver disease.

Clinical bleeding is minimal except in severe liver disease when ecchymoses and epistaxis can occur. Bleeding from local lesions in the GI tract is common. Therapy involves the use of replacement products as needed.

Vitamin K Deficiency

Hepatic cells need vitamin K to complete the post-translational alteration of factors II, VII, IX, and X, PC, and PS (∞ Chapter 30). In the absence of vitamin K, the hepatic cells synthesize precursor proteins, but because γ-carboxyglutamic acid residues are absent, the calcium-binding sites are nonfunctional. Deficiency of vitamin K results in induced functional deficiencies of all of these proteins. If the level of functional proteins falls below 30 U/dL, bleeding symptoms can result, and the PT and/or the APTT is prolonged.

Sources of vitamin K are green, leafy vegetables and synthesis by bacteria in the GI tract. Symptomatic vitamin K deficiency in newborns called **hemorrhagic disease of the newborn (HDN)** is most often seen in the first days of life. Because their livers are still immature, synthesis of the vitamin K-dependent factors in newborns is 30–50% of adult levels. Almost all neonates are vitamin K deficient, presumably as a result of the mother's vitamin K deficiency and/or the lack of colonization of the colon by vitamin K-producing bacteria in the neonate.

HDN is broken into three subtypes: early, classic, and late. Early HDN occurs primarily in infants of mothers who have been on a vitamin K-blocking medication, such as anticonvulsants, and usually occurs within hours to the first week of life. Classic HDN occurs between the first week and first month of life and is largely prevented by prophylactic vitamin K administration at birth. Late HDN occurs from the first month to 3 months after birth.[57] This deficiency is more prevalent in breast-fed babies because human milk contains less vitamin K than cow's milk does. Infants with liver disease can also be susceptible to HDN.

Manifestations of hemorrhagic disease of the newborn are bleeding in the skin or from mucosal surfaces, circumcision, generalized ecchymoses, large intramuscular hemorrhages, and (rarely) intracranial bleeds. In the laboratory, the PT and possibly the APTT are more prolonged than expected at this age. Specific factor assays for factors II, VII, IX, and X are markedly decreased. The BT and the platelet count are within normal limits (Table 32-11).

Hemorrhagic disease of the newborn is prevented in the United States by encouraging administration of vitamin K to all newborns. Although most states have laws requiring its administration, some do not. In countries where this practice has recently been stopped, the disease occurs occasionally.

Causes of vitamin K deficiency in adults include malabsorptive syndromes such as sprue, obstruction of the biliary tract (because bile salts are necessary for absorption), ingestion of vitamin K inhibitors (such as warfarin), and prolonged broad-spectrum antibiotic therapy that abolishes normal flora of the intestine. Vitamin K administration corrects the deficiency within 24 hours.

Acquired Pathologic Inhibitors

Acquired inhibitors of blood coagulation, also called **circulating anticoagulants,** develop pathologically in patients with certain disease states and in some who have no apparent underlying condition. Almost all are immunoglobulins, either IgG or IgM, and can be either alloantibodies or autoantibodies. Two types of inhibitors are described: those directed toward a single coagulation factor and the lupus anticoagulant (LA).

Inhibitors of Single Factors Pathologic inhibitors against most coagulation factors have been reported. They are usually seen in patients with inherited factor deficiencies who have received replacement treatment for bleeding complications, but they are also associated with other conditions such as diseases or drugs and are sometimes seen in patients who are otherwise healthy. With the exception of antibodies to F-VIII and F-IX, they are extremely rare. These inhibitors are recognized because of their interference with or neutralization of clotting factor activity. The following discussion concentrates on the F-VIII and F-IX inhibitors.

Clinical Aspects. Inhibitors to F-VIII and F-IX are observed most often in association with the hemophilias. Approximately 15–20% of patients with severe hemophilia A and 1–3% of patients with severe hemophilia B develop alloantibodies to the respective deficient factor. Inhibitors are neutralizing alloantibodies that render the replacement factor inactive. Twenty-two percent of hemophilia A patients with the inversion mutation described earlier develop F-VIII inhibitors. Most patients with inhibitors have severe hemophilia with very low coagulant levels of the affected factor. All patients also have received replacement therapy for their factor deficiency, and most inhibitors develop within the first 50–100 exposure days to factor, although patients can develop an inhibitor at any time in their life. In hemophilia A patients, the antibody specificity is directed toward the coagulant antigen (VIII:Ag) only, not the VWF portion of the F-VIII/VWF complex. Although most inhibitors develop in severe or moderate forms of hemophilia, they also may be found in some patients with mild forms of hemophilia A.[58]

F-VIII inhibitors (autoantibodies) can also be found in nonhemophilic patients (acquired hemophilia A). Occasionally they develop in otherwise healthy individuals who most often are older patients or females during or following a pregnancy. Disease states associated with F-VIII inhibitors include autoimmune and lymphoproliferative diseases as well as multiple myeloma. Autoantibodies to other clotting factors can appear in similar circumstances as the F-VIII inhibitors.

The clinical course of patients with acquired inhibitors is variable but can resemble that of patients with severe hemophilia and result in fatal consequences in 10–20% of cases. In patients with congenital hemophilia who have not received therapy for 1 to 2 years, the antibody level often decreases, but an anamnestic response can be seen within 2 to 4 days after re-exposure. The antibody can also disappear spontaneously.

Laboratory Evaluation. Laboratory test results in patients with F-VIII or F-IX inhibitors resemble those in patients with severe factor deficiencies. The APTT is markedly prolonged and other screening tests are normal (Table 32-11). Mixing studies (1:1 patient plasma with normal plasma) can be performed as a screening procedure to distinguish between a true factor deficiency and an inhibitor (∞ Chapter 40). If an inhibitor is present, the test on the mixture will remain prolonged. Assays for specific inhibitors can then be performed (∞ Chapter 40).

Therapy for Factors VIII and IX Inhibitors. The type of therapy used for patients with F-VIII inhibitors depends on whether the patient is a low or high responder and on the inhibitor's titer. Low responders (25% of hemophiliacs with inhibitors) are patients with low titer antibodies that do not rise after further exposure to F-VIII. Patients with inhibitors that rise markedly with further exposure to F-VIII (anamnestic response) are known as high responders (~75% of hemophiliacs with inhibitors). For those who are low responders, large amounts of F-VIII that function by "overwhelming" the antibody can be administered successfully to treat or prevent clinical bleeding. If human F-VIII cannot be used because the inhibitor level is too high, F-IX complex products or porcine F-VIII can be used in an attempt to bypass the need for F-VIII. F-IX complex concentrates (PCC) contain prothrombin and factors VII, IX, and X. The mechanism of bypass activity of these concentrates remains unclear, but it has been suggested that their content of activated vitamin K-dependent factors (IIa, Xa, and trace amounts of VIIa and IXa) probably promote thrombin generation in vivo.[33] Recombinant F-VIIa is another bypass agent effective in the treatment of hemophilia patients with inhibitors.[33] Recombinant F-VIIa works by activating F-X and bypassing the need for F-VIII or F-IX in the formation of fibrin and thus is equally effective in both hemophilia A and B patients with inhibitors.

Lupus Anticoagulant The second type of inhibitor of major clinical importance is the **lupus anticoagulant (LA)**, so called because it was first discovered in patients with systemic lupus erythematosus (SLE). Approximately 6–16% of patients with SLE develop LA. The term *LA* is a misnomer because LA is more frequently encountered in patients without lupus and has been associated with a variety of other autoimmune diseases, neoplasias, certain infections, and the administration of drugs such as chlorpromazine or procainamide as well as apparently normal individuals. However, many people still call it the lupus anticoagulant or lupuslike anticoagulant.

LAs are autoantibodies that interact with the phospholipid surfaces of the reagents used in the APTT test (and occasionally the PT), prolonging the test results. They are part of a family of antibodies called *antiphospholipid antibodies* (APL). LAs are usually discovered by finding an unexpectedly prolonged APTT and sometimes PT while performing routine coagulation studies. However, the lupus anticoagulant is a laboratory phenomenon. Although laboratory testing suggests defective hemostasis, most patients do not in fact bleed but rather tend to be hypercoagulable. The pathophysiology, clinical aspects, and laboratory evaluation of LA/APL are discussed in ∞ Chapter 33 with other disorders of hypercoagulability.

ⓔ CASE STUDY *(continued from page 717)*

A TT was performed on Scott, and the results were within the laboratory's reference range. Mixing studies were performed. Scott's plasma was mixed with normal plasma, and the APTT was repeated on the mixture. The result of the APTT on the mixture was 36 sec.

8. What do the results of the APTT on the mixture of Scott's plasma with normal plasma indicate?

9. What test should be performed next?

10. If a F-VIII assay was done with results of <1 U/dL, what molecular studies should be done?

11. What therapy is indicated for this patient?

12. What complications from the therapy are possible?

▶ **FLOW CHARTS**

A flow chart that outlines reflex testing procedures that the laboratory can follow to investigate abnormal hemostatic screening tests is included on this text's Companion Website (Web Figure 32-2■).

▶ **HEMOSTASIS IN THE NEWBORN**

Hemostasis is an evolving process and is age dependent (i.e., it develops or evolves during the process of fetal development and changes with gestational age).[59] Blood coagulation studies in the newborn present special challenges to the laboratory. At birth, hepatic synthesis of several of the clotting proteins is at a lower level than in normal adults, and this makes diagnosing some inherited and acquired hemostatic abnormalities difficult. Some proteins do not reach adult levels until 6–12 months of age. Laboratory screening tests are prolonged (relative to adult normal values) and depend on the child's age and the presence of accompanying diseases. These factors influence the interpretation of the laboratory tests.

Obtaining an adequate blood sample is of utmost importance but technically extremely difficult. Even with maximum attention to quality control, spuriously altered results are possible. A venous sample is preferred to capillary or arterial blood. Obtaining the sample from an indwelling catheter should be avoided because of the danger of heparin contamination.

Adding anticoagulant to the syringe allows one to draw blood more slowly while minimizing the risk of clotting. The amount of anticoagulant must be reduced when the infant's hematocrit is above 55% because of the reduced plasma volume.

Because the total volume of blood in newborns is only 250–350 mL, efforts must be made to minimize the amount of sample drawn (∞ Chapter 40). Some suggestions for minimizing the amount of plasma needed for newborn testing are eliminating duplicate testing when performing the PT and APTT, or running several factor assays using diluted plasma rather than the screening tests.[60] Micro adaptations of several routine procedures, using 5–40 μL of plasma, have been developed.[61]

NORMAL HEMOSTASIS IN THE NEWBORN

Platelets and the proteins of the coagulation and fibrinolytic systems are first detected in fetuses at 10–11 weeks of gestation. Table 32-12 ✪ shows expected values for various laboratory tests for preterm and term infants at birth compared with results in older children and adults as well as the ages when adult levels of the proteins are reached.

Platelet counts reach adult levels by 27 weeks of gestation and, therefore, should be in the normal adult range (and size—i.e., mean platelet volume [MPV]) at birth. As with adults, platelet counts of less than 100×10^9/L should be

considered abnormal. Counts of $100–150 \times 10^9$/L are considered borderline and should be repeated. Platelet structure viewed by electron microscopy appears normal, but the dense body content of serotonin and ADP is <50% of adult levels.[59] Decreased platelet aggregation (relative to adult "normal") with low levels of ADP and with collagen, epinephrine, and thrombin are found at birth but normalize within several weeks. Platelet agglutination with ristocetin, on the other hand, is increased in newborns, which must be considered when diagnosing VWD. Plasma concentration of VWF and the proportion of high molecular weight multimers are increased in newborns (newborns have low levels of the VWF cleaving protease ADAMTS-13).[59] This likely explains the enhanced agglutination with ristocetin. Drugs that affect platelet function such as aspirin when taken by the mother also influence hemostasis in the fetus.

Concentrations of the coagulation proteins for term and preterm infants, older children, and adults are shown in Table 32-13 ✪. Multiple reference ranges are required because the hemostasis system is evolving. The fibrinogen group of factors is at normal adult levels at birth. The concentrations of the proteins of the prothrombin and contact factor groups are decreased at birth due to newborn liver immaturity. They reach adult levels at varying times (Table 32-13). The levels of these clotting factors usually are not low enough to affect hemostasis unless a stressful situation is present. VWF, on the other hand, is increased at birth and gradually decreases over the first 6 months of life.[62]

Natural inhibitors that the liver synthesizes are also decreased in newborns (Table 32-13). Adults with levels of AT equivalent to that of infants are considered at risk for thrombosis. Infants do not have this problem because the procoagulant proteins that are inactivated by AT are also decreased. Levels of PC are very low at birth and remain decreased during the first 6 months of life. Total PS is also decreased, but functional activity is similar to that in adults because it is

✪ TABLE 32-12

Laboratory Tests in Preterm and Term Infants as Compared to those of Adults and Older Children

Test	Preterm Infant (28–31 Weeks) (Day 1)	Preterm Infant (32–36 Weeks) (Day 1)	Term Infant (37–41 Weeks) (Day 1)	Adults and Older Children	Age Adult Level Reached
Platelet count, $\times 10^9$/L	150–430	150–430	174–456	150–450	Before birth
Platelet aggregation	Abnormal	Abnormal	Abnormal	Normal	One month
PT, sec	14.6–16.9*	10.6–16.2†	10.1–15.9*	10.8–13.9*	Comparable at birth
APTT, sec	80–168*	27.5–79.4†	31.3–54.5*	26.6–40.3*	By 6 months
TT, sec		19.0–30.4†	23.5 ± 2.38‡	19.7–30.3†	At birth
FDP		Normal	Normal	Normal	Before birth

PT = prothrombin time; APTT = activated partial thromboplastin time; TT = thrombin time; FDP = fibrin degradation products

*Taken from: Andrew M, Paes B and Johnston M. Development of the Hemostatic System in the Neonate and Young Infant. *Am J Ped Hem/Onc.* 1990;12(1):95–104.

†Taken from: Andrew M, Paes B, Milner R et al. Development of the human coagulation system in the healthy premature infant. *Blood.* 1988;72:1651–57.

‡Taken from: Andrew M, Paes B, Milner R et al. Development of the human coagulation system in the full-term infant. *Blood.* 1987;70:165–72.

✪ TABLE 32-13

Levels of Hemostatic Proteins in Preterm and Term Infants as Compared to Adults and Older Children

Protein	Preterm Infants* (27–31 Weeks) (U/dL)(Day 1)	Term Infants (38–41 Weeks) (U/dL)(Day 1)	Adults and Older Children (U/dL)	Age Adult Level Reached
Coagulant proteins—fibrinogen group				
Fibrinogen, mg/dL	256 ± 70	283 ± 116	278–122	Before birth
Factor V	65 ± 22	72 ± 35	62–150	Before birth
Factor VIII	37–126	50–178	50–149	Before birth
Factor XIII				
A subunit	32–108	27–131	55–155	5 days
B subunit	35–127	30–122	57–137	5 days
Coagulant proteins—prothrombin group				
Factor II (prothrombin)	19–54	26–70	70–146	6 months
Factor VII	24–76	28–104	67–143	5 days
Factor IX	17–20	15–91	55–163	6 months
Factor X	25–64	12–68	70–152	6 months
Coagulant proteins—contact group				
Factor XI	11–33	10–66	67–127	After 6 months
Factor XII	5–35	13–93	52–164	After 6 months
Prekallikrein	15–32	18–69	62–162	After 6 months
HMWK	19–52	6–102	50–136	1 month
Fibrinolytic protein				
Plasminogen	112–248*	195 ± 70	336 ± 88	6 months
Naturally occurring inhibitors				
Antithrombin	20–38	63 ± 24	105 ± 26	3 months
Protein C	12–44	35 ± 18	96 ± 32	After 6 months
Protein S	14–38	36 ± 24	92 ± 32	3 months
Heparin cofactor II	0–60	10–93	96 ± 30	6 months

Taken from: Andrew M, Paes B, and Johnston M. Development of the Hemostatic System in the Neonate and Young Infant. *Am J Ped Hem/Onc.* 1990;12(1):95–104 except as noted (*)

*From: Andrew M, Paes B, Milner R et al. Development of the human coagulation system in the healthy premature infant. *Blood.* 1988;72:1651–57.

completely present in the free (active) form due to the absence of C4BP.[59] Plasminogen levels in infants are decreased, and FDPs are similar to adult values.

The decrease in hemostatic factors in term and preterm infants affects coagulation tests (Table 32-12). The PT is prolonged ~3 seconds compared to that of adults because of the low levels of factors II, VII, and X. However, a PT of more than 17 seconds should be considered abnormal in the newborn.[63] Values in the normal adult range are usually achieved in 3–4 days.

The APTT is also prolonged ~2–3 seconds in term infants and can be significantly prolonged in preterm infants. This test depends on the factors of the intrinsic system and is particularly sensitive to the contact factors. Results of this test are also highly dependent on the reagent used.[60,62] Adult levels can be reached in 4–6 months.[63] The thrombin clotting

time is abnormal although the fibrinogen level is normal due to the presence of a distinct fetal fibrinogen molecule with altered function. The thrombin time becomes normal within a few days after birth.

In general, hemostatic values in preterm infants differ from adults as discussed above. They also differ from term infants but erratically so; however, by 6 months of age, their values are comparable to those of term infants.[64]

COMMON BLEEDING DISORDERS IN THE NEONATE

Although the coagulation systems of the "well" term and preterm infants show low levels of many procoagulant, anticoagulant, and fibrinolytic proteins, hemostasis is usually functionally balanced, and neither thromboses nor hemorrhages occur. However, abnormalities of hemostasis are present in ~1% of newborns. The classification of the most common problems depends on whether the child is considered sick or well. Sick infants include those with prematurity, perinatal infection, respiratory distress syndrome, metabolic derangements, and/or birth asphyxia. Hemostatic abnormalities in babies considered sick are most commonly either DIC, isolated platelet consumption independent of a decrease in clotting factors, or liver failure.

In well babies, the most common abnormalities of hemostasis are immune thrombocytopenia, vitamin K deficiency, hemophilia, and bleeding from a localized vascular lesion. Diagnosing some hereditary bleeding disorders in the neonatal period is difficult, particularly mild or moderate deficiencies of F-IX and VWD. Severe forms of F-VIII or F-IX deficiencies are easier to diagnose. Early onset vitamin K-deficiency bleeding (within the first 24 hours of life) is usually due to placental transfer of maternal drugs that inhibit vitamin K activity in the baby, including Dilantin or other anticonvulsants, antibiotics, and oral anticoagulants.

Bleeding manifestations in babies with DIC are similar to those in other patients with the syndrome and include bleeding from puncture sites, the GI tract, and other locations. The PT and APTT are markedly prolonged, and thrombocytopenia is present in symptomatic babies.

One of the most common causes of death in premature infants is intracranial hemorrhage. Many of these are patients who have severe respiratory distress syndrome or a familial bleeding diathesis (hemophilia or other hereditary coagulation deficiency).

Thrombosis can also occur in infants, particularly those with indwelling catheters, those born to diabetic mothers, or those with predisposing medical conditions (e.g., asphyxia, infection, respiratory distress syndrome). Neonatal hypercoagulability can also be seen in infants with a hereditary thrombophilia (∞ Chapter 33).

SUMMARY

This chapter discusses the conditions associated with abnormal secondary hemostasis encompassing those in which fibrin is formed too slowly or poorly or fibrinolysis proceeds too rapidly so that excessive bleeding results. It also discusses the unique hemostatic status of newborns.

Abnormal fibrin formation occurs in patients with mutations of the genes that code for the circulating procoagulant proteins and result either in decreased synthesis or abnormal function of the protein. The most widely known of these disorders are X-linked deficiencies of F-VIII and F-IX, called the *hemophilias.* von Willebrand factor is complexed with F-VIII in the circulation and when deficient can result in the most common bleeding disorder, von Willebrand disease. More unusual deficiencies of the remaining coagulation factors and of components of fibrinolysis can also result in excessive bleeding. However, in the case of F-XII, prekallikrein, and high molecular weight kininogen, no clinical bleeding symptoms are present in spite of abnormal in vitro laboratory test results. Some patients with deficiencies of these three components can have an increased risk for thrombosis, presumably secondary to impaired fibrinolysis. Laboratory screening tests and specific factor assays establish the diagnosis in disorders associated with coagulant protein deficiencies.

Newborns are at higher risk for bleeding and can have prolonged PTs and APTTs until the vitamin K-producing intestinal bacteria and liver production of the various coagulation factors are established.

REVIEW QUESTIONS

LEVEL I

1. A patient who has a deficiency of a clotting factor could have: (Objective 1)
   a. inherited an abnormal gene from a parent
   b. acquired the deficiency because of another disease present
   c. decreased amount of the particular factor in the blood
   d. all of the above

2. Why do patients who have deficiencies of clotting factors usually have abnormal bleeding? (Objectives 1, 2)
   a. Fibrin formation is slower and less effective than normal.
   b. Platelets do not aggregate normally.
   c. Fibrin is formed too fast and in too large a quantity.
   d. Fibrin is broken down as fast as it is formed.

LEVEL II

1. Referring to the case study for Level I questions 4–6, the results of the platelet aggregation studies indicate that the patient has a defect in which of the following? (Objective 4)
   a. F-VIII
   b. platelet adhesion
   c. fibrinolysis
   d. intrinsic system of fibrin formation

2. What is the usual inheritance pattern of von Willebrand disease? (Objective 3)
   a. autosomal dominant
   b. autosomal recessive
   c. X-linked recessive
   d. not inherited, usually acquired

LEVEL I

3. What clotting factor is deficient in a patient with hemophilia A? (Objective 4)
   a. F-VII
   b. F-VIII
   c. F-IX
   d. F-XIII

Use the following case study to answer questions 4–6.

An 18-year-old female bled profusely following extraction of a tooth. She had a history of sporadically increased menstrual bleeding and nosebleeds. She had had an appendectomy at age 10 with no unusual bleeding. A workup in the coagulation laboratory showed the following:

Laboratory Test	Patient Results	Laboratory Reference Range
Platelet count	312×10^9/L	$150–440 \times 10^9$/L
Bleeding time	9.5 minutes	2–9 minutes
Closure time	Increased	
Prothrombin time	11.5 sec	10–12 sec
Activated partial thromboplastin time	38.0 sec	23–36 sec
F-VIII assay	20 U/dL	50–150 U/dL
F-IX assay	102 U/dL	50–150 U/dL
Platelet aggregation studies	Normal: ADP, collagen, epinephrine Abnormal: ristocetin	

4. Which laboratory tests are outside their reference range? (Objective 2)
   a. all tests shown
   b. platelet aggregation with ristocetin, activated partial thromboplastin time, F-VIII assay
   c. platelet count, prothrombin time, F-IX assay
   d. prothrombin time, activated partial thromboplastin time, F-IX assay

5. The most probable cause of this patient's bleeding is: (Objectives 3, 10)
   a. vascular disorder
   b. F-IX deficiency
   c. von Willebrand disease
   d. disseminated intravascular coagulation

6. What laboratory test that is abnormal in this patient is different from that of a patient with hemophilia A? (Objectives 5, 6)
   a. F-VIII assay
   b. F-IX assay
   c. platelet aggregation studies with ADP
   d. platelet aggregation studies with ristocetin

LEVEL II

3. Which of the following is characteristic of Type I von Willebrand disease? (Objective 4)
   a. decreased amounts of large multimers of VWF
   b. increased amounts of large multimers of VWF
   c. decreased amounts of all VWF multimers
   d. decreased amounts of small VWF multimers only

4. Which laboratory procedure analyzes VWF qualitatively for abnormalities of the molecular structure? (Objective 4)
   a. ristocetin-induced platelet aggregation
   b. F-VIII assay
   c. SDS-page gel electrophoresis
   d. activated partial thromboplastin time

5. What is the cause of von Willebrand disease? (Objective 3)
   a. genetic mutations in the F-VIII gene
   b. genetic mutations in the VWF gene
   c. genetic mutations in the glycoprotein Ib gene
   d. exposure to dyes and chemicals

6. In which of the following conditions would the presence of delayed bleeding and deep muscular hematomas be most likely? (Objectives 1, 5)
   a. a patient with F-VIII deficiency
   b. a patient with F-XII deficiency
   c. a patient who is heterozygous for F-V deficiency
   d. a patient with dysfibrinogenemia

7. In which of the following diseases would you most likely find an abnormal prothrombin time? (Objectives 4, 6)
   a. F-VIII deficiency
   b. F-IX deficiency
   c. disseminated intravascular coagulation
   d. prekallikrein deficiency

8. Which of the following is true concerning acquired circulating pathologic inhibitors to single coagulation factors? (Objective 9)
   a. They do not cause bleeding symptoms.
   b. They cause the same symptoms in the patient as an inherited deficiency of the same factor.
   c. They are often found in patients with von Willebrand disease.
   d. They are antibodies to the phospholipid in the coagulation reagents.

9. Which of the following is true in the condition known as *disseminated intravascular coagulation (DIC)*? (Objective 7)
   a. F-V and F-VIII become increased in activity.
   b. Fibrinolytic activity is absent.
   c. The patient has a single coagulation factor deficiency.
   d. Fibrinogen and platelets become depleted.

REVIEW QUESTIONS (continued)

LEVEL I

7. What result of the platelet count would you expect in a patient with hemophilia A? (Objective 5)
   a. normal
   b. increased
   c. decreased
   d. unpredictable

8. Which is (are) characteristic(s) of a patient with DIC? (Objective 8)
   a. a prolonged PT
   b. a prolonged APTT
   c. a decreased platelet count
   d. all of the above

9. What is the cause of disseminated intravascular coagulation (DIC)? (Objective 8)
   a. an inherited deficiency of F-X
   b. a reaction to another disease that causes the hemostatic system to become activated
   c. a deficiency of vitamin K
   d. an antibody to F-VIII

10. Which result would be expected in a newborn infant? (Objective 9)
    a. a shorter APTT test than that in an adult
    b. a longer APTT test than that in an adult
    c. the lower platelet count than that in an adult
    d. the higher platelet count than that in an adult

LEVEL II

10. What laboratory test is helpful in differentiating primary and secondary fibrin(ogeno)lysis? (Objective 9)
    a. thrombin time
    b. D-dimer test
    c. plasmin-antiplasmin complexes
    d. platelet count

www.pearsonhighered.com/mckenzie

Use this address to access the interactive Companion Website created for this textbook. Find additional information, tables and figures. Evaluate your command of the chapter information using case studies and critical thinking and multiple choice questions.

REFERENCES

1. Sadler JE. Biochemistry and genetics of von Willebrand factor. *Ann Rev Biochem*. 1998;67:395–424.

2. Mazurier C, Ribba AS, Gaucher C, Meyer D. Molecular genetics of von Willebrand disease. *Ann de Genet*. 1997;41:34–43.

3. Von Willebrand EA. Hereditary pseudohemophilia. *Haemophilia*. 1951;5:223–31.

4. Wagner DD, Ginsburg D. Structure, biology, and genetics of von Willebrand factor. In: Hoffman R, Benz EJ Jr, Shatill SJ, Furie B, Cohen HJ, Silberstein LE, eds. *Hematology: Basic Principles and Practice*, 2nd ed. New York: Churchill Livingstone; 1995:1717–25.

5. Federici AB. Diagnosis of von Willebrand disease. *Hemophilia*. 1998;4:654–60.

6. Vischer UM, de Moerloose P. Von Willebrand factor: From cell biology to the clinical management of von Willebrand's disease. *Crit Rev Oncol/Hematol*. 1999;30:93–109.

7. James, AH. More than menorrhagia: A review of the obstetric and gynaecological manifestations of bleeding disorders. *Haemophilia*. 2005;11:295–307.

8. Ginsburg D, Bowie EJW. Molecular genetics of von Willebrand disease. *Blood*. 1992;79:2507–19.

9. Veyradier A, Fressinaud E, Meyer D. Laboratory diagnosis of von Willebrand disease. *Int J Clin Lab Res*. 1998;28:201–10.

10. Favaloro EJ, Facey D, Henniker A. Use of a novel platelet function analyzer (PFA-100) with high sensitivity to disturbances in von Willebrand factor to screen for von Willebrand's disease and other disorders. *Am J Hematol*. 1999;62:165–74.

11. Caron C, Mazurier C, Goudemand J. Large experience with a factor VIII binding assay of plasma von Willebrand factor using commercial reagents. *Br J Haematol*. 2002;117:716–18.

12. Riddell AF, Jenkins PV, Nitu-Walley JC et al. Use of the collagen-binding assay for von Willebrand factor in the analysis of type 2M von Willebrand disease: A comparison with the ristocetin cofactor assay. *Br J Haematol*. 2002;116:187–92.

13. Sadler JE. A revised classification of von Willebrand disease. *Thrombo Haemost*. 1994;71:520–25.

14. Sadler JE et al. Update of the pathophysiology and classification of von Willebrand disease: A report of the Subcommittee on von Willebrand Factor. *J Thromb Haemost* 2006;4:2103–14.

15. Ginsburg D. Molecular genetics of von Willebrand disease. *Thromb Haemost.* 1999;82:585–91.

16. Tefferi A, Nichols WL. Acquired von Willebrand disease: Concise review of occurrence, diagnosis, pathogenesis, and treatment. *Amer J Med.* 1997;103:536–40.

17. van Genderen P, Boerjes RC, van Mourik JA. Quantitative analysis of von Willebrand factor and its propeptide in plasma in acquired von Willebrand syndrome. *Thromb Haemost.* 1998;80:495–98.

18. Sadler JE, Blinder M. Von Willebrand disease: Diagnosis, classification, and treatment. In: Colman RW, Marder VJ, Clowes AW, George JN, Goldhaber SZ, eds. *Hemostasis and Thrombosis. Basic Principles and Clinical Practice,* 5th ed. Philadelphia: Lippincott Williams & Wilkins; 2006:905–21.

19. Pavlovsky A. Contribution to the pathogenesis of hemophilia. *Blood.* 1947;2:185–91.

20. Marder VJ, Mannucci PM, Firkin BG, Hoyer LW, Meyer D. Standard nomenclature for factor VIII and von Willebrand factor: A recommendation by the International Committee on Thrombosis and Haemostasis. *Thromb Haemost.* 1985;54:871–72.

21. Greenberg CS, Orthner CL. Blood coagulation and fibrinolysis. In: Lee GR, Foerster J, Lukens J, Paraskevas F, Greer JP, Rodgers GM, eds. *Wintrobe's Clinical Hematology,* 10th ed. Baltimore: Williams & Wilkins; 1999:684–764.

22. Kaufman RJ, Antonarakis SE, Fay PF. Factor VIII and hemophilia. In: Colman RW, Marder VJ, Clowes AW, George JN, Goldhaber SZ, eds. *Hemostasis and Thrombosis. Basic Principles and Clinical Practice,* 5th ed. Philadelphia: Lippincott Williams & Wilkins; 2006:151–75.

23. Lillicrap D. Molecular diagnosis of inherited bleeding disorders and thrombophilia. *Sem Hematol.* 1999;36:340–451.

24. Kaufman RJ, Antonarakis SE. Structure, biology, and genetics of factor VIII. In: Hoffman R, Benz EJ Jr, Shatill SJ, Furie B, Cohen HJ, Silberstein LE, eds. *Hematology: Basic Principles and Practice,* 2nd ed. New York: Churchill Livingstone; 1995:1633–48.

25. Attali O, Vinciguerra C, Treciak MC et al. Factor IX gene analysis in 70 unrelated patients with haemophilia B: Description of 13 new mutations. *Thromb Haemost.* 1999;82:1437–42.

26. Giannelli F, Green PM, Sommer SS et al. Haemophilia B: Database of point mutations and short additions and deletions, 8th ed. *Nucleic Acids Res.* 1998;26:265–68.

27. Roberts HR, Gray TF III. Clinical aspects of and therapy for hemophilia B. In: Hoffman R, Benz EJ Jr, Shatill SJ, Furie B, Cohen HJ, Silberstein LE, eds. *Hematology: Basic Principles and Practice,* 2nd ed. New York: Churchill Livingstone; 1995:1678–85.

28. Bretter DB, Kraus EM, Levine PH. Clinical aspects of and therapy for hemophilia A. In: Hoffman R, Benz EJ Jr, Shatill SJ, Furie B, Cohen HJ, Silberstein LE, eds. *Hematology: Basic Principles and Practice,* 2nd ed. New York: Churchill Livingstone; 1995:1648–63.

29. Keeney S, Mitchell M, Goodeve A. The molecular analysis of haemophilia A: A guideline from the UK haemophilia doctors' organization haemophilia genetics laboratory network. *Haemophlia.* 2005;11:387–97.

30. Pruthi RK. Hemophilia: A practical approach to genetic testing. *Mayo Clinic Proceedings.* 2005;80(11):1485–99.

31. Giangrande PLF. Management of pregnancy in carriers of haemophilia. *Haemophilia.* 1998;4:779–84.

32. Ponder KP. Gene therapy for hemophilia. *Current Opinion in Hematology.* 2006;13:301–307.

33. Kessler CM, Mariani G. Clinical manifestations and therapy of the hemophilias. In: Colman RW, Marder VJ, Clowes AW, George JN, Goldhaber SZ, eds. *Hemostasis and Thrombosis. Basic Principles and Clinical Practice,* 5th ed. Philadelphia: Lippincott Williams & Wilkins; 2006:887–904.

34. Peyvandi F, Mannucci PM. Rare coagulation disorders. *Thromb Haemost.* 1999;82:1207–14.

35. Moen JL, Lord ST. Afibrinogenemias and dysfibrinogenemias. In: Colman RW, Marder VJ, Clowes AW, George JN, Goldhaber SZ, eds. *Hemostasis and Thrombosis. Basic Principles and Clinical Practice,* 5th ed. Philadelphia: Lippincott Williams & Wilkins; 2006:939–52.

36. Bolton-Maggs PHB et al. The rare coagulation disorders—Review with guidelines for management from the United Kingdom Haemophilia Centre Doctors' Organisation. *Haemophilia.* 2004;10:593–628.

37. Hanss M, Biot F. A database for human fibrinogen variants. *Ann N Y Acad Sci.* 2001;936:89–90. www.geht.org/databaseang/fibrinogen.

38. Mosesson, MW. Hereditary abnormalities of fibrinogen. In: Beutler E, Lichtman MA, Coller BS, Kipps TJ, Seliqsohn U, eds. *William's Hematology,* 6th ed. New York: McGraw-Hill; 2001:1659–71.

39. Roberts HR, Escobar MA. Inherited disorders of prothrombin conversion. In: Colman RW, Marder VJ, Clowes AW, George JN, Goldhaber SZ, eds. *Hemostasis and Thrombosis. Basic Principles and Clinical Practice,* 5th ed. Philadelphia: Lippincott Williams & Wilkins; 2006:923–37.

40. Owren CA, Bowie EJW, Thompson JH. *The Diagnosis of Bleeding Disorders,* 2nd ed. Boston, MA: Little, Brown; 1975.

41. Millar DS, Elliston L, Deex P et al. Molecular analysis of the genotype-phenotype relationship in factor X deficiency. *Human Genetics.* 2000;106:249–57.

42. Peyvandi F, Menegatti M, Santagostino E et al. Gene mutations and three-dimensional structural analysis in 13 families with severe factor X deficiency. *Br. J Haematol.* 2002;117:685–92.

43. Uprichard J, Perry DJ. Factor X deficiency. *Blood Reviews.* 2002;16:97–110.

44. Roberts HR, Hoffman M. Hemophilia and related conditions: Inherited deficiencies of prothrombin (factor II), factor V, and factors VII to XII. In: Beutler E, Lichtman MA, Coller BS, Kipps TJ, eds. *William's Hematology,* 5th ed. New York: McGraw-Hill; 1995:1413–39.

45. Bick RL. *Disorders of Thrombosis and Hemostasis: Clinical and Laboratory Practice.* Chicago: ASCP Press; 1992.

46. Walsh, PN, Gailani D. Factor XI. In: Colman RW, Marder VJ, Clowes AW, George JN, Goldhaber SZ, eds. *Hemostasis and Thrombosis. Basic Principles and Clinical Practice,* 5th ed. Philadelphia: Lippincott Williams & Wilkins; 2006:221–33.

47. Greenberg CS, Sane DC, Lai T-S. Factor XIII and fibrin stabilization. In: Colman RW, Marder VJ, Clowes AW, George JN, Goldhaber SZ, eds. *Hemostasis and Thrombosis. Basic Principles and Clinical Practice,* 5th ed. Philadelphia: Lippincott Williams & Wilkins; 2006:317–34.

48. Katona E, Haramura G, Karpati L, Fachet J, Muszbek L. A simple, quick one-step ELISA assay for the determination of complex plasma factor XIII (A_2B_2). *Thromb Haemost.* 2000;83:268–73.

49. Kaufman RJ, Antonarakis SE, Fay PJ. Factor VIII and hemophilia A. In: Colman RW, Hirsh J, Marder VJ, Clowes AW, George JN, eds. *Hemostasis and Thrombosis: Basic Principles and Clinical Practice,* 4th ed. Philadelphia: Lippincott Williams & Wilkins; 2000:135–56.

50. Colman RW. Contact activation pathway: Inflammation, fibrinolytic, anticoagulant, antiadhesive and antiangiogenic activities. In: Colman RW, Marder VJ, Clowes AW, George JN, Goldhaaber SZ, eds. *Hemostasis and Thrombosis: Basic Principles and Clinical Practice,* 5th ed. Philadelphia: Lippincott Williams & Wilkins; 2006:103–22.

51. Rodgers GM, Greenberg CS. Inherited coagulation disorders. In: Lee GR, Foerster J, Lukens J, Paraskevas F, Greer JP, Rodgers GM, eds. *Wintrobe's Clinical Hematology,* 10th ed. Baltimore: Williams & Wilkins; 1999:1682–1732.

52. Levi M, de Jonge E, van der Poll T, ten Cate H. Disseminated intravascular coagulation. *Thromb Haemost.* 1999;82:695–705.

53. Scherer RU, Spangenberg P. Procoagulant activity in patients with isolated severe head trauma. *Crit Care Med.* 1998;26:149–56.

54. Feinstein DI, Marder VJ, Colman RW. Consumptive thrombohemorrhagic disorders. In: Colman RW, Hirsh J, Marder VJ, Clowes AW, George JN, eds. *Hemostasis and Thrombosis: Basic Principles and Clinical Practice,* 4th ed. Philadelphia: Lippincott Williams & Wilkins; 2000:1197–1234.

55. Baglin T. Disseminated intravascular coagulation: Diagnosis and treatment. *Br Med J.* 1996;312:683–87.

56. Grosset AMB, Rodgers GM. Acquired coagulation disorders. In: Lee GR, Foerster J, Lukens J, Paraskevas F, Greer JP, Rodgers GM, eds. *Wintrobe's Clinical Hematology,* 10th ed. Baltimore: Williams & Wilkins; 1999:1733–80.

57. Zipursky A. Prevention of vitamin K deficiency bleeding in newborns. *Br J Haematol.* 1999;104:430–37.

58. Key, NS. Inhibitors in congenital coagulation disorders. *Br J Haematol.* 2004;127:379–91.

59. Monagle P, Andrew M. Dwevelopmental Hemostasis: Relevance to newborns and infants. In: Nathan DGG, Orkin SH, Ginsburg D, Look AT, eds. *Hematology of Infancy and Childhood,* 6th ed. Philadelphia: WB Saunders; 2003:121–68.

60. Montgomery RR, Marlar RA, Gill JC. Newborn hemostasis. *Clin Haematol.* 1985;14:443–60.

61. Johnston M, Zipursky A. Microtechnology for the study of blood coagulation system in newborn infants. *Can J Med Tech.* 1980; 42:159–64.

62. Andrew M, Paes B, Milner R et al. Development of the human coagulation system in the full-term infant. *Blood.* 1987;70:165–72.

63. Hathaway W, Corrigan J, for the Subcommittee. Normal coagulation data for fetuses and newborn infants. *Thromb Haemost.* 1991; 65:323–25.

64. Andrew M, Paes B, Milner R et al. Development of the human coagulation system in the healthy premature infant. *Blood.* 1988;72: 1651–57.

33

Thrombophilia

Lynne Williams, Ph.D.

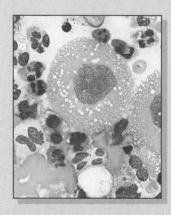

■ OBJECTIVES—LEVEL I

At the end of this unit of study, the student should be able to:

1. Define *hypercoagulability, thrombophilia, thrombus,* and *thrombosis.*
2. Describe the physiological processes involved in hypercoagulability.
3. Explain how a thrombus becomes a thromboembolus.
4. Contrast a white thrombus and a red thrombus, and list the risk factors predisposing to the formation of each.
5. Define *deep vein thrombosis* (DVT); explain how it is diagnosed and what clinical conditions can result.
6. Describe the role of heparin in the neutralization of activated coagulation factors by antithrombin.
7. Diagram the relationship of protein C (PC) and protein S (PS) to the coagulation pathway and explain why a deficiency of either might lead to a thrombotic tendency.
8. Explain why both molecular (antigenic) and functional assays should be performed for diagnosing antithrombin, protein C (PC), or protein S (PS) abnormalities in a patient.
9. Describe activated protein C (APC) resistance (APCR), and explain its contribution to thrombophilia.
10. List two side effects of heparin therapy and what hematology procedures should be monitored to prevent or limit these complications.
11. Contrast unfractionated heparin (UFH) and low molecular weight heparin (LMWH) including anticoagulant mechanisms and monitoring.
12. Discuss how oral anticoagulants such as coumadin decrease a person's risk for thrombosis, and describe the best way to monitor oral anticoagulation.

■ OBJECTIVES—LEVEL II

At the end of this unit of study, the student should be able to:

1. Evaluate the utility of laboratory tests in the differential diagnosis of arterial and venous thrombotic disease.
2. List four clinical manifestations suggestive of an inherited thrombophilia, and explain why many patients are not diagnosed.
3. Explain the differences between type I and type II deficiencies of protein C (PC), protein S (PS), and antithrombin; given values for antithrombin or protein C and S assays, determine the type of deficiency in a patient.

■ OBJECTIVES—LEVEL II (continued)

4. List two deficiencies that can cause warfarin- (coumadin-) induced skin necrosis and give potential treatment options.

5. Justify performing both a clotting and molecular assay for diagnosis of activated protein C resistance (APCR).

6. Describe the two most common mutations leading to hyperhomocysteinemia.

7. Explain how increased levels of prothrombin or fibrinogen might predispose to thrombosis.

8. Describe how deficiencies of plasminogen or plasminogen activator or increased levels of plasminogen activator inhibitor could lead to thrombosis.

9. Identify secondary disorders leading to thrombosis.

10. Describe and explain the treatment of a thrombotic episode.

11. Explain how the INR has standardized prothrombin times.

12. Evaluate the use and monitoring of thrombolytic therapy in treatment of thrombosis.

13. Given a patient history and appropriate laboratory results, interpret the data to determine a probable diagnosis.

KEY TERMS

Activated protein C resistance (APCR)
Antiphospholipid antibody syndrome (APLS)
Deep vein thrombosis (DVT)
Disseminated intravascular coagulation (DIC)
Dysfibrinogenemia
Embolus
Factor-V Leiden (FVL)
Hemolytic uremic syndrome (HUS)
Heparin-induced thrombocytopenia (HIT)
Hypercoagulable
Hyperhomocysteinemia
Low molecular weight heparin (LMWH)
Pulmonary embolism (PE)
Red thrombi
Thromboembolism (TE)
Thrombolytic therapy
Thrombophilia
Thrombophlebitis
Thrombosis
Thrombotic thrombocytopenic purpura (TTP)
Thrombus
Unfractionated heparin (UFH)
White thrombi

BACKGROUND BASICS

Information in this chapter builds on concepts learned in previous chapters. To maximize your learning experience, you should review these concepts before starting this unit of study.

Level I

▶ Describe the mechanisms of platelet activation and the functions of platelets in both primary and secondary hemostasis. (Chapter 29)

▶ Outline the coagulation cascade and the components contributing to fibrin formation. (Chapter 30)

▶ List the components and the function of the fibrinolytic system and the products produced by fibrinolytic action (FDPs). (Chapter 30)

▶ List the mechanisms that maintain normal physiologic control of hemostasis, particularly the inhibitors of both coagulation and fibrinolysis. (Chapter 30)

Level II

▶ Describe the mechanism of activation of serine proteases (complex formation on a phospholipid surface). (Chapter 30)

▶ Summarize the physiologic controls that limit activation of coagulation and fibrinolysis to the sites of vessel injury. (Chapter 30)

▶ Describe the method of activation and physiologic function of the inhibitors of coagulation and fibrinolysis. (Chapter 30)

CASE STUDY

We will address this case study throughout the chapter.

Andrea is a 37-year-old woman recently diagnosed with deep vein thrombosis (DVT) of the right leg. She is dehydrated and on oral contraceptives. She is also on coumadin.

Consider possible factors contributing to the thrombosis in this patient and the laboratory tests that might be used to differentiate and diagnose the cause.

► OVERVIEW

This chapter describes imbalances between procoagulant and anticoagulant processes in the hemostatic system that result in an increased tendency to form thrombi (thrombophilia). The chapter begins with a summary of the factors that influence thrombus formation in the arterial and venous blood vessels and the nature of the resulting thrombi that form in each side of the circulatory system. The chapter defines *thrombophilia* and describes the hereditary and acquired factors that contribute to thrombophilia. It discusses the pathophysiologic basis, clinical manifestations, and laboratory diagnosis for each thrombophilic factor. Emphasis is on the concept of thrombophilia as a multifactorial disease process. For details on laboratory tests mentioned in this chapter, refer to ∞ Chapters 34 and ∞ 40. The chapter ends with a brief discussion of the available therapies for the thrombophilic patient.

► INTRODUCTION

The human hemostatic system represents a balance between procoagulant or thrombogenic factors and anticoagulant and/or fibrinolytic activity. In a normal healthy individual, the two systems are balanced so that neither excessive bleeding nor clotting occurs. When the balance is tipped so that there is more procoagulant or clotting activity (or less anticoagulant activity), the person is said to be **hypercoagulable. Thrombosis** is the formation of a platelet and/or fibrin mass within a vessel, known as a **thrombus** (plural, thrombi). Many conditions can cause hypercoagulability and lead to thrombosis.

The three physiologic components responsible for hemostasis are also the sources of thrombogenic influences: the vascular endothelial cell, platelets, and coagulation proteins (Table 33-1 ✪). The normal intact endothelium is antithrombogenic and does not activate platelets or blood coagulation factors. Damage to vascular endothelial cells can cause the release of prothrombotic substances (e.g., tissue factor, thromboxane [TXA_2], and plasminogen activator inhibitor [PAI-1]) or loss of normally protective antithrombotic functions (e.g., thrombomodulin/protein C activation; heparan

✪ TABLE 33-1

Physiologic Alterations Contributing to Thrombosis

Thrombogenic alterations

- Damage/activation of endothelial cells
- Exposure of subendothelium (loss of endothelial cells)
- Activation of platelets (circulating agonists, interaction with subendothelium)
- Activation of plasma coagulation proteins
- Inhibition of fibrinolysis
- Stasis

Protective mechanisms lost

- Antithrombotic properties of factors released from intact endothelium (prostacyclin, nitric oxide)
- Neutralization of activated coagulation factors by endothelial cell-bound components (thrombomodulin, heparan sulfate)
- Inhibition of activated coagulation factors by naturally occurring plasma protease inhibitors (antithrombin [AT], tissue factor pathway inhibitor [TFPI], heparin cofactor II [HCII])
- Degradation of coagulation factors by inhibiting proteases (activated protein C [APC])
- Dilution of activated clotting factors and disruption of platelet aggregates by unimpeded blood flow
- Breakdown of fibrin thrombi by the fibrinolytic system

(Hirsh J, Colman RW, Marder VJ, George JN, Clowes AW. Overview of thrombosis and its treatment. Hirsh J, Colman RW, Marder VJ, Clowes AW, George JN, eds. In: *Hemostasis and Thrombosis: Basic Principles and Clinical Practice*, 4th ed. Philadelphia: Lippincott Williams & Wilkins; 2000:1071–84.)

sulfate/antithrombin activation; nitric oxide and prostacyclin) (Figure 29-3). Circulating agonists or interaction with exposed subendothelium can activate platelets. Tissue factor (TF) or collagen, resulting from damaged vessels can activate procoagulant plasma proteins. Inadequate control of plasma coagulation can result from decreased activity of protective protease inhibitors or inadequate fibrinolysis. Additionally, stasis, or impaired blood flow, is thrombogenic. Normal unimpeded blood flow dilutes or removes activated clotting factors from their site of activation.

Thrombi can form in any part of the cardiovascular system, including the arteries, veins, heart, and microcirculation. Thrombi are composed of fibrin, platelets, and entrapped cells; the relative proportion of each component is influenced by hemodynamic factors and differs in arterial and venous thrombi. The thrombus is often incorrectly referred to as a *clot;* however, a clot is a mass that forms extravascularly (either in vitro or from blood shed into the tissues or body cavities). Thrombus formation can lead to two major pathologic events. The thrombus can enlarge, causing local obstruction of the blood vessel (ischemia) and resulting in the death of the tissue supplied by that vessel (necrosis). A piece of thrombotic material (an **embolus**) can break off from the thrombus and travel through the circulatory system, lodging at a distant site and obstructing blood flow in that tissue, causing ischemia and necrosis. This obstruction is termed an *embolism.* If the blockage originates from a thrombus, it is referred to as a **thromboembolism (TE).**

▶ THROMBUS FORMATION

ARTERIAL THROMBI

Thrombi formed in arteries where blood flow is rapid are termed **white thrombi.** They are composed primarily of platelets and fibrin with relatively few leukocytes and erythrocytes. Arterial thrombi usually form in regions of disturbed flow, at sites of damage to the endothelium, often in areas of atherosclerotic plaques. Plaques are composed of extracellular lipids, fibrous connective tissue, and foam cells (lipid-filled macrophages and smooth muscle cells). Thrombosis is generally initiated by rupture of the plaque, exposing thrombogenic material in the subendothelium to the blood. Platelet activation and activation of plasma coagulation factors occur, resulting in the formation of fibrin. The activated platelets and fibrin interact to form a thrombus that can extend into the lumen of the vessel, eventually obstructing the artery and inducing ischemia. An embolus often breaks off and lodges in the small vessels of the heart or brain, causing myocardial or cerebral infarction (and tissue death). In addition to endothelial cell loss, more subtle endothelial injury (e.g., exposure to endotoxin, hypoxia, cytokines such as IL-1 or TNF [tumor necrosis factor]) can also promote coagulation. Treatment for arterial thrombi usually involves platelet-inhibiting drugs (e.g., aspirin, clopidogrel, or ticlopidine) or thrombolytic therapy.

Traditional risk factors associated with an increased predisposition to atherosclerosis and the formation of arterial thrombi include hypercholesterolemia, hypertension, smoking, physical inactivity, obesity, and diabetes. Historically, up to one-half of all patients who developed a coronary thrombosis did not have any of these conventional risk factors. Consequently, there was interest in identifying additional laboratory tests that could predict an impending arterial thrombotic event. Standard laboratory tests (prothrombin time [PT], activated partial thromboplastin time [APTT], and thrombin time [TT]) are neither specific nor sensitive for predicting arterial thrombi, and novel risk factors or laboratory tests have thus been sought. While the clinical data for some of these new tests are inconsistent, some do show promise as indicators of an increased thrombotic tendency.[1] These new approaches include tests for hyperhomocysteinemia; elevated lipoprotein (a); fibrinogen; D-dimer; PAI-1; C-reactive protein (CRP); and decreased tPA. None of these tests is specific for arterial thrombosis. Tests suggesting an increase in procoagulant activity (elevated fibrinogen, hyperhomocysteinemia) or decreased fibrinolytic activity (elevated PAI-1) can reflect a thrombotic tendency but not specifically arterial thrombosis.

It was recently recognized that inflammatory processes play a role in the initiation and progression of atherosclerosis (see website, Chapter 33 for further information). Thus, inflammation can be linked to cardiovascular risk, and markers of inflammation can be useful as predictors of preclinical atherosclerosis.[2] CRP is a typical acute phase reactant with elevated serum levels occurring in response to acute injury, infection, or other inflammatory stimuli. The high sensitivity assays for CRP (hs-CRP) are being used to evaluate its role as a sign of chronic vascular inflammation. Clinical data for CRP, fibrinogen, and serum amyloid A (two other acute phase reactant proteins) strongly support a role for inflammation in atherogenesis. Evidence of inflammation can be detected many years in advance of acute thrombosis in apparently healthy men and women, indicating that inflammatory processes occur early and precede vascular occlusion.[3]

VENOUS THROMBI

Thrombi formed in the veins where blood flow is slower are termed **red thrombi.** They are primarily composed of red blood cells trapped in the fibrin mesh with relatively fewer platelets and leukocytes. Such thrombi usually form in regions of slow or disturbed blood flow, often in venous segments that have been exposed to direct trauma.

Although venous thrombi can occur in any vein in the body, they most commonly occur in the lower limbs. Thrombosis of the superficial veins of the legs is usually benign and self-limiting (**thrombophlebitis**). In contrast, involvement of the deep veins of the leg (**deep vein thrombosis [DVT]**) is more serious. Generally, distal thrombi localized to the deep veins of the calf are less serious (and often undergo spontaneous lysis) than those involving the proximal veins (popliteal, femoral, or iliac veins). DVT involving the calf are also less commonly associated with long-term disability or **pulmonary embolism (PE).** The symptoms of venous thrombosis can include localized pain, warmth, redness, and swelling. Embolization of a (deep vein) thrombus to the pulmonary circulation is a serious and potentially life-threatening complication of DVT. A strong association exists between PE and the presence of venous thrombosis in the lower limbs; PE is detected by perfusion lung scanning in ~50% of patients with documented proximal DVT.[4] It has been suggested that DVT and PE are different stages and clinical presentations of the same pathologic process, termed *venous thromboembolism (VTE).*[5]

Like arterial thrombosis, venous thrombosis occurs when activation of blood coagulation exceeds the ability of the natural protective mechanisms (anticoagulants or inhibitors and the fibrinolytic system) to prevent fibrin formation (Table 33-1). Venous thrombosis is associated with the activation of plasma coagulation proteins initiated by vascular trauma or inflammation, the consequences of which are amplified by stasis. Venous stasis predisposes to local thrombosis by impairing the clearing of activated coagulation factors.

VTE can occur spontaneously or be provoked by recognizable clinical risk factors. Clinical risk factors that predispose to venous thrombosis include:

1. *Venous stasis.* Venous return from the legs is enhanced by contraction of calf muscles, which act as a pump to propel blood from the legs toward the heart. Immobility (loss of the pumping action of the contracting muscles), venous obstruction, venous dilation, and increased blood viscosity (polycythemia, dysproteinemia, elevated fibrinogen) all predispose to venous thrombosis.

2. *Vessel wall damage.* The vascular endothelium can be damaged by direct trauma (surgery, severe burns, severe trauma) and by exposure to endotoxin, inflammatory cytokines (IL-1, TNF), thrombin, or hypoxia. Damaged endothelial cells synthesize tissue factor and PAI-1 and internalize thrombomodulin—changes that promote thrombogenesis[6] (Figure 29-3).

3. *Factor V Leiden (FVL) and activated protein C resistance.* Discussed later.

4. *Deficiency of circulating protease inhibitors.* Antithrombin, protein C [PC], protein S [PS], heparin cofactor II (HCII), discussed later.

5. *Elevated prothrombin levels.* Prothrombin 20210, discussed later.

6. *Antiphospholipid antibodies.* Discussed later.

7. *Hyperhomocysteinemia.* Discussed later.

8. *Decreased fibrinolytic activity.* Discussed later. Fibrinolytic activity has been found to be lower in leg veins than in arm veins, which could partly explain the greater tendency for venous thrombosis to occur in the lower extremities.[7]

9. *Malignancy.* The association between venous thrombosis and cancer has been attributed to procoagulant material released from the tumor cells or to complications of chemotherapy.

10. *Miscellaneous.* Other factors associated with increased risk of thrombosis include advanced age, obesity, pregnancy, use of oral contraceptives (OC) and hormone replacement therapy, smoking, hypertension, hyperlipidemia, and a clinical history of previous venous thromboembolism. Blood groups other than Group O (e.g., A, B, AB) have been shown in some studies to have an increased risk of thrombosis[8–13] perhaps the result of higher levels of von Willebrand factor (VWF) in blood groups A, B, and AB.[14]

The diagnosis of DVT can be difficult because similar clinical features and laboratory test results are found in other conditions. It is generally accepted that clinical/laboratory diagnosis of venous thrombosis is unreliable and objective tests are needed to confirm the diagnosis.[15] Objective tests using radiologic procedures to visualize the thrombus can help to identify thrombi.[16] Venography, venous compression ultrasonography (CUS), and spiral computerized tomography (s-CT) can be used to confirm a diagnosis of DVT; pulmonary angiography and ventilation-perfusion lung scanning can be used to confirm PE. Blood tests for biologic markers of thrombin generation and fibrinolysis are often elevated in patients with DVT.[7] Laboratory tests analyzed for their diagnostic utility include prothrombin fragment 1.2, fibrinopeptide A (FPA), thrombin-antithrombin (TAT) complex, soluble fibrin monomer, D-dimer, tPA, and PAI-1. However, these tests are nonspecific and can be abnormal in a number of clinical conditions associated with excessive coagulation and/or fibrinolysis and thus have low specificity for DVT. An appropriately validated quantitative D-dimer assay (different assays have variable sensitivity and specificity) appears to have both high sensitivity and a negative predictive value; thus, a negative result can be used to rule out DVT.[17,18]

✓ **Checkpoint! 1**

Why would defects of fibrinolysis result in hypercoagulability?

▶ **THROMBOPHILIA**

The most common cause of death in the United States is thrombosis; more than 2 million people die from arterial or venous thrombosis every year[19] (Table 33-2 ✪). Thrombotic episodes can be caused by a congenital abnormality and/or an acquired alteration. The proper treatment or prevention of thrombosis depends on careful clinical assessment and extensive testing procedures.

The term **thrombophilia** is used to describe any disorder either inherited or acquired associated with an increased tendency to thrombosis. Although thrombosis at a young age is probably the most important feature of inherited thrombophilia, many patients have their first episode later in life. Women with certain inherited thrombophilic abnormalities have an increased risk of pregnancy loss,

✪ **TABLE 33-2**

Incidence of Thrombosis		
Thrombotic Incident	Incidence per 100,000	U.S. Cases per Year
Deep vein thrombosis (DVT)	159	450,000
Pulmonary embolus (PE)	139	355,000
Fatal pulmonary embolus	94	240,000
Myocardial infarction (MI)	600	1,500,000
Fatal myocardial infarction	300	750,000
Cerebrovascular thrombosis (CVT)	600	1,500,000
Fatal cerebrovascular thrombosis	396	990,000

(Reprinted, with permission, from Bick R, Fareed J. Current status of thrombosis: A multidisciplinary medical issue and major American health problem, beyond the year 2000. *Clin Appl Thromb Hemostasis.* 1997; suppl 1:1–5.)

preeclampsia, and hemolysis, elevated liver enzymes, and low platelet count (HELLP) syndrome whereas some acquired thrombophilic conditions are also associated with recurrent pregnancy loss.[20] Carriers of some inherited thrombophilic defects are prone to other thrombotic complications, such as vitamin K antagonist (warfarin)-induced skin necrosis or heparin resistance. The thrombotic risk of a given hereditary predisposition or an acquired condition varies from low to modest to high risk of VTE (Table 33-3 ✪).

An inherited thrombophilic defect places an individual at risk for but does not inevitably lead to thrombosis. Not all persons with thrombophilia experience a thrombotic event; many will not develop thrombosis unless some other (acquired) risk factor is present. Surgery, pregnancy, immobilization, estrogen therapy, obesity, trauma, and infection can initiate thrombotic events. These conditions can lead to thromboses even in people without an inherited thrombotic tendency, so when a thrombotic episode occurs, it must be decided whether it represents an isolated event or the patient has an underlying genetic predisposition. A thorough personal and family history can help in determining the likelihood of a genetic component. However, other affected family members can be asymptomatic, their condition discovered only after another family member is diagnosed. More than one hemostatic defect or abnormality increases the risk for thrombosis.

HEREDITARY THROMBOPHILIA

Inherited thrombophilia refers to individuals with predisposing genetic defects resulting in a tendency to thrombosis.

Specific inherited alterations associated with TE have been identified (Table 33-4 ✪). Most of these changes involve an increase in procoagulant potential (e.g., activation of the coagulation cascade) or a defect or decrease in natural inhibitors of clotting. Likewise, abnormalities of fibrinolysis or platelet activation can contribute to the thrombotic tendency. An acquired predisposition to thrombosis, such as prolonged immobility or pregnancy, can interact with an underlying hereditary predisposition to precipitate an acute thrombotic event. A combination of more than one hereditary predisposition strongly accelerates and exaggerates the thrombotic process. Thus, thrombosis can occur in susceptible patients having one or more genetic mutations when they are exposed to exogenous prothrombotic stimuli.[21] Their "thrombotic potential" is higher than normal, and generally an additional prothrombotic exposure must occur to push them into an acute thrombotic episode (Figure 33-1 ■). Inherited thrombotic disorders are usually associated with venous thrombosis.

Patients diagnosed with inherited thrombophilia usually present with one or more of the following clinical manifestations:[20]

1. venous thromboembolism at a young age (prior to age 45)
2. recurrent venous thromboembolism
3. family history of venous thromboembolism
4. thrombosis in an unusual site (cervical or visceral veins)

The five most clearly delineated hereditary abnormalities associated with thrombophilia (Factor V Leiden; decreased

✪ TABLE 33-3

Risk of Clinical Venous Thromboembolic Disease

Risk	Hereditary	Acquired
Low	Heterozygous factor V Leiden	General surgery
	Heterozygous prothrombin 20210	Oral contraceptives/pregnancy
	Sickle cell anemia	Long trips
		Elevated F-VIII
Moderate	Heterozygous AT deficiency	Surgery for malignancy
	Heterozygous PC or PS deficiency	Sepsis
		Prolonged immobilization
		Antiphospholipid antibody
		Myeloproliferative syndromes
		Paroxysmal nocturnal hemoglobinuria (PNH)
High	Homozygous factor V Leiden	Total hip or knee replacement
	Homozygous prothrombin 20210	Hip fracture
		Acute promyelocytic leukemia
Excessive	Homozygous or double heterozygous AT, PC, or PS deficiency	Mucin-secreting adenocarcinoma

(Reprinted, with permission, from Marder VJ, Matei DE. Hereditary and acquired thrombophilic syndromes, Colman RW, Hirsch J, Marder VJ, Clowes AW, George JN, eds. In: *Hemostasis and Thrombosis: Basic Principles and Clinical Practice,* 4th ed. Philadelphia: Lippincott Williams & Wilkins; 2000:1243–75.)

⊘ TABLE 33-4

Hereditary Conditions Associated with Thrombosis

Antithrombin deficiency

PC deficiency

PS deficiency

Activated protein C resistance (APCR)

Prothrombin mutation G20210A

HC II deficiency

Tissue factor pathway inhibitor variant

Hyperhomocysteinemia

    Cystathionine beta synthase deficiency

    Methylenetetrahydrofolate reductase deficiency

Dysfibrinogenemia/hyperfibrinogenemia

Elevated F-VIII

F-XII deficiency

Plasminogen deficiency

Plasminogen activator deficiency

Elevated plasminogen activator inhibitor (PAI-1)

or defective protein C, protein S, or antithrombin; and prothrombin 20210 mutation) combined account for ~30% of the initial cases of DVT and are the apparent hereditary defects in 75% of thrombophilic families[22] (Table 33-5 ⊘). In contrast to heterozygous female carriers of a hemophilia gene in whom 50% of normal levels of the clotting factor are sufficient to protect against bleeding, half-normal levels of anticoagulant proteins (AT, PC, PS) are associated with an increased risk of thrombosis.

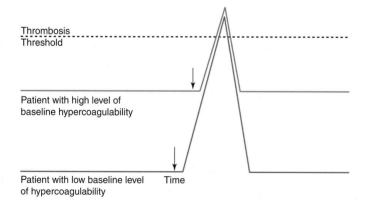

■ **FIGURE 33-1** Interaction of acquired thrombotic triggers with individual baseline hypercoagulability. Individuals with hereditary mutations resulting in thrombophilia have a higher baseline level of hypercoagulability (red line) compared to normal individuals (blue line). As a result, the introduction of an identical acquired prothrombotic stimulus will more easily push the thrombophilia individual into an overt acute thrombotic event (dotted line), compared to a normal individual.

Ⓒ CASE STUDY *(continued from page 733)*

Andrea's mother had had eight children and had experienced no thrombotic events, although two paternal uncles died suddenly of pulmonary embolism. Two of the mother's cousins also had pulmonary emboli: one died suddenly, but the other recovered.

1. What risk factors, if any, are revealed in the patient's history?

Antithrombin Deficiency

Antithrombin (AT) is the major inhibitor of the serine proteases involved in coagulation (∞ Chapter 30; Figure 30-1). AT's relatively weak natural inhibitory function is augmented 1000-fold in the presence of heparin. In vivo, endothelial cell glycosaminoglycans (e.g., heparan sulfate) are the natural catalyst for the inhibitor. Reduction of AT levels to ~50% of normal predisposes to venous thrombosis, because of a decrease in the normal inhibition of the coagulation pathway.

Pathophysiology AT deficiency was the first identified cause of inherited thrombophilia. Described by Egeberg in 1965,[23] AT deficiency is inherited as an autosomal dominant trait. More than 200 different mutations of the AT gene have been identified (www.archive.uwcm.ac.uk/uwcm/mg/hgmd/search.html). Two major types of inherited deficiencies have been described (Table 33-6 ⊘). Type I deficiency is the result of reduced synthesis of a biologically normal protein (i.e., a quantitative deficiency). In this case, the antigenic and functional activities of AT are reduced in parallel. The second type of AT deficiency is produced by a specific molecular defect within the inhibitor (type II, or qualitative deficiency). Functionally, type II mutations involve either the heparin-binding site or the reactive (protease-binding) site of the AT molecule. In this case, the plasma levels of AT functional activity are reduced while AT immunologic activity is essentially normal.

Clinical Findings The prevalence of AT deficiency in the general population is about 0.02% and in patients with VTE is ~1–2%.[22] Heterozygous individuals generally have AT functional activity of 30–60% (reference range 80–120%, or ~140 μg/mL). Homozygous type I deficiency is not compatible with fetal survival. Homozygous type II deficiency is usually associated with severe, life-threatening thrombotic problems in the perinatal period. Affected heterozygous individuals rarely develop thrombotic episodes before puberty, and the risk of thrombosis increases with advancing age. The infrequency of thrombotic events prior to puberty is thought due to the protective effect of α_2-macroglobulin, which is found at higher levels during the first two decades of life than in adults. About 55% of affected patients with familial AT deficiency experience thrombotic episodes (lifetime risk), most commonly involving DVT of the leg and mesenteric veins. About 60% of these individuals develop recurrent thrombotic episodes, and ~40% show clinical signs of PE.[24] Individuals with heparin-binding site defects

⊘ TABLE 33-5

Inherited Thrombophilia: Characteristics of the Five Most Studied Defects

	Factor V Leiden	Prothrombin 20210	Protein C Deficiency	Protein S Deficiency	Antithrombin Deficiency
Occurrence					
General population	4–10%	2–4%	0.2–0.4%	0.07–2.3%	0.02%
First DVT	20%	7%	3%	2–3%	1–2%
Thrombophilic families	40%	18%	6%	4%	4%
Physiologic effect	F-Va resistant to cleavage by APC	↑ Prothrombin	↓ Inactivation of F-Va, F-VIIIa	↓ Cofactor for APC	↓ Inhibition of F-Xa, thrombin
		↑ Thrombin formation	Unregulated coagulation	↓ APC function	Unregulated coagulation
Clinical presentation					
Homozygous	↑↑ Risk VTE (80×)	↑ Risk VTE Possible ↑ arterial TE	Purpura fulminans	Purpura fulminans	Lethal in utero
Heterozygous	↑ Risk VTE (7×)	↑ Risk VTE (3×)	↑ Risk VTE (7×)	↑ Risk VTE (6×)	↑ Risk VTE (10–20×)

DVT = deep vein thrombosis; VTE = venous thromboembolism; APC = activated protein C; ↑ = slightly–moderately increased; ↑↑ = highly increased; ↓ = decreased.
Adapted from Marder VJ, Matei DE. Hereditary and acquired thrombophilic syndromes. In: Colman RW, Hirsh J, Marder VJ, Clowes AW, George JN, eds. *Hemostasis and Thrombosis: Basic Principles and Clinical Practice,* 4th ed. Philadelphia: Lippincott Williams & Wilkins; 2000:1243–75.

generally have significantly less frequent and less severe thrombotic episodes than individuals with defects involving the thrombin-binding site.[25] Among the inherited thrombophilias, AT deficiency, although rare, is generally associated with the most severe clinical manifestations.[26]

Acquired deficiencies of AT occur as well. Healthy newborns have about half the normal adult concentration and gradually reach the adult level by six months of age.[25] A variety of clinical conditions can reduce the concentration of AT in the blood including decreased production of AT (severe hepatic disease), increased consumption of AT (acute thrombosis, DIC), and increased clearance or loss (urinary excretion in the nephrotic syndrome, increased clearance with heparin administration).[27] AT levels are affected by estrogen; premenopausal women have lower levels than men. Also, AT levels are decreased with high-dose (but not low-dose) estrogen OC and in late pregnancy. The low doses of estrogen used in hormone replacement therapy generally do not affect the AT level.[22]

Laboratory Evaluation The two major subtypes of type II AT deficiency are differentiated by two different functional

⊘ TABLE 33-6

Laboratory Classification of Congenital Antithrombin Deficiency

		Functional Activity	
	Concentration	Heparin Cofactor	Progressive AT
Type I	Decreased	Decreased	Decreased
Type II			
Active site defect	Normal	Decreased	Decreased
Heparin-binding site defect	Normal	Decreased	Normal

AT assays. The progressive AT assay quantifies the capacity of AT to neutralize the enzyme activity of a serine protease (e.g., thrombin, or F-Xa) in the absence of heparin, and the heparin cofactor assay measures heparin's ability to catalyze the neutralization of the protease by AT. These two assays combined have identified AT-deficient patients with reductions in heparin cofactor activity without a loss of progressive AT activity (i.e., defects at the heparin-binding site in AT). Other patients exhibit reductions in both functional assays, reflecting mutations near the thrombin-binding site. Immunologic assays (antigen measurements) help distinguish type I and type II defects.

Therapy Patients with AT deficiency can usually be treated successfully with heparin for an acute thrombotic episode, although occasionally higher than usual doses of the drug are required to achieve adequate anticoagulation. If difficulty is encountered in achieving adequate heparinization or recurrent thrombosis is observed despite adequate anticoagulation, AT concentrates are available. Asymptomatic AT-deficient individuals from a thrombophilic kindred are not generally anticoagulated prophylactically unless they are exposed to situations that predispose them to developing thrombosis.[22] Patients with recurrent thrombotic disease may require lifelong antithrombotic treatment with oral anticoagulants (warfarin or coumadin).

Protein C Deficiency

PC is a vitamin K-dependent inhibitor of coagulation (∞ Chapter 30). PC is converted to an activated form (activated protein C [APC]) by thrombin bound to endothelial cell thrombomodulin[28] (Figure 30-18). APC degrades F-Va and F-VIIIa in the presence of its cofactor, PS, and Ca^{2+} (Figure 33-2■). PC in adults is present in plasma at concentrations of about 3–5 μg/mL (70–140%).[29] Term newborns have PC levels of ~25–45% of adult levels, which slowly rise to adult levels during adolescence.[30]

Pathophysiology Reduction of PC levels to ~50% of normal predisposes to venous thrombosis. The diminished capacity to destroy F-Va and F-VIIIa results in an increased production of thrombin, which generates fibrin (a procoagulant effect).

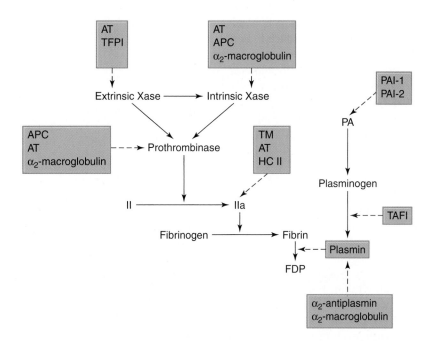

■ **FIGURE 33-2** Physiologic control of the hemostatic process. The extrinsic Xase and intrinsic Xase activate F-X, which forms the prothrombinase complex with F-Va, Ca^{++}, and phospholipid. The prothrombinase complex cleaves prothrombin (II) to form thrombin (IIa). Thrombin cleaves fibrinogen to form fibrin. Plasmin cleaves fibrin and forms fibrin degradation products (FDP). The inhibitors of each of these pathways are depicted in boxes with broken arrows to show the site of inhibition. If there is a defect or deficiency in any of the inhibitors, the hemostatic control mechanism is tipped in favor of thrombosis. AT = antithrombin; TFPI = tissue factor pathway inhibitor; APC = activated protein C; TM = thrombomodulin; HC II = heparin cofactor II; TAFI = thrombin-activatable fibrinolytic inhibitor; PAI = plasminogen activator inhibitor; PA = plasminogen activator

PC deficiency is inherited in an autosomal dominant fashion. Griffin first described the hereditary deficiency of PC in 1981.[31] Similar to AT deficiency, there are two major types of congenital PC deficiency. Type I (the more common form) is characterized by a decrease of both antigen (immunologic) and functional activity to levels of 40–60% of normal (reference range 70–140%). In type II deficiency, there are normal PC antigen levels by immunologic assay but reduced functional levels (a qualitative abnormality of the protein) (Table 33-7 ✪). More than 180 different mutations have been identified for the protein C gene[25] (www.itb.cnr.it/procmd/).

Clinical Findings   Heterozygous PC deficiency is found in ~0.2% of the general population and accounts for about 6% of families with thrombophilia.[22] PC-deficient individuals who develop thrombosis typically present with DVT of the legs and mesenteric veins, often before age 40. About 63% of affected patients develop recurrent venous thrombosis and ~40% exhibit signs of PE.[25] However, many PC-deficient individuals never experience a thrombotic episode unless presented with an additional thrombotic risk factor (either inherited or acquired). Homozygous PC deficiency presents with aggressive thrombotic complications at birth manifest by purpura fulminans (large bruises that become necrotic, histologically similar to warfarin-induced skin necrosis; see below), massive venous thrombosis, and intravascular coagulation.[29] These individuals require replacement of PC and lifetime antithrombotic treatment, usually with oral anticoagulants (warfarin). Liver transplantation has been reported to produce a definitive cure.[32] Acquired PC deficiency is seen in liver disease, severe infection and septic shock, DIC, adult respiratory distress syndrome, and the postoperative state. Oral anticoagulation and vitamin K deficiency also lead to reduced functional PC levels.[25]

Some heterozygous individuals with PC deficiency can experience skin necrosis when treated with warfarin anticoagulants, usually in the first few days of treatment.[33] This warfarin-induced skin necrosis is due to a transient hypercoagulable state, resulting in the formation of fibrin thrombi in the cutaneous vasculature, hemorrhage, and necrosis. With warfarin administration, all vitamin K-dependent clotting factors decrease at a rate that depends on the half-life of the individual factor. PC and F-VII (with the shortest half-lives) decrease within one day with levels of F-II, -IX, and -X falling more slowly over 2–3 days. Individuals with heterozygous PC deficiency who start with PC levels at ~50% quickly develop a transient hypercoagulable state as their levels of PC fall precipitously. The decrease of anticoagulant PC, occurring more rapidly than decreases of most of the procoagulant factors, initially disrupts the delicate hemostatic balance and precipitates a thrombotic event in microvasculature of skin with purpura fulminan symptoms. If this occurs, oral anticoagulation should be stopped immediately, and PC replacement therapy initiated.

Laboratory Evaluation   Various immunologic and functional techniques have been developed to measure PC levels in plasma samples (∞ Chapter 40). Some patients with type II deficiency have normal antigen levels and reduced functional levels in a clotting assay but normal or nearly normal amidolytic activity in chromogenic assays. Therefore, clotting assays are better functional assays for screening for PC deficiency.[34] Testing should not be done while the patient is on oral anticoagulant (coumadin) therapy.

Therapy   Initial treatment for thrombosis associated with PC deficiency is the same as that for most other thrombotic events: heparin followed by oral anticoagulation. Because many heterozygous PC deficient individuals never experience a thrombotic episode, oral anticoagulation may not be needed unless a secondary risk factor is present.[29] PC concentrates are available but usually are used only to treat purpura fulminans in newborns.

Protein S Deficiency

PS is a vitamin K-dependent protein that functions as a cofactor for APC inactivation of F-Va and F-VIIIa (∞ Chapter 30; Figure 30-18). The plasma concentration in normal adults is 65–140% (~23 μg/mL).

Pathophysiology   PS circulates in two forms: an inactive form bound to C4b-binding protein (C4b-BP) (~60% of total) and an unbound or free form (~40% of total). Only free PS has PC cofactor activity. The absolute and relative amounts of PS that are free are influenced by the plasma concentration of C4b-BP. C4b-BP is an acute phase reactant; thus, conditions that increase its production decrease the amount of free PS available to complex with APC. Decreases of free PS contribute to a prothrombotic tendency due to inadequate APC inactivation of F-Va and F-VIIIa. In addition, the direct anticoagulant effect of PS due to its binding to and inhibition of F-Va, F-VIIIa, and F-Xa is decreased in PS deficiency.

First described and linked to a thrombotic tendency in 1984,[35] PS deficiency is inherited in an autosomal dominant manner. The three types of congenital PS deficiency are defined on the basis of total and free PS antigen and APC cofactor activity (Table 33-8 ✪). Type I PS deficiency is characterized by low total antigen and functional activity. Type II deficiency is characterized by normal concentration of both total and free antigen but decreased functional activity (dysfunctional molecule). Type III deficiency is characterized by normal total PS but a decreased free and functional PS concentration (reflecting either a high C4b-BP concentration in plasma or an abnor-

Laboratory Classification of Protein C Deficiency		
	Antigen	Functional Activity
Type I	Decreased	Decreased
Type II	Normal	Decreased

✪ TABLE 33-8

Laboratory Classification of Protein S Deficiency

	Total Protein S	Free Protein S	Protein S Activity
Type I	Decreased	Decreased	Decreased
Type II	Normal	Normal	Decreased
Type III	Normal	Decreased	Decreased

mal binding of PS to this carrier protein).[22] More than 150 mutations causing PS deficiency have been described (www.archive.uwcm.ac.uk/uwcm/mg/hgmd/search.html).

Clinical Findings   The prevalence of PS deficiency in the general population is ~0.7–2.3%, and it accounts for ~6% of cases of familial thrombophilia.[34] The clinical presentation of heterozygous PS deficiency is similar to that of PC deficiency, although PS deficiency has been implicated in some cases of arterial thrombosis.[22] Like PC, PS has been linked with warfarin-induced skin necrosis and in neonatal purpura fulminans when levels approach 0%. Total PS antigen level in healthy full-term newborns is 15–30% of normal adults; however, C4b-BP is also markedly reduced (<20% of adult levels); thus, free PS/functional levels are only slightly reduced compared to those of adults.[36] Acquired PS deficiencies are seen during pregnancy, in association with the use of OC and hormone replacement therapy, in acute TE disease and DIC, in liver disease, in cases of acute bacterial or viral disease (inflammatory states), in vitamin K deficiency, and during oral anticoagulant therapy.[22] Any condition that increases the acute phase reactant C4b-BP decreases free PS and increases the risk of thrombosis.

Laboratory Evaluation   Laboratory evaluation of PS should include assays of both total and free PS (generally immunologic assays) and a functional assay based on the ability of PS to serve as a cofactor for the anticoagulant effect of APC. Plasma level of PS in normal adults is ~23 μg/mL. There is considerable overlap of heterozygous PS deficiency patients and the low normal range; thus, diagnosis can require the performance of multiple assays to establish the diagnosis of PS deficiency.[37] APCR (see below) was reported to cause false positive test results when screening for PS deficiency if clotting (functional) assays are used. However, newer assays using F-V deficient plasma as the substrate have improved the specificity of PS assays.[38]

Therapy   Treatment for PS deficiency is similar to that for PC deficiency. PS concentrates have not yet been developed for clinical use. Coumadin-induced skin necrosis is a rare complication of oral anticoagulation in PS deficiency.

Activated Protein C Resistance

Thrombin activates protein C to APC, which in turn inhibits coagulation by degrading F-Va and F-VIIIa. A novel mecha-

nism for familial thrombophilia was recognized in 1993 with the description of a syndrome characterized by inherited resistance to APC, **activated protein C resistance (APCR)**.[39]

Pathophysiology   APCR is characterized by APC's inability to prolong clotting tests when it is added to the test system. The addition of APC to plasma normally results in a prolongation of the clotting time due to the destruction of F-Va and F-VIIIa. Individuals with APCR exhibit the diminished ability of APC to destroy F-Va. In vivo, inadequate F-Va inactivation can lead to increased production of thrombin and possibly thrombosis. About 90% of cases of APCR are due to a single point mutation of the F-V gene, involving replacement of Arg 506 with Gln (FV^{R506Q}, also called **F-V Leiden [FVL]**). This mutation makes the mutant F-Va molecule resistant to APC inactivation by altering an APC cleavage site.[40]

Studies are currently being conducted in the 10% of individuals with APCR who do not have the FV^{R506Q} mutation.[41] Mutations at Arg 306 (a second APC cleavage site in F-Va) have recently been reported.[42,43] The HR2 F-V haplotype is a recently described polymorphism that also demonstrates low APC sensitivity. However, neither appears to be linked to a thrombotic tendency.[41,43] So far, no genetic abnormalities in the F-VIII gene have been identified as causing APC resistance in humans.[25]

Clinical Findings   The prevalence of heterozygous FVL mutation in Caucasians ranges from 1.0 to 8.5%, depending on the geographic population studied. The mutation is rare in Africans, Asians, Australians, and Native Americans.[44] FVL is seen in as many as 10–30% of patients with venous thrombosis and accounts for about 40% of the cases of familial thrombophilia.[22] Homozygotes are at higher thrombotic risk than heterozygotes as are patients with heterozygous APCR combined with mutations in the genes for PC, PS, or AT.[25] Heterozygotes with FVL are unlikely to develop thromboses unless other acquired risk factors are present (OC, pregnancy, trauma).

Laboratory Evaluation   Laboratory tests for APCR are either clot-based functional tests or molecular techniques. The confirmatory test for FVL is a PCR-based molecular assay. Polymerize chain reaction (PCR) based confirmatory tests for APCR due to mutations other than FVL are available in research laboratories only. Routine clinical diagnosis requires both clotting (screening) tests for APCR and molecular (PCR) tests for FVL because 10% of individuals with APCR do not have the FVL mutation.

Therapy   The management of acute thrombosis in patients with APCR is the same as in other thrombotic patients. Individuals with heterozygous APCR are usually given prophylactic antithrombotic treatment only if they are in a situation of increased thrombotic risk.

Prothrombin Gene Mutation 20210

Prothrombin is cleaved by the activated F-Xa–F-Va complex to form thrombin.

Pathophysiology   In 1996, it was reported that a G → A substitution in the 3′ untranslated region of the prothrombin gene (nucleotide 20210) is associated with a mild elevation of plasma prothrombin levels (115–130% of normal) and an increased risk of venous thrombosis.[45] The prothrombin mutation is the most recent of the hereditary thrombophilias to have a clear-cut genetic mutation defined. The elevated plasma prothrombin level can directly contribute to an increased thrombotic risk by causing increased thrombin generation. Additionally, decreased fibrinolytic activity can occur because of enhanced activation of TAFI.

Clinical Findings   The prevalence of this autosomal dominant gene is ~1–2% among Caucasians, and like FVL, it is infrequent among persons of African, Asian, and Native American origin. It is estimated that ~6% of thrombotic patients are heterozygous for this mutation and that it accounts for about 18% of cases of familial thrombophilia (making it the second most common cause after FVL mutation).[22] A substantial percentage of symptomatic individuals with the prothrombin mutation also had the FVL mutation or another genetic risk factor for thrombosis,[46] supporting the concept that thrombophilia is a multirisk factor disease. Individuals homozygous for the prothrombin mutation have a significantly higher risk of VTE and can have an increased risk of arterial thrombosis.

Laboratory Evaluation   Screening for this mutation using coagulation testing is unreliable because prothrombin levels in these patients overlap with values in the normal population. Molecular testing (PCR) for the single-point mutation at position 20210 in the prothrombin gene is confirmatory.

Therapy   Patients with this disorder are treated the same way other thrombotic patients are. Prophylatic treatment can be given in high-risk situations.

Heparin Cofactor II Deficiency

HC II is a second thrombin inhibitor, and like AT, its action is accelerated by heparin and by dermatan sulfate. In contrast to AT, which inhibits most of the procoagulant serine proteases, HC II inhibits primarily thrombin. HC II deficiency is inherited as an autosomal dominant disorder. Many individuals with this defect are asymptomatic, and it is likely that a partial deficiency (heterozygous state) is a thrombotic risk factor only if it is combined with another thrombophilic risk factor (inherited or acquired).[47,48] Acquired HC II deficiency can be seen in patients with liver disease and in DIC. Several assays are available for measuring HC II, but none is currently FDA approved and thus not available in routine coagulation laboratories. Because both HC II and AT inhibit thrombin, it is recommended that functional assays for AT be based on F-Xa inhibition rather than thrombin inhibition to improve assay specificity for AT.

Tissue Factor Pathway Inhibitor Variant

Tissue factor pathway inhibitor (TFPI) is a natural inhibitor of coagulation that directly neutralizes F-Xa and, in complex with F-Xa, neutralizes the tissue factor:VIIa complex.[49,50] TFPI exists in vivo primarily bound to endothelial cells, and thus measurement of plasma levels (representing ~10–15% of total TFPI) may be uninformative in identifying a deficiency state that could predispose to thrombophilia.[51] A candidate mutation in the TFPI gene resulting in a proline to leucine alteration at position 151 of TFPI has been reported to have an increased risk of VTE.[52]

Hyperhomocysteinemia (HC)

Homocysteine is an amino acid that is metabolized either by transsulfuration to cystathionine or by remethylation to methionine (Figure 33-3 ■). The two main enzymes involved in HC metabolism are cystathionine beta synthase (CBS) and methylene tetrahydrofolate reductase (MTHFR). Normal plasma levels of HC are ~5–15 μmol/L, and HC levels increase with age.

Pathophysiology   Hyperhomocysteinemia (plasma homocysteine level above the normal range) results when homocysteine metabolism is impaired. Severe hyperhomocysteinemia (plasma HC >100 μmol/L) is associated with homocysteinuria and is seen in a group of rare inborn errors of metabolism. The most common causes for homocysteinuria are homozygous mutations in the CBS gene; less commonly mutations occur in the MTHFR gene. Homocysteinuria is associated with premature atherosclerosis (cardiovascular disease and stroke) and venous and arterial thrombosis.[53] More recently, less severe elevations of blood homocysteine levels have also been implicated in VTE.[54]

The mechanisms that link homocysteine to thrombosis are not fully understood, but the major effect is on the vessel wall. Proposed mechanisms include endothelial cell loss, smooth muscle cell proliferation, induction of TF, inhibition of heparan sulfate expression (loss of AT binding), inhibition of nitric oxide (NO) and prostacyclin release, inhibition of tPA binding, and inhibition of thrombomodulin-dependent protein C activation.[25] Mild to moderate homocysteinemia is now recognized to be an independent risk factor for both arterial and venous thrombotic disease. Up to 40% of pa-

Homocysteine Metabolism

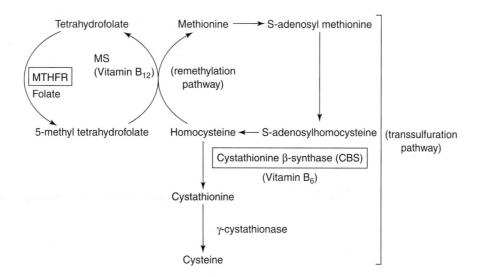

■ FIGURE 33-3   Homocysteine metabolism. Mutations of MTHFR and CBS are associated with hyperhomocysteinemia. Deficiencies of vitamin B_{12}, vitamin B_6, and folate are associated with acquired hyperhomocysteinemia. Hyperhomocysteinemia can lead to increased risk for thrombosis. MTHFR = methylene tetrahydrofolate reductase; MS = methionine synthetase

tients with atherosclerotic coronary or cerebrovascular disease have elevated plasma homocysteine as do 13–18% of patients with an initial episode of VTE prior to age 45.[25]

Clinical Findings   Both inherited and acquired conditions can cause increased HC levels. Multiple genetic mutations of CBS and MTHFR have been identified. Although homozygous CBS deficiency is the most common cause of homocysteinuria, the most common genetic causes of mild homocysteinemia involve mutations of the MTHFR gene. A MTHFR gene polymorphism, nucleotide C677T, which replaces Ala222 by Val, results in a thermolabile molecule with reduced specific activity. This polymorphism appears in homozygous form in 10–20% of the Caucasian population,[55] with 30–40% of the population estimated to be heterozygous for this mutation.[54] This MTHFR mutation is believed to be responsible for the majority of cases of a hereditary predisposition to mild hyperhomocysteinemia.[56] Most heterozygotes do not experience hyperhomocysteinemia or increased risk for vascular disease unless they have other thrombotic risk factors. The most common causes of acquired hyperhomocysteinemia are deficiencies of vitamin B_{12}, folate, or vitamin B_6 (which are cofactors in HC metabolism), smoking, some medications, aging, hypothyroidism, diabetes, and renal disease.[54]

Laboratory Evaluation   HC can be measured by gas chromatography, ion exchange chromatography, and high-performance liquid chromatography. The C677T MTHFR mutation can be identified using molecular assays. MTHFR

heterozygotes or individuals with inadequate vitamin B_6 levels can have normal or only slightly elevated levels of HC. There are significant age and gender differences in HC levels.

Therapy   Treatment of hyperhomocysteinemia usually involves dietary manipulation or vitamin therapy. Administration of vitamin B_6, vitamin B_{12}, or folate often results in normalization of homocysteine levels in these patients, but no clinical efficacy of this approach has been demonstrated in controlled clinical trials.[54]

Fibrinogen Disorders

Fibrinogen is cleaved by thrombin to form fibrin. Fibrinogen can be qualitatively or quantitatively abnormal. Qualitative abnormalities of fibrinogen usually show autosomal dominant inheritance patterns.

Pathophysiology   The **dysfibrinogenemias** are a heterogeneous group of disorders that result in a structurally altered fibrinogen molecule that can lead to altered fibrinogen function. More than 400 different mutations have been identified as causing dysfibrinogenemias.[57] Dysfibrinogenemias can present with no clinical symptoms (~55% of cases), a bleeding diathesis (~25% of cases), or a history of recurrent venous or arterial thromboembolism (~20% of cases).[51] Alterations of fibrinogen predisposing to bleeding include impaired release of fibrinopeptides, defective fibrin polymerization, and abnormal cross-linking by F-XIII$_a$.[58] Two types of thrombotic dysfibrinogenemias appear to be associated with decreased fibrinolytic activity in vivo (thus predisposing to thrombosis): one is abnormally resistant to lysis by plasmin (mutations of plasmin cleavage sites in fibrin), and the other is associated with reduced plasminogen activation (mutations of binding sites for plasminogen or plasminogen activators).[25]

Clinical Findings Patients with thrombotic dysfibrinogenemias are reported to have problems related to pregnancy (spontaneous abortions and postpartum thromboembolism).[59]

Laboratory Evaluation Both quantitative (immunologic assays) and functional tests (thrombin times, reptilase times) for fibrinogen should be performed when dysfibrinogenemia is suspected. Functional fibrinogen measurements are usually significantly lower than antigenic measurements in the plasmas of individuals with dysfibrinogenemia.

Elevated Factor VIII

Individuals with increased plasma levels of F-VIII (>150% of normal) have an increased risk of thrombotic disease possibly due to enhanced thrombin formation[60] or diminished anticoagulant effect of APC.[61] A dose–response relationship appears to exist between F-VIII level and VTE risk.[62] F-VIII levels increase with aging, pregnancy, surgery, chronic inflammation, liver disease, and exercise. Although elevated F-VIII appears to have a hereditary component in some families, a specific molecular basis for the elevated F-VIII levels has not been identified.[63]

Elevated Levels of Other Coagulation Factors

The Northwick Park Heart Study evaluated eight hemostatic measurements as possible thrombogenic risk factors.[64] This study showed a strong positive association between thrombosis and increased levels of F-VII$_a$ and fibrinogen. Elevated fibrinogen can contribute to thrombosis by increasing blood viscosity or thrombin substrate availability. Fibrinogen is an acute phase reactant, and plasma levels of fibrinogen increase in inflammation. Both F-VII$_a$ and fibrinogen levels increase with age. The relative risk for cardiovascular disease is nearly 3 times higher for individuals in the highest quintile of fibrinogen concentration compared to those in the lowest. Increased levels of other factors have been reported to be linked with an increased risk for venous thrombosis.[65] These include F-IX (>129% of normal),[66] and F-XI (>121% of normal).[67]

Factor XII Deficiency

Patients with F-XII deficiency have a prolonged APTT but no clinical bleeding tendency. A number of cases of VTE, myocardial infarction, and stroke have occurred in F-XII-deficient patients.[68] This thrombophilic tendency has been postulated to be related to the role of F-XII in activating fibrinolysis. A number of studies have shown that heterozygous F-XII deficiency does not constitute a major thrombotic risk factor although severe deficiency could be associated with increased thrombotic risk.[22, 23]

Fibrinolytic System Disorders

Hereditary disorders of fibrinolysis are less frequently associated with thrombotic disease than are hereditary anomalies of procoagulants or coagulation inhibitors.[69] Possible causes of abnormalities of fibrinolysis include the structure of fibrin (see dysfibrinogenemias earlier), the amount and function of plasminogen, and the physiology of plasminogen activation (impaired plasminogen activator synthesis or release, increased plasminogen activator inhibitor, or increased levels of TAFI).[70]

Plasminogen Deficiency Plasminogen abnormalities have been classified as either type I (decrease of both protein concentration and functional activity) or type II (normal antigen levels but reduced functional activity [dysplasminogenemia]). Both types have been reported in patients with venous thrombosis.[71,72] However, the association of hypo/dysplasminogenemia as a predisposing factor in VTE is not firmly established. Laboratory tests are available to measure protein levels (immunologic) and functional activity (clot-lysis or chromogenic substrate) of plasminogen.

Tissue Plasminogen Activator (tPA) and Plasminogen Activator Inhibitor (PAI) Inadequate stores or release of tPA or an inappropriate/excess release of PAI could theoretically result in thrombotic events. (Figure 33-1). Several reports have linked defective fibrinolysis associated with decreased release of tPA and/or elevated PAI-1 with familial thrombosis.[73–75] However, two of these families subsequently were shown to have hereditary PS deficiency, the more likely cause of clinical disease in these families.[76,77] It is thought that tPA and PAI-1 likely play a greater role in acquired thrombophilia than in hereditary thrombophilia. Functional (chromogenic assays) and quantitative (ELISA) assays for tPA and PAI-1 are available.

 Checkpoint! 2

Why is thrombotic disease associated with hereditary thrombophilia considered a multigene (or multirisk factor) disease?

 CASE STUDY *(continued from page 737)*

Andrea was initially tested while she had deep vein thrombosis and again six months later after being taken off coumadin. The tests included AT, PC, and PS, fibrinogen, D-dimer, and plasminogen. All test results were in the reference range on both occasions.

2. What other possibilities could explain the thrombotic event in this patient?

ACQUIRED THROMBOPHILIA

The acquired or secondary thrombophilic states include a heterogeneous group of disorders in which an increased risk appears to exist for developing thromboembolic complications. The pathophysiologic basis for the thrombophilic state in most of these situations is complex. Various clinical conditions are associated with a high risk of thrombotic complications (Table 33-9 ✪). As with the hereditary thrombophilias, acquired disorders vary widely in their tendency to cause venous and arterial thrombotic disease (Table 33-3). Acquired defects leading to thrombosis are at least as common as inherited deficiencies and often precipitate the acute thrombotic episode in the patient with an inherited thrombophilia.[2]

Acquired Fibrinolytic Defects

Early studies of fibrinolytic function in patients with thromboembolic disease consistently demonstrated that 30–40% of these patients had an impaired fibrinolytic function.[78] Decreased fibrinolysis has been linked to many acquired conditions including postsurgery, coronary disease, taking OCs, the last trimester of pregnancy, certain infections, aging, radiation therapy, some drugs, and malignancy.[79] Increased plasma PAI-1 level is the most common reason for an impaired fibrinolytic function although this increase is often combined with a decreased capacity to release tPA.[78] Many patients with DVT have a history of a long-lasting inflammatory response, which contributes to an impaired fibrinolytic function by elevating the PAI-1 levels (an acute phase reactant). An increased PAI-1 level in plasma can predict the development of a new thrombotic event (postoperatively, in myocardial infarction, and idiopathic DVT).[78]

Antiphospholipid (aPL) Antibodies/ Antiphospholipid Antibody Syndrome

Antiphospholipid antibody syndrome (aPLS) has multiple clinical manifestations and is the most common cause of acquired thrombophilia.[20] aPL include a broad group of autoantibodies that includes the lupus anticoagulant (LA), anticardiolipin antibodies (ACLA), and several subgroups (antibodies that recognize other phospholipids and phospholipid-binding proteins).[80] These antibodies prolong phospholipid-dependent clotting assays in vitro[23] (∞ Chapter 32).

Phospholipid-reactive antibodies (aPL) were first described in patients with biologic false-positive serologic tests for syphilis and were shown to recognize cardiolipin within the test reagent (i.e., ACLA).[81] The same year, aPL were identified in patients with systemic lupus erythematosus (SLE), subsequently named LA.[82] Other antibodies that reacted with anionic phospholipids other than cardiolipin (e.g., antiphosphatidylserine) were later identified. Before 1990, it was thought that aPL antibodies recognized epitopes within the anionic phospholipids, but it was subsequently demonstrated that many of them recognize proteins (cofactors or antigenic targets) in complex with the phospholipids.[80] These include antibodies recognizing β_2-glycoprotein-1 (β_2GP1), prothrombin, PC, PS, and F-VII. These aPL antibodies can be produced after certain infections (mycobacteria, malaria, and other parasitic organisms), after exposure to certain medications (neuroleptics, chlorpromazine, quinidine, procainamide), and by patients with autoimmune disorders (SLE, Sjögren syndrome, rheumatoid arthritis, immune thrombocytopenic purpura ITP).

Pathophysiology Paradoxically, although these antibodies prolong in vitro coagulation assays (suggestive of defective hemostasis), individuals with aPL antibodies do not suffer from a bleeding diathesis unless other hemostatic defects are present (e.g., thrombocytopenia, hypoprothrombinemia). Rather, the presence of aPL increases the apparent risk of both arterial and venous TE with approximately one-third of patients with such inhibitors having thrombotic events.[25]

The most commonly identified antiphospholipid antibodies, LA and ACLA, behave similarly, and 73% of patients with LA also have ACLA.[83] Immunologically, both LA and ACLA are usually IgG but can be IgM or a mixture of the two. The antibody combines with the phospholipid surfaces

✪ TABLE 33-9

Secondary Disorders and Other Factors Contributing to Acquired Thrombosis

Secondary disorders

Fibrinolytic system defects

Antiphospholipid antibody syndrome

Malignancy

Hip, knee surgery

Hematologic disorders

   Polycythemia vera/myeloproliferative disorders

   Hemolytic anemia

   Sickle cell anemia

   Paroxysmal nocturnal hemoglobinuria

   Acute promyelocytic leukemia

Chronic inflammatory disease

Congestive heart failure

Atrial fibrillation

Nephrotic syndrome

Atherosclerosis

Hyperlipidemia, hypercholesterolemia, increased lipoprotein (a)

Other factors

>50 years of age

Obesity

Diet with inadequate folate, vitamin B_6 or vitamin B_{12}; chronic intake of fatty food

Smoking

Pregnancy, use of OCs, hormone replacement therapy

Stasis/immobilization (prolonged car or air travel; bed rest)

Trauma/postoperative state

of test reagents used in the APTT (and occasionally the PT), prolonging the clotting times. Both LA and ACLA were originally thought to react only with phospholipid. Further studies of antibody specificity revealed, however, that ACLA requires β_2-GPI to be associated with the phospholipid on the surface of the cells to which they bind,[83] and LA were directed against epitopes on prothrombin.

Various mechanisms have been proposed to explain the increased risk of thrombosis with aPL: inhibition of endothelial cell anticoagulant processes and causing cells in the blood (or in contact with the blood) to acquire a procoagulant phenotype.[80] Specific aPL-induced changes include interference with protein C activation or activity (decrease in thrombomodulin expression, decrease in free PS), inhibition of heparin sulfate interaction with AT, inhibition of endothelial cell production or release of prostacyclin, alterations in fibrinolytic mechanisms (decreased tPA and/or increased PAI-1). In addition, aPL can stimulate platelet aggregation and promote tissue factor synthesis by leukocytes.[84]

Clinical Findings The clinical manifestations that are most frequent in these patients include systemic vascular thrombosis (DVT, PE), thrombosis at unusual sites, increased risk of arterial thrombosis (stroke and other neurological complications), and increased risk of adverse pregnancy outcomes (recurrent miscarriages). It is estimated that 5–15% of patients with VTE are positive for LA (aPL) in comparison to 0–2% of the general population.[84] *Secondary aPL syndrome* is a term used to describe when aPL and thrombosis occur in conjunction with an autoimmune condition such as SLE. When aPL occurs as an independent autoimmune disorder, it is referred to as *primary aPL syndrome*.

Laboratory Evaluation No single test identifies every LA/aPL; instead, a combination of tests must be performed. Two types of assays are used to detect aPL antibodies: "LA" are detected by their ability to prolong phospholipid-dependent coagulation reactions, and specific immunoassays, usually ELISA, are used to detect antibodies reactive with cardiolipin, phosphatidylserine, β_2GP1, prothrombin, or F-VII. Table 32-11 in ∞ Chapter 32 shows typical laboratory test results and comparisons to other acquired conditions associated with a prolonged APTT. The sensitivity of the APTT reagent for LA detection varies with different commercial reagents used for the test. Some commercial APTT reagents have been created to be very sensitive to the presence of LA.

The Subcommittee on Lupus Anticoagulant/Antiphospholipid Antibodies of the Scientific and Standardization Committee of the International Society of Thrombosis and Haemostasis has proposed criteria to standardize the diagnosis of LA. Diagnosis requires a four-step approach:

1. prolongation of a phospholipid-dependent coagulation assay (usually the APTT)

2. evidence of inhibitor activity in the patient plasma

3. evidence of the phospholipid-dependance of the inhibitor effect

4. absence of a specific inhibitor against a coagulation factor.

A sequence of suggested tests for evaluating a patient's plasma for the presence of LA is outlined in Table 33-10 ✪.[85]

The first step in identifying LA is that at least one laboratory test that uses phospholipid in the reagent (e.g., the APTT) must be prolonged. This prolonged test must then be repeated on a 1:1 mixture of patient's plasma and normal plasma (NP) to distinguish between an inhibitor and a single-factor deficiency (see mixing studies, ∞ Chapter 40). In the presence of an LA inhibitor, no correction will be noted (the LA usually prolongs the clotting time of the NP immediately after mixing in contrast to inhibitors specific for coagulation factors, which usually require incubation). A specific factor deficiency can also be ruled out by factor assays, if needed.

The possibility that the presence of heparin causes the prolonged APTT must also be eliminated. Heparin can be identified by observing a prolonged thrombin time and a normal reptilase time (∞ Chapter 40). At least one additional abnormal screening test for the LA must be demonstrated.

A confirmatory test is then performed to establish that the antibody/inhibitor is phospholipid dependent. Confirmatory tests are modifications of the screening tests (that were originally abnormal) that alter the amount of phospholipid in the test system. The modifications usually involve ei-

---

✪ TABLE 33-10

Recommended Approach for Identifying the Lupus Anticoagulant (LA)[85]

Screening procedures—two or more using single concentration of phospholipid
1. Demonstrate at least one prolonged phospholipid-based clotting test (e.g., APTT).
2. Demonstrate at least one additional prolonged LA screening test (e.g., dilute Russell's viper venom time [dRVVT], plasma clot time [PCT], kaolin clotting time [KCT])

Confirmatory procedures—modify abnormal screening procedure by altering phospholipid content of the test procedure, which demonstrates that the LA depends on phospholipid
1. Reducing phospholipid concentration in test reagent to accentuate prolonged test (e.g., diluting the test reagent)
2. Neutralizing the effect of the LA by increasing the phospholipid in the test system (e.g., frozen-thawed platelets [platelet neutralization procedure]; platelet vesicles hexagonal phase phospholipid)

Additional requirements for documenting LA
1. Mixing studies with normal platelet free plasma not corrected
2. Exclusion of presence of heparin in the sample (e.g., normal thrombin time/reptilase time)
3. Proof that another coagulopathy is not present or concurrent; specific factor assays to rule out a factor deficiency; detailed clinical history

ther reducing the amount of phospholipid in the reagent or adding an excess of phospholipid to the test system. The most sensitive tests for detecting the inhibitor contain only limited amounts of procoagulant phospholipids (dRVVT, dilute PTT, or perform PT with very dilute tissue factor—the tissue thromboplastin inhibition [TTI] test). When excess phospholipid is added to the test system, there is an overabundance of phospholipid, the antibody is overwhelmed, and the original prolonged test time is shortened to the normal range. The *platelet neutralization procedure* (∞ Chapter 40) is a popular confirmatory test. This test adds washed, frozen, and thawed platelets, an abundant source of phospholipid, to the patient's plasma; the prolonged screening test is corrected. A better confirmatory test is the *hexagonal phase phospholipid test* (Staclot LA by Diagnostica Stago ∞ Chapter 40). The LA can recognize phosphatidylethanolamine in the hexagonal phase array configuration (hexagonal H_{11}) but not in the lamellar phase. Adding H_{11} phase phosphatidyl ethanolamine to an LA patient specimen will correct the prolonged APTT by absorbing the LA antibodies. Unlike the platelet neutralization procedure, the hexagonal phospholipid test does not give false positives with heparin. Figure 33-4 ▪ outlines a flow chart for an approach to the laboratory testing for LA.

Therapy Management of acute VTE in patients with aPLS is similar to that of other individuals with thrombosis. However, the APTT cannot reliably be used to monitor unfrac-tionated heparin dosage without modifications (e.g., the use of an insensitive APTT reagent or the activated coagulation time/ACT test).[25] Low-dose heparin circumvents this problem because it does not require laboratory monitoring (see later section). Patients who develop transient LA/aPL in association with infections do not usually sustain TE episodes. The presence of a persistent LA and/or a high-titer antibody in an asymptomatic patient with no prior thrombotic history is not an indication for anticoagulant therapy unless there are coexisting clinical circumstances (surgery, prolonged immobilization). Corticosteroids can normalize clotting times or reduce aPL antibody titers but might not prevent recurrent thrombosis.[18]

Heparin-Induced Thrombocytopenia (HIT)

Heparin is used to prevent or treat thrombosis. However, its use can cause thrombocytopenia in some patients, generally associated with platelet activation. **H**eparin **a**ssociated **t**hrombocytopenia (HAT) in which the thrombocytopenia results from a direct, nonimmune mediated platelet activation, is not associated with an increased risk of thrombosis. **H**eparin **i**nduced **t**hrombocytopenia (HIT), is due to an autoantibody directed against heparin complexed with platelet factor 4 (PF4).[86] PF4 is released from platelet α-granules during platelet activation, nonspecifically binds to heparin in the circulation, and antibodies are produced to the heparin/PF-4 complex. The antibody/heparin/PF-4

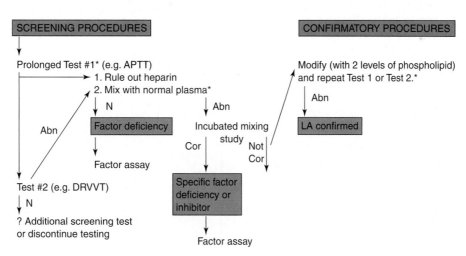

* Plasma samples must be platelet free.

▪ **FIGURE 33-4**   A flow chart for an approach to the diagnosis of the lupus anticoagulant (LA). At least two screening phospholipid-based screening tests (tests using one concentration of phospholipid) must be prolonged. Mixing studies must be uncorrected with normal plasma. The presence of heparin must be ruled out. Confirmatory tests are performed by modifying the abnormal screening tests with two levels of phospholipid. (Adapted from: Brandt JT, Triplett DA, Alving B, Scharrer I. Criteria for the diagnosis of lupus anticoagulants: An update. *Thromb Haemost.* 1995;74:1185–90.) (Cor = corrected; N = normal; Abn = abnormal; LA = lupus anticoagulant; APTT = activated partial thromboplastin time; dRVVT = dilute Russell's viper venom time)

complex then attaches to the platelet surface via the platelet FcγIIa receptors, resulting in increased platelet clearance and thrombocytopenia. The antibody heparin-PF4 complexes occasionally induce platelet activation and aggregation.

The most serious complication of HIT is activation of the clotting system and thrombosis, which can be life threatening. Isolated HIT refers to the patient with thrombocytopenia without thrombosis, whereas HITT is used to refer to patients with HIT and thrombotic complications. It is thought that a number of events contribute to the thrombotic complications including in vivo platelet activation, generation of procoagulant platelet-derived microparticles, and activation of endothelium via HIT antibody recognition of PF4/endothelial heparan sulfate complexes.[86] Thrombocytopenia develops in approximately 3% of patients who receive **unfractionated heparin (UFH)**, and thrombosis occurs in one-third of those.[87] The most common venous thrombotic complications are DVT and PE, and arterial thrombosis most commonly affects the lower limb (acute limb ischemia) or cerebral vessels (thrombotic stroke). Low molecular weight (LMW) heparin can trigger HIT but much less frequently than UFH.[88]

HIT is suspected when a patient receiving heparin demonstrates a thrombocytopenia of $<150 \times 10^9$/L, or a 50% drop in platelet count from baseline. Typically, the onset is 5–14 days after starting any dose, any type, or any route of heparin exposure.[89] A more rapid fall (within hours) in platelet count occasionally occurs if the patient has been treated with heparin within the previous 100 days. Because heparin is generally used in patients who have experienced an acute thrombotic episode or who are at risk of one, other causes of thrombocytopenia must be excluded.

Two types of assays are available to diagnose HIT: functional and antigen assays.[86] Functional assays based on the ability of HIT-IgG to activate platelets are most commonly used. Either ^{14}C-serotonin release or platelet aggregation are used as endpoints in these assays. ELISA assays for HIT-IgG have been developed using the heparin-PF4 target antigen. Most routine hospital laboratories do not offer assays for HIT, but they may be available through reference labs. The HIT antibodies usually remain detectable for only 4–6 weeks. Routine screening for HIT antibodies in patients who are receiving heparin is not recommended because many patients can form HIT antibodies without developing thrombocytopenia or experiencing other adverse events.[86]

Patients receiving UFH should have their platelet counts monitored periodically during therapy, beginning on day 5 of heparin use. If the platelet count falls, heparin should be discontinued and another form of anticoagulant therapy begun (e.g., the heparinoid danaparoid or a direct thrombin inhibitor such as hirudin or argatroban). Although LMWH is a less frequent inducer of HIT, once the antibodies are formed, LMWH cannot be used because it also binds PF4 and the HIT antibody. Oral anticoagulants should not be started until adequate anticoaglation with these alternative agents

has been achieved and the platelet count has returned to the normal range.

Thrombohemorrhagic Disorders

Thrombotic microangiopathies (TMA) The term *thrombotic microangiopathies* has been used to describe clinical disorders characterized by the presence of a microangiopathic hemolytic anemia (see ∞ Chapter 18 for more details on the pathophysiology of the hematologic aspects of these disorders), thrombocytopenia and microvascular thrombotic lesions. **Disseminated intravascular coagulation (DIC), thrombotic thrombocytopenic purpura (TTP), and hemolytic uremic syndrome (HUS)** are TMA disorders. For a number of years, TTP and HUS were considered similar, perhaps overlapping, clinical conditions and were often included in a combined clinical classification of "TTP/HUS." Both conditions are associated with primarily activation of platelets without activation of the coagulation cascade. Platelet aggregates form in the microvasculature and result in a thrombocytopenia. Typically, coagulation assays (PT, APTT, TT) are normal. It has recently been shown that the two disorders are distinct entities with different pathophysiologic causes, laboratory diagnostic approaches, and therapies (Table 33-11 ✪).

Disseminated Intravascular Coagulation   DIC is a syndrome associated with systemic rather than localized activation of coagulation. It is a condition in which the normal balance of hemostasis is altered, resulting in the uncontrolled and inappropriate formation and lysis of fibrin within the blood vessels. It can be triggered by numerous events and can manifest as either a thrombotic or a hemor-

✪ TABLE 33-11

Comparison of TTP and HUS

Feature	TTP	HUS
MAHA	Yes	Yes
Thrombocytopenia	Severe	Moderate to severe
Age	Peak incidence <40	Childhood
Gender	Female	Equal
Epidemic	No	Yes
Recurrence	Common	Rare
Link to *E. coli* O157:H7	Occasional	Yes
Renal failure	Uncommon	Common
Neurologic symptoms	Common	Uncommon
Organ involvement	Multiple	Limited to kidney
VWF multimer	Ultralarge forms present	Smaller multimers predominate
ADAMTS-13 activity	Deficient	Normal

TTP = thrombotic thrombocytopenic purpura; HUS = hemolytic uremic syndrome; MAHA = microangiopathic hemolytic anemia

rhagic hemostatic state. See ∞ Chapter 32 for the full discussion of the pathophysiology and laboratory evaluation of patients with DIC.

Thrombotic Thrombocytopenic Purpura Moschowitz first described TTP in his 1924 report of a 16-year-old female who presented with microangiopathic hemolytic anemia, petechiae, renal failure, and hemiparesis. At autopsy, she was found to have disseminated microvascular thrombi in the terminal arterioles and capillaries of the heart and kidney.[90] For years, TTP was defined by the "classic pentad" of (1) microangiopathic hemolytic anemia, (2) thrombocytopenia, (3) neurologic symptoms, (4) fever, and (5) renal dysfunction.[91] Systemic platelet agglutination produces microvascular thrombosis with variable tissue ischemia and infarction. The thrombi are composed predominantly of platelets with little or no fibrin. The most commonly affected organs are the brain, heart, pancreas, and adrenals; although renal involvement occurs, it rarely progresses to acute renal insufficiency or renal failure.

TTP is now known to be triggered by the presence of ultralarge VWF multimers (ULVWF) in the plasma (∞ Chapter 30).[92,93] VWF is secreted from the Weibel-Palade bodies of activated endothelial cells as ultralarge multimers, larger than the typical large VWF forms that normally circulate. These ultralarge multimers are cleaved by a VWF cleaving protease known as *ADAMTS-13* (**a d**isintegrinlike **a**nd **m**etalloprotease domain with **t**hrombo**s**pondin) type motifs. ADAMTS-13 binds to the surface of endothelial cells and cleaves ULVWF multimers as they are synthesized and released[94,95] (Figure 33-5 ■). When ADAMTS-13 is significantly reduced or absent, the resulting ULVWF multimers adhere to platelets and induce platelet agglutination, resulting in disseminated platelet thrombi.[96]

Familial or inherited TTP is known as the *Upshaw-Shulman Syndrome*.[93] It is a rare autosomal recessive disorder characterized by repeated episodes of TMA during childhood (chronic, relapsing TTP). It is due to a mutation of the ADAMTS-13 gene (9q34), resulting in a deficiency/dysfunction of the enzyme.[97] As a result, these patients have ULVWF in their plasma and a predisposition to forming platelet-rich microvascular thrombi. Treatment is plasma infusion to replace the missing enzyme as needed. Heterozygotes are clinically asymptomatic.

Acquired TTP is an acquired autoimmune deficiency of ADAMTS-13.[93] Also called *idiopathic TTP,* the disorder is more common in females than males (3:2 ratio). Other risk factors for idiopathic TTP are African ancestry and obesity. Of patients, 10–45% have a history of upper respiratory or flulike symptoms within weeks preceding diagnosis. Acquired TTP has also been associated with pregnancy, certain drugs, cancer/chemotherapy, and tissue transplantation. The autoantibodies against ADAMTS-13 block the activity of the VWF cleaving enzyme, producing TTP.[98] Mortality is >90% without treatment. Recommended treatment is plasma exchange (to remove the autoantibody and replacement with functional ADAMTS-13). Most patients (65%) have a single episode of TTP; ~35% have recurrent disease.

Laboratory testing for ADAMTS-13 can be done to confirm the suspected diagnosis, but plasma exchange treatment should begin immediately without waiting for results. Most hospitals rely on reference laboratories for ADAMTS-13 assays. Antibody or inhibitor activity against the protease is measured by a Bethesda-type methodology similar to that used to measure antibodies to F-VIII (∞ Chapter 40).

Hemolytic Uremic Syndrome HUS occurs in two forms, "typical" and "atypical."[93] Typical HUS is associated with bloody diarrhea, fever, and infection by verotoxin-producing *E. coli* (VTEC). Also called *D+ HUS* (diarrhea positive),

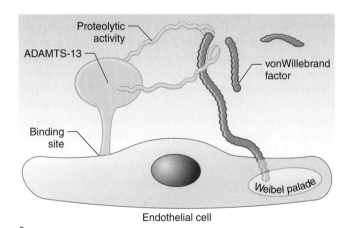

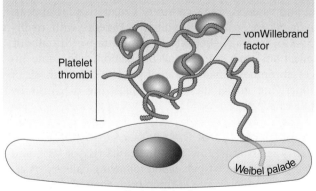

a   b

■ **FIGURE 33-5** VWF Processing by ADAMTS-13. **a.** Normal ADAMTS-13 proteolytically cleaves ultralarge von Willebrand factor (ULVWF) multimers into smaller subunits. **b.** In the absence of ADAMTS-13 activity, ULVWF multimers persist, inducing platelet agglutination and the formation of platelet thrombi. (Reprinted with permission from the American Society for Clinical Laboratory Science (ASCLS), Schneider M, Thrombotic Microangiopathy (TTP and HUS): Advances in Differentiation and Diagnosis, *Clin Lab Sci.* 2007;20(4):216.)

it accounts for 95% of all cases in children. *E. coli* O157:H7 accounts for most of the cases (80%), but other toxin-bearing *E. coli* serotypes, and *Shigella dysenteriae* type 1 have also been linked with HUS.[99]

Thrombocytopenia and neurologic manifestations are less common and less severe in HUS than in TTP. However, renal involvement is more severe than in TTP. Of patients, 60% require renal dialysis, and 40–50% of patients develop chronic renal insufficiency. The pathogenesis of VTEC-HUS is thought to be toxin-induced endothelial damage, primarily in the renal glomeruli, resulting in microvascular thrombi consisting of platelets and fibrin.

Familial (inherited) HUS is a chronic, relapsing clinical condition characterized as a D- or atypical form of HUS.[93] It is usually associated with an inherited abnormality of the complement regulatory system with persistently low levels of complement. Identified abnormalities include homozygous deficiency of complement factor H, membrane cofactor protein (MCP) or factor I.[99,100] However, 50% of the cases of familiar HUS remain unexplained at the molecular level.

Malignancy

The association between thrombosis and malignancy has been recognized for more than 100 years and for a variety of different cancers.[22] TE disease affects 3–25% of cancer patients and is the second most common cause of death.[101] The causes of thrombosis in cancer patients are complex. The three components that play a significant role in thrombogenesis (stasis, activation of blood coagulation, and vascular injury) are present in patients with malignant disease. Patients with cancer are often immobile and bedridden. Tumor cells release coagulation-activating factors including TF and cancer procoagulant protein (a cysteine-containing protease that directly activates F-X). Often malignancies are accompanied by a reduction of natural anticoagulants (AT and PC).[22] Vascular injury can be triggered by surgery, chemotherapy drugs, and vascular access catheters. Chemotherapy appears to augment the risk for thrombosis. Patients with malignancy also have a higher rate of postoperative thrombotic complications than the general population.[25] In some instances, thrombosis manifests itself prior to the diagnosis of an underlying malignancy and predates the diagnosis by several years.[25]

Pregnancy and Oral Contraceptives (OC)

Pregnancy is associated with an increased risk of VTE, and the puerperium (the 6-week period following delivery) is associated with a higher rate of thrombosis than pregnancy itself.[25] Risk factors for thrombosis in pregnancy include advanced maternal age, Cesarean delivery, prolonged immobilization, obesity, prior TE, and one of the inherited thrombophilias. Thrombosis during pregnancy and the puerperium is due to pregnancy-induced alterations in hemostasis as well as venous stasis in the lower extremities. The levels of most coagulation proteins increase during pregnancy (particularly fibrinogen and F-VIII), and there is a significant decline in AT, free and total PS, and fibrinolytic system activity (decreased tPA and increased PAI-1).[25] The net effect of these changes is to promote blood coagulation and may represent a mechanism to control bleeding at the time of placental separation.

Estrogen therapy and high-dose OC have been associated with increased venous and arterial thrombosis related to the estrogen dose.[25] The mechanisms by which OC induce a prothrombotic state are unclear. Its use is associated with changes in the levels of many coagulation proteins including increases of fibrinogen, F-VII, and F-VIII and decreases of AT and PS. Any individual with an inherited thrombophilia or increased thrombotic risk factors should be carefully evaluated before estrogen therapy is begun.

Postoperative State and Trauma

DVT and PE occur with increased frequency in postoperative patients, although the thrombotic risk varies depending on the type of surgery performed. Risk factors associated with increased rates of thrombosis include age (advanced), previous VTE, coexistence of malignancy, inherited thrombophilia, and extended surgical and immobilization times.[25] DVT and PE are also commonly encountered after major trauma. Proposed mechanisms for the activation of the coagulation system include exposure of tissue factor from injured tissue, elevated levels of fibrinogen and VWF, and decreased levels of AT and PC (associated with an acute inflammatory response).

Hematologic Disorders

Several hematologic disorders are associated with thrombosis. Patients with myeloproliferative disorders often experience a predisposition to thrombotic and hemorrhagic complications. Idiopathic myelofibrosis, essential thrombocythemia, and polycythemia vera all are associated with venous and arterial thrombotic events. The mechanisms involved are complex and include the association of vascular occlusive episodes with a high hematocrit and hyperviscosity as well as elevated platelet counts and platelet hyperreactivity (∞ Chapter 22). Sickle cell anemia can lead to thrombosis because of hyperviscosity secondary to sickled erythrocytes. Acute promyelocytic leukemia (APL) is often complicated by a profound coagulopathy due to enhanced procoagulant activity associated with the release of TF from the leukemic cells (∞ Chapter 24). Either diffuse or localized thrombosis can result. Interestingly, with the adoption of all-transretinoic acid as the treatment of choice for APL, patients appear to be more at risk of vascular occlusive disease (thrombosis) than diffuse coagulapathies (DIC).[25] In paroxysmal nocturnal hemoglobinuria (PNH), the chronic intravascular hemolysis is often associated with thrombotic crises (∞ Chapter 15). Membrane vessicles produced by complement-induced hemolysis of the erythrocytes possess prothrombinase-promoting activity and can induce thrombotic events at various vascular sites.[24]

► LABORATORY TESTING IN PATIENTS WITH SUSPECTED THROMBOSIS

When patients are suspected of having an acute thrombotic process or a thrombotic diathesis, it is helpful to ascertain whether they are likely to have an inherited (primary) or an acquired (secondary) thrombophilia. Patients with hereditary defects are at lifelong risk of developing thrombosis, and clinical circumstances (e.g., pregnancy, estrogen use, surgery) can trigger thrombotic episodes in ~50% of such individuals.[25] Taking a complete history is essential including age of onset, location of prior thromboses, circumstances that could have precipitated the event, and particularly a family history of other affected individuals (suggesting a hereditary defect).

Samples for laboratory analysis should not be drawn during a thrombotic episode because the episode itself can affect many laboratory assays. Acute thrombosis is often associated with acquired deficiencies of AT, PC, or PS because these proteins are consumed during thrombosis. Any anticoagulant therapy should be noted because it can affect coagulation tests. Heparin therapy may be associated with up to a 30% decline in AT levels, and warfarin produces a marked drop in the functional activity of PC and PS and a decline to a lesser extent in immunologic levels. Warfarin has also been shown to (rarely) elevate AT levels significantly, sometimes into the normal range in patients with a hereditary deficiency.[25]

Clinical guidelines for thrombotic risk assessment should be based on outcomes assessment. Many institutions have or are preparing testing protocols for effective diagnosis in patients with thrombophilia. The protocol described here varies depending on the patient population, laboratory resources, and other factors (Figure 33-6 ■).

Thrombosis risk testing should begin with screening tests (PT, APTT) to rule out anticoagulant therapy and acquired factor deficiencies and to detect antiphospholipid antibodies that interfere with interpretation of clot-based PS and APCR tests. Additional testing typically includes functional and antigenic (or molecular) measurements of the most common inherited defects: APCR/FVL, prothrombin 20210, MTHFR mutations, PC, PS, and AT. Additional testing for other deficiencies or defects can be performed even if the patient tests positive for one of these initial tests because patients with thrombophilia can have multiple defects.

The best screening tests for deficiencies of AT, PC, and PS are functional assays that detect both quantitative and qualitative defects. Immunologic (antigenic) assays detect only quantitative deficiencies of these proteins. To obtain a definitive diagnosis (differentiate type I and type II deficiencies), thrombotic

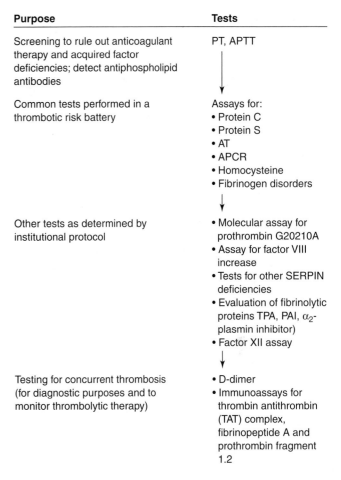

Purpose	Tests
Screening to rule out anticoagulant therapy and acquired factor deficiencies; detect antiphospholipid antibodies	PT, APTT
Common tests performed in a thrombotic risk battery	Assays for: • Protein C • Protein S • AT • APCR • Homocysteine • Fibrinogen disorders
Other tests as determined by institutional protocol	• Molecular assay for prothrombin G20210A • Assay for factor VIII increase • Tests for other SERPIN deficiencies • Evaluation of fibrinolytic proteins TPA, PAI, α_2-plasmin inhibitor) • Factor XII assay
Testing for concurrent thrombosis (for diagnostic purposes and to monitor thrombolytic therapy)	• D-dimer • Immunoassays for thrombin antithrombin (TAT) complex, fibrinopeptide A and prothrombin fragment 1.2

SERPIN-serine proteinase inhibitors (antithrombin, heparin cofactor II); TPA-tissue plasminogen activator; PAI-plasminogen activator inhibitor; AT-antithrombin; PT-prothrombin time; APTT-activated partial thromboplastin time; APCR-activated protein C resistance.

■ **FIGURE 33-6** Protocol for thrombotic risk testing. Testing begins with coagulation screening tests and proceeds according to the protocol established by the institution.

patients need to have both a functional and an antigenic test performed on the hemostatic component in question.

Many thrombotic disorders are difficult to diagnose because individuals can present with borderline laboratory values of a hemostatic component that is not clearly normal or abnormal; multiple testing may be needed. In addition to assays for particular hemostatic proteins associated with hereditary or acquired thrombophilias, assays are available to measure the extent of coagulation enzyme activation in the blood in vivo (e.g., fibrinopeptide A, prothrombin fragment 1.2, thrombin-AT complex, plasmin-antiplasmin complex). Although these assays do not give information regarding the specific *type* of hypercoagulable state that is present, they can provide information supporting the presence of increased activation of the coagulation system. Determining an episode's etiology is important because it suggests specific

TABLE 33-12

Laboratory Tests Used in Diagnosing a Patient with Thrombophilia

	Functional	Antigenic	Molecular
Antithrombin	X	X	
Heparin cofactor II		X	
Protein C	X	X	
Protein S		Total PS	
	Free PS	Free PS	
APCR	X		X
Prothrombin 20210			X
Tissue factor pathway inhibitor			X
Hyperhomocysteinemia			
CBS mutations			X
MTHFR mutations			X
Fibrinogen	X	X	
Factor XII	X		
Plasminogen	X	X	
Tissue plasminogen activator	X	X	
Plasminogen activator inhibitor	X	X	
Antiphospholipid antibodies	Screening with APTT; specific confirmatory tests including platelet neutralization and dilute Russell's viper venom		

APCR = activated protein C resistance; CBS = cystathionine beta synthase; MTHFR = methlene tetrahydrofolate reductase; APTT = activated partial thromboplastin time

and appropriate therapy. All risk factors or possible deficiencies need to be ascertained because they can interact and, in some cases, significantly increase the risk of thrombosis.[102] Table 33-12 ✪ lists some tests that may be useful in diagnosing thrombotic disorders.

✓ **Checkpoint! 3**

Why are both immunologic and functional assays recommended when screening a patient suspected of having a familial thrombophilic defect?

 CASE STUDY *(continued from page 744)*

Initial screening tests left the physician with no clear explanation for the thrombotic events. Several years later, when new tests became available, Andrea, her mother, and two sisters were tested for the factor V Leiden mutation and prothrombin mutation 20210. Results follow:

	Mother	Andrea	Sister 1	Sister 2
FVL mutation	N	Heterozygous	N	N
20210 mutation	Heterozygous	Heterozygous	Heterozygous	Heterozygous

3. Why is Andrea at greater risk for a thrombotic event than her mother or her two sisters?

▶ ANTICOAGULANT THERAPY

The main objective of anticoagulant therapy is to treat or prevent thrombosis. Arterial thrombosis is often caused by the interaction of platelets and vessel wall atherosclerotic plaques and can be treated with antiplatelet drugs. **Thrombolytic therapy** can be useful in treating an acute arterial thrombosis because rapid clot lysis and restoration of blood flow minimize permanent tissue damage. The role of anticoagulant therapy in the treatment of arterial thrombosis is controversial.

Venous thrombosis is often associated with abnormalities in the plasma coagulation system. An acute DVT has historically been treated with heparin for several days followed by oral anticoagulant therapy for 3–6 months. Recently, **low molecular weight heparin (LMWH)** has been found to produce the best results with the lowest risks of adverse complications for many patients with thrombosis.[102]

HEPARIN

Heparin is a heterogeneous group of molecules of sulfated glycosaminoglycans that bind to AT, resulting in rapid inhibition of serine proteases of the coagulation pathway. When administered parenterally, intravenously, or subcutaneously (heparin is not absorbed by the gastrointestinal tract), it produces a potent anticoagulant effect. Heparin does not have a direct effect on blood coagulation but facilitates AT's ability to neutralize serine proteases.

Mechanism of Action

Heparin for therapeutic use is usually extracted from porcine intestinal mucosa or bovine lung. The standard (unfractionated) heparin preparations (UFH) are heterogeneous mixtures of molecules with a mean molecular weight of 12,000 Da (range 5,000–30,000 Da). LMWH preparations (mean molecular weight of 4,500–5,000 Da) are prepared from standard heparin by chemical or enzymatic depolymerization of UFH.

Whereas UFH catalyzes AT inhibition of thrombin, F-Xa and F-IXa, LMWH's major anticoagulant effect is to catalyze the interaction between AT and F-Xa. By inactivating thrombin, heparin prevents fibrin formation, inhibits thrombin-catalyzed activation of F-V and F-VIII, and inhibits thrombin activation of platelets.

The actions of two coagulation inhibitors are accelerated by heparin: AT and HC II. At therapeutic doses of heparin (0.2–0.4 U/mL), F-IXa, F-Xa, and thrombin are inhibited almost exclusively by AT (which has a greater affinity for heparin than does HC II). In the presence of higher concentrations of heparin (or in the presence of dermatan sulfate), thrombin is inhibited primarily by HC II.[103]

Dosage Considerations

The dose of heparin required to produce a therapeutic effect varies from patient to patient because of differences in the plasma concentrations of various heparin-binding proteins (platelet factor 4, histidine-rich glycoprotein, fibronectin, VWF). These proteins bind to and neutralize heparin in the circulation. In some patients, larger doses than normal of heparin are required to achieve a therapeutic effect. The majority of these heparin-resistant patients have high levels of F-VIII and heparin-binding proteins (which are acute phase reactants) in their plasma. Patients with inherited AT deficiency (with AT levels of 40–60% of normal) respond normally to heparin therapy. However, individuals with acquired or inherited AT levels of <25% of normal can be resistant to the anticoagulant effects of heparin.

LMWH is being used with increasing frequency because of its convenience and more reliable pharmacokinetics.[103] The pharmacokinetic profile of UFH varies widely among individuals as a result of binding of heparin to plasma proteins. LMWH does not bind "heparin-binding proteins" in the plasma and thus has a more predictable dose-response profile, nor does it require routine laboratory monitoring. LMWH has a longer half-life and a more predictable anticoagulant effect and is less likely to cause heparin-induced thrombocytopenia and osteoporosis.

Laboratory Monitoring

Several different laboratory tests can be used to determine proper heparin dosage. Individuals' response to heparin varies, so there is no standard dose that provides protection from clotting while preventing adverse side effects. Therapy with standard heparin is usually monitored with a global test of coagulation, such as the activated clotting time (ACT) or the APTT. The PT is not sensitive to heparin and thus is not useful. Usually the heparin dose is adjusted so the APTT is 1.5–2.5 times the patient's baseline value before treatment.[104] Because the sensitivities of APTT reagents and instruments vary widely, each clinical laboratory should determine its own heparin therapeutic range.

LMWH does not produce a predictable prolongation of the APTT at therapeutic doses, so if laboratory monitoring is required, an anti-Xa-based assay using an LMWH standard should be performed.

Complications

Heparin is an effective agent for treating and preventing VTE, but it can have adverse side effects. Excessive bleeding is the most common toxic effect of (high-dose) heparin therapy and has been reported in up to 30% of patients (although fatal bleeding occurred in <0.5% of patients).[103] HIT is suspected when the platelet count falls to <150 × 10^9/L (or platelet count decreases by 50% in patients with preexisting thrombocytopenia). HIT occurs in ~3 % of patients receiving standard heparin but occurs less frequently in patients receiving LMWH (see previous discussion of HIT). Osteoporosis, or bone loss, is sometimes seen with long-term (one month or more) standard heparin therapy. In contrast to warfarin, heparin does not cross the placenta and has not been associated with fetal malformations. Therefore, it is the anticoagulant of choice for prophylaxis and treatment of VTE during pregnancy. In cases of heparin overdose resulting in excessive anticoagulation or bleeding, protamine sulfate can be given to neutralize and reverse the anticoagulant effect of heparin.

In the event that a patient develops HIT or is resistant to heparin, alternate anticoagulants can be used. These include direct anti-Xa inhibitors (fondaparinux and idraparinux) and direct thrombin inhibitors not requiring heparin (argatroban, hirudin, and bivalirudin).[105]

ORAL ANTICOAGULANTS

Oral anticoagulants have been used to treat acute DVT and PE since the 1940s. The coumadin drugs (either sodium warfarin or dicoumarol) are vitamin K antagonists that inhibit coagulation by interfering with vitamin K's action in the liver. Coumadin inhibits hepatic carboxylation of the vitamin K-dependent proteins, resulting in the release of nonfunctional (incompletely γ-carboxylated) molecules to the plasma. These proteins have reduced functional activity relative to their antigenic levels.

Mechanism of Action

Coumadin blocks the epoxide reductase enzyme that converts vitamin K epoxide back to the reduced form of vitamin K, which is the form required as a cofactor for the carboxylation reaction (Figure 30-3). The anticoagulant effect of coumadin depends on the reduced synthesis of biologically active vitamin K-dependent proteins and the normal clearance from the circulation of fully active proteins synthesized before the introduction of the drug. Coumadin inhibits γ-carboxylation of newly synthesized proteins but does not affect the plasma half-life of already circulating proteins. The anticoagulant effect of coumadin (the decrease in plasma activity of the vitamin K-dependent proteins) lags behind the point at which optimal plasma coumadin concentration is reached. The disappearance of biologically active, fully γ-carboxylated factors is determined by the half-life of each. F-VII activity disappears most rapidly ($T_{1/2}\sim6$ hours), F-X and F-IX follow ($T_{1/2}\sim24$ hours), and prothrombin disappears at the slowest rate because of its longer half-life ($T_{1/2}\sim72$ hours).[104] Thus, coumadin does not produce instantaneous anticoagulation but must be administered for 4–5 days before therapeutic anticoagulation is achieved. Coumadin is administered orally, is nearly completely absorbed, and circulates in the blood bound to albumin (97%). Only free coumadin is biologically active. Its plasma half-life is ~44 hours.

Dosage Considerations

Patients who have had a thrombotic incident are normally treated with heparin during the initial phase of anticoagulation because it produces an immediate anticoagulant effect. Because coumadin's full anticoagulant action is achieved only after 4–5 days, coumadin and heparin are given simultaneously during this time. Subsequently, when oral anticoagulation has been achieved, heparin can be discontinued. Coumadin is usually the therapy of choice for chronic anticoagulation to prevent the recurrence of thromboembolic disease. After the treatment of acute TE (DVT or PE), patients are routinely maintained on coumadin for 3–6 months.

Genetic factors can influence coumadin's anticoagulant effect.[105] Coumadin is a racemic mixture of two isomers, the R and S forms that are found in approximately equal proportions. However the S form is five times more potent, and the two forms are cleared by different pathways in the liver. Cytochrome P-450 is the hepatic enzyme responsible for the oxidative metabolism of the S-isomer of coumadin. Mutations of *CYP2C9*, the gene coding for cytochrome P-450, have been associated with hereditary resistance to coumadin resulting from enhanced affinity of the receptor for the drug and accelerated clearance.[105] Patients with genetic coumadin resistance require doses 5- to 20-fold higher than average to achieve an anticoagulant effect. Molecular testing can identify hereditary coumadin resistance.

Laboratory Monitoring

The PT is routinely used to monitor oral anticoagulation. The therapeutic coumadin dosage varies among individuals, and monitoring the anticoagulant effect can be difficult. A major problem has been a variation in the potency of thromboplastins used by different manufacturers. The patient's PT was usually reported as the clotting time in seconds and was compared with the PT of a normal plasma sample. The introduction of a reference standard for thromboplastins by the World Health Organization (ISI—International Sensitivity Index) and the use of the International Normalized Ratio (INR) have reduced the interlaboratory and interhospital variability in monitoring oral anticoagulants (∞ Chapter 40).

Complications

Bleeding complications are observed in 10–20% of patients treated with coumadin; about 50% of these complications occur when the therapeutic range of the PT has been exceeded, but 50% occur despite a PT within the therapeutic range. Although bleeding is usually mild, severe and life-threatening bleeding can occur. Thus, patients receiving oral anticoagulation must be carefully monitored. During the initiation of therapy, PT measurements can be required 2 or 3 times a week; once stabilized, patients generally require a PT every 3 or 4 weeks.[104] The antidote for coumadin overdose is administration of vitamin K. Coumadin crosses the placenta and has been associated with fetal abnormalities; therefore, its use is contraindicated during pregnancy.

THROMBOLYTIC THERAPY

Thrombolytic therapy is a clinical approach to TE disease with the goal of re-establishing vascular perfusion. All currently used thrombolytic agents are plasminogen activators (PA) used to lyse thrombi in vivo. Clinical trials assessing efficacy have been conducted for DVT, PE, peripheral arterial occlusion, acute myocardial infarction (MI), and acute ischemic stroke. The potential clinical benefit of thrombolytic treatment for acute thrombosis is in part determined by the time frame in which treatment should be initiated.[106] For MI or cerebral thromboses, treatment should be started within 4 and 3 hours, respectively, whereas treatment should be initiated for PE within 48 hours. Thrombolytic therapy for DVT maintains efficacy if treatment is initiated within 7 days.

Mechanism of Action

All of the PAs are capable of inducing plasmin lysis of fibrin within a thrombus and are accompanied by a variable degree of plasma fibrinogenolysis (the lytic state). Under normal physiologic conditions, plasminogen and PAs interact when bound to fibrin in the thrombus. Fibrin facilitates the conversion of plasminogen to plasmin because PAI-1 and α_2-antiplasmin (AP) do not efficiently inhibit fibrin-bound PA and plasmin, respectively. Under physiologic conditions, systemic lysis of fibrinogen does not occur because tPA and plasmin are efficiently inhibited by PAI-1 and AP in the circulation. With administration of therapeutic dosages of PA, virtually all of the plasma plasminogen is converted to plasmin, overwhelming the neutralizing capacity of AP and leading to some degree of fibrinogenolysis.

Dosage Considerations

The Food and Drug Administration has approved six plasminogen activators: streptokinase/SK, urokinase/UK, alteplase/tPA, anistreplase, reteplase, and tenecteplase).[106] UK currently is not available in the United States, and anistreplase is rarely used. The major distinctions among the agents relate to their antigenicity, half-life, potential for inducing a lytic state, and hemorrhagic potential. Those PAs derived from a human protein (UK, tPA, alteplase, tenecteplase, and reteplase) are essentially nonantigenic whereas those from a bacterial species can induce antibody formation. The agents' half-life varies from 5 minutes for tPA to 20 minutes for SK to 70 minutes for anistreplase. Several new PAs are in various stages of development or clinical trials. The continued search for new PA variants seeks to develop new agents with greater activity, a longer half-life, or a reduced lytic state.

Laboratory Monitoring

The *lytic state* is due to the systemic conversion of plasminogen to plasmin by circulating PA and the effects of plasmin on components of the circulating blood. Although a number of plasma proteins are involved, the identification of the lytic state is usually a demonstration of a decrease in plasma fibrinogen.[106] This increased degradation of fibrinogen is detected by a prolonged thrombin time test and increased fibrinogen degradation products (FDPs). Other plasma proteins including F-V and F-VIII are also degraded by plasmin. Other potential laboratory tests to monitor the lytic state include a shortened euglobulin lysis time, a quantitative decrease in circulating plasminogen and α_2-antiplasmin, and the generation of plasmin-antiplasmin complexes (P-AP). Free circulating plasmin can be demonstrated using chromogenic assays. Free plasmin also affects platelet function by decreasing aggregation induced by various platelet agonists and by cleaving the platelet membrane receptor for VWF. The lytic state induces a hypocoagulable state due to a combination of decreased clottable fibrinogen and other procoagulant proteins, the generation of FDPs (which inhibit coagulability), and platelet hyporeactivity.[106]

PA dosage regimens are standardized; thus, monitoring thrombolytic therapy is necessary only to document that a lytic state has indeed been achieved.[106] The thrombin time (TT) is sometimes used to monitor fibrinolytic therapy. A baseline TT should be determined and another performed at 3–4 hours after starting therapy. If a lytic state is induced, the TT should become prolonged due to the increased fibrin(ogen) degradation products and decreased fibrinogen level. FDP or D-dimer assays can be used to determine whether the thrombus is lysing.

Complications

The degradation of fibrin produces the beneficial effect of reducing the size of the thrombus (thrombolysis). However, a potential complicating effect can be the lysis of hemostatic plugs and resultant bleeding. Blood hypocoagulability can compound the bleeding tendency due to fibrinogenolysis and platelet dysfunction caused by the increased lytic state. The patient's response to PA therapy is inadequate if the thrombosed vessel does not manifest full reperfusion or if reocclusion quickly follows initial success. Thus, adjunctive treatment with antithrombin and antiplatelet agents is often added to thrombolytic therapy to minimize early reocclusive events.

ANTIPLATELET THERAPY

Various antiplatelet agents are available to reduce or block platelet responsiveness and activation. As with anticoagulant therapy, antiplatelet therapy includes the use of both oral and intravenous agents. Laboratory monitoring generally is not necessary with antiplatelet agents except for the need to monitor platelet counts with some of the drugs that cause thrombocytopenia in a small number of patients.

Aspirin is probably the most common drug used as an antithrombotic/antiplatelet agent in managing arterial thrombosis. Although it has been used for more than a century as an analgesic and antipyretic, it has been used as an antithrombotic only since the 1950s.[100] Aspirin blocks prostaglandin synthesis (TXA_2) in platelets by permanently and irreversibly inhibiting cyclooxygenase (COX-1 enzyme) in them. Aspirin accomplishes this by acetylating serine 520 in human platelet COX-1, blocking the enzyme's ability to interact with its substrate arachidonic acid. As little as a single "baby aspirin" (~30 mg) per day is used as prophylaxis for stroke (far below the dosage used for pain and fever).[101] The unique sensitivity of platelets to aspirin's therapeutic effect is due to the fact that platelets are cytoplasmic fragments from megakaryocytes and lack a nucleus. As a result, the platelet cannot replace its aspirin-acetylated, permanently inhibited COX-1 by synthesis of new proteins and continues to circulate for the rest of its life span in an inactive/inactivatable state (~9–10 days). In spite of the fact that aspirin also inhibits COX-1 in endothelial cells, blocking PGI_2 (platelet inhibitor) production, it has a net antithrombotic effect because these nucleated cells simply synthesize new COX-1 to replace the aspirin-inhibited enzyme. Patients taking aspirin do not have a severe bleeding diathesis, and aspirin exerts only a modest effect on platelet function and bleeding times. The PG-TXA_2 pathway augments platelet aggregation to weak agonists but is not needed for platelet responsiveness to strong agonists such as ADP or thrombin.[107]

The nonsteroidal anti-inflammatory drugs (NSAIDs) excluding aspirin are competitive inhibitors of COX-1 (and COX-2) rather than irreversible inhibitors. Because their actions block enzyme function transiently, they are not generally used as antithrombotic agents alone but sometimes in conjunction with aspirin. NSAIDs include ibuprofen, fluriprofen, and sulfinpyrazone. However, because they do have an antiplatelet effect although transient, surgeons recommend that patients not take these drugs for 7–10 days prior to surgery (as with aspirin). Acetaminophen does not affect platelet function.

ADP receptor antagonists—ticlopidine and clopidogrel—are drugs that block a different platelet activation pathway than do aspirin and other NSAIDs. They modify the ADP receptor, blocking platelet $P2Y_{12}$ receptor activity.[107] Both drugs have been linked to causing TTP in a small number of patients. Ticlopidine is also associated with neutropenia and marrow suppression in a small number of patients (1–2%), which clopidogrel does not. Clopidrogrel also has a lower incidence of TTP and thus is generally the ADP receptor-antagonist drug of choice for most patients.

Dipyridamole inhibits phosphodiesterase, resulting in increased cAMP levels and inhibition of platelet activation. It has been used in patients for decades but has limited antithrombotic effectiveness when used alone. It is often combined with aspirin to improve effectiveness.

Intravenous antiplatelet agents include inhibitors of GP IIb/IIIa. The GPIIb/IIIa platelet membrane receptor interacts with fibrinogen and VWF during platelet activation and aggregation. In contrast to the previously discussed drugs, which block only one of multiple platelet activation pathways, the blockade of GPIIb/IIIa almost completely eliminates platelet function if given in sufficient dosages. *Abciximab (ReoPro)* has been used for a number of years although its use requires the platelet count to be monitored because it causes thrombocytopenia in 1–2% of treated patients. *Eptifibatide (Integrilin)* has also been used and is generally not associated with thrombocytopenia.

 ## Checkpoint! 4

Why should heparin therapy overlap initiation of oral anticoagulant therapy when treating a patient with an acute thrombosis?

SUMMARY

The human hemostatic system normally maintains a balance between procoagulant or thrombogenic factors and anticoagulant or fibrinolytic activity. If this delicate balance is disturbed, the result can be excessive bleeding or unwanted clotting. Arterial and/or venous thrombosis occurs when activation of blood coagulation exceeds the ability of the natural protective mechanisms (anticoagulants/inhibitors and the fibrinolytic system) to prevent or minimize fibrin formation. Clinical risk factors that predispose an individual to either arterial or venous thrombosis have been identified. *Thrombo-philia* refers to any disorder (inherited or acquired) with an increased tendency to venous thromboembolism. Familial thrombophilia generally results from three broad categories of hemostatic abnormalities: (1) accelerated fibrin formation (increased procoagulant activity or diminished natural inhibitor activity), (2) defective fibrinolysis (reduced profibrinolytic factors or increased fibrinolytic inhibitors), or (3) abnormal fibrin (dysfibrinogenemias). An inherited thrombophilic defect places an individual at risk for but does not inevitably lead to thrombosis. Thrombosis occurs in susceptible patients who have one or more genetic mutations when they are exposed to exogenous prothrombotic stimuli. The five most common and most clearly delineated hereditary abnormalities associated with thrombophilia are Factor V Leiden, prothrombin 20210, and decreased or defective antithrombin, PC, and PS.

Patients with a documented thrombotic event need to be carefully evaluated including a complete personal and family history. Any additional risk factors for thrombosis present at the time of the incident (e.g., surgery, pregnancy, stasis) should be assessed. If a positive family history exists, the thrombosis was spontaneous, or multiple thrombotic incidences occurred, a full diagnostic workup should be undertaken to ascertain, if possible, the etiology of the thrombotic event. The evaluation of many of the components that regulate hemostasis (procoagulant proteins, inhibitory proteins, and fibrinolytic regulators) requires both functional (activity) and quantitative (immunologic) assays because both qualitative and quantitative defects of these proteins occur. Definitive diagnosis of some inherited thrombophilic disorders requires molecular analysis of the inherited gene product. The presence of multiple inherited or acquired thrombophilic factors significantly increases the risk for thrombosis. Patients experiencing an acute thrombotic event can be treated with a thrombolytic agent (plasminogen activators), heparin or LMW heparin, or oral anticoagulants. Long-term anticoagulation usually utilizes oral anticoagulants. Antiplatelet therapy can be used to manage arterial thrombosis. These agents block platelet responsiveness and activation. The most common antiplatelet prophylaxis is aspirin. Individuals with inherited thrombophilia usually do not require prophylactic therapy unless an additional prothrombotic clinical risk factor exists (prolonged immobility, surgery, pregnancy, etc.).

REVIEW QUESTIONS

LEVEL I

1. A platelet fibrin mass that forms within a vessel is known as a(n): (Objective 1)
   a. thrombus
   b. embolism
   c. platelet plug
   d. clot

2. Rupture of plaque in an artery may result in: (Objective 4)
   a. formation of a white thrombi
   b. formation of a red thrombi
   c. hyperhomocysteinemia
   d. decreased fibrinolysis

LEVEL II

1. Which of the following clinical manifestations is more likely to be found in a person with an inherited thrombophilia than in a person with an acquired thrombophilia? (Objectives 2, 9)
   a. venous embolism at a young age
   b. absence of a family history of thrombosis
   c. presence of a pulmonary embolism
   d. myocardial infarction in a 50-year-old

REVIEW QUESTIONS (continued)

LEVEL I

3. A patient is diagnosed with DVT. Four days later, a thrombus is found in his lung. This is an example of: (Objectives 3, 5)
   a. a white thrombi
   b. local thrombosis
   c. a thromboembolus
   d. DIC

4. What type of laboratory test results for AT will a patient with a type I deficiency of AT have? (Objective 8)
   a. decreased antigenic and normal functional activity
   b. normal antigenic and normal functional activity
   c. normal antigenic and decreased functional activity
   d. decreased antigenic and decreased functional activity

5. An inherited abnormality in the factor V molecule that renders it resistant to inactivation by protein C is known as: (Objective 9)
   a. AT deficiency
   b. APCR
   c. DIC
   d. prothrombin G20210A

6. A deficiency or defect in protein C can lead to thrombosis due to: (Objective 7)
   a. inability to inactivate protein S
   b. increased platelet activation
   c. inability to neutralize thrombin
   d. inability to inactivate factors Va and VIIIa

7. Patients who receive unfractionated heparin as treatment for a thrombus should be monitored periodically for the complication of HIT. What laboratory test should be used to monitor the patient? (Objective 10)
   a. APTT
   b. PT
   c. thrombin time
   d. platelet count

8. Therapy with low molecular weight heparin is best monitored using what laboratory test? (Objectives 10, 11)
   a. PT
   b. APTT
   c. factor Xa assay
   d. platelet count

9. The best test to monitor coumadin therapy is the: (Objective 12)
   a. PT
   b. APTT
   c. factor Xa assay
   d. platelet count

LEVEL II

2. A patient with thrombophilia has a decreased functional and antigenic activity of protein C. What is the diagnosis? (Objective 3)
   a. APCR
   b. protein S deficiency
   c. type I PC deficiency
   d. type II PC deficiency

3. Why is following up an abnormal clotting assay for APCR with a molecular test recommended? (Objective 5)
   a. the clotting test is not sensitive or specific for APCR
   b. 10% of individuals with APCR do not have the FVL mutation
   c. the clotting test cannot be used for 6 months after a thrombotic episode
   d. the molecular test is inexpensive and more accurate

4. Why does a patient with a thrombotic incident receive both heparin and coumadin for 4–5 days after the incident? (Objective 10)
   a. Heparin is not effective as an anticoagulant without coumadin present.
   b. Coumadin requires heparin for its full anticoagulant effect.
   c. This gives the patient an initial bolus dose of anticoagulant.
   d. Coumadin takes this long to produce its full anticoagulant action.

5. The value of using the INR to report the PT is: (Objective 11)
   a. It reduces interlaboratory variability in monitoring oral anticoagulants.
   b. It can be used to monitor both heparin and coumadin therapy.
   c. Patients on coumadin therapy do not need to be tested as often.
   d. Patients' coumadin dosage does not need to be adjusted as frequently.

6. A patient with a myocardial infarction is admitted to the ER. The physician starts the patient on streptokinase. She calls the laboratory and wants you to suggest a test to ensure that a lytic state is induced by the therapy. What test will you suggest? (Objective 12)
   a. a baseline TT and TT after 3–4 hours of therapy
   b. fibrinogen, plasminogen, and plasmin assays
   c. a PT, APTT, and platelet count
   d. none because no available tests give this information

REVIEW QUESTIONS (continued)

LEVEL I

10. What physiologic protein's anticoagulant effect is accelerated by heparin? (Objective 6)
    a. AT
    b. protein C
    c. protein S
    d. lupus anticoagulant1

LEVEL II

7. A patient has hyperhomocysteinemia. What laboratory test(s) can be helpful in establishing the etiology of his disease? (Objective 6)
    a. APCR clotting assay
    b. AT and PS antigenic assays
    c. molecular tests for MTHFR and CBS
    d. molecular test for prothrombin G20210

8. Which of the following conditions is *not* associated with an increased tendency for thrombosis? (Objective 9)
    a. antiphospholipid antibody syndrome
    b. pregnancy
    c. malignancy
    d. factor VIII deficiency

9. A 30-year-old patient is diagnosed with DVT. This is his third episode of DVTs. He is currently hospitalized and receiving heparin therapy. The physician orders a thrombotic risk battery of tests. What is the most appropriate action that the laboratory should take? (Objective 1)
    a. call the physician and explain that testing will not be accurate during anticoagulant therapy and during the thrombotic episode
    b. perform the battery of tests in the thrombotic risk profile but note that results are not reliable
    c. perform a PT and an APTT and, if prolonged, refuse to do the testing
    d. call the physician and explain that this patient is not a candidate for thrombotic risk testing

10. A patient is on coumadin for treatment of DVT. He returns to the doctor with skin necrosis. What protein deficiency should be tested for after coumadin therapy is finished? (Objective 4)
    a. AT
    b. PC
    c. HC-II
    d. TPAI

www.pearsonhighered.com/mckenzie
Use this address to access the interactive Companion Website created for this textbook. Find additional information, tables and figures. Evaluate your command of the chapter information using case studies and critical thinking and multiple choice questions.

REFERENCES

1. Jackson E, Skerrett PJ, Ridker PM. Epidemiology of arterial thrombosis. In: Colman RW, Hirsh J, Marder VJ, Clowes AW, George JN, eds. *Hemostasis and Thrombosis: Basic Principles and Clinical Practice*, 4th ed. Philadelphia: Lippincott Williams & Wilkins; 2000:1179–96.

2. Ross T. The pathogenesis of atherosclerosis: A perspective for the 1990s. *Nature.* 1993;362:801–9.

3. Ridker PM, Glynn RJ, Henneker CH. C-reactive protein adds to the predictive value of total and HDL cholesterol in determining risk of first myocardial infarction. *Circulation.* 1998;97:2007–11.

4. Doyle DF, Turpic AG, Hirsh J et al. Adjusted subcutaneous heparin or continuous intravenous heparin in patients with acute deep vein thrombosis. A randomized trial. *Ann Intern Med.* 1987;107:441–45.

5. Kearon C, Salzman EW, Hirsh J. Epidemiology, pathogenesis, and natural history of venous thrombosis. In: Colman RW, Hirsh J, Marder VJ, Clowes AW, George JN, eds. *Hemostasis and Thrombosis: Basic Principles and Clinical Practice,* 4th ed. Philadelphia: Lippincott Williams & Wilkins; 2000:1153–77.

6. Hirsh J, Crowther MA. Venous thromboembolism. In: Hoffman R, Benz EJ, Shattil SJ, Furie B, Cohen HJ, Silberstein LE, P McGlave P, eds. *Hematology: Basic Principles and Procedures,* 3rd ed. New York: Churchill Livingstone; 2000:2074–89.

7. Pandolfi M, Robertson B, Isacson S, Nilsson IM. Fibrinolytic activity of human veins in arms and legs. *Thromb Diath Haemorrh.* 1968;20:247–56.

8. Jick H et al. Venous thromboembolic disorder and ABO blood type. A cooperative study. *Lancet.* 1969;1:539–42.

9. Wautrecht JC, Galle C, Motte S, Dereume DP, Dramaix M: The role of ABO blood groups in the incidence of deep vein thrombosis. *Thromb Haemost.* 1998;79:668–69.

10. Larsen TB, Johnsen SP, Gislum M, Moller CA, Larsen H, Sorensen HT. ABO blood groups and risk of venous thromboembolism during pregnancy. *J Thromb Haemost.* 2005;3:300–4.

11. Schleef M, Strobel E, Dick A, Frank J, Schramm W, Spannagl M. Relationship between ABO and secretor genotype with plasma levels of factor VIII and von Willebrand factor in thrombosis patients and control individuals. *Br J Haematol.* 2004;128:100–107.

12. Morelli VM, DeVisser MC, Vos HL, Bertina RM, Rosendaal FR. ABO blood group genotypes and the risk of venous thrombosis: Effect of factor V Leiden. *Thromb Haemost.* 2005;3:183–85.

13. Franchin M, Capra F, Targher G et al. Relationship between ABO blood group and von Willebrand levels: From biology to clinical implications. *Thrombosis Journal.* 2007;5:14–19.

14. Koster T, Blann AD, Briet E, Vandenbroucke JP, Rosendaal FR. Role of clotting factor VIII in effect of von Willebrand factor on occurrence of deep-vein thrombosis. *Lancet.* 1995;345:152–55.

15. Crowther MA, Ginsberg JS. Venous thromboembolism. In: Hoffman R, Benz EJ, Shattil SJ, Furie B, Cohen HJ, Silberstein LE, P McGlave P, eds. *Hematology: Basic Principles and Procedures,* 4th ed. New York: Churchill Livingstone; 2005:2225–40.

16. Lensing AWA, Hirsh J, Ginsberg JS, Buller HR. Diagnosis of venous thrombosis. In: Colman RW, Hirsh J, Marder VJ, Clowes AW, George JN, eds. *Hemostasis and Thrombosis: Basic Principles and Clinical Practice,* 4th ed. Philadelphia: Lippincott Williams & Wilkins; 2000:1277–1301.

17. Bounameaux H, DeMoerloose P, Perrier A, Reber G. Plasma measurement of D-dimer as a diagnostic aid in suspected venous thromboembolism: An overview. *Thromb Haemost.* 1994;71:1–6.

18. Wells PS, Brill-Edwards P, Stevens P et al. A novel and rapid whole-blood assay for D-dimer in patients with clinically suspected deep vein thrombosis. *Circulation.* 1995;91:2184–87.

19. Bick R, Fareed J. Current status of thrombosis: A multidisciplinary medical issue and major American health problem, beyond the year 2000. *Clin Appl Thromb Hemostasis.* 1997;Suppl 1:1–5.

20. Middeldorp S, Buller HR, Prins MH, Hirsh J. Approach to the thrombophilic patient. In: Colman RW, Hirsh J, Marder VJ, Clowes AW, George JN, eds. *Hemostasis and Thrombosis: Basic Principles and Clinical Practice,* 4th ed. Philadelphia: Lippincott Williams & Wilkins; 2000:1085–1100.

21. Schafer AI. Hypercoagulable states: Molecular genetics to clinical practice. *Lancet.* 1994;344:1739–42.

22. Marder VJ, Matei DE. Hereditary and acquired thrombophilic syndromes. In: Colman RW, Hirsh J, Marder VJ, Clowes AW, George JN, eds. *Hemostasis and Thrombosis: Basic Principles and Clinical Practice,* 4th ed. Philadelphia: Lippincott Williams & Wilkins; 2000:1243–75.

23. Egeberg O. Inherited antithrombin deficiency causing thrombophilia. *Thromb Diath Haemorrh* 1965;13:516.

24. Thaler E, Lechner K. Antithrombin III deficiency and thromboembolism. In: Prentice CRM, ed. *Clinics in Haematology,* vol 10. London: Saunders; 1981:369–90.

25. Bauer KA. Hypercoagulable states. In: Hoffman R, Benz EJ, Shattil SJ, Furie B, Cohen HJ, Silberstein LE, P McGlave P, eds. *Hematology: Basic Principles and Procedures,* 3rd ed. New York: Churchill Livingstone; 2000:2009–39.

26. Seligsohn U, Griffin JH. Hereditary thrombophilia. In: Lichtman MA, Beutler E, Kipps TJ et al., eds. *Williams Hematology,* 7th ed. New York: McGraw-Hill; 2006:1981–2007.

27. Vinazzer H. Hereditary and acquired antithrombin deficiency. *Semin Thromb Hemost.* 1999;25:257–63.

28. Esmon CT, Owen WG. Identification of an endothelial cell cofactor for thrombin-catalyzed activation of protein C. *Proc Natl Acad Sci.* 1981;78:2249–52.

29. Esmon CT. Protein C, protein S, and thrombomodulin. In: Colman RW, Hirsh J, Marder VJ, Clowes AW, George JN, eds. *Hemostasis and Thrombosis: Basic Principles and Clinical Practice,* 4th ed. Philadelphia: Lippincott Williams & Wilkins; 2000:335–53.

30. Nizzi F, Kaplan H. Protein C and S deficiency. *Semin Thromb Hemost.* 1999;25:265–72.

31. Griffin J, Evatt B, Zimmerman T, et al. Deficiency of protein C in congenital thrombotic disease. *J Clin Invest.* 1981;68:1370–73.

32. Casella JF, Lewis JH, Bontempo FA et al. Successful treatment of homozygous protein C deficiency by hepatic transplantation. *Lancet.* 1988;1:435–38.

33. McGehee WG, Klotz TA, Epstein P et al. Coumarin necrosis associated with hereditary protein C deficiency. *Ann Int Med.* 1984;101:59–60.

34. Aiach M, Emmerich J. Thrombophilia Genetics. In: Colman RW, Hirsh J, Marder VJ, Clowes AW, George JN, eds. *Hemostasis and Thrombosis: Basic Principles and Clinical Practice,* 5th ed. Philadelphia: Lippincott Williams & Wilkins; 2006:779–93.

35. Comp PC, Nixon RR, Cooper MR, Esmon CT. Familial protein S deficiency is associated with recurrent thrombosis. *J Clin Invest.* 1984;74:2082–88.

36. Schwarz HP, Muntean W, Watzke H et al. Low total protein S antigen but high protein S activity due to decreased C4B-binding protein in neonates. *Blood.* 1988;71:562–65.

37. Bauer KA. Hypercoagulable states. In: Hoffman R, Benz EJ, Shattil SJ, Furie B, Cohen HJ, Silberstein LE, P McGlave P, eds. *Hematology: Basic Principles and Procedures,* 4th ed. New York: Churchill Livingstone; 2005:2197–224.

38. Brunet D, Barthet MC, Morange PE et al. Protein S deficiency: Different biological phenotypes according to the assays used. *Thromb Haemost.* 1998;79:446–47.

39. Dahlbäck B, Carlsson M, Svensson P. Familial thrombophilia due to a previously unrecognized mechanism characterized by poor anticoagulant response to activated protein C. *Proc Natl Acad Sci USA.* 1993;90:1004–8.

40. Dahlbäck B. Activated protein C resistance and thrombosis: Molecular mechanisms of hypercoagulable state due to FVR506Q mutation. *Semin Thromb Hemost.* 1999;25:273–89.

41. Bernard F, Faioni E, Castoldi E et al. A factor V genetic component differing from factor VR506Q contributes to the activated protein C resistance phenotype. *Blood.* 1997;90:1552–57.

42. Williamson D, Brown K, Luddington R et al. Factor V Cambridge: A new mutation (Arg 306 → Thr) associated with resistance to activated protein C. *Blood.* 1998;91:1140–44.

43. Chan WP, Lee CK, Kwong YL et al. A novel mutation of Arg 306 of factor V gene in Hong Kong Chinese. *Blood.* 1998;91:1135–39.

44. Rees DC, Cox M, Clegg JB. World distribution of factor V Leiden. *Lancet.* 1995;346:1133–34.

45. Poort S, Rosendaal F, Reitsma P et al. A common genetic variation in the 3′-untranslated region of the prothrombin gene is associated with elevated plasma prothrombin levels and an increase in venous thrombosis. *Blood.* 1996;88:3698–703.

46. Markis M, Preston FE, Beauchamp NJ et al. Co-inheritance of the 20210 allele of the prothrombin gene increases the risk of thrombosis in subjects with familial thrombophilia. *Thromb Haemost.* 1997; 78:1426–29.

47. Villa P, Azner J, Vaya A et al. Hereditary homozygous heparin cofactor II deficiency and the risk of developing venous thrombosis. *Thromb Haemost.* 1999;82:1011–14.

48. Bernardi F, Legnani C, Micheletti F et al. A heparin cofactor II mutation (HCII Rimini) combined with factor V Leiden or type I protein C deficiency in two unrelated thrombophilic subjects. *Thromb Haemost.* 1996;76:505–9.

49. Rapaport SI. The extrinsic pathway inhibitor: A regulator of tissue factor-dependent blood coaglation. *Thromb Haemost.* 1991;66:6–15.

50. Broze GJ Jr. Tissue factor pathway inhibitor. *Thromb Haemost.* 1995; 74:90–93.

51. Sandset PM. Tissue factor pathway inhibitor (TFPI): An update. *Haemostasis.* 1996;26:154–65.

52. Kleesiek K, Schmidt M, Gotting C et al. The 536C → T transition in the human tissue factor pathway inhibitor (TFPI) gene is statistically associated with a higher risk for venous thrombosis. *Thromb Haemost.* 1999;82:1–5.

53. McCully KS. Vascular pathology of homocysteinemia: Implications for the pathogenesis of arteriosclerosis. *Am J Pathol.* 1969;56: 111–28.

54. Guba S, Fonseca V, Fink L. Hyperhomocysteinemia and thrombosis. *Semin Thromb Hemost.* 1999;253:291–309.

55. Hankey GJ, Eikelboom JW. Homocysteine and vascular disease. *Lancet.* 1999;354:407–13.

56. Frosst P, Blom HJ, Milos R et al. A candidate genetic risk factor for vascular disease: A common mutation in methylenetetrahydrofolate reductase. *Nat Genet.* 1995;10:111–13.

57. Mossesson MW. Hereditary fibrinogen abnormalities. In: Lichtman MA, Beutler E, Kipps TJ et al., eds. *Williams Hematology,* 7th ed. New York: McGraw-Hill; 2006:1909–27.

58. Mosesson M. Dysfibrinogenemia and thrombosis. *Semin Thromb Hemost.* 1999;25:311–19.

59. Haverkate F, Samama M. Familial dysfibrinogenemia and thrombophilia: Report on a study of the SCC subcommittee on fibrinogen. *Thromb Haemost.* 1995;73:151–61.

60. Koster T, Blann AD, Briet E et al. Role of clotting factor VIII in effect of von Willebrand factor on occurance of deep vein thrombosis. *Lancet.* 1995;345:152–55.

61. Kamphuisen PW, Eikenboom JC, Bertina RM. Elevated factor VIII levels and the risk of thrombosis. *Arterioscler Thromb Vasc Biol.* 2001;21:731–38.

62. Kraaijenhagen RA, Pieternella S, Anker PS, Koopman MMW et al. High plasma concentration of factor VIIIc is a major risk factor for venous thromboembolism. *Thromb Haemost.* 2000;83:5–9.

63. Kamphuisen PW, Eikenboom JC, Rosendaal FR, Bertina RM. High factor VIII antigen levels increase the risk of venous thrombosis but are not associated with polymorphisms in the von Willebrand factor and factor VIII gene. *Br J Haematol.* 2001;115:156–58.

64. Meade TW, Mellows S, Brozovic M et al. Haemostatic function and ischaemic heart disease: Principal results of the Northwick Park Heart Study. *Lancet.* 1986;2:533–37.

65. Tripodi A. Levels of coagulation factors and venous thromboembolism. *Haematologica.* 2003;88:705–11.

66. van Hylckama VA, van der Linden IK, Bertina RM, Rosendaal FR. High levels of factor IX increase the risk of venous thrombosis. *Blood.* 2000;95:3678–82.

67. Meijers JC, Tekelenburg WL, Bouma BN et al. High levels of coagulation factor XI as a risk factor for venous thrombosis. *N Engl J Med.* 2000;342:696–701.

68. Goodnough LT, Saito H, Ratnoff OD. Thrombosis or myocardial infarction in congenital clotting factor abnormalities and chronic thrombocytopenias: A report of 21 patients and a review of 50 previously reported cases. *Medicine.* 1983;62:248–55.

69. Seligsohn U, Griffin JH. Hereditary thrombophilia. In: Lichtman MA, Beutler E, Kipps TJ et al., eds. *Williams Hematology,* 7th ed. New York: McGraw-Hill; 2006:1981–2007.

70. Hong J, Kwaan H. Hereditary defects in fibrinolysis associated with thrombosis. *Semin Thromb Hemost.* 1999;253:321–31.

71. Aoki N, Moroi M, Sakata Y et al. Abnormal plasminogen: A hereditary molecular abnormality found in a patient with recurrent thrombosis. *J Clin Invest.* 1978;61:1186–95.

72. Lottenberg R, Dolly FR, Kitchens CS. Recurring thromboembolic disease and pulmonary hypertension associated with severe hypoplasminogenemia. *Am J Hematol.* 1985;19:181–93.

73. Johansson L, Hedner U, Nilsson I. A family with thromboembolic disease associated with deficient fibrinolytic activity in vessel wall. *Acta Med Scand.* 1978;203:477–80.

74. Jorgensen M, Mortensen JZ, Madsen AG et al. A family with reduced plasminogen activator activity in blood associated with recurrent venous thrombosis. *Scand J Haematol.* 1982;29:217–23.

75. Stead NW, Bauer KA, Kinney TR et al. Venous thrombosis in a family with defective release of vascular plasminogen activator and elevated plasma factor VIII/von Willebrand factor. *Am J Med.* 1983; 74:33–39.

76. Bolan CD, Krishnamurti C, Tang DB et al. Association of protein S deficiency with thrombosis in a kindred with elevated levels of plasminogen activator inhibitor-1. *Ann Intern Med.* 1993;119:779–85.

77. Zoller B, Dahlback B. Protein S deficiency in a large family with thrombophilia previously characterized as having an inherited fibrinolytic defect. *Thromb Haemost.* 1993;69:1256 (Abstract).

78. Wiman B. The fibrinolytic enzyme system: Basic principles and links to venous and arterial thrombosis. *Hematol Oncol Clin North Am.* 2000;14:325–38.

79. Fareed J, Hoppensteadt D, Jeske W et al. Acquired defects of fibrinolysis associated with thrombosis. *Semin Thromb Hemost.* 1999;25: 367–74.

80. Rand JH, Senzel L. Antiphospholipid antibodies and the antiphospholipid syndrome. In: Colman RW, Hirsh J, Marder VJ, Clowes AW, George JN, eds. *Hemostasis and Thrombosis: Basic Principles and Clinical Practice,* 5th ed. Philadelphia: Lippincott Williams & Wilkins; 2006:1621–36.

81. Moore JE, Mohr CF. Biologically false positive serological tests for syphilis: Type, incidence, and cause. *J Am Med Assoc.* 1952;150: 467–73.

82. Conley CL, Hartmann RC. A hemorrhagic disorder caused by circulating anticoagulant in patients with disseminated lupus erythematosis. *J Clin Invest.* 1952;31:621.

83. Court EL. Lupus anticoagulants: Pathogenesis and laboratory diagnosis. *Brit J Biomed Sci.* 1997;54:287–98.

84. Rand JH, Senzel L. The antiphospholipid syndrome. In: Lichtman MA, Beutler E, Kipps TJ et al., eds. *Williams Hematology,* 7th ed. New York: McGraw-Hill, 2006:2009–29.

85. Brandt JT, Triplett DA, Alving B, Scharrer I. Criteria for the diagnosis of lupus anticoagulants: An update. On behalf of the Subcommittee on Lupus Anticoagulant/antiphospholipid antibody of the Scientific and Standardization Committee of the ISTH. *Thromb Haemost.* 1995;74:1185–90.

86. Warkentin TE, Chong BH, Greinacher A. Heparin-induced thrombocytopenia: Towards consensus. *Thromb Haemost.* 1998;79:1–7.

87. Warkentin TE. Heparin-induced thrombocytopenia: A ten-year retrospective. *Annu Rev Med.* 1999;50:129–47.

88. Warkentin TE, Levine MN, Hirsh J et al. Heparin-induced thrombocytopenia in patients treated with low-molecular-weight heparin or unfractionated heparin. *N Engl J Med.* 1995;332:1330–35.

89. Warkentin TE, Kelton JG. Temporal aspects of heparin-induced thrombocytopenia. *N Engl J Med.* 2001;344:1286–92.

90. Moschowitz E. Hyaline thrombosis of the terminal arterioles and capillaries: A hitherto undescribed disease. *Proc NY Pathol Soc.* 1924; 24:21–24.

91. Amorosi EL, Ultmann JE. Thrombotic thrombocytopenic purpura: Report of 16 cases and review of the literature. *Medicine.* 1966; 45:139–60.

92. George JN. Thrombotic thrombocytopenic purpura. *N Engl J Med.* 2006;354:1927–35.

93. George JN, Vesely SK, Lammle B. Thrombotic thrombocytopenic purpura-hemolytic uremic syndrome. In: Colman RW, Marder VJ, Clowes AW et al, *Hemostasis and Thrombosis, Basic Principles and Clinical Practice,* 5th ed. Philadelphia: Lippincott Williams & Wilkins; 2006:1613–20.

94. Moake JL, Rudy CK, Troll JH et al. Unusually large plasma factor VIII: von Willebrand factor multimers in chronic relapsing thrombotic thrombocytopenic purpura. *N Eng J Med.* 1982;307:1432–35.

95. Furlan M, Robles R, Lammle B. Partial purification and characterization of a protease from human plasma cleaving von Willebrand factor to fragments produced by in vivo proteolysis. *Blood.* 1996; 878:4223–34.

96. Furlan M, Robles R, Solenthaler M et al. Deficient activity of von Willebrand factor-cleaving protease in chronic relapsing thrombotic thrombocytopenic purpura. *Blood.* 1997;89:3097–103.

97. Levy GG, Nichols WC, Lian EC et al. Mutations in a member of the ADAMTS gene family cause thrombotic thrombocytopenic purpura. *Nature.* 2001;413:488–94.

98. Tsai HM, Lian EC. Antibodies to von Willebrand factor-cleaving protease in acute thrombotic thrombocytopenic purpura. *N Engl J Med.* 1998;339:1585–94.

99. Sadler JE, Poncz M. Antibody-mediated thrombotic disorders: Idiopathic thrombotic thrombocytopenic purpura and heparin-induced thrombocytopenia. In: Lichtman MA, Beutler E, Kipps T et al, eds. *Williams Hematology,* 7th ed. New York: McGraw-Hill; 2006:2031–54.

100. Tarr PI, Gordon CA, Chandler WL. Shiga-toxin-producing Escherichia coli and haemolytic uraemic syndrome. *Lancet.* 2005;365: 1073–86.

101. Green KB, Silverstein RL. Hypercoagulability in cancer. *Hematol Oncol Clin North Am.* 1996;10:499–530.

102. Baker W, Bick R. Treatment of hereditary and acquired thrombophilic disorders. *Semin Thromb Hemost.* 1999;253:387–406.

103. Crowther MA, Ginsberg JS, Tollefsen DM, Blinder MA. Heparin. In: Hoffman R, Benz EJ, Shattil SJ, Furie B, Cohen HJ, Silberstein LE, P McGlave P, eds. *Hematology: Basic Principles and Procedures,* 3rd ed. New York: Churchill Livingstone; 2000:246–56.

104. Furie B. Oral anticoagulant therapy. In: Hoffman R, Benz EJ, Shattil SJ, Furie B, Cohen HJ, Silberstein LE, P McGlave P, eds. *Hematology: Basic Principles and Procedures,* 3rd ed. New York: Churchill Livingstone; 2000:2040–46.

105. Tran HAM, Ginsberg JS. Anticoagulant Therapy for major arterial and venous thromboembolism. In: Colman RW, Hirsh J, Marder VJ, Clowes AW, George JN, eds. *Hemostasis and Thrombosis: Basic Principles and Clinical Practice,* 5th ed. Philadelphia: Lippincott Williams & Wilkins; 2006:1673–88.

106. Marder VJ. Foundations of thrombolytic therapy. In: Colman RW, Hirsh J, Marder VJ, Clowes AW, George JN, eds. *Hemostasis and Thrombosis: Basic Principles and Clinical Practice,* 5th ed. Philadelphia: Lippincott Williams & Wilkins; 2006:1739–51.

107. Roth GJ. Antiplatelet therapy. In: Colman RW, Hirsh J, Marder VJ, Clowes AW, George JN, eds. *Hemostasis and Thrombosis: Basic Principles and Clinical Practice,* 5th ed. Philadelphia: Lippincott Williams & Wilkins; 2006:1725–37.

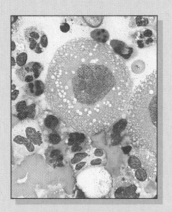

SECTION EIGHT
HEMATOLOGY PROCEDURES

34

Hematology Procedures

Cheryl Burns, M.S.
Aamir Ehsan, M.D.

■ OBJECTIVES—LEVEL I

At the end of this unit of study, the student should be able to:

1. Identify the three anticoagulants used in the hematology laboratory and give examples of laboratory tests that should be performed on blood anticoagulated with each.

2. Explain the mechanism of preventing coagulation for each anticoagulant.

3. Identify equipment and supplies required for phlebotomy.

4. Describe Occupational Safety and Health Administration (OSHA) standards related to phlebotomy.

5. List factors affecting the collection of a blood sample.

6. Determine sequence of draw of phlebotomy collection tubes and correlate the collection technique of a blood sample with potential problems in sample analysis.

7. Describe proper disposal of contaminated equipment and supplies.

8. Identify the component parts of a microscope and explain their functions.

9. Discuss the microscope's preventative maintenance procedures.

10. Describe the peripheral blood smear preparation methods.

11. Identify the characteristics of an optimally prepared peripheral blood smear.

12. Describe the Romanowsky-staining technique.

13. Recognize characteristics of a properly stained peripheral blood smear.

14. Discuss potential causes of improperly stained peripheral blood smears.

15. List the components included in a complete peripheral blood smear examination.

16. Correlate erythrocyte indices, leukocyte count, and platelet count with peripheral blood smear observations.

17. Determine the corrected leukocyte count based on the presence of nucleated erythrocytes.

18. State the principle of each test: cell enumeration by hemacytometer, hemoglobin concentration, hematocrit, erythrocyte sedimentation rate, reticulocyte count, solubility test for hemoglobin S, hemoglobin electrophoresis, acid elution for hemoglobin F, osmotic fragility.

19. For each test listed in Objective 18, describe the procedure, identify potential sources of error, determine appropriateness of use including reflex testing, calculate and interpret results, and explain the clinical significance of the test.

20. Calculate the erythrocyte indices.

21. Correlate erythrocyte indices with CBC data and peripheral blood smear examination.

22. Calculate the reticulocyte count.

23. Identify reference ranges for each test in terms of gender and age.

■ OBJECTIVES—LEVEL II

At the end of this unit of study, the student should be able to:

1. Describe factors that influence brightfield microscopy.

2. Explain the principle of phase contrast microscopy.

3. Choose corrective actions for an improperly prepared or stained peripheral blood smear.

4. Detect abnormalities on peripheral blood smear examination, assess how they can alter cell count results (i.e., presence of nucleated erythrocytes or platelet satellitism), and recommend corrective action to ensure valid results.

5. State the principle of each of the following tests: quantitation of hemoglobin F and hemoglobin A_2, heat denaturation test for unstable hemoglobin, Heinz body stain, sugar-water screening test, Donath-Landsteiner test for PCH, erythropoietin assay, soluble transferrin receptor, and cytochemical stains (e.g., myeloperoxidase).

6. For each test listed in Objective 5, describe the procedure, identify potential sources of error, determine appropriateness of use including reflex testing, interpret results, and explain the clinical significance of the test.

7. For each test discussed in this chapter, correlate abnormal values with clinical conditions.

8. Select the cytochemical stain appropriate for confirming cell lineage and diagnosis in hematopoietic neoplasms.

KEY TERMS

Acute phase reactant
Anticoagulant
Anemia
Beer-Lambert's law
Biphasic antibody
Cold agglutinin disease
Column chromatography
Coverglass smear
Densitometer
Edematous
Hemoconcentration
Isoelectric focusing
Isopropanol precipitation
Leukocyte alkaline phosphatase (LAP)
Mean cell hemoglobin (MCH)
Mean cell hemoglobin concentration (MCHC)
Mean cell volume (MCV)

Multiple myeloma
Optimal counting area
Platelet clump
Platelet satellitism
Polycythemia
Reference interval
Refractive index
Romanowsky-type stain
Rouleaux
Rule of three
Smudge cell
Supernatant
Supravital stain
Tartrate-resistant acid phosphatase (TRAP)
Unique identification number
Wedge smear

The information in this chapter builds on concepts learned in other chapters. To maximize your learning experience, you should review and thoroughly understand these concepts before starting this unit of study.

Level I

▶ Describe normal leukopoiesis. (Chapter 7)

▶ Describe normal erythropoiesis. (Chapter 5)

▶ Summarize the basics of hemoglobin synthesis and structure. (Chapter 6)

▶ Outline the classification systems for the anemias. (Chapter 8)

Level II

▶ Describe potential causes for changes in leukocyte concentrations. (Chapter 7)

▶ Describe potential causes for decreased erythrocyte concentrations. (Chapter 5)

▶ Recognize the erythrocytic morphologic changes associated with size, shape, inclusions, and patterns of distribution. (Chapters 5, 8)

▶ Recognize neutrophil and monocyte morphology and the reactive changes associated with lymphocytes. (Chapter 7)

▶ Recognize and describe the morphologic characteristics of the developing erythrocytes and leukocytes. (Chapters 5, 7)

▶ Recognize and describe normal bone marrow architecture. (Chapter 35)

▶ Describe the hemoglobinopathies including hemoglobin S and hemoglobin C. (Chapter 10)

▶ Compare and contrast alpha thalassemia, beta thalassemia, and hereditary persistance of fetal hemoglobin. (Chapter 11)

▶ Describe anemias characterized by membrane defects: including the pathophysiology of hereditary spherocytosis. (Chapter 15)

▶ Describe immune hemolytic anemias including hemolytic disease of the newborn, transfusion-induced hemolytic anemia, cold hemagglutinin disease, and paroxysmal nocturnal hemoglobinuria. (Chapter 17)

▶ Describe the anemias of disordered iron metabolism and heme synthesis including iron-deficiency anemia and anemia of chronic disease. (Chapter 9)

▶ Describe the etiology, pathophysiology, and classification of:
  ▶ Myeloproliferative disorders (Chapter 22)
  ▶ Acute myelogenous leukemia (Chapter 24)
  ▶ Acute lymphoblastic leukemia (Chapter 25)
  ▶ Lymphoid malignancies (Chapter 26)

▶ OVERVIEW

Hematology tests are some of the most frequently ordered laboratory tests. The results obtained from these laboratory procedures are utilized in the diagnosis of a variety of disorders including anemias, leukemias, infections, and inherited leukocyte disorders. The clinical laboratory professional must be able to perform these tests, verify results, solve problems related to erroneous results, correlate abnormalities with disease states, and suggest reflex tests when appropriate.

The two levels of testing in the hematology laboratory are routine and reflex. *Routine tests* such as the CBC, differential, and reticulocyte count are used as screening tests to determine the presence of a primary disease in the hematopoietic system or to identify hematologic changes that provide clues to the presence of nonhematologic diseases. Analysis of the results of these screening tests with the patient's clinical signs and symptoms help to determine whether further testing is necessary. Algorithms or critical pathways assist in the choice of follow-up testing (reflex testing) to abnormal screening test results. These reflex tests are used to definitively diagnose the patient's disease state. With a definitive diagnosis, the appropriate treatment plan can be implemented and monitored with additional laboratory procedures such as the reticulocyte count. The chapter begins with a discussion of the collection of the sample and care and use of the microscope. Next routine hematology tests are discussed, and the chapter concludes with a discussion of the laboratory procedures used in reflex testing. The principles, procedures, and results of the tests for specific clinical conditions are summarized. Detailed procedures for selected tests are provided on the Companion Website.

▶ SAMPLE COLLECTION: PHLEBOTOMY

The phlebotomy procedure is important to all laboratory testing. The sample's quality dictates the accuracy of its final result. All clinical laboratory professionals should have a thorough understanding of each sample collection technique. This section reviews the various aspects of phlebotomy or sample collection.

ANTICOAGULANTS

Most tests performed in the hematology laboratory involve anticoagulated blood. Once the blood has left the body, a series of reactions occurs causing blood to clot within minutes. To prevent coagulation from occurring, a substance called an **anticoagulant** is mixed with the blood. Three anticoagulants are used in the hematology laboratory: (1) ethylenediaminetetraacetic acid (EDTA), (2) sodium citrate, (3) heparin.[1] Sample collection tubes are color coded by stopper to indicate the type of anticoagulant present in the tube (Table 34-1 ✪).

EDTA is the most commonly used anticoagulant in the routine hematology laboratory. Sample collection tubes can contain one of three different salt forms of EDTA: disodium, dipotassium, or tripotassium. The sample collection tube's stopper is color coded in lavender to indicate the presence of EDTA. EDTA prevents coagulation by chelating calcium, a

TABLE 34-1

Sample Collection Tubes, Their Anticoagulant, and Typical Laboratory Use

Color Code	Anticoagulant	Typical Laboratory Procedure
Red	No anticoagulant	Antibody detection
Light blue	Sodium citrate	PT and APTT
Mottled red	No anticoagulant but contains clot activator and gel to facilitate separation of serum from cells	Cholesterol
Green	Heparin	Osmotic fragility
Purple or lavender	EDTA, K_3 (liquid), or K_2 (spray-coated)	CBC (K_2 EDTA can also be used for routine blood bank procedures; see below)
Pink	EDTA, K_2 (spray coated)	Blood bank procedures and whole blood hematology procedures (different colored stopper for easy distinction of blood bank vs. hematology samples)
Gray	Potassium oxalate and sodium fluoride	Glucose

PT = prothrombin time; APTT = activated partial thromboplastin time

necessary component of the coagulation cascade (∞ Chapter 30). Its removal inhibits the coagulation process. The optimal concentration is 1.5 mg of EDTA per mL blood.

Tests using EDTA samples include complete blood count (CBC), hematocrit, peripheral blood smear examination, platelet count, reticulocyte count, and flow cytometry. Ideally, the sample should be used within 6 hours of collection for the majority of these tests. The sample's stability can be extended to 24 hours with storage at 4°C for certain tests such as the CBC and platelet count. If peripheral blood smears are to be prepared, they should be made within 3 hours of collection. After 3 hours at room temperature, degenerative changes can be observed by examining a Wright-stained blood smear. These changes include leukocytes with vacuoles, irregular cytoplasmic borders, and irregularly shaped nuclei. Also, platelets increase in size. Excess anticoagulant causes erythrocyte shrinkage. Concentrations of more than 2 mg of EDTA per mL blood cause false decreases in the microhematocrit and erythrocyte sedimentation rate (ESR).

Sodium citrate is the recommended anticoagulant for coagulation studies. The Clinical and Laboratory Standards Institute (CLSI) recommends the use of 3.2% sodium citrate.[2] The sample collection tube's stopper is color coded in light blue to indicate the presence of sodium citrate. Sodium citrate prevents coagulation by binding calcium in a soluble complex (∞ Chapter 30). The appropriate ratio of anticoagulant: blood is 1:9. Further discussion of sodium citrate and its use in coagulation studies can be found in ∞ Chapter 40.

Lithium heparin is the CLSI recommended salt of heparin to be used for laboratory testing.[1] The sample collection tube's stopper is color coded in green to indicate the presence of heparin. Heparin's interaction with antithrombin prevents coagulation. The interaction leads to the inhibition of thrombin (∞ Chapter 30). The recommended concentration for sample collection tubes is 15–30 units heparin/mL blood.

Lithium heparin is specifically recommended for the following laboratory tests: ammonia, carboxyhemoglobin, blood gases, zinc, and potassium. In hematology, lithium heparin is the appropriate anticoagulant for the osmotic fragility test. The use of heparin for routine hematology procedures is not appropriate. Heparin can affect the platelets and leukocytes, causing them to clump. In addition, heparin causes morphologic distortion of platelets and leukocytes and tends to cause a bluish discoloration of the background of blood films stained with a Romanowsky stain such as Wright stain.

 Checkpoint! 1

Contrast the mechanisms of anticoagulation for EDTA and heparin.

EQUIPMENT

The equipment needed for blood collection by venipuncture includes sample collection tubes, needles, tube holders or syringes, and a tourniquet. Lancets are used for capillary puncture. Other miscellaneous supplies are described in this section.

Sample Collection Tubes

Evacuated sample collection tubes are sterile and color coded to indicate the type of anticoagulant present or the lack of anticoagulant (Web Figure 34-1 ■, Table 34-1). The Occupational Safety and Health Administration (OSHA) recommends the use of plastic sample collection tubes whenever possible. Collection tubes are manufactured in a variety of sizes to collect different volumes of sample (1 mL, 3 mL, 5 mL, etc.). The variety of volumes available minimizes the removal of excess amounts of blood. Today's hematology and chemistry instruments require only small amounts of sample for analysis. The interior of the sample collection tube is a vacuum. When the stopper is pierced by a needle, the required amount of blood is drawn from the vein into the tube by the vacuum.[1] The tube might not fill properly if the vein collapses or if the needle is displaced from the lumen of the vein.

For capillary punctures, microcollection tubes are available with the same anticoagulants and color coded in the same manner as the evacuated collection tubes, but they do not contain a vacuum. The microcollection tubes contain special features that facilitate the collection of capillary blood into the tubes, such as capillary pipet tips (see Web Figure 34-2■ for examples of microcollection tubes). These adaptations help to decrease the time that it takes to collect the capillary sample and decrease errors related to sample collection (e.g., presence of micro clots or hemolysis).

Needles

Sample collection needles are sterile hollow shafts of stainless steel with a beveled tip. The most common needles used for blood collection are 20- or 21-gauge. The gauge of a needle relates to the diameter of its bore. A small gauge needle has a large diameter. For example, an 18-gauge needle is used to collect donor blood for transfusions because its larger bore diameter permits a more rapid collection of blood and decreases the chance of hemolysis. Special needles are required for sample collection using the evacuated collection tube system. For this system, the needle must be double ended. The needle is screwed into a tube holder. The long end of the needle is inserted into the vein and the short end punctures the collection tube stopper (inside the tube holder) and releases the vacuum allowing for blood collection into the tube.

Tube Holders

The evacuated sample collection tube system requires a tube holder or adapter with a shape similar to a syringe. The needle is threaded into its position in the holder, and sample collection tubes are rested in the holder, semiattached by the shorter needle end (Figure 34-1■). The tube holder also facilitates the insertion of the needle into the vein.

Syringe

The syringe was once the principal method of obtaining a blood sample, but it is now used only for difficult phle-

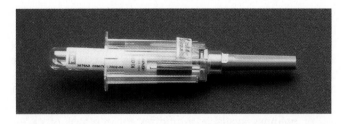

■ FIGURE 34-1 Assembled evacuated collection tube system. The double-ended needle is threaded into the tube holder and the purple top collection tube is secured in the holder by the shorter end of the needle that has partially pierced the stopper. Blood replaces the vacuum in the collection tube when the vein is entered and the stopper is completely pierced.

botomies or the collection of an arterial blood sample. Sterile plastic syringes are available in a variety of sizes (e.g., 1 mL, 5 mL, or 10 mL).

Tourniquet

Various tourniquets including rubber straps, blood pressure cuffs, and rubber tubing are available. Placement of the tourniquet on the patient's upper arm increases the resistance in venous blood flow, resulting in the distension of veins below the tourniquet. The phlebotomist is then able to visualize and/or palpate the veins to identify the "good" vein. The tourniquet should never be left in place longer than 1 minute prior to phlebotomy because this will result in discomfort to the patient and **hemoconcentration** of the blood sample.

Lancets

Various sterile disposable lancets are available for performing capillary puncture. The design of these devices has been improved to minimize the discomfort and maximize the quality of the sample. Disposable lancets provide a controlled incision depth. The selection of a lancet depends on the individual's age. For example, a lancet with an incision depth of 1.8 mm is typically used for neonatal collection to minimize trauma; a device with an incision depth of 2.4 mm is appropriate for older children and adults.

Other Equipment

Other equipment required to perform a phlebotomy includes gloves, safety goggles, alcohol pads, gauze, adhesive bandages, and biohazard sharps containers. Gloves and safety goggles have become important protective equipment for the phlebotomist to prevent exposure to blood-borne pathogens. Alcohol pads are commonly used to cleanse and prepare the phlebotomy site. Gauze with applied pressure is used to stop bleeding after the needle has been removed. Adhesive bandages are used to protect the venipuncture or capillary puncture site. The biohazard sharps container is used for properly disposing of lancets and needles to minimize potential puncture wounds.

VENIPUNCTURE

The venipuncture phlebotomy technique removes blood from a vein for laboratory testing using a sterile needle and an evacuated sample collection tube system.[3] Prior to performing the venipuncture, the phlebotomist must identify the patient. The 2008 National Patient Safety Goals implemented by the Joint Commission on Accreditation of Healthcare Organizations (JCAHO) requires that two patient identifiers be used when collecting blood samples.[4] For example, proper identification can be achieved by comparing the patient's name and **unique identification number** from his or her wrist band to the information written on the requisition form.

Next, the phlebotomist assembles the appropriate equipment for performing the venipuncture. The vein is selected by placing the tourniquet on the patient's upper arm and inspecting the forearm for a prominent vein (see Web Table 34-1 ✪ for considerations in selection of venipuncture site). The median cubital vein is typically used, but the cephalic vein is also appropriate. The vein is cleansed with an alcohol pad and allowed to air dry. The venipuncture is accomplished by inserting the needle into the vein at a 15° angle to the forearm (Web Figure 34-3 ■). A slight release in resistance can be detected when the vein is entered. Blood is collected into the appropriate evacuated collection tubes by pushing the tube until the stopper is punctured with the short end of the needle (see Web Table 34-2 ✪ for the correct collection sequence of evacuated tubes). The vacuum is released as blood enters the collection tube. When blood has been collected in each tube, the tourniquet is released, the needle is withdrawn, and pressure with gauze is applied to the venipuncture site. The needle is immediately discarded into the biohazard sharps container. Collection tubes containing anticoagulant should be thoroughly but gently mixed to prevent clotting of the sample. Each collection tube should be properly labeled with patient's name, unique identification number, and date. Finally, the patient should be checked one last time to verify that bleeding has ceased and an adhesive bandage is applied to the venipuncture site.

CAPILLARY PUNCTURE

The capillary puncture technique allows a small but adequate amount of blood to be obtained for laboratory testing.[5] This is especially important in the pediatric patient (i.e., infant) who has a lower total blood volume. Venipuncture in this patient population can result in anemia. The phlebotomist should properly identify the patient before proceeding with the capillary puncture technique. Selection of the capillary puncture site depends on the individual's age. The side of the heel is used for newborns, and a location slightly to the side of center and perpendicular to the fingerprint of the last segment of the third or fourth finger is chosen for an older child or adult. The puncture site should be warm and not **edematous.** Accumulated interstitial fluid in the edematous area will contaminate the blood sample. Warming the site prior to the capillary puncture increases blood flow through the site, primarily arterial blood flow. With the site identified, appropriate equipment is assembled, and the site is cleansed with an alcohol pad and allowed to air dry. The capillary puncture is made, and the lancet is immediately discarded into a biohazard sharps container. The first drop of blood is wiped away because it likely contains excess interstitial fluid that could result in a diluted blood sample. Subsequent drops of blood are collected into the appropriate microcollection tubes. When sufficient blood has been collected, gauze is placed on the puncture site and slight pressure applied. The microcollection tubes containing anti-

coagulant should be properly mixed to ensure adequate anticoagulation to prevent clot formation. Each microcollection tube should be properly labeled with the patient's name, unique identification number, date, and time of collection. An adhesive bandage is applied to the puncture site.

PHLEBOTOMY SAFETY

OSHA mandates safety guidelines for phlebotomy. The 1992 Occupational Exposure to Bloodborne Pathogens Standard and its 1999 revised directive address this issue thoroughly.[6,7] These standards promote safety through education, good work practices, use of personal protective equipment (PPE), and use of medical devices that minimize exposure risk. Each laboratory should develop an exposure control plan to address these issues. Clinical laboratory professionals should receive instruction as to the potential for exposure to, the methods of preventing exposure to, and the postexposure treatment of blood-borne pathogens such as hepatitis B (HBV), hepatitis C (HCV), and human immunodeficiency virus (HIV).

For the phlebotomist, the educational program should include practical experience using PPE and the new collection systems available to minimize risk of needlesticks. At a minimum, the phlebotomist's PPE should include gloves and goggles to decrease risk of exposure through cuts or abrasions on the skin and exposure through mucous membranes of the eyes. The revised directives require the evaluation and implementation of needlestick systems designed to reduce the risk of needlestick injury (Web Figure 34-4 ■). Disposable lancet devices that retract the lancet into a protective guard after the capillary puncture has been made minimizes risk of a sharps injury due to a lancet. Biohazard sharps containers should be readily available for disposal of lancets and needles.

An additional measure to reduce exposure to blood-borne pathogens is the use of plastic splashguards on the stoppers of sample collection tubes. The splashguards reduce the formation of aerosols that are created when the stopper is removed.

The entire exposure control plan for phlebotomy should be reviewed annually and changed as new devices become available to reduce risk of sharps injury and as new treatments for blood-borne pathogens become available.

 Checkpoint! 2

What are three steps a phlebotomist should take to minimize the risk of exposure to blood-borne pathogens when performing a venipuncture?

▶ MICROSCOPY: THE MICROSCOPE

The compound microscope is an essential instrument in the routine hematology laboratory. Its proper use and regular preventative maintenance are critical to the reliability of the results obtained from its use. Therefore, individuals utilizing the microscope need to be knowledgeable in its basic principles, its operation, and its preventative maintenance.

BRIGHT-FIELD MICROSCOPY

Bright-field microscopy is used extensively to examine stained blood and bone marrow samples. This section describes the components of bright-field microscopy and aberrations that affect the quality of the sample examination.

Principles of the Compound Microscope

Any discussion of the principles of the compound microscope must begin with a review of its components. The components include eyepieces, binocular eyepiece tube, objectives located on the revolving nosepiece, microscope stage, condenser, condenser diaphragm, field diaphragm, and light source (Figure 34-2 ■). The condenser functions to direct the beam of light from the light source onto the sample. As the light rays illuminate the sample, they are altered and light is diffracted. The sample image is produced by a combination of the diffracted light and background light from the light source.[8,9,10]

The magnifying system of the compound microscope uses two sets of lenses to form an enlarged image.[9,10] The first lens system is the objective, which projects a primary image plane to a location approximately 1 cm from the top of the microscope's body. The distance from the back focal plane of the objective to the eyepiece is termed the *optical tube length* (160 mm). The second lens system is the eyepiece located above the primary image plane. The total magnification is the product of the magnification of the first and second lens systems (objective magnification times eyepiece magnification).

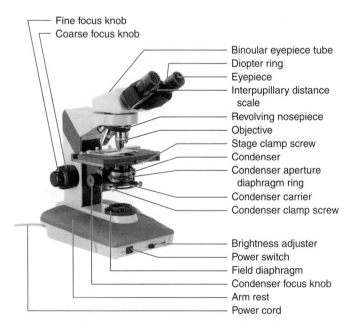

Fine focus knob
Coarse focus knob
Binocular eyepiece tube
Diopter ring
Eyepiece
Interpupillary distance scale
Revolving nosepiece
Objective
Stage clamp screw
Condenser
Condenser aperture diaphragm ring
Condenser carrier
Condenser clamp screw
Brightness adjuster
Power switch
Field diaphragm
Condenser focus knob
Arm rest
Power cord

■ FIGURE 34-2   Basic components of the compound microscope. (Courtesy of Nikon, Inc., Garden City, NY)

✓ Checkpoint! 3

What is the total magnification when a 10× objective is combined with a 10× eyepiece?

The resolving power (resolution) of a lens is its ability to distinguish two separate objects located close to one another and reveal the fine detail in a specimen.[9,10] It is a function of the numerical aperature (NA) of the lens and the wavelength (λ) of the illuminating light. The numerical aperature is a designation of the amount of light entering the objective from the microscope field. The NA of the substage condenser should be equal to or greater than the NA of an objective; otherwise, interference effects will occur. Because the illuminating light remains constant in light microscopy, the numerical aperature determines the resolving power. That is to say, the higher an objective's NA, the greater the resolving power.

Lens Aberrations

An *aberration* is an optical defect that degrades the quality of an image[9,10] Three important types of aberrations are associated with the objectives:

1. *Chromatic aberrations* give rise to color fringes and poor image definition. These aberrations are due to the inability of the lens to bring the different wavelengths of light into focus at a single focal point. For example, blue light is brought to a focal point closer to the lens as compared to red light.

2. *Spherical aberrations* give rise to poor image definition and loss of contrast. In spherical aberrations, the light is refracted by the lens depending on the area (thickness) of the lens it passes through. For example, the light passing through the periphery of the lens is refracted more than light passing through the center. Therefore, the refracted light from the periphery is brought to a shorter focal point than the light passing through the center. This aberration becomes worse as the lens becomes thicker.

3. *Field curvature aberrations* result in the periphery of the field being slightly out of focus when the center is in focus. These aberrations are the result of the image in the focal plane being slightly curved by the objective.

In order to compensate for these aberrations, specialized lenses are employed. The achromat lens will compensate for chromatic aberrations at two colors and spherical aberrations at one color. The apochromat lens will compensate for chromatic aberrations at three colors and spherical aberrations at two colors. The field curvature aberrations may be eliminated with the use of a flat-field (plan) objective lens. A plan apochromat lens is the highest grade, giving exceptional definition, superior color reproducibility, and prominent image flatness. This lens is most useful in the examination of morphologic detail.

Infinity Optical System

Newer microscope models have an infinity optical system. In the infinity optical system, light that passes through the objective becomes a flux of parallel light rays.[11,12] These light rays do not converge to form the primary image until they pass through the tube lens (Figure 34-3 ■). In other words, the infinity objective sends the primary image to "infinity." For comparison, the finite objective projects light rays that converge within the tube length of the microscope to create the primary image (Figure 34-3). Two major advantages of the infinity optical system are the increased sharpness and clarity of the images and the increased flexibility of the microscope system. The increased sharpness and clarity result from higher numerical apertures and longer working distances (i.e., distance from the objective to the surface of the coverslip when the sample is sharply focused).

The infinity space associated with these systems allows for the addition of intermediate attachments without loss of optical performance such as an epi-fluorescence attachment for the evaluation of fluorescent stains.

PHASE-CONTRAST MICROSCOPY

With bright-field microscopy, unstained cells are difficult to the examine due to the lack of absorption differences between cellular structures and undetectable variations in the **refractive index.** Examination of unstained cells can be accomplished using phase-contrast microscopy, which is based on the premise that transparent objects (e.g., unstained cells) cause a change in the phase of transmitted light (i.e., phase shift) due to scattering and deflection of light.[10,12] When the transmitted light is shifted by one-quarter wavelength, these changes can be visualized as differences in light intensity. The two important components of a phase microscope are the annular diaphragm, or annular ring, located in the condenser, and the phase-shifting element, or phase ring, located in the objective. The annular ring directs light through its open circular area creating a hollow cone of light with a dark center that illuminates the sample (Figure 34-4 ■). The phase ring within the objective retards the wavelength of the deflected light by one-quarter wavelength and absorbs the nondiffracted light. This phase shifting occurs in the shaded area (Figure 34-4). As a result, light waves become out of phase. Maximum contrast between the cell and its surroundings is achieved when light waves are out of phase by one-quarter of a wavelength. With phase-contrast microscopy, cellular components that possess a higher refractive index than the surrounding environment appear dark while components that possess a lower refractive index than the surrounding environment appear bright.

For proper operation, the annular ring must be centered to the phase ring.

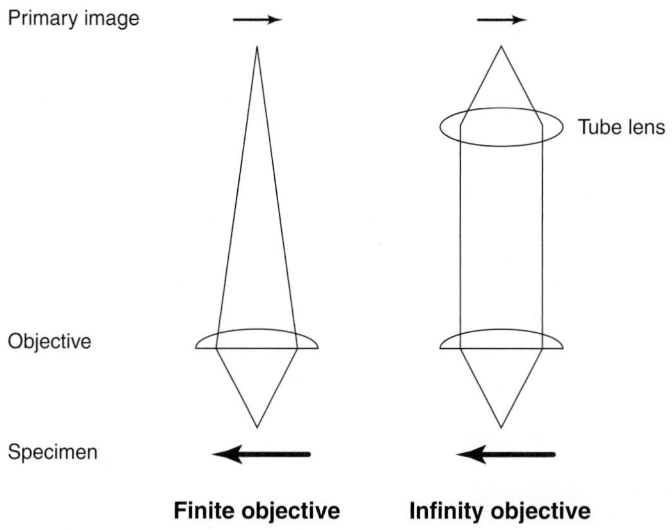

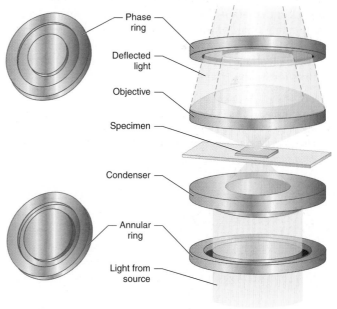

Phase contrast light pathways

Phase ring
Deflected light
Objective
Specimen
Condenser
Annular ring
Light from source

■ FIGURE 34-3 Finite objective vs. infinity objective. In the finite objective, light rays projected from the objective converge to form the primary image within the optical tube. For the infinity objective, light is projected as parallel rays from the objective. These rays converge to form the primary image only after they pass through the tube lens. The infinity space as defined by the distance between the objective and the tube lens can vary from 160 mm to 200 mm.

Primary image
Tube lens
Objective
Specimen
Finite objective   **Infinity objective**

■ FIGURE 34-4 Phase contrast light pathway. The annular ring within the condenser diaphragm creates a hollow cone of light that illuminates the sample. Transmitted light is shifted one-quarter wavelength by the phase-shifting element in the objective, creating maximum contrast between a cell and its surroundings. (Reprinted, with permission, from Molecular Expressions' World Wide Web pages.)

KOEHLER ILLUMINATION

Koehler illumination utilizes a double diaphragm illumination. The two diaphragms are the field diaphragm and the condenser diaphragm. The condenser diaphragm determines the resolution, contrast, and depth of field. Closing the condenser diaphragm increases the contrast and depth of field but decreases the resolution. The field diaphragm determines the illuminated area on the sample surface in relation to the microscope's field of view. In Koehler illumination, the two diaphragms are adjusted to give uniform illumination of the field of view and optimum contrast and resolution of a sample by focusing and centering the light path.[8,9]

The procedure for Koehler illumination varies slightly depending on the microscope manufacturer (see Web Table 34-3 ✪ for this procedure). This procedure should be performed daily before using the microscope, and it should be repeated for each objective, since each objective will have a different light requirement (higher NA objectives require correspondingly higher NA settings on the condenser).

PREVENTATIVE MAINTENANCE

Each laboratory should establish a regular preventative maintenance program. The microscope manufacturer's instruction manual provides a preventative maintenance checklist. Any preventative maintenance program should include the following: (1) clean the oil immersion lens daily with lens tissue and cleaner, (2) dust optical surfaces (eyepieces, condenser, field lens, and filters) using bursts of air or a soft camel's hair brush, (3) clean external surfaces using a mild liquid soap—avoid the use of any organic solvents such as ether, alcohol, or xylene, and (4) periodically inspect objectives for stubborn smudges or scratches.[9,10]

 Checkpoint! 4

How does the examination of a sample by phase-contrast microscopy differ from bright-field microscopy?

PART I

ROUTINE HEMATOLOGY
PROCEDURES

▶ PERIPHERAL BLOOD SMEAR PREPARATION

The morphologic evaluation of hematopoietic cells by light microscopy requires the preparation of a well-stained blood smear.[13–16] The accuracy of the morphologic evaluation depends in part on the quality of the blood smear.

MANUAL METHOD

The two manual methods for preparing blood smears are: the **coverglass smear** and the **wedge smear.** The coverglass smear method provides a smear with even distribution of the leukocytes. The disadvantages of this method are the difficulty in mastering the technique, the fragility of the coverglass, and the difficulty in staining the coverglass. The wedge smear is the method most commonly used in routine laboratory practice but it is subject to poor leukocyte distribution with monocytes and neutrophils being drawn out of the **optimal counting area** to the feather edge. Although the leukocyte distribution is poor, the technique is easily mastered and the smears are less fragile and can be stored for extended periods of time. An advantage of the leukocyte distribution in a wedge smear is that it allows for the identification of abnormal cells that tend to locate on the edges of the smear.

Either EDTA-anticoagulated venous blood or capillary blood is acceptable for the preparation of a blood smear (see Web Table 34-4 ✪ for this procedure). An optimal blood smear has the characteristics listed in Table 34-2 ✪ (see Web Figure 34-5 ■ for examples of properly and improperly prepared blood smears). A common problem associated with blood smears is the failure to dry the blood smear in a timely manner. This results in contraction artifacts of the cells, especially with increased humidity. In certain physiological conditions including **anemia, polycythemia, multiple myeloma,** and **cold agglutinin disease,** making good blood smears is difficult due to the abnormal composition of the blood (Table 34-3 ✪). The thickness or thinness of the blood smear is be regulated by:

- Adjusting the amount of blood used to make the drop
- Altering the speed with which the drop is smeared
- Altering the angle at which the spreader slide is used

Automated Method

Automated methods for preparing blood smears have been developed for nearly all major hematology instruments on the market (∞ Chapter 36). These methods are based on the wedge smear technique. Automated methods that are a component of a hematology instrument combine blood smear preparation and staining. Advantages of these methods include minimal exposure to biohazardous material because many are closed tube systems, increased consistency between blood smears, and increased optimal counting area.

✪ TABLE 34-2

Optimal Blood Smear Characteristics
• Minimum length 2.5 cm
• Gradual transition in thickness from thick to thin
• Straight feather edge
• Margins narrower than slide
• No streaks, waves, or troughs

TABLE 34-3

Resolution of Problems in Preparation of a Blood Smear

Problem	Resolution
Presence of crenated erythrocytes	Dry smear quickly and thoroughly
Thin smear due to anemia	Increase spreader slide angle and increase push speed
Thick smear due to polycythemia	Decrease spreader slide angle and decrease push speed
Presence of agglutinated erythrocytes associated with cold agglutinin disease	Warm blood @ 37°C for 15 minutes prior to preparing smear
Increased viscosity associated with multiple myeloma	Decrease spreader slide angle and decrease push speed

Also available is a portable semiautomated instrument that is not specific for any given hematology instrument. With the semiautomated instrument, the instrument controls the speed and angle of the spreader blade, but the clinical laboratory professional controls the size of the blood drop. Overall advantages and disadvantages of the automated methods are similar to the manual wedge smear method.

✓ **Checkpoint! 5**

A clinical laboratory professional consistently prepares thin blood smears resulting in minimal counting area. What would you suggest this individual do to improve the quality of these blood smears?

▶ **PERIPHERAL BLOOD SMEAR STAINING**

For more than 100 years, **Romanowsky-type stains** have been used in the morphologic classification of hematopoietic cells.[17,18] A Romanowsky-type stained blood smear is extremely important in the hematology laboratory because a wealth of information can be obtained from the evaluation of a well-stained peripheral blood smear.

The combined action of methylene blue and its oxidation products and eosin Y or eosin B produce the Romanowsky staining effect. This yields a purple color to the nuclei of leukocytes and neutrophilic granules and reddish orange color to the erythrocytes. The principal components responsible for this effect are azure B (a methylene blue oxidation product) and eosin Y. The wide variation in purple and red shades seen with Romanowsky staining allows for subtle distinctions in cellular characteristics.

The staining properties of Romanowsky stains depend on the binding of dyes to chemical structures and the interactions between azure B and eosin Y. Acidic groupings of nucleic acids, the proteins of the cell nuclei, and immature or reactive cytoplasm binds azure B, the purplish basic dye. Eosin Y, the reddish acidic dye, binds to the basic groupings of the hemoglobin molecules and the basic proteins within certain granules.

Examples of Romanowsky stains include Wright, Wright-Giemsa, Leishman, May-Grunwald, and Jenner stains. The most commonly used are Wright and Wright-Giemsa stains.

✓ **Checkpoint! 6**

Which component of Wright stain is responsible for staining hemoglobin within erythrocytes?

The staining process begins with the methanol fixation step, which results in the adherence of cellular proteins to the glass microscope slide preventing the cells from being washed away during subsequent steps (see Web Table 34-5 for this procedure). Additional fixation takes place when the blood smear is flooded with Wright's stain. The actual staining begins with the addition of buffer to the Wright's stain resulting in the ionization of the dyes. A properly stained blood smear meets the criteria outlined in Table 34-4 ⊙. Potential causes of an improperly stained blood smear are given in Table 34-5 ⊙.

⊙ **TABLE 34-4**

Characteristics of a Properly Stained Blood Smear by Macroscopic and Microscopic Evaluation

Type of Evaluation	Characteristics
Macroscopic	Smear is pinkish purple in color.
Microscopic	Blood cells are evenly distributed.
	Areas between cells are clear.
	Erythrocytes are orange red.
	Neutrophilic granules are pale purple.
	Eosinophilic granules are red orange.
	Basophilic granules are purplish black.
	Lymphocyte's cytoplasm is blue.
	Leukocyte's nuclei are purple.
	Within nucleus, chromatin and parachromatin are distinct.
	Precipitated stain is minimal or absent.

✪ TABLE 34-5

Potential Causes of Improperly Stained Blood Smear

Problem	Potential Causes
Excessively blue or dark stain	Prolonged staining
	Inadequate washing
	Use of a stain and/or buffer with an alkalinity that is too high
	Thick blood smear
Excessively pink or light stain	Insufficient staining
	Prolonged washing
	Use of a stain and/or buffer with an acidity that is too low
Presence of precipitate	Unclean slides
	Drying during staining process
	Inadequate filtration of stain

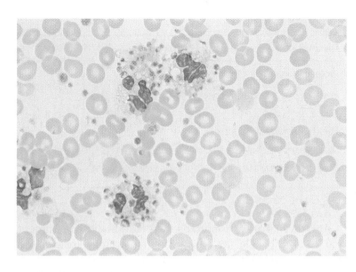

■ FIGURE 34-5   Platelet satellitism. (Peripheral blood, Wright-Giemsa stain; 1000× original magnification)

✓ Checkpoint! 7

If the erythrocytes appear bluish gray and leukocyte nuclei are black, how would you correct this problem?

▶ PERIPHERAL BLOOD SMEAR EXAMINATION

The examination of a well-stained peripheral blood smear is one of the most frequently performed tests in the hematology laboratory.[13,19–21] The thorough examination of a peripheral blood smear may be used (1) as a screening tool to identify illness, (2) for making the definitive diagnosis of certain hematologic and nonhematologic conditions, and (3) to monitor the patient's response to therapy. The peripheral blood smear evaluation includes an estimation of leukocyte and platelet count, detection of abnormal cells and abnormal erythrocyte distribution, review of erythrocyte and platelet morphology, and counting a 100-cell leukocyte differential (see Web Table 34-6 ✪ for a summary of this procedure; the detailed procedure is also provided on the Website ∞ Chapter 34).

On 100× magnification (10× objective), the peripheral blood smear is scanned to ensure even distribution of leukocytes and observe for immature or abnormal cells, **smudge cells, platelet clumps, platelet satellitism**, and abnormal erythrocyte distribution patterns such as **rouleaux** or agglutination (Figure 34-5 ■, Table 34-6 ✪). The leukocyte estimate is obtained by counting the number of leukocytes in each of five fields of view and applying the calculation formula (Figure 34-6 ■). The leukocyte estimate should correlate with the leukocyte count ±25%.

On 1000× magnification (100× objective), platelet morphology is observed, and a platelet estimate is obtained by counting the number of platelets in each of five fields of view and applying a calculation formula similar to that used for the leukocyte estimate (Figure 34-7 ■). The platelet estimate should correlate with the platelet count ±25%. Erythrocyte morphology is evaluated by carefully examining erythrocyte size, shape, color, and observation for the pres-

✪ TABLE 34-6

Abnormalities Detected on Peripheral Blood Smear, Their Effect on Cell Counts, and Corrective Procedures to Take

Abnormality	Effect on Cell Counts	Corrective Action
Smudge cells	No effect on cell counts	Add 1 drop of 22% bovine albumin to 5 drops of blood, mix, and prepare blood smear.
Nucleated erythrocytes	Falsely elevated leukocyte count	Correct leukocyte count for presence of nucleated erythrocytes.
Platelet clumps	Falsely decreased platelet count	If collected in EDTA, recollect using citrate tube. Platelet count should be multiplied by 1.1 to correct for dilutional effect of liquid citrate.
Platelet satellitism	Falsely decreased platelet count	Use correction for platelet clumps.
Erythrocyte agglutination	Falsely decreased erythrocyte count	Warm blood @ 37°C for 15 minutes and retest.
Rouleaux	No effect on cell counts	No correction is available

$$\frac{\text{Total number of leukocytes counted}^*}{5} \times \ 0.2 \times 10^9/\text{L}^{**} = \text{leukocytes} \times 10^9/\text{L}$$

* Total number of leukocytes counted in 5 fields at 100x (10x objective) magnification

** 1 leukocyte = 0.2 x 10⁹/L

Example: If total number of leukocytes counted = 150

$$150/5 \times 0.2 \times 10^9/\text{L} = 6.0 \times 10^9/\text{L}$$

■ FIGURE 34-6 Calculation of leukocyte estimate. This formula is based on performing the estimate at 100× magnification. The estimation factor varies depending on the total magnification used as defined by the ocular and objective magnifications. Thus, each laboratory should determine or validate this factor based on its microscope.

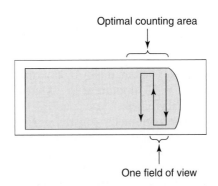

Optimal counting area

One field of view

■ FIGURE 34-8 Pathway for the leukocyte differential. The differential is performed within the optimal counting area where the erythrocytes can be touching but not overlapping. As you approach the opposite side of the smear, the objective is moved into the body of the smear by one field of view. This pattern is followed until 100 leukocytes have been identified.

ence of inclusions. Normal erythrocytes are described as normocytic and normochromic, and this appearance correlates with normal erythrocyte indices. Any change beyond normal variation should be noted because certain variations in the erythrocytes are characteristic of specific hematologic disorders. A detailed discussion of possible morphologic changes can be found in ∞ Chapter 8.

The leukocyte differential is performed by counting 100 cells per slide using the battlement track method for examination (Figure 34-8■). Each leukocyte (∞ Chapter 7) encountered must be identified and placed in the appropriate category; distorted cells are included only if they are clearly identifiable. Nucleated erythrocytes (∞ Chapter 5) are not included within the differential but are tabulated separately. The results of the differential are reported in percentage of each type of leukocyte counted. The nucleated erythrocytes are expressed as number per 100 leukocytes. If 5 or more nucleated erythrocytes are observed, the leukocyte count must be corrected for their presence because they are included in the leukocyte count (Figure 34-9■). Finally, leukocytes are observed for changes in morphology (i.e., Döhle bodies, hypersegmented neutrophils; ∞ Chapters 19 and 20). These changes can be the result of an underlying hematologic disorder, the presence of excess anticoagulant, or the failure to prepare the blood smears within 3 hours of collection. Typical anticoagulant changes include cytoplasmic vacuolization, degranulation, karyorrhexis, karyolysis, and changes in nuclear shape.

The leukocyte differential reference values for children as well as adult males and females can be found in Table B inside the front cover.

✓ **Checkpoint! 8**

In a platelet estimate, 76 platelets were observed in five fields. Calculate the platelet estimate. If the platelet count was 189 × 10⁹/L, would these results correlate? Assume the sample was collected with EDTA.

$$\frac{\text{Total number of platelets counted}^*}{5} \times \ 15 \times 10^9/\text{L}^{**} = \text{Platelets} \times 10^9/\text{L}$$

* Total number of platelets counted in 5 fields at 1000x (100x objective) magnification

** If EDTA-anticoagulated blood, 1 platelet = 15 x 10⁹/L
If capillary blood, 1 platelet = 20 x 10⁹/L

Example: If total number of platelets counted = 100

$$100/5 \times 15 \times 10^9/\text{L} = 300 \times 10^9/\text{L}$$

■ FIGURE 34-7 Calculation of platelet estimate. This formula is based on performing the estimate at 1000× magnification. Refer to Figure 34-6 for a discussion of estimation factor.

$$\frac{\text{Leukocyte count} \times 100}{100 + \text{number of nucleated erythrocytes}^*} = \text{Corrected leukocyte count}$$

*Number of nucleated erythrocytes counted per 100 leukocytes at 1000x (100x objective) magnification

Example: Leukocyte count = 20.0 x 10⁹/L
        Nucleated erythrocytes/100 leukocytes = 10

$$\frac{20.0 \times 10^9/\text{L} \times 100}{100 + 10} = 18.2 \times 10^9/\text{L}$$

■ FIGURE 34-9 Leukocyte count correction for presence of nucleated erythrocytes.

▶ CELL ENUMERATION BY HEMACYTOMETER

Cell counts are performed manually by diluting blood with a diluent, loading a small amount of the diluted sample on a ruled device (hemacytometer), and counting the cells microscopically. The hemacytometer consists of two side-by-side identically ruled glass platforms mounted in a glass holder. Each platform contains a ruled square measuring 3×3 mm (9 mm^2) and is subdivided according to the improved Neubauer ruling (Figure 34-10■). This ruling subdivides the ruled square into 9 large squares, each measuring 1×1 mm (1 mm^2). All 9 squares are used for leukocyte counts. The large center square (1 mm^2) is used for platelet and erythrocyte counts. This center square is divided into 25 smaller squares, each with an area of 0.04 mm^2. The 5 squares labeled R are used in performing the erythrocyte count whereas the entire center square is used in performing the platelet count.

On either side of the two ruled glass platforms is a raised ridge. The coverglass is placed on top of the ridge. The distance between the coverglass and the surface of the ruled area (depth) is exactly 0.1 mm. Thus, the ruled area on each side of the hemacytometer holds a volume of 0.9 mm^3 ($3 \times 3 \times 0.1$).

The unopette system is a fast and accurate method for collecting and diluting blood for cell counts. For each laboratory determination performed, the unopette consists of the following elements: the reservoir, the pipet, and the pipet shield (Figure 34-11■). The reservoir contains a premeasured volume of diluting fluid that is specific for the cell count to be performed.

MANUAL LEUKOCYTE COUNT

Whole blood is diluted with a 1% ammonium oxalate solution, which hemolyzes mature erythrocytes and facilitates leukocyte (white blood cell [WBC]) counting.[22] The standard dilution for leukocyte counts is 1:100. The detailed procedure for the manual leukocyte count is provided on the Website ∞ Chapter 34. With proper light adjustment, the leukocytes should appear as dark dots. The number of leukocytes in all nine squares are counted using the 10× objective. Potential sources of error in performing hemacytometer cell counts are provided in Web Table 34-7 ✪.

The number of leukocytes is calculated per μL ($\times 10^9$/L) of blood. To make this determination, the total number of cells counted must be corrected for the initial dilution of blood and the volume of blood used for counting (Figure 34-12■). Because the dilution of blood for a leukocyte count is 1:100, the reciprocal of the dilution is 100. The volume of blood used is based on the number of squares counted, the area of each square, and the depth of the solution. For the leukocyte count, all nine squares are counted, each square's area is 1 mm^2, and the depth of the solution is 0.1 mm; therefore the volume is 0.9 mm^3. Thus, the number of leukocytes counted in the nine squares is multiplied by 111 (100/0.9) and reported as number of leukocytes per mm^3.

Reference intervals for leukocyte counts in adults and children can be found in Table B on the inside cover. Conditions commonly associated with increased or decreased leukocyte counts are shown in Table 34-7 ✪ (∞ Chapters 7, 19, 20, 22, 24, 25, and 26).

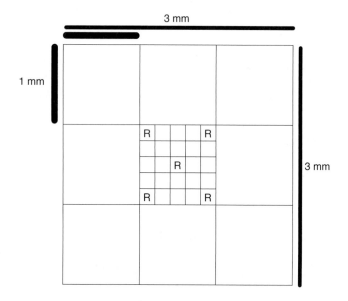

■ FIGURE 34-10   Neubauer hemacytometer counting area. The entire counting area is 9 mm^2 (3 mm × 3 mm) and is divided into 9 squares. Each square is 1 mm^2 (1 mm × 1 mm) in area. Using the 10× objective, 1 square of the counting area (1 mm^2) can be viewed. For the manual leukocyte count, all 9 squares are counted. The center square is further divided and the R squares are used for erythrocyte counts, while the entire center square is used for platelet counts.

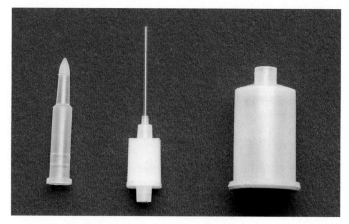

■ FIGURE 34-11   Unopette system (from left to right): pipet shield, pipet, and reservoir.

$$\frac{\text{Total number of cells counted} \times \text{Reciprocal of the dilution}}{\text{Number of squares counted} \times \text{Area of each square} \times \text{Depth of the solution}} = \text{Cells/mm}^3$$

Example:
Total number of cells (one side of hemacytometer)	90
Dilution	1:100
Number of squares counted	9
Area of each square	1 mm^2
Depth of solution	0.1 mm

$$\frac{90 \times 100}{9 \times 1 \text{ mm}^2 \times 0.1 \text{ mm}} = 10,000/\text{mm}^3 \text{ (μL) or } 10.0 \times 10^9/\text{L}$$

■ **FIGURE 34-12** Calculation formula for hemacytometer cell counts.

MANUAL ERYTHROCYTE COUNT

Manual erythrocyte counts are occasionally performed on certain body fluids; therefore they are included in this chapter. Whole blood is diluted with a 0.85% saline solution, which prevents erythrocyte (red blood cell) lysis and facili-

⊘ TABLE 34-7		
Conditions Commonly Associated with Changes in Erythrocyte, Leukocyte, and Platelet Concentrations		
	Increased Concentration	**Decreased Concentration**
Erythrocyte	Polycythemia	Anemia
	Myeloproliferative disorders	Acute leukemia
	Dehydration	Myelodysplastic syndromes
		Hemorrhage
		Hemolysis
Leukocyte	Bacterial infections	Viral infections
	Inflammation	Aplastic anemia
	Metabolic intoxication	Megaloblastic anemia
	Hemolysis	Drug-induced leukopenia
	Hemorrhage	Myelodysplastic syndromes
	Tissue necrosis	
	Strenuous exercise	
	Anxiety or stress	
	Acute leukemia	
	Myeloproliferative disorders	
Platelet	Splenectomy	Immune thrombocytopenic purpura
	Hemorrhage	
	Iron deficiency anemia	Aplastic anemia
	Myeloproliferative disorders	Megaloblastic anemia
		Myelodysplastic syndromes
		Acute leukemia

tates erythrocyte counting.[23] The standard dilution for erythrocyte counts is 1:200. For the manual erythrocyte count, erythrocytes are counted in five of the smaller squares within the large center square (R, Figure 34-10) using the high dry objective (40×). Potential sources of error are listed in Web Table 34-7.

The number of erythrocytes is calculated per μL ($\times 10^{12}$/L) of blood using the calculation formula for hemacytometer cell counts (Figure 34-12). The variations are in the reciprocal of the dilution and the volume. For erythrocyte counts, the reciprocal of the dilution is 200, and the volume is 0.04 mm^3 (10 squares counted, each square's area = 0.04 mm^2; depth = 0.1 mm) when the diluted sample from a single unopette reservior is placed on both ruled areas of the hemacytometer.

The reference intervals for erythrocyte counts in adult males and adult females and children can be found in Table A on the inside cover. The reference intervals vary with age as shown. Conditions commonly associated with increased or decreased erythrocyte counts are shown in Table 34-7 (∞ Chapters 5, 9–13, 15–18, and 21).

MANUAL PLATELET COUNT

Whole blood is diluted with a 1% ammonium oxalate solution (this unopette system is used for manual leukocyte and manual platelet counts).[22] The isotonic balance of the diluent is such that all erythrocytes are lysed while the leukocytes, platelets, and reticulocytes remain intact. The standard dilution for platelet counts is 1:100. The detailed procedure is provided on the Website (∞ Chapter 34). Platelets are counted in the large center square (1 mm^2) using high dry objective (40×). With phase contrast microscopy, the platelets appear as round or oval bodies. Potential sources of error for manual platelet counts are given in Web Table 34-8 ⊘.

The number of platelets is calculated per μL ($\times 10^9$/L) of blood using the calculation formula for hemacytometer cell counts (Figure 34-12). The variations are in the reciprocal of the dilution factor and the volume. For platelet counts, the reciprocal of the dilution is 100 and the volume is 0.2 mm^3 (2 squares counted; each square's area = 1 mm^2; depth = 0.1 mm) when the diluted sample from a single unopette reservoir is placed on both ruled areas of the hemacytometer.

The reference interval for platelet counts is 150 – 440 $\times$ 10^9/L. Conditions commonly associated with increased or decreased platelet counts are shown in Table 34-7 (∞ Chapters 29, 13, 17, 23, 24, 25, and 31).

EOSINOPHIL COUNT

The eosinophil count is performed by diluting whole blood with a staining solution that contains phyloxine B, which stains the eosinophils red; all other leukocytes are preserved but not stained.[24] The detailed procedure is provided on the Website ∞ Chapter 34. Using the low power objective (10×), the eosinophils are counted in the entire ruled area of both counting chambers. Eosinophils appear bright orange-red and are clearly distinguishable from other leukocytes.

The number of eosinophils is calculated per μL ($\times 10^9$/L) of blood using the calculation formula for hemacytometer cell counts (Figure 34-12). The variations will be in the reciprocal of the dilution and the volume. For eosinophil counts, the reciprocal of the dilution for the Unopette system is 32. The volume factor will vary depending on the total area needed to count 100 eosinophils and the depth of the hemacytometer (e.g., Fuchs-Rosenthal hemacytometer = 0.2 mm depth).

The reference interval for adults is $0-0.45 \times 10^9$/L. Conditions associated with an altered eosinophil count are discussed in ∞ Chapters 7, 19 and 22.

✓ Checkpoint! 9

a. *A manual platelet count was performed on an EDTA-anticoagulated blood sample. With the first unopette, 125 platelets were counted. The number of platelets counted from the second unopette was 131. What is this patient's platelet count?*

b. *What are two possible physiologic causes or mechanisms that could lead to a decrease in this patient's platelet count?*

▶ HEMOGLOBIN CONCENTRATION

This procedure dilutes whole blood in cyanmethemoglobin reagent. The diluting fluid hemolyzes the erythrocytes, releasing hemoglobin into the solution. The ferrous ions (Fe^{2+}) of the hemoglobin molecules are oxidized by potassium ferricyanide to ferric ions (Fe^{3+}). This oxidation results in the formation of methemoglobin, which combines with the cyanide ions (CN^-) to form cyanmethemoglobin, a stable compound that can be quantitated using spectrophotometry.[25,26] All hemoglobin derivatives except sulfhemoglobin are converted to cyanmethemoglobin. The detailed procedure is provided on the Website ∞ Chapter 34.

When measured spectrophotometrically at 540 nm, the absorbance of cyanmethemoglobin follows **Beer-Lambert's law** and is directly proportional to the concentration of hemoglobin in the blood. A reference (standard) curve is prepared using cyanmethemoglobin standard solutions of known hemoglobin concentrations (Figure 34-13 ■). The hemoglobin concentration (patient or control) is read from the reference (standard) curve. The reference intervals for hemoglobin vary with age and sex as shown in Table A on the inside cover. Conditions associated with changes in hemoglobin concentration are broadly divided into those associated with decreased levels, the anemias (∞ Chapters 5, 8–13, and 15–18), and those associated with increased levels, the polycythemias (∞ Chapters 5 and 22).

Several physiologic conditions lead to turbidity in the cyanmethemoglobin reagent-patient sample mixture (Table 34-8 ☺).

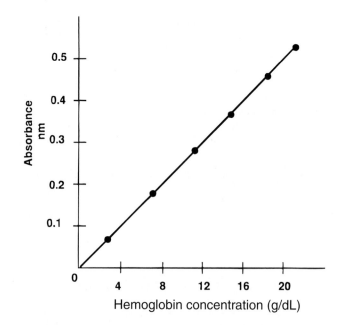

■ **FIGURE 34-13**   Hemoglobin standard calibration curve. When using this standard curve, if the absorbance for a patient's hemoglobin determination is 0.250, the hemoglobin result is 10.0 g/dL.

Any turbidity in the mixture results in falsely elevated values. It is important to recognize the falsely elevated result and take the appropriate corrective action to obtain the true hemoglobin value. A falsely elevated hemoglobin result can be indicated by poor correlation between the patient's hemoglobin and hematocrit result (i.e., hemoglobin × 3 = hematocrit) as will be discussed.

▶ HEMATOCRIT

The hematocrit of a blood sample is the packed cell volume (PCV) denoting the percentage of erythrocytes in a known volume of whole blood.[27,28] It is one of the simplest and most reproducible laboratory tests. The hematocrit is useful in detecting anemia and polycythemia.

In the microhematocrit method, a capillary tube is filled with anticoagulated whole blood and centrifuged in a microhematocrit centrifuge at 10,000–15,000 g for 5 minutes (see Website ∞ Chapter 34 for this detailed procedure). The volume occupied by the erythrocytes is expressed as a percentage of the total volume (packed cell volume). Potential sources of error for this procedure are given in Web Table 34-9 ☺. The reference values vary with age and sex as shown in Table A on the inside cover.

To ensure the accuracy of the hemoglobin and hematocrit a quick mathematical check of hemoglobin × 3 = hematocrit is done. This is called the **rule of three** and works only with normocytic, normochromic erythrocytes. If the calculated hematocrit does not agree within +/−3% of the measured

⊙ TABLE 34-8

Physiologic Conditions Leading to Error in Hemoglobin Determination and Corrective Actions to Take	
Physiologic Condition	**Corrective Action**
Extremely high leukocyte count ($>50.0 \times 10^9$/L)	Centrifuge hemoglobin mixture and use supernatant to determine hemoglobin concentration.
Presence of hemoglobin S or hemoglobin C	Use a 1:2 dilution of the hemoglobin mixture with distilled water to determine hemoglobin concentration (multiply hemoglobin by 2).
Presence of lipemia	Use a patient blank or replace patient's plasma with isotonic saline to determine hemoglobin concentration.
Presence of abnormal globulins (e.g., those found in multiple myeloma or Waldenstrom's macroglobulinemia)	Increase the alkalinity of the cyanmethemoglobin reagent by adding potassium carbonate, and then repeat hemoglobin determination.

hematocrit, a measurement error or instrument malfunction could have occurred, or the patient could have a pathology that requires investigation.

▶ ERYTHROCYTE INDICES

Wintrobe introduced the erythrocyte indices, **mean cell volume (MCV)**, **mean cell hemoglobin (MCH)**, and **mean cell hemoglobin concentration (MCHC)** in 1929. These indices are calculated from the erythrocyte count, hemoglobin concentration, and hematocrit (Table 34-9 ⊙). With the advent of automation in hematology, the erythrocyte indices are measured and/or calculated from data collected by erythrocyte analysis (∞ Chapter 36). The electrical impedance counters measure the MCV by averaging the heights of the voltage pulses. The MCH, MCHC, and hematocrit are calculated from the measured values, MCV, hemoglobin, and erythrocyte count. The automated MCV eliminates the problem of a falsely elevated MCV due to trapped plasma in the centrifuged hematocrit sample. Likewise, the MCHC can also be affected in cases of increased trapped plasma (e.g., sickle cell anemia). The manually cal-

culated MCHC is lower than that obtained from the automated instrument. When the hematocrit is corrected for trapped plasma, the erythrocyte indices calculated from the centrifuged hematocrit agree with those obtained from automated instruments. The erythrocyte indices are used in the morphologic classification of anemias, defining normocytic, microcytic, and macrocytic anemias with the MCV (∞ Chapter 8).

✓ Checkpoint! 10

Given the following erythrocyte data, what is the expected erythrocyte morphology? hemoglobin = 6.2 g/dL; hematocrit = 0.28 L/L; erythrocyte count = 4.10 × 10¹²/L

▶ ERYTHROCYTE SEDIMENTATION RATE

The ESR is a measurement of the rate at which the erythrocytes settle from the plasma. The sedimentation process consists of three phases. Phase 1 occurs within the first 5 to 10

⊙ TABLE 34-9

Erythrocyte Indices		
Calculation	**Example**	**Reference Interval (Conventional)**
$\text{MCV}^* = \dfrac{\text{Hct (\%)}}{\text{RBC } (\times 10^{12}\text{/L})} \times 10$	$\dfrac{42.6}{4.88} \times 10 = 87 \text{ fL}$	80–100 fL
$\text{MCH}^\dagger = \dfrac{\text{Hb (g/dL)}}{\text{RBC } (\times 10^{12}\text{/L})} \times 10$	$\dfrac{14.2}{4.88} \times 10 = 29 \text{ pg}$	28–34 pg
$\text{MCHC}^\ddagger = \dfrac{\text{Hb (g/dL)}}{\text{Hct (\%)}} \times 100$	$\dfrac{14.2}{42.6} \times 100 = 33 \text{ g/dL}$	32–36 g/dL

* If Hct is expressed in L/L, multiply by 1000 instead of 10.
† If Hb is expressed in g/L, do not multiply by 10.
‡ If Hct is expressed in L/L, do not multiply by 100; if Hct is expressed in L/L and Hb in g/L, divide results by 10 and do not multiply by 100.

minutes and represents the aggregation phase when erythrocytes form rouleaux. The second phase is the sedimentation phase when erythrocytes aggregate and the aggregates fall out of solution. The third phase is the packing phase in which the erythrocyte aggregates pack closely together at the bottom of the tube. The rate of erythrocyte settling depends on (1) the protein composition of the plasma, (2) the size and shape of the erythrocytes, and (3) the erythrocyte concentration.[29,30] Increasing levels of plasma proteins (primarily **acute phase reactants** such as C-reactive protein, fibrinogen, alpha globulins, or gamma globulins) result in a decrease of the zeta potential surrounding the erythrocytes. With a lower zeta potential, the erythrocytes are able to join together in rouleaux formation and settle from the plasma at a faster rate. Likewise, the erythrocytes' size and shape affect the rate of fall. Macrocytes settle faster than normal erythrocytes, and microcytes settle slower. Due to their irregular shape, poikilocytes are unable to form rouleaux and settle at a slower rate. The erythrocyte concentration directly affects the ESR (i.e., the higher the erythrocyte concentration, the lower the ESR). An anemic individual will appear to have an increased ESR.

The ESR is used to demonstrate the presence of inflammation and/or tissue destruction. It is a nonspecific test indicating tissue destruction/inflammation but not specifying the cause (i.e., disease state responsible). Table 34-10 ✪ lists a number of conditions associated with an elevated ESR.[31,32]

The CLSI's recommended method is the Westergren method in which EDTA-anticoagulated whole blood is diluted with 0.85% NaCl (see Website ∞ Chapter 34 for the detailed procedure). The diluted blood is aspirated into a calibrated Westergren pipet, and the cells are allowed to settle for a period of exactly 1 hour (Web Figure 34-6 ■) at the end of which the distance in millimeters between the meniscus of the plasma and the top of the sedimented erythrocyte column is read. Potential sources of error in the modified Westergren method for ESR are provided in Web Table 34-10 ✪. The reference interval for ESR varies with age and sex. For adult males and children, the reference interval is 0–10 mm/hr. The reference interval for adult females is 0–20 mm/hr.

Automated methods for determining ESR have been available since the 1990s. The principle of measurement for each instrument is an adaptation of the manual Westergren ESR method that allows determination of ESR in a shorter time period, typically 20 to 30 minutes. The automated methods convert the observed result to "mm/hr" so that reported results are in the conventional unit of measurement for the Westergren ESR. These methods have been verified to provide results comparable to those of the manual Westergren method.[33] The advantage of automated instruments is that they allow standardization of the procedure, increasing accuracy and reproducibility of the results.

One example of an automated ESR instrument is the MINI-VES™ instrument (Diesse Diagnostica Senese, Milan, Italy). It is a compact instrument that simultaneously determines the ESR on 4 samples.[34] The sample is collected in a special vacuum collection tube containing 0.25 mL of 0.105 mol/L sodium citrate. The collection tubes are thoroughly mixed on a laboratory rocker and then placed in the instrument. Within the instrument, the collection tubes are held at an angle of 18°. A photoelectric cell passes up the collection tube and records the height of the erythrocyte column based on the point at which the light transmission is detected, the "initial" reading. After 20 minutes, the process is repeated to obtain the "final" reading. The decrease in height of the erythrocyte column is determined and used to mathematically derive the ESR in mm/hr.

The ESR-Auto Plus™ instrument (Streck, Inc., Omaha, NE) is a random access instrument with 10 ESR tube positions (Figure 34-14 ■).[35] The instrument uses a special vacuum tube containing 3.2% sodium citrate. It is a narrow bore and

✪ TABLE 34-10
Conditions Associated with an Elevated ESR
• Acute and chronic infections
• Acute coronary syndrome
• Multiple myeloma
• Osteomyelitis
• Pelvic inflammatory disease
• Polymyalgia rheumatica
• Pregnancy
• Pulmonary tuberculosis
• Rheumatic fever
• Rheumatoid arthritis
• Systemic lupus erythematosus
• Subacute bacterial endocarditis
• Waldenstrom's macroglobulinemia

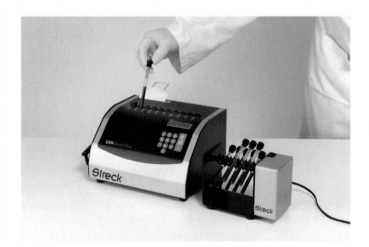

■ FIGURE 34-14   Streck ESR Auto-Plus™ Instrument. (Courtesy of Streck, Inc., Omaha, NE)

100 mm tube, and when filled properly blood is drawn to the 60 mm mark ± 9 mm. Alternatively, an EDTA-anticoagulated sample can be used. In this case, the proper amount of blood is transferred from the EDTA sample to the ESR vacuum tube. The vacuum tubes are thoroughly mixed prior to placing them in the instrument. The vacuum tubes are held in a vertical position at ambient temperature. The instrument scans the tube to determine the height of the packed erythrocyte column at 30 minutes. The observed result is converted to "mm/hr" using a mathematical formula. Using this method, the measurement can be taken at 30 minutes because the majority of samples reach the "packing" phase of the erythrocyte sedimentation process by this time.

C-reactive protein (CRP) determinations by immunologic techniques such as nephelometry or enzyme-linked immunoassays have been introduced as a quantitative replacement for the ESR. CRP is an acute phase reactant that becomes elevated in the same conditions as the ESR. In fact, studies have demonstrated a rise in CRP levels prior to an elevation in the ESR.[36] Normal individuals have low levels of CRP, less than 5 mg/dL. In cases of inflammation, CRP levels can rise to 20–500 mg/dL within 8 hours of the acute inflammatory event.[37] CRP levels provide a quantitative measurement that can be used to monitor individuals with rheumatoid arthritis for better therapeutic management of the disease.[38] However, these assays are not sensitive enough for risk assessment for myocardial infarction or artherosclerosis. The high-sensitivity CRP assay is required if CRP levels are to be used as markers or predictors for those conditions.[39,40]

▶ RETICULOCYTE COUNT

Reticulocytes are immature nonnucleated erythrocytes containing residual RNA (i.e., polychromatophilic erythrocytes). In the erythrocyte maturation sequence, the reticulocyte spends about 2 days in the bone marrow and 1 day in the peripheral blood. As the reticulocyte matures, the amount of RNA decreases. The quantitation of reticulocytes present in the peripheral blood provides a method of evaluating the bone marrow's erythropoietic activity. This evaluation is utilized in the differential diagnosis of anemias and in monitoring a patient's erythropoietic response to therapy (∞ Chapters 5 and 8).[41–44]

Using a **supravital stain** (new methylene blue), residual ribosomal RNA is precipitated within the reticulocytes.[45] The detailed procedure is provided on the Website ∞ Chapter 34. A blood smear is prepared from the mixture of anticoagulated whole blood and supravital stain. The smear is examined microscopically using the oil immersion lens (1000× magnification) fitted with a field-restricted ocular (Figure 34-15 ■). An erythrocyte containing two or more particles of blue-stained material is a reticulocyte (Figure 34-16 ■). The number of reticulocytes is expressed as a percentage of the total number of erythrocytes counted (Web Figure 34-7 ■).

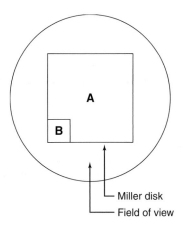

■ FIGURE 34-15 Miller disk. Reticulocyte counting area = A; erythrocyte counting area = B. The B square is one-ninth the area of the A square.

Other erythrocyte inclusions (Pappenheimer bodies, Howell-Jolly bodies, and Heinz bodies; ∞ Chapter 8) can also be stained with new methylene blue and must be distinguished from reticulocytes. Howell-Jolly bodies and Heinz bodies are distinguished from precipitated reticulum by their shape and staining characteristics. Heinz bodies appear as light blue-green inclusions located at the periphery of the erythrocyte. Howell-Jolly bodies are usually one or two round, deep-purple staining inclusions and are visible on Romanowsky stains. Pappenheimer bodies are indistiguishable from reticulum of reticulocytes. If Pappenheimer bodies are suspected, a Prussian-blue iron stain (∞ Chapter 35) should be performed to verify their presence. Reticulum does not stain with the Prussian-blue iron stain.

Misinterpretations can occur when only the percentage of reticulocytes present in the peripheral blood is reported because the reticulocyte percentage is a relative number and depends on the total number of erythrocytes present in the peripheral blood. If the total erythrocyte count is decreased,

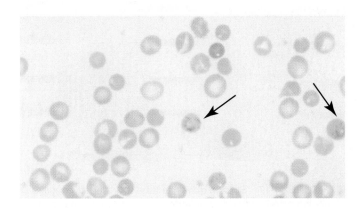

■ FIGURE 34-16 Reticulocytes identified by new methylene blue stain. The reticulocytes are the cells containing bluish purple particulate inclusions. (1000× original magnification)

the reticulocyte percentage does not accurately reflect the bone marrow's production of new erythrocytes. The absolute reticulocyte count, corrected reticulocyte count, and the reticulocyte production index can be used to avoid these interpretation errors. These calculations are discussed in ∞ Chapter 8.

Automation is becoming a more popular method for the determination of the reticulocyte count. The new generation of automated hematology instruments is capable of performing absolute reticulocyte counts and other useful parameters. A thorough discussion can be found in ∞ Chapter 36.

✓ Checkpoint! 11

Morphologic evaluation of a Wright-stained peripheral blood smear reveals the presence of Pappenheimer bodies. How does this affect a reticulocyte count to be performed on the same blood sample? How would you confirm the presence of Pappenheimer bodies?

▶ SOLUBILITY TEST FOR HEMOGLOBIN S

The solubility test is the most commonly used screening test for the presence of hemoglobin S (∞ Chapters 6 and 10). It is based on the relative insolubility of hemoglobin S when combined with a reducing agent (sodium dithionite).[46] Anticoagulated whole blood is mixed with a lysing agent (saponin) and reducing agent. This solution releases the hemoglobin from the erythrocytes and reduces it. If HbS is present, it forms crystals and gives a turbid appearance to the solution (Figure 34-17 ■). A transparent solution is seen with other hemoglobins that are more soluble in the reducing agent (see Website ∞ Chapter 34 for the detailed procedure).

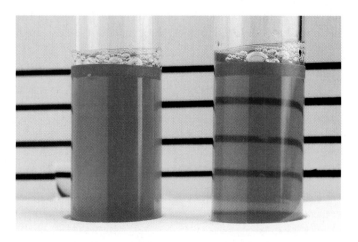

■ **FIGURE 34-17** Sodium dithionite tube test. Negative results are indicated by the clear solution, where the black lines on the reader scale are visible through the test solution (right). Positive results are shown as a turbid solution, where the reader scale is not visible through the test solution (left).

The solubility test does not differentiate hemoglobin S disease from hemoglobin S trait. A hemoglobin electrophoresis procedure should be performed to differentiate these two states. In addition, several abnormal hemoglobin variants can cause sickling and give a positive solubility test. These variants include HbC Harlem, HbS Travis, and HbC Ziguinchor. High-pressure liquid chromatography or **isoelectric focusing** is used to differentiate these variants from HbS.

PART II

REFLEX HEMATOLOGY PROCEDURES

▶ HEMOGLOBIN ELECTROPHORESIS USING CELLULOSE ACETATE

Electrophoresis is the movement of charged molecules in an electric field. Use of this procedure (∞ Chapters 10 and 11)[47] can detect and preliminarily identify hemoglobinopathies and thalassemias. In hemoglobin electrophoresis, hemoglobin A (adult hemoglobin) takes on a net negative charge at an alkaline pH and moves the farthest toward the anode (positive electrode). Many abnormal hemoglobin variants have altered charges due to single amino acid substitutions within their globin chains (∞ Chapter 10). This change in the degree of the negative charge allows for the separation of the majority of abnormal hemoglobin variants from hemoglobin A at an alkaline pH.[48,49] The electrophoretic patterns and hemoglobin percentages of the unknown (patient) samples are compared to those of the control sample containing HbA, -F, -S, and -C, and those of a known adult sample.

In the hemoglobin electrophoresis procedure, EDTA-anticoagulated whole blood is centrifuged to obtain packed erythrocytes. The erythrocytes are washed, and a hemolysate is obtained by lysing them with a hemolysate reagent (e.g., 0.005 M EDTA). The hemolysate (i.e., patient, control, or known adult sample) is applied to a cellulose acetate plate, which is then placed in the electrophoresis chamber. An alkaline buffer, pH 8.6, permits the flow of electrons from the cathode to the anode within the chamber, alters the charge of the hemoglobin molecules based on their amino acid composition, and allows for the migration and separation of the hemoglobin molecules based on the strength of their negative charge. The hemoglobin molecules are allowed to electrophorese (migrate) for 25 minutes. Following the electrophoresis, the cellulose acetate plate is stained with Ponceau S, a protein dye-binding stain. The stained plate is cleared to remove the cellulose acetate and create a transparent plate with the stained hemoglobin bands representing the hemoglobin electrophoretic pattern for each sample. This plate can then be evaluated visually or with a **densitometer** using 525 nm filter to determine the percentage of hemoglobin present in each band or region.

Cellulose acetate electrophoresis allows for the separation of HbA, -F, -S, and -C into distinct bands (Figure 34-18 ■). However, other abnormal hemoglobin variants have the same electrophoretic mobility as HbS and HbC. HbD and HbG have the same mobility as HbS whereas HbE and HbO_Arab have the same mobility as HbC. Thus, additional tests must be used to confirm the presence of these abnormal hemoglobin variants. The solubility test can be used to confirm HbS, and citrate agar electrophoresis can be used to confirm the presence of HbS and HbC.

Citrate agar electrophoresis at pH 6.2 separates HbA, -F, -S, -C into distinct bands (Figure 34-19 ■). Because no other hemoglobin variants travel with HbS and HbC on citrate agar, it is used to confirm their presence.[50] It is also useful in differentiating other hemoglobin variants that travel with HbS and HbC on cellulose acetate electrophoresis; these hemoglobin variants (HbD, HbG, HbE, and HbO_Arab) have the same mobility as HbA on citrate agar. Rare abnormal hemoglobin variants can be positively identified with DNA analysis of the globin genes (∞ Chapter 39).

✓ **Checkpoint! 12**

What is the basis for hemoglobin separation in the hemoglobin electrophoresis procedures?

▶ **QUANTITATION OF HEMOGLOBIN A₂**

HbA₂ is a normal adult hemoglobin present in small amounts (up to 3.5%). Increased amounts of HbA₂ are characteristic of beta thalassemia minor. Therefore, the quantita-

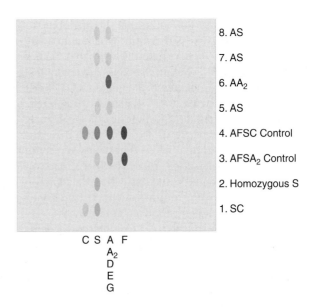

■ **FIGURE 34-19** Electrophoretic mobilities of hemoglobins on citrate agar at pH 6.2, showing separation of hemoglobins S and C from other hemoglobins. (Key: A, A₂, S, F, C, D, E, G = hemoglobin variants)

tion of HbA₂ is useful in its presumptive diagnosis. Slight increases in HbA₂ concentration also have been noted in persons with either HbS trait, HbS disease, unstable hemoglobin variants, or megaloblastic anemia. Decreased HbA₂ concentrations can be seen in iron-deficiency anemia or alpha thalassemia.

Hemoglobin A₂ can be quantitated with anion exchange **column chromatography.** The anion exchange resin is a preparation of cellulose covalently coupled to small positively charged molecules. Thus, the anion exchange resin attracts negatively charged molecules. Hemoglobins, like other proteins, contain positive and negative charges due to the ionizing properties of their component amino acids. In the anion exchange chromatography of hemoglobin A₂, the ionic strength of the buffer and the pH levels are controlled to cause different hemoglobins to possess different net negative charges.[51] These negatively charged proteins are attracted to the positively charged cellulose and bind accordingly. Following binding, the hemoglobins are removed selectively from the resin by altering the pH or ionic strength of the elution buffer. Due to the solubility of hemoglobin A₂ in the elution buffer, hemoglobin A₂ is eluted from the resin as the elution buffer moves through the column. The resin retains the other normal, and most abnormal, hemoglobins. The percentage of hemoglobin A₂ is determined by comparing the absorbance of the hemoglobin A₂ fraction to the absorbance of the total hemoglobin fraction at 415 nm using a spectrophotometer. The CDC National Hemoglobinopathy Laboratory reference interval for HbA₂ is 1.8–3.5%.

Values between 3.5% and 8% are considered indicative of beta thalassemia trait (∞ Chapter 11). Values above 8%

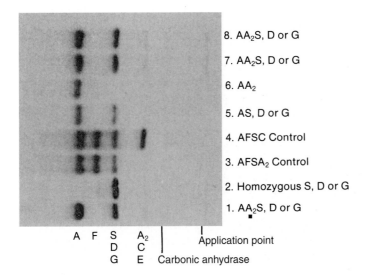

■ **FIGURE 34-18** Electrophoretic mobilities of hemoglobins on cellulose acetate at pH 8.6. (Key: A, A₂, D, G, S, F, C, E = hemoglobin variants) (Courtesy of Helena Laboratories, Beaumont, TX)

indicate the presence of additional hemoglobin variants such as S, C, E, O, D, and S-G hybrid, which elute with HbA$_2$ (∞ Chapter 10). HbA$_2$ cannot be differentiated from several abnormal hemoglobin variants such as hemoglobins C, E, and O, which have a net electrical charge similar to HbA$_2$ at pH 8.6. If abnormal hemoglobin variants are suspected, other hemoglobin electrophoretic techniques or DNA analysis of globin chains should be performed to confirm their presence. HbA$_2$ levels can be normal when iron-deficiency anemia co-exists with beta thalassemia minor. In this situation, HbA$_2$ levels must be considered with family history, laboratory data including serum ferritin, serum iron, total iron-binding capacity, red cell morphology, Hb, Hct, and MCV.

Other techniques can be used to quantitate hemoglobin A$_2$ including high-pressure liquid chromatography and enzyme-linked immunoassay. The enzyme-linked immunoassay utilizes a monoclonal antibody that is directed against the delta-chain, making the assay specific for Hb A$_2$.[52]

The Bio-Rad VARIANT™ II hemoglobin instrument measures Hb A$_{1c}$ levels for glycemic control in diabetic patients and can be used to quantitate Hb A$_2$, HbF, and certain hemoglobin variants.[53–56] For the quantitation of these hemoglobins, this fully automated instrument requires a separate cation-exchange column, specific sodium phosphate buffers and elution program (i.e. Beta-Thal Short program). Within the instrument, a portion of EDTA-anticoagulated blood sample is hemolyzed and diluted and then injected into the cation exchange column. The hemoglobins are separated using a gradient of sodium phosphate buffers of increasing ionic strength for a 6.5 minute elution. The eluted hemoglobins pass through a flow cell where the absorbance is measured at 415 nm with correction at 690 nm. The eluted hemoglobin is identified by its retention time. For example, Hb A$_2$'s retention time is between 3.3 and 3.9 minutes. The concentration of the eluted hemoglobin is determined from its absorbance measurement.

► ACID ELUTION FOR HEMOGLOBIN F

The acid elution test for fetal hemoglobin (HbF) can be used in the differentiation of hereditary persistence of fetal hemoglobin (HPFH) from other conditions associated with high levels of HbF (∞ Chapters 10 and 11). HPFH is characterized by an even or uniform distribution of HbF within the erythrocytes whereas other conditions with high HbF levels are characterized by an uneven or nonuniform distribution of HbF within the erythrocytes. Conditions such as beta thalassemia minor, beta thalassemia major, sickle cell anemia, hereditary spherocytosis, and aplastic anemia are associated with high levels of HbF but nonuniform distribution. This stain can also be used to detect the presence of fetal cells in the maternal circulation (fetal-maternal bleed) during problem pregnancies.

In an acid solution, all hemoglobins are eluted from the erythrocytes except hemoglobin F (fetal hemoglobin).[57]

Blood smears are fixed in 80% ethanol and then incubated in the elution buffer, citrate-phosphate (pH 3.3). The slide is stained with acid hematoxylin and counterstained with eosin. The slide is observed microscopically using the oil immersion lens to determine the distribution of HbF within the erythrocytes and the percentage of HbF-containing erythrocytes. Erythrocytes containing fetal hemoglobin stain bright pink or red with the eosin B stain (Figure 34-20■). The rest of the erythrocytes appear as pale ghosts. Intermediate erythrocytes (pink colored, but not intense) are sometimes seen. The acid hematoxylin stains the leukocyte's nuclei a faint gray purple.

► QUANTITATION OF HEMOGLOBIN F

ALKALI DENATURATION

HbF is resistant to denaturation by strong alkali solutions, but other hemoglobins are not resistant. The addition of a strong alkali solution (1.27 M NaOH) to a hemolysate containing a known concentration of hemoglobin results in hemoglobin denaturation.[58] Adding a saturated solution of ammonium sulfate stops the denaturation process. Ammonium sulfate lowers the pH of the reaction mixture and precipitates all denatured hemoglobins. After filtration, the concentration of the remaining alkali-resistant hemoglobin is determined. The alkali-resistant hemoglobin is expressed as a percentage of the total hemoglobin concentration. The cyanmethemoglobin method determines the hemoglobin concentrations (alkali-resistant and total). The general reference interval for an adult is less than 2%.

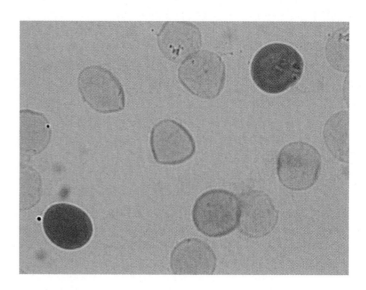

■ FIGURE 34-20   Acid elution test for determination of hemoglobin F. Erythrocytes containing hemoglobin F appear as bright pink staining cells. The light staining cells are erythrocytes that contain adult hemoglobins.

OTHER METHODS

In the clinical laboratory, HbF is typically determined by high-pressure liquid chromatography as discussed previously with HbA$_2$ quantitation or by flow cytometry. In flow cytometry, the cells are permeabilized to allow entry of the fluorescent-conjugated monoclonal antibody directed against HbF into the cell for recognition of HbF. The advantage of flow cytometry is that an increased number of cells (~10,000) are evaluated, thus improving the accuracy of the result. In addition, flow cytometry allows the determination of HbF concentration within individual cells and with the addition of thiazole orange, the differentiation of cells containing HbF such as mature erythrocytes, polychromatophilic erythrocytes or reticulocytes, and nucleated erythrocytes, which can be useful in evaluating certain hematologic diseases (e.g., β-thalassemia).[59]

 Checkpoint! 13

What are the advantages of using flow cytometry to quantitate HbF?

▶ HEAT DENATURATION TEST FOR UNSTABLE HEMOGLOBIN

Unstable hemoglobins are hemoglobin variants that result from a variety of amino acid substitutions or deletions affecting the intramolecular interactions of the hemoglobin molecule (∞ Chapter 10). These hemoglobin variants are susceptible to spontaneous denaturation resulting in Heinz body formation and erythrocyte hemolysis. In the laboratory, blood samples can be manipulated so that unstable hemoglobins become insoluble and form flocculent precipitate at higher temperatures (50°C) whereas normal hemoglobin remains soluble.[60,61] The hemoglobin concentrations for heated and unheated fractions are determined by the cyanmethemoglobin method. The concentration of unstable hemoglobin is expressed as a percentage of the total hemoglobin concentration (unheated fraction). Low concentrations of unstable hemoglobin result in false negative results.

Unstable hemoglobins can cause congenital nonspherocytic hemolytic anemias (∞ Chapter 10). Examples of unstable hemoglobins are hemoglobin Koln, hemoglobin Hammersmith, hemoglobin Zurich, hemoglobin Seattle, and hemoglobin Bristol. A positive heat denaturation test should be confirmed by other test methods that identify unstable hemoglobins, such as tests for erythrocyte inclusions and the **isopropanol precipitation** test. The specific unstable hemoglobin is identified by DNA sequence analysis to determine the hemoglobin mutation followed by HPLC and tandem mass spectrometry analysis to confirm the specific amino acid substitution.

▶ HEINZ BODY STAIN

Heinz bodies represent denatured hemoglobin inclusions that are usually round or oval, appear refractile, and tend to locate adjacent to the erythrocyte membrane. Heinz bodies are visible only on supravital stained smears and are not visible on Wright-stained smears. Heinz bodies can be present in glucose-6-phosphate dehydrogenase deficiency and related enzyme disorders when the individual is exposed to oxidizing agents such as primaquine or sulfanilamide (∞ Chapter 16). In addition, they can be found in individuals with unstable hemoglobins or thalassemias. Heinz bodies are occasionally found in senescent erythrocytes of normal individuals.

A specific dye for Heinz bodies is brilliant green.[62] To visualize Heinz bodies, EDTA-anticoagulated whole blood is first mixed with 0.5% neutral red. The mixture is counterstained with 0.5% brilliant green. Several thick smears are prepared from the final mixture. The smears are observed microscopically for the presence of Heinz bodies. Heinz bodies stain green, reticulocytes and Howell-Jolly bodies stain a deep red, and erythrocytes stain light red. The percentage of erythrocytes containing Heinz bodies can be determined by counting the number of erythrocytes containing Heinz bodies within 500 erythrocytes.

The specificity of the brilliant green dye for Heinz bodies eliminates problems that arise with the use of other supravital stains such as methyl violet or crystal violet. With these other supravital stains, Howell-Jolly bodies, basophilic stippling, and reticulum stain the same as Heinz bodies, often leading to difficulties in interpreting the stain.

▶ OSMOTIC FRAGILITY TEST

In the osmotic fragility test heparin-anticoagulated whole blood is added to increasingly hypotonic solutions of buffered sodium chloride (0.85% to 0.00%) and the solutions incubate for 20 minutes at room temperature.[63] The amount of hemolysis at each concentration is determined by measuring the absorbance of the **supernatants** spectrophotometrically (see Website ∞ Chapter 34 for the detailed procedure). An osmotic fragility graph is prepared by plotting the percentage of hemolysis for each solution against its concentration, and the results are compared to a normal control. In normal individuals, an almost symmetrical sigmoid shaped curve is obtained (Figure 34-21 ■). Normal erythrocytes begin to hemolyze around 0.50% sodium chloride (NaCl) concentration, and hemolysis is complete at 0.30% NaCl. The normal values for osmotic fragility with each sodium concentration are given in Table J in the inside book cover.

In the osmotic fragility test, spherocytes with a decreased surface-area-to-volume ratio have a limited ability to expand in hypotonic solutions. They lyse at higher concentrations of sodium chloride than normal biconcave erythrocytes and

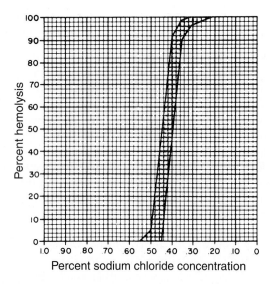

■ FIGURE 34-21 Normal osmotic fragility curve. The osmotic fragility curve of a normal individual would fall within the area defined by the two sigmoid curves. A curve to the left of normal indicates increased fragility and a curve to the right decreased fragility.

are said to have an increased osmotic fragility. Target cells or sickle cells have a large surface-area-to-volume ratio. This increased surface-area-to-volume ratio translates into an increased ability to expand in hypotonic solutions. These cells lyse at lower concentrations of sodium chloride than normal cells and are said to have a decreased osmotic fragility.

An increased osmotic fragility is associated with hemolytic anemias in which spherocytes, particularly hereditary spherocytosis, are present (∞ Chapter 15). Conditions associated with a decreased osmotic fragility include thalassemia, sickle cell anemia, and those conditions in which target cells are observed. Figure 34-22■ depicts the increased osmotic lysis of spherocytes in a hypotonic medium.

An incubated osmotic fragility test is performed to identify patients with mild hereditary spherocytosis in which the standard osmotic fragility test is normal. In the incubated osmotic fragility test, a patient's blood and control blood are incubated for 24 hours at 37°C under sterile conditions. A significantly increased osmotic fragility after incubation is characteristic of hereditary spherocytosis.

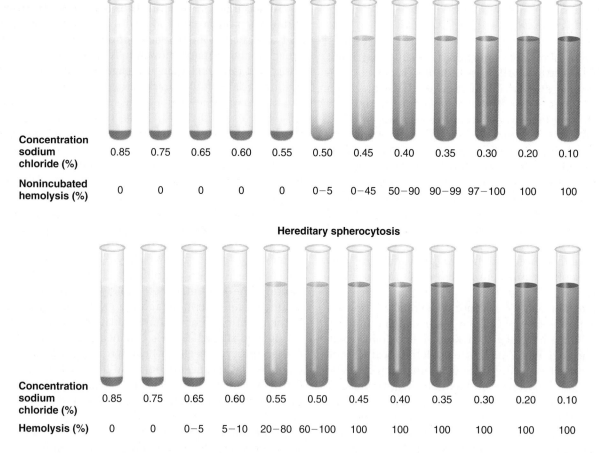

Normal

Concentration sodium chloride (%)	0.85	0.75	0.65	0.60	0.55	0.50	0.45	0.40	0.35	0.30	0.20	0.10
Nonincubated hemolysis (%)	0	0	0	0	0	0–5	0–45	50–90	90–99	97–100	100	100

Hereditary spherocytosis

Concentration sodium chloride (%)	0.85	0.75	0.65	0.60	0.55	0.50	0.45	0.40	0.35	0.30	0.20	0.10
Hemolysis (%)	0	0	0–5	5–10	20–80	60–100	100	100	100	100	100	100

■ FIGURE 34-22 The osmotic fragility test demonstrates the increased osmotic lysis of spherocytes in a hypotonic medium compared with normal erythrocytes. (Key: clear supernatant = no hemolysis; pinkish supernatant = partial hemolysis; red supernatant = complete hemolysis)

✓ Checkpoint! 14

A patient's osmotic fragility test shows beginning hemolysis at 0.60% NaCl and complete hemolysis at 0.50% NaCl. How should these results be interpreted?

▶ SUGAR-WATER SCREENING TEST

A sugar-water solution (10%) provides a low-ionic-strength solution that promotes the attachment of complement to susceptible paroxysmal nocturnal hemoglobinuria erythrocytes.[64] Upon attachment of complement, the erythrocytes hemolyze. Normal erythrocytes do not hemolyze under these conditions. A positive sugar-water test (sucrose hemolysis test) is presumptive evidence for paroxysmal nocturnal hemoglobinuria (PNH) (∞ Chapter 15). In the past, the acidified serum test was used to confirm PNH. However, flow cytometry is now the preferred method because it detects the absence of glycosyl phosphatidylinositol-anchored complement regulatory proteins, CD55 (decay accelerating factor), and CD59 (membrane inhibitor of reactive lysis), which are diagnostic for PNH.[65]

▶ DONATH-LANDSTEINER TEST FOR PCH

The Donath-Landsteiner test is a screening test for paroxysmal cold hemoglobinuria (PCH),[66] which is characterized by the presence of the Donath-Landsteiner antibody, a **biphasic antibody** with anti-P specificity (∞ Chapter 17). This IgG antibody is capable of activating complement resulting in hemolysis. The Donath-Landsteiner test should be performed when an individual presents with hemoglobinuria and a positive direct antiglobulin test due to C3 only with no evidence of autoantibody activity in the serum. In this procedure, a series of test tubes is set up to detect the biphasic nature of complement activation (Table 34-11 ✪). Normal serum serves as a source of complement because individuals with PCH can express low levels of complement. The 50% suspension of group O erythrocytes with P antigen serves as the antibody receptor. Following the appropriate incubation schedule, the tubes are centrifuged and observed for hemolysis. If anti-P is present in the patient's serum, it will bind to the erythrocyte's P antigen during the incubation time in the melting ice bath. During the second incubation time at 37°C, the antibody dissociates from the erythrocytes, and complement is activated leading to hemolysis. Therefore, the test is considered positive for PCH if tubes A1 and/or A2 demonstrate hemolysis and the remaining tubes have no hemolysis. Proper sample collection and processing are essential to this test's outcome. Patient's blood should be allowed to clot at 37°C and the serum separated at this temperature to avoid cold autoabsorption and loss of antibody prior to testing.

▶ ERYTHROPOIETIN

Erythropoietin (EPO) levels are determined by enzyme-linked immunosorbent assay (ELISA). In this procedure, microtiter plate wells are coated with a monoclonal mouse antihuman antibody directed against EPO.[67] This antibody represents the capture antibody because it will bind EPO from the serum, either patient, control, or standard. Following a washing step, the wells are incubated with a polyclonal rabbit anti-EPO that is enzyme-labeled with horseradish peroxidase. This second antibody will bind to the initial antigen–antibody complex. Hence, EPO is sandwiched between two specific antibodies (Web Figure 34-8 ■). A substrate specific for the enzyme label (i.e., tetramethylbenzidine) is added to the microtiter plate wells, and a colorimetric

✪ TABLE 34-11

Schematic Outline of Donath-Landsteiner Test Procedure for Detecting PCH

Incubation Set	Tube 1	Tube 2	Tube 3		Incubation Protocol
A	Patient's serum — 50% group O cells	Patient's serum Normal serum 50% group O cells	— Normal serum 50% group O cells	→	30 minutes in melting ice bath followed by 60 minutes @ 37°C
B	Patient's serum — 50% group O cells	Patient's serum Normal serum 50% group O cells	— Normal serum 50% group O cells	→	90 minutes in melting ice bath
C	Patient's serum — 50% group O cells	Patient's serum Normal serum 50% group O cells	— Normal serum 50% group O cells	→	90 minutes @ 37°C

PCH is indicated if hemolysis occurs in tubes A1 and/or A2 and remaining tubes have no hemolysis. Tubes A3, B3, and C3 represent controls for normal serum complement source and should not demonstrate hemolysis. Tubes B1 and B2 represent controls for the presence of cold-reacting antibodies, and tubes C1 and C2 represent controls for the presence of warm-reacting antibodies. Including these controls to eliminate possible false positive interpretations is important.

reaction occurs. The absorbance of each microtiter well is determined using a microtiter plate reader, an adaptation of a spectrophotometer. The amount of absorbance measured in a given microtiter well is directly proportional to the concentration of EPO in the sample. The control and patient results are determined from a reference (standard) curve that is prepared using known concentrations of EPO. The general reference interval for serum EPO is 3.3–16.6 mIU/mL.

Measurement of EPO levels is useful in diagnosing certain anemias and polycythemia. For example, secondary polycythemias such as chronic obstructive pulmonary disease or cyanotic heart disease are associated with elevated levels of EPO while the myeloproliferative disorder polycythemia vera is associated with normal to low EPO levels (∞ Chapter 22). Decreased levels of EPO are observed in anemia of renal failure, anemia of chronic disease, and anemia of hypothyroidism (∞ Chapters 9 and 13).

▶ SOLUBLE TRANSFERRIN RECEPTOR

Soluble transferrin receptor (sTfR) represents a truncated form of the membrane transferrin receptor that is normally found on the surface of cells that require iron. sTfR levels are determined by ELISA. In this procedure microtiter plate wells are coated with a monoclonal antihuman antibody directed against sTfR.[68] This antibody represents the capture antibody because it will bind sTfR from the serum from either patient, control, or standard. Following a washing step, the wells are incubated with a second monoclonal anti-sTfR that is enzyme labeled with horseradish peroxidase. This second antibody will bind to the initial antigen–antibody complex. Hence, sTfR is sandwiched between two specific antibodies (Web Figure 34-8 for comparison). A substrate specific for the enzyme label is added to the microtiter plate wells, and a colorimetric reaction occurs. The absorbance of each microtiter well is determined using a microtiter plate reader. The amount of absorbance measured in a given microtiter well is directly proportional to the concentration of sTfR in the sample. The control and patient results are determined from a reference (standard) curve that is prepared using known concentrations of sTfR. The general reference interval for serum sTfR is 8.7–28.1 nmol/L.

Measurement of sTfR levels is useful in the differential diagnosis of iron-deficiency anemia from anemia of chronic disease because sTfR levels are elevated in iron-deficiency anemia but are normal in anemia of chronic disease (∞ Chapter 9).

✓ **Checkpoint! 15**

A patient was recently diagnosed with a hypochromic, microcytic anemia. Additional laboratory testing revealed EPO 1.5 mIU/mL and sTfR 15.8 nmol/L. Which anemia is consistent with these results?

▶ CYTOCHEMICAL STAINS

Cytochemical stains are useful in differentiating the cell lineage of malignant cells in the bone marrow. The first stains done usually are the myeloperoxidase and/or Sudan black B to differentiate myeloid cells from lymphoid cells. Additional stains can be required for further differentiation such as differentiating myelocytic from monocytic cells.

MYELOPEROXIDASE

Myeloperoxidase (MPO) is an enzyme capable of catalyzing the oxidation of substances by hydrogen peroxide. The methods using 3,3-diaminobenzidine as the color reagent with Giemsa counterstain or using 3-amino-9-ethylcarbazole provide satisfactory results.[69] This enzyme is present in primary granules of neutrophils, eosinophils, and monocytes. An insoluble dark brown reaction product identifies the sites of MPO activity (Figure 34-23 ■). MPO is the most sensitive and specific stain for granulocytes, which stain intensely. Monocytes stain less intensely than neutrophils. Lymphocytes do not exhibit MPO activity. The MPO is, therefore, useful in the differentiation of acute myelogenous leukemia (AML) from acute lymphocytic leukemia (ALL) and subgrouping of the AMLs (Table 34-12 ✪; Web Table 34-11 ✪). A positive reaction is seen in myeloblasts. Weak staining rarely is seen in monoblasts. Leukemic blasts that are negative for MPO can represent lymphoblasts, AML (minimally differentiated), monoblasts, erythroblasts, and megakaryoblasts or undifferentiated leukemia.[70] The presence of many mature neutrophils with negative MPO staining can indicate a deficiency of MPO.

SUDAN BLACK B

Sudan black B (SBB) is a diazo dye that stains phospholipids, neutral fats, and sterols.[71] Cellular components containing

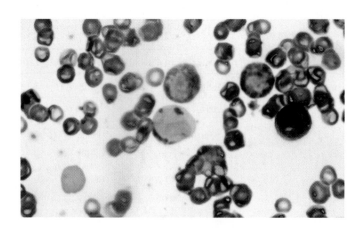

■ FIGURE 34-23   Blasts of AML showing a positive myeloperoxidase stain (brown-black color in cytoplasm). (Bone marrow; MPO stain; 500× magnification)

⊘ TABLE 34-12

Cytochemical Features of Acute Myelogenous Leukemia (AML) Subgroups

Subgroup	Myeloperoxidase or Sudan Black B	Chloroacetate (specific) Esterase	Nonspecific Esterase
AML-minimally differentiated	Negative	Negative	Negative
AML-without maturation	Positive	Positive	Negative
AML-with maturation	Positive	Positive	Negative
Acute promyelocytic leukemia	Positive	Positive	Negative
AML-myelomonocytic	Positive	Positive	Positive*
AML-monoblastic/monocytic	Negative	Negative	Positive*
Acute erythroid leukemia	Positive[†]	Negative	Positive or negative
AML-megakaryoblastic	Negative	Negative	Strongly positive when acetate is used as a substrate

*Monocytic component is positive, and the staining can be inhibited by sodium fluoride incubation. About 20% of AML-monoblastic can be negative for nonspecific esterase
[†]Myeloblasts in AML-erythroid are positive.

lipids stain brown black (Figure 34-24■). SBB stains phospholipids in membranes of primary and secondary granules of the granulocytic series. Auer rods have a rich phospholipid membrane that is identified by the SBB stain. The SBB stain results parallel those seen with the MPO stain in myeloblasts and monoblasts (Table 34-12; Web Table 34-11). Lymphoblasts do not stain with SBB (rare cases are weakly positive). This stain is useful when fresh samples are not available and in unusual cases when myeloblasts have an acquired deficiency of MPO. Therefore, it is useful in the differentiation of AML from ALL. Because of its fat solubility, SBB also can stain marrow fat and some cytoplasmic vacuoles of Burkitt lymphoma cells.[72]

CHLOROACETATE ESTERASE

Several cytochemical methods are available for specific esterase on smears. Chloroacetate esterase (also called *specific esterase*) activity is detected by incubating the sample in naphthol AS-D chloroacetate at an acid pH.[73] As a result of the esterase activity, enzymatic hydrolysis of ester linkages occurs, and free naphthol compounds are liberated. The liberated naphthol immediately couples with a diazonium salt (e.g., fast red violet) forming an insoluble, visible pigment at the site of enzyme activity (Figure 34-25■). Naphthol AS-D chloroacetate is considered specific for the granulocytic series and is present in mast cells. The sites of enzyme activity

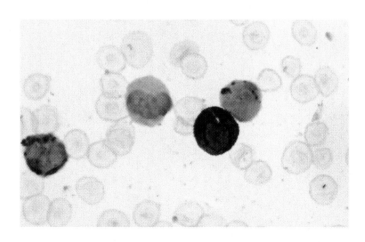

■ **FIGURE 34-24** Blasts of AML showing a positive Sudan black B stain (brown-black color in cytoplasm). (Bone marrow; SBB stain; 500× magnification)

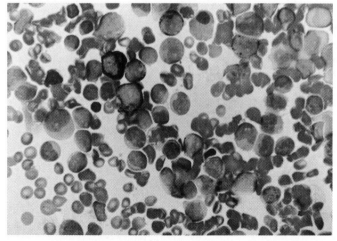

■ **FIGURE 34-25** Blasts of AML showing a positive specific esterase stain (red-magenta color in cytoplasm). (Bone marrow; specific esterase stain; 500× magnification)

show bright red granulation when fast red violet is used. Enzyme activity is weak or absent in monocytes and lymphocytes. Neoplastic eosinophils of acute myelomonoblastic leukemia rarely are positive for chloroacetate esterase. The naphthol AS-D chloroacetate is less sensitive than MPO and SBB, but positive results parallel those seen with the MPO and SBB stains. Therefore, it is useful in the differentiation of AML from ALL (Table 34-12; Web Table 34-11). A combination of chloroacetate esterase and cyanide-resistant peroxidase stains is also helpful in diagnosing acute eosinophilic leukemia, which is characteristically negative for chloroacetate esterase and positive for cyanide-resistant peroxidase.[70]

ALPHA-NAPHTHYL ESTERASE (NONSPECIFIC ESTERASE)

Alpha-naphthyl esterase activity is found primarily in monocytes and macrophages using either α-naphthyl acetate or α-naphthyl butyrate as substrate. Alpha-naphthyl acetate esterase (ANAE) activity is also present in plasma cells, megakaryocytes, hairy cells, and T lymphocytes (dot-like pattern). Similarly, alpha-naphthyl butyrate esterase activity is also present in megakaryocytes (less intense than ANAE) and helper T lymphocytes. The sites of enzyme activity show black granulation and are detected by incubating the sample in α-naphthyl acetate/or butyrate at an alkaline pH (Figure 34-26■). As a result of the esterase activity, enzymatic hydrolysis of ester linkages occurs, and free naphthol compounds are liberated. The liberated naphthol immediately couples with a diazonium salt (e.g., fast blue RR), forming an insoluble, visible pigment at the site of enzyme activity.[73]

Granulocytes are usually negative but can show occasional activity. In addition, enzyme activity can be detected in the erythroblasts of erythroleukemia and focally in lymphoblasts of ALL. Alpha-naphthyl butyrate exhibits strong activity in the monocytic cells but very weak or absent activity in granulocytes, megakaryocytes, and lymphocytes. The combined method for α-naphthyl butyrate esterase and chloroacetate esterase provides an objective means for demonstrating monocytes and granulocytes simultaneously in cytologic preparations and, thus, is useful for differentiating myeloblasts from monoblasts.[74,75]

Alpha-naphthyl esterase is useful in diagnosing acute myelomonocytic and acute monocytic leukemias (Table 34-12; Web Table 34-11).[76] To differentiate monocytes from other cells that occasionally show positivity, sodium fluoride can be added to the incubation mixture. Sodium fluoride inactivates the monocytic enzyme. This is referred to as the *fluoride inhibition test* in which two incubation mixtures are prepared, one without fluoride and the other with fluoride. Slides are incubated in the incubation mixtures, and the staining patterns of the two slides are compared. The slide stained in the incubation mixture containing fluoride shows an inhibition of staining in monocytes but not in other cell lines.

PERIODIC ACID-SCHIFF (PAS)

Periodic acid oxidizes 1,2-glycol groups to dialdehydes. These aldehyde groups combine with Schiff's reagent to produce a magenta product (Figure 34-27■). The stainable compound in the blood cells is primarily glycogen. Cellular components containing polysaccharides, mucopolysaccharides, and glycoproteins possess the 1,2-glycol groups and will be stained.[77] Mature granulocytes (the intensity of staining increases with maturity), platelets, megakaryocytes, and monocytes are stained with PAS. However, the early myeloid cells, the erythroid cells, and many of the lymphoid cells are negative with PAS. Therefore, PAS positivity in these cells can indicate abnormal glycogen metabolism and can be di-

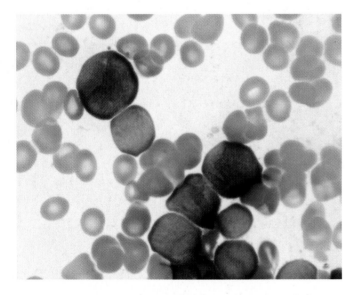

■ FIGURE 34-26   Blasts of acute monoblastic leukemia showing a positive nonspecific esterase (NES) stain (black granulation). (Bone marrow; NSE stain; 500× magnification)

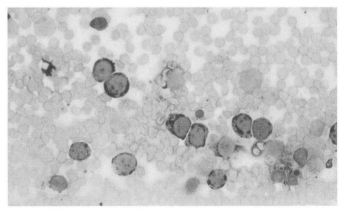

■ FIGURE 34-27   PAS stain showing positive reaction (red-purple cytoplasm) of erythroblasts in acute erythroid leukemia. (Bone marrow; PAS stain; 400× magnification)

agnostically important. The use of this stain in the diagnosing acute leukemias is summarized in Web Table 34-11.

LEUKOCYTE ALKALINE PHOSPHATASE

The determination of **leukocyte alkaline phosphatase (LAP)** activity can be used to differentiate chronic myelogenous leukemia from leukemoid reaction/reactive neutrophilia.[78,79] In this procedure, freshly prepared peripheral blood smears obtained from finger-stick capillary blood or samples anticoagulated with heparin are dried for at least 1 hour prior to fixation in 60% citrate buffered acetone.[78] Fixed slides can be stored overnight in the freezer. The smears are incubated in naphthol AS-MX phosphate at an alkaline pH. The liberated naphthol immediately couples with a diazonium salt (e.g., fast blue RR) forming brown to black particles in the cytoplasm of the cells at the enzyme sites (Figure 34-28 ■). After counterstaining, the smears are evaluated microscopically. Because this enzyme is found within the secondary granules of maturing granulocytes, 100 segmented neutrophils/bands are counted, and each cell is graded using a scale of 0 to 4+ according to the appearance and intensity of the precipitated dye (Table 34-13 ✪). The number of cells counted in each grade is multiplied by that grade, and the products are summed to obtain a total LAP score (Table 34-14 ✪). Improperly stored smears and those prepared from blood anticoagulated with EDTA can give falsely low LAP scores. The range of normal scores is 13–130, although this could vary slightly in each laboratory. The range of possible values is 0–400. A score higher than 160 is generally considered increased and lower than 13 is considered decreased. The LAP scores can be increased in leukemoid reaction (infection, inflammation), polycythemia vera, pregnancy, newborns, stress, oral contraceptives, and medications (steroids, estrogen, lithium, growth factors). In secondary erythrocytosis, idiopathic myelofibrosis and essential thrombocytosis, the enzyme activity is usually normal. LAP scores can be decreased in chronic myelocytic leukemia

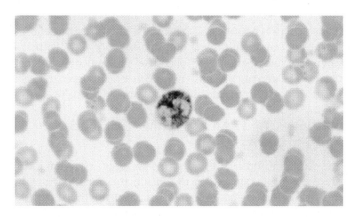

■ **FIGURE 34-28**   LAP stain showing neutrophil with a score of 3+. Note strong dark colored granulation. (Peripheral blood; LAP stain; 500× magnification)

✪ **TABLE 34-13**

Leukocyte Alkaline Phosphatase: Cell Rating and Staining Characteristics

Cell Rating	Amount	Intensity of Staining
0	None	None
1+	<50%	Faint
2+	50–75%	Moderate
3+	75–100%	Strong
4+	100%	Intense

(CML), paroxysmal nocturnal hemoglobinuria, idiopathic thrombocytopenic purpura, and sometimes in myelodysplasia. The LAP score for CML patients in blast crisis or with concurrent infections can be increased.

✓ Checkpoint! 16

A pathology resident is evaluating the peripheral blood smear of a 40-year-old female. The resident suspects CML. To confirm this suspicion, a LAP score is ordered. Do you think that the LAP score will be helpful in making the correct diagnosis?

ACID PHOSPHATASE AND TARTRATE-RESISTANT ACID PHOSPHATASE (TRAP)

Acid phosphatase activity is detected by incubating the sample in naphthol AS-BI phosphoric acid.[80,81,82] Enzyme activity liberates naphthol AS-BI. The liberated naphthol immediately couples with a diazonium salt (e.g., fast garnet) forming an insoluble, visible pigment at the site of enzyme activity. Acid phosphatase activity is present in most normal leukocytes appearing as purplish, dark-red intracellular granules. The acid phosphatase activity in T cell ALL is characteristic, which exhibits focal polarized acid phosphatase activity.

Seven acid phosphatase isoenzymes (0, 1, 2, 3, 3b, 4, and 5) are present in leukocytes. These isoenzymes are cell specific with neutrophils containing isoenzymes 2 and 4, lymphocytes and platelets isoenzyme 3, blasts isoenzyme 3b, and hairy cells isoenzyme 5. All but isoenzyme 5 are sensitive

✪ **TABLE 34-14**

Example of a LAP Score Calculation

Cell Rating	Number of Cells Counted	LAP Score
0	45	0
1+	30	30
2+	15	30
3+	5	15
4+	5	20
		Total LAP score 95

to tartrate inhibition. The hairy cells of hairy cell leukemia exhibit acid phosphatase activity but can be differentiated from other leukocytes using tartrate inhibition.[83,84] Tartrate inhibits the acid phosphatase activity within normal leukocytes, while enzyme activity within hairy cells is resistant to tartrate inhibition (Figure 34-29). Therefore, hairy cell leukemia is said to be strongly **tartrate-resistant acid phosphatase (TRAP)** positive. Weak to moderate TRAP positivity occurs in activated lymphocytes and Sézary cells, a few cases of chronic lymphocytic leukemia, and prolymphocytic leukemia. Mast cells are also TRAP positive, and the morphology of abnormal mast cells on tissue sections is similar to hairy cell leukemia. Toluidine blue stain is helpful in distinguishing mast cells (positive) from hairy cells (negative).

✓ Checkpoint! 17

A 30-year-old male presented to the emergency room complaining of fatigue, weakness, and gum bleeding. The CBC showed anemia, thrombocytopenia, and a WBC of $30 \times 10^9/L$. The peripheral blood smear revealed numerous intermediate to large blasts with fine nuclear chromatin and abundant cytoplasm. The bone marrow biopsy contained 60% blasts. No Auer rods were seen after careful inspection. Several cytochemical stains were then performed. The blasts failed to stain with myeloperoxidase, Sudan black B, and specific esterase; however, the majority of blasts reacted intensely with α-naphthyl esterase. Incubation with sodium fluoride inhibited the staining seen with α-naphthyl esterase. What type of leukemia do you think this patient has?

TERMINAL DEOXYNUCLEOTIDYL TRANSFERASE

Terminal deoxynucleotidyl transferase (TdT) is an intranuclear DNA polymerase responsible for the template-independent addition of deoxyribonucleotides to the 3'-hydroxyl terminus of oligonucleotide primers during immunoglobulin and T cell receptor gene rearrangements. It is normally present in thymus lymphocytes, in pre-B lymphocytes (hematogones), and in 1–3% of normal bone marrow cells (blasts). It is not normally present in peripheral blood lymphocytes or lymph node lymphocytes. Because Tdt is primarily found in lymphoid precursors, its detection is useful in distinguishing ALL from malignant lymphoma.[85,86] However, a positive Tdt result in an acute leukemia should be interpreted with caution because Tdt has been observed in up to 20% of AMLs and specifically in more than 90% of AML-minimally differentiated cases.

In the indirect immunofluorescence technique for detection of Tdt, rabbit anticalf Tdt is applied to the sample (e.g., bone marrow aspirate smear).[87] If the cells' nuclei contain Tdt, this antibody binds to it creating an antibody–antigen complex. Excess anticalf Tdt is washed away. A secondary antibody, fluorescein isothiocyanate-conjugated goat antirabbit IgG antiserum, is used to identify the antibody–antigen complex. The nucleus of cells containing Tdt will fluoresce. Tdt can also be detected by biochemical assays, enzyme immunoassays, and indirect immunoperoxidase or direct immunofluorescence using monoclonal antibodies.

✓ Checkpoint! 18

A pathologist is reviewing the slides from the pleural fluid of a 50-year-old male who has hepatosplenomegaly and minimal lymphadenopathy. It is not clear whether the mononuclear cells are mature lymphoma cells or leukemic blasts. There is not enough material for flow cytometry to do immunophenotyping, but there is enough to make a few extra cytospin smears. Which stain do you think can be useful in this case?

TOLUIDINE BLUE

Toluidine blue is a basic dye that reacts with acid mucopolysaccharides to form red to purple metachromatic granules. Bone marrow trephine sections are stained with 0.1% toluidine blue in ethanol and examined microscopically. A positive reaction is specific for basophils and mast cells. This stain is useful in diagnosing mast cell disease and rare cases of AML with basophilic differentiation.[75,88,89] Because acid mucopolysaccharides can be decreased or absent in neoplastic disorders, a negative reaction does not rule out a neoplasm of these cells.

RETICULIN STAIN AND MASSON'S TRICHROME STAIN

The reticulin and trichrome stains are used to evaluate the presence and extent of fibrosis within the bone marrow. In the Gomori methenamine silver staining method, deparaffinized bone marrow trephine sections are incubated in the following solutions: 0.5% periodic acid, methenamine silver working solution (contains methenamine, silver nitrate, and sodium borate), 0.2% gold chloride, and 3% sodium thiosul-

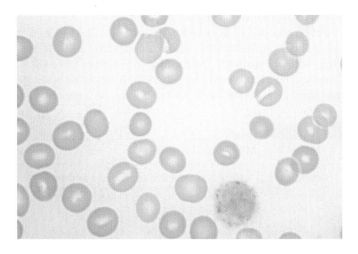

■ **FIGURE 34-29** TRAP stain showing a positive reaction of hairy cell with acid phosphatase that is resistant to tartrate inhibition (reddish granulation). (Peripheral blood; TRAP stain; 500× magnification)

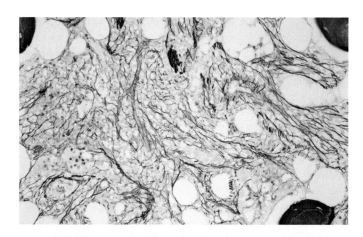

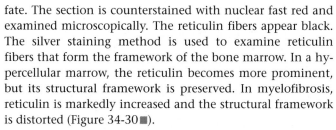

■ FIGURE 34-30   Bone marrow biopsy stained with reticulin stain showing fibrosis (black fibers) in a patient with myelofibrosis. (Bone marrow; paraffin section, reticulin stain; 200× magnification)

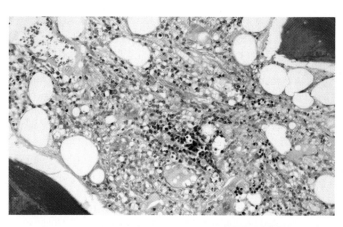

■ FIGURE 34-31   Bone marrow biopsy stained with Masson's trichrome stain showing collagenous fibrosis (fibers are stained light blue) in a patient with myelofibrosis. (Bone marrow; paraffin section, Masson's Trichrome stain; 400× magnification)

fate. The section is counterstained with nuclear fast red and examined microscopically. The reticulin fibers appear black. The silver staining method is used to examine reticulin fibers that form the framework of the bone marrow. In a hypercellular marrow, the reticulin becomes more prominent, but its structural framework is preserved. In myelofibrosis, reticulin is markedly increased and the structural framework is distorted (Figure 34-30 ■).

In the Masson's trichrome stain, deparaffinized bone marrow trephine sections or frozen trephine sections are stained with Weigert's iron hematoxylin working solution and then incubated in the following solutions: Biebrich scarlet-acid fuchsin, phosphomolybdic acid, and aniline blue. The slides are examined microscopically; collagen fibers appear blue, nuclei black, and the background red. The trichrome stain is used to evaluate collagenous fibrosis within the bone marrow. Normally, collagenous fibrosis is focal and perivascular. Increased staining can be observed in myelofibrosis and indicates significant fibrosis (Figure 34-31 ■).

SUMMARY

This chapter reviewed the routine and reflex tests performed within the hematology laboratory. The accuracy and reliability of the results depend on the clinical laboratory professional's knowledge of the test procedure. A thorough understanding of each procedure is necessary to understand the appropriate use, troubleshoot potential sources of error, identify other problems in performing the test, and understand the meaning of test results. Although the majority of the routine hematology tests are performed by automated instrumentation, the basic principles, applications, and potential sources of error hold true for the automated adaptation of each procedure. The results obtained from the routine and reflex test procedures are utilized in diagnosing, prognosing, and therapeutic monitoring a variety of disorders including anemias, leukemias, infections, and inherited leukocyte disorders.

REVIEW QUESTIONS

LEVEL I

1. What is the appropriate sequence to fill sample collection tubes according to top color? (Objective 6)
   a. red, lavender, blue, green
   b. lavender, blue, red, green
   c. blue, red, green, lavender
   d. red, blue, lavender, green

2. The function of a microscope's condenser is to: (Objective 8)
   a. magnify the light beam prior to it striking the sample
   b. collect the diffracted light from the sample
   c. direct the light beam onto the sample
   d. project diffracted light to the objective

LEVEL II

1. In performing a manual platelet count using phase contrast microscopy, identification of the platelets is very difficult. What should be done to improve the identification of the platelets? (Objective 2)
   a. lower the condenser to increase the depth of field
   b. align the annulus with the phase-shifting element
   c. perform Koehler illumination with the 100× objective
   d. decrease the brightness dial to increase resolution

REVIEW QUESTIONS (continued)

LEVEL I

3. A manual leukocyte count was performed on an EDTA-anti-coagulated sample. The sample was diluted 1:100, and a total of 75 leukocytes were counted in all 9 squares of the hemacytometer. What is the leukocyte count? (Objective 19)
   a. 1.3×10^9/L
   b. 3.3×10^9/L
   c. 4.1×10^9/L
   d. 8.3×10^9L

4. Any turbidity in a peripheral blood sample results in a falsely elevated hemoglobin determination. Which of the following is a potential source of turbidity? (Objective 19)
   a. lipemia
   b. leukocyte count $= 18.0 \times 10^9$/L
   c. increased levels of carboxyhemoglobin
   d. presence of hemoglobin F

5. Which of the following is *not* a condition associated with an elevated ESR? (Objective 19)
   a. rheumatoid arthritis
   b. polycythemia vera
   c. multiple myeloma
   d. osteomyelitis

6. Which of the following is observed if a purple top collection tube is underfilled? (Objective 6)
   a. falsely elevated erythrocyte count
   b. falsely decreased microhematocrit
   c. falsely elevated platelet count
   d. falsely decreased hemoglobin

7. In performing a reticulocyte count, the clinical laboratory professional observes suspicious light bluish-green bodies at the periphery of some erythrocytes. What is the appropriate course of action? (Objective 19)
   a. These bodies are aggregated reticulum, and erythrocytes containing them should be tabulated as reticulocytes.
   b. These bodies are iron-containing bodies and should be confirmed using the Prussian-blue stain.
   c. These bodies are aggregated DNA, and erythrocytes containing them should not be tabulated as reticulocytes.
   d. These bodies are denatured hemoglobin, and erythrocytes containing them should not be tabulated as reticulocytes.

8. The laboratory is experiencing problems with the air conditioning system and it is unusually warm. What effect will this temperature change have on the ESRs performed during this time period? (Objective 19)
   a. ESRs will be falsely elevated because higher temperature promotes sedimentation.
   b. ESRs will be falsely decreased because erythrocytes have a higher zeta potential.
   c. ESRs will be unaffected because erythrocyte sedimentation does not depend on temperature.
   d. ESRs will be falsely elevated because erythrocytes will become swollen.

LEVEL II

2. A manual platelet count was performed using the unopette system. A total of 526 platelets were counted on one side of the hemacytometer. Which of the following clinical conditions is associated with this result? (Objective 7)
   a. immune thrombocytopenic purpura
   b. megaloblastic anemia
   c. acute leukemia
   d. iron-deficiency anemia

3. If the solubility test for hemoglobin S is positive, the appropriate reflex test is: (Objective 6)
   a. hemoglobin electrophoresis using cellulose acetate
   b. hemoglobin A_2 by column chromatography
   c. isoelectric focusing with SDS gel
   d. hemoglobin F determination by acid elution

4. While evaluating the erythrocyte morphology on a Wright-stained peripheral blood smear, the clinical laboratory professional observed many crenated erythrocytes. What corrective action will minimize the presence of these cells? (Objective 4)
   a. Allow the sample to stabilize for at least 4 hours and then prepare the blood smear.
   b. Dry the blood smear quickly after its preparation.
   c. Increase the spreader speed to prepare the blood smear.
   d. No corrective action is available.

5. A clinical laboratory professional noted that a patient's platelet count was significantly decreased. In examining the patient's blood smear, platelets appeared to adhere to the neutrophils. How would you obtain an accurate platelet count? (Objective 4)
   a. Recollect sample in citrate and reanalyze platelet count.
   b. Allow sample to set at 25°C for 5 hours and reanalyze platelet count.
   c. Warm sample at 37°C for 15 minutes and reanalyze platelet count.
   d. No corrective action is available.

6. Which screening test can be used if a diagnosis of PNH is suspected? (Objective 6)
   a. hemoglobin electrophoresis
   b. sugar-water test
   c. Donath-Landsteiner test
   d. acid elution test

LEVEL I

9. When examining an acid elution test for hemoglobin F, the clinical laboratory professional observed uniformly stained erythrocytes on the control slide (mixture of adult erythrocytes and cord cells) and on the patient's slide. What is the source of this error? (Objective 19)
   a. fixative
   b. stain
   c. elution buffer
   d. counterstain

10. Electrophoresis using cellulose acetate reveals a band of hemoglobin with HbC mobility. Citrate agar electrophoresis does *not* show a HbC band. The most likely explanation is that the: (Objective 19)
    a. abnormal hemoglobin can be HbE or HbO$_{Arab}$
    b. citrate agar electrophoresis result is erroneous
    c. abnormal hemoglobin can be HbG or HbD
    d. cellulose acetate electrophoresis is not reliable

LEVEL II

7. A patient had the following results:

RBC	2.90×10^{12}/L	MCV	76 fL
Hb	6.2 g/dL	MCH	21 pg
Hct	22.0%	MCHC	28 g/dL
Serum iron	45 μg/dL		
sTfR	28.5 nmol/L		

   With what type of anemia are these results associated? (Objective 7)
   a. iron-deficiency anemia
   b. beta thalassemia minor
   c. anemia of chronic disease
   d. sideroblastic anemia

8. In performing a reticulocyte count, the clinical laboratory professional observes erythrocyte inclusions suggesting denatured hemoglobin. What is the best stain to confirm the identity of these inclusions? (Objective 6)
   a. crystal violet stain
   b. Wright's stain
   c. brilliant green stain
   d. methyl violet stain

9. You are performing several cytochemical stains on a bone marrow sample from a patient recently diagnosed with acute leukemia. You are examining the MPO slide, and the blasts are negative. However, the reagent is nearing its expiration date, and you are not sure whether the stain worked properly. Which cells found in the bone marrow normally express myeloperoxidase and could be used to assess the stain's integrity? (Objective 6)
   a. neutrophils
   b. red cell precursors
   c. megakaryocytes
   d. lymphocytes

10. Based on a patient's CBC and peripheral blood smear examination, a diagnosis of CML is suspected. The physician orders an LAP score to be performed on the current hematology sample (lavender top tube). What should the clinical laboratory professional tell the physician? (Objective 6)
    a. The current hematology sample is acceptable, and the procedure will be completed today.
    b. The current hematology sample is unacceptable because it would result in a falsely decreased LAP score. A new sample must be collected using heparin.
    c. The current hematology sample is unacceptable because it would result in a falsely elevated LAP score. A blood smear should be obtained by capillary puncture.
    d. The current hematology sample is acceptable; however, the LAP score needs to be corrected for the dilutional effect of the anticoagulant.

www.pearsonhighered.com/mckenzie
Use this address to access the interactive Companion Website created for this textbook. Find additional information, tables and figures. Evaluate your command of the chapter information using case studies and critical thinking and multiple choice questions.

REFERENCES

1. Clinical and Laboratory Standards Institute. *Tubes and Additives for Venous Blood Specimen Collection. Approved Standard,* 5th ed. H1-A5. Wayne, PA: CLSI; 2003.

2. Clinical and Laboratory Standards Institute. *Collection, Transport, and Processing of Blood Specimens for Testing Plasma-Based Coagulation Assays and Molecular Hemostasis Assays. Approved Guideline,* 5th ed. H21-A5. Wayne, PA: CLSI; 2008.

3. Clinical and Laboratory Standards Institute. *Procedures for the Collection of Diagnostic Blood Specimens by Venipuncture: Approved Standard,* 6th ed. H3-A6. Wayne, PA: CLSI; 2007.

4. Joint Commission Perspectives. *2008 National Patient Safety Goals.* 2007;27(7).

5. Clinical and Laboratory Standards Institute. *Procedures and Devices for the Collection of Diagnostic Capillary Blood Specimens: Approved Standard,* 5th ed. H4-A5. Wayne, PA: CLSI; 2004.

6. Occupational Safety and Health Administration. *Occupational Exposure to Bloodborne Pathogens Standard.* 29 CFR 1910.1030. U.S. government, Washington DC. 1992.

7. Occupational Safety and Health Administration. Occupational Safety and Health Administration Instruction, CPL 2-2.44D. *Enforcement Procedures for the Occupational Exposure to Bloodborne Pathogens Standard.* 29 CFR 1910.1030. U.S. government, Washington DC. 1999.

8. Nikon, Inc. *Instructions for the Labophot-2.* Garden City, NY: Nikon. 1990.

9. Nikon, Inc. *Introduction to the Microscope: Operation and Preventive Maintenance Using the Nikon Labophot.* Garden City, NY: Nikon. 1981.

10. Murphy DB. *Fundamentals of Light Microscopy and Electronic Imaging.* New York: Wiley-Liss; 2001.

11. Nikon, Inc. *CF160 Optics Overview.* Garden City, NY: Nikon; 2000.

12. Keller E. Light microscopy and cell structure. In DL Spector, RD Goldman, LA Leinwand, eds. *Cells: A Laboratory Manual,* vol. 2. Cold Spring Harbor: Cold Spring Harbor Laboratory Press; 1997.

13. Clinical and Laboratory Standards Institute. *Reference Leukocyte Differential Count (Proportional) and Evaluation of Instrumental Methods: Approved Standard.* 2nd ed. Wayne, PA: CLSI; 2007.

14. Steine-Martin EA. Causes of poor leukocyte distribution in manual spreader slide blood films. *Am J Med Tech.* 1980;46:624–32.

15. Benattar L, Flandrin G. Comparison of the classical manual pushed wedge films with an improved automated method for making blood smears. *Hematol Cell Ther.* 1999;41:211–15.

16. Ryan DH. Examination of the blood. In: Lichtman MA, Beutler E, Kipps TJ, Seligsohn U, Kaushansky K, Pochal JT, eds. *Williams Hematology,* 7th ed. New York: McGraw-Hill; 2006.

17. National Committee for Clinical Laboratory Standards. *Romanowsky Blood Stains.* Villanova, PA: NCCLS; 1986.

18. Marshall PN. Romanowsky staining: State of the art and ideal techniques. In: JA Koepke, ed. *Differential Leukocyte Counting.* Skokie, IL: College of American Pathologists; 1979.

19. Kopecke JA. Standardization of the manual differential leukocyte count. *Lab Med.* 1980;11:371–75.

20. Koepke JA, Dotson MA, Shifman MA. A critical evaluation of manual/visual differential leukocyte counting method. *Blood Cells.* 1985;11:173.

21. Gulati GL, Hyun BH. Blood smear examination. *Hematol Oncol Clin North Am.* 1994;8(4):631–50.

22. *Unopette WBC/Platelet Determination for Manual Methods.* Rutherford, NJ: Becton, Dickinson; 1996.

23. *Unopette Erythrocyte Determination for Manual Methods.* Rutherford, NJ: Becton, Dickinson; 1995.

24. *Unopette Eosinophil Determination for Manual Methods.* Rutherford, NJ: Becton, Dickinson; 1995.

25. Clinical and Laboratory Standards Institute. *Reference and Selected Procedures for the Quantitative Determination of Hemoglobin in Blood,* 3rd ed. H15-A3. Wayne, PA: CLSI; 2000.

26. International Committee for Standardization in Haematology; Expert Panel on Haemoglobinometry. Recommendations for reference method for haemoglobinometry in human blood (ICSH standard 1986) and specifications for international haemiglobincyanide reference preparation, 3rd ed. *Clin Lab Haematol.* 1987;9(1):73–79.

27. Clinical and Laboratory Standards Institute. *Procedure for Determining Packed Cell Volume by the Microhematocrit Method,* 3rd ed. H7-A3. Wayne, PA: CLSI; 2000.

28. International Committee for Standardization in Hematology. Selected methods for the determination of packed cell volume. In: OW van Assendelft, JM England, eds. *Advances in Hematologic Methods: The Blood Count.* Boca Raton, FL: CRC Press; 1982.

29. Clinical and Laboratory Standards Institute. *Reference and Selected Procedure for Erythrocyte Sedimentaion Rate (ESR) Test; Approved Standard,* 4th ed. H2-A4. Wayne, PA: CLSI; 2000.

30. International Committee for Standardization in Hematology. Recommendation for measurement of erythrocyte sedimentation rate. *Am J Clin Pathol.* 1993;46:198.

31. Rabjohn L, Roberts K, Troiano M, Schoenhaus H. Diagnostic and prognostic value of erythrocyte sedimentation rate in contiguous osteomyelitis of the foot and ankle. *J Foot Ankle Surg.* 2007;46 (4):230.

32. Andresdottir MB, Sigfusson N, Sigvaldason H, Gudnason V. Erythrocyte sedimentation rate, an independent predictor of coronary heart disease in men and women, the Reykjavik study. *AJE,* 2003; 158(9):844.

33. Giavarina D, Dall'Olio G, Soffiati G. Method comparison of automated systems for the erythrocyte sedimentation rate. *Am J Clin Pathol.* 1999;112(5):721.

34. Happe MR, Battafarano DF, Dooley DP, Rennie TA, Murphy FT, Casey TJ, Ward JA. Validation of Diesse Mini-Ves Erythrocyte Sedimentation Rate (ESR) Analyzer using the Westergren ESR method in patients with systemic inflammatory conditions. *Am J Clin Pathol.* 2002;118:14.

35. Streck ESR-auto plus operator and technical manual (Part 320440-4). Omaha, NE: Streck; 2005.

36. Gambino R. C-reactive protein—Undervalued, underutilized. *Clin Chem.* 1997;43(11):2017–18.

37. Young B, Gleeson M, Cripps AW. C-reactive protein: A critical review. *Pathology.* 1991;23(2):118.

38. Inoue E, Yamamaka H, Hora M, Tomatsu T, Kamtani N. Comparison of disease activity score (DAS)28—Erythrocyte sedimentation rate and DAS28-C-reactive protein threshold. *Ann Rheum Dis.* 2007; 66:407.

39. Torres JL, Ridker PM. Clinical use of high sensitivity C-reactive protein for the prediction of adverse cardiovascular events. *Curr Opin Cardiol.* 2003;18:471.

40. Roberts WL. CDC/AHA Workshop on Markers of Inflammation and Cardiovascular Disease: Application to Clinical and Public Health Practice - Laboratory Tests Available to Assess Inflammation. *Circulation.* 2004;110:e572.

41. Miyachi H, Asai S, Takemura Y. A cost-effectiveness evaluation of reticulocyte measurement in new outpatients with or without hematologic disorders. *Clin Chem Lab Med.* 2006;44(8):1035.

42. Wiwanitkit V. Comparison of cost effectiveness between measuring the serum erythropoietin level and reticulocyte count for monitoring thalassemic patients: A note in thai beta thalassemia/Hb E subjects. *Hematology.* 2004;9(4):311.

43. Serke S, Riess H, Oettle H, Huhn D. Elevated reticulocyte count: A clue to the diagnosis of haemolytic-uraemic syndrome (HUS) associated with gemcitabine therapy for metastatic duodenal papillary carcinoma: A case report. *Br J Cancer.* 1999;79:1519–21.

44. Bhandari S, Norfolk D, Brownjohn A, Turney J. Evaluation of RBC ferritin and reticulocyte measurements in monitoring response to intravenous iron therapy. *Am J Kid Dis.* 1997;30(6):814–21.

45. Clinical and Laboratory Standards Institute. *Methods for Reticulocyte Counting (Automated Blood Cell Counters, Flow Cytometry, and Supravital Dyes): Approved Standard,* 2nd ed. H44-A2. Wayne, PA: CLSI; 2004.

46. National Committee for Clinical Laboratory Standards. *Solubility Test to Confirm the Presence of Sickling Hemoglobins,* 2nd ed. H10-A2. Villanova, PA: NCCLS; 1995.

47. Beutler E. Disorders of hemoglobin structure: Sickle cell anemia and related disorders. In: Lichtman MA, Beutler E, Kipps TJ, Seligsohn U, Kaushansky K, Prchal JT, eds. *Williams Hematology,* 7th ed. New York: McGraw-Hill Medical; 2006.

48. NCCLS. *Detection of Abnormal Hemoglobin Using Cellulose Acetate Electrophoresis,* 2nd ed. Wayne, PA: NCCLS; 1994.

49. *Hemoglobin Electrophoresis Procedure.* Beaumont, TX: Helena Laboratories; 2001.

50. *SPIFE Acid Hemoglobin Procedure.* Beaumont, TX: Helena Laboratories; 2003.

51. *Beta-Thal HbA$_2$ Quik Column Procedure.* Beaumont, TX: Helena Laboratories; 2004.

52. Ravindran MS, Patel ZM, Khatkhatay MI, Dandekar SP. β-thalassemia carrier detection by ELISA: A simple screening strategy for developing countries. *J Clin Lab Anal.* 2005;19:22–25.

53. Kalleas C, Tentes I, Margaritis D et al. Effect of Hb S in the determination of HbA$_2$ with the Biorad Variant II analyzer. *Clin Biochem.* 2007;40:744–46.

54. Van Kirk R, Sandhaus LM, Hoyer JD. The detection and diagnosis of hemoglobin A$_2$ by high-performance liquid chromatography. *Am J Clin Pathol.* 2005;123:657–61.

55. Riou J, Godart C, Mathis M et al. Evaluation of the Bio-Rad VARIANT™ II HbA2/HbA1c Dual Program for measurement of hemoglobin concentrations and detection of variants. *Clin Chem Lab Med.* 2005;43:237–43.

56. Paleari R, Cannata M, Leto F, Maggio A et al. Analytical evaluation of the Tosoh HLC-723 G7 automated HPLC analyzer for hemoglobin A$_2$ and F determination. *Clin Biochem.* 2005;38:159–65.

57. *Fetal Hemoglobin-Acid Elution: Semi-Quantitative Procedure for Blood Smears.* St. Louis: Sigma-Aldrich Diagnostics; 2005.

58. NCCLS. *Quantitative Measurement of Fetal Hemoglobin Using the Alkali Denaturation Method.* Wayne, PA: NCCLS; 1989.

59. Fibach E. Flow cytometric analysis of fetal hemoglobin in erythroid precursors of β-thalassemia. *Clin Lab Haem.* 2004;26:187–93.

60. Huisman THJ, Jonxis JHP. *The Hemoglobinopathies: Techniques of Identification.* New York: Marcel Decker; 1977.

61. Papassotiriou I, Traeger-Synodinos J, Prome D et. al. Association of unstable hemoglobin variants and heterozygous beta-thalassemia: Example of a new variant Hb acharnes or [β53(D4) Ala → Thr]. *Am J Hematol.* 1999;62:186–92.

62. Schwab ML, Lewis AE. An improved stain for Heinz bodies. *Am J Clin Pathol.* 1969;39:673.

63. *UNOPETTE RBC Osmotic Fragility Determination for Manual Methods Procedure.* Rutherford, NJ: Becton, Dickinson; 1996.

64. Hartmann RC, Jenkins DE. The "sugar-water" test for paroxysmal nocturnal hemoglobinuria. *New Engl J Med.* 1966;275:155.

65. Parker C, Omine M, Richards S et. al. Diagnosis and management of paroxysmal nocturnal hemoglobinuria. *Blood.* 2005;106(12):3699.

66. *American Association of Blood Banks: Technical Manual,* 15th ed. Bethesda, MD: AABB; 2005.

67. *Quantikine IVD Human Epo Immunoassay Procedure.* Minneapolis, MN: R&D Systems; 2003.

68. *Quantikine IVD Human sTfR Immunoassay Procedure.* Minneapolis, MN: R&D Systems; 2004.

69. Sigma-Aldrich, Inc. *Peroxisase (Myeloperoxidase).* St. Louis: Sigma-Aldrich; 2003.

70. Gabbas AG, Li CY. Acute non-lymphocytic leukemia with eosinophilic differentiation. *Am J Hematol.* 1986;21:29–38.

71. Sigma-Aldrich, Inc. *Sudan Black B Staining System.* St. Louis: Sigma-Aldrich; 2003.

72. Stass SA, Pui CH, Melvin S, Rovigatti U, Williams D, Motroni T et al. Sudan black B positive acute lymphoblastic leukaemia. *Br J Haematol.* 1984;57:413–21.

73. Sigma-Aldrich, Inc. *Naphthol AS-D Choloroacetate Esterase and Alpha-Naphthyl Acetate Esterase.* St. Louis: Sigma-Aldrich; 2006.

74. Shibata A, Bennett JM, Castoldi GL. Recommended methods for cytological procedures in hematology. *Clin Lab Haematol.* 1985;7: 55–74.

75. Yam LT, Li CY, Crosby WH. Cytochemical identification of monocytes and granulocytes. *Am J Clin Pathol.* 1971;55:283–90.

76. Li CY. Leukemia cytochemistry. *Mayo Clin Proc.* 1981;56:712–13.

77. Sigma-Aldrich, Inc. *Periodic Acid-Schiff (PAS) Staining System.* St. Louis: Sigma-Aldrich; 2003.

78. Sigma-Aldrich, Inc. *Alkaline Phosphatase.* St. Louis: Sigma-Aldrich; 2003.

79. National Committee for Clinical Laboratory Standards. *Proposed Standard: Histochemical Method for Leukocyte Alkaline Phosphatase.* Villanova, PA: NCCLS; 1984.

80. Sigma-Aldrich, Inc. *Acid Phosphatase, Leukocyte.* St. Louis: Sigma-Aldrich; 2005.

81. Li CY, Yam LT, Lam KW. Acid phosphatase isoenzyme in human leukocytes in normal and pathologic conditions. *J Histochem Cytochem.* 1970;18:473–81.

82. Li CY, Yam LT, Lam KW. Studies of acid phosphatase isoenzymes in human lymphocytes: Demonstration of isoenzyme cell-specificity. *J Histochem Cytochem.* 1970;18:901–10.

83. Yam LT, Li CY, Lam KW. Tartrate-resistant acid phosphatase iso-enzyme in the reticulum cells of leukemic reticuloendotheliosis. *N Engl J Med.* 1971;284:357–60.

84. Yam LT, Janckila AJ, Li CY, Lam KW. Cytochemistry of tartrate-resistant acid phosphatase: Fifteen years' experience. *Leukemia.* 1987; 1:285–88.

85. Bollum FJ. Terminal deoxynucleotidyl transferase as a hematopoietic cell marker. *Blood.* 1979;54:1203–15.

86. Liu L, McGavran L, Lovell MA et. al. Nonpositive terminal deoxynucleotidyl transferase in pediatric precursor B-lymphoblastic leukemia. *Am J Clin Pathol.* 2004;121:810.

87. Sun T, Li CY, Yam LT. *Atlas of Cytochemistry and Immunochemistry of Hematologic Neoplasms.* Chicago: American Society of Clinical Pathologists Press; 1985.

88. Li CY, Yam LT. Cytochemical characterization of leukemic cells with numerous cytoplasmic granules. *Mayo Clin Proc.* 1987;62:978–85.

89. Wick MR, Li CY, Pierre RV. Acute non-lymphocytic leukemia with basophilic differentiation. *Blood.* 1982;60:38–45.

35

Bone Marrow Examination

Aamir Ehsan, M.D.

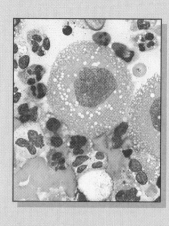

■ OBJECTIVES—LEVEL I

At the end of this unit of study, the student should be able to:

1. Identify the sites for obtaining bone marrow samples.
2. List indications for the need to perform bone marrow studies.
3. Explain the difference between core biopsy and bone marrow aspirate and the use of each.
4. Describe how to perform a bone marrow differential count.
5. Define the *M:E ratio,* and explain what can cause an increase or decrease in it.
6. Describe how to estimate bone marrow cellularity and iron stores and interpret results.
7. Explain the role of the hematology laboratory in bone marrow evaluation.
8. List the reasons that special stains are used on bone marrow specimens.

■ OBJECTIVES—LEVEL II

Upon completion of this unit of study, the student should be able to:

1. Differentiate benign lymphoid aggregates from malignant lymphoma.
2. Evaluate the bone marrow specimen and select the appropriate specimens for ancillary studies.
3. Perform a bone marrow differential count and calculate and interpret the M:E ratio.
4. Estimate and interpret bone marrow cellularity.
5. Correlate results of marrow iron stores with various diseases.
6. Explain the role of the clinical laboratory professional in the bone marrow procedure.
7. Identify key features of a bone marrow report.

KEY TERMS

Dry tap
Granulomatous
Hematogone
Immunohistochemical stain
Ringed sideroblast

BACKGROUND BASICS

The information in this chapter builds on concepts from previous chapters. To maximize your learning experience, you should review these concepts before beginning this chapter.

Level I

▶ Review the development and differentiation of hematopoietic cells. (Chapters 2, 3)
▶ Describe the structure and function of the bone marrow. (Chapter 4)
▶ Describe normal erythropoiesis and leukopoiesis. (Chapters 5, 7)

Level II

▶ Identify the changes that lead to bone marrow hyperplasia or hypoplasia. (Chapter 4)

CASE STUDY

We will refer to this case study throughout the chapter.

Robert, a 32-year-old male, visited his primary care physician with complaints of weakness and fatigue. He had been in good health until two months ago when he noted he was becoming increasingly tired after usual daily work activity. Physical examination reveals no lymphadenopathy, hepatomegaly, or splenomegaly. CBC shows the following:

Hemoglobin	9 g/dL (90 g/L)
Hematocrit	27%
WBC	2.0×10^9/L
Platelet count	30×10^9/L

Evaluate these results and consider additional tests that should be done and a possible diagnosis.

▶ OVERVIEW

Bone marrow examination may be necessary to diagnose, make a prognosis, and/or evaluate therapeutic response for a variety of hematologic and nonhematologic problems. The clinical laboratory professional is responsible for preparing the specimen and performing the preliminary examination of the bone marrow sample. This chapter discusses the indications for performing a bone marrow procedure, as well as the preparation and evaluation of a bone marrow specimen. Emphasis

is on the processing and preparation of the specimen for morphologic study. The evaluation and interpretation of bone marrow findings are discussed. Specimen requirements and indications for ancillary studies are also included. The content of the bone marrow report is described.

▶ INTRODUCTION

Hematopoiesis takes place in different locations during embryogenesis. It begins in the yolk sac as early as 19 days gestation. At about the third month of fetal life, the liver becomes the chief site of hematopoiesis. (To a lesser extent, hematopoiesis occurs in the spleen, kidney, thymus, and lymph nodes.) In the third trimester, after birth, and throughout adult life, the bone marrow is the primary source of hematopoiesis (∞ Chapter 4).

Bone marrow, the hematopoietic compartment of bone, is a highly vascularized loose connective tissue located between the trabeculae of spongy bone. It has a volume of 30–50 mL/kg of body weight. The marrow is composed of two major compartments, hematopoietic and vascular. The hematopoietic compartment includes both hematopoietic cells and stromal cells (supporting cells). It is composed of hematopoietically active red marrow (erythroid and myeloid cells) and hematopoietically inactive yellow marrow. The yellow marrow occupies the central cavity and is composed of adipocytes. The vascular compartment of the bone marrow is composed of the nutrient artery, vein, arterioles, and sinuses (Figure 4-3).

▶ INDICATIONS FOR BONE MARROW EVALUATION

Evaluation of the bone marrow is necessary for diagnosing, managing, making prognoses, and following up a variety of hematologic and nonhematologic disorders (Table 35-1 ✪). The bone marrow should always be evaluated in conjunction with the peripheral blood counts and smear, which often reflect changes in the marrow.

CASE STUDY (continued)

Review of the peripheral blood smear confirms the presence of thrombocytopenia. Red cells are normochromic and normocytic with no increase in reticulocytes. A few teardrop cells are present. White cells show a left shift but no toxic granulation or Döhle bodies. No circulating blasts are seen.

Robert denies any history of alcohol abuse. The test for HIV is negative, and he is not on any medications. Vitamin B_{12} and folic acid levels are normal.

1. Is a bone marrow evaluation indicated in this patient? Why or why not?

⊕ TABLE 35-1

Conditions for Which a Bone Marrow Evaluation Is Indicated

- Primary diagnosis of hematopoietic and lymphoid malignancies
  - Acute leukemias
  - Chronic myeloproliferative disorders
  - Chronic lymphoproliferative disorders
  - Myelodysplastic syndromes
  - Hodgkin and non-Hodgkin lymphomas
  - Plasma cell neoplasms
- Staging of lymphoid malignancies and solid tumors
- Post-treatment follow-up
  - Postchemotherapy and radiation therapy
  - Poststem cell transplant
- Detection of infection and/or source of fever of unknown origin
  - Mycobacterium and fungal infections
  - Granulomas
  - Unknown infectious agents using cultures and special stains
  - Hemophagocytic syndrome
- Primary diagnosis of systemic diseases
  - Metabolic disorders (Gaucher's disease, etc.)
  - Systemic mastocytosis
- Miscellaneous
  - Evaluation of storage iron
  - Evaluation of unexplained cytopenias

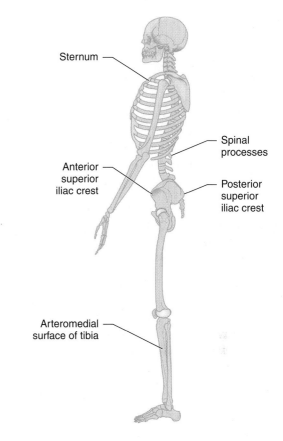

■ **FIGURE 35-1** Sites used for aspiration and biopsy of bone marrow.

► BONE MARROW PROCEDURE

Sites of hematopoiesis also differ by age. At birth, hematopoietic red marrow fills all bone cavities. With age, adipose tissue (fat) replaces hematopoietic tissue in some bones. By adolescence, hematopoietic marrow is only in centrally located bones including the skull, scapulae, ribs, sternum, clavicles, vertebrae, and the proximal ends of the long bones of the arms and legs. In certain disease states (e.g., thalassemia, sickle cell anemia), red marrow in the adult can extend into the long bones. Cellularity within red marrow decreases with age. At birth, red marrow is about 90% cellular. This decreases to about 50% in an elderly adult. This change in sites of hematopoiesis and cellularity has implications for where to sample the bone marrow and how to interpret cellularity. Most marrow specimens are taken from the posterior superior iliac crest (Figure 35-1 ■) after adolescence, although the sternum and anterior iliac crest are occasionally used in adult patients. The anteromedial surface of the tibia is sometimes used in children less than 2 years of age. The spines of the lumbar vertebral bodies L1 and L2 occasionally are used in older children. The composition of marrow obtained from different sites has been shown to be similar (the proportion of different cells at different sites is similar).

The bone marrow aspirates and biopsies are obtained using disposable needles that are modifications of the needle first introduced by Jamshidi.[1] A sterile technique is always used. The skin over the biopsy site is first cleaned with a disinfectant solution, and then 1–2% lidocaine (local anesthetic) is infiltrated into the skin, subcutaneous tissue, and periosteum. Some patients require additional sedation with intravenous or intramuscular medications. A small skin incision is made with a blade to facilitate needle penetration. Performing the biopsy first and then the aspirating to avoid distortion of the marrow architecture in the biopsy specimen is recommended. However, because the aspirate can clot if the biopsy is done first, some institutions prefer performing the aspirate first. When it is done first, performing the biopsy on a different site on the periosteal surface is recommended.[2] In adults, a *trephine core biopsy* commonly uses an 11-gauge cutting needle to obtain a core of marrow tissue. This is followed by aspiration of about 2 mL of marrow using an 18-gauge needle.

Complications of bone marrow biopsy and aspiration are rare, especially when performed by experienced practitioners. The most common complications are localized bleeding or infection. Most patients experience discomfort during the aspiration procedure even with adequate infiltration of local anesthetic. If not carefully performed, going through the entire thickness of the bone and damaging the underlying tissues is possible. This risk is higher with a sternal aspiration. After the biopsy procedure, the patient is advised to lie on the biopsy site. The patient's site should be reevaluated in 15–30 minutes for any bleeding or oozing. The actual procedure usually is performed with the assistance of a clinical laboratory professional. The laboratory professional's responsibility is to determine the adequacy of the samples.

Neither thrombocytopenia, coagulation factor deficiency, or anticoagulant therapy is contraindicated for the bone marrow procedure. Applying pressure at the biopsy site and having the patients lie on their back for 20–30 minutes can control local bleeding in thrombocytopenic patients. Correcting severe coagulation factor deficiencies before the procedure is indicated in hemophiliacs because they can experience intense local bleeding. The only time a bone marrow biopsy should not be performed is when a bone marrow will not assist in diagnosing or evaluating the patient's condition. The indication criteria for performing a bone marrow examination are listed in Table 35-1.

 Checkpoint! 1

A 25-year-old male was recently diagnosed with ALL and received chemotherapy. It is 21 days after the chemotherapy. A bone marrow biopsy has been scheduled to determine whether residual leukemia is present. His platelet count is $10 \times 10^9/L$. Does this patient have a significant risk of bleeding? Is it necessary to cancel the procedure until the platelet count is more than $50 \times 10^9/L$?

▶ BONE MARROW PROCESSING FOR EXAMINATION

A laboratory professional with experience in bone marrow preparation accompanies the physician performing the bone marrow aspirate and biopsy.

BONE MARROW ASPIRATE SMEARS, PARTICLE PREPARATION, AND CLOT SECTIONS

Approximately 1.0–1.5 mL of aspirate is needed to evaluate bone marrow morphology. Although each laboratory has its own preferences for processing the aspirate, a commonly used procedure is described here. Depending on the clinical setting, additional aspirate can be obtained for cytogenetics, flow cytometry, molecular studies, and cultures.

A small amount (about 0.5 mL) of the aspirate is placed on a glass slide and examined to determine whether bone marrow is present in the sample (sometimes it is blood rather than marrow). The presence of particles consisting of fat, granules, and/or small pieces of bone in the aspirate sample that can be

visualized on the slide is evidence that the bone marrow cavity was entered and that marrow was effectively aspirated.[2] The laboratory professional immediately communicates the adequacy of the bone marrow aspirate to the physician. Bone marrow occasionally cannot be aspirated, resulting in a **dry tap.** This can be caused by inadequate technique or more commonly alterations in the bone marrow architecture such as extensive fibrosis (e.g., hairy cell leukemia, chronic idiopathic myelofibrosis) or very increased cellularity (e.g., leukemia). In these cases, bone marrow biopsy is especially important.

Direct smears of bone marrow aspirate are prepared at the bedside using a technique similar to that for preparing peripheral blood smears.[3] Good organization of supplies and speed in making these smears is essential because the aspirate clots quickly. Bone marrow particle crush smears can be prepared by pouring a small amount of marrow aspirate onto a watch glass. Using a glass pipette, the marrow particles are transferred onto several glass slides. A second slide is placed gently on top of the slide with the drop containing the particles. The top slide is pulled apart to evenly distribute the marrow particles. Cell morphology is better appreciated on the aspirate smears, and the architecture and cellularity are assessed on the trephine core biopsy and particle preparation. The clinical laboratory professional usually prepares several aspirate smears for special stains that may be necessary for classifying of acute leukemias and myelodysplastic syndromes and evaluating storage iron. The remaining bone marrow particles can be used for histologic evaluation.

Tissue particles admixed with blood can be left to clot and then fixed in 10% buffered formalin or B-5 (a fixative containing mercury, which is environmentally unfriendly and difficult to dispose of, and is thus rarely used) and processed for histologic sectioning (clot sections). However, better results are obtained if the blood and particles are placed in an ethylenediaminetetraacetic (EDTA) tube and mixed before clotting begins. The blood and particles are filtered through histowrap filter paper, and the concentrated particles on the paper are fixed in 10% buffered formalin. In the histology laboratory, the particles left on paper are collected and embedded in paraffin for further processing.[4]

Some laboratories mix a portion of the marrow aspirate with EDTA. This anticoagulated marrow is placed in a Wintrobe tube and centrifuged. The marrow is separated into four layers: fat and perivascular cells, plasma, buffy coat, and red cells. The ratio between the fat/perivascular and the erythroid/myeloid layers reflects the overall marrow cellularity. Concentrate smears can be prepared from the buffy coat. The direct, concentrate, and particle crush smears are stained with Wright's stain.

TOUCH IMPRINTS AND CORE BIOPSY

Immediately after obtaining the bone marrow core biopsy, touch imprints of the biopsy can be made by gently touching or rolling the tissue several times on 2–4 glass slides.

Some cells from the core specimen will stick to the slide. Some of these slides are stained with Wright's stain, and the rest can be used for special stains in case a good aspirate is not available. After making the touch preparations, the core biopsy specimen is immediately immersed in 10% buffered formalin fixative. The fixed trephine core biopsy, particle, and clot preparations undergo histologic processing including decalcifying, dehydrating, embedding in paraffin blocks, sectioning of 2–3 μm thick sections, and histologic staining with hematoxylin and eosin (H&E). Some laboratories prefer to fix bone marrow particles, clot, and core biopsy in B-5 first followed by 10% buffered formalin fixative. The B-5 fixed samples have better morphologic sections than 10% formalin.

Trephine core biopsies are performed for primary diagnosis as well as for disease staging purposes. When performed for clinical staging of lymphoma, multiple myeloma, and carcinoma, bilateral biopsies are recommended.

▶ MORPHOLOGIC INTERPRETATION OF BONE MARROW

Morphologic review of bone marrow includes cytologic assessment of hematopoietic cells on the aspirate smear as well as histologic assessment of the clot, particle preparation, touch imprint, and core biopsy. Review of these preparations provides a wealth of information about hematopoiesis including estimation of cellularity, details of cell morphology, estimation of the quantity of iron and its distribution, and presence of abnormal cells such as tumor cells.

BONE MARROW ASPIRATE

It is good practice to review the complete blood count (CBC) data and the corresponding peripheral blood smear in conjunction with the bone marrow. The number and appearance of the blood cells guide the morphologist to a differential diagnosis. The bone marrow aspirate is used to evaluate the number, morphology, and maturation process of erythroid and myeloid precursors and megakaryocytes (Figure 35-2 ▦).

The bone marrow aspirate smears are scanned at 100× magnification to determine cellularity and to select a suitable area for examining and performing the differential count. Optimal areas are where the cells are spread out and intact. Areas where the marrow cells are destroyed due to squashing or stripping of their cytoplasm by fibrin thread should be avoided. These areas are characterized by the presence of bare nuclei.

Bone marrow cellularity is determined by estimating the percent of bone marrow space occupied by hematopoietic tissue. The reference range decreases with age. As mentioned, infants have the highest cellularity (90%) and older adults the lowest (50%). While scanning for cellularity, the number and the distribution of the megakaryocytes are usually noted.

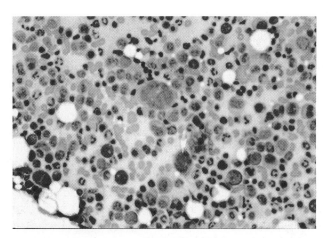

■ FIGURE 35-2 Bone marrow aspirate smear showing normal maturing trilineage hematopoiesis (Bone marrow; Wright-Giemsa stain; 200× magnification)

Megakaryocytes are usually adjacent to a spicule, a fragment of spongy bone along which hematopoietic cells cluster and mature. An optimal aspirate has some spicules present, and most particles should contain at least one megakaryocyte. Direct smears should contain 5–10 megakaryocytes in the readable portion of the slide, and concentrate smears should contain numerous megakaryocytes.[2]

After the initial scan at 100× magnification, the details of nuclear and cytoplasmic maturation are evaluated at higher magnification (500× or 1000×). Evaluation of maturation is an important step when reviewing the marrow aspirate. Abnormal maturation can be seen in any of the three cell lines. For example, abnormal maturation is a diagnostic criteria in the myelodysplastic syndromes (MDS). In MDS, abnormalities of the red cell precursors include multinucleation and nuclear/cytoplasmic dysynchrony (nuclear maturation is delayed compared to cytoplasmic maturation). Myeloid precursors can show abnormal granule development, and megakaryocytes can reveal hypolobulation of the nucleus. Abnormalities in bone marrow that are characteristic of a specific pathology are discussed in ∞ Chapters 8–18 (anemias) and ∞ 21–26 (neoplastic disorders).

Bone Marrow Differential Count
A 500–1000 cell differential (a 500 cell differential can be performed on each of two slides) is usually performed by an experienced clinical laboratory professional or pathologist using 1000× magnification on the direct smear or the crush particle preparation (the morphology is better preserved on these preparations).[2] The concentrate and/or touch imprint is a useful source when the bone marrow is very hypocellular or aspirate could not be obtained (dry tap), although the morphology is not as good as that on direct smears and crush particle preparations. Overall marrow cellularity can be estimated on the particle preparation.

Because the bone marrow composition changes with age, knowing the patient's age when evaluating bone marrow specimens is important. In infants during the first month after birth, dramatic alterations occur in the distribution of the different marrow compartments. Myeloid precursors are usually increased at birth followed (within few weeks) by a predominance of lymphoid cells. These lymphoid cells are called **hematogones** and represent normal immature B cells (Figure 35-3 ■).[5] Morphologically and phenotypically, differentiating hematogones from lymphoblasts is difficult. In young children, lymphocytes can represent about one-third of marrow cellularity, which decreases gradually after puberty.

Bone marrow is not as homogeneous as blood. During the bone marrow procedure, the needle can be placed in an area that has aggregates of erythroid or lymphoid cells. In adult bone marrow, lymphocytes are usually present as interstitial infiltrate and sometimes form lymphoid follicles, which are collections or aggregations of lymphocytes. These lymphocytes can be malignant or benign (see section on benign versus malignant lymphoid aggregates). Depending on the placement of the bone marrow needle, the cells in the follicle can be aspirated. This can give an estimate of markedly increased lymphocytes in the marrow and introduce significant variation in the differential count from sample to sample in the same patient.

Megakaryocytes are not included in the differential count but are evaluated by scanning the smear at 100× because megakaryocytes are not evenly distributed in the marrow or on the smear.

The greatest mass of the adult marrow is composed of granulopoietic and erythropoietic precursors. For the purpose of the differential count, these hematopoietic cells are enumerated within different categories according to their stage of maturation. Cells not normally found in the peripheral blood including macrophages, mast cells, osteoblasts, and osteoclasts can be found in the bone marrow. (These cells are described in ∞ Chapter 4.)

Myeloid to Erythroid Ratio

When adequate numbers of cells are counted (500–1000) and differentiated, the percentage of each category is calculated. The ratio between all granulocytes and their precursors and all nucleated red cell precursors represents the myeloid:erythroid ratio (M:E ratio). This parameter indicates significant changes in the cellularity of the myeloid and erythroid cells. The M:E ratio should always be interpreted in context with the overall cellularity. For instance, a low M:E ratio can mean erythroid hyperplasia or myeloid hypoplasia. If it is known, however, that the bone marrow cellularity is increased, a low M:E ratio means erythroid hyperplasia or ineffective erythropoiesis.

The reference range for the M:E ratio differs depending on whether the segmented neutrophils are included in the counts. If they are considered a part of the bone marrow storage pool and not included in the count, the M:E reference range is between 1.5:1 and 3:1. If segmented neutrophils are included in the count, the M:E reference range is between 2:1 and 4:1.

The granulocytic tissue occupies 2 to 4 times more marrow space than the erythrocytic precursors because of the shorter survival of the granulocytes in the circulation (i.e., neutrophils' 6–10 hours versus erythrocytes' 120 days). Changes in the survival time of granulocytes and erythrocytes are reflected in changes in the M:E ratio. Normal, increased, or decreased M:E ratios are associated with certain disease entities. For example, patients with chronic myelogenous leukemia usually have an increased ratio; in contrast, patients with myelodysplastic syndrome usually have a decreased ratio.

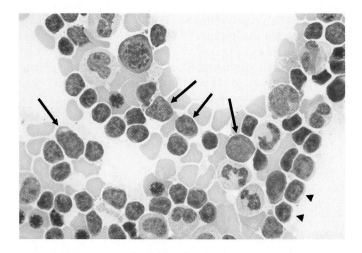

■ **FIGURE 35-3**   A bone marrow aspirate smear from a 21-year-old woman following chemotherapy for acute lymphoblastic leukemia (ALL). Hematogones typically display homogenous chromatin with a smudged appearance, indistinct nucleoli, and scant cytoplasm. Many hematogones (arrows) are indistinguishable from ALL blasts but the morphology of hematogones is variable, reflecting the maturation of the hematogones toward mature lymphocytes (arrows). (Wright stain; 1000× magnification)

✓ Checkpoint! 2

A 60-year-old male complained to his local physician of abdominal fullness. The CBC showed an elevated leukocyte count with absolute neutrophilia and basophilia. The peripheral blood smear revealed numerous myelocytes. A bone marrow biopsy was performed. The bone marrow differential was reported as follows: blasts 1%, myelocytes 35%, metamyelocytes 20%, bands 10%, segmented neutrophils 20%, eosinophils 1%, basophils 3%, pronormoblasts 1%, basophilic normoblasts 3%, polychromatophilic normoblasts 2%, orthochromatic normoblasts 4%, lymphocytes 0%, and monocytes 0%. What is the M:E ratio?

TOUCH IMPRINTS

When the bone marrow is a dry tap secondary to underlying fibrosis (myelofibrosis, hairy cell leukemia) or when the marrow aspirate lacks spicules and is hemodiluted, the touch imprints of the bone marrow biopsy can be the only source for studying the sample's cellular detail and maturation sequence. Sometimes the touch preparations contain enough cells for performing a differential count and cytochemical stains (Figure 35-4 ■).

BONE MARROW PARTICLE PREPARATION, CLOT AND CORE BIOPSY

The advantage of bone marrow biopsy is that it represents a large sample of marrow and bone structures in their natural relationship. Some marrow particles obtained during the aspiration procedure and the biopsy specimen can be processed for histologic examination.

Various other stains also can be used. Iron stain can be performed to evaluate storage iron; however, because of decalcification, the core biopsy might not be good to study marrow iron stores. Iron stores should be evaluated on aspirate smears, particle preparations, or clot sections. Reticulin and trichrome stains are used to evaluate the presence of fibrosis. Acid-fast organisms and fungi in **granulomatous** (a distinctive pattern of chronic reaction in which the predominant cell type is an activated macrophage with an epithelial-like appearance) diseases can be detected quickly with specific stains, offering great advantages in diagnosing these infections. When metastatic tumors and lymphomas are found in the bone marrow, **immunohistochemical stains** can be used on histologic sections to demonstrate specific tumor markers. Immunohistochemical stains use labeled antibodies to identify specific markers (antigens) on cells. Thus, a very precise diagnosis of the origin of a tumor can be made without elaborate, expensive, and more invasive techniques. Immunophenotyping by flow cytometry can be performed only on fresh unfixed bone marrow samples (aspirate or core biopsy); immunophenotyping by immunohistochemistry is performed on paraffin fixed samples.

A disadvantage of the bone marrow biopsy is that it loses fine cellular details in the processing; therefore, it is of little value in diagnosing leukemias and some refractory anemias. In these situations, the touch preparation from the biopsy could supply the missing morphologic details.

Molecular studies can be done on marrow specimens to aid in diagnosing and managing some diseases. Polymerase chain reaction (PCR) can be performed on fresh samples and paraffin embedded formalin fixed marrow biopsy. PCR technology can be used to detect B cell or T cell gene rearrangements, various leukemias, and minimal residual disease and to diagnose infectious diseases (∞ Chapter 39).

Bone Marrow Cellularity

The overall bone marrow cellularity is estimated by comparing the amount of hematopoietic tissue with the amount of adipose (fat) tissue. Fat appears as a clear space. An easy way to determine the normal expected cellularity range in an adult is to subtract the patient's age from 100% and add and substract (+/−) 10%. For example, a normal 70-year-old adult has an overall cellularity between 20% and 40%. Variation in cellularity within the bone marrow can occur. The subcortical and paratrabecular areas are more hypocellular than the deeper medullary area, and variability occurs in cellularity within the sample itself. For these reasons, estimated cellularity is based on an average percentage. If both hypercellular and hypocellular areas are present within the medullary area, the variation should be described in the report because average cellularity can be difficult to estimate.

Although cellularity can be estimated on aspirate smear, clot section, and particle preparation, the bone marrow biopsy is the optimal sample for this purpose and is typically evaluated at 10× objective. After considering the patient's age, bone marrow cellularity is reported as decreased (less than the expected number of hematopoietic cells), normal, or increased (more than the number of expected cells). With experience, reproducible and reliable results can be achieved when evaluating marrow cellularity (Figure 35-5 ■).

BENIGN LYMPHOID AGGREGATES VERSUS MALIGNANT LYMPHOMA

Reactive lymphoid aggregates can be seen in the bone marrow biopsy of elderly individuals. When one sees these aggregates, distinguishing between reactive (benign) versus lymphoma (malignancy) becomes important. Features

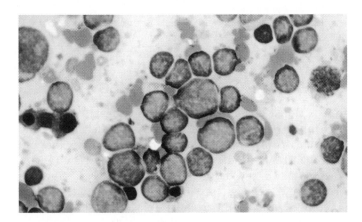

■ FIGURE 35-4   Touch imprint from a case with ALL showing many lymphoblasts. Marrow was inaspirable and therefore was not available for the morphologic review. Cytochemical stains were performed on these imprints, and blasts were negative for all stains. (BM touch imprints; Wright-Giemsa stain; 500× magnification)

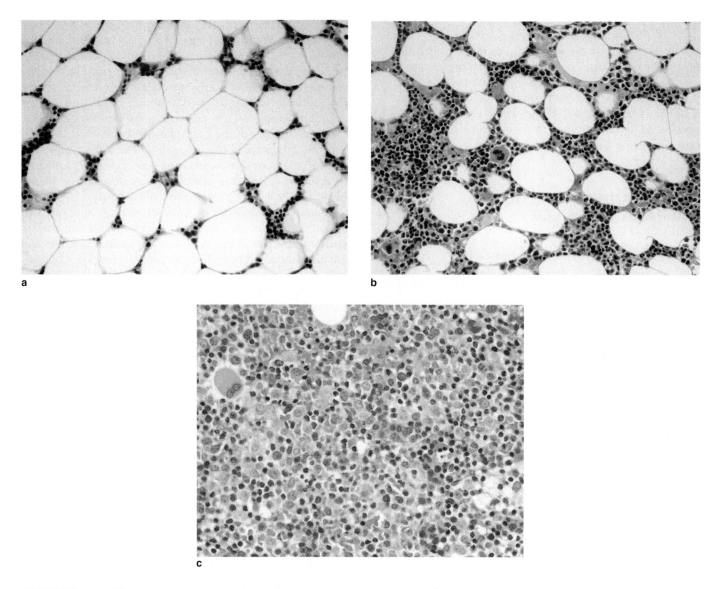

■ FIGURE 35-5   These bone marrow biopsies are from 40-year-old patients **a.** is a hypocellular marrow, **b.** is a normocellular marrow, and **c.** is a hypercellular marrow. (Bone marrow; paraffin section, hematoxylin-eosin stain; 100× magnification)

favoring benign aggregates are nonparatrabecular, single, small, well-defined, polymorphic populations of lymphocytes (small and large lymphocytes) with plasma cells at the periphery and presence of blood vessels within the aggregate (Figure 35-6■). On the contrary, lymphoid aggregates in lymphoma are ill defined, small to large, and composed of monomorphic cells. The malignant aggregates can be paratrabecular or interstial, diffuse, and patchy (Figure 35-7■). In case of doubt, immunohistochemical stains and/or PCR can be performed on the marrow biopsy specimen to differentiate between benign lymphoid aggregates and lymphoma. Presence of an aberrant phenotype or clonal B or T cells would favor lymphoma involving the bone marrow.

BONE MARROW IRON STORES

Iron is stored as ferritin (iron complexed with apoferritin protein) and hemosiderin in reticuloendothelial cells and erythroblasts. The storage iron in the bone marrow that can be visualized is in the form of hemosiderin. On Wright-Giemsa-stained smears, hemosiderin appears as brownish blue granules while on unstained smears, it is golden yellow. To precisely evaluate intracellular storage iron, slides are usually stained with Prussian blue stain.

Prussian Blue Stain for Iron

The Prussian blue stain provides the most direct means for assessing body iron stores. It is designed to demonstrate the

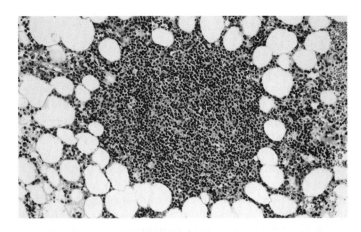

■ FIGURE 35-6   Bone marrow biopsy showing a well circumscribed lymphoid aggregate indicating a benign lymphoid aggregate. (Bone marrow; paraffin section, hematoxylin-eosin stain; 100× magnification)

presence of hemosiderin in histiocytes, erythroblasts (sideroblasts), and/or erythrocytes (siderocytes). The EDTA chelating method should be used to decalcify the bone marrow biopsies if iron studies are being performed. Rapid acid decalcifying solutions extract iron; therefore, these specimens must not be used.

In this staining procedure, a weak acid solution is needed to free the iron from the loose protein bonds present in the hemosiderin molecule. This free iron combines with potassium ferrocyanide to produce ferric ferrocyanide. Free iron appears greenish blue.

Histiocytes contain marrow iron that is usually seen as fine cytoplasmic granules. Sideroblasts are marrow erythroid

precursors that contain iron specks (Figure 35-8 ■). Storage iron can be reported as absent, decreased, adequate, or increased. Some institutions give a numerical value ranging from 0 to 4 (2 representing adequate iron stores in an adult).

Evaluating and grading iron stores can be subjective; thus, for consistency and precision, some guidelines such as increased storage when clumps of iron are easily seen at 100× magnification should be followed; a few specks of iron found after looking at several microscopic fields at 500× or 1000× magnification indicate decreased iron storage. When no stainable iron is detected in the bone marrow smear or tissue sections, iron is depleted or absent. Iron is also stored as intracellular ferritin. All developing normoblasts and reticulocytes contain dispersed ferritin but may not stain with Prussian blue. Small amounts of ferritin enter the blood and can be measured as serum ferritin. The amount of circulating ferritin parallels the concentration of storage iron in the body. Nonspecific increases are associated with chronic infection and inflammation, liver disease, and malignancy. Thus, serum ferritin is not as accurate an indicator of iron sufficiency as hemosiderin in the presence of these conditions.

Use of Bone Marrow Iron Evaluation

Evaluating marrow iron stores is essential in diagnosing anemias, especially in refractory and dyserythropoietic anemias. When the morphologic characteristic of the iron particles in the histiocytes and red cell precursors is an important diagnostic consideration (as in myelodysplastic syndrome), an iron stain is performed on a particle smear. If the overall

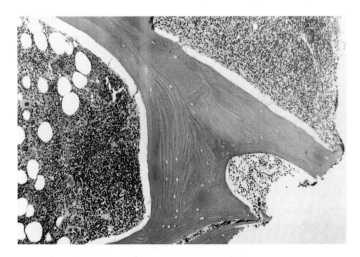

■ FIGURE 35-7   Bone marrow biopsy showing two paratrabecular lymphoid infiltrates suggesting involvement of marrow by a follicle center cell lymphoma. (Bone marrow; paraffin section, hematoxylin-eosin stain; 100× magnification)

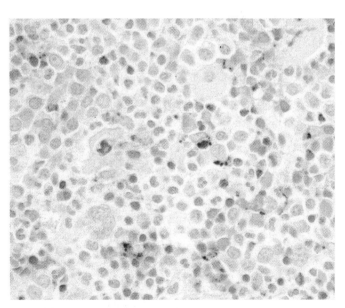

■ FIGURE 35-8   Bone marrow clot section stained with Prussian blue. The bluish granules indicate the presence of iron. (Bone marrow; clot section, Prussian blue stain; 400× magnification)

distribution of the amount of iron is of clinical importance (iron-deficiency anemia, anemia of chronic diseases), then histologic sections of bone marrow particles and marrow clotted particles are stained for iron.

The determination of bone marrow storage iron is useful in the classifying anemias associated with defective hemoglobin synthesis. Storage iron is markedly decreased or absent in iron-deficiency anemia. When storage iron is present in the bone marrow, anemia cannot be a result of iron deficiency unless the patient has been transfused with red cells or treated with iron supplements. Iron stores are normal or increased in anemia of chronic disease and thalassemias. Iron stores are also increased in sideroblastic anemia. The presence of **ringed sideroblasts** is diagnostic for sideroblastic anemia and/or myelodysplastic syndrome. However, ringed sideroblasts can also be seen in myeloproliferative disorders, megaloblastic anemia, alcoholism, and postchemotherapy situations. Ringed sideroblasts are erythroid precursors that have a deposition of excess iron around the nucleus arranged like a necklace. This iron is located within the mitochondria that surround the nucleus.

✓ Checkpoint! 3

A pathologist is evaluating a bone marrow biopsy from a patient suspected of having a myelodysplastic syndrome. Evaluation of the peripheral blood reveals both hypochromic and normochromic red cells. The bone marrow aspirate shows dysplastic (abnormal cell development) changes in the red cell precursors. The pathologist ordered an iron stain on the particle crush preparation. Why is the iron stain useful in this case?

► SPECIAL STUDIES ON BONE MARROW

In most cases, a thorough examination of a well-stained bone marrow aspirate smear and core biopsy provides enough information by which diagnoses of hematopoietic disorders are made. However, several ancillary studies can provide additional information that help support or confirm the morphologic diagnosis. These studies can also provide prognostic information and, in some cases, can predict response to therapy. The most commonly used ancillary studies are flow cytometry, conventional cytogenetics, fluorescent in situ hybridization (FISH), molecular genetic studies, and cytochemical stains (∞ Chapters 34, 37, 38, 39).

FLOW CYTOMETRY

Flow cytometry allows the simultaneous analysis of multiple characteristics of cells in suspension as they pass through a laser light beam. The size and internal complexity of the cells can be estimated, and with the use of fluorochrome-labeled antibodies, the presence of specific cell markers can be determined. Flow cytometry has a wide range of uses in the evaluation of hematologic disorders. It is commonly used to establish the presence of clonality, diagnose and classify malignant lymphomas and leukemias, and detect minimal residual disease after chemotherapy use. The immunophenotyping of peripheral blood, bone marrow, lymph node (and other) tissues, and body fluids is performed only on fresh samples (Table 35-2 ✪) (∞ Chapter 37).

✪ TABLE 35-2

Specimen Requirements for Special Studies on Bone Marrow

Specimen	Flow Cytometry	Cytogenetics	Molecular Studies
Blood	5 mL in EDTA, heparin sodium, or ACD	5 mL preferably in heparin sodium	1–3 mL in EDTA
Bone marrow	1 mL in EDTA, heparin sodium, or ACD	1–3 mL preferably in heparin sodium; bone marrow preferable over blood	1–3 mL in EDTA (preferable over heparin)
Fluids	As much as possible, anticoagulated if contaminated with blood	As much as possible, anticoagulated if contaminated with blood	5–10 mL
Tissue	0.5 cm² fresh in transport media or saline	1 cm² fresh in transport media	3–5 mm² fresh or frozen; fixed specimens good for PCR analysis
All specimens: transport and storage	Should be kept at room temperature and analyzed within 24 hours; up to 72 hours is acceptable in some cases; should be refrigerated if analysis will not occur within 24 hours; frozen or fixed specimens unacceptable	Should be kept at RT and transported to the laboratory within 24 hours; frozen or fixed samples unacceptable	If not analyzed within 24 hours, should be refrigerated (2–8°C) for up to 1 week; samples frozen at −20°C or −70°C should be stored for 2 weeks or 2 years, respectively

EDTA = ethylenediaminetetraacetic acid; ACD = acid citrate dextrose; RT = room temperature

CYTOGENETICS

Chromosome analysis is frequently used in the study of hematopoietic disorders because certain malignancies have characteristic chromosomal alterations. In addition, the presence of some specific chromosomal abnormalities has prognostic implications. Chromosome analysis is routinely used in the primary diagnosis of acute leukemias, malignant lymphomas, myelodysplastic syndromes, and myeloproliferative disorders. Because lymphoma cells are more difficult to grow, adequate clinical history needs to be provided when the sample is sent to the cytogenetics laboratory to allow the cytogenetic technologist to make procedural adjustments. Analysis is performed on fresh samples (Table 35-2). More recent techniques such as FISH have allowed specific cytogenetic questions to be answered more quickly. Triaging the bone marrow samples depends on what clinical answer is

being considered and thus can vary case by case. A guideline is presented (Table 35-3 ✪) that can be modified in any lab depending on the need and/or protocols.

MOLECULAR GENETICS

Although molecular genetic techniques were initially used in research laboratories, they are now performed in clinical laboratories. For hematolymphoid disorders, PCR has emerged as the leading adjunctive technology. The PCR method is used to demonstrate cell clonality and lineage and to identify specific genetic rearrangements. Additionally, PCR can be used to detect minimal residual disease (∞ Chapter 39). Fresh and frozen samples are preferable for PCR; however, samples fixed in formalin or embedded in paraffin are acceptable for PCR analysis (Table 35-2).

✪ TABLE 35-3

Triaging Bone Marrow Samples for Ancillary Studies

Diagnosis/History	Flow Cytometry	Cytogenetics/FISH	Molecular
Acute Leukemia (new, follow-up or post stem cell transplant)	Yes	Yes	Maybe* Post stem cell transplant – Chimerism studies can be performed by PCR
CLL	Yes	Yes	No
CML	No**	Yes	Yes (BCR/ABL mutation)
Chronic myeloproliferative disorders - Polycythemia vera - Essential thrombocythemia - Chronic idiopathic myelofibrosis	No	Yes	Yes (JAK-2 mutation)
Chronic Myelomonocytic leukemia (CMML)	Yes	Yes	No***
Myelodysplasia	No	Yes	No
Multiple myeloma	No	Yes	No
Hodgkin lymphoma	No	No	No
Non-Hodgkin lymphoma	Yes	Maybe****	Maybe****

*Molecular studies are usually not needed (depends upon subtype of acute leukemia) as most genetic abnormalities seen in acute leukemias can be detected by cytogenetics/FISH. However, the distinction between p210 and p190 chimeric protein in ALL with t(9;22) is made by molecular analysis. If uncertain about submitting for molecular studies it's a good idea to store cell pellet with possibility of doing the assay if needed.

**When suspecting CML in blast crisis, send it for flow cytometry.

***Some cases of CMML may need molecular or FISH studies (for example: if suspecting t(5;12) and the cytogenetics are normal)

****When suspecting certain lymphomas (example: Mantle cell, Burkitt's/Burkitt's-like vs large cell lymphomas or anaplastic large cell lymphoma send it for cytogenetics and/or FISH).

When suspecting follicle center cell lymphoma; send it to molecular lab or FISH for Bcl-2 rearrangement.

Note: This table can be modified in any lab depending on the need and/or protocols.

CLL = Chronic Lymphocytic Leukemia; CML = Chronic Myelogeneous Leukemia; FISH = Fluorescence in-situ hybridization.

CASE STUDY *(continued from page 798)*

A bone marrow procedure was performed. The marrow was difficult to aspirate, but the physician was able to obtain some hemodiluted marrow. Bilateral marrow biopsy was also performed. Review of the aspirate smears showed a very hemodiluted sample, but the pathologist was able to see an increased number of blasts. There was not enough aspirate sample to do flow cytometry or cytogenetic and cytochemical stains.

2. How should the marrow evaluation proceed?

CYTOCHEMICAL STAINS

In hematology, *cytochemistry* refers to in vitro staining of cells to allow microscopic examination of the cells' chemical composition. Cells of different lineages have different cytochemical compositions. The staining process does not significantly alter cell morphology. Cytochemical stains are usually performed on specimens from patients who have a neoplasm of hematopoietic cells. These stains help differentiate the lineage of immature cells so that an accurate diagnosis of the type of neoplasm can be made. See Table 34-12.

Smears are usually made from peripheral blood and bone marrow. Although bone marrow aspirate is usually used to make smears for cytochemical stains, the touch imprints from the biopsy can be used if aspirate is insufficient. The smears are incubated with substrates that react with specific cellular constituents (organelle-associated enzymes, carbohydrates, and proteins). If the specific constituent is present in the cell, its reaction with the substrate is confirmed by the formation of a colored product within the cell. The stained slides are evaluated with an ordinary light microscope. Most stains can be performed on air-dried smears. All cytochemical stains should be performed on recently prepared slides. Some cellular constituents are sensitive to heat, light, storage, and processing technique. If stains cannot be performed on recently prepared slides, the unstained smears can be protected from light in the refrigerator. However, a fresh smear is preferred for the myeloperoxidase (MPO) stain (∞ Chapter 34).

▶ BONE MARROW REPORT

The bone marrow report must contain all relevant information and optimally is composed of two components: clinical information and morphologic interpretation. The clinician should provide the patient's biographic data, clinical differential diagnosis, and relevant therapeutic information. The morphology and interpretation by the pathologist and laboratory professional must include site of sampling (e.g., sternum), types of sample obtained, differential counts from both peripheral blood and bone marrow, and morphologic abnormalities in any cell lines in the patient's peripheral blood or bone marrow. The results must be interpreted in conjunction with any additional studies (special stains, flow cytometry, cytogenetics, molecular studies). If the additional studies are significant in establishing the diagnosis but are unavailable when the bone marrow report is written, an addendum report should mention the significance of these studies. The comparison of the current marrow specimen to the previous tissue samples (marrow or other nonmarrow biopsies) is essential in some situations.

Finally, the pathologist's diagnostic interpretation should be rendered within a reasonable period of time. For example, if 50% blasts were present in the blood or the bone marrow, it is reasonable to call the clinician about the preliminary diagnosis of acute leukemia. However, the final diagnosis can be made only after completing the special stains and flow cytometry studies. Comments, if needed, should be concise and relevant to the case and can include a recommendation for additional tests and a possible differential diagnosis.

CASE STUDY *(continued)*

Processing of bone marrow biopsy usually is done overnight.

3. Can a diagnosis be made from tests on the aspirate rather than waiting for the biopsy slides?

SUMMARY

The bone marrow is the primary site of blood cell production after birth. Evaluation of bone marrow is indicated in the diagnosis, management, and follow-up of a variety of hematopoietic disorders including some anemias and malignancies. Bone marrow specimens include aspirates and biopsy. The marrow is processed and evaluated in the laboratory.

Differentiation and classification of acute leukemias depend on accurate identification of the blasts. Because the lineage of the cells is difficult to differentiate using only morphologic characteristics, the immunophenotyping by flow cytometry and/or immunohistochemistry (and cytochemical stain) are used to help identify blast lineage. Cytogenetic analysis is commonly used in diagnosis because certain malignancies have characteristic chromosome abnormalities. Molecular analysis can be used to demonstrate clonality, cell lineage, and genetic abnormalities. It is useful in diagnosing and evaluating minimal residual disease.

REVIEW QUESTIONS

LEVEL I

1. What is the site for bone marrow collection in children under 2 years of age? (Objective 1)
   a. spleen
   b. sternum
   c. tibia
   d. lumbar vertebral bodies

2. Which of the following indicates that a bone marrow biopsy should be performed? (Objective 2)
   a. 20-year-old male with suspected leukemia
   b. 60-year-old female diagnosed with megaloblastic anemia
   c. 30-year-old male diagnosed with HIV
   d. 20-year-old pregnant woman diagnosed with iron-deficiency anemia

3. What site is most commonly used in adults for bone marrow biopsies? (Objective 1)
   a. sternum
   b. posterior iliac crest
   c. anterior iliac crest
   d. tibia

4. The marrow specimen that is best for preserving the architecture of the bone marrow is: (Objective 3)
   a. aspirate
   b. clot section
   c. particle smear
   d. biopsy

5. Which of the following is the best specimen for evaluating the morphology of the hematopoietic precursors? (Objectives 3, 4)
   a. bone marrow aspirate
   b. clot preparation
   c. iliac crest biopsy
   d. none of the above

6. Which of the following diseases is more likely to have a decreased M:E ratio? (Objective 5)
   a. chronic blood loss
   b. granulocytic leukemia
   c. lymphocytic leukemia
   d. chronic infection

7. What is the expected overall cellularity in a bone marrow biopsy of a normal 50-year-old male? (Objective 6)
   a. 80% ± 10%
   b. 100% ± 10%
   c. 50% ± 10%
   d. 30% ± 10%

8. Which of the following stains is used to evaluate the presence of storage iron? (Objective 6)
   a. Wright-Giemsa
   b. Prussian blue
   c. PAS
   d. reticulin

LEVEL II

1. The following is characteristic of a benign lymphoid aggregate: (Objective 1)
   a. The patient has a history of lymphoma.
   b. It is composed predominantly of small lymphocytes.
   c. It is large with ill-defined borders.
   d. It is paratrabecular and lacks plasma cells at the periphery.

2. A hypercellular bone marrow M:E ratio is 10:1. This indicates: (Objective 3)
   a. decreased erythropoiesis
   b. increased erythropoiesis
   c. increased leukopoiesis
   d. decreased leukopoiesis

3. The following is the differential obtained from a patient with a diagnosis of AML: blasts 65%, myelocytes 4%, metamyelocytes 4%, bands 1%, segmented neutrophils 8%, pronormoblasts 2%, basophilic normoblasts 3%, polychromatic normoblasts 3%, orthochromatic normoblasts 3%, lymphocytes 4%, and monocytes 3%. What is the M:E ratio? (Objective 3)
   a. 10:1
   b. 5.4:1
   c. 7.4:1
   d. 1:7.4

4. When evaluating bone marrow biopsy for estimating the marrow cellularity, which ratio is being estimated? (Objective 4)
   a. hematopoietic cells to fat
   b. hematopoietic cells to bony trabeculae
   c. hematopoietic cells to vessels
   d. granulocytes to fat

5. A pathologist is evaluating a bone marrow biopsy from a patient recently diagnosed with lymphoma. The bone marrow evaluation should include which of the following? (Objective 1)
   a. malignant lymphoid aggregate
   b. granulomatous lesions
   c. iron stores
   d. presence of parasites

6. A pathologist is evaluating a bone marrow biopsy in a patient recently diagnosed with Hodgkin lymphoma. Inadvertently, the lab performed an iron stain on a particle crush preparation. The pathologist saw a few ringed sideroblasts but did not see any dysplastic changes suggestive of myelodysplastic syndrome. In which of the following conditions might ringed sideroblasts appear? (Objective 5)
   a. iron-deficiency anemia
   b. thalassemia
   c. alcoholism
   d. Hodgkin's disease

REVIEW QUESTIONS *(continued)*

LEVEL I

9. Why would special stains be performed on a bone marrow specimen? (Objective 8)
   a. to differentiate leukemias
   b. to determine the M:E ratio
   c. to estimate bone marrow cellularity
   d. to identify hematogones

10. The hematology laboratory's role in bone marrow evaluation is to: (Objective 7)
   a. make direct bone marrow smears
   b. perform the bone marrow aspirate procedure
   c. administer the anesthetic before the procedure
   d. determine the appropriate therapy

LEVEL II

7. A clinical laboratory professional evaluating the bone marrow particle preparation of a patient suspected of having acute leukemia identifies a large number of undifferentiated blasts. What ancillary test should be done? (Objective 2)
   a. molecular diagnostics
   b. cytochemical stains
   c. fluorescent in situ hybridization
   d. HIV testing

8. A physician performs a bone marrow biopsy and aspirate on a 65-year-old male. The cellularity is estimated at 80% and the M:E ratio is 0.5 to 1. The correct description of this marrow is: (Objectives 3, 4)
   a. hypercellular with a decreased M:E ratio
   b. hypercellular with an increased M:E ratio
   c. hypocellular with a decreased M:E ratio
   d. hypocellular with an increased M:E ratio

9. A physician performing a bone marrow biopsy on a patient with a possible diagnosis of acute leukemia is unable to obtain any aspirate but was able to obtain two core biopsies. What is the best way for the clinical laboratory professional to use the material obtained? (Objectives 2, 6)
   a. Place both core biopsies in formalin and process one immediately; save the other for ancillary tests.
   b. Place one core biopsy in formalin and freeze the second one at −70°C.
   c. Place one core biopsy in formalin after making touch imprints; put the second in saline.
   d. Place both core biopsies in saline; freeze one at 0°C and process the other immediately.

10. A 20-year-old patient presented with severe headache. A lumbar puncture performed showed a marked increase in atypical mononuclear cells. The differential diagnosis is acute leukemia or malignant lymphoma. What would be most helpful in distinguishing the two diagnoses? (Objective 2)
   a. molecular diagnostic tests
   b. flow cytometry
   c. cytogenetics tests
   d. cytochemical stains

www.pearsonhighered.com/mckenzie
Use this address to access the free, interactive Companion Website created for this textbook. Find additional information, tables and figures. Evaluate your command of the chapter information using case studies and critical thinking and multiple choice questions.

REFERENCES

1. Jamshidi K, Swaim WR. Bone marrow biopsy with unaltered architecture: A new biopsy device. *J Lab Clin Med*. 1971;77:335–42.

2. Ryan DH, Cohen HJ. Bone marrow examination. In: Hoffman R, Benz EJ, Shattil SJ, Furie B, Cohen HJ, Silberstein LE, McGlave P, eds. *Hematology Basic Principles and Practice*, 4th ed. Philadelphia: Elsevier Churchill Livingstone; 2005.

3. Rywlin AM, Marvan P, Robinson MJ. A simple technique for the preparation of bone marrow smears and sections. *Am J Clin Pathol*. 1970;53:389–93.

4. Peterson LC, Brunning RD. Bone marrow specimen processing. In: Knowles D, ed. *Neoplastic Hematopathology*, 2nd ed. Philadelphia: Lippincott Williams & Wilkins; 2001.

5. Longacre TA, Foucar K, Crago S, Chen IM, Griffith B, Dressler L et al. Hematogones: A multiparameter analysis of bone marrow precursor cells. *Blood*. 1989;73:543–52.

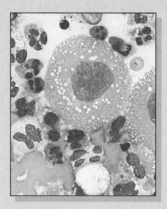

36

Automation in Hematology and Hemostasis

Cheryl Burns, M.S.

■ OBJECTIVES—LEVEL I

At the end of this unit of study, the student should be able to:

1. Cite the electrical impedance principle of cell counting, and identify the instruments that use this technology.

2. Describe the use of radio frequency in cell counting, and identify the instruments that use this technology.

3. State the principles of light scatter used in cell counting, and identify the instruments that use this technology.

4. List the reported parameters for each blood cell–counting instrument.

5. Categorize cell parameters as directly measured and derived from a histogram, scattergram or cytogram, or calculation.

6. Describe the principle of reticulocyte count enumeration by automated blood cell–counting instruments.

7. State the electromechanical principle of clot detection, and identify instruments that use this technology.

8. State the photo-optical principle of clot detection, and identify instruments that use this technology.

■ OBJECTIVES—LEVEL II

At the end of this unit of study, the student should be able to:

1. Compare and contrast the methods of analysis for the described histograms, scatterplots, scattergrams, and cytograms, and interpret the results.

2. Describe and interpret the automated reticulocyte parameters.

3. Describe the application of immunological techniques to coagulation instruments, and identify instruments that use this technology.

KEY TERMS

Aperture

Cellular hemoglobin concentration mean (CHCM)

Cluster analysis

Coincidence

Continuous flow analysis

Contour gating

Hemoglobin distribution width (HDW)

Histogram

Hydrodynamic focusing

Isovolumetric sphering

Mean platelet volume (MPV)

Platelet distribution width (PDW)

Random access

Reagent blank

Reticulated platelet

Scatterplot

Threshold limit

Viscosity

BACKGROUND BASICS

The information in this chapter builds on the concepts learned in previous chapters. To maximize your learning experience, you should review these concepts prior to beginning this unit of study.

Level I

▶ State the principles of cell enumeration by hemacytometer. (Chapter 34)

▶ State the principle of the cyanmethemoglobin method for hemoglobin determination. (Chapter 34)

▶ Calculate the erythrocyte indices. (Chapters 8, 34)

▶ Describe the peripheral blood smear examination process and correlate peripheral blood smear findings with complete blood counts (CBC). (Chapter 34)

▶ Describe and state the principle of the manual reticulocyte count procedure. (Chapter 34)

▶ Describe the basic procedures for evaluation of secondary hemostasis (i.e., prothrombin time and activated partial thromboplastin time). (Chapter 40)

Level II

▶ Summarize the diagnostic use of the reticulocyte count in evaluating hematologic disorders and monitoring various therapies such as iron replacement and bone marrow transplant. (Chapters 8, 9, 27)

▶ OVERVIEW

Automation is firmly established within the hematology/coagulation laboratory. This chapter reviews the fundamental principles of the hematology and coagulation instruments and describes examples of instrumentation that are currently used. The basic principles of operation are discussed, and samples of normal test results are displayed for each instrument.

▶ AUTOMATED BLOOD CELL–COUNTING INSTRUMENTS

The evolution of instrumentation in hematology began in the mid-1950s. Until that time, clinical laboratory professionals performed manual hemacytometer blood cell counts, spun hematocrits, spectrophotometrically determined hemoglobins, and microscopic blood smear evaluations. With the advent of the first single automated blood cell counter, manual hemacytometer blood cell counts for erythrocyte enumeration and leukocyte enumeration were replaced. In general, automated blood cell counters provide data with increased reliability, precision, and accuracy.

With the many advances in hematology instrumentation, automation currently encompasses the primary testing in the hematology laboratory. Automated instruments can perform a complete blood cell count (CBC) including the platelet count, a five-part leukocyte differential, and absolute reticulocyte count. A number of principles for cell counting and differential analysis have been utilized in the past. The two principles of blood cell counting currently used by the hematology instruments are impedance and optical light scattering.

The impedance principle of blood cell counting is based on the increased resistance that occurs when a blood cell with poor conductivity passes through an electrical field. The number of pulses indicate the blood cell count, and the amplitude (i.e., height) of each pulse is proportional to the volume of the cell.[1] Examples of instruments using this principle are the Beckman-Coulter, Sysmex Corporation, and Abbott Diagnostics instruments.

The optical light–scattering principle of blood cell counting is based on light scattering measurements obtained as a single blood cell passes through a beam of light (optical or laser). Blood cells create forward scatter and side scatter that photodetectors detect. The degree of forward scatter is a measurement of cell size, and the degree of side scatter is a measurement of cell complexity or granularity.[2] The Siemens Healthcare (formerly Bayer) instruments utilize this principle for all blood cell counts, and newer models manufactured by Sysmex Corporation and Abbott Diagnostics use this principle for leukocyte enumeration.

The automated reticulocyte count has essentially replaced the manual reticulocyte count for evaluating the bone marrow's erythropoietic activity. Among the hematology instruments, the method of enumeration varies and is discussed with each instrument. These automated methods determine additional reticulocyte parameters including reticulocyte hemoglobin concentration (CHr or Ret He), reticulocyte mean cell volume (MCVr), and immature reticulocyte fraction (IRF). The reticulocyte hemoglobin concentration is determined by directly measuring the reticulocyte's hemoglobin by light-scattering characteristics. The reticulocyte mean cell volume is derived from the reticulocyte cytogram and reflects the average size of the reticulocyte population. The immature reticulocyte fraction, or high-intensity ratio, reflects reticulocytes with an increased amount of RNA or early immature reticulocytes. The presence of increased numbers of immature reticulocytes can be used as an indicator of an erythropoietic response. The reticulocyte hemoglobin concentration is an assessment of iron incorporation into hemoglobin and reflects functional availability of iron to the erythron. Thus, these new parameters can be useful in (1) measuring bone marrow engraftment following transplant, (2) determining bone marrow response to iron or erythropoietin therapy, (3) recognizing the potential cause for poor response to erythropoietin therapy, and (4) diagnosing iron-deficient states in infants and adolescents.[3-7]

This section reviews the basic operating principles of several hematology instruments that are seen in the field. Other instruments use a combination of these principles.

✓ **Checkpoint! 1**

What is the basis of the impedance principle for cell counting?

IMPEDANCE INSTRUMENTS

Four instruments that use the impedance principle in cell counting are described here. Two are Coulter instruments, one is a Sysmex instrument, and one is an Abbott Diagnostics instrument.

Coulter® Gen·S

Introduced by Beckman-Coulter in 1996, the Coulter® Gen·S is a multiparameter blood cell–counting instrument capable of determining a CBC, five-part leukocyte differential, and reticulocyte count.[8] The basic principles of blood cell counting it uses are similar to earlier models such as the Coulter® S-Plus and STKS.[9] However, improvements were made to the determination of the five-part leukocyte differential and enumeration of reticulocytes.[10-14] The ethylenediaminetetraacetic acid (EDTA) anticoagulated blood sample is aspirated by a closed tube system and divided into four aliquots. The first aliquot is delivered to the RBC/platelet dilution chamber where blood cells are diluted in an electrically conductive diluent. Within the dilution chamber is an external electrode and three **apertures,** each of which has an internal electrode (Figure 36-1■). As individual blood cells pass through an aperture, there is an increase in resistance (i.e., pulse height) between the external and internal electrodes that is proportional to the cell volume. A steady stream of diluent flows behind each aperture to prevent cells from reentering the aperture. **Threshold limits** are established

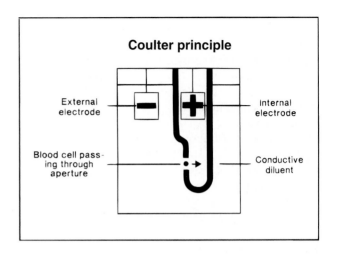

Coulter principle

■ FIGURE 36-1   Coulter principle. Increased electrical resistance, or impedance, occurs when the poorly conductive blood cell passes through the aperture. (Reprinted, with permission, from Pierre R. *Seminar and Case Studies: The Automated Differential.* Hialeah, FL: Coulter Electronics, Inc.; 1985)

for enumerating cells based on cell volume. Particles (cells) of more than 36 fL are counted as erythrocytes. Because three apertures are within the dilution chamber, three erythrocyte (red blood cells [RBC]) counts are obtained. These counts are compared and evaluated by the instrument's data analysis system. If there is agreement, the reported RBC count represents the average of the counts from the three aperatures.

An erythrocyte (RBC) **histogram** (size distribution curve) is created based on cell volume and relative cell number (Figure 36-2■). The RBC histogram allows the visualization of changes in size within the erythrocyte population. For example, a shift to the left of the erythrocyte population correlates with microcytic erythrocytes, and the appearance of two separate peaks correlates with a dual population of erythrocytes (e.g., mixture of microcytic erythrocytes and normocytic erythrocytes). This information can be useful in the diagnosis of certain erythrocyte disorders.

The erythrocyte data obtained from the RBC/platelet dilution includes the RBC count by direct measurement and the mean cell volume (MCV) and red cell distribution width (RDW), which are derived from the RBC histogram (Figure 36-3■). The calculated RBC parameters are the hematocrit (Hct), which is calculated from the MCV and the RBC count (calculated Hct = MCV × RBC); the mean cell hemoglobin (MCH), which is calculated from the RBC count and hemoglobin concentration; and the mean cell hemoglobin concentration (MCHC), which is calculated from the hemoglobin concentration and hematocrit (∞ Chapters 8 and 34). The hemoglobin concentration is obtained from the WBC/hemoglobin dilution chamber.

The platelet count is also obtained from the RBC/platelet dilution chamber. Particles between 2 and 20 fL are counted

Histogram

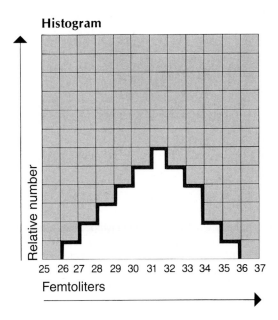

FIGURE 36-2 Histogram, or size distribution curve, allows the visualization of the blood cell population based on the relative cell number and its volume (in fL). (Reprinted, with permission, from *Significant Advances in Hematology.* Hialeah, FL: Coulter Electronics, Inc.; 1983)

as platelets, and a raw platelet histogram is obtained (Figure 36-4 ■). The raw platelet histogram is evaluated to determine whether it is a log normal curve. The raw platelet histogram is electronically smoothed and extrapolated over 0–70 fL. The platelet count is derived from the extrapolated histogram. Two additional parameters are obtained from the platelet histogram: **mean platelet volume (MPV)**, which is analogous to the MCV, and **platelet distribution width (PDW)**, which is analogous to the RDW.

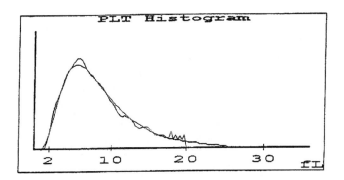

FIGURE 36-4 Normal platelet histogram, Coulter® Gen·S. The jagged line represents the raw data collected from 2–20 fL. The smooth line represents the extrapolated histogram from 0–70 fL.

The second aliquot is delivered to the WBC/hemoglobin dilution chamber where the leukocyte (WBC) count and hemoglobin determinations are made. The WBC count is directly measured by electrical impedance from the leukocyte dilution after lytic agent is added to the dilution. The lytic agent serves to lyse the erythrocytes, convert released hemoglobin to cyanmethemoglobin, and shrink the leukocyte cell membrane and cytoplasm. Therefore, the WBC count represents a measure of the cell volume rather than native cell size as it passes through the aperture. Particles larger than 35 fL are counted as leukocytes. Similar to the RBC count, WBC counts are obtained from the three apertures in the WBC/hemoglobin dilution chamber, and the data analysis system compares and evaluates them. The reported WBC count represents an average of the counts.

The leukocyte (WBC) histogram represents the size distribution curve for the leukocyte data and allows visualization of subpopulations of cells based on their relative sizes. The

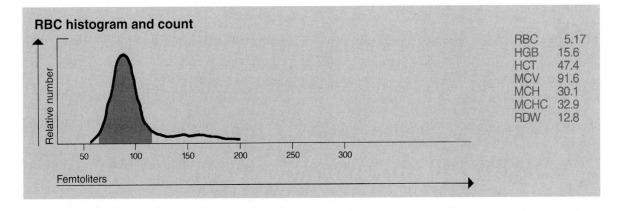

FIGURE 36-3 RBC histogram and count. The shaded area represents those cells used in the RDW (i.e., RDW-CV) calculation. The excluded cells can represent large platelets, platelet clumps, or electrical interference on the left and RBC doublets, RBC triplets, RBC agglutinates, or aperture artifacts on the right. (Reprinted, with permission, from *Significant Advances in Hematology.* Hialeah, FL: Coulter Electronics, Inc.; 1983)

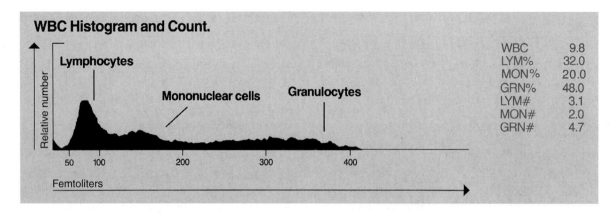

WBC Histogram and Count.

Lymphocytes

Mononuclear cells

Granulocytes

Relative number

50   100   200   300   400

Femtoliters

WBC	9.8
LYM%	32.0
MON%	20.0
GRN%	48.0
LYM#	3.1
MON#	2.0
GRN#	4.7

■ FIGURE 36-5   WBC histogram and count. In a normal patient, the lymphocyte region represents lymphocytes, the mononuclear region represents monocytes, and the granulocyte region represents neutrophils, eosinophils, and basophils. (Reprinted, with permission, from *Significant Advances in Hematology.* Hialeah, FL: Coulter Electronics, Inc.; 1983)

leukocyte histogram is the basis of the three-part differential identifying lymphocytes as cells between 35 and 90 fL, mononuclear cells as cells between 90 and 160 fL, and granulocytes as cells between 160 and 450 fL (Figure 36-5 ■). The instrument's data analysis system examines the WBC histogram for presence of interferences within one or more of the leukocyte populations and using a system of region flags, alerts the clinical laboratory professional (Table 36-1 ✪). The reason for the region flag can be found by careful examination of the peripheral blood smear. For example, presence of nucleated erythrocytes or clumped platelets is associated with a region 1 flag.

The hemoglobin concentration is determined by measuring the absorbance of cyanmethemoglobin in the WBC/hemoglobin chamber at 525 nm. Through the application of Beer's law, this absorbance reading is proportional to the concentration of hemoglobin. Additionally, this instrument utilizes a **reagent blank** at the beginning of each operating

cycle to negate the effect of the reagent alone on the sample's absorbance reading.

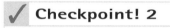

✓ Checkpoint! 2

Why is lytic agent added to the leukocyte dilution?

A third sample aliquot is delivered to the orbital mixing chamber. Within this chamber, blood is mixed by gentle agitation with heated lysing reagent to remove the erythrocytes while leaving the leukocytes in their near native state. A second stabilizing reagent is added to stop the lytic reaction and preserve the integrity of the leukocytes. This dilution is sent to the volume·conductivity·scatter (VCS) flow cell for the determination of the five-part leukocyte differential. The cells pass through the flow cell singly by **hydrodynamic focusing.** As each cell passes through the flow cell, three separate measurements are taken simultaneously. The mea-

✪ TABLE 36-1

Coulter® WBC Histogram Region Flags

Region Flag	Affected Position	Possible Abnormalities
R1	Lymphocyte population does not begin at baseline (~35 fL)	Nucleated erythrocytes, large platelets, clumped platelets, or intracellular parasites (e.g., malaria)
R2	No valley between lymphocyte and mononuclear populations (~90 fL)	Reactive lymphocytes, blast cells
R3	No valley between mononuclear and granulocyte populations (~160 fL)	Eosinophilia, basophilia, immature neutrophils
R4	Granulocyte population does not return to baseline (~450 fL)	Granulocytosis
RM	Interference detected in multiple positions	

Other impedance-based instruments providing three-part leukocyte differentials use a flagging system similar to the Coulter® instruments.

surements include cell volume, cell conductivity, and cell's light scatter characteristics. Cell volume is determined by impedance; cell conductivity that evaluates internal physical and chemical constituents is determined by high-frequency electromagnetic probe; and light scatter characteristics such as cell surface, shape, and reflectivity are determined by a helium-neon laser. The Gen·S instrument's internal system monitors and adjusts reaction characteristics and the data analysis of the VCS-derived characteristics to differentiate the leukocyte cell types.

The Intellikinetics™ application monitors and reacts to changes in the external environment (e.g., changes in ambient room temperature). With this application, the Gen·S system is able to maintain consistent reaction conditions and eliminate cellular analysis problems due to inconsistent location of cells within three-dimensional space. Data analysis is improved through the use of AccuGate™ computer program. The different leukocytes within a sample are identified and classified by **contour gating** that is individualized for each sample (Figure 36-6▪). The advantage of contour gating over traditional linear gating is the ability to differentiate overlapping cell populations (e.g., monocytes from reactive lymphocytes).

In the heated reticulocyte dilution chamber, the fourth aliquot is mixed with new methylene blue reagent. The residual RNA is precipitated within the reticulocytes. The stained sample is then mixed with an acidic, hypotonic solution that (1) elutes hemoglobin from the erythrocytes but permits precipitated RNA to remain and (2) spheres the erythrocytes. This dilution is sent to the VCS flow cell for analysis. The light scatter data generated by flow cytometric examination of sphered erythrocytes and reticulocytes are more reproducible than data generated from non-sphered erythrocytes and reticulocytes. The sphering of mature erythrocytes and reticulocytes eliminates the inherent error in flow cytometric examination of erythrocytes created by irregularly shaped erythrocytes. Contour gating of the VCS-derived characteristics is used to classify reticulocytes versus mature erythrocytes and to identify the immature reticulocyte fraction (Web Figure 36-1▪; ∞ Chapter 8). The reticulocyte parameters obtained by this analysis include absolute reticulocyte count, reticulocyte percentage, immature reticulocyte fraction, and mean reticulocyte volume (i.e., reticulocyte mean cell volume, MCVr).

The computer system compiles all data obtained from the instrument's analysis. For the cell counts, the instrument's computer corrects the counts for **coincidence** (two or more cells passing through the aperture at the same time) and compares the counts for replication (e.g., compares the three RBC counts). If two or three of the counts do not agree, the count (e.g., RBC count) is not reported but recorded as "vote-out." If there is agreement, the reported count represents the average of the counts. The instrument's computer also evaluates the data to detect abnormalities and determines the reported parameters (See Web Table 36-1 ❖ for the reported parameters.). The reported results and selected histograms/**scatterplots** are displayed on the computer screen, printed to a hard copy (Figure 36-7▪), or transferred to the laboratory information system (LIS). If abnormalities are detected, the clinical laboratory professional is alerted by suspect flags (software-generated flags) or user-defined flags (definitive flags). The clinical laboratory professional uses this information to correlate CBC data with peripheral blood morphology to improve the identification and confirmation of abnormalities.

> ### ✓ Checkpoint! 3
>
> *Explain how the* Coulter® Gen·S *determines the five-part leukocyte differential.*

Coulter® LH Series

Like previous models, the LH 750 (introduced in 2003) and the LH 780 (introduced in 2006) provide a CBC, five-part leukocyte differential, and reticulocyte count from a single blood sample aspiration. When the LH SlideMaker and LH SlideStainer are added to the workstation, Wright-stained peripheral smears are prepared and labeled from the same sample decreasing the number of times the sample is handled and the potential for introducing random errors.

The LH series instruments utilize the basic principles of blood cell enumeration, reticulocyte enumeration, and

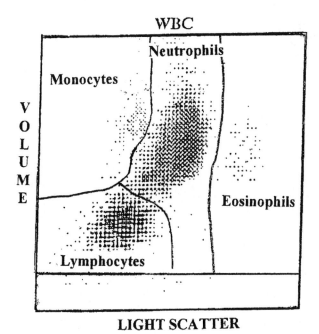

WBC

LIGHT SCATTER

(VOLUME axis on left; labels: Neutrophils, Monocytes, Eosinophils, Lymphocytes)

▪ **FIGURE 36-6** Coulter® Gen·S WBC scatterplot. WBC scatterplot graphs volume versus light scatter and reveals the locations of four leukocyte populations in two-dimensional space. The basophil population is located behind the lymphocytes, but in three-dimensional space is clearly delineated.

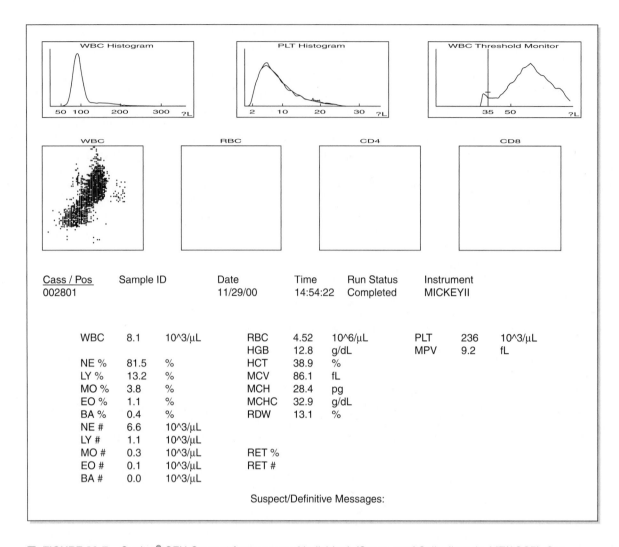

FIGURE 36-7   Coulter® GEN·S report from a normal individual. (Courtesy of Celia Jimeniz, MT(ASCP), San Antonio, TX)

determination of the five-part leukocyte differential that were discussed with the Gen·S instrument.[15] These instruments provide several additional parameters, which are advantageous to the differentiation of normal individuals from individuals with certain disease states. These parameters include the nucleated red blood cell count (NRBC%) and corrected WBC count which were introduced with the LH 750 instrument and the RDW-SD which was introduced with the LH 780 instrument.

If nucleated red blood cells are detected during the analysis of a CBC and differential, the number of nucleated red blood cells (i.e., NRBC%) is determined. Enumeration of nucleated red blood cells begins with their detection on the WBC scatterplot generated by VCS technology (Figure 36-8 ■).[15] If nucleated red blood cells are suspected based on their characteristic signature, the computer system examines the WBC histogram generated by impedance for the presence of cells to the left of the lymphocyte population. If

both plots indicate that nucleated red blood cells could be present, the computer system evaluates the combined information to rule out giant platelets or small lymphocytes. If all data analyses point to the presence of nucleated red blood cells, the number of nucleated red blood cells per 100 leukocytes (NRBC%) is derived from data collected by VCS technology and the application of an algorithm to the WBC count. The NRBC# represents the total number of nucleated red blood cells in the blood sample and is calculated from the NRBC% and the total WBC count (i.e., NRBC# = NRBC% × WBC count). Because increased numbers of nucleated red blood cells falsely increase the total WBC count, this count is corrected for their presence, and the corrected WBC count is reported.

The red cell distribution width-standard deviation (RDW-SD) is determined from the RBC histogram by calculating the width in femtoliters (fL) of the RBC population at the 20% height level on the histogram when the peak height is con-

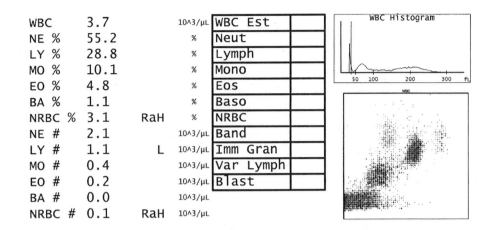

				WBC Histogram
WBC	3.7	10^3/μL	WBC Est	
NE %	55.2	%	Neut	
LY %	28.8	%	Lymph	
MO %	10.1	%	Mono	
EO %	4.8	%	Eos	
BA %	1.1	%	Baso	
NRBC %	3.1	RaH	%	NRBC	
NE #	2.1	10^3/μL	Band	
LY #	1.1	L	10^3/μL	Imm Gran	
MO #	0.4	10^3/μL	Var Lymph	
EO #	0.2	10^3/μL	Blast	
BA #	0.0	10^3/μL		
NRBC #	0.1	RaH	10^3/μL		

■ FIGURE 36-8   Coulter® LH 750 WBC scatterplot and WBC histogram depicting presence of nucleated erythrocytes. On the WBC scatterplot, detection of cells between the lymphocyte population and RBC ghosts is suggestive of nucleated erythrocytes, which are suspected if there is a population of cells to the left of the lymphocyte population on the WBC histogram. The NRBC% is determined if both observations are made and other potential interferences are ruled out (e.g., giant platelets).

sidered 100% (Figure 36-9 ■).[16] Like the RDW-coefficient of variation (CV) (i.e., RDW) the RDW-SD reflects the degree of anisocytosis within the erythrocyte population. The RDW-SD differs from the RDW-CV in that it directly measures the erythrocyte population while the RDW-CV bases its calculation on the population's SD and MCV (RDW = 1 SD/MCV × 100%). Thus, a false RDW-CV can be observed in certain situations. For example, if both the SD and MCV are elevated, the RDW-CV can appear normal when anisocytosis is actually present or if the SD is normal but the MCV is decreased, the RDW-CV can appear increased when in fact there is no anisocytosis. Because the MCV does not affect the RDW-SD, it is potentially a better indicator of the degree of anisocytosis within a given erythrocyte population. The RDW-SD is re-

ported in fL and its reference interval is 39–47 fL in adults. The RDW-SD can be used with other test results in the differentiating iron deficiency anemia from heterozygous beta thalassemia because a low RDW-SD is more closely associated with heterozygous beta thalassemia.[17]

The results generated by an LH instrument are displayed on its computer screen, printed as a hard copy (Figure 36-10 ■), or sent to the LIS for the clinical laboratory professional's review. (See Web Table 36-1 for the reported parameters.) The clinical laboratory professional is alerted to abnormalities by a system of software-generated flags (suspect flags) or user-defined flags (definitive flags). This information can then be used in a more thorough evaluation of the patient's data, examination of a peripheral blood smear, and determination of appropriate reflex tests.

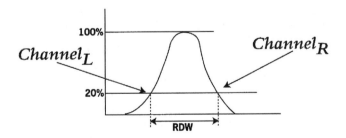

■ FIGURE 36-9   Calculation of RDW-SD. The RDW-SD represents the width of the erythrocyte population at the 20% height level on the RBC histogram and is reported in fL. For example, if Channel$_L$ is 70 fL and Channel$_R$ is 111 fL, the RDW-SD is 41 fL (i.e., 111−70 = 41). (Reprinted, with permission, from Red Cell Distribution Parameters—(1) RDW-SD (2) RDW (CV), Technical Bulletin 9617. Brea, CA: Beckman-Coulter®; 2007)

✓ Checkpoint! 4

The following results were obtained from a blood sample analyzed by the Coulter® LH 750: NRBC# 2.7 × 10⁹/L and corrected WBC 18.1 × 10⁹/L. What was the uncorrected WBC count?

Sysmex XE-2100™

The XE-2100™ is a member of the XE-Series™ of Sysmex instruments currently on the market. This instrument uses four different technologies including impedance (i.e., direct current), radio frequency, absorption spectrophotometry, and flow cytometry with fluorescent dyes to determine CBC, 5-part leukocyte differential, and reticulocyte count.[18–22]

Hemoglobin is measured in a designated channel using the sodium lauryl sulfate (SLS) method. A portion of the

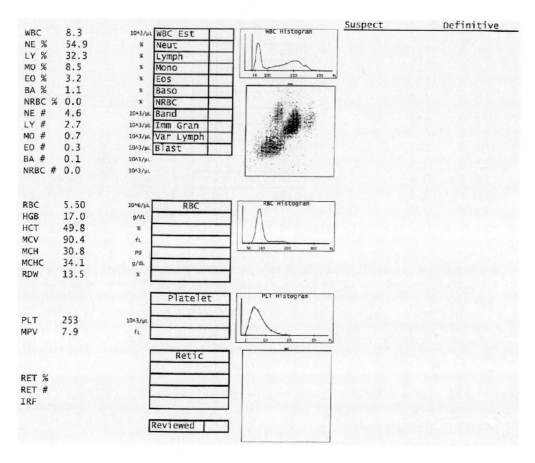

					Suspect	Definitive
WBC	8.3	10^3/µL	WBC Est			
NE %	54.9	%	Neut			
LY %	32.3	%	Lymph			
MO %	8.5	%	Mono			
EO %	3.2	%	Eos			
BA %	1.1	%	Baso			
NRBC %	0.0	%	NRBC			
NE #	4.6	10^3/µL	Band			
LY #	2.7	10^3/µL	Imm Gran			
MO #	0.7	10^3/µL	Var Lymph			
EO #	0.3	10^3/µL	Blast			
BA #	0.1	10^3/µL				
NRBC #	0.0	10^3/µL				

RBC	5.50	10^6/µL	RBC	
HGB	17.0	g/dL		
HCT	49.8	%		
MCV	90.4	fL		
MCH	30.8	pg		
MCHC	34.1	g/dL		
RDW	13.5	%		

			Platelet	
PLT	253	10^3/µL		
MPV	7.9	fL		

		Retic
RET %		
RET #		
IRF		
		Reviewed

■ **FIGURE 36-10** Coulter® LH 750 report from a normal individual. (Courtesy of Charlene A. Ruiz, MT(ASCP), San Antonio, TX)

aspirated blood sample is first diluted with reagent diluent and then SLS-hemoglobin reagent is added. The surfactants within this reagent lyse the erythrocytes and release hemoglobin. Sodium lauryl sulfate converts ferrous iron to ferric iron, forming methemoglobin. Methemoglobin combines with SLS to form the SLS-hemichrome molecule. The absorbance of this molecule is measured at 555 nm to determine the hemoglobin concentration (g/dL) using Beer's law. This method is advantageous for two reasons: (1) free hemoglobin is rapidly converted to detectable chromogen decreasing measurement time and (2) the reagent is cyanide-free.

The erythrocytes and platelets are enumerated using impedance with hydrodynamic focusing. The blood sample is diluted with isotonic diluent and sent to the RBC/PLT sample chamber. A sheath fluid injector piston delivers the diluted blood sample to the direct current (DC) detection block. The blood cells flow through the aperture and resistance (i.e., pulse height) is detected between the internal and external electrodes. The hydrodynamic focusing created by the sheath fluid aligns the blood cells to enter the center of the aperture singly, thus eliminating abnormal cell pulses generated when cells touch the sides of the aperture as they pass through. At the rear of the aperture, blood cells are prevented from drift-

ing back and generating false pulses due to the sweeping flow of the back sheath fluid. From the RBC/PLT dilution, the RBC count and PLT count are directly measured; RBC and PLT histograms are generated; and the hematocrit (HCT) is calculated from the pulse heights of the individual erythrocytes within the erythrocyte population. The pulse height of an individual erythrocyte is directly proportional to its volume.

The RBC and PLT counts are determined from the generated data using automatic discriminators. The RBC count represents the number of cells that fall between a lower discriminator (25–75 fL) and an upper discriminator (200–250 fL). For each blood sample, the data analysis system examines the data to set its specific lower and upper discriminator for this determination. Likewise, the PLT count represents the number of cells that fall between a lower discriminator (2–6 fL) and an upper discriminator (12–30 fL). A fixed discriminator at 12 fL is also used in determining the platelet count to determine whether potential interferences exist that can result in an erroneous platelet count (e.g., presence of erythrocyte fragments). This platelet count is compared to the platelet count determined from the reticulocyte (RET) channel.

Other parameters that are derived or calculated based on data from the RBC/PLT dilution include MCV, MCH, MCHC,

RDW-SD, RDW-CV, and MPV (See Web Table 36-1 for the reported parameters.). The RDW-SD and RDW-CV are determined in the same manner as described for the Coulter® LH 780 instrument.

Two separate channels (i.e., DIFF and WBC/BASO) are used to generate the total leukocyte (WBC) count and five-part leukocyte differential (neutrophils, lymphocytes, monocytes, eosinophils, and basophils). In the DIFF channel, a portion of the aspirated blood sample is diluted with lyse reagent. The lyse reagent removes the erythrocytes and creates "holes" in the cytoplasmic membrane of nucleated cells allowing a polymethine dye (i.e., fluorescent dye) to enter the cell and bind to its DNA and RNA. This dilution is sent to the Optical Detection block. Within the Optical Detection block, the cells pass singly through a laser beam ($\lambda = 633$ nm) emitted by the semiconductor diode laser. Each cell generates forward scatter (reflects cell size), side scatter (reflects cell complexity), and fluorescent intensity (reflects amount of bound fluorescent dye) depending on the cell type. The DIFF scattergram represents a plot of side scatter versus fluorescent intensity. The instrument's adaptive cluster analysis system (ACAS) allows clear separation of the cell populations depicted on DIFF scattergram including RBC ghosts, lymphocytes, monocytes, eosinophils, and neutophils + basophils (Figure 36-11■). By applying the IG Master software to the data generated in the DIFF channel, the immature granulocyte (IG) population is enumerated (Web Figure 36-2■). The IG count includes metamyelocytes, myelocytes, and promyelocytes. Studies indicate that the au-tomated IG count is an acceptable replacement to the manual morphology count for IG, but studies regarding the usefulness of the IG count to screen for sepsis and infection are conflicting.[23–25] Further studies are needed to clarify its use.

In the WBC/BASO channel, the blood sample is diluted, and special lyse reagent that lyses erythrocytes and shears all leukocytes except basophils is added. This dilution is analyzed by the Optical Detection block to capture each cell's forward scatter and side scatter as it passes through the laser beam. The adaptive cluster analysis system evaluates this information to determine a total leukocyte (WBC) count and the basophil count (i.e., basophil percentage and absolute basophil count). The WBC/BASO scattergram (Figure 36-12■) is a plot of side scatter versus forward scatter. On this scattergram, the basophils are easily distinguished from the other leukocytes and RBC ghosts due to their size and complexity (i.e., high forward scatter and high side scatter).

In the IMI channel, reagents act selectively on the lipid membranes of the leukocytes. Mature leukocytes with phospholipid-rich membranes are completely lysed, leaving only bare nuclei. The immature myeloid cells remain intact. In the IMI channel, the cells are analyzed by direct current and radio frequency (reflecting a cell's internal structure and density) to determine the degree of immaturity (Web Figure 36-3■). This channel allows a clear delineation of immature granulocytes and blasts. With the HPC Master software, this channel provides the hematopoietic progenitor cell (HPC) count. Studies have shown that the HPC count correlates well with the CD34$^+$ cell count by flow cytometry.[26] Thus, HPC counts can be used to determine peripheral blood stem cell counts to assess optimal harvesting time following peripheral blood stem cell mobilization (∞ Chapter 27).

This instrument also determines the presence of nucleated erythrocytes in the blood sample and corrects the total leukocyte (WBC) count and lymphocyte count for their presence. The lymphocyte count is affected because nucleated erythrocytes and lymphocytes fall in the same cluster on the DIFF scattergram. Within the NRBC channel, the blood cells are diluted with a lyse plus fluorescent dye reagent. This reagent hemolyzes the erythrocytes, removes the nucleated erythrocytes' cytoplasmic membrane, and shrinks the nucleus. The fluorescent dye binds to the nuclei. For the leukocytes, the reagent perforates only the cytoplasmic membrane allowing fluorescent dye to enter the cell and bind to intracytoplasmic organelles and the nucleus, but the leukocytes' shape is not altered. Thus, leukocytes exhibit stronger fluorescence. As the nuclei of the nucleated erythrocytes and the intact leukocytes pass through the laser beam of the Optical Detection block, they generate forward scatter, side scatter, and fluorescence. This information is used to create the NRBC scattergram, which is a plot of fluorescent intensity versus forward scatter (Figure 36-13■; Web Figure 36-4■). Leukocytes are clearly delineated from the nucleated erythrocytes due to their high fluorescent intensity and high forward scatter (i.e., larger size). This analysis provides a sensitive method to determine NRBC as low as 0.1 NRBC/100 WBCs.

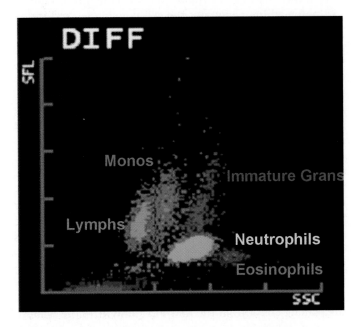

■ FIGURE 36-11   DIFF scattergram, Sysmex XE-2100™. RBC ghosts, lymphocytes, monocytes, eosinophils, and neutrophils + basophils are identified. Basophils are specifically identified in the WBC/BASO scattergram. (Courtesy of Sysmex Corporation, Kobe, Japan)

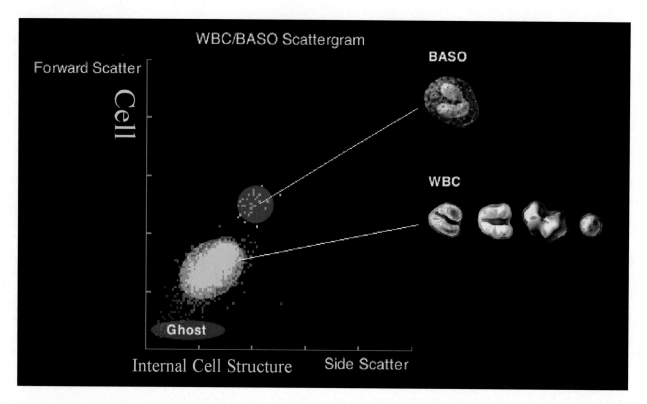

■ FIGURE 36-12   WBC/BASO scattergram, Sysmex XE-2100™. Basophils are clearly distinguished from other leukocytes and RBC ghosts based on their larger size (i.e., forward scatter) and increased complexity (i.e., side scatter). (Courtesy of Sysmex Corporation, Kobe, Japan)

✓ **Checkpoint! 5**

How does the determination of the five-part leukocyte differential for the Coulter® LH 750 instrument and the Sysmex XE-2100™ instrument differ?

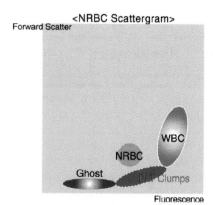

■ FIGURE 36-13   NRBC scattergram, Sysmex XE-2100™. Nucleated erythrocytes are clearly delineated from leukocytes based on their lower fluorescence intensity and smaller size (i.e., less forward scatter) as seen on this schematic pattern. (Reprinted with permission from Rowan RM, Linssen J. A Picture Is Worth a Thousand Words. Sysmex Journal International: 2005;15(1):27–38.)

The reticulocyte count is determined in the RET channel. Within this channel, the fluorescent dye containing oxazine and polymethine penetrates the cell membranes and stains the blood cells. Oxazine binds to residual RNA within the reticulocytes, and polymethine binds to RNA and DNA within nucleated cells. The diode laser of the Optical Detection block evaluates each blood cell and determines its forward scatter and fluorescence. The data analysis system integrates these two characteristics to create the RET scattergram. From this scattergram, cells are classified as mature erythrocytes, reticulocytes and platelets (Figure 36-14 ■). The reticulocytes are further classified based on fluorescent activity to determine reticulocyte maturity (Web Figure 36-5 ■). Reported parameters include absolute reticulocyte count, reticulocyte percentage, low fluorescence ratio (LFR), middle fluorescence ratio (MFR), high fluorescence ratio (HFR), immature reticulocyte fraction (IRF), reticulocyte hemoglobin content (Ret He), and platelet count. The IRF represents the MFR and HFR combined and is reported as a percentage of the total reticulocyte count.

The platelet count from the RET channel is compared to the platelet count from the RBC/PLT dilution. If the platelet count is extremely low, the platelet count from the RET channel is the reported platelet count because it is more accurate due to the additional cellular characteristics that are evaluated. The immature platelet fraction (IPF) is an additional platelet parameter derived from the RET channel that

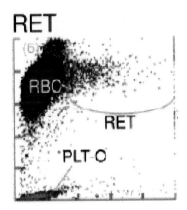

■ FIGURE 36-14   RET scattergram, Sysmex XE-2100™. Mature erythrocytes, reticulocytes, and platelets are identified. (Reprinted with permission from Rowan RM, Linssen J. A Picture Is Worth a Thousand Words. Sysmex Journal International: 2005;15(1): 27–38.)

represents the **reticulated platelets** (Figure 36-15 ■). Reticulated platelets are newly released platelets that possess residual RNA. An increased IPF reflects increased thrombopoiesis, while a decreased IPF reflects decreased platelet production. The IPF is useful in a variety of clinical situations: as an indicator of platelet engraftment following stem cell transplantation; in the diagnosis of thrombocytopenia associated with increased platelet destruction versus bone marrow failure; and as a requirement of platelet transfusion associated with cytotoxic therapy or stem cell transplant.[27–30]

All data, including cell counts, histograms, and scattergrams, are analyzed by the data analysis system. The results are displayed on the computer screen, printed to a hard copy (Figure 36-16 ■), or transferred to the LIS. An extensive flagging program with interpretive comments alerts the clinical laboratory professional to abnormal results. Use of the flag-

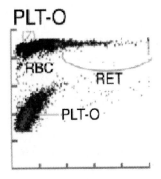

■ FIGURE 36-15   Optical platelet (PLT-O) scattergram, Sysmex XE-2100™. Mature platelets lacking RNA are found in the lower portion of the platelet population while the immature platelet fraction is found in the upper portion of the platelet population due to increased size and higher fluorescence. (Reprinted with permission from Rowan RM, Linssen J. A Picture Is Worth a Thousand Words. Sysmex Journal International: 2005;15(1):27–38.)

ging system and observations of the scattergrams and histograms allow the clinical laboratory professional to focus on specific abnormalities when performing a peripheral blood smear evaluation.

 Checkpoint! 6

Which cellular characteristics are used to determine the immature platelet fraction (IPF) on the Sysmex XE-2100™ instrument?

Abbott CELL-DYN Sapphire®

Like other automated cell counting instruments, the CELL-DYN Sapphire® utilizes a combination of technologies to enumerate erythrocytes, leukocytes, platelets, and reticulocytes and determine a five-part leukocyte differential.[31,32] Flow cytometry, fluorescence staining, and impedance are used to make these determinations.

The instrument aspirates a sample of EDTA anticoagulated blood and sends a portion of this sample to the hemoglobin dilution cup. Hemoglobin reagent dilutes the blood sample, lyses erythrocytes, and converts free hemoglobin to a single chromogen by forming a complex with imidazole. The hemoglobin concentration is determined spectrophotometrically at 540 nm. A reagent blank is used to minimize optical interferences whereas leukocyte interference is minimal because the reagent destroys leukocytes and cellular fragments. This cyanide-free reaction shows good correlation with the cyanmethemoglobin reference method.

In the WBC dilution cup assembly, the sample is diluted for the enumeration of total leukocyte (WBC) count, detection and quantitation of nucleated erythrocytes, and determination of the five-part leukocyte differential. The preheated WBC reagent dilutes the leukocytes, lyses erythrocytes, strips the cytoplasmic membrane from nucleated erythrocytes and fragile leukocytes, and stains DNA of the exposed nuclei with propidum iodide, a fluorescence dye. This dilution is sent to the optical flow cell. Hydrodynamic focusing directs cells through the flow cell in single file. A solid-state laser interacts with each intact cell or exposed nuclei to create light scatter and fluorescence (PI excites @ 488 nm and emits @ 630 nm). Using multi-angle polarized scater separation (MAPSS™) technology, the following light scatter characteristics are determined as follows: (1) 0° light scatter or forward scatter that reflects cell size; (2) 7° light scatter that reflects cell complexity; (3) 90° light scatter or side scatter that reflects nuclear lobularity; and (4) 90° depolarized light scatter that reflects cytoplasmic granularity (Figure 36-17 ■). Data generated by MAPSS technology is used in different ways to classify leukocyte subpopulations and identify certain morphologic flags.[31] For example, discriminant line analysis is used to isolate and identify various cell populations. A histogram is created based on one-dimensional data (e.g., size) or two-dimensional data (e.g., size vs. DNA). The data management system identifies the valley between the cell populations and sets a discriminant line. Scatterplots and contour plots of the data are used to further classify

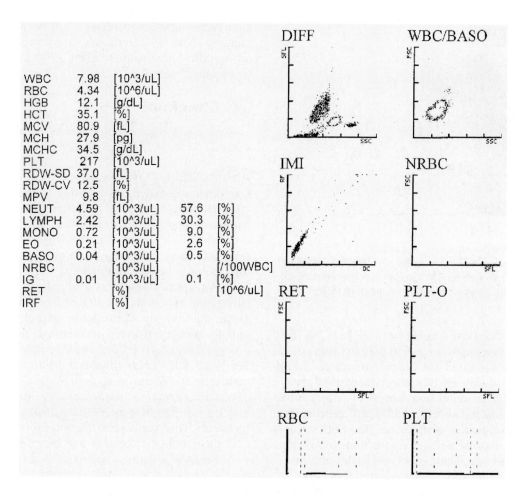

WBC	7.98	[10^3/uL]		
RBC	4.34	[10^6/uL]		
HGB	12.1	[g/dL]		
HCT	35.1	[%]		
MCV	80.9	[fL]		
MCH	27.9	[pg]		
MCHC	34.5	[g/dL]		
PLT	217	[10^3/uL]		
RDW-SD	37.0	[fL]		
RDW-CV	12.5	[%]		
MPV	9.8	[fL]		
NEUT	4.59	[10^3/uL]	57.6	[%]
LYMPH	2.42	[10^3/uL]	30.3	[%]
MONO	0.72	[10^3/uL]	9.0	[%]
EO	0.21	[10^3/uL]	2.6	[%]
BASO	0.04	[10^3/uL]	0.5	[%]
NRBC		[10^3/uL]		[/100WBC]
IG	0.01	[10^3/uL]	0.1	[%]
RET		[%]		[10^6/uL]
IRF		[%]		

■ **FIGURE 36-16**   Sysmex XE-2100™ report from a normal individual (Courtesy of Cynthia Pittman, MT(ASCP)SH, San Antonio, TX)

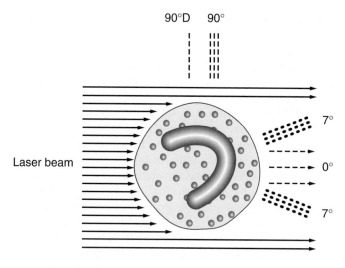

■ **FIGURE 36-17**   Four light scatter measurements from the CELL-DYN Sapphire. The 0° scatter reflects cell size; 7° scatter reflects cell complexity; 90° scatter reflects nuclear lobularity; and 90° depolarized scatter reflects cytoplasmic granularity.

subpopulations of leukocytes. The 0° (size) versus 7° (complexity) scatterplot allows differentiation of neutrophils, monocytes, and lymphocytes (Figure 36-18 ■). Eosinophils are differentiated from neutrophils in the 90°D (granularity) versus 90° (lobularity) scatterplot (Web Figure 36-6 ■). Finally, lymphocytes are separated from basophils based on size and complexity. The data management system analyzes these characteristics to determine the total leukocyte (WBC) count and the five-part leukocyte differential. Additional information obtained from evaluation of this dilution includes the enumeration of nucleated erythrocytes and identification of nonviable or fragile leukocytes, which are based on light scatter characteristics and fluorescence intensity (i.e., DNA content). Because the nucleated erythrocytes are clearly distinguished from leukocytes in this dilution, the total leukocyte count and five-part differential are unaffected by their presence.

Two different dilutions are prepared in the RBC/PLT dilution cup assembly. One dilution represents the erythrocyte/platelet dilution. The diluent dilutes the blood sample and spheres the erythrocytes. Using the principles of

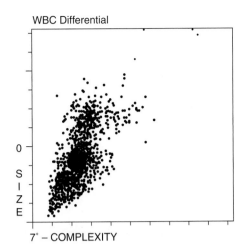

■ FIGURE 36-18 0° (size) vs 7° (complexity) scatterplot, CELL-DYN Sapphire. Neutrophils, monocytes, and lymphocytes are identified. Lymphocytes are located lower left in the scatterplot; the middle cell population is monocytes; and neutrophils are located upper center in the scatterplot.

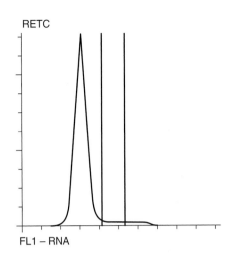

■ FIGURE 36-19 Reticulocyte histogram, CELL-DYN Sapphire. Reticulocytes are found between the two gates. The peak to the left represents mature erythrocytes.

hydrodynamic focusing and impedance, the erythrocytes and platelets are evaluated as they pass singly through the impedance transducer from which the erythrocyte count, erythrocyte size distribution curve (histogram), platelet size distribution curve, and platelet count are obtained. A second portion of the erythrocyte/platelet dilution is sent to the optical flow cell for enumeration of these cells based on light-scatter characteristics. The erythrocyte count from the optical flow cell and the platelet count from the impedance transducer are used as internal quality control checks against the reported erythrocyte count from the impedance transducer and the reported platelet count from the optical flow cell. The second dilution represents the reticulocyte dilution. The blood sample is diluted with the isotonic diluent and nucleic acids are stained with a fluorescence dye (i.e., fluorescein isothiocyanate) that excites @ 488 nm and emits @ 530 nm. This dilution is sent to the optical flow cell, where the number of reticulocytes is determined based on fluorescence intensity and light-scatter characteristics (i.e., 7° light scatter). From this information, a reticulocyte histogram is created that allows the determination of the reticulocyte count and the immature reticulocyte fraction (Figure 36-19 ■).

The data management system analyzes and compiles all data obtained from the instrument and determines the reported parameters (Web Table 36-1). The results are displayed on a computer screen, printed to a hard copy for the clinical laboratory professional's review (Figure 36-20 ■), or transferred to the LIS. System-initiated messages and data flags alert the clinical laboratory professional to potential abnormalities or errors in the results. This information is used to correlate CBC data with peripheral blood morphology to improve the identification and confirmation of abnormalities.

> ### ✓ Checkpoint! 7
>
> a. *Which CELL-DYN scatterplot allows differentiation of eosinophils from neutrophils?*
>
> b. *The CELL-DYN Sapphire's WBC dilution contains propidum iodide, so why don't the neutrophils fluoresce?*

Two additional assays can be performed on the CELL-DYN Sapphire, Immuno T-cell Assay, and ImmunoPlt™ (CD61) assay. Both assays represent fluorescent immunophenotyping methods. The Immuno T-cell Assay uses monoclonal antibodies with different fluorescent labels to identify the T cell population (i.e., fluorescein isothiocyanate labeled anti-CD3) and its two subpopulations, T_{helper} cells (i.e., phycoerythrin labeled anti-CD4) and $T_{cytotoxic}$ cells (i.e., phycoerythrin labeled anti-CD8). Enumeration of these subpopulations is important in evaluating patients with immunodeficiency syndromes and monitoring certain therapeutic interventions.

The Immuno T-cell Assay consists of two reagent tubes, CD3/CD4 and CD3/CD8. The instrument prepares the reaction mixture in each tube by adding the patient sample and the diluent to the tube's monoclonal antibodies. The instrument rocks the reagent tube gently, incubates the reaction mixture for 2 minutes at room temperature, and then aspirates a portion of the reaction mixture from the tube and places it in the WBC dilution cup. WBC reagent is added to create a final dilution of 1:36, which is sent to the optical flow cell for light scatter and fluorescence intensity measurements. Fluorescence intensity, 0° light scatter (i.e., size) and 7° light scatter (i.e., cell complexity) are used to identify and enumerate the different lymphocyte populations. The

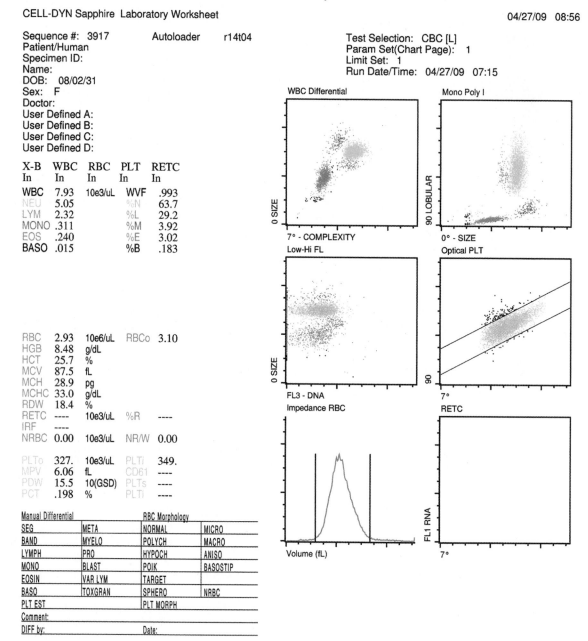

FIGURE 36-20 CELL-DYN Sapphire report depicting WBC differential. (Courtesy of Portneuf Medical Center, Pocatello, Idaho.)

scatterplot of 0° light scatter versus 7° light scatter is used to isolate the lymphocyte population for further examination. The scatterplot of CD3 fluorescence intensity (measured at fluorescein isothiocyanate's emission wavelength of 530 nm) versus CD4 fluorescence intensity (measured at phycoerythrin's emission wavelength of 630 nm) determines the percentage of T_{helper} cells; likewise, the scatterplot of CD3 fluorescence intensity versus CD8 fluorescence intensity determines the percentage of $T_{cytotoxic}$ cells (Web Figure 36-7 ■). The total CD3 fluorescence intensity on a given scatterplot reflects the percentage of T cells present in the patient sample. Comparison of the percentage of CD3 positive cells from each scatterplot can be used as an internal control. The computer system uses established algorithms to process the light scatter and fluorescence measurements and generate the reported parameters. These parameters include total T cell count, percentage of T cells, absolute T_{helper} cell count, percentage of T_{helper} cells, absolute $T_{cytotoxic}$ cell count, percentage of $T_{cytotoxic}$ cells, and the ratio of T_{helper} to $T_{cytotoxic}$ cells. The concentration of these cells can be determined because a CBC is performed on the patient sample prior to preparation of the assay's reagent tubes. This CBC also provides a check of the lymphocyte's viability.

The ImmunoPlt™ (CD61) assay utilizes a platelet-specific monoclonal antibody, anti-CD61 that is labeled with fluorescein isothiocyanate. This assay is useful when a patient's platelet count is very low (e.g., less than 10×10^9/L) or when leukocyte or erythrocyte fragments within the patient sample interfere with platelet enumeration. Because of the specificity of this assay, it provides an accurate platelet enumeration. Like the T-cell assay, the monoclonal antibody is present within a reagent tube. Patient sample and diluent are added to this tube, which are gently mixed. The reagent tube incubates for 1 minute at room temperature. At this point, additional diluent is added to the reagent tube to further dilute the mixture. A portion of this reaction mixture is aspirated into the RBC/PLT dilution cup and diluent is added to create a final dilution of 1:290. A portion of the final dilution is injected into the optical flow cell for measurement. Measurements include 0° light scatter, 7° light scatter, and fluorescence intensity at 530 nm (i.e., fluorescein isothiocyanate's emission wavelength). The instrument's computer system uses established algorithms to process the data generated by these measurements and determines the platelet count. Due to CD61's specificity for platelets, this platelet count is not affected by other cells or cell fragments.

LIGHT-SCATTERING INSTRUMENTS

Technicon Instruments Corporation was important in the development of hematology instrumentation that utilized light scattering technology to enumerate blood cells. Its first instruments were based on **continuous flow analysis** similar to its chemistry instruments. The Hemolog D performed leukocyte differentials based on continuous flow analysis and peroxidase cytochemical staining. The Technicon H-6000 was capable of performing a complete blood cell count and five-part leukocyte differential using continuous flow analysis and an improved cytochemical staining method. The Technicon H*1 was the first of a series of instruments that combined these principles of cell detection and identification with flow cytometry.[33–35] The two instruments described next represent current models whose basic principles of cell enumeration and determination of the leukocyte differential can be traced back to methodologies introduced by the Technicon Instruments Corporation.

Siemens (formerly Bayer) Healthcare ADVIA 120

The ADVIA 120 is capable of performing a CBC, five-part leukocyte differential, and reticulocyte count.[36] It has five measurement channels. The erythrocyte/platelet channel determines the erythrocyte and platelet counts by the light-scattering measurements obtained as diluted cells pass singly through a helium-neon laser beam. The diluent utilized for erythrocyte and platelet counts causes **isovolumetric sphering** of the erythrocytes and platelets. Isovolumetric sphering of erythrocytes eliminates cell volume errors due to variation in erythrocyte shape.[37,38] The erythrocytes are counted and sized by both high-angle (5–15°) and low-angle (2–3°) light-scattering measurements. Individual erythrocyte hemoglobin concentration is determined by the high-angle measurement, and cell volume is determined from the low-angle measurement; thus, the mean cell volume (MCV) and **cellular hemoglobin concentration mean (CHCM)** are obtained. Together, these measurements are used to generate the erythrocyte cytogram, erythrocyte histogram, and hemoglobin histogram (Figure 36-21 ■). The RDW and the **hemoglobin distribution width (HDW)** are derived from these histograms.

Platelets are evaluated simultaneously with the erythrocytes using both high-angle light scatter and low-angle light scatter; however, these signals are amplified for platelet enumeration. This information is used to create a platelet cytogram, and the actual platelet count is obtained by integrated analysis of the platelet cytogram and erythrocyte cytogram to include large platelets while excluding erythrocytes, erythrocyte fragments, and erythrocyte ghosts.

Within the hemoglobin channel, a portion of the EDTA-anticoagulated blood is mixed with the hemoglobin diluent. The erythrocytes are lysed, and free hemoglobin is converted to cyanmethemoglobin. The concentration of cyanmethemoglobin is determined photometrically at 546 nm.

The leukocyte count and five-part leukocyte differential are obtained utilizing two different methods and two separate channels, the peroxidase channel and the basophil/lobularity channel. The peroxidase channel identifies neutrophils, monocytes, and eosinophils by the degree of peroxidase positivity (i.e., increased absorption) and the amount of forward light scatter. Lymphocytes and large unstained cells (LUCs) are identified by the amount of forward light scatter and the fact that they remain unstained by this peroxidase cytochemical–staining method. Erythrocytes are removed prior to the peroxidase staining by lytic action. The amount of forward scatter and degree of peroxidase positivity (i.e., increased absorption) are detected as the cells pass through a tungsten halogen-based flow cell, and this information is used to create the peroxidase cytogram (Web Figure 36-8 ■). Within the basophil/lobularity channel, EDTA-anticoagulated blood is mixed with basophil diluent. The basophil diluent lyses erythrocytes and platelets and strips all leukocytes except basophils of their

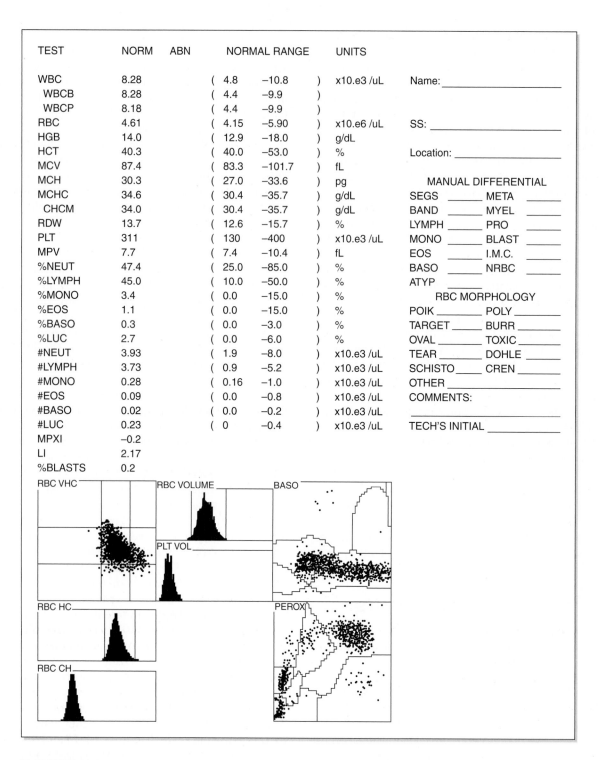

TEST	NORM	ABN	NORMAL RANGE			UNITS
WBC	8.28		(4.8	−10.8	)	x10.e3 /uL
WBCB	8.28		(4.4	−9.9	)	
WBCP	8.18		(4.4	−9.9	)	
RBC	4.61		(4.15	−5.90	)	x10.e6 /uL
HGB	14.0		(12.9	−18.0	)	g/dL
HCT	40.3		(40.0	−53.0	)	%
MCV	87.4		(83.3	−101.7	)	fL
MCH	30.3		(27.0	−33.6	)	pg
MCHC	34.6		(30.4	−35.7	)	g/dL
CHCM	34.0		(30.4	−35.7	)	g/dL
RDW	13.7		(12.6	−15.7	)	%
PLT	311		(130	−400	)	x10.e3 /uL
MPV	7.7		(7.4	−10.4	)	fL
%NEUT	47.4		(25.0	−85.0	)	%
%LYMPH	45.0		(10.0	−50.0	)	%
%MONO	3.4		(0.0	−15.0	)	%
%EOS	1.1		(0.0	−15.0	)	%
%BASO	0.3		(0.0	−3.0	)	%
%LUC	2.7		(0.0	−6.0	)	%
#NEUT	3.93		(1.9	−8.0	)	x10.e3 /uL
#LYMPH	3.73		(0.9	−5.2	)	x10.e3 /uL
#MONO	0.28		(0.16	−1.0	)	x10.e3 /uL
#EOS	0.09		(0.0	−0.8	)	x10.e3 /uL
#BASO	0.02		(0.0	−0.2	)	x10.e3 /uL
#LUC	0.23		(0	−0.4	)	x10.e3 /uL
MPXI	−0.2					
LI	2.17					
%BLASTS	0.2					

Name: _____

SS: _____

Location: _____

MANUAL DIFFERENTIAL

SEGS	_____	META	_____
BAND	_____	MYEL	_____
LYMPH	_____	PRO	_____
MONO	_____	BLAST	_____
EOS	_____	I.M.C.	_____
BASO	_____	NRBC	_____
ATYP	_____		

RBC MORPHOLOGY

POIK	_____	POLY	_____
TARGET	_____	BURR	_____
OVAL	_____	TOXIC	_____
TEAR	_____	DOHLE	_____
SCHISTO	_____	CREN	_____

OTHER _____

COMMENTS:

_____

TECH'S INITIAL _____

RBC VHC

RBC VOLUME

BASO

PLT VOL

RBC HC

PEROX

RBC CH

■ FIGURE 36-21   ADVIA 120 report from a normal individual. (Courtesy of David Teplicek, MT(ASCP), San Antonio, TX)

cytoplasm. The helium-neon laser flow cell measures this dilution and determines the degree of high-angle scatter and low-angle scatter for each cell that is examined. This information is used to create the basophil/lobularity cytogram (Web Figure 36-9 ■). The data management system uses **cluster analysis** to identify individual cell populations within a given cytogram. Each population is identified by its position, area, and density. Thresholds are set, and the number of cells in each population is determined. For the basophil/lobularity cytogram, the normal cell pattern is referred to as the *worm* with the head region representing mononuclear cells and the body region representing polymorphonuclear cells as classified by their high-angle scatter signatures. Basophils have large, low-angle scattered signatures and are located in the region above the worm (Web Figure 36-9). For the peroxidase cytogram, the normal cell pattern depicts the neutrophils in the upper right quadrant, eosinophils in the lower right quadrant, and monocytes in the center triangular region; lymphocytes are located adjacent to the y-axis in the center left quadrant and LUCs are located in the upper left quadrant of the peroxidase cytogram (Web Figure 36-8). The absolute count for each leukocyte population is obtained from the appropriate channel (e.g., absolute neutrophil count from the peroxidase channel and absolute basophil count from the basophil/lobularity channel). The absolute lymphocyte count is obtained by subtracting the absolute basophil count from the absolute lymphocyte count that was obtained from the peroxidase channel. This is necessary because lymphocytes and basophils cannot be differentiated from each other based on analysis of the peroxidase cytogram. The percentage values are calculated from the absolute cell counts. The total leukocyte count is obtained from both channels. The data managment system compares these counts and flags the total leukocyte count if the results do not compare. An advantage of this method of determining cell counts is the capability of performing WBC counts and differentials on samples with very low counts (WBC$<0.1 \times 10^9$/L).

The fifth channel is the reticulocyte channel where cellular RNA of the reticulocytes is stained with oxazine 750, a nucleic acid dye. The helium-neon laser flow cell evaluates the erythroid cells for light-scattering and absorbance characteristics. The high-angle light scatter reflects the hemoglobin concentration within the individual erythroid cells, and low-angle light scatter reflects the size of each cell. Reticulocytes are differentiated from mature erythrocytes based on their RNA content, which is determined by the cell's absorbance reading. Reticulocytes have a higher absorbance compared to mature erythrocytes. In addition to the absolute reticulocyte count and relative reticulocyte percentage, reticulocyte analysis includes a measure of the reticulocyte cellular hemoglobin concentration (CHr™), reticulocyte mean cell volume (MCVr), and the reticulocyte cellular hemoglobin concentration mean.

The ADVIA 120's data management system evaluates the information from the two flow cells, determines the reported parameters, and displays the information on the computer screen (See Web Table 36-1 for the reported parameters.). The results can be printed to hard copy (Figure 36-21) or transferred to the LIS. If abnormalities are detected in cell counts, histograms, or cytograms, the instrument flags the appropriate result(s). The flagging criteria assist the clinical laboratory professional in defining the abnormalities to be reviewed by peripheral blood smear examination.

 Checkpoint! 8

What is the similarity in the reticulocyte methods performed on the ADVIA 120 and XE-2100 instruments?

Siemens Medical ADVIA 2120

The ADVIA 2120 represents the latest model in this series of hematology instruments. The basic principles of blood cell enumeration, reticulocyte enumeration, and determination of the five-part leukocyte differential are the same as those discussed in detail for the ADVIA 120. The hemoglobin determination is a cyanide-free methodology that demonstrates strong correlation with the cyanmethemoglobin method of the ADVIA 120.[39] A disadvantage of the ADVIA 2120 and ADVIA 120 is that neither is currently capable of determining and reporting a nucleated erythrocyte count, although a method is being investigated.[40]

A potential new parameter is the %Hypo or percentage of hypochromic erythrocytes obtained from the red cell erythrogram, a derivation of the erythrocyte cytogram. This parameter is currently designated for "research use only." Studies indicate that the combined use of % Hypo and the CHr™ can be useful in detecting iron deficiency in patients on hemodialysis for chronic renal disease. These patients could experience a superimposed iron deficiency with anemia of chronic disease, which decreases their response to erythropoietin therapy. Early detection of iron deficiency results in appropriate therapeutic intervention to resolve the iron deficiency and, therefore, decrease the poor response rate of hemodialysis patients to erythropoietin therapy.[41,42]

▶ AUTOMATED COAGULATION INSTRUMENTS

Instrumentation was actually introduced into coagulation testing in the early twentieth century. These first instruments, like the majority of instruments utilized today, analyzed the coagulation system through the detection of clot formation.[43,44] The coaguloviscometer developed by Kottman in 1910 determined clotting times by measuring the change in blood **viscosity** as it clotted. The change in viscosity was determined by plotting the voltage against time. Kugelmass introduced a second method of clot detection in 1922. He adapted the nephelometer to coagulation testing. In nephelometry, the clotting time was determined by measuring variations in transillumination as registered by a galvenometer. Baldes and Nygaard introduced the photoelectric technique for determining clotting times in 1936. With their instrument, clotting times were determined by the measurement of increasing optical density as the plasma clotted. Coagulation instrumentation continued to improve, and by the 1960s, semiautomated coagulation instruments began to replace manual techniques in the clinical laboratory. These first instruments were based on electromechanical or optical density methods of clot detection. Coagulation testing evolved in the 1970s with the introduction of fully automated instruments capable of performing multiple coagulation assays.

With the new directions in coagulation testing including chromogenic and immunologic methods, coagulation instruments are now capable of performing these test methods and the clot-based tests. The introduction of instrumentation into coagulation testing has led to increased precision and accuracy and, therefore, improved diagnostic testing and monitoring of therapeutic interventions.

The two principles of clot-based detection currently used by coagulation instruments are electromechanical and optical density. Other available instruments use a combination of these principles.

ELECTROMECHANICAL INSTRUMENTS

These instruments measure the time for a clot to form in plasma by detecting changes in the reaction mixture. One instrument (Fibrometer) detects the completion of an electrical circuit between two electrodes when a clot forms. The other (STArt® 4 Clot Detection) detects a decrease in movement of an iron ball in an electromagnetic field when a clot forms.

BBL FibroSystem

The FibroSystem, a semiautomated coagulation instrument, was introduced in the 1960s. It is composed of a Fibrometer coagulation timer, a thermal prep block to prewarm reagents and samples to 37°C, and an automatic pipet to deliver the appropriate amount of sample or reagent to the test cuvette.[45] The Fibrometer probe, an integral part of the Fibrometer coagulation timer, is the clot detector. The probe consists of two sensory electrodes (stationary and moving) and a probe foot, which is an extension of the moving electrode beyond the base of the probe assembly. In the timing sequence, the moving electrode cycles through the reaction mixture in an elliptical pattern created by raising and lowering the probe foot. The stationary electrode remains in the reaction mixture and is responsible for establishing the electric potential between the two electrodes. The moving electrode becomes electrically active when it is above the reaction mixture. As the fibrin clot is formed, it is picked up by the small hook on the tip of the moving electrode. The electric circuit is completed when the moving electrode becomes activated as it moves out of the reaction mixture; current flows from the stationary electrode through the reaction mixture and fibrin clot to the moving electrode. The creation of this electric circuit causes the timing device to stop, and the clotting time in seconds is recorded. Thus, the principle of clot detection is the electromechanical principle. An advantage of the FibroSystem is that it can be adapted to any coagulation assay that is clot based.

Diagnostica Stago STArt® 4 Clot Detection Instrument

The STArt® 4 Clot Detection instrument is a semiautomated instrument for coagulation testing, a variation of the electromechanical clot detection principle based on the increasing viscosity of plasma as clot formation occurs.[46,47] This stand-alone instrument consists of four independently timed incubation stations with 16 wells, a dispensing pipet, both room temperature and 37°-thermostated reagent storage wells, four measurement channels, and a microprocessor system. The increasing viscosity is detected by the movement of an iron ball located at the bottom of the reaction cuvette. A constant pendular swing of the ball is created by alternating an electromagnetic field on opposite sides of the cuvette utilizing two independent driving coils. As clot formation begins, the plasma viscosity increases with a corresponding decrease in ball movement. The clotting time is determined from an algorithm of the variations in oscillation amplitude. Clotting time results are displayed on the liquid crystal display (LCD) screen, and printed results are obtained from the thermal printer. This instrument can be adapted to any clot-based coagulation assay.

 Checkpoint! 9

Compare the clot detection methods for the Fibrometer system and the STArt 4 system.

OPTICAL DENSITY INSTRUMENTS

Trinity Biotech Coag-A-Mate XM

The Coag-A-Mate XM was first introduced in 1989 by Organon Teknika and is currently supported by Trinity Biotech. According to the January 2008 CAP survey of coagulation instruments, the Coag-A-Mate XM is still utilized in the clinical laboratory.[48] Because it is a good example of a coagulation instrument whose clot detection is optical density, it is discussed here.

The Coag-A-Mate XM is a semiautomated instrument utilizing the change in optical density that occurs with clot formation as its principle of clot detection.[49] The instrument consists of a reagent storage compartment, incubation test plate, photodetection system, and microprocessing system. The test procedures are programmed using the touch entry keypad. Reagents and patient samples are manually pipeted into the test cuvettes. The reaction mixture is warmed to 37°C in the incubation test plate. For determination of the clotting time, the test cuvette is placed in one of two measuring stations. The addition of the final reagent to the test cuvette initiates the timer. The photoelectric cell detects the sudden increase in optical density occurring with fibrin formation, and the timer is stopped. The results are displayed on the LCD panel below each measuring station. This instrument is capable of performing two tests simultaneously. It can perform all clot-based coagulation assays.

CHROMOGENIC/CLOT DETECTION INSTRUMENTS

Several manufacturers currently market coagulation instruments that combine the traditional clot-based detection principle with chromogenic analysis and immunological techniques.

Because the coagulation cascade is a series of enzymatic reactions catalyzed by serine proteases, the activity of these enzymes can be measured by conventional clinical chemistry methods. Chromogenic analysis is an example of a clinical chemistry methodology that has been adapted to coagulation testing. In a chromogenic analysis, the enzyme of interest (e.g., activated coagulation factor) cleaves the chromogenic substrate at a specific site, releasing the chromophore tag. The color intensity is measured spectrophotometrically and is directly proportional to the concentration of the chromophore tag according to Beer's law. Depending on the assay's sequence of reactions, the chromophore tag's concentration is either directly or indirectly related to the concentration (or activity) of the measured substance (e.g., factor VIII activity or antithrombin activity, respectively). Chromogenic assays can be used for testing individual coagulation proteins, biochemical inhibitors, and fibrinolytic proteins based on choice of substrates used in a given assay. In addition to coagulation instruments, chromogenic assays have been adapted for use on a number of spectrophotometric chemistry instruments.

Trinity Biotech AMAX Destiny Plus

The AMAX Destiny Plus is a **random access,** fully automated coagulation instrument capable of performing four different methodologies: electromechanical, optical density, chromogenic, and immunologic.[50] The instrument can perform all methodologies simultaneously. Both samples and reagents are stored at 15°C. A temperature-controlled probe (37°C) is used to transfer the appropriate amount of sample or reagent to the reaction cuvette for measurement.

Electromechanical measurement of clot formation is based on the AMELUNG ball method. The test cuvette contains a stainless steel ball. After sample and reagent (e.g., activated partial thromboplastin reagent) are added to the cuvette, it is placed in a mechanical measurement well. The addition of the starting reagent (e.g., calcium chloride) initiates the rotation of the ball. A magnet holds the rotating ball in a predetermined position within the cuvette. As the fibrin clot forms, fibrin strands draw the ball away from its steady-state position. A sensor detects the change in ball position, stopping the time. The clotting time represents the time elapsed between addition of the starting reagent and detection of the ball movement. The advantage of this measurement is that accurate results are obtained on icteric samples, lipemic samples, and samples from patients on medications that affect optical measurement.

The second method of clot detection available on the AMAX Destiny Plus is optical density. To determine clotting time, sample and reagent (e.g., activated partial thromboplastin reagent) are added to the measuring cuvette, which is moved to the photo-optical measurement position. When the starting reagent (e.g., calcium chloride) is added to the cuvette, the instrument measures the initial absorbance of the reaction mixture at 405 nm and monitors the change in absorbance over time (i.e., creates a clotting curve). The clotting time represents the time elapsed between the addition of starting reagent and the detection of the maximum slope of the clotting curve (Web Figure 36-10■). Because the clotting time is measured as the time difference between the initial absorbance of the reaction mixture and the absorbance at the maximum slope of the clotting curve, the effect of icteria and lipemia on the clotting time is minimized.

The chromogenic assays are performed in the photo-optical measurement well because the final enzymatic reaction in these assays yields paranitroaniline with an absorbance maximum at 405 nm. The temperature-controlled probe delivers the appropriate amount of sample and reagent to the test cuvette. The photodetector cell monitors the optical density over the assay's reaction period at 405 nm. A curve is created by plotting the optical density against time, and the change in optical density (ΔOD) is determined during the linear phase of the reaction. The change in optical density is compared to the assay's calibration curve, and the result is calculated from this comparison and reported in the appropriate units.

The immunologic assays are also performed in the photo-optical measurement well. However, these assays are used not for clot detection but to detect and/or quantitate the presence of certain coagulation proteins or products. For example, immunologic methodology on the AMAX Destiny Plus detects and quantitates D-dimers. In this assay, the reagent is polystyrene microparticles coated with monoclonal antibodies against D-dimer. The temperature-controlled probe delivers the reagent and sample to the test cuvette and the photodetector cell monitors the increase in absorbance at 405 nm that occurs as immune complexes form between the sample's D-dimers and the monoclonal antibodies, thus aggregating the microparticles. The increase in absorbance is directly proportional to D-dimer concentration. Comparison to a standard curve is used to calculate the concentration.

✓ **Checkpoint! 10**

What is the basis of clot detection for the optical density principle?

Diagnostica Stago STA Compact®

Like other automated coagulation instruments, the STA Compact® is a continuous random access instrument that performs clotting assays by electromechanical principle as well as chromogenic and immunological assays.[51] Within this instrument, patient samples and dilution buffers are loaded in the sample drawer and reagents, controls, and calibrators are stored in designated positions within the product drawer maintained at 15–19°C. For the clotting assays (e.g., activated partial thromboplastin time), the sample is aspirated by the sample pipetting needle and placed in a test cuvette containing a stainless steel ball. Then, the reagent (i.e., activated partial thromboplastin) is added by pipetting needle 2. The test cuvette is moved from the measurement station to the incubation area where the temperature of the reaction mixture is warmed to 37°C; the incubation area has 16 positions. After brief incubation, the test cuvette is moved to the measurement area (which has four positions) and pipetting needle 3 adds the starting reagent (i.e., calcium chloride). Together, the alternating electromagnetic field created by two independent driving coils and the rail tracks in the cuvette promote the pendular movement (i.e., oscillation) of the stainless steel ball through the reaction mixture. As the fibrin clot forms, the increasing viscosity of the reaction mixture decreases the ball's oscillation as detected by electromagnetic sensors. The instrument uses an algorithm to calculate the clotting time based on the variations in oscillation amplitude. The clotting times are not affected by lipemic or icteric samples because the determination does not depend on light absorbance.

The chromogenic assays are measured photometrically. The final product of each assay is a chromogen, paranitroaniline with an absorbance maximum of 405 nm. The reaction mixture is set up similarly to that described for the clotting assay. For photometric measurement, monochromatic light is created when incident light from the tungsten-halogen lamp passes through the appropriate interference filter (i.e., 405 nm or 540 nm filter). The monochromatic light then passes through the reaction cuvette, and the chromogen absorbs some of the light. The photodetector measures the amount of absorbance. This absorbance reading is compared to the assay's calibration curve, and the result is calculated from this comparison and reported in the appropriate units.

As previously discussed, the immunological assays are used to detect and/or quantitate the presence of certain coagulation proteins or products (i.e., VWF and D-dimers). For example, STA Compact® measures the concentration of von Willebrand factor (VWF) in plasma using the immunological assay. In this assay, microlatex beads coated with rabbit anti-human VWF are added to a test cuvette containing patient sample. After incubation, the cuvette is moved to the measuring station. The interaction of VWF with its monoclonal antibody causes the microlatex beads to aggregate or clump, thus increasing the absorbance of monochromatic light at 540 nm as measured by the photodetector. This reaction follows Beer's law so that the VWF concentration is directly proportional to absorbance. The VWF concentration is determined by comparison to a standard curve.

SUMMARY

This chapter briefly reviewed the ever-increasing uses of technology for the automated hematology laboratory. The blood cell–counting instruments include those using a combination of technologies such as impedance, light scatter, radio frequency, and fluorescent detection to determine CBC and five-part leukocyte differentials. Most instruments also measure reticulocytes and nucleated erythrocytes. Reticulocyte evaluation includes not only quantitative data but also data on the immaturity of reticulocytes, which indicates the erythropoietic response of the bone marrow to therapy for anemia. The hematology instruments' data analysis systems examine the data for possible interference or abnormalities and if found, the laboratory professional is alerted by suspect or user-defined flags. The laboratory professional uses the flags to correlate the CBC data with peripheral blood morphology and confirm the abnormalities or correct erroneous results. Automated coagulation instruments include those that use electromechanical and/or optical density to detect clot formation in a plasma mixture. In the electromechanical instruments, the formation of a clot completes an electrical circuit between two electrodes. Those instruments using optical density, detect a change in optical density when a clot forms. The addition of chromogenic and immunological assays to these instruments enhances their test assay menus. In chromogenic assays, the activated coagulation factor cleaves a chromogenic substrate, releasing a chromophore tag. The color intensity is measured spectrophotometrically and is related to the factor's concentration. Immunological assays detect coagulation proteins using monoclonal antibodies. The immunologic assay does not measure the protein's functional ability.

To operate these instruments to their fullest potential, it is important that qualified clinical laboratory professionals evaluate the data created by the instrument's analysis of an individual cell's characteristics or clotting characteristics. Through careful review of that data, new applications of these instruments can arise to aid in the early detection of abnormalities. Automation has increased precision and accuracy within the hematology laboratory and shortened the amount of time needed for analysis, but it has also increased the need for the individual laboratory professional's interpretive skills.

REVIEW QUESTIONS

LEVEL I

1. Which instrument uses the optical light scatter method to determine the erythrocyte count? (Objective 3)
   a. GEN·S
   b. XE-2100
   c. CELL-DYN Sapphire
   d. ADVIA 120

2. What is hydrodynamic focusing used for in automated blood cell–counting instruments? (Objective 3)
   a. ensure that only a single cell enters the detection area at any given time
   b. direct the beam of light onto the center of the photodetector
   c. select the appropriate wavelength of light for analysis
   d. focus the beam of light on the detection area

3. Which parameter does the GEN·S instrument calculate? (Objective 5)
   a. erythrocyte count
   b. MCV
   c. reticulocyte percentage
   d. absolute neutrophil count

4. Which dye is used to stain cellular RNA for reticulocyte counting on the ADVIA 120? (Objective 6)
   a. thiazole orange
   b. oxazine 750
   c. new methylene blue
   d. auramine-O

5. For which coagulation instrument is clot formation detected by the flow of current between two sensory electrodes? (Objective 7)
   a. AMAX Destiny Plus
   b. Fibrometer
   c. Coag-A-Mate XM
   d. STArt 4

6. Both electromechanical and photo-optical principles of clot detection are available on this instrument. (Objective 7)
   a. Fibrometer
   b. STA Compact
   c. STArt 4
   d. AMAX Destiny Plus

7. On what is the photo-optical principle of clot detection based? (Objective 8)
   a. observation of increased light transmission as a fibrin clot forms
   b. optical detection of ball movement as a fibrin clot forms
   c. observation of increased absorbance as a fibrin clot forms
   d. photometric detection of an oscillating magnetic force as a fibrin clot forms

LEVEL II

1. What information is needed to create an erythrocyte histogram? (Objective 1)
   a. cell volume and relative cell number
   b. cell size and cell complexity
   c. nuclear size and cellular density
   d. cell forward scatter and cell side scatter

2. Which of the following technologies does the Sysmex XE-2100 *not* use to categorize leukocyte cell types? (Objective 1)
   a. fluorescence
   b. radio frequency
   c. optical light scatter
   d. differential cell lysis

3. Using the ADVIA 120 instrument, which leukocyte cell type is located in the body of the worm of the basophil/lobularity cytogram? (Objective 1)
   a. basophil
   b. monocyte
   c. neutrophil
   d. lymphocyte

4. The Coulter LH 750 five-part leukocyte differential is determined by the analysis of cellular characteristics as defined by: (Objective 1)
   a. light scatter, cytochemical staining, and radio frequency
   b. light scatter and radio frequency
   c. impedance and cytochemical staining
   d. impedance, conductivity, and light scatter

5. The reticulocyte hemoglobin concentration (CHr) is determined by measuring the cell's: (Objective 2)
   a. absorbance and light scatter characteristics
   b. absorbance and radio frequency characteristics
   c. fluorescence intensity and impedance characteristics
   d. fluorescence intensity and conductivity characteristics

6. What does the photodetector measure in the immunological assays performed on the AMAX Destiny Plus? (Objective 3)
   a. decrease in light reflected by antigen-antibody complexes
   b. increase in percent of transmittance because microparticles aggregate
   c. decrease in light scatter because less individual particles are present
   d. increase in absorbance because turbidity accumulates in the reaction mixture

REVIEW QUESTIONS *(continued)*

LEVEL I

8. Which parameter does the CELL-DYN Sapphire directly measure? (Objective 5)
   a. hematocrit
   b. platelet count
   c. relative neutrophil percentage
   d. absolute reticulocyte count

9. Which automated blood cell–counting instrument does *not* use the analysis of fluorescence intensity and light scatter to determine the reticulocyte count? (Objective 6)
   a. XE-2100
   b. ADVIA 120
   c. CELL-DYN Sapphire
   d. LH 750

10. Which parameter does the Sysmex XE-2100 derive from a histogram or scattergram? (Objective 5)
   a. absolute monocyte count
   b. erythrocyte count
   c. mean cell volume
   d. hematocrit

LEVEL II

www.pearsonhighered.com/mckenzie

Use this address to access the interactive Companion Website created for this textbook. Find additional information, tables and figures. Evaluate your command of the chapter information using case studies and critical thinking and multiple choice questions.

REFERENCES

1. Mattern CFT, Brackett FS, Olson B. Determination of number and size of particles by electrical gating: Blood cells. *J Appl Physiol.* 1957; 10:56.

2. Jovin TM et al. Automatic sizing and separation of particles by ratios of light scattering intensities. *J Histochem Cytochem.* 1976; 24:269.

3. Molina FR, Sanchez-Garcia F, Torres A et al. Reticulocyte maturation parameters are reliable early predictors of hematopoietic engraftment after allogeneic stem cell transplant. *Biol Blood Marrow Transplant.* 2007;13:172.

4. Brugnara C, Schiller B, Moran J. Reticulocyte hemoglobin equivalent (Ret He) and assessment of iron-deficient states. *Clin Lab Haem.* 2006;28:303.

5. Stoffman N, Brugnara C, Woods ER. An algorithm using reticulocyte hemoglobin content (CHr) measurement in screening adolescents for iron deficiency. *J Adolescent Health.* 2005;36:529.

6. Tsuchiya K, Ando M, Termura M et al. Monitoring the content of reticulocyte hemoglobin (CHr) as the progression of anemia in nondialysis chronic renal failure (CRF) patients. *Renal Failure.* 2005; 1:59.

7. Buttarello M, Temporin V, Ceravolo R, Farina G, Bulian P. The new reticulocyte parameter (RET-Y) of the Sysmex XE 2100. *Am J Clin Pathol.* 2004;121:489.

8. *Coulter GEN·S System Reference.* Miami, FL: Coulter Corporation; 1996.

9. *Coulter STKS Operator's Guide.* Hialeah, FL: Coulter Corporation; 1991.

10. Allen JK, Batjer JD. Evaluation of an automated method for leukocyte differential counts based on electronic volume analysis. *Arch Path Lab Med.* 1985;109:534.

11. Barnard DF et al. Detection of important abnormalities of the differential count using the Coulter STKR blood counter. *J Clin Path.* 1989;42:772.

12. Corberand JX. Discovery of unsuspected pathological states using a new hematology analyser. *Med Lab Sci.* 1991;48:80.

13. Poulsen KB, Bell CA. Automated hematology: Comparing and contrasting three systems. *Clin Lab Sci.* 1991;4:16.

14. *Clinical Case Studies: Coulter GEN·S System Enhanced VCS Technology.* Bulletin 9165. Brea, CA: Beckman Coulter; 2000.

15. Coulter LH Series System Reference. Brea, CA: Beckman-Coulter; 2003.

16. Red Cell Distribution Parameters—(1) RDW-SD (2) RDW-CV. Bulletin 9617. Brea, CA: Beckman-Coulter; 2007.

17. Lin CK, Lin JS, Chen SY, Jiang ML, Chiu CF. Comparison of hemoglobin and red blood cell distribution width in the differential diagnosis of microcytic anemia. *Arch Pathol Lab Med.* 1992;116(10): 1030.

18. *Sysmex XE-2100 Operator's Manual.* Kobe, Japan: Sysmex; revised 2006.

19. Rowan RM, Linssen J. A picture is worth a thousand words. *Sysmex Journal International.* 2005;15(1):27.

20. Briggs C, Harrison P, Grant D, Staves J, Machin SJ. New quantitative parameters on a recently introduced automated blood cell counter—XE 2100™. *Clin Lab Haem.* 2000;22:345.

21. Ruzicka K, Veitl M, Thalhammer-Scherrer R, Schwarzinger I. The new hematology analyzer Sysmex XE-2100—performance evaluation of a novel white blood cell differential technology. *Arch Pathol Lab Med.* 2001;125:391.

22. Nakul-Aquaronne D, Sudaka-Sammarcelli I, Ferrero-Vacher C, Starck B, Bayle J. Evaluation of the Sysmex XE-2100® Hematology Analyzer in hospital use. *J Clin Lab Anal.* 2003;17:113.

23. Fernandez B, Hamaguchi Y. Automated enumeration of immature granulocytes. *Am J Clin Pathol.* 2007;128:454.

24. Nigro KG, O'Riordan M, Molloy EJ et al. Performance of an automated immature granulocyte count as a predictor of neonatal sepsis. *Am J Clin Pathol.* 2005;123:618.

25. Briggs C, Kunka S, Fujimoto H et. al. Evaluation of immature granulocyte counts by XE-IG master: Upgraded software for XE-2100 automated hematology analyzer. *Lab Hematol.* 2003;9:117.

26. Wang FS, Rowan, RM, Creer M et al. Detecting human CD34+ and CD 34- hematopoietic stem and progenitor cells using a Sysmex automated hematology analyzer. *Lab Hematol.* 2004;10:200.

27. Briggs C, Hart D, Kunka S, Oguni S, Machin SJ. Immature platelet fraction measurement: A future guide to platelet transfusion requirement after haematopoietic stem cell transplantation. *Transfus Med.* 2006;16:101.

28. Abe Y, Wada H, Tomatsu H et al. A simple technique to determine thrombopoiesis level using immature platelet fraction (IPF). *Thromb Res.* 2006;118:463.

29. Briggs C, Kunka S, Hart D, Oguni S, Machin SJ. Assessment of an immature platelet fraction (IPF) in peripheral thrombocytopenia. *Br J Haematol.* 2004;126:93.

30. Takami A, Shibayama M, Orito M, Omote M et al. Immature platelet fraction for prediction of platelet engraftment after allogeneic stem cell transplantation. *Bone Marrow Transplant.* 2007;39:501.

31. *CELL-DYN Sapphire Operator's Manual.* Abbott Park, IL: Abbott Laboratories, Diagnostic Division; November 2007.

32. Muller R, Mellors I, Johannessen B et al. European multi-center evaluation of the Abbott Cell-Dyn Sapphire hematology analyzer. *Lab Hematology.* 2006;12(1):15.

33. Watson JS, Davis RA. Evaluation of the Technicon H*1 Hematology System. *Lab Med.* 1987;18:316.

34. Bollinger PB et al. The Technicon H*1: An automated hematology analyzer for today and tomorrow. *Am J Clin Pathol.* 1987;87:71.

35. Nelson L, Charache S, Wingfield S, Keyser E. Laboratory evaluation of differential white blood cell count information from the Coulter S-Plus IV and Technicon H*1 in patient populations requiring rapid "turnaround" time. *Am J Clin Pathol.* 1989;91:563.

36. *Bayer ADVIA 120 System Operator's Guide.* Tarrytown, NY: Bayer; 1999.

37. Kim YR, Ornstein L. Isovolumetric sphering of erythrocytes for more accurate and precise cell volume measurement by flow cytometry. *Cytometry.* 1983;3:419.

38. Mohandas N et al. Accurate and independent measurement of volume and hemoglobin concentration of individual red cells by laser light scattering. *Blood.* 1986;68:506.

39. Harris N, Jou JM, Devoto G et al. Performance evaluation of the ADVIA 2120 hematology analyzer: An international multicenter clinical trial. *Lab Hematology.* 2005;11(1):62.

40. Kratz A, Maloum K, O'Malley C et al. Enumeration of nucleated red blood cells with the ADVIA 2120 hematology system: An international multicenter clinical trial. *Lab Hematology.* 2006;12(2):63.

41. Wish JB. Assessing iron status: Beyond serum ferritin and transferrin saturation. *CJASN.* 2006;1 Suppl 1:S4.

42. Tessitore N, Solero GP, Lippi G et al. The role of iron status markers in predicting reponse to intravenous iron in haemodialysis patients on maintenance erythropoietin. *Nephrol Dial Transplant.* 2001;16:1416.

43. Ens GE, Jensen R. Coagulation instrumentation review. *Clin Hemostasis Rev.* 1993;7(5):1.

44. Sabo MG. Coagulation instrumentation and reagent systems. In: D. A. Triplett, ed. *Laboratory Evaluation of Coagulation.* Chicago: ASCP Press; 1982.

45. *The FibroSystem Manual.* Cockeysville, MD: Becton Dickinson; June 1976.

46. *STArt-4 Operator's Manual.* Parsipanny, NJ: American Bioproducts; 1990.

47. Ledford MR, Kaczor DA. Evaluation of the ST4 Clot Detection instrument. *Lab Med.* 1992;23:172.

48. College of American Pathologists. Survey of instruments: Coagulation analyzers. *CAP Today.* January 2008.

49. *Coag-A-Mate XM Operations Manual.* Durham, NC: Organon Teknika; 1990.

50. *Amelung AMAX DESTINY Plus Operator's Manual.* Berkeley Heights, NJ: Trinity Biotech USA; 2006.

51. *STA Compact Operator's Manual.* Parsipanny, NJ: Diagnostica Stago; February 2001.

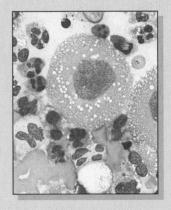

37

Flow Cytometry

Fiona E. Craig, M.D.

■ OBJECTIVES—LEVEL I

At the end of this unit of study, the student should be able to:

1. Describe the components of a flow cytometer and the principles of cell analysis.
2. Illustrate by example the clinical applications of flow cytometry.
3. Appraise the use of fluorochrome-labeled antibodies in immunophenotyping by flow cytometry.
4. Give examples of the clinical applications of immunophenotyping by flow cytometry, and interpret single dot plots.
5. Define *clonality* and identify methods for detecting a monoclonal population of cells by immunophenotyping.
6. List the specimens appropriate for immunophenotyping by flow cytometry.
7. Describe how flow cytometry can be used in cell quantitation.
8. Calculate and interpret the absolute CD4 count.
9. Describe reticulocyte counting by flow cytometry, and define *immature reticulocyte fraction* (IRF).
10. Explain how flow cytometry can be applied to DNA analysis.
11. List the cells positive for CD34, and explain the purpose of a CD34 count.

■ OBJECTIVES—LEVEL II

At the end of this unit of study, the student should be able to:

1. Compare and contrast the immunophenotyping results characteristic of chronic lymphocytic leukemia, hairy cell leukemia, and non-Hodgkin lymphoma.
2. Identify the pitfalls that can be encountered in immunophenotyping mature lymphoid malignancies by flow cytometry, and generate potential solutions.
3. Compare and contrast the immunophenotyping results characteristic of acute lymphoblastic leukemia and acute myelogenous leukemia.
4. Identify the pitfalls that can be encountered in immunophenotyping acute leukemia and lymphoma by flow cytometry, and generate potential solutions.
5. Compare and contrast the usefulness of the sucrose hemolysis test, Ham test, and flow cytometry immunophenotyping in diagnosing paroxysmal nocturnal hemoglobinuria.
6. Select and explain the quality measures that must be enforced in quantitative flow cytometry.
7. Compare and contrast the absolute CD4 count and HIV viral load in the surveillance of HIV infection.

■ OBJECTIVES—LEVEL II (continued)

8. Calculate and interpret the S phase fraction and the DNA index, and give the principle of DNA analysis by flow cytometry.

9. Assess the findings of flow cytometry cell analysis using two or more dot plots, and select the most likely cell represented.

10. Evaluate flow cytometry results to identify problems and generate solutions.

11. Compare reticulocyte counting by flow cytometry with manual methods, and assess the advantages of flow cytometry.

12. Interpret the immature reticulocyte fraction (IRF).

13. Summarize the uses of analysis for the CD34 antigen, and choose recommended procedures to analyze this antigen.

KEY TERMS

Biphenotypic leukemia
CD designation
Compensation
DNA Index (DI)
Flow chamber
Fluorochrome
Forward light scatter
Gating
Hematogone
Hydrodynamic focusing
Immunophenotyping
Minimal residual disease
Photodetector
Side light scatter

BACKGROUND BASICS

The information in this chapter builds on the concepts learned in previous chapters. To maximize your learning experience, you should review these concepts before starting this unit of study.

Level I

▶ Describe the cellular characteristics that differentiate T and B lymphocytes; differentiate the stages of development of granulocytes, lymphocytes, and monocytes. (Chapter 7)

▶ Describe reticulocytes and methods to quantify them. (Chapters 8, 34)

▶ Summarize the classification of malignant leukocyte disorders. (Chapters 21–26)

Level II

▶ Summarize the subtypes of malignant disorders and laboratory tests used to help classify them. (Chapter 21)

▶ Describe the abnormality associated with paroxysmal nocturnal hemoglobinuria (PNH). (Chapter 15)

▶ Outline the cell cycle. (Chapter 2)

▶ Describe the application of immature reticulocyte fraction (IRF). (Chapter 8)

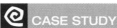
CASE STUDY

We will address this case study throughout the chapter.
Andrew, a 76-year-old male, had a complete blood count (CBC) performed during hospitalization for pneumonia. He was found to have a WBC of 76×10^9/L with 80% lymphocytes. Consider the conditions that are associated with these results and the follow-up testing that might be necessary to confirm a diagnosis.

▶ OVERVIEW

The purpose of flow cytometry is to detect and measure multiple properties of cells so that they can be identified and quantitated. This chapter introduces the principles of flow cytometry and discusses its clinical applications. First, the method of detecting and quantitating particles by flow cytometry is described. This description includes specimen requirements and processing and the concept of gating to isolate cells of interest. The remainder of the chapter addresses the uses of flow cytometry in the clinical laboratory. Flow cytometry is currently used to analyze individual cells for the presence of antigens (immunophenotyping) and to quantitate ribonucleic acid (RNA) or deoxyribonucleic acid (DNA). Immunophenotyping is one of the tools used for diagnosing mature lymphoid malignancies, acute lymphoblastic leukemia (ALL), acute myeloid leukemia (AML), and paroxysmal nocturnal hemoglobinuria (PNH), and monitoring HIV infection. The material in this chapter should be studied with ∞ Chapters 24, 25, and 26 (neoplastic disorders) to obtain a full understanding of where flow cytometry fits into the diagnostic workup of these disorders. This chapter also introduces the application of flow cytometry in reticulocyte counting and DNA analysis.

▶ INTRODUCTION

A *flow cytometer* is an instrument capable of detecting molecules on the surface of or inside individual particles such as cells. Detection of molecules is achieved by isolating single particles/cells and labeling the molecule of interest with a fluorescent marker. Particles/cells that possess the molecule of interest are recognized by the emission of fluorescent light following excitation. Information is acquired from many thousands of particles/cells and stored on a computer for further analysis. The current applications of flow cytometry in the clinical laboratory include immunophenotyping (identifying antigens using detection antibodies) leukocytes and erythrocytes, enumerating reticulocytes, and analyzing DNA (Table 37-1 ✪).

▶ PRINCIPLES OF FLOW CYTOMETRY[1]

ISOLATION OF SINGLE PARTICLES

Flow cytometry is performed on particles in suspension (e.g., cells or nuclei). Leukocytes from peripheral blood and bone marrow specimens are often analyzed after the removal of red blood cells (RBC) by lysis. The cell suspension is aspirated and injected into a **flow chamber** (Figure 37-1 ■), the specimen-handling area of a flow cytometer where cells are forced into single file and directed into the path of a laser beam.

The flow chamber contains two columns of fluid. The particles/cells are contained in an inner column of sample fluid that is surrounded by a column of sheath fluid. The sheath and sample fluids are maintained at different pressures and move through the flow chamber at different speeds. This gradient between the sample and sheath fluid keeps the fluids separate (laminar flow) and is used to control the diameter of the column of sample fluid. The central column of sample fluid is narrowed to isolate single particles/cells that pass through a laser beam (**hydrodynamic focusing**) like a string of beads. Laser light is focused on these single particles/cells and can be measured by **photodetectors** as it is scattered off particles/cells when they pass in front of the beam. If particles/cells have fluorescent molecules attached, the laser light excites the mole-

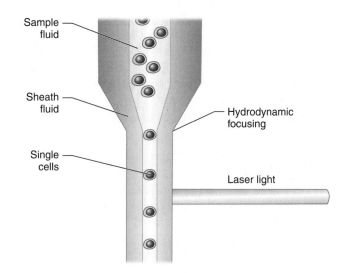

■ FIGURE 37-1   Flow chamber. The sample fluid, containing a suspension of single cells, is injected into a stream of sheath fluid. The stream is narrowed and directed through the laser beam (hydrodynamic focusing).

cules, which then emit light of a specific wavelength, which is also detected.

LIGHT SCATTERING

When the laser beam interacts with a single particle/cell, light is scattered but its wavelength is not altered. The amount of light scattered in different directions can be used to identify the particle/cell because it is related to the physical properties of the particle (size, granularity, and nuclear complexity). Light scattered at a 90° angle (**side light scatter**) is related to the internal complexity and granularity of the particle/cell. Neutrophils produce much side scatter because of their numerous cytoplasmic granules. Light that proceeds in a forward direction (**forward light scatter**) is related to the particle's size. Large cells produce more forward scatter than small cells. Therefore, light scattering can be used to distinguish particles and is currently employed by several hematology analyzers to perform differential counting of leukocytes. (∞ Chapter 36)

> ✓ **Checkpoint! 1**
>
> *Would a lymphocyte or monocyte have more forward light scatter?*

DETECTION OF FLUOROCHROMES

In addition to light scattering, the flow cytometer can be used to detect bound fluorescent markers (**fluorochromes**), which are molecules that are excited by light of one wavelength and emit light of a different wavelength (fluorescent light). Fluorochromes can be used to label detec-

✪ TABLE 37-1
Applications of Flow Cytometry
Immunophenotyping
Lymphoid antigens
Neutrophilic antigens
Monocytic antigens
Terminal deoxynucleotidyl transferase (TdT)
GPI-linked proteins (e.g., CD55 and CD59)
CD4
CD34
Reticulocyte counting
DNA analysis

In the figure:
Sample fluid
Sheath fluid
Single cells
Hydrodynamic focusing
Laser light

tion antibodies or to bind stoichiometrically to DNA or RNA (Table 37-2). Flow cytometers use light of a single wavelength generated by a laser to excite fluorochromes bound to the particle of interest. Light emitted from the fluorochrome is separated from the incident laser light using a combination of filters and mirrors. A photomultiplier tube then detects and quantifies the emitted light.

Clinical flow cytometers usually contain an argon laser that generates light at 488 nm. This single wavelength is often used to excite three different fluorochromes, each emitting light at different wavelengths. Using three different fluorochromes allows detection of three different antigens on the cell. Excitation of additional fluorochromes to detect further antigens usually requires a second laser light source (e.g., helium neon, emission 633 nm). Currently, clinical immunophenotyping studies frequently utilize two laser light sources to identify five or six antigens on each cell analyzed. (Table 37-2). Some flow cytometers used in a research setting are capable of detecting up to 18 different fluorochromes.

A fluorochrome unfortunately does not emit light at a single wavelength. Mirrors, filters, and photodiodes are used to detect the peak wavelength of emitted light from each fluorochrome. However, some overlap between the light emitted from different fluorochromes usually exists. For example, although the peak emissions for the two fluorochromes fluorescein isothiocyanate (FITC) and phycoerythrin (PE) are different, PE emits some light at the wavelength used to detect FITC. The overlap is compensated for either by adjusting the settings on the flow cytometer or by performing a mathematical correction either before or after the data are collected. This process is called **compensation.**

The next section discusses the principles of immunophenotyping, specimen requirements, and techniques for isolating the cells of interest. That discussion is followed by a description of the use of immunophenotyping in identifying abnormal cell populations for diagnosing and classifying leukocyte neoplasms. The last two sections describe the application of flow cytometry to quantitate reticulocytes and to analyze the DNA of solid tumors.

✓ Checkpoint! 2

A laboratory wants to identify cells that have two different antigens. How many laser light sources are needed?

▶ IMMUNOPHENOTYPING BY FLOW CYTOMETRY[2,3,4]

Immunophenotyping is the identification of antigens using detection antibodies. Antibodies are utilized because they bind specifically to antigens and can be labeled with fluorochromes to provide a sensitive and specific detection method. Most immunophenotyping studies involve detecting cell surface antigens. Intracytoplasmic and intranuclear antigens can be detected following permeabilization of cell membranes with detergent and/or alcohol. Detection antibodies can be either polyclonal or monoclonal. Polyclonal antibodies are made by injecting antigen into animals (e.g., rabbit anti-human antibodies). The animal produces many antibodies that are directed against different portions of the antigen. Therefore, the antigen can be recognized even if some parts of it are abnormal. However, polyclonal antibodies are often difficult to standardize and prone to nonspecific binding.

Monoclonal antibodies are directed against a single portion of the antigen. They are produced in myeloma/tumor cell lines and therefore have high purity and reproducibility. Often several different monoclonal or polyclonal antibodies are available from different suppliers to detect a single antigen and can be given a unique company-specific designation. An international workshop has been developed to systematically review antibodies and group those recognizing the same antigen into a cluster of differentiation (**CD designation**). For example, the commercially available antibodies Leu-4 and OKT3 are both designated CD3. Many fluorochrome-labeled detection antibodies are available commercially (Table 37-3 ✪). Combinations of these antibodies are currently used in the clinical laboratory to help identify cells (Table 37-4 ✪).

✪ TABLE 37-2

Example Fluorochromes Used in Flow Cytometry

Application	Fluorochrome	Excitation Wavelength (nm)	Detection Wavelength (nm)
Immunophenotyping	FITC	488	519
Immunophenotyping	PE	488	575
Immunophenotyping	APC	650	660
Immunophenotyping	PerCP-Cy5.5*	488/675	694
Reticulocyte count	Acridine orange	488	530–640
DNA analysis	Propidium iodide	488	617

*PerCP-Cy5.5 is a conjugate of two fluorochromes. PerCP is excited at 488 nm; the emitted signal (675 nm) excites the Cy5.5 component of the molecule.
FITC = fluorescein isothiocyanate; PE = phycherythrin; APC = allophycocyanin.

⊕ **TABLE 37-3**

Antibodies Used for Immunophenotyping by Flow Cytometry

CD Designation	Normal Distribution	Use
CD1a	Immature T cells	Lymphoblastic leukemia/lymphoma
CD2	T cell, NK cell	Lineage of lymphoma or leukemia
CD3	T cell	Lineage of lymphoma or leukemia
CD4	T cell	Lineage of lymphoma or leukemia
CD5	T cell	Lineage of lymphoma/leukemia or aberrant expression on B cell SLL/CLL and mantle cell lymphoma
CD7	T cell, NK cell	Lineage of lymphoma or leukemia
CD8	T cell	Lineage of lymphoma or leukemia
CD11c	Monocytes, lymphoid cells	Hairy cell leukemia: bright+; SLL/CLL: dim+
CD11b	Neutrophils	Myelodysplastic syndrome
CD13	Monocytes	Lineage of leukemia
	Myeloid cells	Myelodysplastic syndrome
CD14	Monocytes	Lineage of leukemia
CD15	Monocytes	Lineage of leukemia
	Myeloid cells	
CD16	NK, NK-like T cells	Large granular lymphocyte leukemia
	Granulocytes	Myelodysplastic syndrome
CD19	B cell	Lineage of lymphoma or leukemia
CD20	B cell	Lineage of lymphoma or leukemia
CD22	B cell	Lineage of lymphoma or leukemia, SLL/CLL: dim+; PLL: bright+
CD23	B cell	SLL/CLL+, mantle cell−
CD25	Many cell types	Hairy cell leukemia bright+
CD33	Monocytes	Lineage of leukemia
	Myeloid cells	
CD34	Stem cells, progenitor cells	Stem cells for transplantation, acute leukemia
CD38	Plasma cells, some lymphocytes, monocytes, myeloid cells	Plasma cell neoplasms
		Prognostic marker in CLL
CD42	Megakaryocytes	Acute megakaryocytic leukemia
CD45	All leukocytes	Lineage of malignancy
		Gating
CD55	GPI-anchored protein	Paroxysmal nocturnal hemoglobinuria
CD56	NK, NK-like T cells	Large granular lymphocyte leukemia
CD57	NK, NK-like T cells	Large granular lymphocyte leukemia
CD59	GPI-anchored protein	Paroxysmal nocturnal hemoglobinuria
CD61	Megakaryocytes	Acute megakaryocytic leukemia
CD79a	B cells (blasts to plasma cells)	Lineage of lymphoma or leukemia
CD103	Subset of intramucosal T cells	Hairy cell leukemia
		Enteropathy associated T cell lymphoma
Glycophorin A	Erythroid	True erythroleukemia
Myeloperoxidase	Myeloid cells	Lineage of leukemia
Kappa	B cell	Maturity, clonality, SLL/CLL dim
Lambda	B cell	Maturity, clonality, SLL/CLL dim

CLL = chronic lymphocytic leukemia; SLL = small lymphocytic lymphoma; PLL = prolymphocytic leukemia; dim = weak intensity of emitted fluorescence; bright = strong intensity of emitted fluorescence; NK = natural killer; GPI = glycosyl phosphatidyl inositol.

TABLE 37-4

Applications of Immunophenotyping by Flow Cytometry

- Diagnosis and classification of mature lymphoid malignancies
- Prognostic markers in chronic lymphocytic leukemia (CD38 and ZAP-70)
- Diagnosis and classification of acute leukemia
- Detection of minimal residual leukemia following therapy
- Diagnosis of paroxysmal nocturnal hemoglobinuria
- Enumeration of T cell subsets (e.g., CD4 counts in HIV)
- Enumeration of CD34+ progenitor cells for transplantation

✓ **Checkpoint! 3**

A cell population is positive with both Leu1 and T1 monoclonal antibodies. As a result, the cell is classified as CD5 positive. Explain.

SPECIMEN REQUIREMENTS AND PREPARATION FOR IMMUNOPHENOTYPING

Immunophenotyping by flow cytometry requires a suspension of individual cells (Table 37-5 ✪). Anticoagulated blood or bone marrow aspirate, body fluid specimens, and fine needle aspiration samples are ideal for immunophenotyping by flow cytometry because they already contain cells in suspension. Leukocytes can be isolated from these samples either by erythrocyte lysis or density gradient centrifugation. Lysis methods are favored because the leukocytes are retained in their original proportions without the risk of losing cell subtypes. Hematopoietic and lymphoid cells can also be isolated from fresh tissue biopsy specimens by manual disaggregation.

Once a suspension of leukocytes without erythrocytes has been prepared, the sample is stained using fluorochrome-labeled antibodies. (In some studies, the leukocytes are stained before the erythrocytes are lysed.) The labeled sample is aspirated into the flow cytometer, and the amount of scattered light and the intensity of each fluorescent signal is recorded for every cell analyzed. The acquired data are then displayed

graphically on histograms or dot plots. Dot plots usually display the intensity of fluorescent light emitted from two fluorochromes (Figures 37-2■ and 37-3■). The plot is divided into quadrants indicating cells labeled with one fluorochrome, the other fluorochrome, or both fluorochromes.

Cells are considered positive for an antigen if they have a fluorescence intensity greater than either the negative control or a negative population of cells present in the same analysis tube (Figures 37-2 and 37-3). The intensity of light emitted is determined by comparison with the known range of intensities for that antibody/fluorochrome combination and divided roughly into three portions: dim or weak intensity, intermediate intensity, and bright or strong intensity. The intensity of emitted light is related to the density of antigens.

ISOLATION OF CELLS OF INTEREST BY GATING

Immunophenotyping requires isolation of the cells of interest (e.g., lymphocytes from monocytes and granulocytes). Cells can be separated either during specimen processing (density gradient centrifugation) or during data analysis (gating). **Gating** is the process of isolating cells by placing an electronic gate around those with the same light-scattering or fluorescence properties. For example, lymphocytes can usually be separated from neutrophils by their location on the forward versus side light scatter dot-plot (Figure 37-2). Fluorescence dot plots can then be set up to display only information obtained from cells falling within the chosen gate. If the gate is too wide, many cell types are included, and identifying the phenotype of the cells of interest becomes difficult. If the gate is too narrow, the cells of interest can be excluded.

The forward versus side light scatter dot plot unfortunately is not always capable of separating the cells of interest. For example, blasts and lymphocytes often appear in the same region on the forward versus side light scatter dot plot. Therefore, a different gating strategy can be required for analyzing acute leukemia. Blasts often have dim CD45 expression while lymphocytes have bright CD45 staining. Therefore, blasts and lymphocytes can be distinguished on a dot plot displaying CD45 intensity versus side angle light scatter (Figure 37-4■). Fluorescence staining can be used for gating only if the chosen antibody (CD45) is present in each analysis tube.

@ **CASE STUDY** *(continued from page 837)*

Flow cytometry immunophenotyping was requested on Andrew.

1. What is the optimal specimen?
2. Which cells are of interest and should be included in the gate?
3. What are the typical forward and side scatter properties of the cells of interest?

✪ **TABLE 37-5**

Specimen Requirements for Immunophenotyping by Flow Cytometry

Specimen type	Requirements	Storage
Peripheral blood	5 mL in EDTA or heparin	<24 hrs, RT
Bone marrow	1 mL in EDTA or heparin	<24 hrs, RT
Fluids	as much as possible	<24 hrs, 4°C
Tissue	Preferably >$\frac{1}{2}$cm³	<24 hrs, 4°C

RT = room temperature; EDTA = ethylenediamine tetraacetic acid.

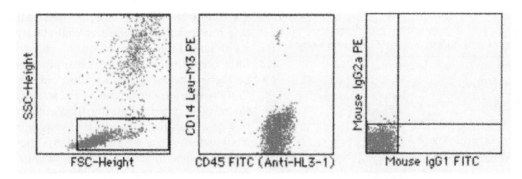

■ FIGURE 37-2   Flow cytometry histograms from analysis of peripheral blood from Andrew, the patient described in the case study. Lymphocytes (green) are included in the rectangular gate. Neutrophils (blue) are excluded from the gate. A few monocytes (red) are included in the gate (i.e., the gate is not pure). The plot of CD45 versus CD14 indicates the gate's composition. Lymphocytes (green) stain strongly with CD45. Monocytes (red) stain with CD14 and CD45. The negative control (Mouse IgG2a versus Mouse IgG1) shows very little nonspecific binding. (Histograms generated using SimulSET software, BD Immunocytometry Systems.) SSC = side scatter; FSC = forward scatter.

✓ **Checkpoint! 4**

Explain why lymphocytes and neutrophils can be separated on a forward versus side light scatter dot plot.

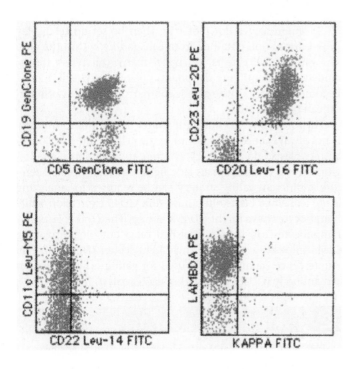

■ FIGURE 37-3   Flow cytometry histograms from the population gated in Figure 37-2. The majority of cells stain for CD19, CD5, CD20, CD23, CD11c (dim), and monoclonal surface immunoglobulin lambda light chain. A few reactive T cells stain for CD5 only. (Histograms generated using SimulSET software, BD Immunocytometry Systems.)

DIAGNOSIS AND CLASSIFICATION OF MATURE LYMPHOID MALIGNANCIES

Flow cytometry immunophenotyping can be used to identify cell lineage (B, T, or natural killer [NK] cell) and the presence of an abnormal population of lymphocytes. This information can assist in detecting malignant cells and identifying a subtype of malignancy. Neoplasms are made up of a population of identical cells (clone). A clone of B lymphocytes can be recognized by uniform expression of one immunoglobu-

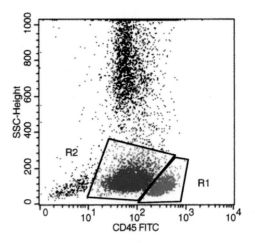

■ FIGURE 37-4   Flow cytometry histogram of CD45 versus side scatter from a case of acute leukemia. The gate R1 (events colored red) includes lymphocytes with bright intensity staining for CD45. The gate R2 (events colored green) includes a population of blasts with dim expression of CD45 and low side scatter. The blasts and lymphocytes have lower side scatter than monocytes and neutrophils. (Histograms generated using CellQuest software, BD Immunocytometry Systems.)

lin light chain (kappa or lambda light chain class restriction). In contrast, a reactive population of B lymphocytes contains a mixture of cells, each with expression of either kappa or lambda immunoglobulin light chain.

Clonality can also be detected by identifying a population of cells that display an abnormal phenotype (aberrant expression of a lymphoid antigen). For example, mature T lymphocytes normally express CD3, CD2, CD5, and CD7. A clone of malignant T lymphocytes could lack detectable CD5 and/or CD7. Another example of an abnormal phenotype is acquisition of an antigen that is not normally present. For example, the T cell marker CD5 is aberrantly expressed on a subset of B cell malignancies (small lymphocytic lymphoma/chronic lymphocytic leukemia and mantle cell lymphoma) (Figure 37-3). Therefore, the presence of CD5-positive B lymphocytes can assist in identifying a lymphoid malignancy and diagnosing a specific subtype. Panels of antibodies are usually selected to separate the common subtypes of lymphoproliferative disorders (Table 37-6 ✪). In addition, flow cytometric immunophenotyping can be used to demonstrate the presence of antigens for directed therapy (for example, CD20 for anti-CD20 monoclonal antibody therapy), identify prognostic markers such as ZAP-70 expression in CLL,[5] and identify a small population of abnormal cells following treatment (**minimal residual disease**).

✪ CASE STUDY *(continued from page 841)*

Flow cytometry revealed the results displayed in Figure 37-3.

4. What is the phenotype?
5. Which features indicate clonality?
6. What is the diagnosis?

Pitfalls Encountered in the Diagnosis of Mature Lymphoid Malignancies

Although immunophenotyping usually provides useful information, potential pitfalls can lead to an incorrect diagnosis. A malignant B cell lymphoproliferative disorder is easily

overlooked if it lacks surface immunoglobulin. Some lymphoid malignancies frequently lack diagnostic surface antigens, including plasma cell neoplasms, HIV associated lymphoma, and mediastinal lymphoma. T cell lymphoma can be difficult to detect because many cases do not demonstrate an abnormal phenotype. Hodgkin lymphoma is difficult to detect by flow cytometry for several reasons: Hodgkin lymphoma lacks many cell surface lymphoid antigens, the neoplastic cells are rare, and a single cell suspension is often difficult to produce because of the presence of fibrosis. Another potential pitfall in flow immunophenotyping is the presence of an abnormal phenotype that is not specific for a single subtype of lymphoid malignancy. For example, CD10 expression can be seen in follicular lymphoma, diffuse large B cell lymphoma and Burkitt lymphoma. Therefore, it is important to interpret immunophenotyping data in conjunction with morphology.

DIAGNOSIS AND CLASSIFICATION OF ACUTE LEUKEMIA[6,7,8,9]

Using the World Health Organization (WHO) classification, a diagnosis of acute leukemia requires manual differential counting to identify more than 20% blasts in the peripheral blood or bone marrow (∞ Chapter 21). Once a diagnosis of acute leukemia has been established, flow cytometry can be used to assist in identifying the subtype of leukemia. Currently most treatment protocols require the distinction of acute lymphoblastic leukemia (ALL) and acute myeloid leukemia (AML). The recognition of Auer rods or the presence of staining with cytochemical stains allows the identification of AML (∞ Chapters 21 and 24). Until the advent of immunophenotyping, all cases of acute leukemia lacking these features were assumed to be ALL. However, immunophenotyping studies have revealed that this assumption is erroneous. Some AML cases lack cytochemical staining and are recognized only by immunophenotyping (AML NOC [not otherwise categorized], minimally differentiated). In addition to the accurate separation of ALL from AML, flow cytometry phenotyping can be used to assist in identifying

---

TABLE 37-6

Characteristic Immunophenotype of Lymphoproliferative Disorders

Diagnosis	CD19	CD5	CD23	CD11c	CD22	CD25	sIg
Chronic lymphocytic leukemia	+	+	+	+/−	+w	+/−	+w/−
Prolymphocytic leukemia	+	−/+	−	−	+	+/−	+
Hairy cell leukemia	+	−	−/+	+br	+br	+	+
Small lymphocytic lymphoma	+	+	+	+/−	+w	+/−	+w/−
Mantle cell lymphoma	+	+	−	−	+	−	+
Follicular lymphoma	+	−	+/−	−	+	−	+

br = bright or strong fluorescence intensity; w = weak or dim fluorescence intensity; + = antigen present; − = antigen absent; +/− = variable expression (often present); −/+ = variable expression (often absent).

subtypes of leukemia that have a different prognosis (e.g., T cell ALL has a worse prognosis in general than B cell ALL) or require an alternate therapeutic regimen (e.g., acute promyelocytic leukemia).

Acute Lymphoblastic Leukemia[6]

Immunophenotyping is essential for the diagnosis of ALL, separation of T and B lineage ALL, and identification of subtypes of B lineage ALL (see Table 25-4, p. 535).

ALL belonging to the B lymphocyte lineage can be divided into subtypes that resemble stages of normal B lymphocyte maturation. During normal maturation in the bone marrow, B cells gain and lose antigens in synchrony until they acquire a mature B cell phenotype (see Table 25-4) (∞ Chapter 7). Normal immature B cell bone marrow precursors at all stages of maturation are referred to collectively as **hematogones** (∞ Chapter 35).

ALL with a precursor B cell phenotype (pre-B and early pre-B) makes up 80% of childhood ALL. B cell lineage is usually defined by the presence of surface CD19 and/or cytoplasmic CD22 expression. Immaturity of the cells is recognized by the presence of CD10 and terminal deoxynucleotidyl transferase (TdT), a template-independent DNA polymerase. However, this phenotype overlaps with a significant proportion of normal bone marrow precursors. Therefore, recognition of small populations of residual ALL cells following treatment often requires identification of cells with an abnormal phenotype. Aberrant expression of a single myeloid antigen (e.g., CD33 or CD13) is found in 30–50% of cases of pre-B cell ALL. Although this abnormal phenotype can be used as a marker of disease, it is not associated with a change in prognosis. Another, more subtle, abnormality is the loss of the synchronous expression of B cell antigens. For example, although CD34 and surface CD22 are both expressed during normal B lymphocyte maturation, they are not usually present together. Cells expressing both surface CD22 and CD34 can be seen in B cell ALL.

CASE STUDY *(continued from page 843)*

7. Which of the flow cytometry results presented in this case indicate that this is a malignancy of mature lymphocytes (chronic lymphocytic leukemia), not acute lymphoblastic leukemia?

ALL with a T cell phenotype is present in 15–20% of cases. The vast majority of cases of T cell ALL express the T cell antigens CD1, CD2, CD3, CD5, and CD7. Unlike mature T cells, T lymphoblasts express CD3 only in the cytoplasm, not on the cell surface. In addition, blasts differ from mature T cells in either expressing both CD4 and CD8 (cortical thymocyte phenotype) or lacking both CD4 and CD8. TdT is present in more than 90% of cases, and CD10 can be present. The phenotype of T cell ALL can be abnormal with loss of one or more of these T cell antigens. Myeloid markers are aberrantly expressed in 25–30% of pre-T cell ALL cases. In general, the prognosis for patients with T cell ALL is worse than for precursor B cell ALL.

 Checkpoint! 5

Why is it important to do immunophenotyping in a case of ALL?

Acute Myeloid Leukemia[7]

The WHO classification scheme recognizes several subtypes of AML (∞ Chapters 21, 24). Most subtypes can be identified using morphology and/or cytogenetics. Immunophenotyping has a limited role in the diagnosis of AML. However, the detection of an abnormal phenotype, such as aberrant expression of a lymphoid antigen, can assist in identifying residual disease following treatment. Immunophenotyping is also required for the diagnosis of AML NOC, minimally differentiated, and is often used for the diagnosis of acute megakaryocytic leukemia. AML NOC, minimally differentiated, is diagnosed when Auer rods are absent and cytochemical stains are negative but there is evidence of nonlymphocytic differentiation by the expression of myeloid antigens. The diagnosis of acute megakaryocytic leukemia relies on identifying megakaryocytic differentiation by immunophenotyping (CD41, CD61) or electron microscopy (platelet peroxidase). Although acute promyelocytic leukemia characteristically lacks staining for CD34 and HLA-DR, this phenotype is not specific. Therefore, morphology in combination with cytogenetic studies still remains the *gold standard for the diagnosis of AML.* In addition to diagnosis and classification, flow cytometry can be used to demonstrate the presence of the antigens for directed therapy, for example the anti-CD33 monoclonal antibody therapy.

Flow cytometry has also been used to identify abnormalities in the phenotype of myeloid populations in myelodysplastic syndromes.[8] Abnormalities include aberrant expression of lymphoid antigens on neutrophilic cells and abnormal gain and loss of antigens as cells mature from promyelocytes to segmented neutrophils.

Pitfalls Encountered in the Diagnosis of Acute Leukemia

Some cases of acute leukemia do not fit neatly into the categories ALL and AML. There may be aberrant expression of antigens (lineage heterogeneity) or a lack of specific antigen expression (undifferentiated leukemia).

Acute Leukemia with Lineage Heterogeneity The term **biphenotypic leukemia** is used when leukemic blasts express several antigens from two different lineages (myeloid and lymphoid). However, identification of lineage requires careful selection of antigens because few are restricted to a single lineage. Myeloperoxidase is found only on cells with myeloid differentiation (restricted to a myeloid lineage). Therefore, the presence of myeloperoxidase indicates myeloid differentiation with a great degree of certainty. By contrast, CD15 is associated with myeloid differentiation but can also be expressed on cells of a T cell lineage. Therefore, CD15 expression does not predict myeloid differentiation with the same degree of certainty as myeloperoxidase. The term *biphenotypic* should be restricted to leukemia that demonstrates equal evidence of differentiation toward more than one lineage. Although scoring systems have been proposed to assist in weighing the phenotypic evidence for each lineage, they do not include all antigens currently evaluated by flow cytometry and do not consider cytochemical and cytogenetic evidence.[9]

Acute Undifferentiated Leukemia Blasts occasionally lack expression of lineage-restricted antigens. For example, the presence of only CD7 does not distinguish T cell ALL from AML. CD7 is normally present on immature T cells and is aberrantly expressed in approximately 10% of AML. Morphologic analysis, cytochemical stains, molecular diagnostic studies, and cytogenetics can assist in determining lineage.

DIAGNOSIS AND SURVEILLANCE OF IMMUNODEFICIENCY DISORDERS

Immunophenotyping by flow cytometry can be used to analyze leukocyte subsets to identify deficiency of a cell type. The most frequent clinical application of flow cytometry is monitoring the immunodeficiency acquired following HIV virus infection (∞ Chapter 37). Less frequently, immunophenotyping is used to detect inherited immunodeficiencies such as the severe combined immunodeficiency disorder (SCID) and X-linked agammaglobulinemia (∞ Chapter 37).

The HIV virus uses the CD4 antigen to infect T lymphocytes and monocytes. After viral fusion, internalization, replication, and dissemination, CD4+ cells are destroyed. The resultant decrease in CD4+ cells leads to immunodeficiency. The absolute number and percentage of CD4+ T lymphocytes present in the peripheral blood can be used to monitor the immune system. HIV surveillance is used to predict the course of disease, decide when to start prophylactic therapy for opportunistic infections, and determine when to commence antiretroviral therapy. An absolute number of CD4+ T lymphocytes less than 200/μL in the peripheral blood also is used to diagnose AIDS in HIV infected individuals.

The CD4 count is determined by staining with fluorescent-tagged antibodies against CD3 (found on T cells but not monocytes) and CD4 followed by whole blood RBC lysis. The percentage of CD4+ lymphocytes is determined by flow cytometry. Gating is critical to avoid exclusion of lymphocytes and contamination by cells other than lymphocytes such as CD4+ monocytes. The absolute CD4 count can be

determined directly by flow cytometry (single platform) by comparing the number of CD4+ cells identified per unit volume analyzed with an absolute number of highly fluorescent beads added to the analysis tube (Figure 37-5 ■). Alternatively, the CD4 count can be calculated from the percentage of CD4+ lymphocytes and the absolute number of lymphocytes determined by a hematology analyzer (dual platform).

> Absolute CD4 count = Absolute lymphocyte count $\times$ Percent CD4+ lymphocytes/100
>
> Absolute lymphocyte count = WBC count ($\times$ 10^9/L) $\times$ Percent lymphocytes from WBC differential/100

A precise and accurate CD4 count is essential (Table 37-7). Results from a patient are often compared with previous results and published diagnostic and therapeutic levels. Therefore, the procedure used for quantitative flow cytometry should attempt to eliminate preanalytical and analytical variables. Preanalytical variables include biologic variability (age, diurnal rhythm, medications), specimen collection, and storage. Analytical variables include sample preparation and errors associated with flow cytometers and hematology analyzers. The CDC publishes guidelines for standardization of CD4 determination. Two levels of stabilized quality control material must be run with each batch of CD4 assays. In addition, proficiency testing for professionals is available through the College of American Pathologists (CAP) surveys.

The HIV viral load is another monitor of HIV infection. Viral load testing measures plasma viral RNA. The CD4 count and the HIV viral load often provide complementary information. The CD4 count is the best indicator of the balance between immune cell production versus destruction and therefore indicates the risk of opportunistic infection or secondary malignancy. The HIV viral load indicates the burden of disease and therefore can be used to monitor response to antiviral therapy and the acquisition of drug resistance.

✓ **Checkpoint! 6**

A patient has 10% CD4+ lymphocytes, a WBC count of 5 $\times$ 10^9/L, and 30% lymphocytes. What is the absolute CD4 count? Is this count compatible with a diagnosis of AIDS in an HIV-infected individual?

CD34 ENUMERATION[10]

CD34 enumeration is used to support bone marrow and peripheral blood stem cell transplantation (∞ Chapter 27). CD34 is an antigen restricted to multipotential hematopoietic stem cells and early progenitors of all lineages. Hematopoietic stem cells are responsible for reconstituting bone marrow function following transplantation. CD34 enumeration is used to determine whether the product collected for transplantation has enough cells. For rapid

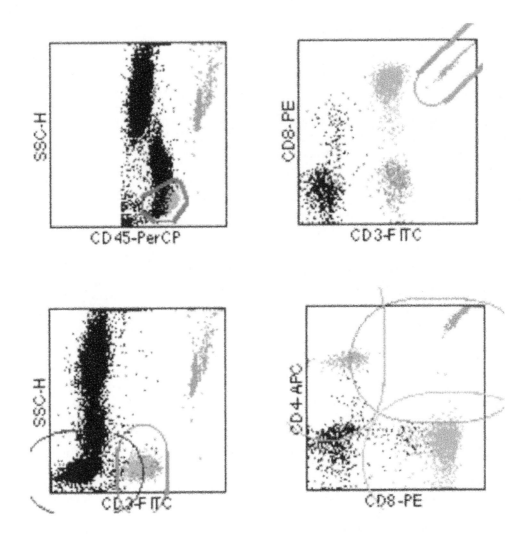

■ FIGURE 37-5   CD4 enumeration. CD4-positive lymphocytes are isolated by gating on cells displaying strong intensity CD45 (within green circle) in top left histogram (all lymphocytes), bright CD3 (red circle) in lower left histogram (all T cells), and CD4 (orange circle) in lower right histogram. The specimen contains a known concentration of fluorescent beads (pink). The absolute CD4 count is determined by comparing the number of CD4-positive events with the number of beads counted (purple circle in upper right histogram). (Histograms generated using MultiSET software, BD Immunocytometry Systems.)

⊙ TABLE 37-7

Procedural Requirements for Quantitative Flow Cytometry

Standardization of procedure

    Patient preparation

    Specimen handling

    Specimen preparation

    Analysis (gating accuracy and purity and precision)

Quality control

Proficiency testing

Documentation of personnel competency

---

engraftment, $2.0–8.0 \times 10^6$ CD34+ cells/kg body weight are needed, and for long-term engraftment, $0.5–2.0 \times 10^6$ CD34+ cells/kg body weight are needed. CD34+ cells can be collected by either bone marrow aspiration or peripheral blood apheresis. Hematopoietic progenitor cells are often mobilized into the peripheral blood using a combination of cytotoxic drugs and growth factors. CD34 enumeration can also be performed on the peripheral blood to determine the optimal time for peripheral blood stem cell collection. CD34 determination is challenging because it needs to be fast, accurate, and precise even at low numbers (0.1% of cells or 5 cells/μL). The European Working Group on Clinical Cell Analysis (EWGCCA) have made recommendations in an attempt to optimize and standardize CD34 determination by flow cytometry (Table 37-8 ✪). Several different analysis protocols (e.g., Milan, ISHAGE, SIHON) exist.

PAROXYSMAL NOCTURNAL HEMOGLOBINURIA (PNH)[11,12]

PNH is a chronic hemolytic disorder caused by an acquired mutation of the *PIG-A* gene (∞ Chapter 15), which encodes an enzyme critical in the synthesis of the glycosylphosphatidylinositol (GPI) anchor that links many proteins to the cell membrane. Flow cytometry can be used to detect the presence of GPI-anchored membrane proteins. In addition, some flow cytometric assays assess the ability of white blood cells to bind a fluorescent-labeled modified toxin (FLAER) that attaches through GPI anchors. Flow cytometric immunophenotyping for CD55 and CD59 on erythroid cells and CD55, CD59, and other GPI-linked antigens on granulocytes appears to be a more sensitive and specific test for diagnosing PNH than the sucrose hemolysis test or Ham test. Erythrocyte immunophenotyping is easier to interpret than analysis of neutrophils but can give a false negative result if hemolysis is active or a transfusion was recently given. Erythrocytes deficient in CD55 and CD59 have also been identified in patients with aplastic anemia and myelodysplastic syndromes and in very small numbers in normal individuals.

▶ RETICULOCYTE COUNTING[13]

Reticulocytes are immature circulating erythrocytes (∞ Chapter 5). They lack a nucleus but contain more RNA than a mature RBC. An increased number of reticulocytes indicates a bone marrow response to anemia (∞ Chapter 8). Manual reticulocyte counting is performed on a blood smear stained with a supravital stain (e.g., new methylene blue). Reticulocytes contain a reticulum of stained precipitated RNA and are counted per 1000 erythrocytes. Automated reticulocyte counting is offered by many hematology analyzers and frequently employs many of the principles of flow cytometry.

✪ TABLE 37-8

Recommendations for CD34 Enumeration (EWGCCA)

- Lyse red cells, do not use wash procedure to avoid centrifugation and possible loss of cell populations.
- Use bright (e.g., PE) fluorochrome conjugates of class II or III monoclonal antibodies that detect all glycoforms of CD34.
- Use vital nuclei acid dye to exclude platelets, unlysed red blood cells, and debris, or 7-amino actinomycin (7-AAD) to exclude dead cells during acquisition.
- Perform dual staining with CD45 to assist in detection of leukocytes.
- Include in the strategy the identification of cells with low levels of CD45 expression and low side scatter.
- Include CD34 bright and dim staining populations.
- Acquire sufficient events to generate at least 100 CD34 positive cells.

✪ TABLE 37-9

Fluorescent Reagents Used in Automated Reticulocyte Counting

- Thiazole orange (Becton Dickinson FACScan flow cytometer)
- New methylene blue (Coulter Beckman, STKS/MAXM, and manual)
- Acridine orange (Coulter Beckman, Gen-S System)
- CD4K530 (Abbott Diagnostics, Cell-Dyn 4000)
- Oxazine 750 (Bayer Diagnostic, Miles H.3/Advia 120)
- Auramine O (Sysmex, R Series, and SE-Avante)

A peripheral blood specimen is stained with a fluorescent dye that binds to RNA (Table 37-9 ✪). The amount of dye bound is proportional to the amount of RNA present. The labeled specimen is passed in front of a laser light source, and cells emitting more than a threshold amount of fluorescent light are counted as reticulocytes (Figure 37-6 ■). This automated method is more precise than the manual method because many more cells are analyzed (usually 30,000 or more). Automated instruments are also capable of determining the maturity of reticulocytes by quantitating the amount of RNA present. The *immature reticulocyte fraction* (IRF) is the proportion of reticulocytes with the highest content of RNA. An increased IRF is the first indication of bone marrow recovery following transplantation or successful replacement therapy with erythropoietin, iron, B_{12}, or folate (∞ Chapters 9,12,13).

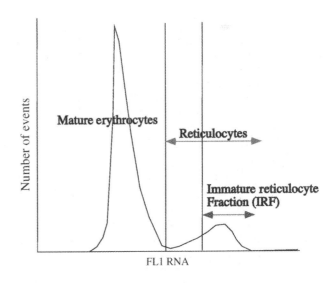

■ FIGURE 37-6 Automated reticulocyte count as performed on the Cell-Dyn 4000. The RNA in reticulocytes reacts with the fluorochrome CD4K530 (Abbott Diagnostics), and the fluorescence is picked up by the FL1 RNA detector. The immature reticulocyte fraction contains more RNA and therefore has a higher fluorescence intensity.

✓ Checkpoint! 7

What are the advantages of automated reticulocyte counting over manual counts?

▶ DNA ANALYSIS

DNA analysis is usually performed on solid tumors to provide prognostic information. Either fresh frozen tissue or a thick section of fixed, paraffin-embedded tissue is processed to produce individual cells or nuclei. The suspension is permeabilized (the cell and/or nuclear membrane is made permeable to allow access of the fluorescent dye to the DNA) and stained with a fluorochrome that binds to DNA. If the fluorescent dye (propidium iodide) binds to both DNA and RNA, RNA is removed by digestion. The amount of fluorochrome bound is proportional to the amount of DNA. The DNA content varies during cell division (proliferation) and is abnormal in cells with numerical chromosome abnormalities (aneuploid) (Figure 37-7■). Computer software uses mathematical formulas to calculate the cells in each phase of the cell cycle, calculate indexes, and identify abnormal populations...

PROLIFERATION

Tumors with an increased number of dividing cells often have a worse prognosis but in some instances are susceptible to therapy directed at dividing cells. The DNA content of cells can be used to determine the proportion of dividing cells. During cell division and prior to mitosis (G2/M phase),

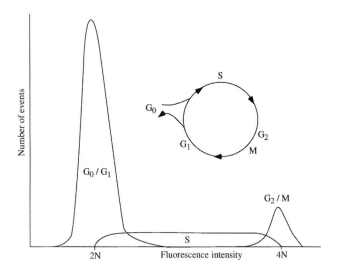

■ FIGURE 37-7　Fluorescence intensity of DNA-bound dye during phases of the cell cycle. Mathematical programs are used to distinguish three areas under the curve (cell cycle phases G_0/G_1, S, and G_2/M).

✪ TABLE 37-10

Calculations for DNA Analysis by Flow Cytometry

- S-phase fraction (SPF) = $100 \times S/(G_0/G_1 + S + G_2/M)$
- Proliferation index (PI) = $100 \times (S + G_2/M)/(G_0/G_1 + S + G_2/M)$
- DNA index = DNA content G_0/G_1 sample/DNA content G_0/G_1 diploid control

the DNA content increases (synthetic, or S, phase) until there are two copies of the entire genome prior to mitosis (G2/M-phase) (Figure 37-7). The *S-phase fraction* is the proportion of all cells (G0/G1 + S + G2/M) that are in the S phase. The proliferative index is the proportion of all cells that are in proliferative phases (S + G2/M) (Table 37-10✪).

PLOIDY

All nondividing, normal human cells contain 46 chromosomes (2 each of 23 chromosomes) and are therefore referred to as being *diploid*. The presence of tumor cells containing an abnormal number of chromosomes is often associated with a worse prognosis. The **DNA Index (DI)** is the DNA content of tumor cells relative to a diploid population of cells. It is calculated as the DNA content of cells in the tumor in the G0/G1 phase of the cell cycle relative to the DNA content of G0/G1 cells in a diploid control. For example, diploid cells have a DI of 1.0. Tetraploid cells (four copies of all chromosomes) have a DI of 2.0, and cells with only one copy of each chromosome (haploid) have a DI of 0.5. *Aneuploidy* is the presence of cells with an abnormal DNA content that is not a multiple of the DNA content of haploid cells, for example, a DI of 1.3.

CLINICAL APPLICATIONS OF DNA ANALYSIS[14]

The clinical utility of DNA analysis remains controversial. One of the most extensively studied tumors is breast carcinoma. A correlation exists between increased S-phase fraction and other markers of a poor prognosis (large breast tumor, the presence of metastatic disease in axillary lymph nodes, high histologic grade, and absence of steroid receptors). However, the main value of DNA analysis in breast carcinoma can be the identification of patients who have a low S-phase fraction and might not require chemotherapy in addition to surgical excision. Interlaboratory variability in methodology and interpretation of results has delayed the routine use of this technique.

SUMMARY

Flow cytometry is a technique that involves the analysis of single particles for their ability to scatter light and fluoresce. This technology is used by stand-alone instruments (flow cytometers) and has also been incorporated into other instruments such as hematology cell analyzers. Flow cytometry is used in the clinical laboratory for immunophenotyping, reticulocyte counting, and DNA analysis. Immunophenotyping uses fluorochrome-labeled detection antibodies to identify cellular antigens. Its primary use is to classify and sub-type leukemia and lymphoma. Reticulocyte and DNA analysis utilize fluorescent dyes that bind to nucleotides. DNA analysis is used to analyze solid tumors. The amount of DNA present helps in making prognosis and treatment decisions.

REVIEW QUESTIONS

LEVEL I

1. Which of the following is a (are) component(s) of a flow cytometer? (Objective 1)
   a. flow chamber
   b. laser light source
   c. light detectors
   d. all of the above

2. Which of the following properties of the cells analyzed by flow cytometry is related to forward angle light scatter? (Objectives 1, 7)
   a. granularity
   b. nuclear complexity
   c. size
   d. shape

3. Which of the following statements explains the use of fluorochromes in immunophenotyping by clinical flow cytometry? (Objectives 3, 5)
   a. All fluorochromes emit light at the same wavelength.
   b. Fluorochromes bind nonspecifically to leukocytes.
   c. The wavelength of the emitted light is the same as that of the incident light.
   d. Several fluorochromes can be excited by light of a single wavelength.

4. Which of the following properties is (are) used for gating in clinical flow cytometry? (Objective 1)
   a. forward angle light scatter
   b. side angle light scatter
   c. intensity of CD45 staining
   d. all of the above

5. Which of the following is a (are) clinical application(s) of flow cytometry? (Objective 2)
   a. DNA quantitation
   b. immunophenotyping
   c. reticulocyte counting
   d. all of the above

6. Which of the following flow cytometry methods is the most appropriate for diagnosing and classifying chronic lymphocytic leukemia? (Objectives 4, 5, 7)
   a. CD34 enumeration
   b. DNA quantitation
   c. immunophenotyping
   d. RNA quantitation

LEVEL II

1. A 45-year-old female presented with pancytopenia. Flow cytometry performed on the peripheral blood revealed the following results:

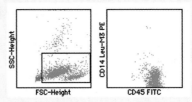

   Which is the predominant cell type in the gate? (Objective 9)
   a. eosinophil
   b. lymphocyte
   c. monocyte
   d. neutrophil

2. Further flow cytometric analysis performed on the sample described in question 1 revealed the following results:

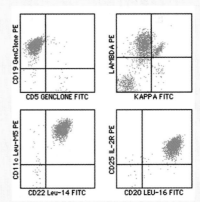

   What is the phenotype of the cells present? (Objective 9)
   a. CD19+, CD5−, CD11+, CD25+
   b. CD19+, CD5+, CD11+, CD25+
   c. CD19+, CD5−, CD11c−, CD25−
   d. CD19−, CD5−, CD11c−, CD25−

REVIEW QUESTIONS (continued)

LEVEL I

7. Which of the following is detected during immunophenotyping by flow cytometry? (Objective 3)
   a. antibodies using detection antigens
   b. antibodies using detection fluorochromes
   c. fluorochromes using detection antibodies
   d. antigens using detection antibodies

8. Which of the following specimens is most appropriate for flow cytometry immunophenotyping? (Objective 6)
   a. formalin-fixed bone marrow aspirate clot
   b. fresh lymph node biopsy
   c. frozen bone marrow biopsy
   d. one-week-old EDTA anticoagulated peripheral blood

9. A peripheral blood sample needs to be shipped to a reference lab for flow cytometry immunophenotyping. Which of the following procedures is most appropriate? (Objective 6)
   a. overnight delivery at room temperature
   b. overnight delivery at 4°C
   c. regular mail service at room temperature
   d. regular mail service at 4°C

10. An 80-year-old male was found to have lymphocytosis. Flow cytometry of the peripheral blood revealed the following results:

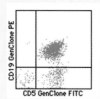

What is the phenotype of the majority of lymphocytes represented in this diagram? (Objective 4)
   a. CD19+, CD5−
   b. CD19+, CD5+
   c. CD19−, CD5−
   d. CD19−, CD5+

LEVEL II

3. Which of the following phenotypes is indicated by the kappa and lambda light chain dot plot displayed in question 2? (Objective 9)
   a. absence of surface immunoglobulin
   b. monoclonal lambda immunoglobulin light chain
   c. monoclonal kappa immunoglobulin light chain
   d. polyclonal immunoglobulin light chains

4. Which of the antigens expressed in question 2 indicates a mature B lymphocyte phenotype? (Objective 1)
   a. CD5
   b. CD11c
   c. CD19
   d. surface immunoglobulin

5. Which of the following is the most likely diagnosis for the case described in question 2? (Objective 1)
   a. acute lymphoblastic leukemia
   b. chronic lymphocytic leukemia
   c. hairy cell leukemia
   d. infectious mononucleosis

6. Flow cytometric analysis of a lymph node fails to reveal an abnormal phenotype. The pathologist is convinced that the node is involved by lymphoma. A touch preparation performed from the specimen received in the laboratory contains numerous large cells that are absent from a cytocentrifuge slide made from the cell suspension prepared for staining. Which of the following is the most likely explanation? (Objective 4)
   a. The sample received for flow cytometry is not representative of the malignancy.
   b. The malignant cells were lost during manual disaggregation of cells.
   c. The malignant cells were excluded from the gate.
   d. The malignant cells have a normal phenotype.

7. Repeat analysis of the case described in question 6 increases the number of large cells present in the suspension stained and analyzed on the flow cytometer. An abnormal phenotype is still not detected. Which of the following neoplasms could be difficult to detect by flow cytometry cell surface antigen studies? (Objective 2)
   a. Hodgkin's disease
   b. T cell lymphoma
   c. plasma cell neoplasms
   d. all of the above

8. A patient presented with circulating blasts. Flow cytometry immunophenotyping performed on the peripheral blood revealed the following phenotype: CD19+, CD10+, surface immunoglobulin IgM kappa. Which of the following is the most likely diagnosis? (Objective 3)
   a. Burkitt lymphoma
   b. acute lymphoblastic leukemia, precursor B cell type
   c. acute lymphoblastic leukemia, precursor T cell type
   d. acute myeloid leukemia

REVIEW QUESTIONS *(continued)*

LEVEL I

LEVEL II

9. Which of the following is the most likely karyotype for the cells described in question 8? (Objective 3)
   a. t(9;22)
   b. t(14;18)
   c. t(8;14)
   d. t(15;17)

10. A patient was found to have circulating blasts. No Auer rods were identified, and all cytochemical stains were negative. Flow cytometry immunophenotyping revealed the presence of myeloid antigens. Which of the following is the most appropriate diagnosis? (Objective 3)
    a. acute lymphoblastic leukemia
    b. acute myeloid leukemia
    c. chronic lymphocytic leukemia
    d. chronic myeloid leukemia

www.pearsonhighered.com/mckenzie

Use this address to access the interactive Companion Website created for this textbook. Find additional information, tables and figures. Evaluate your command of the chapter information using case studies and critical thinking and multiple choice questions.

REFERENCES

1. Givan AL. Principles of flow cytometry: An overview. *Methods in Cell Biology.* 2001;63:19–50.

2. Stelzer GT, Marti G, Hurley A, McCoy P Jr, Lovett EJ, Schwartz A. U.S.-Canadian consensus recommendations on the immunophenotypic analysis of hematologic neoplasia by flow cytometry: Standardization and validation of laboratory procedures. *Cytometry.* 1997;30:214–30.

3. Stewart CC, Behm FG, Carey JL, Cornbleet J, Duque RE, Hudnall SD et al. U.S.-Canadian consensus recommendations on the immunophenotypic analysis of hematologic neoplasia by flow cytometry: Selection of antibody combinations. *Cytometry.* 1997;30:231–35.

4. Borowitz MJ, Bray R, Gascoyne R, Melnick S, Parker JW, Picker L et al. U.S.-Canadian consensus recommendations on the immunophenotypic analysis of hematologic neoplasia by flow cytometry: Data analysis and interpretation. *Cytometry.* 1997;30:236–44.

5. Chen YH, Peterson LC, Dittman D et al. Comparative analysis of flow cytometric techniques in assessment of zap-70 expression in relation to IgVh mutational status in chronic lymphocytic leukemia. *Am J Clin Pathol.* 2007;127:176–81.

6. Khalidi HS, Chang KL, Medeiros LJ, Brynes RK, Slovak ML, Murata-Collins JL, Arber DA. Acute lymphoblastic leukemia: Survey of immunophenotype, French-American-British classification, frequency of myeloid antigen expression and karyotypic abnormalities in 210 pediatric and adult cases. *Am J Clin Pathol.* 1990;111(4):467–76.

7. Khalidi HS, Medeiros LJ, Chang KL, Brynes RK, Slovak ML, Arber DA. The immunophenotype of adult acute myeloid leukemia: High frequency of lymphoid antigen expression and comparison of immunophenotype, French-American-British classification, and karyotypic abnormalities. *Am J Clin Pathol.* 1998;109:211–20.

8. Kussick SJ, Wood BL. Using 4-color flow cytometry to identify abnormal myeloid populations. *Arch Pathol Lab Med.* 2003;127:1140–47.

9. Buccheri V, Matutes E, Dyer MJS, Catovsky D. Lineage commitment in biphenotypic acute leukemia. *Leukemia.* 1993;7:919–27.

10. Gratama JW, Orfao A, Barnett D et al. Flow cytometric enumeration of CD34+ hematopoietic stem and progenitor cells. European Working Group on Clinical Cell Analysis. *Cytometry.* 1998;34:128–42.

11. Richards SJ, Rawstron AC, Hillmen P. Application of flow cytometry to the diagnosis of paroxysmal nocturnal hemoglobinuria. *Cytometry.* 2000;42:223–33.

12. Iwanaga M, Furukawa K, Amenomori T, Mori H, Nakamura H, Fuchigami K, Kamihira S, Nakakuma H, Tomonaga M. Paroxysmal nocturnal haemoglobinuria clones in patients with myelodysplastic syndromes. *Bri J Haematol.* 1998;102:465–74.

13. Koepke JA. Update on reticulocyte counting. *Lab Med.* 1999;30:339–43.

14. Wenger CR, Clark GM. S-phase fraction and breast cancer: A decade of experience. *Breast Canc Res Treat.* 1998;51:255–65.

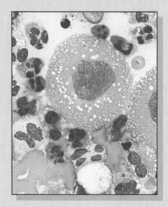

CHAPTER OUTLINE

38

Chromosome Analysis of Hematopoietic and Lymphoid Disorders

Kathleen S. Wilson, M.D, FCAP, FACMG

■ OBJECTIVES—LEVEL I

At the end of this unit of study, the student should be able to:

1. Define *chromosome* and *mitosis*.
2. List the basic steps of cytogenetic analysis, and select the most appropriate type of specimen for analysis of suspected constitutional and neoplastic (acquired) disorders.
3. Identify two major types of chromosome abnormalities, describe how they occur, and use the appropriate terminology to describe them.
4. List the practical uses of cytogenetics in the diagnosis and prognosis of hematolymphoid disorders.

■ OBJECTIVES—LEVEL II

At the end of this unit of study, the student should be able to:

1. Describe chromosome morphology and mitosis.
2. Describe each step of the cytogenetic harvest procedure.
3. Define and compare *aneuploidy, nondisjunction,* and *anaphase lag*.
4. Define and compare *translocation, deletion, inversion,* and *isochromosome*.
5. Identify the general categories of hematopoietic disorders for which cytogenetic analysis is useful for patient care.
6. Correlate diagnostic chromosome aberrations with types of hematolymphoid disorders, and assess their prognostic and therapeutic implications.
7. Assess the prognostic impact of cytogenetic results in acute lymphoblastic leukemia.
8. Explain the clinical utility of cytogenetics in transplantation.
9. Correlate chromosome abnormalities with specific oncogene activation, and assess the role of the oncogene in the neoplasm.

KEY TERMS

Acquired aberration
Acrocentric
Aneuploid
Comparative genomic hybridization (CGH)
Chimerism
Constitutional cytogenetic aberration
Diploid
Endomitosis
Heterologous
Homologous
Hyperdiploid
Hypodiploid
Metacentric
Monosomy
Mosaic
Nondisjunction
Polymorphic variant
Polyploid
Pseudodiploid
Satellite DNA
Submetacentric
Trisomy

BACKGROUND BASICS

The information in this chapter builds on the concepts presented in other chapters relating to cell division and hematopoietic and lymphoid neoplasms. In order to maximize your learning, you should review these concepts before beginning this unit of study.

Level I

▶ Know the stages of the cell cycle, particularly the steps of mitosis. (Chapter 2)
▶ List the major types of neoplastic hematopoietic and lymphoid disorders. (Chapter 21)

Level II

▶ Outline the classification of acute myeloid leukemia and acute lymphoblastic leukemia. (Chapters 24, 25)
▶ Describe the various typical laboratory findings and criteria for classification of myeloproliferative disorders. (Chapter 22)
▶ Describe the typical laboratory findings and classification of the myelodysplastic states. (Chapter 23)
▶ Summarize the chronic lymphoproliferative disorders, list the criteria for distinction of Hodgkin's disease versus non-Hodgkin lymphomas, and define the major classification terminology. (Chapter 26)

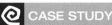 CASE STUDY

We will address this case study throughout the chapter.

Gregory, a healthy 25-year-old man, has a routine physical examination and laboratory studies for new employment. The total white blood cell (WBC) count is 30,000 × 10⁹/L. Consider what conditions may result in this clinical picture and the follow-up studies that should be done.

▶ OVERVIEW

This chapter is designed to give the reader a background for understanding the terminology and application of cytogenetics in diagnosis and treatment of *hematolymphoid neoplasms* (term commonly used to encompass both hematopoietic and lymphoid neoplasms). The chapter begins with a review of chromosome structure and morphology followed by a summary of the procedure used to prepare specimens for chromosome study. Chromosomal abnormalities are discussed, and the terminology used to describe cytogenetic findings is defined. The remainder of the chapter discusses practical uses of cytogenetic analysis in hematolymphoid neoplasms.

▶ INTRODUCTION

Cytogenetics is the study of chromosome structure and number, particularly as they relate to a normal or pathologic state. In 1956, the normal number of chromosomes per human cell was established as 46, and since that time, many chromosome abnormality syndromes have been reported. The use of cytogenetics has markedly improved patient diagnosis and family counseling in the field of constitutional aberrations, including important advances in prenatal diagnosis. Cytogenetic studies are also responsible for major advances in the field of hematolymphoid malignancies and solid tumors. Chromosome analysis of many malignant disorders has become a critical component for patient diagnosis and prognosis as well as for research studies of these disorders.

▶ CHROMOSOME STRUCTURE AND MORPHOLOGY

Nuclear chromatin of human cells is composed of nucleic acid and protein and is organized into 46 chromosomes. The nucleic acids, deoxyribonucleic acid (DNA), and ribonucleic acid (RNA), are composed of polynucleotides. A single nucleotide consists of a phosphate, a sugar (deoxyribose for DNA and ribose for RNA), and a base. The base may be a purine (A = adenine, G = guanine) or a pyrimidine (C = cytosine and T = thymine [DNA] or U = uracil [RNA]). The bases are aligned on the polynucleotide strand in a triplet code so that three bases code for a single amino acid; the succession of bases in the triplet code determines the protein products that will result from transcription of the DNA and translation of the messenger RNA produced. There are approximately 30,000 genes in human cells, each located at a specific site on a specific chromosome (gene locus). The different possible expressions of a gene are known as *alleles*. For example, the gene for the ABO blood group has three major alleles: A, B, and O.

DNA exists as a double-stranded helix with the two polynucleotide strands held together by hydrogen bonds between complementary bases so that G will bind only with C and A only with T (or U for RNA). The bonding of A-T and G-C is called a *base pair*. This double helix has a diameter of approximately 20 Å and is of variable length. For example, the amount of DNA contained in the smallest chromosome, number 21, is composed of approximately 50 million base pairs while the largest chromosome, number 1, has approximately 250 million base pairs. The double helix initially coils around histone proteins resulting in a series of structures called *nucleosomes* (Figure 38-1 ■). These nucleosomes form a superhelix with the six nucleosomes per turn forming a chromatin fiber (called a *solenoid*) with a diameter of 250 Å. These fibers are looped back and forth on a protein-RNA scaffold to form an identifiable chromatid with a diameter of 0.2–0.5 μm. After DNA replication, identical sister chromatids are connected at the centromere giving the final structure of a mitotic chromosome.

The centromere divides chromosomes into short p arms and long q arms (Figure 38-2 ■). If the centromere is in the center of the chromosome so that the length of p = q, it is referred to as a **metacentric** chromosome (chromosomes 1, 3, 16, 19, and 20). If the centromere is not in the center, so that p<q, the chromosome is called **submetacentric** (chromosomes 2, 4, 5, 6–12, 17, 18, and X), and when the centromere is located close to the end of the chromosome so that p is very short, the chromosome is called **acrocentric** (chromosomes 13–15, 21, 22 and Y). The area of the chro-

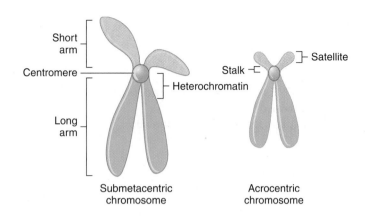

■ FIGURE 38-2 Chromosome structure of a typical submetacentric chromosome and an acrocentric chromosome. short arm = p; long arm = q

mosome around the centromere contains highly repetitive DNA in long clusters of tandem repeats, also known as **satellite DNA,** which is permanently coiled tightly into heterochromatin. Heterochromatic stains darkly and is transcriptionally inactive; euchromatic areas stain lightly and are transcriptionally active during interphase. The heterochromatin on the end of the p arm of acrocentric chromosomes is attached to the rest of the p arm by less tightly coiled chromatin stalks (Figure 38-2).

A normal human cell has 46 chromosomes consisting of 23 pairs. Chromosome pairs 1–22 are autosomes, and the X and Y chromosomes are sex chromosomes. Before banding techniques were developed, the chromosome numbers were assigned by total length of the chromosome beginning with number 1 as the longest and number 22 as the shortest. With the advent of chromosome banding, chromosome 21 was determined to be shorter than 22, but the designations were not changed. A **homologous** chromosome pair consists of two morphologically identical chromosomes that have identical gene loci but can have different alleles at a given locus because one member of a homologous pair is of maternal origin and the other is of paternal origin. For example, a homologous pair consisting of both chromosomes number 9 has the gene locus for the ABO blood group on the long arm. An individual can inherit the allele for blood group A on the maternal number 9 chromosome and the allele for blood group B on the paternal number 9 chromosome. A **heterologous** pair (i.e., the sex chromosomes, X and Y, in a male) consists of morphologically nonidentical chromosomes that have different gene loci.

▶ MITOSIS

Cells that go through a proliferative division do so by a series of stages called the *cell cycle;* it consists of four major phases: G1, S, G2, and mitosis (Figure 38-3 ■) (∞ Chapter 2).

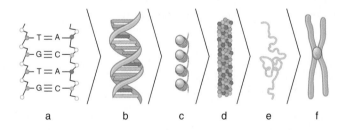

■ FIGURE 38-1 Chromosome morphology and ultrastructure. **a.** Molecular structure of DNA with two polynucleotide chains held together by hydrogen bonding of base pairs (T = thymine, C = cytosine, A = adenine, G = guanine). **b.** Double helical structure of DNA. **c.** Coiling of double helix strand around histone proteins to produce nucleosome. **d.** Superhelix of nucleosome producing chromatin fiber. **e.** Coiling of chromatin fiber to produce chromomere. **f.** Final structure of chromosome consisting of two identical sister chromatids (condensed chromomere) held together at the centromere.

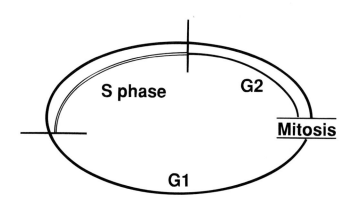

■ FIGURE 38-3   Diagram of the cell cycle beginning with G1, the stage in which the cell is performing its designated duties. The DNA is uncoiled and exists as 46 single chromatids. S phase is the time of DNA synthesis after which the DNA is still uncoiled and consists of 46 chromosomes (sister chromatids joined at the centromere). G2 is a resting phase followed by mitosis.

A cell that is not dividing but is performing its designated function is in interphase. Interphase begins at phase G1 of the cell cycle and continues until the end of phase G2. During G1, the nuclear chromatin is dispersed, and chromo-

some morphology is not identifiable. The next phase, S, is the time of DNA synthesis: The DNA is replicated, and identical sister chromatids are attached at the centromere. This is followed by a short resting phase, G2, after which the cell enters mitosis. The length of time that a cell spends in each phase is quite variable. The average time that a cell spends in mitosis is estimated to be ~45 minutes.

To study human chromosomes, the cells must be mitotically active. *Mitosis* is the process of division of somatic cells by which each daughter cell ends with the same genetic composition as the parent cell. *Prophase* is the first stage of mitosis (Figure 38-4■), during which the DNA begins to coil, chromosome morphology becomes recognizable, and a pair of cytoplasmic organelles known as *centrioles,* which are attached to the mitotic spindle, migrate to opposite poles of the cell. In metaphase, the DNA is tightly coiled and the chromosomes align in the center of the cell (equatorial plate, metaphase plate) while the mitotic spindle apparatus attaches to the kinetochores of the chromosome centromere via microtubules. *Anaphase* begins with the contraction of the spindle fibers pulling apart the sister chromatids so that one sister chromatid migrates to one pole of the cell and the other sister chromatid migrates to the opposite pole of the cell. During *telophase,* the daughter nuclei begin to form at

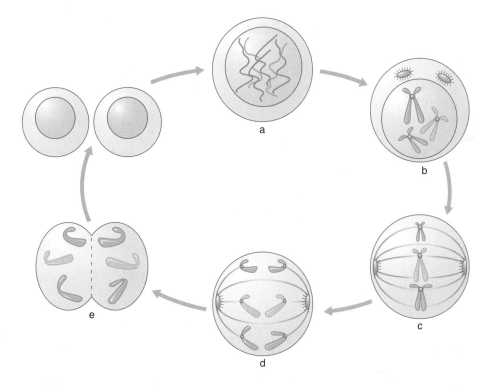

■ FIGURE 38-4   Mitosis. a. Interphase. Chromatin is dispersed. b. Prophase. Chromosome structure is discernible and centrioles begin to migrate. c. Metaphase. Chromosomes are lined up in the center, spindle fibers from the centrioles connect to the centromeres, and the nuclear membrane is not visible. d. Anaphase. Spindle fibers contract and sister chromatids migrate to opposite poles of the cell. e. Telophase. Chromatid migration is complete and the cytoplasmic membrane forms down the center, completing the cell division.

the opposite poles of the cell, and cytokinesis begins. At the end of telophase, *cytokinesis* (the division of the cytoplasm into two daughter cells) completes, and each of the daughter cells then re-enters the G1 phase of the cell cycle. Each resultant daughter cell has the identical genetic composition as the parent cell.

Meiosis is the specialized division of diploid (46 chromosomes) primary gametocytes that results in each gamete (oocyte, and sperm) having a haploid number of chromosomes (23). The understanding of meiosis is critical for the study of constitutional chromosome aberrations and is not discussed in this chapter.

► CYTOGENETIC PROCEDURES

SPECIMEN PREPARATION

Specimens submitted for cytogenetic analysis must have viable cells capable of undergoing mitosis; the choice of appropriate specimens depends on the patient's clinical situation (Table 38-1 ✪). For the evaluation of possible **constitutional cytogenetic aberrations** (aberrations present in every cell in a patient's body, i.e., its constitution), peripheral blood is the most appropriate sample because circulating lymphocytes can be easily manipulated to undergo mitosis by the use of mitogens. For example, phytohemagglutinin (PHA) stimulates predominantly T lymphocytes. If the patient has a lymphocytopenia or if there is a suspicion that cells from different tissue types can have different karyotypes (mosaicism), a punch-biopsy of skin can be obtained for fibroblast culture. When the clinical situation involves a spontaneous abortion (miscarriage), stillbirth, or death shortly after birth, the appropriate sample is fetal tissue (products of conception) or autopsy-acquired organ samples (lung, liver, kidney, diaphragm). A prenatal evaluation requires culturing either amniotic fluid cells or a chorionic villus biopsy processed by direct harvest and tissue culture. These various cultures are harvested at the time of maximal mitotic activity, usually 72–96 hours for peripheral blood and 7–21 days for amniotic fluid and fibroblast cultures.

Acquired aberrations (those happening after birth in a single cell) occur in neoplastic processes such as leukemia, lymphoma, and other tumors. Evaluation of these disorders requires that the neoplastic cells be sampled directly either by peripheral blood, bone marrow, or solid tumor biopsies. These samples are harvested immediately (direct harvest) or by short-term unstimulated cultures to obtain mitoses of the neoplastic cells, not the associated nontumor cells.

The first step of the cytogenetic procedure is to induce cells into mitosis. Once this has been accomplished by any of the methods named, the cells are "harvested." The harvest procedure processes cells that are mitotically active to visualize the chromosomes. The major steps are metaphase inhibition, hypotonic incubation, and fixation.

ℰ CASE STUDY *(continued from page 853)*

The differential WBC count shows 7% blasts, 3% promyelocytes, 25% myelocytes, 10% metamyelocytes, 5% bands, 25% segmented neutrophils, 10% basophils, 5% eosinophils, and 10% lymphocytes. The differential diagnosis includes leukemoid reaction, chronic myelogenous leukemia (CML), and myeloproliferative disorders other than CML. A bone marrow aspirate is performed.

1. What is the most appropriate specimen to submit for cytogenetics, and how should it be processed?

✪ TABLE 38-1

Appropriate Specimens for Cytogenetic Analysis

Clinical Situation	Appropriate Specimen	Type of Processing
Constitutional aberrations	Peripheral blood	Mitogen stimulation of lymphocytes with phytohemagglutinin
	Skin biopsy	Tissue culture
	Autopsy organ samples	Tissue culture
	Products of conception	Tissue culture
	Amniotic fluid	Tissue culture
	Chorionic villus sample	Direct harvest, tissue culture
Neoplastic (acquired) aberrations	Peripheral blood/bone marrow	Direct harvest, unstimulated cultures; stimulated cultures of mature B cell malignancies; all cultures from cell suspension
	Lymph node/spleen	Direct harvest, unstimulated cultures; stimulated cultures of mature B cell malignancies; all cultures from cell suspension
	Solid tumor biopsy	Monolayer and suspension tissue culture

HARVEST PROCEDURE AND BANDING

Mitotically active cells are stopped in metaphase by incubation with agents that disrupt the spindle apparatus, most commonly colchicine or colcemid.[1] The cells are then incubated with a hypotonic solution (frequently 0.075 M KCl) that hemolyzes erythrocytes and partially swells the nucleated cells. Fixation of the cells is then accomplished with Carnoy's fixative, 3:1 methanol:glacial acetic acid. After fixation, a trial slide is prepared by dropping three to four drops of the final cell suspension onto a clean glass slide. The slide is dried and examined by phase microscopy for appropriate spreading and number of mitotic figures. If the first slide does not show optimal quality, the suspension can be concentrated or diluted, or other manipulations can be made to obtain improved chromosome morphology. The remainder of the slides are then prepared and "aged" for banding; this often involves heating the slides in a 60°C oven overnight.

Chromosome banding is obtained by various staining procedures that result in a specific pattern of dark-to-light-stained bands for each homologous chromosome pair. The first chromosome banding technique was reported in 1970 with the use of quinacrine (Q), a fluorescent stain that reveals a pattern of bright and dull bands (Q-bands).[2] Q-banding techniques are relatively simple; however, the banding fades when examined microscopically with ultraviolet illumination, and the resolution of bands is not as detailed as are G-bands (G = Giemsa). Most laboratories routinely analyze G-bands using Giemsa stain and some form of enzyme pretreatment, usually trypsin.[3] These techniques result in a high-quality banding pattern that does not fade with microscopic examination. The pattern of bright or dull Q-bands and dark- or pale-staining G-bands is essentially the same. Reverse banding (R-bands) yields a band pattern opposite to that of Q- and G-bands so that a pale G-band will be dark staining with R-banding. Other banding techniques and special harvest procedures can be helpful for evaluation in certain clinical situations (Table 38-2 ✪).

The study of chromosome morphology has been enhanced by the development of fluorescently labeled DNA probes for

✪ TABLE 38-2

Cytogenetic Banding Techniques and Special Procedures

Type of Banding or Special Procedure	Procedure Description	Result
Q banding	Quinacrine fluorescence A-T rich areas = bright G-C rich areas = dull	Reveals distinct bright and dull band patterns of homologous chromosomes
G banding	Giemsa stain after enzyme pretreatment A-T rich areas = dark G-C rich areas = pale	Reveals distinct dark and pale band patterns of homologous chromosomes identical to Q bands
R banding	A-T rich areas = pale G-C rich areas = dark	Reveals distinct pale and dark band patterns of homologous chromosomes reverse of Q and G bands
C banding	Giemsa stain after acid-alkali denaturation	Stains heterochromatic pericentric regions of chromosomes 1, 9, 16 and long arm of Y chromosome
NOR staining	Silver stain of nucleolar organizing region	Stains stalk region of acrocentric chromosomes 13, 14, 15, 21, and 22
FISH	Fluorescently labeled DNA probes	Depending on probe used, hybridizes with a specific chromosome centromere, arm, whole chromosome, or gene
Synchronization	Synchronization of cells in cell cycle with blocking agent (high dose thymidine)	Increases number of cells in mitosis
High-resolution banding	Cells synchronized and stopped in late prophase or early metaphase	Reveals chromosomes that are less condensed, more toward the prometaphase, and banded at a greater than 800 band stage
Fragile site	Cells cultured with folate/thymidine deprivation	Reveals areas of chromosome gaps, previously used for fra(X)
SCE	Sister chromatid exchange detected by incubation through two cell cycles in BrdU and stained with fluorescent Hoechst-33258	Stains sister chromatids dark or light showing areas of exchange, indicating mutagenicity

FISH = fluorescence in situ hybridization; NOR = nuclear organizing region; SCE = sister chromatid exchange

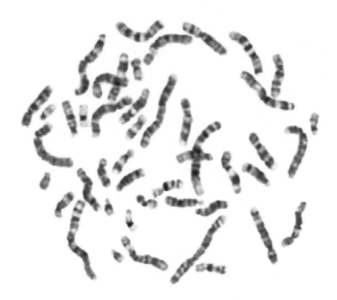

■ FIGURE 38-5   Metaphase spread of chromosomes belonging to a single cell obtained by direct harvest of a bone marrow aspirate. (G-banded, 1000× magnification)

specific chromosome centromeres, whole arms, whole chromosomes, and individual genes (fluorescence in situ hybridization [FISH]).[4] Fluorescent labeled probes allow both specific identification of chromosomes involved in structural or numerical aberrations and analysis of interphase cells. The labeled probe is hybridized directly to cells mounted on glass slides. In this procedure, the morphologic information of the cell with the mutation is preserved. However, the cells must be permeabilized and the DNA denatured for hybridization to occur. The molecular probe is allowed to hybridize to the chromosomes in the tissue specimen on the slide. Probe binding can be visualized using a fluorescent microscope.

CHROMOSOME ANALYSIS

Analysis of chromosomes is best performed microscopically. The adequacy of analysis depends on the mitotic rate of the cells and on banded chromosome morphology. An optimal preparation has mitotic spreads with moderately long chromosomes, few chromosome overlaps, and good quality banding (Figure 38-5 ■). A *karyotype* is a representation of the chromosome makeup of a cell and can now be constructed using a video-computer-linked analysis system. To prepare a karyotype, the chromosomes are grouped initially by size and centromere position and then by the specific pattern of dark-to-light-staining bands (Figure 38-6 ■). The number of

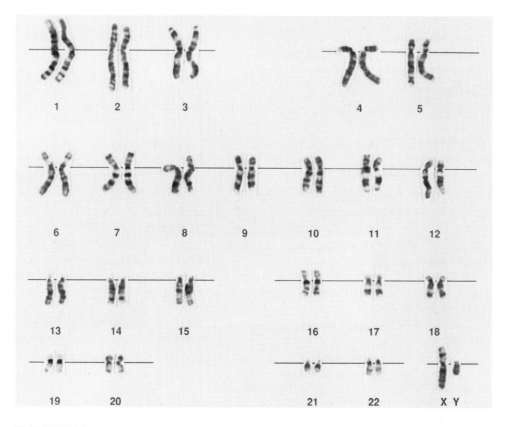

■ FIGURE 38-6   Karyotype of normal male cell with numbered chromosome pairs, G-banded.

cells analyzed per case varies according to the clinical situation. Standardized guidelines for cytogenetic evaluation have been set by accrediting agencies such as the College of American Pathologists (CAP).

✓ **Checkpoint! 1**

A newborn baby boy has multiple congenital malformations, and a chromosome abnormality is suspected as the cause. What is the most appropriate specimen to submit for chromosome analysis, and how should the laboratory professional process the specimen?

▶ **CHROMOSOME ABNORMALITIES**

Chromosome abnormalities are either numerical or structural and can involve the autosomes (1–22) and/or the X and Y sex chromosomes. Constitutional abnormalities are present at the time of birth and are present in all cells if they are inherited from a parent carrier or if they occurred during gametogenesis. Constitutional aberrations can also occur in the embryo shortly after fertilization resulting in a **mosaic:** some cells have the aberration and some are normal. If the aberrations occur some time after birth, they are acquired, and this usually is seen in a single cell line identifying a neoplastic clone.

NUMERICAL ABERRATIONS

A normal human cell with 46 chromosomes is called **diploid.** The word *haploid* is used to designate half the number of chromosomes, 23, and *n* is an abbreviation for the haploid number. Therefore, a cell with 2n (2 × 23) has 46 chromosomes (diploid), and a cell with 3n has 69 chromosomes (triploid). **Aneuploid** refers to a chromosome count other than 46 that is not a multiple of n. If a cell has more than 46 chromosomes, the word **hyperdiploid** is used, and if a cell has fewer than 46 chromosomes, it is called **hypodiploid.**

Most numerical aberrations are thought to be caused by a process of **nondisjunction,** which occurs during meiotic or mitotic cell division when a spindle fiber from the centriole does not connect to the chromosome centromere or when the spindle fiber connects but does not contract (Figure 38-7 ■). This situation results in one daughter cell with an extra chromosome (**trisomy**) and one daughter cell with a chromosome loss (**monosomy**). In most cases, the cell with the chromosome loss does not survive the next cell cycle. Another process, termed *anaphase lag,* results when one chromatid does not completely migrate to the opposite pole but lags behind and gets caught outside the nuclear membrane (Figure 38-8 ■), yielding one daughter cell with a chromosome loss and one daughter cell that is normal.

The word **polyploid** refers to cells that have a chromosome count that is a multiple of the n. Hence, a *tetraploid* cell is polyploid and has a chromosome count of 4n, or 92.

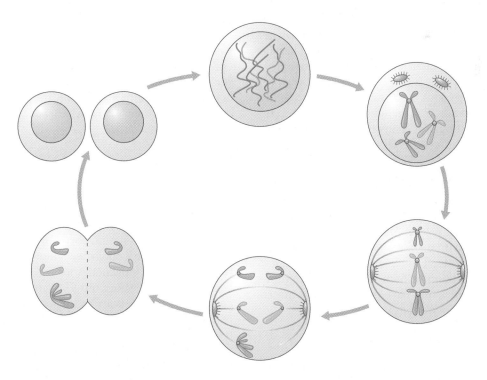

■ FIGURE 38-7   Nondisjunction. During anaphase, the sister chromatids of a chromosome do not disjoin, resulting in one daughter cell with an extra chromosome (trisomy) and the other with a chromosome loss (monosomy).

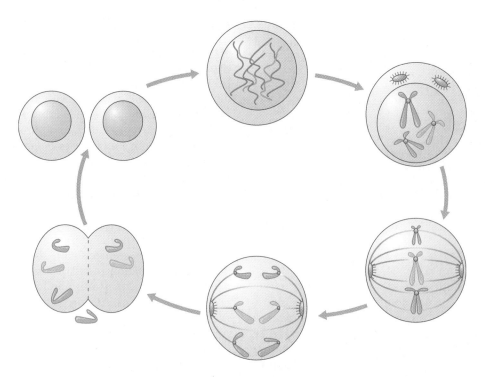

■ FIGURE 38-8   Anaphase lag. Chromatid does not complete migration, resulting in one daughter cell with a normal chromosome count and the other with a chromosome loss.

Endomitosis is the process that results in polyploid cells when there are multiple rounds of S phase (DNA synthesis) without karyokinesis (nuclear division) or cytokinesis (cytoplasmic division). The megakaryocyte is an example of a normal polyploid cell. The word **pseudodiploid** is used when a cell has a chromosome count of 46 but is not normal because of numerical and/or structural aberrations. For example, a cell with a karyotype of 46, XX, +8, −21 is an abnormal cell but has a chromosome count of 46 and therefore is pseudodiploid: it has 46 chromosomes including the 2 sex chromosomes, XX, because although it is missing a number 21 chromosome (−21), it has 3 number 8 chromosomes (+8).

STRUCTURAL ABERRATIONS

Structural chromosome aberrations occur when chromosome breakage occurs and the repair process results in structural loss or in abnormal recombinations. Table 38-3 ✪ lists structural aberrations with a short description and example nomenclature. Any of these can be seen as constitutional or acquired with the exception of homogeneously staining regions and double minutes that have been seen only in neoplastic cells as acquired aberrations.

POLYMORPHIC VARIATION

Morphologic variations are known to occur in certain chromosomes. These variations have no clinical significance but, if present, will be inherited consistently through each generation. **Polymorphic variants** (chromosomes with variant morphology that have no clinical consequence) are easily demonstrated with various banding techniques and can be used to identify maternal versus paternal origin of homologous chromosomes. Some of the more commonly seen polymorphic variants include a pericentric inversion of chromosome 9, variable amounts of pericentric heterochromatin on chromosomes 1, 9, and 16, and a variable amount of heterochromatin on the long arm of the Y chromosome. Also, amounts of satellite material on the short arms of the acrocentric chromosomes can be variable.

▶ CYTOGENETIC NOMENCLATURE

An international committee whose goal is to have one standardized system has established the designation of chromosome number, region, band, and karyotype nomenclature. The International System for Human Cytogenetic Nomenclature (ISCN) has published guidelines including specific rules for cancer cytogenetics for use by clinical and research laboratories.[5] The short and long arms of each chromosome are divided into regions by major landmark bands (Figure 38-9 ■). Each region is further divided into distinct light-, intermediate-, and dark-staining bands. The numbering of regions and bands begins at the centromere and proceeds distally to the terminal portions, *pter* and *qter*. The numbering of bands begins with the number 1 for each region. To designate a specific band of a chromosome, the order is written as chromosome number, arm, region, and band.

TABLE 38-3

Examples of Structural Chromosome Aberration Nomenclature with Explanations

Structural Aberration and Nomenclature	Explanation
Chromosome/chromatid breaks	Break occurs in chromosome/chromatid and is usually repaired. Increased random breaks can be seen with toxins, radiation, and virus exposure.
Dicentric (dic) example: dic(7;8)(q32;q23)	Breaks occur in two chromosomes and the chromosomes—including centromeres—are repaired together resulting in a chromosome with two centromeres; the acentric fragments are lost.
Double minutes (dmin)	Small acentric pieces of DNA, usually paired, indicate gene amplification.
Homogeneously staining region (hsr) example: hsr(11)(q23)	Region of chromosome that stains homogeneously and indicates gene amplification.
Deletion (del), interstitial example: del(7)(q31q32)	Two breaks occur in one arm and material between breaks is lost; break ends are repaired by joining together.
Deletion, terminal example: del(7)(q32)	Break occurs and acentric fragment is lost during mitosis/meiosis.
Duplication (dup) example: dup(7)(q31q32)	Region of a chromosome is duplicated and can be direct or inverted.
Isochromosome (i) example: i(7p) or i(7q)	Centromere splits horizontally and results in chromosome with only short or long arm material. The remaining arm of the chromosome is usually lost.
Inversion (inv), paracentric example: inv(7)(q21q32)	Two breaks occur, and the material between the breaks inverts and then is repaired. When the inversion does not involve the centromere it is referred to as a paracentric inversion.
Inversion, pericentric example: inv(7)(p15q21)	Two breaks occur, and the material between the breaks inverts and then is repaired. When the inversion involves the centromere it is referred to as a pericentric inversion.
Ring chromosome (r) example: r(7)(p21q35)	Breaks occur in the short and long arms, and the broken ends are repaired together; the acentric fragments are lost.
Translocation (t), balanced example: t(7;8)(q32;q23)	Breaks occur in two different chromosomes with fragments repaired (joined) to the opposite chromosome; no loss of DNA occurs.
Derivative (der) chromosome example: der(7)t(7;8)(q32;q23)	This is a structurally rearranged chromosome derived most often from two or more chromosomes. In this example, the derivative, der (7), is the abnormal chromosome 7 that results from a translocation between chromosome 7 and 8 at the designated break points.
Translocation, Robertsonian example: der(14;21)(q10;q10)	A unique type of translocation, breaks occur at or near the centromeres of two acrocentric chromosomes; the centromeric regions fuse, and the short arm/satellite material is lost. The chromosome is derived (der) from the long arms of each chromosome.

A standardized nomenclature system also exists for gene names. The HUGO Gene Nomenclature Committee (HGNC) is the recognized body that approves a gene name and symbol for each known human gene. All approved symbols are stored in the HGNC database. Approved gene names and symbols are readily accessible electronically.[6]

The karyotype of a cell is designated first by the total number of chromosomes followed by the sex chromosomes (XX for female and XY for male). If aberrations are present, sex chromosome abnormalities are listed first followed by abnormalities of autosomes listed in numerical order of the chromosomes involved. Numerical abnormalities are designated by + or − before the chromosome number. Structural abnormalities are listed by the appropriate abbreviation followed by the chromosomes involved in parenthesis and then by the break point band designation in parentheses. Therefore, normal female and normal male karyotypes, respectively, are 46,XX and 46,XY. A male cell with trisomy for chromosomes 8 and 21 is designated: 48, XY, +8, +21. A female cell with trisomy for chromosomes 3, 8, and 15 and a translocation involving chromosomes 9 and 22 is designated 49,XX,+3,+8, t(9;22)(q34;q11.2),+15. The q34;q11.2 refers to the long arms (q), regions 3 and 1, and bands 4 and 1.2, respectively. (See Table 38-3 for other examples of nomenclature.)

▶ CYTOGENETIC ANALYSIS OF HEMATOPOIETIC AND LYMPHOID DISORDERS

Cytogenetic analysis has become an essential part of the diagnostic evaluation of patients with known or suspected neoplasms. Many chromosome aberrations ascertained by either conventional (G-banded) techniques or FISH are now considered diagnostic of or have significant prognostic implications for hematolymphoid malignancies[7] and solid tumors.[8] The cloning of genes at critical chromosome breakpoints in various

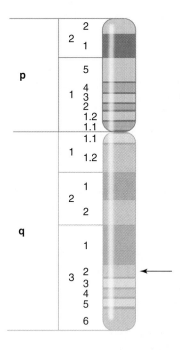

■ FIGURE 38-9   Diagram of bands on chromosome 7 with arm, region, and band designations. The band located at the arrow is designated 7q32.

---

neoplasms has permitted the discovery of the role that these genes play in tumorigenesis and has provided specific DNA sequence targets that can be utilized for the molecular cytogenetic technique of FISH for patient diagnostics. A chromosome aberration found in neoplastic cells is referred to as an *acquired, clonal aberration;* it is an aberration that occurs sometime after birth and is present only in the neoplastic cells.

A clone exists if numerical and/or structural aberrations are identical in at least two cells unless the abnormality is a single chromosome loss (monosomy); then, three cells must have the same chromosome loss. The presence of an abnormal clone is evidence of a neoplasm. Table 38-4 ☼ lists the most common uses of cytogenetic analysis in hematolymphoid disorders.

✓ Checkpoint! 2

Cytogenetic studies were performed on a bone marrow specimen from a female patient with a myelodysplastic state with the following results:

1 cell—47,XX,+8
1 cell—45,XX,−20
5 cells—46,XX,del(5)(q13q34),−7,+21

Which of these aberrations are clonal? What term would apply to the five cells?

Constitutional chromosome aberrations occasionally are found when analyzing neoplastic cells, most often constitutional abnormalities that might not be associated with an ab-

---

☼ TABLE 38-4

Present Applications of Conventional Cytogenetics and Molecular Cytogenetics (FISH) in Hematolymphoid Disorders

- Confirm or establish the diagnosis of a number of leukemias and lymphomas.
- Predict response to specific agents such as tyrosine kinase inhibitors.
- Confirm or predict accelerated phase of chronic myelogenous leukemia (CML).
- Confirm or establish remission and monitor minimal residual disease.
- Aid in the diagnosis and prognosis of myelodysplastic states.
- Evaluate bone marrow transplant for donor versus recipient cells and possible recurrence of original neoplasm.
- Evaluate clonal evolution, which portends a more aggressive phase of disease.

---

normal phenotype. For example, a female patient with acute leukemia and a 47,XXX karyotype could have the +X as an acquired aberration indicative of the malignant cells, or the +X could represent a constitutional abnormality and be present in all of the patient's cells. If the karyotype is 45,XX,−7, however, this is most likely an acquired aberration because monosomy 7 as a constitutional aberration is not compatible with life. The presence of constitutional aberrations must be accurately interpreted and distinguished from acquired clonal aberrations. This is most often accomplished by stimulating peripheral lymphocyte analysis or occasionally by performing skin biopsy fibroblast culture because these cells are not part of the neoplastic clone and any aberrations are constitutional.

PROCESSING OF SPECIMENS

The best sample for cytogenetic analysis of hematolymphoid disorders, excluding lymphomas, is a bone marrow aspirate; even when blast cells are present in the peripheral blood, a higher mitotic rate is usually achieved from the bone marrow sample. These cells are processed by direct harvest and/or unstimulated cultures. The overall cellularity of the marrow aspirate or peripheral blood sample can vary greatly and affects the mitotic yield and chromosome morphology. Therefore, it is best for the cytogenetic laboratory to evaluate the cell count of each specimen, usually with an automated cell counter. Optimal cultures are obtained by inoculating 1 million cells per milliliter of media. The best specimen for study of lymphoma is an involved lymph node. In general, the resolution of chromosomes from an unstimulated peripheral blood or bone marrow/lymph node specimen is not as good as that from a phytohemagglutinin stimulated study, which can reflect an inherent feature of the malignant cells. In fact, cells with particularly poor morphology can represent the abnormal clone whereas the cells with better morphology can be the remaining normal population. Therefore, when working in cancer cytogenetics, the laboratory professional must be careful to analyze each mitotic spread and to evaluate the metaphase preparations with poor resolution and morphology.

Processing cells from lymphoma can include incubation with mitogens in addition to the unstimulated cultures. The neoplastic cells from mature B cell lymphomas often respond to pokeweed or lipopolysaccharide antigens and to stimulation with phytohemagglutinnin in the presence of interleukin-2. A summary of specimen processing is given in Table 38-5 ✪.

CHRONIC MYELOGENOUS LEUKEMIA

The first chromosome abnormality reported to be associated with a malignancy was described in 1960 as an abnormally small chromosome seen in patients with chronic myelogenous leukemia (CML).[9] This abnormality was designated the Philadelphia or Ph[1] (now designated as Ph) chromosome and was believed to be due to a deletion of the long arm of chromosome 22. With the advent of banding techniques, the abnormality was found to actually be a balanced translocation involving chromosomes 9 and 22, t(9;22)(q34;q11.2).[10] This translocation is seen in 90–95% of patients with CML.

Investigators attempted for some time to decipher why a specific chromosome translocation should be so closely associated with a single morphologic type of leukemia. It is now known that the proto-oncogene *ABL1*, normally located at 9q34, is translocated and juxtaposed next to the *BCR* gene at 22q11.2 in the Philadelphia translocation.[11] A proto-oncogene is a normal gene involved in cell division/proliferation and has the capability of becoming an oncogene (∞ Chapter 39). The Ph translocation results in a new chimeric gene consisting of a portion of the *ABL1* from chromosome 9 and a portion of the *BCR* from chromosome 22. The *ABL1* is activated to a functioning oncogene, and a 210 kD (kD = kilo Daltons) polypeptide product of *BCR/ABL1* is present in the leukemic cells.[12] An oncogene is involved in deregulating cell growth

and proliferation and is responsible for neoplastic proliferation usually by mutation, overexpression, or amplification.

Of CML patients, 5–10% lack the classic t(9;22) and instead have a variant translocation involving at least one other chromosome in addition to chromosomes 9 and 22 or a cryptic translocation of chromosomes 9 and 22. *Cryptic translocations* are molecular genetic rearrangements that cannot be identified by conventional cytogenetics and must be evaluated by the molecular techniques of FISH (Figure 38-10 ∎) or the reverse transcriptase polymerase chain reaction (rtPCR) for *BCR/ABL1* gene rearrangement. Patients with variant or cryptic translocations have the same clinical features and prognosis as those with the typical (9;22) translocation (∞ Chapter 39).

In the past, CML was difficult to treat, and patient survival was poor because the t(9;22) and concurrent *BCR/ABL1* gene rearrangement occur in a pluripotent hematopoietic stem cell (HSC) and has the potential to affect all marrow cells derived from that HSC. The identification of the *BCR/ABL1* fusion transcript and the subsequent cloning of these genes permitted an understanding of the endogenous tyrosine kinase activity of *ABL1* and prompted the development of an agent targeted specifically at the protein product of the *ABL1* gene (∞ Chapter 22). This group of agents, called *tyrosine kinase inhibitors* (TKIs), is now a model for the development of novel treatments in various types of cancer because genetic rearrangements of many other hematolymphoid malignancies and solid tumors are known to involve genes also with tyrosine kinase activity. The TKIs have been shown to significantly prolong overall survival in a number of leukemias, lymphomas, and solid tumors and have revolutionized the treatment of these neoplasms by targeting specific genetic loci.[13,14]

When CML patients enter accelerated phase or blast crisis, the majority have a change in the karyotype with chromosome aberrations in addition to the t(9;22) (i.e., clonal evolution). The most frequently observed additional aberrations

✪ TABLE 38-5		
Appropriate Specimens and Type of Processing for Cytogenetic Analysis of Neoplastic Cells		
Possible Diagnosis	**Specimen**	**Processing**
Acute leukemias (myeloid and lymphoid)	Bone marrow at diagnosis	24–72-hour unstimulated cultures; FISH analysis with appropriate probes
Myeloproliferative disorders	Peripheral blood for FISH evaluation to monitor minimal residual disease	
Myelodysplastic syndromes		
Therapy-related myeloid disorders		
Lymphoproliferative disorders	Morphologically involved lymph node, spleen, bone marrow, peripheral blood	Unstimulated cultures; T cell: phytohemagglutinin stimulation; B cell: pokeweed, lipopolysaccharide, PHA, and IL-2
Solid tumor	Morphologically involved tumor tissue	Monolayer and/or suspension cultures
	Effusion (pleural, peritoneal, etc.)	Direct harvest, unstimulated cultures

FISH = fluorescence in situ hybridization; PHA = phytohemagglutinin; IL-2 = interleukin-2

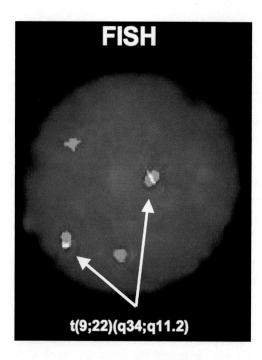

FIGURE 38-10 Identification of the *BCR/ABL1* gene rearrangement with a dual color, dual fusion probe set. The *ABL1* probe is labeled in red and the *BCR* probe in green. One normal *ABL1* gene and one normal *BCR* gene are located on separate chromosomes. The *BCR* and *ABL1* genes are juxtaposed on the two chromosomes involved in the translocation, resulting in two yellow fusion signals.

are an extra Ph [+der(22)t(9;22)], an extra chromosome 8 [+8], an isochromosome for the long arm of chromosome 17 [i(17q)], and an extra chromosome 19 [+19]. This clonal evolution can be detected days or weeks before the actual morphologic transformation to blast crisis is seen in the marrow or peripheral blood, allowing more rapid institution of appropriate treatment.[15]

The t(9;22) is also seen at diagnosis in approximately 15% of cases of acute lymphoblastic leukemia (ALL), more commonly in adults. Although the translocation appears the same cytogenetically as that seen in CML, there is a difference in the site of breakage at the *BCR* locus, resulting in a 190 kD protein. The cases of Ph-positive ALL must be distinguished from a patient presenting in lymphoid blast crisis of CML because the prognosis and treatment are different.

CASE STUDY *(continued from page 856)*

Cytogenetic analysis of bone marrow shows all of the cells to have this karyotype: 46,XY,t(9;22)(q34;q11.2).

2. Is this a constitutional or acquired aberration?

3. Is it a clonal aberration?

4. What is the significance of this finding for the diagnosis?

MYELOPROLIFERATIVE DISORDERS OTHER THAN CML

The other myeloproliferative disorders, polycythemia vera (PV), chronic idiopathic myelofibrosis, and essential thrombocythemia (ET), have acquired clonal chromosome aberrations in approximately 50–60% of cases. Diagnosis of these disorders now requires documented absence of *BCR/ABL1* gene rearrangement.[7] Recurrent aberrations in these myeloproliferative disorders include abnormalities of 1q, +8, +9, del(13q), and del(20q). In addition to negative *BCR/ABL1* gene rearrangement status, molecular genetic evaluation for a particular mutation in the *JAK2* gene, the V617F mutation, has become the standard of care for the diagnosis of these patients (∞ Chapter 22). Patients who have the V617F mutation can definitively be diagnosed with a myeloproliferative disorder, have a high response rate to a particular chemotherapeutic agent called *hydoxyurea,* and have been shown to have shorter overall survivals.[16]

ACUTE MYELOID LEUKEMIA

Approximately 70% of patients with de novo acute myeloid leukemia (AML) have acquired clonal chromosome aberrations in the leukemic cells. These aberrations are present only in the leukemic blasts, not in the other hematopoietic precursors. Therefore, de novo AML appears to be a malignancy of the committed progenitor cell.[17,18] The chromosome abnormalities found can be single, numerical, or structural or complex. Some aberrations such as trisomy 8 occur frequently in AML but are not diagnostic for a specific type of leukemia. Chromosome aberrations when present in the diagnostic specimen can be valuable in following the leukemia's progression or regression. If the original leukemic cells have a clonal aberration, such as +8, a complete remission sample should have only a normal karyotype. In subsequent samples, the presence of even one cell with +8 would indicate an early relapse, which might not be detectable morphologically. Some patients clonally evolve, usually indicating cytogenetic transformation to a more aggressive and treatment-resistant disease.

The World Health Organization (WHO) has established a classification system for AML according to the presence or absence of recurrent cytogenetic abnormalities (∞Chapter 24). Specific cytogenetic aberrations now define particular subtypes of AML that have specific treatment implications. Although these cytogenetic entities are characterized by particular morphologic and clinical features, the primary diagnostic modality is genetic. The WHO AML classification includes the aberrations in Table 38-6 ❂. If a patient with AML lacks one of these recurrent aberrations or other clonal cytogenetic abnormality, classification is based on morphologic categorization established by the French-American-British (FAB) system (∞ Chapter 22).

The t(8;21) and inv(16)/t(16;16) both disrupt the same transcription factor, core binding factor (CBF), and are there-

⊙ TABLE 38-6

Acute Myeloid Leukemia (AML) with Recurrent Cytogenetic Abnormalities

Cytogenetic Aberration	Gene Rearrangement	Comments
t(8;21)(q22;q22)	*ETO(RUNX1T1)/AML1(CBFA or RUNX1)*	Favorable prognosis
inv(16)(p13.1q22) or t(16;16)(p13.1;q22)	*CBFB/MYH11*	Favorable prognosis
t(15;17)(q22;q12)	*PML/RARA*	Responsive to ATRA
Variants		
t(11;17)(q23;q21)	*PLZF(ZBTB16)/RARA*	Resistant to ATRA
t(5;17)(q32;q12)	*NPM1/RARA*	Responsive to ATRA
t(11;17)(q13;q21)	*NUMA1/RARA*	Responsive to ATRA
11q23 abnormalities	*MLL*	Poor prognosis
Complex karyotypes including 5/7 aberrations and 3q21 and 3q26.2 rearrangements	Genes unknown	AML with multilineage dysplasia; abnormal megakaryopoiesis, poor prognosis
Therapy related		
Chromosome 5 and 7 aberrations		Alkylating agent related
11q23 and 21q22 aberrations	*MLL and AML1(RUNX1)*	Topoisomerase-II inhibitor related

ATRA = all transretinoic acid

fore categorized together by the WHO as the Core Binding Factor Leukemias (CBFL). The t(8;21) disrupts the alpha chain of CBF that is encoded by *AML1(RUNX1)*, and the inv(16)/t(16;16) disrupts the beta chain of CBF. The CBFL have relatively favorable prognoses, are more common in younger patients, and can have a unique type of presentation with a particular type of disease called *myeloid sarcoma*, a soft tissue infiltration by the myeloblasts.

The t(8;21), previously reported predominantly in cases of AML-M2 by FAB classification (AML with differentiation) occurs in 5–12% of AML. The protein product of the *ETO(RUNX1T1)/AML1(RUNX1)* gene rearrangement promotes leukemogenesis by blocking myeloid cell differentiation.[19] Frequently seen with the t(8;21) is a loss of a sex chromosome, Y in the male and X in the female. FAB classification previously reported the inv(16)/t(16;16) in cases of AML-M4eo (acute myelomonocytic leukemia with increased marrow eosinophils), which occurs in 10–12% of AML.[7, 20, 21]

The t(15;17) is present in acute promyelocytic leukemia (APL), previously classified as AML-M3 by FAB, and accounts for 5–8% of AML. The translocation results in the fusion of the retinoic acid receptor alpha (*RARA*) gene at 17q12 with the nuclear regulatory factor promyelocytic leukemia (*PML*) gene at 15q22. These patients respond to treatment with all transretinoic acid (ATRA), which induces differentiation of the abnormal promyelocytes followed by chemotherapy with an anthracyclin agent. Three variant translocations also rearrange the RARA gene but involve different partner chromosomes (Table 38-6). Identification of these variant translocations is clinically important because some are resistant to treatment with ATRA while others are responsive.[7]

AML with 11q23 aberrations has monocytic features and is present in 5–6% of AML. The *MLL* gene at band 11q23 is rearranged, and many partner chromosomes are reported. Patients with this aberration have short overall survivals.

The WHO also recognizes an entity of AML with multilineage dysplasia that is characterized by myeloblasts and dysplastic morphologic features in two or more myeloid cell lineages, most commonly including the megakaryocytes. These patients have complex karyotypes often including aberrations of chromosomes 5 and 7 as well as rearrangements at bands 3q21 and 3q26.2. These patients have a poor prognosis with decreased likelihood of achieving complete remission and short overall survival.[7]

SECONDARY (THERAPY-RELATED) LEUKEMIA

Acute myeloid leukemia and myelodysplasia are known to occur with increased incidence in patients who have previously received chemotherapy or radiation therapy. These cases are called *secondary* or *therapy-related myeloid disorders* and are considered as a distinct entity by the WHO. Two major types are recognized based on the causative agent, and each is associated with specific cytogenetic abnormalities. Alkylating agent-related myeloid disorders occur approximately 5–6 years after treatment and are associated with aberrations of chromosomes 5 and 7. Topoisomerase II inhibitor-related myeloid disorders present within 2–3 years of exposure and are associated with break points at band 11q23 and concurrent *MLL* gene rearrangement.[7, 22]

Checkpoint! 3

A 35-year-old man has acute leukemia. Cytogenetic studies of the bone marrow reveal the following: 46,XY,t(15;17)(q22;q12). What type of leukemia does this patient have, and what will cytogenetic studies show after treatment if he achieves complete remission?

MYELODYSPLASTIC SYNDROMES

Myelodysplastic syndromes (MDS) are clonal neoplastic disorders of hematolymphoid stem cells characterized by dysplasia and subsequent ineffective hematopoiesis in two or more myeloid cell lines (∞ Chapter 23). An internationally recognized scoring system for predicting survival of MDS patients and transformation to AML, International Prognostic Scoring System (IPSS), has been developed; its major prognostic variables are the type of cytogenetic abnormality, percentage of blasts, and degree and number of cytopenias. According to the scoring system, good-risk cytogenetics include a normal karyotype, del(5q) as the sole abnormality, del(20q) as the sole abnormality and −Y. Poor-risk cytogenetics include more than or equal to three chromosome aberrations and chromosome 7 abnormalities. Intermediate risk refers to all other abnormalities. These specific cytogenetic aberrations define particular categories of MDS and play a major role in diagnosis, treatment, and management of patients with them.[23]

Checkpoint! 4

Five years ago, a 46-year-old woman received chemotherapy and radiation treatment for breast cancer. She now has pancytopenia. Cytogenetic analysis of the bone marrow is performed and shows 10 of 20 cells with the following: 45,XX,del(5)(q13q34),−7. What is the significance of this finding?

ACUTE LYMPHOBLASTIC LEUKEMIA

Approximately 60–75% of patients with ALL have clonal acquired aberrations of the malignant cells. Cytogenetic findings are a crucial part of the leukemia workup for pediatric cases, and the results are directly related to prognosis. Patients who have the most favorable prognosis have hyperdiploid karyotypes with a chromosome count ranging from 54–65 with concurrent trisomies of chromosomes 4, 10, and 17. Most cases of hyperdiploid ALL have other clinically favorable findings such as 3–7 years of age, total leukocyte count less than 10×10^9/L, and precursor B cell CALLA positive (CD10+) immunophenotype. The t(12;21)(p13;q22) also confers a favorable prognosis: It rearranges the *TEL* (now known as *ETV6*) gene at 12p13 and the *AML1(RUNX1)* gene at 21q22, and it is a cryptic aberration, undetectable in conventional metaphase preparations because the size of the translocated segments are of similar size and staining intensity. To ascertain the presence of this rearrangement, molecu-

lar methods, either FISH or RT-PCR, must be employed. Hypodiploidy, the t(4;11)(q21;q23) that rearranges the *AF4* and *MLL* genes and the t(9;22)(q34;q11.2) that rearranges the *BCR* and *ABL1* genes are associated with a poor outcome.[7, 24, 25]

The patient's age influences the prognostic impact of these cytogenetic aberrations. ALL patients with the t(9;22) ranging in age from 1–18 years have more favorable outcomes than adults. Infants and adults with the t(4;11) have significantly shorter overall survivals than children with the same translocation. See Table 38-7 for some of the more commonly seen aberrations in ALL.

Checkpoint! 5

A 5-year-old girl has fatigue and easy bruising. A CBC shows a leukocyte count of 40×10^9/L with 85% blasts. Bone marrow cytogenetic studies are performed and show all cells with the following karyotype: 53,XX,+X, +4,+6,+10,+18,+20,+21. What is the prognostic significance of this finding?

LYMPHOMA AND LYMPHOPROLIFERATIVE DISORDERS

In recent years, chromosome analysis in lymphoma and lymphoproliferative disorders has added greatly to the understanding of the importance of the gene loci involved in chromosome aberrations seen with specific types of lymphoma. The results of these analyses have also led to the development of molecular probes and their use in the clinical laboratory. The first abnormality described in the lymphomas was the 14q+ seen in Burkitt lymphoma.[26] This was later characterized as t(8;14)(q24.1;q32) and is seen in approximately 75% of cases of Burkitt lymphoma. Two variant translocations, t(2;8)(p11.2;q24.1) and t(8;22)(q24.1;q11.2), have been reported in 10–15% of Burkitt lymphoma. The 14q32 is the site of the gene for the heavy chain of immunoglobulin, and the break at 8q24.1 is just proximal to the site of the proto-oncogene *MYC*. Therefore, the *MYC* gene is translocated to the heavy chain locus at 14q32.[27] This was the first demonstration of a proto-oncogene that was translocated to a location known to be active in B cell lymphoma, resulting in the activation of the oncogene. The t(2;8) results in the juxtaposition of a gene for kappa light chain to *MYC*, and the t(8;22) results in the juxtaposition of a gene for lambda light chain to *MYC*. In cases of Burkitt lymphoma that have the two variant translocations, the tumor cells are found to mark with surface kappa chain when the t(2;8) is found and with lambda chain when the t(8;22) is found.

Many cytogenetic aberrations are now associated with specific types of lymphoma and play a major role in the diagnosis of these entities as well as have prognostic significance. Most of these translocations are known to involve genes that are critical for proliferation of the neoplastic cells or are involved in programmed cell death, apoptosis. Chronic lymphocytic leukemia (CLL) patients with trisomy 12, 11q, or

⊗ TABLE 38-7

Correlation of Chromosome Aberrations in ALL with Immunophenotype, Gene Loci, Prognosis, and Approximate Incidence by Age

ALL Chromosome Phenotype	Known Aberration	Gene Loci	Prognosis	% Incidence In	
				Pediatric	Adult
Precursor B-cell	Hyperdiploid: 54–65 chromosomes		Good	20–25	4
	With trisomies 4, 10 and 17				
CALLA+	Hypodiploid (<44 chr.)		Poor	1	8
	t(12;21)(p13;q22)	TEL(ETV6)/AML1(RUNX1)	Good	30	—
	t(9;22)(q34;q11.2)	BCR/ABL1	Poor	3–4	29
CIg+	t(1;19)(q23;p13.3)	PBX1/E2A(TCF3)	Good with intensive tx	6	3
Biphenotypic & CALLA−	t(4;11)(q21;q23)	AF4/MLL	Poor	2–3 (50% in infant ALL)	4
B cell SIg+	t(8;14)(q24.1;q32)	MYC/IGH @	Good with intensive tx	1–2	5
	t(2;8)(p11.2;q24.1)	IGK@/MYC	Good with intensive tx		
	t(8;22)(q24.1;q11.2)	MYC/IGL@	Good with intensive tx		
T cell	t(8;14)(q24.1;q11.2)	MYC/TRA@ or TRD@	Poor		
	inv(14)(q11.2q32)	TRA@ or TRD@/IGH@	Poor		
	t(v;14)(v;q11.2)	TRA@ or TRD@	Poor		
	t(7;v)(q34;v)	TRB@	Poor		
	t(7;v)(p14;v)	TRG@	Poor		
	t(5;14)(q35;q32)	TLX3/IGH@	Eosinophilia associated		
	9q34 aberration	ABL1 amplification	Good: responsive to TKIs		
	t(11;19)(q23;p13.3)	MLL/MLLT1	Good		

17p aberrations are associated with an atypical morphology and shorter overall survival.[28] The t(11;14) is diagnostic of mantle cell lymphoma in the appropriate morphologic and clinical context, an aggressive entity that requires chemotherapy and transplantation.[29] The presence of the t(11;18) or t(1;14) in extranodal gastric lymphoma of mucosa associated lymphoid tissue (MALT), a type of marginal zone lymphoma, defines it as malignancy and requires treatment with chemotherapy as opposed to antibiotics.[30] Patients with anaplastic large cell lymphoma bearing the t(2;5) have a significantly longer survival than those patients without this aberration.[31] See Table 38-8 ⊗ for the characteristic chromosome aberrations with the lymphoproliferative disorders and gene loci known to be involved in these rearrangements.

BONE MARROW TRANSPLANTATION

Some of the hematolymphoid disorders presented in this chapter are treated by bone marrow or peripheral blood stem cell transplantation, depending on the clinical situation and availability of donors. Cytogenetics, particularly the molecular cytogenetic technique of FISH, is a valuable tool in evaluating the rate of engraftment of the donor cells in opposite sex transplants and monitoring for minimal residual disease. Following successful transplantation, only donor cells should be present. Occasionally, 1–2% of recipient cells are detectable shortly after transplant but then diminish. If recipient cells recur with a normal karyotype, it indicates the development of a **chimerism**, the presence of cells of two different genetic origins in an individual. For example, a female recipient after a male-donated transplant can show 30% XY and 70% XX by FISH analysis with probes for the X and Y centromeres, which is consistent with partial but not complete engraftment. Treatment to promote engraftment, such as increasing the immunosuppression or giving additional donor cells, can thus be employed. If the recipient marrow cells have an initial chromosome aberration, FISH of DNA probes specific for the genes that are rearranged by that aberration can be used to assess the degree of disease burden persisting.

⊘ TABLE 38-8

Correlation of Chromosome Aberrations Seen in Non-Hodgkin lymphoma with Gene Loci Identified

Chromosome Aberration	Lymphoproliferative Disorder	Known Gene Loci
+12	CLL	
del(13)(q14)	CLL	*RB1*
del(11)(q21)	CLL	*ATM*
del(17)(p13)	CLL	*TP53*
t(11;14)(q13;q32)	Mantle cell lymphoma	*CCND1/IGH@*
	Multiple myeloma	*MYEOV/IGH@*
t(11;18)(q21;q21)	Marginal zone B cell lymphoma (including MALT)	*API2/MALT1*
t(1;14)(p22;q32)	Marginal zone B cell lymphoma (including MALT)	*BCL10/IGH@*
t(14;18)(q32;q21)	Follicular lymphoma	*IGH@/BCL2*
t(8;14)(q24.1;q32)	Burkitt lymphoma	*MYC/IGH@*
t(8;22)(q24.1;q11.2)	Burkitt lymphoma	*MYC/IGL@*
t(2;8)(p11.2;q24.1)	Burkitt lymphoma	*IGK@/MYC*
14q11.2 aberration	T cell lymphoma	*TRA@ and TRD@*
7q34 aberration	T-cell lymphoma	*TRB@*
7p14 aberration	T-cell lymphoma	*TRG@*
t(2;5)(p23;q35)	Anaplastic large cell lymphoma (T cell)	*ALK/NPM*

CASE STUDY *(continued from page 864)*

An allogeneic bone marrow transplant is performed with Gregory's sister as the donor. Three months after transplant, the karyotype is 46,XX.

5. What is the significance of this finding?

MOLECULAR CYTOGENETICS

Techniques are now available to evaluate not only the gross chromosome morphology but also the individual gene composition. FISH is an example of such technology, and the role it plays in the diagnosis and prognosis of patients with hematolymphoid disorders has been previously discussed. The advantage of these techniques over conventional cytogenetic studies is that molecular DNA techniques do not require viable cells capable of mitotic activity. Samples of tumor cells can include nonmitosing peripheral blood cells and paraffin embedded tissue. The disadvantage of certain molecular studies, such as FISH, is that they give information only about a single molecular genetic aberration based on the specific probe used, potentially missing other chromosome aberrations that might be present (∞ Chapter 39).

The following scenario illustrates the use of the two different techniques. A 25-year-old man is known to have CML and has received an allogeneic transplant from his sister. The first post-transplant specimen did not have dividing cells in the conventional cytogenetic preparations. FISH of DNA probes that are rearranged in this leukemia, the *BCR* and *ABL1* genes,

was done and was positive in 10 out of 200 interphase nuclei examined, consistent with a low-level persistence of disease. A second sample obtained 3 months later was sufficient for conventional cytogenetics and yielded the following results:

80%	46,XX
10%	46,XY,t(9;22)(q34;q11.2)
10%	47,XY,+8,t(9;22)(q34;q11.2)

In the first sample, the molecular FISH studies were critical to show the persistence of the leukemia. Cytogenetics performed on the second sample was critical to show a cytogenetic transformation toward blast crisis with the additional +8 abnormality. The molecular technique of rtPCR also has significant clinical utility in diagnosing and monitoring patients with hematolymphoid neoplasms including CML (∞ Chapter 39).

Comparative genomic hybridization (CGH) assays can be used to analyze changes in chromosome copy number (copy number variants). Because of the greatly increased resolution that these assays provide, it has been observed that the human genome has much more variability than previously thought with differences found at up to thousands of loci, most of which are not clinically significant. This variability makes interpretation of CGH assays potentially challenging. In addition, CGH assays have been designed to analyze critical regions of the DNA for well-defined genetic abnormalities. DNA from the patient and normal control DNA are labeled using different fluorescent dyes, mixed, and hybridized to normal metaphase chromosomes or to a slide containing hundreds to thousands of defined DNA probes (array CGH).

The color intensity ratio is analyzed along the DNA to detect regions of copy number gain or loss. The current technology is able to detect copy gain and loss of regions that are 50 kb in length.[32]

The use of cytogenetics and/or molecular DNA studies in neoplastic disorders must be well coordinated so to prevent duplication of work and provide minimal cost to the patient.

CASE STUDY *(continued from page 868)*

Six months after transplant, Gregory had bone marrow aspirated for analysis. The mitotic yield of the specimen was not sufficient for routine cytogenetic analysis.

6. What other studies that would be informative as to the status of the donor and recipient cells could be performed?

7. Five years after the transplant, cytogenetic analysis shows the following:

   5 cells—46,XX

   15 cells—47,XY,+8,t(9;22)(q34;q11.2),i(17)(q10)

   What is the significance of these findings?

SUMMARY

Clinical specialists in the hematology laboratory are frequently asked when cytogenic studies are indicated and what specimens are appropriate to submit. For these reasons, it is important for these specialists to have a basic understanding of the specimen requirements, processing, and clinical indications for chromosome analysis. Acquired, clonal chromosome aberrations can be seen in most of the hematolymphoid disorders, including acute and chronic leukemias, myelodysplastic states, myeloproliferative disorders, and lymphomas. These results are used for diagnosis and prognosis in many cases. In addition, cytogenetics can be used to follow the progression or regression of a malignant cell line if the original pretreatment sample revealed a clonal aberration.

The chromosome aberrations found in hematolymphoid disorders are present only in the malignant cells. Many cytogenetic aberrations are now recognized as diagnostic of particular hematolymphoid neoplasms; for example, the t(15;17) is diagnostic of APL. Identification of these specific aberrations with DNA probes has clinical utility for evaluating the patient's response to treatment and degree of residual disease. The identification of these molecular cytogenetic targets has also lead to more effective treatment for many hematolymphoid neoplasms.

REVIEW QUESTIONS

LEVEL I

1. Which of the following is the major component of chromosomes? (Objective 1)
   a. polynucleotides
   b. enzymes
   c. lipids
   d. proteins

2. In which stage of mitosis is the chromosome morphology best observed? (Objective 1)
   a. anaphase
   b. interphase
   c. metaphase
   d. prophase

3. A 4-year-old boy has mental retardation and developmental delay. Which of the following would be the most appropriate specimen for chromosome analysis? (Objective 2)
   a. bone marrow
   b. skin biopsy
   c. peripheral blood
   d. lymph node

4. A 62-year-old man has acute myeloid leukemia. Which of the following would be the most appropriate specimen for chromosome analysis to determine whether there are acquired chromosome aberrations? (Objective 2)
   a. bone marrow
   b. lymph node
   c. peripheral blood
   d. skin biopsy

LEVEL II

Use this case history for questions 1–3.

Stanley, the patient, is a 35-year-old male who presented with a severe nosebleed. He has been previously healthy; however, in the last three weeks, he has noticed easy bruising, and on the day of admission to the hospital, he had a nosebleed that he could not stop. Initial CBC revealed:

Hgb	10 g/dL
Hct	0.30 L/L
MCV	85 fL
WBC	50×10^9/L
Plt ct	20×10^9/L

The peripheral smear showed the majority of cells to have a high nuclear:cytoplasmic ratio, immature chromatin, and cytoplasmic hypergranulation with azurophilic granules. Preliminary cytogenetic analysis performed on bone aspirate revealed 75% of cells to have t(15;17)(q22;q12); 25% of cells have a normal male karyotype.

1. The most likely diagnosis is: (Objective 6)
   a. chronic myeloid leukemia
   b. acute promyelocytic leukemia
   c. acute myeloid leukemia with multilineage dysplasia
   d. secondary (therapy-related) acute myeloid leukemia

LEVEL I

5. Which of the following is a basic criterion of cells that would be processed for chromosome analysis? (Objective 2)
   a. mitotic activity
   b. protein production
   c. presence of nucleolus
   d. presence of mitochondria

6. In the harvest procedure, how are cells stopped in metaphase? (Objective 2)
   a. colchicine/colcemid incubation
   b. incubation with hypotonic solution
   c. fixation with Carnoy's fixative
   d. incubation with phytohemagglutinin

7. The ability to identify individual chromosomes depends on which of the following? (Objective 2)
   a. banding
   b. hypotonic incubation
   c. type of specimen
   d. fixation

8. Which of the following terms is appropriate to describe a human cell that has 47 chromosomes? (Objective 3)
   a. diploid
   b. aneuploid
   c. polyploid
   d. normal

9. Which of the following can result in trisomy? (Objective 3)
   a. anaphase lag
   b. endomitosis
   c. nondisjunction
   d. chromosome breakage

10. Which of the following can result in an abnormal amount of cellular DNA? (Objective 3)
    a. balanced translocation
    b. paracentric inversion
    c. pericentric inversion
    d. isochromosome

LEVEL II

2. The break point on chromosome 17 involves which gene? (Objective 9)
   a. *ABL1*
   b. *MYC*
   c. *BCR*
   d. *RARA*

3. The identification of this cytogenetic aberration (in question 2) in patients has led to their treatment with which of the following? (Objectives 5, 6)
   a. interferon
   b. interleukin
   c. all transretinoic acid
   d. vitamin K

Use this case study for questions 4–7.

A 16-year-old girl has fatigue and increased bruising. A CBC shows the following:

Hb 70g/L

Hct 0.21L/L

WBC 35 × 10^9/L

Platelet count 60 × 10^9//L

Differential, bone marrow aspirate:

   50% blasts with monocytoid features

   15% dysplastic eosinophils with large basophilic granules

   10% myelocytes

   10% metamyelocytes

   13% red blood cell precursors

   2% megakaryocytes

4. Which of the following is most likely to be seen on chromosome analysis of the bone marrow cells? (Objective 6)
   a. t(8;21)
   b. t(15;17)
   c. inv(16)
   d. +8

5. Which of the following genes does the chromosome rearrangement identified in question 4 involve? (Objective 9)
   a. *BCR/ABL1*
   b. *MLL*
   c. *CBFB/MYH11*
   d. *TEL(ETV6)/AML1(RUNX1)*

6. What is the other AML with a recurrent cytogenetic aberration that involves the same transcription factor as identified in question 5? (Objective 9)
   a. t(8;21)
   b. inv(16)
   c. t(15;17)
   d. 11q23 aberration

REVIEW QUESTIONS (continued)

LEVEL I

LEVEL II

7. Which of the following is the most likely diagnosis? (Objective 6)
   a. akylating agent-related AML
   b. core-binding factor leukemia
   c. AML with multilineage dysplasia
   d. AML of ambiguous lineage

8. Which of the following genetic abnormalities is associated with a good prognosis when it is found in ALL? (Objective 7)
   a. chromosome count >54
   b. t(9;22)
   c. t(4:11)
   d. chromosome count <45

9. Which of the following is associated with a poor prognosis when found in ALL? (Objective 7)
   a. chromosome count >54
   b. t(12; 21)
   c. normal karyotype
   d. t(9;22)

10. Which of the following is associated with Burkitt lymphoma? (Objective 6)
    a. t(8;21)
    b. t(14;18)
    c. t(12;21)
    d. t(8;14)

www.pearsonhighered.com/mckenzie

Use this address to access the interactive Companion Website created for this textbook. Find additional information, tables and figures. Evaluate your command of the chapter information using case studies and critical thinking and multiple choice questions.

REFERENCES

1. Barch M, ed. *The AGT Cytogenetics Laboratory Manual*, 3rd ed. New York: Raven Press; 1997.

2. Caspersson T, Lomakka G, Zach L. The fluorescence patterns of the human metaphase chromosomes-distinguishing characters and variability. *Hereditas*. 1971;67:89–102.

3. Seabright, M. A rapid banding technique for human chromosomes. *Lancet*. 1971;2:971–72.

4. Schad C, Kraker W, Tatal S et al. Use of fluorescent in situ hybridization for marker chromosome identification in congenital and neoplastic disorders. *Am J Clin Path*. 1991;96:203–10.

5. Shaffer LG and Tommerup N, eds. *An International System for Human Cytogenetic Nomenclature*. New York: Karger; 2005.

6. HUGO Gene Nomenclature Committee database. www.genenames.org. Accessed July 16, 2007.

7. Jaffe ES, Harris NL, Stein H et al., eds. *World Health Organization Classification of Tumours: Pathology and Genetics, Tumours of Haematopoietic and Lymphoid Tissues*. Lyon, France: IARC Press; 2001.

8. Fletcher CDM, Unni KK, Mertens F, eds. *World Health Organziation Classification of Tumours: Pathology and Genetics of Tumours of Soft Tissue and Bone*. Lyon, France: IARC Press; 2002.

9. Nowell PC, Hungerford DA. A minute chromosome in human, chronic granulocytic leukemia. *Science*. 1960;132:1497.

10. Rowley JD. A new consistent chromosomal abnormality in chronic granulocytic leukemia. *Nature*. 1973;243:290–93.

11. Bartram CR, deKlein A, Groffen J et al. Translocation of C-ABL oncogene correlates with the presence of a Philadelphia chromosome in chronic myelocytic leukemia. *Nature*. 1983;306:239–42.

12. Faderl S, Talpaz M, Kantarjian HM et al. The biology of chronic myeloid leukemia. *N Eng J Med*. 1999;341:164–72.

13. Arora A, Scholar EM. Role of tyrosine kinase inhibitors in cancer therapy. *J Pharmacol Exp Ther* 2005;315:971–79.

14. Droogendijk HJ, Kluin-Nelemans HJC, van Doormaal JJ et al. Imatinib mesylate in the treatment of systemic mastocytosis. *Cancer* 2006;107:345–51.

15. Johansson B, Fioretos T, Mitelman F et al. Cytogenetic and molecular genetic evolution of chronic myeloid leukemia. *Acta Haematol* 2002;107:76–94.

16. Campbell PH, Green AR. The myeloproliferative disorders. *N Engl J Med.* 2006;355:2452–66.

17. Lowenberg B, Downing JR, Burnett A. Acute myeloid leukemia. *N Eng J Med.* 1999;341:1051–62.

18. Willman C. Acute leukemias: A paradigm for the integration of new technologies in diagnosis and classification. *Mod Pathol.* 1999;12: 218–28.

19. Westendorf J, Yamamoto C, Hiebert SW et al. The t(8;21) fusion product, AML-1-ETO, associates with C/EBP-alpha, inhibits C/EBP-alpha-dependent transcription, and blocks granulocytic differentiation. *Mol Cell Biol.* 1998;18:322–33.

20. Marcucci G, Mrozek K, Ruppert AS et al. Prognostic factors and outcome of core binding factor acute myeloid leukemia patients with t(8;21) differ from those of patients with inv(16): A Cancer and Leukemia Group B Study. *J Clin Oncol.* 2005;23:5705–17.

21. Ravindranath Y, Chang M, Steuber CP et al. Pediatric Oncology Group (POG) studies of acute myeloid leukemia (AML): A review of four consecutive childhood AML trials conducted between 1981 and 2000. *Leukemia.* 2005;19:2101–16.

22. Shali W, Helias C, Fohrer C et al. Cytogenetic studies of a series of 43 consecutive secondary myelodysplastic syndromes/acute myeloid leukemias: Conventional cytogenetics, FISH, and multiplex FISH. *Cancer Genet Cytogenet.* 2006;168:133–45.

23. Greenberg P, Cox C, LeBeau MM et al. International scoring system for evaluating prognosis in myelodysplastic syndromes. *Blood.* 1997;89:2079–88.

24. Pui C-H, Evans WE. Treatment of acute lymphoblastic leukemia. *N Engl J Med.* 2006;354:166–78.

25. Van Grotel M, Meijerkink JPP, Beverloo HB et al. The outcome of molecular-cytogenetic subroups in pediatric T-cell acute lymphoblastic leukemia: A retrospective study of patients treated according to DCOG or COALL protocols. *Hematologica.* 2006;91: 1212–21.

26. Menolov G, Manolaova Y. Marker band in one chromosome 14 from Burkitt lymphoma. *Nature.* 1972;237:33.

27. Dalla Favera R, Bregui M, Erickson J, Patterson D, Gallo R, Croce C. Human C-MYC onc gene is located in the region of chromosome 8 that is translocated in Burkitt lymphoma cells. *Proc Natl Acad Sci. USA,* 1982;79:7824–27.

28. Dohner H, Stilgenbauer S, Benner A et al. Genomic aberrations and survival in chronic lymphocytic leukemia. *N Engl J Med.* 2000;343:1910–16.

29. Bertoni F, Zucc E, Cavalli F. Mantle cell lymphoma. *Curr Opin Hematol.* 2004;11:411–18.

30. Farinha P, Gascoyne RD. Molecular pathogenesis of mucosa-associated lymphoid tissue lymphoma. *J Clin Oncol.* 2005;23:6370–78.

31. Jaffe ES. Anaplastic large cell lymphoma: The shifting sands of diagnostic hematopathology. *Mod Pathol.* 2001;14:219–28.

32. Lee C, Iafrate AJ, Brothman AR. Copy number variations and clinical cytogenetic diagnosis of constitutional disorders. *Nat Genet.* 2007;39:S48–54.

39

Molecular Analysis of Hematologic Diseases

Margaret L. Gulley, M.D.

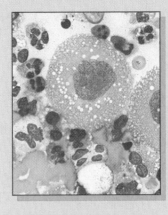

■ OBJECTIVES—LEVEL II

This chapter differs from others in that it has only Level II objectives because the material in this chapter is at the advanced level and requires a background in genetics. At the end of this unit, the student should be able to:

1. Define terms and appropriately use nomenclature associated with molecular pathology.

2. Describe the principles and summarize the procedures for each of the common laboratory tests used in molecular diagnostics.

3. Describe and explain the applications of molecular tests in diagnosing and managing inherited disease, infectious disease, and cancer.

4. Explain the role of genes in acquired versus inherited disorders.

5. Identify common chromosomal translocations and molecular genetic abnormalities associated with chronic myelogenous leukemia, acute leukemia, and lymphoma.

6. Explain how B and T cell malignancies can be differentiated from other conditions by molecular testing.

7. Select the most appropriate molecular test for a given patient condition or provisional diagnosis.

8. Compare and contrast the various molecular methods with regard to diagnostic applications, tissue requirements, and principles.

9. Compare the advantages and disadvantages of molecular tests with other laboratory tests used in diagnosing and managing hematologic disorders.

KEY TERMS

Complementary DNA (cDNA)
DNA sequencing
Fluorescence in situ hybridization (FISH)
Gene
Gene rearrangement
Genome
Genotype
Hybridization
In situ hybridization (ISH)
Locus
Mutation
Nucleotide
Polymerase chain reaction (PCR)
Probe
Real-time PCR
Restriction endonuclease
Southern blot analysis
Transcription
Translation
Translocation

BACKGROUND BASICS

This chapter builds on concepts learned in other chapters of this textbook. The reader should also have a background of genetic principles. To maximize your learning experience, you should review the following material:

▶ Summarize the pathophysiology and etiology of sickle cell anemia. (Chapter 10)

▶ Describe the role of oncogenes in the etiology and pathophysiology of cancer. (Chapters 2, 21)

▶ Describe the application of cytogenetic analysis in diagnosing hematologic disease. (Chapter 38)

▶ Summarize the etiology and pathophysiology of leukemia and lymphoma. (Chapters 21, 22, 24, 25, and 26)

▶ Describe the congenital aberrations that lead to hypercoagulability and venous thrombosis. (Chapter 33)

⊙ CASE STUDY

We will address this case study throughout the chapter.

Carolyn, a 35-year-old female, saw her physician for complaints of fatigue and a 20-pound weight loss in the last 6 months. A complete blood count revealed a white blood cell count of 6.5×10^9/L, hemoglobin of 8 g/dL and platelet count of 25×10^9/L. The leukocyte differential showed 71% blasts. The bone marrow revealed 96% blasts. The blasts were negative for myeloperoxidase, Sudan black B, and combined esterase by cytochemical stains. Cytogenetics revealed t(9;22) (which is characterized by the presence of the Philadelphia chromosome), +8, and +18. Consider the possible disease processes that may be occurring in this patient and laboratory tests that may be helpful in diagnosis and monitoring of her disease.

▶ OVERVIEW

Over the past decade, major advances have been made in applying molecular technology to the practice of laboratory medicine. Nowhere have these applications had more impact than in the field of hematology in which new and improved methods are available to diagnose a wide variety of hematologic diseases. It appears that this revolutionary progress will continue in the coming years as technology advances and new discoveries are brought from the basic science level to their practical realization in clinical laboratories. This chapter introduces molecular analysis of hematologic disorders and describes the most commonly used molecular tests. The application of these tests in selected inherited and malignant hematologic disorders follows.

▶ INTRODUCTION

Molecular diagnostics involves the analysis of deoxyribonucleic acid (DNA) or ribonucleic acid (RNA). DNA is the fundamental substance of heredity that cells use to catalog, express, and propagate information. RNA is the messenger molecule that translates the DNA code so that proteins can be produced. Analysis of DNA and RNA can assist in diagnosing inherited diseases, which by definition have a genetic basis; infectious diseases for which the identification of foreign nucleic acid signals the presence of a particular pathogen; and cancer, which occurs when acquired genetic defects lead to uncontrolled cell proliferation. Laboratory detection of disease-specific genetic alterations is becoming increasingly important for the diagnosis, prognosis, and prediction of response to therapy as well as the monitoring of affected patients.

To understand how DNA technology is implemented in diagnostic laboratories, the basic structure of human DNA first must be reviewed. Each nucleated cell of a person's body contains a complete set of DNA inherited from the person's parents and constituting the person's **genome.** DNA of the human genome is composed of 3 billion pairs of **nucleotides** (one of four building blocks of DNA: A, T, C, G) divided among 46 chromosomes and encoding about 30,000 different genes. Genes are the functional units of DNA that serve as templates for RNA **transcription** (sythesis of RNA from a DNA template) and ultimately protein **translation** (synthesis of protein from an RNA template). The sequence of nucleotides in each gene determines the structure of the encoded protein. In general, every person has two copies of every gene, one that was inherited from the mother and the other from the father. One person's genome differs from another person's by only about 0.2%, or about 1 in every 500 nucleotide pairs. Interestingly, the human genome differs from the chimpanzee genome by only about 1%. Some **gene** sequences are so critical to cell function that they are nearly the same across all species, including bacteria, yeast, and humans. In contrast, other parts

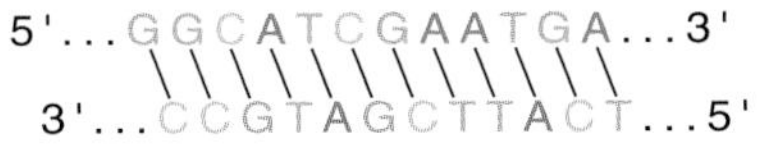

```
5'...GGCATCGAATGA...3'
       \\\\\\\\\\\
3'...CCGTAGCTTACT...5'
```

■ **FIGURE 39-1**   The structure of DNA. DNA is a double-stranded molecule composed of sequences of nucleotides. One strand is bound by hydrogen bonds (shown as diagonal bridges) to its complementary strand. According to the rules of complementary base pairing, the nucleotide adenine (A) is complementary to thymine (T), and guanine (G) is complementary to cytosine (C).

of the genome are highly variable and are exploited in forensic tests to distinguish one person from another.[1] For example, genes of the human leukocyte antigen (HLA) complex are highly variable among populations; genes involved in cell division and in repair of damaged DNA are virtually identical from person to person.

DNA is composed of two complementary strands of nucleotides (Figure 39-1 ■). In living cells, these complementary strands are bound together by hydrogen bonds. In the laboratory, however, the two strands of DNA can be fully dissociated by simply heating to nearly boiling (95°C) or by placing the DNA in an alkaline solution (high pH). Once the strands are separated, a particular nucleotide sequence of interest can be identified using a DNA **probe.** A probe is a single-stranded segment of DNA whose nucleotide sequence is complementary to the target sequence. The probe binds to the target DNA in a process called **hybridization.** This probe hybridization process forms the basis for all of the laboratory tests that have been developed to analyze specific portions of the human genome (Figure 39-2 ■).

► LABORATORY METHODS IN MOLECULAR DIAGNOSTICS

Following are brief descriptions of the most commonly used laboratory tests. They are described in more detail with potential medical applications in the remainder of this chapter.

- **Southern blot analysis** DNA is isolated, cleaved with restriction endonucleases that cut DNA at specific nucleotide sequences, separated by size using gel electrophoresis, transferred to a membrane, and detected with a probe that is complementary to the sequence of interest.
- **Polymerase chain reaction (PCR)** DNA is isolated, and a specific segment of the DNA is copied a billionfold so that it can be more easily detected and, in some cases, further analyzed for structural defects.
- **In situ hybridization (ISH)** DNA or RNA in tissue sections on glass slides is hybridized to a complementary probe and visualized by microscopy. The tissue architecture and cytology are preserved to permit localization of the DNA or RNA to particular cells in the tissue.
- **Fluorescence in situ hybridization (FISH)** Whole chromosomes (metaphase or interphase) are hybridized to a complementary probe labeled with a fluorochrome and visualized by microscopy.
- **DNA sequencing** The nucleotide sequence is determined in a segment of DNA by replicating the DNA strands and monitoring the order in which labeled nucleotides are added to the new strands. DNA sequencing is particularly useful for detecting point mutations located anywhere in the DNA segment.

See Table 39-1 ✪ for the specimen requirements for these procedures.

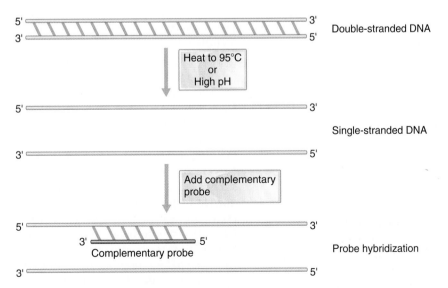

■ **FIGURE 39-2**   The two strands of DNA can be dissociated in vitro by heating them to 95°C or by treating with a solution of high pH. Once separated, the strands can bind to a DNA probe of complementary nucleotide sequence by a process known as *hybridization.*

✪ TABLE 39-1

Specimen Requirements for Molecular Diagnostic Procedures

Procedure	Typical Specimen
Southern blot analysis	Fresh or frozen tissue, fresh body fluid or frozen cell pellet, blood, or marrow
Polymerase chain reaction (PCR)	Fresh, frozen, or paraffin-embedded tissue, blood, or body fluid
In situ hybridization	Paraffin-embedded tissue section
Fluorescence in situ hybridization (FISH)	Fresh cells for metaphase analysis, fixed cells, or tissue sections for interphase analysis
DNA sequencing	Fresh, frozen, or paraffin-embedded tissue, blood, or body fluid

▶ INHERITED DISEASES

In the past few years, molecular biologists have identified specific genetic defects underlying various inherited diseases.[2] By analyzing the DNA from the relevant gene **locus** (specific location on a chromosome), we can now help diagnose a wide variety of diseases.[3] See Table 39-2 ✪ for some of the inherited hematologic diseases for which specific genetic defects have been identified.

The genetic defect responsible for inherited diseases is present in every nucleated cell of a person's body, even if gene expression or clinical manifestation is restricted to only one organ or one stage of development. Because the defect is present in all cells, it can be identified in specimens that are easily collected such as blood or buccal (inside cheek) swabs. Furthermore, the defect can be identified prior to the onset of clinical disease. For example, hemoglobinopathies involving the *HBB* (β-globin) gene can be identified in a fetus even though the *HBB* gene product is not yet expressed nor is there any clinical evidence of disease (∞ Chapter 11).[4]

✪ TABLE 39-2

Inherited or Congenital Hematologic Disorders Amenable to Molecular Genetic Analysis

- Chronic granulomatous disease
- Gaucher disease
- Hereditary hemochromatosis
- Hemoglobinopathies, including sickle cell anemia and thalassemia
- Hemolytic anemias, such as glucose-6-phosphate dehydrogenase deficiency
- Bleeding and thrombotic disorders, including hemophilia
- Immunodeficiencies including adenosine deaminase deficiency, Wiskott-Aldrich syndrome, and X-linked lymphoproliferative disorder
- Myeloperoxidase deficiency
- Porphyrias
- Red cell membrane defects including hereditary spherocytosis

Using correct gene nomenclature in clinical laboratories is important.[5] Note that each human gene has an official name and symbol that can be confirmed on the website www.genenames.org. Gene symbols are displayed in italics, but the corresponding protein symbol is not. The next section describes the application of molecular analysis in two common inherited hematologic diseases, sickle cell anemia and venous thrombosis.

SICKLE CELL ANEMIA

Sickle cell anemia is an autosomal recessive disease that affects 1 in 260 African Americans and almost always shortens their lifespan. The biologic basis of sickle cell anemia is a defect in the HBB (β-globin) protein of hemoglobin. At the DNA level, the defect involves the substitution of a single nucleotide (thymine instead of adenine at the 20th nucleotide in the *HBB* gene), which translates to an amino acid sequence containing valine instead of glutamic acid in the seventh position of the β-globin protein. (*Note:* Because of confusion about numbering, older literature refers to the change as being in the sixth position, but it is actually in the seventh position of the amino acid chain.) That small change in both copies of the *HBB* gene results in a dramatic alteration of hemoglobin molecules so that they tend to polymerize under conditions of dehydration or low oxygen concentration. Hemoglobin polymerization diminishes erythrocyte deformability, thus impairing blood flow through small capillaries. Affected individuals suffer from chronic anemia and recurrent pain as a consequence of small-vessel occlusion and poor oxygen delivery to the tissues.

Laboratory diagnosis of sickle cell anemia traditionally has relied on examination of the blood smear combined with the HbS solubility test and hemoglobin electrophoresis. When these procedures are inconclusive or when prenatal diagnosis is requested, DNA technology is a useful means of identifying or excluding the genetic defect.

Southern Blot Analysis of the Sickle Mutation

To detect the sickle **mutation** by Southern blot analysis, DNA is first extracted from patient blood by (1) detergent solubilization of lipids in cell membranes, (2) protease digestion of proteins, and (3) purification of DNA from the remaining material. The purified DNA is then cleaved with a **restriction endonuclease** that reproducibly cuts the long strands of chromosomal DNA at a specific nucleotide sequence to produce smaller fragments of DNA. These fragments are size fractionated by gel electrophoresis and transferred to a nylon membrane where they are hybridized to a labeled probe targeting the gene of interest, in this case, *HBB*. The pattern of probe hybridization determines whether the sickle mutation is present or absent (Figure 39-3 ■).

The Southern blot assay can be adapted to detect many other disease-associated alterations besides the sickle mutation. Indeed, if a patient's DNA sequence is altered by any mutation, translocation, or small deletion, the number

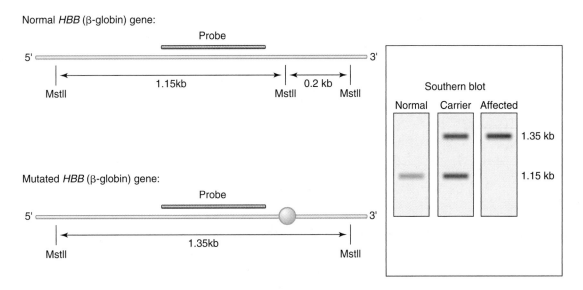

Normal *HBB* (β-globin) gene:

Mutated *HBB* (β-globin) gene:

Southern blot

Normal Carrier Affected

1.35 kb

1.15 kb

■ FIGURE 39-3   Southern blot analysis of the sickle cell mutation is accomplished by first extracting DNA and then cutting it with MstII restriction endonuclease that cleaves DNA at a specific nucleotide sequence (arrows). Because that specific sequence is present many times in the human genome, MstII cuts genomic DNA into many small fragments. The resultant DNA fragments are separated by size using gel electrophoresis, dissociated into single strands by soaking in an alkaline solution, and then transferred to a nylon membrane by a blotting procedure. To identify the fragment containing the *HBB* gene, the membrane is soaked in a radiolabeled DNA probe (bar) that hybridizes to a complementary segment of the *HBB* gene. The pattern of bands recognized by the probe reflects the size of the corresponding restriction fragments measured in kilobases (kb). An *HBB* gene harboring the sickle mutation (shown as a pink circle) fails to cut with MstII, thus altering the band pattern. In this way, a person affected by sickle cell anemia can be distinguished from a carrier (sickle trait) and from a person of normal genotype. *Note:* Restriction endonucleases are naturally occurring enzymes that recognize and cleave specific nucleotide sequences in DNA. Each restriction endonuclease is named for the bacteria from which it was purified. For example, EcoRI is derived from *Escherichia coli* and cleaves DNA having the sequence 5′-GAATTC-3′, whereas HindIII, derived from *Haemophilus influenzae,* cleaves at 5′-AAGCTT-3′. In the example shown here, MstII cleaves the normal DNA when it recognizes the sequence 5′-CCTG**A**GG-3′, but it cannot cleave DNA harboring the sickle mutation 5′-CCTG**T**GG-3′.

and/or size of the resulting restriction fragments will be altered accordingly. The restriction fragment(s) containing the gene of interest is identified by probe hybridization. The probe must be labeled to permit its subsequent detection on the Southern blot. A typical probe is labeled with radionucleotides, permitting its detection by autoradiography. Alternatively, the probe can be labeled with biotin or digoxigenin and detected using colorimetric procedures analogous to what is done in immunoassays of antigen–antibody complexes. Southern blot analysis is a very powerful technology but is also quite labor intensive, so it is used primarily as a backup method in modern molecular laboratories.

Detection of the Sickle Mutation by DNA Amplification Methods such as the Polymerase Chain Reaction

A more common method of detecting the sickle mutation is by DNA amplification, a procedure in which a particular segment of DNA is copied a billionfold. DNA amplification techniques have revolutionized our ability to analyze DNA in the clinical laboratory because we can now examine a rare segment of DNA from a small tissue specimen or even a sin-

gle cell. Several amplification methods have been introduced, but the first and most commonly used method is PCR, which works by enzymatically replicating one particular segment of DNA (typically about 100 nucleotides in length) from among the entire 3 billion base-pair human genome. This process permits rapid, sensitive, and specific identification of a segment of DNA that can then be further tested for a disease-specific genetic defect (Figure 39-4 ■).

Diagnosis of the sickle cell **genotype** can be accomplished by PCR amplification of a segment of the *HBB* gene harboring the sickle mutation site. The amplified DNA is then cleaved with the MstII restriction endonuclease and electrophoresed in an agarose gel. Because MstII differentially cleaves normal DNA compared with sickle DNA, a different electrophorectic band pattern is produced depending on whether the sickle mutation is present or not.

Using an alternate amplification strategy called *allele-specific PCR,* short DNA probes that serve as PCR primers have been designed to preferentially amplify either the normal *HBB* sequence or the defective sickle *HBB* sequence (Figure 39-5 ■). This preferential amplification is based on the premise that mutations interfering with primer hybridization

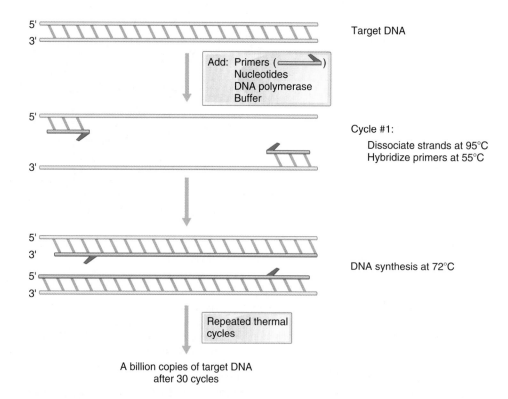

■ FIGURE 39-4   Polymerase chain reaction is a method of enzymatically amplifying a particular segment of DNA through a process of repeated cycles of heating, cooling, and DNA synthesis. First, patient DNA is mixed with the chemicals needed for DNA synthesis. Included are two short DNA probes (called *primers,* shown as half arrows) designed to flank the particular segment of DNA that needs to be amplified. A thermocycler instrument is programmed to sequentially heat and cool the sample. In cycle 1, the sample is heated to 95°C to dissociate complementary strands of DNA and then is cooled to 55°C to permit binding of the short DNA probes that serve as primers for subsequent enzymatic DNA replication at 72°C. This replication generates new complementary strands to produce an exact copy of the original target DNA. In subsequent cycles, the products of previous cycles can serve as templates for DNA replication, allowing an exponential accumulation of DNA copies. After 30 cycles, which takes only several hours, approximately 1 billion copies of the target DNA have been generated.

result in failed amplification reactions. The success or failure of the amplification reaction can be determined while the reaction is occurring by using a strategy called **real-time PCR**, which can be performed in a few hours.

A major advantage of PCR over Southern blot analysis is that PCR can be performed on much smaller specimen volumes because the assay is designed to identify rare target sequences. PCR is also a more rapid laboratory procedure (1–2 days as compared with >4 days for Southern blot analysis), costs relatively less, and is amenable for use on formalin-fixed paraffin-embedded tissues. However, a drawback to PCR is the meticulous attention required to prevent carryover or contamination of laboratory samples by extraneous DNA. To prevent carryover, three separate rooms can be required: one for reagent preparation, one for preamplification steps, and one for postamplification steps.

The sickle cell genotype is relatively easy to diagnose because the specific genetic mutation is identical among all af-fected individuals. Not all inherited diseases are so straight-forward—complex and diverse genetic defects can result in the same clinical syndrome. For example, only about half of all patients with hemophilia A have an identifiable mutation or deletion of the *F8* gene that encodes F8 (also called *FVIII*) protein while the remaining patients presumably have any of several occult genetic defects that somehow inhibit expression of the F8 protein.

INHERITED PREDISPOSITION TO VENOUS THROMBOSIS

Several inherited mutations predispose to venous thrombosis. The most common is a point mutation at position 1601 in the *F5* gene (also called FV_{Leiden}) that interferes with catabolism of the encoded coagulation factor. This mutation is quite common, affecting about 5% of the population; those who inherit it have a sevenfold increased risk of developing

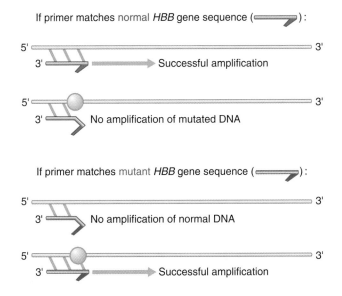

If primer matches normal *HBB* gene sequence (═══➤):

5' ══════════════════════════════ 3'
3' ╱╱╱╱══════➤ Successful amplification

5' ══════════════════════════════ 3'
3' ╱●╲══════╲ No amplification of mutated DNA

If primer matches mutant *HBB* gene sequence (═══➤):

5' ══════════════════════════════ 3'
3' ╱╱╱╲══════╲ No amplification of normal DNA

5' ══════════════════════════════ 3'
3' ══●══════➤ Successful amplification

■ **FIGURE 39-5**   One way that polymerase chain reaction can be used to facilitate detection of the sickle mutation is to design primers (half arrows) that preferentially bind to either normal *HBB* or sickle *HBB* gene sequences. If a primer does not match its target sequence perfectly, particularly at the 5' end of the primer where the DNA polymerase initiates replication, amplification cannot occur. On the other hand, if the primer matches its target, abundant PCR products are generated. If both the normal and mutant primers generate a product, the patient is heterozygous, or a carrier of the sickle trait. (Pink circle represents the *HBB* gene mutation)

thrombosis. The second most common genetic risk factor for venous thrombosis is a point mutation at position 21538 in the *F2* gene encoding prothrombin protein (FII). (*Note:* Older literature referred to this mutation as being at position 20210 and is commonly called *Prothrombin G20210A.* However, the correct standard nomenclature for this mutation is *F2* AF478696.1:g21538G>A).[5] This mutation is found in about 2% of the population and is associated with a three-fold increased risk of venous thrombosis. The *F5* and *F2* gene mutations are readily detectable by real-time PCR followed by melt curve analysis[6,7] (Figure 39-6 ■).

> ✓ **Checkpoint! 1**
>
> *A 40-year-old male is diagnosed with an inherited disease for which a specific point mutation is responsible. His mother died of a similar disease 10 years ago. For purposes of family counseling, the physician wants to know whether she had the same mutation. The histology laboratory has archival paraffin-embedded tissue from the mother. What laboratory method(s) is (are) best for detecting the gene mutation?*

▶ MOLECULAR BASIS OF CANCER

DNA technology is a powerful tool to assist in the diagnosis of cancer.[8] Unlike inherited disease in which every nucleated cell in the body contains defective DNA, cancer results when

one cell acquires genetic defects that stimulate uncontrolled cell division and tumor formation. Virtually all cancers are thought to harbor genetic defects. The specific genes that are altered in tumors and are thereby responsible for tumor formation are called *oncogenes* (∞ Chapters 2, 21). The unaltered counterpart of an oncogene (called a *proto-oncogene*) generally functions to regulate cell growth or differentiation whereas in tumor cells, this function has gone awry as a result of abnormal expression or structural alteration of the gene.

Each time a malignant cell divides, the genetic defect is passed on to its progeny. Therefore, all of the cells within a particular tumor contain the same defective DNA, a concept known as *clonality.* Because cancers harbor clonal genetic defects, cancer cells can be distinguished from normal cells by DNA probe analysis of the defective gene sequences. Certain oncogene defects are highly characteristic of particular types of cancer and can be used to assist in diagnosing and classifying those cancers. This section describes the application of molecular analysis in diagnosing and managing selected leukemias and lymphomas.

CHRONIC MYELOGENOUS LEUKEMIA AND THE *BCR/ABL1* TRANSLOCATION

Traditional cytogenetics demonstrates that hematopoietic neoplasms frequently harbor a characteristic chromosomal **translocation,** as exemplified by the t(9;22) of chronic myelogenous leukemia (CML) (∞ Chapters 22, 38). A translocation is caused by the breakage of DNA from one chromosome and its attachment to (and exchange with) DNA on another locus.

In CML, the characteristic Philadelphia chromosome represents a shortened chromosome 22 resulting from a reciprocal translocation between the *ABL1* gene on chromosome 9 and the *BCR* gene on chromosome 22. This translocation produces a new fusion gene called *BCR/ABL1* that encodes hybrid RNA and hybrid protein. The presence of *BCR* gene elements enhances the potency of the *ABL1* gene product (that functions as a tyrosine kinase enzyme), resulting in uncontrolled cell proliferation.

About 90% of all patients who have clinical and laboratory features of CML have t(9;22) by karyotyping. An additional 5% have an occult (cryptic) translocation that is detectable only by molecular analysis of *BCR/ABL1*. The remaining 5% of tumors suspected of being CML but lacking *BCR/ABL1* do not behave in the same fashion as CML, and these tumors represent other myeloproliferative diseases or myelodysplastic syndromes masquerading as CML. In contrast, those patients with molecular evidence of *BCR/ABL1* share a similar natural history and predisposition to blast crisis. In blast crisis, the transformed acute leukemia cell clone retains the *BCR/ABL1* defect; these cells also have acquired even more genetic defects that account for their more aggressive cytologic appearance and clinical behavior.

While DNA technology is more sensitive than karyotyping for detecting the CML-associated genetic defect, karyotyping has the advantage of revealing other chromosomal

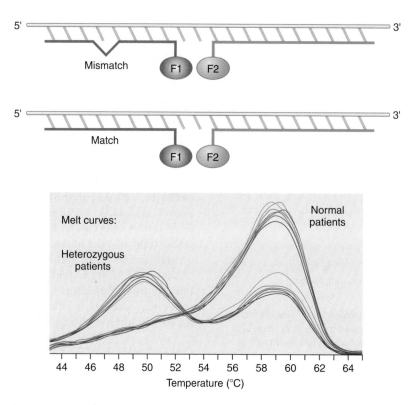

■ **FIGURE 39-6**   Melt curve analysis is a way to determine whether a particular mutation is present by evaluating the temperature at which a labeled probe (shown in red) melts away from its target DNA. To accomplish this, a mixture of probe and target DNA is gradually heated until the probe melts away. Melting occurs at a low temperature if there is a mismatch but at a high temperature if there is a perfect match between the probe and target sequence. The temperature at which dissociation occurs is detected in a real-time PCR instrument that analyzes the interaction between a fluorochrome linked to the probe (shown in red) and another fluorochrome (shown in green) on an adjacent probe. Proximity of the red and green fluorochromes generates a yellowish signal when both probes are bound to the target whereas the red and green fluorochromes floating apart indicates melting has occurred. The above graph depicts melt curves for a series of 20 patients who were tested for the *F2* mutation; those with two normal *F2* genes have a single melt peak at 60°C. In contrast, those patients having one mutant copy and one normal copy of the *F2* gene have two melt peaks, one at 50°C and the other at 60°C, indicating they are heterozygous for the mutation and at increased risk for venous thrombosis.

abnormalities in addition to t(9;22). Therefore, a cost-effective approach to the laboratory workup of suspected CML is first to perform a karyotype and proceed to molecular testing only if the karyotype is nondiagnostic. A white cell pellet can be frozen or stored in Carnoy's fixative in case molecular testing is needed at a later time.

◎ CASE STUDY *(continued from page 874)*

1. What is the classification of this neoplastic hematologic disorder based on the peripheral blood and bone marrow results?

Minimal residual disease (MRD) refers to the post-treatment presence of tumor cells that are not detectable by routine morphologic methods but that result in relapse if they are not eliminated. Amplification strategies such as PCR are exquisitely sensitive for detecting minimal residual disease because abnormal cells are detectable down to 0.01% (1 cell in 100,000 cells) whereas karyotype and FISH typically detect tumor cells at about 1% (1 cell in 100 cells). Another advantage of molecular technology over karyotyping is the capability to analyze cells that are resistant to entering the cell cycle and are therefore difficult to evaluate by traditional cytogenetic methods. For example, neutrophils are fully amenable to DNA analysis, but they are not amenable to karyotyping because they are not capable of dividing.

Molecular Analysis of the *BCR/ABL1* Junction by DNA Amplification

To amplify the *BCR/ABL1* translocation, one typically uses a variant of PCR called *reverse transcriptase PCR* (rtPCR). In this procedure, RNA is extracted from tissues and then converted to **complementary DNA (cDNA)** using an enzyme called *reverse transcriptase*. (The cDNA represents only the exons of the gene because the introns have been removed naturally during the formation of RNA.) The cDNA is then subjected to PCR amplification using primers flanking the transloca-

tion break point, and the product is detected by quantitative real-time PCR (Figure 39-7 ■).[9] This strategy permits an accurate assessment of the amount of *BCR/ABL1* in the patient sample, thus allowing tumor burden to be measured at multiple time points following initiation of treatment.[10] Current treatment regimens typically begin with Gleevec (imatinib mesylate) or similar agents that specifically inhibit the ABL1 tyrosine kinase enzyme activity. Failure to respond to the drug (e.g., increasing tumor levels) could indicate that a mutation-conferring drug resistance has occurred, and such mutations can be characterized by DNA sequencing of the *BCR/ABL1* fusion gene to help predict which drug is most likely to be effective.[11]

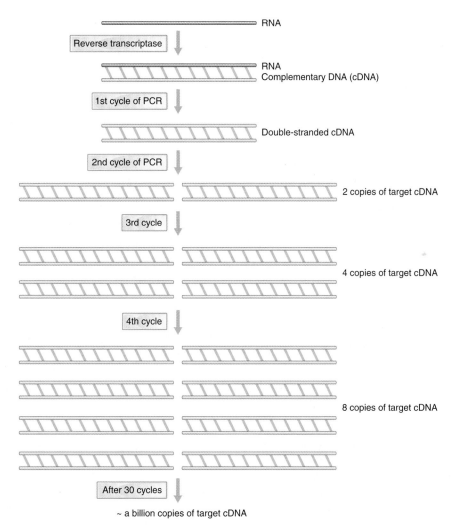

■ FIGURE 39-7   The rtPCR procedure is a means of determining whether a particular RNA transcript is present in a tissue sample. RNA is extracted from the sample and then converted to complementary DNA (cDNA) using the enzyme reverse transcriptase. This cDNA serves as a template for DNA amplification by the polymerase chain reaction. After 30 cycles, about 1 billion copies of the target cDNA sequence have been generated. These abundant copies can then be readily detected or further analyzed to provide valuable information about the RNA in the patient sample.

A unique benefit of rtPCR is the ability to distinguish *BCR/ABL1* break points that are characteristic of CML (called *p210*) from *BCR/ABL1* break points of de novo acute lymphoblastic leukemia (called *p190*).[12] Although these alternate break points appear identical by karyotyping, they are distinct at the molecular level and from a clinical standpoint. They help separate patients with a new diagnosis of acute leukemia from those presenting in blast crisis of CML. Furthermore, detection of *BCR/ABL1* p190 identifies a subset of acute lymphoblastic leukemia patients who are poorly responsive to standard chemotherapy regimens and should be considered for novel or more aggressive therapy.[13]

Another method of detecting the *BCR/ABL1* translocation is by FISH (∞ Chapter 38 for details) using probes targeting the *BCR* and *ABL1* genes.

✓ Checkpoint! 2

A patient with CML was treated with chemotherapy. On subsequent marrow samples, the physician ordered molecular testing to detect residual disease after treatment. The BCR/ABL1 translocation was not detected 3 months after treatment but was detected at the 6th and 7th months after treatment. Interpret this result.

ACUTE PROMYELOCYTIC LEUKEMIA AND THE *PML/RARA* TRANSLOCATION

Refer to Table 39-3 ✪ for the characteristic chromosomal defects of myeloid leukemias. One of the most interesting of these cancers is acute promyelocytic leukemia in which t(15;17) juxtaposes the *PML* gene on chromosome 15 with the retinoic acid receptor alpha (*RARA*) gene on chromosome 17 (∞ Chapter 24). Amazingly, leukemias harboring this genetic defect respond to treatment with retinoic acid derivatives, providing one of the first examples of cancer therapy specifically targeting a gene product thought to be involved in tumorigenesis. Retinoic acid therapy alone unfortunately is insufficient for a cure because the tumor cells eventually

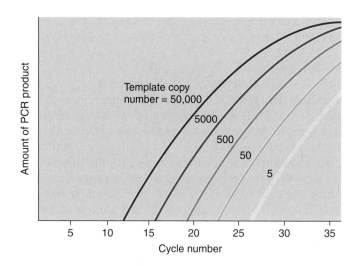

■ **FIGURE 39-8** Tumor burden in acute promyelocytic leukemia patients can be measured using real-time PCR targeting *PML/RARA* transcripts. The higher the tumor burden, the more fusion transcripts are present, so the more template cDNA is present and the earlier the products appear during PCR amplification cycles.

become resistant to its effects. Nevertheless, retinoic acid used in combination with other chemotherapeutic agents appears to improve outcomes in affected patients.[14]

Karyotyping and molecular tests (rtPCR or FISH) are used to detect the characteristic *PML/RARA* translocation.[14] These molecular tests assist in diagnosing and classifying acute leukemia and predict response to retinoic acid therapy. The most sensitive test for monitoring levels of residual tumor burden after therapy is rtPCR, and its results appear to predict which patients will relapse.[15] The rtPCR test converts RNA that has been purified from the patient's blood or marrow to cDNA and uses primers flanking the break point between the *PML* and *RARA* genes to specifically amplify the translocation region. Amplified products can be measured using a real-time PCR instrument (Figure 39-8 ■).

✪ TABLE 39-3

Chromosomal Abnormalities in Selected Subtypes of Myeloid Leukemia

Leukemia	Karyotype	Genes	Clinical Significance
CML	t(9;22)	*BCR/ABL1*	Predisposed to blast crisis, Gleevec responsive
CMML	t(5;12)	*PDGFRB/ETV6*	Gleevec responsive
CEL	t(5;12)	*FIP1L1/PDGFRA*	Gleevec responsive
AML	t(8;21)	*RUNX1/RUNX1T1*	Good response to chemotherapy
APL	t(15;17)	*PML/RARA*	Responds to retinoic acid therapy
AML	inv(16)	*MYH11/CBFB*	Good response to chemotherapy
AML	11q23 defects	*MLL*	Poor response to chemotherapy

CML = chronic myelogenous leukemia; CMML = chronic myelomonocytic leukemia; CEL = chronic eosinophilic leukemia; t = translocation; APL = acute promyelocytic leukemia; inv = inversion; AML = acute myelogenous leukemia

Theoretically, the patient's DNA (rather than RNA) could be used to detect *PML/RARA* by PCR, but the translocation break points vary widely from patient to patient, so multiple primer sets would be needed to detect all possible translocations. In contrast, RNA encoded from the fusion gene is remarkably homogeneous and therefore more amenable for analysis using rtPCR. Keep in mind that RNA is much less stable than DNA and must be handled carefully to avoid degradation.

CASE STUDY (continued from page 880)

2. What molecular defect is consistent with the presence of the Philadelphia chromosome?

3. Would molecular analysis assist in diagnosis? Explain.

4. If molecular analysis is required, which laboratory procedure should be used, and what specimen should be obtained?

ONCOGENE TRANSLOCATIONS IN LYMPHOID LEUKEMIAS AND LYMPHOMAS

Lymphomas and lymphoid leukemias commonly contain chromosomal translocations involving the antigen receptor genes, namely the immunoglobulin (Ig) genes expressed by B cells and the T cell receptor (TR) genes expressed by T cells. Translocations involving these genes are thought to represent errors occurring during physiologic gene rearrangement (to be described in the next section). Any gene located at or near the reciprocal translocation break point is a putative oncogene whose expression can be dysregulated by juxtaposition of the antigen receptor gene.

See Table 39-4 ☉ for the translocations most characteristic of lymphoid neoplasms. In most of these tumors, either Ig or TR genes are juxtaposed with genes that function in regulating cell growth. For example, the *MYC* oncogene of Burkitt lymphoma and the putative *BCL1* oncogene of mantle cell lymphoma encode proteins that promote cell division.[16] In follicular lymphoma, the protein product of the *BCL2* oncogene inhibits cell death. Overexpression of these oncogenes appears to be responsible, at least in part, for the development of lymphoid tumors.

Clonal genetic defects often can be detected by karyotype, Southern blot analysis of the affected oncogene, or PCR amplification of the translocation break point. These types of assays in conjunction with traditional morphologic examination and other laboratory studies are helpful for diagnosing and classifying tumors. Karyotyping and Southern blot analysis are too insensitive to detect minimal residual disease (they detect tumors comprising only 1% or more of a specimen), but PCR assays detect much lower tumor burden and can help predict which patients are likely to relapse following treatment for follicular lymphoma.[17]

In theory, the best treatment for a tumor is to eliminate the genetic defect(s) responsible for its uncontrolled growth.

☉ TABLE 39-4

Chromosomal Abnormalities Characterizing Lymphoma and Lymphoid Leukemia

Lymphoid Neoplasm	Karyotype	Genes*
B cell lymphomas		
Burkitt	t(8;14, 2 or 22)	*MYC/IGH, IGK, or IGL*
Mantle cell	t(11;14)	*BCL1/IGH*
Follicular	t(14;18)	*IGH/BCL2*
Diffuse large cell	t(3;14)	*BCL6/IGH*
MALT	t(11;18)	*BIRC3/MALT1*
B cell leukemias		
Pre-B ALL	t(9;22)	*BCR/ABL1*
Pre-B ALL	t(1;19)	*PBX1/TCF3*
Pre-B ALL	t(12;21)	*ETV6/RUNX1*
Mixed lineage acute	t(various;11)	Various partner genes/*MLL*
T cell leukemias/ lymphomas		
T-ALL	Deletion 1p	*STIL/TAL1*
Anaplastic large cell	t(2;5)	*ALK/NPM1*

*The order of the genes corresponds to the order of the karyotype except for *BCR/ABL1*. ALL = acute lymphoblastic leukemia; MALT = mucosa-associated lymphoid tissue

However, we have not yet succeeded in finding a way to correct the genetic defect that is present in every one of the trillion or so tumor cells that are typically present in a patient's body at the time of diagnosis. Alternatively, if we understood the consequences of a particular genetic defect, it might be possible to wisely intervene in the affected biochemical pathways to thwart tumor growth or trigger tumor cell death. Such has been the case with *BCR/ABL1* and *PML/RARA* inhibitors as described, but progress has been slower in identifying analogous targeted therapies for lymphoid malignancy. As further progress is made in tailoring therapy to specific genetic defects, demands on clinical laboratories to identify these defects in patient samples will increase.

IMMUNOGLOBULIN AND T CELL RECEPTOR GENE REARRANGEMENT

In addition to any translocation that a lymphoid neoplasm may have, B cell tumors have a marker of clonality in their rearranged Ig genes that code for antibody specificity (Figure 39-9 ■). After all, B cell leukemia or lymphoma arises from a single transformed B cell harboring a particular Ig gene rearrangement that is inherited by all tumor cell progeny, resulting in a monoclonal cell population. Therefore, clonal gene rearrangement serves as a marker to distinguish tumor cells from normal cells.[18] Southern blot analysis can evaluate

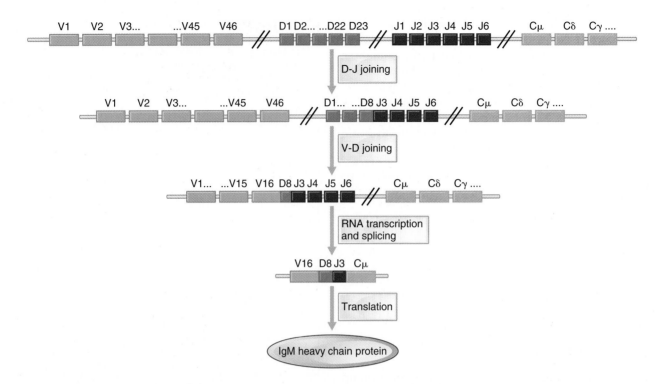

■ FIGURE 39-9   During B cell differentiation, the immunoglobulin heavy chain gene rearranges to produce a unique coding sequence that determines antibody specificity. This occurs through a process of splicing and deletion whereby 1 of 23 diversity (D) regions is juxtaposed with 1 of 6 joining (J) regions and then with 1 of 46 variable (V) regions. Finally, constant (C) region splicing determines antibody isotype (IgM, IgD, IgG, IgA, or IgE). In the example here, V, D, J, and Cμ segments are sequentially spliced together to generate a nucleic acid sequence that encodes IgM heavy chain proteins. These heavy chain proteins complex with kappa or lambda light chain proteins (that are also encoded by rearranged genes) to produce a functional antibody molecule. Each developing B cell has different Ig gene rearrangements, so a population of normal B cells is characterized by polyclonal Ig genes. The diversity of these genes and their encoded antibodies permits immune recognition of many different antigens.

gene rearrangement using a probe targeting the *IGH* gene. *IGH* gene rearrangement also serves as a marker of commitment to the B cell lineage. Information on clonality and lineage is helpful in distinguishing a B cell neoplasm from benign lymphoid hyperplasia.

Analogous to the process by which B cells rearrange their Ig genes, T cells rearrange their TCR genes to encode a unique antigen receptor expressed on the surface of T lymphocytes. TCR gene rearrangement by Southern blot analysis can serve as a clonal marker for T cell tumors analogous to the description for B cell tumors. In the case of T cells, four different TCR genes (called *TRA, TRB, TRD,* and *TRG*) are capable of rearranging. Any particular T cell tumor can exhibit rearrangements of one, two, three, or all four of these TCR genes. In clinical laboratories, assays targeting the *TRB* or *TRG* genes are most commonly used to distinguish monoclonal T cell neoplasms from polyclonal reactive processes.[19]

In recent years, PCR has been implemented as an alternate method of detecting clonal gene rearrangement[18,20] (Figure 39-10■). Current protocols successfully identify clonal *IGH* gene rearrangement in about 95% of B cell neo-

plasms.[21] Although this is less productive than Southern blot assays (which detect virtually 100% of B cell neoplasms), amplification techniques are popular laboratory tools because they are fast, inexpensive, applicable to paraffin-embedded tissue and require a small amount of tissue. Furthermore, the particular rearranged sequence that characterizes each lymphoid tumor can be exploited as a tumor-specific marker to assist in monitoring response to therapy.[22] As with all clinical laboratory tests, appropriate quality control and proficiency testing are essential.

Clinical Utility of Gene Rearrangement Testing
The most valuable contribution of gene rearrangement testing is in distinguishing benign from malignant lymphoproliferations. In general, a malignant lymphoid tumors exhibits clonal antigen receptor **gene rearrangement** while a benign, reactive lymphoid hyperplasia does not.

The converse principle is not always true as exemplified by a few hematopoietic disorders for which clonality does not necessarily imply malignancy. These include large granular lymphocytosis and lymphomatoid papulosis, either of which can harbor clonal gene rearrangement even though they

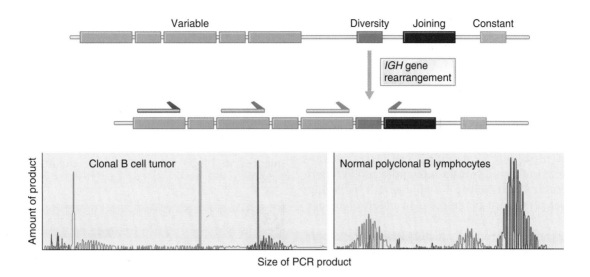

■ FIGURE 39-10   Rearrangement of the immunoglobulin heavy chain (*IGH*) gene involves random splicing of V, D, and J segments to produce a unique coding sequence. This process brings the V and J segments so close together that it becomes possible to PCR-amplify across the rearranged gene by using several primers (shown as half arrows) targeting various V and J segments. In a B cell tumor, all tumor cells contain exactly the same *IGH* rearrangement that was present in the original transformed B cell from which the tumor arose. This tumor-related clonal rearrangement is identified by capillary gel electrophoresis as a spike (representing a single-size PCR product with each primer set). In contrast, benign tissue has normal B lymphocytes whose polyclonal rearrangements appear as multiple different-size PCR products.

often regress without therapy. Because clonality is not always synonymous with malignancy, DNA probe results must be interpreted in the context of clinical information and in correlation with morphologic examination of the tissue to obtain accurate diagnostic and prognostic information.

Although Ig or TCR gene rearrangement can be used to help assign B or T cell lineage to a lymphoid neoplasm, immunophenotypic methods (such as flow cytometry or immunohistochemistry) are more reliable than gene rearrangement tests for assigning the lineage of a hematopoietic neoplasm. Indeed, whenever morphologically equivocal hematopathology specimens are being worked up, immunophenotyping is generally the first-line ancillary laboratory test with gene probe studies reserved as a secondary option.

✓ Checkpoint! 3

An enlarged lymph node was biopsied and sent to the laboratory for molecular anlaysis. Lymphoma was suspected. What molecular test(s) could be done on the specimen to determine whether the lesion is likely to be malignant?

▶ INFECTIOUS DISEASES

Molecular technology has provided new tools for detecting microorganisms based on the unique genetic code of each species.[23] DNA amplification strategies are most useful be-

cause they are sensitive, specific, and rapid for detecting pathogen-specific nucleic acid sequences. Quantitative real-time PCR assays are useful for monitoring the level of organisms during treatment.

Molecular tests are already available for numerous hematology-related pathogens (Table 39-5 ✪). Some organisms exist in the human body as normal flora, and they can eventually cause disease. To investigate this problem, in situ hybridization is helpful for identifying lesion-specific pathogens in biopsy samples.

✪ TABLE 39-5

Pathogens of Hematologic Significance Detectable by Molecular Techniques

- Cytomegalovirus (CMV)
- Epstein-Barr virus (EBV)
- Human herpes virus 8 (HHV8)
- Human immunodeficiency virus (HIV)
- Human T lymphotropic virus type 1 (HTLV1)
- Malaria
- Mycobacteria
- Mycoplasma
- Parvovirus B19
- Toxoplasma

LYMPHOMA-ASSOCIATED VIRUSES

Three viruses have been consistently linked to lymphoid neoplasms: human T lymphotropic virus type 1 (HTLV1), Epstein-Barr virus (EBV), and human herpesvirus 8 (HHV8).[24] HTLV1 infects T helper lymphocytes and causes them to proliferate by upregulation of interleukin 2 and its receptor. Asymptomatic HTLV1 infection is found in 15% of people in Japan and the Caribbean islands. About 0.1% of infected individuals eventually develop adult T cell leukemia/lymphoma characterized by hypercalcemia and a proliferation of peculiar multilobated helper T lymphocytes harboring the virus. Viral cDNA can be detected in blood or tissues using PCR.[25]

EBV infects the oropharyngeal mucosa, where it resides in a subset of B lymphocytes. Virtually all persons are infected before adulthood and, once infected, periodically shed infectious virus in their saliva for the remainder of their lives. EBV is known to cause infectious mononucleosis and is suspected of playing a role in the development of some lymphomas. EBV DNA is found in the majority of immunodeficiency-related lymphomas, 40% of all Hodgkin lymphomas, 20% of sporadic Burkitt lymphomas, and in a small subset of carcinomas and sarcomas. The best analytic test for confirming tumor-associated EBV is in situ hybridization to EBV encoded RNA (EBER).[26] In this procedure, EBV probe hybridizes to viral RNA in paraffin-embedded tissue sections on glass slides. Microscopic visualization allows localization of the virus to particular cells in the lesion, such as the Reed-Sternberg cells of Hodgkin lymphoma (Figure 39-11 ■). In a separate type of procedure performed on whole blood or plasma, EBV viral load measurement by quantitative real-time PCR facilitates diagnosis by virtue of the high circulating levels of EBV DNA in affected patients, and serial viral load measurements are then performed to monitor the efficacy of therapy.[27]

HHV8 rarely causes disease in healthy individuals, but in AIDS patients, it is strongly associated with Kaposi sarcoma, primary effusion lymphoma, and an atypical lymphoproliferative disorder called *multicentric Castleman's disease*. The virus can be detected in lesional tissue by in situ hybridization. Affected patients can be monitored using HHV8 viral load assays that rely on measurement of HHV8 genomic sequences in blood or plasma using quantitative real-time PCR.[28]

@ CASE STUDY *(continued from page 883)*

5. Molecular analysis revealed the *BCR/ABL1* translocation with a p190 break point. What is the most likely diagnosis?

6. Why is this molecular finding helpful in therapeutic decision making?

SUMMARY

DNA technology provides a powerful new tool for laboratory diagnosis of a wide variety of hematologic diseases including inherited disease, infectious disease, and cancer. The laboratory methods commonly used include Southern blot analysis, PCR, in situ hybridization, and FISH. Inherited hematologic diseases that are amenable to molecular diagnosis include sickle cell anemia and venous thrombosis resulting from FV as FII mutations. Leukemias and lymphomas are quite amenable to molecular diagnosis because these malignancies frequently harbor chromosomal translocations or clonal gene rearrangements. All infectious organisms are suitable targets for molecular detection because each species of organism has a unique genome that hybridizes to a complementary

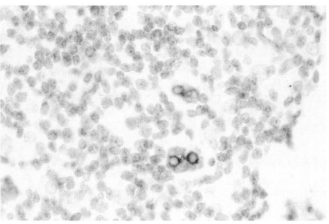

a

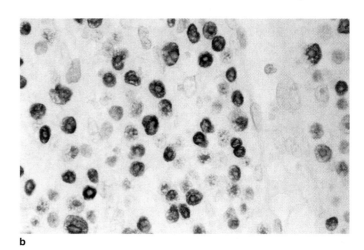

b

■ FIGURE 39-11   In situ hybridization to Epstein-Barr virus EBER transcripts reveals the localization of the virus to Reed-Sternberg cells of Hodgkin's disease (a) and the malignant cells of a diffuse large B cell lymphoma arising in an immunocompromised patient (b). The nuclei of the virus-infected cells are darkly stained as a consequence of a colorimetric reaction occurring at the site of the bound probe.

probe. This facilitates molecular diagnosis of infectious diseases and the virus-associated lymphomas. Newer methods such as DNA sequencing and array technology are now in our toolbox.[29] Automation and manufactured kits are beginning to make molecu- lar testing more accessible and reproducible as well as increasing throughput. The pace of progress is rapid in this exciting corner of the clinical laboratory.

REVIEW QUESTIONS

Use this case history for questions 1 and 2.

A 38-year-old woman complained of dizziness, fatigue, and abdominal pain. On physical examination she appeared pale, and her spleen was enlarged. Laboratory studies revealed anemia and an elevated leukocyte count of 69×10^9/L. A complete spectrum of granulocytic cells from myeloblasts to neutrophils was present in the blood, and the number of basophils was increased. The leukocyte alkaline phosphatase (LAP) score was low. The bone marrow could not be aspirated, but a biopsy revealed that the marrow was packed with myeloid elements. Cytogenetics could not be performed because of the lack of an adequate marrow aspirate and the inability to induce cell division in peripheral blood leukocytes. Blood is submitted for molecular diagnostic testing.

1. Which genetic defect is the most appropriate target for molecular testing to assist in diagnosing the patient's hematologic disorder? (Objective 5)
   a. *PML/RARA*
   b. *BCL2/IGH*
   c. *BCR/ABL1*
   d. *BCL1/IGH*

2. Is there any reason to do molecular testing on the patient at a later date? (Objectives 3, 7)
   a. No, the positive test results are definitive, and nothing more can be accomplished.
   b. Yes, the patient can be monitored to detect residual disease following therapy.
   c. No, but family members should be tested for the same molecular defect.
   d. Yes, the translocation break point must be sequenced to prove which genes are involved.

3. Which of the following reagents is most critical for making a polymerase chain reaction (PCR) reaction specific for the *F5* gene mutation (FV_{Leiden}) as opposed to a prothrombin gene mutation? (Objective 2)
   a. primers
   b. nucleotides
   c. DNA polymerase
   d. buffer

4. All molecular tests that analyze specific portions of the human genome rely on the principle that: (Objective 2)
   a. DNA is different in every cell of a particular individual.
   b. Probes bind to their complementary target sequence through a process called *hybridization.*
   c. Restriction endonuclease cut sites remain the same regardless of any mutations.
   d. Heat or alkaline pH can convert single-stranded DNA to double-stranded DNA.

5. Which of the following assays is most appropriate for detecting a tumor-associated genetic defect that is present in only 0.1% of the cells in a patient sample? (Objective 8)
   a. polymerase chain reaction
   b. Southern blot analysis
   c. karyotype
   d. immunophenotype

6. Polymerase chain reaction (PCR) differs from reverse transcriptase PCR (rtPCR) in the following way(s): (Objectives 2, 8)
   a. Ribonucleotides rather than deoxyribonucleotides are added to the reaction mixture of rtPCR.
   b. Following amplification, PCR generates a DNA product whereas rtPCR generates an RNA product.
   c. RNA rather than DNA serves as the substrate for rtPCR.
   d. All of the above.

7. Immunoglobulin and T cell receptor gene rearrangement studies can be used to: (Objective 6)
   a. distinguish B cell leukemia from B cell lymphoma
   b. determine whether a lymphoid clone is present in a tissue specimen
   c. prove that a tissue sample is benign
   d. detect Epstein-Barr virus in a tissue specimen

8. Which of the following is true about the molecular genetics of cancer? (Objective 3)
   a. Virtually all cancers are thought to harbor genetic defects.
   b. DNA testing can be helpful in making a cancer diagnosis.
   c. The genes responsible for tumor formation are called oncogenes.
   d. All of the above.

9. Which of the following is true about the Southern blot procedure? (Objective 2)
   a. The patient's DNA is cut into fragments using proteinase enzymes.
   b. The electrophoresis step permits the probe to penetrate into the gel.
   c. The probe is labeled so that it can hybridize to its complementary strand.
   d. Interpretation of results relies on visualization of the band pattern.

10. Inherited diseases are characterized by: (Objective 4)
    a. defective DNA having no effect on gene structure or protein function
    b. acquired mutations that are detected only in diseased organs
    c. lack of correlation between genotype and disease status among family members
    d. a genetic defect that is generally present in all tissues of the patient's body

www.pearsonhighered.com/mckenzie
Use this address to access the interactive Companion Website created for this textbook. Find additional information, tables and figures. Evaluate your command of the chapter information using case studies and critical thinking and multiple choice questions.

REFERENCES

1. Butler JM. Genetics and genomics of core short tandem repeat loci used in human identity testing. *J Forensic Sci.* 2006;51:253–65.

2. Ensenauer RE, Reinke SS, Ackerman MJ, et. al. Primer on medical genomics. Part VIII: Essentials of medical genetics for the practicing physician. *Mayo Clin Proc.* 2003;78:846–57.

3. Ansell SM, Ackerman MJ, Black JL, et al. Primer on medical genomics. Part VI: Genomics and molecular genetics in clinical practice. *Mayo Clin Proc.* 2003;78:307–17.

4. Giardine B, van Baal S, Kaimakis P, et al. HbVar database of human hemoglobin variants and thalassemia mutations: 2007 update. *Hum Mutat.* 2007;28:206.

5. Gulley ML, Braziel RM, Halling KC, et al. Clinical laboratory reports in molecular pathology. *Arch Pathol Lab Med.* 2007;131:852–63.

6. Herrmann MG, Durtschi JD, Bromley LK, et al. Amplicon DNA melting analysis for mutation scanning and genotyping: Cross-platform comparison of instruments and dyes. *Clin Chem.* 2006;52: 494–503.

7. Castley A, Higgins M, Ivey J, et al. Clinical applications of whole-blood PCR with real-time instrumentation. *Clin Chem.* 2005;51: 2025–30.

8. Netto GJ, Saad RD. Diagnostic molecular pathology: An increasingly indispensable tool for the practicing pathologist. *Arch Pathol Lab Med.* 2006;130:1339–48.

9. Bustin SA, Mueller R. Real-time reverse transcription PCR (qRT-PCR) and its potential use in clinical diagnosis. *Clin Sci (Lond).* 2005; 109:365–79.

10. van der Velden VH, Hochhaus A, Cazzaniga G, et al. Detection of minimal residual disease in hematologic malignancies by real-time quantitative PCR: Principles, approaches, and laboratory aspects. *Leukemia.* 2003;17:1013–34.

11. Hughes T, Deininger M, Hochhaus A, et al. Monitoring CML patients responding to treatment with tyrosine kinase inhibitors: Review and recommendations for harmonizing current methodology for detecting *BCR-ABL* transcripts and kinase domain mutations and for expressing results. *Blood.* 2006;108:28–37.

12. Nashed AL, Rao KW, Gulley ML. Clinical applications of BCR-ABL molecular testing in acute leukemia. *J Mol Diagn.* 2003;5:63–72.

13. Westbrook CA, Hooberman AL, Spino C, et al. Clinical significance of the BCR-ABL fusion gene in adult acute lymphoblastic leukemia: A Cancer and Leukemia Group B Study (8762). *Blood.* 1992;80: 2983–90.

14. Lo-Coco F, Ammatuna E. Front line clinical trials and minimal residual disease monitoring in acute promyelocytic leukemia. *Curr Top Microbiol Immunol.* 2007;313:145–56.

15. Grimwade D, Lo Coco F. Acute promyelocytic leukemia: A model for the role of molecular diagnosis and residual disease monitoring in directing treatment approach in acute myeloid leukemia. *Leukemia.* 2002;16:1959–73.

16. Kearney L, Horsley SW. Molecular cytogenetics in haematological malignancy: current technology and future prospects. *Chromosoma.* 2005;114:286–94.

17. Lopez-Guillermo A, Cabanillas F, McLaughlin P, et al. Molecular response assessed by PCR is the most important factor predicting failure-free survival in indolent follicular lymphoma: Update of the MDACC series. *Annals of Oncology.* 2000;11:137–40.

18. Evans PA, Pott C, Groenen PJ, et al. Significantly improved PCR-based clonality testing in B-cell malignancies by use of multiple immunoglobulin gene targets. Report of the BIOMED-2 Concerted Action BHM4-CT98-3936. *Leukemia.* 2007;21:207–14.

19. Bruggemann M, White H, Gaulard P, et al. Powerful strategy for polymerase chain reaction-based clonality assessment in T-cell malignancies. Report of the BIOMED-2 Concerted Action BHM4 CT98-3936. *Leukemia.* 2007;21:215–21.

20. van Krieken JH, Langerak AW, Macintyre EA, et al. Improved reliability of lymphoma diagnostics via PCR-based clonality testing: Report of the BIOMED-2 Concerted Action BHM4-CT98-3936. *Leukemia.* 2007;21:201–6.

21. McClure RF, Kaur P, Pagel E, et al. Validation of immunoglobulin gene rearrangement detection by PCR using commercially available BIOMED-2 primers. *Leukemia.* 2006;20:176–79.

22. Cazzaniga G, Biondi A. Molecular monitoring of childhood acute lymphoblastic leukemia using antigen receptor gene rearrangements and quantitative polymerase chain reaction technology. *Haematologica.* 2005;90:382–90.

23. Espy MJ, Uhl JR, Sloan LM, et al. Real-time PCR in clinical microbiology: Applications for routine laboratory testing. *Clin Microbiol Rev.* 2006;19:165–256.

24. Yin CC, Jones D. Molecular approaches towards characterization, monitoring and targeting of viral-associated hematological malignancies. *Expert Rev Mol Diagn.* 2006;6:831–41.

25. Lee TH, Chafets DM, Busch MP, et al. Quantitation of HTLV-I and II proviral load using real-time quantitative PCR with SYBR Green chemistry. *J Clin Virol.* 2004;31:275–82.

26. Gulley ML, Glaser SL, Craig FE, et al. Guidelines for interpreting EBER in situ hybridization and LMP1 immunohistochemical tests for detecting Epstein-Barr virus in Hodgkin lymphoma. *Am J Clin Pathol.* 2002;117:259–67.

27. Fan H, Gulley ML. Epstein-Barr viral load measurement as a marker of EBV-related disease. *Mol Diagn.* 2001;6:279–89.

28. Cohen A, Wolf DG, Guttman-Yassky E, et al. Kaposi's sarcoma-associated herpesvirus: Clinical, diagnostic, and epidemiological aspects. *Crit Rev Clin Lab Sci.* 2005;42:101–53.

29. Fan JB, Chee MS, Gunderson KL. Highly parallel genomic assays. *Nat Rev Genet.* 2006;7:632–44.

40

Laboratory Testing in Coagulation

Carol Hillman-Wiseman, M.S.

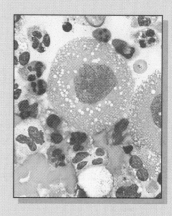

■ OBJECTIVES—LEVEL I

At the end of this unit of study, the student should be able to:

1. Describe special precautions to take regarding specimen collection and processing for coagulation studies, and determine specimen appropriateness.

2. State the principle of each test: bleeding time (BT), prothrombin time (PT), activated partial thromboplastin time (APTT), thrombin time (TT), fibrinogen assay, factor assays, fibrin degradation products (FDP), D-dimer assay, mixing studies.

3. Describe the procedure for determining the bleeding time (BT), prothrombin time (PT), activated partial thromboplastin time (APTT), thrombin time (TT), fibrinogen assay, fibrin degradation products (FDP) and D-dimer assay.

4. Explain the clinical significance of each test listed in Objective 2.

5. Identify the appropriate laboratory procedure for monitoring heparin therapy and oral anticoagulant therapy.

6. Describe the international normalized ratio (INR).

7. Calculate the INR given patient's prothrombin time (PT), mean normal PT, and international sensitivity index (ISI).

8. Interpret the results of routine coagulation testing (i.e., prothrombin time (PT), activated partial thromboplastin time (APTT), fibrinogen assay, thrombin time (TT), fibrinogen degradation products (FDP) and, D-dimer assay).

■ OBJECTIVES—LEVEL II

At the end of this unit of study, the student should be able to:

1. Correlate collection and processing procedures of the blood specimen with potential problems in coagulation testing.

2. Defend the use of 3.2% sodium citrate as an anticoagulant for coagulation studies.

3. State the principle and determine the appropriate utilization for each of the following tests: platelet aggregation studies, reptilase time, prekallikrein screening test, F-XIII screening test, von Willebrand factor activity assay, von Willebrand factor antigen immunoassay, platelet neutralization procedure (PNP), dilute Russell's viper venom time, lupus anticoagulants, F-VIII inhibitor assay, euglobulin lysis, antithrombin (AT), protein C (PC), protein S (PS), plasminogen, antiplasmin, activated protein C resistance (APCR), and F-Xa inhibition.

4. Describe the procedure for each test listed in Level II Objective 3.

■ OBJECTIVES—LEVEL II *(continued)*

5. Interpret results and explain the clinical significance of each test listed in Level II Objective 3.

6. Interpret a set of laboratory results, and suggest the appropriate follow-up or reflex test.

7. Select and defend the most appropriate laboratory tests to monitor anticoagulant therapy, interpret the results, and assess conditions that could affect these tests.

8. Project the potential use of molecular markers in the investigation of a hemostatic problem.

KEY TERMS

Aggregating reagent
Bioavailability
Chromogenic assay
Dilute Russell's viper venom time (dRVVT)
Enzyme-linked immunosorbent assay (ELISA)
Global testing
International normalized ratio (INR)
International sensitivity index (ISI)
Nomogram
Normal pooled plasma
Oral anticoagulant therapy
Pharmacokinetics
Platelet factor 4
Point of care (POC) instrument
Reference interval (RI)
Ristocetin
Ristocetin cofactor (RCoF) assay
Therapeutic range
von Willebrand factor activity (VWF:A)

BACKGROUND BASICS

The information in this chapter builds on the concepts learned in previous chapters. To maximize your learning experience, you should review these concepts before starting this unit of study.

Level I

▶ Describe the vascular contributions to hemostasis. (Chapter 29)

▶ Summarize the steps involved in the formation of the primary platelet plug. (Chapter 29)

▶ List the coagulation factors and the sequence of events involved in the coagulation cascade. (Chapter 30)

▶ Describe the biochemical inhibitors that regulate the coagulation cascade. (Chapter 30)

▶ List the factors and the sequence of events involved in fibrinolysis. (Chapter 30)

Level II

▶ Define the defect and identify the cause of impaired hemostasis in the following disorders of primary hemostasis: Bernard-Soulier syndrome, Glanzmann's thrombasthenia, drug-induced platelet disorders, and immune thrombocytopenic purpura. (Chapter 31)

▶ Define the defect and identify the cause of impaired hemostasis in the following inherited disorders of secondary hemostasis: von Willebrand disease, hemophilia A, and hemophilia B. (Chapter 32)

▶ Summarize the etiology and the pathophysiology of the acquired disorders of secondary hemostasis including disseminated intravascular coagulation, vitamin K deficiency, lupus-like anticoagulant (antiphospholipid antibody), and F-VIII inhibitor. (Chapter 32)

▶ Summarize the effect on the hemostatic system of factor V Leiden, protein C deficiency, antithrombin deficiency, and protein S deficiency. (Chapter 33)

► OVERVIEW

This chapter describes tests performed in the coagulation laboratory that are used to investigate a hemostatic disorder as indicated by either patient history or physical examination. Screening tests are used to place the defect in one of several broad categories followed by more specialized tests to establish a definitive diagnosis. Screening tests for defects of primary hemostasis include a platelet count and/or bleeding time; screening tests for defects of secondary hemostasis are generally the prothrombin time (PT) and the activated partial thromboplastin time (APTT). In some cases, screening tests are performed to assess the patient's hemostatic status before surgery.

Coagulation test results depend highly on the blood specimen's appropriateness and integrity. Thus, this chapter begins with a discussion of specimen collection and processing. The tests discussed are grouped according to the part of the coagulation system that they assess: primary hemostasis, secondary hemostasis, and fibrinolysis. One section of this chapter describes laboratory tests used to assess hypercoagulable states and monitor anticoagulant therapy. A general description of each test includes its theory, procedure summary, and expected results. A detailed procedure for selected tests can be found on the text's Companion Website, which can be downloaded for use in the laboratory component of a hemostasis class. The Website also contains a wealth of information on coagulation testing and refers the reader to other free information.

► INTRODUCTION

The clinical laboratory professional is an integral part of the medical team involved in the diagnosis of bleeding and clotting disorders. The more knowledgeable the individual, the more effectively he or she can interact with other team members to clarify items such as timing of blood draws, medication problems, and test results. The laboratory professional can sometimes solve the diagnostic coagulation mystery before the physician obtains the final results. Extensive knowledge of the physiology of hemostasis and coagulopathies (∞ Chapters 29–33) is needed to understand the testing for the coagulopathies and provide the best care possible for the patient.

A physician should use a stepwise approach (reflexive testing) to diagnose a bleeding problem. When laboratory professionals are aware of the testing sequence, they can assist in determining sample volumes needed for comprehensive testing and work with the physician to prioritize the testing sequence. The stepwise approaches for bleeding problems (Web Figure 32-2) and thrombophilia (Web Figure 33-1) allow the clinical laboratory professional to follow the progression of screening tests ordered according to the rationale as to which specific tests should constitute follow-up testing.

In addition to describing testing for the adult population, this chapter provides additional information for the pediatric population, which includes the newborn, infant, toddler, and children to age 17. Laboratories must be cognizant of the need for smaller sample size (blood sampling and testing) for this group of patients. Because congenital deficiencies are more likely to be discovered and diagnosed in the pediatric age group, tests must be sensitive to the very low levels of the constituent being measured.

The chapter emphasizes the technical information concerning the blood sample(s) needed for the particular test(s). There is a common phrase regarding coagulation: "The result is only as good as the sample." Therefore, to provide meaningful results, the laboratory professional must be knowledgeable in properly drawing, processing, and storing the sample. When the final results on a particular patient do not fit the criteria for reporting a specific result (e.g., duplicates cannot be averaged) or the summary of the test results is not logical, the laboratory professional should consider the sample itself and question its merit. Care should be taken to report only accurate results that reflect the patient's condition.

It is essential that each laboratory establish its own normal range for each coagulation test. The range provided by the commercial company can be a guideline, but every laboratory should do its own testing using normal adults (equal number of males and females) with its own instrument/reagent combination. These normal individuals must be questioned for their medical history: bleeding and/or clotting histories, medications taken (e.g., birth control pills), pregnancy, and bleeding from dental work. Unacceptable sources for normals include blood samples from individuals' pre-employment physicals, presurgery patients, and patients who have tested normal with existing reagents. Testing to establish normal ranges must also be performed over a sufficient number of days (>5 days) to account for the day-to-day variability seen in the specific testing being performed. If normal individuals are not available, commercial companies can provide frozen citrated plasma samples from individuals who have been prescreened (see Website).

Specialized testing can include functional and antigenic measurement of the constituent being evaluated. For available functional assays, the theory is described. The physician needs to know whether the constituent measured is functioning normally. The antigenic assay is performed to determine whether the protein concentration is abnormal. Occasionally, the antigenic assay is normal but the functional assay is abnormal. Historically, antigenic measurement has been available first (e.g., protein C, protein S) and used clinically until functional assays became available. Currently, however, the functional assay usually is ordered when testing for a specific hemostasis constituent. If this functional assay result is decreased and is consistent with the diagnosis, the physician might not request the antigenic determination.

Some tests described in this chapter are not available even in a large hospital setting with an extensive coagulation laboratory. These tests, however, are available from reference laboratories, and phlebotomists must properly collect the blood sample and carefully follow guidelines for transport to the testing site. Laboratory professionals must be familiar with these special assays (purpose, general technique, and details of the blood sample collection) to be able to assist the physician in ordering the correct test and determine when to draw the sample.

This book's Companion Website includes technical information for the clinical laboratory scientist (CLS) and clinical laboratory technician (CLT) working in a coagulation laboratory. The information is practical in nature and is included to improve coagulation testing. The figures and tables there can assist in modifying existing techniques and instituting new protocols (e.g., calculating F-VIII inhibitors, commercial sources of normal plasma for normal ranges).

▶ SPECIMEN COLLECTION AND PROCESSING

The accuracy of coagulation testing relies on properly collecting, processing, and storing the specimen, as discussed here. More technical information as noted is available on the Web.

SPECIMEN COLLECTION

A two-syringe or two-tube technique is preferable when collecting blood with a syringe or an evacuated tube system, with the blood from the second syringe or second tube used for the coagulation specimen.[1,2] This helps to minimize contamination of the sample from tissue factor during phlebotomy. If the second (or third tube) is the coagulation specimen, the prior tube(s) should not contain an anticoagulant or clot-promoting substance because of the possibility of carryover. When certain coagulation studies are requested or in cases of difficult phlebotomy, the two-syringe technique can be the appropriate option. The syringe is filled with sodium citrate so that the final ratio of citrate to blood is the same as in the evacuated tube system. After the sample is drawn, a small amount of air is allowed into the syringe, the needle discarded, and the syringe capped. The sample is then gently mixed to ensure the thorough mixing of citrate and blood. When platelet function testing is to be performed (see the Laboratory Investigation of Primary Hemostasis section), the syringe is the preferred method to obtain the specimen.

Butterfly needles (scalp vein 23 gauge needles with polystyrene tubing that can be attached to a syringe) are used for pediatric patients and with difficult phlebotomies.

When using butterfly needles the two-tube technique alleviates any problem of underfilling the citrate tube. The air in the tubing displaces an equivalent volume of blood in the first tube, causing the first tube not to fill to the proper level. There is no air in the tubing when the second tube is drawn so this tube fills to the proper level. A complete fill is essential to achieve the proper ratio of blood to anticoagulant in the citrate tube.

When drawing blood through an indwelling catheter, care must be taken to avoid heparin contamination of the sample. Heparin is used to keep the catheter line free flowing. To prevent contamination, the catheter line should be flushed with saline, and the first 5 mL (less volume in pediatric patients) of blood should be discarded. If the laboratory suspects heparin contamination of the sample, various commercial absorbants can be added to the plasma to remove the heparin (the absorbent capacity is 2 USP units of unfractionated heparin in 1 mL of citrated plasma)[3] (see Web) and the sample retested. This is a totally separate issue from the patient who is receiving heparin and needs to have the heparin level monitored.

Sodium citrate, 3.2%, is the anticoagulant of choice for coagulation studies.[4] The proper ratio of anticoagulant:whole blood is 1:9. This 3.2% concentration, as opposed to the 3.8% concentration that had been standard, alleviates the problems associated with excess citrate in samples having high hematocrits.[5] However, the Clinical Laboratory Standard Institute (CLSI) guideline recommends adjusting the amount of anticoagulant for the 3.2% concentration as well.[4] A higher hematocrit (>55%) has a smaller volume of plasma relative to the citrate anticoagulant, and the excess free citrate binds the calcium subsequently added in the testing procedure. If the citrate is not adjusted for blood collection, the sample will produce falsely prolonged clotting times because of inadequate recalcification. By adjusting the citrate concentration (lowering the citrate volume in the collection tube and redrawing from the patient), proper test results can be obtained (Web Figure 40-1 ■). Evacuated citrate tubes that draw volumes of 4.5 mL, 2.7 mL, and 1.8 mL are available. A 0.9 mL citrate tube can be prepared in-house for pediatric use and difficult draws if careful guidelines are followed.[6] (See Web.)

Obtaining the proper ratio of 1:9 (citrate:blood) is essential to obtain valid results. If the citrate tube is underfilled, too much calcium can be bound by the excess citrate during the testing procedure, and coagulation tests can be falsely prolonged (affecting the prothrombin time [PT] and the activated partial thromboplastin time [APTT] the most). If the citrate tube is overfilled, insufficient calcium can be bound, and clotting can occur in the tube (i.e., it would contain serum instead of plasma), producing falsely prolonged results as occur in a consumptive coagulopathy.

Accurate labeling of the citrated blood samples is critical (i.e., pre- or postinfusion, time of draw). The coagulation testing can be used to calculate a response to the administration of a specific factor concentrate, establish the baseline level of a factor, or determine which sample of a number of blood draws for the same patient is to be used for each particular test. (See the later section on specific factor inhibitor assay.)

The interactions of the laboratory staff with the health care team are important for obtaining a sample at the proper time. It is beneficial to check the status of the patient's history of receiving blood products because if testing is done within the half-life of the administered clotting factor or platelet products, the tests could measure the transfused component as well as the patient's component. Certain fibrinolytic factors have diurnal variability; therefore, each laboratory needs guidelines on when to draw these samples (see Web, PAI-1). Before performing platelet function testing, the ordering physician, nursing, or laboratory staff must thoroughly question patients regarding medications because some affect the testing for the life of the platelet (7–10 days) (see Web).

SPECIMEN PROCESSING

To obtain plasma for coagulation testing, citrated whole blood is centrifuged. Depending on the test, either platelet-poor or platelet-rich plasma can be required. Properly processing the sample is required to obtain reliable results.

Platelet-Poor Plasma

To obtain platelet-poor plasma (PPP), the citrated specimen is centrifuged for 15 minutes at $2500 \times g$. PPP must have $<10 \times 10^9$/L platelets. Depending on the coagulation instrumentation used, the separated plasma can either be left on top of the packed cells or removed using a plastic pipette and placed in a capped plastic tube. When removing the PPP, leaving a small amount of it on the surface of the packed cells is critical. This ensures that the platelet layer is undisturbed and that platelets have not been resuspended in what should be PPP.

The use of PPP is essential for three technical reasons. One is that platelets contain **platelet factor 4** (PF4), which neutralizes heparin (thus affecting sample's testing for the presence of heparin). Second, platelets contain phospholipids, which affect lupus anticoagulant testing and factor assay testing (especially if the sample is frozen and thawed). Third, platelets contain proteases, which, when released during the thawing of a frozen sample, alter results for von Willebrand factor testing.

A clot of any size in the sample renders it unacceptable. Therefore, after removing the PPP, a wooden applicator stick is twirled into the packed cells to assure that no clot is present. If numerous tests are ordered using the same sample, various aliquots can be prepared and frozen so that on successive days a freshly thawed sample can be tested. The separated plasma can be stored at 18–24°C or 2–8°C for up to 4 hours before testing. If the testing cannot be completed within the 4 hours, the PPP should be stored at −20°C for up to 1 week or −70°C for up to 6 months. Frozen samples must be thawed rapidly at 37°C because excessive heating (>5 minutes) can result in the loss of factor V and F-VIII. Sam-

ples for coagulation testing should never be stored in self-defrosting freezers, because the freeze-thaw cycles will compromise sample integrity.

Specialized testing (e.g., fibrinolytic and thrombotic assays, PF4, β-TG, fibrinopeptide 1+2, tPA), even if not being performed in one's own laboratory, has numerous requirements for processing the sample.[7] Each laboratory must have procedures available for properly handling the citrated sample to ensure valid results when it is sent to reference laboratories.

Platelet-Rich Plasma

Platelet-rich plasma (PRP) is obtained to perform studies of platelet function. If the sample has been drawn into a citrated syringe, the needle should be removed and the sample gently expelled down the side of a polystyrene test tube, capped, and then centrifuged for 10 minutes at $200 \times g$ at room temperature. The PRP should be removed from the packed cells carefully using a plastic pipette and placed in a covered polystyrene tube. PRP usually contains $200–300 \times 10^9$/L platelets. PRP can be stored at room temperature, and testing should be completed within 3 hours.

Citrated Whole Blood

For testing that requires citrated whole blood, the sample is drawn as previously described. This sample type can be used for platelet function testing (i.e., platelet function analyzer [PFA], whole blood aggregation, or one of the global tests of coagulation, such as thromboelastograph [TEG]). To check for clots, the citrated tube or syringe should be carefully scrutinized while mixing, and a wooden applicator stick should be inserted *after* testing has been completed to verify that no clot existed. Because platelets can be activated by foreign surfaces, the sample should not be checked for a clot with the wooden applicator before testing has been completed.

 Checkpoint! 1

Why have most clinical laboratories switched from 3.8% to 3.2% sodium citrate for specimen collection in coagulation studies?

▶ LABORATORY INVESTIGATION OF PRIMARY HEMOSTASIS

Laboratory testing to evaluate primary hemostasis includes tests for platelet concentration and function. The platelet count is described in ∞ Chapter 34. In testing for platelet function, the clinical laboratory scientist must be aware that a wide variety of drugs can affect platelet function for the entire life span of the platelet (7–10 days).[8,9] Each laboratory should have a list of such drugs available so that an extensive platelet function workup is not performed unnecessarily (Web Tables 40-1 ✪, 40-2 ✪, 40-3 ✪). Stress also affects the platelet release reaction.[10] Repeat testing is advisable for abnormal results.

Screening tests for platelet function include the bleeding time (BT) and in vitro testing using the platelet function analyzer (PFA).[11] Definitive testing for platelet function includes PRP and/or whole blood platelet aggregation.

Platelet aggregation depends on the presence of Ca^{2+}. Although sodium citrate binds calcium, the concentration of Ca^{2+} remaining after anticoagulation is sufficient to permit aggregation to occur. Blood drawn in 3.2% sodium citrate shows stronger aggregation than blood collected in 3.8%, presumably due to the increased availability of Ca^{2+}. Therefore, if the normal range is established using 3.2% citrate, all patients must be drawn using that concentration.

Additional testing for platelet function can include flow cytometry and clot retraction. Acquired states of thrombocytopenia such as heparin-induced thrombocytopenia (HIT) and neonatal alloimmune thrombocytopenia (NAIT) require specific testing (∞ Chapters 31 and 33).

BLEEDING TIME

BT is an in vivo measurement of platelet function. In addition to platelet function, the BT is also affected by platelet number and vascular integrity (∞ Chapter 29). The BT measures the time required for bleeding to cease from a superficial skin cut. The testing depends on the temperature; amount of pressure applied to the arm; depth, location, and direction of the incision; movement of the arm (especially wiggling in young children); and the clinical laboratory professional's experience.

Several methods have been used over the years to determine the bleeding time. The oldest method, the Duke bleeding time, utilized a lancet to make a puncture in the ear lobe. In 1941, Ivy improved the BT technique by creating a constant venous pressure with a blood pressure cuff (40 mmHg) and performing the test on the forearm with a lancet. The variability in making the incision has been minimized by using a disposable bleeding time device. The most widely used method today is the modified Ivy BT using a template. Templates for this test are commercially available as sterile disposable devices that use a spring-loaded blade designed to make a skin incision of standard depth and width on the forearm. The general **reference interval** for the BT is 1–9 minutes.[12,13] When screening for von Willebrand's disease (VWD), patients with **von Willebrand factor activity (VWF:A)** >30% generally have normal BT results.[13] The Web describes the BT in detail. Patients with platelet counts <100,000 × 10^9/L usually have a prolonged BT. See Table 40-1 ✪ for conditions associated with prolonged BT (∞ Chapter 31).

PLATELET FUNCTION ANALYZER

The PFA in vitro method for assessing and screening for platelet function is a more standardized technique, eliminat-

---

✪ TABLE 40-1

Conditions Associated with a Prolonged Bleeding Time

- von Willebrand disease
- Bernard-Soulier syndrome
- Glanzmann's thrombasthenia
- Congenital storage pool disease
- Afibrinogenemia
- Severe hypofibrinogenemia
- Certain vascular bleeding disorders such as Ehlers-Danlos syndrome
- Uremia
- Acquired platelet function defects (drug induced)

---

ing the variables discussed with the BT (Web Figure 40-2 ■). The assay measures platelet function in whole blood at a high shear rate. This test adds citrated blood to each of two reservoirs, one with collagen/epinephrine and the other with collagen/adenosine disphosphate (ADP). The instrument aspirates whole blood through a capillary with a 150 μM aperture of a bioactive membrane coated with either collagen/epinephrine or collagen/adenosine diphosphate (ADP). A pressure sensor detects the formation of a platelet plug. The time to occlude the aperture (the "closure time") is a function of platelet count, platelet activity, VWF activity, and hematocrit. This method is sensitive to VWD, aspirin-induced platelet dysfunction, and aggregation defects (all resulting in prolonged or abnormal closure times). A reference range is established for each reservoir using a standardized blood-drawing technique (size of needle, citrate concentration).[11,14]

The expected results with the PFA are:

Condition Reservoir	Normal	Acetyl-salicylic acid (ASA)	VWD	Glanzmann's Thrombasthenia
COL/EPI	Normal	Abnormal	Abnormal	Abnormal
COL/ADP	Normal	Normal	Abnormal	Abnormal

PLATELET AGGREGOMETRY

Platelet aggregation studies are the foundation of platelet function testing in the laboratory. Platelet aggregometry is a challenging technique usually performed in specialized laboratories by experienced laboratory professionals. The testing is time consuming and requires attention to detail regarding sample collection (choice of anticoagulant, check of patient drug history), processing the sample and reagents, pH, time of storage, rate of stirring, and platelet count. A citrated sample is collected and can be used for whole blood testing (measuring luminescence and impedance) or centrifuged slowly for PRP to determine percent aggregation and the curves that are produced (Web Figure 40-3 ■).

Normal Platelet Aggregation Curves

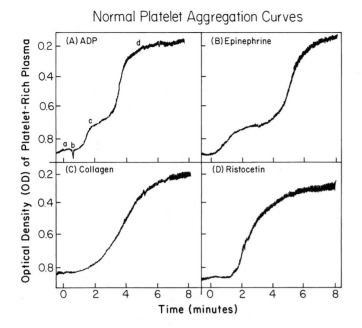

■ **FIGURE 40-1**   Normal platelet aggregation curves. Normal responses to the commonly used aggregating reagents: ADP, epinephrine, collagen, ristocetin. **a.** Baseline before addition of the reagent; **b.** Initial increase in absorbance that occurs immediately following the addition of reagent, representing a change in platelet shape; **c.** the primary wave of aggregation; **d.** secondary wave of aggregation.

Platelet-Rich Plasma (PRP) Aggregation

PRP is carefully prepared from a citrated blood sample by adjusting the platelet count with the patient's own PPP to a standard number (usually 200,000/μL). The sample is stirred, warmed to 37°C in a special photometric device (an aggregometer), and an **aggregating reagent** (agonist) is added. In the presence of the agonist, the platelets begin to aggregate which leads to a change in optical density (OD) of the PRP that the aggregometer records as a graph (curve). Commonly used platelet agonists include ADP, epinephrine, collagen, ristocetin, and arachidonic acid.

Depending on the agonist used and its concentration, a primary and/or secondary wave of aggregation occurs (see Figure 40-1 ■). The primary wave reflects the direct response of the platelets to the aggregating reagent and represents platelet shape change and the formation of small aggregates. The secondary wave represents the complete aggregation response, which occurs as a result of endogenous ADP being released from the activated platelet dense bodies. An aggregating reagent that results in both a primary and secondary wave is said to produce a *biphasic curve*, whereas an aggregating reagent that results in only one wave is said to produce a *monophasic curve*. Changes in platelet aggregation curves are interpreted to identify qualitative platelet disorders (Table 40-2 ✪) (∞ Chapter 31).

✪ TABLE 40-2

Typical Pattern of Response to Aggregating Reagents in Qualitative Platelet Disorders*

Qualitative Platelet Disorders	Aggregating Reagents				
	Collagen	ADP	Epinephrine	Ristocetin	Arachidonic Acid
Normal	Monophasic curve (secondary wave only) representing secondary platelet aggregation associated with release of endogenous ADP	Biphasic curve with 2×10^{-5} M ADP—demonstrating primary and secondary waves of platelet aggregation	Biphasic curve—demonstrating primary and secondary waves of platelet aggregation	Biphasic curve—primary wave resulting from immediate platelet agglutination; secondary wave associated with platelet release induced by platelet agglutination	Monophasic curve (secondary wave only) representing effect of thromboxane A_2 on secondary platelet aggregation
von Willebrand disease	Normal	Normal	Normal	No response	†
Bernard-Soulier syndrome	Normal	Normal	Normal	No response	†
Glanzmann's thrombasthenia	No response	No response	No response	Normal	†
Storage pool disease	No response	Primary wave only	Primary wave only	Normal	Normal
Aspirin ingestion	No response	Primary wave only	Primary wave only	Normal	Suppressed response

*Chapter 31. † Not applicable. Arachidonic acid evaluates the thromboxane A_2 synthetic pathway.

Aggregating reagents produce typical aggregation patterns (Figure 40-1).[15] **Ristocetin** is unique among the agonists in that its action depends on the interaction of plasma VWF and the platelet membrane receptor glycoprotein Ib (GPIb/IX) and technically represents platelet agglutination rather than aggregation (∞ Chapter 29). See the Website for additional information on using lower concentrations of ristocetin to aid in the diagnosis of type IIb VWD (∞ Chapter 32) and Web Figure 40-4 ■. Although ristocetin-induced platelet agglutination (RIPA) can be abnormal in both VWD and Bernard-Soulier syndrome (BSS, a defect of GPIb/IX), plasma ristocetin cofactor activity (VWF:A, discussed later) is usually decreased in VWD but is normal in BSS. Additionally, the RIPA defect observed in VWD can be corrected by adding normal plasma to the patient's PRP because the defect is a deficiency of a plasma protein, not of the platelets. The agglutination defect in BSS is not corrected because it is due to a deficiency of the GPIb/IX complex on the patient's platelet membrane and is not corrected by the addition of normal plasma.

Arachidonic acid (AA) is useful to screen for a patient's ingestion of aspirin or any aspirin-containing products within the previous 7–10 days. This screening can help clarify results when the PRP produces no secondary wave of aggregation with ADP or epinephrine. Platelet release defects or storage pool disease (∞ Chapter 31), which produce results with ADP and epinephrine similar to those seen with aspirin ingestion, can be differentiated by using AA (Table 40-2, Figure 40-2 ■).

Decreasing concentrations of epinephrine, which produce aggregation of patient PRP but not normal control PRP, have been used to diagnose "sticky platelet syndrome" (Web Figure 40-5 ■), a term adopted by E.F. Mammen to describe patients with unexplained arterial vascular occlusions who had platelet hyper-responsiveness to low doses of ADP and/or epinephrine.[16] (See Website.) The precise etiology of this syndrome is presently not known, but abnormal receptors on the platelet surface may be involved. Normal plasma levels of PF4 and beta-thromboglobulin (βTG) suggest that the platelets are not activated at all times. This test is not sensitive for demonstrating this syndrome in pediatric populations.[17]

Aggregometers now have the ability to measure adenosine triphosphate (ATP) secreted from dense granules in PRP and whole blood samples. The luminescence produced improves the diagnosis of storage pool disease because an actual amount of ATP, which is directly proportional to the dense granule content, is measured. This is more accurate than evaluating whether the platelet aggregation curve produced is biphasic.[18,19,20] (See Website Additional Information: Platelet Aggregation Testing.)

Whole Blood Aggregation

The use of whole blood aggregation (Web Figure 40-3) allows for a smaller sample size than is used in PRP aggregation to evaluate platelet function and is a quicker analytic method because PRP does not have to be prepared. However, there also is no standardization of the platelet count because the sample and the control are diluted in saline. The whole blood assay measures electrical resistance across two metal wires (probes). The whole blood sample is initially exposed to a small electric current that coats wires with a monolayer of platelets. Upon the addition of an agonist, platelets form aggregates on the monolayer, adding electrical resistance (ohms) to the circuit. The change in impedance is measured as a function of time. The citrated sample is challenged with ADP, collagen, and thrombin. The use of the agonist thrombin allows for the determination of the content of the dense granules. Thrombin causes dense granules to release ATP, so this testing can efficiently assess whether the patient has δ-storage pool disease. With certain instruments, the sample can also be evaluated for luminescence as was done with PRP.[18]

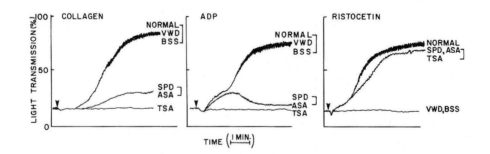

■ FIGURE 40-2   Platelet aggregation patterns in various disorders. Typical tracings obtained using concentrations of collagen, ADP, and ristocetin illustrate the differences between platelet aggregation in normal subjects and that in patients with von Willebrand's disease (VWD), Bernard Soulier syndrome (BSS), thrombasthenia (TSA), storage-pool disease (SPD), and aspirin ingestion and aspirin-like disorders (ASA). Impaired release of ADP accounts for the SPD and ASA defects. VWF corrects the defective ristocetin aggregation in VWD but not in BSS.

ADDITIONAL TESTS EVALUATING PLATELET FUNCTION

Flow Cytometry

New approaches for laboratory diagnosis of the platelet disorders BSS (GPIb/IX deficiency) and Glanzmann's thrombasthenia (GPIIb/IIIa complex deficiency) involve flow cytometry using monoclonal antibodies directed against the platelets' respective glycoproteins. A panel of antibodies that recognize the resting, activated, and ligand-occupied forms of the GPIIb/IIIa complex has been developed.[21] Thus, both the presence and the functional activity of this complex can be measured. Testing can also be performed to evaluate the presence of circulating activated platelets to aid in diagnosing thrombotic syndromes. This specialized testing requires much expertise.[18]

Clot Retraction

The physiologic phenomenon of clot retraction has been described in ∞ Chapter 29. The clot retraction test is performed on blood without anticoagulant. A 1 mL sample of whole blood is placed in a glass tube in a water bath at 37°C and observed for 1–3 hours. Normal blood should clot and begin to retract 30–60 minutes after collection. Retraction should normally occur except in cases of Glanzmann's thrombasthenia, severe hypofibrinogenemia, and thrombocytopenia. To remove the variables of platelet count and fibrinogen level, a PRP retraction can be performed (with a control PRP tested as well). A volume of PRP, APTT reagent, and Ca^{2+} are added in a graduated glass test tube to produce a volume of 1.0 cc. A wooden stick is inserted into the mixture, mixed, and again placed in a 37°C water bath. After 1 hour, the stick is gently removed; the clotted and retracted platelets and fibrin will be attached to it. The test is quantitated by determining the serum remaining in the graduated tube. In Glanzmann's thrombasthenia, there is little or no retraction of the clot; therefore, very little serum is present after removal of the stick.[22]

ACQUIRED STATES OF THROMBOCYTOPENIA

Heparin-Induced Thrombocytopenia (HIT)

Historically, a functional heparin-platelet aggregation assay using normal platelets and the patient's serum was used to screen for HIT. In the presence of HIT immunoglobulins in the patient's plasma, the normal platelets are activated when the heparin used for treatment was added to the PRP. The procedure was time consuming and often resulted in false negatives. The current gold standard for the diagnosis of HIT is a platelet ^{14}C serotonin release assay whose complexity limits its availability to reference laboratories. An **enzyme-linked immunosorbent assay (ELISA)** for detecting antibodies against heparin-PF4 complexes (∞ Chapter 33) is also available. The results obtained with the serotonin release assay and ELISA are generally in agreement in patients with a clinical diagnosis of HIT. However, the ELISA detects antiheparin antibodies in patients who do not have heparin-

induced thrombocytopenia, therefore possibly producing false-positive results if being used to diagnose HIT.[23]

Neonatal Alloimmune Thrombocytopenia (NAIT or NATP)

Neonatal alloimmune thrombocytopenia (NAIT) (∞ Chapter 31) is a syndrome causing transient, isolated, sometimes severe thrombocytopenia in newborns. NAIT results from placental transfer of maternal alloantibodies directed against paternally inherited antigens present on the fetal platelets but absent from maternal platelets. This condition is the platelet counterpart of hemolytic disease of the newborn. NAIT diagnosis is confirmed by serologic or genotypic testing including immunophenotyping of maternal and paternal platelets. The maternal serum also is examined for the presence of antiplatelet antibody. Because of the complexity of this testing, it is usually performed in large reference laboratories or specialized coagulation centers.[23]

 Checkpoint! 2

What effect does aspirin taken daily for a heart condition have on a patient's bleeding time? Explain.

▶ LABORATORY INVESTIGATION OF SECONDARY HEMOSTASIS

Laboratory tests of secondary hemostasis evaluate coagulation factors and inhibitors. The testing of patients for secondary hemostasis starts with screening tests. Following the reflexive chart for guidelines for evaluating bleeding diathesis (Web Figure 32-2), the physician can order the appropriate definitive tests leading to the proper diagnosis. Laboratory professionals should be familiar with the reflexive testing found in the chart. They are occasionally asked to guide the physician who may be unclear concerning which test is most appropriate. The following section includes technical information to help understand the variability within each assay. The ∞ Chapter 40 Website should also be consulted for methodologies, quality control, pediatric considerations, and expanded coverage of the topics.

SCREENING TESTS

The screening tests include the PT, APTT, thrombin time (TT), and quantitative fibrinogen. Abnormalities in any of these tests require further testing. The battery of reflex testing is based on the results of the screening tests (Web Figure 32-2). Poor blood sample integrity can unnecessarily cost time and expense investigating a possible bleeding or clotting disorder.

Prothrombin Time

The PT is an important screening test for the laboratory evaluation of patients with inherited or acquired deficiencies in the extrinsic or common pathway of the coagulation cascade. Historically, it has also been used to monitor oral anticoagulant therapy. In vivo, tissue factor (TF) activates the coagulation cascade via the formation of the TF/F-VIIa complex.[24] In the PT test thromboplastin (TF/calcium mixture) is added to a citrated patient PPP or control PPP, and the time for fibrin formation is recorded. This test is the basis for determining the PT. Numerous commercial sources of thromboplastins (most commonly rabbit brain) are available; they vary in sensitivity to coagulation factor deficiencies. Variabilities result from differences in animal and tissue sources, as well as the method of reagent preparation. Each laboratory must establish its own reference interval (RI) for its reagent/instrument combination.

The procedure for establishing a specific reagent/instrument RI and technical information are on the text's Companion Website. Clot formation can be detected by optical or electromechanical methods using manual, semiautomated, or automated devices. The general reference interval for the PT is 10–13 seconds. See Web Table 40-4 ☉ for potential sources of error for procedures based on clot formation. The PT can be prolonged because of either a deficiency of factors VII, X, V, II (prothrombin), fibrinogen; or the presence of an inhibitor.[22] (Historically the test was called the *prothrombin time* because Professor Armand Quick thought that the test measured only prothrombin.) The PT can be shortened in patients receiving treatment with recombinant factor VIIa concentrate (rF-VIIa), which has been used to produce hemostasis in hemophiliac patients with high-responding inhibitors.[25] As increased levels of rF-VIIa are infused, F-VIIa interacts with TF at the site of vascular injury, activating F-X, which in turn shortens the PT.

The PT is also used to monitor patients on oral anticoagulant therapy (coumadin or warfarin [∞ Chapters 30, 33]). Because of the wide variability among the various PT reagents and instrumentations, the results are usually reported using the international normalized ratio (INR). The PT of a patient on oral anticoagulation is inserted into a formula, which includes the manufacturer's international sensitivity index (ISI) value for its particular thromboplastin. The outcome of this mathematical calculation, the INR, is discussed later in this chapter (Oral Anticoagulant Therapy and the PT). Many current commercial thromboplastins use a recombinant TF and synthetic phospholipids with Ca^{2+}. The goal in making commercial thromboplastins is to obtain a reagent that has an ISI of 1.0 (or close to it). With lower ISI values (the closer to 1.0), the calculation of the INR of a patient being tested in any location worldwide becomes much more reproducible (minimizing interlaboratory and intralaboratory variability). The lot-to-lot variability of the recombinant reagent is believed to be less than that obtained with products prepared from biologic sources. Most recombinant products are associated with a greater prolongation of PT results in patient samples than biologic products.

The same reagent is used for testing patients on oral anticoagulant therapy and patients for specific factor deficiencies. For patients not on oral anticoagulant therapy, usually only the actual PT (in seconds) is reported (the INR value has no additional clinical value).

Prolongation of the PT is also seen with proteins induced by vitamin K-absence or antagonism (PIVKA [∞ Chapter 30]). Factors II, VII, IX, X, protein C, and protein S are vitamin K–dependent coagulation factors. Hepatic production of these proteins in the absence of vitamin K or with vitamin K antagonism (warfarin therapy), dietary deficiency of vitamin K, some types of liver dysfunction, and certain genetic abnormalities (∞ Chapter 32) results in proteins referred to as *PIVKA*. These proteins are immunologically similar to the naturally occurring factors but are dysfunctional because they lack the γ-carboxyglutamic acid residues required for Ca^{2+} and phospholipid binding during clotting. The proteins are also termed non- or descarboxylated proteins. Because PIVKAs lack normal coagulant activity, a prolonged PT results. The testing for PIVKA is by ELISA and is performed only at centralized reference laboratories.[7]

Activated Partial Thromboplastin Time

The APTT is an important screening test for the laboratory evaluation of patients with inherited or acquired deficiencies of proteins in the intrinsic or common pathway of the coagulation cascade. The APTT also can be used as a screening test for the detection of circulating inhibitors of blood coagulation (lupus anticoagulants) (∞ Chapters 30, 32, 33).

The sensitivity of the various commercial APTT reagents to factor deficiencies and to lupus anticoagulants varies greatly. Therefore, each laboratory has to decide which APTT reagent to use depending on its individual needs. The screening tests (PT and APTT) detect a factor deficiency only when the factor decreases to a level of 25–40% of normal (depending on the reagent). A laboratory that wants to determine the sensitivity of its reagent to a particular factor can perform its own evaluation for factor sensitivity.[26] In general, most commercial APTT reagents have good sensitivity for F-VIII deficiency, but their sensitivity for F-IX deficiency is more variable.[27,28,29]

The APTT remains the most common procedure used to monitor the effectiveness of standard (unfractionated) heparin therapy. (See the section on Laboratory Evaluation of Anticoagulant Therapy later in this chapter.) The APTT uses two reagents: an activated partial thromboplastin and Ca^{2+}. The partial thromboplastin reagent simulates activated platelet surfaces by providing phospholipid surfaces on which enzymatic reactions in the coagulation cascade can occur, plus an activator (kaolin, celite, micronized celite, or ellagic acid) that provides the negatively charged surface for the activation of F-XII.[27] After a specific incubation time of citrated plasma (control or patient) with the APTT reagent which allows optimum activation of the contact factors, calcium chloride is added, and the time required for a fibrin clot to form is recorded. Details of this procedure are provided on the text's Companion Website. Clot formation can be detected by optical or electromechanical methods using manual, semiautomated, or automated devices. The general reference interval for adults is 28–35 seconds. See ∞ Chapter 32, Table 32-12, for normal ranges for preterm and term infants.

The APTT also evaluates prekallikrein (PK) and high molecular weight kininogen (HK). Deficiency of F-XII, PK, or HK can result in a markedly prolonged APTT in the absence of clinically significant bleeding.

✓ Checkpoint! 3

Routine coagulation testing was performed on a properly collected and processed specimen. The PT result was prolonged, but APTT was normal. What is the best interpretation of these results?

Thrombin Time

TT has an important role as a screening test because it measures the conversion of fibrinogen to fibrin by adding excess thrombin to undiluted plasma. Because the additional clotting factors previously measured in the PT and APTT have no effect on this test, TT is generally useful for evaluating other parameters affecting the formation of fibrin. There can be interference with the conversion of fibrinogen to fibrin for three major reasons: the presence of hypofibrinogenemia or dysfibrinogenemia (∞ Chapter 32), the presence of heparin, and the presence of fibrin degradation products (FDP). In rare cases, autoantibodies against thrombin (e.g., induced by topical thrombin application or the use of fibrin sealants) and myeloma proteins can also interfere with fibrin formation and result in an abnormal TT.[30] The TT is useful in corroborating an abnormal FDP result and can verify that the citrated blood sample was drawn through an indwelling heparinized catheter that was not well flushed. An extremely prolonged TT usually indicates a heparin effect. If the sample is contaminated with heparin, it can be absorbed with Hepzyme (see Specimen Processing and Website). The testing can then be repeated, or the specimen can be redrawn.

The basic procedure is described on the Web. The general reference interval for the TT is 10–16 seconds. TT's sensitivity can be increased by diluting the thrombin reagent to give a control of 16–18 seconds. The TT in preterm and term infants is longer than the adult reference interval even though the fibrinogen level is within the same normal reference interval (∞ Chapter 32, Table 32-12), which can be explained by the presence of a distinct fetal fibrinogen molecule with altered function. The TT generally becomes normal within a few days after birth.

Quantitative Fibrinogen

Several methods have been used to determine the fibrinogen concentration including turbidimetric precipitation or denaturation methods with some instrumentation calculating a result derived from the slope of the PT. The reference method for fibrinogen determination is the Clauss assay, which is a clot-based functional measurement that adds

thrombin to various dilutions of known concentrations of fibrinogen (reference plasma or calibrator) to produce a thrombin-clotting time in seconds. The clotting times are then plotted on a log/log graph (reference curve), with known concentrations on the x-axis versus clotting time (TT) on the y-axis (Figure 40-3 ■). Thrombin clotting times are performed using appropriate controls (normal and abnormal) and the patient PPP at a 1:10 dilution. The fibrinogen concentration is inversely proportional to the clotting time. If fibrinogen levels are low, more concentrated (i.e., less dilute) dilutions of patient plasma (1:5 or 1:2) are prepared so that fibrinogen can be accurately determined using the reference curve with the result divided by 2 (if a 1:5 dilution) or 5 (if a 1:2 dilution). FDPs do not affect the assay at the normal 1:10 dilution but can when the dilution is lower (i.e., 1:5 or 1:2). The fibrinogen results for the controls and the patient are determined from the reference curve using their respective clotting times. Additional technical information can be found on the Website. In general, the reference interval for fibrinogen (adults and the pediatric population) is 200–400 mg/dL (Chapter 32, Table 32-13).

Decreased levels of fibrinogen occur in acquired disorders such as disseminated intravascular coagulation (DIC), primary and secondary fibrinolysis, liver disease, and congenital disorders such as dysfibrinogenemia and hereditary afibrinogenemia (∞ Chapter 32). When an abnormal fibrinogen is suspected, an antigenic (immunological) test is performed. Increased levels of fibrinogen can occur in inflammatory disorders and pregnancy, and in women receiving oral contraceptives because fibrinogen is an acute phase reactant protein.

TESTS TO IDENTIFY SPECIFIC FACTOR DEFICIENCY

When the PT and/or APTT is prolonged, further testing can be performed to identify the specific cause of the abnormality. To assist in deciding which specific tests should be performed after the screening tests, the reflexive testing in Web Figure 32-2 can be followed. As each of the following specific tests is described, its sensitivity(ies) to decreased levels of clotting factor(s) and whether these levels would be detected in the specific screening test are discussed.

Mixing Studies

Mixing studies (also known as *circulating anticoagulant screen* or *screening test for circulating inhibitor*) are performed to differentiate a factor deficiency from the presence of a circulating inhibitor.[22,31] These studies repeat the screening tests with abnormal results (PT, APTT) using several different dilutions of the patient's PPP mixed with a **normal pooled plasma** (Web Table 40-5 ✪). Because factor levels of ~50% of normal are generally sufficient to produce a normal PT and APTT result, repeating the PT and APTT with dilutions of patient and normal plasmas corrects the prolonged patient result if it is caused by a deficiency of one or more procoagulant factors.

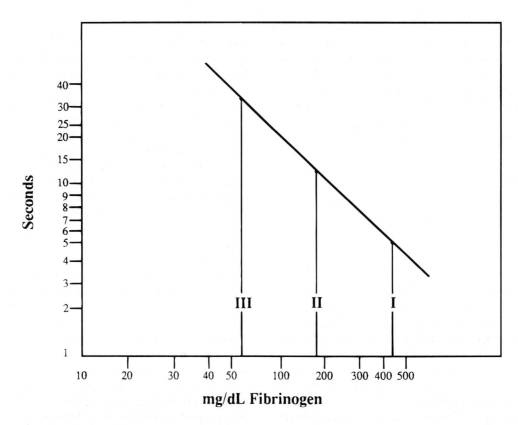

■ FIGURE 40-3   Fibrinogen standard curve. I, II, and III represent reference plasmas of known fibrinogen concentrations. The thrombin time in seconds is on the y-axis, and the fibrinogen concentration in mg/dL is on the x-axis.

The testing is performed immediately and then again after the incubation of the mixture of the patient's PPP and the normal plasma at 37°C. (See the Website Mixing Study for detailed procedures and comprehensive technical information.)

The clotting times for the various dilutions and time intervals are compared to determine whether the patient's prolonged clotting time has been corrected by the addition of normal plasma. Clotting times tend to increase with time and incubation due to the loss of labile factors (F-V and F-VIII); therefore, comparing the patient's diluted sample result with the result obtained from the normal pooled plasma is important. A clotting time is considered prolonged if it is longer than the normal plasma clotting time. The correction of the prolonged test result (PT/APTT) by the normal plasma (Table 40-3 ✪) indicates a factor deficiency. The normal plasma replenishes the deficient factor in the patient's plasma. If a factor deficiency is detected, specific factor assays should be performed to identify and quantitate the specific factor's activity.

The lack of correction of the prolonged test by normal plasma indicates the presence of a circulating or a specific factor inhibitor. A circulating inhibitor inhibits both the coagulation factors in the patient plasma and in the normal plasma with which it is mixed. The detection of a circulating inhibitor (e.g., lupuslike anticoagulant) should be followed by specific tests to identify and verify the type of inhibitor.

✪ TABLE 40-3

Differentiation of Factor Deficiency from Circulating Inhibitors Using the Mixing Study Procedure

Deficiency or Inhibitor	Mixing Study	
	Immediate PT or APTT after Mixing	Mix, Perform PT or APTT after 2-hr Incubation at 37°C
Factor deficiency	Correction	Correction
Lupuslike anticoagulant	No correction	No correction
F-VIII inhibitor	Correction	No correction

Some patient plasmas contain time- and temperature-dependent inhibitors and exhibit correction immediately after mixing them with normal pooled plasma; however, after incubation, the clotting time result is prolonged (Table 40-3). These inhibitors are called *slow acting*, and are characteristic of certain F-VIII inhibitors. These slow-acting, specific inhibitors can be quantitated by performing the F-VIII inhibitor assay (Bethesda assay; see Tests to Evaluate Specific Factor Deficiency). Lupus-like anticoagulants tend to act immediately but are occasionally time dependent.

✓ Checkpoint! 4

Given the following coagulation test results, what is the appropriate follow-up or reflex test?

PT	*Normal*
APTT	*Prolonged*
Mixing studies	*No correction*

Specific Coagulation Factors

Factor assays are performed to confirm a specific factor deficiency and to determine the actual activity of that factor within the plasma. The basis of a factor assay is the ability of the patient's plasma to correct a prolonged PT or APTT of a known factor-deficient plasma (substrate).[32]

Each clotting factor in the extrinsic (F-VII) and common (F-II, -V, and -X) pathways can be measured by using specific one-stage assays based on the PT. A specific factor assay measures the clotting time of a mixture of diluted test plasma (patient or control) and a specific factor-deficient substrate plasma, which supplies normal levels of all factors except the one being measured. TF and calcium chloride (PT reagent) are added to this mixture, and the clotting time is determined.

Each intrinsic pathway factor (F-VIII, F-IX, F-XI, and F-XII) can be measured by one-stage, APTT-based methods. In the case of F-VIII, the assay is referred to as a *factor-VIII:C assay*. As in the testing for extrinsic and common factors the specific factor assay for intrinsic factors measures the clotting time of a mixture of diluted test plasma (patient or control) and a specific factor-deficient substrate plasma, which provides all factors except the one being measured.

For each clotting factor assay based on the PT or APTT test results, the clotting times of factor-deficient substrate plasma containing varying dilutions of a reference pooled plasma (commercially available calibrator that has been assayed against a national or international standard)[33,34] in buffer are used to construct a standard curve (Table 40-4 ✪) (Figure 40-4 ■). Most laboratories use automated instruments to perform the assays, and the data are plotted using the preprogrammed software included with the instrument. The clotting times of the individual dilutions are plotted against the percentage of factor activity of each respective dilution of the assayed standard. The patient's clotting time using at least two dilutions (usually 1:10 and 1:20) with the specific factor-deficient plasma is obtained by performing a PT or APTT test on the mixture. These times are converted to percent of activity from the standard curve. The results of the two dilutions should be linear, showing that no "inhibitory effect" is seen. If the results are not linear, an inhibitory effect, which may be seen with lupus-like anticoagulants, is suspected. The same test is also performed on normal and abnormal controls. For many coagulation factors, the normal factor activity reference range is ~50–150%. (See the Web for factor assays.)

The normal levels of various clotting factors (i.e., F-IX, -XI, and -XII) are quite low at birth (Table 32-13). Therefore, to distinguish newborn factor deficiencies from normal

---

✪ TABLE 40-4

Dilutions for Factor Assays

Tube*	Buffer (mL)	Plasma (mL)	Activity (%)	Dilution
1	0.9	0.1	100.0	1:10
2	1.9	0.1	50.0	1:20
3	0.5	0.5 mL from tube 2	25.0	1:40
4	0.5	0.5 mL from tube 3	12.5	1:80
5	0.5	0.5 mL from tube 4	6.3	1:160
6	0.5	0.5 mL from tube 5	3.2	1:320
7†	0.5	0.5 mL from tube 6	1.6	1:640
8†	0.5	0.5 mL from tube 7	0.8	1:1280

*The example is based on a reference plasma value of 100%. If using a reference plasma with an assayed value other than 100%, the activity would be based on its stated value.

†Additional dilutions are prepared when patient values are possibly less than 1% activity. These dilutions are made and clotting times are determined on each dilution to construct an activity curve. The percent activity is plotted on the x-axis and the clotting time on the y-axis (Figure 40-4).

(Reprinted, with permission, from Brown, BA. *Hematology: Principles and Procedures*, 6th ed. Philadelphia: Lea & Febiger; 1993.)

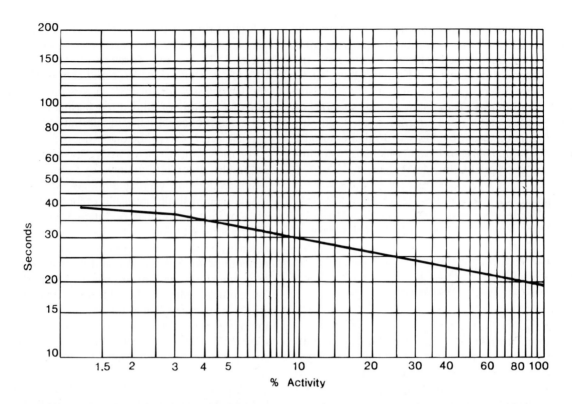

■ FIGURE 40-4   Factor activity curve. The factor activity curve is prepared by plotting the clotting time in seconds for each reference plasma dilution on the y-axis and the percent factor activity for each dilution on the x-axis. (Reprinted, with permission, from Brown BA. *Hematology: Principles and Procedures,* 6th ed. Philadelphia: Lea & Febiger; 1993.)

newborn levels (Table 32-7), the laboratory testing must be accurate when assaying samples with levels <10% of normal. In laboratories where hemophilic patients (F-VIII deficiency) are routinely evaluated, the ability to differentiate between factor levels of <1% and 2–5% is essential.

Commercial chromogenic kits are available to test for F-VIII and other clotting factors. F-VIII exists in the plasma as a complex with VWF. Testing involves its activation by thrombin, with F-VIII acting as a cofactor in the conversion of F-X to F-Xa by F-IXa in the presence of calcium and phospholipid. The amount of F-Xa generated is determined using a specific chromogenic substrate for F-Xa and is directly proportional to the amount of F-VIII in the citrated sample. Currently, these kits are less commonly used in clinical laboratories because of their high cost and the ready availability of the one-stage F-VIII assay. (See Web Figures 40-18a■, 40-18b■, 40-20■). The measurement of antithrombin is also available as a chromogenic assay and can usually be performed with the same instrument.

✓ Checkpoint! 5

What is the function of the factor-deficient substrate reagent and the reference plasma in a factor assay?

Reptilase Time

The reptilase time, which is not affected by the presence of heparin in the sample, is used in conjunction with the thrombin time to detect heparin contamination of the sample and to help differentiate dysfibrinogenemia from the presence of fibrin degradation products (Table 40-5 ✪).

Reptilase is a serine protease found in the venom of the *Bothrops atrox* snake. This thrombin-like enzyme cleaves fibrinopeptide A from fibrinogen, whereas thrombin cleaves both fibrinopeptide A and B.[35,36] The addition of reptilase to PPP initiates clot formation, which can be detected by optical or electromechanical methods using manual, semiauto-

✪ TABLE 40-5

Differentiation of Conditions Associated with a Prolonged Thrombin Time Using the Reptilase Time

Condition	Thrombin Time	Reptilase Time
Heparin contamination	Prolonged	Normal
Dysfibrinogenemia	Prolonged	More prolonged
Presence of fibrin degradation products	More prolonged	Prolonged

mated, or automated devices. The general reference interval for a reptilase time is 18–22 seconds. An increase to 25 seconds or longer is considered significant and indicates dysfibrinogenemia, hypofibrinogenemia, or afibrinogenemia.

Prekallikrein Screening Test

Individuals with a PK deficiency (also known as *Fletcher factor deficiency*) have a prolonged APTT (∞ Chapter 32). Correction of the prolonged APTT of the patient's citrated plasma to normal, or near the upper limit of the normal APTT reference range, after a 10-minute incubation period (before adding calcium chloride) suggests PK deficiency. The longer incubation period increases contact activation of F-XII in the absence of PK. The normal control plasma APTT should remain within or near its control range following the extended incubation period. Kaolin, celite, or silica is the activator of choice for the APTT reagent. Prolonged incubation with ellagic acid might not correct the APTT in PK deficiency.[37,38] PK deficiency can be confirmed by performing a specific factor assay using PK-deficient substrate. As with the F-VIII assay, a quantitative chromogenic substrate assay can quantitate the level of PK in plasma samples.[39]

Factor XIII (Screening Test)

F-XIII activity is necessary for the formation of a stable fibrin clot that occurs by forming covalent bonds between fibrin monomers. Routine screening tests (PT, APTT) detect clot formation, not cross-linking, and thus are not sensitive to F-XIII deficiency. A F-XIII determination should be performed for a patient with clinical symptoms of delayed bleeding or a bruising disorder in whom the screening tests are normal. The screening test for F-XIII deficiency is based on the observation that the fibrin clot has increased solubility because of the lack of cross-linking of the fibrin polymer in the absence of F-XIII.

The patient's PPP is mixed with 0.025M calcium chloride and allowed to clot for 1 hour at 37°C. The clot is removed and placed in another tube containing 5M urea or 1% monochloracetic acid in a 37°C water bath. A normal control plasma is tested at the same time. If the patient's clot dissolves within the 24-hour period, the result indicates a F-XIII activity of less than 1–2% (∞ Chapter 32). The normal control plasma clot resists solubilization by these agents. Patients with levels of 1–2% F-XIII produce clots that typically dissolve within the first 30 minutes,[40,41] the level at which clinical manifestations of F-XIII deficiency occurs.

More accurate quantitative assays for F-XIII that are more sensitive than the screening test described here have been developed. These assays have not gained widespread acceptance because they are relatively infrequently requested and thus are most likely performed in research or reference laboratories.[30]

LABORATORY TESTS FOR VON WILLEBRAND FACTOR (VWF)

The diagnosis of von Willebrand disease (VWD) involves quantitating VWF by both functional and antigenic methods (∞ Chapter 32). A large number of analytical variables affect its accurate determination.

The first variable is the difference over time of laboratory findings in patients with VWD. Serial studies of these patients show variability in VWF results over a 24-month span (see Web Figure 40-6■). Because some VWD patients occasionally have VWF antigen and/or activity (VWF:Ag; VWF:A) levels within the normal reference range, VWD diagnosis cannot be ruled out by a single evaluation.[42]

The second variable is that the results of screening tests (bleeding time and APTT) can be normal in patients with type I VWD. Typically, these patients have factor VIII:C, VWF:A, and VWF:Ag levels of approximately 45–55%, usually producing normal screening test results. Patients with significant bleeding histories should thus be further tested with specific assays (VWF:A and VWF:Ag) even when screening test results are within normal limits. VWD cannot be ruled out on the basis of a normal APTT and bleeding time.[25]

The third variability is the fact that an endogenous release of adrenaline can result in a transient increase in plasma F-VIII and VWF, so a patient who has VWD type I can appear normal. The stress of a difficult phlebotomy, especially in anxious young children, can double or triple the level of VWF, making it impossible to rule out VWD without repeated testing.[25] The patient should be as calm as possible before having the citrated blood sample drawn.

The fourth technical variability is in the processing of the citrated sample. Samples that are centrifuged at 1500 g for 5–10 minutes can have a residual platelet count in the plasma as high as 30,000 to 40,000/mL. Freezing this plasma releases platelet proteases, altering VWF multimeric structure and resulting in an apparent increase in the VWF antigen level and decrease in the VWF activity.[25] Using such samples is inappropriate for von Willebrand testing.

The fifth variability is the reference standard used in the clinical laboratory, which can affect the various assays for VWF. Clinicians sometimes use the ratio of VWF:Ag to VWF:A to subclassify type 2A and 2M variants. Therefore, it is imperative that both of these assays be interpreted against an acceptable and identical reference plasma sample.

The sixth variability is the fact that the patient's blood type affects the VWF plasma level. Individuals with blood group AB have a 60–70% higher level of VWF than those with blood group O. As a result, some laboratories interpret VWF levels referenced to specific normal ranges for blood types.[43] See Table 40-6 ✪ for the mean level of VWF for the various blood groups.

A variety of clinical disorders also can affect the level of VWF.[25] Web Table 40-6 ✪ provides classification of VWF variants for clinical disorders that affect assays for VWF.

⊘ TABLE 40-6

Relationship between Blood Groups and von Willebrand Factor Level

Blood Groups	von Willebrand Factor Level (%)
O	74.8
A	105.9
B	116.9
AB	123.9

The treatment of choice for the classic type (1) of VWD is desmopressin (Desamino-D-arginine vasopression [DDAVP]), which causes a twofold to fourfold increase in a patient's VWF plasma level.[44] A test dose of DDAVP is given to a patient prior to scheduled surgery to measure his or her response to it. Citrated plasma samples are drawn preinfusion as well as 30 minutes and possibly 4 hours postinfusion and are assayed for F-VIII activity, VWF:Ag, and VWF:A. Clinical laboratory professionals must be cautious in handling, centrifuging, and labeling these timed samples.

von Willebrand Factor Activity (VWF:A)

Ristocetin was used as an antibiotic until the early 1970s when it was recognized as causing thrombocytopenia in normal individuals but not in certain individuals with bleeding problems.[45] Although no longer used clinically as an antibiotic, laboratories use it as a diagnostic tool in testing for VWD. The test also is referred to as the **ristocetin cofactor (RCoF) assay**. (See Platelet Aggregometry section.)

In the presence of ristocetin, VWF induces platelet agglutination, which a platelet aggregometer can measure. Decreased RIPA in patient PRP occurs in patients with VWD caused by VWF deficiency or BSS (VWF receptor/GPIb/IX deficiency; ∞ Chapter 31).

The quantitative test for VWF activity uses ristocetin to induce VWF to bind to the glycoprotein Ib/IX receptor (VWF receptor) on formalin-fixed platelets rather than the patient's own platelets. This test system adds ristocetin to formalin-fixed platelets suspended in patient plasma (the source of VWF) and uses a platelet aggregometer to measure the resultant platelet agglutination. The slope of the agglutination is plotted versus the percent activity of a reference plasma. Other modifications of the assay use the time elapsed expressed in millimeters on the graph instead of slope of agglutination.[46]

A reference (standard) curve is prepared by making dilutions of reference plasma (100%, 50%, 25%, and 12.5%) and performing the ristocetin platelet agglutination test on each dilution. The rate of agglutination or the slope of the curve is plotted against each concentration. The control and each patient's sample are tested at two separate dilutions, and the resulting slopes or rates are calculated from the reference curve; the results are averaged and reported as a percentage of activity of VWF:A. Various automated laboratory instru-

ments now available reduce the test variability as a result of the laboratory professional's technical skill. The general reference range for VWF:A is 60–150%. VWF:A is usually decreased in plasma from patients with all three types of VWD and the platelet-type pseudo-VWD (see ∞ Chapter 32, Figure 32-2); type III has the lowest level (Web Table 40-6). Unlike the RIPA that uses patient PRP, which is abnormal in both BSS and VWD, the VWF:A (VWF:RCoF) assay is normal in patients with BSS.

Normal fluctuations occur with the four diagnostic tests used in diagnosing VWD (Web Figure 40-6). Large variations occur in test results in normal individuals as well, stressing the need for commercial reference plasmas to be standardized against international standards in preparing the standard curve for all VWF testing (Web Figures 40-7a ■ and b ■).

The laboratory professional should understand the test results regarding hemophilia versus VWD (Table 32-4) and be able to evaluate each patient's test results, repeat them, and perform verifications as needed. See Web VWF Assays for detailed technical information for this assay.

von Willebrand Factor Antigen Assay (VWF:Ag)

As with clinical testing for most bleeding disorders, the antigenic measurement for VWF:Ag was available before functional assays. Zimmerman[47] used the "rocket" immunoelectrophoresis technique of Laurell[48] to measure the VWF:Ag. (See Web for additional information and Web Figures 40-21 ■, 40-22 ■.)

The Laurell-based assay is an EIA that electrophoreses the plasma sample through an agarose gel containing rabbit antiserum to F-VIII. A rocket-shaped immunoprecipitate forms; its length can be measured and is directly proportional to the amount of VWF:Ag in the plasma sample. The assay is time consuming, and measuring and calculating decreased levels is difficult.

One of the more common current methods for VWF:Ag is an ELISA assay called a *sandwich technique*.[49] Its advantages are increased reproducibility, accuracy at very low levels, and reduced time needed to obtain results. This procedure coats microtiter plate wells with a specific rabbit antihuman VWF antibody (the capture antibody) that will bind VWF:Ag in the test sample. A second rabbit antihuman VWF:Ag antibody is enzyme labeled (alkaline phosphatase or peroxidase) and binds to the initial antigen–antibody complex on free antigenic sites of the VWF:Ag. Hence, the VWF protein is "sandwiched" between two specific antibodies (Figure 40-5 ■). A substrate specific for the enzyme label is added to the microtiter plate wells, causing a colorimetric reaction with the color intensity directly proportional to the concentration of the test sample's VWF. A microtiter plate reader, an adaptation of a spectrophotometer, determines the absorbance of each microtiter well. The assay is made quantitative by preparing a reference curve using a reference plasma calibrated against a national or international standard (as was the VWF:A assay). The controls

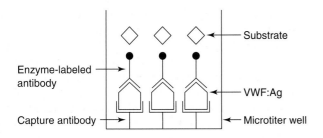

■ FIGURE 40-5   VWF:Ag enzyme-linked immunosorbent assay (ELISA). The capture antibody that is specifically directed against the target antigen, VWF, is fixed to the surface of the microtiter well. Test sample is added to the well. If VWF is present, it will bind to the capture antibody forming an antigen–antibody complex. A second specific antibody to the VWF-antibody complex is then added. This second antibody is enzyme labeled and binds to the VWF-antibody complex if it is present. To determine the presence or concentration of VWF, substrate specific for the enzyme label on the second antibody is added to the well. The enzyme converts the substrate to a colored product whose intensity is directly proportional to the concentration of the VWF in the test sample.

(normal and abnormal) and patient samples are diluted and added to the microtiter wells in the same manner as the reference plasma at various concentrations. The general reference interval for VWF:Ag is 43–150%.

Recently, an immunoturbidimetric assay for VWF:Ag has been developed. The LIA test procedure coats microlatex particles with rabbit antihuman VWF antibodies, producing agglutination when mixed with plasma containing VWF. The extent of agglutination (turbidity) correlates to the level of VWF:Ag present in the citrated plasma sample.[50] The methodology is reliable and easy to automate and produces results in a timely manner. In addition, the methodology is able to detect low levels of antigen, thus improving the ability to diagnose variants of VWD. (See the Web.)

VWF Multimer Analysis

The proper VWD treatment depends on determining the correct disease subtype (∞ Chapter 32). This previously was accomplished by using gel electrophoresis (crossed immunoelectrophoresis, CIE),[51,52] which separated type 2 varients from type 1 VWD, and by using platelet aggregation with varying lower concentrations of ristocetin to separate type 1A from type 2B VWD (described earlier). The crossed immunoelectrophoresis method was limited to a few laboratories because the procedure was technically difficult and labor intensive.

The availability of multimeric analysis has improved VWD diagnosis, resulting in improved treatment of patients. The normal VWF distribution in plasma is as multimers ranging from dimers of approximately 600,000 Daltons (Da) to very large multimers of up to 20 million Da. The use of low concentrations of agarose (0.65 percent) and staining with radiolabeled antibody to VWF allows the full range of multimers to be visualized (by autoradiography or liminog-

raphy). DDAVP is the treatment of choice for type 1 VWD but is less effective in type 2 (see Web Table 40-6). Therefore, establishing the correct subtype of VWD by multimeric analysis is important in determining the appropriate therapeutic approach.[25]

Multimeric analysis is also useful in diagnosing thrombotic thrombocytopenic purpura (TTP) in which unusually large multimers of VWF (UL-VWF) are observed. Normally, ultralarge multimers are cleaved by the VWF protease, ADAMTS-13 (∞ Chapter 33). The presence of UL-VWF indicates a reduced or absent ADAMTS-13 activity.

Because these multimeric analyses are difficult to perform and interpret and require a very pure and specific antibody, specialized reference laboratories or coagulation centers usually perform the multimeric analysis.

Collagen-Binding Assays for VWD

Collagen-binding assays are specialized assays performed on patients to differentiate VWD type 2A and 2B from type 2M. The ELISA assays for collagen binding had initially been considered as potential replacements for the VWF:A (VWF:RCoF assay) because both tests are sensitive to a reduction in high molecular weight multimers of VWF. However, because the collagen-binding assays do not reflect the interaction between VWF and GP1b, they cannot serve as substitute assays. Performing both collagen-binding and VWF:A assays increases the ability to differentiate VWD type 2 variants (discrimination of VWD types 2A or 2B from type 2M).[7,25,53]

ADAMTS-13

The presence of this VWF-cleaving protease can be measured using the ELISA technology. Chronic relapsing TTP, which usually begins in early childhood, is due to mutations in the ADAMTS-13 gene, resulting in markedly decreased protease activity. Both antigenic and activity measurements for ADAMTS-13 are commercially available.[54] The ELISA assay uses a microtiter plate precoated with a monoclonal anti-ADAMTS-13 antibody so that the ADAMTS-13 antigen of the calibrator, controls, and patient samples are measured in citrated plasma samples. Acute TTP, more commonly seen in adults, is usually due to an acquired deficiency in ADAMTS-13 resulting from an IgG autoantibody against the protease. The ELISA assay is highly specific and can differentiate TTP samples from other samples with autoantibodies (e.g., lupus) or high IgG concentrations (e.g., IgG gammopathy).

TESTS TO EVALUATE CIRCULATING INHIBITORS

The most common circulating inhibitors seen in the hemostasis laboratory are lupus-like anticoagulants (LA) or antiphospholipid antibodies (aPL) and F-VIII inhibitors. Various procedures are used in diagnosing antiphospholipid antibodies because no single definitive assay is available.[55] In the pediatric population, the Staclot LA seems to be the most sensitive assay. Because LAs are transient in this population, diagnosing it is often difficult. On repeated tests, the previously abnormal APTT of these patients can be normal.[56] The measurement of the inhibitor to F-VIII is determined with the F-VIII inhibitor assay (Bethesda method).

Lupus-Like Anticoagulants/ Antiphospholipid Antibodies

The inhibitors originally described as *lupus anticoagulants* (LA) are now recognized to be part of a more diverse group of inhibitors collectively referred to as aPL (∞ Chapter 33). They are immunoglobulins, usually of the IgG class, that are directed against the protein component of protein-phospholipid complexes. In vivo, aPL are associated with a thrombotic tendency; in vitro, they prolong phospholipid-dependent clotting assays. Classically, the APTT in these cases is abnormal with a lack of correction in 1:1 mixing studies with normal plasma. The quality of the patient sample (PPP) greatly affects the integrity of the testing. Procoagulant phospholipids (originating from platelets) can be in the patient plasma or in the normal plasma used for the mixing studies. These can neutralize weak lupus-like anticoagulant activities and produce false negative results. Thus, plasma samples should be centrifuged for 10 minutes after which the top two-thirds of the plasma is carefully removed (so as not to disturb the cells) using a plastic transfer pipette. The plasma is transferred to a second tube and recentrifuged for an additional 10 minutes.

APTT is the test generally used to screen for LA/aPLs, although APTT's sensitivity to LA/aPL depends on the reagent.[57,58] Many modifications to the APTT, including the use of lower concentrations of phospholipids in the test reagent, have been recommended in an attempt to increase its sensitivity. Laboratory professionals must evaluate their APTT reagents as to the importance of LA/aPL sensitivity versus the importance of sensitivity to specific factor deficiencies. In cases for which the screening APTT is not prolonged but the patient presents with a positive history of thrombophilia, the physician should proceed with designated testing for LA/aPL. According to the guidelines developed by the International Society on Thrombosis (ISTH), the minimum diagnostic criteria for LA/aPL are the demonstration:

1. of an abnormality of phospholipid-dependent coagulation reactions

2. that the abnormality is due to the presence of an inhibitor rather than a factor deficiency

3. of the phospholipid-dependence of the inhibitor rather than a specific factor inhibitor[59]

Each laboratory must decide which commercially available assay is the most sensitive for its patient population. The presence of heparin as a cause of the abnormal APTT is excluded by a normal thrombin time. The tests that can be used to satisfy the minimum diagnostic criteria for LA/aPL and a brief description of each test follows.

Criterion 1 for diagnosing LA/aPL (demonstration of an abnormality of phospholipid-dependent coagulation reactions) is accomplished by performing a clotting assay using a phospholipid-based reagent. LA/aPL react with anionic phospholipids and therefore can prolong the APTT, the PT (less commonly), or both. Other tests that have been used for this determination include the tissue thromboplastin inhibition test (TTI), the **dilute Russell's viper venom time (dRVVT)**, the kaolin clotting time (KCT), and the PTT-LA.[58] Making an accurate diagnosis can require performing more than one of these phospholipid-based tests because different antiphospholipid antibodies can affect various tests differently. Investigators have found that anticardiolipin antibodies (ACA) prolong the dRVVT to a greater extent than the KCT, whereas LA prolong the KCT to a greater extent than the dRVVT.[59,60] The PT of plasma with aPL usually is only minimally to moderately sensitive to the effect of aPL (typically prolonged 0.5–3.0 seconds).

Criterion 2 for diagnosing LA/aPL (demonstration that the abnormality is due to the presence of an inhibitor rather than a factor deficiency) is accomplished by using mixing studies as described earlier. A correction of a prolonged APTT in a 1:1 mixing study with normal plasma indicates a factor deficiency rather than the presence of an inhibitor. A second tube containing the 1:1 mixture of patient plasma and normal plasma should be incubated for 1–2 hours before testing to rule out the presence of a specific-factor inhibitor.

Criterion 3 for diagnosing LA/aPL (demonstration of the phospholipid-dependence of the inhibitor rather than a specific factor inhibitor) is accomplished by reducing or adding the amount of phospholipids to the test system to demonstrate that the inhibitor is directed at phospholipids rather than a specific coagulation factor.

Tissue Thromboplastin Inhibition (TTI)

The TTI test is a modification of the PT test in which a dilute thromboplastin reagent is compared to the optimal strength reagent. The PT of a plasma with LA/aPL is more prolonged than normal plasma when diluted tissue factor (PT reagent) is used. The ratio of the patient's clotting time with dilute reagent divided by the undiluted reagent clotting time is compared to a normal control. A ratio of >1:3 indicates a positive test. The test is highly sensitive but not specific to LA/aPL because it is also positive in the presence of heparin and when the initial PT is prolonged.

Dilute Russell's Viper Venom (dRVV) Test

The dRVV test, also known as the *Stypven time*, uses a commercial preparation of the venom from the Russell viper (*Daboia*) to activate F-X in a method similar to a routine PT test. The dRVVT test is based on the premise that LA/aPL activity increases in the presence of reduced phospholipids (similar to the TTI test). The reagent contains dilute Russell's viper venom, calcium chloride, and phospholipids. The reagent is added to patient PPP, and RVV activates F-X, resulting in clot formation. If LA/aPL are present, the patient's dRVVT is higher than that of the normal control. The ratio of the patient's clotting time to the clotting time of the normal control is determined. The normal ratio is usually less than 1:2. A confirmatory test also employs Russell's viper venom (RVV) but with a higher phospholipid concentration. The final result is reported as a ratio of the two clotting tests (high and low phospholipid concentration), which is compared with the values of a reference population.[60] The dRVVT appears to be more sensitive to aPL antibodies that react with β2-glycoprotein I (∞ Chapter 33).

Kaolin Clotting Time (KCT)

In the kaolin clotting-time (KCT) test, kaolin, a negatively charged particulate activator, is incubated with test PPP to activate the contact factors and the intrinsic system. The KCT can be a useful screening test for LA/aPL in patients with a normal or minimally abnormal APTT. The KCT appears to be more sensitive in detecting antibodies to prothrombin-phospholipid complexes (∞ Chapter 33).

Platelet Neutralization Proedure (PNP)

LA/aPL have antiphospholipid activity, and tests based on the fact that an excess of phospholipids substantially shortens the prolonged APTT of aPL-containing plasma are important in differentiating aPL from other inhibitors. Ruptured (freeze-thawed) platelets can serve as a source of phospholipids. The patient's PPP is mixed with a suspension of ruptured platelets and an APTT reagent. The addition of calcium chloride activates clot formation. The clotting time is determined and compared with the APTT clotting times of the patient PPP and the saline control (1:2 dilutions of saline and patient PPP). If the aPLs are present, the clotting time with the added phospholipids is significantly shorter than the original APTT and the saline control APTT. False positive results can be seen for patients who are receiving heparin or have extremely high titer inhibitors to other clotting factors.[60]

Hexagonal Phospholipids

The hexagonal phase phospholipids (HPP) test extends the PNP concept but substitutes egg phosphatidylethanolamine in an hexagonal phase configuration for the freeze-thawed platelets. The HPP assay is based on the fact that many aPL antibodies specifically recognize the HPP configuration as an antigenic epitope. Addition of HPP to the reaction mixture neutralizes the inhibitory effect of the aPL antibodies but does not neutralize most factor-specific antibodies.[61] The test (Staclot LA) is performed by incubating the test plasma at 37°C with and without the HPP reagent. An APTT is performed on both of these incubations using an aPL-sensitive reagent. If aPL are present in the test plasma, the HPP would neutralize it resulting in a shortened clotting time for the tube containing it compared to the tube without HPP. By comparing the two clotting times, the presence of aPL antibodies can be identified. This assay has two advantages:

(1) The LA sensitive reagent contains a heparin inhibitor, which makes the test system insensitive to heparin levels up to 1 IU/mL and (2) the Staclot LA procedure adds normal plasma to the test system to correct any prolongation of clotting time due to factor deficiencies that might be present. Reduction of the aPTT result by >8 seconds as the result of adding HPP is consistent with the presence of a phospholipid-dependent inhibitor.

Specific Factor Inhibitor Assay (Bethesda Titer Assay)

A group of hematologists met in Bethesda, Maryland, to create a testing method to standardize the test variables for the factor inhibitor assay and to achieve a uniform definition of an inhibitor unit.[62] The test they developed became known as the *Bethesda titer assay*. Although it was developed to measure F-VIII inhibitors, it can be modified to assay inhibitors of other coagulation proteins. The test is routinely ordered when monitoring the treatment of a severe hemophiliac (F-VIII or F-IX deficiency) twice per year.

Specific inhibitors occur in 10–15% of hemophiliacs at any time after the first infusion of factor concentrate. To detect the presence of an inhibitor in a hemophiliac, the physician must monitor the patient's response to treatment (F-VIII concentrates, both human and recombinant) by requesting F-VIII:C assays.[63] When a particular patient or a family member believes that bleeding has not stopped as it should after an infusion of F-VIII concentrate (calculated to produce a known F-VIII response in that patient), an inhibitor can be suspected. Blood is drawn pre- and postinfusion of concentrate with F-VIII levels performed on each of these citrated blood samples. If the expected response level of F-VIII is not achieved, an inhibitor to the specific factor that the patient lacks is suspected, and an F-VIII inhibitor assay is ordered. Inhibitors can occasionally be found in normal (nonhemophilic) individuals.

Testing for a specific inhibitor is always performed on the preinfusion sample (a trough sample whose F-VIII:C should be <1% F-VIII, usually suggested to be >72 hours after previous infusion). If the patient has an inhibitor, the F-VIII that is infused will be cleared quickly, producing a F-VIII level of <1% at 24 hours or less.[64,65] Presence of residual infused F-VIII can interfere with an inhibitor assay, producing a false negative value. Additionally, in patients with high levels of inhibitors, there may be an effect when assaying other clotting factors. For example, a high F-VIII inhibitor level in a patient who is being tested for F-IX deficiency could cause the F-VIII level in a F-IX deficient reagent plasma to decrease causing an abnormal factor assay result. Thus, it would appear as if the patient had a F-IX deficiency in addition to a F-VIII deficiency even if the F-IX in the patient was within the reference range. (Web Figure 40-9 ■)

The Bethesda titer assay for F-VIII inhibitor uses equal volumes of normal pooled plasma (containing a known F-VIII activity) and patient plasma, which are mixed and incubated for 2 hours at 37°C. Additional tubes are prepared using various dilutions of the patient's plasma in a buffer mixed with normal pooled plasma and are incubated. The control consists of a mixture of normal plasma and a buffer. A F-VIII assay is performed on all incubation mixtures, including the control. If a F-VIII inhibitor is present, it will inactivate the F-VIII in the normal plasma used in the mixtures, and any residual F-VIII can be measured. The patient mixtures are corrected for the amount of F-VIII loss seen in the control (normal plasma + buffer). The residual F-VIII values (F-VIII level in each of the incubated patient dilutions and control) obtained between 25% and 75% activity are then obtained from the standard Bethesda chart (Web Figure 40-8 ■). The resulting units are multiplied by the amount of dilution used and expressed in Bethesda units (BU) (1 BU = 50% residual F-VIII in the incubation mixture)[62] (Web Table 40-7 ✪).

In patients with increased inhibitor levels, multiple dilutions are needed to produce residual activity that can be read from the standard curve. The results are then averaged. When the results show that the inhibitor level appears to rise as the plasma is more diluted (Web Table 40-7, patient C), the patient appears to have complex reaction kinetics, and the inhibitor level is calculated from the lowest dilution that gave a corrected percent residual F-VIII closest to 50%.[66]

An additional option for the treatment of a hemophiliac with an inhibitor is a porcine F-VIII concentrate (Hyate:C®, Speywood Biopharm Ltd, Wrexham, UK). The F-VIII level is monitored often, and the inhibitor assay (Bethesda-type assay for porcine F-VIII) is used to determine the anamnestic response. Instead of using pooled normal plasma (PNP) for the source of F-VIII in the assay, the porcine F-VIII concentrate is diluted with hemophilic plasma to produce a porcine F-VIII plasma with a level of approximately 100% (comparable to PNP); the remaining testing procedure is the same as previously described.[67]

The Bethesda inhibitor assay has been modified with the addition of the Nijmegen modification to improve accuracy for patients with inhibitors of <1.0 BU in the standard Bethesda assay. This modification buffers the PNP to minimize the pH shift and to reduce the F-VIII loss during the 2-hour incubation. It has been shown that patients can demonstrate low levels of inhibitors (<1.0 BU) with the regular Bethesda assay but can be negative with the Nijmegen protocol.[68] These results suggest that the pH changes and F-VIII loss in unbuffered incubation mixtures resulted in low false positive inhibitor levels in some patients. The Nijmegen modification is most likely performed at hemophilia centers where the hematologist must closely monitor patients receiving factor concentrates in order to accurately identify patients with a newly developing inhibitor.

> ✓ **Checkpoint! 6**
>
> *Why are ruptured platelets able to neutralize lupus-like anticoagulants?*

► LABORATORY INVESTIGATION OF THE FIBRINOLYTIC SYSTEM

The thrombin time (TT) may be the only abnormal screening test result in patients with fibrinolytic system abnormalities because the PT and APTT results are often normal. The patient's primary disease and the physician's clinical findings (bleeding or thrombosis) can suggest a fibrinolytic system problem and indicate the need for further laboratory testing. With improvements in diagnostic algorithms and available tests, the use of the D-dimer assay has begun to replace the more generic and less specific test for fibrin degradation products (FDP) and the global assay euglobulin clot lysis.

More specific testing using ELISA and chromogenic assays is also available for fibrinolytic system components that can help evaluate an increased or decreased level of fibrinolysis (∞ Chapter 33). Because these assays are also used to determine a thrombotic tendency, they are described in the text section Laboratory Investigation of Hypercoagulable States (see Web Table 40-8 ✪).

D-DIMER

The D-dimer is a specific marker (fragment) resulting from plasmin degradation (lysis) of the fibrin clot, which has been cross-linked by F-XIIIa (∞ Chapter 30). D-dimer is an excellent marker for disseminated intravascular coagulation (DIC) with secondary fibrinolysis. However, D-dimers are also elevated in pulmonary embolism, deep vein thrombosis, arterial thromboembolism, recent trauma or surgery, cirrhotic liver disease, and renal failure (∞ Chapter 33).

The D-dimer test utilizes monoclonal antibodies against the D-dimer fragment, which can be used in three separate methodologies. The first of these is a semiquatitative assay that utilizes macroscopic latex agglutination. The D-dimer assay should not be used in patients who are taking anticoagulant therapy (heparin or warfarin). The assay can be performed on plasma (citrated, ethylenediaminetetraacetic acid [EDTA], or heparinized) and serum. The extra step of preparing serum (as in the standard FDP test) is avoided because fibrinogen and fibrin do not cross-react with the D-dimer monoclonal antibodies used in these tests. The patient specimen is mixed with latex particles coated with monoclonal antibodies (directed against D-dimer) on a glass slide for a specific amount of time (e.g., 2 minutes). At the end of this time, the laboratory professional observes the reaction mixture macroscopically for the presence of agglutination. Most procedures test both undiluted plasma and a plasma sample, diluted 1:2 in buffer which allows a semiquantitation of results. Lack of macroscopic agglutination in either sample corresponds to a D-dimer level of <0.5 μg/mL. Macroscopic agglutination in the undiluted sample but not in the 1:2 dilution corresponds to a D-dimer of 0.5–1.0 μg/mL. If both samples show agglutination, the result is >1.0 μg/mL. Normal individuals have <0.5 μg/mL.

The second methodology is a more sensitive, quantitative technique using the ELISA format. Although very sensitive and specific for D-dimer, this technique is time consuming (clinically, results are usually needed quickly) and requires the use of specialized equipment and training to perform it.

The third methodology is also based on the concept of microscopic latex agglutination but is an automated procedure and therefore eliminates errors associated with visually reading the agglutination. Antibody-coated latex particles aggregate in the presence of D-dimer, resulting in increased turbidity of the mixture. The increase in scattered light is proportional to the amount of D-dimer in the sample. This assay is extremely sensitive and has an increased detection range. It is considered to have good negative predictive value because a negative test can be used to rule out deep vein thrombosis (DVT), venous thromboembolism (VTE), and pulmonary embolism (PE). The assay, if effectively used, could reduce the use of time-consuming and expensive diagnostic tools such as venography, compression ultrasound, and spiral CT scans for some patients. If the level of D-dimer in the plasma is *not* elevated, no thrombotic process is ongoing, and VTE is not present. However, if the D-dimer level is elevated, a clotting process is occurring, which could be due to VTE as well as other clinical conditions (Table 40-7 ✪). The difficulty with using the D-dimer assay to exclude VTE is establishing the cutoff value. Each laboratory must establish its own cutoff value rather than relying on what the manufacturer provides (Web Table 40-9 ✪). These values need to be developed with input from the clinical staff and re-evaluated periodically.[69] This assay also should not be used in patients on anticoagulant therapy (heparin or warfarin). Studies have demonstrated that anticoagulants decrease circulating D-dimers and could produce a value below the cutoff, masking the presence of VTE.

Most hospitals that utilize the D-dimer assay to confirm DIC also use the D-dimer assay to test for VTE. Because the range of detection necessary for DIC and VTE varies significantly, some institutions provide them as two separate tests (different cutoff values).

FIBRIN DEGRADATION PRODUCTS

The detection of increased levels of fibrin and/or fibrinogen degradation products (FDP) in patient blood samples indicates increased fibrinolytic activity (∞ Chapter 30). The patient's blood sample is collected in a special collection tube containing thrombin (to clot the sample and ensure that all fibrinogen has been removed) and a fibrinolytic inhibitor (to prevent in vitro fibrino[geno]lysis). The patient's serum is mixed with latex particles coated with specific antibodies that recognize FDP on a glass slide for a specific amount of time (e.g., 2 minutes). The reaction mixture is observed macroscopically for the presence of agglutination. The test is semiquantitative with various dilutions made of the patient's serum in buffer. The normal range varies according to the test's manufacturer and sensitivity. Most procedures require the preparation of two dilutions for each sample (i.e., 1:2 and 1:8), which allows a semiquantitative determination of FDP. Macroscopic agglutination in both dilutions corresponds to an FDP level of more than 20 μg/mL. No macroscopic agglutination in either dilution indicates an FDP level less than 5 μg/mL; agglutination observed in the 1:2 dilution but not in the 1:8 dilution corresponds to an FDP level of more than 5 μg/mL but less than 20 μg/mL. Individuals normally have FDP levels less than 5 μg/mL.

The standard FDP assay does not distinguish between fibrin degradation products and fibrinogen degradation products because the antigenic epitopes recognized by the antibodies are expressed on both types of degradation products. Falsely high levels can also occur if the sample is not fully clotted (e.g., due to the presence of a high heparin concentration) and fibrinogen is still present (the antibodies also recognize fibrinogen).

The test is nonspecific because it also is abnormal in the following conditions associated with increased FDPs: liver disease, alcoholic cirrhosis, kidney disease, cardiac disease, postsurgical complications, carcinoma, myocardial infarction, pulmonary embolism, DVT, eclampsia, and DIC.[22]

EUGLOBULIN CLOT LYSIS

A very elementary procedure, euglobulin clot lysis was used before specific antibodies to fibrinolytic products were available. The euglobulin protein fraction is precipitated from plasma in an acid solution (1% acetic acid). The precipitate contains fibrinogen, plasminogen, and plasminogen activators but no fibrinolytic inhibitors (which remain in the supernant). With the removal of the fibrinolytic inhibitors from the test system, the fibrinolytic system's action is more easily demonstrated. The precipitate is redissolved, clotted with thrombin, and observed for clot lysis at 37°C. The fibrin clot generated by thrombin serves as the substrate for plasmin generated from plasminogen by plasminogen activators (also activated by thrombin). The end point is the time in minutes required for complete degradation of the clot into small fibrin strands or particles.[22]

The euglobulin lysis time normally is longer than 90 minutes. Shortened lysis times indicate increased fibrinolytic activity, because of increased levels of the activator or, less commonly, increased levels of plasmin. Shortened lysis

✪ TABLE 40-7	
Partial List of Non-VTE Causes of Elevated D-Dimer	
DIC	Pregnancy
Trauma	Cancer
Surgery	Diabetes
Hematoma	Thrombolytic therapy
Arterial thrombosis	Older age
General hospitalization	

times can occur in fibrinolysis secondary to intravascular co-agulation, in liver disease because of poor clearance of activator, and in thrombolytic therapy because of the therapeutic administration of a plasminogen activator. A fibrinogen level of <100 mg/dL can produce a false positive euglobulin clot lysis test. (See Website.)

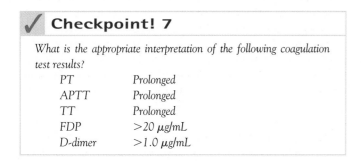

✓ **Checkpoint! 7**

What is the appropriate interpretation of the following coagulation test results?

PT	*Prolonged*
APTT	*Prolonged*
TT	*Prolonged*
FDP	*>20 µg/mL*
D-dimer	*>1.0 µg/mL*

▶ **LABORATORY INVESTIGATION OF HYPERCOAGULABLE STATES**

If individuals have repeated thrombotic episodes, they most likely are in a hypercoagulable state. Laboratory tests can assist in determining whether the thrombosis is due to hereditary or acquired abnormalities of the hemostatic system.

With an improved understanding of hemostasis and the regulatory role of naturally occurring anticoagulants, major advances have been made in identifying some of the hereditary defects associated with hypercoagulability. The first discoveries involved components of the antithrombin and protein C pathways. Infants in general are prone to thrombotic events, and thus the physiological hypercoagulability of the developing hemostatic system has received significant attention (∞ Chapter 32). The newborn infant can be expected to be at greater risk if an underlying hereditary deficiency of an anticoagulant protein also exists. As discussed earlier, provisions must be made to take small sample volumes and for assay sensitivities for components at extremely low levels.

Ideally, all testing should be performed as functional assays. All of the following tests are described as such because they are currently available. If the patient is suspected to have a type 2 deficiency (low activity, but normal antigenic measurement), an antigenic assay (ELISA, or Laurell rocket technique) is required as well. All of the following assays were initially measured in this fashion when an immunoprecipitable antibody became available. These techniques are fully described on the Web, so that the laboratory professional can understand the methodology, problem solve, and learn how to modify assays so that very low levels can be determined if needed. The theory of the chromogenic assay, which has greatly improved diagnostic capabilities of the coagulation laboratory, and LIA testing are also described. (Web Figures 40-18a, 40-18b.)

An important issue is when to test a patient who has had a thrombotic event. If the event was venous, not an arterial

(platelet-derived) thrombosis, the standard accepted approach is to treat the patient appropriately and test later. The diagnostic workup is delayed until the patient is stable and no longer hospitalized with a thrombotic event (which consumes coagulation factors and inhibitors, ∞ Chapter 32) and not receiving warfarin (vitamin K antagonist) or heparin and/or a replacement therapy such as fresh frozen plasma (FFP). Testing for protein C and protein S (vitamin K-dependent proteins) while a patient is taking warfarin or during an active thrombotic process can lead to falsely low activity and/or antigen values and therefore can result in the misdiagnosis of an inherited hypercoagulable state.[70,71] Repeat studies are often needed, and family studies are usually required to confirm a diagnosis.

ANTITHROMBIN

Antithrombin (AT), previously called *antithrombin III,* has powerful and immediate antiprotease action in the presence of heparin. This interaction between AT and heparin is the basis for the poor clinical response to heparin if the patient has significantly decreased levels of AT. AT can be measured by a variety of assays.

The chromogenic assay is a functional two-part assay measuring AT activity in the presence of heparin (Web Figure 40-19 ■). In the first part, plasma is incubated with a known excess of thrombin in the presence of heparin (heparinized buffer). AT neutralizes a proportional amount of the thrombin in the presence of heparin. The second part of the assay determines the residual thrombin activity by its enzymatic activity on an appropriate substrate (fibrinogen tagged with a chromophore, such as p-Nitroanilin [pNA], which when released produces a yellow color that is measured at 405 nm). The amount of thrombin neutralized in the first reaction step is proportional to the amount of AT present in the test sample; thus, the residual amount of thrombin (as measured by the pNA release) is inversely proportional to the test sample's AT level (Web Figure 40-19). A reference (standard) curve is prepared by plotting the AT activity (%) for each reference plasma dilution prepared against its corresponding absorbance. The results for patients and controls are read from this curve using respective absorbance readings. The general reference interval for AT is 80–120%.[72]

The other common functional assay is a clot-based method in which the clotting of fibrinogen rather than the cleavage of a synthetic chromogenic substrate is the endpoint of the assay. Plasma is defibrinogenated (fibrinogen removed) and incubated with heparin and thrombin. Residual thrombin is determined by transfer to a standardized fibrinogen solution, and the time for clotting to occur is measured. As in the chromogenic assay, the clotting time is directly proportional to the concentration of AT in the patient's plasma: The higher the AT level, the higher is the amount of thrombin neutralized in the first step, resulting in a lower level of residual thrombin and a prolonged clotting time in the second step.

Immunological methods measure the concentration of the AT protein using EIA, ELISA (Web Figures 40-21, 40-22, and 40-23 ■), radial immunodiffusion (RID), and micro latex particle immunological assays (LIA tests, automated procedures available) (Web Figure 40-10 ■).

Inherited deficiencies of AT can involve a decrease in the protein (and activity) level or the presence of a dysfunctional protein (∞ Chapter 33). In addition to congenital deficiencies (which are very rare), acquired deficiencies occur in DIC, liver disease due to decreased synthesis, and nephrotic syndrome (the latter as a consequence of urinary protein loss). Healthy newborns have about half the normal adult concentration of AT and gradually reach the adult level by 3–6 months of age (∞ Chapter 32). A number of clinical disorders can be associated with reductions in the plasma concentration of AT, sometimes making it difficult to establish a definitive diagnosis of the hereditary deficiency state. Low levels on an initial screen should be confirmed at a later date. All hereditary deficiencies identified to date have been in heterozygous individuals.

Anticoagulation of patients also affects testing for AT. The administration of heparin decreases plasma AT levels presumably by accelerated clearance of the heparin-antithrombin complex. Thus, the evaluation of plasma samples during heparinization can lead to an erroneous diagnosis of AT deficiency. Plasma AT concentrations are occasionally elevated into the normal range by warfarin in individuals with AT deficiency. Confirmation of the hereditary nature of an AT deficiency may require investigation of other family members. (See Website.)

PROTEIN C/ACTIVATED PROTEIN C (APC)

Functional assays of protein C (PC) have been analyzed by measuring amidolytic activity using a chromogenic substrate or its anticoagulant activity in a clot-based assay. Chromogenic assays can be less informative than clot-based assays when screening for PC defects. Several individuals have been described with normal PC antigen (immunologic) measurements and reduced PC anticoagulant activity in clot-based assays but normal amidolytic activity in chromogenic assays.[73] These individuals could have defects in the ability of activated PC (APC) to interact with platelet membranes or the F-Va or F-VIIIa substrates and thus would not be detected by the amidolytic assay.[73]

APC is an anticoagulant that inactivates F-Va and F-VIIIa. In the assay for PC, a reagent containing snake venom (*Agkistrodon c. contotrix*), protac (a particulate activator for the activation of protein C), and platelet factor 3 activate both PC and the contact factors of the intrinsic pathway. The patient's plasma is incubated with PC-deficient plasma (to compensate for any factor deficiency other than PC), an APTT reagent containing the activator, and then with calcium chloride; the time for clot formation is measured. Activation of PC, resulting in the inactivation of F-Va and

F-VIIIa in the control and patient samples, results in a prolongation of the modified APTT. The longer the modified APTT, the more functional PC is present in the plasma sample. A reference (standard) curve is prepared by plotting the PC activity for each reference plasma dilution assayed in conjunction with the patient samples against its clotting time. The results for patients and controls are obtained from this curve using the respective clotting times (see Website). The general reference interval for PC is 60–150%.[74]

In spite of its limitations as discussed, the chromogenic assay for PC is widely used. In this assay, PC is incubated with a specific activator and the amount of APC measured is based on its enzymatic activity on a chromogenic substrate. The enzymatic activity releases pNA from the chromogenic substrate, and pNA is measured spectrophotometrically at 405 nm. The absorbance of pNA is directly proportional to the amount of APC. A reference (standard) curve is prepared by plotting the protein C activity (%) for each reference plasma dilution against its corresponding absorbance. The results for patients and controls are obtained from this curve using the respective readings.

The PC deficiency diagnosis is complicated for patients on oral anticoagulation therapy. Warfarin therapy reduces functional and, to a lesser extent, immunologic measurements of PC. Several researchers have proposed using the ratios of PC antigen to the F-II or F-X antigen. However, this will not identify patients with type II PC deficiency (low activity, normal antigen). This approach of using ratios can be used only for patients in a stable phase of oral anticoagulation. Other groups have used PC activity assays in conjunction with functional measurements of F-VII (a vitamin K-dependent zymogen with a similar plasma half-life). In practice, investigating individuals suspected of having PC deficiency after oral anticoagulation has been discontinued for at least 1 week and performing family studies are preferable. If discontinuing warfarin therapy is not possible, individuals can be studied while they receive heparin therapy, which does not alter plasma PC levels.[73]

Acquired PC deficiency is found in numerous disease states (∞ Chapter 33). Most individuals with uremia have low levels of PC anticoagulant activity but normal levels of PC amidolytic activity and antigen. This low PC anticoagulant activity has been attributed to a dialyzable moiety in uremic plasma that interferes with most clotting assays for PC activity.[73]

PROTEIN S

Circulating protein S (PS) exists in two forms: free (40%) and bound to C4b binding protein (60%). Only the free protein S serves as a cofactor for APC, enhancing its anticoagulant activity. The functional free form is what clot-based assays measure. Laboratory evaluation of PS also can include assays of total PS antigen (ELISA) and free PS (immunoassays using monoclonal antibody specific for the free form).[75]

Functional PS assay methods are based on the ability of PS to serve as a cofactor for the anticoagulant effect of APC. A typical clot-based procedure for measuring the cofactor activity of PS requires four reagents: (1) PS-deficient plasma to ensure optimal levels of all coagulation factors except PS, (2) purified activated protein C, (3) purified activated F-Va to serve as a substrate for APC, and (4) calcium chloride. Patient PPP is mixed with PS-deficient plasma. APC and activated F-Va reagents are added to this mixture, which is incubated at 37°C. Following incubation, calcium chloride is added to initiate clot formation. The clotting time is proportional to the PS activity in the sample (i.e., the higher the level of PS, the longer is the clotting time).

A reference (standard) curve can be prepared by using dilutions of reference plasma representing 100%, 75%, 50%, and 25% PS activity. The PS activity for each plasma and control is obtained from this curve. The general reference interval for protein S is 66–122%.[76]

Like PC clot-based assays, the presence of factor V Leiden, APC resistance, elevated F-VIII levels, and a lupus anticoagulant can cause false positive PS test results if clotting (functional) assays are used to diagnose PS deficiency.

Inherited deficiencies (autosomal dominant disorder) can involve a decrease in the protein or a dysfunctional protein (∞ Chapter 33). The clot-based procedure for PS detects both quantitative and qualitative deficiencies of PS, but immunologic methods do not detect qualitative deficiencies.

Acquired PS deficiencies are found in numerous disease states (∞ Chapter 33). Although total PS antigen measurements are generally increased in individuals with nephrotic syndrome, functional assays are often reduced because of the loss of free PS in the urine and elevations in C4b-binding protein levels.[73]

ACTIVATED PROTEIN C RESISTANCE (APCR)

APC resistance (APCR) is one of the most common risk factors for thrombosis. The presence of the factor V Leiden (FVL) mutation results in the resistance of F-Va to degradation by APC, commonly referred to as *activated protein C resistance (APCR)*. The molecular testing for FVL (PCR) is described in ∞ Chapter 39.

The clot-based assay is based on the principle that the addition of APC to a plasma sample induces a prolongation of the APTT mediated by the inactivation of F-Va and F-VIIIa in the plasma sample. The sensitivity and specificity of the screening test has been improved by prediluting the patient plasma with F-V–deficient substrate plasma; this permits the evaluation of patients receiving anticoagulants or who have an abnormal APTT due to factor deficiencies other than F-V. The testing proceeds with the performance of an APTT with and without the addition of APC. The APC ratio is calculated using the clotting time of the sample with APC (results

should be prolonged due to the destruction of F-Va and F-VIIIa) divided by the clotting time for the sample without APC. APCR is indicated by an APCR ratio of less than what was established for the laboratory using a particular instrument and reagent combination.[77] (See Web Figure 40-11 for the APCR ratio calculation.) Acquired conditions such as pregnancy, oral conceptive use, elevated F-VIII, and a stroke can also produce APCR.

The APCR functional assay (as described) is a screening, not a diagnostic, test for FVL. Other rare congenital conditions including F-V Cambridge and homozygosity for the HR2 haplotype can result in APCR. Because 10% of individuals with APCR do not have the FVL mutation, clinical diagnosis requires both the clotting and molecular (PCR) tests for the FVL genetic mutation. If FVL mutation is not identified, PCR-based confirmatory tests for APCR due to other genetic mutations are available in research laboratories.

PROTHROMBIN G20210A

Individuals heterozygous for the F-II G20210A mutation (prothrombin 20210) can have prothrombin levels up to 30% higher than noncarriers (∞ Chapter 39). (This mutation is now known to be a mutation in position 21538 of the *F2* gene.) However, because of the overlap with the normal range for F-II, clot-based functional assays for prothrombin are unreliable.[78] Therefore, genetic screening using PCR amplification of the F-II gene is the only reliable way to detect the presence of this phenotype. Detection methods for the amplified product can utilize specific endonucleases, gel electrophoresis, or fluorescent probing. A multiplex PCR-based assay is available for the simultaneous detection of FVL and F-II G20210A.[79]

> ### ✓ Checkpoint! 8
>
> *In diagnostic laboratory evaluation of a hypercoagulable state such as antithrombin deficiency, why is it important to determine the functional activity of the coagulation protein?*

ADDITIONAL TESTING FOR THROMBOSIS

Rare abnormalities in the fibrinolytic system may result in thrombosis. The tests in this section may be performed to assist in diagnosis of these abnormalities. Except for plasminogen, the tests discussed are performed less frequently than those previously described and may require sending samples to a reference laboratory for testing. If only a limited number of these tests are performed at a particular site, they could be prohibitively costly. See ∞ Chapters 30 and 33 and Web Table 40-8 for material related to this topic.

Plasminogen

Plasminogen levels are measured by using a chromogenic assay based on the conversion of plasminogen to plasmin by an excess of streptokinase (SK), which acts as an activator. The first step in this assay involves incubating patient plasma with a known excess of SK, which forms a complex (plasminogen-SK) that causes plasmin-like activity. The second step determines the amount of the complex by its enzymatic activity on a chromogenic substrate. The enzymatic activity results in the release from the chromogenic substrate of pNA, which is measured spectrophotometrically at 405 nm. The pNA absorbance is directly proportional to the plasminogen quantity. A reference (standard) curve is prepared by plotting the plasminogen activity (%) for each reference plasma dilution against its corresponding absorbance. The results for patients and controls are obtained from this curve using the respective absorbance readings. The general reference interval for plasminogen levels is 74–124%.[80]

Inherited deficiencies of plasminogen include quantitative deficiencies characterized by decreased antigenic and functional levels as well as qualitative deficiencies characterized by dysfunctional protein (∞ Chapter 33). Acquired deficiencies are associated with DIC, liver disease, and leukemia. Measuring circulating plasminogen levels is useful in monitoring hepatic regeneration of plasminogen after discontinuation of treatment with SK and in controling and adjusting the rate of infusion of FFP being given to the patient.

Alpha$_2$–Antiplasmin Activity (α_2-antiplasmin)

A chromogenic method to measure α_2-antiplasmin that can be used with microtiter plate, test tube, and automated procedures is available. Incubation of plasma diluted with an excess of plasmin results in a rapid complex formation between the functional plasmin inhibitor (antiplasmin) present in the plasma and the added plasmin. The amount of plasmin activity inhibited is proportional to the amount of plasmin inhibitor in the patient plasma. The residual plasmin hydrolyzes the chromogenic substrate S-2403, liberating the chromophoric group, pNA. The color is observed photometrically at 405 nm.[81] The inhibitor α_2-antiplasmin is important in regulating the fibrinolytic system. Congenital deficiencies are characterized by bleeding occurring some hours after an initial injury. Clotting and wound healing are usually normal, but the hemostatic plug breaks down prematurely. Acquired decreases of α_2-antiplasmin can be observed in liver disease and DIC. Increased levels have been reported during the postoperative period.

Plasmin-α_2-Antiplasmin (PAP) Complex

The plasmin-α_2-antiplasmin (PAP) complex test uses ELISA methodology to detect elevated levels that can occur during thrombotic events, in cases of endogenous hyperfibrinolysis, and during thrombolytic therapy. The blood sample is collected in special precoated plastic tubes containing citrate, aprotinin, and benzamidine.[82] Special specimen processing is required. (See Website.)

Plasminogen Activator Inhibitor (PAI-1)

Both functional[83] and antigenic measurements[84] are available to measure plasminogen activator inhibitor-1 (PAI-1), the primary inhibitor of tissue plasminogen activator (tPA). This inhibitor varies diurnally so attention must be paid to the timing of both collecting the patient sample and obtaining samples for establishing a normal range for the laboratory. An increased plasma level of PAI-1 is associated with impaired fibrinolytic function. Elevated levels of PAI-1 have been observed in thrombolytic disease, acute myocardial infarction, DVT, normal pregnancy, and sepsis (see Website).

Tissue Plasminogen Activator (tPA)

Both functional (chromogenic) and antigenic (ELISA) assays are available to measure tissue plasminogen activator (tPA), an important protein in the fibrinolytic system.[85] The physiologic role of tPA is to activate plasminogen to plasmin, which then degrades fibrin to soluble FDP. Fibrinolysis is regulated by specific interactions between tPA and fibrin and between plasmin and the plasmin inhibitor α_2-antiplasmin. In the assay for tPA, the plasma tPA inhibitor PAI-1 is usually present in large excess and must be prevented from quenching tPA activity. This is accomplished using a special blood collection tube (Biopool Stabilyte tubes, Dia Pharma), which provides mild acidification and stabilization of the sample, blocking the effect of PAI-1.

Thrombin Activatable Fibrinolysis Inhibitor (TAFI)

TAFI induces hypofibrinolysis by decreasing fibrin's ability to bind tPA and plasminogen. High concentrations of TAFI can induce an elevated risk of thrombosis. The TAFI antigen concentration in normal human plasma is usually between 40 and 250%.[86] There are no variations for gender or pregnancy. (See Website.)

Lipoprotein(a)

Lipoprotein(a) interferes with fibrinolytic functions of plasminogen and/or plasmin and can thus promote thrombotic events. The ELISA assay uses serum or citrated plasma.[87] (See Website.)

▶ LABORATORY EVALUATION OF ANTICOAGULANT THERAPY

A critical laboratory function is to monitor patients on anticoagulant therapy. As with diagnostic testing, the same parameters of blood collection, specimen processing, and quality control are essential.

ORAL ANTICOAGULANT THERAPY AND THE PROTHROMBIN TIME—INR VALUE

The clinical laboratory now reports patient values when monitoring **oral anticoagulant therapy** (coumadin, warfarin) using an **international normalized ratio (INR)** value, which is determined from the PT result. This standardization of oral anticoagulant control has greatly improved patient care in this mobile world.

In 1977, the World Health Organization (WHO) introduced an international reference standard for thromboplastins. Since then, several different WHO standard thromboplastins, which represent the different types of commercial thromboplastins, have been established. These standards allow for the calibration of commercial thromboplastins for oral anticoagulant control. Each manufacturer has an in-house standard (a specific lot of its own thromboplastin) that has been carefully calibrated against one of the WHO standards. The **international sensitivity index (ISI)** value is calculated as a specific correction factor for a manufacturer's standard against the WHO reference preparation. The ISI for a particular reagent is instrument dependent. Its value is listed on each package (lot number) of thromboplastin reagent purchased for PT testing (different ISI values are provided for the various types of instrument with which the thromboplastin reagent will be used [i.e., mechanical, optical]).

Commercial manufacturers of thromboplastin reagents are working to produce ISI values close to 1.0. This value that the WHO recommends minimizes discrepancies between labs in reporting the INR value.[88,89,90]

The INR has become the standard for reporting PT results when monitoring long-term oral anticoagulant therapy (∞ Chapter 33). The WHO and the International Committee on Thrombosis and Haemostasis recommended this method of reporting in 1983. Most laboratories currently report both the PT and the INR for a given sample. The advantage of the INR is that it is independent of the reagents and methods used to determine PT and therefore allows better assessment of long-term oral anticoagulant therapy.[88–90] By definition, the INR is the PT ratio equivalent to using the WHO international reference preparation as the source of thromboplastin in the performance of a PT. Each laboratory uses the formula in Figure 40-6 ■ to calculate each INR value from the PT produced for each patient. The PT has thus been improved by standardizing each thromboplastin reagent against reference thromboplastins. The calculation also includes the lab's mean value for at least 20–30 normal control subjects using the specific lot of thromboplastin with a particular type of instrumentation (mean normal PT for the laboratory, not the clotting time of, for example, lyophilized pooled normal plasma). The mean value changes with each new lot of reagent.

By reporting the PT as an INR value, each laboratory is using a standardized unit related to the WHO standards. The INR value has also provided the opportunity to use a com-

$$INR = R^{ISI}$$

Where   R = PT ratio obtained with the working thromboplastin
PT ratio = Patient's PT/Mean normal PT
ISI = International sensitivity index (provided by manufacturer)

Example: Patient's PT = 21.5 seconds
Mean normal PT = 12.0 seconds
ISI = 1.35

$$INR = (21.5/12.0)^{1.35} = 2.2$$

■ FIGURE 40-6   International normalized ratio (INR) calculation formula.

mon unit for defining the **therapeutic ranges** for oral anticoagulant therapy. Patients receiving oral anticoagulants for a hypercoagulable state (arterial or venous thromboembolism) should have an INR between 2.0 and 3.0; occasionally (e.g., with a mechanical valve replacement) the recommended ratio can be higher. Each facility should determine its own therapeutic range.

The efficacy of oral anticoagulants such as warfarin and coumadin is influenced by the patient's body mass, vitamin K content in the diet, drug interactions, wellness, and hepatic function. The INR should be carefully interpreted with regard to the patient's drug regimen (antibiotics or aspirin-containing medication) and dietary changes. The INR was devised to monitor patients on long-term anticoagulant therapy and is thus not meaningful in patients not on anticoagulant therapy. The use of the INR for clinical conditions other than oral anticoagulation has not been validated.

Point-of-care (POC) instruments that determine the individual's INR from a capillary puncture are currently available. The reagent used by these instruments is only thromboplastin; calcium is not required because the blood sample has not been citrated; thus, the calcium is not bound and is available from the patient's whole blood. These instruments determine the PT and calculate the INR. Patients, anticoagulation clinics, and laboratories in physicians' offices use them to monitor and maintain optimal therapeutic levels of oral anticoagulant.

HEPARIN THERAPY

In addition to monitoring patient treatment, physicians must be aware of two phenomena with the use of heparin. The first is the variation in an individual patient's response to heparin due either to a resistance to a specific species of heparin (bovine or porcine) or to variability in heparin-binding proteins and physiologic clearance mechanisms. These mechanisms might not produce the expected clinical results post-treatment. The second phenomenon is a dramatic decrease in the patient's platelet count caused by the heparin infusion (HIT). HIT testing is discussed earlier in this chapter.

ACTIVATED PARTIAL THROMBOPLASTIN TIME (APTT)

Traditionally, the APTT has been the most commonly used procedure to monitor standard (unfractionated) heparin therapy. Heparin response curves previously were prepared by spiking plasma with heparin at various levels and graphing the results. Thus, the patient's APTT at therapeutic levels (0.3 to 0.7 U/mL of heparin) could be determined. The degree of prolongation of the APTT is variable, depending on the APTT reagent, instrument, and even the particular lot of the same reagent (Web Figure 40-12 ■). Some very sensitive reagents do not give measurable clotting times at concentrations of 0.5 U/mL or above, thus eliminating their usefulness in monitoring heparin levels.[30]

Unlike the PT, there is no standardization of the APTT to normalized differences in reagents and test systems. In addition to the sensitivity issues mentioned, complications include the variation in standard heparin preparations, the individuality of a patient's response to heparin due to heparin-binding proteins, and the physiologic clearance mechanisms. For these reasons, two individuals receiving a standard heparin bolus of 5000 units in the same facility can have very different APTT results (one indicating a therapeutic response and the other a supratherapeutic response). Thus, the common practice of 1.5 to 2.5 times the control APTT value is no longer acceptable.

The College of American Pathologists (CAP) requires that clinical laboratories establish a heparin therapeutic range for their APTT procedure.[91] The laboratories determine this range by correlating the APTT results from patients on heparin therapy with the specific test results for F-Xa inhibition from those same samples. Because the therapeutic range for the F-Xa inhibition assay is established as 0.3–0.7 U/mL, the APTT therapeutic range is derived by comparison. A weight-based heparin dosing nomogram should also be provided to the clinicians so they can determine the appropriate dose of heparin to reach and/or maintain a therapeutic range[92,93] (Table 40-8 ✪). Additionally, a variety of factors can impact heparin monitoring (Table 40-9 ✪).

THROMBIN TIME

TT is less commonly used to monitor heparin therapy. Its advantage is that it is not influenced by plasma factor deficiencies.[94,95]

ANTI-XA ASSAY

The APTT might not demonstrate a response to heparin during initial heparin treatment for DVT or PE due to the presence of acute phase reactant proteins as indicated in Table 40-9. In this situation, another heparin assay such as the F-Xa inhibition assay frequently reflects a therapeutic level of heparin and allows proper patient management.

✪ TABLE 40-8

Weight-Based Heparin Dosing Nomogram

| Initial Heparin Dose: | 80 Units/kg Bolus |
| Initial Maintenance Infusion Rate | 18 Units/kg/hr |

Adjustment of maintenance infusion: Perform an APTT 6 hours after the initial heparin bolus and adjust as follows.

APTT, sec*	Bolus	Change in infusion rate of heparin
<40	80 units/kg	Increase infusion by 4 units/kg/hr
40–49	40 units/kg	Increase infusion by 2 units/kg/hr
50–80		No change
81–100		Decrease infusion by 2 units/kg/hr
>100		Stop heparin infusion for 1 hour; then decrease infusion by 3 units/kg/hr

*Based on its established heparin therapeutic range, each laboratory should determine its own APTT ranges for the nomogram.

An APTT should be performed 6 hours after each dosage change and the appropriate changes in dosage applied.

Low molecular weight heparin (LMWH) (∞ Chapter 33) has become a common form of heparin for anticoagulant therapy. It has more reliable **pharmacokinetics** and **bioavailability** than standard heparin and thus does not require routine laboratory monitoring in adults because its dose response is more predictable. For children, monitoring is minimal, although it is critically important in those with poor or nonexistent venous access. LMWH also reduces the risk of heparin-induced thrombocytopenia (∞ Chapter 33

✪ TABLE 40-9

Factors Affecting the Monitoring of Heparin

- Conditions that influence the pharmacokinetics or general bioavailability of heparin: Heparin binds to various plasma proteins (e.g., platelet factor 4, fibrinogen, VWF, fibronectin, and vitronectin), macrophages, and endothelial cells, resulting in decreased bioavailability
- Conditions that alter the characteristics of the APTT dose response to heparin
- Conditions that cause an abnormal baseline APTT (factor deficiency, lupus anticoagulant)
- Patient's body weight
- Antithrombin level
- Specimen collection and processing problems

  Time of collection (minimum of 4 hours needed to achieve steady state with heparin)

  Delayed testing (can result in abnormally prolonged results)

  Failure to achieve PPP (can result in release of PF4 from activation of residual platelets resulting in underestimation of heparin in the sample)

and earlier in this chapter), and probably the risk of osteoporosis with long-term heparin use.

Therapeutic doses of LMWH (enoxaparine [Lovenox®, Sinofi-aventis] and reviparin [Clivarin®, Abbott International, Knoll]) are based on an anti-F-Xa level of 0.5 to 1.0 units/mL. The guideline used for the citrated blood sample is taken 4 to 6 hours after a subcutaneous injection.[93] A standard for performing the anti-F-Xa assay for LMWH is used.

The F-Xa inhibition assay (anti-Xa assay) is also a more specific test for monitoring unfractionated heparin (UFH) therapy. In testing for UFH, a special standard is used. The **chromogenic assay** for both types of heparin uses excess activated F-X (F-Xa), which is added to the patient's PPP and incubated.[96] Heparin present in the patient's PPP inhibits the F-Xa. A chromogenic substrate is added to this mixture, and any residual F-Xa enzymatically cleaves the chromogen, producing a yellow color that is measured spectrophotometrically. A reference (standard) curve is prepared by plotting the various dilutions of known concentrations of heparin against its corresponding absorbance. The results for the patients and controls are obtained from this curve using the respective absorbance readings.[96] The therapeutic range for heparin is 0.3–0.7 U/mL.

ACTIVATED CLOTTING TIME (ACT)

Bedside testing with the ACT has been used in cardiac care units and during cardiac surgery to monitor heparin. The ACT is a traditional whole blood clotting method similar to the APTT principle. The ACT test activates whole blood with a contact activator, and the clot in the sample is detected using a **POC instrument**. The ACT result in seconds is a function of the heparin concentration but is also influenced by factors such as coagulation factors, inhibitors, lysed platelets, increased hemodilution, hypothermia of the patient, and others.[30]

✓ Checkpoint! 9

As seen in Figure 40-6, the patient has a PT of 21.5 seconds (producing an INR of 2.2). In this case, the patient is not on oral coagulation. What is the explanation for not reporting the INR?

▶ ## MOLECULAR MARKERS OF HEMOSTATIC ACTIVATION

A more detailed understanding of the biochemistry of coagulation and fibrinolysis has resulted in the development of a number of sensitive and specific assays that detect molecular markers of platelet activation, generation of coagulation enzymes, and products of intravascular fibrin formation or dissolution[97] (Table 40-10). The availability of testing for molecular markers is useful for the early detection of

⊙ TABLE 40-10		
Immunochemical Markers of Hemostatic Activation		
Coagulation		
Activation peptides	Factor IX activation peptide	
	Factor X activation peptide	
	Prothrombin activation fragment F1+2	
	Protein C activation peptide	
	Fibrinopeptide A, fibrinopeptide B	
Enzyme-inhibitor complexes	Thrombin-antithrombin complex (TAT)	
	Factor Xa-antithrombin complex Factor IXa-antithrombin complex	
	Activated protein C-protein C inhibitor complex	
Fibrinolysis	Bβ1-42 fragment (plasmin cleavage of fibrin)	
	Plasmin–antiplasmin complex (PAP)	
Platelet activation (flow cytometry)	Activated GPIIb/IIIa complex	
	P-selectin (CD62-P)	
	GPIb/IX/V (decrease)	

platelet-driven or coagulation-driven disorders and their use can result in improved medical care for thrombotic and fibrinolytic disease. This testing is not, however, routine and may be available only at large medical centers or reference laboratories.

MARKERS OF FIBRIN FORMATION AND FIBRINOLYSIS

The process of activating coagulation converts a number of zymogens to active serine proteases. Directly measuring the levels of most hemostatic enzymes in vivo (i.e., thrombin, plasmin) is not possible because naturally occurring protease inhibitors rapidly neutralize the majority. However, the activation peptides released on activation of the zymogen can be measured by immunochemical assays (RIA, ELISA). The enzyme-inhibitor complex that forms as a result of zymogen activation can also be measured by similar immunochemical methods. Due to high cost and low volume of test requests, the routine clinical laboratory generally does not offer these assays.

The assays depend on the development of monoclonal or polyclonal antibodies capable of recognizing antigenic determinants on the activation fragment or enzyme-inhibitor complex that are hidden in the parent zymogen or inhibitor. More widely used assays include those for: fibrinopeptide A and/or fibrinopeptide B and prothrombin activation fragment F1+2. Thrombin-antithrombin (TAT) complex and plasmin-antiplasmin (PAP) complex (Table 40-10) testing were described earlier in the chapter.

LABORATORY MARKERS OF PLATELET ACTIVATION

Platelet hyperreactivity or circulating activated platelets have been reported to be associated with several clinical conditions including coronary artery disease, unstable angina, and acute myocardial infarction.[98] The bleeding time, platelet function analyzer, and platelet aggregation tests remain the only standard clinical tests of platelet activation and function, but they are more useful in adults than pediatric patients in assessing platelet hyperreactivity (see earlier section on platelet function testing). A number of additional tests have been developed and are available in specialized coagulation laboratories, including ELISA assays for plasma platelet factor 4 (PF4), β-thromboglobulin (β-TG) and soluble P-selectin (markers of platelet activation and secretion), and urine assays for thromboxane A_2 metabolites (TX-B_2).

Flow cytometry can be used to evaluate platelet activation and function and will likely assume an increasingly important role in the evaluation of in vivo platelet activation.[98] Platelets are labeled with a fluorescent-conjugated antibody, and specific characteristics of a large number of individual platelets can be measured rapidly (1,000–10,000 cells/minute). In the absence of an added (exogenous) platelet agonist, whole blood flow cytometry evaluates the activation state of circulating platelets according to the binding of an activation-dedendent monoclonal antibody. If an exogenous agonist is included in the assay, it is possible to analyze the reactivity of circulating platelets in vitro (i.e., a physiologic assay of platelet function).

Monoclonal antibodies can be used to measure the expression of platelet surface antigens. However, antibodies that detect activation-dependent antigens (i.e., antibodies that bind to activated platelets, not to resting platelets) are particularly useful for assessing platelet hyperreactivity. Monoclonal antibodies that detect an activation-induced conformation change in GPIIb/IIIa appear to be directed against the fibrinogen-binding site of GPIIb/IIIa of activated platelets. P-selectin (CD62-P) (previously referred to as GMP-140 or PADGEM) is a component of the alpha granule membrane of resting platelets and is expressed on the platelet surface after alpha granule secretion. Thus, a P-selectin specific antibody binds only to degranulated, activated platelets, not resting platelets.

The GPIb/IX/V complex (VWF receptor) offers a different approach in evaluating in vivo platelet function. In contrast to activation-dependent monoclonal antibodies (e.g., GPIIb/IIIa), the binding of GPIb/IX/V–specific antibodies to activated platelets is markedly decreased compared to that of resting platelets. This decrease is due to a redistribution of the GPIb/IX/V complex to the membrane of the surface-connected canalicular system with platelet activation. Specific testing for these platelet markers likely is available only in a large clinical flow cytometry laboratory or a university setting.

Evidence of in vivo platelet activation can have significant clinical implications in cardiovascular and thrombotic diseases. Flow cytometric analysis of platelet activation-dependent markers can be used to determine optimal antiplatelet therapy in clinical settings and to measure platelet hyperreactivity in a number of clinical conditions.

GLOBAL TESTING

Hemostasis testing at the POC has become a requirement in the majority of hospitals. Increasing numbers of complex surgical procedures (liver transplantation, coronary bypass graft, and valve repair in patients on the heart-lung machine) have created a demand for the availability of rapid and more comprehensive information on a patient's hemostatic condition. Therapeutic decisions must be made quickly to discriminate between surgical bleeding and a hemostatic disorder.

Unlike typical coagulation tests that are performed in the absence of cellular elements and provide data only on plasma clotting components, thereby overlooking potentially important interactions essential to the clinical evaluation of in vivo hemostasis, **global testing** instruments analyze the entire hemostasis process including coagulation, anticoagulant effects, fibrin formation and stabilization, clot retraction (platelet function), and fibrinolysis. Two of the more commonly used analyzers are described here. Their current uses are primarily in surgery settings where blood product usage can be monitored and in research facilities that wish to improve diagnostic testing and monitor treatment of patients with bleeding and clotting disorders.[30]

Thromboelastography (TEG), a viscoelastic whole blood instrument introduced by Hartert in 1948, is increasingly being used as a near patient testing method for assessing blood coagulability. The instrumentation (thromboelastograph) has become more clinically useful with direct readout of results and shortened reaction times by using activators and inhibitors in the cuvettes. The TEG provides prompt, reliable information to clinicians on the causes of blood loss in critical POC situations. It allows the discrimination between surgical bleeding and hemostasis disorders. The TEG seems to be the most suitable method for the detection of hyperfibrinolysis, an otherwise difficult to analyze coagulopathy that can lead to massive bleeding[30] (Web Figures 40-13 ■, 40-14 ■, 40-15 ■).

The TEG now is also able to assess platelet function in patients who received platelet-inhibiting drugs such as aspirin, clopidogrel, and others. The specialized testing is called *TEG® platelet mapping assay*.[99]

The ROTEM® Haemostasis Whole Blood Analyser is a computerized device based on the TEG. It is designed to be used with appropriate reagents to generate both a qualitative graph and quantitative numerical results. The standardized reagent menu allows for the differentiation of coagulation factor deficiencies, anticoagulant effects, platelet disorders, fibrin polymerization disorders, and hyperfibrinolysis (Web Figures 40-16 ■, 40-17 ■).

 Checkpoint! 10

A patient has a venous thrombotic episode and is to be treated appropriately. When should the blood sample be drawn to perform a thrombotic workup to diagnose an acquired or congenital deficiency? Why?

SUMMARY

This chapter reviewed the laboratory tests performed in the coagulation laboratory and specialized tests available from research or reference laboratories. It highlighted the role of the laboratory professional as an integral part in the diagnosis of bleeding and clotting disorders. The additional technical information provided on this book's Companion Website allows the CLS/CLT to access information to improve coagulation testing so that all intricacies of sample collection, processing, quality control, accuracy, and reproducibility are available for each test.

The tests described were grouped according to the part of the hemostatic system that they assess: primary hemostasis, secondary hemostasis, the fibrinolysis, and hypercoagulable states. A combination of tests from these groups can be selected to screen for a disorder of the hemostatic system. As an example, the PFA, PT, and APTT can be used to identify a defect in either primary or secondary hemostasis. When this defect has been identified, specific laboratory tests can be selected to provide information for making a definitive diagnosis of the coagulation disorder. With the performance of screening tests for fibrinolysis (TT, FDP), further fibrinolytic testing can be performed. Laboratory tests used to evaluate hypercoagulable states (e.g., AT, PC, PS, APCR) and to monitor anticoagulant therapy (e.g., PT/INR, APTT, F-Xa inhibition assay) are some of the most frequently ordered in the coagulation laboratory. Testing is now available to detect activated platelets, coagulation enzymes, and products of intravascular fibrin formation or dissolution. Global testing once used only in the research setting is becoming clinically available.

REVIEW QUESTIONS

LEVEL I

1. The hematology laboratory informs you that the hematocrit on a patient is 57% (0.57 L/L). For the proper anticoagulation of a 5.0 mL sample of the patient's blood, how much 3.2% sodium citrate should be used? (Objective 1)
   a. 0.22 mL
   b. 0.40 mL
   c. 0.57 mL
   d. 0.96 mL

2. What laboratory test is used to monitor oral anticoagulant therapy? (Objective 5)
   a. F-Xa inhibition assay
   b. bleeding time
   c. prothrombin time
   d. activated partial thromboplastin time

3. Which is the specimen of choice for the prothrombin time and activated partial thromboplastin time procedures? (Objective 3)
   a. platelet-rich plasma, citrated
   b. platelet-poor plasma, citrated
   c. serum
   d. plasma, heparinized

4. A physician asks you to recommend a coagulation test for secondary fibrinolysis. Which laboratory test is specific for fibrinolysis? (Objective 4)
   a. D-dimer
   b. fibrin-degradation products
   c. thrombin time
   d. antithrombin

LEVEL II

1. Which laboratory test is *not* used to investigate the hypercoagulable states? (Objectives 3, 5)
   a. antithrombin
   b. activated protein C resistance
   c. plasminogen
   d. activated partial thromboplastin time

2. Platelet aggregation studies revealed normal aggregation curves with collagen, epinephrine, and ADP but an abnormal aggregation curve with ristocetin. Based on these findings, what is the differential diagnosis? (Objective 5)
   a. von Willebrand disease and Bernard-Soulier syndrome
   b. Glanzmann's thrombasthenia and von Willebrand disease
   c. storage pool disease and Glanzmann's thrombasthenia
   d. Bernard-Soulier syndrome and storage pool disease

3. The observation of a normal reptilase time and a prolonged thrombin time indicates what disorder? (Objective 5)
   a. presence of fibrin degradation products
   b. dysfibrinogenemia
   c. hypoplasminogenemia
   d. presence of heparin

4. In performing an activated protein C resistance assay on a patient specimen, you obtained the following results:

Standard APTT	28.4 sec
Modified APTT with APC	71.6 sec

   How would you interpret this assay? (Objective 5)
   a. presence of F-V$_{Leiden}$
   b. increased levels of activated F-VIII
   c. presence of normal F-V
   d. decreased levels of antithrombin

LEVEL I

5. Which of the following methodologies is *not* used to determine fibrinogen concentration? (Objective 3)
   a. chromogenic assay
   b. immunologic assay
   c. precipitation assay
   d. clot-based assay

6. Given the following data, calculate the INR. (Objective 7)

Patient's PT	23.5 sec
Mean normal PT	11.5 sec
ISI	1.15

   a. 2.0
   b. 2.3
   c. 2.5
   d. 1.7

7. The APTT is used as a screen for the laboratory evaluation of inherited and acquired deficiencies in which of the following? (Objective 4)
   a. extrinsic pathway of the coagulation cascade
   b. intrinsic pathway of the coagulation cascade
   c. platelets
   d. vascular system

8. The combination of a prolonged activated partial thromboplastin time and a prolonged test time with the mixing study procedure indicates the presence of what? (Objectives 4, 8)
   a. circulating inhibitor
   b. F-VIII deficiency
   c. antiplatelet antibodies
   d. excessive vitamin K

9. Based on the following data, what is the most likely factor deficiency? (Objective 8)

PT	Normal
APTT	Prolonged
TT	Normal

   a. F-VII
   b. F-II
   c. F-IX
   d. F-XIII

10. Which laboratory test evaluates platelet function? (Objective 2)
    a. bleeding time
    b. reptilase time
    c. prothrombin time
    d. protein C assay

LEVEL II

5. Given the following laboratory results, what is the appropriate reflex test? (Objective 6)

PT	Normal	
APTT	Slightly prolonged	
Platelet aggregation	Collagen	Normal
studies	ADP	Normal
	Ristocetin	Abnormal

   a. ristocetin cofactor assay
   b. F-VIII assay
   c. prekallikrein screen
   d. bleeding time

6. What is the most likely cause of the following laboratory data? (Objective 5)

PT	Normal
APTT	Prolonged
TT	Normal
APTT with 10-minute incubation	Normal

   a. presence of lupuslike anticoagulant
   b. F-XII deficiency
   c. increased levels of tissue plasminogen activator
   d. prekallikrein deficiency

7. Which of the following conditions does *not* have an impact on heparin monitoring? (Objective 7)
   a. patient's body weight
   b. delay in testing
   c. use of citrated platelet-poor plasma
   d. underlying liver disease

8. In monitoring a patient on oral anticoagulant therapy, an INR of 1.3 was obtained. How would you interpret this result? (Objective 7)
   a. The patient is adequately anticoagulated and should be tested again in one month.
   b. The patient is underanticoagulated and should be evaluated for a change in dietary habits.
   c. The patient is overanticoagulated and should receive a vitamin K injection.
   d. Insufficient data to determine status of patient.

9. Based on the following laboratory data, which is the appropriate reflex test? (Objective 6)

PT	Normal
APTT	Prolonged
TT	Normal
Mixing Studies	Correction

   a. dilute Russell's viper venom time
   b. F-XI assay
   c. activated protein C resistance assay
   d. fibrin degradation products assay

REVIEW QUESTIONS (continued)

LEVEL I

LEVEL II

10. Given the following laboratory data, which would you perform to resolve these results? (Objective 6)

PT	Prolonged
APTT	Prolonged
TT	Prolonged
mixing studies	No correction

    a. a reptilase time to confirm heparin contamination

    b. a fibrinogen determination to confirm fibrinogen deficiency

    c. a dilute Russell's viper venom time to confirm lupuslike anticoagulant

    d. a hematocrit to confirm a decreased hematocrit (<20%)

www.pearsonhighered.com/mckenzie

Use this address to access the interactive Companion Website created for this textbook. Find additional information, tables and figures. Evaluate your command of the chapter information using case studies and critical thinking and multiple choice questions.

REFERENCES

1. Jensen R, Fritsma GA. Preanalytical variables in the coagulation laboratory. *Advance.* 2000;9(7):90–94.

2. Adcock DM, Kressin DC, Marlar, RA. Are discard tubes necessary in coagulation studies? *Lab Med.* 1997;28:530–33.

3. Dade Hepzyme package insert, Deerfield, IL: Dade International Inc./IBEX Technologies; December 1997.

4. National Committee for Clinical Laboratory Standards. *Collection, Transport and Processing of Blood Specimens for Coagulation Testing and Performance of Coagulation Assays,* 3rd ed. H21-A3. Villanova, PA: NCCLS; 1998.

5. Adcock DM, Kressin DC, Marlar, RA. The effect of 3.2% vs 3.8% sodium citrate concentration on routine coagulation assays. *Am J Clin Pathol.* 1997;107:105–10.

6. Martinowitz U, Rosner E. Coagulation Laboratory, Hemophilia Center, Chaim Sheba Medical Center, Tel Hashomer, Israel. Personal communication, 1986.

7. Adcock DM, Bethel MA, Macy PA. *Coagulation Handbook.* Austin TX: Esoterix Laboratory Services; 2006.

8. Havertown, PA: Chrono-log; *Instruction Manual for Whole Blood Lumi Aggregation.* January 2003.

9. Hillman CR, Barnhart MI, Lusher JM. Drugs or conditions that alter platelet function. In: Lusher JM, Barnhart M, eds. *Acquired Bleeding Disorders in Children,* vol 4. New York: Masson Publishing, 1981.

10. Arkel YS, Haft JI, Williams R. Alteration in second phase platelet aggregation associated with an emotionally stressful activity. In: Day HJ, Zucker MB, Holmsen H, eds. *Platelet Function Testing.* DHEW Publication No. (NIH) 78-1087. Bethesda, MD: U.S. Department HEW, National Institutes of Health; 1977:705–16.

11. PFA-100® Analyzer. *Getting Started Guide.* Miami, FL: Dade Behring; 1997.

12. Mielke CH. International committee communications: Measurement of the bleeding time. *Thromb Hemostas.* 1984;52:210.

13. National Committee for Clinical Laboratory Standards. *Performance of the Bleeding Time Test,* H43A. Villanova, PA: NCCLS; 1998.

14. Warrier I, Hillman-Wiseman C. Children's Hospital of Michigan, Detroit, MI, Division of Hematology/Oncology. Personal observation. August 2004

15. Weiss HJ. Platelet physiology and abnormalities of platelet function. *N Eng J Med.* 1975;293:531.

16. Mammen EF. Sticky platelet syndrome. *Semin Thromb Hemost.* 1999; 25(4):361–65.

17. Warrier I, Nigro N, Hillman C, Draughn M, Lusher J. Platelet activation with stroke and migraine in children. *Thromb Haemost.* 1991;65(6):351.

18. Ledford-Kraemer MR. The Clotting Times 2004;4(3):2–9. www.clot.ed.com/edit/documents/CTOct2004r.pdf. Accessed 1/19/2009.

19. Hillman CR, Lusher JM, Barnhart MI. Tests of platelet function: Technical points of clinical relevance. In: Lusher JM, Barnhart M, eds. *Acquired Bleeding Disorders in Children,* vol. 4. New York: Masson Publishing; 1981.

20. Harms C. Routine laboratory procedures. In: Triplett DA, ed. *Platelet Function, Laboratory Evaluation and Clinical Application.* Chicago: American Society of Clinical Pathology; 1978.

21. Santoro SA, Eby CS. Laboratory evaluation of hemostatic disorders. In: Hoffman R, Benz EJ, Shattil SJ, Furie B, Cohen HJ, Silberstein LE, McGlave P, eds. *Hematology: Basic Principles and Procedures,* 3rd ed. Philadelphia: Churchill Livingstone, 2000:1841–50.

22. Sirridge MS, Shannon RI. *Laboratory Evaluation of Hemostasis and Thrombosis,* 3rd ed. Philadelphia: Lea & Febiger; 1983.

23. Wilson DB. Acquired platelet defects. In: Nathan DG, Ginsburg D, Look AT, Orkin SH, eds. *Nathan and Oski's Hematology of Infancy and Childhood,* 6th ed. Philadelphia: W.B.Saunders; 2003:1597–1630.

24. National Committee for Clinical Laboratory Standards. *One-Stage Prothrombin Time Test (PT) and Activated Partial Thromboplastin Time (APTT) Test,* HA7-A. Villanova, PA: NCCLS; 1996.

25. Montgomery RR; Gill JC, Scott JP. Hemophila and von Willebrand disease. In: Nathan DG, Ginsburg D, Look AT, Orkin SH, eds.

Nathan and Oski's Hematology of Infancy and Childhood, 6th ed. Philadelphia: W.B. Saunders; 2003.

26. Hillman CRL, Lusher JM. Determining the sensitivity of coagulation screening reagents: A simplified method. *J Lab Med*. 1982; 13:162–65.

27. Hathaway WE, Assmus SL, Montgomery RR et al. Activated partial thromboplastins time and minor coagulopathies. *Am J Clin Path*. 1979;71:22–25.

28. Marlar RA, Bauer PJ, Endres-Brooks JL et al. Comparison of the sensitivity of commercial PTT reagents in the detection of mild coagulopathies. *Am J Clin Pathol*. 1984;82:436–39.

29. Brandt JT, Arkin CF, Bovill EG et al. Evaluation of PTT reagent sensitivity to factor IX and factor IX assay performance. Results from the College of American Pathologists Survey Program. *Arch Pathol Lab Med*. 1990;114:135–41.

30. Kolde HJ. *Haemostasis, Physiology, Pathology Diagnostics*. Basel, Switzerland: Pentapharm; 2004.

31. Triplett DA, Harms CS. Physiological and Pathologic Inhibitors. *Proceedures for the Coagulation Laboratory*. Chicago: American Society of Clinical Pathology; 1981.

32. National Committee for Clinical Laboratory Standards. *Determination of Factor Coagulant Activities*, H48-A. Villanova, PA: NCCLS; 1997.

33. Hultin MB. Coagulation factor assays. In: Beutler E, Lichtman MA, Coller BS et al., eds. *Williams Hematology*, 5th ed. New York: McGraw-Hill; 1995:189–90.

34. Hillman CR. *Techniques for One-Stage Factor Assay*. Monograph by Dade Education. Miami; FL: Baxter Healthcare; 1989.

35. Abbott Diagnostic Systems. *Reptilase-R*. North Chicago, IL: Abbott Laboratories; 1987.

36. Triplett DA, Harms CS. Reptilase time. *Procedures for the Coagulation Laboratory*. Chicago: American Society of Clinical Pathology; 1981.

37. Abildgaard CR, Harrison J. Fletcher factor deficiency: Family study and detection. *Blood*. 1974;43(5):641–44.

38. Triplett DA, Harms, CS. Prekallikrein (Fletcher Factor) confirmatory test. *Procedures for the Coagulation Laboratory*. Chicago: American Society of Clinical Pathology; 1981.

39. Triplett DA, Harms CS. Prekallikrein (Fletcher Factor) synthetic chromogenic substrate assay. *Procedures for the Coagulation Laboratory*. Chicago: American Society of Clinical Pathology; 1981.

40. Triplett DA, Harms CS. Factor XIII. *Procedures for the Coagulation Laboratory*. Chicago: American Society of Clinical Pathology; 1981.

41. Warrier I, Hillman-Wiseman C. Children's Hospital of Michigan, Detroit MI, Division of Hematology/Oncology. Personal observation. August, 1993.

42. Abildgaard CF, Suzuki Z, Harrison J, Jefcoat K, Zimmerman TS. Serial studies in von Willebrand's disease: Variability versus "variants." *Blood*. 1980;56(4):712–16.

43. Gill JC, Endres-Brooks J, Bauer PJ et al: The effect of ABO blood group on the diagnosis of von Willebrand disease. *Blood*. 1987; 69:1691–95.

44. Warrier I, Lusher JM. DDAVP: A useful alternative to blood components in moderate hemophilia A and von Willebrand disease. *J of Ped*. 1983;102:228–33.

45. Howard MA, Firkin BG: Ristocetin: A new tool in the investigation of platelet aggregation. *Thromb Diath. Haemorrh*. 1971;26:362.

46. Triplett DA, Harms CS. Ristocetin cofactor assay. *Procedures for the Coagulation Laboratory*. Chicago: American Society of Clinical Pathology; 1981.

47. Zimmerman TS, Hoyer LW, Dickson L et al. Determination of the von Willebrand's disease antigen (factor VIII related antigen) in plasma by quantitative immunoelectrophoresis. *J Lab Clin Med*. 1975;86:152–59.

48. Laurell CB. Quantitative estimation of proteins by electrophresis on agar gel containing antibodies. *Anal Biochem*. 1966;14:45–52.

49. Cejka AJ. Enzyme immunoassay for factor VIII related antigen. *Clin Chem*. 1982;28:1356.

50. STA®—Liatest® vWF kit package insert. Parsippany, NJ: Diagnostica Stago; 2008.

51. Laurell CB. Antigen-antibody crossed electrophoresis. *Anal Biochem*. 1965;10:358.

52. Sultan Y, Simeon J, Caen JP. Electrophoretic heterogeneity of normal factor VIII/von Willebrand protein, and abnormal electrophoretic mobility in patients with von Willebrand's disease. *J Lab Clin Med*. 1976;87:185.

53. Plumhoff E. *Lab Pointers—Collagen Binding Assay for vWD*. http://www.clot-ed.com/documents/Lpcollagenplumhoff.ppt. #2622, Collagenbindingassay for VWD. Accessed 1/17/09.

54. Technozym ® ADAM-TS-13, Technoclone package insert. April, 2008. West Chester, OH: DiaPharma Group, 2006.

55. Lupus Anticoagulant Working Party, BCSH Hemostasis and Thrombosis Task Force. Guidelines on testing for the lupus anticoagulant. *Am J Clin Pathol*. 1991;44:885.

56. Warrier I, Hillman-Wiseman C. Children's Hospital of Michigan, Detroit, MI, Division of Hematology/Oncology. Personal observation. 1998.

57. Adcock DM, Marlar RA. Activated partial thromboplastins time reagent sensitivity to the presence of the lupus anticoagulant. *Arch Pathol Lab Med*. 1992;116:837.

58. Hoyer LW. Acquired anticoagulants. In: Beutler E, Lichtman MA, Coller BS et al., eds. *Williams Hematology*, 5th ed. New York: McGraw-Hill; 1994.

59. Feinstein DI. Inhibitors of blood coagulation. In: Hoffman R, Benz EJ, Shattil SJ, Furie B, Cohen HJ, Silberstein LE, McGlave P, eds. *Hematology: Basic Principles and Procedures*, 3rd ed. Philadelphia: Churchill Livingstone; 2000.

60. Ledford-Kraemer MR. Ed. *The Clotting Times*. 2005;4(4):2–10. http://www.clot-ed.com/edit/documents/CTJan2005r.pdf. Accessed 1/17/09.

61. Rauch J, Tannenbaum M, and Janoff AS. Distinguishing plasma lupus anticoagulants from antifactor antibodies using hexagonal (II) phase phospholipids. *Thromb Haemost*. 1989;62(3):892–96.

62. Kasper CK, Aledort LM, Counts RB et al. A more uniform measurement of factor VIII inhibitors. *Thromb Haemost*. 1975;34:879–72.

63. Hillman-Wiseman C, Vitali C, Lusher J. Factor VIII inhibitor assay using plasma factor VIII versus recombinant factor VIII—A comparative study. *Thromb Res*. 1994;76(2):221–24.

64. Hillman CRL. Use of quantitative inhibitor assays in treating hemophiliac patients. Check Sample, No. 90-3. Chicago: American Society of Clinical Pathology; 1990.

65. Lusher JM, Hillman CRL. Effect of inhibitors on factor assays. In: Triplett DA, ed. *Advances in Coagulation Testing: Interpretation and Application*. Chicago: American Society of Clinical Pathology; 1986.

66. Kasper CK: Measurement of factor VIII inhibitors. In: Hoyer, LW, ed. *Factor VIII Inhibitors*. New York: Alan R. Liss; 1984.

67. Kasper CK. Laboratory tests for factor VIII inhibitors, their variation, significance and interpretation. *Blood Coagul Fibrinolysis*. 1991;2(1):7–10.

68. Verbruggen B, Novakova I, Wessels H et al. The Nijmegen modification of the Bethesda assay for factor VIII:C inhibitors: Improved specificity and reliability. *Thromb Haemost*. 1995;73(2):247–51.

69. Marlar RA. D-Dimer: Establishing a laboratory assay for ruling out venous thrombosis. *MLO*. 2002;34(11):28–32.

70. Warrier I, Children's Hospital of Michigan, Detroit, MI. Personal communication. 1990.

71. Ledford-Kraemer MR, ed., *Clinical Tidbits*. January, 2007. http://www.clot-ed.com/documents/TBITSPCPSTest.ppt#270,1, When to Test for PC & PS? Accessed 1/24/2009.

72. Stachrom ATIII kit, package insert. Parsippany, NJ: Diagnostica Stago; 2007.

73. Bauer, KA. Inherited disorders of thrombosis and fibrinolysis. In: Nathan DG, Ginsburg D, Look AT, Orkin SH, eds. *Nathan and Oski's Hematology of Infancy and Childhood*, 6th ed. Philadelphia: W.B. Saunders; 2003.

74. Staclot Protein C, package insert. Parsippany, NJ: Diagnostica Stago; 2004.

75. Amiral J, Grosley B, Boyer-Neumann C et al. New direct assay of free protein S antigen using two distinct monoclonal antibodies specific for the free form. *Blood Coagul Fibrinolysis*. 1994;5(2):179–86.

76. Biopool Protein S, package insert. Burlington, Ontario: Biopool; 1996.

77. Coatest APC Resistance, package insert. Molvdale, Sweden: Chromogenix; 2003.

78. Aiach M, Emmerich JE. Thrombophilia genetics. In: Coleman RW, Marder VJ, Clowes AW, George JN, Goldhaber SZ, eds. *Hemostasis and Thrombosis: Basic Principles and Clinical Practice*, 5th ed. Philadelphia: Lippincott Williams & Wilkins; 2006.

79. Endler G, Kyrle PA, Eichinger S et al. Multiplexed mutagenically separated PCR: Simultaneous single-tube detection of the factor V R506Q (G1691A), the prothrombin G20210A, and the methylenetetrahydrofolate reductase A223V (C677T) variants. *Clin Chem.* 2001; 47:333–35.

80. Plasminogen Chromogenix Coamatic Plasminogen, package insert. West Chester, OH: DiaPharma; 2002.

81. DiaPharma, Plasmin Inhibitor, Chromogenix Coamatic Plasmin Inhibitor, package insert. West Chester, OH: 2002.

82. Plasmin-alpha 2-antiploasmin complex (PAP), Technoclone PAP Complex ELISA kit, package insert. Technoclone, West Chester, OH: DiaPharma; 2005.

83. Plasminogen Activator Inhibitor (PAI-1) Spectrolyse pL/PAI-1, Chromogenix Coamatic Plasma Inhibitor, package insert. West Chester, OH: DiaPharma: 2002.

84. Plasminogen Activator Inhibitor (PAI-1) TintElize PAI-1, Biopool, package insert. West Chester, OH: DiaPharma; 2004.

85. Tissue Plasminogen Activator (t-PA) Biopool, Chromolyze tPA, TintElize tPA, package insert. West Chester, OH: DiaPharma; 2002.

86. Thrombin Activatable Fibrinolysis Inhibitor (TAFI) Zymutest TAFI Ag, package insert. West Chester, OH: DiaPharma; 2004.

87. Elitest-Lp(a), Hyphen BioMed. West Chester, OH: DiaPharma; 2001.

88. International Committee for Standardization in Hematology, International Committee on Thrombosis and Haemostasis. ICSH/ICTH recommendations for reporting prothrombin time in oral anticoagulant control. *Thromb. Haemost.* 1985;54:155.

89. Jensen R. Oral anticoagulants and the INR. *Clin Hemostasis Rev.* 1999;13:1–3.

90. Kitchen S, Preston FE. Standardization of prothrombin time for laboratory control of oral anticoagulant therapy. *Semin Thrombo Hemost.* 1999;25:17–26.

91. Hematology and Coagulation: Proposed CAP checklist 2, Question 02:3712. Chicago: College of American Pathologists; November 1999.

92. Berry BB, Geary DL, Jaff MR. A model for collaboration in quality improvement projects: Implementing a weight-based heparin dosing nomogram across integrated health care delivery system. Joint Commission *J Qual Improv.* 1998;24:459–69.

93. Lackie CL, Luzier AB, Donovan JA, Feras HI, Forrest A. Weight-based heparin dosing: Clinical response and resource utilization. *Clin Therapeutics.* 1998;20(4):699–710.

94. Monagle P, Andrews M. Acquired disorders of hemostasis. In: Nathan DG, Ginsberg D, Orkin SH, Look AT, eds. *Nathan and Oski's Hematology of Infancy and Childhood*, 6th ed. Philadelphia: W. B. Saunders; 2003.

95. Penner JA. Experience with the thrombin clotting time assay for measuring heparin activity. *Am J Clin Path.* 1974;61:645.

96. Hoke RA, Carrol RT. Monitoring heparin with an anti-factor X chromogenic assay. *Clin Hemostasis Rev.* 1998;12(9):17–18.

97. Bauer KA, Weitz JI. Laboratory markers of coagulation and fibrinolysis. In: Coleman RW, Hirsh J, Marder VJ, Clowes AW, George JN, eds. *Hemostasis and Thrombosis: Basic Principles and Clinical Practice*, 4th ed. Philadelphia: Lippincott Williams & Wilkins; 2000: 1113–29.

98. Michelson AD. Laboratory markers of platelet activation. In: Coleman RW, Hirsh J, Marder VJ, Clowes AW, George JN, eds. *Hemostasis and Thrombosis: Basic Principles and Clinical Practice*, 4th ed. Philadelphia: Lippincott Williams & Wilkins; 2000.

99. Platelet Mapping™ Assay, TEG Hemostasis Analyzer. package insert. Haemoscope; Niles, IL; 2006.

41

Quality Assessment
in the Hematology Laboratory

Cheryl Burns, M.S.
Lucia More, M.S.

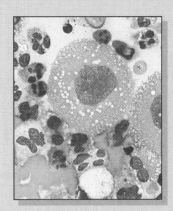

CHAPTER OUTLINE

■ OBJECTIVES—LEVEL I

At the end of this unit of study, the student should be able to:

1. Identify the components of a quality assessment program and match sources of error with component.
2. State the importance of a quality assessment program.
3. State the importance of documentation in a quality assessment program.
4. Describe the use of proficiency testing in the clinical laboratory including required frequency.
5. Given data, employ an appropriate method to determine the reference range for an analyte.
6. Define *universal precautions* and identify their source.
7. Demonstrate knowledge of OSHA standards and their application in the clinical laboratory.
8. Given a material safety data sheet (MSDS), identify critical information.
9. Define *accuracy, precision, control material, mean,* and *standard deviation.*
10. Given the appropriate data, calculate the mean and standard deviation and create a quality control chart.
11. Interpret quality control results utilizing established control charts.
12. Given test results, recognize CBC data and/or histogram variations that indicate the presence of white blood cell (WBC), red blood cell (RBC), and platelet abnormalities.
13. Recognize CBC data that indicate the presence of interfering substances such as lipemia, hemolysis, and icteria.
14. Identify coagulation test results that indicate a problem with sample integrity.

■ OBJECTIVES—LEVEL II

At the end of this unit of study, the student should be able to:

1. Design methods of competency testing.
2. Apply and interpret statistics used in method evaluation.
3. Determine the components and interpret the results of a method evaluation study.
4. Determine and appraise a method's reportable range.
5. Interpret the Westgard rules and their use in evaluating quality control results.

6. Describe the use of moving averages to monitor red blood cell data.

7. Assess the use of patient samples to monitor daily quality control in hematology.

8. Select the appropriate actions to take when abnormalities are detected in hematology or coagulation results.

9. Recommend procedures to correct for the presence of lipemia, hemolysis, and icteria.

10. Demonstrate the ability to use Delta checks in a quality control program.

KEY TERMS

Analytical sensitivity

Analytical specificity

Analytical time

"Blinded" preanalyzed sample

Clinical Laboratory Improvement Amendments of 1988 (CLIA '88)

CLSI

Competency assessment

Correlation coefficient (*r*)

Delta check

Health Insurance Portability and Accountability Act (HIPAA)

Internal quality control program

Linearity

Material safety data sheet (MSDS)

Medical decision level

Outlier

Proficiency testing

Quality control (QC) limit

Random variation

Reference interval (RI)

Reportable range

Slope (*b*)

Split sample

Standard deviation (SD)

Systematic variation

Transcription error

Turnaround time (TAT)

Universal precaution

y-intercept (*a*)

BACKGROUND BASICS

Levels I and II

▶ Describe the sample collection protocol for hematology and hemostasis procedures. (Chapters 34, 40)

▶ Summarize each of the routine hematology procedures, and give potential sources of error. (Chapter 34)

▶ Summarize the characteristics of an optimally stained peripheral blood smear, and give potential sources of error. (Chapter 34)

▶ Summarize each of the screening coagulation tests used in the laboratory, and give potential sources of error. (Chapter 40)

▶ Describe the principles of cell counting used by the automated hematology instruments and principles of clot detection for the automated coagulation instruments. (Chapter 36)

▶ OVERVIEW

One of the most important responsibilities of a clinical laboratory professional is to ensure the quality of test results. To accomplish this, laboratories must establish quality assessment and quality control programs. These programs consist of guidelines designed to ensure accurate testing and reporting of results. A protocol for reviewing patient results to determine whether results can be reported must be included. This chapter discusses components of these programs.

▶ QUALITY ASSESSMENT

Laboratories must have an established quality assessment program as mandated by subpart K—Quality Systems for Nonwaived Testing of the **Clinical Laboratory Improvement Amendments of 1988 (CLIA '88).**[1] A laboratory's quality assessment program should be designed to monitor all aspects related to testing patient samples.[2] The program's goal is to ensure accurate testing and reporting of results from all samples submitted to the laboratory. Accrediting agencies such as the College of American Pathologists (CAP) and the Joint Commission (formerly known as the Joint Commission on Accreditation of Healthcare Organizations [JCAHO]) monitor a program's comprehensiveness and quality. This chapter reviews the various aspects to consider in designing a comprehensive quality assessment program.

BASIC COMPONENTS

A common approach to the development of a quality assessment program is to divide it into three components: (1) pre-examination, which deals with all aspects affecting the test outcome occurring prior to the testing procedure, (2) examination, which incorporates all aspects affecting the testing procedure itself, and (3) postexamination, which deals with aspects affecting the test outcome occurring after the testing procedure (Table 41-1 ✪).

✪ TABLE 41-1

Comprehensive Quality Assessment Program

- Pre-examination components
  - Patient test requisitions
  - Patient preparation
  - Sample collection protocol
  - Sample transport protocol
  - Sample processing protocol
  - Sample acceptability and rejection criteria
  - Sample storage
  - Phlebotomy training
- Examination components
  - Test method/procedure
  - Reagents
  - Internal quality control
  - External quality control (proficiency testing)
  - Maintenance of instrumentation
  - Linearity/reportable range determination
  - Method evaluation (instrument comparison)
  - Reference range determination or verification
  - Personnel requirements
  - Competency testing
  - Continuing education
- Postexamination components
  - Review of patient results
  - Posting of patient results
  - Maintenance of patient records
  - Monitoring of turnaround time
  - Surveying of customer satisfaction
  - Maintaining of all documentation

Pre Examination Component

The testing process begins with the test order. Patient test requisitions should be designed to be user friendly and to provide adequate patient information. At a minimum, this information should include the patient's name or unique patient identifier, age, sex, diagnosis, test to be performed, and source of the sample. The patient should receive appropriate information to prepare for the tests such as being informed to abstain from aspirin or aspirin-like medication prior to platelet function testing. This information should be provided in the laboratory's sample collection procedure manual and in a format easily distributed to and understood by the patient.

One of the most important factors affecting a test's outcome is sample collection (∞ Chapters 34, 40).[3–6] As we often hear, "The test result is only as good as the quality of the sample." Many variables enter into the sample collection process that can effect the outcome (Table 41-2 ✪). The sample collection procedure manual and a thorough educational program for the phlebotomist or the individual designated to perform the phlebotomy (i.e., nursing personnel) should address each potential error. Periodic continuing education should be provided to address sample collection problems or introduce new protocols.

When the sample has been collected, it must be properly labeled and transported to the laboratory for processing and testing. If testing cannot be done immediately, the sample should be properly stored. For example, a sample for routine coagulation testing requires separating plasma from cells and storing the sample at room temperature if testing will be performed within 4 hours (∞ Chapter 40). All of this information should be found within the sample collection procedure manual and vary depending on the test to be performed.

Examination Component

The examination component addresses all issues involving the testing procedure itself. A test method procedure manual should be available in all laboratories. This manual should address each test as to its purpose, principle, sample requirements, reagents, quality control, step-by-step procedure, interpretation of results, and potential sources of error.[7,8]

An **internal quality control program** should be established to monitor the testing process and ensure accurate patient test results. Quality control is addressed in more detail later in this chapter. In addition, overall quality control should be assessed by an external quality control program, also known as **proficiency testing.** Proficiency testing monitors the testing process by comparing the specific laboratory to peer laboratories.[9] This also is addressed in a subsequent section of this chapter.

Maintenance of analytical instruments (e.g., automated blood cell-counting instrument) must be followed as directed by the manufacturer, and documentation of all

⊗ TABLE 41-2

Potential Sources of Errors in Sample Collection and Their Effect on Test Outcome

Source of Error	Effect on Test Outcome
Patient misidentification	Inaccurate test results
Hemolyzed sample	Dilutional effect on analytes, false increase of analytes, and decreased erythrocyte counts
Failure to invert collection tubes that contain anticoagulant properly	Clotted sample and falsely decreased cell counts or prolonged coagulation test results
Failure to fill collection tube properly	Under- or over-anticoagulated sample for coagulation testing with citrate tube
Failure to follow the order of the draw*	Cross-contamination with collection tube additives
Tourniquet application longer than 1 minute	Hemoconcentration of sample
Collection from an IV site	Dilutional effect on analytes
Time of draw	Analyte dependent (e.g., hemoglobin is highest in the morning)
Patient anxiety or crying	Analyte dependent (e.g., increases leukocyte count)

*Order of the draw refers to the suggested order in which different anticoagulant and nonanticoagulant collection tubes are filled from a single venipuncture. For example, a heparin collection tube should be filled prior to an EDTA collection tube to avoid contamination of the heparin collection tube with potassium EDTA (∞ Chapter 34).

maintenance activities must be easily accessible for troubleshooting quality control problems.

Individuals performing the testing procedures must meet the personnel requirements established by CLIA '88, which vary depending on the test procedure. Continuing education is also required to keep testing personnel abreast of changes within the testing procedures and the practice of the profession.

Postexamination Component

The postexamination component addresses factors that can affect the test outcome and its use after the testing process.[10] Procedures should be established for the review of patient results and identification of those results that require further attention. For example, a sample should be repeated if the hemoglobin (Hb) and hematocrit (Hct) do not match (e.g., Hb × 3 = Hct).

Automated instruments can be interfaced with the laboratory information system (LIS) for electronic transfer of patient results. The LIS can also be interfaced with the hospital's or outpatient facility's computer system for reporting of patient results directly to the patient's chart. Electronic transfer of results minimizes **transcription errors.** The records of patient test results should be maintained within the laboratory. Procedures should be established for archiving and retrieving patient test results.

The laboratory is a business enterprise. Therefore, customer (e.g., physician or patient) satisfaction and communication are important issues to be addressed in the quality assessment program. An important factor affecting satisfaction level is **turnaround time (TAT)** for test results. Critical patient care decisions often depend on a laboratory test result. Computerization has made monitoring TAT more manageable. If a TAT problem is identified, laboratory management or the quality assessment committee should investigate it and recommend appropriate action.

In addition, protocols should be established to address customer complaints and other communication issues to minimize customer dissatisfaction. Surveys can be used to assess customer satisfaction and identify areas that need to be addressed. A quality assessment committee should be established to oversee the quality assessment program and determine changes that need to be made and how to implement them.

In accordance with CLIA '88 and the **Health Insurance Portability and Accountability Act (HIPAA)**, the laboratory should establish certain measures that ensure the confidentiality of patient information in each component of the quality assessment program.[1,11] For example, many facilities use unique identifiers rather than patient names or social security numbers to identify a sample and its test requisition. For the postexamination component, the laboratory should have a policy to ensure and document that the appropriate individual receives electronically transmitted test results.

Finally, documented records of all aspects of the quality assessment program should be maintained and retrievable upon request. These documents provide important information regarding the recognition of a problem, the process used to resolve it, and the change that occurred as a result of that process.

 Checkpoint! 1

Explain the importance of each component of the quality assessment program to its ultimate goal.

PROFICIENCY TESTING

Proficiency testing is an external quality control program that monitors the long-term accuracy of the different test systems (e.g., prothrombin time by the Beckman Coulter

ACL TOP instrument) through comparison to peer laboratories. Since the 1960s, many clinical laboratories have participated in proficiency testing surveys such as the survey program of CAP. CLIA '88 mandated however that all clinical laboratories performing nonwaived testing (includes testing methodologies not on the waived test list) participate in a proficiency testing survey at least three times a year.[12] Failure to achieve an acceptable rating for any given analyte (e.g., prothrombin time) in two of three surveys can result in certain sanctions of a laboratory such as delineation of a plan of corrective action for that test procedure or suspension of the certification to perform that test procedure.[13] Sanctions and penalties are issued by the Centers for Medicare and Medicaid Services (CMS). To reinstate a test procedure, the laboratory must obtain an acceptable rating for that analyte in two consecutive proficiency testing surveys.

Clinical laboratories contract with organizations such as CAP or the American Association of Bioanalysts to provide the proficiency testing service. A proficiency testing survey consists of proficiency samples, whole blood, or lypholized serum/plasma representing the full range of values that would be expected in patient samples. These samples are sent to the laboratory at specified time intervals, usually three times per year. Proficiency samples should be tested as part of a typical patient sample run. Results are sent to the survey provider for statistical analysis. The survey provider determines the target value (TV) for each test result through comparison studies with peer laboratories and establishes the acceptable performance (AP) ranges based on CLIA '88 tolerance limit (TL). For example, hemoglobin's tolerance limit is 7%. If the target value for hemoglobin sample 1 is 12.0 g/dL, then the acceptable performance range is 11.2–12.8 g/dL (AP = TV ± TL). The survey provider notifies the clinical laboratory and CMS of its findings.

Each laboratory should have a comprehensive program to respond to an unsatisfactory result. The source of the problem can be identified by checking for changes in the test procedure or reagents, reviewing the instrument's maintenance log and previous quality control results, and identifying changes in testing personnel. With the problem identified, corrective action can be taken to solve it. The laboratory should maintain proficiency testing survey results and documentation of corrective action.

 Checkpoint! 2

If a clinical laboratory loses its certification to perform protein C assays, what is involved in regaining that certification?

COMPETENCY TESTING

An additional requirement under CLIA '88 is **competency assessment** of all personnel performing nonwaived testing. CLIA '88 requires that this assessment take place twice during the first year of employment and annually thereafter.[14,15]

Because the *Federal Register* did not clearly outline the exact mechanisms to evaluate testing personnel's competency, laboratory directors, managers, and supervisors have struggled to determine the appropriate methods to evaluate competency within their laboratories. Clearly, this assessment must be more than a simple evaluation of one's knowledge of the material. The ability to score high on a multiple-choice test regarding laboratory test procedures within one's job description does not evaluate the individual's ability to perform and troubleshoot the test procedures. Direct observation checklists, random assignment of proficiency testing materials, or **"blinded" preanalyzed samples** can be used to evaluate these competencies (see Web Table 41-1 ○ for an example of a direct observation checklist). For each assessment tool, criteria must be established to judge acceptable performance. In the case of a 100-cell leukocyte differential, acceptable criteria might be based on the 95% confidence limits of the expert results (e.g., hematology supervisor or pathologist).[16]

No single method of assessing competency is appropriate for all test procedures. The laboratory supervisor, manager, or director is responsible for choosing appropriate methods for the particular laboratory setting. Additionally, educational materials (i.e., textbooks, selected journal articles, slide study sets, videotapes, or computer-based instruction) should be available to assist clinical laboratory professionals to improve their competency.

 Checkpoint! 3

What is an appropriate method of assessing a clinical laboratory professional's competency in performing prothrombin time (PT) and activated partial thromboplastin time (APTT) using an automated coagulation instrument?

METHOD EVALUATION/ INSTRUMENT COMPARISON

Selection, evaluation, and implementation of a new methodology or instrument in the hematology/hemostasis laboratory should follow an established protocol. Each laboratory should design its own protocol. This section discusses several important components to be included.

Selection

Selection of a new methodology or instrument is a daunting task. In the ideal setting, a committee should be formed to make this selection. For the selection of a new instrument, committee membership can include the hematology/hemostasis supervisor, several clinical laboratory professionals, LIS personnel, the quality assessment supervisor, a biomedical engineer, and the laboratory manager.

The first task of this committee is to determine the desirable characteristics of the new instrument.[17,18] A needs assessment survey could be used for this purpose, it should be completed by those individuals who will be using the instrument and by those individuals who might be affected by the use of that instrument (Web Table 41-2 ⊙). Desirable characteristics identified by this survey can then be used to solicit proposals from vendors (e.g., sales personnel for Beckman-Coulter, Siemens Medical, or Abbott Laboratories) (see Web Table 41-3 ⊙ for these characteristics).

The careful evaluation of the vendor's proposal packet by the selection committee will begin to narrow the selection process to several possible instruments. Members of the selection committee should also seek input from colleagues and the literature with regard to new instrumentation available and other laboratories' experiences with that instrumentation. The in-house evaluation of each instrument is a crucial step in the selection process. At this time, all interested parties would have a hands-on opportunity to assess the actual performance of the instrument in a real-time laboratory. Thus, a more meaningful evaluation can be obtained with regard to whether the instrument meets the laboratory's needs. The more information the committee has on which to base its selection, the better the selection will be. Ultimately, the selection of the instrument comes down to a particular laboratory's needs and the cost of meeting those needs.

The selection process of a new methodology or test system is similar. The selection committee must consider the cost per test, reagents, reagents' shelf-life and storage requirements, quality control program, test's **analytical sensitivity** (the ability to detect small quantities of the analyte), **analytical specificity** (ability to determine only the analyte in question), and **linearity** (range of concentration over which the test method can be used), required instrumentation and equipment, **analytical time,** and sample types that can be analyzed (i.e., whole blood, serum, CSF). Both testing personnel and potential clients should be consulted for their input during the selection process.

Analytical Reliability

With the purchase of a new instrument or the introduction of a new methodology, the laboratory must verify the performance of the instrument and/or method through a series of performance studies. To verify an instrument's analytical reliability, the clinical laboratory professional must evaluate the instrument with regard to **random variation** (variation due to chance) and **systematic variation** (variation within the instrument that alters results but is predictable). Precision studies are used to assess random variation and evaluate the reproducibility of the test method.[19,20] To check within run precision, the clinical laboratory professional should run 10–20 aliquots of a patient sample in the same run. These patient samples should have different concentration levels that correspond to **medical decision levels** of the analyte. For example, to check within run precision for hemoglobin, three patient samples can be chosen: sample 1 Hb = 8.0 g/dL; sample 2 Hb = 12.0 g/dL; sample 3 Hb =

19.0 g/dL. Each sample is separated into 10 aliquots, and each aliquot is analyzed. For each set of data, the mean, **standard deviation (SD),** and coefficient of variation are calculated (Table 41-3 ⊙). Precision can be determined by applying a statistical test called the *F-test* or by comparing the calculated coefficient of variation (CV) to the manufacturer's CV. Within run precision is acceptable if the CV is less than or equal to the manufacturer's CV. If the CV is higher than the manufacturer's CV, the clinical laboratory professional should check the data for **outliers.** Any outlier should be discarded and the data reevaluated. If the CV is still unacceptable, significant random variation exists within this method, or reagent and/or testing personnel errors have affected the study.

Systematic variation is assessed through the methods comparison procedure, which allows comparison of patient results between the new method and a method that is known to be accurate. **Split samples** (division of a single sample into two or more aliquots) are used. The **CLSI** (formerly NCCLS) recommends the use of at least 40 preferably 100, samples.[19-22] The samples should be random so they are representative of the clinical range of samples. Ideally, they should represent different pathologic conditions as well. With the samples identified, each one is split for analysis by each method. The samples are run in duplicate for each

⊙ **TABLE 41-3**

Within Run Precision Study for Hemoglobin Determination by Daman EXCELL-16

	Sample 1	Sample 2	Sample 3
1	7.9	12.0	19.2
2	8.1	12.3	19.4
3	8.0	12.2	19.4
4	8.1	12.2	19.4
5	8.1	12.2	19.3
6	8.0	12.3	19.4
7	8.0	12.3	19.4
8	8.1	12.4	19.5
9	8.1	12.4	19.3
10	8.1	12.3	19.6
Mean	8.1	12.3	19.4
SD	0.07	0.11	0.11
CV	0.86%	0.89%	0.57%
Manufacturer's CV	<1.0%	<1.0%	<1.0%

Three patient samples were chosen, and 10 aliquots of each sample were tested. The mean, standard deviation (SD), and CV were determined for each patient sample. Comparison of each calculated CV to the manufacturer's CV reveals acceptable precision for the hemoglobin procedure because the calculated CV is less than the manufacturer's CV. This procedure demonstrates the reproducibility of this hemoglobin determination. Results are reported in g/dL.

method, but the duplicate run should be done at a different time. All analysis should be completed on the same day, preferably within 4 hours.[22] Several statistical tools are used to analyze the results. The paired *t* test compares the mean of the differences of test results between the two methods and determines whether a statistically significant difference exists between the current method and the new method (see Web Table 41-4 ✪ for an example of a paired *t* test). The calculated *t* value for the two sets of results is compared to the critical *t* value from a statistical table. If the calculated *t* value is less than the critical *t* value, no significant difference exists between the two methods.

Linear regression analysis allows determination of the **y-intercept (a), slope (b),** standard error of the estimate ($s_{y/x}$), **correlation coefficient (r),** and coefficient of determination (r^2) (Figure 41-1 ■). The general formula for the linear regression line is $y = a + bx$, where y is the predicted mean value of y for a given x value. The coefficient of determination evaluates the strength of the relationship between the two methods. For example, an r^2 value of 0.90 for a comparison between current and new methods means that 90%

of the variability in the new method is directly predictable from the variability in the current method. Therefore, a strong relationship exists between the two methods.

Linear regression analysis is also used to detect systematic (constant or proportional) errors and random errors. Constant systematic errors are identified by a change in the y-intercept. A y-intercept with a value other than 0 (y > 0 or y < 0) indicates that a constant difference exists between the new method and the current method regardless of the analyte's concentration. The observation of a constant systematic error usually indicates a calibration problem. Proportional systematic errors are identified by changes in the slope. If there is no difference between the current method and the new method, the slope is 1.00 ± 5%. A change in the slope represents a difference between the new method and the current method that is proportional to the analyte's concentration. That is, the higher the concentration, the greater the difference is between the two methods. A proportional systematic error is most frequently associated with erroneous calibration. Random error can be detected by an increase in the standard error of the estimate. Increased dispersion of results about the regression line results in an increased standard error of the estimate. No standard criteria exist for the interpretation of an acceptable standard error of the estimate. Thus, the result should be evaluated in conjunction with the results of the precision studies.

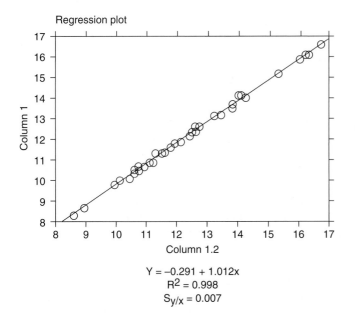

Regression plot

$$Y = -0.291 + 1.012x$$
$$R^2 = 0.998$$
$$S_{y/x} = 0.007$$

■ **FIGURE 41-1** Linear regression analysis for comparison of hemoglobin by automated cell counting instrument (column 1.2) and point-of-care instrument (column 1). Data sets are those given in Web Table 41-4. Interpretation of the linear regression analysis reveals a strong relationship $R^2 = 0.998$ between the automated cell counting instrument's hemoglobin method and the point-of-care instrument's hemoglobin method. No proportional systematic error exists because the slope (1.012) is between 0.95 and 1.05. The y-intercept (−0.291) is slightly less than 0, which indicates a small degree of negative bias or constant systematic error. This can be considered negligible by most laboratories. Random error also is not indicated because the standard error of the estimate (0.007) is nearly 0. Overall, this analysis demonstrates excellent comparison of methods.

✓ Checkpoint! 4

Linear regression analysis was performed on results from a method comparison of the prothrombin time between automated coagulation instrument A and automated coagulation instrument B (Web Figure 41-1 ■). The following results were obtained:

$$\gamma\text{-}intercept = 0.8157$$
$$Slope = 0.9982$$
$$Standard\ error\ of\ the\ estimate = 0.0807$$

What conclusions can be drawn from these results?

Linearity and Reportable Range Determinations

The manufacturer typically determines an instrument's linearity. The linearity of hematology instruments is determined for each directly measured parameter (e.g., leukocyte count, hemoglobin, and mean corpuscular volume [MCV]). Determination of linearity is accomplished by analyzing serial dilutions of a linearity check material multiple times to minimize the effects of imprecision.[23] Regression analysis is used to establish the linear range and the tolerance limits (Table 41-4 ✪). The tolerance limits represent the maximum allowable difference between the measured result and the reference value for a given dilution. A similar procedure is used to determine linearity for coagulation instruments.

Verification of the instrument's **reportable range** must be included within the method evaluation for a new

⊗ TABLE 41-4

Linear Ranges and Tolerance Limits for Abbott Cell-Dyn 4000 Instrument

	Linear Range		
Parameter	SI	USA	Tolerance Limits*
WBC	$0.0–250 \times 10^9$/L	$0.0–250 \times 10^3$/μL	±0.40 or 3.0%
RBC	$0.0–7.50 \times 10^{12}$/L	$0.0–7.5 \times 10^6$/μL	±0.15 or 2.0%
Hb	10.0–250.0 g/L	1.0–25.0 g/dL	±0.3 or 2.0%
MCV[†]	37.0–197.0 fL	37.0–197.0 fL	±2.0 or 2.0%
PLT	$0.0–2000.0 \times 10^9$/L	$0.0–2000.0 \times 10^3$/μL	±5.0 or 4.0%
MPV[†]	2.1–19.0 fL	2.1–19.0 fL	±1.0 or 5.0%
RETIC	$0.0–1500.0 \times 10^9$/L	$0.0–1500.0 \times 10^3$/μL	±18.5 or 3.0%

WBC = white blood cells; RBC = red blood cells; Hb = hemoglobin; MCV = mean corpuscular volume; PLT = platelets; MPV = mean platelet volume; Retic = reticulocyte count.

* The number to be used is the higher of the two at a given count or concentration.

[†] This parameter was tested with standard reference particles.

SI (Systeme International) refers to the internationally recognized unit of measure for each parameter.

USA refers to the conventional unit of measure for each parameter that has been traditionally used in the United States.

(Courtesy of Abbott Laboratories, Abbott Park, IL)

hematology or coagulation instrument or as one of the installation procedures for that new instrument.[24] To verify the reportable range, the clinical laboratory professional should analyze in duplicate at least three different levels of calibrators or linearity check materials that fall within the reportable range.[19] If these results fall within the instrument's defined tolerance limits, the reportable range is verified. In addition, these data can be plotted to visualize the linearity. If the data do not fall within tolerance limits or are nonlinear, the process should be repeated using more calibrators in the affected part of the range. If the data do not verify the instrument's reportable range, the laboratory should modify the reportable range to reflect the instrument's performance characteristics in its current setting.

With the verification of the reportable range, each laboratory should establish its protocol for handling results that exceed the reportable range, either above or below. For example, results above the reportable range may be diluted, reanalyzed, and the result multiplied by the dilution factor to determine the accurate result. Hematology results below the reportable range may require reanalysis of the sample and review of the peripheral blood smear before the result is reported as less than the lower limit of the reportable range.

REFERENCE INTERVAL DETERMINATION

Hematology and coagulation **reference intervals (RI)** are available in various recognized hematology textbooks and hematology/coagulation instrument and reagent manufacturer's manuals. To use these reference intervals, a laboratory must verify that the reference intervals are appropriate for its patient population as CLIA '88 requires.[24] Reference intervals are influenced by the diversity of instrumentation, choice of reagents, and patient population served by the laboratory. The laboratory can choose to validate the manufacturer's reference intervals or establish them for itself. The process of validating a reference interval is less time consuming and more cost effective. The recommended procedure for validation of a reference interval is described in Web Table 41-5 ⊗.[25] Once validated, the reference intervals can be used as representative for the laboratory and its patient population. If the reference intervals are not validated, the more rigorous process of establishing the laboratory's own reference interval should be performed.

Establishing a reference interval is an arduous task. It involves careful planning to define the criteria for subject selection, the process for data acquisition, and the analysis of the data. In the ideal situation, reference intervals should be established based on age and sex stratification of the patient population. For reliable estimates of a reference interval, a minimum of 120 individuals should be tested in each age and sex category.[22,25] One method of categorizing age groups is by decade of life. However, simple mathematical calculation would show the overwhelming number of individuals needed for such a process. Winsten suggests a mechanism to decrease the number of individuals needed by dividing the patient population into four age categories (Table 41-5 ⊗).[26] All subjects should complete brief histories to determine their acceptability for this study and be provided the appropriate instructions to prepare for the blood draw. In addi-

TABLE 41-5

Winsten's Recommended Age Categories for Reference Interval Determination

- Newborns
- Prepubertal individuals
- Adult (includes postpubertal and premenopausal)
- Older adults (includes males >60 years and postmenopausal females)

tion, each subject must sign an institutional review board (IRB) approved consent form. Ideally, 5–10 subjects should be tested per day to minimize possible random introduction of a shift in the reference interval due to instrument or reagent differences.

When all data have been acquired, they must be analyzed. Computer-based spreadsheets facilitate data analysis. CLSI recommends the use of percentile analysis, a nonparametric method,[25] which is appropriate because the analysis does not make any specific assumptions regarding the distribution of data points (e.g., Gaussian or non-Gaussian distribution). Using percentile analysis, the upper and lower limits of the reference interval depend on the ranks of reference data arranged in order of increasing values. The lower limit identifies the estimated 2.5th percentile, and the upper limit identifies the estimated 97.5th percentile, thus defining the 95% reference interval (see Web Table 41-6 ✪ for an example of percentile analysis to determine a reference interval).

✓ Checkpoint! 5

Define the term reference interval.

SAFETY

The laboratory environment includes biohazards, chemical hazards, and physical hazards. All laboratory employees must know the requirements for performing their jobs in a manner that protects them and their coworkers from these hazards. Several governmental agencies have established guidelines and standards for ensuring the safety of the clinical laboratory professional.

Universal Precautions

The Centers for Disease Control (CDC) introduced **universal precautions** in 1982.[27] With the discovery of the human immunodeficiency virus (HIV) and its potential transmission through exposure to infected blood or other body fluids, the CDC recognized the need for preventative guidelines to minimize the potential exposure of health care workers to this virus. Universal precautions state that health care workers should consider all body fluids as potentially infectious. Therefore, health care workers must use the appropriate personal protective equipment (PPE) when handling body fluids to minimize the risk of exposure to biohazardous agents such as HIV, hepatitis B, and other blood-borne pathogens (∞ Chapter 34).

The CDC has updated the original guidelines and continues to do so. Currently, guidelines recommend that all health care workers receive the hepatitis B vaccine. See Web Table 41-7 ✪ for selected recommendations from the CDC and the Occupational Health and Safety Administration (OSHA) designed to minimize the potential exposure to and transmission of blood-borne pathogens to clinical laboratory professionals.[28] Within a health care facility such as a hospital or medical center, the term *standard precautions* is used to define the facility's policies regarding universal precautions and infection control.[29]

OSHA Standards

OSHA regulates many aspects of the clinical laboratory to ensure a safe work environment. The clinical laboratory must meet OSHA's standards for chemical, physical, and fire safety. For biologic safety, OSHA implemented the Blood-borne Pathogen Standards in 1992 (∞ Chapter 34). All OSHA standards require education and training of laboratory employees, an exposure control plan, and a record-keeping mechanism. OSHA's Website (<www.osha.gov>) is a source of additional information and details regarding these standards.

Material Safety Data Sheets

The **material safety data sheet (MSDS)** provides safety information for clinical laboratory professionals who use hazardous materials. Web Figure 41-2■ is an example of an MSDS. It includes pertinent safety information regarding the following for the chemical: proper storage and disposal, precautions that should be taken in handling it, potential health hazards associated with exposure to it, and whether it is a fire or explosive hazard. Under the Hazard Communication Standard, or "Right to Know Law," clinical laboratory professionals must receive training regarding the hazardous chemicals that they work with.[30] This training should include the potential health risks associated with the chemical, interpretation of MSDS and chemical labels, and review of the laboratory's hazard communication program. MSDS must be available at all times to the clinical laboratory professionals.

✓ Checkpoint! 6

If a spill occurred when handling the CELL-DYN Sapphire hemoglobin reagent, what is the appropriate procedure to clean it up? Refer to Web Figure 41-2.

▶ QUALITY CONTROL

The clinical laboratory's quality control program monitors the testing process to ensure that reliable test results are obtained for the patient samples, to detect potential problems within the testing system, and to allow correction of the problem before patient results are affected.

CONTROL MATERIALS

Control materials are assayed samples with predetermined test results. The manufacturer assigns a lot number to each batch of control material. Within a given lot number, the assayed characteristics of the control are the same. For most hematology procedures, stabilized cell suspensions are used. These stabilized cell suspensions closely match the characteristics of human whole blood. The stability of cell suspensions is limited, for most commercially available cell suspensions, the time from a given lot number's start date to its expiration date is 4 months. For coagulation procedures (e.g., PT and APTT), lypholized control materials are used. When reconstituted, the lyophilized control has behavioral characteristics similar to platelet-poor citrated plasma. For these lypholized controls, a given lot number is ordered in sufficient quantities to meet the laboratory's testing needs for 1 year. This is advantageous because it limits the number of times new control limits with the new lot number must be established to once a year, and it provides a continuous monitor of the testing process over reagents and clinical laboratory personnel changes.

ESTABLISHMENT OF QUALITY CONTROL LIMITS

Quality control (QC) limits must be established for each control material prior to its use within the quality control program. Standard protocol for determining quality control limits calls for testing the new control material to collect a minimum of 20 data points (control measurements) over 10 working days.[31] These data points are collected while the current control material is used to monitor the integrity of the testing process and are used to determine the initial control limits. However, as more data points are collected, the limits should be recalculated using all data points to establish truly reliable control limits. The statistics used to establish the QC limits are the mean (x) and standard deviation (SD). Based on the mean and SD, the control limits $\pm 1s$, $\pm 2s$, and $\pm 3s$, are established.

The mean and control limits are then used to establish the QC chart (also known as a *Levey-Jennings chart*) (Figure 41-2■). The QC chart is used to plot the control material results over time to provide a graphical display of the distribution of control results over a given period, usually 1 month.

✓ **Checkpoint! 7**

To establish the control limits for a new lot number of level 1 PT coagulation control, the following data points were collected (results are in seconds): 11.8, 11.6, 12.1, 12.0, 12.3, 12.6, 11.9, 12.2, 12.0, 11.5, 12.7, 12.1, 11.2, 12.3, 12.9, 13.0, 12.3, 11.9, 12.4, 12.5. What are the ±2s control limits?

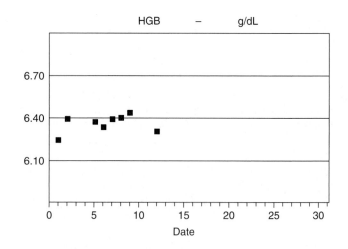

■ FIGURE 41-2   Quality control chart for level 1 hemoglobin control. The ±2SD limits are 6.10–6.70 g/dL with mean = 6.40 g/dL. The quality control results would be interpreted as being in control.

INTERPRETATION OF QUALITY CONTROL CHARTS

Statistically, 95% of the control results should fall within ±2SD, and 99% should fall within ±3SD. Careful and continual evaluation of the QC charts alerts the clinical laboratory professional to potential problems in the testing process before a serious breakdown in the test's integrity occurs. Using the Westgard multirule approach, the problem can be identified and corrected.

Westgard Rules

James O. Westgard, PhD, and colleagues developed the Westgard rules to evaluate control results when two or more levels of control material are used.[32] Table 41-6✪ lists and defines the most commonly used Westgard rules.

Evaluation of Quality Control Charts Using Westgard Multirule Approach

Each laboratory creates its multirule protocol for a given instrument by selecting a combination of Westgard rules. The selection depends on the acceptable level of false rejection (rejection of a control run that is not truly out of control) and error detection (rejection of a control run when a true error is detected) and the number of control levels run on that instrument.[33] The goal of the multirule protocol is to minimize the chance of false rejection of a control run while maximizing the ability to detect true error. For example, the multirule protocol for an instrument using two control levels might be $1_{2s}/1_{3s}/2_{2s}/R_{4s}/4_{1s}/10_x$. The 1_{2s} rule (S is used by Westgard as alternate abbreviation for S.D.) is used as a warning indicating the possibility that a rule has been violated. If a 1_{2s} warning is observed for one of the control results from the current test run, the clinical laboratory profes-

✪ TABLE 41-6

Westgard Rules

Westgard Rule	Definition	Type of Error
1_{2s}	One control result exceeds a 2s limit. This is considered a warning of a potential out-of-control problem.	
2_{2s} for across runs	Two consecutive control results exceed the same 2s limit. Run should be rejected and out-of-control problem investigated.	Systematic
4_{1s} for across runs	Four consecutive control results exceed the same 1s limit. Run should be rejected and out-of-control problem investigated.	Systematic
10_x for across runs	Ten consecutive control results exceed the mean in the same direction (e.g., results are above the mean). Run should be rejected and out-of-control problem investigated.	Systematic
4_{1s} for across runs and between control levels	Two consecutive control results for two control levels exceed the 1s limit in the same direction across the last two control runs. Run should be rejected and out-of-control problem investigated.	Systematic
10_x for across runs and between control levels	Five consecutive control results for two control levels exceed the mean in the same direction across the last five control runs. Run should be rejected and out-of-control problem investigated.	Systematic
2_{2s} for within run	Two consecutive control results for two control levels exceed the 2s limit in the same direction for the current control run. Run should be rejected and out-of-control problem investigated.	Systematic
1_{3s} for within run	One control result exceeds a 3s limit. Run should be rejected and out-of-control problem investigated.	Random
R_{4s} for within run	One control result exceeds +2s limit and the other control result exceeds −2s limit when using two control levels. Run should be rejected and out-of-control problem investigated.	Random

These rules can be applied "across runs" for two or more runs of a single control or both controls or "within run" for a single control or both controls.

sional should evaluate the QC charts, considering previous control results to determine whether a violation has occurred (Figure 41-3 ■).

Depending on the violation, the problem can be classified as a random or systematic error. A random error occurs by chance and can result from missampling or misidentifying the control. Random errors can be identified and corrected by carefully repeating the control. Systematic errors indicate a problem within the testing system, which can result from poor calibration, a change in reagent or an expired reagent, expired or improperly stored control, or deteriorating light source. Review of the daily and periodic maintenance logs for the instrument can help identify the problem. Once the problem has been identified, the correct solution can be implemented.

 Checkpoint! 8

After performing daily quality control on the automated hematology instrument, the clinical laboratory professional observes a 4_{1s} violation for the hemoglobin parameter. What type of error is indicated?

BULL'S TESTING ALGORITHM (MOVING AVERAGES)

Moving averages (continuous statistical analysis on consecutive patient erythrocyte indices by an automated cell counting instrument) is a method of using the erythrocyte indices, MCV, mean corpuscular hemoglobin (MCH), and mean cor-

puscular hemoglobin concentration (MCHC), to monitor the instrument's performance in determining the erythrocyte parameters.[34] The Bull's testing algorithm (X-B analysis) represents a calculation of the moving averages for erythrocyte indices of the patient population. It is based on the premise that the erythrocyte indices within a patient population are stable. Therefore, moving averages can be used to monitor the precision and accuracy of the instrument's performance.

To establish the acceptable ranges for the moving averages, MCV, MCH, and MCHC, the erythrocyte indices on 500 consecutive patient samples are determined and the mean for each index is calculated. The acceptable range is ±3% of the mean; however, each laboratory should determine its acceptable range.[35] These ranges are entered into the instrument's computer. The majority of hematology instruments calculate the moving average from each group of 20 patient samples and determine whether those moving averages fall within the acceptable range (Web Figure 41-3 ■). The instrument alerts the clinical laboratory professional if the moving average exceeds the acceptable range. If a moving average is unacceptable, the clinical laboratory professional should identify the previous 20 samples because this method is sensitive to the patient population. If the previous 20 samples were patients from the renal dialysis clinic or oncology clinic, the change in moving averages could result from the patient population, not an instrument problem. A true alert would indicate an instrumentation problem affecting one or more of the erythrocyte parameters: erythrocyte count, hemoglobin, or hematocrit (∞ Chapters 34, 36).

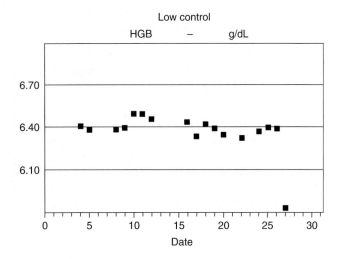

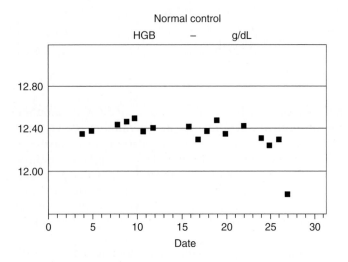

■ FIGURE 41-3   Violation of 2_{2s} rule. Inspection of the current run, day 27, reveals that both control materials exceed the $-2s$ limit, indicating a violation of the 2_{2s} rule within a run. This run should be rejected and the problem resolved before patient samples are run. Because the 2_{2s} violation indicates a systematic error, the clinical laboratory professional should investigate the possibility of a reagent, control, or instrument problem.

MONITORING QUALITY CONTROL WITH PATIENT SAMPLES

Patient samples can be retained and used in conjunction with purchased control materials to monitor the reproducibility of a hematology instrument over a 24-hour period as a result of the stability of cell counts in an ethylenediaminetetracetic acid (EDTA)-anticoagulated sample. For example, four or five patient samples are selected from the morning test run; each sample is analyzed to determine its mean; and the samples are separated into two sets. The first set of separated samples is used to monitor the precision of the instrument during a 24-hour period. This set is tested

every 4 hours. Using the SD and CV for this data, the instrument's precision is evaluated to determine its acceptability. The second set of separated samples is refrigerated for 24 hours. This set is used to monitor precision from day to day. After 24 hours, the second set is analyzed to determine each sample's 24-hour mean. The original mean is compared to the 24-hour mean to determine acceptability. Each laboratory should establish its own limits for acceptability.

Another potential use of retained patient samples is as quality control materials for the laboratory's secondary hematology instrument. Patient samples that are analyzed on the primary hematology instrument, which has been determined to be in control by purchased control materials, can be used to demonstrate that the secondary hematology instrument is in control during the same time interval.

▶ REVIEW OF PATIENT RESULTS

Although automated verification or autoverification of patient results can be utilized in the hematology/hemostasis laboratory, the underlying criteria for the process come from the laboratory's protocol for review of patient results (Web Table 41-8 ⊙).[37] Automated verification allows a faster turnaround time for patient results that meet the established criteria. The clinical laboratory professional is responsible for addressing those patient results that require special attention. This section describes review protocols and certain corrective actions for abnormal results in hematology and hemostasis.

HEMATOLOGY

Clinical laboratory professionals use the review protocol to examine patient data obtained from an automated cell-counting instrument and determine whether the complete blood count (CBC) results can be reported or further action is required.

Detection of Abnormal Test Results

The initial identification of potential abnormalities in the CBC results is accomplished by the instrument's computer system, which is programmed to evaluate the numerical data and histograms and generate suspect flags and user-defined flags (e.g., definitive flags) (∞ Chapter 36). The numerical data, histograms, and alert flags (suspect and user defined) provide information to the clinical laboratory professional that can indicate the presence of interfering substances, abnormal cell morphology, or abnormal cells. Table 41-7 ⊙ reviews common abnormal results or alert flags and their corrective actions.[38]

 Checkpoint! 9

In reviewing a patient's CBC results, the clinical laboratory professional notes an MCHC of 37 g/dL. What corrective action should be taken?

⊗ **TABLE 41-7**

Common Abnormal Results or Alert Flags and Their Corrective Actions

Abnormal Result/Alert Flag	Confirmation/Corrective Action	Rationale
Hemoglobin <7.0 g/dL	Confirm on alternate instrument.	A hemoglobin <7.0 g/dL is a critical value and should be confirmed before it is reported.
Hemoglobin × 3 does not equal hematocrit ±3	Confirm on alternate instrument or perform manual hematocrit.	This rule applies to normal individuals only and is used to identify common interfering substances in hematocrit determination (MCV) or hemoglobin determination (see MCHC below).
MCHC >36 g/dL	1. Perform manual hematocrit. 2. Check for presence of cold agglutinins, lipemia, or icteria.	Poor correlation between hemoglobin and hematocrit and an MCHC >36 g/dL is associated with cold agglutinins, lipemia, and icteria. Cold agglutinins cause erythrocyte clumping and result in falsely elevated MCV, falsely decreased red blood cells, falsely decreased hematocrit, and MCHC >36 g/dL. Lipemia causes a falsely elevated hemoglobin because of the increased turbidity of sample and MCHC >36 g/dL. Corrective actions are discussed within the text.
Platelet count <50 × 10⁹/L	1. Perform platelet estimate on peripheral blood smear and examine feather edge for platelet clumps. 2. Examine for grapelike cluster clumps of platelets associated with EDTA–dependent agglutination. If present, recollect using sodium citrate anticoagulant and multiply result by 1.1 (dilution factor). 3. Examine for platelet satellitism.	Presence of platelet clumps or platelet satellitism results in falsely decreased platelet counts. Platelet satellitism and platelet clumps can be EDTA dependent. Therefore, use of sodium citrate as the anticoagulant circumvents the mechanism of platelet clumping and platelet satellitism and allows determination of the platelet count.
WBC <2.0 × 10⁹/L or >30.0 × 10⁹/L	Perform leukocyte estimate on peripheral blood smear. Leukocyte estimate should agree within ±25% of the leukocyte count.	Poor correlation between leukocyte estimate and leukocyte count can be caused by instrument errors or sample collection error.
MCV <70 fL, >110 fL (adult), >120 fL pediatrics	Review peripheral blood smear for microcytosis or macrocytosis.	Clinically significant changes in MCV are associated with nutritional deficiencies and thalassemias.
Automated differential flagged	Perform manual differential.	Confirm presence of abnormal cells or abnormal erythrocyte morphology.
Platelets >900 × 10⁹/L	Perform platelet estimate on peripheral blood smear. Platelet estimate should agree within ±25% of the platelet count. Examine for presence of erythrocyte fragments.	Poor correlation between platelet estimate and platelet count could be caused by the presence of erythrocyte fragments that are similar in size and volume to platelets. Erythrocyte fragments can cause a falsely elevated platelet count.
Automated differential vote out	Perform manual differential.	Due to the presence of abnormal cells, the instrument is unable to properly classify the cells and determine the automated differential. The leukocyte differential must be obtained by performing a manual differential.
MCHC >36 g/dL, no correction after warming to 37°C	Examine peripheral blood smear for presence of spherocytes.	Spherocytes have a decreased surface area-to-volume ratio and typically have an MCHC >36 g/dL. After ruling out the possibility of cold agglutinins, the presence of spherocytes should be suspected.
Microcytic/fragmented red blood cell flags	1. Review erythrocyte morphology on peripheral blood smear. 2. Perform platelet estimate on peripheral blood smear.	Microcytic erythrocytes or erythrocyte fragments are similar in size and volume to platelets. Therefore, the presence of microcytic cells/fragments can result in a falsely elevated platelet count. Poor correlation between the platelet estimate and platelet count is associated with this observation.
WBC, RBC, or platelets > upper limit of established reportable range (or +++++)	Perform a 1:2 or 1:3 dilution of the sample with diluent. Run the sample and multiply the result by the dilution factor. Report the elevated parameter from the diluted sample only.	Cell counts that exceed the upper limit of their reportable range require a dilution of that sample to lower the number of cells present and bring the diluted cell count into the instrument's reportable range. The actual cell count is then obtained by multiplying the diluted sample's cell count by the dilution factor.

WBC = white blood cells; RBC = red blood cells; MCV = mean corpuscular volume; MCH = mean corpuscular hemoglobin; MCHC = mean corpuscular hemoglobin concentration

On occasion, spurious CBC results are obtained (e.g., results at first appear accurate but on review are invalid). These results might not be grossly abnormal or flagged by the instrument's computer, but the results do fall significantly outside the reference interval. The clinical laboratory professional should be alert for this possibility because spurious results can indicate a problem with the sample itself. Before these CBC results can be reported, the sample should be examined for potential sources of error (i.e., clots, lipemia, and agglutination). Table 41-8 ❂ reviews the spurious hematol-

❂ TABLE 41-8

Spurious Hematology Results, Underlying Problems, and Possible Causes

Erroneous Parameter	Underlying Problem	Possible Cause
Pseudoleukocytosis	Abnormal precipitant	Fibrin strands, cryoglobulinemia, cryofibrinogenemia, paraproteinemia
	Unlysed erythrocytes	Cold agglutinins, presence of abnormal hemoglobins such as hemoglobin S (HbS) or hemoglobin C (HbC)
	Platelet abnormalities	Platelet clumps, giant platelets, EDTA-dependent platelet aggregation
	Extraneous cell type or intracellular parasites	Nucleated erythrocytes, malarial parasites
	Carryover	Extreme leukocytosis in previous sample
Pseudoleukopenia	Cell lysis	Storage artifact, leukemia (esp. chronic lymphocytic leukemia [CLL]), uremia, immunosuppression
	Aggregates counted as single cells	Cold agglutinins, other antibody-related aggregation, aggregation related to presence of mucopolysaccharide
Pseudoincreased hemoglobin	Inappropriate dilution	Overfilled collection tubes
	Interference at 540 nm	Carboxyhemoglobin
	Turbidity	High leukocyte count, lipemia, abnormal hemoglobin (e.g., HbS and HbC), icteria (hyperbilirubinemia), cryoglobulinemia, paraproteinemia
Pseudodecreased hemoglobin	Interference at 540 nm	Sulfhemoglobin
Pseudoincreased RBC count	Other cells/particles counted	High leukocyte count, high platelet count, giant platelets, presence of cryofibrinogen or cryoglobulin
Pseudodecreased RBC count	Aggregates counted as single cells	Warm agglutinin, cold agglutinin, EDTA-dependent agglutination
	Absent/very small erythrocytes	In vitro hemolysis with microcytic erythrocytes or erythrocyte fragments (MCV <50 fL)
Pseudoincreased MCV	Other cells/particles	High leukocyte count
	Aggregates sized as single cells	Warm agglutinin, cold agglutinin, EDTA-dependent agglutination
	Osmotic swelling	Storage artifact, hyperglycemia, hypernatremia, hyperosmolar states
Pseudodecreased MCV	Instrument-related artifact	Hypochromic erythrocytes
	Other cells/particles	Giant platelets, cryoglobulinemia, cryofibrinogenemia
Pseudoincreased hematocrit, automated	Artificial increase in MCV	High leukocyte count ($>50,000/\mu L$), hyperosmolar states, erythrocyte agglutination
	Artificial increase in erythrocyte count	Cryoglobulin, cryofibrinogen, giant platelets
Pseudodecreased hematocrit, automated	Artificial reduction in MCV	Hyperosmolar states
	Artificial reduction in erythrocyte count	In vitro hemolysis, microcytic erythrocytes, cold agglutinin
Pseudoincreased hematocrit, manual	Increased plasma trapping	Polycythemia, microcytosis, sickle cell trait/disease, spherocytosis
	Decreased erythrocyte flexibility	Prolonged storage
Pseudodecreased hematocrit, manual	Decreased plasma trapping	Prolonged centrifugation, increased centrifugal force
	Increased cell shrinkage	Excess EDTA; K_3EDTA rather than K_2EDTA or Na_2EDTA
Pseudoincreased MCH	Spuriously high hemoglobin	(See hemoglobin)
	Spuriously low erythrocyte count	(See erythrocyte count)

⊘ TABLE 41-8

Spurious Hematology Results, Underlying Problems, and Possible Causes (continued)

Erroneous Parameter	Underlying Problem	Possible Cause
Pseudodecreased MCH	Spuriously low hemoglobin	(See hemoglobin)
	Spuriously high erythrocyte count	(See erythrocyte count)
Pseudoincreased MCHC	Spuriously high hemoglobin	(See hemoglobin)
	Spuriously low hematocrit or product of MCV × erythrocyte count	(See hematocrit)
Pseudodecreased MCHC	Spuriously low hemoglobin	(See hemoglobin)
	Spuriously high hematocrit or product of MCV × erythrocyte count	(See hematocrit)
Pseudothrombocytosis, automated	Very small erythrocytes or RBC fragments	In vitro hemolysis with microcytes or erythrocyte fragments (MCV <50 fL)
	Cytoplasmic fragments of nucleated cells	Cytoplasmic fragmentation of blasts in acute leukemia or leukemic cells in certain lymphomas
	Microorganisms, bacteria, or fungi	Bacterial septicemia; infection with *Candida sp.* that are similar in size to platelets
	Other particles	Cryoglobulinemia
Pseudothrombocytopenia, automated	Aggregates counted as single cell or aggregates exceed upper threshold and are not counted	EDTA-dependent agglutination
	Platelet satellitism	Platelets surround WBCs, EDTA-dependent process
	Giant platelets that exceed upper threshold for platelet count	Myeloproliferative disorders or myelodysplastic syndromes associated with abnormally large platelets
Pseudoincreased reticulocyte count, automated	Inaccurate gating of RBCs	Platelet clumps, giant platelets, WBC fragments, nucleated RBCs
	Other RBC inclusions	Howell-Jolly bodies, Pappenheimer bodies, Heinz bodies, basophilic stippling
	Intraerythrocytic parasites	Plasmodium, Babesia
	Other particles	Cold agglutinins, paraproteinemia
	Autofluorescence of RBCs	Porphyria, certain drugs

(Adapted, with permission, from Brigden ML, Dalal BI, Sprouts BI. Spurious and artifactual test results I: Cell counter-related abnormalities. *Lab Med.* 1999; 30(5):325–34. © 1999 American Society of Clinical Pathologists.)

ogy results that can be encountered in the clinical laboratory including the underlying problem that led to the erroneous parameter and the possible causes.[39–41]

Use of Delta Checks

Delta checks rely on consecutive testing of a particular patient. Comparison of current hematology results to the most recently reported previous result for a given patient allows the detection of certain random errors.[42] This method of error detection is termed the **delta check** and has been one of the greatest benefits of the LIS (Web Figure 41-4 ■).

Limits can be defined to determine the allowable difference among consecutive results of a specific test (e.g., hemoglobin) over an established time interval. The limits define when the LIS will flag a result. The delta check difference can be calculated as either a difference in the absolute value or as a percentage of the difference. Regardless of the method used, the delta limit should be set so that true changes in test results are not flagged as delta check failures.

If the time limit between comparisons and the maximum allowable differences have been carefully set, correct results will not be flagged. Therefore, the most likely causes of a delta check is a sample mislabeling or random testing error.

In the hematology laboratory, certain tests have very little intraindividual variation, especially the erythrocyte indices, platelet counts, PT, and other coagulation studies. When a delta check occurs for one of these parameters, an investigation should be undertaken before any results are reported (see Web Table 41-9 ⊘ for the investigation process).

Correction for Interfering Substances

The presence of lipemia, icterus, or hemolysis in the plasma of an EDTA-anticoagulated blood sample can cause an artificial elevation of the hemoglobin because of increased absorbance. The presence of interfering substances is commonly detected by the application of the Rule of 3, or hemoglobin × 3 = hematocrit ±3. To correct for the presence of these substances, an aliquot of the well-mixed blood sample is placed in another test tube and centrifuged at 1500 rpm for 5 minutes. A hemoglobin determination is performed on the plasma (supernatant). The corrected hemoglobin is calculated by subtracting the plasma hemoglobin result from the whole blood hemoglobin result (Hemoglobin$_{corrected}$ = Hemoglobin$_{original}$ − Hemoglobin$_{supernatant}$). Alternatively, the plasma can be removed from the centrifuged sample and replaced with an equal volume of saline. The cells are resuspended in the saline, and the corrected hemoglobin is obtained by performing a hemoglobin determination on this sample. The MCH and MCHC need to be recalculated using the corrected hemoglobin result and initial red blood cell count and hematocrit regardless of the correction method used for the hemoglobin.

Certain patients develop IgM antibodies or cold agglutinins directed against erythrocyte antigens. As the blood sample cools, these antibodies begin to agglutinate erythrocytes. The automated cell-counting instrument evaluates the agglutinated erythrocytes as one cell, resulting in a decreased erythrocyte count, increased MCV, decreased hematocrit, and MCHC >36 g/dL. Incubation of the blood sample at 37°C for 15 minutes disrupts the antigen–antibody reaction and dissociates the agglutinated erythrocytes. The warmed sample should be mixed thoroughly and analyzed immediately; its results are reportable unless the platelet count decreases by more than 50×10^9/L. Warming the sample occasionally causes loss of platelets. If this occurs, the original platelet count should be reported. Some patients exhibit a strong cold agglutinin titer, and the results may not correct after extended warming. In this situation, a manual hematocrit is performed, and the following additional results are reported from the original sample: white blood count, hemoglobin, and platelet count. The other CBC parameters cannot be reported.

HEMOSTASIS

As in hematology, patient results for coagulation tests should be reviewed for accuracy. This includes ensuring correct procurement of samples, checking for interfering substances, and using delta checks.

Overanticoagulation/Underanticoagulation

As discussed in ∞ Chapter 40, the proper ratio of blood: anticoagulant is 9:1 for the coagulation sample. All sample tubes should be examined visually to ensure that they have been properly filled. Comparison tubes can be prepared by adding water to empty collection tubes up to the expected fill level. Coagulation sample collection tubes containing less than 90% of the expected volume must be rejected because the sample is overanticoagulated due to a decrease in the 9:1 ratio.

For coagulation testing, the samples should have a hematocrit between 20% and 55%. If the hematocrit is below 20%, the amount of citrate will be insufficient to anticoagu-

late the sample, resulting in falsely shortened clotting times (e.g., prothrombin time). A hematocrit result of more than 55% results in an overanticoagulated sample and falsely prolonged clotting times. This effect on clotting times (i.e., PT and APTT) has been observed with the use of 3.2% sodium citrate as an anticoagulant.[43] The formula to adjust the blood-to-anticoagulant ratio for samples with low or high hematocrits is given in Web Figure 41-5 .

> ✓ **Checkpoint! 10**
>
> *The clinical laboratory professional observes that the 3.2% sodium citrate tube for a PT and APTT is only two-thirds full. Explain the effect this will have on the patient's coagulation results.*

Interfering Substances

Hemolyzed samples are unacceptable for coagulation testing because thromboplastin-like substances will have been released, resulting in shortened clotting times. Coagulation instruments based on photo-optical detection could be unable to test samples that contain interfering substances such as lipemia or icteria because these substances affect the endpoint detection (e.g., absorbance). An electromechanical (∞ Chapter 36) or manual clot detection method should be used to obtain accurate results from these samples.

Use of Delta Checks

Each laboratory must determine appropriate limits for delta checks in the hemostasis laboratory. In general, a change in the PT of ±5 seconds or in the APTT of ±15 seconds from a sample tested in the previous 24 hours could indicate a mislabeled sample.

SUMMARY

This chapter reviewed the components of a laboratory's quality assessment program. These can be divided into three components: pre-examination, examination, and postexamination. The pre-examination component includes all aspects that occur before testing that could affect the results including such things as sample collection and handling as well as test requisition. The examination component includes all testing aspects including proficiency testing and personnel competency. Proficiency testing monitors the reliability of a laboratory's test results by comparison to those of its peers and provides a good indication of a test method's long-term accuracy. Competency testing ensures that clinical laboratory professionals are proficient in the performance, interpretation, and troubleshooting of test procedures within their assigned area of the laboratory. The postexamination includes aspects that occur after the testing is performed that could affect the results. This includes review of patient results and turn around time.

When a new instrument or method is introduced to the laboratory, method evaluation studies must be performed to compare the new method to the current method, assess for random and systematic variation, and validate the reportable range. Precision studies allow the assessment of random variation, and linear regression analysis assesses systematic variation. A laboratory that chooses to use the manufacturer's reference intervals must validate them so they can be used for that laboratory and patient population. The laboratory can choose to establish its own reference interval. OSHA and other federal and state agencies mandate safety procedures. Each laboratory must adhere to those standards.

The laboratory's quality control program including the use of Westgard rules and moving averages monitors the day-to-day reliability of a test method and provides an early indicator of potential problems with it. Each laboratory creates its multirule protocol for an instrument by selecting a combination of Westgard rules.

Review of patient results is necessary to ensure that results reflect the patient's condition. This review is a very important component of the quality assessment program. The clinical laboratory professional's ability to recognize and take corrective action when abnormal patient results occur is at the heart of the clinical laboratory science profession. Review and recognition of abnormal patient results followed by corrective action represent the final steps before a test result is reported. The physician uses the reported test results to make critical decisions in a patient's diagnosis and treatment or management of disease. Therefore, a good quality assessment program directly affects patient care.

REVIEW QUESTIONS

LEVEL I

1. Which source of error represents a pre-examination factor? Failure to: (Objective 1)
   a. refrigerate the thromboplastin reagent
   b. correct the platelet count when using sodium citrate
   c. invert collection tubes properly
   d. perform daily maintenance on cell counting instrument

2. Under CLIA '88, how frequently should proficiency testing be performed? (Objective 4)
   a. once a year
   b. twice a year
   c. three times a year
   d. four times a year

3. When validating a manufacturer's reference interval, what is the minimum number of subject samples that should be used? (Objective 5)
   a. 10
   b. 20
   c. 60
   d. 120

4. Which governmental organization implemented universal precautions? (Objective 6)
   a. Occupational Safety and Health Administration (OSHA)
   b. Centers for Disease Control (CDC)
   c. Food and Drug Agency (FDA)
   d. Centers for Medicare and Medicaid Services (CMS)

5. Which of the following is an OSHA recommendation to be followed in the clinical laboratory? (Objective 7)
   a. Gloves should be worn when working with blood but are not required when performing a venipuncture.
   b. Safe needle devices should be used when performing a venipuncture or capillary puncture.
   c. Mouth pipetting is acceptable for transferring liquid reagents (e.g., saline or deionized water).
   d. Hand washing is necessary only if hands become contaminated with blood or other body fluids.

LEVEL II

1. Which is the first step in the selection of a new instrument? (Objective 3)
   a. conducting a needs assessment survey
   b. determining the cost per test
   c. performing an in-house evaluation of the instrument
   d. evaluating the quality control program

2. Which performance study in the method evaluation process assesses random variation? (Objective 3)
   a. precision study
   b. method comparison study
   c. linearity study
   d. calibration study

3. Given the following linear regression results, which is the appropriate interpretation? (Objective 2)

y-intercept	0.869
Slope	1.027
Standard error of the estimate	0.014

   a. No significant difference exists between the new method and current method results.
   b. A proportional systematic error exists between the new method and current method results.
   c. A random error exists between the new method and current method results.
   d. A constant systematic error exists between the new method and current method results.

LEVEL I

6. Which critical information regarding a chemical is found on its MSDS? (Objective 8)
   a. expiration date
   b. lot number
   c. storage requirements
   d. intended use

7. You are responsible for determining the control limits for the low fibrinogen control. The data points were collected and the mean ($x = 64$ mg/dL) and SD ($s = 3.0$ mg/dL) determined. What are the 3SD limits? (Objective 10)
   a. 61.0–67.0 mg/dL
   b. 58.0–70.0 mg/dL
   c. 55.0–73.0 mg/dL
   d. 52.0–76.0 mg/dL

8. How should the clinical laboratory professional interpret the PT control results for the current control run if the $\pm$2SD control limits are 11.80–14.20 seconds for Level I and 25.00–28.00 seconds for Level II? (Objective 11)

Current Run	Level I	11.6 seconds
	Level II	24.6 seconds

   a. acceptable
   b. unacceptable

9. Which of the following parameters will be affected by the presence of lipemia? (Objective 13)
   a. RBC, Hb, Hct, MCV, MCH, MCHC
   b. RBC, Hct, MCV, MCHC
   c. Hb, MCH, MCHC
   d. Hct, MCV, MCHC

10. In interpreting a patient's CBC results, the clinical laboratory professional notes that the platelet count is 25×10^9/L. Which of the following could be associated with this finding? (Objective 12)
    a. observation of erythrocyte fragments on the blood smear
    b. presence of cryoglobulins
    c. observation of platelet clumps at the feather edge of the blood smear
    d. presence of intracellular parasites such as malaria

LEVEL II

4. A clinical laboratory professional performed a procedure to verify the hemoglobin reportable range on the Cell-Dyn 4000. The highest level of linearity check material was 22.0 g/dL. This material was run several times with 21.2 g/dL representing the mean. How should this finding be interpreted? (Refer to Table 41-4) (Objective 4)
   a. The result is within the tolerance limits, and the reportable range is verified.
   b. The result exceeds the tolerance limits and the procedure should be repeated with new check material.
   c. The result exceeds the tolerance limits, and additional check material should be run in the upper limits of the reportable range.
   d. The result exceeds the tolerance limits, and the verification of reportable range should be repeated after the instrument is recalibrated.

5. After performing daily quality control on the automated hematology instrument, the clinical laboratory professional observes a 2_{2s} violation for the hemoglobin, MCH, and MCHC parameters. All other parameters were in control. What type of error is indicated? (Objective 5)
   a. random
   b. systematic

6. Regarding question 5, which is the most likely cause of the error? (Objective 5)
   a. failure to adequately mix the control materials
   b. improper storage of the control materials
   c. depleted supply of lysing reagent
   d. expired diluting fluid

7. For the automated hematology instruments, moving averages can be used to monitor the instrument's performance in determining which parameters: (Objective 6)
   a. leukocyte
   b. erythrocyte
   c. platelet
   d. reticulocyte

8. Initial interpretation of a patient's CBC results showed an MCHC of 38 g/dL. The clinical laboratory professional warmed the sample to 37°C and reanalyzed it. No change was observed. What is the appropriate course of action? (Objective 8)
   a. observe the blood smear for the presence of spherocytes
   b. replace patient's plasma with equal volume of saline and reanalyze.
   c. recollect patient sample using sodium citrate and analyze
   d. examine the blood smear for the presence of nucleated erythrocytes

REVIEW QUESTIONS *(continued)*

LEVEL I

LEVEL II

9. The following coagulation test results were obtained: PT = 7.5 seconds and APTT = 20 seconds. How should the clinical laboratory professional approach these findings? (Objective 8)
   a. report results to patient's chart
   b. observe sample for the presence of hemolysis
   c. check sample for small clots
   d. examine collection tube to determine whether it was underfilled

10. Which source of error would be detected by a delta check? (Objective 10)
   a. depleted reagent supply
   b. improper calibration of the instrument
   c. deteriorating light source
   d. failure to correctly label the patient's sample

www.pearsonhighered.com/mckenzie

Use this address to access the interactive Companion Website created for this textbook. Find additional information, tables and figures. Evaluate your command of the chapter information using case studies and critical thinking and multiple choice questions.

REFERENCES

1. Medicare, Medicaid, and CLIA Programs: Laboratory Requirements Relating to Quality Systems and Certain Personnel Qualifications; Final Rule, 42 CFR Part 493, Subpart K (493.1200). *Federal Register* 2003;68(16):3704–13.

2. Carver CJ. Establishing a thorough quality assurance program. *Advance for Medical Laboratory Professionals.* 2000;12(9):6.

3. Stankovic AK, Smith S. Elevated serum potassium values: The role of preanalytical variables. *Am J Clin Pathol.* 2004;121(Suppl 1): S105–S112.

4. Tarapchak P. Identify, eliminate the "error" of your ways. *Advance for Administrators of the Laboratory.* 2000;10(3):64–71.

5. King D. A variety of variables. *Advance for Medical Laboratory Professionals.* 2000;12(24):14–17.

6. Drew N. Monitoring specimen collection errors. *Advance for Medical Laboratory Professionals.* 2000;12(15):12–15.

7. CLSI. *Laboratory Documents: Development and Control; Approved Guideline,* 5th ed. GP2-A5. Wayne, PA: CLSI; 2006.

8. Medicare, Medicaid, and CLIA Programs: Laboratory Requirements Relating to Quality Systems and Certain Personnel Qualifications; Final Rule, 42 CFR Part 493, Subpart K (493.1251). *Federal Register.* 2003;68(16):3706.

9. Shahangian S, Holmes EH, Taylor RN. Toward optimal PT use. *MLO.* 2000;32(4):32–43.

10. Carver C. A closer look at post-analytical policies and procedures. *Advance for Medical Laboratory Professionals.* 2000;12(7):6.

11. Centers for Disease Control and Prevention. HIPAA privacy rule and public health. Guidance from CDC and the U.S. Department of Health and Services. *MMWR.* 2003;52:1–20.

12. Medicare, Medicaid, and CLIA Programs: Laboratory Requirements Relating to Quality Systems and Certain Personnel Qualifications;

Final Rule, 42 CFR Part 493, Subpart H (493.800) and Subpart I (493.900). *Federal Register.* 2003;68(16):3702–3703.

13. Ehrmeyer SS, Laessig RH. Has compliance with CLIA requirements really improved quality in US clinical laboratories? *Clinica Chimica Acta.* 2004;346(1):37–43.

14. Medicare, Medicaid, and CLIA Programs: Laboratory Requirements Relating to Quality Systems and Certain Personnel Qualifications; Final Rule, 42 CFR Part 493, Subpart K (493.1235). *Federal Register.* 2003;68(16):3705.

15. Sharp, SE, Elder BL. Competency assessment in the clinical microbiology laboratory. *Clin Microbiol Rev.* 2004;17(3):681–94.

16. Leach AP, Haun DE. Assessing competence in finding and reporting abnormal morphologic features while scanning peripheral blood smears. *Clin Lab Science.* 2000;13(3):160–65.

17. James E. Automated analyzer selection: Strategies for success. *Advance for Medical Laboratory Professionals.* 2004;16(2):20–22.

18. Barglowski M. The instrument selection process: Beyond the sales pitch. *MLO.* 2001;33(2):45–51.

19. Polancic J, Roncancio G. *Method Verification and Instrument Selection Procedures.* Springfield: The Laboratory Consultants, Inc. of Illinois; October 1994.

20. Plaut D. Analytical accuracy: Verifying performance. *MT Today.* 1994;14–16.

21. CLSI. *Method Comparison and Bias Estimation Using Patient Samples; Approved Guidelines,* 2nd ed. EP9-A2. Wayne, PA: CLSI, 2002.

22. Cembrowski GS, Martindale RA. Quality control and statistics. In: Bishop ML, Fody EP, and Schoeff, L eds. *Clinical Chemistry: Principles, Procedures, Correlations,* 5th ed. Philadelphia: Lippincott Williams & Wilkins; 2005.

23. *CELL-DYN 4000 System Operator's Manual.* Abbott Park, IL: Abbott; March 1999:4–12.

24. Medicare, Medicaid, and CLIA Programs: Laboratory Requirements Relating to Quality Systems and Certain Personnel Qualifications; Final Rule, 42 CFR Part 493, Subpart K (493.1253). *Federal Register.* 2003;68(16):3707.

25. CLSI. *How to Define and Determine Reference Intervals in the Clinical Laboratory; Approved Guideline,* 2nd ed. C28-A2. Wayne, PA: CLSI; 2000.

26. Winsten S. The ecology of normal values in clinical chemistry. *Crit Rev Clin Lab Sci.* 1976;6:319.

27. Centers for Disease Control. Acquired immunodeficiency syndrome (AIDS): Precautions for clinical and laboratory staffs. *MMWR.* 1982; 31:577–80.

28. Centers for Disease Control. Updated U.S. Public Health Service guidelines for the management of occupational exposures to HIV and recommendations for postexposure prophylaxis. *MMWR.* 2005; 54(RR-9):1–17

29. Duerink DO, Farida H, Nagelkerke NJD et al. Preventing nosocomial infections: improving compliance with standard precautions in an Indonesian teaching hospital. *J Hosp Infect.* 2006;64:36–43.

30. Occupational Safety and Health Administration Hazard Communication; Final Rule, 29 CFR, *Federal Register.* 1994;59:6126–84.

31. Westgard JO. QC: The calculations. In: Westgard JO, ed. *Basic QC Practices: Training in Statistical Quality Control for Healthcare Laboratories,* 2nd ed. Madison, WI: Westgard Quality Corporation; 2002.

32. Westgard JO, Barry PL, Hunt MR, Groth T. A multi-rule Shewhart chart for quality control in clinical chemistry. *Clin Chem.* 1981; 27:493–501.

33. Westgard JO. QC: The multirule procedure. In: Westgard JO, ed. *Basic QC Practices: Training in Statistical Quality Control for Healthcare Laboratories,* 2nd ed. Madison, WI: Westgard Quality Corporation; 2002.

34. Bull BS, Elashoff RM, Heilbron DC et al. A study of various estimators for the derivation of quality control procedures from patient erythrocyte indices. *Am J Clin Pathol.* 1974;61:473–81.

35. *CELL-DYN 4000 System Operator's Manual.* Abbott Park, IL: Abbott; March 1999:11-53–11-57.

36. Dotson MA. Methods to monitor and control systematic error. In: Stiene-Martin EA, Lotspeich-Steininger CA, Koepke JA, eds. *Clinical Hematology: Principles, Procedures, Correlations,* 2nd ed. Philadelphia: J. B. Lippinocott; 1998.

37. CLSI. *Autoverification of Clinical Laboratory Test Results; Approved Guideline.* AUTO10-A. Wayne, PA: CLSI; 2006.

38. Cornbleet J. Spurious results from automated hematology cell counters. *Lab Med.* 1983;14(8):509–14.

39. Brigden ML, Dalal BI. Spurious and artifactual test results I: Cell counter-related abnormalities. *Lab Med.* 1999;30(5):325–34.

40. Zandecki M, Genevieve F, Gerard J, Godon A. Spurious counts and spurious results on haematology analysers: A review. Part 1: Platelets. *Int Jnl Lab Hem.* 2007;29:4–20.

41. Zandecki M, Genevieve F, Gerard J, Godon A. Spurious counts and spurious results on haematology analysers: A review. Part II: White blood cells, red blood cells, haemoglobin, red cell indices and reticulocytes. *Int Jnl Lab Hem.* 2007;29:21–41.

42. Houwen B, Duffin D. Delta checks for random error detection in hematology tests. *Lab Med.* 1989;20(6):378–81.

43. Marlar RA, Potts RM, Marlar AA. Effect on routine and special coagulation testing values of citrate anticoagulant adjustment in patients with high hematocrit values. *Am J Clin Pathol.* 2006;126: 400–5.

APPENDIX A
Answers to Case Study Questions

CHAPTER 1

Case Summary: Aaron had clinical signs of infection and a past history of ear infections. The CBC results revealed a high WBC count consistent with an infectious process. The diagnosis of otitis media usually can be made by history and physical examination. Laboratory tests are not required.

Question:

1. If Aaron was diagnosed with otitis media, what cellular component(s) in his blood would be playing a central role in fighting this infection?

Explanation:

The leukocytes, or white blood cells, are the cells that are central in fighting infection.

Question:

2. Aaron's physician ordered a CBC. The results are Hb 11.5 g/dL; Hct 0.34L/L; RBC 4.0×10^{12}/L; WBC 18×10^9/L. What parameters, if any, are outside the reference range? Why do you have to take Aaron's age into account when evaluating these results?

Explanation:

The WBC count is increased. The upper reference range for WBC in a 2-year-old is 17×10^9/L. It is important to consider Aaron's age because the reference ranges for blood cell concentrations are different in children of various ages and are different from those in adults.

CHAPTER 4

Case Summary: Francine had an acute lymphocytic leukemia. This is a type of leukemia that is characterized by a malignant proliferation of immature lymphocytic cells.

Question:

1. Refer to the tables on the inside cover of the book and determine which blood cell parameters, if any, are abnormal.

Explanation:

The hemoglobin is decreased. The WBC is normal, but the platelets are markedly decreased.

Question:

2. Describe Francine's bone marrow as normal, hyperplastic, or hypoplastic.

Explanation:

The bone marrow is hyperplastic. Normal bone marrow cellularity varies with age. A rule of thumb is that cellularity is 100% minus the age of the individual. This applies to marrow cellularity in the range of 30–90%.

Question:

3. What conditions can cause this bone marrow finding?

Explanation:

Conditions associated with an increased celluarity of bone marrow may include anemia and leukemia.

Question:

4. What do you think is the cause of the splenomegaly?

Explanation:

The splenomegaly could be due to extramedullary hematopoiesis. Malignant cells may be proliferating in the spleen.

Question:

5. Why might the peripheral blood reveal changes associated with hyposplenism when the spleen is enlarged?

Explanation:

Tumor cells can incapacitate the spleen, causing functional hyposplenism.

Question:

6. What might explain the lymphadenopathy?

Explanation:

The malignant lymphocytic cells may be proliferating in the lymph nodes causing enlargement.

CHAPTER 5

Case Summary: This is a case of Stephen, a 28-year-old Caucasian male of Italian descent with an acute hemolytic anemia. An initial diagnosis of malaria was presumptively made. The patient, however, was negative for malaria. He was eventually diagnosed as having G6PD deficiency and a hemolytic anemia induced by the antimalarial drug primaquine.

Question:

1. Predict Stephen's reticulocyte count: low, normal, or increased.

Explanation:

From the erythrocyte count, HGB, and HCT, we know the patient is moderately anemic. The increase of polychromatic erythrocytes on a blood smear suggests an increased number of reticulocytes.

Question:

2. What is the cellular mechanism that results in hemolysis due to a deficiency in G6PD?

Explanation:

In the hexose monophosphate shunt, the reduction of NADPH and glutathione depends on the enzyme glucose-6-phosphate dehydrogenase (G6PD). When this enzyme is deficient, hemoglobin denatures under oxidant stress, and intracellular hemoglobin precipitates form.

Question:

3. Explain how Heinz body inclusions cause damage to the erythrocyte membrane.

Explanation:

Hemoglobin precipitates known as Heinz bodies form along the inner surface of the erythrocyte membrane. This results in a loss of membrane flexibility, cell lysis, and splenic trapping.

Question:

4. Would you predict Stephen's serum erythropoietin levels to be low, normal, or increased? Why?

Explanation:

Hemolytic anemias result from factors outside the marrow. Erythroid production and maturation are normal. The loss of erythrocytes results in a systemic decrease in cellular oxygen tension. This stimulates EPO production from the kidneys, which in turn stimulates erythropoiesis in the marrow.

Question:

5. Stephen's haptoglobin level is 25 mg/dL. Explain why Stephen has a low haptoglobin value.

Explanation:

The oxidant stress caused by the malarial drug primaquine was out of balance due to the patient's erythrocyte deficiency of G6PD. This resulted in hemoglobin precipitation (Heinz bodies) and cell destruction. Some of the hemoglobin is released into the peripheral blood and is bound by haptoglobin. The haptoglobin reserves become depleted quickly.

 CHAPTER 6

Case Summary: Jerry lost a substantial amount of blood from the fractures and surgery. If his hemoglobin had been normal before the accident (14–16 g/dL), he lost about one-half of the volume of his blood. With the loss of this much blood, he also lost a substantial amount of iron. Although he was given iron supplements, it will take time for his hemoglobin to reach normal again. He had symptoms of anemia with lethargy and pallor. They result from a loss of hemoglobin and, hence, a decrease in the amount of oxygen delivered to the tissue. The blood transfusions will bring his hemoglobin concentration up more rapidly and give his body the energy it needs to repair itself.

Question:

1. If Jerry is iron deficient, what is the effect on synthesis of ALAS, transferrin receptor, and ferritin?

Explanation:

The iron regulatory protein (IRP) is the primary physiologic iron sensor and plays a role in regulating the synthesis of molecules involved in hemoglobin synthesis. Lack of iron results in decreased synthesis of ALAS, increased synthesis of transferrin receptor, and decreased synthesis of ferritin.

Question:

2. What was the rationale for giving Jerry the iron?

Explanation:

Because Jerry had lost the blood through bleeding, he also lost a substantial amount of iron. Even if body storage of iron is normal, iron supplements are often given, in this case to provide the iron needed for rapid and increased hemoglobin synthesis.

Question:

3. Explain why Jerry may have these symptoms.

Explanation:

Jerry's hemoglobin was very low, which means that his tissues were not getting the oxygen they needed. This leads to a decrease in metabolic activity and, consequently, a decrease in energy. Pallor is a classic sign of anemia because blood is preferentially circulated to critical areas of the body including the brain, heart, and so on. The skin's blood supply decreases, causing a loss of the pinkish color of the skin, especially apparent in Caucasians.

Question:

4. Explain why Jerry may have had more energy after the transfusions.

Explanation:

The transfusions boosted Jerry's hemoglobin level and, thus, increased the amount of oxygen that could be transported to the tissues for critical metabolic processes.

CHAPTER 7

Case Summary: Harry had a physical as a prerequisite for buying a life insurance policy. His results were within the reference range for his sex and age except for the WBC count, which was above the reference range.

Question:
1. Are any of these results outside the reference range? If yes, which one(s)?

Explanation:
The WBC count is above the reference range.

Question:
2. If this were a newborn, would you change your evaluation? Why?

Explanation:
Newborns have a higher reference range for WBC; therefore, if this were a newborn, the WBC count would fall within the reference range.

Question:
3. Are any of the WBC concentrations outside the reference range (relative or absolute)?

Explanation:
All results, both percents and absolute values, are within the reference range.

Question:
4. Is there a need for reflex testing on Harry? Explain your answer.

Explanation:
Although Harry's WBC count is slightly above the reference range, his absolute individual white cell numbers are within it. Given the fact that he has no symptoms, the physical examination was normal, and no abnormal cells were noted on the blood smear, there is probably no need to do additional testing. The reference range is usually set by calculating the mean and adding and subtracting two standard deviations. This range includes 95% of normal individuals. About 5% of individuals have a result outside this range but are still normal. This may be the case with Harry.

 CHAPTER 8

Case Summary: George had a severe macrocytic, hyperchromic anemia as revealed by the red cell indices. The anemia developed slowly over time, which gave his body the opportunity to adapt to a low hemoglobin level. The probability of shock and death of a patient who had lost this much blood quickly would have been high. The yellowness of the eyes suggests a high bilirubin concentration, which is typical of a hemolytic anemia. This patient had a test that revealed antibodies and complement on his red blood cells. This supports the diagnosis of an immune hemolytic anemia. The presence of spherocytes supports this diagnosis because they are a sign that the spleen has removed antibody/antigen complexes from the cell membrane. Note that the MCHC is increased, which is typical of spherocytes. The high reticulocyte count and presence of polychromatophilic erythrocytes indicate the bone marrow is responding appropriately by increasing output of erythrocytes. The high reticulocyte count is probably responsible for the increased MCV.

Question:
1. Calculate the erythrocyte indices. Does the information given suggest acute or chronic blood loss? What is the significance of the RDW?

Explanation:
MCV 113 fL; MCH 43.7 pg; MCHC 38.8 g/dL. The case history suggests chronic blood loss. The hemoglobin is very low, and the patient probably would be in shock if he had lost this much blood suddenly. The RDW suggests significant anisocytosis.

Question:
2. Calculate the absolute reticulocyte count. His RBC count is $0.71 \times 10^{12}/L$, and the reticulocyte count is 22%. Is this increased, decreased, or normal?

Explanation:
The absolute reticulocyte count is

$$22\% \times 0.71 \times 10^{12}/L = 0.156 \times 10^{12}/L = 156 \times 10^{9}/L$$

This is at the high end of the reference range.

Question:
3. George's blood smear revealed marked spherocytosis. Explain the importance of this finding.

Explanation:
Spherocytes are cells that have lost membrane. They are significant in this case because they indicate a hemolytic anemia.

Question:
4. Explain George's abnormal indices.

Explanation:
The indices are all elevated: MCV 113 fL; MCH 43.6 pg; MCHC 38.8 g/dL. The increased MCV may be due to the high reticulocyte count. The MCH is elevated due to the presence of these large cells that are able to hold more hemoglobin than a smaller cell. The MCHC is elevated due to the marked spherocytosis.

Question:
5. Classify George's anemia morphologically and functionally.

Explanation:

George's anemia is morphologically classified as macrocytic, hyperchromic. Functionally, it is classified as a survival defect. It appears that the cells are being destroyed by an immune hemolytic process. The bone marrow has increased production of cells as the increased reticulocyte count indicates.

CHAPTER 9

Case Summary: Jose is suffering from IDA due to chronic blood loss from the GU tract. He has the typical blood picture of microcytic, hypochromic erythrocytes. His iron studies reveal a lack of total body iron. The serum iron and % transferrin saturation are low.

Question:

1. How would you describe his anemia morphologically?

Explanation:

MCV = 63 fL; MCH = 19.5 pg. The anemia is microcytic, hypochromic.

Question:

2. Calculate % saturation.

Explanation:

Serum iron/TIBC = 4%. The serum iron is low and the TIBC increased resulting in a low % saturation.

Question:

3. Is this value normal, decreased, or increased?

Explanation:

Decreased. Less than 15% saturation is considered decreased.

Question:

4. What disease, if any, is suggested by this value?

Explanation:

Iron deficiency (ID). The percent saturation of transferrin is decreased in ID, usually to less than 10%.

Question:

5. How do the iron study results of our patient help in differentiating the diagnosis of iron deficiency from ACD?

Explanation:

In ACD, the serum iron is low, and the TIBC and % saturation are normal or decreased. In ACD, the total body iron is normal to increased. In ID, total body iron is decreased.

Question:

6. What additional iron test that was not done would be most helpful in this case?

Explanation:

Serum ferritin is a good indicator of iron stores and is less invasive than a bone marrow. The drawback to serum ferritin is that it is an acute phase reactant.

Question:

7. Do the iron studies in Jose (serum iron 17 μg/dL, TIBC 425 μg/dL) suggest sideroblastic anemia?

Explanation:

No, iron studies in this patient reveal a lack of total body iron. Sideroblastic anemia has a defect in the incorporation of iron into the porphyrin ring. Iron accumulates in the red cell and macrophage. Thus, the total body iron is increased in sideroblastic anemia.

Question:

8. Do Jose's laboratory test results and clinical history indicate that a bone marrow examination is necessary?

Explanation:

No, adequate information is present from other laboratory tests. The CBC and iron studies give important clues to a diagnosis of ID anemia. A bone marrow may be performed in difficult cases but is usually not necessary.

CHAPTER 10

Case Summary: Shane, previously diagnosed with a hemoglobinopathy, was admitted to the hospital with symptoms of vaso-occlusive crisis. Testing revealed he had pneumonia and sickle cell disease. The infection was probably responsible for precipitating the crisis.

Question:

1. Identify a laboratory test needed to determine Shane's hemoglobinopathy.

Explanation:

Hemoglobin electrophoresis is needed to identify a hemoglobinopathy. HPLC may be done to quickly identify the percentage of HbS.

Question:

2. What is the abnormal hemoglobin causing this Shane's disease?

Explanation:

HbS.

Question:

3. Is Shane heterozygous or homozygous for the disorder?

Explanation:

We can assume that the patient is homozygous because of the very high concentration of HbS present and lack of HbA.

Question:

4. What is this disorder called?

Explanation:

This disorder is referred to as *sickle cell disease* or *sickle cell anemia*.

Question:

5. What physiological condition does Shane have that could lead to sickling of his erythrocytes?

Explanation:

This patient has fever, suggesting infection or inflammation. The chest radiograph indicated pneumonia. It is possible that the infection is causing hypoxia and other physiological alterations that promote sickling.

Question:

6. What is the cause of this Shane's pain and acute distress?

Explanation:

The patient is experiencing a vaso-occlusive crisis as a result of sickling of erythrocytes in the microvasculature. (Physicians refer to this as a "pain crisis.") It is possible he is also experiencing acute chest syndrome.

Question:

7. Why might Shane be more susceptible to pneumonia than an individual without sickle cell disease?

Explanation:

It is likely that he has functional asplenia as a result of repeated sickling episodes in the spleen. Without a functioning spleen, he is more susceptible to certain bacterial infections. Often sickle cell patients are treated with prophylactic antibiotics to prevent infections.

Question:

8. Which of Shane's hematologic test results are consistent with a diagnosis of sickle cell anemia?

Explanation:

His hemoglobin is markedly reduced and in the range typically seen in sickle cell disease. Also, leukocytes and platelets are increased, which are common findings. The presence of sickle cells and other findings on the blood smear are all consistent with a diagnosis of sickle cell disease.

Question:

9. What does the presence of polychromatophilic erythrocytes signify?

Explanation:

Polychromatophilic erythrocytes are actually reticulocytes. This indicates that the bone marrow is attempting to compensate for the deficit of erythrocytes in the peripheral blood by releasing these slightly immature cells.

Question:

10. Why is the absolute neutrophil count elevated?

Explanation:

Bacterial infection is associated with neutrophilia.

Question:

11. What is the significance of ovalocytes on the blood smear?

Explanation:

These cells are probably irreversibly sickled cells.

Question:

12. What is the significance of Howell–Jolly bodies on the smear?

Explanation:

The patient's spleen is not functional and is incapable of removing these inclusions from the erythrocytes.

Question:

13. What is the significance of Shane's elevated LD?

Explanation:

Lactic dehydrogenase is an enzyme found in high concentration in erythrocytes. Elevated LD levels are associated with increased hemolysis of erythrocytes, a typical finding in sickle cell disease.

CHAPTER 11

Case Summary: John had the typical symptoms of anemia. His CBC revealed a microcytic, hypochromic anemia. Tests for iron deficiency were negative. Hemoglobin electrophoresis was abnormal with the presence of hemoglobins H and Bart's. These hemoglobins indicate a deficiency of α-chains. The presence of some HbA, HbA$_2$, and HbF indicate that some α-chains are being produced. This suggests the presence of α-thalassemia. The parents also exhibit symptoms of anemia and should be tested to determine whether they have a form of α-thalassemia. This will help confirm the child's diagnosis.

Question:

1. Based on the indices, classify the anemia morphologically.

Explanation:

Microcytic, hypochromic

MCV = 69 fL

MCH = 21 pg

MCHC = 29.2 g/dL

The MCV is below the lower limit of normal (80 fL) indicating the presence of microcytic erythrocytes. The MCHC is the best indicator of hemoglobin content and is below the lower limit of normal (32 g/dL), suggesting hypochromasia. The below normal MCH (<27 pg) corroborates the decreased hemoglobin content.

Question:

2. Name the dominant poikilocyte observed in this peripheral blood smear.

Explanation:

The dominant poikilocytes are target cells.

Question:

3. Name three disorders that frequently present with the same poikilocyte that dominates in this peripheral blood smear.

Explanation:

Thalassemia

Hemoglobinopathy

Iron-deficient anemia

Liver disease

Question:

4. List two additional lab tests that would help confirm the diagnosis and predict the results of each.

Explanation:

Disorder	Hb Electrophoresis	Hb Solubility Test	Iron Panel
Thalassemia (α)	HbH Hb Bart's ↓ HbA, A$_2$, and F	Negative	Normal
Thalassemia (β)	Hb Bart's ↓ HbA ↑HbA$_2$ and HbF	Negative	Normal
Hemoglobinopathy	HbS or HbC or HbE, etc. ↓ HbA	Positive with some (HbS, etc.)	Normal
Iron deficiency anemia	Normal	Negative	↓ Serum iron ↓Ferritin ↓% Saturation ↓BM iron ↑ TIBC

Question:

5. Is the hemoglobin electrophoresis normal or abnormal?

Explanation:

Abnormal.

Question:

6. If abnormal, list hemoglobins that are elevated, decreased, or abnormally present.

Explanation:

Elevated	Decreased	Abnormal
None	HbA	Hb Bart's
	HbF	HbH
	HbA$_2$	

Question:

7. If abnormal, which globin chain(s) is(are) decreased?

Explanation:

α-chains and all α-chain containing hemoglobins (HbA, F, and A$_2$) are decreased.

Question:

8. If abnormal, which globin chain(s) is (are) produced in excess?

Explanation:

β-chain containing HbH and γ-chain containing Hb Bart's are elevated, ruling out a β-, γ-, $\delta\beta$-, and $\gamma\delta\beta$-thalassemia.

Question:

9. Is the iron panel normal or abnormal?

Explanation:

Normal.

Question:

10. If the iron test results are abnormal, list those outside the normal range and indicate whether they are elevated or decreased.

Explanation:

Normal, so nonapplicable.

Question:

11. If abnormal, state the disorder(s) consistent with the abnormal iron panel.

Explanation:

An abnormal iron panel usually presents with a pattern consistent with one of the iron metabolism disorders (i.e., iron deficiency, lead poisoning, anemia of chronic disease, sideroblastic anemia). A normal iron panel, as is the case here, rules out iron deficiency anemia.

Question:

12. Given all the data supplied, what is the definitive diagnosis of John's anemia?

Explanation:

A microcytic, hypochromic anemia with target cells suggests a thalassemia, hemoglobinopathy, or iron-deficiency anemia. The other microcytic, hypochromic anemias involving abnormal iron metabolism are also possibilities but usually do not present with significant numbers of target cells. The normal iron panel rules out iron deficiency anemia and the other disorders of iron metabolism. The negative hemoglobin solubility rules out some hemoglobinopathies. The abnormal hemoglobin electrophoresis confirms the diagnosis by further ruling out iron deficiency (which shows a normal Hb electrophoresis) and hemoglobinopathies by absence of structural hemoglobin variants that have an amino acid substitution (i.e., HbS, HbC, HbE). The decreased concentration of all three α-containing hemoglobins, HbA, HbA$_2$, and HbF, suggest an α-thalassemia. The presence of the abnormal hemoglobins, HbH and Hb Bart's, rule out a β- and γ-thalassemia, respectively. The severity of the symptoms, the inherited nature of the disease, the early age of onset, the microcytic, hypochromic peripheral blood picture with target cells, and the presence of HbH and Hb Bart's on Hb electrophoresis indicate a severe form of α-thalassemia called *HbH disease*.

 CHAPTER 12

Case Summary: This is the case of Kathy, a 36-year-old female with a megaloblastic anemia. An initial diagnosis of moderate anemia, jaundice, and neurological complications was made. Based on the patient's laboratory test results, she was diagnosed as having a vitamin B$_{12}$ deficiency. The Schilling test demonstrated that the deficiency was due to the absence of intrinsic factor. This patient can be diagnosed with a megaloblastic anemia due to a lack of intrinsic factor. The patient is suffering from the adult form of pernicious anemia with demonstrated anti-intrinsic factor antibodies.

Question:

1. What is the morphologic classification of the patient's anemia?

Explanation:

It is macrocytic. The morphologic classification of anemia includes normocytic, microcytic, and macrocytic. Macrocytic is the classification when the MCV >100 fL.

Question:

2. Based on the information obtained so far, what is the most likely defect?

Explanation:

There is a vitamin B$_{12}$ deficiency. The patient was admitted with signs of a moderate hemolytic anemia and neurological symptoms. Her CBC shows she has a macrocytic anemia. Her leukocyte and platelet counts are at the lower end of the normal range, indicating a developing pancytopenia. The blood smear revealed hypersegmented neutrophils, ovalocytes, and Howell-Jolly bodies. Her bilirubin values support a diagnosis of hemolysis due to an increased indirect bilirubin. On a differential diagnosis, neurological symptoms typically accompany vitamin B$_{12}$ deficiency rather than a folate deficiency. Based on her serum vitamin B$_{12}$ and folate results, she can be definitively diagnosed as having a megaloblastic anemia due to a vitamin B$_{12}$ deficiency.

Question:

3. What is the significance of the AST/ALT results?

Explanation:

There is no liver disease. These are both liver enzymes. Because they are normal, liver disease is ruled out as a source of jaundice or the macrocytic anemia.

Question:

4. What further testing can be done to obtain a definitive diagnosis?

Explanation:

Testing for methymalonic acid (MMA) and homocysteine are helpful to identify a vitamin B$_{12}$ deficiency. Both are increased in Vitamin B$_{12}$ deficiency. To help determine whether the deficiency is due to an absence of intrinsic factor, tests for intrinsic factor antibodies, the Schilling test, and/or gastric analysis may be done. A common cause of vitamin B$_{12}$ deficiency in a patient with no previous gastrointestinal history is pernicious anemia.

Question:

5. What is this patient's definitive diagnosis?

Explanation:

She has pernicious anemia. The Schilling test result in Part I showed less than 7% of the initial radioactively tagged dose of oral vitamin B$_{12}$ in the urine 24 hours later. When the test was repeated with intrinsic factor, a larger amount of the B$_{12}$ dose was found in the urine after 24 hours. Gastric analysis provides stomach pH levels. The diagnosis of pernicious anemia is supported by the finding of intrinsic factor blocking antibodies in her blood.

Question:

6. How would the diagnosis change if the special testing results were as follows?
Schilling Test:
Part I, before intrinsic factor: 1%
Part II, after intrinsic factor: 3%
Instrinsic factor-blocking antibodies: Negative

Explanation:

The diagnosis is not pernicious anemia. The vitamin B$_{12}$ deficiency is due to some other malabsorption disorder. An abnormal Schilling test result following Part II with oral intrinsic factor and the absence of autoantibodies suggest that her vitamin B_{12} deficiency was due to some sort of malabsorption disorder such as Crohn's disease or bowel blind-loop syndrome.

Question:

7. What would you predict this patient's reticulocyte count to be?

Explanation:

It is normal to low. The patient's reticulocyte count would probably be normal to decreased. Megaloblastic anemia results from ineffective erythropoiesis with intramedullary hemolysis, which blunts the number of reticulocytes in the marrow storage pool. In addition, polychromasia was *not* found on the patient's blood smear, which is a sign of reticulocytosis.

CHAPTER 13

Case Summary: Rachael had symptoms of anemia and a bleeding disorder when she was first seen by her physician. Her past medical history was significant in that she had recently recovered from a viral infection. Her laboratory results revealed pancytopenia and a low reticulocyte count. Bone marrow examination showed hypoplasia. These findings suggest acquired aplastic anemia associated with past viral infection.

Question:

1. Select laboratory tests appropriate for screening for aplastic anemia.

Explanation:

The CBC is an important screening test for all anemias.

Question:

2. Justify the selection of laboratory screening tests based on Rachael's clinical signs and symptoms.

Explanation:

It is important to know the patient's hemoglobin and hematocrit because anemia may be one cause of her weakness and shortness of breath. A low platelet count may explain the presence of petechiae and bruises.

Question:

3. Evaluate the relationship between Rachael's age and the likelihood of having aplastic anemia.

Explanation:

Because approximately 25% of cases occur in persons younger than age 20, it is possible she may have aplastic anemia. Overall, however, the incidence of aplastic anemia is quite low.

Question:

4. If aplastic anemia is present, would you expect her to have an idiopathic or secondary form? Explain your answer.

Explanation:

It is difficult to estimate whether she has an idiopathic or secondary form without a more complete history. Idiopathic forms are more common in this age group, however. Approximately 50–70% of all cases of aplastic anemia cannot be linked to a specific cause.

Question:

5. What aspect of this patient's history may be associated with the occurrence of aplastic anemia?

Explanation:

Our knowledge of the previous infection with hepatitis is helpful. Some data suggest an association between aplasia and infections with viruses.

Question:

6. Is it likely that Rachael has a constitutional form of aplastic anemia? Explain your answer.

Explanation:

It is unlikely that a constitutional form of aplastic anemia would be detected at such an advanced age. Fanconi's anemia is first observed in much younger children who typically have other congenital abnormalities.

Question:

7. Correlate these clinical findings with her laboratory screening test results.

Explanation:

The patient's weakness and shortness of breath are related to the degree of anemia indicated by her decreased hemoglobin and hematocrit. Petechiae and bruising are caused by her severe thrombocytopenia. Recurrent fevers are suggestive of infection. She is severely neutropenic and, therefore, at high risk for infection.

Question:

8. Evaluate each of the patient's laboratory results by comparing them to reference ranges.

Explanation:

All CBC parameters are below reference range for a person of this age.

Question:

9. Which of the patient's routine laboratory results are consistent with those expected for aplastic anemia?

Explanation:

All are consistent with expected results for patients with aplastic anemia.

Question:

10. Classify the morphologic type of anemia.

Explanation:

The patient's MCV is 100 fL and MCHC is 29. The anemia is macrocytic, normochromic. This finding is consistent with aplastic anemia.

Question:

11. Calculate the absolute lymphocyte count. Are her lymphocytes truly elevated as suggested by the relative lymphocyte count?

Explanation:

The absolute lymphocyte count is 1.1×10^9/L, which is slightly decreased. The relative lymphocyte count (94%) is very high because the patient is severely neutropenic. Thus, examining the relative count without considering the total leukocyte count can be very misleading.

Question:

12. Correct the reticulocyte count. Why is this step important?

Explanation:

The patient's corrected reticulocyte count is 0.4%, which is below reference range. All reticulocyte counts need to be corrected when anemia is present in order to assess the bone marrow's degree of compensation for the anemia.

Question:

13. Calculate the absolute reticulocyte count.

Explanation:

The patient's absolute reticulocyte count is 17×10^9/L, which is consistent with a diagnosis of aplastic anemia.

Question:

14. Compare these results with those expected for a person with aplastic anemia.

Explanation:

A markedly hypocellular marrow is consistent with a diagnosis of aplastic anemia. The hematopoietic material was insufficient to aspirate an adequate sample.

Question:

15. Interpret the significance of the lack of malignant cells and hematopoietic blasts.

Explanation:

If malignant cells were present in the marrow, a diagnosis of metastatic disease or lymphoma rather than aplastic anemia would have been likely. Bone marrows of patients with leukemias and myelodysplastic syndromes typically are hyperplastic with increased numbers of hematopoietic blasts present. Aplastic anemia vs hypoplastic MDS is a very difficult differential diagnosis.

Question:

16. Suggest a means of improving the validity of bone marrow examination results for this patient.

Explanation:

When aplastic anemia is suspected, it may be advisable to sample multiple areas of the bone marrow.

Question:

17. Appraise the prognosis for Rachael.

Explanation:

Prognosis is rather poor for patients with aplastic anemia unless a compatible donor can be found for bone marrow transplant.

Question:

18. Predict a treatment regimen.

Explanation:

Treatment would consist of supportive therapy using blood components. A platelet transfusion would probably be ordered immediately. Antithymocyte globulin (ATG) will most likely be administered. If the aplasia did not resolve, a bone marrow transplant would be considered.

Question:

19. What other hematologic conditions must be ruled out for this patient?

Explanation:

Other causes of pancytopenia of the peripheral blood include myelodysplastic syndromes (MDS) and megaloblastic anemia.

Question:

20. What laboratory test is most beneficial in differentiating aplastic anemia from these other disorders? Compare the expected results for aplastic anemia with those of the other disorders.

Explanation:

Serum B_{12} and folic acid levels could be used to rule out anemia due to a deficiency of one of these nutrients. However, a bone marrow examination is essential to make a diagnosis in this case. If the patient had megaloblastic anemia, megaloblastic changes would be evident in the hematopoietic cells. Myelodysplastic changes, increased numbers of myeloblasts, and cytogenic abnormalities would support a diagnosis of MDS.

CHAPTER 14

Case Summary: Sashi had a severe drop in her hemoglobin after pancreatic surgery. Thinking that she was bleeding internally, the physician was ready to take her back to surgery. Laboratory tests revealed a high reticulocyte count indicating that her bone marrow was producing erythrocytes at an accelerated rate. Her bilirubin was increased indicating accelerated hemolysis. The blood smear revealed the presence of spherocytes, which suggests cell membrane damage and grooming by the spleen. Patient history revealed that the patient had received multiple transfusions for previous illness as well as several units during this hospitalization. Workup for a delayed transfusion reaction revealed the presence of alloantibodies and suggested that the spherocytes were due to antigen–antibody complexes on the cell membrane. Based on laboratory results, the decision was made that the patient was not bleeding internally but that her low hemoglobin was due to extravascular hemolysis of red cells.

Question:

1. What type of anemia is suggested by the laboratory results and clinical history?

Explanation:

Decreased survival is suggested by the laboratory results. This is most probably an immune hemolytic anemia because spherocytes are present. The bone marrow's production of cells is increased as indicated by reticulocytosis (285×10^9/L, RPI >2).

Question:

2. Do the laboratory test results indicate intravascular or extravascular hemolysis? Explain.

Explanation:

It is extravascular as suggested by laboratory results and presence of spherocytes on the blood smear. The haptoglobin is probably decreased because of severity of hemolysis.

Question:

3. Is this anemia due to an intrinsic or extrinsic erythrocyte defect?

Explanation:

It is extrinsic. Patient history suggests an acquired defect. Presence of spherocytes, a positive DAT, and presence of antibodies suggest immune hemolytic anemia, probably as a result of the transfusions given.

CHAPTER 15

Case Summary: Jack is a 12-year-old with a lifelong history of hemolytic crises suggesting a hereditary condition. Laboratory results reveal a microcytic anemia with an increased MCHC. The blood smear shows a variety of poikilocytes suggestive of hemolysis. The osmotic fragility test is increased. The test that is most helpful in this case is the thermal sensitivity test. The cells are heat sensitive, which with the other laboratory results and clinical history suggests hereditary pyropoikilocytosis.

Question:

1. Calculate the erythrocyte indices.

Explanation:

$$MCV = \frac{29.2 \times 10}{4.0} = 73 \text{ fL} \qquad MCH = \frac{10.8 \times 10}{4.0} = 27 \text{ pg}$$

$$MCHC = \frac{10.8 \times 100}{29.2} = 37 \text{ g/dL}$$

Question:

2. Based on the calculated indices, describe the patient's red blood cells.

Explanation:

The patient's erythrocytes are microcytic, hyperchromic. The term *hyperchromic* is technically correct, but most laboratory professionals use this term sparingly. This term signifies that the erythrocytes have too much hemoglobin when in essence that is not true. Instead, these erythrocytes have lost part of their membrane, which causes a decrease in the surface-area-to-volume ratio. This changes the erythrocyte from a discocyte to a spherocyte. The only erythrocyte that will reflect an MCHC of >36g/dL is the spherocyte.

Question:

3. What additional lab tests should be ordered?

Explanation:

This patient has a hemolytic type of anemia with erythrocytes that are microcytic. Erythrocyte morphology on the peripheral smear revealed elliptocytes, spherocytes, and fragmented erythrocytes. It is important to know whether this problem is the result of a stimulated immune system (antibodies present). A DAT test should be ordered to determine whether this is true. If the DAT is negative, the patient may have an inherited erythrocyte membrane defect. Lab tests that could be used to differentiate the erythrocyte membrane disorders include the osmotic fragility test and the thermal sensitivity test.

Question:

4. Interpret the results of the osmotic fragility test.

Explanation:

The patient's erythrocytes lysed at a higher NaCl concentration than the control cells. This signifies that the patient's erythrocytes cannot take on as much water as normal cells and, thus, they are said to have increased osmotic fragility.

Question:

5. What do the results of the thermal sensitivity test reveal about the patient's red blood cells?

Explanation:

The results of the thermal sensitivity test reveal that the patient's erythrocytes are abnormally heat sensitive. Normal erythrocytes will not fragment until heated to 49°–50°C.

Question:
6. What disorder is suggested by the patient's lab findings?

Explanation:
The patient has a hemolytic anemia that is not a result of a stimulated immune system. The erythrocyte morphology reveals microcytosis, spherocytes, elliptocytes, teardrop cells, and micropoikilocytes. The osmotic fragility is increased and the thermal sensitivity test shows that the erythrocytes are heat sensitive. These findings suggest that the patient has hereditary pyropoikilocytosis.

 CHAPTER 16

Case Summary: Henry, a 25-year-old black male experienced fever, chills, and general malaise 3 days after receiving prophylactic primaquine. Laboratory testing revealed that he was anemic and the bilirubin was increased. In addition, haptoglobin was decreased. Review of the blood smear revealed bite cells and spherocytes. A Heinz body stain was positive. Based on these results, a hemolytic anemia was suspected. He received two units of packed red blood cells. A test for G6PD was performed and results were borderline low. Follow-up testing revealed a low G6PD.

Question:
1. What test should be considered after finding bite cells on a blood smear?

Explanation:
The appearance of bite cells on a blood smear suggests physical damage to the RBCs as the spleen attempts removal of Heinz bodies. Therefore, a Heinz body stain can be employed to reveal their presence as a cause of the anemia.

Question:
2. Why was the initial G6PD test result normal and the repeat test abnormal?

Explanation:
The initial test for G6PD was normal for two reasons. First, the older, more deficient erythrocytes were selectively destroyed during the hemolytic crisis, leaving younger cells with more normally functioning enzyme. Second, the patient had been transfused, and therefore any blood sample would not be representative of his own cells but would contain G6PD contributed by the donor erythrocytes.

Question:
3. What was the precipitating cause of the patient's anemia?

Explanation:
The patient developed anemia because of treatment with the oxidant drug primaquine. Oxidant damage to hemoglobin due to lack of reducing power supply by G6PD in the hexose-monophosphate shunt leads to erythrocyte destruction.

 CHAPTER 17

Case Summary: Nancy's data demonstrate reactions seen in warm autoimmune hemolytic anemia secondary to systemic lupus erythematosus. Spherocytes indicate extravascular hemolysis, and reticulocytosis suggests compensation by increased bone marrow production of erythrocytes. The positive DAT (anti-IgG) is a clue that the cell destruction is immune mediated. Her serum reacts with all antibody screening cells and panel cells after addition of antihuman globulin. The diagnosis of systemic lupus erythematosus (SLE)—an autoimmune disease characteristically diagnosed in women between the ages of 24 and 40—provides additional support for the secondary nature of the immune mediated hemolysis. Patients with SLE often develop not only antibodies against nuclear components of all cells in the body but also to erythrocytes, as demonstrated in this patient. Treatment would begin initially with steroids, and if the patient was nonresponsive, other modalities would be considered. Transfusion is discouraged unless the hemoglobin value drops to a very low level.

Question:
1. What are some reasons that she could have a low hemoglobin value?

Explanation:
Low hemoglobin may be due to iron deficiency, occult bleeding, or extravascular hemolysis.

Question:
2. What is the significance of the spherocytes?

Explanation:
They indicate damage to the cell membrane and extravascular hemolysis.

Question:
3. Based on these results, what do you suspect is going on with this patient? Explain.

Explanation:
Some type of immune-mediated hemolysis is occurring due to the presence of IgG on the erythrocyte.

Question:
4. What type of antibody appears to be present in this patient? Explain.

Explanation:
It is an autoantibody. The patient's serum is reacting with her own cells, which indicates that the antigen is present on her own cells.

Question:
5. What is the relationship of the patient's primary disease, systemic lupus erythematosus, and her anemia?

Explanation:

SLE is an autoimmune disease in which the patient often develops a WAIHA secondary to the disease.

Question:

6. How would knowing that the patient had not been transfused in the last several months help you make a decision on the underlying cause of the antibody?

Explanation:

If the patient had been transfused, the foreign antigens on the transfused cells could have stimulated an alloantibody. However, the alloantibody would not be reacting with the patient's own cells.

Question:

7. What would you tell the clinician about giving a transfusion?

Explanation:

Transfusions are discouraged in WAIHA because the transfused cells contain an antigen that will react with the antibody and be destroyed just as the patient's own cells are. If the patient's oxygen carrying capacity is low and the patient is demonstrating symptomatic anemia, transfusion should not be denied, as the red cells will provide increased oxygen carrying capacity even if their survival is reduced.

Question:

8. What kind of therapy might be used?

Explanation:

The most common therapy is the use of corticosteroids, which depress the immune reaction. If the patient does not respond to this drug, other cytotoxic drugs or splenectomy may be indicated.

 CHAPTER 18

Case Summary: This case demonstrates the sequence of testing that might be used to determine the cause of microangiopathic hemolytic anemia. The presence of schistocytes may be seen in a number of conditions, but additional laboratory tests such as platelet count and coagulation studies will help in identifying the underlying cause. In addition, medical history such as age, diarrheal episodes, pregnancy status, or other physical conditions (acquired or inherited) will help in differential diagnosis and in deciding a sequence of additional testing. In this case, age and lack of diarrheal prodrome rule out HUS. The low platelet count but normal coagulation tests help rule out DIC. The most likely condition is TTP. The lack of an identifiable precipitating condition and the adult age onset indicate that this is most likely of the single episode, nonrecurring type.

Question:

1. What are some conditions that result in the presence of schistocytes?

Explanation:

Some conditions that result in the presence of schistocytes include disseminated intravascular coagulation, hemolytic uremic syndrome, thrombotic thrombocytopenic purpura, mechanical trauma due to artificial heart valves, malignant hypertension, and burns (thermal injury).

Question:

2. What is the significance of these results?

Explanation:

The platelet count indicates a thrombocytopenia, which correlates with the patient's increased tendency to bruising. Her reticulocyte count was elevated and indicates a response by the bone marrow.

Question:

3. Why might the clinician order coagulation tests?

Explanation:

The presence of unexplained bruises may indicate an abnormality in the hemostatic mechansim. This can be screened for by coagulation tests.

Question:

4. What do these findings indicate about the underlying problem?

Explanation:

The PT and APTT showed slightly prolonged levels, and the fibrinogen was only slightly decreased. This rules out DIC because with DIC, you would expect greatly prolonged PT and APTT values, decreased fibrinogen, increased FDP, and positive D-dimer.

Question:

5. Based on these results, what is the most likely condition associated with these clinical and laboratory results? Explain.

Explanation:

It is most likely TTP. The patient's age, normal urinary volume, and lack of diarrheal prodrome help rule out HUS. The neurological symptoms in concert with the other laboratory values point to TTP.

Question:

6. What therapy might be used?

Explanation:

Plasma exchange with either fresh frozen plasma (FFP) or with cryopoor FFP can be used.

CHAPTER 19

Case Summary: This trauma patient had surgery to repair bone fractures. After surgery, his WBC count was elevated with a predominance of bands. The platelet count and hemoglobin were also below the reference range for his age and sex. Although a bacterial infection was suspected based on the CBC, cultures were negative. Despite the high WBC count and shift to the left, there were no toxic changes of the leukocytes. After further review, it was determined that Dennis had Pelger-Huët anomaly. The bands were actually mature neutrophils whose nucleus failed to segment.

Question:

1. What results, if any, are abnormal?

Explanation:

The white blood count and number of bands are elevated.

Question:

2. What is the most likely reason for these results?

Explanation:

The most likely reason for an elevated white count and left shift on a trauma patient who has had emergency surgery is a bacterial infection acquired either from the original trauma or during surgery. Leukocytosis without toxic changes present or a shift to the left may occur in postsurgical patients.

Question:

3. Given the leukocyte morphology and cultures, what additional condition must now be considered?

Explanation:

Because the cultures are all negative and there are no other indications of a reactive process, such as toxic granulation, Döhle bodies, or vacuoles, it is unlikely the patient has an infection. Pelger-Huët anomaly is a benign inherited condition in which the neutrophils have hyposegmentation. The nuclei are shaped like dumbbells or wire-rimmed eyeglasses and have very condensed chromatin.

Question:

4. Explain the clinical significance of the nuclear anomaly described in this patient.

Explanation:

Pelger-Huët anomaly is benign, and the neutrophils appear to function normally. The greatest significance of this disorder is that it be recognized and cells not mistakenly identified as bands leading to an incorrect diagnosis of infection. In this case, the patient had additional tests (the cultures) performed that probably were not necessary had the condition been diagnosed previously.

Question:

5. Why is the white count elevated?

Explanation:

Pelger-Huët does not typically present with leukocytosis unless it is accompanied by another condition. The white count is probably in-

creased due to tissue damage from the accident trauma and/or the surgery. Also, although the patient's hemoglobin is only low normal, it is likely that a young previously healthy man had a higher value before the accident. He could have lost blood from the accident and/or during the surgery. Acute blood loss and surgery are associated with leukocytosis.

CHAPTER 20

Case Summary: Heidi has had recurrent infections since birth. Her WBC was normal but there was an absolute lymphocytopenia. Further investigation suggested an immune deficiency disorder and led to additional laboratory tests. These tests revealed high levels of erythrocyte adenosine and deoxyadenosine indicating a deficiency in adenosine deaminase. This deficiency occurs from a gene deletion resulting in an autosomal inherited severe combined immunodeficiency. Normal immune function is restored when (1) toxic metabolites are cleared, (2) a normal adenosine deaminase gene is inserted into the patient's lymphocytes, or (3) the patient has a bone marrow transplant.

Question:

1. Does this patient have a leukocytosis or leukopenia? Explain.

Explanation:

No, she does not have a leukocytosis or leukopenia. The WBC count is within normal range.

Question:

2. Does this patient have an abnormal lymphocyte count? Explain.

Explanation:

The absolute lymphocyte count = 7.6×10^9/L $\times$ 0.04 = 0.304 $\times$ 10^9/L. This is abnormally low because the reference range at this age is $2.5 - 16.5 \times 10^9$/L.

Question:

3. What is the absolute lymphocyte count?

Explanation:

At 54 days, the absolute lymphocyte count is only 12.3×10^9/L $\times$ 0.01 = 0.123 lymphocytes $\times$ 10^9/L, a condition of lymphocytopenia.

Question:

4. What possible causes exist for these opportunistic infections?

Explanation:

Two causes of immunodeficiency are suspected with opportunistic infection and severe lymphocytopenia: (1) AIDS and (2) severe combined immunodeficiency syndrome.

Question:

5. Is this child more likely to have a congenital or acquired immune deficiency?

Explanation:

A congenital immune deficiency is more probable as the child has had recurrent infections and lymphocytopenia since birth.

Question:

6. If she has a congenital immune deficiency, is it more likely she has X-linked or autosomal SCIDS?

Explanation:

Autosomal SCIDS is more likely. Females who carry the abnormal X-linked SCIDS gene have normal immunity. Only normal X chromosomes are found in the lymphocytes of females who carry the abnormal X-linked SCIDS gene.

Question:

7. Are the lymphocytes more likely to be morphologically heterogeneous or homogeneous? Why?

Explanation:

They are more likely homogeneous. The congenital immune deficiency disorders are characterized by normal appearing lymphocytes, but the lymphocytes are either defective or decreased in concentration or both. Heterogeneous lymphocytes are normally reactive lymphocytes. They are stimulated by infectious agents.

Question:

8. What confirmatory test is indicated?

Explanation:

A test to determine a decreased adenosine deaminase level or increased purine metabolites of deoxyadenosine triphosphate and deoxyguanosine triphosphate confirm an enzyme deficiency.

CHAPTER 21

Case Summary: Agnes has chronic lymphocytic leukemia. The patient is elderly and had been in good health, and the symptoms of the leukemia had progressed slowly. The predominant cell present on the peripheral blood smear is a mature lymphocyte. The patient's prognosis should be good, with a life span of 5 years or more with supportive therapy.

Question:

1. Given the patient's laboratory results, would this most likely be considered an acute or chronic leukemia? Explain.

Explanation:

It is likely chronic leukemia. The peripheral blood shows an accumulation of mature lymphocytic cells with an increased white blood cell count.

Question:

2. What group of leukemia (cell lineage) is suggested by the patient's blood cell differential results?

Explanation:

Lymphocytic leukemia is suggested. The patient exhibits an increased percentage of mature lymphocytes with an increased white blood cell count and a lack of myelocytic cells.

Question:

3. What would you expect the blast count on the bone marrow to be?

Explanation:

It would be <20% under the WHO definition. In acute leukemias, blasts constitute more than 20% of the nonerythroid marrow nucleated cells; in MDS, MPD, and chronic leukemia, blasts compose less than 20% (WHO) of the marrow cells.

Question:

4. Would you expect Agnes to survive more than 3 years or succumb fairly quickly after treatment?

Explanation:

She should survive more than 3 years. Chronic leukemias progress slowly, and the course of the disease is measured in years rather than months as is typical for the acute leukemias.

Question:

5. Is Agnes a suitable candidate for a bone marrow transplant? Why or why not?

Explanation:

She is not. The highest rate of success with bone marrow transplants has occurred in those younger than 40 years of age in a first remission with a closely matched donor. Because this patient is 72 years old and CLL patients usually do well with supportive therapy, it is unlikely that she would be a candidate for a bone marrow transplant.

Question:

6. What types of treatment are available for our patient Agnes?

Explanation:

Chemotherapy, radiation, bone marrow transplant, immunotherapy are available. Permanent remission in CLL is rare. Treatment is conservative and usually reserved for patients with more aggressive forms of the disease.

CHAPTER 22

Case Summary: The clinical findings of abdominal discomfort, increasing splenomegaly, weakness, and bone pain are consistent with chronic myeloproliferative disorders. The laboratory findings of increased uric acid, left shift, increased platelet count, difficult bone marrow aspiration, dacryocytes on peripheral blood smear, and cytogenetic abnormalities are all characteristic of CIMF (chronic idiopathic myelofibrosis). Malignant stem cells give rise to abnormal leukocytes, erythrocytes, and megakaryocytes. The megakaryocytes secrete excessive PDGFs that stimulate fibroblasts to lay down excessive reticulin and collagen in the bone marrow cavity. This fibrosis leads to the extramedullary hematopoiesis causing splenomegaly and hepatomegaly.

In this case, the peripheral blood film with a leukoerythroblastic picture of immature myeloid cells, nucleated red blood cells, and dacryocytes should rule out causes of marrow infiltration by nonhematopoietic tumor cells, granulomas, or fungus.

The diagnosis of this case is CIMF. Myelofibrosis can evolve into any of the chronic myeloproliferative disorders or acute leukemia. A moderate leukocytosis (WBC <30.0 ×10^9/L), leukoerythroblastosis, dry tap, and lack of the Philadelphia chromosome distinguish CIMF from the other myeloproliferative disorders.

Question:

1. What are Roger's MCV and MCHC?

Explanation:

MCV = 35/3.6 × 10 = 97 fL and MCHC = 11.6/35 × 100 = 33%

Question:

2. How would you classify his anemia morphologically?

Explanation:

The patient has a normochromic, normocytic anemia.

Question:

3. Based on Roger's history and current laboratory data, what other tests should be performed?

Explanation:

Because of the hepatosplenomegaly and laboratory results, a bone marrow and Philadelphia chromosome analysis should be considered. *BCR/ABL1* gene rearrangement is also necessary.

Question:

4. What diagnoses are suggested?

Explanation:

All MPD (CML, essential thrombocytosis, polycythemia vera, or CIMF) can produce a leukocytosis and fibrotic bone marrow.

Question:

5. Give a reason for the unsuccessful, dry-tap, bone marrow aspiration.

Explanation:

Increased fibrosis in the bone marrow makes aspiration difficult. Excess PDGF and TGF-β stimulate collagen proliferation and reticulin fibrosis in the bone marrow. Dry taps may also result from improper placement of the needle into the marrow cavity, a marrow that is hypocellular, or one that is packed tightly with neoplastic cells.

Question:

6. What characteristic peripheral blood morphologies correlate with the bone marrow picture and physical exam?

Explanation:

You would expect to see dacryocytes and should look for micromegakaryocytes in the peripheral blood.

Question:

7. What is the most likely explanation for the increased splenomegaly?

Explanation:

The progressive bone marrow fibrosis causes anemia, resulting in extramedullary hematopoiesis in the spleen and liver. This increases splenic blood flow, red cell pooling, and enlargement of the spleen.

Question:

8. What are possible outcomes of this disorder?

Explanation:

CIMF can show progressive fibrosis or evolve into polycythemia vera, essential thrombocythemia, CML, or acute leukemia.

CHAPTER 23

Case Summary: Hancock had bicytopenia (anemia and thrombocytopenia) with a shift to the left and dysplastic erythrocyte and granulocyte features. The bone marrow was hypercellular with an increased M:E ratio. There was trilineage dysplasia. Based on the WHO criteria for subgrouping the MDS, he most probably has RAEB.

The results of the CBC on Hancock were:

RBC: 1.60×10^{12}/L

Hb: 5.8 g/dL

Hct: 0.17 L/L

WBC: 10.5×10^9/L

Platelets: 39×10^9/L

Reticulocyte count: 0.8%

Differential: 44% segmented neutrophils

7% band neutrophils

6% lymphocytes

28% eosinophils

1% metamyelocytes

1% myelocytes

9% promyelocytes

4% blasts

The neutrophilic cells show marked hyposegmentation and hypogranulation. RBC morphology included anisocytosis and poikilocytosis, teardrop cells, ovalocytes, and schistocytes.

Question:

1. Cytopenia is present in what cell lines?

Explanation:

Cytopenia is present in the erythrocytic and megakaryocytic cell lines (RBCs and platelets are decreased).

Question:

2. What abnormalities are present in the differential?

Explanation:

The abnormalities present in the differential are a shift to the left including metamyelocytes, myelocytes, promyelocytes, and a few blasts as well as a marked increase in eosinophils.

Question:

3. What evidence of dyspoiesis is seen in the leukocyte morphology?

Explanation:

Hyposegmentation and hypogranulation in the leukocyte morphology are evidence of dyspoiesis.

Question:

4. Calculate the MCV. What peripheral blood findings are helpful to rule out megaloblastic anemia?

Explanation:

The MCV is calculated as 106 fL (170/1.6). The following peripheral blood findings help to rule out megaloblastic anemia: hyposegmentation of neutrophils rather than hypersegmentation, WBC count slightly elevated rather than decreased as is typical in megaloblastic anemia, and shift to the left with blasts that is not characteristic of megaloblastic anemia.

Question:

5. What features of the differential resemble CML? What helps to distinguish this case from CML?

Explanation:

Increased eosinophils and all stages of granulocytes in the peripheral blood are found in both MDS and CML. However, the WBC count is too low for typical CML; the RBC and platelet counts are not usually decreased to this extent in CML.

Question:

6. Which of the hematopoietic cell lines exhibit dyshematopoiesis in the bone marrow?

Explanation:

All three cell lines (myeloid, erythroid, and megakaryocytic) exhibit dyshematopoiesis in the bone marrow.

Question:

7. How would you classify the bone marrow cellularity?

Explanation:

The bone marrow shows increased cellularity for a 65 year old; normal cellularity for a 65 year old would be approximately 35%.

Question:

8. What does the M:E ratio indicate?

Explanation:

The M:E ratio indicates myeloid hyperplasia; a normal M:E ratio is 3:1 or 4:1.

Question:

9. Identify at least two features of the bone marrow that are compatible with a diagnosis of MDS.

Explanation:

Features in the bone marrow compatible with a diagnosis of MDS are increased blasts in the bone marrow ($<20\%$), dyserythropoiesis, dysleukopoiesis, dysmegakaryopoiesis, and hypercellularity.

Question:

10. What chemistry tests would be helpful to rule out megaloblastic anemia?

Explanation:

Testing for vitamin B_{12} and folate levels would be helpful to rule out megaloblastic anemia; values should be normal to increased, not decreased as would be seen in megaloblastic anemia. Early megaloblastic changes may be detected by testing for methylmalonic acid (MMA) and homocysteine levels. These components are intermediaries in folate and vitamin B_{12} metabolism and are elevated early in functional vitamin deficiencies.

Question:

11. What is the most likely MDS subgroup based upon what criteria?

Explanation:

The most likely MDS subgroup is RAEB1 based upon the following criteria: <5% blasts in the peripheral blood, 5–19% blasts in the bone marrow, cytopenia in at least two cell lines, and qualitative abnormalities in all cell lines.

Question:

12. Using the International Prognostic Scoring System (IPSS), what is the prognosis for this patient?

Explanation:

Use of the International Prognostic Scoring System (IPSS) on this patient is 2 cytopenias = 0.5; 12% blasts in bone marrow = 1.5; complex karyotype with multiple abnormalities = 1.0. Total = 3.0 (high risk—median survival 0.4 year).

@ CHAPTER 24

Case Summary: Guillermo had bleeding symptoms when he was seen in the emergency room. A CBC was performed and revealed leukocytosis, anemia, and thrombocytopenia. The differential was abnormal with blasts and promyelocytes present. A bone marrow was performed. The M:E ratio was elevated at 7.8:1. The predominant cell was an abnormal promyelocyte. These cells had very heavy granulation and multiple Auer rods. The diagnosis is AML-M3 of the hypergranular type.

Question:

1. What clues do you have that this patient may have an acute leukemia?

Explanation:

There are anemia, increased WBC, decreased platelets, and, most significantly, blasts and promyelocytes on the peripheral blood smear.

Question:

2. Based on the presenting data, what additional testing might be of value?

Explanation:

A bone marrow should be performed. Other tests could include cytogenetics, molecular testing for the RAR-α/PML translocation, and FISH for translocation (15:17).

Question:

3. Based on the peripheral blood examination, what cytochemical stain results would you expect to find on Guillermo's neoplastic cells?

Explanation:

Myeloperoxidase, Sudan black B, and specific esterase should be positive because these cells are myeloid in origin.

Question:

4. If the cells from Guillermo's bone marrow were immunophenotyped, which of the following would be positive? CD13, CD33, CD34, CD2, CD7, CD10, CD19.

Explanation:

Because these are promyelocytes, the cells should be positive for CD13 and CD33. The CD34 is generally negative in APL. CD2, CD7, CD10, CD19 are lymphocyte markers and should be negative.

Question:

5. Based on the morphology and cytochemical staining of these cells, what is the most likely AML classification?

Explanation:

It most likely belongs to the group acute myeloid leukemias with recurrent genetic abnormalities and the subgroup acute promyelocytic leukemia.

Question:

6. What is the major complication associated with this leukemia?

Explanation:

Disseminated intravascular coagulation (DIC) is common due to the release of large numbers of granules from the promyelocytes, which have procoagulant activity.

Question:

7. What chromosome abnormality is associated with this leukemia?

Explanation:

The t(15;17) karyotype is diagnostic of acute promyelocytic leukemia. At the molecular level, the RAR-α/PML is found.

Question:

8. If this patient were treated with all transretinoic acid and 2 weeks later the blood count was repeated, what would you expect to find?

Explanation:

The peripheral blood count would be increased because the promyelocytes mature into granulocytes with this therapy.

@ CHAPTER 25

Case Summary: Dan had nonspecific but typical symptoms and clinical findings of an acute lymphocytic leukemia. His CBC revealed anemia, thrombocytopenia, and leukocytosis. The differential showed that the majority of peripheral blood leukocytes were lymphoblasts. A bone marrow, immunophenotyping, and cytogenetics should be done for treatment and prognostic information.

Question:

1. Based on this data, what would be the initial interpretation of Dan's presentation?

Explanation:

These results are characteristic of acute lymphoblastic leukemia.

Question:

2. What is the correct choice of tests that should be used as the initial follow up in this case?

Explanation:

A bone marrow should be done, and the peripheral blood specimen should be sent for immunophenotyping to determine the T or B cell lineage of the blasts.

Question:

3. If the flow cytometry pattern showed a positive CD10, what would be the classification of this acute leukemia?

Explanation:

The CD10 antigen is found on a pre-B acute leukemia and is called *common acute lymphocytic leukemia antigen,* or *CALLA.* This identifies a subgroup of ALL known as common ALL or CALLA positive ALL.

Question:

4. In this situation, would the therapeutic outcome be considered favorable or bleak? Why?

Explanation:

CALLA positive ALL is the most common ALL found in children in the Western world, and it has the most favorable outcome of the immunologic subtypes.

CHAPTER 26

Case Summary: Julia, a 56-year-old female, had painless lymphadenopathy. Her laboratory results revealed a leukocytosis with a relative and absolute lymphocytosis. The lymphocytes were mature with clumped chromatin and irregular nuclear outline. The lymphocytes were CD10 positive, characteristic of circulating lymphoma cells. A biopsy of the lymph node showed infiltration with neoplastic lymphocytes. The diagnosis of low-grade, non-Hodgkin lymphoma, follicular type was made. She received chemotherapy. Two years later, she returned with expanding lymph nodes in her neck. A biopsy was performed, and a diagnosis of diffuse large cell lymphoma was made. The second lymphoma was probably a transformation of the previous low-grade lymphoma.

Question:

1. What is the differential diagnosis?

Explanation:

The differential diagnosis for a lymphocytosis composed of mature cells includes all chronic leukemia lymphoproliferative disorders discussed: chronic lymphocytic leukemia, prolymphocytic leukemia, hairy cell leukemia, large granular lymphocyte leukemia, Sézary's syndrome, and circulating lymphoma. The nuclear irregularities and history of lymphadenopathy are both suggestive of circulating lymphoma.

Question:

2. What studies could be performed to establish the diagnosis?

Explanation:

Flow cytometry immunophenotyping performed on the peripheral blood may help to establish a diagnosis. Chronic lymphocytic leukemia, hairy cell leukemia, large granular lymphocyte leukemia, and Sézary's syndrome all have a characteristic immunophenotype. Circulating lymphoma may either have a generic, monoclonal B cell phenotype or express antigens specific for the subtype of lymphoma such as CD10 expression in follicular lymphoma. The case described was CD10 positive. This information and the appearance of the lymphocytes suggest the presence of non-Hodgkin lymphoma, follicular type. Biopsy of a lymph node would be of value in confirming this interpretation.

Question:

3. What is the cause of the lymphadenopathy?

Explanation:

The lymphadenopathy is due to the presence of non-Hodgkin lymphoma. Neoplastic lymphoid cells have replaced the normal cells of the lymph node. The lack of tingible body macrophages and mitotic figures distinguishes the neoplastic nodules from benign germinal centers.

Question:

4. Is this process low grade or high grade?

Explanation:

This non-Hodgkin lymphoma has characteristics of a low-grade lymphoma: nodular growth, small cells, lack of apoptosis (tingible body macrophages), and absence of mitotic figures. The diagnosis of follicular lymphoma, grade 1 was established.

Question:

5. What is the diagnosis?

Explanation:

The diagnosis is diffuse large B-cell lymphoma.

Question:

6. What is the relationship of this disease to the previous diagnosis?

Explanation:

This disease probably represents transformation from the previously diagnosed follicular lymphoma.

 CHAPTER 27

Case Summary: Brandon, a 35-year-old male (weight 80 kg) was recently diagnosed with AML with maturation and received induction chemotherapy. Day 21 after chemotherapy, the bone marrow reveals no evidence of residual leukemia. Two weeks later circulating blasts were seen in the peripheral blood. He was evaluated for a stem cell transplant. He was given a PBSCT from a sibling and developed what appeared to be GVHD after 3 months.

Question:

1. Is Brandon a candidate for stem cell transplant?

Explanation:

Yes, these findings indicate that he may have a relapse of his leukemia.

Question:

2. If yes, what form of transplant is required for him?

Explanation:

Circulating blasts in the peripheral blood are a poor prognostic sign and indicate that this patient is probably having a relapse of his leukemia. A bone marrow examination is definitely indicated. If this patient has residual leukemic blasts, the patient is a candidate for a stem cell transplant (if the donor is immediately available). The patient has AML, so an allogeneic SCT is an appropriate option.

Question:

3. What testing should be done on Brandon to proceed with the transplant?

Explanation:

HLA typing should be performed on the patient, and the search for HLA-matched siblings should be done.

Question:

4. There is an HLA-matched sibling who has agreed to be a donor for Brandon. Should the source of stem cells be peripheral blood or bone marrow? Why?

Explanation:

To harvest bone marrow stem cells, the donor has to undergo general anesthesia while stem cells from peripheral blood can be collected by apheresis after mobilizing the stem cells from the marrow by administration of G-CSF to the donor. In addition, studies have shown that the PBSCs engraft earlier than the bone marrow stem cells and have less degree of GVHD. Given these facts, peripheral blood should be the source of stem cells.

Question:

5. PBSCs were collected by apheresis. Enumeration of CD34 count indicates that the total CD34+ cells collected are 6×10^6/kg. Is this an adequate dose for SCT?

Explanation:

Yes, for allogeneic SCT, the total CD34+ cells should be more than 2×10^6/kg.

Question:

6. Stem cells were collected and frozen for Brandon. Does he need to undergo any form of therapy before the transplant?

Explanation:

Yes, the patient should receive myeloablative chemotherapy and/or irradiation, and then the stem cells can be infused later with the hope of complete engraftment.

Question:

7. Brandon received stem cells from his HLA-matched sibling that were successfully engrafted. Three months later, he developed diarrhea, skin rash, and jaundice. What could be the possible cause for this?

Explanation:

Because the patient received allogeneic SCT, the presence of diarrhea, skin rash, and jaundice most likely represents GVHD. However, opportunistic infections and drug reactions should also be considered.

 CHAPTER 28

Case Summary: Radiologic studies show a large effusion in the right pleural cavity. A thoracentesis is performed and 1 L of thick, yellow fluid is aspirated. Laboratory studies show a total protein of 4.5 g/dL (serum = 6 g/dL), lactate dehydrogenase 40 U/L (serum = 50 U/L), and total leukocyte count of 20,000/μL with 90% segmented neutrophils, 10% histiocytes, and many degenerating cells.

Question:

1. Is this a transudate or exudate?

Explanation:

This is an exudate because the protein fluid/serum = 0.75, the fluid LD/serum LD = 0.80, and the WBC is >1000 m/L.

Question:

2. Is this a chylous fluid?

Explanation:

No, this is not chylous because the predominant cell is not a lymphocyte. Because of its appearance, it may be considered pseudochylous.

Question:

3. What would be an appropriate next step to determine whether the material seen is debris or true organism?

Explanation:

The quickest and easiest procedure is to make another slide and perform a Gram stain. If there is not a sufficient amount of fluid remaining, a Gram stain can be performed on the original unstained slide. The material seen is degenerating neutrophils.

Question:

4. How should this be interpreted?

Explanation:

In fluids that have findings of severe infection, the reactive changes of the mesothelial cells can be striking, and caution should be taken not to overinterpret them. Also, degenerative changes can simulate changes of malignancy with what appears to be an irregular nuclear membrane.

Question:

5. Is this an exudate or transudate?

Explanation:

This is an exudate because the protein fluid/serum = 0.78, the fluid LD/serum LD = 0.83, and the WBC is >1000 μ/L.

Question:

6. What is the most appropriate interpretation of these findings?

Explanation:

Most of the infection is resolved and the tissue cells show changes suggestive of malignancy, most likely an adenocarcinoma. This needs to be verified by cytology.

Question:

7. What is the most appropriate interpretation of these cells?

Explanation:

These cells initially appear as mesothelial cells; however, the CSF does not have mesothelial cells, and the patient is an adult with no history of recent brain surgery or CSF shunt or reservoir. Therefore, this most likely represents a metastatic carcinoma. This should be verified by cytology.

Question:

1. Does Michael have a defect in primary or secondary hemostasis?

Explanation:

He has a defect in primary hemostasis as a result of thrombocytopenia.

Question:

2. If Michael were given TPO, how would you expect his bone marrow and peripheral blood picture to change?

Explanation:

Because TPO influences megakaryocytes to proliferate, you would expect to see an increase in megakaryocytes in the bone marrow and an increase in platelets in the peripheral blood.

Question:

3. The physician explained to Michael that the reddish-purple spots on his legs and ankles were tiny pinpoint hemorrhages into the skin. Explain the relationship of these hemorrhages to the platelet count.

Explanation:

The platelet count is severely decreased. Thus, there is a defect in the formation of the primary hemostatic plug allowing blood to leak from small vessels.

Question:

4. What is the most likely cause of Michael's pancytopenia?

Explanation:

Acute leukemia is associated with thrombocytopenia and anemia. The WBC may be normal or increased. Treatment for leukemia includes chemotherapy, which destroys not only leukemic cells but also normal hematopoietic cells.

Question:

5. Why would the administration of growth factors such as EPO and TPO be considered in this case?

Explanation:

EPO and TPO stimulate the proliferation of erythroblasts and megakaryoblasts, respectively, in the bone marrow. This will increase the number of red blood cells and platelets in the peripheral blood.

@ CHAPTER 29

Case Summary: Michael was diagnosed with ALL and received chemotherapy as a part of his treatment regimen. His CBC showed pancytopenia after several treatments. He had pinpoint hemorrhages on his legs and ankles as a result of the severe thrombocytopenia.

@ CHAPTER 30

Case Summary: Shawn, a 10-year-old boy, had recurrent nosebleeds and anemia. Epistaxis began when he was about 18 months old. The nosebleeds occurred one or two times a month and began spontaneously. He bruised easily. The family history indicated that the boy's grandparents were cousins. The patient had a brother who died at 10 years of age of intracranial hemorrhage. Laboratory testing revealed a prolonged PT but an APTT in the reference range. This suggests a defect in one of the coagulation factors in the extrinsic pathway.

Question:

1. What do the results of the screening tests platelet count, bleeding time, prothrombin time (PT), and activated partial thromboplastin time (APTT) indicate?

Explanation:

Screening tests indicate the platelet compartment (primary hemostasis) is likely normal. The problem probably is a defect of the plasma proteins (secondary hemostasis).

Question:

2. What component of the hemostatic mechanism is most likely affected?

Explanation:

A normal APTT and a prolonged PT indicate a defect of the extrinsic pathway.

Question:

3. What evidence exists to indicate that Shawn has a hereditary bleeding disorder?

Explanation:

This patient's bleeding history began when he was just 18 months old and has occurred regularly since that time. Nosebleeds begin spontaneously (in the absence of trauma), and the patient has a history of easy bruisability. One brother also had a bleeding diathesis and died of intracranial hemorrhage at age 10.

Question:

4. Are the nosebleeds significant in considering a diagnosis?

Explanation:

Nosebleeds in the absence of trauma are significant; although they often indicate a platelet defect, platelet screening tests in this patient were normal.

Question:

5. What coagulation factors are included in the extrinsic pathway?

Explanation:

F-VII and tissue factor.

Question:

6. What factors are included in the intrinsic pathway?

Explanation:

F-XII, F-XI, prekallikrein, high molecular weight kininogen, F-IX, and F-VIII are included.

Question:

7. What factors are included in the common pathway?

Explanation:

F-X, F-V, prothrombin, and fibrinogen are included.

Question:

8. An abnormal PT and a normal APTT would indicate a problem with which factor?

Explanation:

F-VII.

Question:

9. Does any evidence exist to indicate a problem with Shawn's fibrinolytic system?

Explanation:

No.

Question

10. Why were liver function tests done on Shawn?

Explanation:

They were done to rule out an acquired deficiency of coagulation proteins.

Question

11. What is the significance of normal results in a patient with hemostatic disease?

Explanation:

Deficiency of one or more coagulation factors in the absence of liver disease or overt clinical thrombosis suggests a genetic deficiency of the factor being evaluated.

Question

12. Do these findings explain the patient's bleeding history?

Explanation:

Yes, the boy has a homozygous F-VII deficiency, and his parents are heterozygous. Because homozygosity for F-VII is rare, the family history proved to be significant. The nosebleeds (more commonly associated with platelet dysfunction) are probably due to the reduction of thrombin generation upon hemostatic activation and the resultant loss of thrombin-catalyzed platelet activation.

CHAPTER 31

Case Summary: Mohammed experienced increased bleeding from superficial wounds acquired from an automobile accident. Petechiae were also noted. With these symptoms, a platelet disorder is most likely. His laboratory tests confirmed this. His platelet count was slightly decreased but not so low as to cause his bleeding symptoms. His bleeding and closure times were prolonged, which indicated a platelet function disorder. Coagulation factor screening tests were normal. Platelet aggregation studies showed abnormal aggregation with ristocetin that was not corrected by vWf. This confirmed that his disorder was Bernard-Soulier disease.

Question:

1. What laboratory tests, hematology, and hemostasis would likely be ordered immediately that would be most informative in interpreting the cause of the patient's bleeding?

Explanation:

Platelet count, prothrombin time, and activated partial thromboplastin time are the screening tests ordered most often. These tests will detect the presence of a problem either in the platelet numbers or in fibrin formation in most patients with hemorrhagic symptoms.

Question:

2. Does the patient most likely have a disorder of primary or of secondary hemostasis? Why?

Explanation:

The patient most likely has a disorder of primary hemostasis. The presence of petechiae and excess bleeding from superficial cuts are seen in primary hemostatic disorders and are unlikely in disorders of secondary hemostasis.

Question:

3. Explain how these laboratory tests confirm that the patient's bleeding is related to a problem in primary hemostasis rather than secondary hemostasis.

Explanation:

Most disorders of secondary hemostasis are ruled out when the results of the prothrombin time and activated partial thromboplastin time are within the reference ranges (see Table E, inside cover). The platelet count is slightly decreased.

Question:

4. Is the bleeding more likely related to problems with the vascular system or with platelets? Why?

Explanation:

Both hereditary and acquired vascular disorders have characteristic abnormalities that are not included in the history, and therefore we will assume them to be absent. A platelet problem is most likely.

Question:

5. Is this profuse bleeding with the presence of petechiae consistent with the platelet count? Why?

Explanation:

Profuse bleeding and petechiae are not usually evident until the platelet count is below 50×10^9/L. Therefore, the amount of bleeding is not consistent with the platelet count.

Question:

6. What additional testing would be helpful in identifying the cause of the patient's excess bleeding?

Explanation:

The patient should be questioned for recent ingestion of drugs that affect platelet function, for example, aspirin or aspirin-containing products. In the absence of a history of ingestion of drugs, platelet aggregation testing to identify abnormal platelet function would likely be ordered.

Question:

7. Is there a possibility that the patient's platelet count is spuriously increased or decreased? Why?

Explanation:

This is unlikely because the patient's peripheral smear report does not indicate platelet satellitism, platelet agglutination, or the presence of abnormally small erythrocytes or other features that could cause a spuriously increased platelet count.

Question:

8. Is this patient's problem more likely acquired or inherited? Why?

Explanation:

The patient's problem is most likely inherited because he has had bleeding problems all of his life.

Question:

9. What is the significance of these platelet function tests?

Explanation:

Both the bleeding time and closure time are prolonged, which indicates abnormal platelet function. The platelet aggregation studies with ristocetin are abnormal, but aggregation is normal with other agonists. Abnormal aggregation with ristocetin is characteristic of either von Willebrand disease or Bernard-Soulier disease.

Question:

10. What is the most likely condition?

Explanation:

The patient's platelet aggregation studies were not corrected with the addition of von Willebrand factor. This indicates that the problem is unlikely to be von Willebrand disease. Because the patient had large platelets on the blood smear and typical platelet aggregation studies, the most likely diagnosis is Bernard-Soulier disease.

Question:

11. What additional testing would be considered?

Explanation:

DNA studies may be done in a research facility to determine the molecular abnormality or flow cytometry to demonstrate reduction of the GPIb/IX complex on the platelet membrane.

CHAPTER 32

Case Summary: Scott was seen in the ER for severe bleeding in the knee after a slight fall. There is a family history of similar bleeding in males on the maternal side of the family. A prothrombin time and thrombin time on Scott were normal, but the APTT was prolonged. The APTT was corrected when patient's plasma was mixed with normal plasma, suggesting a factor deficiency. An F-VIII assay showed a severe decrease. Scott was diagnosed with hemophilia A.

Question:

1. What term is used to describe the type of bleeding from minor cuts that the mother is describing?

Explanation:

The type of bleeding in this patient indicates delayed bleeding and joint bleeding (hemarthrosis).

Question:

2. Does this history seem to be typical of a platelet disorder or of a coagulation factor disorder? Why?

Explanation:

These bleeding symptoms are characteristic of coagulation factor disorders (disorders of secondary hemostasis) rather than platelet disorders (disorders of primary hemostasis).

Question:

3. What type of inheritance is most probably present in this family?

Explanation:

X-linked inheritance is most probable in this family.

Question:

4. Is this history typical of that of a patient with von Willebrand disease? Why?

Explanation:

No, the inheritance pattern seems to be X-linked. The inheritance of vWD is usually autosomal dominant, although inheritance of the severe form of vWD is described as autosomal recessive.

Question:

5. What could have caused the patient's great uncle to have acquired HIV infection?

Explanation:

The uncle's HIV infection could have been acquired prior to 1984 from preparations of F-VIII concentrate that he received to control bleeding (prior to current protocols that include a viral-inactivation step in the production of the concentrate).

Question:

6. Name the coagulation factor deficiencies that are possible with these laboratory results.

Explanation:

When the APTT is abnormal and the PT is normal, the possible deficiencies are F-VIII, F-IX, F-XI, F-XII, prekallikrein, and high molecular weight kininogen.

Question:

7. What is the most likely factor deficiency? Why?

Explanation:

The most likely factor deficiency is F-VIII because it is the most common.

Question:

8. What do the results of the APTT on the mixture of Scott's plasma with normal plasma indicate?

Explanation:

The results of the mixing studies indicate that normal plasma corrected the patient's result. This indicates a factor deficiency rather than an inhibitor.

Question:

9. What test should be performed next?

Explanation:

An F-VIII assay should be performed next.

Question:

10. If an F-VIII assay was done with results of <1 U/dL, what molecular studies should be done?

Explanation:

Molecular studies for the inversion mutation in intron 22 should be done for all patients with severe F-VIII deficiency.

Question:

11. What therapy is indicated for this patient?

Explanation:

Therapy for F-VIII deficiency includes heat-inactivated F-VIII concentrates and recombinant F-VIII.

Question:

12. What complications from the therapy are possible?

Explanation:

A complication of therapy that occurs in patients with hemophilia A, particularly those with the inversion mutation in intron 22, is the development of an inhibitor.

 CHAPTER 33

Case Summary: Andrea is a 37-year-old female who was diagnosed with deep vein thrombosis of the leg. She is dehydrated. She is on oral contraceptives and coumadin. Her family history revealed that paternal uncles and maternal cousins had thrombotic episodes. Testing for AT, PC, PS, fibrinogen, D-dimer, and plasminogen was done during the DVT episode and again 6 months after she was off coumadin. All tests were within the reference range. Several years later, she was tested and found to be heterozygous for both F-V $_{Leiden}$ and prothrombin G20210.

Question:

1. What risk factors, if any, are revealed in the patient's history?

Explanation:

This patient had several risk factors for thrombosis including dehydration and oral contraceptives. There is also a strong family history of thrombosis, suggesting a hereditary component in the etiology of her acute thrombotic event.

Question:

2. What other possibilities could explain the thrombotic event in this patient?

Explanation:

She was initially tested twice because testing during an acute thrombotic episode or while on coumadin is not as informative as testing after the episode has resolved or when the patient is no longer taking anticoagulants. Unfortunately, based on the available tests, neither set of tests helped establish a diagnosis. Additional causes of hereditary thrombophilia could include activated protein C resistance; prothrom-

bin mutation 20210; hyperhomocysteine; deficiencies of heparin cofactor II, TFPI, t-PA, or F-XII; and elevated fibrinogen, F-VIII, or PAI-1.

Question:

3. Why is Andrea at higher risk for a thrombotic event than her mother or her two sisters?

Explanation:

Specific molecular assays of the family were subsequently done, and they revealed both the V $_{Leiden}$ and prothrombin 20210 mutations. The fact that both these mutations were found in the same family probably accounts for the strong family history. The patient had inherited two different genetic mutations, both of which carry an increased risk of thrombosis. In addition, she had several other clinical risk factors, probably contributing to her thrombotic event. Because the mother and sisters had a single genetic mutation, their risk of thrombosis was probably less than that of Andrea. The patient was taken off oral contraceptives and put back on coumadin.

 CHAPTER 35

Case Summary: Robert was pancytopenic. Clinical history and further laboratory tests revealed no cause for the pancytopenia. A bone marrow aspirate and a biopsy were obtained. Evaluation revealed the presence of many blasts. The diagnosis based on bone marrow testing was acute myelocytic leukemia.

Question:

1. Is a bone marrow evaluation indicated for this patient? Why or why not?

Explanation:

CBC data indicate that the patient is pancytopenic. Presence of pancytopenia in a young patient is worrisome. The common causes of pancytopenia in a young patient include HIV infection, alcoholism, medications, and B $_{12}$ and folic acid deficiency. Presence of teardrop cells with pancytopenia indicates marrow fibrosis or marrow infiltration by leukemia, lymphoma, or granulomas. Bone marrow evaluation for this patient is definitely indicated. The patient does not have lymphadenopathy, hepatomegaly, or splenomegaly, so the chance of lymphoma involving the marrow is very unlikely.

Question:

2. How should the marrow evaluation proceed?

Explanation:

Fortunately, the laboratory professional made several touch imprints from the biopsy. There is no reason for doing cytochemical stains on the aspirate smear if one has a good quality and good number of touch imprint slides. These touch imprints were of good quality and showed many blasts. The touch imprints were stained with cytochemical stains. No differentiation was present among these blasts. The cells stained consistent with myeloblasts. The hemodiluted marrow was sent for flow cytometry and cytogenetics. The aspirate can be sent for flow cytometry because flow is more sensitive in detecting the lineage of blasts. Flow cytometry was positive for myeloid markers and negative for lymphoid markers. The remainder of the aspirate was sent for cytogenetics with a hope that some cells might be able to grow and show any specific cytogenetic abnormality.

Question:

3. Can a diagnosis be made from tests on the aspirate rather than waiting for the biopsy slides?

Explanation:

Yes, the presence of many blasts in the bone marrow aspirate smears and on the touch imprints indicates acute leukemia. The lineage of blasts can be determined based on cytochemical stains and/or flow cytometry. Bone marrow biopsy in this case would not provide any added information.

 CHAPTER 37

Case Summary: The case is an example of chronic lymphocytic leukemia involving the peripheral blood. It demonstrates the technique of gating the cells of interest, determining a phenotype, and using of a characteristic phenotype in establishing a diagnosis of a subtype of lymphoid malignancy.

Question:

1. What is the optimal specimen?

Explanation:

The CBC revealed peripheral blood lymphocytosis. Therefore, flow cytometry of the peripheral blood would be appropriate. An EDTA anticoagulated specimen is ideal. The CBC sample could be used if it was processed within 24 hours of being drawn. Other anticoagulants (e.g., heparin and ACD) are adequate.

Question:

2. Which cells are of interest and should be included in the gating?

Explanation:

The cells of interest are the lymphocytes.

Question:

3. What are the typical forward and side scatter properties of the cells of interest?

Explanation:

Lymphocytes have low side scatter (granularity) and variable forward scatter (size).

Question:

4. What is the phenotype?

Explanation:

The majority of the lymphocytes have the following abnormal phenotype: CD45+, CD19+, CD20+, CD23+, CD5+, lambda+, kappa−.

Question:

5. Which features indicate clonality?

Explanation:

Expression of only one immunoglobulin light chain (lambda, but not kappa) and the aberrant expression of CD5 indicate a clonal population of B cells.

Question:

6. What is the diagnosis?

Explanation:

The diagnosis is chronic lymphocytic leukemia, B cell (CLL), or small lymphocytic lymphoma (SLL). CD5-positive B cells are characteristic of CLL, SLL, or mantle cell lymphoma (MCL). CD23 expression is found in CLL and SLL but not MCL. Although lymphoma primarily involves the lymph nodes and other lymphoid organs, there may be secondary involvement of the peripheral blood and bone marrow.

Question:

7. Which of the flow cytometry results presented in this case indicate that this is a malignancy of mature lymphocytes (chronic lymphocytic leukemia), not acute lymphoblastic leukemia?

Explanation:

The strong expression of CD45, presence of surface immunoglobulin, and absence of CD34 and CD10 expression all indicate a mature B lymphocyte phenotype.

 CHAPTER 38

Case Summary: Gregory had leukocytosis and a shift to the left when initially seen. The differential diagnosis was important in order to determine whether this abnormal blood picture was due to a benign or neoplastic process. Cytogenetic studies revealed an acquired clonal aberration t(9;22) diagnostic of CML. Gregory had a bone marrow transplant with his sister's donated cells. Five years later, cytogenetic studies revealed a relapse and impending blast crisis.

Question:

1. What is the most appropriate specimen to submit for cytogenetic analysis, and how should it be processed?

Explanation:

The most appropriate specimen to submit for chromosome analysis of CML is a bone marrow sample. If the bone marrow is not aspirable, peripheral blood can be used but sometimes will not yield mitoses. The processing must be performed by direct harvest and/or unstimulated cultures.

Question:

2. Is this a constitutional or acquired aberration?

Explanation:

This is an acquired aberration that is present only in the hematopoietic cells—RBC precursors, WBC precursors, megakaryocytes, and some lymphocytes.

Question:

3. Is it a clonal aberration?

Explanation:

This is a clonal aberration because it is present in more than one cell (in this case, it was present in 100% of cells analyzed, which is typical for CML).

Question:

4. What is the significance of this finding for the diagnosis?

Explanation:

The finding of the t(9;22) confirms the diagnosis of CML.

Question:

5. What is the significance of this finding?

Explanation:

This finding confirms the engraftment of female donor cells in the recipient bone marrow. While no cells with the t(9;22) are found by cytogenetic methods, molecular studies may show the presence of the BCR/ABL1 gene rearrangement because these techniques are more sensitive than routine cytogenetics.

Question:

6. What other studies could be performed that would be informative as to the status of the donor and recipient cells?

Explanation:

FISH analysis can be performed on the interphase nuclei using probes for the X and Y chromosome to demonstrate the sex of the cells present. In addition, probes for the t(9;22) can be used if male cells are present to determine whether they are leukemic cells. Molecular studies can also be obtained for the BCR gene rearrangement.

Question:

7. What is the significance of these findings?

Explanation:

The cytogenetic results performed at 5 years posttransplant show not only a relapse of the CML, but also a cytogenetic transformation indicative of pending blast crisis as evidenced by the +8 and i(17)(q10) that were not seen in the original leukemic cells.

CHAPTER 39

Case Summary: This patient had a high blast percentage in the peripheral blood and bone marrow that is typical of acute leukemia. However, she also had the t(9;22) with Philadelphia chromosome, which is associated with chronic myelogenous leukemia (CML). This translocation of BCR/ABL1 implies this patient could be suffering from a blast crisis of CML. There are times when the chronic phase of CML may not be diagnosed before blast crisis. The other possibility here is that the patient has de novo acute leukemia. These leukemias also may harbor a Philadelphia chromosome, but the break points in the BCR gene at the molecular level are often different from the break points in CML. This patient had the de novo form of acute lymphocytic leukemia (ALL) as molecular analysis revealed BCR/ABL1 with a p190 rather than a p210 breakpoint.

Question:

1. What is the classification of this neoplastic hematologic disorder based on the peripheral blood and bone marrow results?

Explanation:

This patient has an acute leukemia as indicated by the blast count, which is >20% in both the peripheral blood and bone marrow.

Question:

2. What molecular defect is consistent with the presence of the Philadelphia chromosome?

Explanation:

The BCR/ABL1 translocation is the molecular equivalent of the Philadelphia chromosome. There is a reciprocal translocation between the ABL1 gene on chromosome 9 and the BCR gene on chromosome 22. The Philadelphia chromosome represents the shortened chromosome 22. This fusion gene produces a new protein having increased tyrosine kinase activity.

Question:

3. Would molecular analysis assist in diagnosis? Explain.

Explanation:

Molecular analysis would assist in diagnosis. This patient has the Philadelphia chromosome associated with CML but has a peripheral blood and bone marrow picture of acute leukemia. Thus, she may be in the blast crisis of CML or have a de novo acute leukemia. In de novo acute leukemia, the break point in the BCR gene is often different, producing a fusion gene encoding a p190 protein.

Question:

4. If molecular analysis is required, which laboratory procedure should be used, and what specimen should be obtained?

Explanation:

The rt-PCR analysis of *BCR/ABL1* should be done. A bone marrow specimen or peripheral blood may be used.

Question:

5. The molecular analysis revealed *BCR/ABL1* translocation consistent with a p190 break point. What is the most likely diagnosis?

Explanation:

This defect is found in some cases of de novo ALL, and this is the most likely diagnosis.

Question:

6. Why is this molecular finding helpful in therapeutic decision making?

Explanation:

It identifies a set of patients who are less responsive to standard chemotherapy, and the prognosis is poor compared to Philadelphia-negative ALL.

Answers to Checkpoints

✓

Chapter 1

Checkpoint! 1
What cellular component of blood may be involved in disorders of hemostasis?

Answer
The platelets are involved in hemostasis.

Checkpoint! 2
Is reflex testing suggested by these results?

Answer
The girl has a decreased hemoglobin and increased WBC count. Reflex testing is suggested to help identify the cause of these abnormal results. A differential will identify the types of leukocytes that are present in increased concentrations and give clues to the diagnosis. Further laboratory testing can also help identify the cause of the anemia.

Chapter 2

Checkpoint! 1
What is meant by the phrase "lipid asymmetry" when describing cell membranes?

Answer
The phospholipid's content of the inner (cytoplasmic) half of the lipid bilayer differs from the phospholipid's content of the outer (external) half of the lipid bilayer. Phosphotidylethanolamine (PE) and phosphatidylserine (PS) occur in the inner layer while phosphatidylcholine (PC) and sphingomyelin (SM) occur predominantly in the outer layer.

Checkpoint! 2
Explain the difference between densely staining chromatin and lighter staining chromatin when viewing blood cells under a microscope.

Answer
Densely staining chromatin represents tightly twisted or folded regions of chromatin that are transcriptionally inactive. Lighter staining chromatin represents unwound or loosely twisted regions of chromatin that are transcriptionally active.

Checkpoint! 3
What is the difference between a "polymorphism" and a "mutation"?

Answer
Polymorphism describes a change in the nucleotide sequence of a gene that occurs with a frequency of >1% of the population. Mutation describes a change in the nucleotide sequence of a gene that results in an abnormality of function of that gene or gene product.

Checkpoint! 4
A cell undergoing mitosis fails to attach one of its duplicated chromosomes to the microtubules of the spindle apparatus during metaphase. The cell's metaphase checkpoint malfunctions and does not detect the error. What is the effect (if any) on the daughter cells produced?

Answer
If one of the paired (duplicated) sister chromatids fails to attach to the mitotic spindle during metaphase, the duplicated chromosomes will not separate during anaphase and telophase. If the cell does not catch this mistake, and cytokinesis still completes, one daughter cell will have two copies of that chromosome and the other daughter cell will have none. Both cells are said to be *aneuploid* (i.e., have an abnormal number of chromosomes).

Checkpoint! 5
What would be the effect on the hematopoietic system homeostasis if the expanded clone of antigen-activated B lymphocytes failed to undergo apoptosis after the antigenic challenge was removed?

Answer
The result would be an accumulation of excess lymphocytes and a progressive lymphocytosis.

Checkpoint! 6
Mutations of proto-oncogenes predisposing to malignancy are said to be dominant mutations while mutations of antioncogenes are said to behave as recessive mutations, requiring the loss of both alleles. Explain this difference in behavior of the gene products.

Answer
The products of proto-oncogenes are usually proteins that are important in regulating cell growth, differentiation, or apoptosis in their wild-type state. Mutations resulting in enhanced cell growth or in defective or deficient differentiation or apoptosis generally are capable of exerting an effect on the indicated process whenever the aberrant protein is produced (i.e., a single allele resulting in the production of some quantity of the indicated protein). In contrast, antioncogenes or tumor suppressor genes produce protein products that inhibit cell growth or promote apoptosis. Because the human genome carries two copies of all genes carried on the autosomes, a mutation of one tumor-suppressor allele resulting in a loss of function will still leave the other allele producing a wild-type protein product. Both alleles must be knocked out before the cell experiences complete loss of that protein effect.

Chapter 3

Checkpoint! 1

Hematopoietic stem cells that have initiated a differentiation program are sometimes described as undergoing death by differentiation. Explain.

Answer

When a hematopoietic stem cell makes the commitment to differentiate, it begins a maturation process that will culminate in what we call *terminally differentiated cells* (i.e., cells that have lost the capacity to divide and have a finite [limited] life span). Thus, the process of differentiation "dooms" the cell to eventual death.

Checkpoint! 2

Explain the difference in the nomenclature used to label progenitor cells from that used to label maturing cells within the hematopoietic hierarchy of cells.

Answer

Because progenitor cells are not morphologically recognizable, they are identified by the progeny they produce when grown in in vitro cultures. Thus, they are identified as colony-forming units (CFU) or burst-forming units (BFU) with the types of cells in the colony indicated by the corresponding appended letter (e.g., CFU-E = produce a colony of erythroid cells). The maturing cells, which are morphologically recognizable, are described using the root of the lineage (e.g., erythro) with appropriate prefix and suffix to indicate stage of development (e.g., proerythroblast).

Checkpoint! 3

Cytokine control of hematopoiesis is said to be characterized by redundancy and pleiotrophy. What does this mean?

Answer

Redundancy refers to the fact that many different cytokines do the same thing (i.e., GM-CSF and IL-3 have overlapping [nearly identical] activities. IL-11 and TPO both stimulate platelet production [although TPO is the more important cytokine, physiologically]). Redundancy is a good thing because it assures the organism that if a mutation knocks out a regulatory gene, there are additional cytokines that can take over and substitute for the lost activity. At least part of the explanation for redundancy may be the "shared receptor chains" that have been identified for certain groups of cytokines.

Pleiotrophy refers to the fact that a single cytokine often has multiple activities, often on multiple target cells.

Checkpoint! 4

Individuals with congenital defects of the γ-chain of the IL-2 receptor suffer from profound defects of lymphopoiesis far greater than individuals with congenital defects of the α-chain of the IL-2 receptor. Why?

Answer

The γ-chain of the IL-2 receptor is shared with five other cytokines, all important in regulating lymphopoiesis—IL-4, IL-7, IL-9, IL-11, and IL-15. Thus, a disabling mutation of the γ-chain results in loss of physiologic activity of all six cytokines, whereas mutations affecting the α-chain compromise only the physiologic activity of a single cytokine, IL-2.

Chapter 4

Checkpoint! 1

Describe the bone marrow stromal location of erythrocyte, granulocyte, platelet, and lymphocyte differentiation.

Answer

Erythrocytes develop in erythroblastic islands located near the sinuses. The more mature cells are at the periphery of the island, and the more immature are closer to the center. Granulocytes are produced in nests that are close to trabeculae and arterioles but distant from venous sinuses. Platelets are produced from the cytoplasm of megakaryocytes, which are located next to the vascular sinus.

Checkpoint! 2

Describe the process by which a blood cell moves from the marrow to the vascular space.

Answer

New blood cells move along adventitial cells to the abluminal surface of venous sinuses. Spaces between reticular cells allow hematopoietic cells to contact the abluminal side of vascular endothelium, and a receptor-mediated process forces the abluminal and luminal sides of the endothelial cell to touch where the new blood cell is located. These two portions of the endothelial membrane fuse and create a pore through which the blood cell enters the vascular space.

Checkpoint! 3

Describe how old or damaged erythrocytes are removed from circulation by the spleen.

Answer

Old or damaged erythrocytes circulating through the slow transit compartment of the red pulp encounter a toxic (hypoxic, hypoglycemic, acidic) environment and become identifiable to macrophages in the red pulp cords as cells that need to be removed from the circulation. The macrophages phagocytose these undesirable cells before they exit the spleen.

Checkpoint! 4

List 3 causes each of workload and infiltrative splenic hypertrophy.

Answer

Workload splenic hypertrophy is a form of secondary hypersplenism. It is associated with inflammatory and infectious diseases that increase the defensive function of the spleen. This is thought to be caused by an increase in the number of macrophages or an increase in lymphoid cells. Blood disorders in which cells are intrinsically abnormal or are coated with antibody lead to removal of these cells by the splenic macrophages.

Additional cells or metabolic by-products in the spleen can cause infiltrative hypertrophy. This includes disorders in which macrophages accumulate large amounts of undigestable substances, neoplasms in which tumor cells infiltrate the spleen, myelofibrosis in which the spleen contains foci of extramedullary hematopoiesis and in congestive splenomegaly following liver cirrhosis.

Chapter 5

Checkpoint! 1

What is meant by the term "erythron"?

Answer

Erythron refers to the summation of stages of erythrocytes in the marrow, peripheral blood, and within vascular areas of specific organs such as the spleen. Erythropoiesis involves the entire erythron.

Checkpoint! 2

What is the first stage of red cell maturation that has visible cytoplasmic evidence of hemoglobin production on a Romanowsky-stained smear?

Answer

The basophilic normoblast stage may have patches of newly synthesized hemoglobin. The RNA in the young cell stains dark blue, but the hemoglobin stains pink. In the next stage, polychromatophilic normoblast, a mix of the blue and pink stains give the cytoplasm a bluish gray, or polychromatic, staining appearance.

Checkpoint! 3

How would an increase in RBC membrane permeability affect intracellular sodium balance?

Answer

A cation pump within the membrane controls the intracellular balance of sodium (Na^+) and potassium (K^+). Sodium is maintained at a low intracellular concentration while potassium is kept concentrated inside the cell at 25 times more than the concentration of sodium. The biconcave disc shape of an RBC is vital to the cell's function and longevity of the cell. Maintaining this shape depends on the membrane structure providing an exact permeability to ions on either side of the membrane. Even a slight increase in membrane permeability can cause an inflow of sodium resulting in a defective membrane and an alteration of shape.

Checkpoint! 4

Compare and ocontrast the placement of lipids in the erythrocyte membrane and their function.

Answer

Approximately 95% of the lipid content of the membrane consists of equal amounts of unesterified cholesterol and phospholipids. The remaining lipids are free fatty acids and glycolipids. Membrane cholesterol exists in free equilibrium with plasma cholesterol. The phospholipids' molecules are arranged with polar heads directed to the inside and outside of the cell and the hydropholbic tails directed to the interior of the bilayer. The mobility of phospholipids within the membrane contributes to membrane fluidity. A small portion of membrane lipids are glycolipids in the form of glycosphingolipid. Glycolipids are responsible for some antigenic properties of the membrane.

Checkpoint! 5

Compare placement in the membrane and function of peripheral and integral membrane erythrocyte proteins.

Answer

Integral proteins span the entire thickness of the cell membrane whereas peripheral proteins are on the inner side (cytoplasmic) of the membrane. The integral proteins carry the erythrocyte antigens and attach the skeletal lattice to the bilipid layer of the membrane. The peripheral proteins form a skeletal support for the membrane lipid layer.

Checkpoint! 6

Uncontrolled oxidation of hemoglobin results in what RBC intracellular inclusion?

Answer

The erythrocyte normally maintains a large ratio of NADPH to $NADP^+$. When the RBC metabolic pathways fail to reduce oxidized hemoglobin, hemoglobin sulfhydryl groups (-SH) are oxidized, which leads to denaturation and precipitation of hemoglobin in the form of Heinz bodies. Heinz bodies attach to the inner surface of the cell membrane, decreasing cell flexibility.

Checkpoint! 7

Which erythrocyte metabolic pathway is responsible for providing the majority of cellular energy? For regulating oxygen affinity? For maintaining hemoglobin iron in the reduced state?

Answer

About 90–95% of the cell's glucose breakdown occurs in the Embden-Meyerhof pathway. Two moles of ATP are generated from each mole of glucose metabolized. ATP is the primary energy source of the erythrocyte. The Rapoport-Leubering shunt produces 2,3-DPG, which affects oxygen affinity. The hexose-monophosphate shunt and methemoglobin reductase pathways help maintain hemoglobin iron in the reduced state.

Checkpoint! 8

Why are there different reference intervals for hemoglobin concentration in male and female adults but not in male and female children?

Answer

The male hormone, testosterone, stimulates erythropoiesis indirectly by stimulating EPO production in the kidney. This results in about a 1–2 gm increase in hemoglobin in males. Testosterone production increases significantly in adolescence.

Checkpoint! 9

What would the predicted serum EPO levels be in a patient with an anemia due to end-stage kidney disease?

Answer

End-stage renal disease results in a primary decrease in EPO production and, therefore, decreased serum EPO levels. Because EPO is the primary stimulator of erythropoiesis, low levels result in marrow erythroid hypoplasia and a moderate to severe anemia.

Checkpoint! 10

What are the laboratory tests that would diagnose an increase in RBC destruction (i.e., hemolysis) and what would be the expected results?

Answer

The lab tests that should be done include the total bilirubin, haptoglobin, and the hemoglobin/hematocrit (H&H). If hemolysis is significant, the indirect bilirubin would increase and the hematocrit and hemoglobin would decrease. The haptoglobin would be decreased because it removes extracellular hemoglobin dimers. Respiratory carbon monoxide could also be measured as an indicator of heme catabolism, but this is rarely done. When present in large quantity, methemalbumin and hemopexin-heme complexes impart a brownish color to the plasma. So, in addition, a Schumm's test could be performed to detect these abnormal compounds spectrophotometrically.

Chapter 6

Checkpoint! 1

Describe the quaternary structure of a molecule of hemoglobin. How may a mutation in one of the globin chains at the subunit interaction site affect hemoglobin function?

Answer

Hemoglobin is composed of four subunits, each of which is composed of a heme group nestled in a globin chain. There are two pairs of globin chains. The four subunits are held together by salt bonds, hydrophobic contacts, and hydrogen bonds in a tetrahedral formation giving the hemoglobin molecule a nearly spherical shape. An oxygen molecule can attach to each of the four subunits. In the deoxyhemoglobin form, 2,3-DPG combines in the central cavity of the molecule.

Because there is considerable movement between chains when ligands such as oxygen bind to a hemoglobin molecule, mutations in globin genes may affect subunit or dimmer pair interactions. These could result in altered oxygen affinity or hemoglobin instability.

Checkpoint! 2

What globin chains are produced in the adult?

Answer

The chains, produced are α, β, δ, γ. The chains pair up to form HbA, HbA_2 and HbF.

Checkpoint! 3

What are the names and globin composition of the embryonic, fetal, and adult hemoglobins?

Answer

Embryonic	$\xi_2\gamma_2$	Hb Portland
	$\xi_2\varepsilon_2$	Hb Gower I
	$\alpha_2\varepsilon_2$	Hb Gower II
Fetal	$\alpha_2\gamma_2$	HbF (also found in adult)
Adult	$\alpha_2\beta_2$	HbA
	$\alpha_2\delta_2$	HbA_2

Checkpoint! 4

A patient has an anemia caused by a shortened RBC life span (hemolysis). How would this affect the HbA_{1c} measurement?

Answer

The red cells are being destroyed at an increased rate and are being replaced with new cells that have no HbA_{1c}. The red cell lifespan decreases and the amount of HbA_{1c} depends on a time-averaged concentration of glucose with older cells having more HbA_{1c} than younger cells. The HbA_{1c} is not a good indication of glucose control in this case. This same phenomenon also could occur in patients treated with erythropoietin. Additionally, if abnormal forms of hemoglobin are present such as in sickle cell anemia (HbS), there is no HbA and therefore there is no HbA_{1c}.

Checkpoint! 5

What factors influence an increase in the amount of oxygen delivered to tissue during an aerobic workout?

Answer

During an aerobic workout, a buildup of lactic acid and CO_2 occurs in the tissues. This leads to a shift to the right in affinity of hemoglobin for oxygen, resulting in an increase of oxygen delivered to the tissues.

Checkpoint! 6

A 2-year-old child was found to have 15% methemoglobin by spectral absorbance at 630 nm. What tests would you suggest to help differentiate whether this is an inherited or acquired methemoglobinemia, and what results would you expect with each diagnosis?

Answer

Tests that should be done include NADPH-reductase activity and hemoglobin electrophoresis. See Table 5-7 for expected results.

Chapter 7

Checkpoint! 1

An adult patient's peripheral blood smear revealed many myelocytes, metamyelocytes, and band forms of neutrophils. Is this a normal finding?

Answer

No, metamyelocytes and myelocytes are not normal findings in the peripheral blood. They indicate a shift to the left in granulocytes and can be seen in infection, inflammation, and other conditions. (See ∞ Chapter 21 for a complete list.)

Checkpoint! 2

An adult patient's WBC count is 10×10^9/L, and there are 90% neutrophils. What is the absolute number of neutrophils? Is this in the reference range for neutrophils, and if not, what term would be used to describe it?

Answer

The absolute count for neutrophils is 9×10^9/L. This indicates an increase in neutrophils referred to as *neutrophilia*.

Checkpoint! 3

A patient with life-threatening recurrent infections is found to have a chromosomal mutation that results in a loss of active integrin molecules on the neutrophil surface. Why would this result in life-threatening infections?

Answer

This is known as *leukocyte adhesion deficiency-1 (LAD-1)*, an inability of the neutrophils to "tightly adhere" to the vascular endothelial surface. If the neutrophils cannot do this, they have difficulty moving to the site of infection, and therefore, a patient with this condition would be at risk for infections.

Checkpoint! 4

A patient has a compromised ability to utilize the oxygen-dependent pathway in neutrophils. What two important microbial killing mechanisms could be affected?

Answer

Production of the respiratory burst and generation of cytotoxic reactive oxygen intermediates would be abnormal.

Checkpoint! 5

Indicate which of the granulocytes will be increased in the following conditions: a bacterial infection, an immediate hypersensitivity reaction, and an asthmatic reaction.

Answer

Neutrophils are increased in a bacterial infection. Basophils are increased in an immediate hypersensitivity reaction. Eosinophils are increased in an asthmatic reaction.

Checkpoint! 6

An adult patient's neutrophil count and monocyte count are extremely low ($<0.50 \times 10^9$/L and $<0.050 \times 10^9$/L, respectively). What body defense mechanism is at risk?

Answer

Phagocytosis and/or the innate immune system is compromised when the neutrophil and monocyte concentrations are decreased.

Checkpoint! 7

How would you morphologically differentiate a reactive lymphocyte from a plasma cell on a peripheral blood smear?

Answer

A reactive lymphocyte's size is usually increased, 16 to 30 μm, and the N:C ratio is decreased. The nuclear chromatin pattern may be dispersed, and nucleoli may be visible. The cytoplasm is frequently abundant, very basophilic, and foamy. The cytoplasmic membrane may have scalloped edges due to indentations made by surrounding erythrocytes. Azurophilic granules may be present. A plasma cell ranges in size from 14 to 20 μm and has a decreased N:C ratio. The small nucleus is eccentrically placed in the cell. The nuclear chromatin may have a spoke wheel pattern. The cytoplasm is nongranular and has a deep basophilic color.

Checkpoint! 8

A young adult patient's blood smear reveals 70% reactive lymphocytes and 10% nonreactive lymphocytes in a 10×10^9/L WBC count. What is the absolute concentration of total lymphocytes and reactive lymphocytes? What is a probable cause of these findings?

Answer

The counts indicate 8×10^9/L total lymphocytes and 7×10^9/L reactive lymphocytes. A viral infection is a probable cause of these results. (See ∞ Chapter 22 for specific causes of increased reactive lymphocytes.)

Chapter 8

Checkpoint! 1

Calculate the indices and describe the erythrocytes given the following information: Hb = 7.1g/dL, Hct = 0.23L/L, RBC = 3.59×10^{12}/L.

Answer

MCV = 64 fL; MCH = 19.8 pg; MCHC = 30.8 g/dL. The cells are microcytic and hypochromic.

Checkpoint! 2

A patient has an MCV of 130 fL and an RDW of 14.5. Review of the blood smear reveals anisocytosis. Explain the discrepancy between the blood smear finding and the RDW.

Answer

The RDW is calculated by dividing the standard deviation of erythrocyte size by MCV. If the SD is abnormally high but the MCV is also high, an RDW in the normal range may be calculated.

Checkpoint! 3

Is it possible to have an increased relative reticulocyte count and an absolute reticulocyte count in the normal interval? Explain.

Answer

Yes. If the patient is very anemic, the ratio of reticulocytes to total number of erythrocytes is not a very accurate indicator of bone marrow production. For example, a reticulocyte count in a patient with a decreased erythrocyte count may be calculated to be an increased percentage of reticulocytes. However, calculating the absolute number of reticulocytes will reveal that the number of reticulocytes is actually in the reference interval. Of course, a reticulocyte count in the reference interval in the presence of anemia is not an adequate response.

Checkpoint! 4

What laboratory test is the least invasive and most cost efficient to evaluate erythrocyte production in the presence of anemia?

Answer

The reticulocyte count is an informative index of erythropoietic activity. It requires a peripheral blood specimen and is easy to perform. Calculation of the absolute reticulocyte count or RPI provides more information. The IRF is provided by some instruments and is very helpful in providing a reticulocyte maturity index.

Chapter 9

Checkpoint! 1

A patient's iron studies revealed: serum iron 100 μg/dL; TIBC 360 μg/dL. Calculate % saturation and UIBC. Are these values normal or abnormal?

Answer

% saturation = serum iron/TIBC
% saturation = 100/360 = 28%
UIBC = TIBC − serum iron
UIBC = 360 − 100 = 260
Normal results

Checkpoint! 2

A 30-year-old female and a 25-year-old male both had a bleeding ulcer. Assume that each acquired the ulcer at the same time, was losing about the same amount of blood, had equal amounts of storage iron to begin with, and was taking in about 15 mg dietary iron each day. Would you expect that the woman and man would develop ID at the same time? Explain.

Answer

The woman would probably develop ID sooner because she is also losing about 20 mg of iron per month through menstruation.

Checkpoint! 3

How does the peripheral blood picture in ACD differ from that seen in IDA?

Answer

In IDA, the erythrocytes are usually microcytic, hypochromic. In ACD, the erythrocytes are usually normocytic, normochromic; normocytic, hypochromic; or in long-standing cases, microcytic, hypochromic.

Checkpoint! 4

What is the risk of population genetic screening for HH? What is the benefit of population genetic screening for HH?

Answer

The risks are that individuals who have the mutated gene may be discriminated against by health insurance companies and that all of those who test positive may not develop the disease as disease penetrance has not yet been determined. The benefit is that individuals who have the mutated gene can be identified early before they develop clinical signs of the disease. Therapy by phlebotomy can then prevent chronic disease associated with HH.

Chapter 10

Checkpoint! 1

Why can't all structural hemoglobin variants be identified by hemoglobin electrophoresis?

Answer

Not all point mutations in the hemoglobin molecule change its electrical charge. If the charge is not changed, the variant hemoglobin will travel as a normal hemoglobin.

Checkpoint! 2

What is meant by the term silent carrier *when referring to a hemoglobinopathy?*

Answer

The patient has an abnormal hemoglobin but it does not cause any symptoms of disease.

Checkpoint! 3

What functional effect would this have on the hemoglobin molecule?

Answer

It increases oxygen affinity. The R structure is the oxygenated form of hemoglobin while the T form is the deoxygenated form.

Checkpoint! 4

Why don't newborns with sickle cell anemia experience episodes of vaso-occlusive crisis?

Answer

The predominant hemoglobin in newborns is HbF, which does not sickle. HbS does not become the predominant hemoglobin until after the first 6 months of life.

Checkpoint! 5

Outline the treatment options that might be used for a patient with HbS disease, pneumonia, and vaso-occlusive crisis. Discuss how each would affect his clinical condition.

Answer

In the short term, the patient's pain would be managed and he would be hydrated. He would be given antibiotics and respiratory therapy for the pneumonia. Long-term therapy might include transfusions to reduce symptoms of anemia. He might be placed on hydroxyurea therapy to increase the amount of HbF, thus reducing the frequency of vaso-occlusive crises. If he has not suffered severe organ damage and a compatible donor can be found, he might be a candidate for bone marrow transplant to correct the genetic defect–causing sickle cell disease.

Checkpoint! 6

Explain these results and suggest further testing that may help in diagnosis.

Answer

In sickle cell trait, the amount of HbS is usually less than 50% while in sickle cell anemia, it is typically >90%. The presence of some HbA suggests sickle cell trait in this patient. The patient may have inherited another abnormal hemoglobin gene such as thalassemia. Electrophoresis at acid pH should be performed to eliminate the possibility of hemoglobins with similar mobilities at alkaline pH. DNA testing may provide evidence of thalassemia. A microcytic hypochromic anemia is also a clue to the presence of thalassemia.

Checkpoint! 7

What is the functional abnormality of HbC and HbS? Why do these two abnormal hemoglobins have the same altered functions?

Answer

The HbS and HbC have decreased solubility and tend to crystallize. They both have a point mutation in the $\beta 6$ position where a nonpolar amino acid replaces glutamine.

Checkpoint! 8

Explain the results and suggest a follow-up test to determine a diagnosis.

Answer

The patient may have another abnormal hemoglobin that migrates similar to HbS. Electrophoresis on citrate agar at pH 6.0 should be performed to allow distinction of this hemoglobin from HbS.

Checkpoint! 9

What laboratory test might differentiate these two conditions?

Answer

Hemoglobin electrophoresis. HbE shows an abnormal band, but β-thalassemia has no abnormal hemoglobins present.

Checkpoint! 10

a. Explain why patients with an unstable hemoglobin variant usually experience acute hemolysis only after administration of certain drugs or with infections.
b. If a patient is suspected of having a congenital Heinz body hemolytic anemia but hemoglobin electrophoresis is normal, why is it necessary to perform additional tests?

Answer

a. The hemoglobin becomes unstable when the normal red blood cell environment changes to a more acidic or hypoxic environment.
b. The abnormal hemoglobin may have an electrophoretic mobility identical to that of normal hemoglobin, thereby masking the presence of the abnormal hemoglobin.

Checkpoint! 11

Why should red cell enzymes be measured and hemoglobin electrophoresis be performed on a patient with congenital cyanosis?

Answer

The defect may be due either to inheritance of HbM, which could be detected by hemoglobin electrophoresis or to a defect in the methemoglobin reduction system, which can be detected by enzyme analysis.

Chapter 11

Checkpoint! 1

Differentiate the etiology of thalassemias and hemoglobinopathies.

Answer

Thalassemia results from deletional or nondeletional mutations in one or more globin genes that reduce or eliminate synthesis of the corresponding globin chain(s). Hemoglobinopathy is a qualitative hemoglobin disorder caused by a point mutation in a globin gene, usually the β-gene, that results in an amino acid substitution in the corresponding globin chain and alters hemoglobin stability and function.

Checkpoint! 2

What are the most common genetic mutations associated with α-thalassemia?

Answer

Gene deletions.

Checkpoint! 3

Why do α- and β-thalassemia result in more clinically severe disease than other types of thalassemia?

Answer

HbA is composed of α- and β-chains and constitutes 97% of adult hemoglobin. Thus, a reduction in either α- or β-chains decreases the concentration of the most abundant normal adult hemoglobin. The other globin chains are associated with hemoglobins that are either low in concentration in adult blood or are designed to function in embryonic or fetal life.

Checkpoint! 4

Which of the three normal adult hemoglobins would be affected in hydrops fetalis?

Answer

Hydrops fetalis occurs when there is a deletion in all 4 α-genes; therefore, all three normal adult hemoglobins, HbA, HbA_2, and HbF, are affected because each contains α-chains.

Checkpoint! 5

Compare oxygen binding characteristics of HbH relative to HbA and myoglobin.

Answer

The allosteric interactions of the two α-chains and the two β-chains confer on HbA cooperative oxygen binding characteristics called *heme/heme interaction*. As a deoxygenated HbA molecule binds an oxygen molecule, hemoglobin incurs an increased affinity for oxygen at the other three available sites. Oxygen affinity continues to increase with each subsequent molecule bound. By virtue of the binding of hydrogen atoms and 2,3-DPG to oxyhemoglobin in the tissues, HbA releases oxygen molecules in an incremental fashion regulated by the oxygen, carbon dioxide, and hydrogen ion concentration in the tissue. The incremental binding and release of oxygen is expressed as a sigmoidal oxygen dissociation curve. HbH, by virtue of its four β-chain composition, does not exhibit heme/heme interaction and therefore functions as four separate subunits with identical oxygen affinities. The oxygen dissociation curve is therefore expressed as a hyperbolic curve similar to that of monomeric myoglobin.

Checkpoint! 6

Why do the symptoms of β-thalassemia major delay until approximately the sixth month of life?

Answer

β-thalassemia major is characterized by an absence or significant reduction in the synthesis of β-chains. Although the synthesis of β-chains begins at approximately the third trimester of fetal development, quantities sufficient to assemble significant amounts of HbA do not occur until approximately 6 months of age. Therefore, the lack of production of β-chains and the resultant lack of HbA is not manifested until 6 months of age when HbA synthesis is expected. The major hemoglobin at birth is HbF.

Checkpoint! 7

In β-thalassemia, what erythrocyte parameter from the CBC differs significantly from that found in iron deficiency?

Answer

The erythrocyte count in thalassemia is normal or high for the degree of anemia, but in iron deficiency, it is decreased. Both iron deficiency and thalassemia are characterized by microcytic, hypochromic anemia with target cells.

Checkpoint! 8

Why is $\gamma\delta\beta$-thalassemia more severe than $\delta\beta$-thalassemia and CS thalassemia?

Answer

All normal adult hemoglobin contains α-chains with either γ- (HbF), δ- (HbA_2), or β- (HbA) chains. A reduction or absence of all three chains in $\gamma\delta\beta$-thalassemia decreases the production of all three adult hemoglobins. $\delta\beta$-thalassemia can partially compensate by producing γ-chains (HbF). Patients with CS thalassemia bear some normal α-genes and can therefore make all adult hemoglobins, albeit at a reduced rate.

Checkpoint! 9

In combination disorders of structural Hb variants and thalassemia, why is the severity less when α-thalassemia is inherited with sickle cell trait than when β-thalassemia is coexpressed with sickle cell trait?

Answer

The severity of symptoms associated with HbS is related to the concentration of HbS. The combination of one HbS β-gene (β^s-gene) and one β-thalassemia-gene results in little to no HbA formation because both of the β-genes are mutated. In contrast, an α-gene mutation reduces the number of α-chains that can combine with β^s-chains, reducing the amount of the abnormal structural hemoglobin (HbS) and thus reducing the symptoms associated with the abnormal hemoglobin.

Checkpoint! 10
Which laboratory tests should be done first to differentiate thalassemia and iron deficiency?

Answer
The most cost-efficient and diagnostically effective studies should be done first. In this case, iron studies should be done first because iron deficiency is the most common cause of microcytic hypochromic anemia. The iron studies include serum ferritin, serum iron, TIBC, and percent saturation. If the iron studies do not reveal iron deficiency, hemoglobin electrophoresis should be done.

Chapter 12

Checkpoint! 1
Explain why patients with B$_{12}$ or folate deficiency have megaloblastic maturation.

Answer
The megaloblastic anemias are the result of abnormal DNA synthesis (a nuclear maturation defect). As a result, the delayed nuclear development prevents cell division. RNA synthesis and cytoplasmic maturation are not affected. The result is production of large cells with nuclear cytoplasmic asynchrony. The basis for the nonmegaloblastic anemias may be related to an increase in membrane lipids.

Checkpoint! 2
Patients with megaloblastic anemia often present with a yellow or waxy pallor. What is the diagnostic significance of this clinical symptom?

Answer
Ineffective erythropoiesis in the marrow is due to nuclear/cytoplasmic asynchrony of cell development as a result of the lack of thymidine and a diminished DNA synthesis. The abnormal cells are hemolyzed in the marrow. If intramedullary hemolysis is significant, all classic signs of hemolysis will accompany the megaloblastosis. Plasma unconjugated bilirubin levels will increase and result in jaundice, which results in a yellow and waxy skin pallor.

Checkpoint! 3
Why are abnormalities of leukocytes and platelets present in megaloblastic anemia?

Answer
Granulocytes and platelets may also show changes evident of abnormal hematopoiesis (nuclear maturation defect). Hypersegmented neutrophils (more than five nuclear lobes) may be found in megaloblastic anemia even in the absence of macrocytosis. This finding is considered highly sensitive and specific for megaloblastic anemia. Giant metamyelocytes and bands with loose, open chromatin in the nuclei are diagnostic. The myelocytes show poor granulation as do more mature stages. Megakaryocytes may be decreased, normal, or increased. Maturation, however, is distinctly abnormal. Some larger

than normal forms can be found with separation of nuclear lobes and nuclear fragments.

Checkpoint! 4
What abnormal morphological findings on a stained blood smear comprise the triad in megaloblastic anemia?

Answer
Macroovalocytes, Howell-Jolly bodies, and hypersegmentation of PMNs

Checkpoint! 5
Hal Jones had small bowel resection due to carcinoma. Explain why he is at high risk for folate deficiency.

Answer
Dietary folate must be deconjugated in the small intestine for absorption to occur. Intestinal villi in the small intestine contain receptors for folate binding and absorption into the body. An individual with a small bowel resection would require ongoing folate therapy because absorption is impaired. Pharmacological doses of folate are given periodically intramuscularly to maintain normal levels.

Checkpoint! 6
What is the most common cause of folate deficiency and in what groups of individuals is it usually found?

Answer
Nutritional insufficiency is the most common cause of folate deficiency. Body stores of folate are sufficient to maintain minimal body requirements for only 3–6 months. Folate deficiency develops more rapidly than B$_{12}$ deficiency. Once a negative folate balance occurs, serum folate values can begin to decrease within 2 weeks. In developed countries, the elderly, alcoholics, and pregnant women are considered high-risk groups for folate deficiency.

Checkpoint! 7
A patient has the following results: vitamin B$_{12}$: 50 pg/mL, serum folate: 4 ng/dL, and RBC folate: 100 ng/mL. Interpret these results.

Answer
Normal serum B$_{12}$ values range from 247–800 pg/ml in adults and 160–1200 pg/ml in newborns. Normal serum reference interval for serum folate is 2.5–20 ng/ml and for RBC folate is 160–700 ng/ml. These results indicate the patient is vitamin B$_{12}$ deficient with an accompanying decrease in RBC folate. Serum folate is normal. The RBC and serum folate are not good indicators of folate status in vitamin B$_{12}$ deficiency; a deficiency of vitamin B$_{12}$ impairs methionine synthesis and leads to the accumulation of methyl-THF in the serum. In addition, vitamin B$_{12}$ is required for normal transfer of methyl-THF to the cells and for conjugating the folate to keep it in the cell. Thus, serum folate may be falsely increased and erythrocyte folate may be falsely decreased in vitamin B$_{12}$ deficiency. In this case, the patient appears to have a vitamin B$_{12}$ deficiency. Even though the RBC folate is low, it is not a good indicator of folate deficiency. Homocysteine and MMA tests may help define the deficiency.

Checkpoint! 8

Explain why there is a megaloblastic anemia in transcobalamin II deficiency when the serum vtiamin B_{12} concentration is normal.

Answer

Although transcobalamin II is only about 5% saturated, it is the primary transport protein for vitamin B_{12}. Transcobalamin II binds 90% of the newly absorbed vitamin B_{12}. Congenital deficiency of transcobalamin II produces a severe megaloblastic anemia in infancy. However, serum vitamin B_{12} concentration in this condition is normal. This is most likely due to the fact that transcobalamin I serves as a passive reservoir that is in equilibrium with liver stores of the vitamin. Transcobalamin I normally binds 75% of the recycled endogenous vitamin B_{12} in the body but it is only about 50% saturated. With a deficiency of transcobalamin II, more vitamin B_{12} is bound by trancobalamin I.

Checkpoint! 9

Explain why severe B_{12} deficiency sometimes presents with neurological disease.

Answer

In vitamin B_{12} deficiency, a defect in degradation of propionyl CoA to methylmalonyl CoA and, finally, to succinyl CoA occurs. As propionyl CoA accumulates, it is used as a primer for fatty acid synthesis replacing the usual primer acetyl CoA. It is probable that demyelination (destruction, removal, or loss of the lipid substance that forms a myelin sheath around the axons of nerve fibers), a characteristic finding in vitamin B_{12} deficiency, is a result of this erroneous fatty acid synthesis. Because of the defective fatty acid degradation, a critical feature of demyelination in vitamin B_{12} deficiency is neurological disease. Peripheral nerves are most often affected, presenting as motor and sensory neuropathy. The brain and spinal cord may also be affected leading to dementia, spastic paralysis, and other serious neurological disturbances.

Checkpoint! 10

Explain why some believe that pernicious anemia is an autoimmune disorder.

Answer

Pernicious anemia is often associated with autoimmune disease. Antibodies directed against the patient's own cells or proteins are found. Autoantibodies found in pernicious anemia (PA) are of two types, blocking and binding. Blocking antibodies prevent the formation of the intrinsic factor/B_{12} complex, and binding antibodies prevent attachment and absorption of B_{12} into the ileum mucosal epithelial cell. Antibodies against intrinsic factor are detected in up to 75% of PA patients. The majority of PA patients demonstrate antibodies against the parietal cells in the floor of the stomach. Patients with PA can have one or both types of antibodies.

Checkpoint! 11

What two lab tests are the most specific indicators of B_{12} deficiency?

Answer

A specific test that measures the increased excretion of methylmalonic acid (MMA) in the urine indirectly indicates decreases in vitamin B_{12} concentration. Homocysteine increases in the plasma of patients with vitamin B_{12} or folate deficiency. Monitoring serum levels can serve as an early detector of vitamin B_{12} deficiency. Many recent studies have concluded that MMA and homocysteine are the most sensitive and specific indicators of vitamin B_{12} deficiency.

Checkpoint! 12

Which clinical type of CDA gives a HAM test result and presents with a normoblastic marrow?

Answer

With CDA-II, bone marrow precursors are normoblastic but are typically multinucleated with up to seven nuclei. Type II is distinguished by a positive acidified serum test (Ham test) but a negative sucrose hemolysis test. In the Ham test, only about 30% of normal sera are effective in lysing CDA II cells.

Checkpoint! 13

What is the main cause of nonanemic macrocytosis?

Answer

Alcohol abuse is one of the most common causes of nonanemic macrocytosis. The macrocytosis associated with alcoholism is usually multifactorial and may be megaloblastic. In up to 60% of cases, anemia does not accompany macrocytosis.

Checkpoint! 14

What are three clinical or laboratory findings (besides assessing the marrow) that can distinguish a nonmegaloblastic(normoblastic) macrocytic anemia from a megaloblastic anemia?

Answer

A normoblastic macrocytic anemia does not present with pancytopenia. Granulocytes and platelet counts are usually normal. Hypersegmented neutrophils are not found in nonmegaloblastic macrocytosis, and the abnormal RBC morphology is less pronounced. In addition, symptoms commonly found in megaloblastic anemia such as jaundice, glossitis, and neuropathy are absent in nonmegaloblastic anemia.

Chapter 13

Checkpoint! 1

An anemic patient has a corrected reticulocyte count of 1.5%, hemoglobin of 10.0 g/dL, hematocrit of 0.30 L/L, total neutrophil count of $0.4 \times 10^9/L$, and a platelet count of $30 \times 10^9/L$. Is it likely that this patient has aplastic anemia?

Answer

No, it is unlikely that this patient has aplastic anemia. Two of the peripheral blood findings are inconsistent with the diagnostic criteria.

Chapter 14

Checkpoint! 1

A patient is suspected of having a hemolytic disease. The reticulocyte count is increased, but the hemoglobin, serum bilirubin, and haptoglobin are within the normal range. Explain.

Answer

The patient may have compensated hemolytic disease, which explains the normal hemoglobin. Serum bilirubin is not a sensitive test for hemolysis and is not always increased in hemolytic disease.

Haptoglobin is an acute phase reactant and may be normal if the patient has concurrent infection, inflammation, or malignancy.

Checkpoint! 2

Explain why it is helpful for the laboratory professional to know whether a particular hemolytic anemia is characterized by intravascular or extravascular hemolysis.

Answer

By knowing whether there is intravascular or extravascular hemolysis, one can recommend laboratory tests to help define the etiology of the hemolysis and evaluate laboratory test results accordingly. Hemoglobinuria, hemoglobinemia, and hemosidinuria are present only if there is intravascular hemolysis.

Checkpoint! 3

Why is it helpful for the laboratory professional to know the clinical history and suspected cause of a hemolytic anemia?

Answer

It will assist in making recommendations for reflex and confirmatory laboratory tests and evaluation of test results. For instance, a spherocytic hemolytic anemia could be due to an intrinsic erythrocyte abnormality (hereditary spherocytosis, HS) or to an immune process. HS is a chronic anemia and can often be found in other family members. Test follow-up for HS should include osmotic fragility. Testing to determine the deficient or defective protein include SDS-PAGE, densitometry, ELISA, PCR and flow cytometry. Immune hemolytic anemia is usually an acute problem. Follow-up for an immune hemolytic anemia is a DAT (AHG) test to confirm the presence of antibodies on the erythrocyte.

Chapter 15

Checkpoint! 1

List various factors related to changes in the erythrocyte that may lead to a decrease or increase in the MCV in hereditary spherocytosis.

Answer

Erythrocyte factors that may cause a change in the MCV include spherocytes, polychromasia, and depleted iron stores or folate levels. Many densely stained spherocytes on the peripheral smear may cause a decrease in the MCV. Increased polychromasia may lead to an increase in the MCV. Chronic hemolysis can lead to depleted iron stores and folate levels. Low iron stores will lead to microcytic erythrocytes and thus a decreased MCV; depleted folate levels will lead to the formation of macrocytes and an increased MCV.

Checkpoint! 2

Interpret the results of the following osmotic fragility test:

	Patient	Control
Initial hemolysis	0.35 % NaCl	0.45 % NaCl
Complete hemolysis	0.25 % NaCl	0.30 % NaCl

Answer

The osmotic fragility test reveals that the patient's erythrocytes lysed at a lower concentration of NaCl than the control cells. This indicates that the patient's erythrocytes are more resistant to hemolysis or less osmotically fragile than the control cells. Target cells and sickle cells are able to resist hemolysis in hypotonic saline solutions longer than normal cells.

Checkpoint! 3

Why do the elliptocytes in HE demonstrate normal osmotic fragility?

Answer

The elliptocytes in HE demonstrate a normal osmotic fragility curve because the defect does not lead to a change in the surface-area-to-volume ratio of the erythrocyte. The elliptocyte can take on as much fluid as a normal cell and lyse at the same concentration of hypotonic saline as a normal cell.

Checkpoint! 4

Interpret the results of the following thermal sensitivity test. Patient's erythrocytes: Marked erythrocyte fragmentation after 10-minute incubation at 46°C. Normal control: No significant change in erythrocyte morphology after 10-minute incubation at 46°C.

Answer

The patient's erythrocytes are demonstrating an increased sensitivity to heat by fragmenting at 46°C. Normal erythrocytes do not fragment until heated to 49–50°C. Hereditary pyropoikilocytosis is an inherited disorder that demonstrates erythrocytes that are sensitive to heat.

Checkpoint! 5

Determine the type of erythrocyte membrane disorder based on the following lab results—retic count: 4%; osmotic fragility: increased; autohemolysis: increased; bilirubin: increased; peripheral smear: 30% stomatocytes present.

Answer

The erythrocyte membrane disorder that best fits these lab results is hereditary overhydrated stomatocytosis. Key features include a large percentage of stomatocytes and an increased osmotic fragility test. The patient's bilirubin level is elevated, which signifies increased erythrocyte hemolysis. Other disorders presenting with an increased number of stomatocytes include acute alcoholism, liver disease, and cardiovascular disease. These disorders, however, show little hemolysis.

Checkpoint! 6

Explain why the osmotic fragility is decreased in DHS.

Answer

The erythrocytes in DHS are dehydrated. They can take on more water than a normal erythrocyte and display complete lysis at a lower concentration of hypotonic saline than normal erythrocytes.

Checkpoint! 7

Compare the membrane lipid abnormalities seen in LCAT deficiency, spur cell anemia, and abetalipoproteinemia and explain how they may result in hemolysis of the cell.

Answer

Spur cell anemia—increase in serum lipoproteins, increase in membrane cholesterol, but normal membrane concentration of phospholipid. As the ratio of the membrane cholesterol to phospholipid increases, the cell is flattened and loses deformability. After repeated splenic passages, portions of membrane fragment, and the cell acquires the spur shape resulting in eventual hemolysis.

Abetalipoproteinemia—absence of serum β-lipoprotein, low serum cholesterol, triglycerides, phospholipids. There is an increase in the ratio of cholesterol to phospholipid. Erythrocyte membrane cholesterol is normal, but sphingomyelin is increased. Membrane fluidity is decreased because of increased sphingomyelin. As the cell ages, the degree of distortion increases, resulting in hemolysis.

LCAT deficiency—LCAT catalyzes formation of cholesterol esters from cholesterol. In LCAT deficiency, increased levels of cholesterol, phospholipids, and triglycerides in serum occur. High-density lipoproteins are decreased. Increased serum cholesterol results in increased cholesterol in the erythrocyte. Target cells are formed with high cholesterol levels. Hemolysis is mild.

Checkpoint! 8
Explain why immunophenotyping with CD14, CD55 and CD59 is used to establish a diagnosis of PNH.

Answer
PNH is characterized by a deficiency of GPI necessary to link a variety of proteins to the cell. CD55, CD59, and CD14 are GPI linked proteins. CD55 and CD59 are found on neutrophils. CD59 is found on erythrocytes, and CD14 is found on monocytes. These proteins are linked to the cell membrane by GPI. It is recommended that at least two different antibodies be used to detect different kinds of GPI anchored proteins.

Chapter 16

Checkpoint! 1
Transfusion of red blood cells in a patient with chronic nonspherocytic, hemolytic anemia due to an erythrocyte enzyme deficiency does not reverse or prevent the recipient's condition. However, a transfusion does help to raise the patient's hemoglobin. If tests are performed to quantitate the enzyme after a transfusion, the results may be within the normal reference interval. Explain.

Answer
Presence of transfused cells contribute to a falsely normal test result because these cells are normal and contain a normal amount of the enzyme.

Checkpoint! 2
Oxidant compounds are harmful because they result in production of harmful peroxides or other oxygen radicals that overwhelm the body's natural mechanisms to scavenge them. Why is the mechanism of protection against oxidants easily compromised in G6PD deficiency?

Answer
Protection from oxidants is easily overcome in G6PD deficiency because the enzyme cannot supply enough NADPH to keep glutathione in the reduced state. Reduced glutathione is the cell's primary protection from oxidants.

Checkpoint! 3
Erythrocyte morphology should always be examined carefully. The ability to pick up subtle clues as to the cause of a disease process can be acquired from a comprehensive evaluation of abnormal erythrocyte morphology. How is this likely to aid the diagnosis of G6PD deficiency?

Answer
Careful evaluation of a blood smear and reporting of bite cells will alert the health care practitioner as to the mechanism of cell destruction. When the mechanism of destruction is considered, this will lead to the selection of more diagnostically effective definitive tests to find the root cause of the anemia.

Checkpoint! 4
What are the differentiating characteristics of PK and G6PD deficiencies found on the peripheral blood smear?

Answer
PK deficiency has echinocytes and irregularly contracted cells; G6PD deficiency has bite cells and spherocytes. After splenectomy, additional cell abnormalities may be found.

Chapter 17

Checkpoint! 1
What are the three major categories of immune hemolytic anemia, and how is antibody production stimulated in each type?

Answer
Autoimmune—alteration of self-antigen or immune system regulation dysfunction
Alloimmune—response to foreign erythrocyte antigen
Drug induced—immune response to epitope on drug in combination with erythrocyte antigen

Checkpoint! 2
Explain how the class of immunoglobulin, amount of antibody bound, and thermal reactivity of the antibody affect hemolysis.

Answer
IgM is able to activate complement efficiently causing intravascular hemolysis. IgG is less able to activate complement, and the coated cells are removed in the spleen (extravascular) via interaction with Fc receptors on splenic macrophages.

Because a minimum amount of antibody molecules must be bound for hemolysis to occur, the more antibody molecules on the cell, the more likely it is that hemolysis will occur.

IgG antibodies typically have optimal reactivity at 37°C (body temperature) whereas IgM antibodies have an optimal thermal amplitude of 20–25°C.

Checkpoint! 3
Compare the mechanisms of IgG mediated hemolysis with those of IgM mediated hemolysis.

Answer
IgM mediated hemolysis has two possible outcomes. The first occurs when the IgM molecule fixes complement and the complement cascade goes to completion (C1–C9). This results in intravascular hemolysis. If, however, the IgM molecule fixes complement but the cascade does not go to completion, the C3b molecules that remain on the erythrocytes interact with C3b receptors on macrophages resulting in extravascular hemolysis.

In IgG mediated hemolysis, complement is infrequently activated and most hemolysis is extravascular. The Fc portion of the attached IgG molecule reacta with Fc receptors on splenic macrophages. The cell may be completely phagocytized by the macrophage or portions of the membrane may be removed resulting in spherocytes.

Checkpoint! 4

Compare the purpose of the DAT and the IAT and state the type of specimen used for each test.

Answer

DAT is used to detect *erythrocytes* that have been coated with antibody or complement fragments in vivo. The specimen used is serum or plasma collected in EDTA anticoagulant. The IAT is used to detect the presence of antibodies in the patient's *serum*. The specimen used is EDTA plasma or serum.

Checkpoint! 5

What are the clinical findings and the immune stimuli for WAIHA?

Answer

Clinical findings—symptoms related to anemia including weakness, jaundice, pallor. Idiopathic WAIHA: no identifiable cause. *Secondary WAIHA*—associated with disease such as lymphoproliferative diseases including CLL, neoplasms, and autoimmune disorders such as SLE, chronic inflammatory diseases, and viral/bacterial infections.

Checkpoint! 6

What is the DAT pattern in WAIHA? Explain why spherocytes are commonly seen in WAIHA.

Answer

The most common pattern is reaction with:

Polyspecific AHG	positive
anti-IgG	positive
anti-C3	negative

In some cases, the anti-C3 is positive.

Spherocytes are seen because the erythrocyte is coated with IgG, and as it passes through the spleen, the splenic macrophages (with Fc receptors) interact with the cell and remove portions of the erythrocyte membrane. As more portions are removed, the cell becomes round (spherocyte).

Checkpoint! 7

Describe the mechanism of cell destruction in CHD.

Answer

The antibody in CHD is usually an IgM that is capable of activating complement and causing intravascular hemolysis. The IgM activates complement in the cooler portions of the circulation. As the erythrocytes move into warmer parts of the circulation, IgM leaves the cell and complement cascade goes through C9. In other instances, the IgM antibody fixes complement but the cascade does not go to completion. Cells are then destroyed via the C3b receptors on macrophages.

Checkpoint! 8

Explain why MCV, MCH, and MCHC may be falsely increased when blood from someone with CHD is tested using an automated counter.

Answer

If the blood is cool, the IgM antibodies cause agglutination of the cells. As these clumps of cells are measured for MCV, they are measured as a single cell and thus appear macrocytic.

Hematocrit (which is calculated) is incorrect because of the incorrect erythrocyte count. Hemoglobin is correct because this parameter is determined by lysis of the cells. The erythrocyte count is falsely decreased because the clumps are counted as one cell.

MCH, which is derived from the hemoglobin and erythrocyte count, then is falsely elevated as is the MCHC, which is derived from the hemoglobin and hematocrit values.

Checkpoint! 9

Compare the DAT findings and the antibody specificity in WAIHA and CHD.

Answer

	WAIHA	CHD
Polyspecific AHG:	+	+
Anti-IgG:	+	−
Anti-C3:	− or +	+
Antibody specificity:	directed to a complex Rh antigen molecule	anti-I

Checkpoint! 10

Compare the antibody specificity and the confirmatory test for PCH and CHD.

Answer

	PCH	CHD
Antibody specificity:	anti-P	anti-I
Confirmatory test:	Donath-Landsteiner test	Cold agglutinin test

Checkpoint! 11

Compare the different types of drug-induced hemolysis including the type of hemolysis, the drug usually associated with the mechanism, and the DAT profile.

Answer

	Drug adsorption	Immune complex	Autoantibody
Hemolysis	Extravascular	Intravascular	Extravascular
Drug	Penicillin	Quinidine	Aldomet
DAT profile:			
Poly	Positive	Positive	Positive
Anti-IgG	Positive	Negative	Positive
Anti-C3	Negative	Positive	Negative

Checkpoint! 12

Compare the underlying mechanisms, pathophysiology, and clinical symptoms of an acute hemolytic transfusion reaction and a delayed one.

Answer

	Acute	Delayed
Mechanism	IgM (usually ABO system)	IgG (usually Kidd system)
	Intravascular hemolysis	Extravascular hemolysis
Pathophysiology	Naturally occuring; ABO antibodies react immediately with foreign antigen on transfused cells	Immune stimulated; Secondary exposure to foreign antigen causes antibody titer to increase
Clinical symptoms	Chills, fever, hypotension; Difficulty in breathing; Increased pulse rate	Malaise, fever, drop in hemoglobin, dark or red urine, usually one week post-transfusion

Checkpoint! 13

What are the required laboratory tests for investigating a suspected transfusion reaction? Compare the characteristic laboratory findings in acute hemolytic transfusion reactions and delayed transfusion reactions.

Answer

Required tests are clerical check, DAT, and comparison for visible hemoglobin between the pretransfusion and posttransfusion specimens.

	Acute	Delayed
DAT	Positive but may be weak because of intravascular hemolysis; sometimes negative	Positive (may take 12–24 hours)
Visible hemoglobin	Positive	Negative

Checkpoint! 14

Compare the pathophysiology and clinical findings in ABO-HDFN and Rh-HDFN.

Answer

ABO-HDFN—usually occurs when mother is Group O and baby is Group A or B.

Pathophysiology—The naturally occurring IgG anti-A, anti-B or anti-A,B is able to cross the placenta and coats the fetal cells. Does not require previous sensitization.

Clinical findings—Generally mild anemia (or none) present in newborn. May present with jaundice 24–48 hours after birth, but kernicterus resulting from high levels of bilirubin is rare.

Rh-HDFN—occurs when mother is Rh negative and baby is Rh positive.

Pathophysiology—Occurs when mother has been previously sensitized to the Rh (D) antigen through previous pregnancy or transfusion. As the fetal erythrocytes containing the D antigen (Rh positive) enter maternal circulation, they serve as a secondary immune stimulus and increase titer of anti-D. This is an IgG-class antibody that crosses the placenta and coats the baby's cells.

Clinical findings—Anemia may be mild to severe. Baby may become jaundiced in first 24 hours after birth. Hepatosplenomegaly may be present. As level of unconjugated bilirubin rises due to increased hemolysis of erythrocytes, it may reach toxic levels and deposit in the brain causing kernicterus.

Checkpoint! 15

Compare the laboratory findings including the peripheral blood smear findings and the DAT for infants born with ABO-HDFN and those with Rh-HDFN.

Answer

	ABO-HDFN	Rh-HDFN
DAT	Weakly positive with polyspecific AHG and anti-IgG	Positive with polyspecific AHG and anti-IgG
Blood smear	Spherocytes (severe cases)	Macrocytic, normochromic (rare spherocyte)
	Polychromatophilia	Polychromatophilia
	Nucleated erythrocytes (severe cases)	Nucleated erythrocytes
		Increased leukocytes with shift to the left

	Increased reticulocytes	Increased reticulocytes
Hemoglobin	Normal to slight decrease	Moderate to severe decrease
Bilirubin	Slight increase	Moderate to significant increase

Chapter 18

Checkpoint! 1

Microangiopathic hemolytic anemia is characterized by what abnormal erythrocyte? How is this cell formed?

Answer

The abnormal erythrocytes are schistocytes. As erythrocytes are forced through the fibrin deposits in the blood vessels, the membranes may be sliced open. When the membrane reseals itself, abnormal forms such as the schistocytes result.

Checkpoint! 2

What are the two types of HUS, and what organisms or diseases are most commonly associated with each type?

Answer

Diarrhea positive HUS is due primarily to Shigalike toxin I and II from *Escherichia coli* O157:H7 but is occasionally due to Shiga toxin of *Shigella dysenteriae*.

Diarrhea negative HUS is caused by *Streptococcus pneumoniae*.

Checkpoint! 3

Explain how infection with E. coli O157:H7 results in intravascular hemolysis.

Answer

There is damage to the intestinal mucosa from the Shigalike toxins of *E. coli* O157:H7, and this allows toxin and inflammatory mediators to enter the circulation. Toxins attach to receptors on the endothelial cells of the vessels. Platelet aggregating substances are released and cause platelet activation and formation of thrombi. As erythrocytes pass through the thrombi, the membrane is damaged.

Checkpoint! 4

What are the typical erythrocyte morphology and coagulation test results in children with HUS?

Answer

Schistocytes, spherocytes, and burr cells may be present. There may be polychromasia. The PT may be normal or slightly prolonged, the APTT is normal, and the fibrin split products are slightly elevated.

Checkpoint! 5

How does the clinical presentation of TTP differ from that of HUS? How is it similar?

Answer

The conditions share four traits: thrombocytopenia, central nervous system abnormalities, renal dysfunction, and presence of schistocytes. The degree of renal dysfunction in HUS is more severe; in TTP, the neurologic symptoms are more severe. The diagnosis of TTP requires only two criteria: microangiopathic hemolytic anemia (schistocytes) and thrombocytopenia. The entire range of symptoms is rarely seen.

Checkpoint! 6

Explain how DIC can be differentiated from TTP and HUS based on co-agulation tests.

Answer

In DIC, the PT, APTT, and thrombin time are prolonged. There is an increase in fibrin degradation products and a decrease in fibrinogen. In HUS and TTP, the PT is usually normal or only slightly prolonged; the APTT is normal. Any increase in fibrin degradation products is slight.

Checkpoint! 7

Why do malaria and babesiosis result in anemia?

Answer

Both organisms (Plasmodium sp. and Babesia sp.) are intraerythrocytic parasites. After they have completed part of the life cycle within an erythrocyte, the organism causes rupture of the cell, resulting in intravascular hemolysis. High levels of parasitemia and chronic infection result in anemia. Some cells containing the organisms may also be removed in the spleen, resulting in extravascular hemolysis.

Chapter 19

Checkpoint! 1

Calculate the absolute number of each cell type. Is each of these relative and absolute cell counts normal or abnormal?

Answer

Neutrophils—$0.60 \times 5.0 = 3.0 \times 10^9$/L
Lymphocytes—$0.35 \times 5.0 = 1.8 \times 10^9$/L
Monocytes—$0.05 \times 5.0 = .25 \times 10^9$/L
All of the cell counts are normal. If the total leukocyte count and the relative differential percents are normal, the absolute counts are also normal.

Checkpoint! 2

How can CML be distinguished from a leukemoid reaction?

Answer

The white cell count is usually higher and there are more immature cells in CML. Eosinophils and basophils are often elevated in CML but not in leukemoid reaction. Other cell counts (red and platelet) are more likely to be abnormal in CML. The LAP (low in CML and high or normal in leukemoid reaction) and Philadelphia chromosome (positive in CML) can be helpful. Patient demographic and symptoms follow: CML is usually a disease of middle age adults and presents with systemic symptoms such as enlarged spleen and nodes and bone pain due to bone marrow expansion; leukemoid reaction from a reactive process usually presents with fever or symptoms related only to the primary condition.

Checkpoint! 3

What is the difference between a leukemoid reaction and a leukoerythroblastic reaction?

Answer

A leukemoid reaction occurs when a leukocytosis with a shift to the left in circulating granulocytes occurs. It is a transient condition that happens in response to a stimulus-like infection or inflammation. A leukoerythroblastic reaction is characterized by a shift to the left in granulocytes and nucleated RBCs in the peripheral blood. The total WBC count can be increased, normal, or decreased. It is found in myeloproliferative conditions and leukemia.

Checkpoint! 4

How can the correct white count be determined when neutrophils clump in the presence of EDTA?

Answer

If neutrophils clump in the presence of EDTA, the blood for the white count and differential must be collected by a method without its presence. Manual or automated counts can be performed using fingerstick or capillary collection. Blood collected in a different anticoagulant also may be used for selected tests. Heparin provides an accurate white cell count, but the erythrocytes are distorted. Citrate can be used if corrections are made for the dilutional affects of the increased volume of anticoagulant in a blue top tube.

Checkpoint! 5

Describe the difference between hypersegmented neutrophils, hyposegmented neutrophils, and pyknotic nuclei. In what conditions is each seen?

Answer

Hypersegmented neutrophils have six or more nuclear segments and are associated with megaloblastic anemia. Hyposegmented neutrophils are mature cells with one or two nuclear segments and are associated with Pelger-Huët anomaly and some leukocyte malignancies. Be aware that bands, metamyelocytes, and myelocytes have one or two segments as well but are immature cells. Pyknotic nuclei are smooth nuclear fragments seen when the cell is dying. Disintegrating cells can be seen in blood but more often are found in infectious body fluids.

Checkpoint! 6

Explain how you can distinguish if toxic granulation and vacuoles are due to the patient's condition or to artifact.

Answer

Toxic granulation and vacuoles are associated with infection. Thus, you should correlate these findings with other signs of infection. A high WBC count and a shift to the left may be present in an infectious state. The patient's history may also be important. A comparison to other blood smears stained with the same stain is helpful if it is suspected that the large dark granules are due to precipitated stain. If due to staining artifact, the toxic granulation is present on other blood smears as well. The time the blood was collected should be checked; blood stored in EDTA might show vacuoles in PMNs.

Checkpoint! 7

Why is the basophil and eosinophil count important when assessing the benign or neoplastic nature of a disorder?

Answer

Basophils and eosinophils are rarely increased in benign disorders but are commonly increased in neoplastic disorders. Evaluated together with other hematologic data and the patient's clinical history, the eosinophil and basophil count may provide important clues to the disorder assessment.

Chapter 20

Checkpoint! 1

A patient with lymphocytosis showing reactive lymphocyte morphology with large, basophilic cells, fine chromatin, and a visible nucleolus has a negative infectious mononucleosis serologic test. What is a possible cause for this altered lymphocyte morphology?

Answer

Causes of reactive lymphocyte morphology are other viral infections, particularly hepatitis or cytomegalovirus, and reactions to drugs or toxoplasmosis. If the patient is under 10 years of age, the child may not produce heterophil antibodies in increased quantities and thus yield a negative serologic test when infected with EBV. Some adults do not produce a positive serologic test either even though they are infected with EBV.

Checkpoint! 2

Why is lymphocytopenia a concern if there is no accompanying leukopenia.

Answer

A decrease in lymphocytes impairs the body's immune response and makes the patient more susceptible to disease.

Checkpoint! 3

Why does infection with HIV result in an increased chance for opportunistic infections?

Answer

HIV-1 gains access to cells through the CD4 protein receptor on the cell surface. Some T lymphocytes, monocytes, and macrophages express this receptor. Once in the cell, it destroys the T lymphocyte, compromising the cell-mediated immune system and allowing opportunistic infections to cause disease.

Checkpoint! 4

Would you expect female carriers of X-linked SCIDS to be more susceptible to infection than the normal population?

Answer

No, all of their lymphocytes have the normal X chromosome activated.

Checkpoint! 5

What laboratory findings suggest WAS in a child, and how is the diagnosis confirmed?

Answer

Thrombocytopenia, lack of blood group reverse typing, decreased IgM levels but increased IgE and IgA levels suggest WAS. Diagnosis for WAS is substantiated by flow cytometry and molecular analysis. A positive PCR test revealing the gene mutation confirms the presence of the disease.

Chapter 21

Checkpoint! 1

A patient has 50% monoblasts in the bone marrow. Which of the four major types of leukemia does he have, AML, CML, ALL, or CLL?

Answer

A patient with 50% monoblasts in the bone marrow has AML. ALL and CLL can be eliminated due to their lymphoid lineage, and CML <20% blasts in the bone marrow.

Checkpoint! 2

A 62-year-old male presents with an elevated leukocyte count, mild anemia, and a slightly decreased platelet count. His physician suspects leukemia. Explain why the erythrocytes and platelets would be affected.

Answer

Leukemia is a stem cell disorder in which all cell progeny are involved. If the patient has the suspected leukemia, he would experience an unregulated production of neoplastic cells. As the neoplastic cell population increases, the concentration of normal cells, such as the platelets and erythrocytes, decreases.

Checkpoint! 3

Does a 3-year-old child with Down syndrome have an increased risk of developing leukemia? Why or why not?

Answer

Yes, some individuals with congenital abnormalities associated with karyotypic abnormalities have a markedly increased risk of developing acute leukemias.

Checkpoint! 4

Why is the finding of Auer rods an important factor in the diagnosis of leukemia?

Answer

Auer rods can be found in the blast cells and promyelocytes of some acute myeloid leukemias. The finding of Auer rods can help establish the diagnosis because these unique, pink-staining inclusions are not found in ALL. Auer rods are fused lysosomes.

Checkpoint! 5

A patient has 35% blasts in the bone marrow. They do not show any specific morphologic characteristics that will allow them to be classified according to cell lineage. What are the next steps that the CLS should take with this specimen?

Answer

Cytochemistry can help establish cell lineage as myeloid or lymphoid. An immunologic analysis provides information on what specific membrane antigens are on the blast cells. By using a panel of monoclonal antibodies, the cells' lineage can usually be determined because specific surface markers are characteristically found on each particular cell line. Genetic analysis can also be performed because some cytogenetic chromosome karyotypes are commonly found in certain types of leukemia.

Chapter 22

Checkpoint! 1

In essential thrombocythemia, all hematopoietic lines have increased cell proliferation. Which lineage has the most increase?

Answer

The megakaryocytic cell line is the one most increased in essential thrombocythemia.

Checkpoint! 2

A patient has the CML phenotype, but the genetic karyotype does not show the Philadelphia chromosome. If this is truly a CML, what should molecular analysis show?

Answer

Molecular analysis would show a BCR/ABL gene rearrangement in a new fused hybrid gene.

Checkpoint! 3

Describe the peripheral blood differential of a CML patient.

Answer

There is a shift to the left in granulocytes with high numbers of myelocytes and promyelocytes. If blasts are present, they compose less than 20% of cells.

Checkpoint! 4

What clinical, peripheral blood, and genetic features differentiate CML from an infectious process?

Answer

An extreme peripheral blood leukocytosis—segmented neutrophils with a left shift showing many myelocytes, some promyelocytes, and blasts are found in CML. Age of the patient and absence of infection, low LAP score, and presence of the Philadelphia chromosome or BCR/ABL translocation all are hallmarks for CML that differentiate it.

Checkpoint! 5

What one feature separates other forms of MPD from CML?

Answer

The Philadelphia chromosome occurs in CML.

Checkpoint! 6

What growth factors are primarily responsible for stimulating fibrogenesis in the bone marrow?

Answer

Platelet-derived growth factor (PDGF), transforming growth factor-beta (TGF-β), and epidermal growth factor (EGF) are increased and associated with marrow fibrosis.

Checkpoint! 7

What erythrocyte morphologic feature is a hallmark for myelofibrosis?

Answer

The finding of dacryocytes (teardrop erythrocytes) is a hallmark for myelofibrosis with myeloid metaplasia.

Checkpoint! 8

Which of the following conditions are associated with an absolute increase in red cell mass? Iron deficiency, smoking, emphysema, pregnancy, or dehydration.

Answer

Smoking, emphysema, and pregnancy are conditions in which additional red cells are needed to prevent a physiologic anemia. Iron deficiency prevents the formation of additional red cells. Dehydration causes a relative red cell mass increase due to decreased plasma volume.

Checkpoint! 9

Renal tumors may produce an inappropriate amount of EPO, resulting in what type of polycythemia?

Answer

Secondary polycythemia, or increase of red cell mass due to an identifiable cause.

Checkpoint! 10

Is a patient who has a platelet count of 846 $\times$ 10^9/L, splenomegaly, and abnormal platelet function tests of hyperaggregation likely to have reactive or essential thrombocytosis?

Answer

This patient is likely to have essential thrombocytosis. Patients with reactive thrombocytosis rarely have platelet counts higher than 1,000 $\times$ 10^9/L nor would they have splenomegaly or thrombotic complications.

Chapter 23

Checkpoint! 1

How does the typical peripheral blood picture in MDS differ from aplastic anemia?

Answer

The typical blood picture in aplastic anemia is pancytopenia, a significant decrease in all three cell populations (∞ Chapter 13). In MDS, cytopenia is present in the peripheral blood in one cell line or more. Pancytopenia has been estimated to occur in only 19% of cases of MDS. Both MDS and aplastic anemia can be macrocytic. MDS exhibits more frequent qualitative abnormalities indicating dyspoiesis, such as anisocytosis, poikilocytosis, basophilic stippling, Howell-Jolly bodies, and nucleated RBCs. The neutrophils often show abnormal granulation and pseudo–Pelger-Huët cells. Giant and hypogranular platelets may be seen. The bone marrow is the best way to differentiate the two syndromes. A hypoplastic bone marrow is typical in aplastic anemia. MDS usually shows a hypercellular marrow, but if it is hypocellular, it may be difficult to differentiate from aplastic anemia.

Checkpoint! 2

Why is serum vitamin B_{12}, serum folate level, or bone marrow iron stain important in the diagnosis of MDS?

Answer

Some features of the blood picture in MDS resemble the megaloblastic anemias (macrocytosis, megaloblastoid changes in erythrocytic precursor cells). A normal serum vitamin B_{12} and/or folate level rule out megaloblastic anemia. An iron stain on the bone marrow allows assessment of the presence of ringed sideroblasts, which may be seen in RA and are necessary for a diagnosis of RARS.

Checkpoint! 3

Why is it important to correctly identify the number of blasts when evaluating the peripheral blood or bone marrow smear of a patient suspected of having MDS?

Answer

The number of blasts is used to classify the MDS into different subtypes and to predict prognosis and treatment. It is also used to differentiate MDS from acute leukemia.

Chapter 24

Checkpoint! 1

What results would you expect to find on the CBC and differential in a suspected case of acute leukemia?

Answer

You would expect a normocytic, normochromic anemia; decrease in platelets with some large forms present; neutropenia; monocytosis; and on the differential blast cells, an increase in eosinophils and basophils.

Checkpoint! 2

What is the major difference between the FAB and WHO classification systems in differentiating acute leukemia from the other neoplastic hematologic disorders?

Answer

In the WHO classification, the minimum blast count compatible with AL is 20%; in the FAB classification, the minimum was 30%.

Checkpoint! 3

Explain why molecular analysis is not performed on all suspected cases of AL.

Answer

The molecular aberrations are not known for all AL and, thus, probes are not available. Those in which an aberration is commonly present and can be probed for are APL and the ALL.

Checkpoint! 4

Why is it important to do molecular studies on patients with acute promyelocytic leukemia?

Answer

The RAR-α/PML abnormality is diagnostic of APL. Those with this translocation respond to therapy with all transretinoic acid. If the translocation disappears after therapy and then reappears, relapse can be predicted.

Checkpoint! 5

What hematologic feature helps differentiate AML minimally differentiated from AML without maturation?

Answer

Cytochemical stains in AML without maturation are negative, but some of the blasts in AML minimally differentiated have a positive reaction with myeloperoxidase and/or Sudan black B. Both have myeloid antigens, CD13 and CD33.

Checkpoint! 6

A patient with AML has a peripheral blood differential that includes 91% myeloblasts, 3% promyelocytes, 3% granulocytes, and 3% monocytes. Which category of AML is the most likely diagnosis? Explain.

Answer

This is an AML minimally differentiated. There are >90% myeloblasts. AML with differentiation has <90% myeloblasts.

Checkpoint! 7

What is the differentiating hematologic feature of acute erythroid leukemia that allows it to be subgrouped?

Answer

More than 50% of the bone marrow cells are erythroid and 20% or more of the remaining cells are blasts.

Checkpoint! 8

Predict the peripheral blood picture of a patient on antifolate chemotherapy.

Answer

There would be a megaloblastic blood picture including pancytopenia with a macrocytic anemia.

Chapter 25

Checkpoint! 1

Compare the typical age groups in which AML and ALL are found.

Answer

The AMLs are characteristically found in adults in contrast to the ALLs, which are typically found in children. The AML minimally differentiated is most common in adults and in infants less than 1 year of age.

Checkpoint! 2

Contrast the malignant neoplastic cells in ALL with those found in AML.

Answer

Myeloblasts are generally larger than lymphoblasts. They have more abundant grayish cytoplasm. The nucleus has fine chromatin and prominent nucleoli. Lymphoblasts have scant, blue cytoplasm. The nucleus has coarser chromatin, and the nucleoli are inconspicuous. The ALL and AML blasts cannot be definitively identified by morphology alone because considerable heterogeneity occurs from that just described. Cytochemistry is helpful in determining cell lineage. The myeloperoxidase and Sudan black B are positive in myeloblasts and negative in lymphoblasts. Immunophenotyping is helpful also. The myeloblasts are positive for CD13 and CD33; lymphoblasts are negative for these antigens.

Checkpoint! 3

Why is it necessary to immunophenotype the lymphoblasts in ALL if they have been identified as lymphoblasts morphologically?

Answer

The lymphoblasts should be immunophenotyped to determine whether they are of T or B cell origin. This information has treatment and prognostic implications.

Checkpoint! 4

A patient has 50% blasts in his bone marrow. Cytochemical stains are negative with peroxidase, and Sudan black B. Immunophenotyping is CD19-positive, but CD20-, CD2-, CD10-, and CD7-negative. What additional testing may be helpful in distinguishing the immunologic subgroup of this leukemia?

Answer

These appear to be lymphoblasts by cytochemistry results. The cells have the B cell antigen CD19 but are negative for other B cell markers, CD10 and CD20. Cells are negative for the T cell markers CD2 and CD7. This may be a very early progenitor B ALL. Testing for the CD34 marker and the presence of TdT would be helpful.

These are markers of very early cells. Molecular testing for the rearrangement of the immunoglobulin genes may also help determine whether these are B cells.

Checkpoint! 5
Contast the morphology of blasts found in the two subtypes of ALL.

Answer
Lymphoblasts are typically small, up to twice the size of a small lymphocyte, with scant to moderate amounts of light basophilic or blue-grey cytoplasm. The nucleus is round or slightly indented with finely granular to slightly clumped chromatin and inconspicuous or absent nucleoli. The two subtypes of ALL in the WHO classification are precursor B cell leukemia and precursor T cell leukemia. Morphologically, the T and B lymphoblasts cannot be differentiated. T lymphoblasts are similar to B lymphoblasts, although there is more likely to be variability in size, and cytoplasmic vacuoles may be present. The chromatin pattern may vary from case to case but is homogeneous within cases. The cytochemistry is also similar to that seen in B ALL, but acid phosphatase may show focal intense positivity in T ALL.

Checkpoint! 6
A 3-year-old patient has 45% lymphoblasts in the bone marrow. The blasts are slightly larger than lymphocytes and appear to be a homogeneous population. The nuclear membrane is regular, and nucleoli are not prominent. There is a small amount of moderately basophilic cytoplasm. What is the most likely WHO group of this leukemia? If the cells tested positive for CD19, CD10, and CD34, what is the most likely immunologic subgroup? Why should cytogenetics be done on this patient?

Answer
The description of the blasts best fits the precursor B cell leukemia subgroup. These markers suggest the early pre-B immunologic subgroup. Cytogenetics is important in ALL to provide prognostic information.

Checkpoint! 7
A patient with acute leukemia has two morphologically different types of blasts. One population is positive for CD7 and CD2. The other is positive for CD33 and CD13. What is the most appropriate classification of this leukemia?

Answer
This is most likely an acute leukemia with lineage heterogeneity. Beause the lineage-associated markers are found on two different sets of blasts, it is most likely a bilineage acute leukemia. The blasts appear by immunophenotype to be myeloblasts and T lymphoblasts.

Chapter 26

Checkpoint! 1
How does the bcl-2 gene rearrangement differ from most other oncogenes?

Answer
The bcl-2 gene rearrangement leads to persistence of cells due to an inhibition of apoptosis rather than uncontrolled cell proliferation.

Checkpoint! 2
How does staging differ from grading in defining and classifying the lymphoid malignancies?

Answer
Staging determines the extent and distribution of disease; *classifyng* separates grades of lymphoma and often uses a combination of morphology, phenotype, and genotype.

Checkpoint! 3
The chronic lymphoid leukemic malignancies are a heterogeneous group. What characteristics allow them to be grouped together?

Answer
The chronic lymphoid leukemic malignancies are grouped together because the malignant cell is a mature lymphocyte, a cell found in the blood and bone marrow (leukemic distribution).

Checkpoint! 4
What cell characteristically distinguishes Hodgkin lymphoma from non-Hodgkin lymphoma? Describe this cell.

Answer
The Reed-Sternberg cell characteristically distinguishes Hodgkin lymphoma from non-Hodgkin lymphoma. It has two or more nuclear lobes containing inclusionlike nucleoli and an area of peri-nucleolar clearing (owl's eye appearance).

Checkpoint! 5
What clinical finding differentiates multiple myeloma from other plasma cell neoplasms?

Answer
The presence of multiple lytic bone lesions differentiates multiple myeloma from other plasma cell neoplasms.

Chapter 27

Checkpoint! 1
A physician is evaluating a 28-year-old patient with a history of acute lymphoblastic leukemia for PBSC transplantation. The laboratory professional found circulating leukemic blasts in the peripheral blood. Is this patient a candidate for an autologous PBSC transplant?

Answer
Presence of circulating blasts in a patient who is being evaluated for the autologous PBSC is not a good sign. Because PBSCs are collected from the person's peripheral blood by apheresis technology, the stem cell product in this patient would definitely contain leukemic blasts. It would be almost impossible to separate these leukemic blasts from the normal stem cells even by purging. Therefore, autologous PBSC transplant is not an option for this patient at least at this point. The search for the matched allogeneic stem cell donor should be made.

Checkpoint! 2
A patient with CML needs a stem cell transplant. What would be the best form of transplant for him, and what antigen type needs to be matched?

Answer
CML is a stem cell disorder, which means the patient's own stem cells are affected by the disease. Therefore, the best form of transplant for this patient is an allogeneic stem cell transplant. For this allogeneic transplant, the patient and donor should be matched for

HLA-A, -B and -DR antigens. ABO antigens are tested for both donor and patient; however, the matching is not required for the allogeneic stem cell transplant.

Checkpoint! 3

You receive a peripheral blood specimen in the hematology laboratory with a request for a mononuclear cell count and analysis of CD34+ cells. Without any further information, why should you consider this a STAT request?

Answer

The volume of cells necessary to achieve a successful engraftment may be determined indirectly by the MNC count or the CD34+ count. A clinical decision can be made to collect more cells depending on these counts. The timing of the collection of the stem cells also may be determined based on these counts.

Checkpoint! 4

A physician wants to evaluate the engraftment on a male patient who received SCT from his brother 4 months ago. What laboratory tests should be performed to make this assessment?

Answer

To evaluate the long-term engraftment of HSCs, various laboratory methods have evolved. Currently, the most widely used tests are in situ hybridization (ISH) with sex chromosome and typing of variable number tandem repeat (VNTR) polymorphism by DNA amplification. The ISH is applicable when the donor and recipient are of different sex. In this case, the VNTR polymorphism by DNA amplification to distinguish donor and recipient cells must be performed.

Checkpoint! 5

A CMV-seronegative patient requires SCT. Two HLA-matched donors are available. Is it important to know the CMV status of the stem cell donor? If the stem cell donor is CMV-seronegative and the patient requires red cell transfusion during the peritransplant period, what blood components (in terms of CMV status) would you select for this patient?

Answer

The CMV-seropositive person (i.e., a subject who shows serologic evidence of prior CMV exposure) can be an SCT donor to a CMV-seronegative recipient. However, if two HLA-compatible donors are available for a CMV-seronegative patient, the preference is given to the donor who is seronegative for CMV. The rationale is that CMV infection can be fatal in the peritransplant setting. However, if the CMV-seronegative donor is not available but a matched CMV-seropositive donor is available, transplant can still be performed. Most transplant physicians believe that a CMV-seronegative recipient should receive CMV-seronegative cellular blood components if the stem cells' donor is also CMV-seronegative. If the CMV-negative blood component is not available, transfusing a leukocyte-reduced filtered component may effectively prevent the transmission of CMV disease.

Chapter 28

Checkpoint! 1

To obtain a sample of cerebrospinal fluid for anlaysis, the needle must be inserted into what area of the central nervous system?

Answer

Subarachnoid space.

Checkpoint! 2

A 32-year-old woman has right-sided chest pain and shortness of breath that has worsened over a 2-week period. Chest radiologic studies reveal a right pleural effusion, and a thoracentesis is performed. The pleural fluid specimen on a cytocentrifuged, Wright-stained slide reveals cells similar to that seen in Figure 28-7. What is the best interpretation of this finding? If there is a strong concern that this may represent a low-grade lymphoma, what would be the best way to determine whether these are benign or malignant lymphocytes?

Answer

These cells are benign lymphocytes with the artifact of a pale staining area resembling nucleoli. These are not blasts because of the mature chromatin. Immunophenotyping by flow cytometry of the pleural fluid would be the best way to determine whether this is a benign or malignant population of lymphocytes.

Checkpoint! 3

When examining a cytocentrifuged, Wright-stained slide of a body fluid specimen, what are the best features to use in determining whether tissue cells are benign or malignant?

Answer

Nuclear features are the best to use to distinguish benign and malignant cells. These include nuclear membrane (smooth or irregular), chromatin pattern (regular or irregular distribution), and nucleoli (present or absent, nucleolar membrane smooth or irregular).

Checkpoint! 4

A 47-year-old man is found comatose at home by his wife. During examination in the emergency room a spinal tap is performed and grossly bloody spinal fluid is obtained. The total red blood cell count in the first tube is the same as that in the third tube. A cytocentrifuged, Wright-stained slide shows findings similar to that seen in Figure 28-54. What is the most appropriate interpretation?

Answer

There has been a true subarachnoid hemorrhage.

Checkpoint! 5

A 57-year-old man has an acutely swollen, painful, reddened joint in his left great toe. Joint fluid is aspirated, and a photomicrograph is taken (Figure 28-69). This picture is taken with polarized light using a quartz compensator. What is the most appropriate interpretation of this finding?

Answer

Both monosodium urate and calcium pyrophosphate crystals are present.

Chapter 29

Checkpoint! 1

Think about the last time that you injured your finger with a paper cut. Did your finger bleed immediately? If not, what might have prevented immediate bleeding?

Answer

No, vasoconstriction of the blood vessels prevented it.

Checkpoint! 2

What actions of the endothelial cells prevent clotting from occurring within the blood vessels?

Answer

Their negatively charged surface repels clotting factors and platelets in the normal peripheral blood circulation. They synthesize heparan sulfate and thrombomodulin, which inhibit fibrin formation. They synthesize PGI_2, which inhibits platelet activation. They synthesize tPA and PAI-1, which control fibrinolysis.

Checkpoint! 3

What would be the effect on the platelet count if a patient had a mutation in the gene for thrombopoietin that resulted in inability of the gene to code for functional mRNA?

Answer

The platelet count would be decreased.

Checkpoint! 4

If a patient has a mutation in the gene for thrombopoietin that resulted in inability of the gene to code for mRNA, how would you expect the number of megakaryocytes seen on bone marrow smears to be affected?

Answer

The number of megakaryocytes in the bone marrow would be decreased.

Checkpoint! 5

If a patient inherited a mutation of the gene for glycoprotein IIIa that resulted in its absence, what two platelet antigens would be decreased or absent?

Answer

The HPA-1 and HPA-3 would be decreased or absent.

Checkpoint! 6

If a patient with Bernard-Soulier disease or von Willebrand disease cut a finger, would you expect bleeding to stop as fast as the bleeding stops when you cut your own finger? Why?

Answer

No, because their platelets would be unable to adhere to collagen and the primary hemostatic plug would take longer to form to halt the bleeding.

Checkpoint! 7

Your finger is still bleeding at this point, but the platelets are aggregating to form the primary hemostatic plug. Let's review the key events:
a. To what do platelets first adhere?
b. What bridge and what platelet membrane receptor are needed for platelet adhesion?
c. What bridge and what platelet membrane receptor are needed for platelets to attach to one another?
d. What is the attachment of platelets to one another called?

Answer

a. Collagen
b. Von Willebrand factor and glycoprotein Ib/IX
c. Fibrinogen and glycoprotein IIb/IIIA
d. Platelet aggregation

Checkpoint! 8

Your finger has now stopped bleeding. Outline the steps of primary hemostasis that have occurred.

Answer

The blood vessels have undergone vasoconstriction and are by now possibly beginning to dilate. Platelet adhesion, platelet secretion, platelet aggregation, and formation of the primary hemostatic plug have occurred.

Chapter 30

Checkpoint! 1

What is the major distinction between the so-called extrinsic and intrinsic pathways?

Answer

Both pathways require enzymes and protein cofactors originally present in plasma; however, the extrinsic pathway also requires an activator (tissue factor) that is not found in the blood under normal circumstances.

Checkpoint! 2

Will a patient who is vitamin K-deficient produce any of the vitamin K-dependent factors? Why is vitamin K so vital to the formation of coagulation complexes?

Answer

A patient who is vitamin K-deficient still synthesizes the proteins but fails to attach the extra carboxyl group to the γ-carbon of glutamic acid residues in the GLA domains of the protein, which is required for full functional activity of the proteins. The γ-carboxy form of the proteins is required for Ca^{2+}-mediated interaction with phospholipid surfaces, which is required for forming the coagulation activation complexes.

Checkpoint! 3

Why are the domains of the serine proteases involved in blood clotting so important in the hemostatic mechanism?

Answer

The catalytic domain of the protease cleaves the substrate(s) of this protease. The various noncatalytic domains of the serine proteases contain the regulatory elements of the proteins and are responsible for conferring the specificity of activation and activity of each enzyme. They bind calcium and promote interaction with phospholipids, cofactors, receptors, and substrates.

Checkpoint! 4

Which components of the intrinsic pathway are believed to be essential for in vivo hemostasis?

Answer

Factors IX, VIII, and possibly factor XI are the components. Factor XII, prekallikrein, and HMW kininogen are not essential for normal in vivo hemostasis.

Checkpoint! 5

Historically, the major importance for initiating coagulation was assigned to either the intrinsic or the extrinsic pathway. What are some observations that suggest that the classic concepts were not accurate?

Answer

Thrombin can activate factor XI, bypassing the need for contact activation by factor XII/kallikrein/HK. Factor IX can be activated by factor VIIa as well as factor XIa (again, bypassing the need for contact activation). Thus, initiation of coagulation by tissue factor/factor VII is sufficient to initiate activation of both pathways. However, full escalation of the coagulation system requires proteins of both pathways.

Checkpoint! 6

What are the three steps in the formation of an insoluble fibrin clot?

Answer

(1) Proteolytic *cleavage* of fibrinopeptides A and B by thrombin, forming a fibrin monomer, (2) spontaneous *polymerization* of fibrin monomers to form fibrin polymers, and (3) *stabilization* of the fibrin polymers by F-XIIIa.

Checkpoint! 7

Why is the process of fibrinolysis a vital part of the hemostatic mechanism? Why must it be closely regulated and controlled?

Answer

Fibrinolysis is needed to restore the blood vessel structure and function to normal when the fibrin clot is no longer needed. It is essential to balance the activity of the procoagulant proteins. If activity of fibrinolysis is deficient, the result is thrombosis; if fibrinolysis is excessive, the result is hemorrhage.

Checkpoint! 8

Why are the plasmin degradation products of fibrinogen and fibrin different?

Answer

Plasmin cleaves at the same place on molecules of either fibrin or fibrinogen (at the coiled regions, midway between the terminal D domains and the C-central domain). In fibrinogen, this produces separate D and E fragments. However, because fibrin monomers have been covalently crosslinked by F-XIIIa, complexes of various combinations (particularly the so-called D-dimer) are formed. The presence of D-dimer confirms that both the procoagulant system (thrombin) and the fibrinolytic system (plasmin) have been activated.

Checkpoint! 9

Why are naturally occurring inhibitors important in the hemostatic mechanism?

Answer

Naturally occurring inhibitors help control the activity of the coagulation and fibrinolytic proteases. They are inactive when distant from a site of vessel damage, helping to limit clot formation to areas of vessel injury. They are essential in preventing unwarranted initiation or excessive amplification of the coagulation cascade.

Chapter 31

Checkpoint! 1

Assume that you are the clinical laboratory scientist collecting a blood specimen from a patient with a suspected bleeding disorder. You noticed petechiae and several bruises on the patient's arm. What screening tests would the physician likely have ordered? What results of these tests would you expect (normal or abnormal) in this patient?

Answer

The physician would likely have ordered a platelet count, prothrombin time, and activated partial thromboplastin time as screening tests. The presence of petechiae indicates a platelet abnormality, the most common of which is thrombocytopenia. Therefore, you would expect the platelet count to be decreased. The prothrombin and activated partial thromboplastin times are normal in platelet abnormalities that are not complicated or accompanied by abnormalities of fibrin formation.

Checkpoint! 2

If you observed an average of 14 platelets on a peripheral blood smear prepared from the needle tip and your laboratory allowed correlation between the direct instrument count and the blood smear estimate of 20%, what range would you expect the instrument count to be? Is this platelet estimate within an acceptable reference range?

Answer

Average of 14 platelets $\times$ 15 $\times$ 10⁹/L = 210 $\times$ 10⁹/L. An acceptable range of the instrument count would be 168–252 $\times$ 10⁹/L. Yes, this is within the acceptable reference range.

Checkpoint! 3

How many platelets per 1000$\times$ field would you expect to observe on the peripheral smear of a patient with acute ITP?

Answer

You would expect to see an average of fewer than six platelets per field. It can be difficult to find platelets on the blood smear of some ITP patients.

Checkpoint! 4

A 6-year-old boy was brought to his pediatrician because the mother noticed small pinkish spots on the boy's legs. Upon examination he also had several bruises on his arms and legs. Laboratory tests were ordered. His platelet count was 20 $\times$ 10⁹/L and PT and APTT were within normal limits. The CBC was normal except for the low platelet count. There was no previous history of bleeding. The mother said she noted the spots after he was given the hepatitis vaccine. What is the most probable type of thrombocytopenia? Should other coagulation tests be performed at this time?

Answer

The most probable type of thrombocytopenia experienced by this patient is an immune type of increased destruction, which is reportedly associated with viral infections in some children. Other coagulation tests are not necessary.

Checkpoint! 5

What is the pathophysiology of the thrombocytopenia in megaloblastic anemia?

Answer

Thrombocytopenia occurs in megaloblastic anemia because of ineffective production of all myeloid cell lines in the bone marrow.

Checkpoint! 6

Explain why primary thrombocytosis is often associated with abnormal platelet function while secondary thrombocytosis is not.

Answer

Primary thrombocytosis is associated with the myeloproliferative disorders, which are clonal disorders of the pluripotential stem cell. The abnormal clone grows autonomously and not in response to normal regulatory factors. It is likely that abnormalities in platelet function are acquired along with the ability to grow autonomously. In secondary thrombocytosis, the platelets are increased because of the normal regulatory routes in response to a need for more platelets.

Checkpoint! 7

Compare the results of platelet aggregation studies in platelet adhesion, aggregation, and secretion disorders.

Answer

Platelet adhesion to collagen requires that the von Willebrand factor attached to platelet GPIb/IX receptors bridge the platelet to the collagen fiber. Platelet aggregation studies are abnormal with ristocetin in these disorders because it takes the place of collagen in the test. Other routine agonists require the platelet GPIIb/IIIa receptor and fibrinogen as the bridge to attach one platelet to another platelet. Platelet aggregation disorders involve abnormalities in the GPIIb/IIIa receptor or in fibrinogen. Therefore, platelet aggregation studies will be abnormal with all agonists except ristocetin. In platelet secretion disorders, platelets are able to respond to agonists in the primary wave of aggregation but are unable to release their own ADP and manufacture their own thromboxane A_2, so that the secondary wave of aggregation seen with ADP and epinephrine and the wave of aggregation with collagen are abnormal.

Checkpoint! 8

Why are the bleeding time test and the closure time abnormal for up to 7 days following ingestion of aspirin?

Answer

Aspirin inhibits the platelet enzyme cyclooxygenase, which is necessary for production of thromboxane A_2. TXA_2 is necessary in the activated platelet for secretion of granule contents and, therefore, the function of the platelets is impaired. The defective platelets continue to circulate for their normal life span, which is about 10 days. Because they are circulating, the bone marrow is not stimulated to produce new platelets to replace the defective ones.

Chapter 32

Checkpoint! 1

a. Why do patients with type 1 VWD have 25–50% of VWF in their plasma?
b. Why do they have a corresponding decrease in F-VIII in their plasma?

Answer

a. Type 1 VWD is inherited as an autosomal dominant characteristic. Patients have symptoms with abnormalities of only one gene. The second gene is still functional. Theoretically, 50% of VWF would be present but other variations such as the blood type O may result in less than 50% in some patients.
b. Patients with type 1 VWD have a corresponding decrease in F-VIII in their plasma because F-VIII requires the presence of VWF to be present in the plasma.

Checkpoint! 2

a. If a patient with VWD has an equal decrease in F-VIII assay, VWF:RCo, and VWF:Ag assay, does this more likely indicate that there is a true decrease in the amount of or does it indicate that the patient has a type of VWD that is characterized a functional abnormality of F-VIII. Support your answer.
b. What type of VWD is most likely in a patient with these laboratory test results?

Answer

a. A true quantitative decrease in the amount of F-VIII occurs because the tests for function and immunologic activity are both decreased.
b. These results are characteristic of VWD, type 1.

Checkpoint! 3

What abbreviation is acceptable for:
a. the antigenic properties of VWF?
b. the functional activity of F-VIII?
c. the complex of F-VIII and VWF?

Answer

a. VWF:Ag
b. F-VIII:C
c. F-VIII/VWF complex

Checkpoint! 4

Referring to Table 32-3, explain the reason why the platelet function tests are abnormal in VWD and not in F-VIII or F-IX deficiencies.

Answer

Platelet function tests are abnormal in VWD because VWF is necessary for platelets to adhere to collagen. This affects the closure time, the bleeding time, and platelet aggregation studies with ristocetin. Ristocetin takes the place of collagen in the platelet aggregation test system. In the absence of VWF, platelets do not adhere and do not aggregate. VWF is not needed for platelets to aggregate with other agonists. F-VIII and F-IX deficiencies have a decrease in these coagulation proteins that affects fibrin formation, but platelets are normal and VWF is present.

Checkpoint! 5

Explain why the thrombin time will be abnormal in patients with afibrinogenemia and dysfibrinogenemia.

Answer

The thrombin time depends on the adequate conversion of soluble fibrinogen to fibrin. Patients with afibrinogenemia have no fibrinogen to convert to fibrin, and patients with dysfibrinogenemia have fibrinogen with an abnormal ability to convert to fibrin.

Checkpoint! 6

Explain why the prothrombin time but not the APTT is prolonged in F-VII deficiency.

Answer

F-VII is activated by tissue thromboplastin, which is the first step in fibrin formation via the "extrinsic pathway." The reagent for the prothrombin time is tissue thromboplastin; therefore, when the F-VII is deficient, fibrin formation is delayed. In the APTT, tissue thromboplastin is not present in the test system. Instead, fibrin is formed by activating the contact factor system and F-VII is bypassed.

Checkpoint! 7

Explain why the laboratory screening tests are normal in patients with F-XIII deficiency.

Answer

All laboratory screening tests depend on fibrin formation in the test container and are not influenced by whether or not the fibrin was covalently cross-linked. F-XIII functions after fibrin formation to stabilize the fibrin in vivo. It is not necessary to produce the end-point (fibrin formation) in the in vitro assays.

Checkpoint! 8

a. Why is thrombocytopenia usually present in a patient with DIC?
b. Which hemostasis laboratory screening tests (PT and APTT), if any, will the following affect?

> *Decreased F-V?*
> *Decreased F-VIII?*
> *Decreased fibrinogen?*
> *Decreased antithrombin?*

c. Which laboratory test results would distinguish DIC from hemophilia A?

Answer

a. Thrombocytopenia is usually present because platelets are consumed in DIC. They are activated by thrombin and are incorporated into the fibrin clots within the circulation.
b. Decreased F-V—PT and APTT
  Decreased F-VIII—APTT
  Decreased fibrinogen—PT and APTT
  Decreased antithrombin—neither
c. The APTT is abnormally prolonged and the F-VIII assay is decreased in hemophilia A. All other tests are normal. In DIC, all factors and inhibitors that are consumed as blood clots are abnormal, and fibrinolytic products are increased because blood is clotting and lysing in DIC. This affects all of the hemostasis tests that are routinely performed as well as the platelet count.

Chapter 33

Checkpoint! 1

Why would defects of fibrinolysis result in hypercoagulability?

Answer

Under normal conditions, hemostasis depends on a delicate balance between clot-promoting factors (procoagulant influences) and clot-inhibiting factors (anticoagulants and fibrinolysis). Defects in fibrinolysis result in hypercoagulability because the delicate balance has been disturbed, and the clot-promoting factors dominate the clinical picture.

Checkpoint! 2

Why is thrombotic disease associated with hereditary thrombophilia considered a multigene (or multirisk factor) disease?

Answer

Individuals who have inherited a thrombophilia gene generally do not experience thrombotic episodes unless they have a second genetic or acquired predisposing factor. Thus, many individuals who carry thrombophilia genes do not have acute thrombotic events and may be diagnosed only when family screening is done for another family member who has had a thrombosis.

Checkpoint! 3

Why are both immunologic and functional assays recommended when screening a patient suspected of having a familial thrombophilic defect?

Answer

Inherited defects of the hemostatic proteins involved in familial thrombophilia can be either quantitative or qualitative. Immunologic assays for total protein will fail to diagnose qualitative defects (dysfunctional proteins), which typically give normal antigen levels but reduced functional levels. Functional assays are generally considered the better screening assay if a familial thrombophilia is suspected.

Checkpoint! 4

Why should heparin therapy overlap initiation of oral anticoagulant therapy when treating a patient with an acute thrombosis?

Answer

Oral anticoagulants (vitamin-K antagonists) decrease functional levels of procoagulant proteins F-II, F-VII, F-IX, and F-X, as well as the anticoagulant proteins PC and PS. However, this action is not immediate (as is the anticoagulant effect of heparin), and the decrease in activity of each of these proteins varies, depending on the half-life of each in the circulation. Because PC has a relatively short half-life, clearance of biologically active molecules (presynthesized before oral anticoagulants were begun) occurs more quickly for PC than for the procoagulant protein factors F-II, F-IX, and F-X. Thus, for the first few days after initiating coumadin therapy, there is an imbalance between clot-inhibiting influences (PC) and clot-promoting influences (F-II, F-VII, and F-X). The net effect is a period of hypercoagulability before the full anticoagulant effect of coumadin is realized. For a patient who already has a hemostatic system that is presumably not in balance, this could further aggravate it. Thus, heparin anticoagulant therapy should be continued through the first 4–5 days of oral anticoagulant therapy until the full effect of coumadin is achieved.

Chapter 34

Checkpoint! 1

Contrast the mechanisms of anticoagulation for EDTA and heparin.

Answer

EDTA prevents blood coagulation by chelating calcium. Because calcium is an important component of several enzymatic reactions in the coagulation cascade, its removal blocks fibrin formation. Heparin prevents blood coagulation by enhancing antithrombin activity. Antithrombin, in turn, inhibits thrombin and blocks fibrin formation.

Checkpoint! 2

What are three steps a phlebotomist should take to minimize the risk of exposure to blood-borne pathogens when performing a venipuncture?

Answer

Steps to minimize exposure to blood-borne pathogens include (1) wearing gloves, (2) using goggles, (3) performing venipuncture with a safe needle tube holder, (4) disposing of the needle in a biohazard sharps container, and (5) washing the hands following the removal of gloves.

Checkpoint! 3

What is the total magnification when a 10× objective is combined with a 10× eyepiece?

Answer

The total magnification is $(10\times) \times (10\times) = 100\times$.

Checkpoint! 4

How does the examination of a sample by phase-contrast microscopy differ from bright-field microscopy?

Answer

(1) Bright-field microscopy requires a stained sample to examine cellular details; phase-contrast microscopy allows examination of unstained cells. (2) Phase-contrast microscopy requires a condenser with an annular ring and objective with phase ring. These components must be matched. Bright-field microscopy uses a standard condenser and objectives.

Checkpoint! 5

A clinical laboratory professional consistently prepares thin blood smears resulting in minimal counting area. What would you suggest this individual do to improve the quality of these blood smears?

Answer

Because the blood smears are consistently too thin, the clinical laboratory professional should try increasing the angle of the spreader slide and increasing the speed. This will achieve a thicker blood smear.

Checkpoint! 6

Which component of Wright stain is responsible for staining hemoglobin within erythrocytes?

Answer

Eosin, the acidic dye, binds to basic groups on the hemoglobin molecule.

Checkpoint! 7

If the erythrocytes appear bluish gray and leukocyte nuclei are black on a stain, how would you correct this problem?

Answer

Two common causes for excessive blue appearance are prolonged staining and use of a buffer or stain with too alkaline pH. Therefore, try decreasing the staining time to see if the problem resolves or check the pH of the buffer and stain to verify whether one or both are too alkaline. If the pH is the problem, make the appropriate adjustments to lower the pH or try a new bottle of reagent.

Checkpoint! 8

In performing the platelet estimate, 76 platelets were observed in five fields. Calculate the platelet estimate. If the platelet count was 189×10^9/L, would these results correlate? Assume the sample was collected with EDTA.

Answer

The platelet estimate is 228×10^9/L. Yes, the estimate is within 25% of the platelet count (189×10^9/L $\times 0.25 = 47 \times 10^9$/L).

Checkpoint! 9

a. A manual platelet count was performed on an EDTA-anticoagulated blood sample. With the first unopette, 125 platelets were counted. The number of platelets counted from the second unopette was 131. What is this patient's count?

b. What are two possible physiologic causes or mechanisms that could lead to a decreased in this patient's platelet count?

Answer

a. The first unopette is $125 \times 100 \times 1/0.2 = 62.5 \times 10^9$/L; the second unopette is $131 \times 100 \times 1/0.2 = 65.5 \times 10^9$/L. The patient's platelet count equals (62.5×10^9/L + 65.5×10^9/L)/2, or 64×10^9/L. *Note:* Each unopette was used to charge both ruled areas of the hemacytometer so that the area counted was 0.2 mm². b. This patient's decreased platelet count may be the result of decreased production of platelets in the bone marrow (e.g., aplastic anemia) or increased destruction of the platelets (e.g., immune thrombocytopenic purpura).

Checkpoint! 10

Given the following erythrocyte data, what is the expected erythrocyte morphology? hemoglobin = 6.2 g/dL; hematocrit = 0.28 L/L; erythrocyte count = 4.10×10^{12}/L

Answer

Based on the erythrocyte data, the erythrocyte indices are MCHC = 22 g/dL; MCV = 68 fL; MCH = 15 pg. These indices are lower than their respective reference intervals. Therefore, the expected erythrocyte morphology would be the presence of hypochromic microcytic erythrocytes.

Checkpoint! 11

Morphologic evaluation of a Wright-stained peripheral blood smear reveals the presence of Pappenheimer bodies. How will this affect a reticulocyte count to be performed on the same blood sample? How would you confirm the presence of Pappenheimer bodies?

Answer

The presence of Pappenheimer bodies could falsely elevate the reticulocyte count because both Pappenheimer bodies and reticulum will stain with new methylene blue. Prussian blue stain is used to confirm the presence of Pappenheimer bodies: It stains iron but not reticulum.

Checkpoint! 12

What is the basis for hemoglobin separation in the hemoglobin electrophoresis procedures?

Answer

The net charge of hemoglobin molecules can be altered by the pH of the buffer. When placed in an electric field, the hemoglobin molecules will be separated based on their net charge. For example, at pH 8.6, hemoglobin molecules have a net negative charge with hemoglobin A possessing the strongest net negative charge and traveling the fastest.

Checkpoint! 13

What are the advantages of using flow cytometry to quantitate HbF?

Answer

Flow cytometry allows the evaluation of large numbers of erythrocytes, thus increasing the significance of the HbF result. In addition, the HbF concentration within individual erythrocytes is observed to demonstrate the distribution of HbF within the patient's erythrocyte population. Flow cytometry can also be used to demonstrate HbF concentration in polychromatophilic erythrocytes (i.e., reticulocytes) and nucleated erythrocytes. These findings may be useful in diagnosing certain erythrocyte disorders such as beta-thalassemia major because it is characterized by an uneven distribution of HbF within its erythrocyte population.

Checkpoint! 14

A patient's osmotic fragility test shows beginning hemolysis at 0.60% NaCl and complete hemolysis at 0.50% NaCl. How should these results be interpreted?

Answer

These results indicate increased osmotic fragility that is associated with hereditary spherocytosis.

Checkpoint! 15

A patient was recently diagnosed with a hypochromic, microcytic anemia. Additional laboratory testing revealed EPO 1.5 mIU/mL and sTfR 15.8 nmol/L. Which anemia is consistent with these results?

Answer

These results are consistent with anemia of chronic disease. A normal sTfR level but decreased EPO are characteristic findings in this anemia.

Checkpoint! 16

A pathology resident is evaluating the peripheral blood smear of a 40-year-old female. The resident suspects CML. To confirm this suspicion, a LAP score is ordered. Do you think that the LAP score will be helpful in making the correct diagnosis?

Answer

Yes, the LAP score can be used to differentiate CML from a leukemoid reaction because the LAP score in patients with CML is usually decreased. However, patients with CML in blast crisis with high numbers of circulating blasts can have an increased score. Therefore, LAP scores should always be interpreted in conjunction with the morphologic examination of the sample.

Checkpoint! 17

A 30-year-old male presented to the emergency room complaining of fatigue, weakness, and gum bleeding. The CBC showed anemia, thrombocytopenia, and a WBC of 30 × 10⁹/L. The peripheral blood smear revealed numerous intermediate to large blasts with fine nuclear chromatin and abundant cytoplasm. The bone marrow biopsy contained 60% blasts. No Auer rods were seen after careful inspection. Several cytochemical stains were then performed. The blasts failed to stain with myeloperoxidase, Sudan Black B, and specific esterase; however, the majority of blasts reacted intensely with the α-naphthyl esterase. Incubation with sodium fluoride inhibited the staining seen with α-naphthyl esterase. What type of leukemia do you think this patient has?

Answer

Alpha-naphthyl esterase stains primarily monocytes and its precursors; therefore, it is useful in the diagnosis of acute leukemias with a monocytic component such as acute monocytic and myelomonocytic leukemias. However, other bone marrow elements can also show staining with α-naphthyl esterase. Therefore, the fluoride in-

hibition test is recommended. In this test, sodium fluoride is added to the α-naphthyl esterase incubation mix. Sodium fluoride inhibits the monocytic enzyme. In our patient, the blasts failed to stain in the mix containing the fluoride, confirming the monocytic differentiation. The predominance of staining with α-naphthyl esterase and the absence of staining with myeloperoxidase, Sudan black B, and specific esterase indicate that this patient most likely has acute monocytic leukemia (AML).

Checkpoint! 18

A pathologist is reviewing the slides from the pleural fluid of a 50-year-old male who has hepatosplenomegaly and minimal lymphadenopathy. It is not clear if the mononuclear cells are mature lymphoma cells or leukemic blasts. There is not enough material for flow cytometry to do immunophenotyping, but there is enough to make a few extra cytospin smears. Which stain do you think can be useful in this case?

Answer

A TdT stain will be very useful. TdT is a DNA polymerase found in the nuclei of immature lymphocytes and is present in the majority of ALL cases. TdT is a primitive cell marker and is of value in distinguishing ALL from malignant lymphoma. It is also helpful in defining leukemic cells in body fluids.

Chapter 35

Checkpoint! 1

A 25-year-old male was recently diagnosed with ALL and received chemotherapy. It is 21 days after chemotherapy. A bone marrow biopsy has been scheduled to determine if residual leukemia is present. His platelet count is 10 × 10⁹/L. Does this patient have a significant risk of bleeding? Is it necessary to cancel the procedure until the platelet count is over 50 × 10⁹/L?

Answer

Bone marrow biopsies can be performed in thrombocytopenic patients. Applying pressure at the biopsy site and having the patient lie on the back for 20–30 minutes can control the local bleeding seen in thrombocytopenic patients. Evaluating this patient's marrow is more important than delaying because of the risk of local bleeding.

Checkpoint! 2

A 60-year-old male complained to his local physician of abdominal fullness. The CBC showed an elevated leukocyte count with absolute neutrophilia and basophilia. The peripheral blood smear revealed numerous myelocytes. A bone marrow biopsy was performed. The bone marrow differential was reported as follows: blasts 1%, myelocytes 35%, metamyelocytes 20%, bands 10%, segmented neutrophils 20%, eosinophils 1%, basophils 3%, pronormoblasts 1%, basophilic normoblasts 3%, polychromatophilic normoblasts 2%, orthochromatic normoblasts 4%, lymphocytes 0%, and monocytes 0%. What is the M:E ratio?

Answer

The myeloid precursors include blasts, myelocytes, metamyelocytes, bands, segmented neutrophils, eosinophils, and basophils. Thus, the total number of myeloid cells is 90 (1 + 35 + 20 + 10 + 20 +

1 + 3). The nucleated red cell precursors include pronormoblasts, basophilic normoblasts, polychromatic normoblasts, and orthochromatic normoblasts. The sum of erythroid precursors is 10(1 + 3 + 2 + 4), which produces an M:E ratio of 9:1. This elevated M:E ratio with the clinical history and peripheral blood findings suggests chronic myelogenous leukemia.

Checkpoint! 3

A pathologist is evaluating a bone marrow biopsy from a patient suspected of having a myelodysplastic syndrome. Evaluation of the peripheral blood reveals both hypochromic and normochromic red cells. The bone marrow aspirate shows dysplastic (abnormal cell development) changes in the red cell precursors. The pathologist ordered an iron stain on the particle crush preparation. Why is the iron stain useful in this case?

Answer

The pathologist is most probably looking for the presence of ringed sideroblasts, nucleated red cells in which one-third of the nucleus is encircled by iron granules. The presence of ringed sideroblasts is diagnostic for sideroblastic anemia and/or myelodysplastic syndrome. However, ringed sideroblasts can also be seen in myeloproliferative disorders, megaloblastic anemia, and alcoholism as well as following chemotherapy.

Chapter 36

Checkpoint! 1

What is the basis of the impedance principle for cell counting?

Answer

The impedance principle is based on the fact that blood cells are poorly conductive particles. Increased resistance is observed when a poorly conductive particle passes through an electrical field.

Checkpoint! 2

Why is lytic agent added to the leukocyte dilution?

Answer

Lytic agent is added to the leukocyte dilution for several reasons. First, the lytic agent will lyse the erythrocytes and eliminate their interference with the WBC count (i.e., falsely elevated WBC count). The lytic agent also perforates the leukocyte's membrane and shrinks the membrane around the nucleus. This allows the instrument to measure each leukocyte's cell volume and create the WBC histogram. Finally, the lytic agent converts the released hemoglobin to cyanmethemoglobin for the measurement of hemoglobin concentration.

Checkpoint! 3

Explain how the Coulter® Gen·S determines the five-part leukocyte differential.

Answer

The Coulter® Gen·S utilizes impedance, conductivity, and light scatter to determine the leukocyte differential. Impedance identifies each cell's volume and is traditionally used to generate a three-part differential. With the additional data generated for each cell by conductivity (i.e., cell's internal conductivity) and light scatter (i.e., cell's size and granularity) and the use of contour gating to analyze the data in three-dimensional space, the five-part leukocyte differ-

ential can be determined (i.e., neutrophil, lymphocyte, monocyte, eosinophil, and basophil).

Checkpoint! 4

The following results were obtained from a blood sample analyzed by the Coulter® LH 750: NRBC# 2.7 × 10⁹/L and corrected WBC 18.1 × 10⁹/L. What was the uncorrected WBC count?

Answer

Since the corrected WBC count is the uncorrected WBC count—the absolute number of nucleated red blood cells (NRBC)—the uncorrected WBC count is 20.8 × 10⁹/L.

Checkpoint! 5

How does the determination of the five-part leukocyte differential differ between the Coulter® LH 750 instrument and the Sysmex XE-2100™ instrument?

Answer

The Sysmex XE-2100™ instrument utilizes fluorescent staining of nucleic acids and forward/side scatter characteristics to determine lymphocytes, monocytes, eosinophils, and neutrophils + basophils. The basophils are separated from the neutrophils in a second dilution utilizing a specific lyse reagent that leaves the basophils intact. The light scatter characteristics of the basophils versus other leukocytes allows clear delineation of basophils. For the Coulter® LH 750 instrument, a combination of impedance, conductivity, and forward/side scatter characteristics is used to determine the five-part leukocyte differential.

Checkpoint! 6

Which cellular characteristics are used to determine the immature platelet fraction (IPF) on the Sysmex 2100™ instrument?

Answer

During the reticulocyte analysis, the immature platelet fraction is isolated based on the size of the immature platelets and their fluorescence intensity. The fluorescence intensity is due to oxazine binding to the residual RNA within these platelets.

Checkpoint! 7

a. Which CELL-DYN scatterplot allows differentiation of eosinophils from neutrophils?
b. The CELL-DYN Sapphire's WBC dilution contains propidum iodide. Why don't the neutrophils fluoresce?

Answer

a. The 90°D versus 90° scatterplot allows differentiation of eosinophils from neutrophils based on their different granularity and lobularity characteristics.
b. Propidium iodide binds specifically to DNA within the cell but is unable to pass through inact cell membranes. As a result, the neutrophils and other intact leukocytes do not fluoresce because the propidium iodide was unable to enter the cell and bind to its DNA.

Checkpoint! 8

What is the similarity in the reticulocyte methods performed on the Advia 120 and XE-2100 instruments?

Answer

Both methods use oxazine for the detection of residual RNA. (Yes, they both use flow cytometric analysis, but that is common to all instruments discussed in this chapter.)

Checkpoint! 9

Compare the clot detection methods for the Fibrometer system and STArt 4 system.

Answer

For the Fibrometer system, the completion of an electric circuit between two electrodes by the fibrin strand indicates clot formation. The STArt 4 system detects clot formation by a decrease in the iron ball's movement as plasma viscosity increases.

Checkpoint! 10

What is the basis of clot detection for the optical density principle?

Answer

Detection of clot formation is based on an increase in absorbance (i.e., optical density) or decreased transmittance as measured by a photodetector.

Chapter 37

Checkpoint! 1

Would a lymphocyte or monocyte have more forward light scatter?

Answer

Forward light scatter depends on cell size; larger cells have more forward scatter. A monocyte is larger than a lymphocyte and would have more forward light scatter.

Checkpoint! 2

A laboratory wants to identify cells that have two different antigens. How many laser light sources are needed?

Answer

One laser light source is needed because a single wavelength can excite up to three fluorochromes.

Checkpoint! 3

A cell population is positive with both Leu1 and T1 monoclonal antibodies. As a result the cell is classified as CD5 positive. Explain.

Answer

The Leu1 and T1 antibodies detect the same antigen. This antigen has been given the cluster of differentiation designation CD5.

Checkpoint! 4

Explain why lymphocytes and neutrophils can be separated on a forward versus side light dot-plot.

Answer

Granulocytes have more side light scatter than lymphocyes because of their granularity.

Checkpoint! 5

Why is it important to do immunophenotyping in a case of ALL?

Answer

Immunophenotyping is necessary to differentiate T cell ALL from B cell ALL, and mature B cell ALL from precurser B cell ALL. Treatment and prognosis in these different subtypes differ.

Checkpoint! 6

What is the absolute CD4 count? Is this count compatible with a diagnosis of AIDS in an HIV infected individual?

Answer

$5 \times 10^9/L \times 0.30 = 1.5 \times 10^9/L \times 10\% = 0.15 \times 10^9/L (150/\mu L)$
A CD4 count less than $200/\mu L$ is diagnostic of AIDS in an HIV infected individual.

Checkpoint! 7

What are the advantages of automated reticulocyte counting over manual counts?

Answer

Many more cells are counted in automated counts than in manual counts. Automated counts by flow cytometry can determine the cells' maturity.

Chapter 38

Checkpoint! 1

A newborn baby boy has multiple congenital malformations, and a chromosome abnormality is suspected as the cause. What is the most appropriate specimen to submit for chromosome analysis? How should the laboratory professional process the specimen?

Answer

The most appropriate specimen to determine the presence of a constitutional aberration is peripheral blood. The specimen should be processed by culture stimulated with phytohemagglutinin to stimulate mitosis of the circulating lymphocytes.

Checkpoint! 2

Cytogenetic studies were performed on a bone marrow specimen from a female patient with a myelodysplastic state with the following results:

    one cell—47,XX,+8
    one cell—45,XX,−20
    five cells—46,XX,del(5)(q13q34),−7,+21

    Which of these aberrations are clonal? What term would apply to the five cells?

Answer

The clonal aberrations are the del(5), −7, and +21. The +8 and −20 are seen in only one cell each and are therefore nonclonal. The five abnormal cells would be referred to as *pseudodiploid*.

Checkpoint! 3

A 35-year-old man has acute leukemia. Cytogenetic studies of the bone marrow reveal the following: 46,XY,t(15;17)(q22;q12). What type of leukemia does this patient have, and what will cytogenetic studies show after treatment if he achieves complete remission?

Answer

The t(15;17) is diagnostic for acute promyelocytic leukemia, AML-M3. If the patient achieved complete remission, cytogenetic analysis of bone marrow cells would show a normal male karyotype.

Checkpoint! 4

Five years ago a 46-year-old woman received chemotherapy and radiation treatment for breast cancer. She now has pancytopenia. Cytogenetic analysis of the bone marrow is performed and shows 10 of 20 cells with the following: 45,XX,del(5)(q13q34),−7. What is the significance of this finding?

Answer

These results show clonal acquired aberrations indicative of a neoplastic cell line. The del(5) and −7 are consistent with a secondary myelodysplastic state/acute leukemia.

Checkpoint! 5

A 5-year-old girl has fatigue and easy bruising. A CBC shows a leukocyte count of 40×10^9/L with 85% blasts. Bone marrow cytogenetic studies are performed and show all cells with the following karyotype: 53,XX,+X,+4,+6,+10,+18,+20,+21. What is the prognostic significance of this finding?

Answer

This karyotype in a pediatric patient with acute lymphoblastic leukemia would correlate with a good prognosis.

Chapter 39

Checkpoint! 1

A 40-year-old male is diagnosed with an inherited disease for which a specific point mutation is responsible. His mother died of a similar disease 10 years ago. For purposes of family counseling, the physician wants to know if she had the same mutation. The histology laboratory has archival paraffin-embedded tissue from the mother. What laboratory method(s) are best for detecting the gene mutation?

Answer

PCR and DNA sequencing are often used to detect point mutations in paraffin-embedded tissue. In most cases, this tissue is not amenable to Southern blot analysis. In situ hybridization and FISH are not good choices for detecting point mutations.

Checkpoint! 2

A patient with CML was treated with chemotherapy. On subsequent marrow samples, the physician ordered molecular testing for residual disease after treatment. The BCR/ABL1 translocation was not detected 4 months after treatment but was detected at the 8th and 9th months after treatment. Interpret this result.

Answer

The *BCR/ABL1* translocation may be detected for several months after successful therapy, presumably because some of the tumor cells have not died. However, the longer after therapy it is found and if it is persistent over several tests or if it reappears after previous negative testing, the higher is the likelihood of relapse.

Checkpoint! 3

An enlarged lymph node was biopsied and sent to the laboratory for molecular analysis. Lymphoma was suspected. What molecular test(s) could be done on the specimen to determine if the node is likely to be malignant?

Answer

Detection of clonal immunoglobulin or TR gene rearrangement by PCR or Southern blot can be used to differentiate clonal from polyclonal proliferation. Clonal gene rearrangement is characteristic of malignant lymphoid tumors. B cell tumors usually have clonal rearrangements of Ig heavy chain and kappa light chain genes. T cell tumors usually have clonal rearrangement of TRB and TRG genes. Further classification of a lymphoma is aided by molecular tests for translocations such as *BCL1/IGH* in mantle cell lymphoma, *BCL2/IGH* in folicular lymphoma, or MYC translocation in Burkitt lymphoma.

Chapter 40

Checkpoint! 1

Why have most clinical laboratories switched from 3.8% to 3.2% sodium citrate for specimen collection in coagulation studies?

Answer

The use of 3.2% sodium citrate minimizes the chances of overanticoagulating a specimen due to a high hematocrit or an inadequately filled collection tube.

Checkpoint! 2

What effect does aspirin taken daily for a heart condition have on the bleeding time of a patient? Explain.

Answer

Aspirin irreversibly inhibits cyclooxygenase, which is responsible for thromboxane A_2 synthesis. Thromboxane A_2 is required for platelet aggregation; therefore, the bleeding time is prolonged. Because aspirin's action is irreversible, the platelet is affected for its life span ($\sim$7–10 days).

Checkpoint! 3

Routine coagulation testing was performed on a properly collected and processed specimen. The PT was prolonged, but APTT was normal. What is the best interpretation of these results?

Answer

These results indicate an F-VII deficiency. The PT evaluates factors in the extrinsic and common pathways, and the APTT evaluates factors in the intrinsic and common pathways. Because only the PT is prolonged, the factor deficiency must be in the extrinsic pathway.

Checkpoint! 4

Given the following coagulation test results, what is the appropriate follow-up or reflex test?

PT	normal
APTT	prolonged
Mixing studies	no correction

Answer

The appropriate follow-up or reflex test is the platelet neutralization procedure, dilute Staclot LA, or Russell's viper venom time. Any of these tests would identify the presence of lupuslike anticoagulant.

Checkpoint! 5

What is the function of the factor deficient substrate reagent and the reference plasma in a factor assay?

Answer

The factor deficient substrate reagent ensures that all coagulation factors except the coagulation factor to be assayed are at optimal activity levels. In this way, only the activity level of a single coagulation factor is evaluated. Reference plasma contains a known activity level for each coagulation factor and is used to establish the factor activity curve from which the patient's factor activity can be determined (similar to a standard curve).

Checkpoint! 6

Why are ruptured platelets able to neutralize lupus-like anticoagulants?

Answer

Platelet membrane phospholipids are exposed when platelets rupture. Because lupuslike anticoagulants are antiphospholipid antibodies, they will bind to the exposed phospholipids and will no longer interfere with the test reagent phospholipids.

Checkpoint! 7

What is the appropriate interpretation of these coagulation test results?

PT	prolonged
APTT	prolonged
TT	prolonged
FDP	>20 μg/mL
D-dimer	>1.0 μg/mL

Answer

These coagulation test results indicate disseminated intravascular coagulation (DIC). D-dimer is a specific indicator of fibrin clot degradation as is observed in DIC.

Checkpoint! 8

In diagnostic laboratory evaluation of a hypercoagulable state such as antithrombin deficiency, why is it important to determine the functional activity of the protein?

Answer

Several hypercoagulable states are characterized by a normal antigenic level of protein but have decreased functional activity. In other words, the hypercoagulable state is the result of a dysfunctional coagulation protein. The diagnosis would be missed if only the antigenic level was assessed.

Checkpoint! 9

As seen in Figure 40-6, the patient has a PT of 21.5 seconds (producing an INR of 2.2). In this case the patient is not on oral anticoagulation. What is the explanation for not reporting the INR?

Answer

The INR reflects the standardization of the thromboplastin reagent for a certain PT to a standardized reference thromboplastin using the same type of instrumentation. It does not reflect the level of deficiency present in the sample. Therefore, only the PT should be reported.

Checkpoint! 10

A patient has a venous thrombotic episode, and is to be treated appropriately. When should the blood sample be drawn to perform a thrombotic work-up in order to diagnose an acquired or congenital deficiency? Why?

Answer

To properly diagnose a thrombotic deficiency, the patient must be off treatment. If the sample is drawn too early, the consumptive process that occurred may produce decreased levels of coagulation proteins as well as conflicting results due to anticoagulation treatment and possible supplemental treatment with FFP. This may lead to misdiagnosis of a deficiency in one or more factors. If the patient is tested while hospitalized and the results conflict, repeat studies should then be performed. Family studies also should be considered.

Chapter 41

Checkpoint! 1

Explain the importance of each component of the quality assessment program to its ultimate goal.

Answer

The preexamination component is critical to the quality assessment (QA) program because the test outcome is only as good as the sample from which it is determined. The QA program must ensure proper collection and handling of samples prior to testing. The examination component represents all factors that impact the testing system. The test outcome will be affected if a breakdown in the testing system occurs due to lack of a proper QA program. A breakdown in the QA program within the postexamination component affects the recording/reporting of the test outcome. This may delay appropriate treatment for the patient.

Checkpoint! 2

If a clinical laboratory loses its certification to perform protein C assays, what is involved in regaining that certification?

Answer

The clinical laboratory professional should determine the reason for the failure, correct the problem, and document the process. Following the corrective action, successful participation in two consecutive proficiency testing surveys for protein C would result in the laboratory's recertification to perform protein C assays.

Checkpoint! 3

What is an appropriate method of assessing a clinical laboratory professional's competency in performing the prothrombin time (PT) and partial thromboplastin time (APTT) using an automated coagulation instrument?

Answer

A combination of direct observation checklist and blinded preanalyzed samples provides an appropriate method of assessing competency in performing PT and APTT.

Checkpoint! 4

Linear regression analysis was performed on results from a method comparison of the prothrombin time between automated coagulation instrument A and automated coagulation instrument B (Web Figure 41-1). The following results were obtained:

y-intercept = 0.8157
slope = 0.9982
standard error of the estimate = 0.0807

What conclusions can be drawn from these results?

Answer

Based on the linear regression results, a constant difference occurs between the automated instrument A and the automated instrument B because the y-intercept is more than zero. That is, the automated instrument A gives consistently higher results than the automated instrument B. Therefore, a constant systematic error exists. The slope between 0.95 and 1.05 indicates there is no proportional systematic error between the two methods . There is no random error because the standard error of estimate is nearly zero, indicating very little dispersion of results about the linear regression line.

Checkpoint! 5

Define the term reference interval.

Answer

For a given analyte, the *reference interval* represents the usual results for a healthy population. For example, the reference interval for hemoglobin in the adult male population is 13.3–17.7 g/dL.

Checkpoint! 6

If a spill occurred when handling the CELL-DYN Sapphire hemoglobin reagent, what is the appropriate procedure to clean it up? Refer to Web Figure 41-2.

Answer

According to the MSDS sheet, absorb the spill reagent with a liquid-binding material such as sand and use a neutralizing agent. Then, wash the spill area with appropriate cleaning material. The contaminated materials should be disposed of in accordance with federal, state, and local regulations.

Checkpoint! 7

To establish the control limits for a new lot number of level 1 PT coagulation control, the following data points were collected (results are in seconds): 11.8, 11.6, 12.1, 12.0, 12.3, 12.6, 11.9, 12.2, 12.0, 11.5, 12.7, 12.1, 11.2, 12.3, 12.9, 13.0, 12.3, 11.9, 12.4, 12.5. What are the $\pm 2s$ control limits?

Answer

The first step to determine these control limits is to calculate the mean and standard deviation for these results. Based on these data points, the mean is 12.2 seconds and the standard deviation is 0.50. Therefore, the $\pm 2s$ control limits would be 11.20–13.20 seconds.

Checkpoint! 8

After performing daily quality control on the automated hematology instrument, the clinical laboratory professional observes a 4_{1s} violation for the hemoglobin parameter. What type of error is indicated?

Answer

The 4_{1s} violation indicates a systematic error that may be due to an expired lysing reagent or a deteriorating hemoglobin lamp.

Checkpoint! 9

In reviewing a patient's CBC results, the clinical laboratory professional notes an MCHC of 37 fL. What corrective action should be taken?

Answer

The clinical laboratory professional must first determine the cause of the falsely elevated MCHC. The presence of cold agglutinins, lipemia, icteria, or spherocytes in a patient sample has been associated with an MCHC of more than 36 fL. Lipemia and icteria are substances that cause falsely elevated hemoglobin and consequently falsely elevated MCHC. Centrifuging the sample and examining the plasma can identify these substances. If either is present, the saline replacement procedure is performed to obtain an accurate hemoglobin and MCHC. If cold agglutinins are suspected, the hematocrit will be falsely decreased (i.e., MCV × RBC = Hct), and consequently, the MCHC falsely elevated. A manual hematocrit may quickly identify this problem. If cold agglutinins are present, the sample is warmed to 37°C for 15 minutes to dissociate the agglutinated cells prior to analysis to obtain accurate results. If other possibilities are ruled out, the peripheral blood smear is examined for the presence of spherocytes. No corrective action is needed if spherocytes are present.

Checkpoint! 10

The clinical laboratory professional observes that the 3.2% sodium citrate tube for a PT and APTT is only two-thirds full. Explain the effect this will have on the patient's coagulation results.

Answer

If the sample collection tube is only two-thirds full, excess anticoagulant is present and the plasma is overanticoagulated. Therefore, the coagulation results are falsely prolonged.

APPENDIX C

Answers to Review Questions

CHAPTER 1
1. a
2. d
3. a
4. c
5. b
6. a
7. c
8. b
9. d
10. d

CHAPTER 2
Level I
1. b
2. c
3. d
4. c
5. a
6. a
7. b
8. c
9. a
10. d

Level II
1. d
2. b
3. c
4. b
5. a
6. d
7. a
8. d
9. b
10. b

CHAPTER 3
Level I
1. b
2. c
3. d
4. a
5. d
6. a
7. b
8. c
9. b
10. c

Level II
1. c
2. a
3. c
4. b
5. a
6. d
7. d
8. a
9. b
10. c

CHAPTER 4
Level I
1. a
2. b
3. a
4. d
5. a

Level II
1. a
2. a
3. d
4. a
5. b

CHAPTER 5
Level I
1. a
2. b
3. b
4. c
5. a
6. c
7. d
8. d
9. c
10. b

Level II
1. a
2. d
3. c
4. d
5. d
6. b
7. c
8. a
9. a
10. c

CHAPTER 6
Level I
1. a
2. b
3. b
4. c
5. d
6. c
7. b
8. d
9. c
10. a

Level II
1. d
2. b
3. a
4. c
5. b
6. d
7. b
8. b
9. a
10. b

CHAPTER 7
Level I
1. c
2. b
3. b
4. b
5. c
6. b
7. a
8. a
9. b
10. c

Level II
1. a
2. d
3. a
4. b
5. b
6. d
7. d
8. d
9. c
10. c

Level II
1. b
2. c
3. c
4. a
5. a
6. c
7. b
8. c
9. c
10. b

CHAPTER 8

Level I
1. d
2. a
3. b
4. b
5. a
6. c
7. a
8. d
9. a
10. b

Level II
1. c
2. d
3. c
4. d
5. a
6. c
7. d
8. b
9. a
10. d

CHAPTER 9

Level I
1. b
2. a
3. c
4. c
5. d
6. d
7. d
8. b
9. d
10. c

Level II
1. a
2. d
3. b
4. c
5. b
6. c
7. b
8. a
9. b

10. a
11. c
12. b

CHAPTER 10

Level I
1. b
2. a
3. c
4. c
5. b
6. d
7. d
8. b
9. a
10. c

Level II
1. a
2. d
3. b
4. c
5. d
6. d
7. a
8. b
9. a
10. c

CHAPTER 11

Level I
1. c
2. a
3. d
4. a
5. d
6. c
7. b
8. a
9. c
10. b

Level II
1. a
2. c
3. a
4. a
5. d
6. b
7. b
8. d
9. a
10. a

CHAPTER 12

Level I
1. b
2. a
3. c

4. c
5. d
6. a
7. b
8. c
9. a
10. c

Level II
1. b
2. d
3. c
4. b
5. a
6. a
7. b
8. d
9. c
10. b

CHAPTER 13

Level I
1. b
2. a
3. d
4. a
5. c
6. c
7. d
8. a
9. d
10. b

Level II
1. c
2. b
3. c
4. d
5. a
6. c
7. a
8. d
9. b
10. c

CHAPTER 14

Level I
1. d
2. b
3. b
4. a
5. c

Level II
1. c
2. a
3. d
4. a
5. b

CHAPTER 15

Level I

1. a
2. c
3. d
4. b
5. b
6. d
7. c
8. c
9. d
10. b

Level II

1. c
2. b
3. c
4. a
5. a
6. c
7. a
8. d
9. c
10. b

CHAPTER 16

Level I

1. d
2. b
3. c
4. d
5. c
6. a
7. a
8. c
9. a
10. d

Level II

1. c
2. b
3. a
4. b
5. a
6. c
7. a
8. d
9. d
10. a

CHAPTER 17

Level I

1. b
2. c
3. a
4. a
5. d
6. c
7. c

8. b
9. c
10. b

Level II

1. b
2. b
3. a
4. a
5. d
6. d
7. c
8. a
9. c
10. d

CHAPTER 18

Level I

1. b
2. d
3. a
4. d
5. c
6. d
7. a
8. a
9. c
10. a

Level II

1. a
2. c
3. d
4. b
5. a
6. c
7. d
8. b
9. c
10. d

CHAPTER 19

Level I

1. b
2. d
3. a
4. b
5. a
6. b
7. a
8. d
9. c
10. c

Level II

1. d
2. c
3. d
4. b
5. c

6. a, b, d, e
7. a, b, c, d, e
8. a, d, e
9. a, b, d, e
10. a, c, d
11. a, d

CHAPTER 20

Level I

1. c
2. b
3. c
4. c
5. a
6. c
7. c
8. d
9. d
10. c

Level II

1. d
2. b
3. a
4. a
5. a
6. a
7. c
8. d
9. a
10. a

CHAPTER 21

Level I

1. a
2. a
3. b
4. b
5. b
6. d
7. b
8. a
9. d
10. b
11. a
12. d

Level II

1. a
2. c
3. d
4. c
5. a
6. b
7. c
8. b
9. d
10. b
11. a
12. c

13. a
14. c

CHAPTER 22
Level I
1. b
2. a
3. b
4. d
5. a
6. b
7. d
8. a
9. c
10. b

Level II
1. b
2. a
3. c
4. b
5. c
6. d
7. d
8. c
9. d
10. a

CHAPTER 23
Level I
1. a
2. c
3. d
4. a
5. c
6. c
7. d
8. a
9. b
10. c

Level II
1. d
2. d
3. a
4. b
5. a
6. d
7. d
8. a
9. b
10. c

CHAPTER 24
Level I
1. b
2. b
3. b
4. b

5. a
6. c
7. a
8. c
9. d
10. d

Level II
1. a
2. d
3. a
4. c
5. a
6. a
7. c
8. a
9. d
10. c

CHAPTER 25
Level I
1. b
2. d
3. c
4. a
5. c
6. b
7. d
8. d
9. c
10. b

Level II
1. d
2. d
3. a
4. b
5. b
6. c
7. d
8. a
9. b
10. c

CHAPTER 26
Level I
1. d
2. b
3. d
4. d
5. c
6. a
7. d
8. b
9. d
10. a

Level II
1. a
2. c

3. a
4. c
5. a
6. b
7. a
8. a
9. a
10. a

CHAPTER 27
Level I
1. d
2. d
3. b
4. c
5. b
6. a
7. a
8. d
9. c
10. b

Level II
1. c
2. c
3. a
4. d
5. d
6. d
7. b
8. b
9. c
10. a

CHAPTER 28
Level I
1. d
2. c
3. d
4. d
5. a
6. d
7. d
8. d
9. d
10. a

Level II
1. d
2. a
3. b
4. a
5. b
6. a
7. c
8. a
9. c
10. c

CHAPTER 29

Level I
1. b
2. c
3. d
4. c
5. c
6. b
7. d
8. d
9. b
10. d

Level II
1. b
2. c
3. a
4. d
5. a
6. c
7. b
8. d
9. a
10. b

CHAPTER 30

Level I
1. b
2. a
3. c
4. c
5. b
6. b
7. b
8. c
9. c
10. a

Level II
1. a
2. d
3. d
4. c
5. b
6. b
7. d
8. a
9. b
10. a

CHAPTER 31

Level I
1. d
2. d
3. a
4. b
5. a
6. c
7. d
8. d

9. d
10. b

Level II
1. c
2. a
3. c
4. a
5. b
6. d
7. c
8. d
9. c
10. a

CHAPTER 32

Level I
1. d
2. a
3. b
4. b
5. c
6. d
7. a
8. d
9. b
10. b

Level II
1. b
2. a
3. c
4. c
5. b
6. a
7. c
8. b
9. d
10. b

CHAPTER 33

Level I
1. a
2. a
3. c
4. d
5. b
6. d
7. d
8. c
9. a
10. a

Level II
1. a
2. c
3. b
4. d
5. a
6. a

7. c
8. d
9. a
10. b

CHAPTER 34

Level I
1. c
2. c
3. d
4. a
5. b
6. b
7. d
8. a
9. c
10. a

Level II
1. b
2. d
3. a
4. b
5. a
6. b
7. a
8. c
9. a
10. b

CHAPTER 35

Level I
1. c
2. a
3. b
4. d
5. a
6. a
7. c
8. b
9. a
10. a

Level II
1. b
2. c
3. c
4. a
5. a
6. c
7. b
8. a
9. c
10. b

CHAPTER 36

Level I
1. d
2. a

3. d
4. b
5. b
6. d
7. c
8. b
9. d
10. c

Level II
1. a
2. b
3. c
4. d
5. a
6. d

CHAPTER 37
Level I
1. d
2. c
3. d
4. d
5. d
6. c
7. d
8. b
9. a
10. b

Level II
1. b
2. a
3. b
4. d
5. c
6. b
7. d
8. a
9. c
10. b

CHAPTER 38
Level I
1. a
2. c

3. c
4. a
5. a
6. a
7. a
8. b
9. c
10. d

Level II
1. b
2. d
3. c
4. c
5. c
6. a
7. b
8. a
9. d
10. d

CHAPTER 39
Level II
1. c
2. b
3. a
4. b
5. a
6. c
7. b
8. d
9. d
10. d

CHAPTER 40
Level I
1. b
2. c
3. b
4. a
5. a
6. b
7. b

8. a
9. c
10. a

Level II
1. d
2. a
3. d
4. c
5. a
6. d
7. c
8. b
9. b
10. a

CHAPTER 41
Level I
1. c
2. c
3. b
4. b
5. b
6. c
7. c
8. b
9. c
10. c

Level II
1. a
2. a
3. d
4. c
5. b
6. c
7. b
8. a
9. b
10. d

GLOSSARY

A

Abetalipoproteinemia (hereditary acanthocytosis) - rare, autosomal recessive disorder characterized by the absence of serum β-lipoprotein, low serum cholesterol, low triglyceride, and low phospholipid and an increase in the ratio of cholesterol to phospholipid.

Acanthocyte - abnormally shaped erythrocyte with spicules of varying length irregularly distributed over the cell membrane's outer surface; also known as *spur cell*. There is no central area of pallor.

Achlorhydria - absence of hydrochloric acid in stomach gastric secretions.

Acquired aberration - chromosome aberration (either numerical or structural) that occurs at some time after birth and involves only one cell line.

Acquired immune deficiency syndrome (AIDS) - disease caused by infection with human immunodeficiency virus type I (HIV-1). The virus selectively infects helper T lymphocytes (CD4+) causing rapid depletion of these cells. This causes a deficiency in cell-mediated immunity. The patients have repeated infections with multiple opportunistic organisms and an increase in malignancies.

Acquired inhibitors - *See* Circulating anticoagulants.

Acrocentric - description of a chromosome that has the centromere close to the terminal end so that the short arm is much shorter than the long arm. The short arm consists only of a stalk and a small amount of DNA called a *satellite*.

Acrocyanosis - *See* Raynaud's phenomenon.

Activated partial thromboplastin time (APTT) - screening test used to detect deficiencies in the intrinsic and common pathway of the coagulation cascade.

Activated lymphocyte - *See* Reactive lymphocyte.

Activated protein C resistance (APCR) - condition in which activated protein C is not able to inactivate F-V, which may cause or contribute to thrombosis. In most cases, it is due to a mutation in F-V in which Arg 506 is replaced with Gln (F-V$_{Leiden}$).

Acute leukemia - malignant hematopoietic stem cell disorder characterized by proliferation and accumulation of immature and nonfunctional hematopoietic cells in the bone marrow and other organs.

Acute lymphocytic leukemia (ALL) - malignant lymphoproliferative disorder characterized by proliferation and accumulation of lymphoid cells in the bone marrow. Peripheral blood smear reveals the presence of many undifferentiated or minimally differentiated cells.

Acute myeloid leukemia (AML) - malignant myeloproliferative disorder characterized by proliferation and accumulation of primarily undifferentiated or minimally differentiated myeloid cells in the bone marrow.

Acute phase reactant - plasma protein that rises rapidly in response to inflammation, infection, or tissue injury.

Acute undifferentiated leukemia (AUL) - acute leukemia in which the morphology, cytochemistry, and immunophenotype of the proliferating blasts lack sufficient information to classify them as myeloid or lymphoid origin.

ADAMTS-13 - metalloprotease enzyme responsible for cleavage of the ultralarge multimers of VWF released from endothelial cells into the VWF multimer sizes normally found in the circulation.

Adaptive immune response - interaction of the T lymphocyte, B lymphocyte, and macrophage in a series of events that allows the body to attack and eliminate foreign antigens.

ADCC - antibody-dependent cell cytotoxicity that describes the recognition and lysis of cells by NK cells. This occurs by binding IgG to the NK cell CD 16 receptor. Any target cell coated with IgG can be bound to NK cells and lysed. Monocytes, macrophages, and neutrophils also have this receptor and act in a similar manner.

Adipocyte - cell whose cytoplasm is largely replaced with a single fat vacuole; fat cell.

Adsorbed plasma - platelet-poor plasma that is adsorbed with either barium sulfate or aluminum hydroxide to remove the coagulation factors II, VII, IX, X (the prothrombin group). Factors V, VIII, XI, XII, and fibrinogen (I) are present in adsorbed plasma. This plasma is one of the reagents used in the substitution studies to determine a specific factor deficiency.

Afibrinogenemia - condition in which there is absence of fibrinogen in the peripheral blood. It may be caused by a mutation in the gene controlling the production of fibrinogen or by an acquired condition in which fibrinogen is pathologically converted to fibrin.

Aged serum - serum that lacks coagulation factors fibrinogen (I), prothrombin (II), V, VIII. Aged serum is prepared by incubating normal serum for 24 hours at 37°C. Factors VII, IX, X, XI, and XII are present in aged serum. This serum is one of the reagents used in the substitution studies to determine a specific factor deficiency.

Agglutinate - clumping together of erythrocytes as a result of interactions between membrane antigens and specific antibodies.

Aggregating reagent - chemical substance (agonist) that promotes platelet activation and aggregation by attaching to a receptor on the platelet's surface.

Agonist - chemical substance that can attach to a platelet membrane receptor and activate platelets causing them to aggregate (e.g., collagen, ADP). These agonists are used in the laboratory to test platelet function using a platelet aggregometer or platelet function analyzer.

Agranulocytosis - absence of granulocytes in the peripheral blood.

AIDS related complex (ARC) - second recognized clinical stage of a person infected with the HIV virus. Immune-compromised patients with mild symptoms of weight loss, fever, lymphadenopathy, thrush, chronic rash, or intermittent diarrhea are included in this category.

Alder-Reilly anomaly - benign condition characterized by the presence of leukocytes with large purplish granules in their cytoplasm when stained with a Romanowsky stain. These cells are functionally normal.

Aleukemic leukemia - disorder in which the abnormal malignant cells are found only in the bone marrow.

Allele - one of two or more genes that correspond to the same trait and occupy the same position on paired chromosomes.

Alloantibodies - antibodies produced in one individual in response to the antigens of another individual of the same species.

Allogeneic - pertaining to an allograft in which donor and host belong to the same species but are not genetically identical.

Allogeneic stem cell transplantation - transplantation of stem cells between genetically dissimilar animals of the same species.

Alloimmune hemolytic anemia - hemolytic disorder generated when blood cells from one person are infused into a genetically unrelated person. Antigens on the infused donor cells are recognized as foreign by the recipient's lymphocytes, stimulating the production of antibodies. The antibodies react with donor cells and cause hemolysis.

Alpha granules - platelet storage granules containing a variety of proteins that are released into an area after platelet activation.

Analytical sensitivity - ability to detect small amounts of the analyte.

Analytical specificity - ability to detect only the analyte in question.

Analytical time - period between specimen entry into the test system and the reporting of the result by the instrument.

Anemia - disorder characterized by decrease in the normal concentration of hemoglobin or erythrocytes. This may be caused by increased erythrocyte loss or decreased erythrocyte production. Anemia may result in hypoxia.

Aneuploid - number of chromosomes per cell that does not equal a multiple of the haploid number, n, for example, in human cells a chromosome count of 45, 47, 48, etc.

Anisocytosis - term used to describe a general variation in erythrocyte size.

Antibody - immunoglobulin produced in response to an antigenic substance.

Anticardiolipin antibody (ACA) - autoantibody directed against negatively charged phospholipids. *See* Antiphospholipid antibody.

Anticoagulant - chemical substance added to whole blood to prevent blood from coagulating. Depending on the type of anticoagulant, in vitro coagulation is prevented by the removal of calcium (EDTA) or the inhibition of the serine proteases such as thrombin (heparin).

Antigen - any foreign substance that evokes antibody production (an immune response) and reacts specifically with that antibody.

Antigen-dependent lymphopoiesis - development of immunocompetent lymphocytes into effector T and B lymphocytes that mediate the immune response through production of lymphokines and antibodies. The process is initiated when mature lymphocytes come into contact with an antigen. This process occurs in secondary lymphoid tissue.

Antigen-independent lymphopoiesis - development of lymphoid stem cells into immunocompetent T and B lymphocytes (virgin lymphocytes). This process occurs in the primary lymphoid tissue under the regulation of hematopoietic growth factors.

Antigen presenting cell (APC) - term used to describe the macrophage in the immune response; the macrophage phagocytizes substances foreign to the host and presents its antigenic determinants on its membrane to antigen-dependent T lymphocytes.

Antihuman globulin (AHG) - globulin used in a laboratory procedure that is designed to detect the presence of antibodies directed against erythrocyte antigens on the erythrocyte membrane.

Antioncogene - gene that codes for a normal substance that suppresses tumor formation. Maturation and/or absence of both alleles allows tumor growth. Also called *tumor-suppressor gene.*

Antiphospholipid antibody - autoantibody directed against antigens that consist of a negatively charged phospholipid. Clinically important antiphospholipid antibodies include anticardiolipin antibody (ACA) and lupus anticoagulant (LA). In some individuals, these antibodies are associated with thrombosis and other hemostatic defects.

Antiphospholipid antibody syndrome - clinical condition characterized by the presence of high titers of antiphospholipid antibodies, thrombocytopenia, and recurrent arterial and venous thromboses, often affecting young males.

Aperture - small opening through which blood cells are drawn into an electronic cell counter. Electrodes are located on either side of the aperture, and electrical resistance is detected as the cell passes through the aperture.

Apheresis - separation or removal. Whole blood is withdrawn from the donor or patient and separated into its components. One of the components is retained, and the remaining constituents are recombined and returned to the individual.

Aplasia - failure of hematopoietic cells to generate and develop in the bone marrow.

Aplastic anemia - anemia characterized by peripheral blood pancytopenia and hypoplastic marrow. It is considered a pluripotential stem cell disorder.

Aplastic crisis - abrupt, transient cessation of erythropoiesis that occurs in some hemolytic anemias and infections.

Apoferritin - cellular protein that combines with iron to form ferritin. It is found attached only to iron, not in the free form.

Apoptosis - programmed cell death resulting from activation of a predetermined sequence of intracellular events; "cell suicide."

APSAC - anisoylated plasminogen streptokinase activator complex; a modification of the enzyme streptokinase that is a chemically altered complex of streptokinase and plasminogen and is used as a thrombolytic agent in the treatment of thrombosis.

APTT - laboratory test that measures fibrin-forming ability of coagulation factors in the intrinisic coagulation cascade.

Arachidonic acid (AA) - unsaturated essential fatty acid, usually attached to the second carbon of the glycerol backbone of phospholipids, released by phospholipase A_2 and a precursor of prostaglandins and thromboxanes.

Arachnoid mater - delicate membrane that covers the central nervous system; middle layer of the meninges.

Artificial oxygen carrier (AOC) - two groups of AOCs including hemoglobin-based oxygen carriers (HBOCs) in solution and perfluorocarbons (PFCs). The HBOCs consist of purified human or bovine hemoglobin and recombinant hemoglobin. The oxygen dissociation curve of HBOCs is similar to that of native human blood. Hemoglobin tests based on colorimetric analysis could give erroneous results. PFCs are fluorinated hydrocarbons with high gas-dissolving capacity. They do not mix in aqueous solution and must be emulsified. In contrast to HBOCs, a linear relationship exists between pO_2 and oxygen content in PFCs. Thus, relatively high O_2 partial pressure is required to maximize delivery of O_2 by PFCs.

Ascites - effusion and accumulation of fluid in the peritoneal cavity.

Ascitic fluid - fluid that has abnormally collected in the peritoneal cavity of the abdomen.

Atypical lymphocyte - *See* Reactive lymphocyte.

Auer rods - reddish-blue staining needlelike inclusions within the cytoplasm of leukemic myeloblasts that occur as a result of abnormal cytoplasmic granule formation. Their presence on a Romanowsky-stained smear is helpful in differentiating acute myeloid leukemia from acute lymphoblastic leukemia.

Autoantibodies - antibodies in the blood capable of reacting with the subject's own antigens.

Autohemolysis - lysis of the subject's own erythrocytes by hemolytic agents in the subject's serum.

Autoimmune hemolytic anemia (AIHA) - anemia that results when individuals produce antibodies against their own erythrocytes. The antibodies are usually against high-incidence antigens.

Autologous stem cell transplantation - transplantation or infusion of a person's own stem cells.

Autosome - chromosome that does not contain genes for sex differentiation; in humans, chromosome pairs 1–22.

Autosplenectomy - extensive splenic damage secondary to infarction. This is often seen in older children and adults with sickle cell anemia.

Azurophilic granules - granules (primary granules) within myelocytic leukocytes that have a predilection for the aniline component of a Romanowsky-type stain. These granules appear bluish purple or bluish black when observed microscopically on a stained blood smear. They first appear in the promyelocyte.

▶ **B**

Backlighting - highlighting a parameter that falls outside its reference interval or a user-defined action limit. Backlighting alerts the clinical laboratory professional of a potential problem or error that requires further investigation.

Band neutrophil - immediate precursor of the mature granulocyte. This cell type can be found in either the bone marrow or peripheral blood. The nucleus is elongated and nuclear chromatin is condensed. The cytoplasm stains pink, and there are many specific granules. The cell is 9–15 μm in diameter. Also called *stab* or *unsegmented neutrophil*.

Basophil - mature granulocytic cell characterized by the presence of large basophilic granules. These granules are purple blue or purple black with Romanowsky stain. The cell is 10–14 μm in diameter, and the nucleus is segmented. Granules are cytochemically positive with periodic acid-schiff (PAS) and peroxidase. The granules contain histamine and heparin peroxidase. Basophils constitute $<0.2 \times 10^9$/L or 0–1% of peripheral blood leukocytes. The basophil functions as a mediator of inflammatory responses. The cell has receptors for IgE.

Basophilia - increased concentration of circulating basophils.

Basophilic normoblast - nucleated precursor of the erythrocyte that is derived from a pronormoblast. The cell is 10–16 μm in diameter. The nuclear chromatin is coarser than the pronormoblast, and nucleoli are usually absent. Cytoplasm is more abundant, and it stains deeply basophilic. The cell matures to a polychromatophilic normoblast. Also called *prorubricyte*.

Basophilic stippling - precipitating ribonucleoproteins and mitochondrial remnants that compose erythrocyte inclusions. Observed on Romanowsky-stained blood smears as diffuse or punctate bluish-black granules in toxic states such as drug (lead) exposure. Diffuse, fine basophilic stippling may occur as an artifact.

B cell ALL - immunologic type of ALL in which the neoplastic cell is a B lymphoid cell. There are subtypes.

B cell receptor (BCR) - specific antigen receptor on the B lymphocyte membrane.

bcl-2 **gene** - gene on chromosome 18 producing bcl-2 protein. The translocation t(14;18) found in follicular lymphoma leads to bcl-2 overexpression and inhibition of lymphocyte cell death.

Beer Lambert's law - law that forms the mathematical basis for colorimetry. The equation is $A = C \times L \times K$. A is absorbance, C is the concentration of the colored substance, L is the depth of the solution through which the light travels, and K is a constant.

Bence-Jones protein - excessive immunoglobulin light chain in the urine.

Benign - Description of tissue that is nonmalignant. Formed from highly organized, differentiated cells that do not spread or invade surrounding tissue.

Bernard-Soulier disease - rare hereditary platelet disorder characterized by a genetic mutation in the gene coding for platelet glycoprotein Ib resulting in platelets' inability to adhere to collagen.

BFU-E - burst forming unit-erythroid; a committed erythroid progenitor cell. It gives rise to the unipotential CFU-E stem cell. It is relatively insensitive to EPO except in high concentrations. GM-CSF stimulates it to enter the cell cycle.

Bilineage leukemia - leukemia that has two separate populations of leukemic cells, one of which phenotypes as lymphoid and the other as myeloid.

Bilirubin - breakdown product of the heme portion of the hemoglobin molecule. Initial steps in the degradation of hemoglobin result in a lipid-soluble form (unconjugated or indirect bilirubin) that travels in the blood stream to the liver, where it is converted into a water-soluble form (conjugated or direct bilirubin) that can be excreted into the bile.

Bioavailability - degree and rate at which a free drug is available to produce its effect.

Biphasic antibody - antibody that binds to erythrocytes at room temperature or below and causes hemolysis when the blood warms to 37°C.

Biphenotypic leukemia - acute leukemia that has myeloid and lymphoid markers on the same population of neoplastic cells.

Birefringent - description of a substance that can change the direction of light rays that are directed at the substance; can be used to identify crystals.

2,3-bisphosphoglycerate (2,3-BPG) - product of the glycolytic pathway that affects the oxygen affinity of hemoglobin. It serves in the biochemical feedback system that regulates the amount of oxygen released to the tissues. As the concentration of 2,3-BPG increases, hemoglobin's affinity for oxygen decreases and more oxygen is released to the tissue. Also referred to as 2,3-*diphosphoglycerate (2,3-DPG)*.

Bite cells - erythrocytes with a portion of the cell missing; seen in G6PD deficiency and drug-induced oxidant hemolysis.

Bleeding time and PFA 100 - screening test that measures platelet function.

Blinded preanalyzed samples - previously analyzed samples that are integrated randomly into a specimen run and possess no identifying feature (e.g., number or designation) to indicate that they are different from current patient specimens. These samples used as a part of a quality control program can be identified only by the individual who selected and relabeled them.

Blister cell - cell with a clear area next to the membrane on one side of the cell. It is thought to be formed when the phagocyte removes a Heinz body in the cell and is seen in G6PD deficiency.

Blood coagulation - formation of a blood clot, usually considered a normal process.

Bohr effect - effect of pH on hemoglobin-oxygen affinity. This is one of the most important buffer systems in the body. As the H^+ concentration in tissues increases, the affinity of hemoglobin for oxygen is decreased, permitting unloading of oxygen.

Bone marrow aspirate - fluid withdrawn from the bone marrow by aspiration using a special needle (e.g., Jamshidi needle) and syringe. It represents the specialized soft tissue that fills the medullary cavities between the bone trabeculae. Examination of the bone marrow aspirate is useful in evaluating hematopoietic cellular morphology, distribution, and development; observing for presence of abnormal cells; and estimating cellularity.

Bone marrow trephine biopsy - removal of a small piece of the bone marrow core that contains marrow, fat, and trabeula. Examination of the trephine biopsy is useful in observing the bone marrow architecture and cellularity and allows interpreting the spatial relationships of bone, fat, and marrow cellularity.

Bordetella pertussis - gram-negative aerobic coccobacilli that is the cause of whooping cough. The hematologic picture in whooping cough is leukocytosis with lymphocytosis. The lymphocytes are small cells with folded nuclei.

Buffy coat - layer of white blood cells and platelets that lies between the plasma and erythrocytes in centrifuged blood sample.

Burkitt cell - lymphoblast that is found in Burkitt's lymphoma.

Butt cell - circulating neoplastic lymphocyte with a deep indentation (cleft) of the nuclear membrane. Butt cells may be seen when follicular lymphoma involves the peripheral blood.

 C

Cabot ring - reddish-violet erythrocyte inclusion resembling the figure 8 on Romanowsky-stained blood smears that can be found in some cases of severe anemia.

Capitated payment - reimbursement method for health care by third-party payers in which the insurer contracts with certain health care providers who agree to provide services for a defined population on a per-member fee schedule. The insurer determines who the providers will be.

Carboxyhemoglobin - compound formed when hemoglobin is exposed to carbon monoxide; it is incapable of oxygen transport.

Carboxylation - addition of a carboxyl group to a coagulation factor (II, VII, IX, X, Proteins C, S, Z). This occurs in the liver. The factor is not functional until it is carboxylated. Vitamin K is required for this reaction.

Cardiac tamponade - critical clinical condition in which the pericardial sac fills with fluid and restricts the heartbeat and venous return to the heart.

Caspase - cysteine protease responsible for cell alterations in apoptosis.

Catalytic domain - molecular area of a molecule that is common to all serine proteases involved in blood clotting. Cleavage of a peptide bond occurs here and converts the proenzyme to its active form.

CD designation - cluster of differentiation; refers to a group of monoclonal antibodies recognizing the same protein marker antigen on a cell. The antibodies are used to classify cell types and stages of maturation.

Cell cycle - biochemical and morphological stages a cell passes through leading up to cell division; includes G1, S, G2, and M phases.

Cell cycle checkpoint - point in the cell cycle at which progress through the cycle can be halted until conditions are suitable for the cell to proceed to the next stage.

Cell-mediated immunity - immune response mediated by T lymphocytes. The event requires interaction between histocompatible T lymphocytes and macrophages with antigen. At least three important T lymphocyte subsets are involved: helper, suppressor, and cytotoxic.

Cellular hemoglobin concentration mean (CHCM) - erythrocyte index that represents the average hemoglobin concentration of the individual cells analyzed. CHCM is derived from the hemoglobin histogram. Interference with the hemoglobin determination due to turbidity or lipemia can be identified by comparing the CHCM to the MCHC.

Central nervous system (CNS) - part of the nervous sytem that consists of the brain and spinal cord.

Centriole - cytoplasmic organelle that is the point of origin for the contractile protein known as *spindle fiber*.

Centromere - primary constriction that attaches sister chromatids in a chromosome, dividing the chromatids into long and short arms.

Cerebrospinal fluid (CSF) - fluid that is normally produced to protect the brain and spinal cord. Produced by the choroid plexus cells and absorbed by the arachnoid pia, it circulates in the subarachnoid space.

CFU-E - colony-forming unit–erythroid; unipotential stem cell derived from the BFU-E. It has a high concentration of EPO membrane receptors and with EPO stimulation transforms into the earliest recognizable erythroid precursor, the pronormoblast.

CH50 - functional hemolytic titration assay to measure lysis, the endpoint of complement activation. It measures the amount of patient serum required to lyse 50% of a standardized concentration of antibody-sensitized SRBC. Because all complement proteins are required for lysis to occur, any single complement factor deficiency causes a negative reaction (no lysis).

Charcot-Leyden crystals - crystals formed from eosinophil granules; found in tissues with large numbers of eosinophils.

Cheidak-Higashi anomaly - multisystem disorder inherited in an autosomal recessive fashion and characterized by recurrent infections, hepatospleomegaly, partial albinism, and CNS abnormalities; neutrophil chemotaxis and killing of organisms is impaired. There are giant cytoplasmic granular inclusions in leukocytes and platelets.

Chemotaxins - chemical messengers that cause migration of cells in one direction. Also called *chemokines*.

Chimerism - state of being of cells from two different zygotes expressed in one individual.

Chloride shift - phenomenon in which a plasma Cl- diffuses into the erythrocyte when a free bicarbonate iron diffuses out of the erythrocyte into the plasma.

Cholecystitis - inflammation of the gallbladder.

Cholelithiasis - formation of calculi or bilestones in the gallbladder or bile duct.

Chromatid - structure of DNA during G_0 and G_1 of the cell cycle. After S-phase, DNA has replicated, and the chromosome consists of two parallel, identical chromatids held together at the centromere.

Chromogenic assay - spectrophotometric measurement of an enzyme's activity based on the release of a colored pigment following enzymatic cleavage of the pigment-producing substrate (chromogen).

Chromosome - nuclear structure seen during mitosis and meiosis consisting of supercoiled DNA with histone and nonhistone proteins. It consists of two identical (sister) chromatids attached at the centromere.

Chronic basophilic leukemia - rare myeloproliferative disease (MPD), also referred to as *atypical MPD*. There is an extreme increase in basophils in the peripheral blood. Cell of origin is a bipotential progenitor cell capable of differentiation into either basophil or eosinophil lineages or differentiation into basophil or mast cell lineages

Chronic eosinophilic leukemia - clonal eosinophilia with an HES phenotype. It is Ph chromosome and has a persistent eosinophilia of $>1.5 \times 10^9$/L. There is no evidence of clonality or $> 2\%$ blasts in the peripheral blood.

Chronic idiopathic thrombocytopenic purpura (ITP) - immune form of thromboyctopenia that occurs most often in young adults and lasts longer than 6 months.

Chronic lymphocytic leukemia (CLL) - lymphoproliferative disorder characterized by a neoplastic growth of lymphoid cells in the bone marrow and an extreme elevation of these cells in the peripheral blood. It is characterized by leukocytosis, $<20\%$ blasts, and a predominance of mature lymphoid cells.

Chronic idiopathic myelofibrosis (CIMF) - myeloproliferative disorder characterized by excessive proliferation of all cell lines as well as progressive bone marrow fibrosis and blood cell production at sites other than the bone marrow, such as the liver and spleen. Also called *agnogenic myeloid metaplasia, myelofibrosis with myeloid metaplasia, and primary myelofibrosis*.

Chronic myelogenous leukemia (CML) - myeloproliferative disorder characterized by a neoplastic growth of primarily myeloid cells in the bone marrow and an extreme elevation of these cells in the peripheral blood. There are two phases to the disease: chronic and blast crisis. In the chronic phase, there are less than 20% blasts in the bone marrow or peripheral blood, whereas in the blast crisis phase, there are more than 20% blasts. Individuals with this disease have the BCR/ABL translocation, which codes for a unique P210 protein. Also referred to as *chronic granulocytic leukemia (CGL)*.

Chronic myelomonocytic leukemia (CMML) - subgroup of the myelodysplastic syndromes. There is anemia and a variable total leukocyte count. An absolute monocytosis ($>1 \times 10^9$/L) is present;

immature erythrocytes and granulocytes may also be present. There are less than 5% blasts in the peripheral blood. The bone marrow is hypercellular with proliferation of abnormal myelocytes, promonocytes, and monoblasts, and there are $<20\%$ blasts.

Chronic neutrophilic leukemia - myeloproliferative disorder (MPD) characterized by a sustained increase in neutrophils in the peripheral blood with a slight shift to the left. The Ph chromosome and BCR/ABL translocation are absent.

Chronic nonspherocytic hemolytic anemia - group of chronic anemias characterized by premature erythrocyte destruction. Spherocytes are not readily found when differentiating these anemias from hereditary spherocytosis.

Chylous - body effusion that has a milky, opaque appearance due to the presence of lymph fluid and chylomicrons.

Circulating inhibitor (anticoagulant) - acquired pathologic protein, primarily immunoglobulins (IgG or IgM) with antibody specificity toward a factor involved in fibrin formation. Circulating inhibitors interfere with the activity of the factor. The inhibitors are associated with a number of conditions, such as hemophilia, autoimmune diseases, malignancies, certain drugs, and viral infections.

Circulating leukocyte pool - population of neutrophils actively circulating within the peripheral blood stream.

Clinical Laboratory Improvement Amendments (CLIA) - regulations that mandate standards in clinical laboratory operations and testing signed into federal law in 1988.

Clonality - presence of identical cells derived from a single progenitor. It can be detected by the identification of only one of the immunoglobulin light chains (kappa or lambda) on B cells or the presence of a population of cells with a common phenotype.

Clonogenic - giving rise to a clone of cells.

Clot - extravascular coagulation whether occurring in vitro or in blood shed into the tissues or body cavities.

Clot retraction - cohesion of a fibrin clot that requires adequate, functionally normal platelets. Retraction of the clot occurs over a period of time and results in the expression of serum and a firm mass of cells and fibrin.

Cluster analysis - analysis in which floating thresholds cluster specific cell populations together based on size and staining or absorption characteristics. With cluster analysis, an instrument is able to accommodate for shifts in abnormal cell populations from one sample to another sample.

CLSI - organization whose mission is "to develop best practices in clinical and laboratory testing and promote their use throughout the world using a consensus-driven process that balances the viewpoints of industry, government, and the healthcare professions." (http://www.clsi.org/Content/NavigationMenu/AboutCLSI/VisionMissionandValues/Vision_Mission_Value.htm)

Coagulation factors - soluble inert plasma proteins that interact to form fibrin after an injury.

Cobalamin - cobalt-containing complex that is common to all subgroups of the vitamin B_{12} group.

Codocytes - *See* Target cell.

Codon - sequence of three nucleotides that encodes a particular amino acid.

Coefficient of determination (r^2) - statistic that represents the square of the correlation coefficient. It is a measure of the strength of the relationship between two data sets.

Coefficient of variation - relative standard deviation or standard deviation expressed as a percentage of the mean for a set of data.

Cofactor - a substance of coagulation factors V and VII that function as cofactors. It is required for the conversion of specific zymogens to the active enzyme form.

Coincidence - in an electronic cell counter, a phenomenon of two or more cells crossing the sensing zone at the same time and evaluated as only one cell.

Cold agglutinin disease - condition associated with the presence of cold-reacting autoantibodies (IgM) directed against erythrocyte surface antigens. This causes clumping of the red cells at room or lower temperatures.

Colony-forming unit - visible aggregation (seen in vitro) of cells that developed from a single stem cell.

Colony-stimulating factor - cytokine that stimulates the growth of immature leukocytes in the bone marrow.

Column chromatography - laboratory separation method based on the differential distribution of a liquid or gaseous sample (mobile phase) that flows through a column of specific substance (stationary phase). Depending on the chemical characteristics of the stationary phase, the substance of interest may bind to the stationary phase and remain in the column or directly pass through the column and remain in the mobile phase. If the substance remains in the column, a second mobile phase (elution buffer) is used to release the substance from the stationary phase and allow it to pass through the column.

Committed/progenitor cells - parent or ancestor cells that differentiate into one cell line.

Common coagulation pathway - one of the three interacting pathways in the coagulation cascade. The common pathway includes three rate-limiting steps: (1) activation of factor X by the intrinsic and extrinsic pathways, (2) conversion of prothrombin to thrombin by activated factor X, and (3) cleavage of fibrinogen to fibrin.

Comparative genomic hybridization (CGH) - assay that can be used for the analysis of changes in chromosome copy number (copy number variants); also designed to analyze critical regions of the DNA for well-defined genetic abnormalities.

Compensated hemolytic disease - disorder in which the erythrocyte life span is decreased but the bone marrow is able to increase erythropoiesis enough to compensate for the decreased erythrocyte life span; anemia does not develop.

Compensation - process of adjusting the settings on the flow cytometer or performing a mathematical correction for overlap of light emitted by several fluorochromes. The is done either before or after the data are collected.

Competency assessment - mechanism of assessing the requisite ability of testing personnel to perform a given laboratory procedure. This includes recognition of specimen collection errors, interpretation of test results to detect possible instrument or specimen problems, interpretation of quality control results, troubleshooting of instrument or specimen problems, and proper reporting of results.

Complement - any of the 11 serum proteins that causes lysis of the cell membrane when sequentially activated.

Complementary DNA - synthetic DNA transcribed from an RNA template by the enzyme reverse transcriptase. Also known as *cDNA*.

Complete blood count (CBC) - hematology screening test that includes the white blood cell (WBC) count, red blood cell (RBC) count, hemoglobin, hematocrit, and, often, platelet count. It may also include red cell indices.

Compression syndrome - altered physiological function of an organ or tissue due to impingement by an abnormal mass.

Compound heterozygote - individual possessing two different abnormal alleles of a gene.

Conditioning regimen - high-dose chemotherapy and/or irradiation given to the patient before stem cell transplantation.

Congenital - present at birth.

Congenital aberration - chromosome aberration (either numerical or structural) that is present at the time of birth in all cell lines or in several cell lines in the case of mosaicism.

Congenital amegakaryocytic thrombocytopenia (CAMT) - condition present at birth with decreased marrow megakaryocytes and peripheral blood thrombocytopenia, which eventually converts into bone marrow failure and aplastic anemia. Most cases are caused by mutations of the gene for the thrombopoietin receptor (c-*mpl*).

Congenital Heinz body hemolytic anemia - inherited disorder characterized by anemia due to decreased erythrocyte life span. Erythrocyte hemolysis results from the precipitation of hemoglobin in the form of Heinz bodies, which damage the cell membrane and causes cell rigidity.

Congenital thrombocytopenia with radioulnar synostosis (CTRUS) - congenital disorder presenting with decreased marrow megakaryocytes and peripheral blood thrombocytopenia, which eventually converts into bone marrow failure and aplastic anemia. Most cases caused by mutations within the *HOXA11* gene (which codes for a regulatory protein involved in the development of hematopoietic and bone tissue).

Consolidation therapy - second phase of cancer chemotherapy whose function is to damage or kill those malignant cells that were not destroyed during the induction phase.

Constitutional aberrations - genetic aberrations present in every cell in a patient's body.

Consumption coagulopathy - *See* Disseminated intravascular coagulation

Contact group - group of coagulation factors in the intrinsic pathway involved with the initial activation of the coagulation system. It requires contact with a negatively charged surface for activity. These factors include factors XII, XI, prekallikrein, and high-molecular-weight kininogen.

Continuous flow analysis - automated method of analyzing blood cells that allows measurement of cellular characteristics as the individual cells flow singly through a laser beam.

Contour gating - subclassification of cell populations based on two characteristics such as size (x-axis) and nuclear density (y-axis) and the frequency (z-axis) of that characterized cell type. This information is used to create a three-dimensional plot. A line is drawn along the valley between two peaks to separate two cell populations.

Correlation coefficient (r) - determines the distribution of data about the estimated linear regression line.

Coverglass smear - blood smear prepared by placing a drop of blood in the center of one cove glass, then placing a second cover glass on top of the blood at a 45° angle to the first cover glass. The two cover glasses are pulled apart, creating two cover glass smears.

CRM– - cross-reacting material negative; a clotting factor that is defective and can be identified both by abnormal functional and immunologic tests.

CRM + - cross-reacting material positive; a functionally defective clotting factor that can, however, be identified by immunologic means.

Crossover - reciprocal exchange of genetic material between chromatids that normally occurs in meiosis to increase the diversity of the species.

Cryoprecipitate - preparation of proteins containing fibrinogen, von Willebrand factor, and factor VIII prepared by freezing and thawing plasma and used for replacement therapy in patients with hemophilia A and von Willebrand disease.

Cryopreservation - maintenance of the viability of cells by storing them at very low temperatures.

Cryosupernatant - product that lacks large VWF multimers that are present in fresh frozen plasma yet still contains the VWF cleaving protease missing in thrombotic thrombocytopenic purpura (TTP) patients.

Culling - filtering and destroying senescent/damaged red cells by the spleen.

Cyanosis - bluish color of the skin and mucous membranes that develops as a result of excess deoxygenated hemoglobin in the blood.

Cyclins/Cdks - kinase proteins that regulate the transition between the various phases of the cell cycle.

Cytochemistry - chemical staining procedures used to identify various constituents (enzymes and proteins) within white blood cells. It is useful in differentiating blasts in acute leukemia, especially when morphologic differentiation on Romanowsky-stained smears is impossible.

Cytogenetic remission - absence of recognized cytogenetic abnormalities associated with a given neoplastic disease (previously identified in a patient) after therapy.

Cytokine - protein produced by many cell types that modulates the function of other cell types. The group includes interleukins, colony-stimulating factors, and interferons.

Cytomegalovirus (CMV) - herpes virus that replicates only in human cells. The virus has a widespread distribution and is spread by close contact with an infected person.

Cytoplasm - protoplasm of a cell outside the nucleus.

 D

DcytB - duodenal cytochrome –B reductase; ferric reductase that reduces ferric iron to the ferrous state at the enterocyte brush border.

D-dimer - cross-linked fibrin degradation product that is the result of plasmin's proteolytic activity on a fibrin clot. The presence of D-dimers is specific for fibrinolysis.

Decay accelerating factor - regulating complement protein found on cell membranes that accelerates decay (dissociation) of membrane bound complement (C3bBb). An absence of this factor leads to excessive sensitivity of these cells to complement lysis.

Deep vein thrombosis (DVT) - formation of a thrombus, or blood clot, in the deep veins (usually a leg vein).

Delayed bleeding - symptom of severe coagulation factor disorders in which a wound bleeds a second time after initial stoppage of bleeding. This occurs because the primary hemostatic plug is not adequately stabilized by the formation of fibrin.

Delta check - comparison of current hematology results to the most recently reported previous result for a given patient. This check helps detect certain random errors.

Delta (δ) storage pool disease - autosomal dominant disease characterized by a decrease in dense granules in the platelets.

Demarcation membrane system - cytoplasmic membrane system in the megakaryocyte that separates small areas of the cell's cytoplasm. These areas eventually become the platelets.

Demyelination - destruction, removal, or loss of the lipid substance that forms a myelin sheath around the axons of nerve fibers. It is a characteristic finding in vitamin B_{12} deficiency.

Dense bodies - platelet storage granules containing nonmetabolic ADP, calcium, and serotonin along with other compounds that are released from activated platelets.

Dense tubular system (DTS) - membrane in the platelet that originates from the smooth endoplasmic reticulum of the megakaryocyte. It is one of the storage sites for calcium ions within platelets. The channels of the DTS do not connect with the surface of the platelet.

Densitometry - laboratory testing method that determines the pattern and concentration of protein fractions separated by electrophoresis. It measures the amount of light absorbed by each dye-bound protein fraction as the fraction passes a slit through which light is transmitted. The amount of light absorbed (optical density) is directly proportional to the protein's concentration.

Deoxyhemoglobin - hemoglobin without oxygen.

Diamond-Blackfan anemia - congenital, progressive erythrocyte hypoplasia that occurs in very young children. There is no leukopenia or thrombocytopenia.

Diapedese - passage of blood cells through the unruptured capillary wall. For leukocytes, this involves active locomotion.

Differentiation - appearance of different properties in cells that were initially equivalent.

2,3-diphosphoglycerate (2,3-DPG) - product of the glycolytic pathway that affects the oxygen affinity of hemoglobin. It serves in the biochemical feedback system that regulates the amount of oxygen released to the tissues. As the concentration of 2,3-DPG increases, hemoglobin's affinity for oxygen decreases and more oxygen is released to the tissue. See *2,3-bisphosphoglycerate (2,3-BPG)*.

Diploid - number of chromosomes in somatic cells that is 2n. For human cells, 2n = 46.

Direct antiglobulin test (DAT) - laboratory test used to detect the presence of antibody and/or complement that is attached to the erythrocyte. The test uses antibody directed against human immunoglobulin and/or complement. Also called the antihuman globulin (AHG) test.

Disseminated intravascular coagulation (DIC) - complex condition in which the normal coagulation process is altered (resulting in systemic rather than localized activation) by an underlying condition. Resulting complications may include thrombotic occlusion of vessels, bleeding, and ultimately organ failure. DIC is initiated by multiple triggers, most involving damage to the endothelial lining of vessels.

DMT1 - integral membrane protein that transports ferrous iron across the apical enterocyte plasma membrane.

DNA (deoxyribonucleic acid) - blueprint that cells use to catalog, express, and propagate information. DNA is the fundamental substance of heredity that is carried from one generation to the next. It is a double-stranded molecule composed of complementary nucleotide sequences. The two strands of DNA are held together by hydrogen bonds formed according to the following rules of complementary nucleotide pairing: G bonds with C; A bonds with T; other combinations cannot bond.

DNA index (DI) - DNA content of tumor cells relative to a diploid population of cells. It is calculated as the DNA content of cells in the tumor in the G0/G1 phase of the cell cycle relative to the DNA content of G0/G1 cells in a diploid control.

DNA sequencing - Determining the nucleotide sequence in a segment of DNA by replicating the DNA strands and monitoring the order in which labeled nucleotides are added to the new strands.

Döhle bodies - oval aggregates of rough endoplasmic reticulum that stains light gray blue (with Romanowsky stain) found within the cytoplasm of neutophils and eosinophils. It is associated with severe bacterial infection, pregnancy, burns, cancer, aplastic anemia, and toxic states.

Donath-Landsteiner antibody - biphasic IgG antibody associated with paroxysmal cold hemoglobinuria. The antibody reacts with erythrocytes in capillaries at temperatures below 15°C and fixes complement to the cell membrane. Upon warming, the terminal complement components on erythrocytes are activated, causing cell hemolysis.

Downey cell - outdated term used to describe morphologic variations of the reactive lymphocyte.

Drug-induced hemolytic anemia - hemolytic anemia precipitated by ingestion of certain drugs. The process may be immune mediated or nonimmune mediated.

Dry tap - description of situation when bone marrow cannot be aspirated. This can be caused by inadequate technique or alterations in the bone marrow architecture such as extensive fibrosis or very increased cellularity.

Dura mater - dense membrane covering the central nervous system; outermost layer of the meninges.

Dutcher bodies - intranuclear membrane-bound inclusion bodies found in plasma cells. The body stains with periodic acid-Schiff (PAS) indicating it contains glycogen or glycoprotein. The appearance is finely distributed chromatin, nucleoli, or intranuclear inclusions.

Dysfibrinogenemia - hereditary condition in which the fibrinogen molecule has a structural alteration.

Dyshematopoiesis - abnormal formation and/or development of blood cells within the bone marrow.

Dyspepsia - symptoms due to abnormalities in the process of digestion.

Dysplasia - abnormal cell development.

Dyspoiesis - abnormal development of blood cells frequently characterized by asynchrony in nuclear to cytoplasmic maturation and/or abnormal granule development.

 E

Ecchymosis - bruise (bluish-black discoloration of the skin) that is larger than 3mm in diameter caused by bleeding from arterioles into subcutaneous tissues without disruption of intact skin.

Echinocyte - spiculated erythrocyte with short, equally spaced projections over the entire outer surface of the cell.

Edematous - the swelling of body tissues due to the accumulation of tissue fluid.

Effector lymphocytes - antigen-stimulated lymphocytes that mediate the efferent arm of the immune response.

Efficacy - ability to produce the desired effect (e.g., anticoagulation).

Effusion - abnormal accumulation of fluid.

Egress - act of going out or exiting. The term is used to describe the exit of blood cells from the blood to the tissue.

ELISA (Enzyme linked immunosorbent assay) - immunological examination that employs an enzyme linked to an antibody or antigen as a marker for the detection of a specific protein. When a substrate specific for the enzyme label is added to the test system, the colored product that results is proportional to the concentration of the protein in the test sample.

Elliptocyte - abnormally shaped erythrocyte. The cell is an oval to elongated ellipsoid with a central area of pallor and hemoglobin at both ends. Also known as *ovalocyte, pencil cell,* and *cigar cell.*

Embolism - blockage of an artery by embolus, usually by a portion of blood clot but can be other foreign matter, resulting in obstruction of blood flow to the tissues.

Embolus - piece of blood clot or other foreign matter that circulates in the blood stream and usually becomes lodged in a small vessel obstructing blood flow.

Endomitosis - rounds of nuclear DNA synthesis without nuclear or cytoplasmic division.

Endoplasmic reticulum (ER) - cytoplasmic organelle in eukaryocytic cells that consists of a network of interconnected tubes and flattened membranous sacs. If the ER has ribosomes attached, it is known as *granular* or *rough endoplasmic reticulum (RER)*, and if ribosomes are not attached, it is known as *smooth endoplasmic reticulum (SER)*.

Endosteum - membrane that lines the bone medullary cavity that contains the bone marrow.

Endothelial cells - flat cells that line the cavities of the blood and lymphatic vessels, heart, and other related body cavities.

Endothelial cell protein C receptor (EPCR) - receiver on the membrane of endothelial cells of larger vessels that binds and immobilizes protein C, augmenting the activation of protein C by the thrombin:thrombomodulin complex.

Engraftment - homing of infused stem cells into the bone marrow microenvironment resulting in hematopoietic recovery.

Enzyme - protein that catalyzes a specific biochemical reaction but is not itself altered in the process.

Eosinophil - mature granulocyte cell characterized by the presence of large acidophilic granules. These granules are pink to orange pink with Romanowsky stains. The cell is 12–17 μm in diameter, and the nucleus has 2–3 lobes. Granules contain acid phosphatase, glycuronidase cathepsins, ribonuclease, arylsulfatase, peroxidase, phospholipids, and basic proteins. Eosinophils have a concentration of less than 0.45×10^9/L in the peripheral blood. The cell membrane has receptors for IgE and histamine.

Eosinophilia - increase in the concentration of eosinophils in the peripheral blood ($>0.5 \times 10^9$/L). It is associated with parasitic infection, allergic conditions, hypersensitivity reactions, cancer, and chronic inflammatory states.

Epigenetics - heritable changes in gene expression not due to changes in DNA sequence.

Epistaxis - hemorrhage from the nose.

Epitope - structural portion of an antigen that reacts with a specific antibody. Also called *antigenic determinant.*

Epstein-Barr virus (EBV) - agent that attaches to B lymphocytes by a specific receptor designated CD21 on the B lymphocyte membrane surface.

Error detection - laboratory's multirule quality control procedure to detect a true error in the testing system and reject the control run.

Erythroblastic island - composite of erythroid cells in the bone marrow that surrounds a central macrophage. These groups of cells are usually disrupted when bone marrow smears are made but may be found in erythroid hyperplasia. The central macrophage is thought to transfer iron to the developing cells. The least mature cells are closest to the center of the island and the more mature cells are on the periphery.

Erythroblastosis fetalis - hemolytic anemia occurring in newborns as a result of fetal-maternal blood group incompatibility involving the Rh factor of ABO blood groups. It is caused by an antigen–antibody reaction in the newborn when maternal antibodies traverse the placenta and attach to antigens on the fetal cells.

Erythrocyte - red blood cell (RBC) that has matured to the nonnucleated stage. The cell is about 7 μm in diameter. It contains the respiratory pigment hemoglobin, which readily combines with oxygen to form oxyhemoglobin. The cell develops from the pluripotential stem cell in the bone marrow under the influence of the hematopoietic growth factor erythropoietin and is released to the peripheral blood as a reticulocyte. The average life span is about 120 days, after which the cell is removed by cells in the mononuclear-phagocyte system. The average concentration is about 5×10^{12}/L for males and 4.5×10^{12}/L for females.

Erythrocytosis - abnormal increase in the number of circulating erythrocytes as measured by the erythrocyte count, hemoglobin, or hematocrit.

Erythron - summation of the stages of erythrocytes in the marrow, peripheral blood, and within vascular areas of specific organs such as the spleen.

Erythrophagocytosis - phagocytosis of an erythrocyte by a histiocyte; the erythrocyte can be seen within the cytoplasm of the histiocyte as a pink globule or, if digested, as a clear vacuole on stained bone marrow or peripheral blood smears.

Erythropoiesis - formation and maturation of erythrocytes in the bone marrow. It is under the influence of the hematopoietic growth factor erythropoietin.

Erythropoietin - hormone secreted by the kidney that regulates erythrocyte production by stimulating the stem cells of the bone mar-

row to mature into erythrocytes. Its primary effect is on the committed stem cell CFU-E.

Essential thrombocythemia - myeloproliferative disorder affecting primarily the megakaryocytic element in the bone marrow. There is extreme thrombocytosis in the blood (usually $>1,000 \times 10^9$/L). Also called *primary thrombocythemia, hemorrhagic thrombocythemia,* and *megakaryocytic leukemia.*

Euchromatin - region of the chromosome that contains genetically active DNA, is lighter staining, and replicates early in S phase of the cell cycle. *See* heterochromatin.

Evan's syndrome - condition characterized by a warm autoimmune hemolytic anemia and concurrent severe thrombocytopenia.

Exchange transfusion - simultaneous withdrawal of blood and infusion with compatible blood.

Exon - protein-coding DNA sequence of a gene.

Extracellular matrix - noncellular components of the hematopoietic microenvironment in the bone marrow.

Extramedullary erythropoiesis - red blood cell production occurring outside the bone marrow.

Extramedullary hematopoiesis - formation and development of blood cells at a site other than the bone marrow.

Extravascular - occurring outside of the blood vessels.

Extrinsic pathway - one of the three interacting pathways in the coagulation cascade. The extrinsic pathway is initiated when tissue factor comes into contact with blood and forms a complex with factor VII. The complex activates factor X. The term *extrinsic* is used because the pathway requires tissue factor, a factor extrinsic to blood.

Extrinsic Xase - complex of tissue factor and factor VIIa that forms when a vessel is injured.

Exudate - effusion that is formed by increased vascular permeability and/or decreased lymphatic resorption. This indicates a true pathologic state in the anatomic region, usually either infection or tumor.

 F

FAB classification - current internationally accepted scheme for the classification of the acute leukemias. Cell identification is based on cell identification by a combination of bright-light microscopy and cytochemical testing. (FAB = French-American-British)

Factor V$_{Leiden}$ - mutant form of F-V in which Arg 506 is replaced with Gln. This makes the molecule resistant to inactivation by activated protein C.

Factor VIII:C assay - method that determines the amount of F-VIII.

Factor VIII concentrate - lyophilized preparation of concentrated F-VIII used for replacement therapy of F-VIII in patients with hemophilia A.

Factor VIII inhibitor - IgG immunoglobulin with antibody specificity to F-VIII. The inhibitor inactivates the factor. The antibodies are time and temperature dependent. F-VIII inhibitors are associated with hemophilia.

Factor VIII/vWF complex - plasma form of VWF associated with F-VIII.

Faggot cell - cell in which there is a large collection of Auer rods and/or phi bodies.

False rejection - rejection of a control run that is not truly out of control. The result falling outside the control limits or violating a Westgard rule is due to the inherent imprecision of the test method.

Fanconi anemia (FA) - autosomal recessive disorder characterized by chromosomal instability. Patients have a complex assortment of congenital anomalies in addition to a progressive bone marrow hypoplasia.

Favism - sensitivity to a species of bean, *Vicia faba*. The condition is commonly found in Sicily and Sardinia in individuals who have inherited glucose-6-phosphate dehydrogenase deficiency. It is characterized by fever, acute hemolytic anemia, vomiting, and diarrhea after ingestion of the bean or inhalation of the plant pollen.

Fee for service - payment method for health care in which consumers choose their own health care providers and the provider determines the fees for the services. The fees may be paid by the patient or a third-party payer.

Ferritin - iron-phosphorus-protein compound formed when iron complexes with the protein apoferritin. It is a storage form of iron found primarily in the bone marrow, spleen, and liver. Small amounts can be found in the peripheral blood proportional to that found in the bone marrow.

Ferroportin - basolateral tranporter protein of ferrous iron across the basolateral membrane (also known as *IREG1*). It is the only known cellular exporter of iron.

Fibrin degradation products (FDP) - breakdown products of fibrin or fibrinogen that are produced when plasmin's proteolytic action cleaves these molecules. The four main products are fragments X, Y, D, and E. The presence of fibrin degradation products indicates either fibrinolysis or fibrinogenolysis.

Fibrin monomer - structure resulting when thrombin cleaves the A and B fibrinopeptides from the α and β chains of fibrinogen.

Fibrinogen group - group of coagulation factors that are activated by thrombin and are consumed during the formation of fibrin and therefore absent from serum. It includes factors I, V, VIII, and XIII. Also called *consumable group*.

Fibrinolysis - breakdown of fibrin.

Fibrin polymer - complex of covalently bonded fibrin monomers. The bonds between glutamine and lysine residues are formed between terminal domains of γ chains and polar appendages of α chains of neighboring residues.

Fibronectin - extracellular-matrix glycoprotein capable of binding heparin.

Fibrosis - abnormal formation of fibrous tissue.

Flame cell - plasma cell with reddish-purple cytoplasm. The red tinge is caused by the presence of a glycoprotein and the purple by ribosomes.

Flow chamber - specimen handling area of a flow cytometer where cells are forced into single file and directed in front of the laser beam.

Fluorescence in situ hybridization (FISH) - technique in which whole chromosomes (metaphase or interphase) are hybridized to a complementary probe that is labeled with a fluorochrome and visualized by microscopy.

Fluorochrome - molecule excited by light of one wavelength and emits light of a different wavelength.

Forward light scatter - laser light scattered in a forward direction in a flow cytometer. Forward light scatter is related to particle size (e.g., large cells produce more forward scatter).

Free erythrocyte protoporphyrin (FEP) - protoporphyrin within the erythrocyte that is not complexed with iron. The concentration of FEP increases in iron-deficient states. It is now known that in the absence of iron, erythrocyte protoporphyrin combines with zinc to form zinc protoporphyrin (ZPP).

Fresh frozen plasma (FFP) - colorless fluid portion of blood that is frozen at –18° C or colder within 6 hours of collection. It is formed by removal of all cellular components.

F-test - statistical tool used to compare features of two or more sets of data.

Functional hyposplenism - reduced splenic function due not to the loss of splenic tissue but to the accumulation of cells sequestered in the spleen.

▶ **G**

Gammopathy - abnormal condition in which there is an increase in serum immunoglobulins.

Gating - in flow cytometry, isolating cells with the same light scattering or fluorescence properties by placing a gate around them electronically.

Gene - functional segment of DNA that serves as a template for RNA transcription and protein translation. Regulatory sequences control gene expression so that only a small fraction of the estimated 100,000 genes is ever transcribed by a given cell.

Gene cluster - group of closely linked genes that can be affected as a group.

Gene promoter - DNA sequence that RNA polymerase binds to in order to begin transcription of a gene.

Gene rearrangement - process in which segments of DNA are cut and spliced to produce new DNA sequences. During normal lymphocyte development, rearrangement of the immunoglobulin genes and the T cell receptor genes results in new gene sequences that encode the antibody and surface antigen receptor proteins necessary for immune function.

Gene therapy - introduction of a normally functioning gene into the appropriate target cell of an affected individual.

Genome - total aggregate of inherited genetic material. In humans, the genome consists of 3 billion base pairs of DNA divided among 46 chromosomes including 22 pairs of autosomes numbered 1–22 and the two sex chromosomes.

Genomics - study of all nucleotide sequences, including structural genes, regulatory sequences, and noncoding DNA segments, in the chromosomes of an organism.

Genotype - genetic constitution of an individual, often referring to a particular gene locus.

Germinal center - lightly staining center of a lymphoid follicle where B cell activation occurs.

Germline - cell lineage that consists of germ cells.

Glanzmann's thrombasthenia - rare hereditary platelet disorder characterized by a genetic mutation in one of the genes coding for the glycoproteins IIb or IIIa and resulting in the inability of platelets to aggregate.

Global testing - specialized global instrumentation that provides analysis on the entire hemostatic process including coagulation, anticoagulant effects, fibrin formation and stabilization, clot retraction, and fibrinolysis on a whole blood sample.

Globin - protein portion of the hemoglobin molecule.

Glossitis - inflammation of the tongue.

Glucose-6-phosphate-dehydrogenase (G6PD) - enzyme within erythrocytes that is important in carbohydrate metabolism. It dehydrogenates glucose-6-phosphate to form 6-phosphogluconate in the hexose monophosphate shunt. This reaction produces NADPH from NADP and provides reducing power to the erythrocyte, protecting the cell from oxidant injury.

Glutathione - tripeptide that takes up and gives off hydrogen and prevents oxidant damage to the hemoglobin molecule. A deficiency of glutathione is associated with hemolytic anemia.

Glycocalin - portion of glycoprotein Ib of the platelet membrane that is external to the platelet surface and contains binding sites for von Willebrand factor and thrombin.

Glycocalyx - amorphous coat of glycoproteins and mucopolysaccharides covering the surface of cells, particularly the platelets and endothelial cells.

Glycolysis - anaerobic conversion of glucose to lactate and pyruvic acid resulting in the production of energy (ATP).

Glycoprotein Ib - glycoprotein of the platelet surface that contains the receptor for von Willebrand factor and is critical for initial adhesion of platelets to collagen after an injury.

Glycoprotein IIb/IIIa complex - complex of membrane proteins on the platelet surface that is functional only after activation by agonists and then becomes a receptor for fibrinogen and von Willebrand factor. It is essential for platelet aggregation.

Glycosylated hemoglobin - hemoglobin that has glucose irreversibly attached to the terminal amino acid of the beta chains. Also called *HbA$_{1c}$*.

Golgi apparatus - cytoplasmic organelle composed of flattened sacs or cisternae arranged in stacks. In secretory cells, it functions in concentrating and packaging secretory products. It does not stain with Romanowsky stains and appears as a clear area usually adjacent to the nucleus.

Gower hemoglobin - embryonic hemoglobin detectable in the yolk sac for up to 8 weeks gestation. It is composed of two zeta (ζ) chains and two epsilon (ε) chains.

Graft-versus-host disease (GVHD) - tissue injury secondary to HLA-mismatch grafts resulting from immunocompetent donor T lymphocytes that recognize HLA antigens on the host cells and initiate a secondary inflammatory response.

Graft versus leukemia - favorable effect seen when immunocompetent donor T cells present in the allograft destroy the recipient's leukemic cells.

Granulocytopenia - decrease in granulocytes below 1.8×10^9/L.

Granulocytosis - increase in granulocytes above 7.0×10^9/L. It is usually seen in bacterial infections, inflammation, metabolic intoxication, drug intoxication, and tissue necrosis.

Granulomatous - distinctive pattern of chronic reaction in which the predominant cell type is an activated macrophage with epithelial-like (epithelioid) appearance.

Gray platelet syndrome (alpha storage pool disease) - rare hereditary platelet disorder characterized by the lack of platelet alpha granules.

 H

Hairy cell - neoplastic cell of hairy cell leukemia characterized by circumferential, cytoplasmic, hairlike projections.

Ham test - specific laboratory test for paroxysmal nocturnal hemoglobinuria (PHN). When erythrocytes from a patient with PNH are incubated in acidified serum, the cells lyse due to complement activation. Also called *acid-serum lysis test*.

Haploid - number of chromosomes in a gamete that is n; consists of one of each of the autosomes and one of the sex chromosomes. For human cells, n = 23.

Haplotype - one of the two alleles at a genetic locus.

Haptoglobin - serum α_2-globulin glycoprotein that transports free plasma hemoglobin to the liver.

HDFN - *See* hemolytic disease of the fetus and newborn.

Health Insurance Portability and Accountability Act (HIPAA) - law that mandates health care entities to establish measures that ensure the confidentiality of patient information.

Heinz bodies - inclusions in the erythrocyte composed of denatured or precipitated hemoglobin. It appears as purple-staining body on supravitally stained (crystal violet) smears.

HELLP syndrome - obstetric complication characterized by hemolysis (H), elevated liver enzymes (EL), and a low platelet count (LP). The etiology and pathogenesis are not well understood.

Helmet cell - abnormally shaped erythrocyte with one or several notches and projections on either end that look like horns. The shape is caused by trauma to the erythrocyte. Also called *keratocyte* and *horn-shaped cells*.

Hematocrit - packed cell volume of erythrocytes in a given volume of blood following centrifugation of the blood. It is expressed as a percentage of total blood volume or as a liter of erythrocytes per liter of blood (L/L). Also referred to as *packed cell volume* (PCV).

Hematogones - precursor B lymphocytes present normally in the bone marrow.

Hematologic remission - absence of neoplastic cells in the peripheral blood and bone marrow and the return to normal levels of hematologic parameters.

Hematology - study of formed cellular blood elements.

Hematoma - localized collection of blood under the skin or in other organs caused by a break in the wall of a blood vessel.

Hematopoiesis - production and development of blood cells normally occurring in the bone marrow under the influence of hematopoietic growth factors.

Hematopoietic microenvironment - specialized, localized environment in hematopoietic organs that supports the development of hematopoietic cells.

Hematopoietic progenitor cell - hematopoietic precursor cell developmentally located between stem cells and the morphologically recognizable blood precursor cells; includes multilineage and unilineage cell types.

Hematopoietic stem cell - hematopoietic precursor cell capable of giving rise to all lineages of blood cells.

Heme - nonprotein portion of hemoglobin and myoglobin that contains iron nestled in a hydrophobic pocket of a porphyrin ring (ferroprotoporphyrin). It is responsible for the characteristic color of hemoglobin.

Hemochromatosis - clinical condition resulting from abnormal iron metabolism characterized by accumulation of iron deposits in body tissues.

Hemoconcentration - increased concentration of blood components due to loss of plasma from the blood.

Hemoglobin - intracellular erythrocyte protein that is responsible for the transport of oxygen and carbon dioxide between the lungs and body tissues.

Hemoglobin distribution width - measure of the distribution of hemoglobin within an erythrocyte population. It is derived from the hemoglobin histogram generated by the Bayer/Technicon instruments.

Hemoglobin electrophoresis - method of identifying hemoglobins based on differences in their electrical charges.

Hemoglobinemia - presence of excessive hemoglobin in the plasma.

Hemoglobinopathy - disease that results from an inherited abnormality of the structure or synthesis of the globin portion of the hemoglobin molecule.

Hemoglobinuria - presence of hemoglobin in the urine.

Hemojuvelin (HJV) - glycosylphosphatidylnositol-anchored protein that has been shown to regulate hepcidin expression.

Hemolysis - destruction of erythrocytes resulting in the release of hemoglobin. In hemolytic anemia, this term refers to the premature destruction of erythrocytes.

Hemolysis, elevated liver enzymes and low platelet (HELLP) syndrome - severe form of preeclampsia characterized by hemolysis, elevated liver enzymes, and low platelet count. It may be a cause of microangiopathic hemolytic anemia.

Hemolytic anemia - disorder characterized by a decreased erythrocyte concentration due to premature destruction of the erythrocyte.

Hemolytic disease of the fetus and newborn (HDFN) - alloimmunne disease characterized by fetal red blood cell destruction as a result of incompatibility between maternal and fetal blood groups.

Hemolytic transfusion reaction - interaction of foreign (nonself) erythrocyte antigens and plasma antibodies due to the transfusion of blood. There are two types of transfusion reactions: immediate (within 24 hours) and delayed (occurring 2 to 14 days after transfusion).

Hemolytic uremic syndrome (HUS) - disorder characterized by a combination of microangiopathic hemolytic anemia, acute renal failure, and thrombocytopenia.

Hemopexin - plasma glycoprotein (β-globulin) that binds the heme molecule in plasma in the absence of haptoglobin.

Hemophilia A - sex-linked (X-linked) hereditary hemorrhagic disorder caused by a genetic mutation of the gene coding for coagulation F-VIII.

Hemophilia B - sex-linked (X-linked) hereditary hemorrhagic disorder caused by a genetic mutation of the gene coding for coagulation F-IX.

Hemorrhage - loss of a large amount of blood either internally or externally.

Hemorrhagic disease of the newborn - severe bleeding disorder in the first week of life caused by deficiencies of the vitamin K-dependent clotting factors due to vitamin K deficiency.

Hemosiderin - water insoluble, heterogeneous iron–protein complex found primarily in the cytoplasm of cells (normoblasts and histocytes in the bone marrow, liver, and spleen); the major long-term storage form of iron. It is readily visible microscopically in unstained tissue specimens as irregular aggregates of golden yellow to brown granules. It may be visualized with Prussian-blue stain as blue granules. The granules are normally distributed randomly or diffuse.

Hemosiderinuria - presence of iron (hemosiderin) in the urine as a result of intravascular hemolysis and disintegration of renal tubular cells.

Hemostasis - localized, controlled process that results in arrest of bleeding after an injury.

Heparin - polysaccharide that inhibits coagulation of blood by preventing thrombin from cleaving fibrinogen to form fibrin. It is commercially available in the form of a sodium salt for therapeutic use as an anticoagulant.

Heparin associated thrombocytopenia (HAT) - thrombocytopenia associated with heparin therapy in some patients due to a nonimmune-mediated direct platelet activation effect.

Heparin-induced thrombocytopenia (HIT) - thrombocytopenia associated with heparin therapy in some patients due to an immune-mediated destruction of platelets due to heparin-dependent platelet-activating IgG antibodies produced against the platelet factor 4 (PF4)-heparin complex.

Hepcidin - master iron-regulating protein that regulates iron recycling/balance via interaction with ferroportin 1. It is a negative regulator of intestinal iron absorption.

Hephaestin - facilitates export of iron and oxidizes Fe^{++} iron to Fe^{+++} for binding to apotransferrin.

Hereditary elliptocytosis - autosomal-dominant condition characterized by the presence of increased numbers of elongated and oval erythrocytes. The abnormal shape is due to a horizontal interaction defect with abnormal spectrin, deficiency, or defect in band 4.1 or deficiency of glycophorin C and abnormal band 3.

Hereditary erythroblastic multinuclearity with positive acidified serum test (HEMPAS) - type II congenital dyserythropoietic anemia (CDA). CDA is characterized by both abnormal and ineffective erythropoiesis. Type II is distinguished by a positive acidified serum test but a negative sucrose hemolysis test.

Hereditary pyropoikilocytosis (HPP) - rare but severe hemolytic anemia inherited as an autosomal recessive disorder. It is characterized by marked erythrocyte fragmentation. The defect is most likely a spectrin abnormality in the erythrocyte cytoskeleton.

Hereditary spherocytosis - chronic hemolytic anemia caused by an inherited erythrocyte membrane disorder. The vertical interaction defect is most commonly due to a combined spectrin and ankyrin deficiency. The defect causes membrane instability and progressive membrane loss. Secondary to membrane loss, the cells become spherocytes and are prematurely destroyed in the spleen. The condition is usually inherited as an autosomal dominant trait.

Hereditary stomatocytosis - rare hemolytic anemia inherited in an autosomal dominant fashion. The erythrocyte membrane is abnormally permeable to sodium and potassium. The cell becomes overhydrated, resulting in the appearance of stomatocytes. The specific membrane abnormality has not been identified.

Hereditary xerocytosis - hereditary disorder in which the erythrocyte is abnormally permeable to sodium and potassium with an increased potassium efflux. The erythrocyte becomes dehydrated and appears as either target or spiculated cells. The cells are rigid and become trapped in the spleen.

Heterochromatin - region of the chromosome that contains genetically inactive DNA, is dark staining, and replicates late in S phase of the cell cycle.

Heterologous - refers to morphologically nonidentical chromosomes that have different gene loci.

Heterophile antibodies - antibodies that can react against a heterologous antigen that did not stimulate the antibody's production. In infectious mononucleosis, heterophile antibodies are produced in response to infection with Epstein-Barr virus and react with sheep, horse, and beef erythrocytes.

Heterozygous - different genes at a gene locus.

Hexose-monophosphate shunt - metabolic pathway that converts glucose-6-phosphate to pentose phosphate. This pathway couples oxidative metabolism with the reduction of nicotinamide adenine dinucleotide-phosphate (NADPH) and glutathione. This provides the cell with reducing power and prevents injury by oxidants.

HFE - transmembrane protein that associates with beta2-microglobulin. It binds to the transferrin receptor (TfR) on cells and regulates the interaction of the receptor with transferrin. When bound to TfR, it reduces the affinity of the receptor for iron-bound transferrin (Tf-Fe) by 5- to 10-fold. Mutations are associated with hereditary hemochromatosis.

Histogram - graphical representation of the number of cells within a defined parameter such as size.

HIV-I (human immunodeficiency virus type-I) - virus that causes acquired immunodeficiency syndrome (AIDS).

Hodgkin lymphoma (disease) - malignancy that most often arises in lymph nodes and is characterized by the presence of Reed-Sternberg cells and variants with a background of varying numbers of benign lymphocytes, plasma cells, histiocytes, and eosinophils. The origin of the malignant cell is still controversial.

Homologous - having two morphologically identical chromosomes that have identical gene loci but may have different gene alleles because one member of a homologous pair is of maternal origin and the other is of paternal origin.

Homozygous - identical genes at a gene locus.

Horizontal interactions - side-by-side interactions involving the proteins of the erythrocyte membrane.

Howell-Jolly bodies - erythrocyte inclusions composed of nuclear remnants (DNA). On Romanowsky-stained blood smears, they appear as a dark purple spherical granule usually near the periphery of the cell. They are commonly associated with megoblastic anemia and splenectomy.

Humoral immunity - immunity imparted as a result of B lymphocyte activation. The B lymphocyte differentiates to a plasma cell that produces antibodies specific to the antigen that stimulated the response.

Hybridization - process in which one nucleotide strand binds to another strand by formation of hydrogen bonds between complementary nucleotides.

Hydrodynamic focusing - phenomenon that allows cells/particles to flow in a single column due to differences in the pressures of two columns of fluid in a flow chamber of a flow cytometer. The particles are contained in an inner column of sample fluid that is surrounded by a column of stream sheath fluid. The gradient between the sample and sheath fluid keeps the fluids separate (laminar flow) and is used to control the diameter of the column of sample fluid. The central column of sample fluid is narrowed to isolate single cells that pass through a laser beam like a string of beads.

Hydrops fetalis - genetically determined hemolytic disease (thalassemia) resulting in production of an abnormal hemoglobin (hemoglobin Bart's, γ_4) that is unable to carry oxygen. No alpha(α) globin chains are synthesized.

Hypercoagulable state - condition associated with an imbalance between clot-promoting and clot-inhibiting factors. This leads to an increased risk of developing thrombosis.

Hyperdiploid - number of chromosomes per cell that is more than 2n. For human cells, this would be >46.

Hypereosinophilic syndrome - persistent blood eosinophilia over 1.5×10^9/L with tissue infiltration, absence of clonal genetic aberrations, and no apparent cause of the increase in eosinophils.

Hyperhomocysteinemia - elevated levels of homocysteine in the blood as a result of impaired homocysteine metabolism. It can be due to acquired or congenital causes. It is associated with premature atherosclerosis and arterial thrombosis.

Hyperplasia - increase in the number of cells per unit volume of tissue. This can be brought about by an increase in the number of cells replicating, an increase in the rate of replication, or prolonged survival of cells. The cells usually maintain normal size, shape, and function. The stimulus for the proliferation may be acute injury, chronic irritation, or prolonged, increased hormonal stimulation. In hematology, a hyperplastic bone marrow is one in which the proportion of hematopoietic cells to fat cells is increased.

Hypersplenism - disorder characterized by enlargement of the spleen and pancytopenia in the presence of a hyperactive bone marrow.

Hypocellularity - decreased cellularity of hematopoietic precursors in the bone marrow.

Hypochromic - lack of color; used to describe erythrocytes with an enlarged area of pallor due to a decrease in the cell's hemoglobin content. The mean corpuscular hemoglobin concentration (MCHC) and mean corpuscular hemoglobin (MCH) are decreased.

Hypodiploid - number of chromosomes per cell that is less than 2n. For human cells, this would be <46.

Hypofibrinogenemia - condition in which there is an abnormally low fibrinogen level in the peripheral blood. It may be caused by a mutation in the gene controlling the production of fibrinogen or an acquired condition in which fibrinogen is pathologically converted to fibrin.

Hypogammaglobulinemia - condition associated with a decrease in resistance to infection as a result of decreased γ-globulins (immunoglobulins) in the blood.

Hypoplasia - condition of underdeveloped tissue or organ usually caused by a decrease in the number of cells. A hypoplastic bone marrow is one in which the proportion of hematopoietic cells to fat cells is decreased.

Hypoproliferative - decreased production of any cell type.

Hypoxia - deficiency of oxygen to the cells.

 I

Idiopathic - pertaining to disorders or diseases in which the pathogenesis is unknown.

Idiopathic (or immune) thrombocytopenic purpura (ITP) - acquired condition in which the platelets are destroyed by immune mechanisms faster than the bone marrow is able to compensate. Platelets are decreased.

Immature reticulocyte fraction (IRF) - index of reticulocyte maturity provided by flow cytometry. The IRF may be helpful in evaluating bone marrow erythropoietic response to anemia, monitoring anemia, and evaluating response to therapy.

Immune hemolytic anemia - disorder caused by premature, immune-mediated destruction of erythrocytes. Diagnosis is confirmed by the demonstration of immunoglobulin (antibodies) and/or complement on the erythrocytes.

Immune thrombocytopenic purpura (ITP) - autoimmune disorder in which autoreactive antibodies bind to platelets, shortening the platelet life span.

Immune response - body's defense mechanism that includes producing antibodies to foreign antigens.

Immunoblast - T or B lymphocyte that is mitotically active as a result of stimulation by an antigen. The cell is morphologically characterized by a large nucleus with prominent nucleoli, a fine chromatin pattern, and an abundant, deeply basophilic cytoplasm.

Immunocompetent - having the ability to respond to stimulation by an antigen.

Immunoglobulin - molecule produced by B lymphocytes and plasma cells. It reacts with antigen. It consists of two pairs of polypeptide chains: two heavy and two light chains linked together by disulfide bonds. Also called *antibody*.

Immunohistochemical stains - stains applied using immunologic principles and techniques to study cells and tissues. Usually a labeled antibody is used to detect antigens (markers) on a cell.

Immunophenotyping - identifying antigens using detection antibodies.

Immunosuppressed - suppressed ability to produce antibodies to antigens.

Immunotherapy - form of therapy in which different immune cells are manipulated in vivo or in vitro and later infused to alter the immune function of other cells.

Indirect antiglobulin test (IAT) - laboratory test used to detect the presence of serum antibodies against specific erythrocyte antigens.

Induction therapy - initial phase of cancer chemotherapy. Its function is to rapidly drop the tumor burden and induce a remission back to a normal state.

Ineffective erythropoiesis - premature death of erythrocytes in the bone marrow preventing release into circulation.

Infectious lymphocytosis - A condition found in young children. The most striking hematologic finding is a leukocytosis of $40-50 \times 10^9$/L with 60–97% small, normal-appearing lymphocytes. It is thought to be a reactive immune response to a viral infection and is no longer considered a unique disease.

Infectious mononucleosis - self-limiting lymphoproliferative disease caused by infection with Epstein-Barr virus (EBV). The usually increased leukocyte count is related to an absolute lymphocytosis. Various forms of reactive lymphocytes are present. Serologic tests to detect the presence of heterophil antibodies are helpful in differentiating this disease from more serious diseases. Also known as the *kissing disease*.

Innate immune response - body's first response to common classes of invading pathogens. It is rapid but limited. The leukocyte receptors that participate in it are always available and do not require cell activation in order to be expressed. Once a pathogen is recognized, effector cells can attack, engulf, and kill it. Neutrophils, monocytes, and macrophages play a major role in the innate immune system.

In situ hybridization - detection of specific DNA or RNA sequences in tissue sections or cell preparations using a labeled complementary nucleic acid sequence or probe.

Integral proteins - proteins embedded between phospholipids within a cell membrane.

Internal quality control program - system designed to verify the validity of laboratory test results that is followed as part of the daily laboratory operations. Typically, it is monitored using Levey-Jennings plots and Westgard rules.

International normalized ratio (INR) - method of reporting prothrombin time results when monitoring long-term oral anticoagulant therapy. Results are independent of the reagents and methods used.

International Sensitivity Index (ISI) - value provided by the manufacturer of thromboplastin reagents. It indicates the responsiveness of the particular lot of reagent compared to the international reference thromboplastin.

Intrinsic coagulation pathway - one of the three interacting pathways in the coagulation cascade. The intrinsic pathway is initiated by exposure of the contact coagulation factors (F-XII, F-XI, prekallikrein, and high-molecular-weight kininogen) with vessel subendothelial tissue. The intrinsic pathway activates F-X. The term *intrinsic* is used because all intrinsic factors are contained within the blood.

Intrinsic factor - glycoprotein secreted by the parietal cells of the stomach that is necessary for binding and absorption of dietary vitamin B_{12}.

Intrinsic Xase - complex of F-IXa, F-VIIIa, phospholipid, and calcium that assembles on membrane surfaces.

Intron - DNA base sequence interrupting the protein coding sequence of a gene; this sequence is transcribed into RNA but is cut out of the message before it is translated into protein.

IRE - stem-loop-stem structure in either the 5' or 3' noncoding regions of mRNA recognized and bound by iron-binding proteins

(IRE-BP or IRP). The binding affinity of IRP for the IRE is determined by the amount of cellular iron. The IRP binds to the IRE region when iron is scarce and dissociates when iron is plentiful. When bound, the IRP modulates the translation of the mRNA. The translation of the proteins involved in iron metabolism including ferritin, ferroportin, ALA synthase2, transferrin, and DMT1 are regulated by this mechanism.

IRP - protein that binds to a stem-loop structure of ferritin and transferrin receptor mRNA. The stem-loop structure of mRNA is known as the iron-responsive element (IRE). It is also referred to as *IRE-BP* (*iron-responsive element-binding protein*). The binding affinity of IRE-BP for the IRE is determined by the amount of cellular iron. The IRE-BP is involved in the regulation of transferrin receptors and ferritin.

Irreversibly sickled cells (ISC) - rigid cells that have been exposed to repeated sickling events and cannot revert to a normal discoid shape. They are ovoid or boat-shaped and have a high MCHC and low MCV.

Ischemia - deficiency of blood supply to a tissue caused by constriction of the vessel or blockage of the blood flow through the vessel.

Isoelectric focusing - technique of moving charged particles through a support medium with a continuous pH gradient. Individual proteins will move until they reach the pH that is equal to their isoelectric point.

Isopropanol precipitation - technique that identifies the presence of unstable hemoglobins due to their insolubility in isopropanol as compared to normal hemoglobins.

Isovolumetric sphering - method employed by the Bayer/Technicon instruments in which a specific buffered diluent is used to sphere and fix the blood cells without altering their volume.

 J

JAK2 gene - Janus kinase 2, codes for a tyrosine kinase closely associated with cytokine receptors. A gain in function mutation that gives the cell a proliferative advantage is common in the myeloproliferative disorders, especially polycythemia vera.

Jaundice - condition characterized by yellowing of the skin, mucous membranes, and the whites of the eye caused by accumulation of bilirubin.

Juvenile myelomonocytic leukemia - clonal hematopoietic neoplasm of childhood characterized by proliferation of the granulocytic and monocytic lineages. There is a peripheral blood monocytosis ($>1 \times 10^9$/L), with <20% blasts (including promonocytes).

 K

Karyolysis - destruction of the nucleus.

Karyorrhexis - disintegration of the nucleus resulting in the irregular distribution of chromatin fragments within the cytoplasm.

Karyotype - systematic display of a cell's chromosomes that determines the number of chromosomes present and their morphology.

Kernicterus - toxic buildup of bilirubin in brain tissue; associated with hyperbilirubinemia.

Keratocytes - abnormally shaped erythrocytes with one or several notches and projections on either end that look like horns. Also

called *helmet cells* and *horn-shaped cells*. The shape is caused by trauma to the erythrocyte.

Killer cell - population of cytolytic lymphocytes identified by monoclonal antibodies. Involved in several activities such as resistance to viral infections, regulation of hematopoiesis, and activities against tumor cells.

Knizocytes - abnormally shaped erythrocyte that appears on stained smears as a cell with a dark stick-shaped portion of hemoglobin in the center and a pale area on either end. The cell has more than two concavities.

 L

L&H/popcorn cell - *See* Popcorn cell.

Lacunar cell - neoplastic cell variant found in NS Hodgkin lymphoma characterized by abundant pale-staining cytoplasm. It is also characterized by cytoplasmic clearing and delicate, multilobated nuclei.

Large granular lymphocyte - null cell with a low nuclear-to-cytoplasmic ratio, pale blue cytoplasm, and azurophilic granules. It does not adhere to surfaces or phagocytose.

Latex immunoassay (LIA) test - immuno-turbidimetric assay using microlatex particles coated with specific antibodies. In the presence of the antigen to be tested, the particles agglutinate producing an adsorption of light proportional to the antigen level present in the sample.

Laurell "rocket" technique (EIA-Electroimmunoassay) - agarose plates containing antibody are electrophoresed with an antigen (in PPP) until a "rocket" of precipitated antigen–antibody forms (measured following the staining of the gel). The height of the rocket is proportional to the quantity of antigen present in the PPP.

Lecithin:cholesterol acyl transferase (LCAT) deficiency - rare autosomal disorder that affects metabolism of high-density lipoproteins. It is characterized by a deficiency of an enzyme that catalyzes the formation of cholesterol esters from cholesterol. Its onset is usually during young adulthood.

Leptocyte - abnormally shaped erythrocyte that is thin and flat with hemoglobin at the periphery. It is usually cup shaped.

Leukemia - progressive, malignant disease of the hematopoietic system characterized by unregulated, clonal proliferation of the hematopoietic stem cells. The malignant cells eventually replace normal cells. It is generally classified as chronic or acute, and lymphoid or myelogenous.

Leukemic hiatus - gap in the normal maturation pyramid of cells with many blasts and some mature forms but very few intermediate maturational stages. Eventually, the immature neoplastic cells fill the bone marrow and spill over into the peripheral blood producing leukocytosis (e.g., acute leukemia).

Leukemic stem cell - rare cell with infinite proliferative potential that drives the formation and growth of tumors.

Leukemoid reaction - transient, reactive condition resulting from certain types of infections or tumors characterized by an increase in the total leukocyte count to more than 25×10^9/L and a shift to the left in leukocytes (usually granulocytes).

Leukocyte - white blood cell (WBC) of which there are five types: neutrophils, eosinophils, basophils, lymphocytes, and monocytes.

The function of these cells is to defend against infection and tissue damage. The normal reference range for total leukocytes in peripheral blood is $4.5–11.0 \times 10^9$/L.

Leukocyte alkaline phosphatase (LAP) - enzyme present within the specific (secondary) granules of granulocytes (from the myelocyte stage onward). It is useful in distinguishing leukemoid reaction/reactive neutrophilia (high LAP) from chronic myelogenous leukemia (low LAP).

Leukocytosis - increase in WBCs in the peripheral blood; WBC count over 11×10^9/L.

Leukoerythroblastic reaction - condition characterized by the presence of nucleated erythrocytes and a shift to the left in neutrophils in the peripheral blood; often associated with myelophthisis.

Leukopenia - decrease in leukocytes below 4×10^9/L.

Leukopoiesis - production of leukocytes.

Linearity - range of concentration over which the test method can be used without modifying the sample (i.e., diluting the sample).

Linearity check material - commercially available matter with known concentrations of the analytes and no interfering substances or conditions. Linearity check material is used to determine an instrument's or method's linearity.

Linear regression analysis - statistical tool used to determine a single line through a data set that describes the relationship between two methods, X and Y. General equation is $Y = a + bx$, where a denotes the y-intercept; b is the slope; and Y is the predicted mean value of Y for a given x value.

Linkage analysis - process of following the inheritance pattern of a particular gene in a family based on its tendency to be inherited with another locus on the same chromosome.

Locus - specific position on the chromosome.

Low-molecular-weight heparin (LMWH) - heparin molecules of M.W. 2,000–12,000 Daltons.

LRP receptor (LDL receptorlike protein) - receiver on hepatocytes that removes plasmin/antiplasmin, plasminogen activator/plasminogen activator inhibitor, and thrombin/antithrombin complexes from the circulation.

Lupuslike anticoagulant - circulating substance that arises spontaneously in patients with a variety of conditions (originally found in patients with lupus erythematosus) and directed against phospholipid components of the reagents used in laboratory tests for clotting factors. *See* Antiphospholipid antibody.

Lymphadenopathy - abnormal enlargement of lymph nodes.

Lymphoblast - lymphocytic precursor cell found in the bone marrow. The cell is 10–20 μm in diameter and has a high nuclear/cytoplasmic ratio. The nucleus has a fine (lacy) chromatin pattern with one or two nucleoli. The cytoplasm is agranular and scant. It stains deep blue with Romanowsky stain. The cell contains terminal deoxynucleotidyltransferase (TdT) but no peroxidase, lipid, or esterase.

Lymphocyte - mature leukoctye with variable size depending on the state of cellular activity and amount of cytoplasm. The nucleus is usually round with condensed chromatin and stains deep, dark purple with Romanowsky stains. The cytoplasm stains a light blue. Nucleoli are usually not visible. A few azurophilic granules may be present. These cells interact in a series of events that allow the body to attack and eliminate foreign antigen. They have a peripheral blood concentration in adults from 1.0 to 4.8×10^9/L (20–40% of leukocytes). The concentration in children less than 10 years old is higher.

Lymphocytic leukemoid reaction - response characterized by an increased lymphocyte count with the presence of reactive or immature appearing lymphocytes. It is associated with whooping cough, chicken pox, infectious mononucleosis, infectious lymphocytosis, and tuberculosis.

Lymphocytopenia - decrease in the concentration of lymphocytes in the peripheral blood ($<1.0 \times 10^9$/L). Also called *lymphopenia*.

Lymphocytosis - increase in peripheral blood lymphocyte concentration ($>4.8 \times 10^9$/L in adults or $>9 \times 10^9$/L in children).

Lympho-epithelial lesion - infiltration of epithelium by groups of lymphocytes. Infiltration of mucosal epithelium by neoplastic lymphocytes is characteristic of MALT lymphoma.

Lymphoid follicle - sphere of B cells within lymphatic tissue.

Lymphokines - substances released by sensitized lymphocytes and responsible for activation of macrophages and other lymphocytes.

Lymphoma - malignant proliferation of lymphocytes. Most cases arise in lymph nodes, but it can begin at many extranodal sites. The lymphomas are classified as to B or T cell and low, intermediate, or high grade.

Lymphoma classification - process of dividing (grading) lymphomas into groups, each with a similar clinical course and response to treatment. Current schemes use a combination of morphologic appearance, phenotype, and genotype.

Lyonization - process in which all but one X chromosome in a cell are randomly inactivated.

Lypholized - serum or plasma sample that has been freeze dried. The sample is reconstituted with a diluent, typically distilled or deionized water.

Lysosmal granules - granules containing lysosomal enzymes.

Lysosome - membrane-bound sacs in the cytoplasm that contain various hydrolytic enzymes.

▶ M

Macrocyte - abnormally large erythrocyte. The MCV is >100 fL. Oval macrocytes are characteristically seen in megaloblastic anemia.

Macro-ovalocyte - abnormally large erythrocyte with an oval shape. This cell is characteristically seen in megaloblastic anemia.

Macrophage - large tissue cell (10–20 μm) derived from monocytes. The cell secretes a variety of products that influence the function of other cells. It plays a major role in both nonspecific and specific immune responses.

Maintenance therapy - third and final phase of cancer chemotherapy whose function is to prevent the repair and/or return of the malignant clone, thus allowing the normal immune system to clear away all remaining disease.

Malignant neoplasm - clone of identical, anaplastic (dedifferentiated), proliferating cells. Malignant cells can metastasize.

Marginating pool - population of neutrophils that are attached to or marginated along the vessel walls and not actively circulating. This is about one-half of the total pool of neutrophils in the vessels.

Material safety data sheet (MSDS) - document that provides safety information for clinical laboratory professionals who use hazardous materials; includes pertinent safety information regarding the proper storage and disposal of a chemical, precautions that should be taken in handling the chemical, potential health hazards associated with exposure to it, and whether the chemical is a fire or explosive hazard.

Mastocytosis - heterogeneous group of mast cell diseases characterized by the abnormal proliferation of mast cells in one or more organ systems. It is suggested that mast cell disorders be classified as myeloproliferative disorders. Two major groups of mast cell disorders are cutaneous and systemic.

Maturation - process of attaining complete development of the cell.

Maturation index - mathematical expression that attempts to separate AML-M5 and AML-M1 with and without maturation.

Mean cell hemoglobin (MCH) - indicator of the average weight of hemoglobin in individual erythrocytes reported in picograms. The reference interval for MCH is 28–34 pg. This parameter is calculated from the hemoglobin and erythrocyte count: MCH (pg) = Hemoglobin (g/dL) ÷ Erythrocyte count ($\times 10^{12}$/L) × 10.

Mean cell hemoglobin concentration (MCHC) - measure of the average concentration of hemoglobin in grams per deciliter of erythrocytes. The reference interval is 32–36 g/dL. The MCHC is useful when evaluating erythrocyte hemoglobin content on a stained smear. This parameter correlates with the extent of chromasia exhibited by the stained cells and is calculated from the hemoglobin and hematocrit. MCHC (g/dL) = hemoglobin (g/dL) ÷ hematocrit (L/L).

Mean cell volume (MCV) - average volume of individual erythrocytes reported in femtoliters. The reference interval for MCV is 80–100 fL. This parameter is useful when evaluating erythrocyte morphology on a stained blood smear. The MCV usually correlates with the diameter of the erythrocytes observed microscopically. The MCV can be calculated from the hematocrit and erythrocyte count: MCV (fL) = Hematocrit (L/L) ÷ Erythrocyte Count ($\times 10^{12}$/L) × 1000.

Mean platelet volume - mean volume of a platelet population; analogous to the MCV of erythrocytes.

Medical decision level - concentration of an analyte indicating that medical intervention is required for proper patient care.

Medullary hematopoiesis - blood cell production and development in the bone marrow.

Megakaryocyte - large cell found within the bone marrow characterized by the presence of large or multiple nuclei and abundant cytoplasm. It gives rise to the blood platelets.

Megaloblastic - asynchronous maturation of any nucleated cell type characterized by delayed nuclear development in comparison to the cytoplasmic development. The abnormal cells are large and are characteristically found in pernicious anemia and other megaloblastic anemia.

Metacentric - chromosome that has the centromere near center so that the short arm and long arms are equal in length.

Meninges - three membranes covering the brain and spinal cord.

Metamyelocyte - granulocytic precursor cell normally found in the bone marrow. The cell is 10–15 μm in diameter. The cytoplasm stains pink and there is a predominance of specific granules. The nucleus is indented with a kidney bean shape. The nuclear chromatin is condensed and stains dark purple.

Methemoglobin - hemoglobin with iron that has been oxidized to the ferric state (Fe^{+++}); is incapable of combining with oxygen.

Methemoglobin reductase pathway - metabolic pathway that uses methemoglobin reductase and NADH to maintain heme iron in the reduced state (Fe^{++}).

Microangiopathic hemolytic anemia (MAHA) - any hemolytic process that is caused by prosthetic devices or lesions of the small blood vessels.

Microcyte - abnormally small erythrocyte. The MCV is typically less than 80 fL and its diameter is less than 7.0 μm on a stained smear.

Microenvironment - unique environment in the bone marrow where orderly proliferation and differentiation of precursor cells take place.

Micromegakaryocyte - small, abnormal megakaryocyte sometimes found in the peripheral blood in MDS and the myeloproliferative syndromes.

Microtubule - cylindric structure (20–27 μm in diameter) composed of protein subunits. It is a part of the cytoskeleton, helping some cells maintain shape. Microtubules increase during mitosis and form the mitotic spindle fibers. They also assist in transporting substances in different directions. In the platelet, a band of tubules located on the circumference is thought to be essential for maintaining the disc shape in the resting state.

Minimal (minimum) residual disease - condition with the presence of malignant cells detected by molecular tests when all other tests are negative.

Mitotic pool - population of cells within the bone marrow that is capable of DNA synthesis. Also called *proliferating pool*.

Mixed lineage acute leukemia - acute leukemia that has both myeloid and lymphoid populations present or blasts that possess myeloid and lymphoid markers on the same cell.

Molecular remission - absence of detectable molecular abnormalities using PCR or related molecular technologies in patients who had identifiable abnormalities before therapy. This is the most sensitive test for detecting minimal residual disease.

Monoblast - monocytic precursor cell found in bone marrow. It is about 14–18 μm in diameter with abundant agranular, blue-gray cytoplasm. The nucleus may be folded or indented. The chromatin is finely dispersed, and several nucleoli are visible. The monoblast has nonspecific esterase activity that is inhibited by sodium fluoride.

Monoclonal gammopathy - alteration in immunoglobulin production that is characterized by an increase in one specific class of immunoglobulin.

Monocyte - mature leukocyte found in bone marrow or peripheral blood. Its morphology depends on its activity. The cell ranges in size from 12–30 μm with an average of 18 μm. The blue-gray cytoplasm is evenly dispersed with fine dustlike granules. There are two types of granules. One contains peroxidase, acid phosphatase, and arylsulfatase. Less is known about the content of the other granule. The nuclear chromatin is loose and linear forming a lacy pattern. The nucleus is often irregular in shape.

Monocytopenia - decrease in the concentration of circulating monocytes ($<0.1 \times 10^9$/L).

Monocytosis - increase in the concentration of circulating monocytes ($>0.8 \times 10^9$/L).

Mononuclear phagocyte (MNP) system - collection of monocytes and macrophages found both intravascularly and extravascularly. It plays a major role in initiating and regulating the immune response.

Monosomy - one daughter cell with a missing chromosome (one copy instead of two).

Morulae - basophilic, irregularly shaped granular, cytoplasmic inclusions found in leukocytes in an infectious disease called *ehrlichiosis*.

Mosaic - process that occurs in the embryo shortly after fertilization, resulting in congenital aberrations in some cells and some normal cells.

Mott cell - pathologic plasma cell whose cytoplasm is filled with colorless globules. These globules most often contain immunoglobulin (Russell bodies) and form as a result of accumulation of material in the RER, SER, or Golgi complex due to an obstruction of secretion. The cell is associated with chronic plasmocyte hyperplasia, parasitic infection, and malignant tumors. Also called *grape cell*.

Multimer analysis - analysis that determines the structure of VWF multimers.

Multiple myeloma - plasma cell malignancy characterized by increased plasma proteins.

Mutation - any change in the nucleotide sequence of DNA. In instances in which large sequences of nucleotides are missing, the alteration is referred to as a *deletion*.

Myeloblast - first microscopically identifiable granulocyte precursor. It is normally found in the bone marrow. The cell is large (15–20 μm) with a high nuclear/cytoplasmic ratio. The nucleus has a fine chromatin pattern with a nucleoli. There is moderate amount of blue, agranular cytoplasm.

Myelocyte - granulocytic precursor cell normally found in the bone marrow. The cell is 12–18 μm in diameter with a pinkish granular cytoplasm. Both primary and secondary granules are present.

Myelodysplastic syndromes (MDS) - group of primary neoplastic pluripotential stem cell disorders characterized by one or more cytopenias in the peripheral blood with prominent maturation abnormalities (dysplasia) in the bone marrow.

Myelodysplastic/myeloproliferative diseases - category of neoplasms in the WHO classification but not found in the FAB classification system. It includes clonal hematopoietic neoplasms that have some clinical, laboratory, or morphologic findings of both a myelodysplastic syndrome (MDS) and a chronic myeloproliferative disease (MPD).

Myeloid-to-erythroid ratio (M:E ratio) - ratio of granulocytes and their precursors to nucleated erythroid precursors derived from performing a differential count on bone marrow nucleated hematopoietic cells. Monocytes and lymphocytes are not included. The normal ratio is usually between 1.5:1 and 3.5:1, reflecting a predominance of myeloid elements.

Myeloid/NK cell acute leukemia - acute leukemia in which the neoplastic cells coexpress myeloid antigens (CD33, CD13, and/or CD15) and NK cell-associated antigens (CD56, CD16, CD11b), while they lack HLA-DR and T lymphocyte associated antigens CD3 and CD8.

Myeloperoxidase - enzyme present in the primary granules of myeloid cells including neutrophils, eosinophils, and monocytes.

Myelophthisis - replacement of normal hematopoietic tissue in bone marrow by fibrosis, leukemia, or metastatic cancer cells.

Myeloproliferative disorders (MPD) - group of neoplastic clonal disorders characterized by excess proliferation of one or more cell types in the bone marrow.

▶ N

Natural killer cell - type of lymphoid cell that has the capacity for spontaneous cytotoxicity for various target cells. Its cytotoxicity is non-MHC restricted. It possesses CD16 (the FcγIII receptor for IgG) and CD56. NK cells constitute about 15% of the circulating lymphocytes in the peripheral blood.

Necrosis - pathologic cell death resulting from irreversible damage; "cell murder."

Neonatal alloimmune thrombocytopenia (NAIT) - thrombocytopenia due to immune destruction of platelets that occurs in newborns due to the transfer of maternal alloantibodies.

Neoplasm - abnormal formation of new tissue (such as a tumor) that serves no useful purpose; may be benign or malignant.

Neutropenia - decrease in neutrophils below 1.8×10^9/L.

Neutrophil - mature white blood cell with a segmented nucleus and granular cytoplasm. This cell constitutes the majority of circulating leukocytes. The absolute number varies between 1.8 and 7.0×10^9/L. Also called *granulocytes* or *segs*.

Neutrophilia - increase in neutrophils over 7.0×10^9/L. It is seen in bacterial infections, inflammation, metabolic intoxication, drug intoxication, and tissue necrosis.

Nondisjunction - error in segregation that occurs in mitosis or meiosis so that sister chromatids do not disjoin. A spindle fiber malfunction results in one daughter cell with an extra chromosome (trisomy) and one daughter cell with a missing chromosome (monosomy).

Nonspecific granules - large, blue-black granules found in promyelocytes. The granules have a phospholipid membrane and stain positive for peroxidase.

Nonthrombocytopenic purpura - condition in which platelets are normal in number but purpura are present; purpura is considered to be caused by damage to the blood vessels.

Normal pooled plasma - platelet-poor plasma collected from at least 20 individuals for coagulation testing. Plasmas should give PT and APTT results within the laboratory's reference interval. The plasma is pooled and used in mixing studies to differentiate a circulating inhibitor from a factor deficiency.

Normoblast - nucleated erythrocyte precursor in the bone marrow. Also known as *erythroblast*.

Normogram - chart that displays the relationship between numerical variables.

Nuclear-cytoplasmic asynchrony - condition in which the cellular nucleus matures more slowly than the cytoplasm, suggesting a disturbance in coordination. As a result, the nucleus takes on the appearance of a nucleus associated with a younger cell than its cytoplasmic development indicates. This is a characteristic of megaloblastic anemias.

Nuclear-to-cytoplasmic ratio (N:C ratio) - ratio of the volume of the cell nucleus to the volume of the cell's cytoplasm. This is usually estimated as the ratio of the diameter of the nucleus to the diameter of the cytoplasm. In immature hematopoietic cells, the N:C ratio is usually higher than in more mature cells. As the cell matures, the nucleus condenses and the cytoplasm expands.

Nucleolus (pl: nucleoli) - spherical body within the nucleus in which ribosomes are produced. It is not visible in cells that are not synthesizing proteins or that are not in mitosis or meiosis. It stains a lighter blue than the nucleus with Romanowsky stains.

Nucleotide - basic building block of DNA composed of nitrogen base (A = adenine, T = thymine, G = guanine, or C = cytosine) attached to a sugar (deoxyribose) and a phosphate molecule.

Nucleus (pl: nuclei) - characteristic structure in the eukaryocytic cell that contains chromosomes and nucleoli. It is separated from the cytoplasm by a nuclear envelope. The structure stains deep bluish-purple with Romanowsky stain. In young, immature hematopoietic cells, the nuclear material is open and dispersed in a lacy pattern. As the cell becomes mature, the nuclear material condenses and appears structureless.

Null cell - *See* Large granular lymphocytes.

 O

Oncogene - altered gene that contributes to the development of cancer. Most oncogenes are altered forms of normal genes that function to regulate cell growth and differentiation. The normal gene counterpart is known as a proto-oncogene.

Open canalicular system (OCS) - membrane system in the platelet forming twisted channels that lead from the platelet surface to the interior of the platelet. It is a remnant of the demarcation membrane system of the megakaryocyte. Also called *surface connected canalicular system* (*SCCS*).

Opportunistic organisms - organisms that are usually part of the normal flora but can cause disease if there is a significant change in host resistance or within the organism itself.

Opsonin - antibody or complement that coats microorganisms or other particulate matter found within the blood stream so that the foreign material may be more readily recognized and phagocytized by leukocytes.

Optimal counting area - area of the blood smear where erythrocytes are just touching but not overlapping; used for morphologic evaluation and identification of cells.

Oral anticoagulant - group of drugs (e.g., coumadin, warfarin) that prevent coagulation by inhibiting the activity of vitamin K, which is required for the synthesis of functional prothrombin group coagulation factors.

Orthochromatic normoblast - nucleated precursor of the erythrocyte that develops from the polychromatophilic normoblast. It is the last nucleated stage of erythrocyte development. The cell normally is found in the bone marrow.

Osmotic fragility - laboratory procedure employed to evaluate the ability of erythrocytes to withstand different salt concentrations; this depends on the erythrocyte's membrane, volume, surface area, and functional state.

Osteoblast - cell involved in formation of calcified bone.

Osteoclast - cell involved in resorption and remodeling of calcified bone.

Outlier - data point that falls outside the expected range for all data. An outlier is not considered to be part of the population that was sampled.

Oxygen affinity - ability of hemoglobin to bind and release oxygen. An increase in CO_2, acid, and heat decreases oxygen affinity, while an increase in pO_2 increases oxygen affinity.

Oxyhemoglobin - compound formed when hemoglobin combines with oxygen.

▶ **P**

P_{50} value - partial pressure of oxygen at which 50% of hemoglobin is saturated with oxygen.

P53 gene - normally functions as an antioncogene by preventing proliferation of DNA-damaged cells, promoting apoptosis of these damaged cells, and preventing unwanted DNA amplification. When mutated, this gene may lose its tumor suppressive effect.

Paired *t*-test - statistical tool used to compare the difference between two paired data sets. Paired *t*-test determines whether a statistically significant difference exists between the two paired data sets.

Pancytopenia - marked decrease of all blood cells in the peripheral blood.

Panhypercellular - increase in all blood cells in the peripheral blood.

Panmyelosis - panhypercellularity in the bone marrow.

Pappenheimer bodies - iron-containing particles in mature erythrocyte. On Romanowsky stain, they are visible near the periphery of the cell and often occur in clusters.

Paroxysmal cold hemoglobinuria (PCH) - autoimmune hemolytic anemia characterized by hemolysis and hematuria upon exposure to cold.

Paroxysmal nocturnal hemoglobinuria (PNH) - stem cell disease in which the erythrocyte membrane is abnormal, making the cell more susceptible to hemolysis by complement. There is a lack of decay accelerating factor (DAF) and C8 binding protein (C8bp) on the membrane, which are normally responsible for preventing amplification of complement activation. The deficiency of DAF and C8bp is due to the lack of glycosyl phosphatidyl inositol (GPI), a membrane glycolipid that serves to attach (anchor) proteins to the cell membrane. Intravascular hemolysis is intermittent.

Passenger lymphocyte syndrome - immune hemolytic following solid organ, bone marrow, or stem cell transplant . The donor B lymphocytes that are transplanted with the organ or the bone marrow produce antibodies against recipient's blood group antigens. Hemolysis is primarily due to ABO incompatibility between donor and recipient (Group O donor and Group A or B recipient). Although ABO is the most frequent antigen system involved, Rh, Kell, Kidd, or other blood group systems may be involved.

Pelger-Huët anomaly - inherited benign condition characterized by the presence of functionally normal neutrophils with a bilobed or round nucleus. Cells with the bilobed appearance are called *pincenez cells*.

Percent saturation - portion of transferrin that is complexed with iron.

Pericardial cavity - body cavity that contains the heart.

Pericardium - membrane that lines the pericardial cavity.

Peripheral membrane protein - protein that is attached to the cell membrane by ionic or hydrogen bonds but is outside the lipid framework of the membrane.

Peritoneal cavity - space between the inside abdominal wall and outside of the stomach, small and large intestines, liver, superior aspect of the bladder, and uterus.

Peritoneum - lining of the peritoneal cavity.

Pernicious anemia - megaloblastic anemia resulting from a lack of intrinsic factor. The intrinsic factor is needed to absorb cobalamin (vitamin B_{12}) from the gut.

Petechiae - small, pinhead-size purple spots caused by blood escaping from capillaries into intact skin. These are associated with platelet and vascular disorders.

Phagocytosis - cellular process of cells engulfing and destroying a foreign particle through active cell membrane invagination.

Phagolysosome - digestive vacuole (secondary lysosome) formed by the fusion of lysosomes and a phagosome. The hydrolytic enzymes of the lysosome digest the phagocytosed material.

Phagosome - formation of an isolated vacuole within the process of opsonization.

Pharmacokinetics - quantitative study of a drug's disposition in the body over time.

Phase microscopy - type of light microscopy in which an annular diaphragm is placed below or in the substage condenser, and a phase-shifting element is placed in the rear focal plane of the objective. This causes alterations in the phases of light rays and increases the contrast between the cell and its surroundings. This methodology is used to count platelets.

Phenotype - physical manifestation of an individual's genotype, often referring to a particular genetic locus.

Phi body - smaller version of the Auer rod.

Photomultiplier tube - light detector used in flow cytometers and other analytical instruments.

Pia mater - thin membrane directly covering the central nervous system; middle layer of the meninges.

Pica - perversion of appetite that leads to bizarre eating practices; a clinical finding in some individuals with iron deficiency anemia.

Pitting - removal of abnormal inclusions from erythrocytes by the spleen.

PIVKA (protein-induced by vitamin-K absence or antagonist) - these factors are the nonfunctional forms of the prothrombin group coagulation factors. They are synthesized in the liver in the absence of vitamin K and lack the carboxyl (COOH) group necessary for binding the factor to a phospholipid surface.

Plasma cell - transformed, fully differentiated B lymphocyte normally found in the bone marrow and medullary cords of lymph nodes. It may be seen in the circulation in certain infections and disorders associated with increased serum γ-globulins. The cell is characterized by the presence of an eccentric nucleus containing condensed, deeply staining chromatin and deep basophilic cytoplasm. The large Golgi apparatus next to the nucleus does not stain, leaving an obvious clear paranuclear area. The cell has the PC-1 membrane antigen and cytoplasmic immunoglobulin.

Plasma cell neoplasm - monoclonal neoplasm of immunoglobulin secreting cells.

Plasma exchange - removal of patient plasma and replacement with donor plasma.

Plasmacytoid lymphocyte - an intermediate cell in immunoblast development between the B lymphocyte and the plasma cell. It has morphologic similarity to the lymphocyte but has marked cytoplasmic basophila similar to that of plasma cells. It is occasionally seen in the peripheral blood of patients with viral infection.

Plasmacytosis - presence of plasma cells in the peripheral blood or an excess of plasma cells in the bone marrow.

Plasmin - proteolytic enzyme with trypsinlike specificity that digests fibrin or fibrinogen as well as other coagulation factors. Plasmin is formed from plasminogen.

Plasminogen - β-globulin, single-chain glycoprotein that circulates in the blood as a zymogen. Large amounts of plasminogen are absorbed with the fibrin mass during clot formation. Plasminogen is activated by intrinsic and extrinsic activators to form plasmin.

Plasminogen activator inhibitor-1 (PAI-1) - primary inhibitor of tissue plasminogen activator (t-PA) and urokinaselike plasminogen activator (tcu-PA) released from platelet α granules during platelet activation.

Plasminogen activator inhibitor-2 (PAI-2) - inhibitor of tissue plasminogen activator and urokinaselike plasminogen activator. Secretion of PAI-2 is stimulated by endotoxin and phorbol esters. Increased levels impair fibrinolysis and are associated with thrombosis.

Platelet - round or oval disc-shaped structure in the peripheral blood formed from the cytoplasm of megakaryocytes in the bone marrow. Platelets play an important role in primary hemostasis by adhering to the ruptured blood vessel wall and aggregating to form a platelet plug over the injured area. Platelets are also important in secondary hemostasis by providing platelet phospholipids important for the activation of coagulation proteins. The normal reference range for platelets is $150–450 \times 10^9/L$.

Platelet activation - stimulation of a platelet that occurs when agonists bind to the platelet's surface and transmit signals to the cell's interior. Activated platelets form aggregates known as the *primary platelet plug*.

Platelet adhesion - platelet attachment to collagen fibers or other nonplatelet surfaces.

Platelet aggregation - platelet-to-platelet interaction that results in a clumped mass; may occur in vitro or in vivo.

Platelet clump - aggregation of platelets; may occur when blood is collected by capillary puncture (due to platelet activation) and when blood is collected in EDTA anticoagulant (due to unmasking of platelet antigens that can react with antibodies in the serum).

Platelet distribution width (PDW) - coefficient of variation of platelet volume distribution; analogous to RDW.

Platelet factor 4 - protein present in platelet's alpha granules that is capable of neutralizing heparin.

Plateletpheresis - procedure in which platelets are removed from the circulation.

Platelet-poor plasma (PPP) - citrated plasma containing less than 15×10^9/L platelets. It is prepared by centrifugation of citrated whole blood at a minimum RCF of $1000 \times g$ for 15 minutes. PPP is used for the majority of coagulation tests.

Platelet procoagulant activity - property of platelets that enables activated coagulation factors and cofactors to adhere to the platelet surface during the formation of fibrin.

Platelet-rich plasma (PRP) - citrated plasma containing approximately 200–300×10^9/L platelets. It is prepared by centrifugation of citrated whole blood at an RCF of $150 \times g$ for 10 minutes. PRP is used in platelet aggregation studies.

Platelet satellistism - adherence of platelets to neutrophil membranes in vitro; this can occur when blood is collected in EDTA anticoagulant.

Platelet secretion - release of the contents of the platelet alpha granules and dense bodies during platelet activation.

Platelet-type pseudo-VWD - platelet disorder characterized by an increased affinity of the platelet GPIb/IX receptor for VWF , resulting in spontaneous binding of the large VWF multimers to the platelet. It resembles VWD clinically and often presents with similar laboratory test results but is not associated with genetic mutations involving the *VWF* gene and thus is not considered "true" VWD.

Pleura - lining of the pleural cavities.

Pleural cavity - space between the chest wall and the lungs.

Plethora - excess of blood.

Plumbism - lead poisoning.

Pluripotential cell - cell that differentiates into many different cell lines. It has the potential to self-renew, proliferate, and differentiate into erythrocytic, myelocytic, monocytic, lymphocytic, and megakaryocytic blood cell lineages.

Poikilocytosis - term used to describe the presence of variations in the shape of erythrocytes.

Point of care (POC) instrument - instrument that allows for analytical testing of patient specimens outside the laboratory setting (e.g., home testing or physician's office testing).

Polychromatophilia - quality of being stainable with more than one portion of the stain; the term is commonly used to describe erythrocytes that stain with a grayish or bluish tinge with Romanowsky stains due to residual RNA, which takes up the blue portion of the dye.

Polychromatophilic erythrocyte - erythrocyte with a bluish tinge when stained with Romanowsky stain; contains residual RNA. If stained with new methylene blue, these cells show reticulum and are identified as reticulocytes.

Polyclonal - arising from different cell clones.

Polyclonal gammopathy - alteration in immunoglobulin production that is characterized by an increase in immunoglobulins of more than one class.

Polycythemia - condition associated with increased erythrocyte count.

Polycythemia vera - myeloproliferative disorder associated with an increased proliferation of erythroid cells.

Polymerase chain reaction - procedure for copying a specific DNA sequence many times.

Polymorphic variants - variant morphology of a portion of a chromosome that has no clinical consequence.

Polymorphonuclear neutrophil (PMN) - mature granulocyte found in bone marrow and peripheral blood. The nucleus is segmented into 2 or more lobes. The cytoplasm stains pinkish and there is abundant specific granules. This is the most numerous leukocyte in the peripheral blood (1.8–7.0×10^9/L). Its primary function is defense against foreign antigens. It is active in phagocytosis and killing microorganisms. Also called *segmented neutrophil* or *seg.*

Polyploid/polyploidy - number of chromosomes per cell that is a multiple of *n* (23) other than 1 or 2 (e.g., 3n[69], 4n[92]).

Popcorn cell (L&H cell) - neoplastic cell variant found in LP Hodgkin lymphoma characterized by a delicate multilobated nucleus and multiple, small nucleoli. The L&H cell has a B cell phenotype: LCA+ (leukocyte common antigen), CD20+, CD 15.

Porphyrins - highly unsaturated tetrapyrrole ring bonded by four methane ($-CH=$) bridges. Substituents occupy each of the eight peripheral positions on the four pyrrole rings. The kind and order of these substituents determine the type of porphyrin. Porphyrins are metabolically active only when they are chelated.

Portland hemoglobin - embryonic hemoglobin found in the yolk sac and detectable up to 8 weeks gestation. It is composed of two zeta (ζ) and two gamma (γ) chains.

Postmitotic pool - neutrophils in the bone marrow that are not capable of mitosis. These cells include metamyelocytes, bands, and segmented neutrophils. Cells spend about 5–7 days in this compartment before being released to the peripheral blood. Also called *maturation-storage pool.*

Post translational modification - process occuring in eukaryotic cells that modify the protein product produced by ribosomal translation; it may involve the addition of sugar groups (glycosylation) and phosphate groups (phosphorylation) or other modifications to amino acids (e.g., gamma carboxylation of coagulation proteins).

Primary aggregation - earliest association of platelets in an aggregate that is reversible.

Primary fibrinogenolysis - clinical situation that occurs when there is a release of excessive quantities of plasminogen activators into the blood in the absence of fibrin clot formation. Excess plasmin degrades fibrinogen and the clotting factors, leading to a potentially dangerous hemorrhagic condition.

Primary hemostasis - initial arrest of bleeding that occurs with blood vessel/platelet interaction.

Primary hemostatic plug - aggregate of platelets that initially halts blood flow from an injured vessel.

Primary thrombocytosis - increase in platelets that is not secondary to another condition. It usually refers to the thrombocytosis that occurs in neoplastic disorders.

Probe - tool for identifying a particular nucleotide sequence of interest. A probe is composed of a nucleotide sequence that is complementary to the sequence of interest and is therefore capable of hybridizing to that sequence. Probes are labeled in a way that is detectable, such as by radioactivity.

Procoagulant - inert precursor of a natural substance that is necessary for blood clotting or a property of anything that favors formation of a blood clot.

Proficiency testing - utilizing unknown samples from an external source (e.g., College of American Pathologists) to monitor the quality of a given laboratory's test results.

Progenitor cell - parent or ancestor cells that differentiate into mature, functional cells.

Prolymphocyte - immediate precursor cell of the lymphocyte; normally found in bone marrow. It is slightly smaller than the lymphoblast and has a lower nuclear to cytoplasmic ratio. The nuclear chromatin is somewhat clumped, and nucleoli are usually present. The cytoplasm stains light blue and is agranular.

Promonocyte - monocytic precursor cell found in the bone marrow. The cell is $14-18\ \mu$m in diameter with abundant blue-gray cytoplasm. Fine azurophilic granules may be present. The nucleus is often irregular and deeply indented. The chromatin is finely dispersed and stains a light purple blue. Nucleoli may be present. Cytochemically, the cells stain positive for nonspecific esterase, peroxidase, acid phosphatase, and arylsulfatase. The cell matures to a monocyte.

Promyelocyte - granulocytic precursor cell normally found in the bone marrow. The cell is $15-21\ \mu$m in diameter. The cytoplasm is basophilic, and the nucleus is quite large. The nuclear chromatin is lacy, staining a light purple blue. Several nucleoli are visible. The distinguishing feature is the presence of large blue-black primary (azurophilic) granules. The granules have a phospholipid membrane that stains with Sudan black B. The granules contain acid phosphatase, myeloperoxidase, acid hydrolases, lysozyme, sulfated mucopolysaccharides, and other basic proteins. The promyelocyte matures to a myelocyte. Also called *progranulocyte*.

Pronormoblast - precursor cell of the erythrocyte. The cell is derived from the pluripotential stem cell and is found in the bone marrow. The cell is $12-20\ \mu$m in diameter and has a high nuclear-cytoplasmic ratio. The cytoplasm is deeply basophilic with Romanowsky stains. The nuclear chromatin is fine, and there is one or more nucleoli. The cell matures to a basophilic normoblast. Also called *rubriblast*.

Proteomics - study of the structure and function of proteins in a cell or tissue at a specific time under certain predefined conditions; includes information on the way the proteins function and interact with each other inside cells.

Proteosome - eukaryotic assembly of proteins that degrades other proteins.

Prothrombinase complex - complex formed by coagulation factors Xa and V, calcium, and phospholipid. This complex activates prothrombin to thrombin.

Prothrombin group - group of coagulation factors that are vitamin K dependent for synthesis of their functional forms and that require calcium for binding to a phospholipid surface. Includes factors II, VII, IX, and X. Also known as *vitamin K-dependent factors*.

Prothrombin time (PT) - screening test used to detect deficiencies in the extrinsic and common pathway of the coagulation cascade and to monitor the effectiveness of oral anticoagulant therapy.

Prothrombin time ratio - proportion calculation derived by dividing the patient's prothrombin time result by midpoint of the laboratory's normal range and used to calculate the International Normalized Ratio (INR).

Prourokinase - immature, single-chain form of urokinase that is prepared from urine and by recombinant DNA techniques and can be activated to a two-chain form by plasmin.

Pseudochylous - fluid that appears chylous due to the presence of many inflammatory cells; does not contain lymph fluid or chylomicrons.

Pseudodiploid - cell that has a chromosome count of $2n$ (46) but with a combination of numerical and/or structural aberrations (e.g., 46, XY, -5, -7, 2D8, 2D21).

Pseudoneutrophilia - increase in the concentration of neutrophils in the peripheral blood ($>7.0 \times 10^9$/L) occurring as a result of cells from the marginating pool entering the circulating pool. The response is immediate but transient. This redistribution of cells accompanies vigorous exercise, epinephrine administration, anesthesia, convulsion, and anxiety states. Also called *immediate* or *shift neutrophilia*.

Pseudo–Pelger-Huët cells - acquired condition in which neutrophils display a hyposegmented nucleus. Unlike the real Pelger-Huët anomaly, the nucleus of this cell contains a significant amount of euchromatin and stains more lightly. A critical differentiation point is that all neutrophils are equally affected in the genetic form of Pelger-Huët anomaly, but only a fraction of neutrophils are hyposegmented cells in the acquired state. It is associated with MDS and MPD and may also be found after treatment for leukemias.

Pulmonary embolism - obstruction of the pulmonary artery or one of its branches by a clot or foreign material that has been dislodged from another area by the blood current.

Pure red cell aplasia (PRCA) - anemia with selective decrease in erythrocyte precursors in the marrow.

Purging - technique by which undesirable cells that are present in the blood or bone marrow products are removed.

Purpura - (1) purple discoloration of the skin caused by petechiae and/or ecchymoses; (2) a diverse group of disorders that are characterized by the presence of petechiae and ecchymoses.

Pyknotic - pertaining to degeneration of the nucleus of the cell in which the chromatin condenses to a solid, structureless mass and shrinks.

▶ **Q**

Quality control limit - expected range of results. These limits are used to determine whether a test method is in control and to minimize the chance of inaccurate patient results. If the test method is out of control, an intervention is required to reconcile the problem.

Quebec platelet disorder - storage pool disorder of platelets due to abnormal proteolysis of alpha granule proteins due to increased levels of urinary-type plasminogen activator.

Quiescence (G_0) - phase in a cell that has exited the cell cycle and is in a nonproliferative state.

▶ **R**

R (relaxed) structure - conformational change in hemoglobin that occurs as the molecule takes up oxygen.

Radar chart - graphical representation of eight CBC parameters: WBC, RBC, Hb, Hct, MCV, MCH, MCHC, and PLT. Lines are drawn to connect the parameters; the chart resembles a radar oscilloscope. Changes in the shape of the radar chart indicate different hematologic disorders.

Radial immunodiffusion - diffusion technique in which antibody is incorporated into agarose gel and antigen is placed into wells in the gel. The antigen is quantitated by the size of a precipitin ring that forms as antigen diffuses from a sample well into the gel.

Random access - capability of an automated hematology instrument to process specimens independently of one another; may be programmed to run individual tests (e.g., Hb or platelet counts) or a panel of tests (e.g., CBC with reticulocyte count) without operator intervention.

Random variation - variation within an instrument or test method that is due to chance. This type of variation can be either positive or negative in direction and affects precision.

Rapoport-Leubering shunt - metabolic pathway in which 2,3-bis-phosphoglycerate (2,3-BPG) is synthesized from 1,3-bisphospho-glycerate. 2,3-BPG facilitates the release of oxygen from hemoglobin in the erythrocyte. Also referred to as *2,3-DPG* (*diphosphoglycerate*).

Raynaud's phenomenon - secondary disorder resulting from vaso-arterial spasms in the extremities of the body when exposed to the cold. It is characterized by blanching of the skin, followed by cyanosis, and finally redness when the affected area is warmed. Also referred to as *acrocyanosis*.

RBC indices - indices that help classify the erythrocytes as to their size and hemoglobin content. The values for hemoglobin, hematocrit, and erythrocyte are used to calculate the three indices: mean corpuscular volume (MCV), mean corpuscular hemoglobin concentration (MCHC), and mean corpuscular hemoglobin (MCH). The indices give a clue as to what the erythrocytes should look like on a stained blood film.

Reactive lymphocyte - antigen-stimulated lymphocyte that exhibits a variety of morphologic features. The cell is usually larger than the resting lymphocyte and has an irregular shape. The cytoplasm is more basophilic. The nucleus is often elongated and irregular with a finer chromatin pattern than that of the resting lymphocyte. Often this cell is increased in viral infections. Also called *virocyte,* or *stimulated, transformed, atypical, activated,* or *leukocytoid lymphocyte.*

Reactive neutrophilia - increase in the concentration of peripheral blood neutrophils ($>7.0 \times 10^9$/L) as a result of reaction to a physiologic or pathologic process.

Reagent blank - measurement of absorbance due to reagent alone; eliminates false increase in sample absorbance due to reagent color.

Red thrombus - thrombus composed mostly of red blood cells; so named because of its red coloration.

Reed-Sternberg cell - cell found in the classic form of Hodgkin lymphoma. It is characterized by a multilobated nucleus and large inclusion-like nucleoli.

Reference interval - test value range that is considered normal. Generally the range is determined to include 95% of the normal population.

Reflex testing - follow-up testing that is performed based on results of screening tests.

Refractive Index - degree to which a transparent object will deflect a light ray from a straight path.

Refractory - pertains to disorders or diseases that do not respond readily to therapy.

Refractory anemia - subgroup of the myelodysplastic syndromes. Anemia refractory to all conventional therapy is the primary clinical finding. Blasts constitute <1% of nucleated peripheral blood cells. The bone marrow shows signs of dyserythropoiesis.

Refractory anemia with excess blasts (RAEB) - subgroup of the myelodysplastic syndromes. There are usually cytopenias and signs of dyspoiesis in the peripheral blood with <5% blasts. The bone marrow is usually hypercellular with dyspoiesis in all hematopoietic cell lineages. Bone marrow blasts vary from 5% to 20%.

Refractory anemia with excess blasts in transformation (RAEB-T) - subgroup of the myelodysplastic syndromes. There is(are) cytopenia(s) in the peripheral blood with more than 5% blasts. The bone marrow is usually hyperceullular with dyspoiesis and 20–30% blasts. In the WHO classification, this would be considered acute leukemia (>20% blasts).

Refractory anemia with ringed sideroblasts (RARS) - subgroup of the myelodysplastic syndromes characterized by <1% blasts in the peripheral blood, anemia, and/or thrombocytopenia and/or leukopenia. There are more than 15% ringed sideroblasts and <5% blasts in the bone marrow.

Refractory cytopenia with multilineage dysplasia (RCMD) - category in the WHO classification system for patients with dysplastic features in at least 10% of the cells in two or more cell lines, less than 5% blasts in the bone marrow, and less than 1% blasts in the peripheral blood.

Remission - diminution of the symptoms of a disease.

Replication - process by which DNA is copied during cell division. Replication is carried out by the enzyme DNA polymerase, which recognizes single-stranded DNA and fills in the appropriate complementary nucleotides to produce double-stranded DNA. Synthesis is initated at a free 5′ end where double-stranded DNA lies adjacent to single-stranded DNA, and replication proceeds in the 5′ direction. In the laboratory, DNA replication can be induced as a means of copying DNA sequences as exploited in the polymerase chain reaction.

Reportable range - range that is defined by a minimum value and a maximum value of calibration material.

Reticulated platelet - platelet newly released from the bone marrow and that possesses residual RNA.

Restriction endonuclease - enzyme that cleaves double-stranded DNA at specific nucleotide sequences. For example, HindIII cleaves DNA only where the sequence 5′-AAGCTT-3′ is present. Various other enzymes are known to cut various specific target sequences. Examples of common restriction endonucleases are BamH1, EcoR1, Mnl1, MstII, Pst1, and Xba1.

Restriction point - point that occurs in late G1; point when cell cycle progression becomes autonomous.

Reticular cell - one of the three major types of cell in the bone marrow stroma. It is also found in the spleen and lymph nodes. These cells branch to form reticular fibers. Also called *fibroblasts.*

Reticulocyte - first nonnucleated stage of erythrocyte development in the bone marrow. It contains RNA that is visualized as granules or filaments within the cell when stained supravitally with new methylene blue. Normally, reticulocytes constitute approximately 1% of the circulating erythrocyte population.

Reticulocyte production index (RPI) - indicator of the bone marrow response in anemia. The calculation corrects the reticulocyte count for the presence of marrow reticulocytes in the peripheral blood. It is calculated as follows:

(Patient hematocrit [L/L] ÷ 0.45 [L/L]) × reticulocyte count (%) × (1 ÷ maturation time of shift reticulocytes) = RPI

Reticulocytosis - presence of excess reticulocytes in the peripheral blood.

Rh null disease - disorder associated with the lack of the Rh antigen on erythrocytes.

Rhopheocytosis - energy- and temperature-dependent process by which iron enters cells.

Ribosomes - cellular particle composed of ribonucleic acid (RNA) and protein whose function is to synthesize polypeptide chains from amino acids. The sequence of amino acids in the chains is specified by the genetic code of messenger RNA. Ribosomes appear singly or in reversibly dissociable units and may be free in the cytoplasm or attached to endoplasmic reticulum. The cytoplasm of blood cells that contain a high concentration of ribosomes stains bluish purple with Romanowsky stains.

Richter's transformation - transformation from CLL to another disease, usually large B cell lymphoma.

Ringed sideroblasts - erythroblasts with abnormal deposition of excess iron within mitochondria resulting in a ring formation around the nucleus.

Ristocetin - aggregating reagent that specifically evaluates VWF interaction with glycoprotein Ib on platelets.

Ristocetin induced platelet aggregation (RIPA) - measures ability of patient's VWF to bind to normal platelets, inducing platelet aggregation in a platelet aggregation assay.

RNA (ribonucleic acid) - single-stranded molecule composed of ribonucleotides (A, C, G, and U). RNA is produced by transcription of genes from a DNA template; RNA in turn serves as a template for protein translation.

Romanowsky-type stain - any stain consisting of methylene blue and its oxidation products and eosin Y or eosin B.

Rouleaux - erythrocyte distribution characterized by erythrocytes stacked like a roll of coins. This is due to abnormal coating of the cell's surface with increased plasma proteins, which decreases the zeta potential between cells.

Russell bodies - globule filled with immunoglobulin found in pathologic plasma cells called Mott cells. *See* Mott cell.

Russell's viper venom - venom that possesses thromboplastin-like activity and activates factor X.

▶ **S**

Satellite DNA - DNA containing many tandem repeats. Morphologically, it appears as a small ball-like structure making up the short arm of acrocentric chromosomes. This is the locus of the nucleolar organizing region.

Scatterplot - dot-plot histogram of two cellular characteristics. Together, the two characteristics allow definition of the leukocyte subpopulations.

Schilling test - definitive test useful in distinguishing vitamin B_{12} deficiency due to malabsorption, dietary deficiency, or absence of IF. It measures the amount of an oral dose of radioactively labeled crystalline B_{12} that is absorbed in the gut and excreted in the urine.

Schistocyte - fragment of an erythrocyte. A schistocyte may have a variety of shapes including triangle, helmet, and comma.

Scott syndrome - rare platelet disorder characterized by abnormal $Ca++$ induced phospholipids scrambling in which platelet membranes fail to support plasma procoagulant protein activation.

Secondary aggregation - irreversible aggregation of platelets that occurs over time.

Secondary fibrinolysis - clinical condition characterized by excessive fibrinolytic activity in response to disseminated intravascular clotting.

Secondary hemostasis - formation of fibrin that stabilizes a primary platelet plug.

Secondary hemostatic plug - primary platelet aggregate that has been stabilized by fibrin formation during secondary hemostasis.

Secondary thrombocytosis - increase in platelet concentration in the blood. The increase is in response to stimulation by another condition.

Secretion - energy-dependent discharge or release of products usually from glands in the body but also pertaining to the contents of platelet granules that are released after stimulation of the platelets by agonists; also product that is discharged or released.

Self-renewal - property of regenerating the same cells.

Sequestration crisis - sudden splenic pooling of sickled erythrocytes that may cause a massive decrease in erythrocyte mass within a few hours

Serine protease - family of serine proteases includes thrombin, factors VIIa, IXa, Xa, XIa, XIIa, and the digestive enzymes chymotrypsin and trypsin. They selectively hydrolyze arginine- or lysine-containing peptide bonds of other zymogens converting them to serine proteases. Each serine protease involved in the coagulation cascade is highly specific for its substrate.

Serpin - family of serine protease inhibitors that inhibit target molecules by formation of a 1:1 stoichiometric complex.

Severe combined immunodeficiency syndrome (SCIDS) - heterogeneous group of disorders based on diverse genetic origins, different inheritance patterns, and severity of clinical manifestations. The disease may be inherited either as a sex-linked trait or as an autosomal-recessive trait. This is the most severe immune deficiency disease.

Sézary's cell - circulating neoplastic cell found in Sézary's syndrome characterized by a very convoluted (cerebriform) nuclear outline.

Shelf life - time period for which a reagent or control is stable given appropriate storage conditions. Shelf life changes once the reagent or control is reconstituted if lypholyzed or opened if liquid.

Shift neutrophilia - *See* Pseudoneutrophilia.

Shift to the left - appearance of increased numbers of immature leukocytes in the peripheral blood.

Sickle cell (drepanocyte) - elongated crescent shaped erythrocyte with pointed ends. Sickle cell formation may be observed in wet preparations or in stained blood smears from patients with sickle cell anemia.

Sickle-cell anemia - genetically determined disorder in which hemoglobin S is inherited in the homozygous state. No hemoglobin A is present. Hemoglobins S, F, A$_2$ are present.

Sickle cell trait - genetically determined disorder in which hemoglobin S is inherited in the heterozygous state. The patient has one normal β-globin gene and one β^S-globin gene. Both hemoglobin A and hemoglobin S are present.

Side light scatter - laser light scattered at a 90° angle due to internal complexity and granularity of the particle (e.g., neutrophils produce much side scatter because of their numerous cytoplasmic granules).

Sideroacrestic - defect in iron utilization.

Siderocyte - erythrocyte that contains stainable iron granules.

Sideropenic - lack of iron.

Single nucleotide polymorphism (SNP) - change in which a single base in the DNA differs from the usual base at that position

Slope - angle or direction of the regression line with respect to the x and y axes. The slope is used to identify the presence of proportional systematic error.

Small lymphocytic lymphoma (SLL) - condition identical to CLL but primarily involves the lymph nodes. The two disorders appear to belong to one disease entity with differing clinical manifestations.

Smooth endoplasmic reticulum (SER) - *See* Endoplasmic reticulum.

Smudge cell - cell whose cytoplasmic membrane has ruptured, leaving a bare nucleus. Increased numbers of smudge cells are observed in lymphoproliferative disorders such as chronic lymphocytic leukemia. It can also be seen in reactive lymphocytosis and in other neoplasms.

Southern blot - procedure first described by Ed Southern for determining DNA structure. In this procedure, DNA is cleaved with restriction endonucleases that cut DNA at specific nucleotide sequences. The resulting DNA fragments are electrophoresed in an agarose gel to separate them by size and then treated with a solution of high pH that separates double-stranded DNA into two single-stranded parts. The single-stranded fragments are then transferred to a membrane where they can be hybridized to a complementary labeled probe. Probe hybridization permits identification of the DNA fragments containing the sequence of interest. The size and number of those fragments reflects the structure of the DNA.

Specificity - ability of a test method to determine only the analyte meant to be detected or measured.

Specimen run - interval, period of time, or number of specimens for which the accuracy and precision of the laboratory procedure is expected to remain stable.

Spectrin - predominant peripheral membrane protein found in the erythrocyte membrane. It is composed of dimeric chains, α and β, that associate to form tetramers.

Spent phase - stage in polycythemia vera in which after a period of 2–10 years, the patient may develop bone marrow failure accompanied by an increase in splenomegaly. Anemia and bleeding may be the primary clinical findings, secondary to a decreased platelet count and decreasing hematocrit. This phase is often a transition to AML.

Spherocyte - abnormally round erythrocyte with dense hemoglobin content (increased MCHC). The cell has no central area of pallor because it has lost its biconcave shape.

Splenectomy - removal of the spleen.

Splenomegaly - abnormal enlargement of the spleen.

Split sample - division of a single sample into two or more aliquots for the purpose of testing on two or more instruments within the same time period or retesting the sample at another time.

Spur cell anemia - acquired hemolytic condition associated with severe hepatocellular disease such as cirrhosis, in which there is an increase in serum lipoproteins, leading to excess of erythrocyte membrane cholesterol. The total phospholipid content of the membrane, however, is normal. The predominant poikilocyte is an erythrocyte with irregular points and no area of central pallor (acanthocytes).

Stab - *See* Band.

Stage - stage of a neoplasm indicates the extent and distribution of disease. Determining the stage of disease usually involves radiologic studies, peripheral blood examination, bone marrow aspiration, and biopsy.

Standard deviation - distribution of a set of data about the mean.

Standard error of the estimate (S$_{y/x}$) - measure of the variation in the regression line. The S$_{y/x}$ is used to identify random error.

Starry sky - morphologic appearance characteristic of high-grade lymphoma produced by numerous tingible body macrophages (stars) and a diffuse sheet of neoplastic cells (sky).

Stomatocyte - abnormal erythrocyte shape characterized by a slit-like area of central pallor. This cell has a uniconcave, cup shape.

Streptokinase - bacterial enzyme derived from group C-beta hemolytic steptococci that activates plasminogen to plasmin and is used as a thrombolytic agent in the treatment of thrombosis.

Stroma - extracellular matrix or microenvironment that supports hematopoietic cell proliferation in the bone marrow.

Stromal cells - cellular elements of the hematopoietic microenvironment in the red portion of bone marrow.

Submetacentric - chromosome that has the centromere positioned off center so that the short arm is shorter than the long arm.

Sucrose hemolysis test - screening test to identify erythrocytes that are abnormally sensitive to complement lysis. In this test, erythrocytes, serum, and sucrose are incubated together. Cells abnormally sensitive to complement will lyse. The test is used to screen for paroxysmal nocturnal hemoglobinuria. Also called *sugar-water test*.

Sulfhemoglobin - stable compound formed when a sulfur atom combines with each of the four heme groups of hemoglobin; it is incapable of carrying oxygen.

Supernatant - clear liquid remaining on top of a solution after centrifugation of the particulate matter.

Supravital stain - stain used to stain cells or tissues while they are still living.

Syngeneic stem cell transplantation - transplantation of stem cells between genetically identical twins.

Synovium - continuous membrane that lines the bony, cartilaginous, and connective tissue surfaces of a joint.

Systematic variation - variation within an instrument or test method that occurs in one direction and can be predicted. This type of variation affects accuracy.

▶ T

Target cell - abnormally shaped erythrocyte. The cell appears as a target with a bull's-eye center mass of hemoglobin surrounded by an achromic ring and an outer ring of hemoglobin. The osmotic fragility of this cell is decreased. Also called *Mexican hat cell* and *codocyte*.

Tartrate resistant acid phosphatase (TRAP) - acid phosphatase staining following tartrate incubation.

T cell ALL - immunologic subgroup of ALL. There are two types: early precursor T-ALL and T-ALL. T-ALL is differentiated using two CD markers, CD7 (gp40 protein) and CD2 (E-receptor), and TdT.

T cell receptor (TCR) - antigen receptor on immunocompetent T lymphocytes

Teardrop (dacryocytes) - erythrocyte that is elongated at one end to form a teardrop or pear-shaped cell. Teardrop may form after erythrocytes with cellular inclusions have transversed the spleen. A teardrop cell cannot return to its original shape because it has either been stretched beyond the limits of deformability of the membrane or has been in the abnormal shape for too long a time.

Telangiectasia - persistent dilation of superficially located veins.

Thalassemia - group of genetically determined microcytic, hypochromic anemias resulting from a decrease in synthesis of one or more globin chains in the hemoglobin molecule. The disorder may occur in the homozygous or heterozygous state. Heterozygotes may be asymptomatic but homozygotes typically have a severe, often fatal, disease. Thalassemia occurs most frequently in populations from the Mediterranean area and Southeast Asia.

Therapeutic range - level of a drug that is beneficial but not toxic to the individual.

Transcription error - error made in reporting test results when copying results manually from the instrument to a paper or typing them into a computer.

Threshold limit - level above which voltage pulses of particles are counted. Adjusting the threshold limit allows different types of cells to be counted.

Thrombin activatable fibrinolysis inhibitor (TAFI) - inhibitor of fibrinolysis activated by the thrombin-thrombomodulin complex, which inhibits fibrinolysis by cleaving free lysine groups on fibrin

Thrombocyte - *See* Platelet.

Thrombocytopenia - decrease in the number of platelets in the peripheral blood below the reference range for an individual laboratory (usually below 150×10^9/L).

Thrombocytopenia with absent radii (TAR) - inherited condition characterized by isolated hypoplasia of the megakaryocytic lineage, thrombocytopenia, and bilateral radial aplasial.

Thrombocytosis - increase in the number of platelets in the peripheral blood above the reference range for an individual laboratory (usually over 450×10^9/L).

Thromboembolism - blockage of a small blood vessel by a blood clot that was formed in the heart, arteries, or veins, dislodged and moved through blood vessels until reaching a smaller vessel and blocking further blood flow.

Thrombogenic - tendency to thrombose.

Thrombolytic therapy - therapy designed to dissolve or break down a thrombus.

Thrombomodulin - intrinsic membrane glycoprotein present on endothelial cells that serves as a cofactor with thrombin to activate protein C. It forms a 1:1 complex with thrombin inhibiting thrombin's ability to cleave fibrinogen to fibrin but enhances thrombin's ability to activate protein C.

Thrombophilia - tendency to form blood clots abnormally. Also referred to as *hypercoagulability.*

Thrombophlebitis - thrombosis within a vein that is accompanied by an inflammatory response, pain, and redness of the area.

Thrombopoietin - cytokine that regulates the maturation of megakaryocytes and the production of platelets.

Thrombosis - formation of a blood clot or thrombus, usually considered to be under abnormal conditions within a blood vessel.

Thrombotic thrombocytopenia purpura (TTP) - acute disorder characterized by microangiopathic anemia, decreased number of platelets, and renal failure as well as neurological symptoms. TTP is due to decreased activity of ADAMTS-13, resulting in the presence of ultralarge molecules of VWF in the circulation and platelet agglutination.

Thrombus - blood clot within the vascular system.

TIBC - total iron binding capacity; refers to the total amount of iron that transferrin can carry, about 250–450 μg/dL.

Tingible body macrophage - macrophage phagocytosing fragments of dying cells. It is found in areas of extensive apoptosis (reactive germinal centers and high-grade lymphoma).

Tissue factor - coagulation factor present on subvascular cells that forms a complex with factor VII when the vessel is ruptured. This complex activates factor X. Tissue factor is an integral protein of the cell membrane.

Tissue factor pathway inhibitor (TFPI) - intrinsic pathway inhibitor that inhibits both F-VIIa and F-Xa by forming a quarternary complex of TFPI-FXa-TF-FVIIa.

Tissue homeostasis - maintenance of an adequate number of cells to carry out the functions of the organism. Homeostasis is controlled by cell proliferation, cell differentiation, and cell death (apotosis).

Tissue plasminogen activator (t-PA) - serine protease that activates plasminogen to plasmin. It forms a bimolecular complex with fibrin increasing the catalytic efficiency of t-PA for plasminogen activation.

Toxic granules - large, dark blue-black primary granules in the cytoplasm of neutrophils that are present in certain infectious states. They are usually seen in conjunction with Döhle bodies.

Toxoplasmosis - condition that results from infection with *Toxoplasma gondii.* Acquired infection may be asymptomatic, or symptoms may resemble infectious mononucleosis. There is a leukocytosis with relative lymphocytosis or rarely an absolute lymphocytosis and the presence of reactive lymphocytes.

Trabecula - projection of calcified bone extending from cortical bone into the marrow space; provides support for marrow cells.

Transcription - synthesis of RNA from a DNA template.

Transcription factor - protein that controls when genes are switched on or off (i.e., whether genes are transcribed or not).

Transcription factors bind to regulatory regions in the genome and help control gene expression.

Transferrin - plasma β_1-globulin responsible for binding iron and its transport in the bloodstream. Each gram of transferrin can bind 1.25 mg of iron. The capacity of transferrin to bind iron is functionally measured as the total iron-binding capacity (TIBC).

Transglutaminase - F-XIIIa is the only coagulation protein with transglutaminase activity. It catalyzes the formation of isopeptide bonds between glutamine and lysine residues on fibrin, forming stable covalent crosslinks.

Transient erythroblastemia of childhood (TEC) - temporary suppression of erythropoiesis that frequently occurs after a viral infection in infants and children. Therapy is supportive, and patients usually recover within 2 months.

Translation - synthesis of protein from an RNA template.

Translocation - abnormal chromosomal rearrangement whereby part of one chromosome breaks off and becomes attached to another chromosome. The site of juxtaposition between the two chromosomes is referred to as the breakpoint.

Transplancental idiopathic thrombocytopenic purpura - form of ITP that is present in newborns because of maternal transfer of platelet-destroying antibodies.

Transudate - effusion that is formed due to increased hydrostatic pressure or decreased osmotic pressure; does not indicate a true pathologic state in the anatomic region.

Trisomy - one daughter cell with an extra chromosome (three copies instead of two).

T-structure (tense) - conformational change in a hemoglobin molecule that occurs when oxygen is released from hemoglobin.

Turnaround time - time between specimen collection and reporting of a test result.

Type 1 VWD (classic VWD) - quantitative decrease of structurally normal VWF.

Type 2 VWD - qualitative disorder of VWF; has four possible subtypes: 2A, 2B, 2M, and 2N.

Type 3 VWD - severe, rare quantitative deficiency of VWF.

Type I myeloblasts - classic description of myeloblasts. These cells contain no granules and have a highly immature nucleus.

Type II myeloblasts - more mature than the type I myeloblasts; cells that can contain Auer rods, phi bodies, and/or primary granules.

Type III myeloblasts - similar to type II myeloblasts but have >20 granules in the cytoplasm.

Tyrosine kinase protein - protein that regulates metabolic pathways and serves as receptor for growth factors.

▶ **U**

Ubiquitin - protein found in all eukaryotic cells that becomes covalently attached to certain residues of other proteins, tagging a protein for intracellular proteolytic destruction.

UIBC (unsaturated iron binding capacity) - portion of transferrin that is not complexed with iron. (TIBC-serum iron = UIBC).

Unfractionated heparin - heterogeneous mixture of sulfated glycosaminoglycans (range 5000–30,000 daltons) obtained from extraction of porcine intestinal mucosa or bovine lung.

Unique identification number - number assigned to a patient admitted to the hospital that can be used to identify them. It is printed on the patient's arm band.

Universal precautions - preventative guidelines to minimize the potential exposure of health care workers to blood-borne pathogens. These guidelines include the use of gloves whenever handling any body fluid.

Untranslated region (UTR) - portion of DNA on a chromosome whose bases are not involved in protein synthesis.

Urokinase (urokinase-type plasminogen activator– uPA) - enzyme found in urine and plasma that activates plasminogen to plasmin and is used as a thrombolytic agent in the treatment of thrombosis.

Urokinase-type plasminogen activator receptor (uPAR) - endothelial cell membrane receptor that binds uPA and facilitated plasminogen activation.

▶ **V**

Variable number tandem repeats - DNA sequences that are tandemly repeated in a genome and that can vary among different individuals.

Vascular permeability - property of endothelial cells of blood vessels that selectively allows for exchange of gases, nutrients, and waste products.

Vasculitis - inflammation of a blood vessel.

Vasoconstriction - narrowing of the lumen of blood vessels that occurs immediately following an injury.

Vaso-occlusive crisis - acute event caused by spontaneous blockage of microvasculature by rigid sickle cells. The crisis may be triggered by infection, dehydration, decreased oxygen pressure, or slow blood flow. Often the crisis occurs without a known cause.

Vertical interactions - up-and-down interactions involving the skeletal lattice and proteins of the erythrocyte membrane. These interactions stabilize the lipid bilayer membrane.

Viral load - measuring the number of copies of HIV-1 RNA indicates a patient's viral load.

Viscosity - resistance to flow; physical property dependent on the friction of component molecules in a substance as they pass one another.

Vitamin K-dependent factors - *See* Prothrombin group.

Vitronectin - serum or extracellular-matrix glycoprotein capable of binding heparin.

von Willebrand disease - autosomal dominant hereditary bleeding disorder in which there is a lack of von Willebrand factor (VWF). This factor is needed for platelets to adhere to collagen. Platelet aggregation is abnormal with ristocetin. The bleeding time is also abnormal. The APTT may be prolonged due to a decrease in the F-VIII molecule secondary to a decrease in VWF.

von Willebrand factor (VWF) - plasma factor needed for platelets to adhere to collagen. It binds to the platelet glycoprotein Ib. It is synthesized in megakaryocytes and endothelial cells. The VWF is a molecule of multimers. It is noncovalently linked to F-VIII in plasma.

von Willebrand factor (VWF) activity (VWF:RCo; VWF:A) - test that determines the ability of VWF to function in platelet adhesion. VWF :RCo measures the ability of the patient's VWF to support agglutination of normal platelets by ristocetin in a platelet aggregometer.

von Willebrand factor (VWF):Ag assay - immunologic test that determines the quantity of VWF protein.

von Willebrand factor (VWF) multimer - VWF molecule consisting of multiple copies of identical subunits linked together.

 W

Warm autoimmune hemolytic anemia - anemia resulting from the presence of IgG autoantibodies that are reactive at 37°C with antigens on subject's erythrocytes. The antibody–antigen complex on the cell membrane sensitizes the erythrocyte, which is removed in the spleen or liver.

Wedge smear - blood smear prepared on a glass microscope slide by placing a drop of blood at one end and with a second slide pulling the blood the length of the slide.

White thrombus - thrombus composed mostly of platelets and fibrin that appears light gray.

Wiskott-Aldrich Syndrome/X-linked Thrombocytopenia (WAS/ XLT) - WAS is a disorder of small platelets, thrombocytopenia, and severe immune dysregulation. XLT is a disorder involving mutations of the *WAS* gene, which manifests as isolated thrombocytopenia without immune dysfunction.

World Health Organization (WHO) classification - classification system for the neoplastic blood disorders. It uses newer diagnostic techniques to categorize neoplasms including genetics and flow cytometry.

▶ **Y**

y-intercept - point where the regression line intersects the y-axis. The y-intercept is used to identify the presence of constant systematic error.

▶ **Z**

Zymogen - inactive precursor that can be converted to the active form by an enzyme, alkali, or acid. The inert coagulation factors are zymogens. Also called *proenzyme*.

Index